VOLUME 5

3rd Edition

DIAGNOSIS OF BONE AND JOINT DISORDERS

Donald Resnick, M.D.

Professor of Radiology
University of California, San Diego
Chief of Osteoradiology Section
Veterans Administration Medical Center
San Diego, California

With the Editorial Assistance of Catherine F. Fix
With the Technical Assistance of Debra J. Trudell

W.B. SAUNDERS COMPANY
A Division of Harcourt Brace & Company
Philadelphia   London   Toronto   Montreal   Sydney   Tokyo

W.B. SAUNDERS COMPANY
A Division of
Harcourt Brace & Company

The Curtis Center
Independence Square West
Philadelphia, Pennsylvania 19106

Library of Congress Cataloging-in-Publication Data

Resnick, Donald

Diagnosis of bone and joint disorders / Donald Resnick.—3rd ed.

p.   cm.

Includes bibliographical references and indexes.

ISBN 0–7216–5066–X (set)

1. Musculoskeletal system—Diseases—Diagnosis.   2. Bones—Diseases—
   Diagnosis.   3. Joints—Diseases—Diagnosis.   4. Diagnostic
   imaging.   I. Title.

[DNLM: 1. Bone Diseases—diagnosis.   2. Joint Diseases—diagnosis.
3. Diagnosis Imaging.   WE 300 R434d 1995]

RC925.7.R47 1995

616.7′1075—dc20

DNLM/DLC   93–48321

Diagnosis of Bone and Joint Disorders, 3rd edition

Volume One	ISBN	0–7216–5067–8
Volume Two	ISBN	0–7216–5068–6
Volume Three	ISBN	0–7216–5069–4
Volume Four	ISBN	0–7216–5070–8
Volume Five	ISBN	0–7216–5071–6
Volume Six	ISBN	0–7216–5072–4
Six Volume Set	ISBN	0–7216–5066–X

Last digit is the print number: 9   8   7   6   5   4   3   2   1

CONTENTS

▼

SECTION

XIV

▼

Traumatic, Iatrogenic, and Neurogenic Diseases

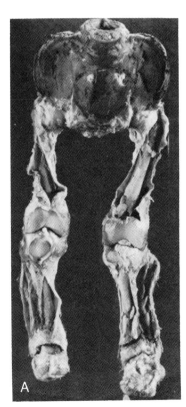 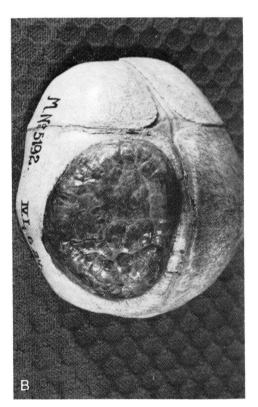

A Scurvy: Findings include subperiosteal hematomas (the periosteal membranes have been opened) and transmetaphyseal fractures.
B Ossifying hematoma (cephalhematoma): The hematoma is located in the parietal bone and does not cross the sutural line in this infant.

67

Physical Injury: Concepts and Terminology

Donald Resnick, M.D.,
Thomas G. Goergen, M.D., and Gen Niwayama, M.D.

No other facet of musculoskeletal disease occupies a more fundamental or important role than that related to physical abuse. The evaluation of the complications of trauma is an integral part of orthopedic surgery, a large part of the practice of emergency room medicine, and the most common indication for skeletal radiography. Complete textbooks are devoted to a discussion of the consequences of such trauma both in the child and in the adult.

Physical injury contributes to a wide variety of alterations in the bones, joints, and soft tissues. In addition to fractures, dislocations, subluxations, and capsular, tendinous, muscular, and ligamentous tears, trauma can affect the growth plate of the immature skeleton as well as the hyaline cartilaginous and fibrocartilaginous joint structures. Further complications of trauma include reflex sympathetic dystrophy (see Chapter 51), osteolysis (see Chapter 94), osteonecrosis (see Chapter 80), many of the osteochondroses (see Chapter 81), neuropathic osteoarthropathy (see Chapter 78), infection (see Chapters 64 to 66), and heterotopic bone formation (Figs. 67–1 and 67–2) (see Chapter 95). Trauma also has been implicated in the development of certain neoplasms, such as aneurysmal bone cysts. Nonmechanical trauma to the musculoskeletal system can result from thermal and electrical injury (see Chapter 72), irradiation (see Chapter 73), and chemical substances (see Chapters 74 to 76).

This chapter represents an overview of the subject of physical trauma. It is not meant to compete with the standard references in the field,[1–8] nor to replace the tens of

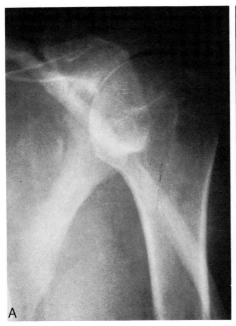
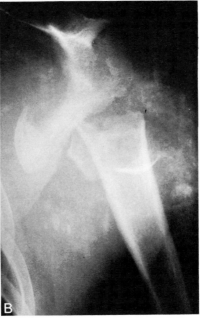

FIGURE 67–1. Complications of physical injury: Neuropathic osteoarthropathy. Radiographs obtained 2 weeks apart reveal the rapid development of neuropathic osteoarthropathy after an anterior dislocation of the glenohumeral joint. The initial radiograph **(A),** obtained as part of a venogram, shows an anterior glenohumeral joint dislocation. Subsequently **(B),** fragmentation of the entire humeral head is apparent. (Courtesy of E. Johnson, M.D., Denver, Colorado.)

thousands of scientific articles that describe specific musculoskeletal injuries. Rather, emphasis is placed on the general principles governing the analysis of fractures and dislocations in both the adult and the child, the consequences of injuries to joints and soft tissues, and certain conditions in which radiographic manifestations simulate those associated with nontraumatic skeletal disorders. Subsequent chapters describe specific physical injuries in the appendicular and axial skeleton, internal derangements of joints, and sports-related injuries.

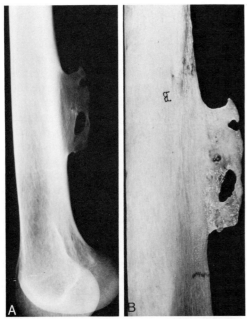

FIGURE 67–2. Complications of physical injury: Heterotopic bone formation. Radiograph **(A)** and corresponding photograph **(B)** of a femoral specimen reveals the osseous excrescence arising from the surface of the bone that may be the residua of "myositis ossificans."

AVAILABLE DIAGNOSTIC TECHNIQUES

Plain film radiographic examination is well suited to the evaluation of most skeletal injuries. Obtaining an adequate radiologic examination in emergency room patients can be extremely difficult, however.[9] These patients frequently are uncooperative because of pain and restricted motion, and their consciousness may be altered. Despite these difficulties, it is imperative that both the technologist and the radiologist be patient and thorough. Immediate review of the radiographs must be accomplished while the patient is still in the radiology department so that inadequate or suboptimal films can be identified and repeat films can be obtained without delay. When the patient's condition limits maneuverability, alternative projections can be substituted for more standard views (see Chapter 1). Fluoroscopy can be a useful adjunct to the initial radiographic examination, as the patient can conveniently be turned to the proper obliquity to visualize a possible abnormality (see Chapter 3).

The sensitivity as well as the availability of conventional radiography has led to its routine use in the delineation of skeletal injuries. Unfortunately, the radiographic examination also has been used for a diagnostic screening test, serving as a replacement for a careful and thorough history and physical examination, especially in hospitals with a busy or understaffed emergency room. The result has been an increasing number of unnecessary radiographic procedures, a situation made worse by medicolegal issues, patients' expectations, and a lack of objective screening guidelines.[10] Although critical analyses of the efficacy of emergency radiography of the skull,[11–15] ribs,[16, 17] and extremities[10] have led, in some instances, to the establishment of specific criteria for the examinations, uniform acceptance of such criteria has not occurred. As an example, high yield criteria for skull radiography, based on information from the patient's history and physical and neurologic examinations, were developed by Bell and Loop in 1971,[18] abridged

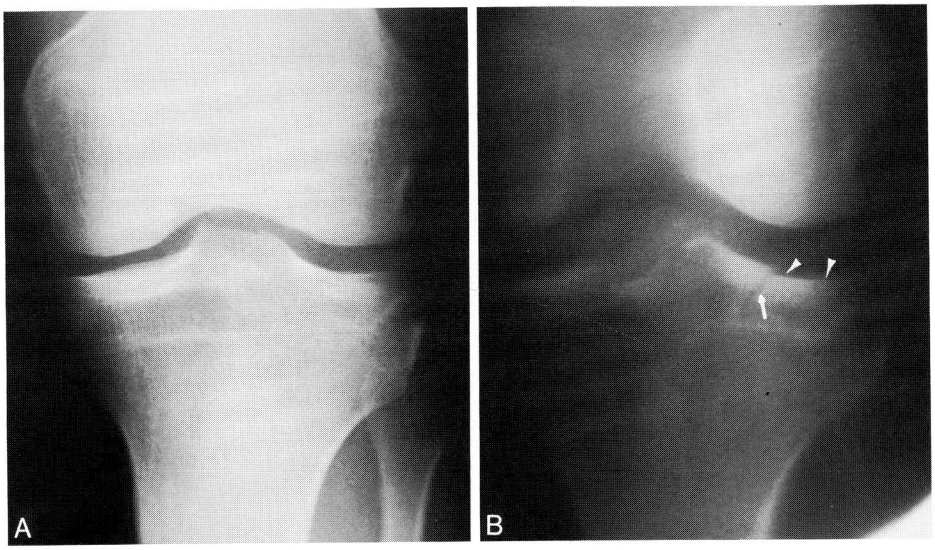

FIGURE 67–3. Physical injury: Use of conventional tomography. The fracture line (arrow) and the slight depression of the articular surface (arrowheads) are evident only on the conventional tomogram.

by Phillips in 1978,[19] and further modified in subsequent years.[11–14] Although it might be suggested that under ideal circumstances, clinical criteria could be formulated that would restrict the radiographic examination of the skull or other regions only to those patients who would have positive findings, a negative study is an unnecessary one only if the radiographic result could have been predicted or, at the very least, does not affect treatment.[10] Furthermore, even a positive radiographic examination may not be essential if the findings do not influence subsequent therapeutic decisions (as in the case of a rib fracture in which the pulmonary complications delineated on a chest film are those that truly influence therapy).[17] Finally, the proper assessment of emergency radiography requires also an analysis of alternative imaging techniques, such as CT or MR imaging, that may allow assessment of soft tissue as well as osseous structures (for example, in the patient with skull trauma in whom intracranial sequelae are most important).

In the evaluation of trauma in children, a debate has existed regarding the need to obtain comparison radiographs of the opposite extremity. Although this practice generally has been advocated in available textbooks,[20–22] a survey of members of the Society for Pediatric Radiology indicated that fewer than 30 per cent of these persons routinely used comparison views and that the additional radiographs provided important information in fewer than 5 per cent of cases.[23] McCauley and associates,[24] in a review of 300 cases of childhood injury, noted that when pediatric radiologists were initially interpreting the films, comparison films rarely were indicated. These investigators concluded that comparison views should be obtained selectively, not routinely, if the diagnosis is in doubt. Most typically, such a situation arises in the evaluation of Salter-Harris type 1 growth plate injuries and hip trauma. Radiographs of the opposite side also may be helpful in the assessment of bowing fractures and injuries about the elbow.

Specialized radiographic techniques such as conventional tomography (see Chapter 7) and magnification radiography (see Chapter 4) generally are not necessary for proper diagnosis in cases of skeletal trauma. Occasionally, such techniques allow identification of subtle fracture lines when initial radiographs are normal, examples including fractures of the carpal scaphoid bone, tibial plateaus, and femoral neck (Figs. 67–3 and 67–4), but routine use of these techniques is not indicated. When the clinical suspicion of a bone infraction is great, the patient can be treated as if a definite fracture had been identified, even when initial radiographs are normal. Radiographs obtained 2 or 3 weeks later may reveal callus formation, substantiating the presence of a fracture.

Xeroradiography (see Chapter 6) and low KV radiography (see Chapter 5) can be helpful in the evaluation of trauma, especially when a soft tissue injury is suspected. Stereoradiography, too, may be of aid. Such supplementary methods, however, have assumed a lesser role in the evaluation of musculoskeletal injury owing to the increasing availability of CT and MR imaging.

Radiographs obtained during the application of manual stress can be used effectively in certain situations to uncover an articular injury that is not apparent on initial radiographs (Fig. 67–5). This technique is employed most commonly in instances of injury to the acromioclavicular joint, knee, and ankle, although similar analysis can be applied to the evaluation of the consequences of trauma to the hip, glenohumeral joint, small joints of the hand and foot, and other sites. Stress radiography should be accomplished soon after the traumatic event, prior to the appearance of significant muscle spasm that may make the technique less rewarding. Local anesthesia may be required for successful application of manual stress to an injured joint, and correct application of the stress is mandatory. Comparison views of the opposite (uninjured) side are of diagnostic value in many cases.

The role of CT in the area of skeletal trauma has been summarized in Chapter 8. In general, this technique is able to define the presence and extent of certain fractures or dislocations, to detect intra-articular abnormalities, including cartilage damage and osteocartilaginous bodies, and to assess the nearby soft tissues. Its application to traumatic abnormalities in regions of complicated anatomy, such as the spine, the bones in the face and pelvis, the glenohumeral and sternoclavicular joints, and the midfoot and hindfoot, is especially noteworthy (Fig. 67–6), and the facts that the examination is accomplished with a greater degree of pa-

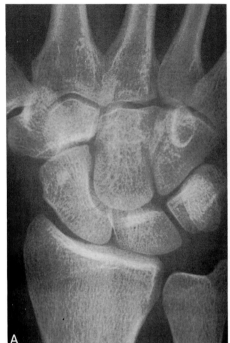 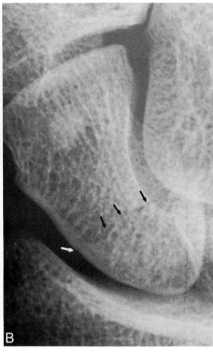

FIGURE 67–4. Physical injury: Use of radiographic magnification. Although both the conventional radiograph and the magnified projection reveal a scaphoid fracture, its extent (arrows) is better determined with magnification.

FIGURE 67–5. Physical injury: Use of stress radiography. Injuries involving the ligaments about the ankle may not be detected on routine radiographs. Radiographs obtained during the application of manual stress may allow their detection. In this case, such radiographs obtained during varus stress of the plantar flexed foot **(A)** and anterior stress **(B)** clearly demonstrate displacements of the talus with respect to the tibia, indicative of an injury of the anterior talofibular ligament.

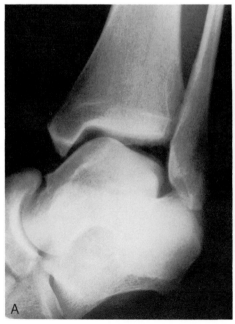 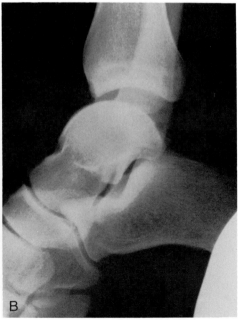

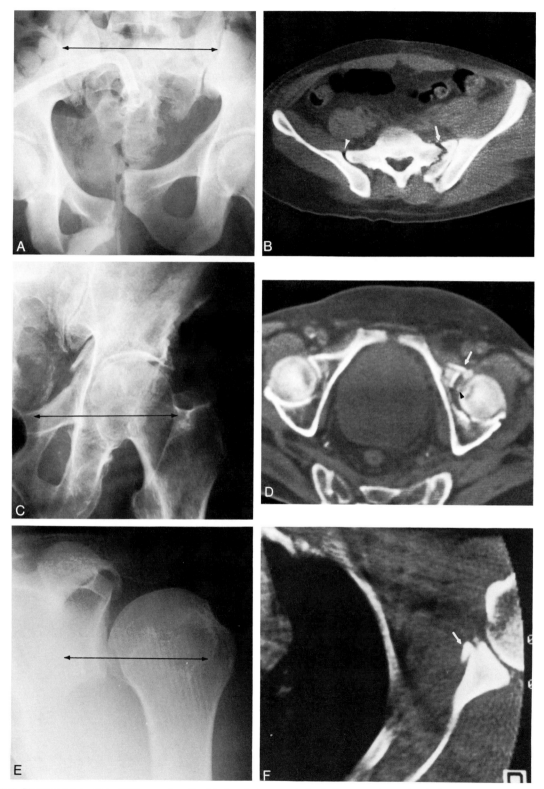

FIGURE 67–6. Physical injury: Use of CT scanning. Double-headed arrows indicate the approximate level of the transaxial scan in each case.
  A, B Osseous pelvis. Although the initial radiograph shows symphyseal diastasis and a fracture of the sacrum, the latter (arrow) is better demonstrated with CT, which also reveals diastasis of the contralateral sacroiliac joint with a vacuum phenomenon (arrowhead).
  C, D Acetabulum. Complex fractures in this region are well evaluated with CT, which, in this case, shows comminution of the anterior rim of the acetabulum (arrow) and an intra-articular fragment (arrowhead).
  E, F Glenohumeral joint. In this patient with a previous anterior dislocation of the glenohumeral joint, note the osseous Bankart lesion (arrow), which is readily apparent on CT but poorly seen with conventional radiography.

tient comfort than with routine radiography and that plaster casts are not accompanied by significant deterioration of the image quality also are important. The relative advantages of CT over conventional tomography in instances of skeletal trauma are debated and are dependent on the specific anatomic site that is being evaluated.[25] In certain regions, such as the hip, the inability to obtain initial CT images in a coronal or sagittal plane is a disadvantage. In comparison to conventional tomography, however, CT provides far better assessment of soft tissue structures, and secondary findings such as a lipohemarthrosis,[26] which can be detected by CT, are diagnostically important.

After trauma to the musculoskeletal system, the important indication for arteriography is the identification of vascular abnormalities, including disruption and occlusion of major vessels, arteriovenous fistulae, and aneurysms, in patients whose physical examination indicates signs such as ischemia, pulse deficit, or bleeding that are compatible with a significant injury to the blood vessels.[27–29] Peripheral pulses may be palpable even with complete transection of an artery, however, and absent distal pulses may occur secondary to hypovolemia, preexisting atherosclerosis, or vasospasm.[30] Therefore, the proximity of major vessels to the site of a fracture or dislocation is used by some investigators as an indication for arteriography, even in patients whose clinical examination does not provide evidence of vascular injury.[30] With regard to the extremities, the vessels that are injured most commonly are in close proximity to a bone and held in a relatively fixed position by fascial or muscular attachment; the subclavian artery may be injured by the distal fragment of a clavicular fracture; the axillary artery may be damaged in shoulder dislocations owing to the injury itself or to attempts at reduction of the humeral head; the brachial artery may be injured by a fracture of the humerus or a dislocation of the elbow; the radial or ulnar artery may be lacerated by fractures of the radius and ulna; the femoral artery in the adductor canal and the popliteal artery throughout its course are vulnerable in fractures or dislocations of contiguous bones; the anterior tibial artery

or, less commonly, the posterior tibial artery may be compromised by fractures of the tibia; and the posterior tibial and dorsalis pedis arteries may be affected in fractures or dislocations of the ankle or foot.[31–34] The mechanisms leading to the vascular injury include a tear due to the presence of a sharp bone fragment, compression related to a hematoma or swelling within a tight fascial compartment, a shearing type of injury, and entrapment in the fracture fragments with angulation and occlusion.[32] With regard to injuries of the bony pelvis, bleeding may result from laceration or tearing of one or more vessels and may be massive; the identification of the site of arterial compromise can be accomplished with arteriography.[35]

Scintigraphy also is useful in the evaluation of patients with skeletal trauma. This role is perhaps best exemplified in the diagnosis of stress fractures (see later discussion), although scintigraphy may be helpful in detecting subtle acute fractures when radiographs are normal (e.g., in the carpal bones,[36–39] ribs,[40] foot,[39, 41] and bones of the pelvis and hip[37]) or in excluding fractures in the presence of significant clinical findings.[42] It also can be used to evaluate the healing response. The vast majority of fractures are detected by bone scintigraphy within hours of the injury (Fig. 67–7), with some delay in scintigraphic abnormality (24 hours) encountered in older patients, particularly those with osteoporosis. The radionuclide alterations are not specific for fracture, occurring also in soft tissue, synovial, and ligamentous injuries. The scintigraphic pattern of fractures changes over a period of time, with three somewhat distinct stages being evident[43, 44]: The acute stage persists for approximately 2 to 4 weeks after the injury and is characterized by a diffuse area of increased tracer accumulation about the fracture site; the subacute stage persists for approximately 8 to 12 weeks and is characterized by a well-defined linear abnormality at the site of fracture; and the healing stage is characterized by a gradual diminution in the intensity of the abnormality until the scan returns to normal. Difficulty arises in determining the age of a fracture because of considerable variability in the time required for

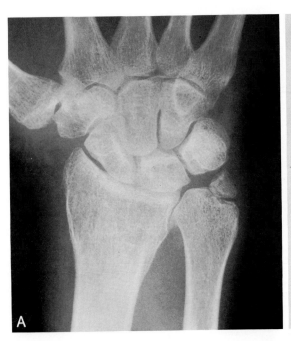

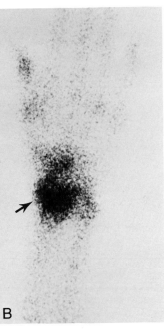

FIGURE 67–7. Physical injury: Use of bone scintigraphy. This 54 year old man was involved in an automobile accident, injuring his wrist. The same wrist had been injured several years previously.

A An initial radiograph shows an old fracture of the ulnar styloid process and, possibly, an acute fracture of the radial styloid process.

B Approximately 12 hours after the accident, a bone scan shows intense radionuclide activity in the distal portion of the radius (arrow), consistent with an acute fracture, with a lesser degree of abnormal activity in the carpus and ulna. Two weeks later, a radiograph of the wrist (not shown) demonstrated the new fracture of the radius.

fracture sites to return to normal on bone scintigraphy. It is evident that abnormal radionuclide activity persists beyond the time necessary for clinical or even radiographic healing and that surgery, the use of orthopedic fixation devices, and old age prolong this period of radionuclide recovery.[43] The minimal time required for the bone scan to return to normal after fracture appears to be about 5 to 7 months, and in 90 per cent of cases the scan is normal by 2 years following the injury.[44]

A knowledge of the scintigraphic patterns that are characteristic of normal fracture healing is required for the accurate diagnosis of delayed healing or nonunion by radionuclide techniques. Nonunion of a fracture, which is particularly common in the tibia, femur, and, to a lesser extent, humerus, radius, ulna, and clavicle, has been divided into two types according to the amount of metabolic activity at the fracture site: an atrophic nonunion in which radioactivity at the fracture site diminishes in comparison to the expected intensity of radiotracer concentration, and a reactive nonunion in which the radionuclide concentration is normal or increased.[43] In instances of atrophic nonunion, a generalized decrease in radioactivity may be accompanied by a focal zone of photopenia, indicative of a pseudarthrosis, interposition of soft tissues, a region of avascularity, or infection.[43] Previous investigations that have attempted to differentiate reliably among normal healing, delayed union, and nonunion on the basis of the scintigraphic appearance at the fracture site have met with varying degrees of success.[45–51]

As discussed in Chapter 80, scintigraphy also has been used to delineate early avascularity of bone after fracture, especially in the proximal portion of the femur. A region of decreased accumulation of the bone-seeking radiopharmaceutical agent is compatible with interruption of blood supply related either to the fracture itself or to attempts at fracture reduction.

MR imaging is assuming ever-increasing importance in the analysis of many musculoskeletal disorders, including injury. The initial and pessimistic view that bone was invisible on MR images was both simplistic and inaccurate. The unique signal intensity characteristics of marrow allow MR imaging to provide a unique perspective with regard to abnormalities, including traumatic ones, that involve the interior of a bone and, indeed, new terms such as bone marrow edema and bone bruise have been developed to describe some of the alterations visible on MR images (see later discussion). Furthermore, in an indirect fashion, MR imaging provides information regarding the bone cortex. Although compact cortical bone is devoid of signal on MR images, its interruption or violation by tumor, infection, or fracture may be evident during the MR imaging examination, and the accompanying response of the periosteal membrane also may be visible. The physician should understand, however, that it is the ancillary findings such as marrow and soft tissue edema and hemorrhage accompanying the fracture that are displayed more dramatically than the fracture line itself on the MR images. By no means should MR imaging be considered a suitable substitute for routine radiography or, perhaps, even CT or conventional tomography in the assessment of complex fractures when information regarding the precise relationship of fracture fragments is required. Finally, MR imaging is unparalleled in the investigation of traumatically induced internal de-

rangements of joints, providing diagnostic information related to the integrity of articular cartilage, menisci, labra, and intra-articular ligaments; to periarticular ligamentous and tendinous injuries; and to injury-related abnormalities of muscles and other soft tissues (see also Chapter 70). In a similar fashion, MR imaging is of unique value in the assessment of injury to the spinal cord (see Chapter 69).

The extreme sensitivity of MR imaging to bone (and cartilage) injury makes it an indispensable supplementary technique in some patients whose initial routine radiographs after acute trauma either are negative or reveal equivocal results (Fig. 67–8). In this regard, MR imaging competes favorably with bone scintigraphy, even single photon emission computed tomography (SPECT). The sensitivities of MR imaging and bone scintigraphy in the diagnosis of occult fractures after acute injury appear to be similar, but the MR imaging examination enjoys far greater specificity. An abbreviated MR imaging study whose cost is not unlike that of scintigraphy may be sufficient for diagnosis of occult fractures of the femoral neck, about the knee, or elsewhere.[52–54] Additionally, modifications in MR imaging technique such as fat suppression, intravenous administration of gadolinium contrast agent, and short tau inversion recovery (STIR) imaging,[55] while increasing the duration and the expense of the examination, may provide even greater sensitivity for fracture detection. The MR imaging examination also is well suited to the assessment of osteochondral and stress fractures (see later discussion). Although it has invaded the territory once held firm by bone scintigraphy, MR imaging has not eliminated altogether the need for scintigraphic analysis of musculoskeletal injury. MR imaging is far better when employed to evaluate a single region of the body, whereas bone scintigraphy is more effective as a general surveyor of the skeleton, which assumes clinical importance in cases of multiple injuries or of child abuse (see later discussion).

RADIOGRAPHIC REPORTING

The formulation of an accurate, timely, and concise radiographic report is an important responsibility of the radiologist and yet one that commonly is ignored.[56] Orthopedic surgeons and trauma physicians sometimes have complained of incomplete descriptions, inaccurate terminology, inappropriate remarks, and omission of helpful radiographic recommendations.[57] Although the report is not meant to eliminate the need for the film review by the referring physician, it should describe the characteristics of the injury accurately through the use of precise and accepted terminology so that the subsequent review of the radiographs does not disclose findings that are completely unexpected. Furthermore, the radiologist should avoid clinical conclusions regarding the adequacy of fracture reduction or treatment; statements such as ''an unsatisfactory reduction'' or ''an unacceptable fixation'' are guaranteed to attract the attention of the referring physician, and, perhaps, the legal profession as well.

The initial report necessarily must be more detailed than subsequent reports, which are concerned primarily with interval changes related to treatment and healing (Figs. 67–9 and 67–10). It should be divided into an *introduction* (containing comments regarding the body part being examined, the radiographic projections that are available, the radio-

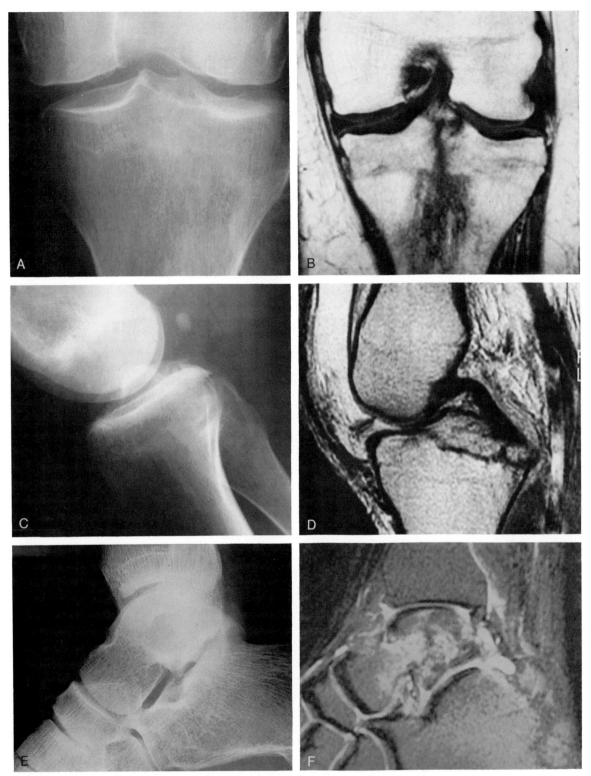

FIGURE 67–8. Physical injury: Use of MR imaging.

A, B Proximal portion of the tibia. The initial radiograph **(A)** reveals minimal sclerosis beneath the tibial eminences but was interpreted as normal. A coronal T1-weighted (TR/TE, 750/20) spin echo MR image **(B)** vividly displays the fracture.

C, D Proximal portion of the tibia. With routine radiography **(C),** a subtle fracture line is evident. A sagittal proton density (TR/TE, 2000/30) spin echo MR image **(D)** displays the fracture of the posterior portion of the tibial plateau as a region of low signal intensity. Note subtle surrounding marrow edema of higher signal intensity and the attachment of an intact posterior cruciate ligament to the fragment. A joint effusion is present.

E, F Talus. A fracture is not seen on the plain film **(E),** nor was it detected with conventional tomography (not shown). A sagittal T2-weighted (TR/TE, 2050/80) spin echo MR image **(F)** clearly shows the fracture of the body of the talus with bone marrow edema and joint effusions.

(E, F, Courtesy of G. Greenway, M.D., Dallas, Texas.)

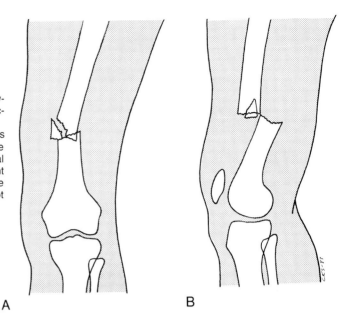

FIGURE 67–9. Physical injury: Initial radiographic report. Line drawings of radiographs show anteroposterior **(A)** and lateral **(B)** projections of the left femur.

Body of Report: Portable anteroposterior and lateral radiographs of the left femur show a comminuted transverse fracture of the midshaft with a separate butterfly fragment arising from the medial aspect. With respect to the distal fragment, posterior displacement with moderate anterolateral angulation and slight overriding are seen. No significant rotatory component is seen, but the hip has not been included on the radiograph.

Conclusion: Comminuted midshaft fracture, left femur.

logic technique that is employed [such as the use of portable equipment], the presence of partially obscuring splints, casts, or dressing material, and the timing of the examination); *general description of the injury* (containing comments regarding the configuration and location of the fracture or dislocation); *closing statements* (containing pertinent observations based on the foregoing description and any recommendations for additional radiographic projections or

imaging studies); and the *conclusion* or *impression* (in which the most important radiographic features are summarized).[58] The conclusion actually can be placed at the beginning of the report, presenting the most relevant information first.[57]

The first radiographic report after the treatment of a fracture or dislocation must be more detailed and complete than subsequent reports, in which emphasis is placed on the analysis of any change in position or alignment of the fragments (in cases of fracture) or the articular surfaces (in cases of subluxation or dislocation) and of interval healing. This first radiographic report after initiation of treatment should have the same organization as the initial report. The introductory comments again should describe the radiographic projections that are available, the presence of a cast or related material, and the timing of the examination relative to that of the injury. When a series of films has been obtained either after multiple attempts at closed reduction or during the course of an operative reduction, the reports should reflect the total number of films, but the emphasis is directed toward the interpretation of the final set of radiographs. With regard to the general description of the injury, only pertinent features need be repeated in the posttreatment radiographic report. The type of fixation device (pins, screws, nails, or plates) and the effect of the reduction on position and alignment of the bones and joints are noted (Table 67–1). Closing statements should reflect the status

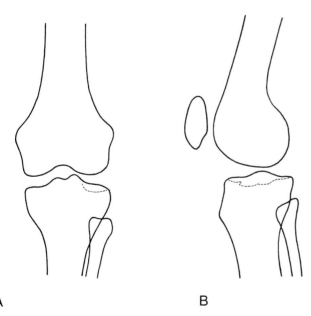

FIGURE 67–10. Physical injury: Initial radiographic report. Line drawings of radiographs showing anteroposterior **(A)** and lateral **(B)** projections of the left knee. Oblique radiographs also were obtained.

Body of Report: Standard radiographs of the left knee show an effusion with a fat-fluid level and a fracture of the articular surface of the lateral tibial plateau. The maximum depression of the fracture fragment measures 4 mm. Remaining osseous structures are normal. Conventional tomography may be helpful in accurately assessing the degree of depression and comminution of the articular surface.

Conclusion: Depression fracture, lateral plateau of left tibia.

TABLE 67–1. Some Situations That Require Absolute Measurements of Reduction

General Situations
    Varus or valgus angulation
    Distraction or overriding
    Angular deformity or displacement on stress radiographs
    Distraction of fragments at an articular surface
Specific Situations
    Dorsal angulation of the distal portion of the radius
    Subluxation or kyphosis of vertebrae
    Depression of an impacted fracture of the tibial plateau
    Angulation and displacement of a supracondylar fracture of the humerus

of healing (unless the injury is acute) and, as in the initial report of the injury, the conclusion should be concise.

FRACTURES

Epidemiology

The likelihood, location, and configuration of a fracture after an injury depend on a number of factors, including the age and sex of the person, the type and mechanism of the injury, and the presence of any predisposing factors that might alter the bones or soft tissues of the musculoskeletal system. Birth-related trauma in the newborn, sports-related activities in the adolescent or young adult, occupation-related stresses in the mature adult, and normal activities in the elderly are typical situations leading to skeletal injury. In men, the frequency of fractures is greatest in the second and third decades of life and in old age; in women the frequency is less than that in men until the age of approximately 45 or 50 years, after which fractures become more common in women than in men.

Fractures of the small bones of the hands and feet, the tubular bones of the extremities (tibia and humerus), and the clavicle predominate in adolescents and young adults owing to their participation in recreational or occupational activities; fractures of the proximal portions of the femur and humerus, the distal part of the radius, and the pelvis are especially common in elderly persons, particularly women, reflecting the locations vulnerable to trauma in a skeleton weakened by metabolic diseases, such as osteoporosis. The physeal and metaphyseal regions in children, the epiphyses in teenagers, the diaphyses in young adults, and the epiphyses and metaphyses in elderly persons are sites in the tubular bones that often are injured. Such site selection relates to changing patterns of skeletal strength and weakness as well as mechanisms of injuries. Even an identical type of injury, such as a fall on the outstretched hand, will lead to musculoskeletal consequences that differ among the various age groups, however: a supracondylar fracture of the humerus in the young child; a metaphyseal fracture of the distal portion of the radius in the older child; an epiphyseal separation of the radius in the adolescent; a carpal injury in the young adult; a Colles' type fracture of the distal portion of the radius in the middle-aged person; and a fracture of the surgical neck of the humerus in the elderly patient.[2]

Motor vehicle accidents represent a leading cause of injury and death at all ages and, in fact, are the major cause of death in the United States in persons between the ages of 5 and 34 years.[2] Patterns of skeletal injury among those involved in such accidents vary according to the type of terrain, the speed of the vehicle, the type of vehicle, the age of the person, and his or her location in the vehicle (e.g., driver, passenger); these patterns are modified further according to whether safety restraints were being used and the type of restraint that was employed. Spinal fractures and dislocations, hip dislocations, patellar fractures, sternal injuries, and injuries of the foot and ankle are among the skeletal abnormalities that are seen.

Terminology

A *fracture,* in its most simple definition, is a break in the continuity of bone or cartilage, or both. Each fracture is

TABLE 67–2. Radiographic Signs of Open Fractures

Soft tissue defect
Bone protruding beyond soft tissues
Subcutaneous or intra-articular gas
Foreign material beneath skin
Absent pieces of bone

associated with soft tissue injury, the character and the degree of which have additional therapeutic implications. Conversely, in an attempt to emphasize the soft tissue component, a fracture might be defined as a soft tissue injury in which there is a break in bone or cartilage. A *transchondral fracture* is one that involves a cartilaginous surface. If the cartilage alone is involved, the term *chondral fracture* is used; a fracture composed of cartilage and subjacent bone is termed an *osteochondral fracture.*

In a *closed (simple) fracture* the skin is intact, which prevents communication between the fracture and the outside environment. An *open fracture* allows communication between the fracture and the outside environment due to disruption of the skin. Bone fragments may or may not protrude through the cutaneous defect. Although closed and open fractures are distinguishable clinically, findings indicating an open fracture may be further apparent on the radiographs (Table 67–2), confirming the severity of the injury and the poorer prognostic implications.[59] Open fractures have a higher rate of disturbances in healing, in part related to an increased frequency of infection. Furthermore, as they are associated more often with high impact trauma, the severity of soft tissue and bone injury prolongs healing. Systems used to classify open fractures and to gauge their ultimate prognosis are based on the size of the wound.[60, 61] Type I open fractures are associated with an opening in the skin of 1 cm or less in length with minimum stripping of soft tissue; type II open fractures are associated with a laceration more than 1 cm long with moderate soft tissue damage; type IIIA open fractures are associated with extensive soft tissue damage and crushing but also with adequate soft tissue coverage of the fractured bone; type IIIB open fractures are characterized by extensive soft tissue injury with periosteal stripping and exposure of bone, usually associated with massive contamination; and type IIIC open fractures are associated with an arterial injury requiring operative repair.

A *complete fracture* occurs when the entire circumference (tubular bone) or both cortical surfaces (flat bone) of a bone have been disrupted. In an *incomplete fracture* a break in the cortex does not extend completely through the bone. The lack of a complete break imparts some degree of stability, which may be advantageous in the management of a nondisplaced fracture. When angular deformity is present, the intact cortex may prevent satisfactory realignment, and it may be necessary to convert the incomplete fracture to a complete one to achieve an acceptable reduction. Incomplete fractures occur in the resilient elastic bones of children and young adults. They may be classified further into various types, including bowing, greenstick, and torus fractures (see later discussion).

The descriptive nomenclature of fractures may be amplified by the use of terms denoting the direction of the fracture line with reference to the shaft (long bones) or cortex

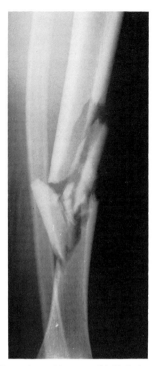

FIGURE 67–11. Comminuted fracture. Multiple fracture fragments of the tibia are evident.

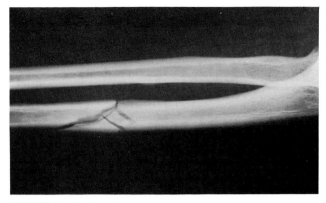

FIGURE 67–12. Butterfly fracture fragment. A comminuted fracture of the midportion of the shaft of the ulna contains a wedge-shaped butterfly fragment.

(irregular bones). The direction of the fracture line reflects the vector of the applied force (see later discussion). Four basic types of linear fractures involving the shaft of a tubular bone may be recognized: *transverse, oblique, oblique-transverse,* and *spiral.* With an increasing magnitude of applied force, fracture comminution may result, and the primary configuration (and mechanism of injury) may be obscured. In many comminuted fractures, however, this mechanism still may be deduced by careful analysis of the radiographs.

A *comminuted fracture* (Fig. 67–11) is one with more than two fracture fragments, regardless of the total number of such fragments. Comminuted fractures may result from a variety of different mechanisms, but, in general, the greater the applied force and the more rapid its application, the greater is the energy absorption by the bone and the severity of comminution. Crush fractures result in severe comminution and associated soft tissue injury.

Certain distinctive subtypes of comminuted fractures exist. A *butterfly fragment* (Fig. 67–12) is a wedge-shaped fragment arising from the shaft of a long bone at the apex of the force input. The most common sites of butterfly fragments are the femoral and humeral diaphyses. The therapeutic implication of this type of fragment, particularly if large, concerns the difficulty in achieving and maintaining reduction owing to the oblique nature of the fracture and the lack of fixation of the osseous fragment. A *segmental fracture* (Fig. 67–13) is one in which the fracture lines isolate a segment of the shaft of the tubular bone. Segmental fractures have special implications regarding adequacy of the blood supply and healing rate, depending on their size and location within the bone. A segmental fracture may be missed, particularly if signs and symptoms related to one of the fracture sites predominate; the clinical manifestations

of a femoral shaft fracture may overshadow those related to a fracture of the ipsilateral femoral neck.

Descriptions of the location of a fracture relate to its anatomic position within the bone. A tubular bone may be divided roughly into thirds, and a fracture may be described as arising in the proximal, middle, or distal third or at the junction of the proximal and middle or middle and distal thirds. A fracture approximately equidistant from the ends of a bone may be called a midshaft fracture. Fractures in other regions are described by additional anatomic reference points (e.g., metacarpal base, metacarpal head, supracondylar or subtrochanteric region).

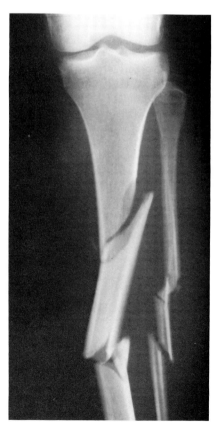

FIGURE 67–13. Segmental fracture. A segment of the shaft of the tibia and a portion of the fibula have been isolated in this injury.

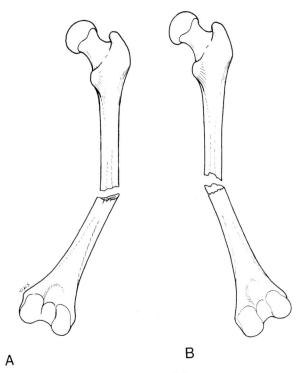

FIGURE 67–14. Varus and valgus angulation.
  A Varus angulation. The distal fragment is angulated toward the midline.
  B Valgus angulation. The distal fragment is angulated away from the midline.

The *alignment* of a fracture refers to the longitudinal relationship of one fragment to another. If there is no significant angulation, the fracture is said to be in anatomic or near anatomic alignment. By convention, angulation of the distal fragment is described in relationship to the proximal one. Such angulation may be medial or lateral, dorsal or ventral, or, in the forearm, radial or ulnar. The terms *varus* and *valgus* often are used, although they are confusing and modern usage actually is opposite from their derivation.[62] By current convention, varus refers to angulation of the distal fracture fragment toward the midline of the body; valgus refers to angulation of the distal fracture fragment away from the midline of the body (Fig. 67–14). Alternatively, terms describing the angulation at the fracture site may be used, although these do not allow either ideal conceptualization of the direction in which the distal fragment must be moved to correct the alignment or integration of specific angular measurements. *Anterior angulation* at the fracture site means that the apex of the fracture is directed anteriorly (ventrally). Conversely, *posterior angulation* at the fracture site indicates that the apex of the fracture site is directed posteriorly (dorsally).[1022]

Fracture position describes the relationship of the fracture fragments, exclusive of angulation, compared with the normal anatomic situation (Fig. 67–15). Deviation from anatomic position is called displacement; terminology descriptive of displacement includes apposition and rotation. Thus, a fracture may be displaced without deviation of alignment or angulated without displacement of fragments. *Apposition* considers the degree of bone contact at the fracture site. A fracture with complete or 100 per cent apposition usually is described as *undisplaced*. Partial degrees of

surface contact may be quantitated roughly using percentages (e.g., 25, 50, or 75 per cent apposition). If the fracture surfaces are separated, the amount of *distraction* may be measured. Overlapping fracture surfaces with resultant shortening are described as a bayonet deformity (Fig. 67–16).

Rotatory displacement of a fracture (i.e., rotation about the long axis of a bone) may be extremely difficult to determine radiographically, yet reduction of rotatory displacement appears to be more important functionally than reduction of angulation. Radiographic evaluation of rotation is facilitated by including the joints both proximal and distal to the fracture on the film, as well as by comparison views in one or both planes (Fig. 67–17). In the absence of comminution, whenever the diameter of a long bone changes abruptly across the fracture site, a rotational displacement must be considered. This difference in diameter has been termed the "disparate diameter sign" and can be applied only when the cross section of the bone at the fracture site is not circular.[63]

An *avulsion fracture* occurs when an osseous fragment is pulled from the parent bone by a tendon or ligament (Fig. 67–18). Such fractures often are located at sites of bony prominences. In the case of a ligamentous avulsion fracture, the term "sprain-fracture" may be used. The term "chip fracture" should not be applied to an avulsion fracture, as it incompletely describes the nature of the injury, which involves disruption of the muscle or ligament attachment. In the assessment of an avulsion fracture, the effect of this soft tissue disruption on joint stability must be considered.

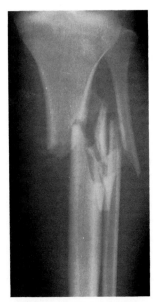

FIGURE 67–15. Fracture position. A comminuted fracture of the proximal portion of the tibial diaphysis and an oblique fracture of the proximal portion of the fibular diaphysis are present. Lateral displacement of the tibia distal to the fracture site is seen with approximately 20 per cent apposition of the major fragments at the fracture site. No rotation or angulation of the tibial fracture has occurred. With regard to the fibular fracture, the distal fragment is displaced medially with respect to the proximal fragment, without evidence of rotation. No apposition of the fracture fragments is seen. Medial angulation of the distal fibular fragment with respect to the proximal one (or, alternatively, lateral angulation at the fracture site) is observed.

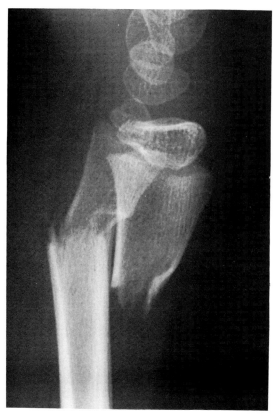

FIGURE 67–16. Bayonet deformity. Observe fractures of the distal portions of the radius and ulna. The radial fragment is displaced dorsally with overriding, a bayonet deformity.

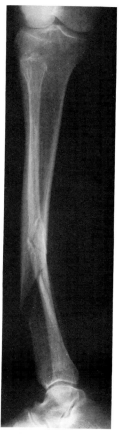

FIGURE 67–17. Rotatory displacement. This radiograph of the lower portion of the leg reveals that the knee is in an oblique position and the ankle is in a lateral attitude. Fractures of the shafts of the tibia and fibula are observed, with marked lateral rotation of the distal fragments.

Complete evaluation may require stress radiography, MR imaging, or arthrography.

An *impaction fracture* results when one fragment of bone is driven into an apposing fragment (Fig. 67–19). Most impaction fractures involve cancellous bone, as the softer structure allows telescoping of fragments. Although impaction of bone fragments usually imparts a degree of stability, it is difficult to assess this stability accurately radiographically.

Two specific types of impaction fractures are recognized. A *depression fracture* results when impacting forces occur between one hard bone surface and an apposing softer surface. A common depression fracture occurs when the hard surface of the femoral condyle is driven into the relatively softer tibial plateau (Fig. 67–20). A *compression fracture* is a type of impaction fracture characteristically involving vertebral bodies. Forceful flexion of the spine may result in a wedge fracture of a vertebral body caused by its mechanical compression between the adjacent vertebral bodies with depression of the endplate(s) within the spongy bone of the vertebral centrum (Fig. 67–21). A vertebral compression fracture is distinguished from other types of vertebral fractures that result from vertical compression forces, such as the Jefferson fracture of the atlas and burst fractures (see Chapter 69).

Additional types of fractures, including stress and pathologic fractures, are discussed later in this chapter.

Fracture Healing

After a fracture, a remarkable series of events (Fig. 67–22) occurs that leads to osseous healing in the majority of

cases.[64–69] Three indistinctly separated phases of healing are recognized: an inflammatory phase (representing approximately 10 per cent of the entire time of fracture healing); a reparative phase (representing about 40 per cent of this time); and a remodeling phase (the longest phase, representing as much as 70 per cent of the time).[64] Initially, bleeding takes place from the damaged ends of the bones

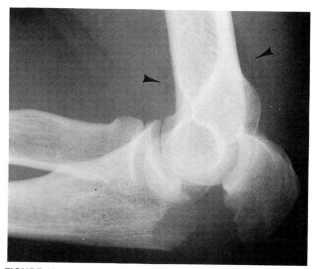

FIGURE 67–18. Avulsion fracture. The triceps tendon is attached to the large fracture fragment. A joint effusion is noted (arrowheads).

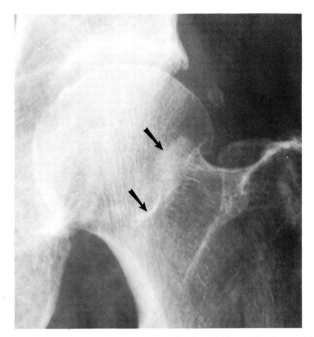

FIGURE 67–19. Impaction fracture. A sclerotic line extends across the lateral aspect of the subcapital region (arrows).

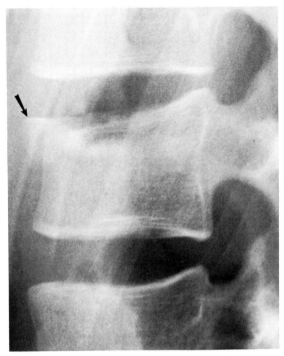

FIGURE 67–21. Compression fracture. A compression fracture of the superior surface of the second lumbar vertebral body is present, with a small comminuted corner fragment (arrow).

and from the neighboring soft tissues. Formation of a hematoma within the medullary canal, between the fracture ends, and beneath the elevated periosteum is followed by clot formation. Interruption of blood vessels produces osteocytic death, and the necrotic material induces an intense,

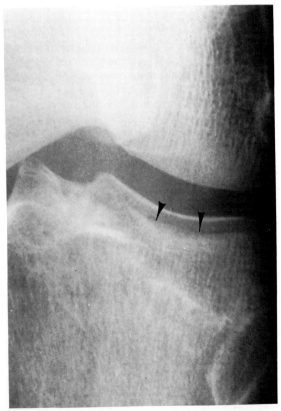

FIGURE 67–20. Depression fracture. The double contour of the lateral tibial plateau has resulted from a depressed fracture (arrowheads).

acute inflammatory response. Vasodilation, exudation of plasma and leukocytes, and infiltration of polymorphonuclear leukocytes, histiocytes, and mast cells are identified.

A reparative phase begins with organization of the fracture hematoma and invasion by fibrovascular tissue, which replaces the clot and lays down the collagen fibers and the matrix, which later will become mineralized to form the woven bone of the provisional or primary callus.[69] Participation of cells in the periosteum, endosteum, and granulation tissue can be recognized in the healing process, although the site and type of cellular activity[70] and the amount of new bone that is formed are variable and influenced by the nature of the bone that is affected. Callus envelops the bone ends rapidly, producing increasing stability at the fracture site. In some areas, particularly at the periphery of the callus, cartilage appears and is converted to bone by the process of endochondral ossification. The bone ends gradually become enveloped in a fusiform mass of callus whose internal and external components lead to increasing immobilization of the fracture fragments.[64]

During the process of repair, a remodeling phase also can be identified, which is associated with resorption of unnecessary segments of the callus and proliferation of trabeculae along lines of stress. The exact location of osteoblastic and osteoclastic activity apparently is mediated by electrical mechanisms.[64, 71, 72] The fate of the dead bone at the fracture site is influenced by mechanical factors. It may be resorbed or incorporated into the bony mass, providing osseous continuity and stability.

The three phases of fracture healing—inflammatory, reparative, and remodeling—overlap, and cellular activity at a fracture site, which can be outlined using radioisotopic studies, persists long after the radiographic changes appear static;[64] for example, it has been estimated that increased

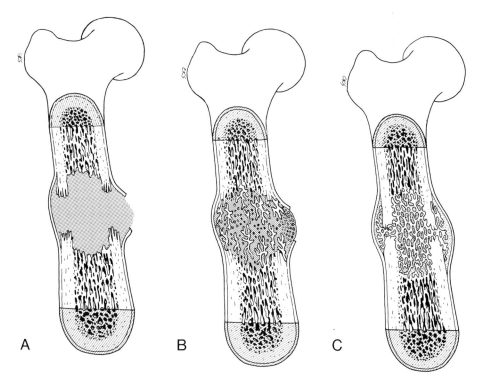

FIGURE 67–22. Normal fracture healing.

A After the injury, bleeding is related to osseous and soft tissue damage. A hematoma followed by clot formation develops within the medullary canal between the fracture ends and beneath the periosteal membrane, which itself may have been torn.

B Callus formation takes place, consisting of external bridging callus at the periosteal surface, intramedullary callus, and primary callus at the ends of the fracture fragments.

C The callus envelops the bone ends rapidly, producing increasing stability at the fracture site.

A   B   C

activity is present at the site of a tibial fracture for a period of 6 to 9 years. Many local factors can modify the healing process: the degree of trauma (retarded healing is expected in fractures associated with extensive osseous and soft tissue injury); the degree of bone loss (retarded healing occurs when the bone loss is substantial); the type of bone involved (cancellous bone unites rapidly at sites of osseous contact, whereas cortical bone may unite with or without extensive external callus, depending on the degree of apposition of the fragments); the extent of immobilization (improper immobilization may lead to delayed union or nonunion); the presence of infection (retarded bone healing occurs when infection is present); the presence of an underlying pathologic process (neoplastic, metabolic, and other disorders delay the healing process); use of radiation therapy (irradiated bone unites at a slower rate); the presence of extensive osteonecrosis (avascular bone impedes fracture healing); and the occurrence of intra-articular extension (fibrinolysins in the synovial fluid may destroy the initial clot, producing a delay in fracture union).[64] Systemic factors such as the age of the patient (healing is more rapid in the immature skeleton) and the presence of abnormal serum levels of certain hormones (corticosteroids inhibit fracture healing) also can be influential in fracture repair.

The orderly sequence of events terminating in complete healing of a fracture does not invariably take place as described. In some instances, the healing process is markedly slowed (delayed union) or arrested altogether (nonunion). As the rate of fracture healing depends on many local and systemic factors, there is no uniformly accepted definition of delayed union, although the clinical application of the term implies that the healing attempt is proceeding at a pace that is slower than that which is expected in a given bone. The histologic characteristics of a delayed union are similar to those of normal union, although the conversion of fibrocartilage to bone at the fracture site is delayed or

may cease temporarily. Such conversion may start anew either spontaneously or after some type of orthopedic intervention. Protracted or permanent cessation of fibrocartilage mineralization results in a nonunion. Nonunion generally indicates that the fracture site has failed to heal completely during a period of approximately 6 to 9 months after the injury and that a typical *pseudarthrosis* (consisting of a synovium-lined cavity and synovial fluid typically related to persistent motion at the nonunion site) or a fibrous union has developed, in which the ends of the bone are either osteoporotic and atrophic or sclerotic.[64]

Milgram[73] has suggested that only two terms, nonunion (Fig. 67–23) and pseudarthrosis (Fig. 67–24), should be applied to improper fracture healing, and that the latter term is appropriate only when a false joint cavity separates the ends of a bone at a fracture site. Such pseudarthroses are expected at fracture sites, such as those of the humerus, in which bending stresses are great. Pseudarthroses developing at a fracture site of the femoral neck also are common. Gross pathologic findings of a pseudarthrosis include a space containing fluid at the fracture site and cartilage-like tissue over the bone ends. Pseudarthroses in extra-articular sites probably result from transformation of fibrocartilage in the region of a nonunion. Pseudarthroses in intra-articular sites may develop as a primary phenomenon. In the latter situation, the morphology of the pseudarthrosis is more reminiscent of that of a true joint.

Thus, nonunions of fractures may occur with or without the formation of a pseudarthrosis. Nonunion of a scaphoid, tibial, or femoral fracture is encountered most commonly, whereas nonunion occurring after a fracture of the humerus,[74–76] radius, ulna, and clavicle[77] is somewhat less frequent (Figs. 67–25 to 67–27). Nonunion of a type 2 odontoid fracture leads to an os odontoideum (Fig. 67–28). The causes of nonunion include open, comminuted, segmental, or pathologic fractures, insufficient immobilization of the

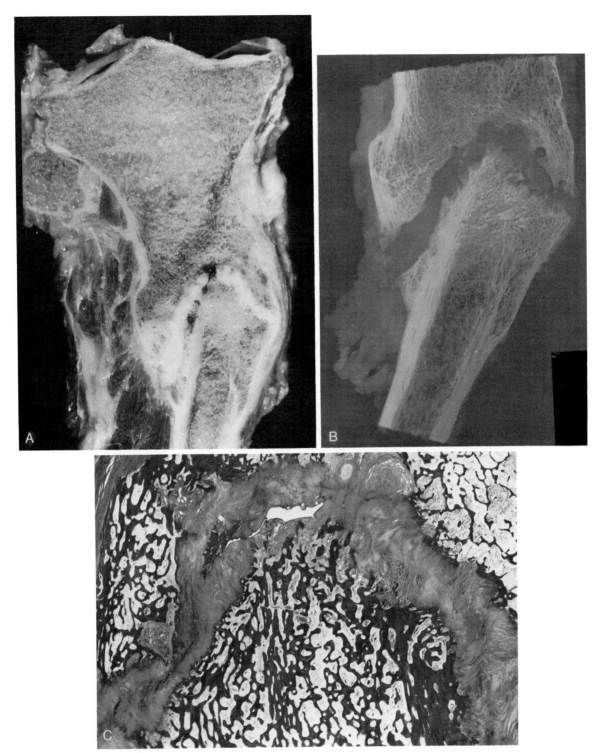

FIGURE 67–23. Abnormal fracture healing: Nonunion.

A A photograph of a coronal section of the proximal portion of the tibia is shown, in which a nonunion of a fracture of over 1 year's duration had occurred. An angulated position of the fractured tibia is shown, in which white fibrous tissue separates the fractured ends. The callus forming around the proximal fragment has created a large concave cup of old and new bone.

B A specimen radiograph of another section of tissue from the same tibia shows tiny buds of new bone extending into the radiolucent zone.

C A histologic preparation reveals fibrous tissue with considerable chondroid differentiation of the cells. One small cleft is visible within the area of nonunion, which, if extended, would represent a true pseudarthrosis. The ends of the bone are sclerotic. Focal fragments of necrotic bone are visible. (×5, hematoxylin and eosin.)

(From Milgram JW: Clin Orthop *268:*203, 1991.)

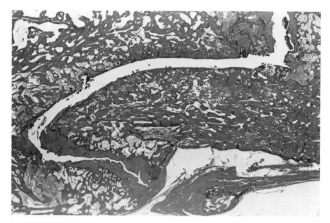

FIGURE 67–24. Abnormal fracture healing: Pseudarthrosis. Note a Z-shaped fracture line of a long tubular bone. Although reactive fibrocartilage lines the fracture fragments, a space is seen between the apposing surfaces of bone. Sclerotic bone is evident. (×5.5, hematoxylin and eosin.) (From Milgram JW: Clin Orthop *268:*203, 1991.)

osseous fragments, infection, interposition of soft tissue between the edges of the fractured bone, inadequate blood supply, poor nutritional status, and metabolic bone disease.

Although radiographs are used routinely to monitor the stage of healing of a fracture, the diagnosis of delayed union or nonunion requires clinical assessment. The gradual obliteration of a fracture line generally is regarded as a favorable radiographic finding, but it is one that can be created also by varying the orientation of the x-ray beam with respect to the injured bone. Furthermore, clinical evidence of solid union at a fracture site may occur at a time when routine radiographs show clear evidence of a persistent fracture line. Ancillary imaging techniques such as bone scintigraphy, CT, and MR imaging may be used in the assessment of fracture healing and in the diagnosis of delayed union, nonunion, or pseudarthroses, although data

regarding the efficacy of these techniques are incomplete and, in some cases, conflicting.[78, 79]

Delayed unions and nonunions of fractures should be distinguished from *malunions*. A malunited fracture is one that has healed in an improper position (e.g., excessive angular or rotational deformity). Malunion of a fracture in an adult may lead to a deformity that is readily apparent on clinical examination and one that may require surgical correction. Malunion of a fracture in a child may be a temporary phenomenon that disappears spontaneously with further skeletal growth.

Special Types of Fractures

Pathologic Fractures. A pathologic fracture is one in which the bone is disrupted at a site of preexisting abnormality, frequently by a stress that would not have fractured a normal bone. Any process that weakens the osseous tissue structurally, particularly if it involves cortical bone, can result in a pathologic fracture. The most common underlying abnormalities are tumors and osteoporosis, although infectious, articular, and metabolic processes all can be manifested in this fashion. The term "insufficiency fracture" has been used to describe disruption occurring at sites of nontumorous lesions. Of the tumorous causes of pathologic fractures, skeletal metastasis predominates, followed, in order of frequency, by benign lesions (such as simple bone cysts, enchondromas, and giant cell tumors) and pri-

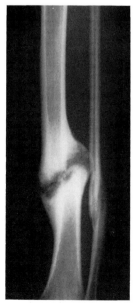

FIGURE 67–25. Abnormal fracture healing: Nonunion. Tibia. A classic hypertrophic nonunion is evident. Prominent external callus and irregular bone ends are seen. The adjacent fibular fracture has healed.

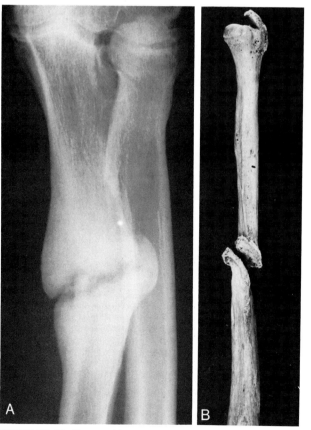

FIGURE 67–26. Abnormal fracture healing: Nonunion. Ulna.
 A Note the typical features of a hypertrophic nonunion. Deformity of the proximal portion of the radius also is evident.
 B Note the pointed and atrophic appearance of the bone about the fracture site.

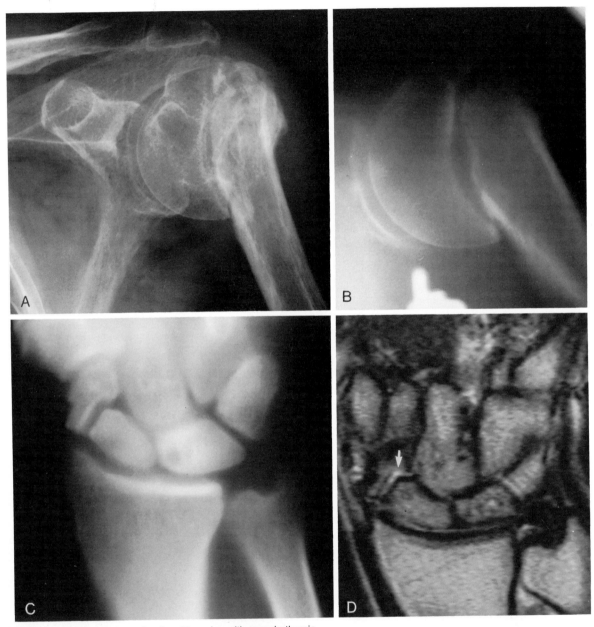

FIGURE 67–27. Abnormal fracture healing: Nonunion with pseudarthrosis.

A, B Humerus. A nonunion with a pseudarthrosis developed after a displaced fracture of the proximal humerus had occurred. Conventional radiography **(A)** and tomography **(B)** show smooth, sclerotic fracture lines. Fluoroscopy documented considerable motion at the fracture site with movement of the arm.

C, D Scaphoid bone of the wrist. The conventional tomogram **(C)** reveals sclerotic fracture lines with smooth margins in the scaphoid bone. Cystic and sclerotic changes in the lunate bone are consistent with Kienbock's disease. A coronal T2-weighted (TR/TE, 2500/60) spin echo MR image **(D)** shows fluid of high signal intensity (arrow) in the fracture gap as well as increased signal intensity in the lunate bone.

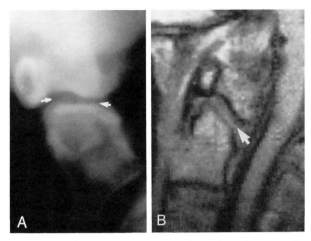

FIGURE 67–28. Abnormal fracture healing: Nonunion. Os odontoideum. This patient had had a remote fracture of the base of the odontoid process.

A Conventional tomography confirms the presence of a nonunion at the fracture site (arrows). The apposing surfaces of the bone are sclerotic.

B A sagittal T1-weighted (TR/TE, 680/21) spin echo MR image also shows the site of nonunion (arrow) with low signal intensity on either side of the fracture, consistent with sclerotic bone.

mary osseous malignancies (including plasma cell myeloma, histiocytic lymphoma, Ewing's sarcoma, and osteosarcoma). Large and aggressive lesions are more likely to produce pathologic fractures than are small, nonaggressive

processes. The propensity and the time required for spontaneous healing of pathologic fractures related to tumors depend on many factors, including the specific type of neoplasm. Fractures related to plasma cell myeloma, for example, heal more frequently than those related to carcinoma of the breast, lung, or kidney. Pathologic fractures in certain sites, such as the femoral neck, tend to heal slowly or not at all.

The identification of a lesion at risk for fracture is a subject of considerable interest and importance. Such a lesion may require prophylactic orthopedic surgery, depending on its nature and precise site, the activity level of the patient, and the prognosis of the disease process. Although the size of the lesion and, more important, the extent of cortical destruction generally are believed to be fundamental factors influencing the likelihood of pathologic fracture, routine radiography represents an inadequate technique in evaluating such factors.[80] Conventional tomography and, particularly, CT with its transaxial image display are superior methods in this evaluation.

The radiographic distinction between a pathologic and a nonpathologic fracture is not always easy. This differentiation is not difficult when a fracture line traverses a large area of osseous destruction or when the adjacent or distant bones are riddled with additional lesions (Fig. 67–29). When a smaller lesion is present, the fracture itself may obscure the area of lysis or sclerosis, especially in the presence of displacement at the fracture site. The absence of a history of trauma or fracture pain and the presence of

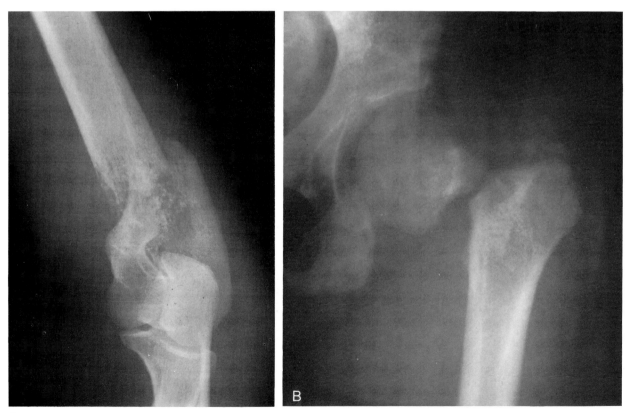

FIGURE 67–29. Pathologic fracture.

A A transverse fracture line through a metastatic focus from bronchogenic carcinoma can be detected in the distal portion of the humerus. Note the osteolysis, cortical irregularity, and soft tissue swelling.

B In this example, a pathologic fracture of the femoral neck relates to renal osteodystrophy, which had led to considerable resorption of the femur, predisposing to its fracture.

symptoms and signs of preexisting abnormality, such as angular deformity, painless swelling, or generalized bone pain, are clinical aids to the diagnosis of a pathologic fracture. The radiographic diagnosis is substantiated by the presence of bone destruction, altered architecture or density, and deformity. A transverse fracture line, particularly one that is not located in the diaphysis of a tubular bone, and an inability to reconstruct the entire bone mentally by "piecing together" the fracture fragments are additional radiographic clues. Diagnostic difficulty may be encountered in the patient who has a nonpathologic fracture that is days to weeks old, as resorption, osteolysis, or rotation about the fracture site may create the illusion of an underlying lesion. This is especially true with fractures of the femoral neck, pubic rami, and distal portion of the clavicle (see Chapter 94).

Pathologic fractures related to certain types of tumors may be associated with characteristic radiographic features. Displacement of a cortical fracture fragment into the interior of a fluid-filled cystic lesion of bone (e.g., simple bone cyst) may be followed by migration of the fragment to a dependent portion of the lesion (fallen fragment sign). Depressed fractures of an expansile osteolytic lesion (e.g., giant cell tumor, aneurysmal bone cyst) may be accompanied by comminution of the thin cortical shell, resulting in a cracked eggshell appearance.[2] Classic imaging characteristics, such as the patterns of signal intensity on MR images, in these and other types of tumors are altered in the presence of a pathologic fracture, owing to the presence of hemorrhage.

Trabecular Microfractures (Bone Bruises). With the application of MR imaging to the evaluation of musculoskeletal injuries has come the identification of intraosseous regions of altered signal intensity that have been designated occult intraosseous fractures[81, 82] or bone bruises.[53] These injuries, which typically are located close to a joint surface, are believed to result from compression or impaction forces, although there are no correlative histologic data to confirm this belief. Their frequent association with other traumatic abnormalities such as cruciate and collateral ligament injuries of the knee[54, 83] is consistent with the occurrence of trabecular microfractures with resultant hyperemia, hemorrhage, and edema in the bone marrow. Arthroscopy in cases in which bone bruises are evident on MR examination fails to reveal corresponding lesions, documenting that the adjacent articular surface is normal.[53] The presence of similar changes in the signal intensity of the bone marrow on MR images in patients with osteochondral lesions supports the concept of injury in the pathogenesis of bone bruises, and histologic data that indicate marrow edema in cases of transient osteoporosis of periarticular bone (in which these same signal intensity changes are observed) are further evidence that intraosseous fluid accumulation accompanies these bone bruises. It appears likely that the trabecular alterations that characterize bone bruise are very similar if not identical to those associated with stress fractures, although in the former situation an acute episode of trauma rather than chronic repetitive stress is the initiating event. Whether bone bruises themselves are symptomatic is not clear, although their occurrence as an isolated finding in patients with local pain supports the possibility. Resolution of the MR imaging abnormalities associated with bone bruises generally occurs over a period of 1 to several months and may coincide with decrease or disappearance of the patient's symptoms.[53]

The characteristics of these trabecular microfractures on MR images are remarkably constant and have been described most completely with regard to distal femoral and proximal tibial lesions about the knee (Fig. 67–30). The findings are those of marrow fluid, with low signal intensity regions on T1-weighted spin echo MR images and high signal intensity regions on T2-weighted spin echo and short tau inversion recovery (STIR) images. The bone bruises are displayed most prominently on the STIR images,[84] which even may lead to overestimation of their size, and they also may be vividly apparent when fat suppression techniques with or without the use of intravenous administration of gadolinium contrast agent are employed.[85] Bone bruises typically are poorly defined and speckled in appearance, although linear areas of altered signal intensity also may be observed. Such linear areas, however, are more characteristic of stress fractures. As amorphous regions of low signal intensity on T1-weighted spin echo MR images that characterize bone bruises may be difficult to differentiate from similar regions of low signal intensity resulting from normal trabeculae, the increased signal intensity of bone bruises on T2-weighted spin echo and STIR images assumes diagnostic importance. Furthermore, the detection of bone bruises at specific anatomic sites provides secondary evidence that other injuries may be present; examples of this include the occurrence of bone bruises in the lateral femoral condyle and posterolateral portion of the tibia in patients with injuries of the anterior cruciate ligament[54, 83, 86]; of bone bruises in the lateral femoral condyle in persons with injuries of the medial collateral ligament of the knee; and of bone bruises in the lateral femoral condyle and medial portion of the patella in patients with lateral patellar dislocation[87] (Fig. 67–31). Indeed, as the pathogenesis of bone bruises appears to include compression or impaction forces, their sites of occurrence about the knee or elsewhere are entirely predictable on the basis of an understanding of mechanisms of subluxation or dislocation of joints or other injuries (see Chapter 70).

Stress Fractures. Stress fractures can occur in normal or abnormal bone that is subjected to repeated cyclic loading, with the load being less than that which causes acute fracture of bone.[88–92] Two types of stress fractures can be recognized: a *fatigue fracture,* resulting from the application of abnormal stress or torque to a bone with normal elastic resistance; and an *insufficiency fracture,* occurring when normal stress is placed on a bone with deficient elastic resistance. Both fatigue and insufficiency fractures can occur in the same person if an abnormal stress is placed on an abnormal bone.

Fatigue fractures frequently share the following features: The activity is new or different for the person; the activity is strenuous; and the activity is repeated with a frequency that ultimately produces symptoms and signs.[71, 88, 93] Rarely, fatigue fractures are asymptomatic.[94] Typical examples are the fatigue fractures that occur in the metatarsal bones of military recruits ("march" fractures),[90, 91, 95–97] and in the lower extremities in athletes, joggers, and dancers,[98–100] although other strenuous activities can produce similar infractions at these and additional sites.[101–114] Both recreational and competitive runners are prone to fatigue fractures of the proximal posteromedial surface of the tibia, the distal

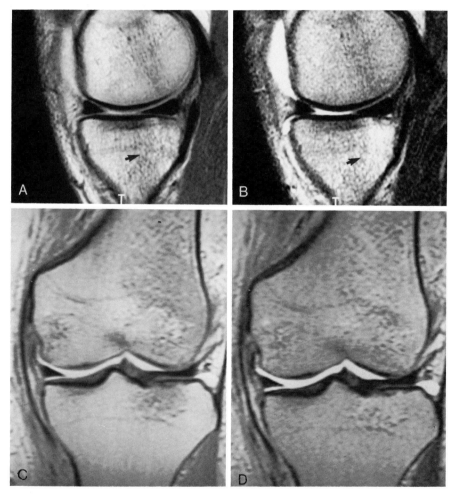

FIGURE 67–30. Trabecular microfractures (bone bruises).

A, B Sagittal proton density (TR/TE, 2200/30) **(A)** and T2-weighted (TR/TE, 2200/80) spin echo MR images show the characteristic finding of a bone bruise (arrows), which in this case involves mainly the posterior portion of the medial tibial plateau. The lesion is of high signal intensity in **B.** Note the joint effusion.

C, D Similar abnormalities of signal intensity in a different patient are evident on coronal proton density (TR/TE, 2500/20) **(C)** and T2-weighted (TR/TE, 2500/60) **(D)** spin echo MR images. The bone bruises are located in the lateral portions of the distal femur and proximal tibia and, to a lesser extent, in the medial femoral condyle. They are of higher signal intensity in **D** and are associated with a partial tear of the medial collateral ligament and a joint effusion.

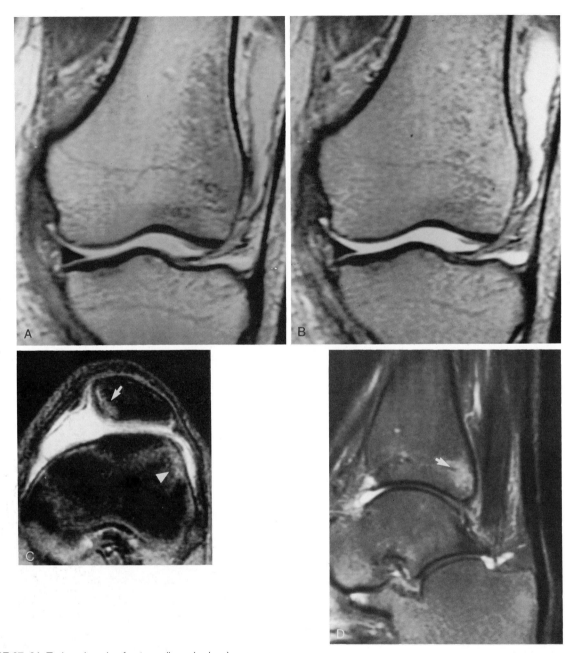

FIGURE 67–31. Trabecular microfractures (bone bruises).

A, B Medial collateral ligament injury. Coronal proton density (TR/TE, 2500/20) **(A)** and T2-weighted (TR/TE, 2500/60) **(B)** spin echo MR images show a bone bruise in the lateral femoral condyle, of high signal intensity in **B,** associated with a complete tear of the medial collateral ligament of the knee. A joint effusion is evident.

C Patellar dislocation. A transaxial multiplanar gradient recalled (MPGR) MR image (TR/TE, 500/11; flip angle, 15 degrees) shows high signal intensity in the medial portion of the patella (arrow) and lateral femoral condyle (arrowhead) related to trabecular microfractures occurring during a lateral dislocation of the patella. The medial retinaculum is attenuated, and a large joint effusion is present.

(C, Courtesy of S. K. Brahme, M.D., La Jolla, California.)

D Posterior portion of tibia. In a 24 year old hockey player a sagittal T2-weighted (TR/TE, 3000/84) fast spin echo MR image, obtained with fat suppression technique, shows a bone bruise (arrow) of high signal intensity in the posterior malleolus. This patient had had additional injuries, which required surgical repair of lateral ankle ligaments.

(D, Courtesy of D. Witte, M.D., Memphis, Tennessee.)

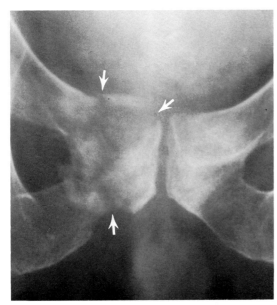

FIGURE 67–32. Insufficiency fractures: Rheumatoid arthritis and osteoporosis. In parasymphyseal bone, such fractures (arrows) are accompanied by osteolysis, osteosclerosis, and bone fragmentation.

shaft of the fibula, the navicular bone of the foot, and the femoral neck; leaping activities such as may occur in basketball can lead to fatigue fractures of the anterior surface of the tibia and the calcaneus.[93]

The causes of insufficiency fractures are diverse[88] and include rheumatoid arthritis,[115–117] osteoporosis,[118–122] Paget's disease,[71] osteomalacia or rickets,[123] hyperparathyroidism, renal osteodystrophy,[1023] osteogenesis imperfecta, osteopetrosis, fibrous dysplasia, and irradiation.[71] Of these causes, rheumatoid arthritis and osteoporosis deserve emphasis. In patients with the former disease, predisposing factors include osteopenia owing to disuse, corticosteroid therapy and osteomalacia, angular deformities in the extremities, and arthroplasties allowing new physical activities; the insufficiency fractures predominate in the bones of the legs and pelvis (Fig. 67–32). In patients with osteoporosis, such fractures occur in the sacrum, pubic rami, and lower extremities as well as other sites (Fig. 67–33). In Paget's disease, the convex aspect of the tubular bones, especially the femur, is affected (Fig. 67–34). Fatigue and insufficiency fractures are not infrequent after certain surgical procedures that result in altered stress or an imbalance of muscular force on normal or abnormal bones. Common examples are noted in the metatarsal bones after bunion surgery,[124–126] in the lower extremities following arthrodesis or arthroplasty,[116] in the pubic rami after hip[127, 128] or knee[129, 130] surgery, and in the clavicles after radical mastectomy or neck dissection[131–132] (Fig. 67–35). Fatigue and insufficiency fractures also are observed in the distal portion of the tibia or in the bones of the foot in patients with healing or healed gross traumatic fractures of a more proximal portion of the tibia, fibula, or femur after they begin weightbearing.[133, 134]

Although routine radiography plays an essential role in the diagnosis of stress fractures (see following discussion), it is the radionuclide examination that provides not only one means of early detection,[135–150] but also a visual account of the biomechanical properties of bone that are fundamen-

tal to the pathogenesis of stress fractures. Roub and colleagues[89] have provided an excellent summary of these properties (Fig. 67–36). When a bone is stressed, osteonal remodeling or osteonization takes place, in which resorption of circumferential lamellar bone and its subsequent replacement by dense osteonal bone are identified.[151–154] Because of this process, a vulnerable period exists after a stressful occurrence, in which the cortical bone is less capable of withstanding further stress and in which the foci of osseous resorption may be transformed into sites of microfracture. This complication is especially likely to occur when unusual and unaccustomed activity leads to increased tone and strength of a muscle in a relatively short period of time while the increased strength of the bone lags behind.[88] The stress fracture begins as a small cortical crack, which progresses as the stress continues or becomes more exaggerated[155, 156]; such progression is characterized by the appearance of subcortical infraction in front of the advancing main crack in the bone.[157] If the stress is eliminated, the sequence is interrupted or slowed so that new bone formation "catches up" to the increased demand, and a state of increased bone strength then is reached.[158] Increasing physical activity under controlled circumstances can produce osseous hypertrophy without evidence of microfracture. Exercise programs of the professional athlete are designed to allow the bone to compensate for the exaggerated muscular stresses that are encountered; bony hypertrophy is well recognized in the lower extremities of long distance runners and ballet dancers[100] as well as in the upper extremities of baseball pitchers and tennis players.[159, 160] This is radiologic evidence of Wolff's law at work.[161]

The biomechanical properties of bone that have been outlined have their scintigraphic counterparts.[89] The stressed and "painful" bone undergoing accelerated remodeling produces an abnormal radionuclide image in

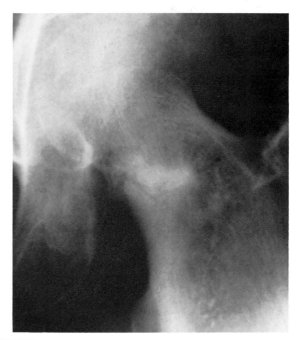

FIGURE 67–33. Insufficiency fractures: Osteoporosis. This elderly woman developed bilateral insufficiency fractures of the femoral necks. Observe a bandlike pattern of bone sclerosis in the medial portion of the femoral neck. (Courtesy of R. Sweet, M.D., Pomona, California.)

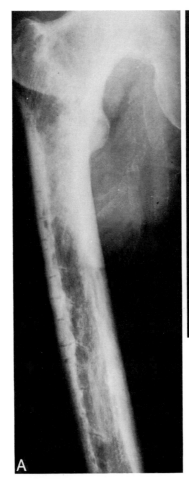

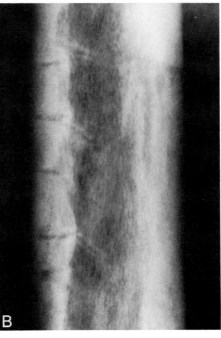

FIGURE 67–34. Insufficiency fractures: Paget's disease. Multiple radiolucent fracture lines are seen in the lateral aspect of the diaphysis. Note osseous thickening in the endosteal margin of the cortex at the sites of fracture. (Courtesy of C. Wackenheim, M.D., and Y. Dirheimer, M.D., Paris, France.)

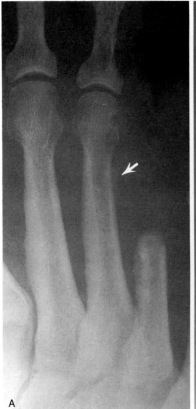

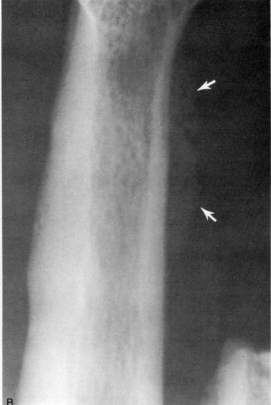

FIGURE 67–35. Fatigue fractures after surgical procedures.

A, B This diabetic patient developed osteomyelitis that required surgical resection of the fourth and fifth digits of the foot. Subsequently, activity-related foot pain occurred, which was due to a stress fracture of the shaft of the third metatarsal bone (arrows), characterized by periostitis, which is best delineated on a magnification radiograph **(B).** No evidence of infection was apparent.

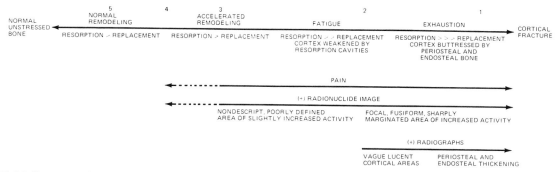

FIGURE 67–36. Stress reaction in bone. A comparison of the histologic, clinical, scintigraphic, and radiologic responses. (From Roub LW, et al: Radiology *132:*431, 1979.)

which nondescript, poorly defined areas of increased accumulation of bone-seeking pharmaceutical agents are observed in the absence of radiographic findings. Appropriate modification of the physical activity may allow osseous "healing" without the appearance of cortical infraction. If the strenuous activity continues, the painful bone may reveal focal fusiform, sharply marginated areas of increased radionuclide activity that can be associated with radiolucent cortical areas and periosteal and endosteal thickening on the roentgenogram, and a diagnosis of a true stress fracture is substantiated (Fig. 67–37). Thus, a stress fracture appears to represent one end of the spectrum of bony response to stress.

The identification of abnormal scintigraphic patterns in athletic persons who subsequently do not develop stress fractures has led to a redefinition of some of the conditions that had formerly been considered together as osseous stress injuries. Shin splints represents one of these conditions, in which a specific abnormality has been identified during bone scintigraphy, especially if three-phase studies (angiographic, blood pool, and delayed phases) are performed.[149, 150] In patients with shin splints, radionuclide angiograms and blood pool images are normal, whereas on delayed images, a longitudinally oriented area of increased radionuclide accumulation is seen in the posteromedial cortex of the tibia (Fig. 67–38). This pattern of abnormality differs from that typically seen in an acute stress fracture (in which all phases of the radionuclide examination are abnormal and a more fusiform area of augmented activity is apparent) and is consistent with the belief that shin splints represent periosteal disruptions of varying length, possibly caused by rupture of the Sharpey's fibers that extend from the muscle through the periosteum into the cortical structure of bone.[150] The location of the scintigraphic abnormality suggests that abnormal excursion of the soleus muscle and, perhaps, other muscle-tendon complexes is responsible for the clinical manifestations. An equivalent lesion occurring in the anteromedial portion of the cortex in the upper or middle region of the femur, corresponding in location to the insertion site or sites of one or more adductor muscle groups, has been designated thigh splints.[137]

Three-phase bone scintigraphy also allows monitoring of the healing stress fracture. As such healing progresses, first the radionuclide angiogram and then the blood pool images revert to normal; the intensity of uptake on the delayed images decreases over 3 to 6 months, although minor abnormalities may persist for 8 to 10 months.[150] The configuration of the abnormal radiopharmaceutical uptake changes from fusiform to a narrower, less defined focus during this period of observation.[150]

Although CT[162, 163] and even ultrasonography[164] also have been used to evaluate stress fractures, their role is limited. CT may reveal a linear radiolucent line as well as periosteal and endosteal bone formation. Increased density in the medullary canal and soft tissue swelling represent additional, although nonspecific, CT abnormalities.[165] A peculiar variety of stress fracture of the tibia characterized by a longitudinal rather than a transverse or oblique course is well evaluated with this imaging method (see Fig. 67–41).[166–169]

MR imaging represents a diagnostic method with comparable sensitivity and superior specificity with respect to bone scintigraphy in the assessment of stress fractures.[53, 170–173] Stress fractures appear most typically as a linear zone of low signal intensity surrounded by a broader, poorly defined area of slightly higher (although still low) signal intensity on T1-weighted spin echo MR images and as a linear area of low signal intensity surrounded by a broader region of high signal intensity on T2-weighted spin echo images[53] (Fig. 67–39). High signal intensity on STIR images and after the intravenous administration of gadolinium contrast agent also may be observed (Fig. 67–40). Less typically, the MR imaging abnormalities of a stress fracture are identical to those of a bone bruise (see previous discussion). Occasionally, a long segment of a tubular bone is involved (Fig. 67–41). Soft tissue edema may be an associated abnormality.

The clinical findings of stress fractures are characteristic. Activity-related pain that is relieved by rest is typical. Localized tenderness and soft tissue swelling also can be observed. Almost any bone in the body can be affected, and the specific site of involvement is influenced by the type of physical activity that is being undertaken. The bones in the lower extremity are affected more frequently than those in the upper extremity. More than one site can be involved simultaneously, more than one stress fracture can occur in a single bone, and symmetric changes are not unusual.[174]

The radiographic abnormalities are influenced by the location of the fracture and the interval between the time of injury and that of the radiographic examination. Certain features are more characteristic of stress fractures in the diaphysis of a tubular bone, whereas others are encountered in stress fractures in the end of a tubular bone (e.g., the tibial plateau) or in areas that are predominantly cancellous

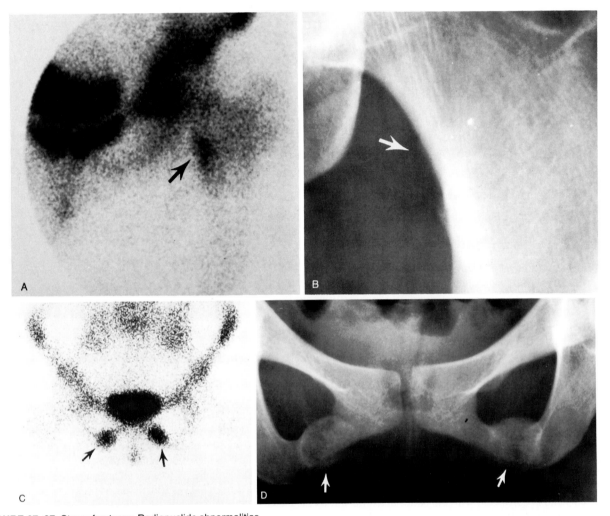

FIGURE 67–37. Stress fractures: Radionuclide abnormalities.

A, B An athletic young woman developed persistent hip pain aggravated by activity. A radionuclide examination reveals a focal, sharply marginated area of increased activity in the femoral neck (arrow). A radiograph of the hip delineates a minimal amount of indistinct new bone formation along the medial aspect of the femoral neck (arrow).

C, D This 24 year old female jogger developed exercise-related pain in the symphysis pubis and the foot. Bilateral stress fractures of the inferior pubic rami are evident on scintigraphic and radiographic examination (arrows). A metatarsal stress fracture also was evident.

(C, D, Courtesy of P. Kaplan, M.D., Charlottesville, Virginia.)

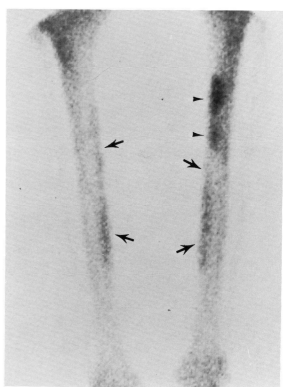

FIGURE 67–38. Stress changes: Shin splints. A 19 year old female athlete who was running 3 miles each day for 3 months developed pain in both calves. On a frontal view of the lower legs during the delayed portion of a bone scan, longitudinally oriented areas of increased tracer accumulation are apparent in the medial cortex of the midportion of the tibiae (arrows). Two localized areas of increased radionuclide activity in the left tibia (arrowheads) may represent stress fractures.

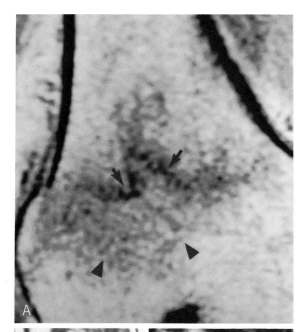

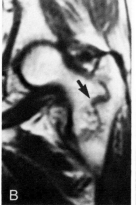

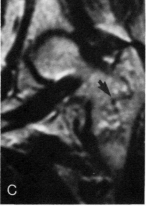

FIGURE 67–39. Stress fractures: MR imaging abnormalities.

A Fatigue fracture of femur. A coronal T1-weighted (TR/TE, 900/20) spin echo MR image reveals the fracture line (arrows) of low signal intensity, surrounded by a broader area of slightly higher but still diminished signal intensity (arrowheads), representing edema. The latter area revealed high signal intensity on a gradient echo sequence (not shown). (Courtesy of S. Fernandez, M.D., Mexico City, Mexico.)

B, C Insufficiency fracture of femur. In a 90 year old woman, coronal proton density (TR/TE, 1800/20) **(B)** and T2-weighted (TR/TE, 1800/80) **(C)** spin echo MR images show the fracture (arrows) in the intertrochanteric region of the femoral neck. Observe some adjacent areas of high signal intensity in **C.** (Courtesy of S. K. Brahme, M.D., La Jolla, California.)

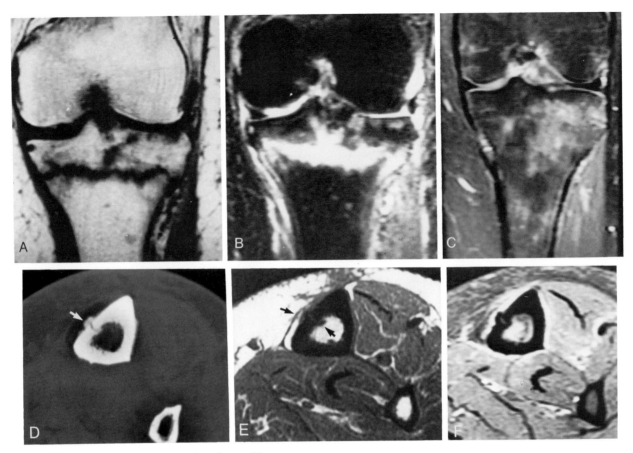

FIGURE 67–40. Stress fractures: MR imaging abnormalities.

A, B Insufficiency fracture of tibia. In this 72 year old woman, coronal T1-weighted (TR/TE, 500/20) **(A)** and short tau inversion recovery (STIR) (TR/TE, 2500/40; inversion time, 160 msec) **(B)** MR images reveal the horizontal and vertical fracture lines in the proximal portion of the tibia. In **B**, note high signal intensity in and about the fracture. A joint effusion is present.

C Fatigue fracture of tibia. This 42 year old woman developed left knee pain after starting a new jogging program. A coronal T1-weighted (TR/TE, 550/20) spin echo MR image obtained with chemical presaturation of fat (ChemSat) and after intravenous administration of a gadolinium contrast agent shows a broad area of high signal intensity in the lateral tibial plateau and lateral portion of the tibial metaphysis. The findings are consistent with a stress fracture.

D–F Insufficiency fracture of tibia. In a 73 year old woman, transaxial CT **(D)** and T1-weighted (TR/TE, 683/17) spin echo MR image **(E)** reveal the site of cortical violation (arrows). This finding as well as adjacent marrow and soft tissue edema, of high signal intensity, is better seen in a transaxial T1-weighted (TR/TE, 683/17) spin echo image obtained with fat suppression and after intravenous administration of a gadolinium contrast agent **(F)**. **(D–F,** Courtesy of D. Levey, M.D., Corpus Christi, Texas.)

bone (e.g., the tarsus). In a diaphysis, a linear cortical radiolucent area frequently is associated with periosteal and endosteal cortical thickening (Fig. 67–42). In some cases, multiple radiolucent striations that extend partially or completely across the cortex are seen[175] (Fig. 67–43). The degree of bone formation can be extreme, obscuring the radiolucent defect(s) within the cortex. Magnification radiography and conventional tomography can outline the linear or bandlike nature of the radiolucent area and the disruption of the osseous surface, findings that then can be differentiated from those of an osteoid osteoma (circular or elliptical cortical radiolucent area with or without calcification in an area of sclerosis) and an abscess (circular or oval radiolucent area without calcification with surrounding sclerosis). In an epiphyseal or metaphyseal location or in a cancellous area, focal sclerosis representing condensation of trabeculae is the typical finding, and periostitis is not prominent (Fig. 67–44). With healing at either site, the sclerosis may become more diffuse, and eventually it and the fracture line can disappear.

Biomechanical principles can be applied to the explanation of stress fractures in various sites of the body.[88] A few specific examples are included in Table 67–3.

1. Calcaneal or other tarsal stress fracture. Fatigue fracture of the calcaneus is not uncommon in military recruits,[176, 177] and insufficiency fractures in this site can accompany rheumatoid arthritis, neurologic disorders, and other diseases[178] (Fig. 67–45). The failure of bone is related to the antagonistic action of the Achilles and plantar tendons and is accentuated when osteoporosis or spastic muscular tension is present.

Stress fractures in other tarsal bones are less common. Those in the tarsal navicular bone have been observed in physically active persons, especially in basketball players and runners,[179–187] and are a known complication of competitive racing in greyhound dogs.[188] Characteristically, the stress fracture in humans is oriented in the sagittal plane and is located dorsally and in the central one third of the bone (Fig. 67–46). It may extend partially or completely through the navicular and only rarely is evident on routine

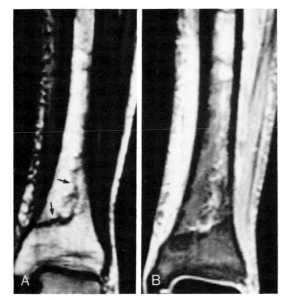

FIGURE 67–41. Stress fractures: MR imaging abnormalities. Fatigue fracture (longitudinal type) of the tibia. In a 58 year old man who jogged regularly, a coronal proton density (TR/TE, 1800/22) spin echo MR image **(A)** shows a stress fracture of the distal end of the tibia with both horizontal and vertical limbs (arrows). A coronal STIR MR image (TR/TE, 2000/20; inversion time, 140 ms) reveals high signal intensity in the tibial metaphysis and diaphysis. Soft tissue edema also is present.

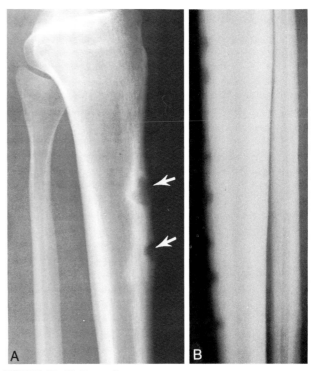

FIGURE 67–43. Stress fractures: Radiographic abnormalities in diaphyses.
 A Note the irregular radiolucent areas (arrows) in the anterior cortex of the proximal portion of the tibia. Periosteal and endosteal new bone formation about the fractures is evident. (Courtesy of M. Dalinka, M.D., Philadelphia, Pennsylvania.)
 B In a different patient, at least seven such areas can be seen. (Courtesy of P. Kaplan, M.D., Charlottesville, Virginia.)

radiographs, requiring for diagnosis a high index of clinical suspicion, scintigraphy, CT,[189] and conventional tomography (performed in an anatomic anteroposterior plane).[194, 195] Stress fractures of other portions of the navicular bone,[190] of the talus,[1012] of the os peroneum,[259] and of the cuneiforms[191–193] and cuboid[194, 195] bone (Fig. 67–47) are relatively rare.

2. Fibular stress fracture. In the act of running, the calf musculature is active in flexion and extension of the ankle and in closer approximation of the tibia and fibula. The

magnitude of the muscular activity is influenced by the type of ground surface, increasing in the presence of hard turf. Changing muscular stresses can result in the "runner's fracture."[88, 118] Jumping also can produce fibular stress fractures; classically, the proximal portion of the bone is affected in jumping, whereas the distal portion may be altered in running[196–198] (Fig. 67–48). In children and adolescents, ballet dancing may lead to fibular stress fractures,[199, 200] and bowing of the bone may be an associated abnormality.[199]

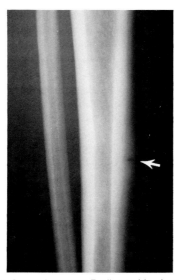

FIGURE 67–42. Stress fractures: Radiographic abnormalities in diaphyses. A horizontally oriented, linear cortical lucent area with surrounding periosteal proliferation (arrow) is typical of a stress fracture of the diaphysis of the tibia.

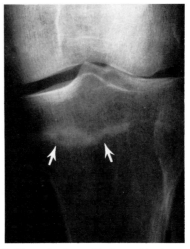

FIGURE 67–44. Stress fractures: Radiographic abnormalities in metaphyses and epiphyses. Bandlike focal sclerosis (arrows) is typical of a stress fracture in the proximal portion of the tibia.

TABLE 67–3. Locations of Stress Fracture by Activity*

Location	Activity or Event
Sesamoids of metatarsal bones	Prolonged standing
Metatarsal shaft	Marching; stamping on ground; prolonged standing; ballet; postoperative bunionectomy
Navicular	Stamping on ground; marching; long distance running
Calcaneus	Jumping; parachuting; prolonged standing; recent immobilization
Tibia: Midshaft and distal shaft	Long distance running
Proximal shaft (children)	Running
Fibula: Distal shaft	Long distance running
Proximal shaft	Jumping; parachuting
Patella	Hurdling
Femur: Shaft	Ballet; long distance running
Neck	Ballet; marching; long distance running; gymnastics
Pelvis: Obturator ring	Stooping; bowling; gymnastics
Lumbar vertebra (pars interarticularis)	Ballet; lifting heavy objects; scrubbing floors
Lower cervical, upper thoracic spinous process	Clay shoveling
Ribs	Carrying heavy pack; golf; coughing
Clavicle	Postoperative radical neck
Coracoid of scapula	Trapshooting
Humerus: Distal shaft	Throwing a ball
Ulna: Coronoid	Pitching a ball
Shaft	Pitchfork work; propelling wheelchair
Hook of hamate	Holding golf club, tennis racquet, baseball bat

*Modified from Daffner RH: Skel Radiol 2:221, 1978.

Fibular stress fractures also may occur subsequent to traumatic tibiofibular synostosis.[201]

3. *Tibial stress fracture.* Stress fracture of the proximal diaphysis of the tibia can occur during running,[202] particularly in children,[203–205] and stress fracture of the middle and distal tibial diaphysis can take place during long-distance running, marching, and ballet dancing.[100, 104, 200, 206–213, 1014] The posteromedial portion of the cortex is affected more frequently than the anterolateral portion (Fig. 67–49). These fractures, which occasionally may proceed to nonunion,[211, 214] should be differentiated from shin splints, which are related to periostitis provoked by muscle and fascia tension (see previous discussion).[215, 216] Stress fractures involving the medial malleolus also may be encountered in young athletes.[217, 218] Subtle fissures develop at the junction of the medial malleolus and tibial plafond, and small osteolytic foci also may develop[218] (Fig. 67–50). Stress fractures of the tibia (or the fibula) may be associated with golfing[1013] and with osteoarthritis of the knee.[219, 220]

4. *Femoral stress fracture.* Stress fracture of the shaft or neck of the femur (Figs. 67–51 and 67–52) can result from numerous activities, including long-distance running, ballet dancing, and marching.[100, 104, 221–240] Although both adults and children can be affected, stress fractures of the femoral neck are rare in children with open capital physeal growth plates.[102, 241, 242] In this area, Devas[243] has described two types of stress fracture: a transverse type, more frequent in older patients, appearing as a small radiolucent area in the superior aspect of the femoral neck and becoming displaced in some situations; and a compression type, more common in younger patients, appearing as a haze of callus in the inferior aspect of the neck and being stable in most cases. The propensity for some femoral stress fractures to become complete and even displaced deserves emphasis.[244, 245]

5. *Metatarsal stress fracture.* The metatarsal bones are very frequent sites of stress fracture, which may accompany marching, ballet dancing, prolonged standing, foot deformities, and surgical resection of adjacent metatarsal bones.[90, 91, 95–97, 246–253] The middle and distal portions of the shafts of the second and third metatarsal bones are affected most often,[494] but any metatarsal bone (Fig. 67–53), including the first (Fig. 67–54), may be involved. In the last location, it is the base of the bone that is altered, and periostitis, a frequent finding at other metatarsal sites, is relatively uncommon. The base of the second metatarsal bone (or, rarely, other metatarsal bones) also may be affected.[247] If the stressful activity is not discontinued, recurrent fractures are observed.[246] These recurrent stress fractures usually occur at a different anatomic site.[254]

Occasionally, stress fractures involve the metatarsal heads, leading to sclerosis and flattening of the subchondral bone (Fig. 67–55). The findings resemble those of Freiberg's infraction or diabetic neuropathic osteoarthropathy.

6. *Other lower extremity stress fractures.* Stress fractures of the patella are either transverse or longitudinal, occur in both children and adults, and are associated with physical activities that include hurdling, running, walking, soccer, and fencing.[255–257] In some instances the resulting radiographic abnormalities resemble those associated with a bipartite patella, suggesting that the latter, when painful, may be of traumatic cause. Stress fractures of the phalangeal and sesamoid bones in the foot also have been described.[258–262]

7. *Public rami and symphysis stress fracture.* Stress fractures of the pubic arch and parasymphyseal bone are encountered in pregnant women, joggers, long-distance runners, or marathoners,[263–266] although similar fractures occur in patients with osteoarthritis of the hip,[267] in those who have undergone hip arthroplasty, and in association with osteoporosis (Fig. 67–56) and rheumatoid arthritis.[268–270] Complications of such stress fractures include osteolysis simulating malignancy, delayed union, refracture, and, in patients with osteoporosis, additional fractures elsewhere in the bony pelvis (ilium, sacrum). Avulsive injuries leading to abnormalities of the symphysis pubis are discussed later.

8. *Other pelvic stress fractures.* Although fatigue fractures of the sacrum have been described in children and athletes (Fig. 67–57) and in pregnant women,[271–273] it is the occurrence of insufficiency fractures of the sacrum and other pelvic sites in patients with postmenopausal or senile osteoporosis or rheumatoid arthritis, and in those who have received corticosteroid medications or radiation therapy (Fig. 67–58), that has been given far more emphasis.[274–281] Such insufficiency fractures are important for the following reasons: they may lead to significant clinical manifestations, including severe low back or groin pain, that simulate those associated with skeletal metastasis; routine radiographic findings often are subtle and easily overlooked; bone dis-

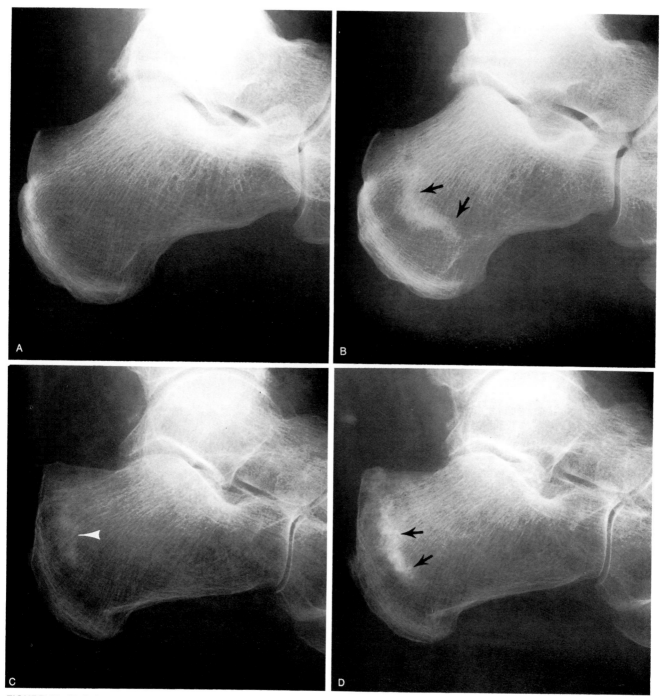

FIGURE 67–45. Calcaneal stress fractures.

A, B Examinations obtained 2 months apart reveal an initially normal radiograph and, subsequently, a meandering vertically oriented sclerotic line (arrows). This illustrates the typical location and appearance of a stress fracture in this bone.

C, D In a different patient, radiographs obtained several weeks apart delineate an initially poorly defined area of sclerosis (arrowhead), which, on subsequent examination, becomes better delineated (arrows).

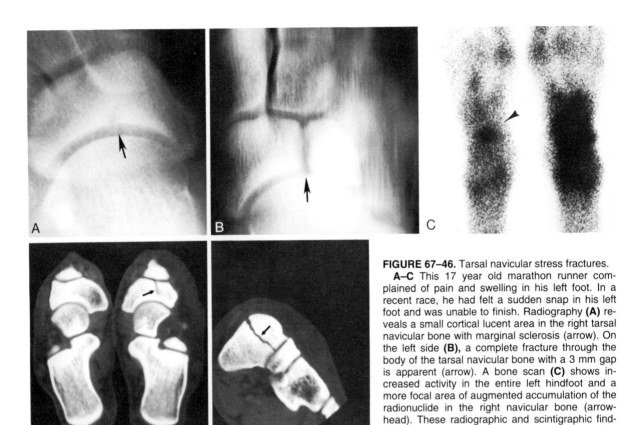

FIGURE 67–46. Tarsal navicular stress fractures.

A–C This 17 year old marathon runner complained of pain and swelling in his left foot. In a recent race, he had felt a sudden snap in his left foot and was unable to finish. Radiography **(A)** reveals a small cortical lucent area in the right tarsal navicular bone with marginal sclerosis (arrow). On the left side **(B),** a complete fracture through the body of the tarsal navicular bone with a 3 mm gap is apparent (arrow). A bone scan **(C)** shows increased activity in the entire left hindfoot and a more focal area of augmented accumulation of the radionuclide in the right navicular bone (arrowhead). These radiographic and scintigraphic findings are diagnostic of bilateral stress injuries with a complete fracture in the left foot.

(**A–C,** From Goergen TG, et al: AJR *136:*201, 1981. Copyright 1981, American Roentgen Ray Society.)

D, E In a professional basketball player, direct transverse **(D)** and coronal **(E)** CT scans show a stress fracture in the tarsal navicular bone that has progressed to a complete fracture (arrows).

(**D, E,** Courtesy of L. Rogers, M.D., Chicago, Illinois.)

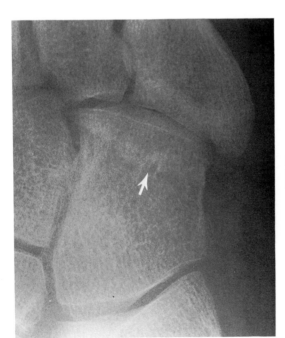

FIGURE 67–47. Cuboid stress fractures. Note the transverse band of sclerosis in the distal portion of the cuboid bone (arrow). (Courtesy of M. Dalinka, M.D., Philadelphia, Pennsylvania.)

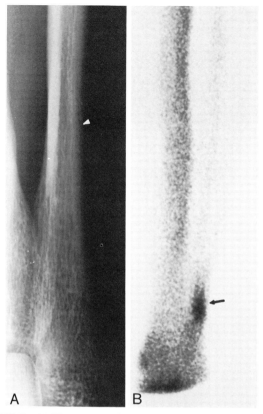

FIGURE 67–48. Fibular stress fractures.

　A A subtle oblique radiolucent line extends across the cortex of the distal segment of the fibula (arrowhead).

　B Accumulation of the bone-seeking radionuclide (arrow) in the same area is evident.

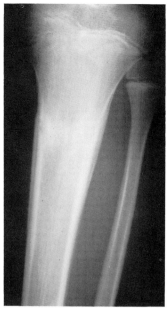

FIGURE 67–49. Tibial stress fracture. In a 12 year old boy, observe a band of sclerosis across the proximal metadiaphysis of the bone with periostitis. (Courtesy of K. Van Lom, M.D., San Diego, California.)

placement at the fracture site may occur in neglected cases; and biopsy (which rarely is necessary) may provide a tissue sample whose histologic features, including the cellularity associated with a healing fracture, may resemble those of a malignant tumor such as osteosarcoma or chondrosarcoma.

　Sacral insufficiency fractures involve one or both sides of the bone with vertical fracture lines typically located close to the sacroiliac joint or joints. These vertically oriented fractures may lead to subtle interruption of the superior cortical surface or arcuate lines of the sacrum. Horizontal fracture lines also may be evident. Bone scintigraphy reveals accumulation of the radionuclide at the fracture sites, sometimes producing an "H" pattern of increased radiotracer uptake in the sacrum (Fig. 67–59). The transaxial displays provided by CT and MR imaging are well suited to the detection of sacral insufficiency fractures (Fig. 67–59). MR images (Fig. 67–60) usually reveal low signal intensity in the involved marrow on T1-weighted spin echo images and high signal intensity in this marrow on T2-weighted spin echo images,[282] and they can be used to monitor fracture healing and a decrease in adjacent bone marrow edema.[283] Sacral insufficiency fractures may occur as an isolated finding, although they frequently are associated with other insufficiency fractures of the pelvis, especially after radiation,[277] that lead to instability of the pelvic ring. Other involved sites include the para-acetabular bone (Fig. 67–61) and the ilium, in addition to the parasymphyseal location that was noted earlier.[279, 284, 285]

　9. Upper extremity stress fracture. These fractures are far less frequent than stress fractures in the bones of the lower extremity. Typical sites include the ribs in golfers, rowers, and tennis players[103, 286]; the coracoid process of the scapula in trapshooters[102]; the ulnae of rodeo riders, tennis players,[287, 1015] baseball pitchers,[288] volleyball players, weightlifters,[289] and patients using wheelchairs[497]; the hook of the hamate in tennis players, golfers, and baseball players[290, 291]; the olecranon process in baseball pitchers and javelin throwers[292–293]; the phalangeal tufts in guitar players[110, 294]; the phalanges of the hand in bowlers[295]; and the inferior edge of the glenoid fossa in baseball pitchers.[296] Additional

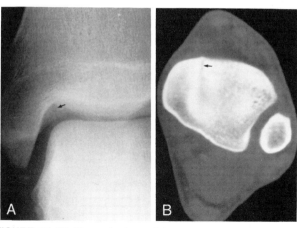

FIGURE 67–50. Stress fracture of the medial malleolus. This 20 year old man developed the gradual onset of pain over the medial malleolus, especially during athletic activities. The routine radiograph **(A)** shows a small vertical fissure (arrow) at the junction between the medial malleolus and tibial plafond. Transaxial CT scan **(B)** at the level of the plafond reveals a small sagittal fissure (arrow) with adjacent bone sclerosis. (From Schils JP, et al: Radiology *185:*219, 1992.)

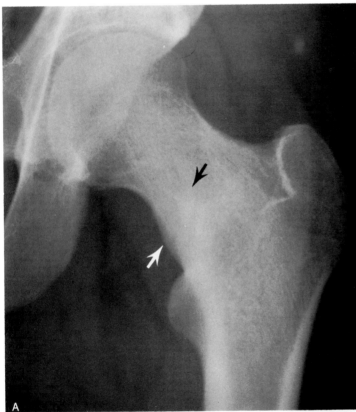

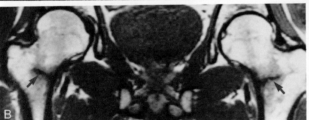
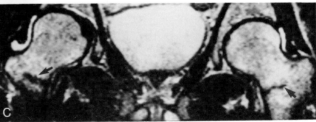

FIGURE 67–51. Femoral stress fractures: Femoral neck.

A In the medial portion of the femoral neck, observe buttressing and sclerosis (arrows).

B, C In this 18 year old male soldier, intense physical activity led to bilateral hip pain. Coronal proton density (TR/TE, 2000/20) **(B)** and T2-weighted (TR/TE, 2000/80) **(C)** spin echo MR images reveal bilateral fatigue fractures (arrows) in the medial portion of the femoral neck. In **B,** the fracture itself and the surrounding marrow edema are of low signal intensity. In **C,** the edema reveals high signal intensity and the fracture remains of low signal intensity.

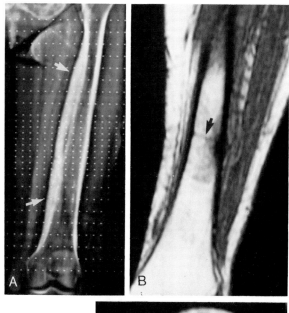

FIGURE 67–52. Femoral stress fractures: Femoral shaft.

A A scout CT scan of the femur in a 56 year old woman with a 10 year history of thigh pain shows diffuse, mature periosteal bone formation (arrows) along the medial portion of the entire diaphysis. The findings are consistent with a stress reaction. (Courtesy of A. Newberg, M.D., Boston, Massachussetts.)

B, C In a 76 year old woman with exercise-related thigh and leg pain, a coronal T1-weighted (TR/TE, 550/25) spin echo MR image **(B)** shows a linear region of low signal intensity (arrow) compatible with a stress fracture, a broader region of diminished signal intensity consistent with marrow edema, and cortical thickening. On a transaxial T2-weighted (TR/TE, 2100/70) spin echo MR image **(C),** observe high signal intensity in the edematous bone marrow of the femur and adjacent soft tissues. (Courtesy of T. Broderick, M.D., Orange, California.)

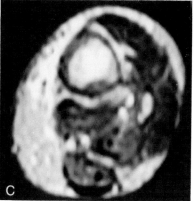

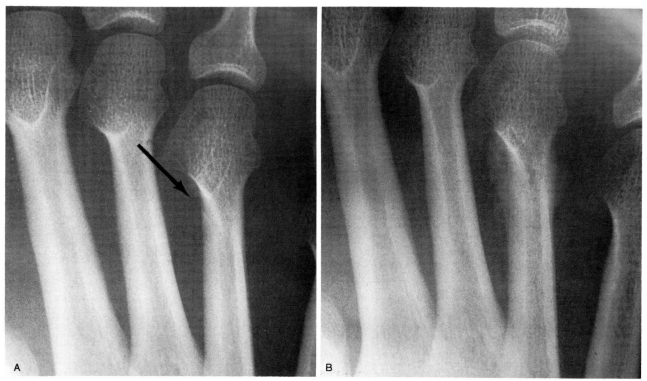

FIGURE 67–53. Metatarsal stress fractures: Lateral metatarsal bones.

In a military recruit, the initial radiograph **(A)** delineates an oblique linear radiolucent line through the distal shaft of the fourth metatarsal bone (arrow). Several weeks later **(B),** considerable new bone formation can be seen.

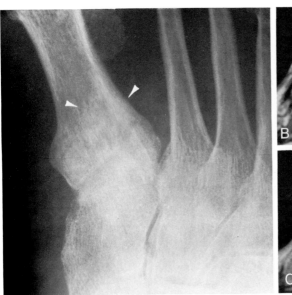

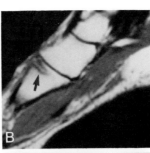

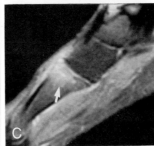

A

FIGURE 67–54. Metatarsal stress fractures: First metatarsal bone.

A In this patient with rheumatoid arthritis, recent pain at the base of the first metatarsal bone was accompanied by a changing radiographic appearance in which patchy bone sclerosis is identified (arrowheads). The findings are compatible with an insufficiency type of stress fracture.

B, C In a different patient, a sagittal T1-weighted (TR/TE, 650/20) spin echo MR image **(B)** shows a stress fracture (arrow) involving the dorsal aspect of the base of the first metatarsal bone. A sagittal T1-weighted (TR/TE, 400/15) spin echo MR image obtained with chemical presaturation of fat (ChemSat) and after intravenous administration of a gadolinium contrast agent **(C)** reveals high signal intensity in the bone and adjacent soft tissues (arrow).

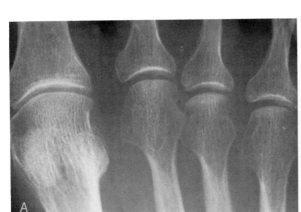

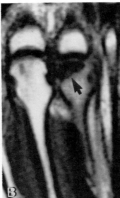

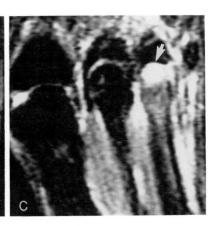

FIGURE 67–55. Metatarsal stress fractures: Metatarsal heads.

A In this 56 year old female jogger, note subtle sclerosis of the subchondral bone in the second, third, and fourth metatarsal heads.

B, C In a 46 year old man with a 6 month history of foot pain during running, a transverse T1-weighted (TR/TE, 500/17) spin echo MR image **(B)** shows an area of low signal intensity (arrow) in the head of the third metatarsal bone. A transverse short tau inversion recovery (STIR) image (TR/TE, 2000/43; inversion time, 140 msec) **(C)** reveals high signal intensity in this region (arrow) and fluid in the first and second metatarsophalangeal joints.

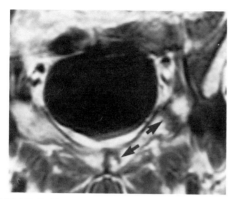

FIGURE 67–56. Pubic rami stress fractures. In this 80 year old man, a coronal T1-weighted (TR/TE, 600/11) spin echo MR image shows two fractures (arrows) appearing as linear regions of low signal intensity in the iliopubic bone column of the pelvis. (Courtesy of S. K. Brahme, M.D., La Jolla, California.)

sites of stress fracture include the humerus,[297–300] the radius,[301–305] the metacarpal bones,[306] the acromion,[307] and the carpal scaphoid[308, 309] and pisiform[310] (Fig. 67–62).

10. Stress fracture of bones in the thorax. Stress fractures of the ribs (related to physical activity or coughing),[103, 311–314] the clavicle,[315] and the sternum (related to osteoporosis, thoracic kyphosis, and pulmonary disease)[316–318] have been described. Specific physical activities leading to stress fractures of the ribs were noted earlier. Additional causes of stress reaction in the ribs are costovertebral joint arthrosis[1005] and prolonged vibrator chest physiotherapy.[1006]

11. Stress fracture of the neural arch of the vertebra (spondylolysis). Spondylolysis represents a defect in the pars interarticularis of the vertebra. It may or may not be associated with a slippage of one vertebral body onto the adjacent one, the slippage being termed spondylolisthesis.[319] Spondylolysis is observed most frequently in the lumbar region of the spine, although reports of cervical spondylolysis are numerous (these cervical abnormalities may

have a different pathogenesis).[320–330] In the cervical spine, the defect occurs most typically at the sixth vertebral level, usually is bilateral, and commonly is accompanied by spina bifida, suggesting a congenital predisposition or cause; defects in the upper cervical spine are rare, usually occur at the level of the axis (Fig. 67–63) or the fourth cervical level, and may be traumatic or congenital.[331] Defects at the seventh cervical vertebral level or at multiple cervical levels are extremely rare. Cervical spondylolysis may or may not be accompanied by spondylolisthesis and neurologic deficits, and it should be distinguished from congenital absence of a cervical pedicle, which is an innocuous condition.[328] In the lower portion of the spine, the fifth lumbar vertebra is affected most commonly (approximately 67 per cent of cases) (Fig. 67–64), and the frequency of spondylolysis diminishes on proceeding cephalad in the lumbar region (L4, 15 to 30 per cent; L3, 1 to 2 per cent). Spondylolysis rarely is encountered in the first or second lumbar vertebra.[332, 333] Multiple levels of involvement in the lumbar spine of a single patient (Fig. 67–65) are reported.[334, 335] Symptoms and signs may be absent, although back and radicular pain, tenderness, gait abnormality, and neurologic deficits can be observed.[336, 337]

The considerable attention that has been focused on defects in the neural arch of the lumbar vertebrae is not surprising in view of the overall frequency of spondylolysis in the general population. It has been estimated that 3 to 7 per cent of vertebral columns reveal at least one area of spondylolysis.[338–341] This rate of occurrence may be greater in Japanese subjects,[342] in Eskimos,[343] and in whites than in blacks.[340, 344] The frequency of spondylolysis appears to be greater in athletes, particularly those involved in gymnastics, diving, weight-lifting, pole-vaulting, and American football.[345] Most series demonstrate a male predominance, with the ratio of affected men to affected women being between 2 to 1 and 4 to 1.[340, 346, 347] Typically, spondylolysis is discovered in childhood or early adulthood, and the frequency of the abnormality does not increase after the age of 20 years.[340] Radiologic and anatomic studies confirm the

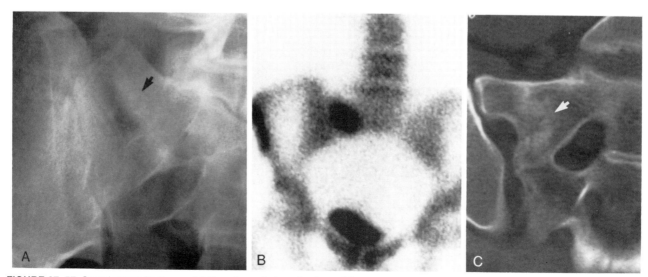

FIGURE 67–57. Sacral stress fractures: A fatigue type of stress fracture of the sacrum developed in this 20 year old woman who was an avid runner and bicyclist. The routine radiograph **(A)** shows subtle bone sclerosis (arrow) in the right side of the sacrum. Increased accumulation of the bone-seeking radionuclide is observed at the site of fracture **(B)**. Transaxial CT scan **(C)** reveals the sacral fracture (arrow). (Courtesy of W. Murray, M.D., Boise, Idaho.)

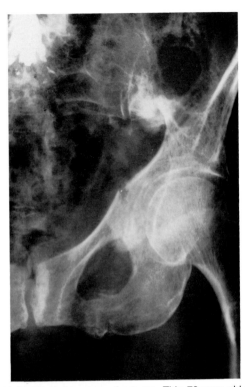

FIGURE 67–58. Pelvic stress fractures. This 78 year old woman who had undergone radiation therapy for a metastatic lesion of the left ilium developed insufficiency fractures of the pubic rami as well as a similar fracture of the ilium, adjacent to the sacroiliac joint, that extends through the metastatic focus. A parasymphyseal fracture also is evident, leading to sclerosis adjacent to the symphysis pubis. Although a sacral insufficiency fracture was present, it is not well shown on this radiograph. Myelography had been performed previously.

rarity of pars interarticularis defects in infants,[348, 349] although documented cases of spondylolysis in infants between the ages of 3 and 8 months have appeared.[344, 350, 351] The frequency of these defects rises precipitously between the ages of 5 and 7 years.[352]

The cause of lumbar spondylolysis has long been debated. Conflicting opinions have related the osseous defects to congenital or traumatic factors, although the current consensus strongly supports an acquired traumatic lesion originating sometime between infancy and early adult life.[344, 353–362] It is the type of fracture—fatigue versus acute—that is not clear. It seems probable that spondyloly-

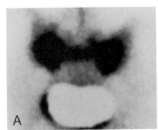 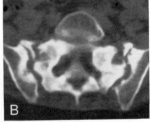

FIGURE 67–59. Sacral stress fractures. The typical imaging features of insufficiency fractures of the sacrum, as shown in a 65 year old woman, include an "H" pattern of radionuclide uptake on a bone scan **(A)** and comminuted fracture lines with sclerosis on transaxial CT **(B)**. In this case, the ilium adjacent to both sacroiliac joints also is involved. (Courtesy of G. Greenway, M.D., Dallas, Texas.)

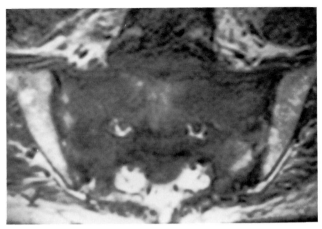

FIGURE 67–60. Sacral stress fractures. The typical MR imaging features of an insufficiency fracture of the sacrum, as shown in this 67 year old woman, include low signal intensity on a transaxial T1-weighted (TR/TE, 500/13) spin echo MR image. The normal appearance of the marrow in the ilii makes the diagnosis of skeletal metastasis less likely.

sis results most frequently from a fatigue fracture occurring after repeated trauma rather than from an acute fracture after a single traumatic episode,[344, 363] although an acute pathogenesis is supported by some observers.[364] The pars interarticularis appears to be the vulnerable point when repetitive stresses act on the vertebral arch.[356, 365] An increase in lumbar lordosis as well as a more vertical attitude of the top of the sacrum may accentuate the stresses placed on this arch.[345, 366] Radiographic and scintigraphic abnormalities have been detected in the area of the pars interarticularis (as well as in the region of the pedicles) in athletes, presumably related to chronic stress,[367–370] and spondylolysis has developed in patients with scoliosis and after spinal fusion.[371–373] Furthermore, spondylolysis virtually is non-

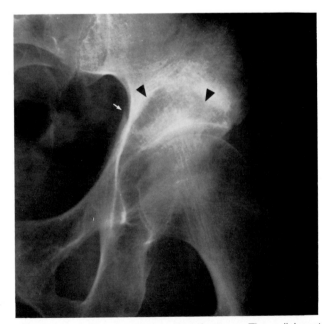

FIGURE 67–61. Para-acetabular stress fractures. The radiolucent band (arrowheads) with surrounding sclerosis is typical of an acetabular insufficiency fracture. It resembles the findings encountered in cases of parasymphyseal insufficiency fractures. Note disruption (arrow) of the iliopubic bone column in this 76 year old man.

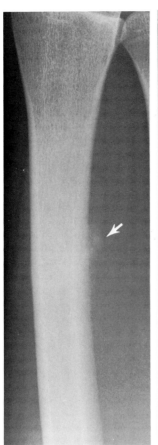
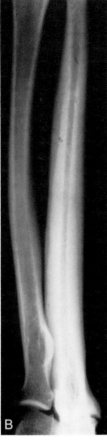

FIGURE 67–62. Upper extremity stress fractures.

A Radial stress fracture. This 22 year old "hustler" made his living playing billiards several hours each day. He was reputed to have a distinctive twisting motion that produced an effective spin of the ball. A stress fracture of the radius, manifested as a cortical radiolucent line and periostitis (arrow), temporarily ended his success at the billiard table.

B Ulnar stress reaction. Diffuse cortical thickening of the ulna is evident in this 27 year old professional rodeo rider.

(**B,** Courtesy of G. Greenway, M.D., Dallas, Texas.)

existent in patients who have never walked.[374] Yet, there are differences between spondylolysis and other types of fatigue fractures: Spondylolysis frequently develops at an earlier age than other fatigue fractures; there is a hereditary predisposition; the fluffy periosteal callus formation that commonly is noted at sites of other stress fractures rarely is observed in spondylolysis; it develops after minor trauma; and the defect in the pars interarticularis commonly persists.[344] These differences are not present uniformly. For example, some patients do recall a single traumatic event that initiated the back complaints. Furthermore, callus and healing with disappearance of the defect can be noted in some cases,[344, 358, 375–377] although fibrous union and a pseudarthrosis can be detected on histologic examination of the defect in others.[376]

Genetic influences are important in this condition. Spondylolytic families can be discovered in which over 25 per cent of persons demonstrate a defect in the pars interarticularis.[349, 378] Furthermore, patients have an increased frequency of nearby congenital anomalies of the spine, such as transitional vertebrae and spina bifida.[341] These findings may indicate not that the defect itself is

inherited but rather that there is a genetic influence on the strength of the bone of the pars interarticularis that predisposes certain persons to stress fracture. Local dysplastic osseous changes have not been demonstrated histologically, and it is possible that the genetic influences in some cases are being confused with environmental and occupational factors (e.g., the occurrence of spondylolysis in the athletic child of athletic parents).[338]

The experimental production of spondylolysis also supports a traumatic rather than a genetic origin. Lamy and associates[364] produced fractures through the pars interarticularis in approximately 35 per cent of cadaveric lumbar vertebrae that were stressed in flexion, whereas Cyron and coworkers[355] were able to create spondylolytic-type fractures in lumbar vertebrae by causing strains in extension. The fractures commenced in the anterolateral cortical layers of the pars interarticularis, an area of relatively thick bone.[358, 379] These studies and others underscore the importance of trauma in the pathogenesis of spondylolysis.

It is possible that either a single traumatic episode or repeated trauma can result in spondylolysis; thus, acute fractures or stress fractures conceivably can produce the same radiographic findings. Using this assumption, Wiltse and colleagues[380] have classified lumbar spondylolysis and spondylolisthesis into five types:

Type I: Dysplastic, with associated congenital abnormality of the upper sacrum and the arch of the lumbar vertebra.

Type II: Isthmic, with a defect in the pars interarticularis that may be (a) a fatigue fracture, (b) an elongated but intact pars, or (c) an acute fracture.

Type III: Degenerative, resulting from long-standing intersegmental instability.

Type IV: Traumatic, caused by fractures in areas of the posterior elements other than the pars interarticularis.

Type V: Pathologic, owing to generalized or localized bone disease.

Radiographic alterations of spondylolysis are diagnostic[359, 381, 382] (Figs. 67–64 and 67–65), although specialized techniques occasionally are required[383, 384] and radiolucent lines resembling true osseous defects are encountered.[385] Spondylolysis usually is evident in the lateral radiographic projection; however, oblique views are particularly helpful. The spine has a "Scottie dog" appearance on oblique pro-

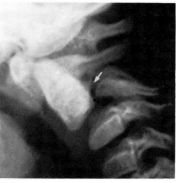

FIGURE 67–63. Spondylolysis in the cervical spine: Axis. Note the site of the defect (arrow) and vertebral displacement and angulation of the spine at the C2-C3 level during flexion of the child's neck. (Courtesy of S. K. Brahme, M.D., La Jolla, California.)

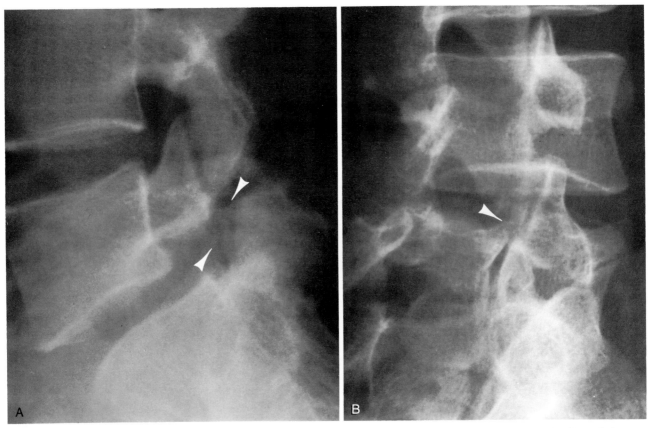

FIGURE 67–64. Spondylolysis in the lumbar spine: L5. Lateral **(A)** and left posterior oblique **(B)** projections reveal a defect through the pars interarticularis (arrowheads). The spine has a "Scottie dog" appearance on oblique views. The resulting lucent lesion has produced a break in the "neck" of the "Scottie dog" on the oblique projection. A grade I spondylolisthesis of L5 on S1 can be noted on the lateral radiograph.

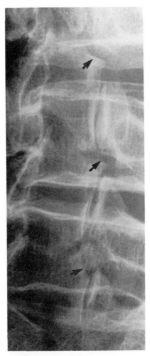

FIGURE 67–65. Spondylolysis at multiple levels in the lumbar spine. The left posterior oblique projection reveals defects (arrows) in the pars interarticularis of L3, L4, and L5. The opposite side was affected similarly. (Courtesy of A. G. Bergman, M.D., Stanford, California.)

jections. A unilateral or bilateral radiolucent area through the neck of the "Scottie dog" is well demonstrated. Reactive sclerosis about the radiolucent band may be seen, although true callus is unusual. On frontal radiographs, laminar fragmentation may be seen.[386] Slippage, or spondylolisthesis, may be encountered in some cases, a phenomenon that is more obvious if radiographs are obtained with the patient in a standing position[387, 388] or under stress with 30 pounds of weight on the shoulders. Wedging and hypoplasia of the fifth lumbar vertebra in association with spondylolysis may create a radiographic appearance of spondylolisthesis when true slippage is not present.[389] In cases of unilateral spondylolysis, hypertrophy and reactive sclerosis as well as fracture of the contralateral pedicle and lamina may be detected as a physiologic response to the presence of an unstable neural arch[390–392] (Figs. 67–66 and 67–67). Differentiation of the sclerotic bone from that which occurs in an osteoid osteoma must be accomplished, as excision of an eburnated pedicle associated with contralateral spondylolysis will create painful instability. Similarly, the sclerotic bone accompanying a contralateral spondylosis should be differentiated from that which occurs contralateral to a congenitally absent pedicle, lamina, or articular facet.[393–396] Additional radiographic abnormalities detected on frontal projections[397] and on flexion and extension films[398] in cases of spondylolysis with or without spondylolisthesis aid in differential diagnosis.

Arthrography with the introduction of contrast material

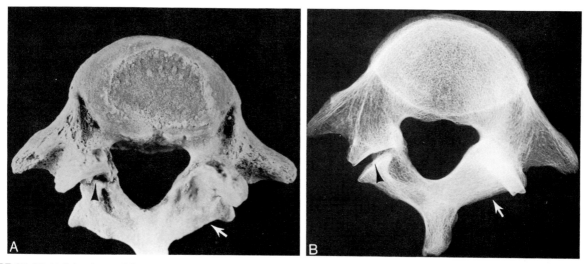

FIGURE 67–66. Unilateral spondylolysis with contralateral bony hypertrophy and reactive sclerosis. On a specimen photograph and radiograph, observe the defect in the posterior arch (arrowheads) and the contralateral osseous enlargement (arrows).

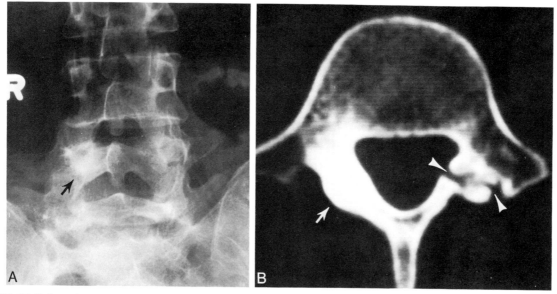

FIGURE 67–67. Unilateral spondylolysis with contralateral bony hypertrophy and reactive sclerosis. This 35 year old man had chronic back pain.

A The predominant abnormality on the frontal radiograph of the lumbar spine is osteosclerosis in the region of the right pedicle of the fifth lumbar vertebra (arrow). The left transverse process of this vertebra is smaller than that on the right.

B A transaxial CT scan of this vertebra reveals spondylolysis (arrowheads) and contralateral bone hypertrophy (arrow).

(Courtesy of J. A. Amberg, M.D., San Diego, California.)

into an adjacent apophyseal joint demonstrates communication with the adjacent ipsilateral apophyseal joint through the fracture of the pars interarticularis and, occasionally, with the contralateral joint via the retrodural space.[399] Although the findings serve to document that the pars defects may contain synovial fluid, perhaps explaining why such defects frequently do not heal, arthrography is not considered an important method in the diagnosis of spondylolysis.

Scintigraphy can be a helpful diagnostic method in cases of low back pain of obscure cause in which a definite pars interarticularis defect cannot be verified. Increased uptake of bone-seeking radiopharmaceutical agents may indicate increasing stress in the pars interarticularis with or without a definite fracture.[400–402] It has been suggested that scintigraphy allows the detection of more recently acquired and symptomatic spondylolyses, as such defects will accumulate the bone-seeking radiotracer, whereas older and non-symptomatic spondylolyses will not[403–408] (Fig. 67–68). Investigators also have suggested that the absence of focal accumulation of the bone-seeking radionuclide in patients with radiographically confirmed spondylolysis is consistent with the presence of a nonunion at the fracture site with little therapeutic benefit expected from immobilization,[409] and that single photon emission computed tomography

(SPECT) is more reliable than standard bone scintigraphy in the assessment of spondylolysis and related conditions.[400]

CT represents an additional imaging technique that has been used to delineate areas of spondylolysis.[410] On trans-axial scans, differentiation of the defect in the pars interarticularis from the nearby apophyseal joint may be difficult unless serial images are studied carefully.[411] Multiplanar reconstruction of the image data aids in this differentiation and in the delineation of foraminal encroachment and indentation of the neural canal from soft tissue or bone callus formation.[410] CT also allows detection of other clefts in the neural arch that are rarer than those in the pars interarticularis[412] (Figs. 67–68 and 67–69).

The role of MR imaging as a method of diagnosing spondylolysis appears to be limited. Rather, MR imaging is more suited to the assessment of some of the complications of spondylolysis such as spondylolisthesis, nerve root impingement, and disc degeneration and herniation.[413–416] The sagittal plane is more useful than the transaxial plane in demonstrating the entire pars interarticularis. Although the signal intensity of the pars defect generally differs from that of the adjacent bone marrow, it varies considerably according to whether fluid, fat, cartilage, or fibrous tissue occupies the defect and according to the presence and degree of

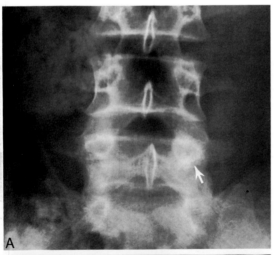

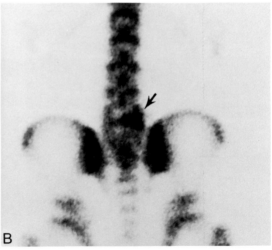

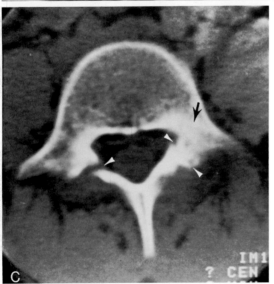

FIGURE 67–68. Spondylolysis: Use of scintigraphy. This man complained of chronic low back pain.

A The anteroposterior radiograph of the lumbar spine reveals a radiodense left pedicle of the fifth lumbar vertebra (arrow).

B Bone scintigraphy shows accumulation of the radiotracer in the vicinity of this pedicle (arrow). No increase in radionuclide activity is evident in the opposite side.

C A transaxial CT scan at this level confirms the presence of bilateral spondylolysis (arrowheads). Reactive sclerosis in the pedicle, transverse process, and lamina on the left side (arrow) explains the scintigraphic appearance.

(Courtesy of P. VanderStoep, M.D., St. Cloud, Minnesota.)

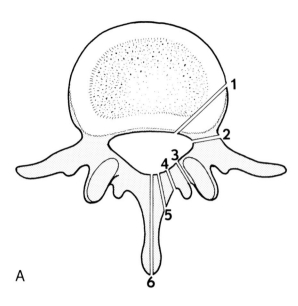

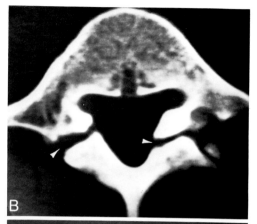

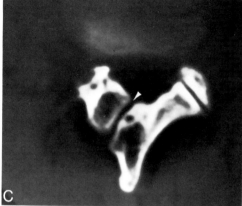

FIGURE 67–69. Clefts in the neural arch.

A 1, Persistent neurocentral synchondrosis; 2, pediculate or retrosomatic cleft; 3, pars interarticularis cleft, or spondylolysis; 4, retroisthmic cleft; 5, paraspinous cleft; 6, spinous cleft.

(**A,** From Johansen JG, et al: Radiology *148:*447, 1983.)

B Pars interarticularis clefts (arrowheads).

C Retroisthmic cleft (arrowhead).

(**C,** Courtesy V. Vint, M.D., San Diego, California.)

adjacent bone sclerosis.[414] A cortical defect or cortical discontinuity is a reliable MR imaging finding of spondylolysis, but it is one shown equally well by CT.

Spondylolisthesis is discussed in Chapter 40; however, a few additional comments are appropriate here owing to the association of this entity with spondylolysis. It is difficult to predict which patients with spondylolysis will develop spondylolisthesis. Although anatomic factors, including the shape of the fifth lumbar vertebra and the dome of the sacrum, have been suggested to play an important role in the development of vertebral slippage, these changes in vertebral shape are more likely the result of the slip rather than its cause.[341] A sagittal orientation of the L4-L5 facet joints also has been emphasized as a causative factor of spondylolisthesis, although this may be more important in cases of degenerative spondylolisthesis than of spondylolytic spondylolisthesis.[417] Progressive slippage in association with spondylolysis potentially can occur at any time[418] but generally is seen prior to the age of 16 years and typically is asymptomatic.[341] Rather, spondylolisthesis usually is demonstrable at about the same time that spondylolysis is discovered. Progression of vertebral slippage is a finding that is much more common in the dysplastic type of spondylolysis than in the isthmic type.[419]

A variety of methods for measuring the degree of spondylolisthesis have been proposed[319] (Fig. 67–70). The reliability of such methods has been questioned, however,[420] and radiographs obtained with the patient standing for a prolonged period of time or with the application of axial compression may reveal a greater degree of spondylolisthesis than that demonstrated on routine radiographs.[421] Other diagnostic techniques, such as CT, myelography, discography, and MR imaging, are useful in evaluating spinal stenosis, disc degeneration, or other spinal complications of isthmic spondylolisthesis.[418, 422–425]

Greenstick, Torus, and Bowing Fractures. In the immature skeleton, fractures that do not completely penetrate the entire shaft of a bone are not infrequent. The main types of incomplete fractures, in addition to stress fractures, are greenstick, torus, and bowing fractures.

A *greenstick (hickory stick, willow) fracture* is one that perforates one cortex and ramifies within the medullary bone[152] (Fig. 67–71). The name is derived from the resemblance of these fractures to a young branch of a tree, which, when broken, is disrupted on its outer surface but remains intact on its inner surface. Greenstick fractures result from angular force and commonly become converted to complete fractures because of the exaggeration of the deformity as the bone continues to grow. Typical locations of greenstick fractures are the proximal metaphysis or diaphysis of the tibia and the middle third of the radius and ulna. In the healing stage of these fractures, well-defined subperiosteal defects containing fat may be observed (Fig. 67–72).[426–429] These defects may result from the inclusion of medullary fat drops in the subperiosteal hematoma.[427, 430]

A *torus (buckling) fracture* results from an injury insufficient in force to create a complete discontinuity of bone but sufficient to produce a buckling of the cortex[431] (Fig. 67–73). A longitudinal compression force generally is involved.[432] Torus fractures are common in metaphyseal regions and in patients with osteoporosis. Significant clinical abnormalities may accompany these fractures, and the

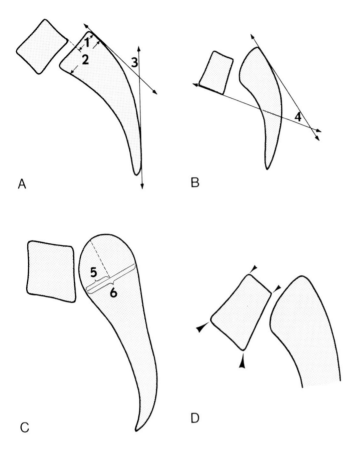

FIGURE 67–70. Spondylolisthesis: Methods of measurement.

A The degree of anterior displacement of the fifth lumbar vertebra with respect to the sacrum is expressed as the percentage obtained by dividing the amount of displacement (1) by the maximum anteroposterior diameter of the first sacral vertebra (2) and multiplying this value by 100. Sacral inclination is calculated by drawing a line along the posterior border of the first sacral vertebra and measuring the angle created by this line intersecting a true vertical line (angle at 3).

B Sagittal rotation is determined by extending a line along the anterior border of the body of the fifth lumbar vertebra until it intersects a line drawn along the posterior border of the first sacral vertebra. The angle of intersection of these lines (4) is measured.

C Percentage of rounding of the top of the sacrum is determined from a series of radiographs by dividing line 5 by line 6 and multiplying by 100.

D The degree of wedging of the slipped vertebra is expressed as a percentage determined by dividing the posterior height of the vertebral body (between small arrowheads) by the anterior height (between large arrowheads) and multiplying this value by 100.

(From Wiltse LL, Winter RB: J Bone Joint Surg [Am] *65:*768, 1983.)

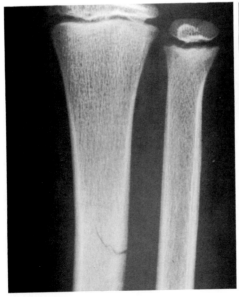

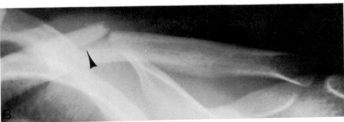

FIGURE 67–71. Greenstick fractures.

A Observe that the fracture involves one side of the radius and extends incompletely through the bone.

B A complete break of the superior cortex of the clavicle is seen, with extension of the fracture line along the longitudinal axis of the bone (arrowhead).

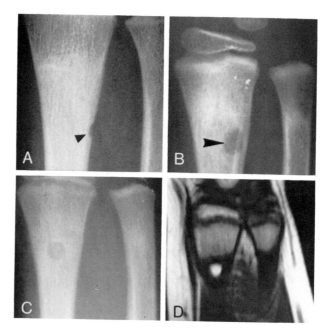

FIGURE 67–72. Greenstick fractures: Posttraumatic cysts.

A Three months after a greenstick fracture of the radius, a small subperiosteal cyst (arrowhead) can be identified in this 7 year old girl.

B Two months after a similar type of fracture of the radius (and ulna) in a different child, a larger cyst (arrowhead) is seen. (Courtesy of A. Newberg, M.D., Boston, Massachusetts.)

C, D Routine radiography **(C)** and a coronal T1-weighted (TR/TE, 650/25) spin echo MR image **(D)** show a fat-containing posttraumatic cyst of the radius in a 7 year old girl. Note its high signal intensity in **D.** The ulna also had been fractured. (Courtesy of S. K. Brahme, M.D., La Jolla, California.)

radiographs may be interpreted as normal unless subtle bulging of the cortex is identified. Oblique and lateral radiographs commonly are more helpful than frontal projections. Follow-up examination confirms the presence of a torus fracture and may reveal transverse bands of increased radiodensity, indicating osseous impaction.

With the application of both compressive and angular forces, a combination of the greenstick and torus fractures may result, the *lead pipe* fracture (Fig. 67–74).

Bowing fractures are a plastic response, usually to longitudinal stress in a bone.[433–444] They virtually are confined to children and most typically are apparent in the radius and the ulna, although their presence in neonates and adults[440, 445–447] and involvement of other areas, such as the clavicle, ribs, tibia, humerus, fibula, and femur,[440–443, 448–451] are encountered.

Experimental data have indicated specific patterns of bony deformation related to longitudinal compression

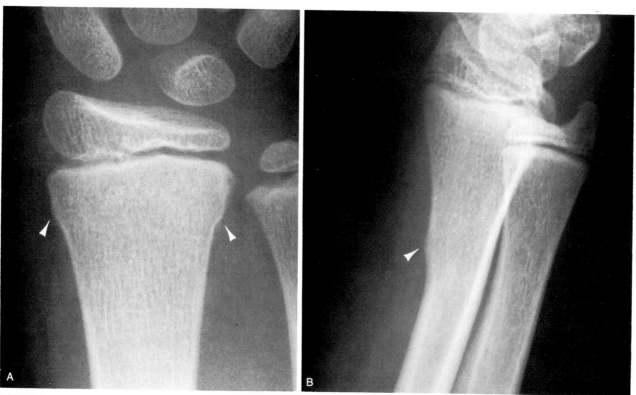

FIGURE 67–73. Torus fractures. Two examples of torus fractures of the distal end of the radius in children. Note the buckling of the cortex (arrowheads).

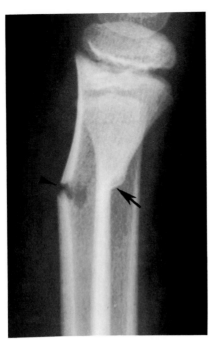

FIGURE 67–74. "Lead pipe" fracture. Note a torus fracture of the dorsal surface of the radius (arrow) and a greenstick fracture of the volar surface (arrowhead).

forces[155, 161] (Fig. 67–75). An initial zone of elastic deformation of bone is characterized by bowing that disappears with release of the offending force. With greater force, plastic deformation occurs, which results in permanent bowing of the bone. Still further increase in stress will lead to fracture. Histologic analysis of the bowed bone will reveal cortical fatigue lines and microfractures. These experimental results can be applied to the analysis of bowing fractures in humans. The deforming force usually is longitudinal without a shear component, particularly with regard to bowing fractures of the radius or ulna, although a direct blow can lead to a bowing fracture of the fibula; the deforming force must be greater than the maximal strength of the bone (approximately 100 to 150 per cent of body weight); and the duration of the force must be shorter than the time necessary to reach the point of fracture.[437] Commonly, bowing is identified in one of two neighboring bones (e.g., radius and ulna; fibula and tibia), and a fracture of the adjacent bone is evident. The latter fracture usually is diaphyseal in location and may allow dispersion of enough of the stress to prevent a similar fracture of the bowed bone. Similarly, dislocation of one bone can be associated with bowing of the adjacent one; an example of this is a dislocation of the radial head in association with a bowed ulna. Bowing also may involve one bone without an abnormality of an adjacent one or may affect both bones simultaneously.

Radiographic analysis of bowing deformities reveals lateral or anteroposterior bending of the affected bone (Fig. 67–76). The abnormality may be subtle, necessitating comparison radiographs of the opposite side for correct diagnosis. Sequential radiographs of a plastic bowing deformity usually reveal no evidence of periostitis, although thickening of the involved cortex may be detected. Scintigraphy may identify increased uptake of bone-seeking pharmaceutical agents even when radiographic findings are only

equivocal.[452] A bowed bone generally remains bowed, resists attempts at reduction, holds an adjacent fracture in angulation, and prevents relocation of an adjacent dislocation.[437] The force necessary to reduce a plastic deformity is equivalent in magnitude to that required to create it. In the neonate, periostitis and rapid and complete remodeling represent features of bowing fractures that differ from those in older children.[447]

The principles that govern the appearance of bowed fractures in children can be applied to these lesions in other clinical settings.[437] In the adult, the range of plastic deformation is narrower than in the child or adolescent, although a longitudinal force of the correct magnitude and duration can create a bowed bone. Similar deformities may appear in pathologic bone, as in fibrous dysplasia, Paget's disease, and osteogenesis imperfecta.

Birth Injuries. A number of specific musculoskeletal injuries related to birth may be encountered. Epiphyseal displacement involving the proximal portion of the femur and proximal and distal portions of the humerus, leading to a radiographic appearance simulating that of dislocation, is described later in this chapter. Such injury as well as fractures at certain characteristic sites may be related to several factors, including abnormal intrauterine position, difficult or prolonged labor, large fetal size, and the requirement of cesarean section.

Depressed fractures of the skull have been described in the newborn infant, in some instances related to cesarean section or abnormal presentation.[453, 454] Additional causative factors for these fractures may be compression of the fetal head against the sacrum, pubic symphysis, or ischial spines and excessive pressure of the obstetrician's hands or of forceps used during the delivery.[455] Clavicular fractures occurring during birth have been associated with prolonged labor, large fetal size, and shoulder dystocia.[456, 457] Such fractures may result from contact of the fetal shoulder with the mother's symphysis pubis in a cephalic delivery or the pressure of the obstetrician's hands in an attempt to depress the shoulder in a breech delivery.[2] The usual site of clavic-

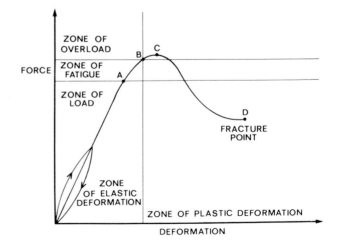

FIGURE 67–75. Graphic relationship of bony deformation (bowing) and force (longitudinal compression), after Chamay and Tschantz.[156, 161] The linear response in the zone of elastic deformation and the weakening of bone in the zone of plastic deformation are demonstrated. (From Borden S IV: Roentgen recognition of acute plastic bowing of the forearm in children. AJR *135*:524, 1975. Copyright 1975, American Roentgen Ray Society.)

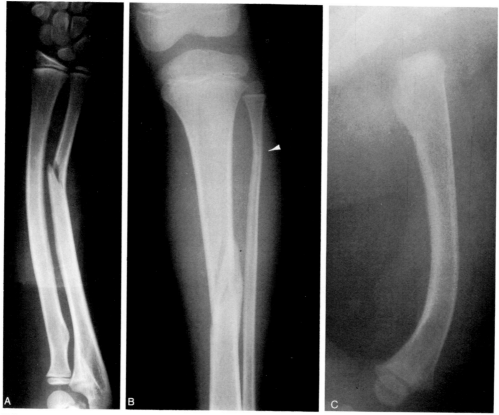

FIGURE 67–76. Bowing deformities of bone.
A Note the bowing of the radius associated with a fracture of the adjacent ulna.
B Observe subtle bowing of the proximal portion of the fibula (arrowhead) associated with a tibial fracture.
C Prominent bowing of the femur is evident.

ular fracture is at the junction of the middle and lateral thirds of the bone. Routine radiography or ultrasonography allows accurate diagnosis.[458] The major differential diagnostic consideration is clavicular pseudarthrosis (see Chapter 90).

Fractures of tubular bones also may be seen in the neonate. The femur and the humerus are involved most frequently.[459–461] Risk factors for such fractures are obstetric maneuvers, breech presentation, uterine malformation in a primiparous mother, and cesarean section.[455]

Toddler's Fractures. Infants and toddlers frequently show a limp of acute onset without a clear history of specific injury.[2] Because of their activities that include stumbling, tripping, or falling, these children are prone to develop a number of specific injuries, all of which can be manifested in this fashion. The classic toddler's fracture is a nondisplaced, oblique fracture of the distal diaphysis of the tibia[462] (Fig. 67–77). Although this is the most common pattern of injury, other causes for these clinical manifestations are occult fractures of the fibula, femur, metatarsal bones (particularly the first), and less commonly the calcaneus (Fig. 67–78), cuboid bone, pubic rami, or patella.[2, 463–468] The majority of toddler's fractures first occur between the ages of 1 and 3 years, and the remainder occur below the age of 1 year.[466] Femoral fractures generally are seen at a younger age than tibial fractures. Diaphyseal and metaphyseal injuries predominate, and physeal abnormalities are uncommon.[2] Radiographs initially may be entirely negative

or reveal only subtle alterations. Scintigraphy represents a sensitive test for the diagnosis of toddler's fractures.[464, 465] The major differential diagnostic consideration is child abuse (see later discussion). The solitary nature of the injury, the infrequency of physeal abnormality, and the absence of signs of soft tissue bruising in toddler's injuries generally allow accurate diagnosis.[2]

Acute Chondral and Osteochondral Fractures. Shearing, rotational, or tangentially aligned impaction forces generated by abnormal joint motion may produce fractures of one or both of the two apposing joint surfaces.[2] Acute injuries can produce fragments consisting of cartilage alone (chondral fractures) or cartilage and underlying bone (osteochondral fractures)[469–472] (Fig. 67–79). In general, the fracture line parallels the joint surface, and it is the depth of the lesion that defines the cartilaginous and osseous components of the fragment. Obviously, a purely cartilaginous fragment creates no direct radiographic abnormalities, whereas one containing calcified cartilage and bone becomes apparent owing to a varying degree of radiodensity (Fig. 67–80). Secondary radiographic signs consisting of soft tissue swelling and a joint effusion can be apparent with either chondral or chondro-osseous fragments. Fluoroscopy and arthrography with or without conventional tomography or CT scanning may be used to define the nature and location of the fracture more accurately; defects in the cartilaginous surface, contrast filling of an osseous excavation, and intra-articular chondral and osseous bodies may

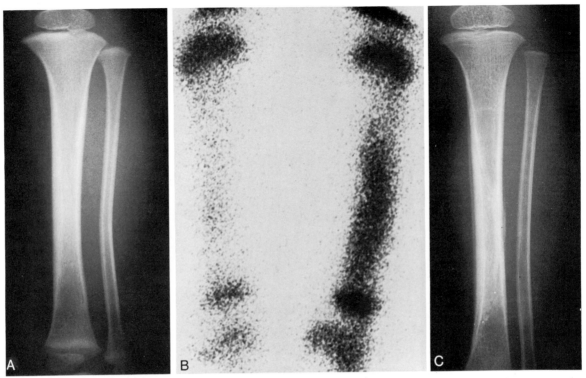

FIGURE 67–77. Toddler's fracture: Tibia. The initial radiograph **(A)** reveals a normal tibia and a bowing fracture of the fibula. The bone scan **(B)**, accomplished at the same time, reveals abnormal accumulation of the radionuclide in the lower leg. Three weeks later, the radiograph **(C)** shows a fracture and periostitis in the tibia.

be recognized (see Chapter 13).[473, 474] Furthermore, MR imaging plays a unique role in the assessment of these injuries (see later discussion).

After the injury, the detached portion of the articular surface can remain in situ, be slightly displaced, or become loose, or free, within the joint cavity (Figs. 67–81 and 67–82). In many cases, the osteocartilaginous fragments attach to the synovial lining at a distant site and become reabsorbed. If a fragment maintains some attachment to its site of origin, it can undergo revascularization and new bone formation, and radiographically evident growth and trabeculation can be seen. Free chondral or osteochondral fragments can undergo (1) proliferation of new layers of cartilage and bone, (2) resorption due to surface osteoclasis, or

(3) degenerative calcification of cartilage in both the original cartilage and the cartilage of the layers that have formed about the initial nidus or fragment.[469] These histologic findings have radiographic counterparts; free bodies may become more visible with time owing to proliferation of new cartilage and bone or secondary degenerative calcification, or both. With the proliferation of new cartilage and bone, a laminated appearance is identified, whereas with secondary degenerative calcification, a more or less homogeneous increase in radiodensity is seen.

The radiographic identification of loose osteocartilaginous bodies or those attached to the synovial lining requires a careful search of the recesses and dependent portions of the joint. Common sites of localization of such bodies in-

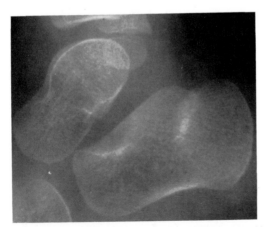

FIGURE 67–78. Toddler's fracture: Calcaneus. This 2 year old child with a limp has an oblique fracture of the calcaneus.

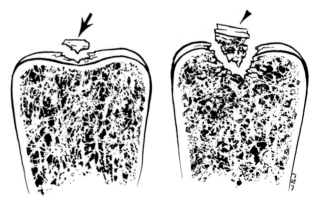

FIGURE 67–79. Acute chondral and osteochondral fractures: Components of fragments (schematic drawing). Fragments can consist of cartilage alone (arrow) or both cartilage and bone (arrowhead).

FIGURE 67-80. Acute chondral and osteochondral fractures: Lateral femoral condyle. Observe a defect in the lateral condyle (arrow) of the femur with a large, displaced bone fragment (arrowheads). An effusion is present.

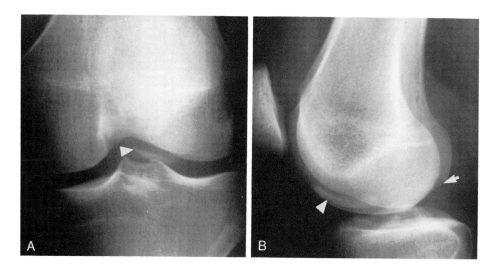

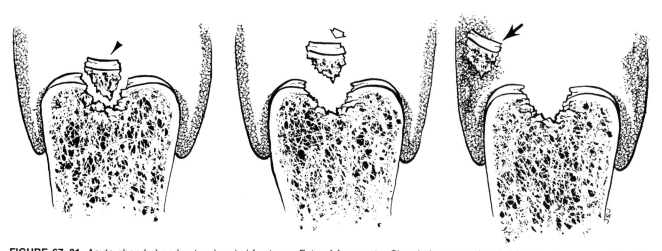

FIGURE 67-81. Acute chondral and osteochondral fractures: Fate of fragments. Chondral or osteochondral fragments can remain in situ (arrowhead), be displaced slightly or loose in the articular cavity (open arrow), or become embedded at a distant synovial site, evoking a local inflammatory reaction (solid arrow).

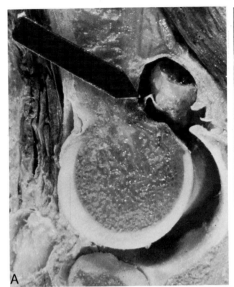
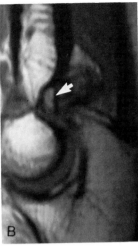

FIGURE 67–82. Acute chondral and osteochondral fractures: Fate of fragments. Olecranon fossa of humerus. A photograph of a section of the elbow **(A)** shows typical location of an intra-articular body (arrow) in the olecranon fossa. A sagittal T1-weighted (TR/TE, 800/20) spin echo MR image of the elbow **(B)** shows such a body (arrow). (**A,** Courtesy of M. Pitt, M.D., Birmingham, Alabama.)

clude the olecranon fossa in the elbow, the axillary and subscapular recesses in the glenohumeral joint, and the posterior regions in the knee (Fig. 67–82). The detection of osteocartilaginous bodies should stimulate a search for their site of origin. A relatively small defect in the articular surface may be the only evidence of the initial fracture location, even in the presence of multiple and large intra-articular bodies. Special views and conventional tomograms or CT scans may be required for identification of the fracture site. Such identification is important, as single or multiple chondral or osseous bodies can accompany a variety of other conditions, including idiopathic synovial (osteo)chondromatosis and articular disorders such as neuropathic osteoarthropathy, crystal-induced arthropathy, degenerative joint disease, and osteonecrosis. In idiopathic synovial (osteo)chondromatosis, radiographic clues include the presence of multiple opaque areas of approximately equal size scattered throughout the articular cavity, confined to one segment of the joint, or even within a synovial cyst, and the absence of evidence of an underlying articular disorder or trauma. The diagnosis of idiopathic synovial (osteo)chondromatosis is substantiated by the pathologist, who frequently notes metaplasia of synovial lining cells into cartilage and bone.

Osteochondral injuries are a well recognized component of a variety of momentary or persistent subluxations and dislocations (see Chapter 68). Classic examples include injuries of the glenoid region of the scapula and humeral head with dislocations of the glenohumeral joint (Fig. 67–83); of the patella and lateral femoral condyle with dislocations of the patella (Fig. 67–84); and of the femoral head with dislocations of the hip. Osteochondral injuries may occur in countless other locations, however, accompanying a variety of subluxations, dislocations, and periarticular fractures that allow impaction of apposing joint surfaces (e.g., about the ankle and elbow). Indeed, MR imaging has provided direct evidence of the frequency of these osteochondral injuries and, in doing so, has given new insight regarding their pathogenesis.

Numerous descriptions exist of subchondral and intraosseous foci of altered signal intensity, especially about the knee, during MR imaging examinations of patients with a history of injury, frequently acute, although the terminology applied to these lesions and theories regarding their pathogenesis have not been consistent.[53, 81–83, 86, 87, 475, 476] Some of the lesions are located at a distance from the chondral surface and are consistent with trabecular microfractures, or bone bruises (see previous discussion), whereas others, on the basis of clinical or imaging data, appear to represent stress fractures or avulsion injuries (e.g., the Segond fracture of the lateral portion of the tibia[477]). What remains in these descriptions are a number of subchondral abnormalities, frequently extending to the joint surface. Mink and Deutsch,[53] in an assessment of MR imaging examinations of the knee, divided these latter abnormalities into two types: (1) plateau and femoral fractures and (2) osteochondral fractures. The first of these two categories of injury was characterized by single or multiple areas of decreased signal intensity that extended vertically to involve the articular surfaces on both T1- and T2-weighted images. Osteochondral fractures were described as either displaced (in which the cartilage and often a small underlying segment of bone were fractured and at least partially displaced from their site of origin) or impacted (in which the overlying

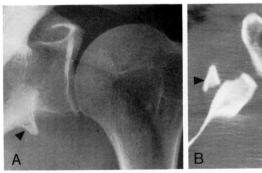

FIGURE 67–83. Acute chondral and osteochondral fractures: Anterior glenohumeral joint dislocation. Routine radiography **(A)** and transaxial CT **(B)** show a large osteochondral fragment (arrowheads) arising from the glenoid surface in a patient with an acute anterior glenohumeral joint dislocation that has been reduced. (Courtesy of J. Schils, M.D., Cleveland, Ohio.)

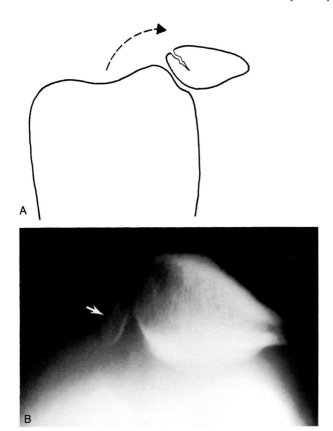

FIGURE 67–84. Acute chondral and osteochondral fractures: Lateral patellar dislocation.

A Lateral dislocation of the patella can be associated with an osteochondral fracture on the medial aspect of the patella or the lateral margin of the lateral femoral condyle, or at both sites.

B Note the fracture of the medial margin of the patella (arrow) and the lateral subluxation of the patella on this axial radiograph.

cartilage and the subchondral bone were impacted into the medullary cavity, and no large, free fragments were generated). Displaced osteochondral fractures arose from the patella or from either the medial or lateral femoral condyle, and all were confirmed at arthroscopy; impacted osteochondral fractures were encountered almost invariably in the lateral femoral condyle. The impacted fractures were characterized by a very marked decrease in signal intensity at the site of injury on T1- and T2-weighted MR images and by surrounding marrow edema, with an increase in signal intensity on T2-weighted MR images.

Vellet and associates,[475] in a study of patients with acute posttraumatic hemarthrosis of the knee, detected occult subcortical femoral and tibial fractures in 72 per cent of patients. Lesions were divided into two types, depending on their appearance on T1-weighted spin echo MR images: occult, including reticular, geographic, linear, impaction, and osteochondral fractures; and overt, including osteochondral and frank fractures. Occult fractures predominated in the lateral compartment of the knee, consistent with the occurrence of valgus forces at the time of injury. On the basis of the observation that occult fractures in the lateral femoral condyle often were accompanied by similar fractures in the posterolateral portion of the tibia, a mechanism of anterior dislocation of the tibia relative to the femur was proposed. Significant osteochondral sequelae of these occult fractures frequently were observed at the time of MR imaging 6 to 12 months later.

On the basis of the results of these and other investigations, MR imaging appears to be extremely sensitive in the detection of a heterogeneous group of acute posttraumatic lesions of the knee (and of other sites) that escape detection with routine radiography (Fig. 67–85). Some of these clearly involve the articular surfaces and are best considered various forms of osteochondral fractures, whereas others appear to be located at a distance from these surfaces. They may represent a spectrum of injury whose precise manifestations in any individual patient are dictated primarily by the mechanism and magnitude of the injury. At one end of the spectrum is the bone bruise, a self-limited, benign abnormality with no osteochondral sequelae[478]; at the other end of the spectrum is the overt, or frank, fracture that may or may not involve the osteochondral surface. In between these two are a number of other traumatic lesions, varying in location with respect to the articular surface, frequently occult without routine radiographic abnormality, and sometimes associated with significant late sequelae.

The location of osteochondral and subchondral lesions, as detected by MR imaging, in patients with acute trauma provides important information with regard to mechanism of injury and associated abnormalities. Occult injuries of the posterolateral portion of the tibia and midportion of the lateral femoral condyle (Fig. 67–86A), frequently occurring together, are associated with complete disruption of the anterior cruciate ligament and appear to represent a response to impaction of these two regions during anterior translation of the tibia and relative external rotation of the femur.[83, 86] A deep lateral femoral notch (Fig. 67–86B) identifiable on routine lateral projections of the knee appears to represent the radiographic counterpart of these MR imaging abnormalities.[479, 480] Occult injuries of the lateral femoral condyle and patella, including osteochondral fractures, may accompany transient lateral dislocations of the patella.[84, 87, 481] Numerous other patterns of bone injury (i.e., bone bruise, osteochondral fracture) are encountered regularly in the assessment of the knee, shoulder, hip, ankle, and other locations in which signal intensity changes in the marrow not only confirm a structural cause of the patient's pain but also delineate precisely the impaction forces accompanying abnormal joint motion (see Chapter 70).

Osteochondritis Dissecans. Osteochondritis dissecans indicates fragmentation and possible separation of a portion of the articular surface. The clinical manifestations are variable, related to the specific site of involvement. The age of onset varies from childhood to middle age, but an onset in adolescence is most frequent. Patients may be entirely asymptomatic; however, pain aggravated by movement, limitation of motion, clicking, locking, and swelling may be apparent. Single or multiple sites can be affected. Although the role of trauma is undeniable in most locations, a familial history has been evident in some cases, especially in osteochondritis of the knee,[482–491] and an autosomal dominant mode of inheritance has been suggested.[492] Major alterations associated with familial cases of osteochondritis dissecans are short stature, endocrine dysfunction, Scheuermann's disease, Osgood-Schlatter disease, tibia vara, and the carpal tunnel syndrome, and it also is possible that a separate variety of osteochondritis dissecans occurs in the juvenile patient owing to irregularities of ossification.[493]

Despite the existence of reports that emphasize genetic factors or growth disturbances in the pathogenesis of osteo-

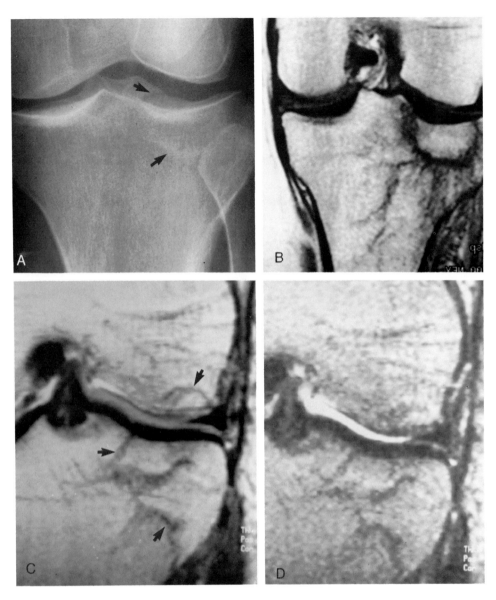

FIGURE 67–85. Acute chondral and osteochondral fractures: Various types.

A, B Lateral tibial plateau. A routine radiograph **(A)** shows a subtle fracture (arrows) of the lateral tibial plateau. A coronal T1-weighted (TR/TE, 450/19) spin echo MR image **(B)** reveals a curvilinear fracture line in the lateral tibial plateau with radiating fracture lines in the adjacent tibial metaphysis.

C, D Lateral tibial plateau and lateral femoral condyle. A coronal proton density (TR/TE, 1800/20) spin echo MR image **(C)** reveals fractures (arrows) in both the lateral femoral condyle and the lateral tibial plateau. With T2 weighting (TR/TE, 1800/90) **(D)**, hyperintensity in the affected bone marrow is seen. A tear of the medial collateral ligament of the knee also was present.

FIGURE 67–86. Acute chondral and osteochondral fractures: Association with deficiency of the anterior cruciate ligament of the knee.

A A sagittal T1-weighted (TR/TE, 600/20) spin echo MR image reveals bone marrow edema of low signal intensity in the posterolateral portion of the tibia (arrow) and midportion of the lateral femoral condyle (arrowhead). The adjacent condylar notch appears enlarged. The pattern of bone injury almost is diagnostic of disruption of the anterior cruciate ligament, a finding that was confirmed at the time of arthroscopy.

B In a different patient, note deepening and widening of the lateral condylar notch (arrowhead) of the femur, indicative of disruption or deficiency of the anterior cruciate ligament.

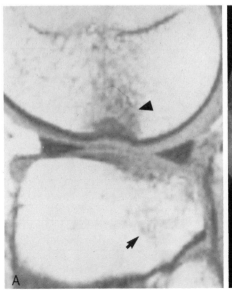
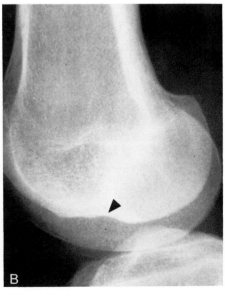

chondritis dissecans, the condition generally is believed to be the eventual result of an osteochondral fracture that initially was caused by shearing, rotatory, or tangentially aligned impaction forces.[469, 472] Because of the insensitivity of subchondral bone, with the absence of recognizable symptoms and signs in many cases, it is not always possible to define the exact time and mechanism of the injury, or even to determine if more than one injury has occurred,[495] nor is it possible to exclude the etiologic contributions of nontraumatic factors.[496] Although numerous descriptions of the histologic abnormalities in osteochondritis dissecans exist, they are not uniform, leading to differing interpretations of the findings.[469–471, 493, 496, 499] Fragments of cartilage or cartilage and bone are observed, but the cartilage may appear hypertrophied, with or without laminar calcification,[500] and the subchondral bone commonly is avascular, often with evidence of early repair.[496] A similar healing response is observed in the bony bed at the site of detachment. Various components of this histologic picture are emphasized by proponents of the traumatic, ischemic, or defective ossification schools of thought as supporting their particular point of view with regard to the cause of osteochondritis dissecans (Fig. 67–87).

A uniformly accepted classification system for the morphologic changes of osteochondritis dissecans does not exist. Arthroscopic findings confirm the existence of a spectrum of abnormalities ranging from intact overlying cartilage to cartilage disruption with a displaced fragment. The precise management of osteochondritis dissecans likewise is not agreed on, and the patient's age, clinical manifestations, and level of physical activity, as well as the specific anatomic location of the lesion and the experience and preference of the orthopedic surgeon, all influence the choice of therapy. Considerable interest has developed concerning the determination of the stability of the fragment (i.e., stable or unstable [or loose]). Those fragments that are ballotable but are associated with intact overlying cartilage, sometimes referred to as loose in situ fragments, may be fixed surgically; those that are grossly loose may be removed. With this in mind, orthopedic surgeons have attempted to identify noninvasive or minimally invasive imaging examinations that would provide information about the lesion similar to that apparent on arthroscopic assessment. There are many such examinations from which to choose, including routine radiography, conventional tomography or CT scanning with or without arthrography, standard arthrography, scintigraphy, MR imaging, and MR arthrography. None is ideal.

Mesgarzadeh and colleagues[501] used conventional radiography, bone scintigraphy, and MR imaging in assessing mechanical stability of osteochondritis dissecans, mainly in the femoral condyles. Employing arthroscopy as a means of verification of the findings, lesions that were large (particularly when greater than 0.8 cm² in area) or associated with a broad sclerotic margin (especially when greater than 3 mm thick) on routine radiographic examination tended to be loose grossly. Significant accumulation of the bone-seeking radionuclide during the flow, blood-pool, and late phases of the radionuclide examination generally indicated the presence of a loose fragment. MR imaging findings of loose fragments included displacement from its bed of origin and the presence of fluid at the interface of the fragment and its parent bone. The signal intensity of the fragment

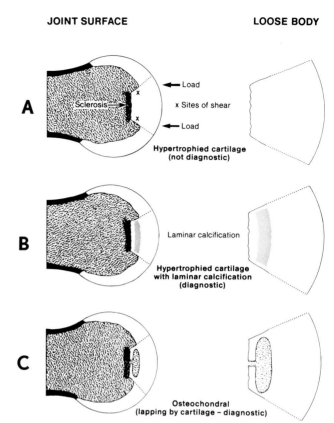

JOINT SURFACE　　　　　　　　**LOOSE BODY**

FIGURE 67–87. Osteochondritis dissecans: Components of fragments (schematic drawing). These diagrams emphasize the importance of defective ossification in the pathogenesis of osteochondritis dissecans.

A Arrest of bone growth has led to a subchondral band of sclerosis. The overlying cartilage is thicker than normal. Surface load is converted to shear at the shoulder of the defects so that separation occurs first on the deep surface. The detached fragment may consist only of hypertrophied cartilage.

B In some instances, a plate of laminar calcification develops in the detached fragment, a finding that is considered diagnostic of the condition by some observers.

C In other instances, a small focus of ossification possesses a bridge to the main portion of the epiphysis, a finding that also is regarded as diagnostic.

(From Barrie HJ: J Rheumatol *11*:512, 1984.)

itself, which usually increased on T2-weighted MR images, was not a useful indicator of the stable or unstable nature of the lesion.

Although subsequent studies using MR imaging to evaluate osteochondritis dissecans noted its value in delineating the status of the overlying cartilage,[502, 503] it was the investigations of De Smet and coworkers on osteochondritis dissecans of the femoral condyles[504] and talus[505] that next focused mainly on the signal intensity characteristics of the zone between the lesion and the parent bone. High signal intensity, indicative of fluid or granulation tissue, in this zone on T2-weighted MR images proved to be strong but not infallible evidence of an unstable lesion, whereas the presence of fluid encircling the fragment or focal cystic areas beneath the fragment were the best indicators of such instability (Fig. 67–88). Similarly, the absence of a zone of high signal intensity at the interface of the fragment and the parent bone was a reliable sign of lesion stability.

The intravenous[506] or intra-articular[507] administration of a gadolinium contrast agent has been used as a supplementary

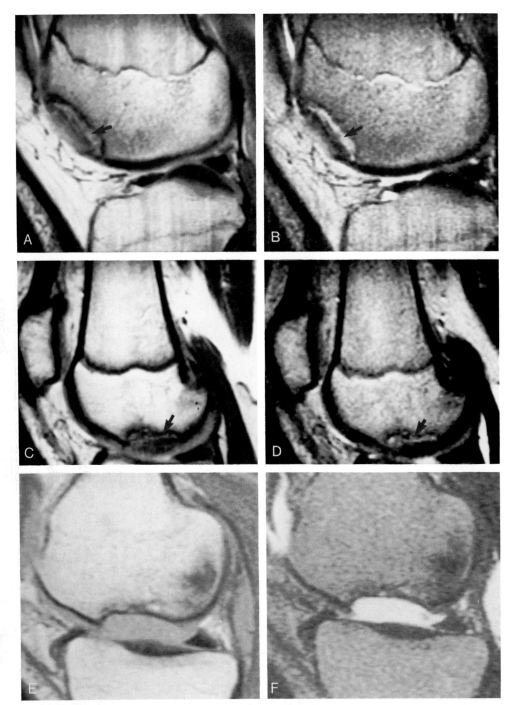

FIGURE 67–88. Osteochondritis dissecans: MR imaging. Femoral condyles. Various stages of disease.

A, B Lateral femoral condyle. In this 17 year old man, sagittal proton density (TR/TE, 2200/30) **(A)** and T2-weighted (TR/TE, 2200/80) **(B)** spin echo MR images reveal the lesion involving the anterior surface of the lateral condyle. The fragment is ossified, and the junction between it and the parent bone (arrows) demonstrates intermediate signal intensity in **A** and high signal intensity in **B**. The abnormalities are consistent with granulation tissue or fluid in this junctional area. Although the overlying cartilage is not seen well, the MR imaging findings suggest the presence of an unstable lesion. (Courtesy of J. Blassinghame, M.D., San Diego, California.)

C, D Medial femoral condyle. In this 12 year old boy, sagittal proton density (TR/TE, 2000/20) **(C)** and T2-weighted (TR/TE, 2000/80) **(D)** spin echo MR images show features similar to those in **A** and **B**. The junctional tissue (arrows) shows higher signal intensity in **D** than in **C**. A small joint effusion is present. Although the findings are consistent with the presence of an unstable fragment, the patient responded well to conservative therapy. (Courtesy of D. Gershuni, M.D., San Diego, California.)

E, F Lateral femoral condyle. Sagittal proton density (TR/TE, 3000/20) **(E)** and T2-weighted (TR/TE, 3000/80) **(F)** spin echo MR images in this 35 year old man show a large condylar defect containing fluid in continuity with the joint effusion. No fragment is evident within this osseous bed, and the overlying cartilage is absent. An intra-articular osteochondral fragment was present elsewhere in the joint.

MR imaging method in the assessment of osteochondritis dissecans. With intravenous administration, the gadolinium agent has led to enhancement of signal intensity in the zone between the fragment and the parent bone, which corresponded to histologic evidence of a loose fragment and subjacent granulation tissue; absence of such enhancement corresponded to histologic findings of a stable fragment with subjacent trabeculae and without granulation tissue.[506] When compared to standard T1-weighted spin echo and gradient echo MR imaging techniques, the administration of intra-articular gadolinium contrast agent (MR arthrography) prior to using such techniques resulted in an improvement in accurate assessment of the overlying articular cartilage.[507]

Although the available data would appear to indicate a role for MR imaging in the analysis of lesion stability in cases of osteochondritis dissecans, its advantages when compared to those of other methods, particularly arthroscopy, require further analysis. The finding of fluid at the base of the osteochondral fragment represents indirect but reliable evidence that the overlying cartilage is not intact, and it is a finding that corresponds to the presence of radiopaque contrast material or air that collects in this re-

gion when arthrographic methods are used to study osteochondritis dissecans. The likelihood of fluid extending through the cartilaginous defect and into the base of the fragment depends not only on the extent of the chondral damage but also on the amount of joint fluid that is present. In this regard, the use of MR arthrography appears to have merit owing to the large amounts of fluid that may be introduced into the joint (Fig. 67–89). Also, the sensitivity of MR imaging to the detection of fluid at the interface between the fragment and the parent bone varies according to the precise methods that are employed and may be greater when volumetric acquisition and thin sections are employed. Furthermore, the differentiation of fluid and granulation tissue in this interface with MR imaging techniques may be challenging. A theoretical value exists with respect to the direct analysis of the cartilage surface with MR imaging, but specific imaging parameters that are most suited to this analysis still are evolving (see Chapter 70). Finally, the choice of an appropriate diagnostic method may depend on the specific anatomic site that is involved. Because of this, a survey of the most typical locations of osteochondritis dissecans is appropriate.

Femoral Condyles. The most typical location of osteo-

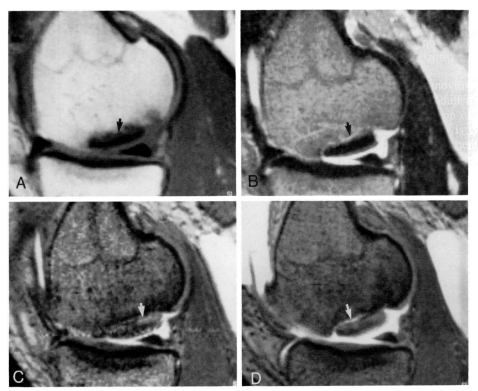

FIGURE 67–89. Osteochondritis dissecans: MR imaging. Femoral condyles—various MR imaging techniques. This patient developed osteochondritis dissecans in the medial femoral condyle. A posterior synovial cyst (popliteal cyst) was palpable.

A On a sagittal T1-weighted (TR/TE, 700/15) spin echo MR image, a large osteochondral lesion is present. The junctional tissue (arrow) between the fragment and parent bone is of the same signal intensity as that of muscle. The cartilaginous surface is seen poorly. A synovial cyst is present posteriorly.

B On a sagittal T2-weighted (TR/TE, 2500/90) spin echo MR image, a large joint effusion is apparent. The junctional tissue (arrow) shows slight hyperintensity, consistent with fluid or granulation tissue. Disruption of the articular cartilage posteriorly is evident.

C On a sagittal gradient echo (fast imaging steady precession—FISP) image (TR/TE, 40/10; flip angle, 40 degrees) obtained with volumetric acquisition, the posterior defect in the articular cartilage again is evident. No fluid is apparent in the junctional zone (arrow).

D After the intra-articular administration of a gadolinium contrast agent, a sagittal FISP gradient echo volumetric image with the same imaging parameters as in **C** shows fluid in the junctional zone (arrow) and disruption of articular cartilage. This method provides the most complete information in this case.

(Courtesy of J. Kramer, M.D., Vienna, Austria.)

chondritis dissecans is the condylar surfaces of the distal portion of the femur.[508–518] Men are affected more frequently than women, and the average age at onset of symptoms and signs is 15 to 20 years, although the age range is highly variable. Unilateral changes predominate over bilateral changes in a ratio of approximately 3 to 1. A significant history of knee trauma can be elicited in about 50 per cent of cases. Pain and swelling may be prominent. The possible locations of the osteochondral defect have been summarized by Aichroth,[508] who, in an analysis of over 100 patients, determined that the medial condyle was affected in approximately 85 per cent of cases and the lateral condyle in 15 per cent. A classic defect on the inner (lateral) aspect of the medial femoral condyle occurred in 69 per cent of cases, whereas an extended classic or inferocentral medial condylar lesion was evident in 6 per cent and 10 per cent of cases, respectively (Figs. 67–90 and 67–91). Other investigators have detected a somewhat higher frequency of lateral condylar lesions, of approximately 30 per cent.[513, 514] Such lateral lesions may involve the inferior or anterior surface of the femoral condyle.[519] The posterior portions of the condyles[520] and even the tibial plateaus[521] may be affected.

The pathogenesis of osteochondritis dissecans of the femoral condyles is not agreed on. Although a juvenile form of the disease, characterized by a familial history,

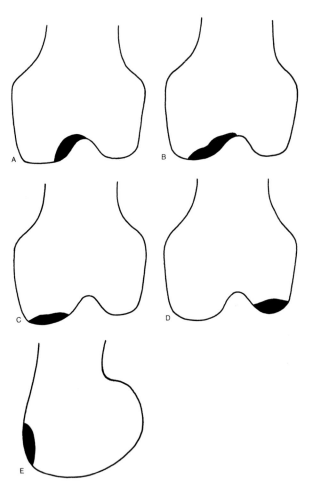

FIGURE 67–90. Osteochondritis dissecans of the femoral condyles: Sites of occurrence. **A,** Classic (medial condyle): **B,** extended classic (medial condyle); **C,** inferocentral (medial condyle); **D,** inferocentral (lateral condyle); **E,** anterior (lateral condyle).

involvement of multiple sites, and irregularities of ossification, has been described,[322–324] the fact that bone necrosis may be recognized on histologic evaluation of some of the lesions in most cases is undeniable. Rather, it is the cause of the osteonecrosis and the role of trauma that have been debated. Milgram's observation that some of the fragments originating from the joint surface in this disease contain articular cartilage alone, with no evidence of necrotic subchondral bone,[509] an observation also confirmed by other investigators,[512, 525–527] would support a primary traumatic cause. Even fragments with osseous components can reveal evidence of bone marrow viability.[509, 526, 528] Furthermore, examination of specimens of bone at the femoral origin of the fragments has not shown evidence of bone infarction.[509, 527, 529] These pathologic observations appear to underscore the importance of trauma in initiating this condition. The mechanism of the traumatic event is not clear but may be related to rotatory forces acting on the fixed weight-bearing knee. Shearing forces, direct blows, and ligamentous avulsions could produce osteochondral fragments.[515, 530, 531] The trauma may be major or minor, and the relative insensitivity of cancellous bone would account for the absence of acute symptoms and signs in some patients.[509, 526] The presence and degree of displacement of the chondral or osteochondral fragment apparently can vary; some bodies may be torn free immediately, whereas others remain attached and undergo remodeling owing to retained blood supply from adjacent soft tissue structures.[509] Subsequent trauma could lead to progressive disruption, and motion may induce the formation of cartilaginous callus in the cleft within the subchondral bone.

The radiographic characteristics of osteochondritis dissecans in situ of the femoral condyles have been well summarized by Milgram.[509] Purely chondral lesions require arthrography (Fig. 67–92), CT arthrography, MR imaging, or arthroscopy for accurate diagnosis.[532, 533] The osseous component of an osteochondral lesion is detectable with routine radiography or standard CT (Fig. 67–93). A small osseous lesion may be separated from the normal or sclerotic base of the femoral defect by a radiolucent crescentic zone. Fragmentation and collapse of the partially separated body can be recognized. Disruption and displacement of the osteochondral fragment produce a loose or synovium-embedded intra-articular osseous body (Fig. 67–94). The site of origin on the femur gradually may be remodeled, although a slightly flattened or irregular articular surface frequently can be detected for decades.[498] Secondary degenerative joint disease has been described in long-term follow-up examinations of those patients with osteochondritis dissecans of the knee who have had the first manifestation of the disorder after the closure of the growth plate[513]; the pattern of degenerative joint disease in these persons has been described as atypical in that it begins about 10 years earlier in life than does usual osteoarthritis of the knee, more commonly involves the three compartments of the knee, and frequently is associated with loose bodies. Osteoarthritis has been reported to be more frequent in cases in which the initial lesion of osteochondritis dissecans was large and involved the weight-bearing surface of the condyle.[534] In some of the reported cases of degenerative joint disease occurring after osteochondritis dissecans, the initial lesion may have represented spontaneous osteonecrosis about the knee (see Chapter 80).

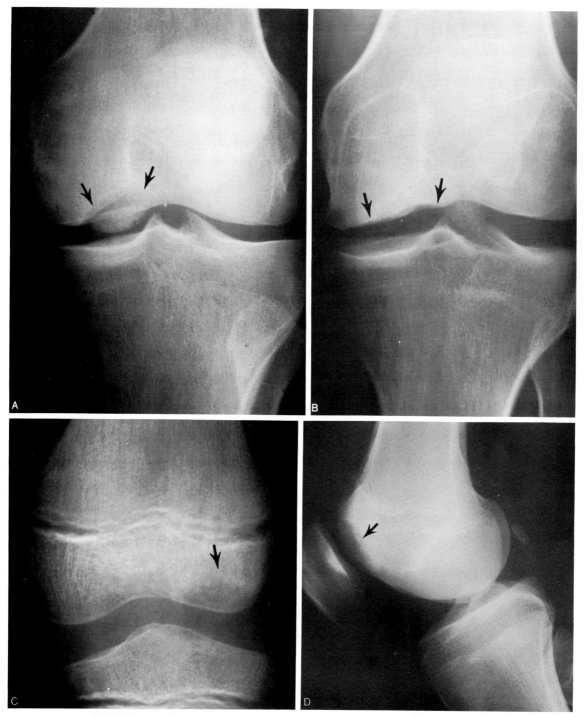

FIGURE 67–91. Osteochondritis dissecans of the femoral condyles: Sites of occurrence.
A Classic defect of medial condyle (arrows).
B Extended classic defect of medial condyle (arrows).
C Inferocentral lesion of lateral condyle (arrow).
D Anterior lesion of lateral condyle (arrow).

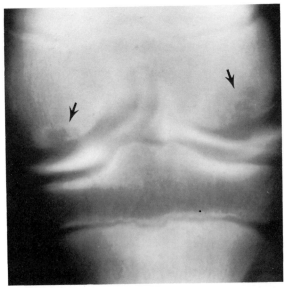

FIGURE 67–92. Osteochondritis dissecans of the femoral condyles: Arthrotomography. This 12 year old boy had a long history of bilateral knee pain. Symmetric abnormalities in both knees were evident on radiographic examination. Arthrotomography using radiopaque contrast material alone confirms the presence of the osseous defects (arrows) in both the medial and the lateral condyles and the integrity of the articular cartilage. (Courtesy of J. Eglehoff, M.D., and R. Towbin, M.D., Cincinnati, Ohio.)

The major differential diagnosis of the radiographic features of condylar osteochondritis dissecans is spontaneous osteonecrosis of the knee. This lesion occurs in older persons, is associated with the sudden onset of clinical manifestations, and almost invariably involves the weight-bearing portion of the medial femoral condyle. It appears to represent a true osteonecrosis, although the cause of the necrosis is not certain. Osteochondritis dissecans of the knee also must be differentiated from the fragmentation that may accompany neuropathic osteoarthropathy and from the normal grooves that appear on the medial and lateral femoral condyles on lateral radiographs (see Chapter 22).

Patella. In comparison to osteochondritis dissecans of the femoral condyles, that of the patella is rare.[535–542] Unilateral involvement predominates; however, bilateral cases are encountered.[1016] Men are affected more frequently than women, and the age of clinical onset usually is between 15 and 20 years. Familial cases are rare.[543] The typical site of the lesion is the medial facet of the patella. Involvement of the lateral facet occurs in approximately 30 per cent of cases, and the most medial or "odd" facet generally is spared. The middle or lower portion of the bone is affected almost universally, whereas the superior portion is uninvolved.

The cause of the lesion appears to be traumatic,[544] although support for primary ischemic necrosis does exist[545] despite the rich blood supply to the subchondral patellar bone.[546] Although a history of an injury may not be elicited, it is well recognized that the articular surface is exposed repeatedly to trauma, and a tangential shearing force may be responsible for the lesion. Historically, patients frequently note pain, originating when the knee was flexed under load, supporting the concept of a shearing fracture. An association with ligamentous laxity and lateral patellar subluxation also supports this concept of a traumatic cause.[539] The lesions are identified optimally on lateral and axial radiographs, appearing as osseous defects near the convexity between the condylar articular surfaces of the

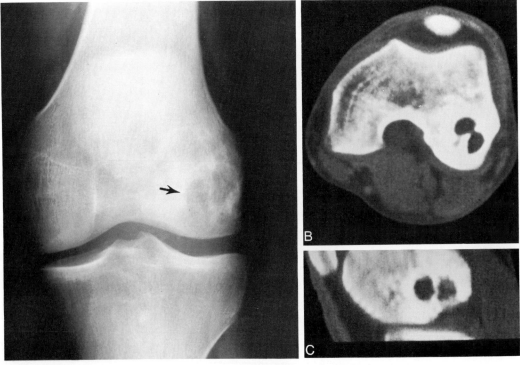

FIGURE 67–93. Osteochondritis dissecans of the femoral condyles: CT.
A In this 20 year old man, a large radiolucent lesion of the lateral femoral condyle is evident (arrow).
B, C Its precise size, configuration, and relationship to the articular surface are well shown on transaxial and sagittal CT images.

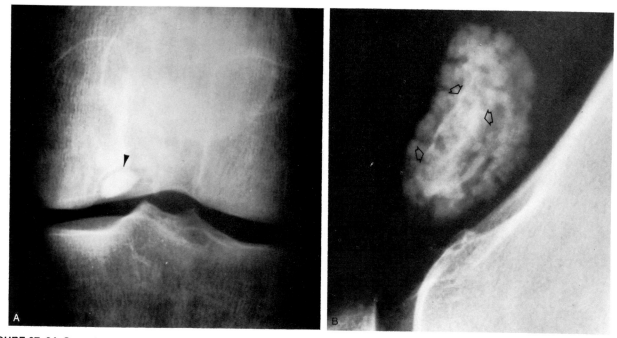

FIGURE 67–94. Osteochondritis dissecans of the femoral condyles: Fate of fragments.

A Fragment remaining in situ: Note the osseous dense area (arrowhead), indicating a fragment that remains in its bed in the medial femoral condyle.

B Loose body with proliferation of new cartilage. Note the layered appearance as calcification has occurred about the original nidus (open arrows) in the suprapatellar pouch.

patella (Fig. 67–95). Single or multiple intra-articular osseous bodies also may be recognized. Arthrography can identify the chondral component of the injury. CT rarely is necessary in the evaluation of this lesion.[547] MR imaging may provide information regarding the viability and stability of the osteochondritic fragment[548] (Fig. 67–96).

The major differential diagnoses are chondromalacia patellae, dorsal defect of the patella, and osteochondral fractures related to direct injury or recurrent dislocation. Chondromalacia patellae usually is confined to the cartilaginous layer of the bone. Radiographs may be entirely normal, although local subchondral sclerosis and detached flakes of calcified cartilage have been recognized. The dorsal defect of the patella is a benign lesion associated with a round and lytic defect with well-defined margins in the superolateral aspect of the bone[549, 550] (Fig. 67–97). Arthrography reveals intact cartilage in almost all cases.[551] This defect occurs in both sexes, may be bilateral, and is unassociated with symptoms and signs (with rare exceptions).[552] It appears to represent an anomaly of ossification and may be part of the spectrum of a bipartite or multipartite patella.[553, 554]

Dislocation of the patella is associated with an osteochondral fracture at the medial side of the patella and, less frequently, at the lateral margin of the lateral femoral condyle.[555–560] Although this diagnosis is obvious if the patient is seen when the patella is dislocated, the patella may become reduced spontaneously, and the patient may not volunteer a history that is appropriate for the injury. Thus, identification of the typical fractures is important in the accurate diagnosis of this condition. The radiographic abnormalities are characteristic, appearing on axial views of the patella. The findings relate both to true fracture of the patella and femur and to calcification and ossification of

adjacent hematomas.[559] Patellar and femoral fractures are caused by the contraction of the quadriceps muscle during relocation, driving the patella into the lateral femoral condyle.[494] MR imaging may show changes in signal intensity of the bone marrow in both bones.[87]

Although tumors and infection also may affect the patella, the resulting radiographic picture does not resemble that of osteochondritis dissecans. Osteoarthritis of the patellofemoral compartment in the knee leads to irregularity and erosion of cartilage and bone (Fig. 67–98).

Talus. Osteochondritis dissecans also is recognized in the talar dome.[561–577] The middle third of the lateral border of the talus and the posterior third of the medial border are the two most common sites of injury, and they are involved with approximately equal frequency.[561] Men are affected more often than women, and the patients usually are in the second to fourth decades of life. Clinical and experimental evidence confirms the traumatic nature of these lesions, particularly the lateral one, although the exact mechanism of injury has not been agreed on.[561, 578, 579] The lateral talar lesion appears to relate to an inversion injury of the ankle[561] (Figs. 67–99 and 67–100). As the foot is inverted, the lateral border of the talar dome is compressed against the fibula. Further inversion ruptures the lateral collateral ligament and results in an avulsion of a small piece of the dome. This osteochondral fragment may remain in place or be displaced by continued inversion. The fragment may invert or rotate[571] or lodge in the inferior tibiofibular joint.[570] If the injury is mild and the lateral ligament remains intact, clinical manifestations may be relatively mild; more severe injury with ligamentous tear is associated with pain and swelling. The medial talar dome lesion, which generally but not invariably is considered to be traumatic in pathogenesis,

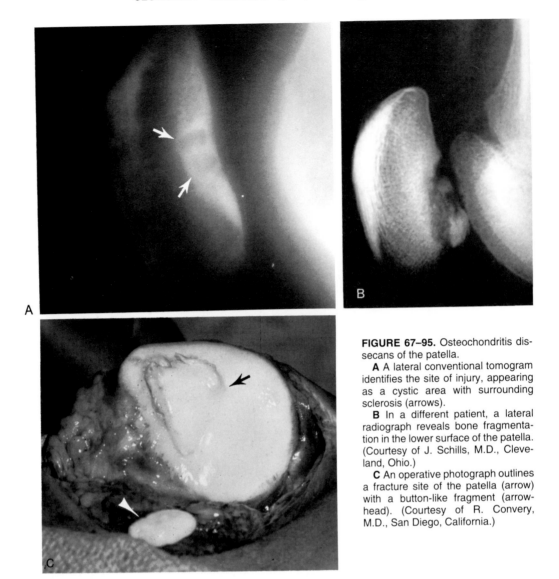

FIGURE 67–95. Osteochondritis dissecans of the patella.

A A lateral conventional tomogram identifies the site of injury, appearing as a cystic area with surrounding sclerosis (arrows).

B In a different patient, a lateral radiograph reveals bone fragmentation in the lower surface of the patella. (Courtesy of J. Schills, M.D., Cleveland, Ohio.)

C An operative photograph outlines a fracture site of the patella (arrow) with a button-like fragment (arrowhead). (Courtesy of R. Convery, M.D., San Diego, California.)

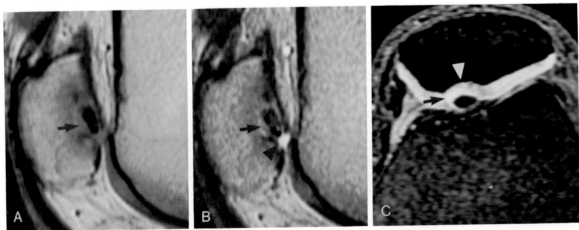

FIGURE 67–96. Osteochondritis dissecans of the patella. In this 30 year old man, a sagittal proton density (TR/TE, 2200/20) spin echo MR image **(A)** shows the patellar defect containing a bone fragment of low signal intensity. The junctional region (arrow) is of intermediate signal intensity. The patellar articular cartilage is not well evaluated. A sagittal T2-weighted (TR/TE, 2200/80) spin echo MR image **(B)** reveals higher signal intensity of the junctional region (arrow). Fluid arising from the joint has collected in a defect (arrowhead) in the patellar articular cartilage. A transaxial spoiled gradient recalled acquisition in the steady state (SPGR) MR image (TR/TE, 58/10; flip angle, 60 degrees), obtained with volumetric acquisition and chemical presaturation of fat (ChemSat) **(C)**, shows the bone fragment, adjacent high signal intensity (arrow) in the junctional zone, and the osseous bed (arrowhead) in the patella. The articular cartilage of the patella is thinned or absent at the site of the bone fragment.

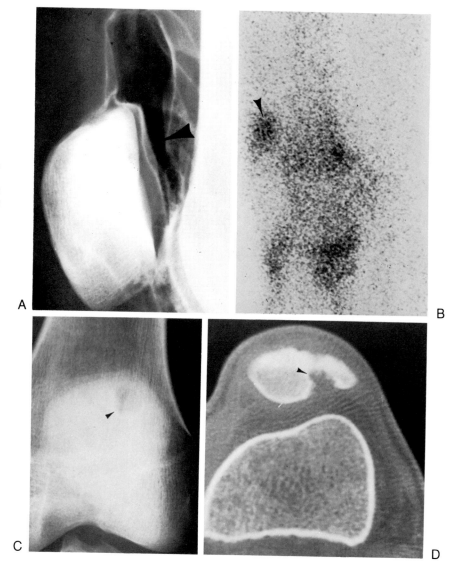

FIGURE 67–97. Dorsal defect of the patella (DDP).

A In a patient with a DDP, an arthrogram reveals intact patellar cartilage with slight thinning of the chondral surface over the upper pole (arrowhead), a normal finding.

B In a symptomatic 18 year old patient with a DDP, a lateral view of a bone scan after injection of technetium pyrophosphate shows diffuse increased patellar activity (arrowhead). Normal growth plate activity also is noted.

C, D In another patient, routine radiography **(C)** and transaxial CT **(D)** show a DDP (arrowheads). In **D,** note the extension of the lesion to the posterior aspect of the bone and the irregularity of the adjacent anterior patellar surface.

(C, D, Courtesy of J. Martin, M.D., San Diego, California.)

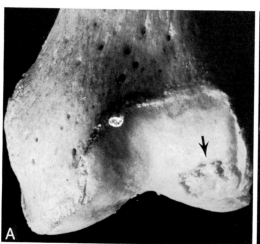

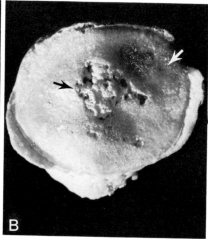

FIGURE 67–98. Osseous abnormalities in the patellofemoral compartment. Observe bone erosion in the lateral femoral condyle, the lateral facet of the patella, and the ridge between the lateral and medial patellar facets (arrows). The precise cause of these changes is unknown, although they resemble those associated with osteoarthritis. (Courtesy of D. Ortner, M.D., Washington, D.C.)

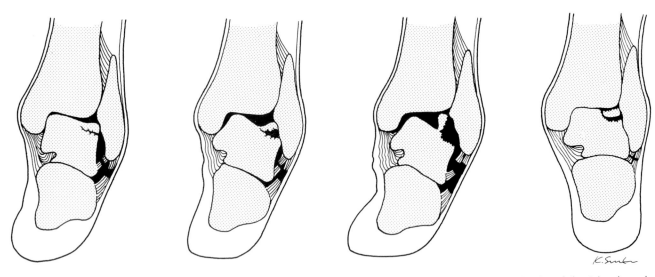

FIGURE 67–99. Osteochondritis dissecans of the talus: Lateral lesion. As the foot is inverted, the lateral border of the talar dome is compressed against the face of the fibula. Although initially the adjacent ligaments may remain intact, further inversion can produce rupture of these ligaments, with avulsion of the osteochondral fragment. This fragment can remain in situ, become inverted, or be displaced. (After Berndt AL, Harty M: J Bone Joint Surg [Am] *41:*988, 1959.)

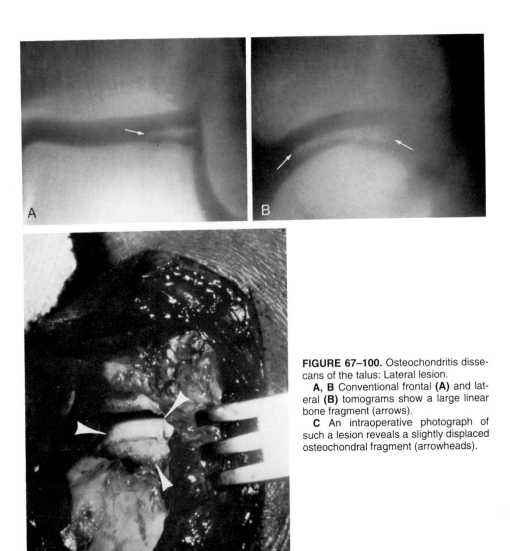

FIGURE 67–100. Osteochondritis dissecans of the talus: Lateral lesion.

A, B Conventional frontal **(A)** and lateral **(B)** tomograms show a large linear bone fragment (arrows).

C An intraoperative photograph of such a lesion reveals a slightly displaced osteochondral fragment (arrowheads).

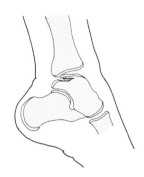
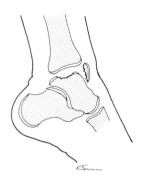

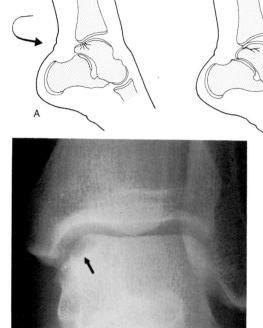

FIGURE 67–101. Osteochondritis dissecans of the talus: Medial lesion.

A Plantar flexion of the foot, inversion, and rotation may produce a small area of talar compression. Greater forces lead to "gouging out" of an osteochondral fragment owing to the presence of the adjacent tibia. This fragment may remain in situ or become displaced.

B In this patient, note the lucent lesion of the medial talar dome (arrow), the site of an osteochondral fragment.

(**A** After Berndt AL, Harty M: J Bone Joint Surg [Am] *41:*988, 1959.)

may be related to plantar flexion of the foot with inversion, followed by rotation of the tibia on the talus[561] (Fig. 67–101). This combination of forces produces compression of the talus while the collateral ligaments remain intact. Greater force causes the posteroinferior lip of the tibia to ride medially across the everted medial margin of the talus, producing an osteochondral fragment that may remain in situ or become partially or completely displaced. The same force can injure portions of the deltoid and lateral collateral ligaments. The medial talar fracture frequently is cup-shaped, deeper, and larger than the lateral talar lesion, which may be shallow and wafer-shaped.[567] Although unilateral alterations predominate, bilateral changes involving the medial talar dome, the lateral talar dome, or both domes are encountered (Fig. 67–102). A variety of classification systems have been used to describe the extent of either the lateral or medial lesions.[561, 580, 581]

Carefully obtained radiographs usually can delineate the site of injury. Anteroposterior, lateral, internal oblique, and external oblique projections should be obtained. These

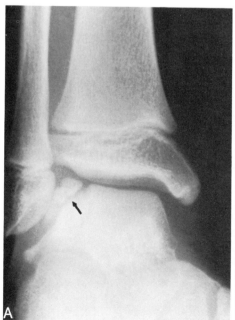
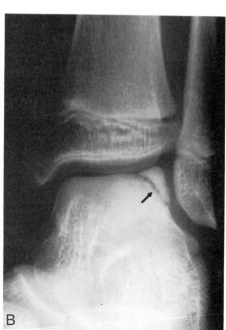

FIGURE 67–102. Osteochondritis dissecans of the talus: Bilateral lateral lesions. This 10 year old female gymnast developed bilateral ankle pain. The lateral talar defects (arrows) almost are symmetric in appearance and location. (Courtesy of G. Greenway, M.D., Dallas, Texas.)

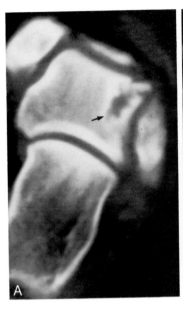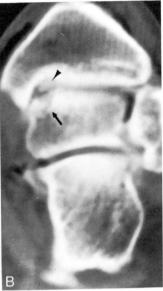

FIGURE 67–103. Osteochondritis dissecans of the talus: CT.

A Coronal CT reveals a large lateral talar lesion (arrow) with a partially displaced bone fragment.

B In a different patient, a coronal CT scan shows an osseous lesion (arrow) and an inverted fragment in the joint space (arrowhead).

(Courtesy of R. Kerr, M.D., Los Angeles, California.)

views may be supplemented by radiographs taken with the ankle in stress and with varying degrees of plantar flexion and dorsiflexion of the ankle, and by fluoroscopy and conventional tomography or CT scanning (Fig. 67–103).[562, 564, 565, 581, 582] The osseous defects may be quite subtle, consisting of slight irregularity of the articular surface, shallow excavations with or without adjacent sclerosis, and small "flake" fracture fragments. Frequently, they appear larger on lateral radiographs and tomograms. Arthrography and conventional or computed arthrotomography are indicated in some cases to delineate the fracture site better, to define the condition of the overlying chondral coat, and to detect intra-articular osseous and cartilaginous bodies.[583, 584] MR imaging (Fig. 67–104) also has been used to define the extent of the lesion,[503, 505, 585] although its precise role is not yet clear[581] (see previous discussion). Precise identification of the location and the extent of injury are important in determining the need for surgery and the specific surgical approach that must be used.[586–588]

Gross pathologic findings confirm the disruption of the articular surface; histologic analysis indicates viability of the cartilaginous portion of the lesion and, in some cases, a potential to heal (Fig. 67–105).

Other Sites. Posttraumatic osteochondral fractures, osteochondritis dissecans, and necrosis can be identified at other sites (see Chapter 81), including other tarsal bones[574, 589] and the tibia (Fig. 67–106), the humeral head,[590] the glenoid cavity,[591, 592] the acetabulum,[593] the elbow,[594–600] and the wrist.[601] Osteochondritis dissecans about the elbow usually involves the capitulum[602, 603] (Fig. 67–107), although the trochlear region of the humerus also may be affected.[604] A history of acute injury or chronic stress, as occurs in gymnastics, is frequent. As in other sites, MR imaging (Fig. 67–108) has been used in a preliminary fashion to evaluate the lesion.[605, 606] The major differential diagnostic consideration in cases of capitular involvement is Panner's disease (see Chapter 81).

Fractures of the Shafts of the Long Tubular Bones

It is the application of an abnormal force to a bone, a process termed loading, that results in an injury. The likelihood of a fracture as well as its specific configuration during such an injury depends on the precise characteristics of the load (its type, magnitude, and rate) and those of the

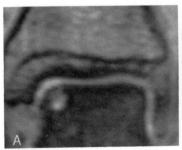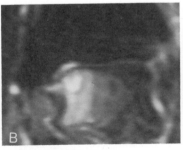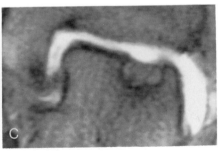

FIGURE 67–104. Osteochondritis dissecans of the talus: MR imaging.

A, B In a 19 year old woman, a coronal multiplanar gradient recalled (MPGR) MR image (TR/TE, 267/15; flip angle, 25 degrees) **(A)** shows a medial talar lesion of high signal intensity. This finding is compatible with fluid in the lesion. No alterations in signal intensity in the remainder of the talus can be seen. A coronal short tau inversion recovery (STIR) MR image (TR/TE, 2500/40; inversion time, 160 msec) **(B)** reveals the hyperintense lesion. Also note increased signal intensity around the lesion, consistent with marrow edema, and a small amount of joint fluid.

C In a second patient, a coronal T1-weighted (TR/TE, 500/20) spin echo MR image, obtained with chemical presaturation of fat (ChemSat) and after the intra-articular injection of a gadolinium contrast agent, shows a lateral talar lesion with loss of the overlying articular cartilage.

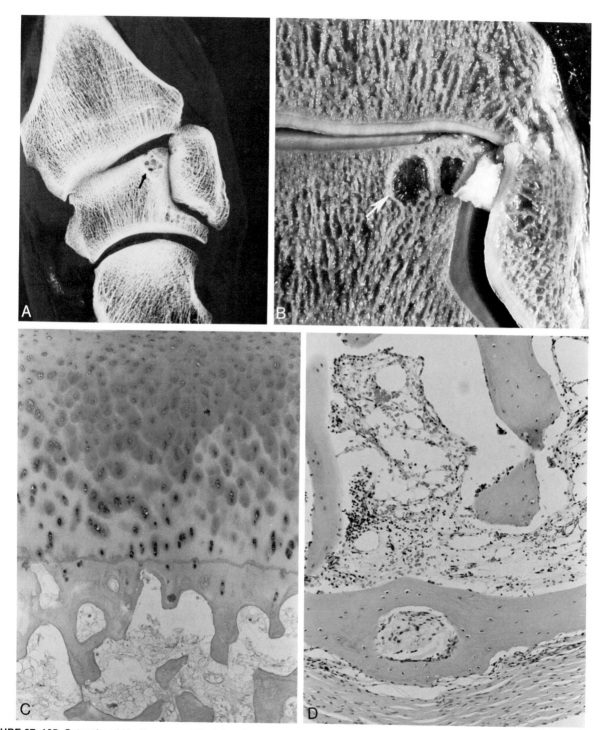

FIGURE 67–105. Osteochondritis dissecans of the talus: Gross pathologic and histologic abnormalities.
  A, B A radiograph and photograph of a coronal section of the ankle reveal a typical lateral talar dome lesion (arrows). Note the disruption of the articular cartilage over the lesion and the sclerotic bone.
  C Observe the necrosis of the subchondral bone and viable articular chondrocytes.
  D In a specimen from a different patient, the subchondral bone is viable, and a fibrous capsule is identified.
  (**C, D,** From Flick AB, Gould N: Foot Ankle 5:165, 1985. Copyright 1985, American Orthopaedic Foot Society.)

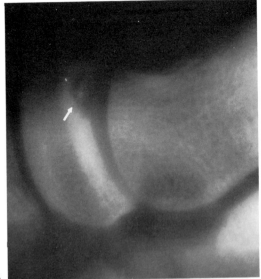

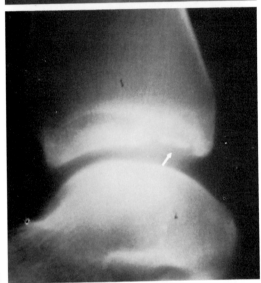

FIGURE 67–106. Osteochondritis dissecans of other tarsal bones and the tibia.
A Tarsal navicular bone in a 33 year old male athlete (arrow).
B Tibia in a young male runner (arrow).
(**B,** Courtesy of V. Vint, M.D., San Diego, California.)

target bone (its material and structural properties).[607] Important properties of bone that determine its ability to withstand loading include energy-absorbing capacity, elasticity, fatigue strength, and density.[608] The ability of bone to absorb energy varies with the person's age, sex, and metabolic status, the integrity of surrounding tissues, and the specific bone that is being considered. The impressive ability of the femur to resist compressive force owing to its highly developed trabecular system is well recognized, as is the weakening of the femur that occurs in osteoporosis and Paget's disease. The bones of children are more plastic (ductile) than the more brittle bones of adults, a fact that contributes to the occurrence of incomplete and bowing fractures in the pediatric age group, injuries that almost never are seen in adults. Additional factors that contribute to the production of a fracture are the presence of a preexisting lesion and a previous surgical procedure. A break in the cortex of the bone related to either of these factors results in an area of

weakness; this weakening effect increases exponentially when the size of the defect becomes greater than 30 per cent of the diameter of the bone. Cortical bone graft donor sites and pin tracts are at risk for fracture. Metallic implants also affect the biologic properties of bone; they increase the stiffness of the bone containing the implant, which, in turn, results in an area of increased stress at the transition point between the metallic device and the adjacent bone (termed a stress riser), an area subject to fracture.

Four basic types of load can be applied to an object such as a long tubular bone: *tension* (or traction) forces act perpendicular to the cross section of the bone, pulling apart trabeculae; *compression* forces act in a similar perpendicular direction, pressing together trabeculae; *torsion* (or rotational) forces are twisting in nature; and *bending* forces lead to angulation. Of these types of force, compression, torsion, and bending working independently or in combination are common causes of bone injury; tension forces usually result in soft tissue rather than osseous alterations.

The energy-absorbing capacity of bone, including its ability to change shape under external forces, also must be considered in the production of fractures. The external forces (load) cause a *stress* on the bone, and the resultant distortion of the bone is called a *strain*. As has been described previously (see Fig. 67–75), this relationship between stress and strain may be plotted graphically. The first portion of the curve is linear, with the resulting strain being directly proportional to the applied stress. In this zone of elastic deformation, removal of the load will allow the object to return to its original shape. The slope of the curve is an indication of the stiffness of the material; the steeper the slope, the stiffer the material. At the point where the slope changes (yield point or limit of proportionality), strain increases more rapidly with increasing stress. In this part of the curve, termed the zone of plastic deformation, the object does not return completely to its original shape after removal of the stress. This portion of the curve is a measure of brittleness. The more ductile the material, the greater its ability for plastic deformity. With continued application of stress, the object eventually reaches the point of fracture (failing point).

Such stress-strain diagrams vary with the biologic characteristics of the material. For example, brittle materials (adult bones) are stronger in resisting compression than in resisting tension; conversely, ductile materials (young bones) are stronger in resisting tension than in resisting compression. Each time a material is subjected to a stress, there is some release of energy.[609] The application of chronic repetitive stresses, with each stress event being below the tensile strength of the material, ultimately may lead to failure. This principle of fatigue strength may be considered in the production of stress (fatigue) fractures in bone. The principle is more complex in biologic systems than in material technology owing to the healing (repair) capacity of bone and supporting soft tissues.

The fracture configuration or pattern depends on the interaction of a particular load and a specific bone. Several types are recognized (Fig. 67–109) (Table 67–4):

1. *Transverse fracture* (mechanism: bending, or angular, forces in long bones; tensile, or traction, forces in short bones). A transverse fracture line, occurring at a right angle to the shaft, usually is the result of a bending force. Tensile

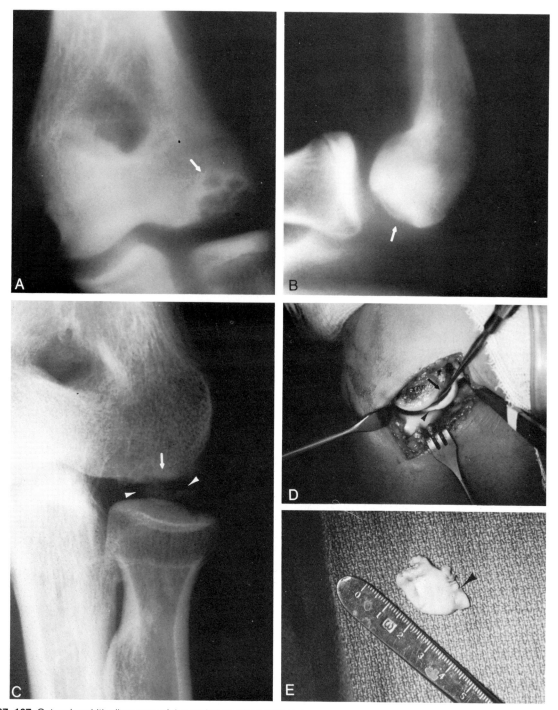

FIGURE 67–107. Osteochondritis dissecans of the capitulum of the humerus.

A, B Elbow pain in this 12 year old gymnast had resulted from osteochondritis dissecans of the capitulum (arrows). (Courtesy of G. Greenway, M.D., Dallas, Texas.)

C A similar lesion (arrow) in a 29 year old man has resulted in an intra-articular osseous body (arrowheads). (Courtesy of V. Vint, M.D., San Diego, California.)

D, E Operative findings in a third patient reveal a fragment of cartilage and bone (arrowheads) arising from the capitulum (arrow). The radial head also is visible in the operative photograph. (Courtesy of J. Fronek, M.D., San Diego, California.)

TABLE 67–4. Biomechanics of Fractures in Long Tubular Bones*

Fracture Pattern	Mechanism of Injury	Location of Soft Tissue Hinge	Energy Load	Common Sites
Transverse	Bending	Concavity	Low	Diaphyses
Oblique	Compression, bending, and torsion	Concavity (often destroyed)	Moderate	Radius, ulna, tibia, fibula
Oblique-transverse	Compression and bending	Concavity or side of butterfly fragment	Moderate	Femur, tibia, humerus
Spiral	Torsion	Vertical segment	Low	Tibia, humerus
Diaphyseal impaction	Compression	Variable	Variable	Humerus, femur, tibia
Comminuted	Variable	Destroyed	High	Variable

*From Gonza ER, Harrington IJ: Biomechanics of Musculoskeletal Injury. © 1982, Williams & Wilkins Co, Baltimore, pp 2, 21.

failure of the bone takes place on its convex side (opposite to the input force) with subsequent compressive failure of bone on its concave side.[310, 311] Often, the cortex on the compressive side fails before the transverse fracture is complete, resulting in cortical splintering. A soft tissue hinge may be preserved on the side of the input force. Transverse fractures also may be caused by traction forces at sites of tendon or ligament insertion in bone.

2. *Oblique fracture* (mechanism: a combination of compression, bending, and torsion forces). Combined forces consisting of compression and torsion and, to a lesser extent, bending typically lead to an oblique fracture[610] (Fig. 67–110). Such a fracture resembles a spiral fracture superficially (see later discussion), although differentiation between the two is important, as the former (oblique fracture) has a higher frequency of nonunion and the latter (spiral fracture) usually heals uneventfully.[607] In an oblique fracture, the ends of the bones are short and blunt, a vertical segment is not identified, and a clear space may be seen; in a spiral fracture, long, sharp, and pointed ends and a vertical segment are characteristic, and, unless the fracture is distracted, no clear space is evident on radiographs obtained in any projection. An oblique fracture most commonly involves the paired bones of either the forearm or the lower leg. A simple transverse or oblique fracture, often involving only one bone of the forearm or lower leg, is the result of a "tapping" force, a force of dying momentum applied over a linear area. As the force is absorbed almost totally by one bone, the companion bone is spared and there is minimal soft tissue damage.

3. *Oblique-transverse fracture* (mechanism: a combination of axial compression and bending forces). This combination of forces can lead to several different types of fracture: If the compression forces are larger than the bending forces, an oblique fracture is produced; if the bending forces are sufficiently large, a purely transverse fracture is seen; if both the compression and the bending forces are of sufficient magnitude, an oblique-transverse fracture results[607] (Fig. 67–111). The last type is a common fracture configuration,[610] particularly in the tibia, femur, and humerus, and its frequency indicates that pure compression or pure angular forces are less common than combined forces. Either the oblique or the transverse component may dominate, depending on the magnitude of the respective forces.

A butterfly fragment may be an added component of the oblique-transverse fracture pattern (see Fig. 67–12). As the fracture fragments continue to angulate owing to the bending load, the fragment containing the beak or oblique segment is impacted against the other fragment, leading to shearing of a piece of bone, the butterfly fragment.[607] Thus, this fragment occurs on the compression side of the bone on which the force impacts. Such fragments commonly are identified in fractures of the tubular bones of the lower extremity in pedestrians injured by automobiles.[607]

4. *Spiral fracture* (mechanism: torsion force). Spiral fractures, which are relatively uncommon and which result from twisting or rotational forces, perhaps combined with axial compression, usually are observed in the humerus and the tibia[610, 612] (Fig. 67–112). The short, straight longitudinal portion of a spiral fracture represents the initial site of bone failure, which subsequently propagates both proximally and distally.[613] Spiral fractures may be further classified as being either right-handed or left-handed.[614] This classification system depends on the identification of a dominant spiral and distinguishing it from the vertical or oblique connecting element. It has been suggested that a correlation exists between the side of the body and the direction of the spiral. Whether this pattern reflects the action of muscle

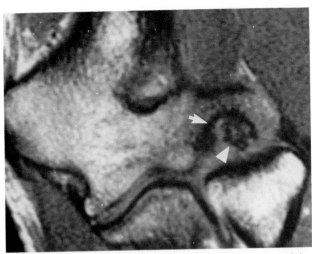

FIGURE 67–108. Osteochondritis dissecans of the capitulum of the humerus. A coronal proton density (TR/TE, 2000/20) MR image in a 16 year old man reveals the capitular lesion (arrow) containing a bone fragment (arrowhead). The overlying articular cartilage is not well seen.

(Courtesy of M. Schweitzer, M.D., Philadelphia, Pennsylvania.)

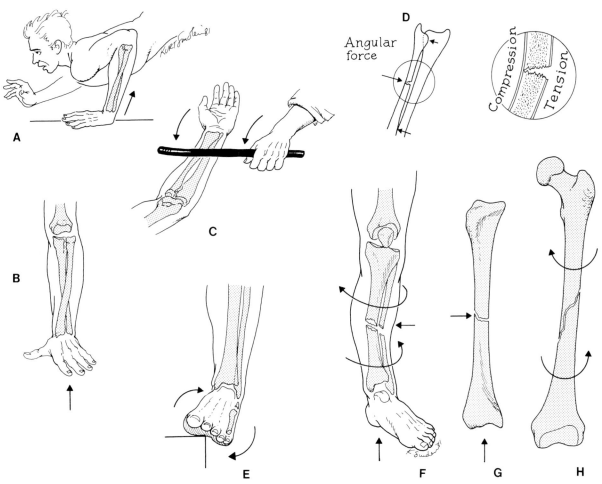

FIGURE 67–109. Biomechanics of fractures in long tubular bones.

A, B Application of longitudinal compression force (axial compression). Loading of a long bone in this manner may cause an incomplete (bowing or torus) fracture in a child or an impaction of the diaphysis into the metaphysis in an adult (e.g., an intercondylar fracture of the distal portion of the humerus or femur).

C, D Application of angular force (bending). This may result in a greenstick fracture in a child or a transverse fracture in an adult. Cortical bone is stronger in compression than in tension, so that the bone fails initially on the tension side (opposite to the input force) and the fracture propagates transversely to the long axis of the bone. The periosteum may be preserved on the side of the input force.

E Traction force (tension) at the site of a tendon or ligament insertion may result in a transverse (avulsion) fracture.

F The oblique fracture configuration results from a combination of multiple forces, including longitudinal compression and angular and rotational forces.

G An oblique-transverse fracture results from a combination of angular and axial compression forces. The direction of the fracture line is determined by the relative magnitude of the two forces: When axial compression force predominates, the oblique component is larger; conversely, a predominantly angular force results in a more transverse fracture configuration. The oblique fragment may separate in a butterfly configuration.

H A spiral fracture results from rotational forces. The fracture line approximates an angle of 40 to 45 degrees, and the direction of the spiral denotes that of the rotational forces.

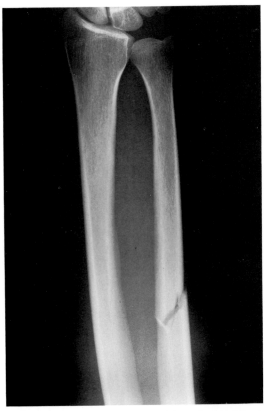

FIGURE 67–110. Oblique fracture. An oblique (tapping) fracture of the midshaft of the ulna has resulted from a direct blow. The radius is intact.

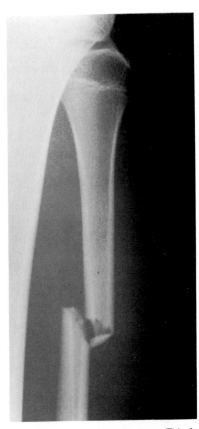

FIGURE 67–111. Oblique-transverse fracture. This fracture of the fibula is slightly comminuted.

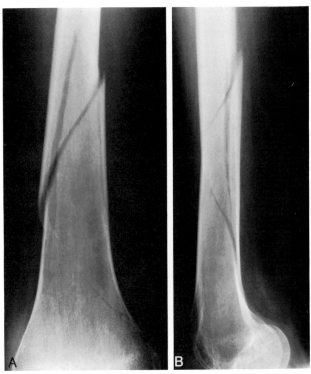

FIGURE 67–112. Spiral fracture. Anteroposterior **(A)** and lateral **(B)** radiographs reveal the fracture of the femoral diaphysis.

pull in the production of a spiral fracture or is related to the anatomic structure of the bone, which leads to biomechanically weak points, is uncertain. From these data, it seems that most tibial fractures would be reduced by internal rotation of the foot (and opened by external rotation). Manipulation of the fracture initially in the proper direction is desirable clinically for reduction, as further opening of a fracture might allow interposition of soft tissue and increased displacement, making subsequent reduction more difficult.

5. *Diaphyseal impaction fracture* (mechanism: axial compression force). In certain locations such as the humerus, femur, and tibia, an axially applied load will drive the diaphyseal bone, with its thick and rigid cortex, into the thin metaphyseal bone; examples of this injury are the supracondylar fracture of the femur and the comminuted fracture of the tibial plateaus.[607]

6. *Comminuted fracture* (mechanism: variable). Indirect or direct application of force, usually of high energy, leads to multiple osseous fragments of varying size. When two or more bones are located close to each other, as in the forearm, lower leg, hand, or foot, they usually are all involved.

In addition to the type of load, its magnitude and rate of application are important determinants in fracture configuration. In general, the greater the magnitude of the load, the more extensive is the destruction of tissue and the more complex is the fracture pattern.[615] Oblique, oblique-transverse, butterfly, and comminuted fractures are examples of high energy injuries. With respect to the load rate, bone is a viscoelastic material whose mechanical properties vary according to how rapidly the forces are applied. This characteristic exerts an important influence on fracture biomechanics, as the likelihood of a specific fracture will be influenced significantly by the rate at which the bone is loaded.[607]

DISLOCATIONS

Terminology

A *dislocation* results when there is complete loss of contact between two osseous surfaces that normally articulate. A *subluxation* represents a partial loss of this contact. A closed subluxation or dislocation exists when the skin and soft tissues remain intact over the injured joint; an open dislocation or subluxation exists if there is associated soft tissue injury that exposes the joint to the outside environment (Fig. 67–113).

Subluxations and dislocations usually are caused by physical trauma, although they also may occur when congenital or acquired conditions produce musculature imbalance (e.g., developmental dysplasia of the hip, neurologic disorders) or when articular disorders produce incongruities of the joint surfaces and instability (e.g., rheumatoid arthritis). Dislocations of the glenohumeral joint and other sites such as the hip may occur during seizures. Many dislocations and subluxations related to trauma are associated with fractures of a neighboring bone.[616] Although the radiographic diagnosis of a dislocation or a subluxation is not difficult when the bones remain malaligned after the injury, spontaneous reduction can occur. In these cases, characteristic fractures in periarticular bone can confirm the presence of a previous dislocation. Typical examples of such fractures are the Hill-Sachs lesion of the humeral head after an

anterior dislocation of the glenohumeral joint, fractures of the femoral head that accompany either anterior or posterior dislocations of the hip, and the medial patellar fracture after lateral dislocation of the patella. Furthermore, these fractures may predispose the joint to future dislocations.

Accurate radiographic diagnosis of subluxations and dislocations requires that films be obtained in more than a single projection. Ideally, at least two projections oriented at right angles to each other should be used and, frequently, supplementary radiographs may be necessary. Radiographs exposed during stress or weight-bearing (e.g., for the ankle or acromioclavicular joint) and comparison views of the uninvolved side (e.g., for the child's elbow) can be useful.

An accurate description of a dislocation or subluxation varies with the anatomic complexity of the involved joint. When the joint is composed of two bones, the joint injury derives its name from that joint (e.g., dislocation of the hip, glenohumeral, or interphalangeal joint). When the joint comprises more than two bones, the dislocation still is named after the involved articulation if it affects the two major bones. If the smallest bone of the three is dislocated, the injury is named after that bone (e.g., a dislocation of the patella).

A third type of joint derangement is termed a *diastasis* (Fig. 67–114). This term refers to abnormal separation of a joint that normally is only slightly moveable (e.g., the distal tibiofibular syndesmosis, the symphysis pubis, or the sacroiliac joint).

Biomechanics

Conventional classification schemes define four types of joint motion: gliding and angular movements, circumduction, and rotation.[617] These may occur independently or, far more frequently, in various combinations. In any location, the precise characteristics of joint movement are governed principally by the shape of the articular surfaces[618] (Table 67–5). When movement is limited, the reciprocal articular surfaces approach each other in size, but when movement is free the bone that habitually is more mobile possesses the larger surface.[617] Spheroidal (ball-and-socket) joints, such as the hip and glenohumeral joint, allow movement in

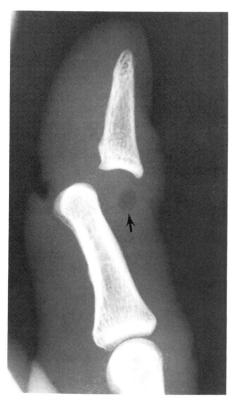

FIGURE 67–113. Open dislocation. Dorsal dislocation of the terminal phalanx at the interphalangeal joint of the thumb is associated with a soft tissue defect in the volar surface of the finger and soft tissue air (arrow).

TABLE 67–5. Morphologic Classification of Synovial Joints*

Type of Joint	Motion	Examples
Plane	Uniaxial	Intermetatarsal, intercarpal
Hinge	Uniaxial	Humeroulnar, interphalangeal
Pivot	Uniaxial	Proximal radioulnar, median atlantoaxial
Bicondylar	Uniaxial (minimal movement also in a second axis)	Knee, temporomandibular
Ellipsoid	Biaxial	Radiocarpal, metacarpophalangeal
Sellar	Biaxial	First carpometacarpal, ankle, calcaneocuboid
Spheroidal	Triaxial	Hip, glenohumeral

*Adapted from Williams PL, Warwick R: Gray's Anatomy, 36th British Ed. Philadelphia, WB Saunders Co, 1980, p 430.

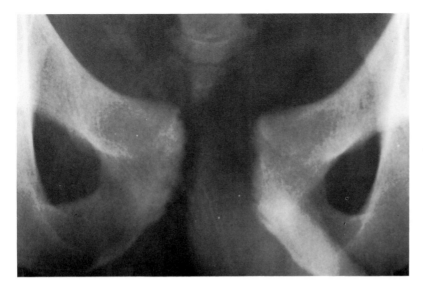

FIGURE 67–114. Diastasis. Abnormal widening of the symphysis pubis is apparent.

three axes (three degrees of freedom); hinged joints, such as the interphalangeal and humeroulnar joints, and bicondylar articulations, such as the knee, are restricted to movement primarily in one axis (one degree of freedom), and the sides of the joints typically are provided with strong collateral ligaments.[617] In general, increasing freedom of movement is achieved at the expense of joint stability.[618]

The stability of an articulation can be influenced by both intrinsic factors (which in turn relate to the shape of the apposing articular surfaces) and extrinsic factors (which include the existence, location, and strength of surrounding ligaments and muscles). Closely fitted or highly congruous articular surfaces, such as exist in the hip, are inherently stable; poorly fitted or loosely packed articular surfaces, such as exist in the knee, are inherently unstable and depend on the stability provided by the strong ligaments and muscles that connect their components.[618]

Traumatic dislocation of a joint implies that the joint capsule and protective ligaments have been damaged. A tear in these tissues may permit the extrusion of the articular end of the bone. Alternatively, the capsule may be stripped from one of its osseous sites of attachment, or a stretched ligament may lead to avulsion of a bone fragment. Although trauma may produce a dislocation of any articulation, the most commonly involved sites are the glenohumeral joint, elbow, ankle, hip, and interphalangeal joints.

TRAUMA TO SYNOVIAL JOINTS

Traumatic Synovitis and Hemarthrosis

After a blow or abnormal stress, joint swelling and pain may develop. A joint effusion appearing within the first few hours after trauma usually is related to a hemarthrosis; nonbloody effusions usually appear 12 to 24 hours after injury.[619, 620]

Experimental evidence indicates that trauma may produce a subtle increase in vascular permeability owing to mechanisms other than gross disruption of vessels, suggesting that the genesis of traumatic effusions, including bloody ones, is multifactorial.[621] Pain and, occasionally, fever may

be apparent in cases of hemarthrosis, and in all such cases, occult fractures or ligamentous injury must be excluded by careful clinical and radiologic examination.[622, 623] In addition to injuries, hemarthrosis also may be associated with hemophilia, and other bleeding disorders, pigmented villonodular synovitis, neuropathic osteoarthropathy, crystal deposition diseases, chronic renal failure, and intra-articular tumors.

Bloody or nonbloody effusions occurring after trauma are associated with radiographic findings that are related to displacement of intra-articular fat pads and edema of extra-articular fat planes. Typical examples of these findings are widening of the suprapatellar pouch in cases of knee trauma; ventral and posterior displacement of the fat pads about the distal end of the humerus (Fig. 67–115A) and distortion of the fat planes overlying the supinator muscle in cases of elbow trauma; displacement and obliteration of the fat plane overlying the pronator quadratus muscle (Fig. 67–115B) and about the carpal scaphoid in cases of wrist trauma; displacement and distortion of fat planes anterior and posterior to the distal portion of the tibia in cases of ankle trauma (Fig. 67–115C); and "bulging" of the "capsular" fat in cases of hip trauma in children.[624–629] In general, the displacement and distortion of many of these fat planes indicate only the presence of fluid or a mass in the joint and may be evident in a variety of articular processes; however, in the clinical setting of trauma, detection of these changes should encourage a thorough search for a subtle fracture or subluxation. Similarly, widening of the articular space owing to accumulation of fluid can follow intra-articular trauma[630] (Fig. 67–115D) but also may be observed in other articular conditions. Chronic accumulation of blood in the joint, as in cases of hemophilia and pigmented villonodular synovitis, may lead to hemosiderin deposition in the synovial membrane and increased radiodensity of the distended joint. This finding, however, generally is subtle. More useful in documenting the presence of hemosiderin deposition in the synovial tissues is MR imaging. On spin echo and particularly on gradient echo MR images, hemosiderin accumulation is characterized by low signal intensity. Similar low signal intensity may be apparent in the presence of intra-articular gas, calcification,

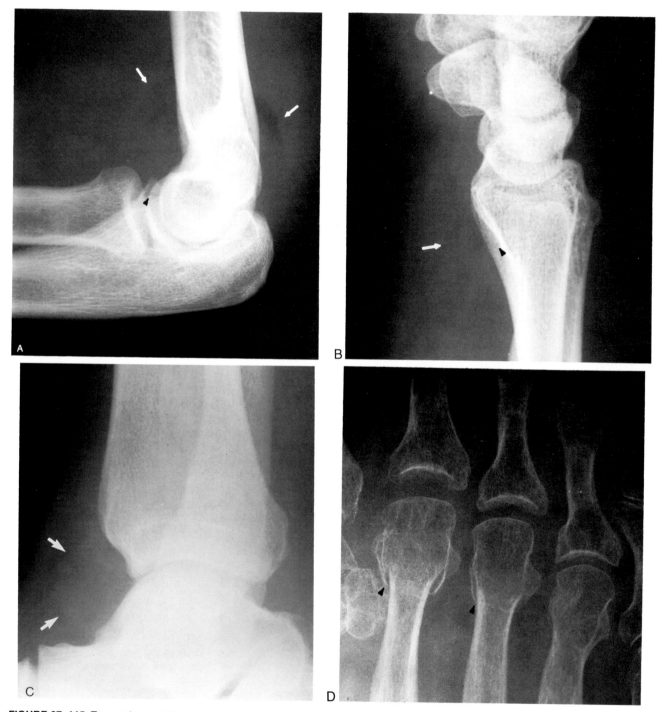

FIGURE 67–115. Traumatic synovitis, hemarthrosis, and soft tissue edema.

A Displacement of the anterior and posterior fat pads (arrows) about the elbow after trauma usually indicates intra-articular fluid or blood. Note the fracture of the coronoid process of the ulna (arrowhead).

B Obliteration of the fat plane about the pronator quadratus muscle (arrow) is associated with a subtle fracture (arrowhead).

C Observe distention of the anterior capsule (arrows), indicative of a large posttraumatic hemarthrosis in the ankle.

D Widening of the second and third metatarsophalangeal joints accompanies fractures of the metatarsal heads (arrowheads) and may be related to synovitis, hemarthrosis, or osseous shortening.

or ossification and after deposition of amyloid, monosodium urate crystals, or metallic debris.

Careful evaluation of synovial fluid in some joints may document the presence of "wear particles" consisting of chondral fragments and debris.[631] Their presence in a traumatized joint, such as the knee, may indicate damage to the fibrocartilaginous meniscus. The particles are identified more readily in the absence of a hemarthrosis, as they may be obscured by abundant erythrocytes in the synovial fluid.

Lipohemarthrosis

Bloody synovial fluid containing fat droplets can be noted grossly and microscopically after trauma to a joint.[632–634] The discovery of intra-articular fat, when combined with bone marrow spicules, is reliable evidence of an intra-articular fracture, the fat being released from the marrow after cortical violation. Frequently, however, a hemorrhagic effusion containing fat may be observed in patients without fracture, probably related to significant cartilaginous or ligamentous injury.[635–637] As fat also is present in the synovium, it is possible that damage to the synovium alone can release fat into the synovial fluid.[637] Other sources of lipids in the synovial fluid include the rich vascular bed between the adjacent cells and the joint and intra-articular fat pads (as in the elbow).[638] The amount of fat in the synovial fluid is directly proportional to the severity of the joint injury.[635] Although fat globules are seen occasionally in many other types of effusion, their accumulation is much greater in cases of trauma. In fact, joint effusions containing large amounts of lipids (chylous effusions) without blood (and sometimes without an associated fracture) are described.[639, 640] After trauma, synovitis with synovial fluid leukocytosis may result as a response to intra-articular lipid droplets and may be associated with intracellular (leukocytes) accumulation of the lipids owing to phago-

cytosis.[637, 641] The findings may simulate those of a septic arthritis.

Radiographic examination using horizontal beam technique may demonstrate a fat-blood fluid level after injury to the joint[633, 636, 642–647] (Fig. 67–116). Most commonly, this finding is seen in a knee or a shoulder (Fig. 67–117), although it also may be noted in other joints, including the elbow.[648] In the knee, subtle tibial plateau fractures may be the source of the fat, requiring careful radiography and tomography for detection,[649–651] although fat also may originate from fibular, femoral, or patellar fractures as well as from soft tissue injury to cartilage, ligaments, fat pads, or synovium.[652] Small amounts of fat and blood in this joint may not be sufficient to produce a fat-blood fluid level on cross-table radiography, although large amounts will reveal a typical radiopaque straight line at the interface of the fat above and the blood below. Occasionally, routine lateral knee films taken without horizontal beam technique in patients with significant intra-articular fat will allow visualization of the capsule as a water-dense linear structure outlined on both sides by fat.[653] In the shoulder and the elbow, radiographically evident fat-blood fluid levels can accompany fractures, dislocations, and, perhaps, injuries to the synovium or surrounding soft tissue structures.[643, 645, 648]

Lipohemarthroses also may be detected with CT[26] or MR imaging[654] (Fig. 67–118). The former method allows assessment of small amounts of intra-articular fat that may escape detection with standard radiographic techniques and is useful in the diagnosis of occult fractures about the hip, shoulder, and knee. With MR imaging, the appearance of a lipohemarthrosis is more complex as several layers and interfaces are evident with signal intensity characteristics dependent on the specific imaging sequences that are employed. The most superior zone contains floating fat, a central zone contains serum, and an inferior zone contains dependent red blood cells.[654] A signal void, representing

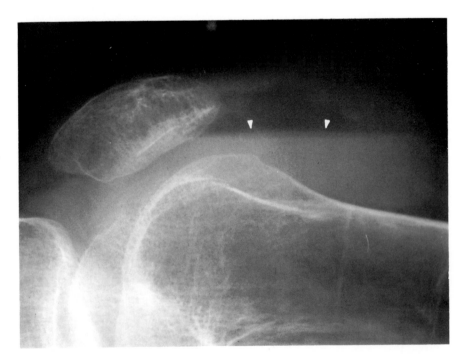

FIGURE 67–116. Lipohemarthrosis. On a cross-table lateral radiograph, a straight radiodense fluid line (arrowheads) at a fat-blood interface can be a helpful clue to an underlying yet subtle fracture.

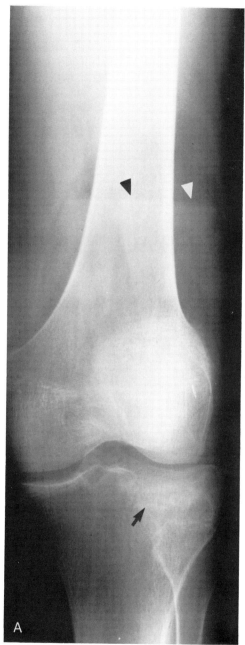

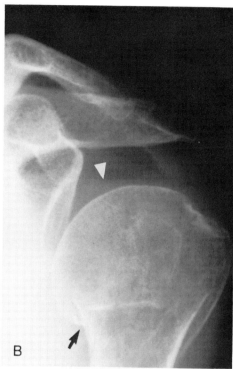

FIGURE 67–117. Lipohemarthrosis.

A Knee. On a frontal radiograph obtained with the patient standing, a fat-fluid level (arrowheads) is a useful finding in the detection of a fracture of the lateral tibial plateau (arrow).

B Shoulder. On a frontal radiograph of the shoulder in an upright patient, a fat-fluid level (arrowhead) has resulted from a fracture (arrow) of the surgical neck of the humerus. Note inferior displacement, or drooping, of the humeral head.

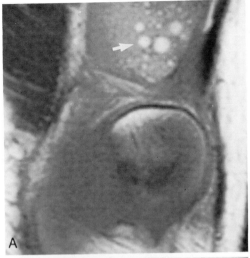

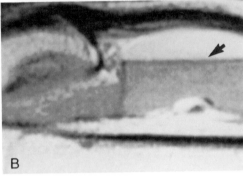

FIGURE 67–118. Lipohemarthrosis.

A On a coronal T1-weighted (TR/TE, 500/20) spin echo MR image of the knee, globules of fat (arrow) in the suprapatellar pouch, above the patella, are of high signal intensity. The bloody joint effusion is of intermediate signal intensity. (Courtesy of R. Reinke, M.D., Long Beach, California.)

B This sagittal T1-weighted (TR/TE, 900/30) spin echo MR image shows a dominant fluid level (arrow) at the interface of fat (above) and serum (below). The image has been rotated 90 degrees to simulate the orientation of a cross table radiograph. (Courtesy of R. Stiles, M.D., Atlanta, Georgia.)

chemical shift artifact, may be visible at the interface of fat and serum.

TRAUMA TO SYMPHYSES

Traumatic insult to symphyses, including the symphysis pubis, manubriosternal joint, and intervertebral disc, is not infrequent. Subluxation (i.e., diastasis) or dislocation of the symphysis pubis leads to a single break in the pelvic ring and commonly is combined with a second injury with pelvic disruption, such as a fracture of the ilium or sacrum or a diastasis of the sacroiliac joint. Minor degrees of instability in this location may be discovered during radiographic examination performed with the patient standing first on one leg, then on the other. Exaggerated movement at the articulation indicates violation of its integrity, although, under normal circumstances, some motion at the symphysis pubis may be observed, especially in pregnant women (see Chapter 58). Subluxation or dislocation of the manubriosternal joint usually indicates significant trauma and may be seen after automobile accidents in which the chest strikes the steering wheel. Similar displacement at this site occasionally occurs spontaneously in association with exaggerated thoracic kyphosis as in generalized osteoporosis, osteomalacia, renal osteodystrophy, and plasma cell myeloma.

Violation of the intervertebral disc may be combined with fractures of the vertebral bodies and posterior elements, leading to spinal instability. One example of an injury that can lead to disruption of both the intervertebral disc (plus surrounding bone) and the posterior spinal structures is the seat-belt fracture (Fig. 67–119). During an automobile accident, the trunk flexes over the seat belt. A horizontal fracture of a vertebral body (Chance fracture) or tearing of the intervertebral disc can be combined with laminal and spinous process fractures or ligamentous tear (see Chapter 69).

Trauma to the discovertebral junction can result from obvious or occult injury. In either situation, violation of the cartilaginous endplate and subchondral bone plate of the

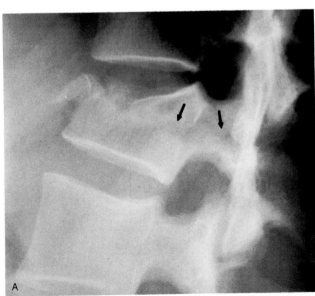

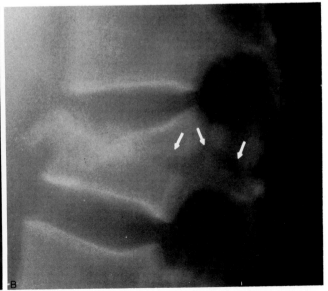

FIGURE 67–119. Seat-belt injury. After an automobile accident, a transverse fracture of an upper lumbar vertebra is sometimes associated with a transverse fracture through the pedicles and laminae (arrows).

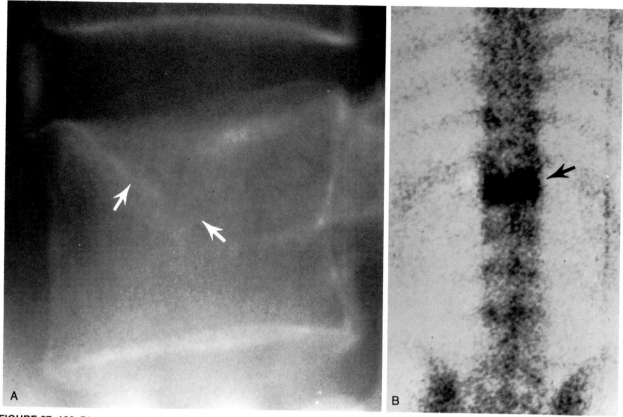

FIGURE 67–120. Discovertebral trauma. Acute compression fracture.
A After an injury with axial loading of the spine, intraosseous displacement of discal material (cartilaginous node) (arrows) can be seen.
B A radionuclide study with technetium pyrophosphate reveals increased accumulation of isotope at the site of injury (arrow).

vertebral body may allow intraosseous displacement of discal material (cartilaginous or Schmorl's nodes)[655–659] (Figs. 67–120 and 67–121). Cartilaginous nodes may appear in acute injuries in which excessive axial loading of the spine occurs. This can result in obvious compression fracture of the vertebral body or subtle injury at the discovertebral junction. With axial loading, nuclear pressure increases. Fracture of the cancellous bone of the vertebral body and disruption of the cartilaginous endplate allow discal material to enter the vertebral body. Typically, the cranial disc protrudes into the vertebra, although both cranial and caudal discs may be involved. In the latter instance, the invading cranial and caudal discal tissue may split the vertebral body, producing a burst fracture of the vertebra (see Chapter 69). This sequence of events requires the presence of a relatively normal nucleus pulposus; compression injuries in patients with intervertebral (osteo)chondrosis (see Chapter 40) produce uniform flattening of the vertebral body.[660]

The intravertebral discal material may be associated with surrounding osseous compression and reactive bone formation. Radiographs reveal one or more radiolucent areas, with bony sclerosis in the vertebral body that may be combined with intervertebral disc space loss. The radiographic appearance may simulate that of infection or tumor. CT and MR imaging may clarify the nature of the abnormalities (Fig. 67–122).

Another type of injury of the discovertebral junction occurs at the site of attachment of the anulus fibrosus to the rim of the vertebral body. At this site, fibrous extensions of the anulus are attached firmly to the vertebral rim. In the developing skeleton, this union is far more solid than that between the cartilage in the vertebral rim and the ossified portion of the vertebral body.[661] Thus, in the young patient, injury with prolapse of the contiguous intervertebral disc can lead to displacement of the ossified portion of the vertebral rim owing to separation of the osteocartilaginous junction between the rim and the remaining vertebral body. This may occur either anteriorly[659] (Fig. 67–123A,B) or posteriorly, the latter associated with the displacement of a bony ridge into the spinal canal[662–666] (Fig. 67–123C,D). The posterior injury may involve the cervical or lumbar (Fig. 67–124) segment of the spine and is discussed in detail in Chapter 69. In the mature skeleton, osseous union between the rim and vertebral body occurs, producing a much stronger connection. Even in the adult, however, injury can lead to osseous avulsion at the site of attachment of anulus fibers. Hyperextension injury to the cervical spine can be associated with a small bony flake at this site.

TRAUMA TO SYNCHONDROSES (GROWTH PLATES)

Mechanisms and Classification

The growth plate of the immature skeleton is especially vulnerable to injury; approximately 6 to 15 per cent of fractures of the tubular bones in children under the age of 16 years involve the growth plate and neighboring bone.[667–683] Forces that produce ligamentous tear or joint dislocation in the adult may lead to growth plate injury in the child and

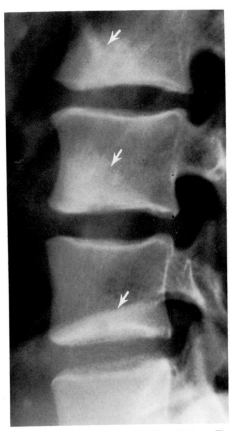

FIGURE 67–121. Discovertebral trauma: Occult injury. The reactive sclerosis of the inferior surfaces of multiple lumbar vertebrae (arrows) may represent the sequela of intraosseous discal displacements (cartilaginous nodes), although, in some cases, the precise cause of the abnormality is unclear.

adolescent, as the joint capsule and ligamentous structures are approximately two to five times stronger than the cartilaginous plate.[674] Four types of stress may produce growth plate injury; shearing or avulsive forces account for approximately 80 per cent of injuries, and splitting or compressive stresses account for the remainder.[670] Sites that are affected most typically are the distal tibial, fibular, ulnar, and radial growth plates and the proximal humeral growth plate. Growth plate injuries may occur acutely as a result of a single episode of trauma or chronically as a consequence of prolonged stress, particularly that associated with athletics (e.g., gymnastics). Subtle clinical findings may follow the acute traumatic insult; pain, swelling, tenderness, and limitation of motion may be encountered. Identification of the abnormality of the growth plate on the radiograph in such instances also may be difficult. The irregular bandlike radiolucency of the normal cartilaginous plate can obscure minor degrees of separation or diastasis. Well-coned radiographs and multiple projections are mandatory, and conventional tomograms also may be necessary. Early diagnosis and treatment can prevent significant growth disturbance and deformity. With chronic stress, widening and irregularity of the physis and metaphyseal sclerosis are observed (see later discussion and Chapter 71). Rare causes of growth plate injury include immobilization, neuropathic osteoarthropathy, ischemia, metabolic and infectious disorders, and thermal insult (e.g., thermal and electrical burns, frostbite).

Of the various regions of the growth plate, it is the hypertrophic zone that is most vulnerable to shearing and avulsive injuries (Fig. 67–125). The germinal cells usually are spared, and growth will continue as long as there has been no interference with the blood supply.[675] The vulnerability of the blood supply varies with the specific region of the body that is traumatized (Fig. 67–126). In certain locations, such as the proximal portion of the femur, the growth plate is situated intra-articularly, and the vascular supply to the epiphysis is applied closely to the periphery of the plate, increasing its susceptibility to injury.[670] In these areas and others, growth disturbance can ensue, and the degree of deformity depends on the potential for future growth of the undamaged segment of the growth cartilage.[671] The younger the patient, the longer the period of growth and the greater the potential for future deformity. Once a deformity has appeared, its progression may be stimulated by abnormal mechanical forces.

The vulnerability of the hypertrophic zone of the growth plate to shearing injury appears to be influenced by the rate of growth.[672, 676] An increase in the thickness of this zone during periods of rapid growth may promote epiphyseal separations. Other factors also influence the susceptibility of the growth plate to shearing forces, however.[672] Furthermore, compression forces produce failure of the metaphysis rather than the growth plate in most instances. This may be observed in the normal skeleton as well as in certain pathologic states, such as scurvy.[677] Metaphyseal failure is more common at the sites at which the metaphysis is not protected from compression stress; one example is the vertebral endplate, where a compression fracture can produce a cartilaginous node. Metaphyseal fragility also is accentuated by any condition associated with osseous weakening, be it related to the osteoclastosis of hyperparathyroidism or the hypervascularity of the normal growth spurt.

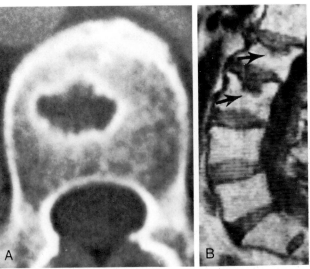

FIGURE 67–122. Cartilaginous nodes: CT and MR imaging.

A CT. A transaxial scan reveals the typical appearance of a cartilaginous node. It generally is well defined, circular or lobulated, close to the discovertebral junction, and accompanied by a rim of bone sclerosis.

B MR imaging. A sagittal T1-weighted (TR/TE, 600/20) spin echo MR image shows the location and the appearance of cartilaginous nodes in the lumbar spine (arrows).

(**B**, Courtesy of M. Solomon, M.D., San Jose, California.)

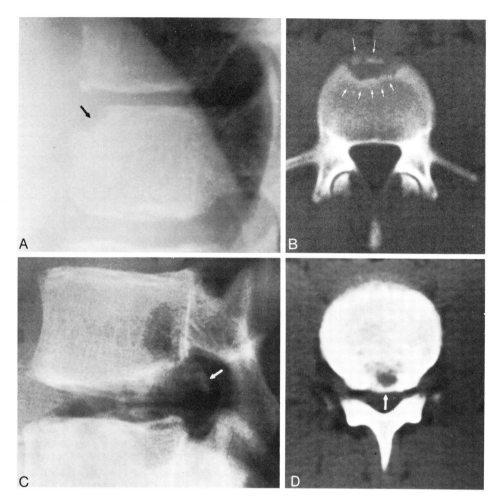

FIGURE 67–123. Cartilaginous nodes: Anterior and posterior prolapse.

A, B Anterior prolapse leading to limbus vertebra. On a radiograph **(A)** in this young child, a radiolucent area in the vertebral body (arrow) has resulted from a cartilaginous node. This finding in combination with loss of height of the intervertebral disc simulates infection. (Courtesy of A. D'Abreu, M.D., Porto Alegre, Brazil.) In a different patient, transaxial CT **(B)** shows the characteristics of a limbus vertebra. A radiolucent area is accompanied by bone spicules anteriorly, representing a portion of the ossified vertebral rim, and bone sclerosis posteriorly (arrows). (Courtesy of R. Yagan, M.D., Cleveland, Ohio.)

C, D Posterior prolapse leading to intraspinal bone displacement. In an 18 year old weight-lifter with the acute onset of back and leg pain, a lateral radiograph **(C)** shows displacement of a portion of the ring apophysis (arrow) into the spinal canal. Transaxial CT **(D)** reveals the location of the displaced bone (arrow). (Courtesy of G. Greenway, M.D., Dallas, Texas.)

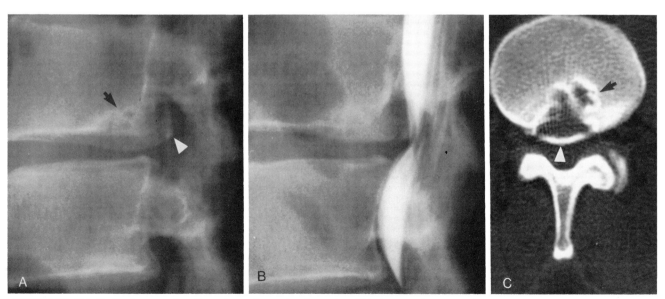

FIGURE 67–124. Cartilaginous nodes: Posterior prolapse. Lumbar spine. This 37 year old man, with a history of seizures since childhood, had increasing low back pain. The routine radiograph **(A)** shows a posterior cartilaginous node (arrow) involving the inferior surface of the third lumbar vertebral body and intraspinal displacement of a fragment (arrowhead) of the posterior rim of the vertebral body. The L3-L4 intervertebral disc is narrowed. Myelography **(B)** shows a large extradural defect at this level, compatible with disc herniation. The transaxial CT scan **(C)** shows the cartilaginous node (arrow) and curvilinear bone fragment (arrowhead).

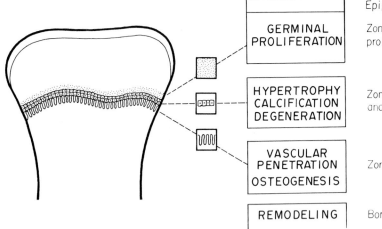

FIGURE 67–125. Growth plate injuries: Histology of normal physis. It is the zone of hypertrophy that is most vulnerable to shearing and avulsive injuries.

Avulsion injury to the growth plate commonly is observed at sites of apophyses. Examples include the lesser trochanter, the medial epicondyle of the distal portion of the humerus, the tibial tubercle, the spinous process of a vertebra, and the base of the fifth metatarsal bone.[672, 678] At some sites, notably the calcaneus, the iliac crest, and the vertebral body, irregularity of the metaphysis provides some degree of protection against avulsion injury.[679] The vulnerability of any specific apophysis to avulsion injury is governed by its development and maturation and, specifically, depends on the time of appearance and fusion of the apophysis. The avulsed cartilage may continue to demonstrate osteogenesis, producing small or large bony ossicles.[680, 681]

A splitting injury of the growth plate produces a fracture that crosses the entire epiphyseal complex, perpendicular to the growth plate. With healing, callus formation may take place across the plate, anchoring the epiphysis to the metaphysis.[669] Cessation of growth occurs at this focus, and as the remainder of the epiphyseal complex continues to grow, angular deformity may ensue.

After an injury to the growth plate, repair is initiated quickly, unless an injury to the germinal layer of the cartilage or to the vascular supply of the epiphysis has occurred.[670] Initially, a transient increase in the thickness of the growth plate occurs, which reaches a peak in approximately 10 days. Fibrin appears within the line of cleavage; the cartilage cells continue to grow, and the physeal plate thickens as the cellular columns lengthen.[669] In about 3 weeks, dissolution and resorption of fibrin are observed and normal growth resumes.[675] Radiographically evident residua of growth disturbance related to prior physeal injury may be observed, however. Such residua include transphyseal linear ossific striations[682] and growth recovery lines that are modified in appearance according to sites of arrest of physeal growth.[683] Large physeal bars, or bridges, also may be detected (Fig. 67–127).

Although several classification systems of growth plate injuries have been proposed, that of Salter and Harris is accepted most widely.[675] This system separates the lesions into five types according to their radiographic appearance (Fig. 67–128). In recent years, modification and expansion of the Salter and Harris classification scheme have occurred as a response to new observations regarding the effects of physical injury to the epiphysis, metaphysis, diaphysis, zone of Ranvier, and perichondrial ossification groove.[684, 685, 1024]

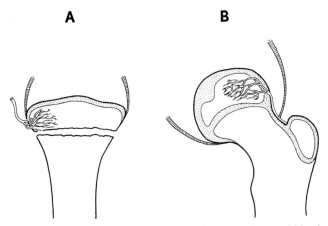

FIGURE 67–126. Growth plate injuries: Anatomy of normal blood supply to epiphysis. In most locations (A), the articular capsule inserts directly into the epiphysis so that the growth plate is extra-articular. The epiphyseal vessels penetrate the periosteum of the epiphysis at a site remote from the growth plate. Less commonly (B), the physis is intra-articular owing to the attachment of the joint capsule to the metaphysis. The epiphyseal vessels enter the epiphysis after crossing the edge of the growth plate and are at risk for injury when growth plate disruption occurs.

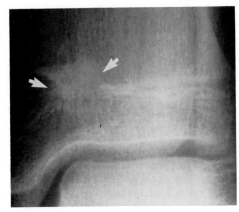

FIGURE 67–127. Growth plate injuries: Physeal bar. An ossific bridge (arrows) involves the medial aspect of the distal tibial physis, having resulted from a previous Salter-Harris type II injury of this physis (which was associated with a displaced distal fibular fracture).

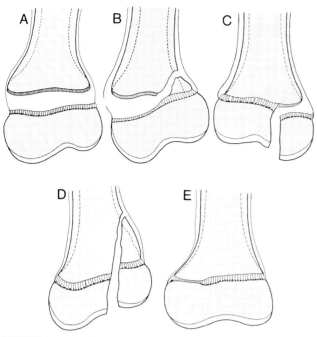

FIGURE 67–128. Growth plate injuries: Classification system.

A Type I: A split in the growth plate occurs through the zone of hypertrophic cells. The periosteum is intact.

B Type II: The growth plate is split and the fracture enters the metaphyseal bone, creating a triangular fragment. The periosteum about the fragment is intact, whereas that on the opposite side may be torn.

C Type III: A vertical fracture line extends through the epiphysis to enter the growth plate. It then extends transversely across the hypertrophic zone of the plate.

D Type IV: A fracture extends across the epiphysis, growth plate, and metaphysis. Note the incongruity of the articular surface and the violation of the germinal cells of the growth plate.

E Type V: Compression of portion of the growth plate may be unassociated with immediate radiographic abnormalities.

Type I (6 per cent). Type I represents a pure epiphyseal separation, with the fracture isolated to the growth plate itself (Fig. 67–129A). A shearing or avulsion force causes a cleavage through the zone of hypertrophic cells. This type of injury has a favorable prognosis and becomes apparent at a relatively young age, at a time when the growth plate is wide; it is especially frequent in children younger than 5 years old and as a result of birth injury.[686] The proximal portions of the humerus and femur and distal portion of the humerus are the sites affected most commonly. Similar lesions occur in children with rickets or scurvy and in adolescents with epiphysiolysis in the proximal portion of the femur.[2] Radiographic recognition of this injury is not difficult when the growth plate is wide and when the epiphysis remains displaced. In many instances, however, spontaneous reduction of the separation takes place, and the radiographic diagnosis is more difficult. Helpful signs are soft tissue swelling, particularly when centered at the physeal level, and minimal widening or irregularity of the growth plate. Comparison radiographs of the opposite (uninvolved) side are of further diagnostic help.

A subgroup of type I injuries has been identified (type IB) in children with certain underlying disorders that affect metaphyseal ossification, such as leukemia and thalassemia.[684] Injuries in these children may localize to weakened trabeculae in the metaphysis and, in the absence of control

of the primary disease process, physeal destruction and osseous bridging may ensue. One additional subgroup (type IC) of these injuries has been described in infancy, usually before or immediately after the appearance of the ossification center; a localized marginal region of the germinal cell layer is crushed against the metaphysis as a result of the force produced by the displaced cartilaginous nucleus.[684] Injury to the cells of the germinal layer may lead to growth disturbance, although years may pass before this disturbance becomes evident radiographically.

Type II (75 per cent). Type II, the most common type of growth plate injury, results from a shearing or avulsion force that splits the growth plate for a variable distance before entering the metaphyseal bone, separating a small fragment of the bone, the Thurston Holland[687] or "corner sign" (Fig. 67–129B). The periosteum on the side of the metaphyseal fracture remains intact, but that on the opposite side is disrupted in conjunction with growth plate separation. Because of the intact periosteum, the fracture fragment usually is reduced easily. The usual age of injury is 10 to 16 years, and the common sites of involvement are the distal ends of the radius, tibia, fibula, femur, and ulna, in order of decreasing frequency. The predilection is for areas with large ossification centers. The prognosis after this injury generally is good owing to the absence of subsequent growth disturbance. In anatomic sites at which the physis normally is more undulating in configuration, as in the distal portion of the femur, a localized abnormality of growth occasionally is encountered.[1089] A variation of this injury (type IIB) results in a free metaphyseal fragment, leading to problems in reduction and stabilization.[684]

A relatively common variation of the type II lesion (type IIC) results when a thin layer of the metaphysis that lies parallel to the growth plate is fractured with or without the usual triangular metaphyseal fragment. This pattern of injury is common in the phalanges of the hands (Fig. 67–130). Finally, a type IID lesion has been proposed in which a localized compressive injury to the germinal cells takes place. This may occur if the corner of the fractured metaphysis is driven into the physis. The most common sites of type IID lesions are the distal portions of the femur and fibula, followed in frequency by the proximal portions of the humerus and tibia. A type II fracture in these regions, particularly if displaced, may be associated with a protracted growth problem, manifested by the formation of a localized osseous bridge between the epiphysis and the metaphysis. As a classic type II lesion cannot be distinguished from a type IID lesion by radiographic techniques, the decision for closer long-term follow-up observation is based on an increased suspicion owing to the location and the displacement of the fracture.

Type III (8 per cent). In the type III variety of injury, the fracture line extends vertically through the epiphysis and growth plate to the hypertrophic zone and then horizontally across the growth plate itself, usually on one side or the other (Fig. 67–129C). Type III injuries are especially common in children between the ages of 10 and 15 years and in the medial or lateral portion of the distal part of the tibia, with less frequent involvement of the proximal end of the tibia and distal part of the femur. Radiography usually allows prompt recognition of the fracture, although multiple projections and stress views sometimes are necessary. Displacement generally is minimal, and if care is exercised in

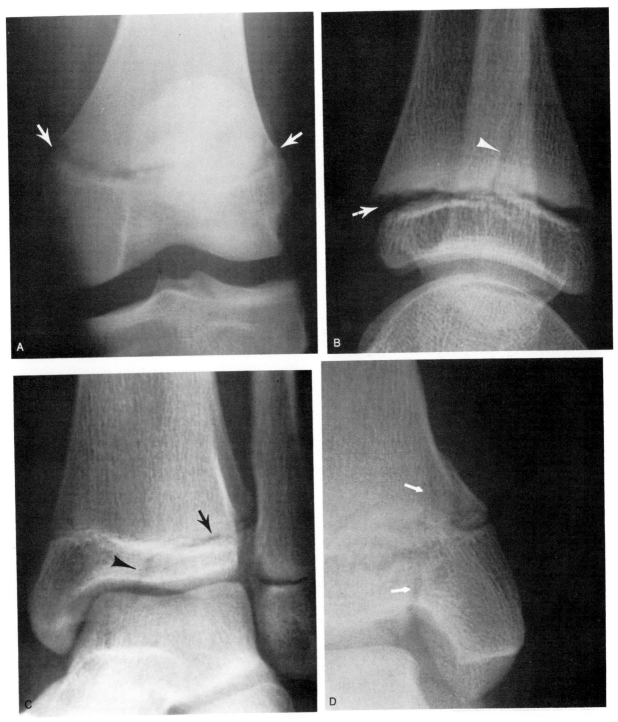

FIGURE 67–129. Growth plate injuries: Different types of fractures.
   A Type I: Note the widening (arrows) of the growth plate of the distal end of the femur.
   B Type II: Observe the widening of the growth plate (arrow) and the metaphyseal fracture (arrowhead).
   C Type III: The epiphyseal fracture line (arrowhead) and growth plate violation (arrow) can be recognized.
   D Type IV: Observe the fracture line extending vertically through the epiphysis and metaphysis (arrows).

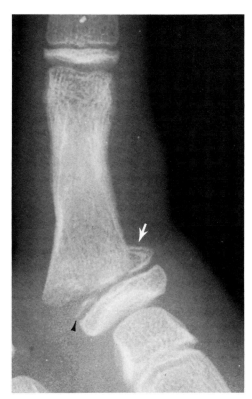

Figure 67–130. Growth plate injuries. Variation of type II lesion. In addition to the triangular metaphyseal fragment (arrow) that usually accompanies a type II lesion, a thin layer of the metaphysis (arrowhead) has been separated from the remaining metaphyseal bone.

the reduction of the fracture, growth arrest and deformities are rare. If reduction is not complete, the gap in the growth plate may become replaced with bone.[671]

Two additional type III injuries have been defined.[684] A type IIIB lesion results when a thin layer of primary spongiosa arising from the metaphysis accompanies the epiphyseal fragment. A type IIIC lesion is nonarticular in nature, as might occur in the convex ischial tuberosity. In this instance, avulsive forces may cause separation of a large portion of the cartilaginous apophysis and the adjacent fibrocartilaginous symphysis pubis. This injury may affect the growth region between these contiguous cartilaginous structures.

Type IV (10 per cent). A vertically oriented splitting force can produce a fracture that extends across the epiphysis, the growth plate, and the metaphysis, producing a fragment that consists of a portion of both the epiphysis and the metaphysis (Fig. 67–129D). This injury most frequently is encountered in the distal portions of the humerus (in children younger than 10 years of age) and tibia (in those over 10 years of age). The radiographic diagnosis is facilitated by the presence of considerable metaphyseal and epiphyseal bone within the fragment; however, in younger children in whom the epiphysis is unossified or only partially ossified, the injury may be mistaken for a type II growth plate fracture. This is an important distinction, as the prognosis in type II and type IV injuries is different. A type II injury is easily reduced and is associated with a good prognosis, whereas a type IV injury may require open reduction and careful realignment so that growth arrest and joint deformity are not encountered at a later date. When there is radiographic evidence of a triangular metaphyseal fracture

fragment in a location in which the epiphyseal ossific center is small, a type IV lesion should be suspected. Arthrography and MR imaging can further define the specific nature of the injury.

A type IVB lesion represents a combination of a type III and a type IV injury. Most often it occurs at the time of skeletal maturity. A type IVC lesion, the counterpart of the type IIIC fracture, is an injury through the metaphysis, the adjacent nonarticular growth plate, and the nonarticular apophysis. Finally, a type IVD lesion is caused by a violent traumatic episode in which comminution of the metaphysis and the formation of additional fracture fragments occur.

Type V (1 per cent). A crushing or compressive injury to the end of a tubular bone can lead to the rare type V growth plate fracture. Injury to the vascular supply in the germinal cells of the plate occurs without any immediate radiographic signs; there is no irregularity or widening of the growth plate. Subsequent radiographic examination may indicate focal areas of diminished or absent bony growth, which, in the presence of normal development in adjacent areas, can lead to angular deformity. Premature osseous fusion of the injured portion of the plate may be identified, particularly when tomographic techniques or MR imaging is used (see later discussion). This injury is more prominent in older children and adolescents, particularly those between the ages of 12 and 16 years. The physes of the distal portions of the femur and tibia and proximal portion of the tibia are affected more typically. Associated fractures of the diaphysis of the femur or tibia and fibula may be seen.[2]

Ozonoff[670] and Ogden[684] have emphasized several additional types of injury to the growth plate or neighboring bone, or to both.

Type VI. An injury (e.g., physical trauma, burn, or infection) to the perichondrium can produce reactive bone formation external to the growth plate. The resultant osseous bridge may act as a barrier to growth of the adjacent portion of the plate so that progressive osseous angulation may appear.

Type VII. Type VII, a relatively common type of injury, is associated with epiphyseal alterations in the absence of involvement of the growth plate or metaphysis. Transchondral fractures and osteochondritis dissecans are examples of type VII injuries. The fragment may be purely cartilaginous or may consist of both cartilage and bone. Complications include irregularity of the articular surface with secondary degenerative joint disease and intra-articular osteocartilaginous bodies.

Type VIII. A type VIII injury affects metaphyseal growth and remodeling mechanisms in the immature skeleton, related primarily to effects on the blood supply. A metaphyseal fracture may alter the vascularity to the region of ossification significantly, temporarily slowing this process.

Type IX. An injury to the periosteum of the diaphysis in rare circumstances may result in disruption of normal diaphyseal growth and remodeling. Segmental comminuted fractures, wringer injuries, and severe burns are examples of the type of trauma that may lead to this kind of injury. When paired bones of the forearm or lower leg are involved, synostosis eventually may occur.[688]

Approximately 25 to 30 per cent of patients with growth plate injuries develop some degree of growth deformity, and in 10 per cent of patients, this deformity is quite significant.[670] The prognosis is related to the age of the patient, the anatomy of the vascular supply to the region, the type of injury, and the immediacy and adequacy of the reduction. In general, the younger the patient at the time of injury, the poorer the prognosis for residual deformity. Types I, II, and III injuries have a relatively good prognosis, whereas type IV injuries carry a guarded prognosis, and types V and VI injuries have a poor prognosis. Late sequelae include growth impairment, premature growth plate fusion, epiphyseal malposition and rotation, and osteonecrosis.[670]

Premature partial arrest of growth is produced by a bridge of bone, or bone bar, that extends from the metaphysis to the epiphysis across a portion of the physis (Fig. 67–131). The remaining portion of the physis continues to grow, resulting in increasing angular deformity.[689, 690] In the knee, for example, genu valgum, varum, or recurvatum indicates closure of the lateral, medial, or anterior portion of the physis, respectively, and, with central closure of the growth plate, "cupping" of the metaphysis is seen.[689] Although acute physical injury is a typical cause of a bone bar, thermal injury, irradiation, infection, neoplasm, iatrogenic events (e.g., insertion of a metal plate across the physis, extravasation of an intravenous infusion), and chronic stress (e.g., Blount's disease) are additional causes.[689, 1017] It is the type IV injury that most characteristically leads to closure of a portion of the physis; a type V injury may result in premature closure of the entire growth plate. Of interest, it has been suggested that symmetric

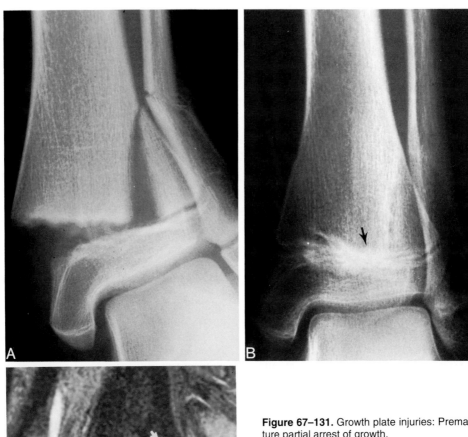

Figure 67–131. Growth plate injuries: Premature partial arrest of growth.

A, B Initially **(A),** a type II physeal injury in the distal portion of the tibia (as well as a fibular fracture) is seen. Subsequently **(B),** a bone bar (arrow) has led to premature closure of a portion of the tibial physis.

C This 9 year old boy had had an injury involving the distal femoral metaphysis two years previously that had been treated surgically. A local infection then developed and, subsequently, progressive deformity of the bone occurred. In a sagittal multiplanar gradient recalled (MPGR) MR image (TR/TE, 700/20; flip angle, 40 degrees) a physeal bar (arrow) is evident, accounting for the deformity. **(C,** Courtesy of D. Witte, M.D., Memphis, Tennessee.)

premature closure of a physis after trauma is more likely related to ischemia than to physeal compression.[691]

The majority of bone bars are located in the proximal portion of the tibia and the distal portion of the femur, and accurate diagnosis often requires the use of conventional tomography, CT scanning, scintigraphy, or MR imaging (see following discussion) as a supplement to routine radiography.[692–695, 1019, 1020]

MR imaging has been used clinically and experimentally to investigate traumatic abnormalities of the growth plate, and its role in such investigation is expected to become more prominent in the years ahead. Both spin echo and gradient echo MR imaging techniques have been employed. Some investigators regard the latter technique as being superior for delineation of the cartilage of the growth plate,[696] whereas others indicate that although gradient echo methods are optimal for differentiating between cartilage and bone, they are suboptimal for distinguishing among the zones of the cartilaginous epiphysis.[697] With either type of method, the appearance of the growth plate varies with its stage of development and, hence, the age of the patient, and regional factors dependent on the specific anatomic site that is studied are encountered. In a study of the normal knee, Harcke and colleagues[696] divided the MR imaging characteristics into four stages, based primarily on the extent of physeal development. MR imaging findings in children less than 2 years of age, in whom the distal femoral and proximal tibial epiphyses were composed primarily of cartilage, represented the first of these stages. The cartilage of the physes had intermediate signal intensity on T1-weighted spin echo MR images and high signal intensity on gradient echo images. The developing ossification centers initially were of low signal intensity on both types of images, owing to the presence of calcification, and subsequently revealed fat-containing bone marrow with high signal intensity on these MR images. MR imaging findings in children between the ages of 2 and 12 years, representing stage II, were characterized by thinning of the physes owing to enlargement of the ossifying epiphyses. The signal intensity of the cartilage in the growth plates varied according to the type of imaging sequence that was employed in a fashion similar to that in stage I. After children had reached the age of 12 years, MR imaging findings (stage III) were characterized by incomplete visualization of the cartilaginous physeal plates, particularly their central portion, designated the drop-out sign, which was more apparent on spin echo than on gradient echo MR images. As physeal closure commenced, spin echo images failed to demonstrate intermediate signal intensity cartilage in larger portions of the physis, although gradient echo images often depicted a thin, hyperintense band of cartilage. Finally, at the time of complete closure of the physes, MR imaging findings (stage IV) consisted of a single hypointense band between the metaphysis and epiphysis, representing the thick physeal ghost comprising dense osseous metaphyseal and epiphyseal plates. The authors concluded that the drop-out sign, which may relate to technical or anatomic factors, could simulate the appearance of premature closure of the physis. Furthermore, its central location was similar to that of traumatically induced closure of the physis, creating further diagnostic difficulty. Comparison MR imaging studies of the opposite extremity might be helpful.

Despite these potential diagnostic pitfalls, MR imaging may prove useful in the analysis of acute physeal injury or delayed posttraumatic complications of such injury. Such imaging may allow definition of the plane or planes of acute injury to physeal cartilage and neighboring bone and, in so doing, provide more accurate information than that displayed on routine radiographs (Fig. 67–132), particularly in infants and young children, in whom large portions of the epiphyses are unossified. MR imaging data in such instances may lead to a change in the classification of the physeal injury (e.g., type II injury to type IV injury) and indicate the coexistence of ligamentous or other soft tissue damage.[697] Horizontal tears of the physeal cartilage may appear as regions of low signal intensity on MR images,[697] and increased vascularity and edema of marrow in areas of injury (or physeal bar formation) typically are demonstrated as regions of high signal intensity on T2-weighted spin echo and certain gradient echo MR images and of enhanced signal intensity after the intravenous administration of a gadolinium contrast agent.[698] In experimental investigations, MR imaging also has provided information regarding disturbances of physeal growth after epiphyseal and metaphyseal injury.[699] Injury to the epiphyseal vessels produces ischemic damage to the proliferative zone of the growth plate, and resulting bone bridges or focal curving of the growth plate may be observed on MR images; injury to the metaphyseal vessels blocks normal endochondral ossification, and thickening of the growth plate and tonguelike extensions of physeal cartilage into the metaphysis may be evident on such images.[699] Although much of the data related to the delineation of growth disturbances after physeal injury using MR imaging have been derived from experimental studies in animals, results of preliminary investigations in humans also have been encouraging with regard to the detection with MR imaging of premature partial growth arrest after such injury.[700, 701] This detection may be easier when peripheral rather than central portions of the physis are involved, and the failure to demonstrate a physeal bar by MR imaging in cases in which a bridge is suspected radiographically may have prognostic importance[697] and may affect therapeutic planning dramatically.

Several principles are of importance in the management of epiphyseal and growth plate injuries.[675]

1. Epiphyseal displacement should be reduced promptly as reduction becomes progressively more difficult with increasing delay. After 10 days, types I and II lesions are better left unreduced, as the forces required for reduction are likely to damage the germinal cells of the growth plate.

2. Absolute anatomic reduction aimed at achieving articular surface congruity is essential in types III and IV lesions and may require open reduction and pinning. Anatomic reduction of types I and II lesions is less critical.

3. Smooth Kirschner wires are used when internal stabilization is necessary, and threaded pins or screws are never placed across a growth plate. These fixation devices are removed after an adequate period of healing.

4. All growth plate injuries need long-term follow-up examinations, the period of observation being dictated by such factors as the type of injury, the site involved, the potential for future growth, the epiphyseal blood supply, the method of reduction, and whether the injury is open or closed.

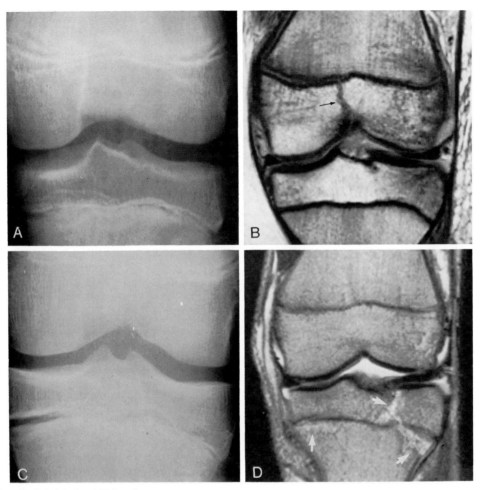

Figure 67–132. Growth plate injuries: MR imaging.

A, B In a 13 year old boy, a frontal radiograph **(A)** reveals no significant abnormalities. A coronal T1-weighted (TR/TE, 800/20) spin echo MR image **(B)** shows a vertical fracture line (arrow) in the distal femoral epiphysis, indicative of a Salter-Harris type III physeal injury. Bone bruises appear as regions of diminished signal intensity in the metaphysis and epiphysis of the distal part of the femur and in the epiphysis of the proximal end of the tibia. (Courtesy of S. K. Brahme, M.D., La Jolla, California.)

C, D This young boy suffered an injury to the knee while playing soccer. A routine radiograph **(C)** shows widening of the medial portion of the proximal tibial physis, suggesting a Salter-Harris type I injury. A coronal T2-weighted (TR/TE, 2000/80) spin echo MR image **(D)** reveals high signal intensity (arrows) in the tibia, consistent with a Salter-Harris type IV injury, in a bone bruise of the lateral portion of the distal femoral epiphysis, and in and about the medial collateral ligament, indicating ligamentous disruption and soft tissue edema. An effusion is present. (Courtesy of A. Newberg, M.D., Boston, Massachusetts.)

Specific Injuries

Slipped Capital Femoral Epiphysis. Slippage of the capital femoral epiphysis is a well-recognized occurrence in children and adolescents. It is observed most typically between the ages of 10 and 17 years in boys and 8 and 15 years in girls, with the average age of onset being 13 or 14 years in boys and 11 or 12 years in girls.[702–708] Rarely, a slipped epiphysis occurs in a younger child or neonate who has had severe trauma[709–714] or another disorder, such as malnutrition, developmental dysplasia of the hip, Legg-Calvé-Perthes disease, or tuberculosis,[706, 715, 716] and in an older adolescent or adult with delayed skeletal maturation.[704, 705, 715, 717, 718] A familial history of the disease has been noted in some reports.[719] Rarely, the condition is observed in identical twins, and an increased prevalence of the human leukocyte antigen (HLA) B27 in this condition has been reported.[1018] Boys are affected more frequently than girls, although the ratio of male to female cases varies from one series to another. The frequency of slipped capital femoral epiphysis is greater in black patients than in whites[715, 720, 721] and is especially high in overweight children.[706, 707] The occurrence of slipped capital femoral epiphysis in tall, thin children is unusual. The left side is affected almost twice as frequently as the right side in male patients,[722] whereas among female patients, both hips are affected with equal frequency. About 20 to 35 per cent of patients with slipped capital femoral epiphysis have bilateral involvement,[705, 706, 723, 1025] an occurrence that is more frequent in girls. The contralateral femoral head may be involved late, just prior to skeletal maturity, and its displacement may lead to minimal symptoms.[724–726]

A variety of contributing factors have been emphasized in the pathogenesis of slipped capital femoral epiphysis.

1. Trauma. Although trauma is an important precipitating event in slipped epiphyses in infants and young children, it appears to have only a minor contributing role in older persons. Fewer than 50 per cent of patients have a history of significant injury. Transphyseal fractures of the proximal portion of the femur that occur after an acute injury are considered to be unrelated to slipped capital femoral epiphyses.[727, 728, 1026]

2. Adolescent Growth Spurt. The association of slipped capital femoral epiphysis with the adolescent growth spurt is well recognized.[729] Experimental observations in animals have indicated that a minimal amount of shearing stress is necessary to displace the epiphysis when the growth plate is relatively wide, as during periods of rapid growth.[730] The vulnerability of the growth plate during this period is further accentuated by its change in configuration from a horizontal to an oblique plane, increasing the shearing stresses.[706] A higher frequency of this disorder in boys than in girls may be related to a greater and longer growth spurt in the former.[731]

3. Hormonal Influences. The relationship of slipped capital femoral epiphysis to periods of rapid growth has led to speculation regarding the influence of various hormones in the pathogenesis of this condition.[706, 732, 733] Experimental observations have indicated that a deficit of sex hormones relative to growth hormone can produce a widening of the growth plate and a reduction of the shearing force necessary to displace the epiphysis[730, 734, 735]; a delay in skeletal maturation, which is associated with a higher frequency of slipped capital femoral epiphysis, may accentuate this imbalance between growth and sex hormonal levels by lengthening the period of vulnerability due to the late closure of the growth plate. Despite these observations, however, no clear evidence, exists that levels of growth hormone are abnormal in patients with slipped capital femoral epiphysis. Yet, the list of endocrine diseases that have been associated with this femoral disorder is impressive indeed and includes hypothyroidism, hypoestrogenic states, acromegaly, gigantism, cryptorchidism, and pituitary and parathyroid tumors.[733]

4. Weight and Activity. One of the most striking characteristics of patients with slipped capital femoral epiphysis is a tendency to be overweight.[736] Obesity increases the shearing stress on the growth plate (which may be accentuated by changes in the orientation of the physis[737, 738]) and can lead to slippage even during usual activity. The propensity for epiphyseal slippage appears to be greater in physically active adolescents than in those who are less active, probably related to their exposure to greater shearing forces during strenuous activity.[739] An increased frequency of such slippage that has been reported to occur in summer months[740] also may relate to increased physical activity in that season.

The stresses about the hip that are most likely to produce growth plate shear are those of abduction and external rotation.[670] With the exception of the adductor group, the muscles about this joint insert laterally into the region below the greater trochanter and thus pull the femoral shaft laterally and anteriorly in external rotation. The femoral head seated in the acetabulum is located in a posterior and medial direction with respect to the remainder of the femur. Although a posteromedioinferior "slippage" of the capital femoral epiphysis is typical,[741] other directions in which the epiphysis can "move" are anteriorly[742] and superiorly or in a valgus orientation.[743, 744] Histologic studies after slippage have indicated a fracture or cleft through the hypertrophic cells of the growth plate, widening of the growth plate, formation of cartilage clusters and bars divided by longitudinally arranged eosinophilic septa, and islands of unorganized cartilage dispersed irregularly in the proximal metaph-

ysis.[745–747] Mickelson and coworkers[647, 648] observed a change in composition of cartilage matrix in the distal region of the growth plate that might predispose that region to slippage. Other authors have noted diminished cellularity, severe disorientation and misalignment of chondrocytes, and findings suggesting a deficiency in collagen[749, 750] (Fig. 67–133).

Although other diagnostic methods such as conventional tomography, CT scanning (Fig. 67–134), scintigraphy, MR imaging (Fig. 67–134), and ultrasonography have been employed,[751, 752] the radiographic analysis remains essential to the diagnosis of slipped capital femoral epiphysis.[670, 753–757] Both anteroposterior and frog-leg or lateral projections are mandatory; abnormalities on the frontal projection alone may be quite subtle, even in the presence of significant epiphyseal displacement. Comparison radiographs of the opposite side can be very useful. In acute or subacute stages of this disorder, several radiographic signs may be apparent. On the anteroposterior view, osteoporosis of both the femoral head and the femoral neck is common (Fig. 67–135A). The margin of the metaphysis may appear blurred or indistinct, and the growth plate may appear increased in width. The epiphyseal height frequently is reduced. A tangential line along the lateral border of the femoral neck may fail to intersect any part of the epiphysis or may cross only a small portion of it. The metaphysis may appear to be displaced from the acetabulum so that no overlap exists between the medial third of the metaphysis and the posterior margin of the acetabulum.[758] On the true lateral view or frog-leg view (this last view sometimes is not recommended as it may lead to further displacement of the femoral epiphysis[759]), the degree of epiphyseal displacement usually is quite easy to ascertain (Fig. 67–135B,C). The anterior or posterior margins of the epiphysis and metaphysis fail to correspond to each other.[670] The degree of slippage can be estimated by dividing the amount of displacement by the total width of the metaphysis.

In chronic stages of slipped capital femoral epiphysis, reactive bone formation appears along the medial and posterior portions of the femoral neck, a buttressing phenomenon that is similar to that which occurs in degenerative joint disease.[670] Premature fusion of the growth plate may result in femoral shortening. Rarely, spontaneous reduction of the slipped epiphysis may occur.[760]

Sequelae of slipped capital femoral epiphysis include severe varus deformity, shortening and broadening of the femoral neck, osteonecrosis, chondrolysis, and degenerative joint disease. Osteonecrosis has been described in 6 to 15 per cent of patients with this disorder[670, 761–765] (Fig. 67–136A). This complication results from an insult to the precarious blood supply to the proximal portion of the femur and is accentuated after acute severe slippage, closed or delayed manipulation, open reduction, and a femoral neck osteotomy.[766] Clinical findings include persistent or exacerbated pain after treatment of the slippage. Typical radiologic and scintigraphic[752, 767] abnormalities of ischemic necrosis of bone are present. Chondrolysis may be observed in as many as 40 per cent of patients with epiphyseal slippage and is more frequent in black than in white patients, in women than in men, and in persons with severe slippage.[768] It usually occurs within 1 year of the slippage, may be evident in untreated or treated persons, may affect the contralateral, uninvolved hip in patients with unilateral

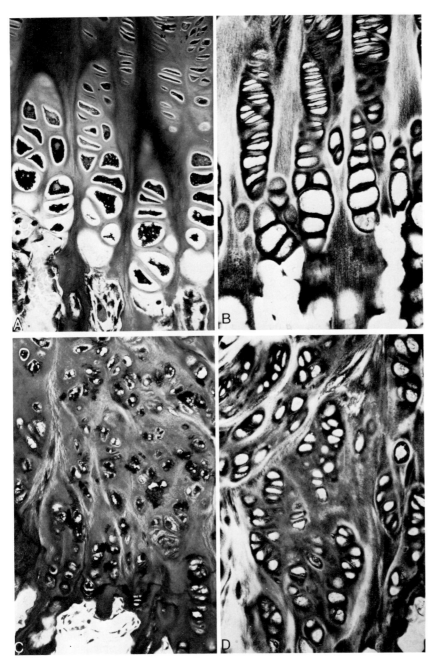

Figure 67–133. Slipped capital femoral epiphysis: Histologic abnormalities.

A Normal physis. Positive (dark) staining of the extraterritorial matrix indicates higher glycoprotein content than in the chondrocyte islands (periodic acid-Schiff, 250×).

B Normal physis. The chondrocyte islands (territorial matrix) stain positively (dark), indicating high proteoglycan content. The extraterritorial matrix shows a lower proteoglycan content. This pattern of staining is the opposite of that in **A** and relates to the type of stain that is used ("Stains All," 250×).

C Slipped epiphysis. Severe distortion of the architecture and irregular glycoprotein staining are seen (periodic acid-Schiff, 150 ×).

D Slipped epiphysis. Severe misalignment and distortion of the architecture with irregular patterns of staining are seen ("Stains All," 50×).

(From Agamanolis DP, et al: Slipped capital femoral epiphysis: A pathological study. II. A light microscopic and histiochemical study. J Pediatr Orthop 5:40, 1985.)

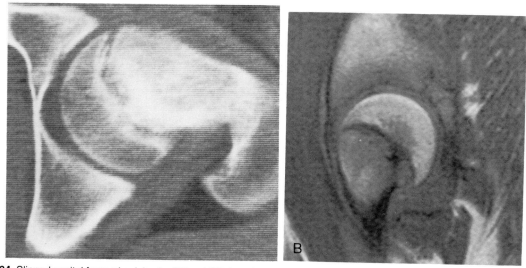

Figure 67–134. Slipped capital femoral epiphysis: CT and MR imaging abnormalities.
A A transaxial CT scan shows that the femoral head is displaced posteriorly with respect to the femoral neck. This display may provide information that helps the orthopedic surgeon plan the surgical procedure. (From Busch MT, et al: Orthop Clin North Am *18:*637, 1987.)
B In a sagittal T1-weighted (TR/TE, 800/20) spin echo MR image, note posterior displacement and tilting of the femoral epiphysis. (**B,** Courtesy of S. Eilenberg, M.D., San Diego, California.)

slipped capital femoral epiphysis, and may appear in conjunction with osteonecrosis[670, 769–774] (see Chapter 94). Radiographs outline osteoporosis, concentric narrowing of the interosseous space, and eburnation and osteophytosis of apposing osseous margins. Some recovery in the joint space may be seen after a period of months in approximately one third of patients.[769, 775] Its cause is unknown,[776] although chondrolysis may be initiated by synovial inflammation in which immunologic mechanisms play an important role.[773, 777] Synovitis in fact may be fundamental to the slippage of the epiphysis itself.[777] Degenerative joint disease occurring after a slipped capital femoral epiphysis can produce a narrowed interosseous space associated with typical displacement of the femoral head (Fig. 67–136).[778] This appearance should not be confused with the "tilt deformity" of the femoral head that is common in patients with osteoarthritis who have not had a previous epiphysiolysis (see Chapter 39).

Growth Plate Injuries About the Knee. Growth plate trauma in the distal portion of the femur may be related, in many cases, to birth, athletic, or automobile injuries.[779–783] Examples include the wagon-wheel fracture resulting when children catch their legs between the spokes of wagon or bicycle wheels[781] and the clipping injury of adolescent football players.[783, 784] Type II and type III (Fig. 67–137) Salter-Harris injuries are especially common, although other types, including triplane fractures (Fig. 67–138), may be evident. The prognosis is guarded in many instances because of the possible sequelae of shortening and angulation.

Injury to the proximal tibial physis is relatively rare,[785–787] as the collateral ligaments attach distal to the growth plate, the medial on the tibial shaft and the lateral on the fibula.[669] Any type of Salter-Harris injury can be encountered, including triplane fractures,[1011] although type III lesions predominate,[673] and stress radiographs frequently are required for accurate diagnosis.[786] Approximately 20 per cent of patients develop partial or complete arrest of growth.[673] A serious early complication is neurovascular compromise; popliteal artery injuries typically are associated with type I

or type II lesions.[788] One additional example of a physeal injury in the proximal portion of the tibia is an avulsion fracture of the tibial tubercle.[678, 789]

Growth Plate Injuries About the Ankle. Injuries to the growth plate in the distal portion of the tibia are common. Although all of the classic Salter-Harris lesions are observed, the type II injury is most frequent, followed in order of decreasing frequency by types III, IV, and I lesions.[790–793] A rare complication of the type II injury is interposition of the anterior tibial neurovascular bundle between the displaced epiphysis and the lower end of the tibia, which prevents fracture reduction and may compromise the blood supply to the foot.[794] Ten to 12 per cent of physeal injuries in this site are followed by growth disturbances.[673]

The triplane fracture of the distal portion of the tibia represents approximately 5 to 10 per cent of all injuries in this location[673, 790] and deserves special consideration.[795–803] It sometimes is referred to as a transitional fracture of the distal part of the tibia owing to its typical occurrence in adolescents at the time of the transition to adulthood, when physiologic closure of the distal tibial physis is occurring.[798] This closure is initiated at the anterolateral aspect of the circumference of the medial malleolus and spreads posteriorly and laterally; the anterolateral quadrant of the physis is the last to be obliterated.[798] The primary mechanism of injury appears to be external rotation of the foot, although plantar flexion also has been suggested.[797] The resulting injury has several variations, including a two-plane fracture pattern (Tillaux or Kleiger fracture, which involves only the epiphysis) or three-plane fracture patterns (in which an additional metaphyseal fracture is present).[798]

In the descriptions of the classic triplane injury, the sagittal, transverse, and coronal components of the fracture with involvement of a portion of the growth plate, the articular surface, and the metaphysis have been emphasized (Fig. 67–139). Radiographically, a triplane fracture presents the appearance of two different types of Salter-Harris injuries (a type III lesion on the anteroposterior radiograph and a type II lesion on the lateral radiograph), although, in

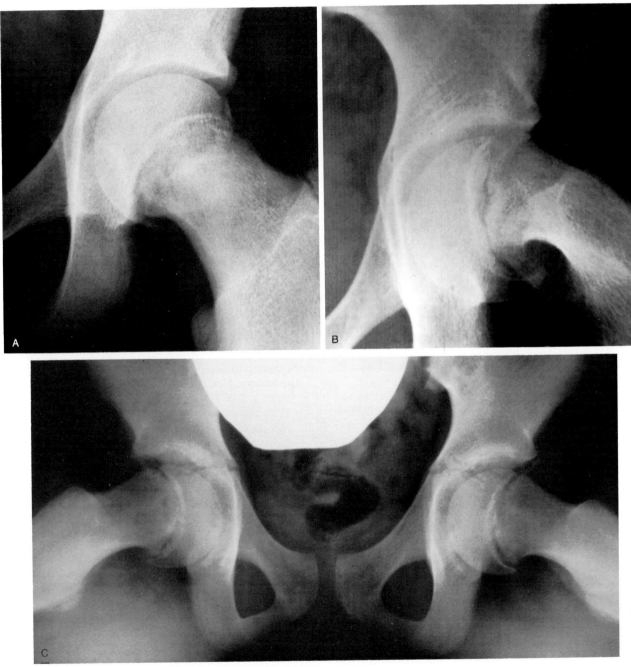

Figure 67–135. Slipped capital femoral epiphysis: Radiographic abnormalities.
  A Anteroposterior view. Subtle findings include mild osteoporosis of the proximal portion of the femur and an indistinct metaphyseal margin.
  B Frog-leg view. The degree of posterior slippage is readily apparent. Note the widened growth plate.
  C Frog-leg view. Bilateral slipped epiphyses are present, with the right side being involved more severely.
  (**C,** Courtesy of B. Howard, M.D., Charlotte, North Carolina.)

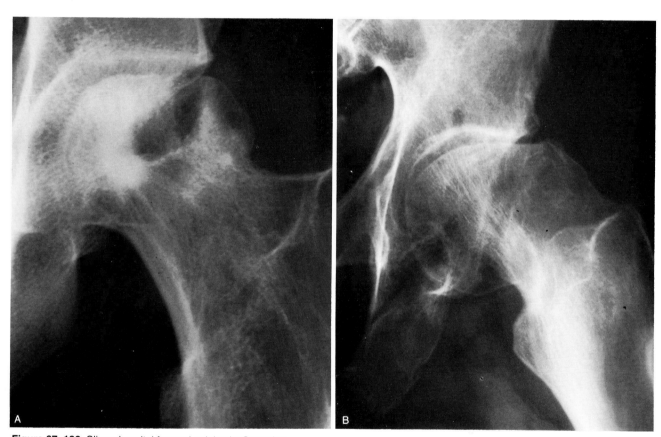

Figure 67–136. Slipped capital femoral epiphysis: Sequelae.
  A Osteonecrosis. Note the collapsed and fragmented epiphysis with irregular articular margin. Buttressing of the femoral neck is prominent.
  B Degenerative joint disease. Observe the malalignment of the femoral head and neck indicating the presence of a previous epiphysiolysis. The joint space is narrowed superiorly, and buttressing of the medial portion of the femoral neck is observed. The absence of a curvilinear radiodense line on the medial aspect of the femoral head distinguishes this appearance from that seen in the tilt deformity of osteoarthritis.

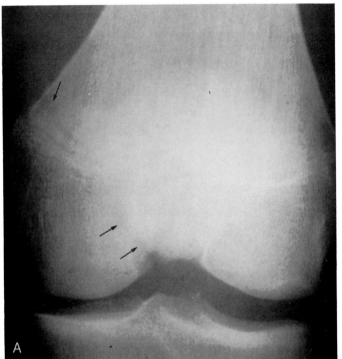

FIGURE 67–137. Growth plate injuries: Knee—type III injury of the distal end of the femur.

A A radiograph of the knee of a 15 year old boy who was injured while playing American football shows a type III physeal injury (arrows) of the distal end of the femur.

B, C In this 16 year old patient with a similar history, coronal proton density (TR/TE, 2200/16) **(B)** and T2-weighted (TR/TE, 2200/80) **(C)** spin echo MR images show a type II physeal injury (arrows) of the distal portion of the femur. Note the prominent bone marrow edema with high signal intensity in **C**.

(Courtesy of G. Greenway, M.D., Dallas, Texas.)

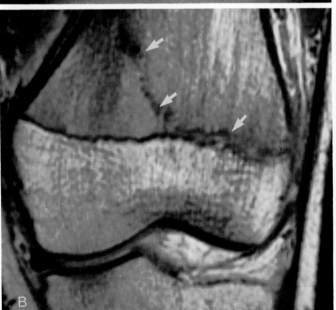

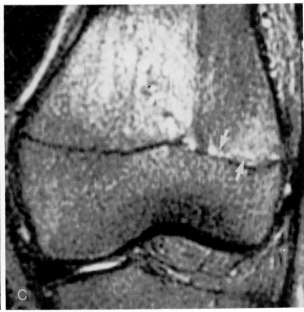

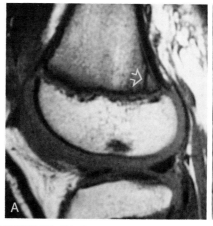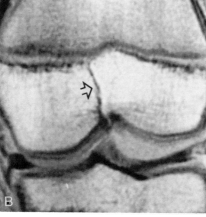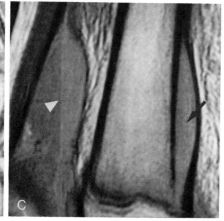

FIGURE 67–138. Growth plate injuries: Knee—triplane fracture of the distal end of the femur. An 11 year old girl was injured on a trampoline. The sagittal T1-weighted (TR/TE, 717/13) spin echo MR image **(A)** demonstrates a coronally oriented fracture (open arrow) of the distal metaphysis of the femur and physeal widening posteriorly. A large joint effusion is present. On a coronal proton density (TR/TE, 2000/16) spin echo MR image **(B)**, the sagittally oriented epiphyseal fracture (open arrow) is evident, with widening of the physis. A sagittal proton density (TR/TE, 2000/13) spin echo MR image of the lower part of the femur **(C)** shows a fluid level (arrowhead) and a subperiosteal hematoma (solid arrow). (Courtesy of G. Greenway, M.D., Dallas, Texas.)

reality, it represents a variation of a type IV injury pattern (Fig. 67–140). Two, three, or four fragments may result, with two fragments being most common. Owing to the complexity of the injury, CT represents an excellent technique for delineating the site and extent of involvement[797, 801, 802] (Fig. 67–141). MR imaging may be used for the same purpose (Fig. 67–142). Although early closure of the traumatized physis is expected, significant shortening of the involved limb is infrequent. Complications appear to be more common in injuries with multiple fragments and in those with an associated fibular fracture.

An isolated vertical fracture of the distal tibial epiphysis also is evident in the adolescent age group.[804–806] This injury, often designated the juvenile fracture of Tillaux, in its

classic form involves the lateral portion of the distal tibial epiphysis and conforms to a Salter-Harris type III injury owing to extension of the fracture laterally through the open physis (Fig. 67–143). The mechanism of injury relates to either lateral rotation of the foot or medial rotation of the leg on the fixed foot, producing an avulsion fracture attributable to the pull of an intact distal anterior tibiofibular ligament. The adult counterpart of this injury, in which a triangular rather than a quadrilateral piece of bone is separated from the remaining portion of the epiphysis, relates to an avulsion fracture of the anterior distal tibial tubercle, or tubercle of Chaput.[806] The prognosis of the juvenile fracture of Tillaux is good if articular congruity is restored.[807]

Other types of physeal injuries of the distal part of the

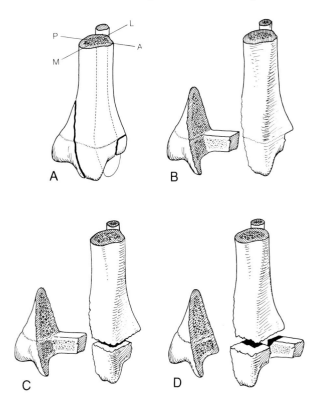

FIGURE 67–139. Growth plate injuries: Ankle—triplane fracture. (A, anterior; P, posterior, M, medial; L, lateral.)

A, B Two-part triplane fracture in place **(A),** and separated **(B)** as viewed from the medial side.

C Three-part triplane fracture.

D Four-part triplane fracture.

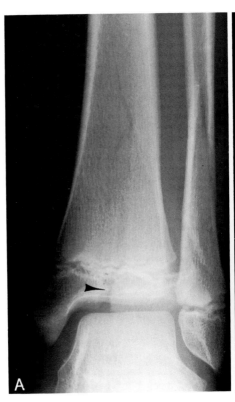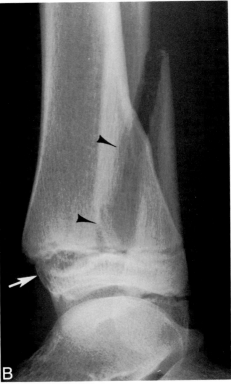

FIGURE 67–140. Growth plate injuries: Ankle—triplane fracture.
A The anteroposterior radiograph shows an injury that has the appearance of a type III lesion (arrowhead).
B On the lateral radiograph, a type II lesion is apparent (arrowheads). Note posterior displacement of the distal tibial epiphysis (arrow) and an oblique fibular fracture.

tibia, including those that involve the medial side of the physis and medial malleolus,[808, 809] frequently are associated with more complex injuries of the ankle.

Growth Plate Injuries About the Shoulder. Disruption of the epiphysis and physis in the proximal portion of the humerus is relatively infrequent.[810, 811] It usually is observed in boys between the ages of 11 and 16 years, although children and infants may be affected[812] (Fig. 67–144). The mechanism responsible for the injury is variable, including indirect (fall on the outstretched hand with the wrist, shoulder, and elbow fully extended) or direct (posterolateral shearing force) trauma. Its occurrence in adolescent baseball pitchers as an epiphysiolysis is termed the little league shoulder syndrome[813, 814] (Fig. 67–145). Potentially these physeal injuries, which account for about 3 per cent of all such lesions,[811] have considerable importance owing to the significant amount of growth that takes place at this site. Residual shortening (1 to 3 cm) of the extremity may be evident in approximately 10 per cent of patients.

Separation of the proximal humeral epiphysis may result from an injury during birth, particularly with prolonged labor, breech presentation, or other causes of difficult delivery.[2, 815, 816] Clinically and radiographically, an incorrect diagnosis of glenohumeral joint dislocation may seem likely. As ossification of the epiphyseal center of the proximal end of the humerus is not apparent at birth, radiographic misdiagnosis relates to improper interpretation of the cause of the laterally displaced humeral shaft. As traumatic dislocation of the glenohumeral joint rarely, if ever, occurs at birth, a physeal injury represents a far better diagnosis.[2] Arthrography,[815] ultrasonography,[816] and (probably) MR imaging can be used to substantiate the presence of a physeal separation.

The epiphysis of the inner margin of the clavicle is the last one in the body to merge with the adjacent shaft of the bone. This epiphysis ossifies at approximately 18 to 20 years of age and, with the closure of the growth plate, merges with the shaft of the clavicle at approximately 25 years of age. Investigators[817] have emphasized that injury to the medial end of the clavicle in the immature skeleton can produce an epiphyseal separation that may be misdiagnosed as a sternoclavicular joint dislocation. Failure to recognize partial ossification of the epiphysis may lead to this erroneous diagnosis in the young adult; prior to the initial appearance of ossification of the epiphyseal center, it is impossible to differentiate epiphyseal separation of the medial end of the clavicle and dislocation of the sternoclavicular joint on conventional radiography, although MR imaging or arthrography potentially would allow such differentiation. The epiphyseal injury may be of Salter-Harris type I or II. The periosteal cloak may remain in place, allowing gradual replacement and repair of the medial portion of the clavicle.

Physeal injuries about the shoulder may account for pseudodislocations of the acromioclavicular joint in children. Such injuries include displacement of the distal portion of the clavicle from its periosteal sleeve and avulsion of the epiphysis of the coracoid process.[818] The coracoclavicular ligaments remain intact (also see Chapter 68).

Physeal injury at the base of the coracoid process may occur acutely or as a response to chronic stress (Fig. 67–146).

Growth Plate Injuries About the Elbow. The accurate diagnosis of elbow injury in the immature skeleton is complicated by the presence of multiple ossification centers.[670, 819] Although comparison views of the opposite elbow may be helpful,[670, 819] some degree of asymmetry can occur in the normal person. Thus, it is necessary to know

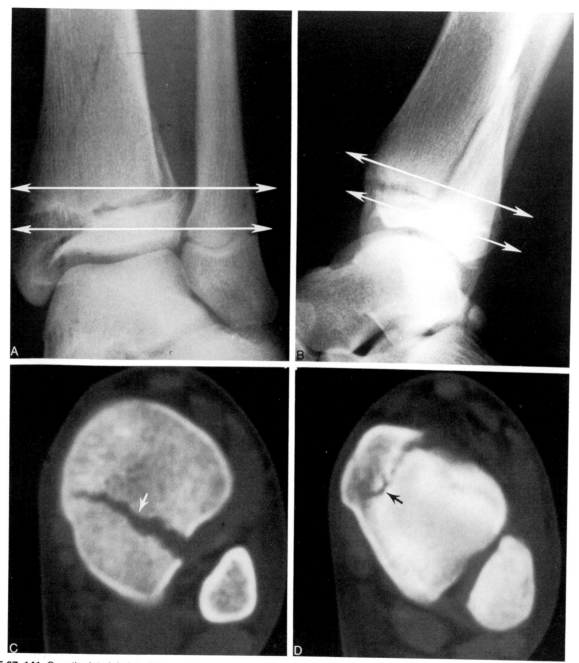

FIGURE 67–141. Growth plate injuries: Ankle—triplane fracture. CT.

  A, B The typical features of a triplane fracture of the distal portion of the tibia are evident in the frontal and lateral radiographs. A type III physeal lesion is suggested in **A** and a type II lesion in **B**.

  C, D Transaxial CT scans at the approximate levels indicated in **A** and **B** are shown. In **C**, a transaxial scan through the metaphysis, a coronally oriented fracture is seen (arrow). In **D**, a transaxial scan through the epiphysis, the fracture line (arrow) is oriented sagitally.

  (Courtesy of G. Greenway, M.D., Dallas, Texas.)

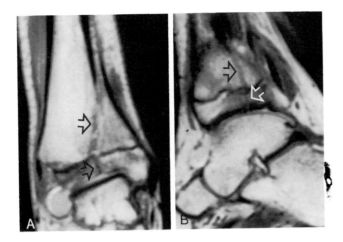

FIGURE 67–142. Growth plate injuries: Ankle—triplane fracture. MR imaging. A coronal T1-weighted (TR/TE, 700/20) spin echo MR image **(A)** and a sagittal T1-weighted (TR/TE, 600/20) spin echo MR image **(B)** show complex fractures (open arrows) of the distal tibial epiphysis and metaphysis that resemble Salter-Harris type IV injuries in each plane. (Courtesy of J. Kirkham, M.D., Minneapolis, Minnesota.)

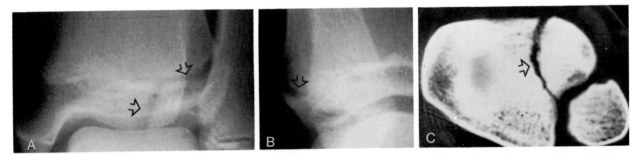

FIGURE 67–143. Growth plate injuries: Ankle—juvenile fracture of Tillaux. Frontal **(A)** and lateral **(B)** radiographs and a transaxial CT image **(C)** show the injury (open arrows) involving the anterolateral portion of the epiphysis. It represents a type III Salter-Harris injury.

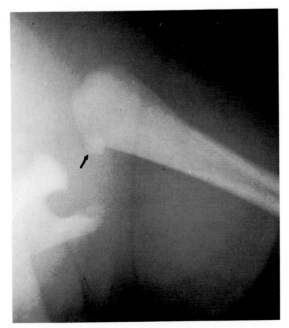

FIGURE 67–144. Growth plate injuries: Shoulder. A type I physeal injury of the proximal portion of the humerus is typical of obstetric trauma. Note the position of the partially ossified epiphysis (arrow).

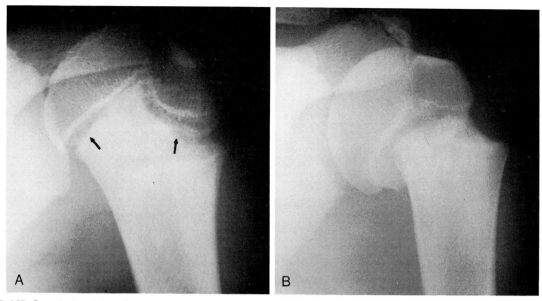

FIGURE 67–145. Growth plate injury: Shoulder—little league shoulder syndrome.
  A This 13 year old left-handed baseball pitcher developed progressive, exercise-related left shoulder pain. Note widening and irregularity of the humeral physis (arrows) on the left side **(A)**. This is a type I growth plate injury. (Courtesy of G. Greenway, M.D., Dallas, Texas.)
  B A more severe example of this injury is shown in which a greater degree of displacement is evident.

the time and the pattern of ossification of the various epiphyseal centers (Fig. 67–147). At birth, the entire distal portion of the humerus is cartilaginous, and no centers of ossification are present. The first distal humeral ossification center to appear is the capitulum, which ossifies during the first year of life. The medial epicondyle appears at approximately 5 to 7 years of age, followed by the trochlea at ages 9 to 10 years and, finally, by the lateral epicondyle at ages 9 to 13 years.[819] These centers fuse with the shaft between the ages of 14 and 16 years, except for the medial epicondyle, which may not fuse until 18 or 19 years of age. The ossification center of the radial head appears at ages 3 to 6 years, and the olecranon center of the ulna appears at ages 6 to 10 years. An acronym that may be used as an aid in remembering the sequence of appearance of some of these ossification centers is CRIT: C, capitulum; R, radial head; I, internal or medial epicondyle; T, trochlea.[820]

In general, ossification centers develop as single, smooth radiodense collections, although certain vagaries in their appearance have been described.[821–824] The ossification center of the capitulum is situated anteriorly on the lateral radiograph and initially reveals a normal downward tilting configuration.[821] With further ossification, the capitulum demonstrates a relatively straight superior border with slight widening of the adjacent posterior aspect of the growth plate. If not recognized as a normal finding, this widening may be falsely attributed to separation of the epiphysis. By the age of 14 years, the capitulum generally reveals complete fusion. The precise pattern of fusion is variable; it may fuse with the trochlea and the lateral epicondyle before uniting with the humerus.[821] With regard to the medial epicondyle, ossification generally proceeds from a single smooth, round, or oval nucleus, although normal ossification may be multicentric in appearance, producing a fragmented developing center that can simulate a fracture.[822] Furthermore, it occupies a medial or posteromedial location with respect to the distal end of the humerus, which can be accentuated on radiographic projections that are exposed in an off-lateral (steep oblique) position.

The normal appearances of the developing radial head

FIGURE 67–146. Growth plate injury: Shoulder-coracoid process. This 13 year old boy injured his shoulder while trapshooting.
  A Transaxial CT shows widening of the physis (open arrow) at the base of the coracoid process.
  B A sagittal oblique T1-weighted (TR/TE, 700/15) MR image, obtained with chemical presaturation of fat and after intravenous administration of a gadolinium contrast agent, shows hyperintensity (open arrows) at this site. The tip of the coracoid process is indicated with an arrowhead.
  (Courtesy of G. Applegate, M.D., Van Nuys, California.)

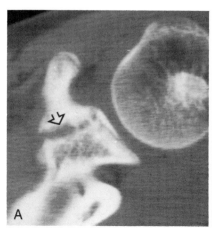

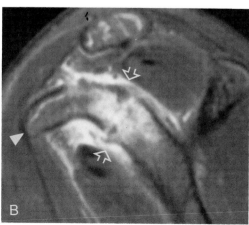

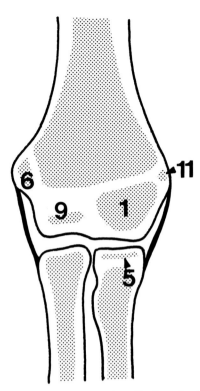

FIGURE 67–147. Normal pattern of ossification about the elbow. Numbers indicate approximate age in years at which the center begins to ossify (see text).

and neck readily are misinterpreted as evidence of trauma because (1) the radial neck of an infant is slightly angulated medially in the frontal projection, simulating a dislocation of the radial head; (2) the early physis of the proximal portion of the radius is wedge-shaped, mimicking an avulsion fracture of the head; and (3) notches and clefts in the metaphysis of the proximal portion of the radius may closely resemble posttraumatic abnormalities.[823]

Normally, the metaphysis of the distal portion of the humerus and capitulum are anteverted about 140 degrees relative to the shaft of the humerus. A line drawn along the anterior cortex of the humerus on the lateral radiograph, the anterior humeral line, should intersect the middle third of the capitular ossification center.[825] In the presence of supracondylar fractures of the humerus, the most common fracture about the elbow in children, posterior displacement or angulation of the distal fragment will allow the anterior humeral line to pass through the anterior third of the ossification center or even anterior to the capitulum (Fig. 67–148).

Many types of epiphyseal injuries affect the child's elbow.[826–835] A fracture of the medial condyle of the humerus is rare. If this injury occurs prior to ossification of the trochlea, diagnosis on the basis of routine radiographs is difficult, although a small piece of bone separated from the adjacent humeral metaphysis may be evident.[836] A fracture of the lateral condyle is frequent and represents a Salter-Harris type IV injury.[834] The fracture line splits the epiphysis and separates a portion of the adjacent metaphysis and the capitulum. Because the extensors of the forearm are attached to the fragment, it commonly is displaced posteriorly and inferiorly by muscle traction.[819] Separation of the medial epicondyle ossification center is the result of stress

placed on the flexor pronator tendon that attaches to this site. It represents approximately 10 per cent of all elbow injuries and leads to a transverse fracture or inferior displacement of the epicondyle.[837] In some instances, the epicondyle may become entrapped within the joint[838] (Figs. 67–149 and 67–150). In this situation, the displaced epicondylar ossification center can simulate a normal trochlear center, and the diagnosis may be missed; however, the appearance of a "trochlear" center without a medial epicondylar center, with rare exception,[839] is inconsistent with the normal sequence of ossification about the distal portion of the humerus, a fact that facilitates proper diagnosis of the injury in some patients. The posterior location of the ossific focus on the lateral projection of the elbow is another useful sign.

Separation with or without fracture of the entire distal humeral epiphysis may be mistaken for a fracture of the lateral humeral condyle or a dislocation of the elbow,[840–844] (Fig. 67–151). A fracture-separation of the distal humeral epiphysis occurs below the usual level of a supracondylar fracture. This injury typically results from a fall on the outstretched hand or from lifting the infant by grasping the forearm. Shearing stresses develop on the distal portion of the humerus, producing the fracture-displacement of the entire epiphysis. In most cases, a Salter-Harris type I or II injury is present. Differentiation between these two types of epiphyseal displacement requires visualization of the metaphyseal osseous fragment that accompanies the type II injury. Anteroposterior and lateral radiographs usually reveal a normal alignment of the radial shaft and capitellar ossification center, normal alignment of the radius and ulna, and malalignment of these bones with the humerus as well as soft tissue swelling. Typically, the radius and ulna are displaced in a posterior and medial direction with respect to the humerus. Cubitus varus deformity may result.

Other Growth Plate Injuries. Similar injuries may involve the triradiate cartilage of the acetabulum[852, 853] and may appear about the wrist, hands (Fig. 67–152), feet, and even the bones of the axial skeleton.[845–851, 1021] These have been well summarized by Rogers.[669] The relative frequency of some physeal injuries is indicated in Table 67–6.

Chronic Stress Injuries

As discussed in Chapter 71, a variety of musculoskeletal manifestations occur in professional and recreational athletes that are related to the chronic application of stress. Indeed, as indicated earlier in this chapter, fatigue fractures of bone represent one type of skeletal response to the stress of vigorous and repetitious physical activity, and diffuse bone hypertrophy and avulsion injuries (see later discussion) are additional manifestations of such stress. Although similar manifestations may be observed in children and adolescents, the open physes of the developing skeleton provide an additional anatomic site at which stress-related abnormalities may appear. The growth plates in the distal portions of the radius and ulna, the proximal portion of the humerus, the distal aspect of the femur, and the distal aspect of the tibia are affected most commonly in a variety of athletic endeavors that include gymnastics, soccer, baseball, basketball, American football, and swimming. Although the specific type of physical activity will dictate which anatomic region will be altered, the general radiographic ab-

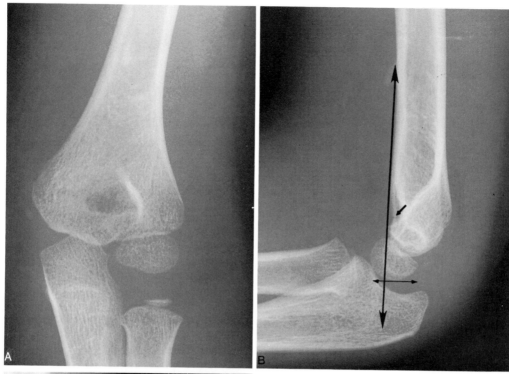

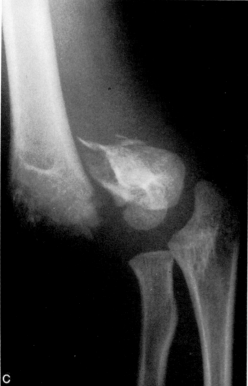

FIGURE 67–148. Elbow injuries: Supracondylar fracture of the humerus.

A, B The frontal radiograph **(A)** shows no obvious abnormality. On the lateral radiograph **(B),** elevation of the intracapsular fat pads and a subtle supracondylar fracture line (arrow) are seen. A line drawn along the anterior cortex of the humerus intersects the anterior third of the capitular ossification center. This indicates minimal posterior displacement at the fracture site.

C A markedly displaced and comminuted supracondylar fracture is demonstrated.

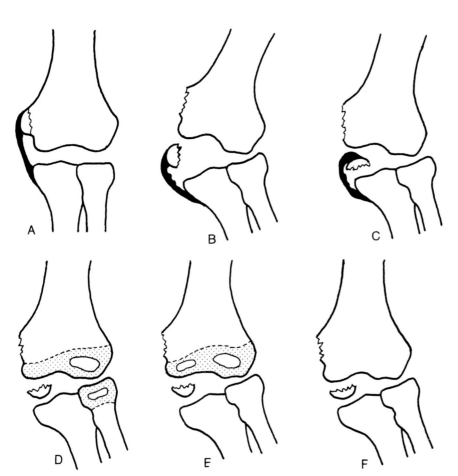

FIGURE 67–149. Injuries of the medial epicondyle of the humerus.

A The initial site of fracture is indicated.

B, C After a valgus stress with temporary opening of the medial aspect of the elbow joint, the epicondyle is avulsed, and it may be drawn into the joint by traction from its attached flexor pronator muscle group and the ulnar collateral ligament. When the force is relieved, the joint closes, entrapping the medial epicondyle.

D–F The radiographic appearance depends on the age of the patient at which the injury occurs. When entrapment takes place before ossification of the trochlear center **(D)**, the entrapped medial epicondyle may be mistaken for a "normal" trochlea. If the entrapment occurs at a slightly older age **(E)**, the medial epicondyle usually is visualized between the trochlea and the coronoid process of the ulna in the anteroposterior projection. If it lies slightly posterior to the trochlea, identification may be possible only on the lateral view. In the older adolescent **(F)**, the entrapped epicondyle is located between the coronoid process of the ulna and the site of fusion between the trochlea and distal humeral metaphysis.

(From Chessare JW, et al: AJR *129*:49, 1977. Copyright 1977, American Roentgen Ray Society.)

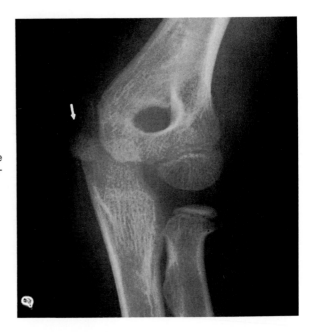

FIGURE 67–150. Injuries of the medial epicondyle of the humerus. Note the position of the avulsed epicondyle (arrow), which corresponds to that illustrated in 67–149**B.**

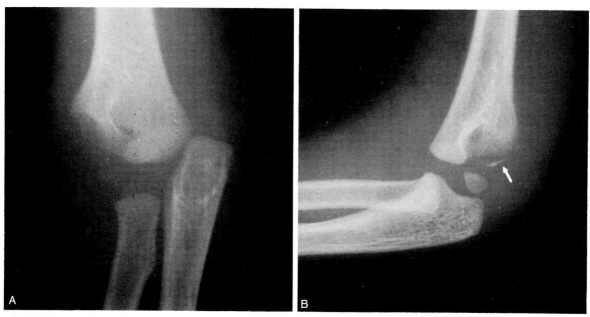

Figure 67–151. Growth plate injury of the distal portion of the humerus. Although the anteroposterior radiograph **(A)** appears to delineate a dislocation of the elbow with medial displacement of the ulna and the radius, the lateral radiograph **(B)** identifies the metaphyseal ossific flake (arrow) and the normal alignment of the radius and capitulum, indicating that a separation of the distal humeral growth plate has occurred.

FIGURE 67–152. Growth plate injury in the terminal phalanx of the hand. This injury results from hyperflexion in which the epiphysis with its extensor tendon attachment remains undisplaced. The remainder of the phalanx is flexed acutely by the unopposed flexor profundus tendon. Dorsal protrusion of the metaphysis through the skin may appear, explaining, in part, why such injuries are significant. A similar injury may occur in the foot.

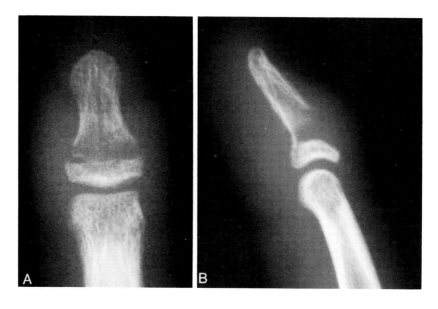

TABLE 67–6. Relative Frequency of Some Physeal Injuries*

	Frequency (Per Cent)	Typical Age† (Years)	Age Range (Years)
Distal portion of radius	49.9	9–14	
Distal portion of humerus‡	16.7	birth–5§	
		6‖	3–10
Distal portion of tibia	11.0	12	8–13
Distal portion of fibula	9.1		
Distal portion of ulna	5.7		
Proximal portion of radius	4.2	9–10	8–13
Proximal portion of humerus	3.1	14–15	10–16
Distal portion of femur	1.2	11–12	10–15
Proximal portion of ulna	0.7		
Proximal portion of tibia	0.5	13–15	
Proximal portion of femur	0.1	2–6	
		12–15	
Other	0.8		

*From Shapiro F: Orthopedics 5:720, 1982.
†Girls, owing to earlier skeletal maturity and advanced skeletal age relative to boys, have injuries at an average age 1 to 2 years younger than boys.
‡The majority of these fractures are lateral condyle lesions.
§Distal humeral fracture-separations.
‖Lateral humeral condyle fracture-separations.

normalities accompanying the chronic stress are similar in each of these locations. Part or all of the physis appears widened and irregular with accompanying sclerosis of varying degree in the adjacent metaphysis (Fig. 67–153). Superficially, these radiographic abnormalities resemble those occurring in rickets, hypophosphatasia, or metaphyseal dysplasias. The unilateral or asymmetric distribution of the changes in some cases, however, provides an important diagnostic clue which, when coupled with a thorough history and physical examination, ensures accurate assessment of the findings.

The radiographic abnormalities occurring about the physes of the distal part of the radius and the distal end of the ulna in gymnasts serve as an appropriate prototype of this type of injury. Although participation in gymnastics may lead to significant alterations at additional skeletal sites such as the olecranon and other regions about the elbow[854–857] and the knee,[858] it is the changes about the wrist in this sport that have received the most attention.[859–864] Unlike most other sports, in gymnastics the upper extremities are used as weight-bearing limbs.[863] In many of the specific gymnastic events, both compression and rotational forces are applied to the wrist and are borne mainly by the distal end of the radius. The resulting physeal changes usually occur first and are more prominent in the radius than in the ulna, but both bones commonly are involved. The injury appears to represent a Salter-Harris type I or type II lesion, but repetitive forces may result in subtle but permanent sequelae. Complications include symmetric or asymmetric retardation of or halted growth at the affected site or sites, positive ulnar variance, and abnormalities of the distal radioulnar joint.[862, 863] Although the prevalence of stress-related changes about the wrist in gymnasts is not clear, the injuries appear to be related to advanced levels of training and competition.[863]

TRAUMA TO SUPPORTING STRUCTURES, SYNDESMOSES, AND ENTHESES

Tendon and Ligament Injury and Healing

Tendons connect bone to muscle, whereas ligaments connect bone to bone. Tendons generally have large parallel collagen fiber bundles that insert uniformly into bone; ligaments have smaller diameter collagen fibers that can be either parallel, as in the collateral ligaments of the knee, or branching and interwoven, as in the cruciate ligaments of the knee.[865] The sites of insertion of tendons or ligaments into bone reveal functional adaptations to allow dissipation of forces. Two types of insertion into bone are seen: The more common type of insertion (direct) crosses the miner-

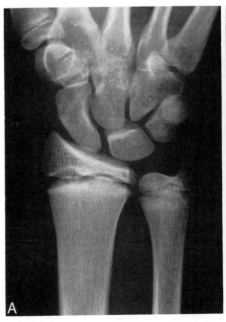
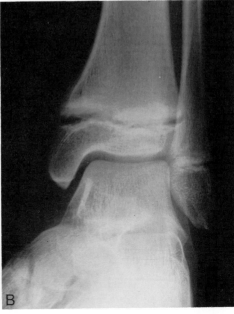

FIGURE 67–153. Growth plate injury: Chronic stress in athletics.

A Wrist involvement in gymnastics. Note subtle physeal widening and irregularity in the radius and in the ulna. (Courtesy of R. Dussault, M.D., Charlottesville, Virginia.)

B Ankle involvement in judo. The physes of the distal end of the tibia and, to a lesser extent, the distal portion of the fibula show minor degrees of widening and irregularity, with metaphyseal sclerosis.

alization front and progresses from fibrocartilage to mineralized fibrocartilage to bone; the second, less common type of insertion (indirect) is characterized by oblique fibers that are anchored into the periosteum of the bone.[865]

In an intact musculotendinous system, complete with its bony attachment, the muscle belly itself is the weakest point; in a tendon-bone preparation, the bone-tendon junction is the weakest point.[64, 866] The ultimate strength of such a system depends on many factors, including the rate of loading. Tendons derive their nutrition from a mesotenon that brings a vascular network in an arcade comparable to that in the mesentery of the gut.[64] A tendon deprived of blood supply degenerates and dies.

Tendons most typically tear at their insertion sites into bone with or without avulsion of a small osseous fragment. Tears also may develop at the musculotendinous junction and, rarely, within the substance of the tendon.[2] Intrasubstance ligament tears are encountered, however. After injury, tendon healing is related to fibroblastic infiltration from surrounding soft tissues.[867, 868] Proliferating connective tissue penetrates between the ends of sutured tendons and deposits collagen fibers that reveal progressive orientation, finally forming tendon fibers identical to those in normal tendons.[64, 869] The healing response of tendons, however, depends on the extent of the injury. A partial rupture of the tendon initiates an intrinsic healing response in which inactive tenocytes are transformed into active tenocytes; with complete rupture of a tendon, the overlying paratenon and surrounding connective tissue are fundamental to tendon healing. An effective healing process requires close approximation of the ends of the divided tendon; complete tendon ruptures leading to separation of tendon ends will not heal unless they are closely applied to each other so that collagenous tissue from the periphery can proliferate and penetrate the injured areas. Similarly, healing of ligaments is characterized by stages of hemorrhage, proliferation of vascular granulation tissue, progressive fibrosis, and scar formation with maturation.[865] Such healing is encouraged by direct apposition of the divided surfaces; collagenation about closely applied or sutured pieces of ligament can result in repair and restoration of a relatively normal ligamentous apparatus[870, 871] (Fig. 67–154). Early motion appears to be beneficial for ligament healing and proper function.

Tendon tears or ruptures can appear at virtually any site in the body. Typical examples are injuries of the tendons in the hands and feet and of the patellar, triceps, peroneal, quadriceps, rotator cuff, and Achilles tendons[872–878] (Fig. 67–155). In most cases, significant trauma initiates the tendon injury, although spontaneous ruptures have been documented,[1007] especially in patients with rheumatoid arthritis and systemic lupus erythematosus and in those receiving local corticosteroid injection (see Chapters 25, 26, 33, and 74). Radiographic diagnosis of a purely soft tissue injury can be difficult, although soft tissue swelling, changes in tendon contour, and bone displacement may be detected. Additional diagnostic techniques such as xeroradiography, low KV radiography, ultrasonography, and arthrography can be helpful (see Chapters 5, 6, 10, 11, and 13). The gold standard for the imaging of tendons is MR imaging, and its role is discussed in detail in Chapter 70 (Fig. 67–156).

Ligament tears or ruptures also are widely distributed and are particularly noteworthy about the wrist, ankle, elbow, and knee.[879–883] In these cases, plain film radiography may require supplementation with stress radiography and arthrography. Stress radiographs are especially helpful in the investigation of ligamentous injuries of the knee[884–889] and the ankle[890–892]; application of force during radiography can outline displacement or tilting of the apposing articular surfaces. Difficulty in interpreting stress radiographs relates to incomplete or inappropriate force application and to mild displacement that may occur in normal persons. Arthrography, as in the ankle, the knee, and the articulations of the hand (e.g., the first metacarpophalangeal joint), performed after ligamentous injury may indicate abnormal leakage or extravasation of contrast media. Similarly, contrast opacifi-

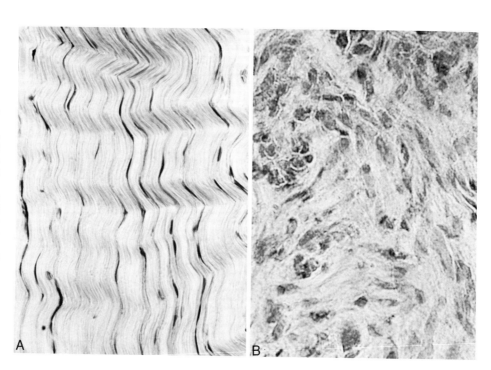

FIGURE 67–154. Injury and repair of ligaments.

A Normal ligament. Note undulating appearance, called "crimp," of longitudinally oriented cells and collagen matrix (hematoxylin and eosin, 310×).

B Injured ligament. Twenty-one days after injury, there is random orientation of plump fibroblasts, producing equally random matrix (hematoxylin and eosin, 310×).

(From Frank C, et al: Clin Orthop *196*:15, 1985.)

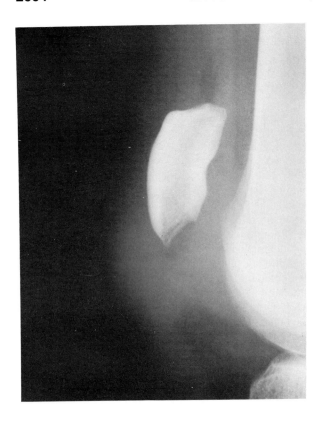

FIGURE 67–155. Tendon injuries: Patellar tendon. In this example, acute rupture of the patellar tendon is associated with soft tissue swelling, loss of the normal tendinous contour, and superior displacement of the patella (although the latter finding is better evaluated with the patient's knee flexed).

cation of tendon sheaths (tenography) or tendons themselves (tendinography) may reveal abnormal patterns in patients with tendon or ligament tears.[893, 894] Once again, however, it is MR imaging that holds the greatest promise in noninvasive assessment of ligaments (see Chapter 70).

Posttraumatic ossification of injured ligaments is well recognized, especially in the knee (Fig. 67–157).

Avulsion Injuries

Abnormal stress on ligaments and tendons may lead to characteristic avulsions at their sites of attachment to bone.[895, 896] For example, avulsion of a portion of the calcaneus, the patella, or the ulnar olecranon may accompany exaggerated pull of the Achilles, quadriceps, or triceps tendon, respectively (Fig. 67–158).[897, 898] Avulsion injuries of the proximal portion of the humerus, occurring generally during a dislocation of the glenohumeral joint, may involve either of the tuberosities and are related to tendinous traction provided by the various components of the rotator cuff. Avulsion also may accompany cruciate ligament injuries and spinal trauma (e.g., clay-shoveler's fracture of the spinous processes of the lower cervical and upper thoracic vertebrae) or shoulder trauma.[899] Indeed, virtually any skeletal site of attachment of a tendon or ligament may be affected by an avulsion injury, occurring either as an isolated phenomenon (Fig. 67–159) or as part of a more complex fracture or dislocation. Cartilaginous or cartilaginous and bony fragments may be avulsed. The size of the avulsed fragment is quite variable; in the adult, only small osseous flecks may be pulled from the parent bone, whereas in the child or adolescent, an entire apophysis may undergo avulsion. The degree of displacement of the fragment also is variable.

Although the detection of avulsion injuries in adults may be difficult as a result of the small size or minimal displacement of the bone fragment, proper identification of such injuries in children provides even greater diagnostic challenges owing primarily to the presence of unossified portions of the immature skeleton. Because the tendinous, ligamentous, and capsular tissue is much stronger than the physeal cartilage, forces that might produce a ligamentous or tendinous injury or dislocation in an adult may lead to physeal avulsion in a child. Such injuries commonly involve the apophyses of the skeleton. The apophyses are not involved in longitudinal growth but are responsible for the development of bone protuberances to which a tendon is attached or from which muscles arise or insert.[2] What appears to be a minor injury in the young child with a small avulsed piece of bone in reality may represent an avulsion of the entire apophysis. In the older child or adolescent with more extensive ossification of the skeleton, the size of the displaced bone fragment may be larger, facilitating proper diagnosis and interpretation of the injury. Apophyseal avulsions may occur at many different skeletal sites, although those of the pelvis and hips are encountered most frequently.

Several avulsion injuries about the pelvis and the hips in young athletes have characteristic radiographic features.[900–904, 1003] These include (1) avulsion injuries of the anterior superior iliac spine, which occur in sprinters as the result of stress at the origin of the tensor fasciae femoris or the sartorius muscle (Fig. 67–160); (2) avulsion injuries of the anterior inferior iliac spine and of a groove just above the superior aspect of the acetabular rim, which relate to stress at the origins of the straight and reflected heads of the rectus femoris (Fig. 67–161A); (3) avulsion injuries of the apophysis of the lesser trochanter owing to stress of the

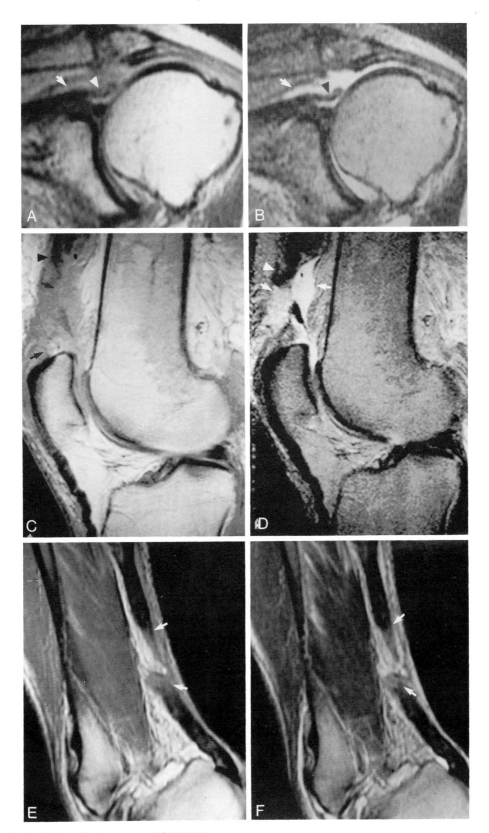

FIGURE 67–156. Tendon injuries: Various sites—MR imaging.

A, B Supraspinatus tendon of the rotator cuff. Coronal proton density (TR/TE, 2000/30) **(A)** and T2-weighted (TR/TE, 2000/80) **(B)** spin echo MR images reveal a massive tear of the supraspinatus tendon. The tendon is retracted medially (arrowheads), fluid is present both in the glenohumeral joint and in the subacromial portion (arrows) of the subacromial-subdeltoid bursa, and the humeral head is elevated.

C, D Quadriceps tendon. On sagittal proton density (TR/TE, 1800/20) **(C)** and T2-weighted (TR/TE, 1800/80) **(D)** spin echo MR images, note disruption of the quadriceps tendon (arrowheads) with fluid in the tendinous gap (arrows). The patella is low in position (patella baja), and the patellar tendon has a wrinkled appearance. (Courtesy of R. Kerr, M.D., Los Angeles, California.)

E, F Achilles tendon. Sagittal proton density (TR/TE, 2000/20) **(E)** and T2-weighted (TR/TE, 2000/60) **(F)** spin echo MR images show complete disruption (between arrows) of the Achilles tendon.

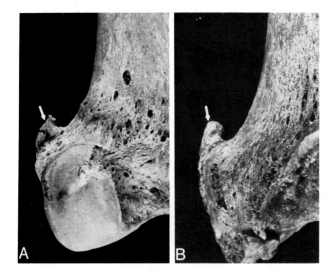

FIGURE 67–157. Ligament injuries: Heterotopic ossification. Posttraumatic ossification in the medial collateral ligament of the knee (arrows) is termed Pelligrini-Stieda disease.

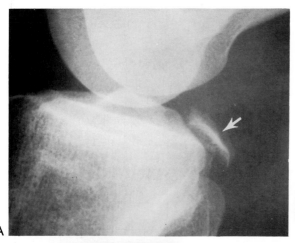

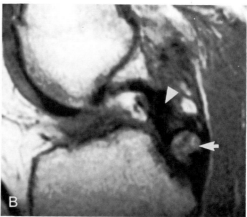

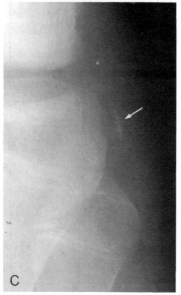

FIGURE 67–158. Avulsion injuries: Tibia.

A Cruciate ligament avulsion. Observe the posterior bony fragment (arrow), resulting from an old posterior cruciate injury.

B Cruciate ligament avulsion. A sagittal proton density (TR/TE, 1000/40) spin echo MR image shows a tibial avulsion fracture (arrow) related to the site of attachment of the posterior cruciate ligament (arrowhead).

C Lateral capsular avulsion (Segond injury). Note the small linear avulsion fracture (arrow), which generally is indicative of an associated injury to the anterior cruciate ligament.

(**B,** Courtesy of M. Schweitzer, M.D., Philadelphia, Pennsylvania.)

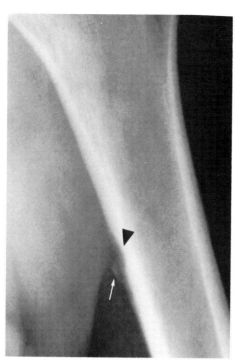

FIGURE 67–159. Avulsion injuries: Humerus. This internal rotation view of the shoulder of a body builder shows a small avulsion fracture (arrow) at the site of insertion of the pectoralis major tendon. Note the cortical irregularity (arrowhead).

psoas major during strenuous hip flexion (Fig. 67–162); (4) avulsion injuries of the apophysis of the ischial tuberosity due to violent contraction of the hamstring muscles (Fig. 67–163), often occurring in hurdlers; (5) avulsion injuries of the greater trochanter of the femur produced by gluteal muscle contraction; (6) avulsion of the apophysis of the iliac crest due to severe contraction of the abdominal muscles associated with abrupt directional change during running; and (7) avulsion injuries near the symphysis pubis related to adductor muscle (adductor longus, adductor brevis, gracilis) insertion sites[904–909] (Fig. 67–161B). Clinical findings accompanying these avulsion injuries include local pain, tenderness, and swelling. The fracture line may extend directly through the physeal cartilage or extend into the subjacent bone or ossifying apophysis, or both. The resulting radiographic abnormalities are variable, dependent on the precise orientation of the fracture line, the stage of development of the apophysis, and the amount of apophyseal displacement. Hence, radiographs may appear almost entirely normal or may reveal irregularity at the site of avulsion and displaced pieces of bone of variable size. Follow-up radiographs may show considerable new bone formation or healing with incorporation of the fragment into the parent bone, which, in some cases, is associated with bizarre skeletal overgrowth or deformity simulating neoplasm (Fig. 67–164).

Another type of avulsion injury that is confined to the immature skeleton is the sleeve fracture. This injury has been described with respect to the patella,[910–912] although similar injuries conceivably may occur at other skeletal sites. The chondrosseous junction of the developing patella is affected in this avulsion injury. Although avulsion injuries of the tibial tuberosity have been observed in children and adolescents,[913,914] those involving the site of attachment of the patellar tendon to the inferior margin of the patella are more typical (Fig. 67–165). An extensive sleeve of cartilage may be pulled away from the main portion of the patella, together with an osseous fragment from its distal pole.[912] A similar lesion may affect the superior portion of the patella or the medial margin of the bone (owing to acute lateral dislocation of the patella). Indeed, the bipartite patella or dorsal defect of the patella (both involving the lateral side of the bone) and the Sinding-Larsen-Johansson lesion (affecting the inferior portion of the patella) may represent chronic sequelae of this type of injury.[912] In the acute stage, a radiographically visible small bone fragment may lead to an underestimation of the size and significance of the patellar sleeve fracture. The avulsion becomes more obvious when progressive ossification of the fragment develops later. Weakening of the quadriceps mechanism and involvement of articular cartilage are important complications of the injury.

As is discussed in Chapter 90, many skeletal alterations that generally are classified as normal variations of growth in actuality represent acute or chronic injuries of developing chondro-osseous centers. In some instances, ossicles develop, perhaps as a result of a ligamentous avulsion fracture. The ossicles that commonly are observed in the medial or lateral malleolus of the tibia are examples of this phenomenon[915] (see Chapter 90).

Diastasis

The term diastasis implies a separation of normally joined bony elements; it frequently is applied to syndesmoses and, specifically, to injuries of the ligaments that extend between the lower tibia and the lower fibula.[916] Complete or partial diastasis can appear, depending on the extent of damage to the tibiofibular and interosseous ligaments. Radiographs may reveal abnormal separation of the tibia and fibula in which the space (la ligne claire) between the medial cortex of the fibula and the posterior edge of the peroneal groove is greater than 5.0 or 5.5 mm in the anteroposterior radiograph.[916, 917] Fractures of the neighboring bones also may be evident, although these may occur at some distance from the site of diastasis. Soft tissue ossification and even ankylosis between the tibia and the fibula may occur subsequently (Fig. 67–166).

The term diastasis likewise is applied to separation of apposing bone surfaces about symphyses (e.g., symphysis pubis), although such injuries also are designated subluxations or dislocations.

TRAUMA TO SKELETAL MUSCLE

Muscle cells are derived mainly from mesenchymal cells. Further differentiation of these progenitor cells allows them to be divided into three distinct categories. Two of these, skeletal muscle and cardiac muscle, are striated. Skeletal muscle sometimes is referred to as voluntary muscle because contractions may be under voluntary control in some situations. Cardiac muscle is involuntary and is confined to the myocardium of the heart. The third category is termed nonstriated muscle, or smooth involuntary muscle, is able to effect prolonged tonic contractions, and is located in

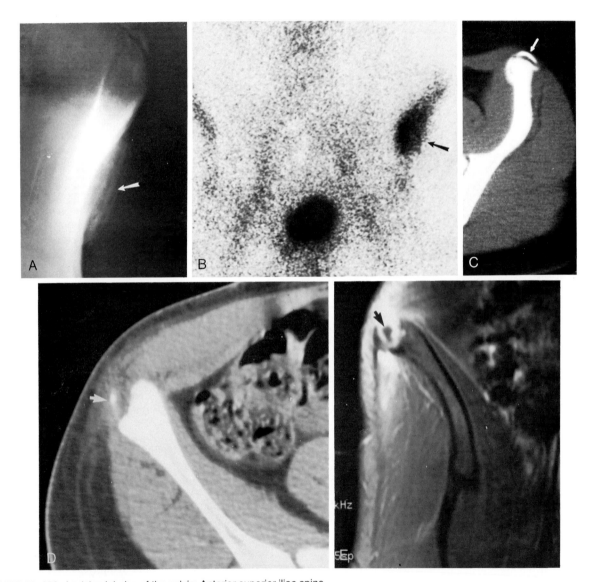

FIGURE 67–160. Avulsion injuries of the pelvis: Anterior superior iliac spine.
  A Observe bone irregularity at the origin of the sartorius muscle (arrow).
  B The bone scan shows increased accumulation of the radionuclide at this site (arrow).
  C Transaxial CT demonstrates the avulsion to good advantage (arrow).
  (A–C Courtesy of G. Greenway, M.D., Dallas, Texas.)
  D, E In a different patient, transaxial CT **(D)** and a coronal T1-weighted (TR/TE, 816/11) spin echo MR image obtained with fat suppression and after the intravenous injection of a gadolinium compound **(E)** show the site of avulsion (arrows). Note associated high signal intensity in **E. (D, E,** Courtesy of D. Levey, M.D., Corpus Christi, Texas.)

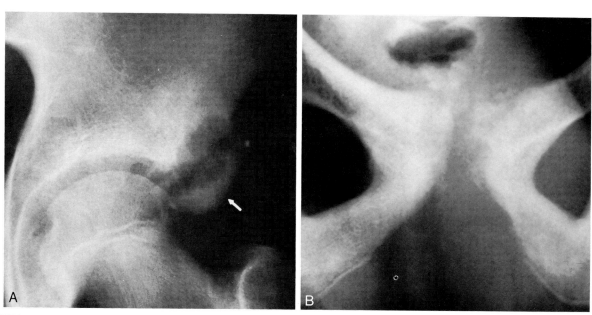

FIGURE 67–161. Avulsion injuries of the pelvis.
 A Anterior inferior iliac spine. The avulsed fragment (arrow) is related to stress at the origin of the rectus femoris muscle.
 B Symphysis pubis and inferior pubic ramus. The osseous irregularity may result from avulsion injuries due to stress in the adductor brevis, adductor longus, and gracilis muscles.
 (**B,** From Schneider R, et al: Radiology *120*:567, 1976.)

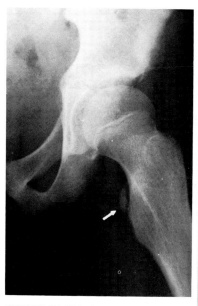

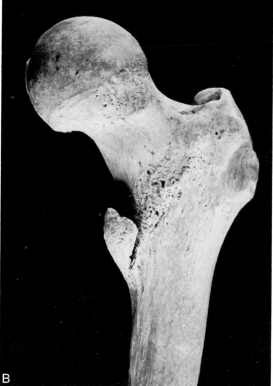

FIGURE 67–162. Avulsion injuries of the femur: Lesser trochanter.
 A Note displacement of the apophysis of the lesser trochanter (arrow) owing to the pull of the iliopsoas muscle.
 B A specimen photograph shows a similar lesion.

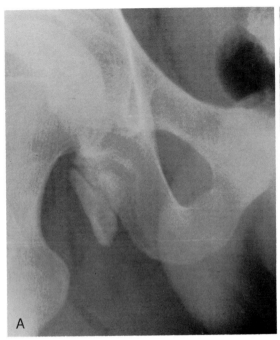

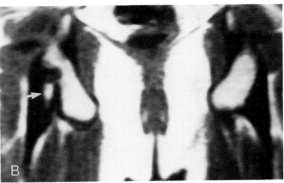

FIGURE 67–163. Avulsion injuries of the pelvis: Ischial tuberosity. The routine radiograph **(A)** reveals a well-defined bone fragment adjacent to an irregular ischial tuberosity, consistent with an old avulsion injury. A coronal T1-weighted (TR/TE, 600/20) spin echo MR image **(B)** shows the location of the bone fragment (arrow). (Courtesy of H. S. Kang, M.D., Seoul, Korea.)

various anatomic sites, including the walls of blood vessels and those of the genitourinary and alimentary tracts.

Any discussion of physical injury would be incomplete if injury to skeletal muscle was not given consideration. Such injury can occur as an isolated abnormality or as part of a more complex situation in which fractures, dislocations, and other soft tissue abnormalities are present. Trauma to skeletal muscle may result from any type of accidental injury, but it is encountered most often in the setting of physical exertion, particularly that of athletic endeavors. Intense and prolonged exercise, especially in a person who is not properly trained or conditioned, can produce a muscle strain or pull, related to rapid and violent contraction of the muscle, but this is but one of a spectrum of injuries that affect skeletal muscle. Accurate assessment of the type and extent of injury previously had been the sole responsibility of the examining physician who, on the basis of clinical history and careful physical examination, arrived at his or her conclusion on the nature and significance of the muscle abnormalities. With the introduction and refinement of MR imaging as a diagnostic technique that can be applied effectively to the analysis of skeletal muscle, the examining physician, should he or she choose, has an additional method to judge the severity of the injury.

Skeletal muscles do not act independently. Rather, they transmit their contractile forces to adjacent structures through tendinous attachments. The muscle serves as the active element in this action, and the tendon is the passive element. The junctional region between the muscle fibers and the tendinous attachment is termed the myotendinal, or musculotendinous, junction. At this junction, muscle fibers of variable shape thicken and become continuous with the fibrous bundles of the tendon. Many, if not most, of the injuries to muscle in fact occur at the myotendinal junction. In the discussion that follows, physical injury to skeletal muscle, including the myotendinal junction, is addressed. An excellent review of this subject is provided by Mink,[918] many of whose observations are included here. Neuromus-

cular disorders (Chapter 77) and inflammatory (Chapter 35), infectious (Chapter 64), and neoplastic (Chapter 95) disorders of skeletal muscle are considered elsewhere in this book.

Muscle Anatomy and Physiology

The basic units of skeletal muscle are the fibers themselves, each of which is a single cell containing many hundreds of nuclei.[919] These fibers are arranged in bundles, or fasciculi, of various sizes within the muscle. Connective tissue located between muscle fibers, around a fasciculus, or about the entire muscle is designated endomysium, perimysium, or epimysium, respectively. Each fiber is elongated, stretching either from one end of the muscle to the other or through part of the length of the muscle (and ending in tendinous or other connective tissue insertions that penetrate the body of the muscle).[919] The cytoplasm, or sarcoplasm, of the muscle cell is divided into longitudinal threads, or myofibrils. The myofibrils, in longitudinal section, are traversed by striations that differ in their chemical and optical properties and are termed the I (isotropic), A (anisotropic), Z (Krause's membrane), and H (Hensen's line) bands.[919] Myofilaments are smaller structures within each myofibril. Two types of myofilaments exist: fine ones consisting of actin, and thicker ones composed of myosin. Each of the myofilaments is crossed by Z bands, creating regions known as sarcomeres. During muscle contraction, the actin filaments slide toward the center of the sarcomere, bringing Z bands closer together, and producing shortening of the entire muscle unit.[918]

Most muscles show a mixture of two types of fibers, known as type I, or slow, fibers and type II, or fast, fibers. Histochemical differences are used to distinguish between these types of fibers. Type I fibers are characterized by the presence of low myofibrillar adenosine triphosphatase (ATPase) activity, whereas type II fibers have high ATPase activity. Furthermore, type I fibers have abundant mito-

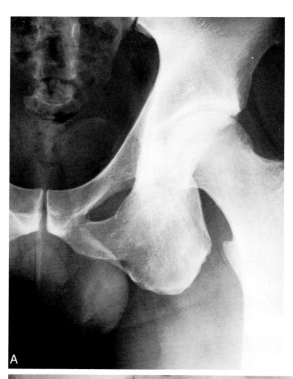

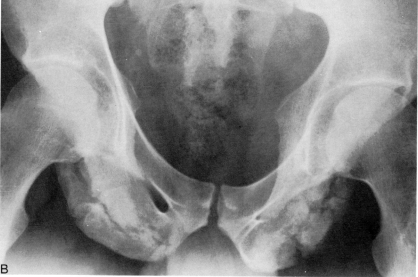

FIGURE 67–164. Avulsion injuries of the pelvis: Ischial tuberosity. In both patients, observe osseous enlargement and, in **B,** fragmentation. These findings relate to old avulsion injuries.

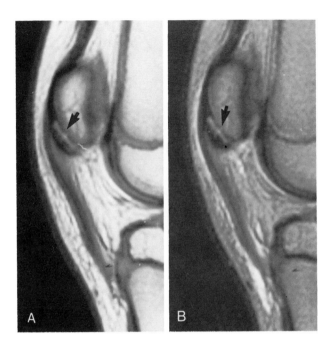

FIGURE 67–165. Avulsion injuries of the patella: Sleeve fracture. In this 9 year old girl, sagittal proton density (TR/TE, 2000/30) **(A)** and T2-weighted (TR/TE, 2000/80) **(B)** spin echo MR images show avulsion (arrows) of the inferior portion of the developing chondro-osseous patella with adjacent edema.

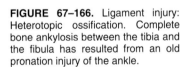

FIGURE 67–166. Ligament injury: Heterotopic ossification. Complete bone ankylosis between the tibia and the fibula has resulted from an old pronation injury of the ankle.

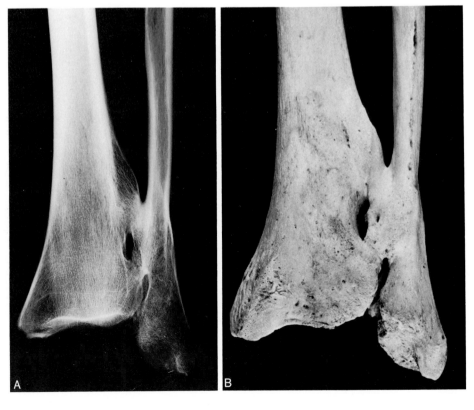

chondria and bulky sarcomeres, whereas type II fibers have fewer mitochondria and more extensive sarcoplasmic reticulum.[918, 919] Type II fibers obtain energy primarily by glycolytic respiration, whereas type I fibers also have a well-developed aerobic metabolism.[919] Type I fibers are better suited to a relatively slow but repetitive type of contraction, such as the tonic forces characteristic of postural muscles, and are more resistant to fatigue than type II fibers. Hence, type I fibers are more involved in endurance activities than those requiring speed and strength of short duration. Type II fibers, in contrast, are adapted to produce rapid phasic forces that are operational in large-scale movements of the human body.[919] Type I fibers have been designated as slow twitch and type II fibers as fast twitch fibers.[918]

Muscle Injury and Repair

Skeletal muscle contracts as a response to injury. Such contraction leads to an increase of pressure in the muscle. The sheath that encloses the muscle, the epimysium, and the overlying fascia, serves as a relatively rigid tissue and gives counterpressure to the forces of muscular contraction.[920, 921] As a consequence, large intracompartmental hematomas can develop within the muscle tissue before the transmural pressure is high enough to prevent further intramuscular fluid expansion.[920] The anatomic arrangement of muscle tissue within surrounding sheaths contributes to the frequent development of compartment syndromes after trauma (see later discussion).

Skeletal muscle is capable of limited regeneration. Fibers on each side of a damaged zone break up into nucleated cylinders of cytoplasm, macrophages enter the necrotic area, and they engulf dead materials but leave the basement membrane intact.[919] The muscle fiber cylinders then fuse and grow inside the original basement membrane to form a myotube. Eventual fusion of the two undamaged ends and hypertrophy and maturation lead to a creation of the new intact fiber.[919] With extensive muscle damage, however, such regeneration is not possible, and connective tissue is formed to replace the injured muscle, with resultant loss of function. In certain situations, such as after laceration, healing of skeletal muscle is associated with extensive scarring and ossification.[920]

Direct Muscle Injury

Muscle Laceration. Muscle lacerations result from penetrating injuries. The typical healing response results in the formation of a scar composed of dense connective tissue.[918] Owing to the presence of limited muscle regeneration and the absence of extensive reinnervation of the distal portion of the muscle, restoration of function of the muscle is not complete. MR imaging in cases of lacerated muscle is characterized by a defect, often transverse, with interruption of the continuity of the muscle and changes in signal intensity reflecting the presence of blood and edema[918] (Fig. 67–167).

Muscle Contusion. Compression of a muscle from direct trauma leads to a contusion. The force necessary to produce a contusion is not infrequent in certain contact sports, such as American football, and the term ''charleyhorse'' sometimes is used to describe the injury. The blow results in capillary rupture and interstitial hemorrhage (bleeding between the fibers of the damaged connective tissue) followed

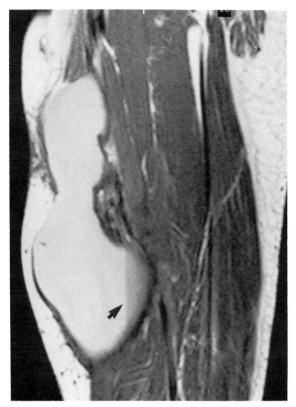

FIGURE 67–167. Skeletal muscle injury: Laceration. This young man lacerated his thigh while on a motorcycle. A soft tissue mass developed and enlarged quickly. It followed the course of the sartorius muscle. A sagittal T1-weighted (TR/TE, 650/20) spin echo MR image shows high signal intensity within the superficial intramuscular mass, with a fluid-debris level (arrow), findings consistent with a recently formed hematoma. (Courtesy of S. Eilenberg, M.D., San Diego, California.)

by edema and an inflammatory mass.[918] Contusions vary in severity, although the muscle still is able to function, even in severe cases.

There are four basic MR imaging characteristics of a muscle contusion[918]: (1) The affected muscle usually is slightly increased in girth; (2) edema leads to an increase in signal intensity on T2-weighted spin echo and short tau inversion recovery (STIR) MR images and, owing to its isointensity with muscle, is not well seen on T1-weighted spin echo images; (3) a feathery, interstitial pattern is evident that relates to the dispersion of inflammatory fluid within and between the muscle fibers; and (4) there is no evidence of disruption of muscle fibers (Fig. 67–168).

Soft tissue ossification, often designated myositis ossificans traumatica, may occur subsequent to muscle contusion. This subject is discussed in Chapter 95.

Indirect Muscle Injury

Indirect injuries to muscle occur from overzealous use during physical exercise. Certain muscles are prone to develop exercise-related, or exertional, muscle injury, in part because of the specific type of muscle contraction that they exhibit. Such muscle contractions are divided into two basic types: Isometric contraction produces tension without a change in muscle length; isotonic contraction produces tension associated with a change in muscle length.[918] Isotonic

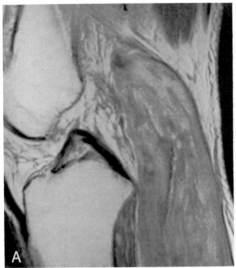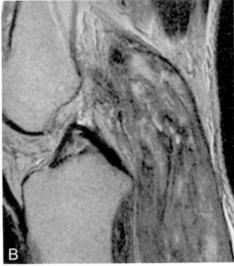

FIGURE 67–168. Skeletal muscle injury: Contusion. This 29 year old man suffered a direct blow to the back of the knee and calf. Sagittal proton density (TR/TE, 2000/30) **(A)** and T2-weighted (TR/TE, 2000/80) **(B)** spin echo MR images show enlargement of the medial head of the gastrocnemius muscle. The muscle is inhomogeneous in signal intensity in both images and generally is of higher signal intensity than normal.

contraction is divided further into two types: Concentric action occurs when the muscle shortens during contraction; eccentric action occurs when the muscle lengthens during contraction. As muscles produce greater tension during stretching than when shortening, eccentric contractions, as occur when a weight in the hand is lowered parallel to the thorax, lead to greater tension than concentric contractions and are considered the primary cause of exertional muscle injury.[918]

Injury-prone muscles show several typical characteristics.[918] First, such muscles commonly perform eccentric actions (e.g., hamstring muscles). Second, the muscles commonly act across two joints (e.g., biceps brachii and gastrocnemius muscles). Third, muscles having type II or fast fibers and involved in activities requiring sudden acceleration or deceleration typically are affected (e.g., hip flexors and adductors, rectus femoris muscle).

MR imaging has been employed to evaluate physiologic and pathologic alterations in skeletal muscle after physical exertion.[922–927] After moderate exercise, T2 relaxation times increase regardless of the type of exercise performed, although the T2 values are significantly higher in those muscles performing concentric actions than those performing eccentric actions.[918] Resulting increases in signal intensity within muscles on T2-weighted spin echo MR images and STIR images correlate strongly with the mean force exerted during the exercise.

Similar alterations in signal intensity are observed after acute muscle strains. Such strains are defined as painful stress-induced injuries resulting from the application of a single violent force.[918] Whereas contusions produce injury at the point of impact, strains lead to injury at the musculotendinous junction. The precise MR imaging findings are influenced by the severity of the strain and its duration[928] (Figs. 67–169 to 67–171). Minor, or grade 1, strains produce MR imaging findings similar to those of a muscle contusion. With moderate, or grade 2, muscle strains, a focal masslike lesion or a stellate defect, or both, can be observed on the MR images.[918] The signal intensity of the involved muscle or muscles reflects the presence of edema or blood. Serial MR imaging in cases of grade 1 or 2 muscle strain reveals initial alterations in the center of the affected muscle, subsequent involvement of the entire muscle, and, finally, resolution of the abnormalities.[918] With severe, or grade 3, muscle strains, discontinuity of the muscle is evident, and blood collects between the torn edges. A true hematoma may form.

Delayed onset muscle soreness (DOMS) represents another response to physical exertion. Clinical findings, consisting of muscle soreness and tenderness to palpation, occur within 1 to several days after muscle exertion. MR imaging findings in DOMS resemble those of grade 1 muscle strains, and the conspicuity of these findings generally follows the clinical course and correlates with histologic and ultrastructural changes in the involved musculature.[926]

Muscle Herniation

Focal herniation of muscle through a defect in its enclosing fascia may occur as a complication of local blunt trauma or as a result of muscle hypertrophy.[929, 930] Typically, the lower leg, especially its anterior tibial compartment, is involved, and the tibialis anterior muscle is affected most frequently. A soft tissue mass that becomes tense and decreases in size during muscle contraction is a common clinical finding. MR imaging represents an effective diagnostic technique when such herniation is suspected.[930] Surgical repair with closure of the fascial defect may lead to an anterior compartment syndrome.

Rhabdomyolysis

Rhabdomyolysis is a relatively common syndrome of muscle injury that alters the integrity of the cell membrane, allowing the escape of cellular contents into the general circulation.[931, 932] Causative factors include burns, crush injuries, prolonged muscular compression, exposure to toxins, seizures, and extremely intense exercise, especially in hot climates.[918] Although multiple intracellular enzymes may be released, creatine kinase is the most sensitive to muscle injury.[932] Myoglobulin can be detected in the urine. Clinical findings include fever and intense pain and weakness; among the complications that may be encountered are tetany, acute renal failure, compartment syndrome, and dis-

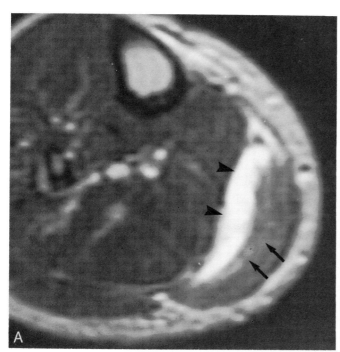

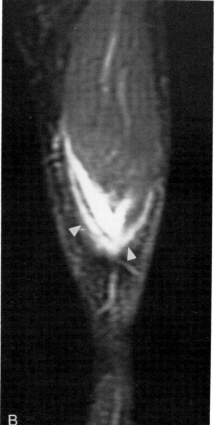

FIGURE 67–169. Skeletal muscle injury: Grade 1 strain. A transaxial T2-weighted (TR/TE, 2000/80) spin echo MR image **(A)** reveals an increase in signal intensity of the gastrocnemius muscle (arrows) and a perifascial fluid collection (arrowheads). A coronal short tau inversion recovery (STIR) MR image (TR/TE, 2200/35; inversion time, 160 msec) **(B)** defines the fluid collection (arrowheads) just deep and distal to the gastrocnemius muscle. (From Deutsch AL, Mink JH, Kerr R: MRI of the Foot and Ankle. New York, Raven Press, 1992.)

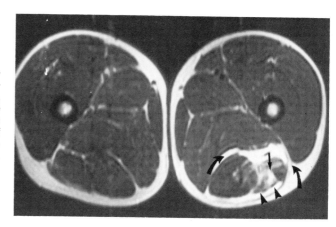

FIGURE 67–170. Skeletal muscle injury: Grade 2 strain. This professional football player suffered an acute hamstring strain during push-off from the line of scrimmage. On a transaxial T2-weighted (TR/TE, 2000/80) spin echo MR image, note that the biceps femoris muscle demonstrates edema throughout its substance (arrowheads) with several small focal areas perhaps representing limited interruption of muscle fibers (small arrow). Perifascial edema (large arrows) is striking. (From Deutsch AL, Mink JH, Kerr R: MRI of the Foot and Ankle. New York, Raven Press, 1992.)

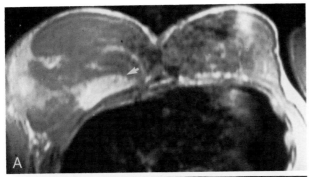

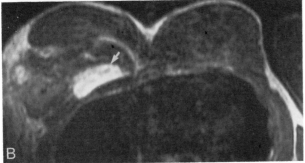

FIGURE 67–171. Skeletal muscle injury: Rupture and retraction. During bench pressing, this weight-lifter ruptured his right pectoralis muscle. On transaxial T1-weighted (TR/TE, 600/20) **(A)** and T2-weighted (TR/TE, 2000/80) **(B)** spin echo MR images, note distortion of muscle anatomy with localized edema and a focal hematoma (arrows) of high signal intensity in both images. (From Fleckenstein JL, Shellock FG: Top Magn Reson Imaging 3:50, 1991.)

seminated intravascular coagulation. Ultrasonography,[933] CT,[932, 934] scintigraphy,[935] and MR imaging[918] may be used to investigate this condition and its complications. Swelling and regions of low attenuation in muscles are typical CT findings of rhabdomyolysis.[932] MR imaging reveals increased intramuscular signal intensity on T2-weighted spin echo and STIR images.[918]

Compartment Syndrome and Myonecrosis

Compartment syndrome is a condition characterized by elevated pressure within an anatomically confined space leading to irreversible damage to the contents (i.e., muscle and neurovascular components) of the closed space.[936] Any condition that increases the contents of a compartment or that reduces the volume of a compartment may lead to a compartment syndrome. Common causes are trauma with hemorrhage, fractures, increased capillary permeability after thermal burns, and intense physical activity. Regardless of the precise cause, elevation of intracompartmental pressure leads to some degree of venous obstruction; pressure within the involved compartment may continue to rise until the low intramuscular arteriolar pressure is exceeded.[936] With further increase in the intracompartmental pressure, muscle and nerve ischemia results, and the changes become irreversible. The current explanation for the development of a compartment syndrome is the theory of the arteriovenous gradient; an increase in tissue pressure reduces the local arteriovenous gradient and therefore local perfusion.[920] If perfusion is reduced to the degree that metabolic needs are not met, a compartment syndrome will

result. In cases of acute compartment syndrome, pressure within the compartment never rises sufficiently to totally counter the systolic or diastolic pressure in the major artery traversing the compartment.[937]

The list of potential causes of this syndrome is impressive indeed. A decrease in the size of the compartment, which may lead to the compartment syndrome, may result from the application of a tight cast, constrictive dressings, or pneumatic antishock garments.[936] An increase in the contents of the compartment, which likewise may lead to this syndrome, may be related to hemorrhage (fractures of the tibia, femur, bones of the forearm, or those about the elbow) or to edema (postischemic swelling after arterial injury or restoration of arterial flow after arterial thrombosis).[936] Additional causes are bleeding disorders, anticoagulant therapy, excessive skeletal traction, and osteotomy.

The clinical manifestations of a compartment syndrome may be acute or chronic. Typical acute findings are pain out of proportion to the extent of the injury, weakness and pain on passive stretching of the extremity, hypoesthesia in the distribution of the nerves traversing the compartment, and the presence of a tense, swollen compartment.[918] Pulses always are palpable in cases of acute compartment syndrome. Chronic compartment syndromes are associated with prolonged and repetitive physical exertion, and they can lead to exercise-related pain in recreational or professional athletes. Techniques allowing direct measurement of intracompartmental pressure provide evidence of elevated pressure and permit accurate diagnosis, particularly in acute cases. If not diagnosed and treated early, an acute compartment syndrome subsequently may be associated with muscle necrosis and permanent neurologic damage with fibrous contracture (e.g., Volkmann's contracture).

MR imaging findings in patients with an acute compartment syndrome include swelling of the affected extremity and abnormalities of signal intensity in the muscles of the involved compartment and, less commonly, other compartments.[918] Similar and often transient MR imaging abnormalities may accompany chronic compartment syndromes. Complications such as myonecrosis may be delineated with MR imaging, and even routine radiography may reveal significant, and sometimes diagnostic, findings in cases of long-standing compartment syndrome (Fig. 67–172). One such finding is sheetlike calcification involving the anterolateral portion of the lower leg, commonly associated with dysfunction of the peroneal nerve.

Although myonecrosis is a recognized complication of the ischemia that results from a compartment syndrome, it occurs in other situations as well. Infectious myonecrosis may relate to a variety of microorganisms, including clostridia, Bacteroides, Enterococcus, Staphylococcus, Pseudomonas, Aerobacter, Klebsiella, diptheroids, *Serratia marcescens,* Rhizopus, Mucor, and Absidia species (see Chapter 66). Trichinosis, cysticercosis, toxoplasmosis, and leptospirosis also can lead to infective myonecrosis. Additional causes of myonecrosis are vascular disease or occlusion (as in sickle cell anemia and diabetes mellitus) and coma or prolonged sleep from drug overdose, in which prolonged compression of a tissue compartment may be the responsible factor. Although gas formation in involved muscles and other soft tissues in instances of infective myonecrosis may be noted on routine radiographs, more subtle

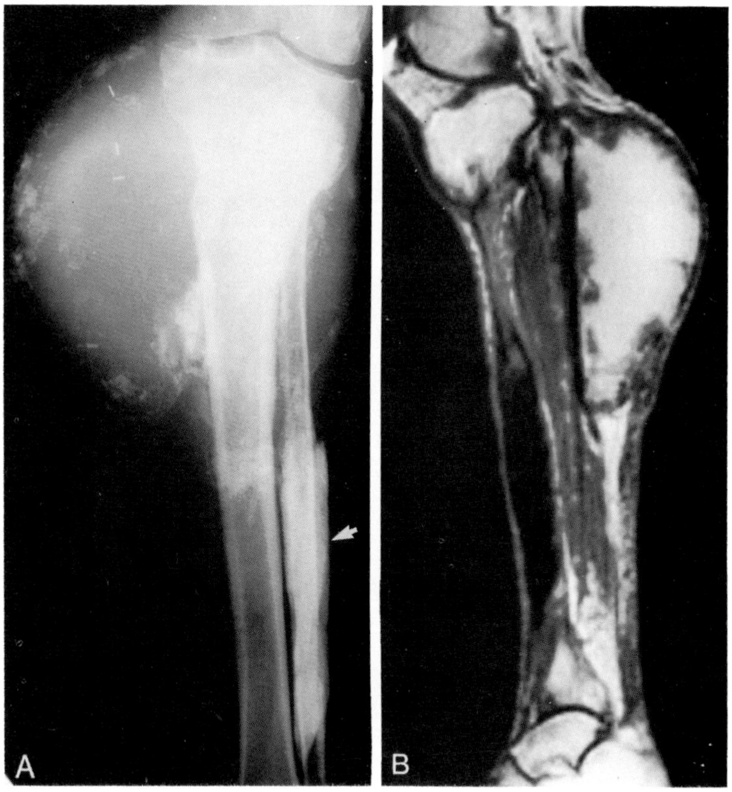

FIGURE 67–172. Skeletal muscle injury: Compartment syndrome and myonecrosis. In this patient, a chronic compartment syndrome in the lower leg that occurred after a tibial fracture has led to enlargement and calcification of the gastrocnemius muscle, evident with routine radiography **(A)**. Also note sheetlike calcification (arrow) in the anterolateral compartment of the leg. A sagittal proton density (TR/TE, 2000/15) spin echo MR image **(B)** shows the enlarged muscle with central high signal intensity. Cystic degeneration of the gastrocnemius muscle had produced these findings. The calcification with its signal void is seen in the anterior soft tissues and periphery of the gastrocnemius muscle. (Courtesy of J. Spaeth, M.D., Albuquerque, New Mexico.)

findings of myonecrosis are detected with bone scintigraphy, CT, and MR imaging.[938, 939]

TRAUMATIC ABUSE OF CHILDREN (ABUSED CHILD SYNDROME)

A great deal of attention has been directed toward the problem of deliberate child abuse.[940–963] It has been estimated that as many as 200,000 incidents are reported each year in the United States.[670] Furthermore, approximately 2500 children per year die from physical abuse (usually related to head or abdominal injuries),[964] and 10 per cent of children under the age of 5 years who are seen by emergency room physicians for trauma have inflicted injuries.[957] Child abuse is assumed to be the greatest single cause of death in the United States in infants between 6 and 12 months of age.[965] Boys and girls are affected in equal numbers, and most children are younger than 6 years old, with 25 per cent of the children being under the age of 2 years. Radiographic abnormalities can be detected in 50 to 70 per cent of cases. Although these abnormalities may involve multiple systems in the body, it is the skeletal alterations that have received a great deal of emphasis.

Traumatic insult to the child's skeleton can produce elevation of the periosteal membrane, which is loosely attached to the diaphysis of tubular bones. The vascularity of the osteogenic layer of the periosteum is responsible for the appearance of a subperiosteal hematoma. Although the resultant periostitis is a delayed radiographic finding (Fig. 67–173A), it has been emphasized repeatedly that the firm attachment of the periosteal membrane to the metaphyses of the tubular bones can lead to an immediate radiographic abnormality—single or multiple metaphyseal bone frag-

ments (Fig. 67–173B). Even though it does not discount the importance of metaphyseal fractures in the diagnosis of child abuse, one investigation has provided histologic and radiographic data that indicate transmetaphyseal disruption of trabeculae, rather than avulsion, is the cause of the corner fractures and bucket-handle osseous fragments that are seen in this syndrome.[966] The resultant fragments consist of a disc of bone and calcified cartilage. Reactive bone formation with sclerosis can be a prominent change associated with periostitis and metaphyseal fracture. Physeal injuries also occur, especially when a massive force is applied with traction, compression, or rotation, and can lead to epiphyseal separation.[964] An increase in the thickness of the hypertrophic cell zone of the growth plate cartilage occurs with healing of the metaphyseal fractures and physeal injuries. Radiolucent zones appear in the metaphyses with such healing.[967, 968]

The proper workup of a child suspected of having been physically abused includes a radiographic survey of all of the long bones, the pelvis, the spine, the ribs, and the skull.[670, 962] A single radiograph of the entire skeleton is inadequate diagnostically.[969] Scintigraphy with bone-seeking pharmaceutical agents also may be a useful adjunct to the radiographic examination[970–975] (Fig. 67–174), demonstrating sites of visceral and soft tissue injury as well,[976] although false-negative radionuclide studies have been noted,[977] and these latter examinations are more invasive and time-consuming than conventional radiography.[1004] Radiographic findings include single or multiple fractures, especially in the ribs (Fig. 67–173C), but also involving, in order of descending frequency, the humerus, the femur, the tibia, the small bones of the hand and foot, and the skull. Skull fractures that are multiple and those that are bilateral

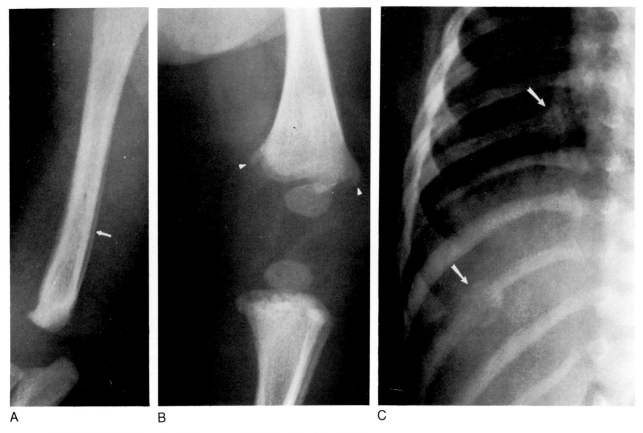

FIGURE 67–173. Abused child syndrome: Radiographic abnormalities.
  A Periostitis (arrow) is a delayed radiographic sign of trauma.
  B Metaphyseal irregularity and corner fractures (arrowheads) are more immediate radiographic clues to child abuse.
  C Rib fractures (arrows) are frequent in the abused child.
  (Courtesy of D. Edwards, M.D., San Diego, California.)

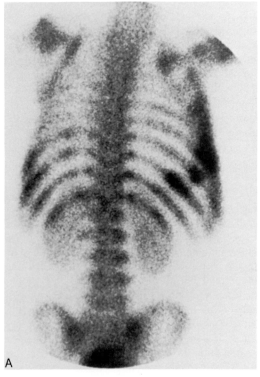

FIGURE 67–174. Abused child syndrome: Scintigraphic abnormalities. The bone scan in this 5 year old child shows increased accumulation of the radionuclide in the ribs, left ulna, metacarpal bones, and phalanges. (Courtesy of P. Garver, M.D., San Diego, California.)

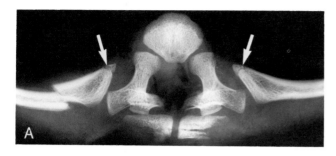

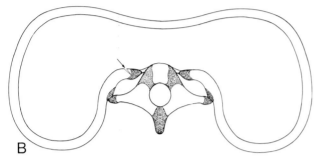

FIGURE 67–175. Abused child syndrome: Involvement of the heads of the ribs.

A A sectional radiograph of the costovertebral joints of the eighth ribs in an abused infant (2½ months of age) who died as a result of his injuries shows bilateral fractures (arrows) of the heads of the ribs. A fracture of the right rib at the costotransverse joint with periostitis also is evident.

B The mechanism of injury appears to be anteroposterior compression. The posterior portions of the ribs are levered over the transverse processes, resulting in mechanical failure and fracture of the rib head (arrow).

(From Kleinman PK, et al: Radiology *185*:119, 1992.)

and cross sutures are suggestive of child abuse.[978] Pelvic fractures are rare. Diaphyseal or metaphyseal fractures, most commonly transverse,[979] can be seen in various stages of healing.[963] The metaphyseal infractions may be quite subtle, requiring multiple projections for adequate visualization. "Unusual" fractures such as those of the sternum, the lateral aspect of the clavicle, the scapula, and the vertebral bodies (especially the anterior portions) and posterior osseous elements[954, 975, 980, 981] should arouse suspicion of abuse. Other clues to correct diagnosis include overabundant callus formation, bilateral acute fractures, and fractures in the lower extremities in infants and young children who are not walking.[963, 982] Rib fractures that are bilateral and paravertebral[983] or involve the head of the rib[984] (Fig. 67–175) and those that conform in distribution to the size of an adult's fist are suggestive of child abuse. Injury of the spinal cord may accompany vertebral trauma.

Subperiosteal bone formation may be apparent between 7 to 14 days after the injury. It varies in appearance from focal, thin periosteal deposits to massive bone formation. Periostitis with intramedullary foci of necrosis also may represent the sequela of traumatically induced pancreatitis in the abused child.[943] Late skeletal findings include metaphyseal cupping, growth disturbances, subluxation, and diaphyseal widening due to subperiosteal apposition.

Extraosseous alterations may include cutaneous lesions, myositis, malnutrition with decrease in subcutaneous fat, pulmonary contusion and laceration with pneumothorax, gastrointestinal hemorrhage with mass formation and obstruction, pancreatitis, hepatic and renal injuries, mucosal

alterations in the mouth and palate, ocular lesions such as retinal detachment, and intracranial and subdural hematomas.[960, 964] Retinal hemorrhage is a consistent finding in those abused infants who have been shaken repeatedly and violently (the shaken baby syndrome), and is associated with elevated intracranial pressure related to intracranial and subdural hematomas.[985, 986]

The accurate diagnosis of the abused child syndrome is facilitated by radiographic changes that include multiple and unusual fractures in different stages of healing, metaphyseal infractions, and subperiosteal hemorrhage with periostitis. Disorders or conditions that must be differentiated from this syndrome are the normal periostitis of infancy, metaphyseal changes of normal growth,[987, 988] osteogenesis imperfecta,[989–992] types of congenital insensitivity to pain, spondylometaphyseal and metaphyseal dysplasias,[993, 994] and infantile cortical hyperostosis. The most helpful clues to distinguishing osteogenesis imperfecta from child abuse are the presence of blue sclerae or abnormal teeth, a family history of disease, the detection of wormian bones, and the absence of those types of fractures that are typical of child abuse.[1669] None of these features allows absolute differentiation between these two conditions, however, and children with osteogenesis imperfecta also may be abused.[991] Metaphyseal avulsion fractures similarly may accompany abnormal copper metabolism in the kinky hair syndrome (Menkes' syndrome).[995–999] Metaphyseal changes in a variety of other congenital disorders and scurvy may resemble those in the abused child syndrome.[1000]

Several other points of differential diagnosis should be mentioned. The typical age range of children with nonaccidental trauma is 1 to 4 years; after this age, children generally are able to escape the abusing parent or, at the very least, verbalize what has occurred. The usual accidental injuries in the young child are torus fractures of the distal portion of the radius, spiral fractures of the tibia (toddler's fractures), and clavicular and skull fractures. Accidental fractures of tubular bones require that the child be able to accelerate himself or herself; thus, an infant alone cannot break a humerus and a crawling child cannot break a femur. Rarely, passive exercise or physical therapy in premature children can result in injuries that simulate those of child abuse.[1001, 1002]

SUMMARY

In addition to such complications as reflex sympathetic dystrophy, osteolysis, osteonecrosis, many of the osteochondroses, neuropathic osteoarthropathy, heterotopic bone formation, and infection, physical trauma may lead to a variety of radiographic abnormalities. Radiologic characteristics of the fractures in the various skeletal sites are explained on the basis of biomechanical principles. Special types of injuries include pathologic, stress, greenstick, torus, bowing, and transchondral fractures, trabecular microfractures, and osseous infractions accompanying subluxations and dislocations. The precise cause of osteochondritis dissecans is not clear, but trauma is suspected. Trauma to synovial joints may lead to synovitis, hemarthrosis, and lipohemarthrosis; trauma to symphyses may result in intraosseous cartilaginous displacements (cartilaginous nodes); trauma to synchondroses may cause variable patterns of acute or chronic growth plate injury; and trauma to supporting structures, syndesmoses, and entheses may lead to tendinous and ligamentous laceration and disruption, avulsion, and diastasis. A variety of alterations occur in skeletal muscle related to physiologic stress and acute or chronic injury. Characteristic skeletal abnormalities also appear in the abused child.

References

1. Rockwood CA, Green DP: Fractures in Adults, 2nd Ed. Philadelphia, JB Lippincott Co, 1984.
2. Rogers LF: Radiology of Skeletal Trauma. 2nd Ed. New York, Churchill Livingstone, 1992.
3. Harris JH, Harris WH: The Radiology of Emergency Medicine. Baltimore, Williams & Wilkins Co, 1975.
4. Tachdjian MO: Pediatric Orthopedics. Philadelphia, WB Saunders Co, 1972.
5. Ayella RJ: Radiologic Management of the Massively Traumatized Patient. Baltimore, Williams & Wilkins Co, 1978.
6. Bowerman JW: Radiology and Injury in Sport. New York, Appleton-Century-Crofts, 1977.
7. Berquist TH: Imaging of Orthopedic Trauma. 2nd Ed. New York, Raven Press, 1991.
8. Browner BD, Jupiter JB, Levine AM, et al: Skeletal Trauma. Fractures, Dislocations, Ligamentous Injuries. Philadelphia, WB Saunders Co, 1992.
9. Resnick D: Skeletal aches and pains. Radiol Clin North Am 16:37, 1978.
10. Brand DA, Frazier WH, Kohlhepp WC, et al: A protocol for selecting patients with injured extremities who need x-rays. N Engl J Med 306:333, 1982.
11. DeSmet AA, Fryback DG, Thornbury JR: A second look at the utility of radiographic skull examination for trauma. AJR 132:95, 1979.
12. Thornbury JR, Campbell JA, Masters SJ, et al: Skull fracture and the low risk of intracranial sequelae in minor head trauma. AJR 143:661, 1984.
13. MacEwan DW, Bristow GK, Gordon WL: Managed reduction of unnecessary skull radiography. J Can Assoc Radiol 35:287, 1984.
14. Baker SR, Gaylord GM, Lantos G, et al: Emergency skull radiography: The effect of restrictive criteria on skull radiography and CT use. Radiology 156:409, 1985.
15. Freed HA: Posttraumatic skull films: Who needs them? Ann Emerg Med 15:233, 1986.
16. Thompson BM, Finger W, Tonsfeldt D, et al: Rib radiographs for trauma: Useful or wasteful. Ann Emerg Med 15:261, 1986.
17. DeLuca SA, Rhea JT, O'Malley TO: Radiographic evaluation of rib fractures. AJR 138:91, 1982.
18. Bell RS, Loop JW: The utility and futility of radiographic skull examination for trauma. N Engl J Med 284:236, 1971.
19. Phillips LA: A study of the effect of high yield criteria for emergency room skull radiography. Washington, DC: US Department of Health, Education, and Welfare Publication No. 73-8069, 1978.
20. Caffey J: Pediatric X-Ray Diagnosis. 5th Ed. Chicago, Year Book Medical Publishers, 1967.
21. Poznanski AK: Practical Approaches to Pediatric Radiology. Chicago, Year Book Medical Publishers, 1976.
22. Rang M: Children's Fractures. Philadelphia, JB Lippincott Co, 1974.
23. Merten D: Comparison radiographs in extremity injuries of childhood: Current application in radiological practice. Radiology 126:209, 1978.
24. McCauley RGK, Schwartz AM, Leonidas JC, et al: Comparison views in extremity injury in children: An efficacy study. Radiology 131:95, 1979.
25. Strange-Vorgnsen HH, Neergaard K, Schantz K: CT scan compared to tomography in suspected hip fracture. Arch Orthop Trauma Surg 111:132, 1992.
26. Egund N, Nilsson LT, Wingstrand H, et al: CT scans and lipohaemarthrosis in hip fractures. J Bone Joint Surg [Br] 72:379, 1990.
27. Halpern M, Freiberger RH: Arteriography in orthopedics. AJR 94:194, 1965.
28. McDonald EJ, Goodman PC, Winestock DP: The clinical indication for arteriography in trauma to the extremity. A review of 114 cases. Radiology 116:45, 1975.
29. Piyachon C, Arthachinta S: Arteriography in trauma of the extremities. AJR 119:580, 1973.
30. Chervu A, Quinones-Baldrich WJ: Vascular complications in orthopedic surgery. Clin Orthop 235:275, 1988.
31. Louis DS, Ricciardi JE, Spengler DM: Arterial injury: A complication of posterior elbow dislocation. A clinical and anatomical study. J Bone Joint Surg [Am] 56:1631, 1974.
32. Pradhan DJ, Juanteguy JM, Wilder RJ, et al: Arterial injuries of the extremities associated with fractures. Arch Surg 105:582, 1972.
33. Gainor BJ, Metzler M: Humeral shaft fracture with brachial artery injury. Clin Orthop 204:154, 1986.
34. Hall RF Jr, Gonzales M: Fracture of the proximal part of the tibia and fibula associated with an entrapped popliteal artery. A case report. J Bone Joint Surg [Am] 68:941, 1986.
35. Ring EJ, Athanasoulis C, Waltman AC, et al: Arteriographic management of hemorrhage following pelvic fracture. Radiology 109:65, 1973.
36. Jorgensen TM, Andresen JH, Thommesen P, et al: Scanning and radiology of the carpal scaphoid bone. Acta Orthop Scand 50:663, 1979.
37. Batillas J, Vasilas A, Pizzi WF, et al: Bone scanning in the detection of occult fractures. J Trauma 21:564, 1981.
38. Deininger HK: Die Skelettszintigraphie als Erganzung der traumatologischen Röntgendiagnostik. Radiologe 21:35, 1981.
39. Jung H, Schlenkhoff D, Barry BA, et al: Die Knochenszintigraphie mit 99mTechnetium-Phosphat-Komplexen in der Diagnostik von Frakturen spongiöser Knochen. Unfallheilkunde 83:103, 1980.
40. Fogelman I: Lesions in the ribs detected by bone scanning. Clin Radiol 31:317, 1980.
41. Hisada K, Suzuki Y, Iimori M: Technetium 99m pyrophosphate bone imaging in the evaluation of trauma. J Clin Nucl Med 1:18, 1976.
42. Rosenthall L, Hill RO, Chuang S: Observation on the use of 99mTc-phosphate imaging in peripheral bone trauma. Radiology 119:637, 1976.
43. Matin P: Bone scintigraphy in the diagnosis and management of traumatic injury. Semin Nucl Med 13:104, 1983.
44. Matin P: The appearance of bone scans following fractures, including immediate and long-term studies. J Nucl Med 20:1227, 1979.
45. Auchincloss JM, Watt I: Scintigraphy in the evaluation of potential fracture healing: A clinical study of tibial fractures. Br J Radiol 55:707, 1982.
46. Jacobs RR, Jackson RP, Preston DF, et al: Dynamic bone scanning in fractures. Injury 12:455, 1981.
47. O'Reilly RJ, Cook DJ, Gaffney RD, et al: Can serial scintigraphic studies detect delayed fracture union in man? Clin Orthop 160:227, 1981.
48. Gumerman LW, Fogel SR, Goodman MA, et al: Experimental fracture healing: Evaluation using radionuclide bone imaging: Concise communication. J Nucl Med 19:1320, 1978.
49. Hadjipavlou A, Lisbona R, Rosenthall L: Difficulty of diagnosing infected hypertrophic pseudarthrosis by radionuclide imaging. Clin Nucl Med 8:45, 1983.
50. Lund B, Lund JO, Sorensen OH, et al: Evaluation of fracture healing in man by serial 99mTc-Sn-pyrophosphate scintimetry. Acta Orthop Scand 49:435, 1978.
51. Desai A, Alavi A, Dalinka M, et al: Role of bone scintigraphy in the evaluation and treatment of nonunited fractures: Concise communication. J Nucl Med 21:931, 1980.
52. Quinn SF, McCarthy JL: Prospective evaluation of patients with suspected hip fracture and indeterminate radiographs: Use of T1-weighted MR images. Radiology 187:469, 1993.
53. Mink JH, Deutsch AL: Occult cartilage and bone injuries of the knee: Detection, classification, and assessment with MR imaging. Radiology 170:823, 1989.
54. Berger PE, Ofstein RA, Jackson DW, et al: MRI demonstration of radiographically occult fractures: What have we been missing? RadioGraphics 9:407, 1989.
55. Meyers SP, Wiener SN: Magnetic resonance imaging features of fractures using the short tau inversion recovery (STIR) sequence: Correlation with radiographic findings. Skel Radiol 20:499, 1991.
56. Orrison WW, Nord TE, Kinard RE, et al: The language of certainty: Proper terminology for the ending of the radiologic report. AJR 145:1093, 1985.
57. Pitt MJ, Speer DP: Radiographic reporting of orthopedic trauma. Med Radiogr Photogr 58:14, 1982.
58. Daves ML: Language of certainty. AJR 147:209, 1986.
59. Olerud S, Karlstrom GK, Danckwardt-Lilliestron G: Treatment of open fractures of the tibia and ankle. Clin Orthop 136:212, 1978.
60. Gustillo RB, Anderson JT: Prevention of infection in the treatment of one thousand and twenty-five open fractures of long bones. Retrospective and prospective analyses. J Bone Joint Surg [Am] 58:453, 1976.
61. Gustillo RB, Mendoza RM, Williams DN: Problems in the management of type III (severe) open fractures: A new classification of type III open fractures. J Trauma 24:742, 1984.
62. Houston CS, Swischuk LE: Varus and valgus—no wonder they are confused. N Engl J Med 302:471, 1980.
63. Naimark A, Kossoff J, Leach RE: The disparate diameter—a sign of rotational deformity in fractures. J Can Assoc Radiol 34:8, 1983.
64. Cruess RL, Dumont J: Healing of bone, tendon and ligament. In CA Rockwood Jr, DP Green (Eds): Fractures. Philadelphia, JB Lippincott, 1975, p 97.
65. Mûlholland MC, Pritchard JJ: The fracture gap (Abstr). J Anat 93:590, 1959.
66. McClements P, Templeton RW, Pritchard JJ: Repair of a bone gap (Abstr). J Anat 95:616, 1961.
67. Ham AW: A histological study of the early phases of bone repair. J Bone Joint Surg 12:827, 1930.
68. Lindholm R, Lindholm S, Liukko P, et al: The mast cell as a component of callus in healing fractures. J Bone Joint Surg [Br] 51:148, 1969.
69. McKibbin B: The biology of fracture healing in long bones. J Bone Joint Surg [Br] 60:150, 1978.
70. Simmons DJ: Fracture healing perspectives. Clin Orthop 200:100, 1985.
71. Collins PC, Paterson DC, Vernon-Roberts B, et al: Bone formation and impedance of electrical current flow. Clin Orthop 155:196, 1981.
72. Black J: Tissue response to exogenous electromagnetic signals. Orthop Clin North Amer 15:15, 1984.
73. Milgram JW: Radiologic and Histologic Pathology of Nontumorous Diseases of Bones and Joints. Northbrook, IL, Northbrook Publishing Co, 1990, p. 385.
74. Trotter DH, Doboz W: Nonunion of the humerus: Rigid fixation, bone grafting, and adjunctive bone cement. Clin Orthop 204:162, 1986.
75. Healy WL, White GM, Mick CA, et al: Nonunion of the humeral shaft. Clin Orthop 219:206, 1987.

76. Rooney PJ, Cockshott WP: Pseudarthrosis following proximal humeral fractures: A possible mechanism. Skel Radiol 15:21, 1986.
77. Manske DJ, Szabo RM: The operative treatment of mid-shaft clavicular nonunions. J Bone Joint Surg [Am] 67:1367, 1985.
78. Oni OOA, Graebe A, Pearse M, et al: Prediction of the healing potential of closed adult tibial shaft fractures by bone scintigraphy. Clin Orthop 245:239, 1989.
79. Wallace AL, Strachan RK, Best JJK, et al: Quantitative early phase scintigraphy in the prediction of healing of tibial fractures. Skel Radiol 21:241, 1992.
80. Keene JS, Sellinger DS, McBeath AA, et al: Metastatic breast cancer in the femur. A search for the lesion at risk of fracture. Clin Orthop 203:282, 1986.
81. Lee JK, Yao L: Occult intraosseous fracture: Magnetic resonance appearance versus age of injury. Am J Sports Med 17:620, 1989.
82. Yao L, Lee JK: Occult intraosseous fracture: Detection with MR imaging. Radiology 167:749, 1988.
83. Murphy BJ, Smith RL, Uribe JW, et al: Bone signal abnormalities in the posterolateral tibia and lateral femoral condyle in complete tears of the anterior cruciate ligament: A specific sign? Radiology 182:221, 1992.
84. Lance E, Deutsch AL, Mink JH: Prior lateral patellar dislocation: MR imaging findings. Radiology 189:905, 1993.
85. Kapelov SR, Teresi LM, Bradley WG, et al: Bone contusions of the knee: Increased lesion detection with fast spin-echo MR imaging with spectroscopic fat saturation. Radiology 189:901, 1993.
86. Kaplan PA, Walker CW, Kilcoyne RF, et al: Occult fracture patterns of the knee associated with anterior cruciate ligament tears: Assessment with MR imaging. Radiology 183:835, 1992.
87. Kirsch MD, Fitzgerald SW, Friedman H, et al: Transient lateral patellar dislocation: Diagnosis with MR imaging. AJR 161:109, 1993.
88. Daffner RH: Stress fractures: Current concepts. Skel Radiol 2:221, 1978.
89. Roub LW, Gumerman LW, Hanley EN Jr, et al: Bone stress: A radionuclide imaging perspective. Radiology 132:431, 1979.
90. Wilson ES Jr, Katz FN: Stress fractures. An analysis of 250 consecutive cases. Radiology 92:481, 1969.
91. Savoca CJ: Stress fractures. A classification of the earliest radiographic signs. Radiology 100:519, 1974.
92. Gilbert RS, Johnson HA: Stress fractures in military recruits—review of twelve years' experience. Milit Med 131:716, 1966.
93. Daffner RH, Pavlov H: Stress fractures: Current concepts. AJR 159:245, 1992.
94. Groshar D, Lam M, Even-Sapir E, et al: Stress fractures and bone pain: Are they closely associated? Injury 16:526, 1985.
95. Zatzkin HR: Trauma to the foot. Semin Roentgenol 5:419, 1970.
96. Protzman RR, Griffis CG: Stress fracture in men and women undergoing military training. J Bone Joint Surg [Am] 59:825, 1977.
97. Levy JM: Stress fractures of the first metatarsal. AJR 130:679, 1978.
98. Newberg AH, Kalisher L: Case report: An unusual stress fracture in a jogger. J Trauma 18:816, 1978.
99. Miller EH, Schneider HJ, Bronson JL, et al: A new consideration in athletic injuries. The classical ballet dancer. Clin Orthop 111:181, 1975.
100. Schneider HJ, King AY, Bronson JL, et al: Stress injuries and developmental change of lower extremities in ballet dancers. Radiology 113:627, 1974.
101. Miller F, Wenger DR: Femoral neck stress fracture in a hyperactive child. A case report. J Bone Joint Surg [Am] 61:435, 1979.
102. Sandrock AR: Another sports fatigue fracture. Stress fracture of the coracoid process of the scapula. Radiology 117:274, 1975.
103. Rasad S: Golfer's fractures of the ribs. Report of 3 cases. AJR 120:901, 1974.
104. Hallel T, Amit S, Segal D: Fatigue fractures of tibial and femoral shaft in soldiers. Clin Orthop 118:35, 1976.
105. Cohen HR, Becker MH, Genieser NB: Fatigue fracture in Hare Krishna converts. New group at risk. NY State J Med 74:1998, 1974.
106. Provost RA, Morris JM: Fatigue fracture of the femoral shaft. J Bone Joint Surg [Am] 51:487, 1969.
107. Brower AC, Neff JR, Tillema DA: An unusual scapular stress fracture. AJR 129:519, 1977.
108. Engber WD: Stress fractures of the medial tibial plateau. J Bone Joint Surg [Am] 59:767, 1977.
109. Lecestre P, Benoit J, Dabos N, et al: Les fractures de fatigue. A propos de 8 cas. Rev Chir Orthop 63:815, 1977.
110. Young RS, Bryk D, Ratner H: Selective phalangeal tuft fractures in a guitar player. Br J Radiol 50:147, 1977.
111. Meuerman KOA: Stress fracture of the pubic arch in military recruits. Br J Radiol 53:521, 1980.
112. Sammarco GJ: Diagnosis and treatment in dancers. Clin Orthop 187:176, 1984.
113. Sullivan DS, Warren RF, Pavlov H, et al: Stress fractures in 51 runners. Clin Orthop 187:188, 1984.
114. Greaney RB, Gerber FH, Laughlin RL, Kmet JP, Metz CD, Kilcheski TS, Rao BR, Silverman ED: Distribution and natural history of stress fractures in U.S. Marine recruits. Radiology 146:339, 1983.
115. Rappoport AS, Sosman JL, Weissman BN: Spontaneous fractures of the olecranon process in rheumatoid arthritis. Radiology 119:83, 1976.
116. Schneider R, Kaye JJ: Insufficiency and stress fractures of the long bones occurring in patients with rheumatoid arthritis. Radiology 116:595, 1975.
117. Miller B, Markheim HR, Towbin MN: Multiple stress fractures in rheumatoid arthritis. J Bone Joint Surg [Am] 49:1408, 1967.
118. Devas M: Stress Fractures. London, Churchill Livingstone, 1975.
119. Bauer G, Gustafsson M, Mortensson W, et al: Insufficiency fractures in the tibial condyles in elderly individuals. Acta Radiol (Diagn) 22:619, 1981.
120. Manco LG, Schneider R, Pavlov H: Insufficiency fractures of the tibial plateau. AJR 140:1211, 1983.
121. DeSmet AA, Neff JR: Pubic and sacral insufficiency fractures: Clinical course and radiologic findings. AJR 145:601, 1985.
122. Cooper KL, Beabout JW, Swee RG: Insufficiency fractures of the sacrum. Radiology 156:15, 1985.
123. Milkman LA: Pseudofractures (hunger osteopathy, late rickets, osteomalacia). Report of a case. AJR 24:29, 1930.
124. Ford LT, Gilula LA: Stress fractures of the middle metatarsals following the Keller operation. J Bone Joint Surg (Am) 59:117, 1977.
125. Michetti ML: March fracture following a McBride bunionectomy. A case report. J Am Podiatry Assoc 60:286, 1970.
126. Frede TE, Lee JK: Compensatory hypertrophy of bone following surgery on the foot. Radiology 146:347, 1983.
127. Oh I, Hardacre JA: Fatigue fracture of the inferior pubic ramus following total hip replacement for congenital hip dislocation. Clin Orthop 147:154, 1980.
128. Resnick D, Guerra J Jr: Stress fractures of the inferior pubic ramus following hip surgery. Radiology 137:335, 1980.
129. Torisu T: Fatigue fracture of the pelvis after total knee replacements: Report of a case. Clin Orthop 149:216, 1980.
130. Gaucher A, Pourel J, Wiederkehr P, et al: Stress fractures after tibial osteotomy. Rev Rhum Mal Osteoartic 49:204, 1982.
131. Cummings CW, First R: Stress fracture of the clavicle after a radical neck dissection. Case report. Plast Reconstr Surg 55:366, 1975.
132. Baumgarten C, Koischwitz D: Die "fehlende" Clavicula—Ein spezifischer knochenszintigraphischer Befund nach Ablatio mammae. Nuklearmedizin 21:262, 1982.
133. Zlatkin MB, Bjorkengren A, Sartoris D, et al: Stress fractures of the distal tibia and calcaneus subsequent to acute fractures of the tibia and fibula. AJR 149:329, 1987.
134. Schultz E: Case report 624. Skel Radiol 19:391, 1990.
135. Markey KL: Stress fractures. Clinics Sports Med 6:405, 1987.
136. Nagle CE, Freitas JE: Radionuclide imaging of musculoskeletal injuries in athletes with negative radiographs. Physician Sportsmed 15:147, 1987.
137. Charkes ND, Siddhivarn N, Schneck CD: Bone scanning in the adductor insertion avulsion syndrome ("thigh splints"). J Nucl Med 28:1835, 1987.
138. Milgrom C, Chisin R, Liebergall M: Bone Scintigraphic findings in recruits after short periods of nonweight-bearing ambulation. A report of two cases. Orthop Review 17:187, 1988.
139. Zwas ST, Elkanovitch R, Frank G: Interpretation and classification of bone scintigraphic findings in stress fractures. J Nucl Med 28:452, 1987.
140. Prather JL, Nusynowitz ML, Snowdy HA, et al: Scintigraphic findings in stress fractures. J Bone Joint Surg [Am] 59:869, 1977.
141. Geslien GE, Thrall JH, Espinosa JL, et al: Early detection of stress fractures using 99mTc-polyphosphate. Radiology 121:683, 1976.
142. Wilcox JR Jr, Moniot AL, Green JP: Bone scanning in the evaluation of exercise-related stress injuries. Radiology 123:699, 1977.
143. Mills GQ, Marymont JH III, Murphy DA: Bone scan utilization in the differential diagnosis of exercise-induced lower extremity pain. Clin Orthop 149:207, 1980.
144. Meuerman KOA, Elfving S: Stress fractures in soldiers: A multifocal bone disorder. Radiology 134:483, 1980.
145. Spencer RP, Levinson ED, Baldwin RD, et al: Diverse bone scan abnormalities in "shin splints." J Nucl Med 20:1271, 1979.
146. Saunders AJS, Sayed TF, Hilson AJW, et al: Stress lesions of the lower leg and foot. Clin Radiol 30:649, 1979.
147. Norfray JF, Schlachter L, Kernahan T Jr, et al: Early confirmation of stress fractures in joggers. JAMA 243:1647, 1980.
148. Rosen PR, Micheli LJ, Treves S: Early scintigraphic diagnosis of bone stress and fractures in athletic adolescents. Pediatrics 70:11, 1982.
149. Holder LE, Michael RH: The specific scintigraphic pattern of "shin splints in the lower leg": Concise communication. J Nucl Med 25:865, 1984.
150. Rupani HD, Holder LE, Espinola DA, et al: Three-phase radionuclide bone imaging in sports medicine. Radiology 156:187, 1985.
151. Sweet DE, Allman RM: Stress fracture. RPC of the month from the AFIP. Radiology 99:687, 1971.
152. Johnson LC: Morphologic analysis in pathology: The kinetics of disease and general biology of bone. In HH Frost (Ed): Bone Biodynamics. Henry Ford Hospital International Symposium, Boston, Little, Brown and Co, 1964, p 607.
153. Burr DB, Milgrom C, Boyd RD, et al: Experimental stress fractures of the tibia. Biological and mechanical aetiology in rabbits. J Bone Joint Surg [Br] 72:370, 1990.
154. Mori S, Burr DB: Increased intracortical remodeling following fatigue damage. Bone 14:103, 1993.
155. Brooks DB, Burstein AH, Frankel VH: The biomechanics of torsional fractures: The stress concentration of a drill hole. J Bone Joint Surg [Am] 52:507, 1970.
156. Chamay A: Mechanical and morphological aspects of experimental overload and fatigue in bone. J Biomech 3:263, 1970.
157. Wright TM, Hayes WC: The fracture mechanics of fatigue crack propagation in compact bone. J Biomed Mater Res 10:637, 1976.
158. Li G, Zhang S, Chen G, et al: Radiographic and histologic analyses of stress fracture in rabbit tibias. Am J Sports Med 13:285, 1985.

159. Jones HH, Priest JD, Hayes WC, et al: Humeral hypertrophy in response to exercise. J Bone Joint Surg [Am] 59:204, 1977.

160. Torg JS, Pollack H, Sweterlitsch P: The effect of competitive pitching on the shoulders and elbows of preadolescent baseball pitchers. Pediatrics 49:267, 1972.

161. Chamay A, Tschantz P: Mechanical influence in bone remodeling. Experimental research on Wolff's law. J Biomech 5:173, 1972.

162. Murcia M, Brennan RE, Edeiken J: Computed tomography of stress fracture. Skel Radiol 8:193, 1982.

163. Somer K, Meuerman KOA: Computed tomography of stress fractures. J Comput Assist Tomogr 6:109, 1982.

164. Howard CB, Lieberman N, Mozes G, et al: Stress fracture detected sonographically. AJR 159:1350, 1992.

165. Yousem D, Magid D, Fishman EK, et al: Computed tomography of stress fractures. J Comput Assist Tomogr 10:92, 1986.

166. Lequesne M, Coulomb R, Kahn MF: Fractures "de fatigue" longitudinale du tibia. Rev Rhum Mal Osteoartic 30:30, 1963.

167. Allen GJ: Longitudinal stress fractures of the tibia: Diagnosis with CT. Radiology 167:799, 1988.

168. Miniaci A, McLaren AC, Haddad RG: Longitudinal stress fracture of the tibia: Case report. J Can Assoc Radiol 39:221, 1988.

169. Goupille P, Quintrec J-SGL, Job-Deslandre C, et al: Longitudinal stress fractures of the tibia: Diagnosis with CT. Radiology 171:583, 1989.

170. Stafford SA, Rosenthal DI, Gebhardt MC, et al: MRI in stress fracture. AJR 147:553, 1986.

171. Froelich JW: Imaging of fractures: Stress and occult. J Rheumatol 18:4, 1991.

172. Lee JK, Yao L: Stress fractures: MR imaging. Radiology 169:217, 1988.

173. Martin SD, Healey JH, Horowitz S: Stress fracture. MRI. Orthopedics 16:75, 1993.

174. Matheson GO, Clement DB, McKenzie DC, et al: Stress fractures in athletes. A study of 320 cases. Am J Sports Med 15:46, 1987.

175. Daffner RH: Anterior tibial striations. AJR 143:651, 1984.

176. Winfield AC, Dennis JM: Stress fractures of the calcaneus. Radiology 72:415, 1959.

177. Hullinger CW: Insufficiency fracture of the calcaneus similar to march fracture of the metatarsal. J Bone Joint Surg 26:751, 1944.

178. Stein RE, Stelling FH: Stress fracture of the calcaneus in a child with cerebral palsy. J Bone Joint Surg [Am] 59:131, 1977.

179. Goergen TG, Venn-Watson EA, Rossman DJ, et al: Tarsal navicular stress fractures in runners. AJR 136:201, 1981.

180. Hunter LY: Stress fracture of the tarsal navicular. More frequent than we realize? Am J Sports Med 9:217, 1981.

181. Torg JS, Pavlov H, Cooley LH, et al: Stress fractures of the tarsal navicular. A retrospective review of twenty-one cases. J Bone Joint Surg [Am] 64:700, 1982.

182. Pavlov H, Torg JS, Freiberger RH: Tarsal navicular stress fractures: Radiographic evaluation. Radiology 148:641, 1983.

183. Campbell G, Warnekros W: A tarsal stress fracture in a long-distance runner. A case report. J Am Podiatry Assoc 73:532, 1983.

184. Hulkko A, Orava S, Peltokallio P, et al: Stress fracture of the navicular bone. Nine cases in athletes. Acta Orthop Scand 56:503, 1985.

185. Graff KH, Krahl H, Kirschberger R: Stressfrakturen des Os Naviculare Pedis. Z Orthop 124:228, 1986.

186. Ting A, King W, Yocum L, et al: Stress fractures of the tarsal navicular in long-distance runners. Clinics Sports Med 7:89, 1988.

187. Fitch KD, Blackwell JB, Gilmour WN: Operation for non-union of stress fracture of the tarsal navicular. J Bone Joint Surg [Br] 71:105, 1989.

188. Bateman JK: Broken hock in the greyhound. Repair methods and the plastic scaphoid. Vet Rec 70:621, 1958.

189. Kiss ZS, Khan KM, Fuller PJ: Stress fractures of the tarsal navicular bone: CT findings in 55 cases. AJR 160:111, 1993.

190. Orava S, Karpakka J, Hulkko A, et al: Stress avulsion fracture of the tarsal navicular. Am J Sports Med 19:392, 1991.

191. Meurman KOA, Elfving S: Stress fractures of the cuneiform bones. Br J Radiol 53:157, 1980.

192. Meurman KOA: Less common stress fractures in the foot. Br J Radiol 54:1, 1981.

193. Creighton R, Sonoga A, Gordon G: Stress fracture of the tarsal middle cuneiform bone. A case report. J Am Podiatr Assoc 80:489, 1990.

194. Chen JB: Cuboid stress fracture. A case report. J Am Podiatr Assoc 83:153, 1993.

195. Nicastro JF, Haupt HA: Probable stress fracture of the cuboid in an infant. A case report. J Bone Joint Surg [Am] 66:1106, 1984.

196. Symeonides PP: High stress fractures of the fibula. J Bone Joint Surg [Br] 62:192, 1980.

197. Orava S, Jormakka E, Hulkko A: Stress fractures in young athletes. Arch Orthop Trauma Surg 98:271, 1981.

198. Springer H-H, Brucki R: Ermudungsbruche der Fibula beim Jogging. Z Orthop 120:735, 1982.

199. Kozlowski K, Azouz M, Hoff D: Stress fracture of the fibula in the first decade of life. Report of eight cases. Pediatr Radiol 21:381, 1991.

200. Nussbaum AR, Treves ST, Micheli L: Bone stress lesions in ballet dancers: Scintigraphic assessment. AJR 150:851, 1988.

201. Kottmeier SA, Hanks GA, Kalenak A: Fibular stress fracture associated with distal tibiofibular synostosis in an athlete. A case report and literature review. Clin Orthop 281:195, 1992.

202. Orava S, Puranen J, Ala-Ketola L: Stress fractures caused by physical exercise. Acta Orthop Scand 49:19, 1978.

203. Devas M: Stress fractures in children. J Bone Joint Surg [Br] 45:528, 1963.

204. Pilgaard S, Poulsen JO, Christensen JH: Stress fractures. Acta Orthop Scand 47:167, 1976.

205. Daffner RH, Martinez S, Gehweiler JA Jr, et al: Stress fractures of the proximal tibia in runners. Radiology 142:63, 1982.

206. Singer M, Maudsley RH: Fatigue fractures of the lower tibia: A report of five cases. J Bone Joint Surg [Br] 36:647, 1954.

207. Burrows HJ: Fatigue infraction of the middle of the tibia in ballet dancers. J Bone Joint Surg [Br] 38:83, 1956.

208. Giladi M, Ahronson Z, Stein M, et al: Unusual distribution and onset of stress fractures in soldiers. Clin Orthop 192:142, 1985.

209. Orava S, Hulkko A: Stress fracture of the mid-tibial shaft. Acta Orthop Scand 55:35, 1984.

210. Davies AM, Evans N, Grimer RJ: Fatigue fractures of the proximal tibia simulating malignancy. Br J Radiol 61:903, 1988.

211. Rettig AC, Shelbourne D, McCarroll JR, et al: The natural history and treatment of delayed union stress fractures of the anterior cortex of the tibia. Am J Sports Med 16:250, 1988.

212. Nielsen MB, Hansen K, Hølmer P, et al: Tibial periosteal reactions in soldiers. A scintigraphic study of 29 cases of lower leg pain. Acta Orthop Scand 62:531, 1991.

213. Giladi M, Milgrom C, Simkin A, et al: Stress fractures and tibial bone width. A risk factor. J Bone Joint Surg [Br] 69:326, 1987.

214. Green NE, Rogers RA, Lipscomb AB: Nonunions of stress fractures of the tibia. Am J Sports Med 13:171, 1985.

215. Mubarak SJ, Gould RN, Lee YF, et al: The medial tibial stress syndrome. A cause of shin splints. Am J Sports Med 10:201, 1982.

216. Michael RH, Holder LE: The soleus syndrome. A cause of medial tibial stress (shin splints). Am J Sports Med 13:87, 1985.

217. Shelbourne KD, Fisher DA, Rettig AC, et al: Stress fractures of the medial malleolus. Am J Sports Med 16:60, 1988.

218. Schils JP, Andrish JT, Piraino DW, et al: Medial malleolar stress fractures in seven patients: Review of the clinical and imaging features. Radiology 185:219, 1992.

219. Satku K, Kumar VP, Pho RWH: Stress fractures of the tibia in osteoarthritis of the knee. J Bone Joint Surg [Br] 69:309, 1987.

220. Satku K, Kumar VP, Chacha PB: Stress fractures around the knee in elderly patients. A cause of acute pain in the knee. J Bone Joint Surg [Am] 72:918, 1990.

221. Giladi M, Milgrom C, Stein M, et al: External rotation of the hip. A predictor of risk for stress fractures. Clin Orthop 216:131, 1987.

222. Bédard D, Dussault RG, Jean J-P, et al: Fractures de fatigue du col fémoral. J Can Assoc Radiol 39:209, 1988.

223. Johansson C, Ekenman I, Törnkvist H, et al: Stress fractures of the femoral neck in athletes. The consequence of a delay in diagnosis. Am J Sports Med 18:524, 1990.

224. Pouilles JM, Bernard J, Tremollières F, et al: Femoral bone density in young male adults with stress fractures. Bone 10:105, 1989.

225. Ihmeidan IH, Tehranzadeh J, Oldman SA, et al: Case report 443. Skel Radiol 16:581, 1987.

226. Levin DC, Blazina ME, Levine E: Fatigue fractures of the shaft of the femur: Simulation of malignant tumor. Radiology 89:883, 1967.

227. Devas MB: Stress fractures of the femoral neck. J Bone Joint Surg [Br] 47:728, 1965.

228. Haggert GE, Eberle HJ: Bilateral stress fractures of the neck of the femur. A case report. Lahey Clin Bull 10:15, 1956.

229. Branch HE: March fractures of the femur. J Bone Joint Surg 26:387, 1944.

230. Hajek MR, Noble HB: Stress fractures of the femoral neck in joggers. Case reports and review of the literature. Am J Sports Med 10:112, 1982.

231. Butler JE, Brown SL, McConnell BG: Subtrochanteric stress fractures in runners. Am J Sports Med 10:228, 1982.

232. Lombardo SJ, Benson DW: Stress fractures of the femur in runners. Am J Sports Med 10:219, 1982.

233. Skinner HB, Cook SD: Fatigue failure stress of the femoral neck. A case report. Am J Sports Med 10:245, 1982.

234. Meurman KOA, Lamminen A: Strebfrakturen des Femurs bei Soldaten. ROFO 134:528, 1981.

235. Erne P, Burckhardt A: Femoral neck fatigue fracture. Arch Orthop Trauma Surg 97:213, 1980.

236. Blatz DJ: Bilateral femoral and tibial shaft stress fractures in a runner. Am J Sports Med 9:322, 1981.

237. Luchini MA, Sarokhan AJ, Micheli LJ: Acute displaced femoral-shaft fractures in long-distance runners. Two case reports. J Bone Joint Surg [Am] 65:689, 1983.

238. Milgrom C, Giladi M, Stein M, et al: Stress fractures in military recruits. A prospective study showing an unusually high incidence. J Bone Joint Surg [Br] 67:732, 1985.

239. Vento JA, Slavin JD Jr, O'Brien JJ, et al: Bilateral "simultaneous" femoral neck fractures following minimal stress. Clin Nucl Med 11:411, 1986.

240. Annan IH, Buxton RA: Bilateral stress fractures of the femoral neck associated with abnormal anatomy—a case report. Injury 17:164, 1986.

241. Meaney JEM, Carty H: Femoral stress fractures in children. Skel Radiol 21:173, 1992.

242. Wolfgang GL: Stress fracture of the femoral neck in a patient with open

capital femoral epiphyses. A case report. J Bone Joint Surg [Am] 59:680, 1977.

243. Devas MB: Compression stress fractures in man and the greyhound. J Bone Joint Surg [Br] 43:540, 1961.

244. Aro H, Dahlström S: Conservative management of distraction-type stress fractures of the femoral neck. J Bone Joint Surg [Br] 68:65, 1986.

245. Tountas AA, Waddell JP: Stress fractures of the femoral neck. A report of seven cases. Clin Orthop 210:160, 1986.

246. Milgrom C, Giladi M, Chisin R, Dizian R: The long-term followup of soldiers with stress fractures. Am J Sports Med 13:398, 1985.

247. Micheli LJ, Sohn RS, Solomon R: Stress fractures of the second metatarsal involving Lisfranc's joint in ballet dancers. J Bone Joint Surg [Am] 67:1372, 1985.

248. Eisele SA, Sammarco GJ: Fatigue fractures of the foot and ankle in the athlete. J Bone Joint Surg [Am] 75:290, 1993.

249. Anderson EG: Fatigue fractures of the foot. Injury 21:275, 1990.

250. Kitaoka HB, Cracchiolo A III: Stress fracture of the lateral metatarsals following double-stem silicone implant arthroplasty of the hallux metatarsophalangeal joint. Clin Orthop 239:211, 1989.

251. Drez D Jr, Young JC, Johnston RD, et al: Metatarsal stress fractures. Am J Sports Med 8:123, 1980.

252. DeLee JC, Evans JP, Julian J: Stress fracture of the fifth metatarsal. Am J Sports Med 11:349, 1983.

253. Black JR: Stress fractures of the foot in female soldiers: A two year survey. Milit Med 147:861, 1982.

254. Giladi M, Milgrom C, Kashtan H, et al: Recurrent stress fractures in military recruits. One-year follow-up of 66 recruits. J Bone Joint Surg [Br] 68:439, 1986.

255. Dickason JM, Fox JM: Fracture of the patella due to overuse syndrome in a child. A case report. Am J Sports Med 10:248, 1982.

256. Iwaya T, Takatori Y: Lateral longitudinal stress fracture of the patella: A report of three cases. J Pediatr Orthop 5:73, 1985.

257. Jerosch JG, Castro WHM, Jantea C: Stress fracture of the patella. Am J Sports Med 17:579, 1989.

258. Shiraishi M, Mizuta H, Kubota K, et al: Stress fracture of the proximal phalanx of the great toe. Foot Ankle 14:28, 1993.

259. Crain MR, El-Khoury GY: Stress fracture of the os peroneum. AJR 152:430, 1989.

260. Van Hal ME, Keene JS, Lange TA, et al: Stress fractures of the great toe sesamoids. Am J Sports Med 10:122, 1982.

261. Hulkko A, Orava S, Pellinen P, et al: Stress fractures of the sesamoid bones of the first metatarsophalangeal joint in athletes. Acta Orthop Trauma Surg 104:113, 1985.

262. Yokoe K, Mannoji T: Stress fracture of the proximal phalanx of the great toe. A report of three cases. Am J Sports Med 14:240, 1986.

263. Pavlov H, Nelson TL, Warren RF, et al: Stress fractures of the pubic ramus. A report of twelve cases. J Bone Joint Surg [Am] 64:1020, 1982.

264. Noakes TD, Smith JA, Lindenberg G, et al: Pelvic stress fractures in long distance runners. Am J Sports Med 13:120, 1985.

265. Latshaw RF, Kantner TR, Kalenak A, et al: A pelvic stress fracture in a female jogger. A case report. Am J Sports Med 9:54, 1981.

266. Mikawa Y, Watanabe R, Yamano Y, et al: Stress fracture of the body of pubis in a pregnant woman. Case report. Arch Orthop Trauma Surg 107:193, 1988.

267. Resnick D, Guerra J Jr: Stress fractures associated with adjacent osteoarthritis. J Rheumatol 8:161, 1981.

268. Gaucher A, Raul P, Wiederkehr P, et al: Fractures de contrainte des branches pubiennes. J Radiol 63:471, 1982.

269. Davies AM, Evans NS, Struthers GR: Parasymphyseal and associated insufficiency fractures of the pelvis and sacrum. Br J Radiol 61:103, 1988.

270. Jackson JE, Henderson BL, Lavender JP: Bone scintigraphy in parasymphyseal insufficiency fractures. Br J Radiol 61:859, 1988.

271. Czarnecki DJ, Till EW, Minikel JL: Unilateral sacral stress fracture in a runner. AJR 151:1255, 1988.

272. Hoang T-A, Nguyen TH, Daffner RH, et al: Case report 491. Skel Radiol 17:364, 1988.

273. Grier D, Wardell S, Sarwack J, et al: Fatigue fractures of the sacrum in children: Two case reports and a review of the literature. Skel Radiol 22:515, 1993.

274. Blomlie V, Lien HH, Iversen T, et al: Radiation-induced insufficiency fractures of the sacrum: Evaluation with MR imaging. Radiology 188:241, 1993.

275. Renner JB: Pelvic insufficiency fractures. Arthritis Rheum 33:426, 1990.

276. Hauge MD, Cooper KL, Litin SC: Insufficiency fractures of the pelvis that simulate metastatic disease. Mayo Clin Proc 63:807, 1988.

277. Abe H, Nakamura M, Takahashi S, et al: Radiation-induced insufficiency fractures of the pelvis: Evaluation with ^{99m}Tc-methylene diphosphonate scintigraphy. AJR 158:599, 1992.

278. Stroebel RJ, Ginsburg WW, McLeod RA: Sacral insufficiency fractures: An often unsuspected cause of low back pain. J Rheumatol 18:117, 1991.

279. Davies AM, Bradley SA: Iliac insufficiency fractures. Br J Radiol 64:305, 1991.

280. Khorasani R, Nagel JS, Tumeh SS: Radiologic vignette. Arthritis Rheum 34:1387, 1991.

281. Newhouse KE, El-Khoury GY, Buckwalter JA: Occult sacral fractures in osteopenic patients. J Bone Joint Surg [Am] 74:227, 1992.

282. Brahme SK, Cervilla V, Vint V, et al: Magnetic resonance appearance of sacral insufficiency fractures. Skel Radiol 19:489, 1990.

283. Lien HH, Blomlie V, Talle K, et al: Radiation-induced fracture of the sacrum: Findings on MR. AJR 159:227, 1992.

284. La Roche M, Rousseau H, Jacquemier J-M, et al: Unusual stress fracture on the roof of the acetabulum: Magnetic resonance imaging. J Rheumatol 18:115, 1991.

285. Davies AM, Evans NS, Struthers GR: Parasymphyseal and associated insufficiency fractures of the pelvis and sacrum. Br J Radiol 61:103, 1988.

286. Holden DL, Jackson DW: Stress fracture of the ribs in female rowers. Am J Sports Med 13:342, 1985.

287. Rettig AC: Stress fracture of the ulna in an adolescent tournament tennis player. Am J Sports Med 11:103, 1983.

288. Mutoh Y, Mori T, Suzuki Y, et al: Stress fracture of the ulna in athletes. Am J Sports Med 10:365, 1982.

289. Patel MR, Stricevic M: Stress fracture of the ulnar diaphysis: Review of the literature and report of a case. J Hand Surg [Am] 11:443, 1986.

290. Stark HH, Jobe FW, Boyes JH, et al: Fracture of the hook of the hamate in athletes. J Bone Joint Surg [Am] 59:575, 1977.

291. Carter PR, Eaton RG, Littler JW: Ununited fracture of the hook of the hamate. J Bone Joint Surg [Am] 59:583, 1977.

292. Torg JS, Moyer RA: Non-union of a stress fracture through the olecranon epiphyseal plate observed in an adolescent baseball pitcher. J Bone Joint Surg [Am] 59:264, 1977.

293. Nuber GW, Diment MT: Olecranon stress fractures in throwers. A report of two cases and a review of the literature. Clin Orthop 278:58, 1992.

294. Destouet JM, Murphy WA: Guitar player acro-osteolysis. Skel Radiol 6:275, 1981.

295. Fakharzadeh FF: Stress fracture of the finger in a bowler. J Hand Surg [Am] 14:241, 1989.

296. Bennett GE: Shoulder and elbow lesions of the professional baseball pitcher. JAMA 117:510, 1941.

297. Allen ME: Stress fracture of the humerus. A case study. Am J Sports Med 12:244, 1984.

298. Rettig AC, Beltz HF: Stress fracture in the humerus in an adolescent tennis tournament player. Am J Sports Med 13:55, 1985.

299. Bartsokas TW, Palin WD, Collier BD: An unusual stress fracture site: Mid-humerus. Physician Sportsmed 20:119, 1992.

300. Sterling JC, Calvo RD, Holden SC: An unusual stress fracture in a multiple sport athlete. Med Sci Sports Exercise 23:298, 1991.

301. Weigl K, Amrami B: Occupational stress fracture in an unusual location: Report of a case in the distal end of the shaft of the radius. Clin Orthop 147:222, 1980.

302. Farquharson-Roberts MA, Fulford PC: Stress fracture of the radius. J Bone Joint Surg [Br] 62:194, 1980.

303. Moss GD, Goldman A, Sheinkop M: Case report 219. Skel Radiol 9:148, 1982.

304. Perry CR, Perry HM III, Burdge RE: Stress fracture of the radius following a fracture of the ulna diaphysis. Clin Orthop 187:193, 1984.

305. Orloff AS, Resnick D: Fatigue fracture of the distal part of the radius in a pool player. Injury 17:418, 1986.

306. Howard RS II, Conrad GR: Ice cream scooper's hand. Report of an occupationally related stress fracture of the hand. Clin Nucl Med 17:721, 1992.

307. Schils JP, Freed HA, Richmond BJ, et al: Stress fracture of the acromion. AJR 155:1140, 1990.

308. Hanks GA, Kalenak A, Bowman LS, et al: Stress fractures of the carpal scaphoid. A report of four cases. J Bone Joint Surg [Am] 71:938, 1989.

309. Manzione M, Pizzutillo PD: Stress fracture of the scaphoid waist. A case report. Am J Sports Med 9:268, 1981.

310. Israeli A, Engel J, Ganel A: Possible fatigue fracture of the pisiform bone in volleyball players. Int J Sports Med 3:56, 1982.

311. Gurtler R, Pavlov H, Torg JS: Stress fracture of the ipsilateral first rib in a pitcher. Am J Sports Med 13:277, 1985.

312. Lankenner PA Jr, Micheli LJ: Stress fracture of the first rib. A case report. J Bone Joint Surg [Am] 67:159, 1985.

313. Sacchetti AD, Beswick DR, Morse SK: Rebound rib: Stress-induced first rib fracture. Ann Emerg Med 12:177, 1983.

314. Roberge RJ, Morgenstern MJ, Osborn H: Cough fracture of the ribs. Am J Emerg Med 2:513, 1984.

315. Kaye JJ, Nance EP Jr, Green NE: Fatigue fracture of the medial aspect of the clavicle. An academic rather than athletic injury. Radiology 144:89, 1982.

316. Mitchell EA, Elliot RB: Spontaneous fracture of the sternum in a youth with cystic fibrosis. J Pediatr 97:789, 1980.

317. Keating TM: Stress fracture of the sternum in a wrestler. Am J Sports Med 15:92, 1987.

318. Chen C, Chandnani V, Kang HS, et al: Insufficiency fracture of the sternum caused by osteopenia: Plain film findings in seven patients. AJR 154:1025, 1990.

319. Wiltse LL, Winter RB: Terminology and measurement of spondylolisthesis. J Bone Joint Surg [Am] 65:768, 1983.

320. Sheikholeslamzadeh S, Aalami-Harandi B, Fateh H: Spondylolisthesis of the cervical spine. Report of a case. J Bone Joint Surg [Br] 59:95, 1977.

321. Moseley I: Neural arch dysplasia of the sixth cervical vertebra. "Congenital cervical spondylolisthesis." Br J Radiol 49:81, 1976.

322. Bellamy R, Lieber A, Smith SD: Congenital spondylolisthesis of the sixth cervical vertebra. Case report and description of operative findings. J Bone Joint Surg [Am] 56:405, 1974.

323. Charlton OP, Gehweiler JA Jr, Martinez S, et al: Spondylolysis and spondylolisthesis of the cervical spine. Skel Radiol 3:79, 1978.

324. Kosnik EJ, Johnson JC, Scoles PV, et al: Cervical spondylolisthesis. Spine 4:203, 1979.

325. Ferriter PJ, O'Leary P, Block J, et al: Cervical spondylolisthesis. A case report. Spine 9:830, 1984.

326. Hasue M, Kikuchi S, Matsui T, et al: Spondylolysis of the axis. Report of four cases. Spine 8:901, 1983.

327. Karasick S, Karasick D, Wechsler RJ: Unilateral spondylolysis of the cervical spine. Skel Radiol 9:259, 1983.

328. Edwards MG, Wesolowski D, Benson MT, et al: Computed tomography of congenital spondylolisthesis of the sixth cervical vertebra. Clin Imaging 15:191, 1991.

329. Forsberg DA, Martinez S, Vogler JB III, et al: Cervical spondylolysis: Imaging findings in 12 patients. AJR 154:751, 1990.

330. Coughlin WF, McMurdo SK: CT diagnosis of spondylolysis of the axis vertebra. AJR 153:195, 1989.

331. Nordström REA, Lahdenranta TV, Kaitila II, et al: Familial spondylolisthesis of the axis vertebra. J Bone Joint Surg [Br] 68:704, 1986.

332. Lowe J, Libson E, Ziv I, et al: Spondylolysis in the upper lumbar spine. A study of 32 patients. J Bone Joint Surg [Br] 69:582, 1987.

333. Ravichandran G: Upper lumbar spondylolysis. Int Orthop (SICOT) 5:31, 1981.

334. Ravichandran G: Multiple lumbar spondylolyses. Spine 5:552, 1980.

335. Mathiesen F, Simper LB, Seerup A: Multiple spondylolyses and spondylolistheses. Br J Radiol 57:338, 1984.

336. Porter RW, Hibbert CS: Symptoms associated with lysis of the pars interarticularis. Spine 9:755, 1984.

337. Edelson JG, Nathan H: Nerve root compression in spondylolysis and spondylolisthesis. J Bone Joint Surg [Br] 68:596, 1986.

338. Eisenstein S: Spondylolysis. A skeletal investigation of two population groups. J Bone Joint Surg [Br] 60:488, 1978.

339. Willis TA: The separate neural arch. J Bone Joint Surg 13:709, 1931.

340. Roche MB, Rowe GG: The incidence of separate neural arch and coincidental bone variations. Anat Rec 109:233, 1951.

341. Fredrickson BE, Baker D, McHolick WJ, et al: The natural history of spondylolysis and spondylolisthesis. J Bone Joint Surg [Am] 66:699, 1984.

342. Hasebe K: Die Wirbelsäule der Japaner. Z Morphol Anthropol 15:259, 1912.

343. Stewart TD: The age incidence of neural-arch defects in Alaskan natives, considered from the standpoint of etiology. J Bone Joint Surg [Am] 35:937, 1953.

344. Wiltse LL, Widell EH Jr, Jackson DW: Fatigue fracture: The basic lesion in isthmic spondylolisthesis. J Bone Joint Surg [Am] 57:17, 1975.

345. Merbs CF: Spondylolysis: Its nature and anthropological significance. Int J Anthropol 4:163, 1989.

346. Meyerding AW: Low backache and sciatic pain associated with spondylolisthesis and protruded intervertebral disc: Incidence, significance, and treatment. J Bone Joint Surg 23:461, 1941.

347. Nathan H: Spondylolysis. J Bone Joint Surg [Am] 41:303, 1959.

348. Batts M Jr: The etiology of spondylolisthesis. J Bone Joint Surg 21:879, 1939.

349. Wiltse LL: The etiology of spondylolisthesis. J Bone Joint Surg [Am] 44:539, 1962.

350. Borkow SE, Kleiger B: Spondylolisthesis in the newborn. A case report. Clin Orthop 81:73, 1971.

351. Wertzberger KL, Peterson HA: Acquired spondylolysis and spondylolisthesis in the young child. Spine 5:437, 1980.

352. Baker DR, McHollick W: Spondyloschisis and spondylolisthesis in children. J Bone Joint Surg [Am] 38:933, 1956.

353. Farfan HF, Osteria V, Lamy C: The mechanical etiology of spondylosis and spondylolisthesis. Clin Orthop 117:40, 1976.

354. Hadley LA: Stress fracture with spondylolysis. Am J Roentgenol 90:1258, 1963.

355. Cyron BM, Hutton WC, Troup JDG: Spondylolytic fracture. J Bone Joint Surg [Br] 58:462, 1976.

356. Cyron BM, Hutton WC: The fatigue strength of the lumbar neural arch in spondylolysis. J Bone Joint Surg [Br] 60:234, 1978.

357. Cyron BM, Hutton WC: Variations in the amount and distribution of cortical bone across the partes interarticulares of L5. A predisposing factor in spondylolysis? Spine 4:163, 1979.

358. Krenz J, Troup JDG: The structure of the pars interarticularis of the lower lumbar vertebrae and its relation to the etiology of spondylolysis, with a report of a healing fracture in the neural arch of a fourth lumbar vertebra. J Bone Joint Surg [Br] 55:735, 1973.

359. Fullenlove TM, Wilson JG: Traumatic defects of the pars interarticularis of the lumbar vertebrae. AJR 122:634, 1974.

360. Rowe GG, Roches MB: The etiology of separate neural arch. J Bone Joint Surg [Am] 35:102, 1953.

361. Dietrich M, Kurowski P: The importance of mechanical factors in the etiology of spondylolysis. A model analysis of loads and stresses in human lumbar spine. Spine 10:532, 1985.

362. Hensinger RN: Spondylolysis and spondylolisthesis in children and adolescents. J Bone Joint Surg [Am] 71:1098, 1989.

363. Pfeil E: Experimentelle Untersuchugen zur Frage der Entstehung der Spondylolyse. Z Orthop 109:231, 1971.

364. Lamy C, Eng B, Bazergui A, et al: The strength of the neural arch and the etiology of spondylolysis. Orthop Clin North Am 6:215, 1975.

365. Schulitz KP, Niethard FU: Strain on the interarticular stress distribution. Arch Orthop Trauma Surg 96:197, 1980.

366. Swärd L, Hellström M, Jacobsson B, et al: Spondylolysis and the sacrohorizontal angle in athletes. Acta Radiologica 30:359, 1989.

367. Ireland ML, Micheli LJ: Bilateral stress fracture of the lumbar pedicles in a ballet dancer. A case report. J Bone Joint Surg [Am] 69:140, 1987.

368. Traughber PD, Havlina JM Jr: Bilateral pedicle stress fractures: SPECT and CT features. J Comput Assist Tomogr 15:338, 1991.

369. Jackson DW, Wiltse LL, Dingeman RD: Stress reactions involving the pars interarticularis in young athletes. Am J Sports Med 9:304, 1981.

370. Abel MS: Jogger's fracture and other stress fractures of the lumbosacral spine. Skel Radiol 13:221, 1985.

371. Mau H: Scoliosis and spondylolysis-spondylolisthesis. Arch Orthop Trauma Surg 99:29, 1981.

372. Brunet JA, Wiley JJ: Acquired spondylolysis after spinal fusion. J Bone Joint Surg [Br] 66:720, 1984.

373. Friedman RJ, Michelli LJ: Acquired spondylolisthesis following scoliosis surgery. A case report. Clin Orthop 190:132, 1984.

374. Rosenberg NJ, Bargar WL, Friedman B: The incidence of spondylolysis and spondylolisthesis in nonambulatory patients. Spine 6:35, 1981.

375. Murray RO, Colwill MR: Stress fractures of the pars interarticularis. Proc R Soc Med 61:555, 1968.

376. Zippel H, Runge H: Pathologische Anatomie und Pathogenese von Spondylolyse und Spondylolisthesis im Kindesalter. Z Orthop 114:189, 1976.

377. Rabushka SE, Apfelbach H, Love L: Spontaneous healing of spondylolysis of the fifth lumbar vertebra. Case report. Clin Orthop 93:256, 1973.

378. Shahriaree H, Sajadi K, Rooholamini SA: A family with spondylolisthesis. J Bone Joint Surg [Am] 61:1256, 1979.

379. Troup JDG: The etiology of spondylolysis. Orthop Clin North Am 8:57, 1977.

380. Wiltse LL, Newman PH, Macnab I: Classification of spondylolysis and spondylolisthesis. Clin Orthop 117:23, 1976.

381. Leger J-L, Bouchard R, Maltais R: Étude radiologique de 305 cas de spondylolyse avec ou sans spondylolisthesis. J Can Assoc Radiol 30:86, 1979.

382. Epstein BS, Epstein JA, Jones MD: Lumbar spondylolisthesis with isthmic defects. Radiol Clin North Am 15:261, 1977.

383. Lisbon E, Bloom RA: Anteroposterior angulated view. A new radiographic technique for the evaluation of spondylolysis. Radiology 149:315, 1983.

384. Dubowitz B, Friedman L, Papert B: The oblique cranial tilt view for spondylolysis. J Bone Joint Surg [Br] 69:421, 1987.

385. El-Khoury GY, Yousefzadeh DK, Kathol MH, et al: Pseudospondylolysis. Radiology 139:72, 1981.

386. Amato M, Totty WH, Gilula LA: Spondylolysis of the lumbar spine: Demonstration of defects and laminal fragmentation. Radiology 153:627, 1984.

387. Lowe RW, Hayes TD, Kaye J: Standing roentgenograms in spondylolisthesis. Clin Orthop 117:80, 1976.

388. Leger JL, Bouchard R, Maltais R: Etude radiologique de 305 cas de spondylolyse avec ou sans spondylolisthesis. J Can Assoc Radiol 30:86, 1979.

389. Saraste H, Brostrom L-A, Aparisi T: Radiographic assessment of anatomic deviations in lumbar spondylolysis. Acta Radiol (Diagn) 25:317, 1984.

390. Sherman FC, Wilkinson RH, Hall JE: Reactive sclerosis of a pedicle and spondylolysis in the lumbar spine. J Bone Joint Surg [Am] 59:49, 1977.

391. Aland C, Rineberg BA, Malberg M, et al: Fracture of the pedicle of the fourth lumbar vertebra associated with contralateral spondylolysis. Report of a case. J Bone Joint Surg [Am] 68:1454, 1986.

392. O'Beirne JG, Horgan JG: Stress fracture of the lamina associated with unilateral spondylolysis. Spine 13:220, 1988.

393. Segal D, Franchi AV: Congenital absence of lumbar facets as a cause of lower-back pain. Spine 11:78, 1986.

394. Degesys GE, Miller GA, Newman GE, et al: Absence of a pedicle in the spine. Metastatic disease versus aplasia. Spine 11:76, 1986.

395. Downey EF Jr, Whiddon SM, Brower AC: Computed tomography of congenital absence of posterior elements in the thoracolumbar spine. Spine 11:68, 1986.

396. Lederman HM, Kaufman RA: Congenital absence and hypoplasia of pedicles in the thoracic spine. Skel Radiol 15:219, 1986.

397. Ravichandran G: A radiologic sign in spondylolisthesis. AJR 134:293, 1980.

398. Penning L, Blickman JR: Instability in lumbar spondylolisthesis: A radiologic study of several concepts. AJR 134:293, 1980.

399. McCormick CC, Taylor JR, Twomey LT: Facet joint arthrography in lumbar spondylolysis: Anatomic basis for spread of contrast medium. Radiology 171:193, 1989.

400. Bellah RD, Summerville DA, Treves ST, et al: Low-back pain in adolescent athletes: Detection of stress injury to the pars interarticularis with SPECT. Radiology 180:509, 1991.

401. Oakley RH: Review of spondylolisthesis and spondylolysis in paediatric practice. Br J Radiol 57:877, 1984.

402. Jackson DW, Wiltse LL, Cirincione RJ: Spondylolysis in the female gymnast. Clin Orthop 117:68, 1976.

403. Lowe J, Schachner E, Hirschberg E, et al: Significance of bone scintigraphy in symptomatic spondylolysis. Spine 9:653, 1984.

404. Gelfand MJ, Strife JL, Kereiakes JG: Radionuclide bone imaging in spondylolysis of the lumbar spine in children. Radiology 140:191, 1981.

405. Collier BD, Johnson RP, Carrera GF, et al: Painful spondylolysis or spondylolisthesis studied by radiography and single-photon emission computed tomography. Radiology 154:207, 1985.

406. Papanicolaou N, Wilkinson RH, Emans JB, et al: Bone scintigraphy and radiography in young athletes with low back pain. AJR 145:1039, 1985.

407. Pennell RG, Maurer AH, Bonakdarpour A: Stress injuries of the pars interarticularis: Radiologic classification and indications for scintigraphy. AJR 145:763, 1985.

408. Elliott S, Hutson MA, Wastie ML: Bone scintigraphy in the assessment of spondylolysis in patients attending a sports injury clinic. Clin Radiol 39:269, 1988.

409. van den Oever M, Merrick MV, Scott JHS: Bone scintigraphy in symptomatic spondylolysis. J Bone Joint Surg [Br] 69:453, 1987.

410. Rothman SLG, Glenn WV Jr: CT multiplanar reconstruction in 253 cases of lumbar spondylolysis. Am J Neuroradiol 5:81, 1984.

411. Langston JW, Gavant ML: "Incomplete ring" sign: A simple method for CT detection of spondylolysis. J Comput Assist Tomogr 9:728, 1985.

412. Johansen JG, McCarty DJ, Haughton VM: Retrosomatic clefts: Computed tomographic appearance. Radiology 148:447, 1983.

413. Lang PH, Genant HK, Chafetz NI, et al: Magnetre sonanztumographie bei Spondylolyse und Spondylolisthese. Z Orthop 126:651, 1988.

414. Grenier N, Kressel HY, Schiebler ML, et al: Isthmic spondylolysis of the lumbar spine: MR imaging at 1.5 T. Radiology 170:489, 1989.

415. Johnson DW, Farnum GN, Latchaw RE, et al: MR imaging of the pars interarticularis. AJR 152:327, 1989.

416. Jinkins JR, Matthes JC, Sener RN, et al: Spondylolysis, spondylolisthesis, and associated nerve root entrapment in the lumbosacral spine: MR evaluation. AJR 159:799, 1992.

417. Grobler LJ, Robertson PA, Novotny JE, et al: Etiology of spondylolisthesis. Assessment of role played by lumbar facet joint morphology. Spine 18:80, 1993.

418. Heggeness MH, Esses SI, Kostuik JP: Acquisition of lytic spondylolisthesis in the adult. J Spinal Dis 4:486, 1991.

419. McPhee IB, O'Brien JP, McCall IW, et al: Progression of lumbosacral spondylolisthesis. Australas Radiol 25:91, 1981.

420. Danielson B, Frennered K, Irstam L: Roentgenologic assessment of spondylolisthesis. I. A study of measurement variations. Acta Radiol Diagn 29:345, 1988.

421. Kälebo P, Kadziolka R, Swärd L, et al: Stress views in the comparative assessment of spondylolytic spondylolisthesis. Skel Radiol 17:570, 1989.

422. Schlenzka D, Seitsalo S, Poussa M, et al: Premature disc degeneration: Source of pain in isthmic spondylolisthesis in adolescents? J Pediatr Orthop 1:153, 1993.

423. Annertz M, Holtäs S, Cronqvist S, et al: Isthmic lumbar spondylolisthesis with sciatica. MR imaging vs myelography. Acta Radiol Diagn 31:449, 1990.

424. Birch JG, Herring JA, Maravilla KR: Splitting of the intervertebral disc in spondylolisthesis: A magnetic resonance imaging finding in two cases. J Pediatr Orthop 6:609, 1986.

425. Henson J, McCall IW, O'Brien JP: Disc damage above a spondylolisthesis. Br J Radiol 60:69, 1987.

426. Pfister-Goedek L, Braune M: Cyst-like cortical defects following fractures in children. Pediatr Radiol 11:93, 1981.

427. Malghem J, Maldague B: Transient fatty cortical defects following fractures in children. Skel Radiol 15:368, 1986.

428. Moore TE, King AR, Travis RC, et al: Post-traumatic cysts and cyst-like lesions of bone. Skel Radiol 18:93, 1989.

429. Davids JR, Graner KA, Mubarak SJ: Post-fracture lipid inclusion cyst. A case report. J Bone Joint Surg [Am] 75:1528, 1993.

430. Phillips CD, Keats TE: The development of post-traumatic cyst-like lesions in bone. Skel Radiol 15:631, 1986.

431. Silverman FN: Problems in pediatric fractures. Semin Roentgenol 13:167, 1978.

432. Light TR, Ogden DA, Ogden JA: The anatomy of metaphyseal torus fractures. Clin Orthop 188:103, 1984.

433. Naga AH, Broadrick GL: Traumatic bowing of the radius and ulna in children. NC Med J 38:452, 1977.

434. Crowe JE, Swischuk LE: Acute bowing fractures of the forearm in children: A frequently missed injury. AJR 128:981, 1977.

435. Rydholm U, Nilsson JE: Traumatic bowing of the forearm. A case report. Clin Orthop 139:121, 1979.

436. Borden S IV: Traumatic bowing of the forearm in children. J Bone Joint Surg [Am] 56:611, 1974.

437. Borden S IV: Roentgen recognition of acute plastic bowing of the forearm in children. AJR 125:524, 1975.

438. Manoli A II: Traumatic fibular bowing with tibial fracture: Report of two cases. Orthopedics 1:145, 1978.

439. Voumard C, Lopez J, Queloz J, et al: Les fractures plastiques de l'avant-bras chez l'enfant. Ann Radiol 21:551, 1978.

440. Cook GC, Bjelland JC: Acute bowing fracture of the fibula in an adult. Radiology 131:637, 1979.

441. Martin W III, Riddervold HO: Acute plastic bowing fractures of the fibula. Radiology 131:639, 1979.

442. Cail WS, Keats TE, Sussman MD: Plastic bowing fracture of the femur in a child. AJR 130:780, 1978.

443. Stenström R, Gripenberg L, Bergius A-R: Traumatic bowing of forearm and lower leg in children. Acta Radiol (Diagn) 19:243, 1978.

444. Sanders WE, Heckman JD: Traumatic plastic deformation of the radius and ulna. A closed method of correction of deformity. Clin Orthop 188:58, 1984.

445. Greene WB: Traumatic bowing of the forearm in an adult. Clin Orthop 168:31, 1982.

446. Golimbu C, Firooznia H, Rafii M, et al: Acute traumatic fibular bowing associated with tibial fractures. Clin Orthop et al: 182:211, 1984.

447. Zionts LE, Leffers D, Oberto MR, et al: Plastic bowing of the femur in a neonate. J Pediatr Orthop 4:749, 1984.

448. Tetiz CC, Carter DR, Frankel VH: Problems associated with tibial fractures with intact fibulae. J Bone Joint Surg [Am] 62:770, 1980.

449. Bowen A: Plastic bowing of the clavicle in children. A report of two cases. J Bone Joint Surg [Am] 65:403, 1983.

450. Orenstein E, Dvonch V, Demos T: Acute traumatic bowing of the tibia without fracture. Case report. J Bone Joint Surg [Am] 67:965, 1985.

451. Caro PA, Borden S IV: Plastic bowing of the ribs in children. Skel Radiol 17:255, 1988.

452. Miller JH, Osterkamp JA: Scintigraphy in acute plastic bowing of the forearm. Radiology 142:742, 1982.

453. Tavarez LA, Kottamasu SR, Ezhuthachan SG, et al: Neonatal skull depression: Review of four cases. J Perinatol 9:423, 1989.

454. Saunders BS, Lazoritz S, McArtor RD, et al: Depressed skull fracture in neonate. Report of three cases. J Neurosurg 50:512, 1976.

455. Nadas S, Gudinchet F, Capasso P, et al: Predisposing factors in obstetrical fractures. Skel Radiol 22:195, 1993.

456. Joseph PR, Rosenfeld W: Clavicular fractures in neonates. Am J Dis Child 144:165, 1990.

457. Cohen AW, Otto SR: Obstetric clavicular fractures: A three-year analysis. J Reprod Med 25:119, 1980.

458. Katz R, Landman J, Dulitsky F, et al: Fracture of the clavicle in the newborn. An ultrasound diagnosis. J Ultrasound Med 7:21, 1988.

459. Hägglund G, Hanson LI, Wiberg G: Correction of deformity after femoral birth fracture: 16 year follow-up. Acta Orthop Scand 59:333, 1988.

460. Madsen ET: Fractures of the extremities in the newborn. Acta Obstet Gynecol Scand 34:41, 1955.

461. Kellner KR: Neonatal fracture and cesarean section. Am J Dis Child 136:865, 1982.

462. Dunbar JS, Owen HF, Nogrady MB, et al: Obscure tibial fracture of infants—the toddler's fracture. J Can Assoc Radiol 15:136, 1964.

463. Starshak RJ, Simons GW, Sty JR: Occult fracture of the calcaneus—another toddler's fracture. Pediatr Radiol 14:37, 1984.

464. Park H, Kernek CB, Robb JA: Early scintigraphic findings of occult femoral and tibial fractures in infants. Clin Nucl Med 13:271, 1988.

465. Moss EH, Carty H: Scintigraphy in the diagnosis of occult fractures of the calcaneus. Skel Radiol 19:575, 1990.

466. Oudjhane K, Newman B, Oh KS, et al: Occult fractures in preschool children. J Trauma 28:858, 1988.

467. Conway JJ, Poznanski AP: Acute compression injuries of bone, or the toddler's fracture revised. Pediatr Radiol 17:85, 1987.

468. Gross RH: Causative factors responsible for femoral fractures in infants and young children. J Can Assoc Radiol 15:136, 1983.

469. Milgram JW, Rogers LF, Miller JW: Osteochondral fractures: Mechanisms of injury and fate of fragments. AJR 130:651, 1978.

470. Milgram JW: The classification of loose bodies in human joints. Clin Orthop 124:282, 1977.

471. Milgram JW: The development of loose bodies in human joints. Clin Orthop 124:292, 1977.

472. Tomatsu T, Imai N, Takeuchi N, et al: Experimentally produced fractures of articular cartilage and bone. The effects of shear forces on the pig knee. J Bone Joint Surg [Br] 74:457, 1992.

473. Hudson TM: Joint fluoroscopy before arthrography: Detection and evaluation of loose bodies. Skel Radiol 12:199, 1984.

474. Sartoris DJ, Kursunoglu S, Pineda C, et al: Detection of intra-articular osteochondral bodies in the knee using computed arthrotomography. Radiology 155:447, 1985.

475. Vellet AD, Marks PH, Fowler PJ, et al: Occult posttraumatic osteochondral lesions of the knee: Prevalence, classification, and short-term sequelae evaluated with MR imaging. Radiology 178:271, 1991.

476. Stallenberg B, Gevenois PA, Sintzoff SA Jr, et al: Fracture of the posterior aspect of the lateral tibial plateau: Radiographic sign of anterior cruciate ligament tear. Radiology 187:821, 1993.

477. Weber WN, Neumann CH, Barakos JA, et al: Lateral tibial rim (Segond) fractures: MR imaging characteristics. Radiology 180:731, 1991.

478. Deutsch AL, Mink JH: Magnetic resonance imaging of musculoskeletal injuries. Radiol Clin North Am 27:983, 1989.

479. Warren RF, Kaplan N, Bach BR: The lateral notch sign of anterior cruciate ligament insufficiency. Am J Knee Surg 1:119, 1988.

480. Cobby MJ, Schweitzer ME, Resnick D: The deep lateral femoral notch: An indirect sign of a torn anterior cruciate ligament. Radiology 184:855, 1992.

481. Virolainen H, Visuri T, Kuusela T: Acute dislocation of the patella: MR findings. Radiology 189:243, 1993.

482. Pick M: Familial osteochondritis dissecans. J Bone Joint Surg [Br] 37:142, 1955.

483. Stougaard J: Familial occurrence of osteochondritis dissecans. J Bone Joint Surg [Br] 46:542, 1964.

484. Stougaard J: The hereditary factor in osteochondritis dissecans. J Bone Joint Surg [Br] 43:256, 1961.

485. Hanley W, McKusick VA, Barranco FT: Osteochondritis dissecans with as-

sociated malformations in two brothers: A review of familial aspects. J Bone Joint Surg [Am] 49:925, 1967.

486. Auld CD, Chesney RB: Familial osteochondritis dissecans and carpal tunnel syndrome. Acta Orthop Scand 50:727, 1979.

487. Andrew TA, Spivey J, Lindebaum RH: Familial osteochondritis dissecans and dwarfism. Acta Orthop Scand 52:519, 1981.

488. Kozlowski K, Middleton R: Familial osteochondritis dissecans: A dysplasia of articular cartilage? Skel Radiol 13:207, 1985.

489. Phillips HO, Grubb SA: Familial multiple osteochondritis dissecans. Report of a kindred. J Bone Joint Surg [Am] 67:155, 1985.

490. Paes RA: Familial osteochondritis dissecans. Clin Radiol 40:501, 1989.

491. Fonseca AS, Keret D, MacEwen GD: Familial osteochondritis dissecans. Orthopedics 13:1259, 1990.

492. Robinson RP, Franck WA, Carey EJ Jr, et al: Familial polyarticular osteochondritis dissecans masquerading as juvenile rheumatoid arthritis. J Rheumatol 5:2, 1978.

493. Barrie HJ: Hypothesis—a diagram of the form and origin of loose bodies in osteochondritis dissecans. J Rheumatol 11:512, 1984.

494. Delahaye RP, Doury P, Pattin S, et al: Les fractures des métatarsiens. Rev Rhum Mal Osteoartic 43:707, 1976.

495. Barrie HJ: Osteochondritis dissecans 1887–1987. A centennial look at König's memorable phrase. J Bone Joint Surg [Br] 69:693, 1987.

496. Pappas AM: Osteochondrosis dissecans. Clin Orthop 158:59, 1981.

497. Evans DL: Fatigue fracture of the ulna. J Bone Joint Surg [Br] 37:618, 1955.

498. Bradley J, Dandy DJ: Osteochondritis dissecans and other lesions of the femoral condyles. J Bone Joint Surg [Br] 71:518, 1989.

499. Clanton TO, DeLee JC: Osteochondritis dissecans. History, pathophysiology and current treatment concepts. Clin Orthop 167:50, 1982.

500. Barrie HJ: Hypertrophy and laminar calcification of cartilage in loose bodies as probable evidence of an ossification abnormality. J Pathol 132:161, 1980.

501. Mesgarzadeh M, Sapega AA, Bonakdarpour A, et al: Osteochondritis dissecans: Analysis of mechanical stability with radiography, scintigraphy, and MR imaging. Radiology 165:775, 1987.

502. Lehner K, Heuck A, Rodammer G, et al: MRI bei der Osteochondrosis dissecans. ROFO 147:191, 1987.

503. Yulish BS, Mulopulos GP, Goodfellow DB, et al: MR imaging of osteochondral lesions of the talus. J Comput Assist Tomogr 11:296, 1987.

504. De Smet AA, Fisher DR, Graf BK, et al: Osteochondritis dissecans of the knee: Value of MR imaging in determining lesion stability and the presence of articular cartilage defects. AJR 155:549, 1990.

505. De Smet AA, Fisher DR, Burnstein MI, et al: Value of MR imaging in staging osteochondral lesions of the talus (osteochondritis dissecans): Results in 14 patients. AJR 154:555, 1990.

506. Adam G, Bühne M, Prescher A, et al: Stability of osteochondral fragments of the femoral condyle: Magnetic resonance imaging with histopathologic correlation in an animal model. Skel Radiol 20:601, 1991.

507. Kramer J, Stiglbauer R, Engel A, et al: MR contrast arthrography (MRA) in osteochondrosis dissecans. J Comput Assist Tomogr 16:254, 1992.

508. Aichroth P: Osteochondritis dissecans of the knee. A clinical study. J Bone Joint Surg [Br] 53:440, 1971.

509. Milgram JW: Radiological and pathological manifestations of osteochondritis dissecans of the distal femur. A study of 50 cases. Radiology 126:305, 1978.

510. Linden B, Telhag H: Osteochondritis dissecans. A histologic and autoradiograph study in man. Acta Orthop Scand 48:682, 1977.

511. Lipscomb PR Jr, Lipscomb PR Sr, Bryan RS: Osteochondritis dissecans of the knee with loose fragments. Treatment by replacement and fixation with readily removed pins. J Bone Joint Surg [Am] 60:235, 1978.

512. Chiroff RT, Cooke CP: Osteochondritis dissecans: A histologic and microradiographic analysis of surgically excised lesions. J Trauma 15:689, 1975.

513. Linden B: Osteochondritis dissecans of the femoral condyles. A long-term follow-up study. J Bone Joint Surg [Am] 59:769, 1977.

514. Linden B: The incidence of osteochondritis dissecans in the condyles of the femur. Acta Orthop Scand 47:664, 1976.

515. Aichroth P: Osteochondral fractures and their relationship to osteochondritis dissecans of the knee. An experimental study in animals. J Bone Joint Surg [Br] 53:448, 1971.

516. Matthewson MH, Dandy DJ: Osteochondral fractures of the lateral femoral condyle. A result of indirect violence to the knee. J Bone Joint Surg [Br] 60:199, 1978.

517. Mollan RAB: Osteochondritis dissecans of the knee. A case report of an unusual lesion on the lateral femoral condyle. Acta Orthop Scand 48:517, 1977.

518. Mansat CH, Mansat M, Douroureau L, et al: Ostéochondrite disséquante du genou. Rev Rhum Mal Osteoartic 45:177, 1978.

519. Cayea PD, Pavlov H, Sherman MF, et al: Lucent articular lesion in the lateral femoral condyle: source of patellar femoral pain in the athletic adolescent. AJR 137:1145, 1981.

520. Outerbridge RE: Osteochondritis dissecans of the posterior femoral condyle. Clin Orthop 175:121, 1983.

521. Towbin J, Towbin R, Crawford A: Osteochondritis dissecans of the tibial plateau. A case report. J Bone Joint Surg [Am] 64:783, 1982.

522. Mubarak SJ, Carroll NC: Familial osteochondritis dissecans of the knee. Clin Orthop 140:131, 1979.

523. Mubarak SJ, Carroll NC: Juvenile osteochondritis dissecans of the knee: etiology. Clin Orthop 157:200, 1981.

524. Cahill B: Treatment of juvenile osteochondritis dissecans and osteochondritis dissecans of the knee. Clin Sports Med 4:367, 1985.

525. Nagura S: The so-called osteochondritis dissecans of Konig. Clin Orthop 18:100, 1960.

526. Phemister DB: The causes of and changes in loose bodies arising from the articular surface of the joint. J Bone Joint Surg 6:278, 1924.

527. Fisher AGT: A study of loose bodies composed of cartilage or of cartilage and bone occurring in joints, with special reference to their pathology and etiology. Br J Surg 8:493, 1921.

528. Fairbank HAT: Osteochondritis dissecans. Br J Surg 21:67, 1933.

529. Campbell CJ, Ranawat CS: Osteochondritis dissecans: The question of etiology. J Trauma 6:201, 1966.

530. Rosenberg NJ: Osteochondral fractures of the lateral femoral condyle. J Bone Joint Surg [Am] 46:1013, 1964.

531. Kennedy JC, Grainger RW, McGraw RW: Osteochondral fractures of the femoral condyles. J Bone Joint Surg [Br] 48:436, 1966.

532. Gilley JS, Gelman MI, Edson M, et al: Chondral fractures of the knee. Arthrographic, arthroscopic, and clinical manifestations. Radiology 138:51, 1981.

533. Dory MA: Chondral fracture of the anterior intercondylar groove of the femur. Clin Rheumatol 2:175, 1983.

534. Twyman RS, Desai K, Aichroth PM: Osteochondritis dissecans of the knee. A long-term study. J Bone Joint Surg [Br] 73:461, 1991.

535. Pantazopoulos T, Exarchou E: Osteochondritis dissecans of the patella. Report of four cases. J Bone Joint Surg [Am] 53:1205, 1971.

536. Rombold C: Osteochondritis dissecans of the patella. J Bone Joint Surg 18:230, 1936.

537. Rideout DF, Davis S, Navani SV: Osteochondritis dissecans patellae. Br J Radiol 39:673, 1966.

538. Kleinberg S: Bilateral osteochondritis dissecans of the patella. J Bone Joint Surg [Am] 31:185, 1949.

539. Edwards DH, Bentley, G: Osteochondritis dissecans patellae. J Bone Joint Surg [Br] 59:58, 1977.

540. Orava S, Weitz H, Holopainen O: Osteochondritis dissecans patellae. Z Orthop 117:906, 1979.

541. Herzberger M, Schuler P, Rossak K: Osteochondrosis dissecans patellae. Z Orthop 120:268, 1982.

542. Pattin S, Lechat S, Bouvier B, et al: L'ostéochondrite disséquante de la rotule. Rev Rhum Mal Osteoartic 51:131, 1984.

543. Livesley PJ, Milligan GF: Osteochondritis dissecans patellae. Is there a genetic predisposition? Int Orthop (SICOT) 16:126, 1992.

544. Desai SS, Patel MR, Michelli LJ, et al: Osteochondritis dissecans of the patella. J Bone Joint Surg [Br] 69:320, 1987.

545. Smillie IS: Osteochondritis Dissecans. Edinburgh, E & S Livingstone Ltd, 1960.

546. Scapinelli R: Blood supply of the human patella. J Bone Joint Surg [Br] 49:563, 1967.

547. Howie JL: Computed tomography in osteochondritis dissecans of the patella. J Comput Assist Tomogr 36:197, 1985.

548. Pfeiffer WH, Gross ML, Seeger LL: Osteochondritis dissecans of the patella. MRI evaluation and a case report. Clin Orthop 271:207, 1991.

549. Haswell DM, Berne AS, Graham CB: The dorsal defect of the patella. Pediatr Radiol 4:238, 1976.

550. Goergen TG, Resnick D, Greenway G, et al: Dorsal defect of the patella (DDP): A characteristic radiographic lesion. Radiology 130:333, 1979.

551. Hunter LY, Hensinger RN: Dorsal defect of the patella with cartilaginous involvement. A case report. Clin Orthop 143:131, 1979.

552. Gamble JG: Symptomatic dorsal defect of the patella in a runner. Am J Sports Med 14:425, 1986.

553. van Holsbeeck M, Vandamme B, Marchal G, et al: Dorsal defect of the patella: Concept of its origin and relationship with bipartite and multipartite patella. Skel Radiol 16:304, 1987.

554. Ho VB, Kransdorf MJ, Jelinek JS, et al: Dorsal defect of the patella: MR features. J Comput Assist Tomogr 15:474, 1991.

555. Milgram JE: Tangential osteochondral fracture of the patella. J Bone Joint Surg 25:271, 1943.

556. Morscher E: Cartilage-bone lesions of the knee joint following injury. Reconstr Surg Traumatol 12:2, 1971.

557. Ahstrom JP: Osteochondral fracture in the knee joint associated with hypermobility and dislocation of the patella. J Bone Joint Surg [Am] 47:1491, 1965.

558. Frandsen PA, Kristensen H: Osteochondral fracture associated with dislocation of the patella: Another mechanism of injury. J Trauma 19:195, 1979.

559. McDougall A, Brown JD: Radiological sign of recurrent dislocation of the patella. J Bone Joint Surg [Br] 50:841, 1968.

560. Hammerle C-P, Jacob RP: Chondral and osteochondral fractures after luxation of the patella and their treatment. Arch Orthop Trauma Surg 97:207, 1980.

561. Berndt AL, Harty M: Transchondral fracture (osteochondritis dissecans) of the talus. J Bone Joint Surg [Am] 41:988, 1959.

562. Smith GR, Winquist RA, Allan TNK, et al: Subtle transchondral fractures of the talar dome: A radiological perspective. Radiology 124:667, 1977.

563. Scharling M: Osteochondritis dissecans of the talus. Acta Orthop Scand 49:89, 1978.

564. Yvars MF: Osteochondral fractures of the dome of the talus. Clin Orthop 114:185, 1976.

565. Newberg AH: Osteochondral fractures of the dome of the talus. Br J Radiol 52:105, 1979.

566. Yuan HA, Cady RB, DeRosa C: Osteochondritis dissecans of the talus associated with subchondral cysts. Report of three cases. J Bone Joint Surg [Am] *61:*1249, 1979.

567. Canale ST, Belding RH: Osteochondral lesions of the talus. J Bone Joint Surg [Am] *62:*97, 1980.

568. McCullough CH, Venugopal V: Osteochondritis dissecans of the talus: The natural history. Clin Orthop *144:*264, 1979.

569. Alexander AH, Lightman DM: Surgical treatment of transchondral talar-dome fractures (osteochondritis dissecans). J Bone Joint Surg [Am] *62:*646, 1980.

570. Wray DG, Muddu BN: Lateral dome fracture of the talus. J Trauma *21:*818, 1981.

571. Kenny CH: Inverted osteochondral fracture of the talus diagnosed by tomography. A case report. J Bone Joint Surg [Am] *63:*1020, 1981.

572. Flick AB, Gould N: Osteochondritis dissecans of the talus (transchondral fractures of the talus): Review of the literature and new surgical approach for medical dome lesions. Foot Ankle *5:*165, 1985.

573. Mannis CI: Transchondral fracture of the dome of the talus sustained during weight training. Am J Sports Med *11:*354, 1983.

574. Burkus JK, Sella EJ, Southwick WO: Occult injuries of the talus diagnosed by bone scan and tomography. Foot Ankle *4:*316, 1984.

575. Zilch H, Friedebold G: Diagnostik und Therapie chondraler und osteochondraler Frakturen im Bereich des oberen Sprunggelenkes. Unfallheilkunde *86:*153, 1983.

576. Thompson JP, Loomer RL: Osteochondral lesions of the talus in a sports medicine clinic. A new radiographic technique and surgical approach. Am J Sports Med *12:*460, 1984.

577. Meisler K, Sherman G, Frankel R, et al: Osteochondritis dissecans of the talus (transchondral fractures of the talus): Review of the literature and case reports. Curr Podiatr Med, Nov-Dec 1990, p 9.

578. DeGinder WL: Osteochondritis dissecans of the talus. Radiology *65:*590, 1955.

579. Roden S, Tillegard P, Unander-Scharin L: Osteochondritis dissecans and similar lesions of the talus. Report of fifty-five cases with special reference to etiology and treatment. Acta Orthop Scand *23:*51, 1953.

580. Loomer R, Fisher C, Lloyd-Smith R, et al: Osteochondral lesions of the talus. Am J Sports Med *21:*13, 1993.

581. Anderson IF, Crichton KJ, Grattan-Smith T, et al: Osteochondral fractures of the dome of the talus. J Bone Joint Surg [Am] *71:*1143, 1989.

582. Zinman C, Wolfson N, Reis ND: Osteochondritis dissecans of the dome of the talus. Computed tomography scanning in diagnosis and follow-up. J Bone Joint Surg [Am] *70:*1017, 1988.

583. Heare MM, Gillespy T III, Bittar ES: Direct coronal computed tomography arthrography of osteochondritis dissecans of the talus. Skel Radiol *17:*187, 1988.

584. Davies AM, Cassar-Pullicino VN: Demonstration of osteochondritis dissecans of the talus by coronal computed tomographic arthrography. Br J Radiol *62:*1050, 1989.

585. Nelson DW, DiPaola J, Colville M, et al: Osteochondritis dissecans of the talus and knee: Prospective comparison of MR and arthroscopic classifications. J Comput Assist Tomogr *14:*804, 1990.

586. Pritsch M, Horoshovski H, Farine I: Arthroscopic treatment of osteochondral lesions of the talus. J Bone Joint Surg [Am] *68:*862, 1986.

587. Pettine KA, Morrey BF: Osteochondral fractures of the talus. A long-term follow-up. J Bone Joint Surg [Br] *69:*89, 1987.

588. Bauer M, Jonsson K, Lindén B: Osteochondritis dissecans of the ankle. A 20-year follow-up study. J Bone Joint Surg [Br] *69:*93, 1987.

589. Richter R, Richter T, Nübling W: Kasuistischer Beitrag zur Osteochondrosis dissecans des Os naviculare pedis. ROFO *143:*728, 1986.

590. Anderson WJ, Guilford WB: Osteochondritis dissecans of the humeral head. An unusual cause of shoulder pain. Clin Orthop *173:*166, 1983.

591. Shanley DJ, Mulligan ME: Osteochondrosis dissecans of the glenoid. Skel Radiol *19:*419, 1990.

592. Hall FM: Osteochondrosis dissecans and avascular necrosis of bone. Skel Radiol *20:*272, 1991.

593. Hardy Ph, Hinojosa JF, Coudane H, et al: L'ostéochondrite disséquante du cotyle. A propos d'un cas. Rev Chir Orthop *78:*134, 1992.

594. Roberts N, Hughes R: Osteochondritis dissecans of the elbow joint: A clinical study. J Bone Joint Surg [Br] *32:*348, 1950.

595. Woodward AH, Bianco AJ Jr: Osteochondritis dissecans of the elbow. Clin Orthop *110:*35, 1975.

596. Lerner HH, Watkins MB, Resnick B: Osteochondritis dissecans of the supratrochlear septum of the humerus. AJR *55:*717, 1946.

597. Martel W, Abell MR: Case report 46. Skel Radiol *2:*173, 1978.

598. Lindholm TS, Osterman K, Vankka E: Osteochondritis dissecans of elbow, ankle and hip: A comparison survey. Clin Orthop *148:*245, 1980.

599. Mitsunaga MM, Adishian DA, Bianco AJ Jr: Osteochondritis dissecans of the capitellum. J Trauma *22:*53, 1982.

600. Burmester E, Mendoza AS, Gmelin E: Computertomographie des Ellbogengelenkes. ROFO *143:*671, 1986.

601. Meves H, Schneider-Sickert F: Gibt es eine Osteochondrosis dissecans am Kahnbein der Hand? Z Orthop *113:*424, 1975.

602. Bauer M, Jonsson K, Josefsson PO, et al: Osteochondritis dissecans of the elbow. A long-term follow-up study. Clin Orthop *284:*156, 1992.

603. Maffulli N, Chan D, Aldridge J: Derangement of the articular surfaces of the elbow in young gymnasts. J Pediatr Orthop *12:*344, 1992.

604. Vanthournout I, Rudelli A, Valenti Ph, et al: Osteochondritis dissecans of the trochlea of the humerus. Pediatr Radiol *21:*600, 1991.

605. Murphy BJ: MR imaging of the elbow. Radiology *184:*525, 1992.

606. Jawish R, Rigault P, Padovani JP, et al: Osteochondritis dissecans of the humeral capitellum in children. Eur J Pediatr Surg *3:*97, 1993.

607. Gozna ER: Biomechanics of long bone injuries. In ER Gozna, IJ Harrington (Eds): Biomechanics of Musculoskeletal Injury. Baltimore, Williams & Wilkins Co, 1982, p 1.

608. Evans FG: Relation of the physical properties of bone to fracture. AAOS Instructional Course Lectures *18:*110, 1961.

609. Evans FG: Mechanical Properties of Bones. Springfield, Ill, Charles C Thomas, 1973.

610. Alms M: Fracture mechanics. J Bone Joint Surg [Br] *43:*162, 1961.

611. Curry JD: Mechanical properties of bone. Clin Orthop *73:*210, 1970.

612. Böstman OM: Spiral fractures of the shaft of the tibia. Initial displacement and stability of reduction. J Bone Joint Surg [Br] *68:*462, 1986.

613. Renner RR, Mauler GG, Ambrose JL: The radiologist, the orthopedist, the lawyer, and the fracture. Semin Roentgenol *13:*7, 1978.

614. Rosenthal DI, Christensen J, Emerson RH: "Handedness" of spiral fractures of the tibia. Skel Radiol *11:*128, 1984.

615. Reilly DT, Burstein AH: The mechanical properties of cortical bone. J Bone Joint Surg [Am] *56:*1001, 1974.

616. Perkins G: The Ruminations of an Orthopaedic Surgeon. London, Butterworths, 1970.

617. Williams PL, Warwick R (Eds): Gray's Anatomy. 36th British Ed. Philadelphia, WB Saunders Co, 1980, p 430.

618. Harrington IJ: Biomechanics of joint injuries. In ER Gozna, IJ Harrington (Eds): Biomechanics of Musculoskeletal Injury. Baltimore, Williams & Wilkins Co, 1982, p 31.

619. Davie B: The significance and treatment of haemarthrosis of the knee following trauma. Med J Aust *1:*1355, 1969.

620. Wilkinson A: Traumatic haemarthrosis of the knee. Lancet *2:*13, 1965.

621. Weinberger A, Schumacher HR: Experimental joint trauma: Synovial response to blunt trauma and inflammatory reaction to intraarticular injection of fat. J Rhematol *8:*380, 1981.

622. Noyes FR, Bassett RW, Grood ES, et al: Arthroscopy in acute traumatic hemarthrosis of the knee. J Bone Joint Surg [Am] *62:*687, 1980.

623. Eiskjaer S, Larsen ST, Schmidt MB: The significance of hemarthrosis of the knee in children. Arch Orthop Trauma Surg *107:*96, 1988.

624. Butt WP, Lederman H, Chuang S: Radiology of the suprapatellar region. Clin Radiol *34:*511, 1983.

625. MacEwan DW: Changes due to trauma in the fat plane overlying the pronator quadratus muscle: A radiologic sign. Radiology *82:*879, 1964.

626. Rogers SL, MacEwan DW: Changes due to trauma in the fat plane overlying the supinator muscle: A radiologic sign. Radiology *92:*954, 1969.

627. Bledsoe RC, Izenstark JL: Displacement of fat pads in disease and injury of the elbow: A new radiographic sign. Radiology *73:*717, 1959.

628. Bohrer SP: The fat pad sign following elbow trauma. Its usefulness and reliability in suspecting "invisible fractures." Clin Radiol *21:*90, 1970.

629. Hunter RD: Swollen elbow following trauma. JAMA *230:*1573, 1974.

630. Weston WJ: Joint space widening with intracapsular fractures in joints of the fingers and toes of children. Australas Radiol *15:*367, 1971.

631. Sedgwick WG, Gilula LA, Lesker PA, et al: Wear particles: Their value in knee arthrography. Radiology *136:*11, 1980.

632. Lawrence C, Seife B: Bone marrow in joint fluid: A clue to fracture. Ann Intern Med *74:*740, 1971.

633. Kling DH: Fat in traumatic effusions of the knee joint. Am J Surg *6:*71, 1929.

634. Berk RN: Liquid fat in the knee joint after trauma. N Engl J Med *277:*1411, 1967.

635. Gregg JR, Nixon JE, DiStefano V: Neutral fat globules in traumatized knees. Clin Orthop *132:*219, 1978.

636. Holmagren BS: Flussiges fett in Kniegelenk nach Trauma. Acta Radiol *23:*131, 1942.

637. Graham J, Goldman JA: Fat droplets and synovial fluid leukocytes in traumatic arthritis. Arthritis Rheum *21:*76, 1978.

638. Rabinowitz JL, Gregg JR, Nixon JE: Lipid composition of the tissues of human knee joints. II. Synovial fluid in trauma. Clin Orthop *190:*292, 1984.

639. Reginato AJ, Feldman E, Rabinowitz JL: Traumatic chylous knee effusion. Ann Rheum Dis *44:*793, 1985.

640. White RE, Wise CM, Agudelo CA: Post-traumatic chylous joint effusion. Arthritis Rheum *28:*1303, 1985.

641. Baer AN, Wright EP: Lipid laden macrophages in synovial fluid: A late finding in traumatic arthritis. J Rheumatol *14:*848, 1987.

642. Peirce CB, Eaglesham DC: Traumatic lipohemarthrosis of the knee. Radiology *39:*655, 1942.

643. Saxton HM: Lipohaemarthrosis. Br J Radiol *35:*122, 1962.

644. Nelson SW: Some important diagnostic and technical fundamentals in radiology of trauma, with particular emphasis on skeletal trauma. Radiol Clin North Am *4:*241, 1966.

645. Arger PH, Oberkircher PE, Miller WT: Lipohemarthrosis. AJR *121:*97, 1974.

646. Feldman F, Ellis K, Green WM: The fat embolism syndrome. Radiology *114:*535, 1975.

647. Schwegler N, Hug I: Fettflussigkeitsspiegel bei Tibiakopf-Impressions-fraktur. ROFO *122:*301, 1975.

648. Yousefzadeh DK, Jackson JH Jr: Lipohemarthrosis of the elbow joint. Radiology 128:643, 1978.

649. Fagerberg S: Tomographic analysis of depressed fractures within the knee joint, and of injuries to the cruciate ligaments. Acta Orthop Scand 27:219, 1958.

650. Chuinard EG: Fractures of the condyles of the tibia. Clin Orthop 37:115, 1964.

651. Newberg AH, Greenstein R: Radiographic evaluation of tibial plateau fractures. Radiology 126:319, 1978.

652. Train JS, Hermann G: Lipohemarthrosis: Its occurrence with occult cortical fracture of the knee. Orthopedics 3:416, 1980.

653. Sacks BA, Rosenthal DI, Hall FM: Capsular visualization in lipohemarthrosis of the knee. Radiology 122:31, 1977.

654. Kier R, McCarthy SM: Lipohemarthrosis of the knee: MR imaging. J Comput Assist Tomogr 14:395, 1990.

655. Resnick D, Niwayama G: Intravertebral disk herniations: Cartilaginous (Schmorl's) nodes. Radiology 126:57, 1978.

656. Hilton RC, Ball J, Benn RT: Vertebral end-plate lesions (Schmorl's nodes) in the dorsolumbar spine. Ann Rheum Dis 35:127, 1976.

657. Martel W, Seeger JF, Wicks JD, et al: Traumatic lesions of the discovertebral junction in the lumbar spine. AJR 127:457, 1976.

658. Williams JL, Moller GA, O'Rourke TL: Pseudoinfections of the intervertebral disc and adjacent vertebrae. AJR 103:611, 1968.

659. McCall IW, Park WM, O'Brien JP, et al: Acute traumatic intraosseous disc herniation. Spine 10:134, 1985.

660. Roaf R: A study of the mechanics of spinal injuries. J Bone Joint Surg [Br] 42:810, 1960.

661. Keller RH: Traumatic displacement of the cartilaginous vertebral rim: A sign of intervertebral disc prolapse. Radiology 110:21, 1974.

662. Handel SF, Twiford TW Jr, Reigel DH, et al: Posterior lumbar apophyseal fractures. Radiology 130:629, 1979.

663. Techakapuch S: Rupture of the lumbar cartilage plate into the spinal canal in an adolescent. A case report. J Bone Joint Surg [Am] 63:481, 1981.

664. Laredo J-D, Bard M, Chretien J, et al: Lumbar posterior marginal intra-osseous cartilaginous node. Skel Radiol 15:201, 1986.

665. Callahan DJ, Pack LL, Bream RC, et al: Intervertebral disc impingement syndrome in a child. Report of a case and suggested pathology. Spine 11:402, 1986.

666. Fujita K, Shinmei M, Hashimoto K, et al: Posterior dislocation of the sacral apophyseal ring. A case report. Am J Sports Med 14:243, 1986.

667. Sakakida K: Clinical observations on the epiphyseal separation of long bones. Pacif Med Surg 73:108, 1965.

668. Larson RL, McMahon RO: The epiphyses and the childhood athlete. JAMA 196:607, 1966.

669. Rogers LF: The radiography of epiphyseal injuries. Radiology 96:289, 1970.

670. Ozonoff MB: Pediatric Orthopedic Radiology. Philadelphia, WB Saunders Co, 1979.

671. Siffert RS: The effect of trauma to the epiphysis and growth plate. Skel Radiol 2:21, 1977.

672. Alexander CJ: Effect of growth rate on the strength of the growth plate-shaft junction. Skel Radiol 1:67, 1976.

673. Shapiro F: Epiphyseal growth plate fracture-separations. A pathophysiologic approach. Orthopedics 5:720, 1982.

674. Harsha WN: Effects of trauma upon epiphyses. Clin Orthop 10:140, 1957.

675. Salter RB, Harris WR: Injuries involving the epiphyseal plate. J Bone Joint Surg [Am] 45:587, 1963.

676. Salter RB, Harris WR: Injuries of the growth plate. In M Rang (Ed): The Growth Plate and Its Disorders. London, E & S Livingstone, 1969, p 132.

677. Park EA, Guild HG, Jackson D, et al: The recognition of scurvy with especial reference to the early x-ray changes. Arch Dis Child 10:265, 1935.

678. Chow SP, Lam JJ, Leong JCY: Fracture of the tibial tubercle in the adolescent. J Bone Joint Surg [Br] 72:231, 1990.

679. Alexander CJ: The etiology of juvenile spondyloarthritis (discitis). Clin Radiol 21:178, 1970.

680. Berry JM: Fracture of the tuberosity of the ischium due to muscular action. JAMA 59:1450, 1912.

681. Stayton CA: Ischial epiphysiolysis. AJR 76:1161, 1956.

682. Ogden JA: Transphyseal linear ossific striations of the distal radius and ulna. Skel Radiol 19:173, 1990.

683. Hynes D, O'Brien T: Growth disturbance lines after injury of the distal tibial physis. Their significance in prognosis. J Bone Joint Surg [Br] 70:231, 1988.

684. Ogden JA: Injury to the growth mechanisms of the immature skeleton. Skel Radiol 6:237, 1981.

685. Speer DP: Collagenous architecture of the growth plate and perichondrial ossification groove. J Bone Joint Surg [Am] 64:399, 1982.

686. Haliburton RA, Barber JR, Fraser RL: Pseudodislocation: An unusual birth injury. Can J Surg 10:455, 1967.

687. Holland CT: Radiographical note on injuries to the distal epiphysis of the radius and ulna. Proc R Soc Med 22:695, 1929.

688. Vince KG, Miller JE: Cross-union complicating fracture of the forearm. Part II. Children. J Bone Joint Surg [Am] 69:654, 1987.

689. Peterson HA: Partial growth plate arrest and its treatment. J Pediatr Orthop 4:246, 1984.

690. Langeskold A: Surgical treatment of partial closure of the growth plate. J Pediatr Orthop 1:3, 1981.

691. Peterson HA, Burkhart SS: Compression injury of the epiphyseal growth plate: Fact or fiction? J Pediatr Orthop 1:377, 1981.

692. Young JWR, Bright RW, Whitley NO: Computed tomography in the evaluation of partial growth plate arrest in children. Skel Radiol 15:530, 1986.

693. De Campo JF, Boldt DW: Computed tomography of partial growth plate arrest: initial experience. Skel Radiol 15:526, 1986.

694. Murray K, Nixon GW: Epiphyseal growth plate: Evaluation with modified coronal CT. Radiology 166:263, 1988.

695. Harcke HT, Zapf SE, Mandell GA, et al: Angular deformity of the lower extremity: Evaluation with quantitative bone scintigraphy. Work in progress. Radiology 164:437, 1987.

696. Harcke HT, Snyder M, Caro PA, et al: Growth plate of the normal knee: Evaluation with MR imaging. Radiology 183:119, 1992.

697. Jaramillo D, Hoffer FA: Cartilaginous epiphysis and growth plate: Normal and abnormal MR imaging findings. AJR 158:1105, 1992.

698. Jaramillo D, Shapiro F, Hoffer FA, et al: Post-traumatic growth-plate abnormalities: MR imaging of bony-bridge formation in rabbits. Radiology 175:767, 1990.

699. Jaramillo D, Laor T, Zaleske DJ: Indirect trauma to the growth plate: Results of MR imaging after epiphyseal and metaphyseal injury in rabbits. Radiology 187:171, 1993.

700. Havránek P, Lizler J: Magnetic resonance imaging in the evaluation of partial growth arrest after physeal injuries in children. J Bone Joint Surg [Am] 73:1234, 1991.

701. Gabel GT, Peterson HA, Berquist TH: Premature partial physeal arrest. Diagnosis by magnetic resonance imaging in two cases. Clin Orthop 272:242, 1991.

702. Howorth MB: Slipping of the upper femoral epiphysis. Surg Gynecol Obstet 73:723, 1941.

703. Burrows HJ: Slipped upper femoral epiphysis. J Bone Joint Surg [Br] 39:641, 1957.

704. Jerre T: A study in slipped upper femoral epiphysis. Acta Orthop Scand (Suppl) 6:1, 1950.

705. Sorensen KH: Slipped upper femoral epiphysis, clinical study on aetiology. Acta Orthop Scand 39:499, 1968.

706. Kelsey JL: Epidemiology of slipped capital femoral epiphysis: A review of the literature. Pediatrics 51:1042, 1973.

707. Kelsey JL, Acheson RM, Keggi KJ: The body build of patients with slipped capital femoral epiphysis. Am J Dis Child 124:276, 1972.

708. Ninomiya S, Nagasaka Y, Tagawa H: Slipped capital femoral epiphysis. A study of 68 cases in the eastern half area of Japan. Clin Orthop 119:172, 1976.

709. Towbin R, Crawford AH: Neonatal traumatic proximal femoral epiphysiolysis. Pediatrics 63:456, 1979.

710. Milgram JW, Lyne ED: Epiphysiolysis of the proximal femur in very young children. Clin Orthop 110:146, 1975.

711. Lindseth RE, Rosene HA: Traumatic separation of the upper femoral epiphysis in a newborn infant. J Bone Joint Surg [Am] 53:1641, 1971.

712. Ogden JA, Gossling HR, Southwick WO: Slipped capital femoral epiphysis following ipsilateral femoral fracture. Clin Orthop 110:167, 1975.

713. Wojtowycz M, Starshak RJ, Sty JR: Neonatal proximal femoral epiphysiolysis. Radiology 136:647, 1980.

714. Ogden JA, Lee KE, Rudicel SA, et al: Proximal femoral epiphysiolysis in the neonate. J Pediatr Orthop 4:285, 1984.

715. Kelsey JL, Keggi KJ, Southwick WO: The incidence and distribution of slipped capital femoral epiphysis in Connecticut and Southwestern United States. J Bone Joint Surg [Am] 52:1203, 1970.

716. Graziano GP, Kernek CB, DeRosa GP: Coexistent Legg-Calvé-Perthes disease and slipped capital femoral epiphysis in the same child. J Pediatr Orthop 7:61, 1987.

717. Moore RD: Aseptic necrosis of the capital femoral epiphysis following adolescent epiphyseolysis. Surg Gynecol Obstet 80:199, 1945.

718. Al-Aswad BI, Weinger JM, Schneider AB: Slipped capital femoral epiphysis in a 35 year old man. A case report. Clin Orthop 134:131, 1978.

719. Hägglund G, Hansson LI, Sandström S: Familial slipped capital femoral epiphysis. Acta Orthop Scand 57:510, 1986.

720. Henrikson B: The incidence of slipped capital femoral epiphysis. Acta Orthop Scand 40:365, 1969.

721. Bishop JO, Oley TJ, Stephenson CT, et al: Slipped capital femoral epiphysis. A study of 50 cases in Black children. Clin Orthop 135:93, 1978.

722. Hagglund G, Hansson LI, Ordeberg G: Epidemiology of slipped capital femoral epiphysis in southern Sweden. Clin Orthop 191:82, 1984.

723. Loder RT, Aronson DD, Greenfield ML: The epidemiology of bilateral slipped capital femoral epiphysis. A study of children in Michigan. J Bone Joint Surg [Am] 75:1141, 1993.

724. Busch MT, Morrissy RT: Slipped capital femoral epiphysis. Orthop Clin North Am 18:637, 1987.

725. Hägglund G, Hansson LI, Ordeberg G, et al: Bilaterality in slipped upper femoral epiphysis. J Bone Joint Surg [Br] 70:179, 1988.

726. Jensen HP, Steinke MS, Mikkelsen SS, et al: Hip physiolysis. Bilaterality in 62 cases followed for 20 years. Acta Orthop Scand 61:419, 1990.

727. Schwarz N: Secondary displacement of an undetected transphyseal femoral neck fracture. J Bone Joint Surg [Br] 73:521, 1991.

728. Walls JP: Hip fracture-dislocation with transepiphyseal separation. Case report and literature review. Clin Orthop 284:170, 1992.

729. Hägglund G, Hansson LI, Hansson V, et al: Growth of children with physiolysis of the hip. Acta Orthop Scand 58:117, 1987.

730. Morscher E: Strength and morphology of growth cartilage under hormonal influence of puberty. Reconstr Surg Traumatol *10:*3, 1968.

731. Hillman JW, Hunter WA Jr, Barrow JA III: Experimental epiphysiolysis in rats. Surg Forum *8:*566, 1957.

732. Jayakumar S: Slipped capital femoral epiphysis with hypothyroidism treated by nonoperative method. Clin Orthop *151:*179, 1980.

733. McAfee PC, Cady RB: Endocrinologic and metabolic factors in atypical presentations of slipped capital femoral epiphysis. Report of four cases and review of the literature. Clin Orthop *180:*188, 1983.

734. Harris WR: The endocrine basis for slipping of the upper femoral epiphysis. An experimental study. J Bone Joint Surg [Br] *32:*5, 1950.

735. Oka M, Miki T, Hama H, et al: The mechanical strength of the growth plate under the influence of sex hormones. Clin Orthop *145:*264, 1979.

736. Brenkel IJ, Dias JJ, Davies TG, et al: Hormone status in patients with slipped capital femoral epiphysis. J Bone Joint Surg [Br] *71:*33, 1989.

737. Gelberman RH, Cohen MS, Shaw BA, et al: The association of femoral retroversion with slipped capital femoral epiphysis. J Bone Joint Surg [Am] *68:*1000, 1986.

738. Pritchett JW, Perdue KD: Mechanical factors in slipped capital femoral epiphysis. J Pediatr Orthop *8:*385, 1988.

739. Murray RO, Duncan C: Athletic activity in adolescence as an etiological factor in degenerative hip disease. J Bone Joint Surg [Br] *53:*406, 1971.

740. Loder RT, Aronson DD, Bollinger RO: Seasonal variation of slipped capital femoral epiphysis. J Bone Joint Surg [Am] *72:*378, 1990.

741. Howorth B: History of slipping of the capital femoral epiphysis. Clin Orthop *48:*11, 1966.

742. Kampner SL, Wissinger HA: Anterior slipping of the capital femoral epiphysis. Report of a case. J Bone Joint Surg [Am] *54:*1531, 1972.

743. Finch AD, Roberts WM: Epiphyseal coxa valga. J Bone Joint Surg *28:*869, 1946.

744. Skinner SR, Berkheimer GA: Valgus slip of the capital femoral epiphysis. Clin Orthop *135:*90, 1978.

745. LaCroix P, Verbrugge J: Slipping of the upper femoral epiphysis. A pathological study. J Bone Joint Surg [Am] *33:*371, 1951.

746. Ponseti IV, McClintock R: The pathology of slipping of the upper femoral epiphysis. J Bone Joint Surg [Am] *38:*71, 1956.

747. Mickelson MR, Ponseti IV, Cooper RR, et al: The ultrastructure of the growth plate in slipped capital femoral epiphysis. J Bone Joint Surg [Am] *59:*1076, 1977.

748. Ippolito E, Mickelson MR, Ponseti IV: A histochemical study of slipped capital femoral epiphysis. J Bone Joint Surg [Am] *63:*1109, 1981.

749. Agamanolis D, Weiner DS, Lloyd JK: Slipped capital femoral epiphysis: A pathological study. I. A light microscopic and histochemical study of 21 cases. J Pediatr Orthop *5:*40, 1985.

750. Agamanolis D, Weiner DS, Lloyd JK: Slipped capital femoral epiphysis: A pathological study. II. An ultrastructural study of 23 cases. J Pediatr Orthop *5:*47, 1985.

751. Castriota-Scanderbeg A, Orsi E: Slipped capital femoral epiphysis: Ultrasonographic findings. Skel Radiol *22:*191, 1993.

752. Smergel EM, Harcke T, Pizzutillo PD, et al: Use of bone scintigraphy in the management of slipped capital femoral epiphysis. Clin Nucl Med *12:*349, 1987.

753. Loyd RD, Evans JP: Acute slipped capital femoral epiphysis. South Med J *68:*857, 1975.

754. Bloomberg TJ, Nuttall J, Stoker DJ: Radiology in early slipped femoral capital epiphysis. Clin Radiol *29:*657, 1978.

755. Aadalen RJ, Weiner DS, Hoyt W, et al: Acute slipped capital femoral epiphysis. J Bone Joint Surg [Am] *56:*1473, 1974.

756. Scham SM: The triangular sign in the early diagnosis of slipped capital femoral epiphysis. Clin Orthop *103:*16, 1974.

757. Steel HH: The metaphyseal blanch sign of slipped capital femoral epiphysis. J Bone Joint Surg [Am] *68:*920, 1986.

758. Jacobs P: A note on the diagnosis of early adolescent coxa vara (slipped epiphysis). Br J Radiol *35:*619, 1962.

759. Crawford AH: Slipped capital femoral epiphysis. J Bone Joint Surg [Am] *70:*1422, 1988.

760. Clarke NMP, Harrison MHM: Slipped upper femoral epiphysis. A potential for spontaneous recovery. J Bone Joint Surg [Br] *68:*541, 1986.

761. Mickelson MR, El-Khoury GY, Cass JR, et al: Aseptic necrosis following slipped capital femoral epiphysis. Skel Radiol *4:*129, 1979.

762. Dalinka MK, Alavi A, Forsted DH: Aseptic (ischemic) necrosis of the femoral head. JAMA *238:*1059, 1977.

763. Lowe HG: Avascular necrosis after slipping of the upper femoral epiphysis. Bone Joint Surg [Br] *43:*688, 1961.

764. Hall JE: The results of treatment of slipped femoral epiphysis. J Bone Joint Surg [Br] *39:*659, 1957.

765. Boyer DW, Mickelson MR, Ponseti IV: Slipped capital femoral epiphysis. Long-term follow-up study of one hundred and twenty-one patients. J Bone Joint Surg [Am] *63:*85, 1981.

766. Lynch GJ, Stevens DB: Slipped capital femoral epiphysis. Treatment by pinning in situ. Clin Orthop *221:*260, 1987.

767. Gelfand MJ, Strife JL, Graham EJ, et al: Bone scintigraphy in slipped capital femoral epiphysis. Clin Nucl Med *8:*613, 1983.

768. Vrettos BC, Hoffman EB: Chondrolysis in slipped upper femoral epiphysis. Long-term study of the aetiology and natural history. J Bone Joint Surg [Br] *75:*956, 1993.

769. Lowe HG: Necrosis of articular cartilage after slipping of the capital femoral epiphysis. Report of six cases with recovery. J Bone Joint Surg [Br] *52:*108, 1970.

770. Gage JR, Sundberg AB, Nolan DR, et al: Complications after cuneiform osteotomy for moderately or severely slipped capital femoral epiphysis. J Bone Joint Surg [Am] *60:*157, 1978.

771. Cruess RL: The pathology of acute necrosis of cartilage in slipping of the capital femoral epiphysis. A report of two cases with pathological sections. J Bone Joint Surg [Am] *45:*1013, 1963.

772. Tillema DA, Golding JSR: Chondrolysis following slipped capital femoral epiphysis in Jamaica. J Bone Joint Surg [Am] *53:*1528, 1971.

773. Ingram AJ, Clarke MS, Clark CS Jr, et al: Chondrolysis complicating slipped capital femoral epiphysis. Clin Orthop *165:*99, 1982.

774. Miller RK, Menelaus MB: Bilateral chondrolysis with unilateral slipped capital femoral epiphysis. J Bone Joint Surg [Br] *73:*523, 1991.

775. Hartman JT, Gates DJ: Recovery from cartilage necrosis following slipped capital femoral epiphysis. A seven year study of 166 cases. Orthop Rev *1:*33, 1972.

776. Sternlicht AL, Ehrlich MG, Armstrong AL, et al: Role of pin protrusion in the etiology of chondrolysis: A surgical model with radiographic, histologic, and biochemical analysis. J Pediatr Orthop *12:*428, 1992.

777. Morrissy RT, Steele RW, Gerdes MH: Localized immune complexes and slipped upper femoral epiphysis. J Bone Joint Surg [Br] *65:*574, 1983.

778. Cooperman DR, Charles LM, Pathria M, et al: Post-mortem description of slipped capital femoral epiphysis. J Bone Joint Surg [Br] *74:*595, 1992.

779. Larson RL: Epiphyseal injuries in the adolescent athlete. Orthop Clin North Am *4:*839, 1973.

780. Smith L: A concealed injury to the knee. J Bone Joint Surg [Am] *44:*1659, 1962.

781. Cassebaum WH, Patterson AH: Fractures of the distal femoral epiphysis. Clin Orthop *41:*79, 1965.

782. Stephens DC, Louis DS: Traumatic separation of the distal femoral epiphyseal cartilage plate. J Bone Joint Surg [Am] *56:*1383, 1974.

783. Rogers LF, Jones S, Davis AR, et al: "Clipping injury" fracture of the epiphysis in the adolescent football player: An occult lesion of the knee. AJR *121:*69, 1974.

784. Torg JS, Pavlov H, Morris VB: Salter-Harris type-III fracture of the medial femoral condyle occurring in the adolescent athlete. J Bone Joint Surg [Am] *63:*586, 1981.

785. Aitken AP, Ingersoll RE: Fractures of the proximal tibial epiphyseal cartilage. J Bone Joint Surg [Am] *38:*787, 1956.

786. Shelton WR, Canale ST: Fractures of the tibia through the proximal tibial epiphyseal cartilage. J Bone Joint Surg [Am] *61:*167, 1979.

787. Burkhart SS, Peterson HA: Fractures of the proximal tibial epiphysis. J Bone Joint Surg [Am] *61:*996, 1979.

788. Rivero H, Bolden R, Young LW: Proximal tibial physis fracture and popliteal artery injury. Radiology *150:*390, 1984.

789. Henard DC, Bobo RT: Avulsion fractures of the tibial tubercle in adolescents. A report of bilateral fractures and review of the literature. Clin Orthop *177:*182, 1983.

790. MacNealy GA, Rogers LF, Hernandez R, et al: Injuries of the distal tibial epiphysis: Systematic radiographic evaluation. AJR *138:*683, 1982.

791. Salter RB: Injuries of the ankle in children. Orthop Clin North Am *5:*147, 1974.

792. Vahvanen V, Aalto K: Classification of ankle fractures in children. Arch Orthop Trauma Surg *97:*1, 1980.

793. Cass JR, Peterson HA: Salter-Harris type-IV injuries of the distal tibial epiphyseal growth plate, with emphasis on those involving the medial malleolus. J Bone Joint Surg [Am] *65:*1059, 1983.

794. Grace DL: Irreducible fracture-separations of the distal tibial epiphysis. J Bone Joint Surg [Br] *65:*160, 1983.

795. Dias LS, Giegerich CR: Fractures of the distal tibial epiphysis in adolescence. J Bone Joint Surg [Am] *65:*438, 1983.

796. Peiro A, Aracil J, Martos F, et al: Triplane distal epiphyseal fracture. Clin Orthop *160:*196, 1981.

797. Cone RO III, Nguyen V, Flournoy JG, et al: Triplane fracture of the distal tibial epiphysis: Radiographic and CT studies. Radiology *153:*763, 1984.

798. Von Laer L: Classification, diagnosis and treatment of transitional fractures of the distal part of the tibia. J Bone Joint Surg [Am] *67:*687, 1985.

799. Spiegel PG, Mast JW, Cooperman DR, et al: Triplane fractures of the distal tibial epiphysis. Clin Orthop *188:*74, 1984.

800. Denton JR, Fischer SJ: The medial triplane fracture: Report of an unusual injury. J Trauma *21:*991, 1981.

801. Clement DA, Worlock PH: Triplane fracture of the distal tibia. A variant in cases with an open growth plate. J Bone Joint Surg [Br] *69:*412, 1987.

802. Feldman F, Singson RD, Rosenberg ZS, et al: Distal tibial triplane fractures: Diagnosis with CT. Radiology *164:*429, 1987.

803. Ertl JP, Barrack RL, Alexander AH, et al: Triplane fracture of the distal tibial epiphysis. Long-term follow-up. J Bone Joint Surg [Am] *70:*967, 1988.

804. Kump WL: Vertical fractures of the distal tibial epiphysis. AJR *97:*676, 1966.

805. Kleiger B, Mankin HJ: Fracture of the lateral portion of the distal tibial epiphysis. J Bone Joint Surg [Am] *46:*25, 1964.

806. Simon WH, Florus R, Schoenhaus H, et al: Juvenile fracture of Tillaux. A distal tibial epiphyseal fracture. J Am Podiatr Med Assoc *79:*295, 1989.

807. Manderson EL, Ollivierre CO: Closed anatomic reduction of a juvenile Tillaux

fracture by dorsiflexion of the ankle. A case report. Clin Orthop 276:262, 1992.

808. Beaty JH, Linton RC: Medial malleolar fracture in a child. A case report. J Bone Joint Surg [Am] 70:1254, 1988.

809. Kennedy JP, Weiner DS: Avascular necrosis complicating fracture of the distal tibial epiphysis. J Pediatr Orthop 11:234, 1991.

810. Smith FM: Fracture-separation of the proximal humeral epiphysis. Am J Surg 91:627, 1956.

811. Neer CS II, Horwitz BS: Fractures of the proximal humeral epiphyseal plate. Clin Orthop 41:24, 1965.

812. Kleinman PK, Akins CM: The ''vanishing'' epiphysis: Sign of Salter Type I fracture of the proximal humerus in infancy. Br J Radiol 55:865, 1982.

813. Hansen NM Jr: Epiphyseal changes in the proximal humerus of an adolescent baseball pitcher. Am J Sports Med 10:380, 1982.

814. Barnett LS: Little league shoulder syndrome: Proximal humeral epiphysiolysis in adolescent baseball pitchers. A case report. J Bone Joint Surg [Am] 67:495, 1985.

815. White SJ, Blane CE, DiPietro MA, et al: Arthrography in evaluation of birth injuries of the shoulder. J Can Assoc Radiol 38:113, 1987.

816. Broker FHL, Burbach T: Ultrasonic diagnosis of separation of the proximal humeral epiphysis in the newborn. J Bone Joint Surg [Am] 72:187, 1990.

817. Denham RH Jr, Dingley AF Jr: Epiphyseal separation of the medial end of the clavicle. J Bone Joint Surg [Am] 49:1179, 1967.

818. Havránek P: Injuries of the distal clavicular physis in children. J Pediatr Orthop 9:213, 1989.

819. Rogers LF: Fractures and dislocations of the elbow. Semin Roentgenol 13:97, 1978.

820. Poznanski A: Personal communication, 1979.

821. Silberstein MJ, Brodeur AE, Graviss ER: Some vagaries of the capitellum. J Bone Joint Surg [Am] 61:244, 1979.

822. Silberstein MJ, Brodeur AE, Graviss ER, et al: Some vagaries of the medial epicondyle. J Bone Joint Surg [Am] 63:524, 1981.

823. Silberstein MJ, Brodeur AE, Graviss ER: Some vagaries of the radial head and neck. J Bone Joint Surg [Am] 64:1153, 1982.

824. Silberstein MJ, Brodeur AE, Graviss ER: Some vagaries of the lateral epicondyle. J Bone Joint Surg [Am] 64:444, 1982.

825. Rogers LF, Malave S Jr, White H, et al: Plastic bowing, torus and greenstick supracondylar fractures of the humerus: Radiographic clues to obscure fractures of the elbow in children. Radiology 128:145, 1978.

826. Fowles JV, Kassab MT: Displaced fractures of the medial humeral condyle in children. J Bone Joint Surg [Am] 62:1159, 1980.

827. Peiro A, Mut T, Aracil J, et al: Fracture-separation of the lower humeral epiphysis in young children. Acta Orthop Scand 52:295, 1981.

828. Harrison RB, Keats TE, Frankel CJ, et al: Radiographic clues to fractures of the unossified medial humeral condyle in young children. Skel Radiol 11:209, 1984.

829. Brodeur AE, Silberstein MJ, Graviss ER, et al: The basic tenets for appropriate evaluation of the elbow in pediatrics. Curr Probl Diagn Radiol 12:6, 1983.

830. Peterson HA: Triplane fracture of the distal humeral epiphysis. J Pediatr Orthop 3:81, 1983.

831. Papavasiliou VA: Fracture-separation of the medial epicondylar epiphysis of the elbow joint. Clin Orthop 171:172, 1982.

832. Beghin JL, Bucholz RW, Wenger DR: Intercondylar fractures of the humerus in young children. A report of two cases. J Bone Joint Surg [Am] 64:1083, 1982.

833. D'Ambrosia R, Zink W: Fractures of the elbow in children. Pediatr Ann 11:541, 1982.

834. Rutherford A: Fractures of the lateral humeral condyle in children. J Bone Joint Surg [Am] 67:851, 1985.

835. Fowles JV, Kassab MT, Moula T: Untreated intra-articular entrapment of the medial humeral epicondyle. J Bone Joint Surg [Br] 66:562, 1984.

836. De Boeck H, Casteleyn PP, Opdecam P: Fracture of the medial humeral condyle. Report of a case in an infant. J Bone Joint Surg [Am] 69:1442, 1987.

837. Chessare JW, Rogers LF, White H, et al: Injuries of the medial epicondylar ossification center of the humerus. AJR 129:49, 1979.

838. Tayob AA, Shively RA: Bilateral elbow dislocations with intra-articular displacement of the medial epicondyles. J Trauma 20:332, 1980.

839. Resnik CS, Hartenberg MA: Ossification centers of the pediatric elbow: A rare normal variant. Pediatr Radiol 16:254, 1986.

840. Mizuno K, Hirohata K, Kashiwagi D: Fracture-separation of the distal humeral epiphysis in young children. J Bone Joint Surg [Am] 61:570, 1979.

841. DeLee JC, Williams KE, Rogers LF, et al. Fracture-separation of the distal humeral epiphysis. J Bone Joint Surg [Am] 62:46, 1980.

842. Holda ME, Manoli A II, La Mont RL: Epiphyseal separation of the distal end of the humerus with medial displacement. J Bone Joint Surg [Am] 62:52, 1980.

843. De Jager LT, Hoffman EB: Fracture-separation of the distal humeral epiphysis. J Bone Joint Surg [Br] 73:143, 1991.

844. Ruo GY: Radiographic diagnosis of fracture-separation of the entire distal humeral epiphysis. Clin Radiol 38:635, 1987.

845. Manoli A II: Irreducible fracture-separation of the distal radial epiphysis. Report of a case. J Bone Joint Surg [Am] 64:1095, 1982.

846. Samuel AW: Epiphyseal plate injuries in the hand. Injury 12:503, 1981.

847. Aitken AP: The end results of the fractured distal radial epiphysis. J Bone Joint Surg 17:302, 1935.

848. Godshall RW, Hansen CA: Incomplete avulsion of a portion of the iliac epiphysis. An injury of young athletes. J Bone Joint Surg [Am] 55:1301, 1973.

849. Yellin JA, Towbin RB, Kaufman RA: Stubbed finger osteomyelitis. J Trauma 25:808, 1985.

850. Roy S, Caine D, Singer KM: Stress changes of the distal radial epiphysis in young gymnasts. A report of twenty-one cases and a review of the literature. Am J Sports Med 13:301, 1985.

851. Torre BA: Epiphyseal injuries in the small joints of the hand. Hand Clin 4:113, 1988.

852. Scuderi G, Bronson MJ: Triradiate cartilage injury. Report of two cases and review of the literature. Clin Orthop 217:179, 1987.

853. Heeg M, Visser JD, Oostvogel HJM: Injuries of the acetabular triradiate cartilage and sacroiliac joint. J Bone Joint Surg [Br] 70:34, 1988.

854. Chan D, Aldridge MJ, Maffulli N, et al: Chronic stress injuries of the elbow in young gymnasts. Br J Radiol 64:1113, 1991.

855. Maffulli N, Chan D, Aldridge MJ: Overuse injuries of the olecranon in young gymnasts. J Bone Joint Surg [Br] 74:305, 1992.

856. Wilkerson RD, Johns JC: Nonunion of an olecranon stress fracture in an adolescent gymnast. A case report. Am J Sports Med 18:432, 1990.

857. Hotchkiss RN: Common disorders of the elbow in athletes and musicians. Hand Clinics 6:507, 1990.

858. Bak K: Separation of the proximal tibial epiphysis in a gymnast. Acta Orthop Scand 62:293, 1991.

859. Carter SR, Aldridge MJ: Stress injury of the distal radial growth plate. J Bone Joint Surg [Br] 70:834, 1988.

860. Yong-Hing K, Wedge JH, Bowen CVA: Chronic injury to the distal ulnar and radial growth plates in an adolescent gymnast. A case report. J Bone Joint Surg [Am] 70:1087, 1988.

861. Carter SR, Aldridge J, Fitzgerald R, et al: Stress changes of the wrist in adolescent gymnasts. Br J Radiol 61:109, 1988.

862. Albanese SA, Palmer AK, Kerr DR, et al: Wrist pain and distal growth plate closure of the radius in gymnasts. J Pediatr Orthop 9:23, 1989.

863. Caine D, Roy S, Singer KM, et al: Stress changes of the distal radial growth plate. A radiographic survey and review of the literature. Am J Sports Med 20:290, 1992.

864. Dobyns JH, Gabel GT: Gymnast's wrist. Hand Clinics 6:493, 1990.

865. Woo S L-Y, Young EP: Structure and function of tendons and ligaments. In VC Mow, WC Hayes (Eds): Basic Orthopaedic Biomechanics. New York, Raven Press, 1991, p 199.

866. Welsh RP, MacNab I, Riley V: Biomechanical studies of rabbit tendon. Clin Orthop 81:171, 1971.

867. Peacock EE: Biological principles in the healing of long tendons. Surg Clin North Am 45:461, 1965.

868. Peacock EE: A study of the circulation in normal tendons and healing grafts. Ann Surg 149:415, 1959.

869. Minns RJ, Stevens FS: Local denaturation of collagen fibers during the mechanical rupture of collagenous fibrous tissue. Ann Rheum Dis 39:164, 1980.

870. Clayton ML, Weir GL Jr: Experimental investigations of ligamentous healing. Am J Surg 98:373, 1959.

871. Tipton CM, Schild RJ, Flatt AE: Measurement of ligamentous strength in rat knees. J Bone Joint Surg [Am] 49:63, 1967.

872. Mornet J, Doliveux P: La maladie des tendons d'achille et sa complication: La rupture. Rev Rhum Mal Osteoartic 40:607, 1973.

873. Reveno PM, Kittleson AC: Spontaneous Achilles tendon rupture. Radiology 93:1341, 1969.

874. Margles SW, Lewis MM: Bilateral spontaneous concurrent rupture of the patellar tendon without apparent associated systemic disease: A case report. Clin Orthop 136:186, 1978.

875. Newberg A, Wales L: Radiographic diagnosis of quadriceps tendon rupture. Radiology 125:367, 1977.

876. Kamali M: Bilateral traumatic rupture of the infrapatellar tendon. Clin Orthop 142:131, 1979.

877. Donati RB, Cox S, Echo BS, et al: Bilateral simultaneous patellar tendon rupture in a female collegiate gymnast. A case report. Am J Sports Med 14:237, 1986.

878. Andersen E: Triceps tendon avulsion. Injury 17:279, 1986.

879. Staples OS: Ruptures of the fibular collateral ligaments of the ankle. Result study of immediate surgical treatment. J Bone Joint Surg [Am] 57:101, 1975.

880. Moore TM, Meyers HM, Harvey JP Jr: Collateral ligament laxity of the knee. Long-term comparison between plateau fractures and normal. J Bone Joint Surg [Am] 58:594, 1976.

881. Liljedahl S-O, Lindvall N, Wetterfors J: Early diagnosis and treatment of acute ruptures of the anterior cruciate ligament. A clinical and arthrographic study of forty-eight cases. J Bone Joint Surg [Am] 47:1503, 1965.

882. Van de Berg A, Collard A: Diagnosis of the disorders of the knee ligaments. A radiological measurement of laxity. J Belge Radiol 62:49, 1979.

883. Seligson D, Gassman J, Pope M: Ankle instability: Evaluation of the lateral ligaments. Am J Sports Med 8:39, 1980.

884. Jacobsen K: Demonstration of rotatory instability in injured knees by stress radiography. Acta Orthop Scand 49:195, 1978.

885. Jacobsen K: Stress radiographic measurements of post-traumatic knee instability. A clinical study. Acta Orthop Scand 48:301, 1977.

886. Jacobsen K: Stress radiographical measurement of the anteroposterior, medial and lateral stability of the knee joint. Acta Orthop Scand 47:335, 1976.

887. Sylvin LÉ: A more exact measurement of the sagittal stability of the knee joint. Acta Orthop Scand 46:1008, 1975.

888. Kennedy JC, Fowler PJ: Medial and anterior instability of the knee. J Bone Joint Surg [Am] 53:1257, 1971.

889. Hastings DE: Knee ligament instability—a rational anatomical classification. Clin Orthop 208:104, 1986.

890. Freeman MAR: Instability of the foot after injuries to the lateral ligament of the ankle. J Bone Joint Surg [Br] 47:669, 1965.

891. Rubin G, Witten M: The talar tilt angle and the fibular collateral ligaments. J Bone Joint Surg [Am] 42:311, 1960.

892. Johannsen A: Radiological diagnosis of lateral ligament lesion of the ankle. A comparison between talar tilt and anterior drawer sign. Acta Orthop Scand 49:295, 1978.

893. Grevsten S, Eriksson K: Tendinography for diagnosing injuries of tendons and ligaments. Acta Radiol (Diagn) 20:447, 1979.

894. Blanshard KS, Finlay DBL, Scott DJA, et al: A radiological analysis of lateral ligament injuries of the ankle. Clin Radiol 37:247, 1986.

895. Tehranzadeh J, Serafini AN, Pais MJ: Avulsion and Stress Injuries of the Musculoskeletal System. Basel, Karger Press, 1989.

896. Tehranzadeh J: The spectrum of avulsion and avulsion-like injuries of the musculoskeletal system. RadioGraphics 7:945, 1987.

897. Farrar EL III, Lippert FG III: Avulsion of the triceps tendon. Clin Orthop 161:242, 1981.

898. Tiger E, Mayer DP, Glazer R: Complete avulsion of the triceps tendon: MRI diagnosis. Computer Med Imaging Graphics 17:51, 1993.

899. White GM, Riley LH Jr: Isolated avulsion of the subscapularis insertion in a child. A case report. J Bone Joint Surg [Am] 67:635, 1985.

900. Metzmaker JN, Pappas AM: Avulsion fractures of the pelvis. Am J Sports Med 13:349, 1985.

901. Fernbach SK, Wilkinson RH: Avulsion injuries of the pelvis and proximal femur. AJR 137:581, 1984.

902. Vazelle F, Rochcongar P, Lejeune JJ, et al: Le syndrome d'algie pubienne du sportif (pubialgie). J Radiol 63:423, 1982.

903. Tehranzadeh J, Kurth LA, Elyaderani MK, et al: Combined pelvic stress fracture and avulsion of the adductor longus in a middle-distance runner. A case report. Am J Sports Med 10:108, 1982.

904. Schneider R, Kaye JJ, Ghelman B: Adductor avulsive injuries near the symphysis pubis. Radiology 120:567, 1976.

905. Stayton CA: Ischial epiphysiolysis. AJR 76:1161, 1956.

906. Symeonides P: Isolated traumatic rupture of the adductor longus muscle of the thigh. Clin Orthop 88:64, 1972.

907. Ellis R, Greene A: Ischial apophyseolysis. Radiology 87:646, 1966.

908. Krahl H, Rompe G: Ermüdungsbruch der pars symphysica des Schambeines. Beitrag zur Differentialdiagnose der Uberlastungsschaaden am vordern Beckenring. Z Orthop 111:216, 1973.

909. Lombardo SJ, Retting AC, Kerlan RK: Radiographic abnormalities of the iliac apophysis in adolescent athletes. J Bone Joint Surg [Am] 65:444, 1983.

910. Houghton GR, Ackroyd CE: Sleeve fracture of the patella in children. J Bone Joint Surg [Br] 61:165, 1979.

911. Bishay M: Sleeve fracture of upper pole of patella. J Bone Joint Surg [Br] 73:339, 1991.

912. Grogan DP, Carey TP, Leffers D, et al: Avulsion fractures of the patella. J Pediatr Orthop 10:721, 1990.

913. Lepse PS, McCarthy RE, McCullough FL: Simultaneous bilateral avulsion fracture of the tibial tuberosity. A case report. Clin Orthop 229:232, 1987.

914. Frankl U, Waisilewski SA, Healy WL: Avulsion fracture of the tibial tubercle with avulsion of the patellar ligament. Report of two cases. J Bone Joint Surg [Am] 72:1411, 1990.

915. Ogden JA, Lee J: Accessory ossification patterns and injuries of the malleoli. J Pediatr Orthop 10:306, 1990.

916. Sclafani SJA: Ligamentous injury of the lower tibiofibular syndesmosis: Radiographic evidence. Radiology 156:21, 1985.

917. Husfeldt E: Significance of roentgenography of ankle joint in oblique projection in malleolar fractures. Hospitalstid 80:788, 1937.

918. Mink JH: Muscle injuries. In AL Deutsch, JH Mink, R Kerr (Eds): MRI of the Foot and Ankle. New York, Raven Press, 1992, p 281.

919. Warwick R, Williams PL: Gray's Anatomy. 35th British Ed. Philadelphia, WB Saunders Co, 1973, p 474.

920. Nerlich ML, Tscherne H: Biology of soft tissue injuries. In BD Browner, JB Jupiter, AM Levine, et al (Eds): Skeletal Trauma. Fractures, Dislocations, Ligamentous Injuries. Philadelphia, WB Saunders Co, 1992, p 77.

921. Letho M, Alanen A: Healing of muscle trauma. Correlation of sonographical and histological findings in an experimental study in rats. J Ultrasound Med 6:425, 1987.

922. Fleckenstein JL, Canby RC, Parkey RW, et al: Acute effects of exercise on MR imaging of skeletal muscle in normal volunteers. AJR 151:231, 1988.

923. Fleckenstein JL, Weatherall PT, Parkey RW, et al: Sports-related muscle injuries: Evaluation with MR imaging. Radiology 172:793, 1989.

924. Shellock FG, Fukunaga T, Mink JH, et al: Exertional muscle injury: Evaluation of concentric versus eccentric actions with serial MR imaging. Radiology 179:659, 1991.

925. Shellock FG, Fukunaga T, Mink JH, et al: Acute effects of exercise on MR imaging of skeletal muscle: Concentric vs eccentric actions. AJR 156:765, 1991.

926. Nurenberg P, Giddings CJ, Stray-Gundersen J, et al: MR imaging–guided muscle biopsy for correlation of increased signal intensity with ultrastructural change and delayed-onset muscle soreness after exercise. Radiology 184:865, 1992.

927. Fleckenstein JL, Shellock FG: Exertional muscle injuries: Magnetic resonance imaging evaluation. Top Magn Res Imaging 3:50, 1991.

928. De Smet AA: Magnetic resonance findings in skeletal muscle tears. Skel Radiol 22:479, 1993.

929. Wolfort FG, Mogelvang LC, Filtzer HS: Anterior tibial compartment syndrome following muscle hernia repair. Arch Surg 106:97, 1993.

930. Zeiss J, Ebraheim NA, Woldenberg LS: Magnetic resonance imaging in the diagnosis of anterior tibialis muscle herniation. Clin Orthop 244:249, 1989.

931. Gabow PA, Kaehy WD, Kelleher SP: The spectrum of rhabdomyolysis. Medicine 61:141, 1982.

932. Barloon TJ, Zachar CK, Harkens KL, et al: Rhabdomyolysis: Computed tomography findings. CT 12:193, 1988.

933. Kaplan GN: Ultrasonic appearance of rhabdomyolysis. AJR 134:375, 1980.

934. Mangano FA, Zaontz M, Pahira JJ, et al: Computed tomography of acute renal failure secondary to rhabdomyolysis. J Comput Assist Tomogr 9:777, 1985.

935. Ludmer LM, Chandeysson P, Barth WF: Diphosphonate bone scan in an unusual case of rhabdomyolysis: A report and literature review. J Rheumatol 20:382, 1993.

936. Rorabeck CH: Compartment syndromes. In BD Browner, JB Jupiter, AM Levine, et al (Eds): Skeletal Trauma. Fractures, Dislocations, Ligamentous Injuries. Philadelphia, WB Saunders Co, 1992, p 285.

937. Rorabeck CH: The treatment of compartment syndromes in the leg. J Bone Joint Surg [Br] 66:93, 1984.

938. Farmlett EJ, Fishman EK, Magid D, et al: Computed tomography in the assessment of myonecrosis. J Can Assoc Radiol 38:278, 1987.

939. Timmons JH, Hartshorne MF, Peters VJ, et al: Muscle necrosis in the extremities: Evaluation with Tc-99m pyrophosphate scanning—a retrospective review. Radiology 167:173, 1988.

940. Kogutt MS, Swischuk LE, Fagan CJ: Patterns of injury and significance of uncommon fractures in the battered child syndrome. AJR 121:143, 1974.

941. Spackman TJ: Pediatric trauma: Medical abuse of infants. Radiol Clin North Am 11:633, 1973.

942. Akbarnia B, Torg JS, Kirkpatrick J, et al: Manifestations of the battered-child syndrome. J Bone Joint Surg [Am] 56:1159, 1974.

943. Slovis TL, Berdon WE, Haller JO, et al: Pancreatitis and the battered child syndrome. Report of 2 cases with skeletal involvement. AJR 125:456, 1975.

944. Hiller HG: Battered or not—a reappraisal of metaphyseal fragility. AJR 114:241, 1972.

945. Silverman FN: Unrecognized trauma in infants, the battered child syndrome, and the syndrome of Ambroise Tardieu. Radiology 104:337, 1972.

946. Caffey J: Some traumatic lesions in growing bones other than fractures and dislocations: Clinical and radiological features. Br J Radiol 30:225, 1957.

947. O'Neill JA Jr, Meacham WF, Griffin PP, et al: Patterns of injury in the battered child syndrome. J Trauma 13:332, 1973.

948. Tröger J: Das misshandelte Kind. Radiologe 18:233, 1978.

949. Swischuk LE: Spine and spinal cord trauma in the battered child syndrome. Radiology 92:733, 1969.

950. Faure C, Steadman C, Lalande G, et al: La vertèbre vagabonde. Ann Radiol 22:96, 1979.

951. Cullen JC: Spinal lesions in battered babies. J Bone Joint Surg [Br] 57:364, 1975.

952. Rao KS, Hyde I: Digital lesions in non-accidental injuries in children. Br J Radiol 57:259, 1984.

953. English PC, Grossman H: Radiology and the history of child abuse. Pediatr Ann 12:870, 1983.

954. Kleinman PK, Zito JL: Avulsion of the spinous processes caused by infant abuse. Radiology 151:389, 1984.

955. Radkowski MA: The battered child syndrome: Pitfalls in radiological diagnosis. Pediatr Ann 12:894, 1983.

956. Ben-Youssef L, Schmidt TL: Battered child syndrome simulating myositis. J Pediatr Orthop 3:392, 1983.

957. Radkowski MA, Merten DF, Leonidas JC: The abused child: Criteria for radiologic diagnosis. RadioGraphics 3:262, 1983.

958. Merten DF, Kirks DR, Ruderman RJ: Occult humeral epiphyseal fracture in battered infants. Pediatr Radiol 10:151, 1981.

959. Kleinman PK, Raptopoulos VD, Brill PW: Occult nonskeletal trauma in the battered-child syndrome. Radiology 141:393, 1981.

960. Kirks DR: Radiological evaluation of visceral injuries in the battered child syndrome. Pediatr Ann 12:888, 1983.

961. Greinacher I, Troger J: Das sogenannte ''battered-child-syndrom'' aus der sicht der Kinderrontgenologen. Radiologe 22:342, 1982.

962. Merten DF, Radkowski MA, Leonidas JC: The abused child: A radiological reappraisal. Radiology 146:377, 1983.

963. Galleno H, Oppenheim WL: The battered child syndrome revisited. Clin Orthop 162:11, 1982.

964. Caniano DA, Beaver BL, Boles ET Jr: Child abuse. An update on surgical management in 256 cases. Ann Surg 203:219, 1986.

965. Kottmeier PK: The battered child. Pediatr Ann 16:343, 1987.

966. Kleinman PK, Marks SC, Blackbourne B: The metaphyseal lesion in abused infants: a radiologic-histopathologic study. AJR 146:895, 1986.

967. Kleinman PK, Marks SC Jr, Spevak MR, et al: Extension of growth-plate cartilage into the metaphysis: A sign of healing fracture in abused infants. AJR 156:775, 1991.

968. Osier LK, Marks SC Jr, Kleinman PK: Metaphyseal extensions of hypertro-

phied chondrocytes in abused infants indicate healing fractures. J Pediatr Orthop 13:249, 1993.

969. Merten DF, Carpenter BLM: Radiologic imaging of inflicted injury in the child abuse syndrome. Pediatr Clin North Am 37:815, 1990.

970. Fordham EW, Ramachandran PC: Radionuclide scanning of osseous trauma. Semin Nucl Med 4:411, 1974.

971. Marty R, Denney JD, McKamey MR, et al: Bone trauma and related benign disease: Assessment by bone scanning. Semin Nucl Med 6:107, 1976.

972. Jaudes PK: Comparison of radiography and radionuclide bone scanning in the detection of child abuse. Pediatrics 73:166, 1984.

973. Haase GM, Ortiz VN, Sfakianakis GN, et al: The value of radionuclide bone scanning in the early recognition of deliberate child abuse. J Trauma 20:873, 1980.

974. Sty JR, Starshak RJ: The role of bone scintigraphy in the evaluation of the suspected abused child. Radiology 146:369, 1983.

975. Smith FW, Gilday DL, Green MD: Unsuspected costo-vertebral fractures demonstrated by bone scanning in the child abuse syndrome. Pediatr Radiol 10:103, 1980.

976. Howard JL, Barron BJ, Smith GG: Bone scintigraphy in the evaluation of extraskeletal injuries from child abuse. RadioGraphics 10:67, 1990.

977. DeSmet AA, Kuhns LR, Kaufman RA, et al: Bony sclerosis and the battered child. Skel Radiol 2:39, 1977.

978. Meservy CJ, Towbin R, McLaurin RL, et al: Radiographic characteristics of skull fractures resulting from child abuse. AJR 149:173, 1987.

979. King J, Diefendorf D, Apthorp J, et al: Analysis of 429 fractures in 189 battered children. J Pediatr Orthop 8:585, 1988.

980. Kleinman PK, Marks SC: Vertebral body fractures in child abuse. Radiologic-histopathologic correlates. Invest Radiol 27:715, 1992.

981. Carty HML: Fractures caused by child abuse. J Bone Joint Surg [Br] 75:849, 1993.

982. Leventhal JM, Thomas SA, Rosenfield NS, et al: Fractures in young children. Distinguishing child abuse from unintentional injuries. Am J Dis Child 147:87, 1993.

983. Kleinman PK, Marks SC, Adams VI, et al: Factors affecting visualization of posterior rib fractures in abused infants. AJR 150:635, 1988.

984. Kleinman PK, Marks SC, Spevak MR, et al: Fractures of the rib head in abused infants. Radiology 185:119, 1992.

985. Duhaime A-C, Genarelli TA, Thibault LE, et al: The shaken baby syndrome. A clinical, pathological, and biochemical study. J Neurosurg 66:409, 1987.

986. Kleinman PK: Diagnostic imaging in infant abuse. AJR 155:703, 1990.

987. Kleinman PK, Belanger PL, Karellas A, et al: Normal metaphyseal radiologic variants not to be confused with findings of infant abuse. AJR 156:781, 1991.

988. Oestrich AE, Ahmad BS: The periphysis and its effect on the metaphysis: I. Definition and normal radiographic pattern. Skel Radiol 21:283, 1992.

989. Kleinman PK: Differentiation of child abuse and osteogenesis imperfecta: Medical and legal implications. AJR 154:1047, 1990.

990. Ablin DS, Greenspan A, Reinhart M, et al: Differentiation of child abuse from osteogenesis imperfecta. AJR 154:1035, 1990.

991. Carty H: Differentiation of child abuse from osteogenesis imperfecta. AJR 156:635, 1991.

992. Dent JA, Paterson CR: Fractures in early childhood: Osteogenesis imperfecta or child abuse? J Pediatr Orthop 11:184, 1991.

993. Langer LO, Brill PW, Ozonoff MB, et al: Spondylometaphyseal dysplasia, corner fracture type: A heritable condition associated with coxa vara. Radiology 175:761, 1990.

994. Kleinman PK: Schmid-like metaphyseal chondrodysplasia simulating child abuse. AJR 156:576, 1991.

995. Gerdes AM, Tonnesen T, Pergament E, et al: Variability in clinical expression of Menkes syndrome. Eur J Pediatr 148:132, 1988.

996. Wesenberg RL, Gwinn JL, Barnes GR Jr: Radiological findings in the kinky-hair syndrome. Radiology 92:500, 1969.

997. Menkes JH: Kinky hair disease. Pediatrics 50:181, 1972.

998. Adams PC, Strand RD, Bresnan MJ, et al: Kinky hair syndrome: Serial study

999. Kirschner RH, Stein RJ: The mistaken diagnosis of child abuse. A form of medical abuse? J Am Dis Child 139:873, 1985.

1000. Horan FT, Beighton PH: Infantile metaphyseal dysplasia or "battered babies"? J Bone Joint Surg [Br] 62:243, 1980.

1001. Pickett WJ III, Johnson F, Enzenauer RW: Case report 192. Skel Radiol 8:85, 1982.

1002. Helfer RE, Scheurer SL, Alexander R, et al: Trauma to the bones of small infants from passive exercise: A factor in the etiology of child abuse. J Pediatr 104:47, 1984.

1003. Sundar M, Carty H: Avulsion fractures of the pelvis in children: A report of 32 fractures and their outcome. Skeletal Radiol 23:85, 1994.

1004. Diament MJ: Should the radionuclide skeletal survey be used as a screening procedure in suspected child abuse victims. Radiology 148:573, 1983.

1005. Macones AJ Jr, Fisher MS, Locke JL: Stress-related rib and vertebral changes. Radiology 170:117, 1989.

1006. Wood BP: Infant ribs: Generalized periosteal reaction resulting from vibrator chest physiotherapy. Radiology 162:811, 1987.

1007. Stern RE, Harwin SF: Spontaneous and simultaneous rupture of both quadriceps tendons. Clin Orthop 147:188, 1980.

1008. Pritsch M, Horoshovski H, Farine I: Arthroscopic treatment of osteochondral lesions of the talus. J Bone Joint Surg [Am] 68:862, 1986.

1009. Haller J, Kindynis P, Resnick D, et al: Fatigue fracture of the sacrum: A case report. J Can Assoc Radiol 40:277, 1989.

1010. Volpin G, Milgrom C, Goldsher D, et al: Stress fractures of the sacrum following strenuous activity. Clin Orthop 243:184, 1989.

1011. Piétu G, Cistac C, Letenneur J: Triplane fractures of the upper end of the tibia. Report of two cases. Fr J Orthop 5:104, 1991.

1012. Black KP, Ehlert KJ: A stress fracture of the lateral process of the talus in a runner. J Bone Joint Surg [Am] 76:441, 1994.

1013. Gregori ACP: Tibial stress fractures in two professional golfers. J Bone Joint Surg [Br] 76:157, 1994.

1014. Milgrom C, Finestone A, Shlamkovitch N, et al: Youth is a risk factor for stress fracture. A study of 783 infantry recruits. J Bone Joint Surg [Br] 76:20, 1994.

1015. Bollen SR, Robinson DG, Crichton KJ, et al: Stress fractures of the ulna in tennis players using a double-handed backhand stroke. Am J Sports Med 21:751, 1993.

1016. Renu JMA, Bou CV, Portet RV, et al: Osteochondritis dissecans of the patella. 12 cases followed for 4 years. Acta Orthop Scand 65:77, 1994.

1017. Sanpera L Jr, Fixsen JA, Hill RA: Injuries to the physis by extravasation. A rare cause of growth plate arrest. J Bone Joint Surg [Br] 76:278, 1994.

1018. Mullaji AB, Emery RJH, Joysey VC, et al: HLA and slipped capital femoral epiphysis. J Orthop Rheumatol 6:167, 1993.

1019. Wioland M, Bonnerot V: Diagnosis of partial and total physeal arrest by bone single-photon emission computed tomography. J Nucl Med 34:1410, 1993.

1020. Snyder M, Harcke HT, Bowen JR, et al: Evaluation of physeal behavior in response to epiphyseodesis with the use of serial magnetic resonance imaging. J Bone Joint Surg [Am] 76:224, 1994.

1021. Noonan KJ, Saltzman CL, Dietz FR: Open physeal fractures of the distal phalanx of the great toe. A case report. J Bone Joint Surg [Am] 76:122, 1994.

1022. Green SA, Gibbs P: The relationship of angulation to translation in fracture deformities. J Bone Joint Surg [Am] 76:390, 1994.

1023. Vande Berg BC, Malghem J, Goffin EJ, et al: Transient epiphyseal lesions in renal transplant recipients: Presumed insufficiency stress fractures. Radiology 191:403, 1994.

1024. Rogers LF, Poznanski AK: Imaging of epiphyseal injuries. Radiology 191:297, 1994.

1025. Keenan WNW, Clegg J: Idiopathic bilateral slipped upper femoral epiphysis in a child under six years of age. J Bone Joint Surg [Am] 76:495, 1994.

1026. Hughes LO, Beaty JH: Fractures of the head and neck of the femur in children. J Bone Joint Surg [Am] 76:283, 1994.

of radiological findings with emphasis on the similarity to the battered child syndrome. Radiology 112:401, 1974.

68

Physical Injury: Extraspinal Sites

Donald Resnick, M.D., and Thomas G. Goergen, M.D.

In the previous chapter, concepts and terminology related to physical injury of bones, joints, and soft tissues (i.e., tendons, ligaments, and muscles) were addressed. Some types of injuries, such as those of the synchondroses (growth plates), that are unique to the immature skeleton and others, such as greenstick, torus, and bowing fractures, that virtually are confined to the immature skeleton were addressed as well. In this chapter and the next, specific injuries to extraspinal and spinal sites are summarized. Emphasis here is placed on articular subluxations, dislocations, and diastases and on fractures of periarticular bone, although important injuries of the long and short tubular, flat, irregular, and small bones also are discussed. The role of routine radiography, justifiably, receives foremost attention, as it frequently represents the initially (and, sometimes, solely) employed diagnostic method. Other imaging techniques such as CT and MR imaging are discussed, but these receive more emphasis in Chapters 67 and 69 and, particularly, in Chapter 70, in which a variety of internal derangements of joints are described.

This survey of physical injuries of extraspinal sites begins in the upper extremity, proceeding in a proximal to distal direction, then considers the lower extremity, again in a proximal to distal direction, and finally extends to the bony pelvis and thoracic cage. It is not meant to compete with standard references in the field[1–6] but rather to provide an overview of the more important physical injuries occurring in extraspinal sites. Furthermore, a discussion of injuries of the cranium and facial bones is beyond the scope of this chapter. The interested reader should refer to the excellent summary of such injuries provided by Rogers.[2]

UPPER EXTREMITY

Shoulder

Injuries about the shoulder are among the most commonly encountered traumatic abnormalities, although their precise patterns vary according to the person's age. Fractures of the clavicle and physeal injuries of the proximal humerus are encountered at birth; clavicular fractures also are frequent in the child; dislocations of the glenohumeral and acromioclavicular joints typically are seen in young adults; and fractures of the proximal portion of the humerus dominate in elderly persons.

Glenohumeral Joint Dislocation. The glenohumeral joint is relatively unstable. The glenoid cavity has an articular surface that is approximately one third as large as that of the humeral head, and the stability of the articulation is provided in large part by surrounding capsular and ligamentous structures.[7] Such structures include the muscles and tendons of the rotator cuff, the glenoid labrum, the glenohumeral ligaments, and the coracoacromial arch (see Chapter 70). Because of these anatomic characteristics and the frequency of injury to the shoulder region, dislocations of this joint occur often. These dislocations can be classified into anterior, posterior, superior, and inferior types.

Anterior dislocation is by far the most frequent, representing over 95 per cent of such injuries (Fig. 68–1). Anterior dislocations are further classified as subcoracoid (the most common type) (Fig. 68–2A), subglenoid (second in frequency) (Fig. 68–2B), and subclavicular and intrathoracic (rare types of anterior dislocation) (Fig. 68–3). Anterior dislocations (as well as posterior dislocations of the glenohumeral joint) are best evaluated radiographically by the inclusion of a lateral scapular projection or an axillary projection, or both, in addition to the standard frontal views of the shoulder (Fig. 68–4).

Anterior dislocations are associated with a compression fracture on the posterolateral aspect of the humeral head that is produced by impaction of the humerus against the anterior rim of the glenoid fossa. This osseous defect of the humerus has been recognized for a century,[8] although the report of Hill and Sachs in 1940[9] of the humeral lesion was the first review of the subject in the English language. Because of this, the osseous defect frequently is termed the Hill-Sachs lesion (Fig. 68–5).

This lesion is observed in many cases of anterior dislocation of the glenohumeral joint. It frequently is larger in

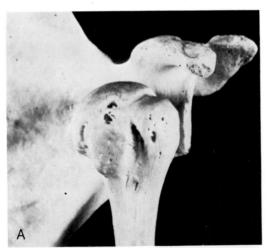

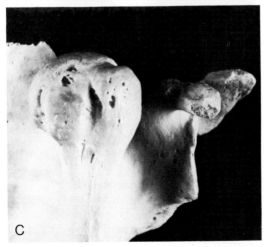

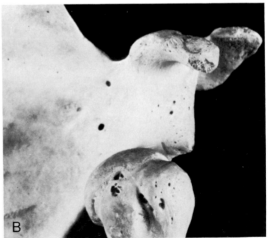

FIGURE 68–1. Glenohumeral joint: Types of anterior dislocation.

A Subcoracoid type. This is the most common variety of anterior dislocation, resulting from a combination of indirect abduction, extension, and external rotation forces. The head of the humerus is displaced anteriorly and is situated inferior to the coracoid process.

B Subglenoid type. This is the second most common type of anterior dislocation of the glenohumeral joint. The head of the humerus is displaced in an anterior and inferior direction owing to an abduction force that is stronger than the external rotation force. Fracture of the greater tuberosity of the humerus and tearing of the rotator cuff are well-recognized complications of this pattern of dislocation.

C Subclavicular type. This rare type of anterior glenohumeral joint dislocation is characterized by the addition of a lateral force that drives the humeral head medial to the coracoid process and below the midportion of the clavicle.

(**A-C,** From Greenway GD, et al: Med Radiogr Photogr *58*:22, 1982.)

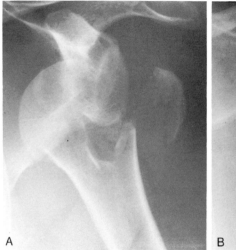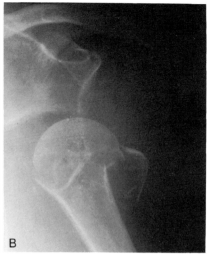

FIGURE 68-2. Glenohumeral joint: Anterior dislocation—subcoracoid and subglenoid types.
   A Subcoracoid type. Note the anterior and medial displacement of the humeral head and fracture of the greater tuberosity.
   B Subglenoid type. The humeral head is displaced anteriorly and inferiorly, and the greater tuberosity is fractured.

those cases that are dislocated for a considerable period of time, those that are recurrent, and those in which the direction of dislocation is anteroinferior rather than purely anterior.[10] The reported frequency of the lesion has varied considerably. Hill and Sachs detected it in 27 per cent of 119 cases of acute anterior dislocation and in 74 per cent of 15 cases of recurrent anterior dislocation.[9] Other investigators have noted the Hill-Sachs defect in 50 to 100 per cent of cases of recurrent dislocations.[11–16] Much of this variation is related to the difference in the radiographic technique used to investigate patients with glenohumeral joint dislocation.[10, 17, 18] In fact, many different radiographic projections have been described in this clinical setting (see Chapter 1). Films obtained in various degrees of internal rotation are mandatory, as such rotation of the humerus will produce a tangential view of the osseous lesion (Fig. 68–6). Fluoroscopy also can be helpful in equivocal cases. The role of CT in allowing identification of the Hill-Sachs lesion has not been defined precisely, although it is certainly less important than the role of computed arthrotomography (and

MR imaging) in delineating associated abnormalities of the glenoid labrum[19–24] (see following discussion and Chapters 13 and 70). The radiographic detection of a Hill-Sachs lesion is important, as it delineates the nature of a shoulder injury that may be obscure clinically, implies a propensity for recurrent dislocation, and influences the necessity for and choice of a surgical procedure (Fig. 68–7).

A second type of fracture accompanying anterior dislocation of the humeral head involves the glenoid fossa and is called the Bankart lesion[25] (Figs. 68–8 and 68–9). When osseous fragmentation of the anterior glenoid rim occurs, the abnormality may be apparent on plain film radiographs in frontal or axillary projections, or both.[26] Specialized radiographic projections such as the Didiee and the West Point views are of further diagnostic help.[18] Although large osseous fractures of the glenoid are apparent occasionally,[27] the fracture may include only the cartilaginous surface of the bone, and an arthrogram may be necessary to detect the changes (see Chapter 13). Double contrast arthrography (air and contrast media) using the axillary projection is helpful in delineating the cartilaginous Bankart lesion, and this technique also allows identification of the large anterior recesses of the glenohumeral joint that are produced by single or recurrent dislocation. Conventional[28] or computed[29] arthrotomography and standard MR imaging or MR arthrography represent the methods of choice in the detection of alterations of the glenoid labrum, however (see Chapter 70).

A number of other osseous and nonosseous injuries accompany anterior dislocations of the glenohumeral joint. An avulsion fracture of the greater tuberosity of the humerus occurs in 10 to 15 per cent of cases. It is variable in size, and the resulting abnormal contour of the humeral head may simulate that seen with a Hill-Sachs lesion. Disruption of the rotator cuff may complicate anterior dislocation of the glenohumeral joint, particularly in patients who are older than 40 years of age.[30, 31] Various portions of the cuff, including the supraspinatus, infraspinatus, and subscapularis tendons, may be affected, and resulting clinical manifestations (i.e., inability to abduct the arm after reduction of the dislocation) may be falsely attributed to an injury of the axillary nerve. Indeed, injuries to the brachial plexus occur in 7 to 45 per cent of anterior glenohumeral joint

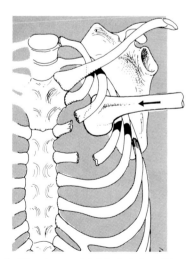

FIGURE 68-3. Glenohumeral joint: Anterior dislocation—intrathoracic type. This extremely rare variety of anterior dislocation of the glenohumeral joint is characterized by medial displacement of the humeral head, which is driven between the ribs, entering the thoracic cavity.

Text continued on page 2700

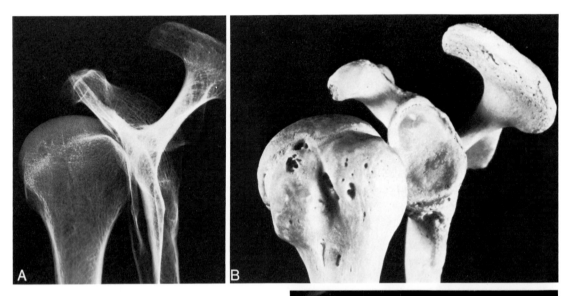

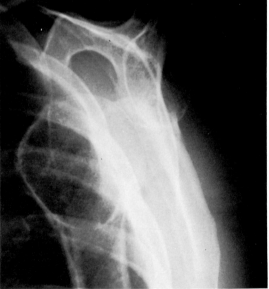

FIGURE 68–4. Glenohumeral joint: Anterior dislocation—use of lateral scapular projection.

A, B A tangential radiograph of the scapula reveals the displaced humeral head, which now lies in front of the glenoid cavity beneath the coracoid process. (From Greenway GD, et al: Med Radiogr Photogr *58*:22, 1982.)

C In this patient, the tangential scapular projection reveals the abnormal position of the humeral head, which is located in front of the glenoid cavity.

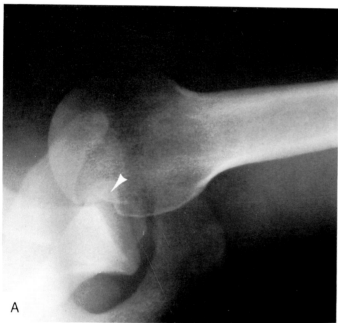

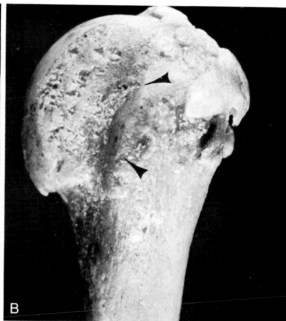

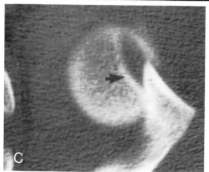

FIGURE 68–5. Glenohumeral joint: Anterior dislocation—Hill-Sachs lesion.

   A An axillary radiograph reveals an anterior dislocation of the humeral head. Note the impaction of the anterior glenoid process and the posterolateral aspect of the humeral head, producing a Hill-Sachs lesion (arrowhead). Although the dislocation is well shown on this radiograph, axillary projections are difficult to obtain while the humeral head is still displaced.

   B A photograph of the posterior surface of the humeral head demonstrates the characteristics of a Hill-Sachs lesion (arrowheads).

   C Transaxial CT shows an anterior dislocation with a Hill-Sachs lesion (arrow).

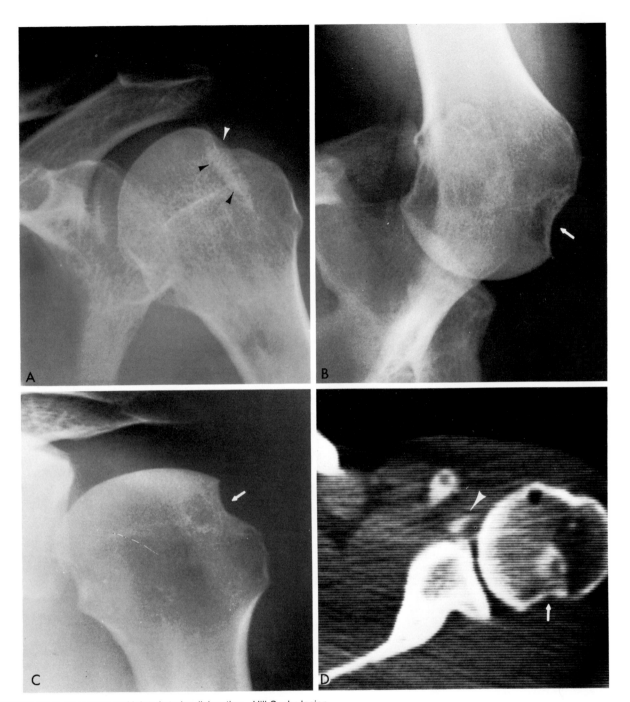

FIGURE 68–6. Glenohumeral joint: Anterior dislocation—Hill-Sachs lesion.

A In a patient with a previous anterior dislocation, the internal rotation view reveals the extent of the Hill-Sachs lesion (arrowheads).

B–D In a different patient, a large Hill-Sachs lesion is evident on both the notch **(B)** and Didiee **(C)** views (arrows). Note its presence on the CT **(D)** (arrow) in association with fragmentation of the anterior glenoid rim (arrowhead).

POSTERIOR

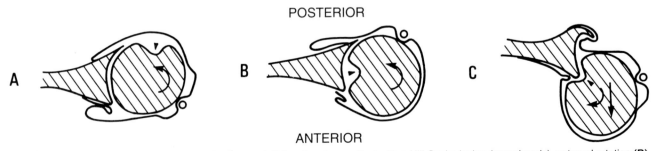

ANTERIOR

FIGURE 68–7. Hill-Sachs lesion: Propensity for recurrent dislocation. In a patient with a Hill-Sachs lesion (arrowheads), external rotation **(B)** may allow the lesion to engage the glenoid process so that during subsequent internal rotation **(C)**, the humeral head is levered out of the glenoid fossa, producing an anterior dislocation. (**A**, Neutral position.) (Courtesy of G. Greenway, M.D., Dallas, Texas.)

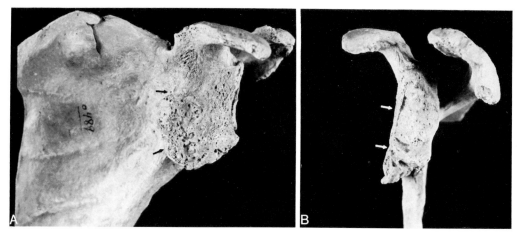

FIGURE 68–8. Glenohumeral joint: Anterior dislocation—Bankart lesion. An exaggerated Bankart-type lesion has resulted from a chronic unreduced anterior dislocation. A large osseous lesion (arrows) is well seen on frontal and tangential photographs of this scapular specimen.

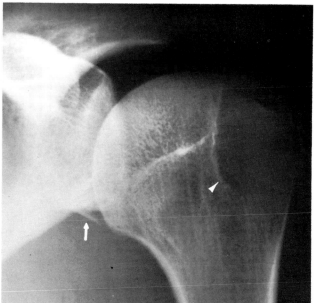

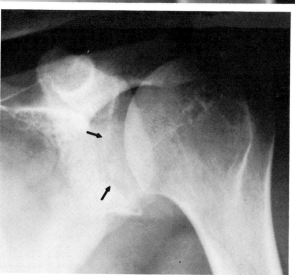

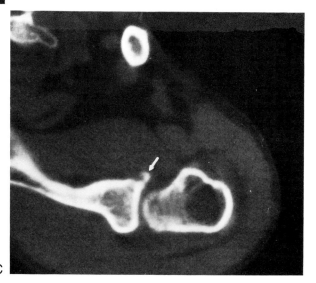

FIGURE 68–9. Glenohumeral joint: Anterior dislocation—Bankart lesion.
　A In addition to the Hill-Sachs lesion (arrowhead), note the fragmentation of the glenoid rim (arrow).
　B In a different patient, disruption of the anterior margin of the glenoid fossa is seen (between arrows).
　C Transaxial CT shows a typical osseous Bankart lesion (arrow).

dislocations, and such injuries may occur with or without rotator cuff disruption.[899]

Approximately 40 per cent of anterior glenohumeral joint dislocations are recurrent.[2] Recurrent dislocations are more likely in cases of subcoracoid and subglenoid dislocations and in younger persons. Chronic unreduced anterior dislocations with massive Hill-Sachs and Bankart-like lesions also are encountered[32] (Fig. 68–8).

Many types of surgical procedures have been advocated for the treatment of patients with recurrent anterior glenohumeral joint dislocations. Some of these are listed in Table 68–1.

Posterior dislocation of the glenohumeral joint is rare, constituting approximately 2 to 4 per cent of all shoulder dislocations. Specific types of posterior dislocation include the subacromial (the most common type) and the subglenoid and subspinous (rare injuries) varieties (Fig. 68–10). Over 50 per cent of these cases are unrecognized on initial evaluation, despite the presence of a history of trauma, pain, swelling, and limitation of motion. The diagnosis of adhesive capsulitis (frozen shoulder) often is suggested in such cases.[33, 34] Many cases of posterior dislocation result from convulsions, and in these instances, bilateral dislocations may be evident[35–37] (Fig. 68–11). Physical examination reveals a posteriorly displaced humeral head that is held in internal rotation.[38] Absence of external rotation and limitation of abduction are present in virtually all cases of posterior dislocation. Associated injuries include stretching of the posterior capsule, fracture of the posterior aspect of the glenoid rim, an avulsion fracture of the lesser tuberosity of the humerus, and a stretched or detached subscapularis tendon.

Radiographs are diagnostic; the routine examination must include a lateral view of the scapula (Fig. 68–12) or an axillary view of the shoulder, or both, and additional projections also may be helpful.[39] On an anteroposterior radiograph, posterior dislocation of the humeral head distorts the normal elliptical radiodense area created by the overlapping of the head and the glenoid fossa (Fig. 68–13). An empty or vacant glenoid cavity is a second radiographic sign of dislocation in this projection; the posterior displacement of the humeral head may create a space between the anterior rim of the glenoid and the humeral head that frequently is

greater than 6 mm.[40] In addition, the normal parallel pattern of the articular surfaces of the glenoid concavity and the humeral head convexity is lost. Other radiographic signs of posterior dislocation on frontal radiographs include a fixed position of internal rotation of the humerus and a second cortical line, the trough line, parallel and lateral to the subchondral articular surface of the humeral head.[41] This line represents the margin of a troughlike impaction fracture of the humeral head (Fig. 68–14) created when this structure contacts the posterior glenoid rim during the dislocation.[42] As such, it is analogous to the Hill-Sachs lesion that is seen in association with anterior glenohumeral joint dislocation and is quite diagnostic of a posterior dislocation. The medially located lesser tuberosity that appears during marked internal rotation in the normal shoulder should not be misinterpreted as a trough or as a site of impaction fracture, however.

A tangential view of the glenoid normally demonstrates no overlapping of the humeral head and glenoid rim.[43] In patients with posterior glenohumeral joint dislocation, the humeral head is displaced medially, and abnormal overlapping may be seen. An axillary or lateral scapular projection directly delineates the posterior position of the humeral head with respect to the glenoid. The degree of displacement of the humeral head as evident on these two projections in patients with posterior dislocations of the glenohumeral joint, particularly when associated with large trough fractures of the humeral head, may be less than in those patients with anterior dislocations of the glenohumeral joint, producing some diagnostic difficulty.

CT represents an additional imaging technique that can be used to evaluate patients with acute (or chronic) dislocations of the glenohumeral joint[32] (Figs. 68–15 and 68–16). This method also is useful in the evaluation of posterior subluxation (without frank dislocation) of the glenohumeral joint.[44]

Owing to a delay in accurate diagnosis of posterior dislocations of the glenohumeral joint,[45] secondary osteoarthritis in this location is not infrequent.[46] Radiographic findings, including joint space narrowing, osteophytosis, and deformity of the humeral head, simulate those of calcium pyrophosphate dihydrate crystal deposition disease, hydroxyapatite crystal deposition disease, ischemic necrosis of bone, and ochronosis. In untreated chronic dislocations, deformity of the posterior portion of the scapula is seen (Fig. 68–17).

Superior dislocation of the glenohumeral joint is rare[47] (Fig. 68–18). An extreme forward and upward force on the adducted arm can produce extensive damage to the rotator cuff, capsule, biceps tendon, and surrounding musculature and fracture of the acromion, clavicle, coracoid process, or humeral tuberosities. Without such fractures, the radiographic appearance of a superior dislocation of the humeral head is identical to that of a primary, massive rotator cuff tear. *Inferior dislocation* of the glenohumeral joint (luxatio erecta) also is rare[48–54] (Fig. 68–19). A direct axial force on a fully abducted arm or a hyperabduction force leading to leverage of the humeral head across the acromion is responsible for this type of dislocation.[54] Following this injury, the superior aspect of the articular surface of the humeral head is directed inferiorly and does not contact the inferior glenoid rim. As a result, the arm is held over the patient's head, the inferior aspect of the capsule is torn, and associ-

TABLE 68–1. Some Types of Surgical Procedures Used for Recurrent Anterior Glenohumeral Joint Dislocations

Procedure	Technique
Bankart[25]	Repair of anterior capsular mechanism using drill holes and sutures
Putti-Platt[253]	Shortening of the anterior capsule and subscapularis muscle
Magnuson-Stack[254]	Transfer of the subscapularis tendon from lesser tuberosity to greater tuberosity
Eden-Hybbinette[255, 256]	Bone graft to anterior glenoid region
Oudard[257]	Bone graft to coracoid process
Trillat[258]	Osteotomy with displacement of coracoid process
Bristow-Helfet[259]	Transfer of coracoid process with its attached tendons to neck of the scapula

Text continued on page 2705

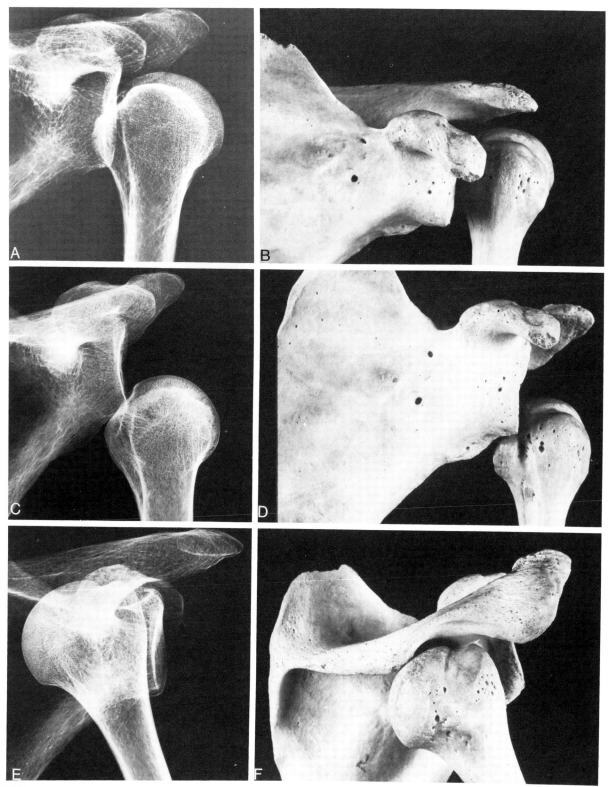

FIGURE 68–10. Glenohumeral joint: Types of posterior dislocation.

A, B Subacromial type. This is the most common pattern of posterior dislocation of a glenohumeral joint. The articular surface of the humeral head is directed posteriorly and is behind the glenoid fossa and beneath the acromion process. Note the internal rotation of the humerus.

C, D Subglenoid type. This is a less common pattern of injury in which the humeral head is displaced posteriorly and inferiorly with respect to the glenoid fossa.

E, F Subspinous type. In this rare injury, the humeral head becomes situated medial to the acromion process, inferior to the scapular spine, and posterior to the glenoid process. (From Greenway GD, et al: Med Radiogr Photogr *58*:22, 1982.)

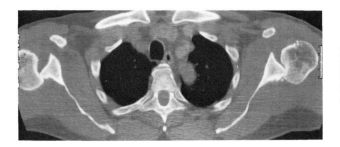

FIGURE 68–11. Glenohumeral joint: Posterior dislocation—bilateral recurrent dislocations. Transaxial CT shows posterior displacement of both humeral heads and trough fractures of the medial surface of the humeral heads. (Courtesy of M. Schweitzer, M.D., Philadelphia, Pennsylvania.)

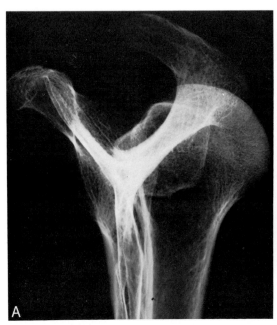

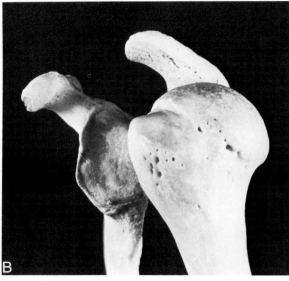

FIGURE 68–12. Glenohumeral joint: Posterior dislocation— use of lateral scapular projection. The lateral projection of the scapula outlines the posterior position of the humeral head, which is located beneath the acromion process. The degree of humeral displacement in cases of posterior glenohumeral joint dislocation is variable; in many instances, it is subluxed rather than truly dislocated. (From Greenway GD, et al: Med Radiogr Photogr 58:22, 1982).

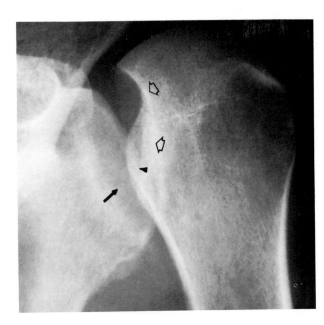

FIGURE 68–13. Glenohumeral joint: Posterior dislocation. An anteroposterior radiograph in a patient with a posterior glenohumeral joint dislocation. Findings include distortion of the normal elliptical radiodense region created by overlying of the humeral head and glenoid fossa (arrowhead), a "vacant" glenoid cavity (solid arrow), loss of parallelism between the articular surfaces of the glenoid cavity and humeral head, internal rotation of the humerus, and an impaction fracture (open arrows).

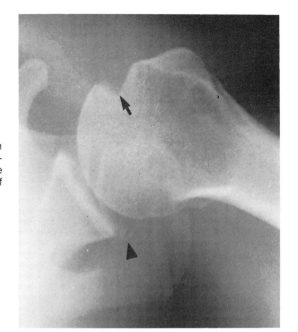

FIGURE 68–14. Glenohumeral joint: Posterior dislocation—trough fracture. An axillary radiograph reveals this fracture (arrow) involving the anteromedial portion of the humeral head, indicative of a previous posterior dislocation of the glenohumeral joint. Note fragmentation (arrowhead) of the posterior aspect of the glenoid rim.

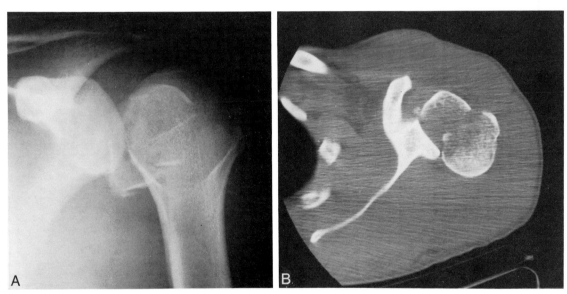

FIGURE 68–15. Glenohumeral joint: Posterior dislocation—use of CT in acute injuries. In a 23 year old man, the frontal radiograph **(A)** demonstrates an abnormal relationship of the humeral head and glenoid fossa, an empty glenoid cavity, and avulsion and fragmentation of the lesser tuberosity of the humerus. A transaxial CT scan **(B)** shows a posterior dislocation of the glenohumeral joint and the avulsed tuberosity.

FIGURE 68–16. Glenohumeral joint: Posterior dislocation—use of CT in chronic injuries. This 38 year old man had a long history of shoulder pain with decreased motion of the glenohumeral joint. Movement of this articulation was associated with crepitus. The frontal radiograph **(A)** shows a humerus that is internally rotated, irregularity of the glenoid region of the scapula, and deformity of the medial aspect of the humeral head. A transaxial CT scan **(B)** reveals a chronic posterior dislocation of the glenohumeral joint, a trough fracture of the humeral head (open arrow), and excavation of the posterior surface of the scapula (arrowhead).

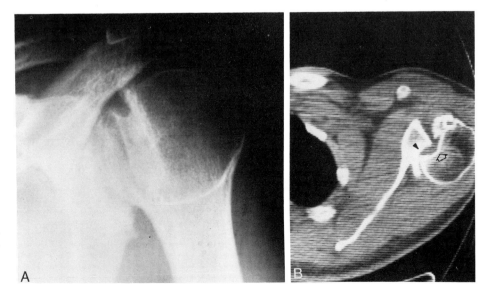

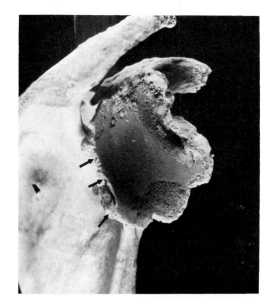

FIGURE 68–17. Glenohumeral joint: Posterior dislocation—scapular deformity. Note the deformity of the posterior portion of the glenoid fossa (arrows). This finding relates to the long-standing abutment of the posteriorly dislocated humeral head and glenoid cavity.

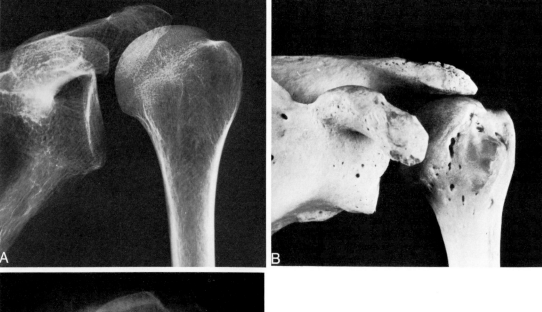

FIGURE 68–18. Glenohumeral joint: Superior dislocation.

A, B In this unusual pattern of dislocation, the humeral head is displaced in a superior direction. Damage to the soft tissues, including the joint capsule, the rotator cuff, the biceps tendon, and the surrounding muscles, is seen. Fractures associated with this dislocation also may be apparent. (From Greenway GD, et al: Med Radiogr Photogr *58*:22, 1982).

C An example of an acute superior dislocation of the glenohumeral joint is shown. Note the elevation of the humeral head with respect to the glenoid cavity.

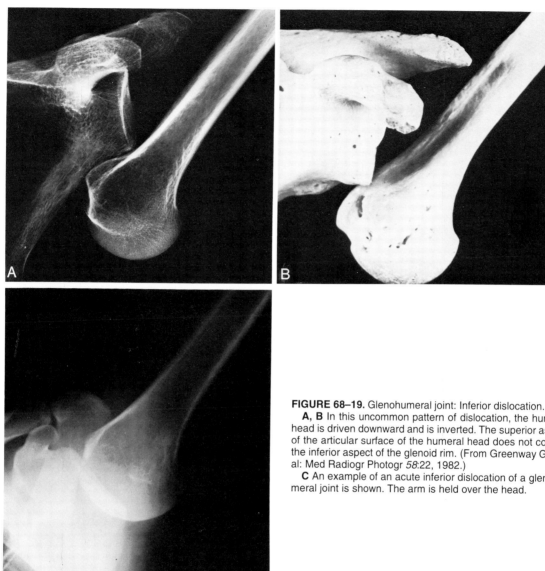

FIGURE 68–19. Glenohumeral joint: Inferior dislocation.
   A, B In this uncommon pattern of dislocation, the humeral head is driven downward and is inverted. The superior aspect of the articular surface of the humeral head does not contact the inferior aspect of the glenoid rim. (From Greenway GD, et al: Med Radiogr Photogr *58*:22, 1982.)
   C An example of an acute inferior dislocation of a glenohumeral joint is shown. The arm is held over the head.

ated injuries, including a fracture of the greater tuberosity of the humerus, of the acromion process, of the coracoid process, of the clavicle, or of the inferior glenoid margin, may be seen. A lesion of the humeral head, simulating a Hill-Sachs lesion, may accompany luxatio erecta, although it is located more superiorly and laterally.[54] Complications of inferior dislocation of the glenohumeral joint include injuries of the axillary artery and brachial plexus and, later, recurrent subluxation or dislocation and adhesive capsulitis.

In addition to traumatic glenohumeral joint dislocation, *voluntary subluxation or dislocation* may be encountered, especially in adolescents.[55, 56] In these cases, spontaneous displacements of the humeral head on one or both sides occur anteriorly or, more frequently, posteriorly. Although it has been proposed that developmental anomalies of the glenoid cavity or generalized ligamentous laxity may be responsible for this phenomenon[57, 58] and that some patients also may reveal genu valgum and weak arches, widespread abnormalities generally are not evident in patients with

voluntary dislocation of the glenohumeral joint.[56] This condition has a favorable prognosis.[889]

A special type of inferior displacement of the humeral head is termed the *drooping shoulder*[59–62] (Fig. 68–20). It can be associated with uncomplicated fractures of the surgical neck of the humerus. The pathogenesis of the displacement is not clear, although relaxation or stretching of the supporting musculature, detachment of the capsule, and hemarthrosis have each been proposed as possible mechanisms. The appearance of a similar displacement in patients with neurologic injuries of the brachial plexus, especially those involving the axillary nerve, supports the view that muscular alterations produce the subluxation, whereas the detection of a drooping shoulder in patients with various articular disorders (e.g., hemophilia) may indicate that joint effusion also can lead to inferior displacement of the humeral head. The degree of inferior displacement of the humeral head is variable. In some cases, only subtle widening of the superior portion of the joint space is visible,

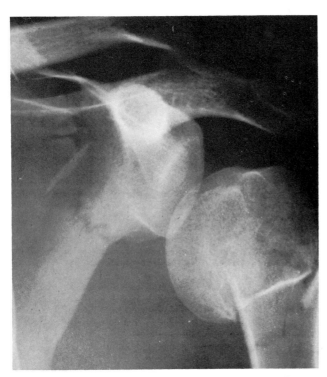

FIGURE 68–20. Glenohumeral joint: Drooping shoulder. A fracture of the surgical neck of the humerus is associated with inferior subluxation of the head with respect to the glenoid cavity. Observe an associated scapular fracture.

whereas in others gross displacement is seen. Recognition of this condition will eliminate erroneous diagnosis of fracture-dislocation of the proximal humerus, and conservative therapy will lead to disappearance of the drooping shoulder over a period of weeks.

Acromioclavicular Joint Dislocation. Subluxation or dislocation of the acromioclavicular joint is a common injury,[63–65] representing approximately 10 per cent of all dislocations involving the shoulder. Acromioclavicular joint injury is observed most commonly in patients between the ages of 16 and 40 years. The abnormality is rare in children,[66] in whom an apparent dislocation of the acromioclavicular joint can represent, in reality, a displaced fracture of the distal portion of the clavicle (see Chapter 67). Injury to the acromioclavicular joint can result from indirect or direct forces. An upward indirect force produced by a fall on the outstretched hand can be transmitted from its point of application in the upper extremity along the humerus to the acromioclavicular articulation. With the arm in a position of moderate flexion and abduction, the force traverses the glenohumeral joint and is concentrated on the acromion.[67] The scapula is forced in a superior and medial direction. Resulting injuries may include superior dislocation of the glenohumeral joint, acromial fracture, and acromioclavicular capsular stretching and tear. The last-named abnormality, which usually is unassociated with an injury to the coracoclavicular ligament, leads to an acromioclavicular joint sprain or subluxation. A second pattern of indirect injury to the acromioclavicular articulation results from a downward force applied by a pull on the upper extremity. A direct injury to the acromioclavicular joint is produced by a fall on the shoulder at a time when the arm is held in adduction, close to the body. In this most common mecha-

nism of injury, the scapula and the clavicle are driven downward. The clavicle may be impacted against the first rib, preventing its further descent. Resulting injuries can include a fracture of the first rib or of the clavicle or, in the absence of such a fracture, injury to the acromioclavicular articulation. The degree of disruption of the acromioclavicular and coracoclavicular ligaments varies; the initial injury is to the acromioclavicular ligaments followed by damage to the coracoclavicular ligament.

Injuries of the acromioclavicular joint are classified in several ways (one of which is described here), according to the extent of ligamentous damage[68–70] (Fig. 68–21). A type I injury, indicative of a mild sprain, is associated with stretching or tearing of the fibers of the acromioclavicular ligaments; the acromioclavicular joint remains stable, and the clavicular position is normal. A type II injury, indicative of a moderate sprain, is associated with disruption of the acromioclavicular ligaments and the aponeurosis of the deltoid and trapezius muscle attachments to the distal portion of the clavicle. The coracoclavicular ligament may be strained but otherwise is intact, and the distal aspect of the clavicle may sublux in a posterior or superior direction. With this type of injury, minor elevation of the distal portion of the clavicle or widening of the acromioclavicular joint, or both, may be evident on radiographs. A type III injury, representing a severe sprain, is characterized by disruption of both the acromioclavicular and coracoclavicular ligaments along with the muscle aponeurosis; on radiographs, elevation of the distal aspect of the clavicle with respect to the acromion is detected. This injury produces an unstable clavicle. Occasionally, the coracoclavicular ligaments remain intact, and an avulsion fracture or epiphyseal separation of the coracoid process is evident[71–74] (Fig. 68–22).

Type I injuries are diagnosed clinically rather than radiographically, although there may be soft tissue swelling and minimal widening of the acromioclavicular joint. The radiographic diagnosis of type II and type III injuries is based on the detection of displacement of the distal portion of the clavicle with relation to the acromion and on the degree of displacement that is evident (Fig. 68–23). Special radiographs may be required, including an angulated frontal projection[75] and films obtained with weight held in the hand (stress radiographs). The stress radiograph should include both shoulders to facilitate comparison between the uninvolved and involved joints (Fig. 68–24). Widening of the acromioclavicular joint without superior displacement of the distal clavicle may be the sole radiographic feature of an injury. Although comparison of the joint width of the injured side with that on the opposite side or of the width of the injured acromioclavicular joint on the routine and stress radiographs may provide diagnostic help, some articular laxity may occur in asymptomatic and noninjured patients. Upward displacement of the distal clavicle provides more definitive evidence of an acromioclavicular joint injury. A difference of 3 to 4 mm in the distance between the superior aspect of the coracoid process and the inferior or superior aspect of the clavicle in the two shoulders indicates an acromioclavicular subluxation or dislocation in which the injured distal clavicle moves superiorly.[76] A complete coracoclavicular ligament disruption is suggested by an increase of the coracoclavicular distance by 40 to 50 per cent.[77] Rarely, inferior dislocation of the clavicle at the

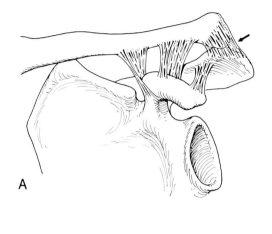

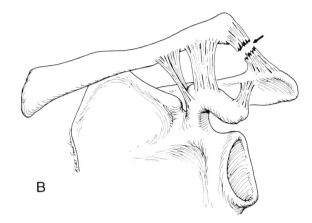

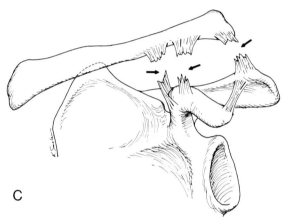

FIGURE 68–21. Acromioclavicular joint: Classification of injuries.

A Type I injury. Stretching or tearing of the fibers of the acromioclavicular ligaments (arrow) constitutes a mild sprain. The relationship between the distal portion of the clavicle and the acromion remains normal.

B Type II injury. Disruption of the acromioclavicular ligaments (arrow) constitutes a part of this injury, which is classified as a moderate sprain. The coracoclavicular ligament may be strained but otherwise is intact. Minor elevation of the distal portion of the clavicle or widening of the acromioclavicular joint, or both, is the anticipated radiographic abnormality.

C Type III injury. This is a severe sprain and is characterized by disruption of both the acromioclavicular and the coracoclavicular ligaments (arrows) with dislocation of the acromioclavicular joint.

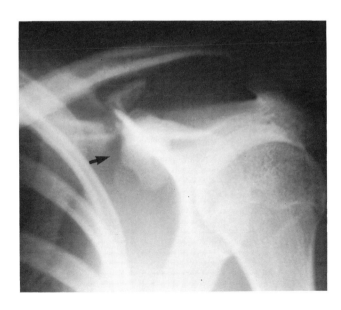

FIGURE 68–22. Acromioclavicular joint dislocation: Type III injury. In this child, the distal portion of the clavicle is elevated, and a fracture (arrow) at the base of the coracoid process is seen.

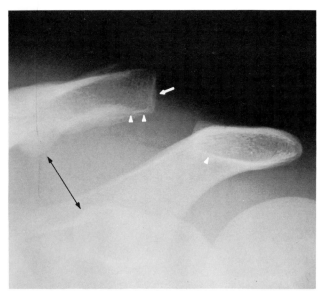

FIGURE 68–23. Acromioclavicular joint dislocation: Type III injury. Observe superior displacement of the clavicle (arrow) with respect to the acromion. The inferior margin of the clavicle no longer is aligned with the inferior margin of the acromion (arrowheads). There is widening of the acromioclavicular joint and an increased distance between the clavicle and the coracoid process (double-ended arrow).

acromioclavicular joint occurs in which the bone is forced beneath the acromion or coracoid process.[78] Other rare patterns of injury include a type III acromioclavicular joint dislocation with superior entrapment of the clavicle above the acromion, preventing reduction,[79] simultaneous dislocations of both the acromioclavicular and sternoclavicular joints (floating clavicle),[80–82] and pseudodislocation of the acromioclavicular articulation owing to a longitudinal rupture in the periosteal envelope of the clavicle.[83]

Certain complications can be noted following subluxation or dislocation of the acromioclavicular joint. Coracoclavicular ligamentous calcification or ossification can appear after the injury regardless of the type of treatment that is initiated[84, 85] (Fig. 68–25). The radiodense collections may occur within a period of weeks following the traumatic episode, can be prominent in as many as 70 per cent of cases, and do not appear to influence the eventual prognosis of the patient.

As discussed in Chapter 94, posttraumatic osteolysis of the distal portion of the clavicle is another complication of acute or repetitive injury to the acromioclavicular joint or

adjacent bones. Progressive resorption of the outer end of the bone follows the injury after a variable period of time (weeks to months) and leads to initial soft tissue swelling and disappearance of the subchondral bone followed by more extensive osseous destruction. Similar changes may appear on the acromion, and the articular surface may widen and become indistinct, simulating an infection. The nature of the injury that initiates the osteolysis can be minor, without radiographic findings. The natural course of the osteolytic process is variable. In general, osteolysis continues for a period of 12 to 18 months, resulting in loss of 0.5 to 3 cm of clavicular bone. Following stabilization of the lytic phase, reparative changes occur over a period of 4 to 6 months, during which cortical reconstitution may be evident. The acromioclavicular articulation may remain widened indefinitely. The pathogenesis of posttraumatic osteolysis is not clear; autonomic nervous system dysfunction, vascular insufficiency, hyperemia, and synovitis have each been suggested as important contributing factors.

Osteoarthritis of the acromioclavicular joint represents one additional complication of dislocation or subluxation.

Sternoclavicular Joint Dislocation. Sternoclavicular joint injuries are rare compared with those of the glenohumeral or acromioclavicular joint, representing only about 2 to 3 per cent of all shoulder dislocations. Anterior dislocations predominate over posterior (retrosternal) dislocations, although the seriousness of posterior dislocations has resulted in many reports of this injury.[86–88] Almost all cases of sternoclavicular subluxation and dislocation are traumatic, although congenital[89] and spontaneous[90] displacements have been recorded. Radiographic analysis is facilitated by a variety of special projections (see Chapter 1) and may be supplemented with conventional or computed tomography in some instances.[19, 91, 92] The latter represents the most important technique in the diagnosis of dislocation of the sternoclavicular articulation.

Traumatic dislocation of the sternoclavicular joint requires a direct or indirect force of great magnitude.[93, 94] Dislocation related to a direct force, the less frequent mechanism of injury, occurs when a force is applied directly to the anteromedial aspect of the clavicle, producing a posterior dislocation of the sternoclavicular joint; anterior sternoclavicular joint dislocation does not occur by direct mechanisms. An indirect force transmitted to the sternoclavicular articulation along the longitudinal axis of the clavicle from the shoulder can produce either an anterior or a posterior sternoclavicular joint dislocation. As indicated previously, panclavicular dislocation with displacement of

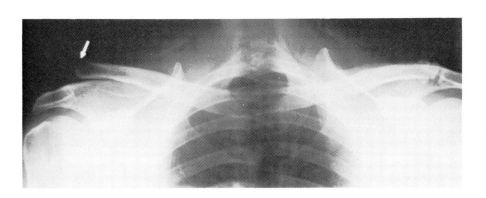

FIGURE 68–24. Acromioclavicular joint dislocation: Type III injury—stress radiography. Compare the radiographic findings on the normal left side and the abnormal right side. The involved clavicle (arrow) is elevated, with an increased distance between the coracoid process and the inferior surface of the clavicle.

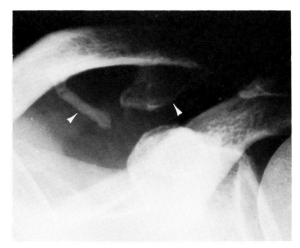

FIGURE 68–25. Acromioclavicular joint dislocation: Coracoclavicular ligament ossification. Observe ligamentous ossification (arrowheads) in a patient who had a type III injury of the acromioclavicular joint.

both the sternoclavicular and the acromioclavicular articulations is a rare injury.

Prompt recognition of the less common posterior sternoclavicular joint dislocation is required because the displaced clavicle may impinge on the trachea, the esophagus, the great vessels, or the major nerves in the superior mediastinum, leading to vascular compromise, cough, dysphagia, and dyspnea. Death may ensue in unrecognized or severe injuries.[94]

Anterior, or presternal, dislocations (Fig. 68–26) are caused by forces that move the shoulder backward and outward or downward. As the distal clavicle is displaced posteriorly, its sternal end, using the first rib and thorax as a fulcrum, springs anteriorly, tearing the sternoclavicular ligaments. An avulsion fracture of the inferior margin of the clavicle may be seen. On physical examination, a prominent anteriorly displaced medial end of the clavicle is visible and palpable and, in the presence of disruption of the costoclavicular ligaments, may be displaced superiorly. Serious complications are rare following this type of dislocation, although a "cosmetic bump" may remain indefinitely.

Posterior, or retrosternal, dislocations of the sternoclavicular joint are an uncommon injury, representing approximately 5 per cent of all of the dislocations at this site (Fig. 68–27). As indicated previously, severe pain may be accompanied by signs related to clavicular impingement on adjacent neurovascular structures and airways. A depression of the skin overlying the displaced medial end of the clavicle may be identified. A pneumothorax or hemothorax may be an associated finding.

An additional injury of the medial end of the clavicle is an epiphyseal fracture or separation. The growth plate at this site is among the last to become obliterated during skeletal maturation, disappearing at approximately 25 years of age. Various types of injuries to the growth plate can occur.[95, 96] Before the medial clavicular epiphysis ossifies at

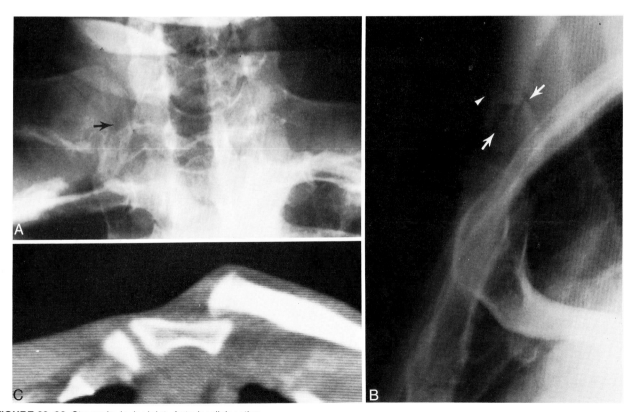

FIGURE 68–26. Sternoclavicular joint: Anterior dislocation.
A, B A lordotic projection **(A)** shows a fracture of the right clavicle (arrow). The superior position of the injured clavicle, in comparison to that of the opposite clavicle, indicates an anterior dislocation of the sternoclavicular joint. In the Heinig view **(B)**, the fracture (arrows) and anterior dislocation (arrowhead) are again visible.
C In a different patient, transaxial CT shows an anterior dislocation of the left sternoclavicular joint.

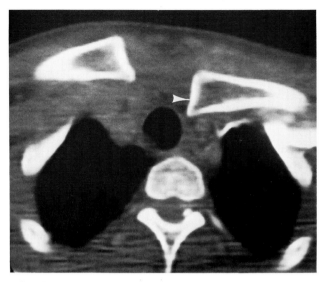

FIGURE 68–27. Sternoclavicular joint: Posterior dislocation. A transaxial CT scan reveals the posterior position of the injured clavicle (arrowhead) and its relationship to the trachea.

the age of about 18 years, it is extremely difficult to differentiate between a dislocation of the sternoclavicular joint and a fracture through the growth plate.

Fractures of the Proximal Portion of the Humerus. The type of injury that is encountered in the proximal portion of the humerus is dependent, to a large extent, on the age of the person. In the neonate, physeal separation or, less commonly, fracture of the proximal portion of the humerus may result from birth injury. In the immature skeleton of the child and adolescent, physeal separation with or without associated fractures is encountered; and in the young adult, glenohumeral joint dislocations or subluxations predominate (see previous discussion). It is in middle-aged adults, over the age of 45 years, and in the elderly that fractures of the proximal portion of the humerus typically are seen (Table 68–2). They are more frequent in women than in men, and—in common with fractures of the vertebral bodies, proximal portion of the femur, and distal portion of the radius—their likelihood following injury is very much dependent on the severity of osteopenia.[97]

The classification of fractures of the proximal region of the humerus on the basis of the level of disruption or the mechanism of injury[98] has been replaced in large part by a scheme proposed by Neer[99] that emphasizes the presence or the absence of significant displacement of one or more of the four major osseous segments of this part of the humerus (Fig. 68–28A). These segments are the articular segment containing the anatomic neck; the greater tuberosity; the lesser tuberosity; and the shaft and surgical neck. Approximately 80 per cent of fractures of the proximal portion of the humerus are undisplaced, owing to the protection afforded by the periosteum, joint capsule, and rotator cuff. A displaced fracture exists if any of the four segments is separated by more than 1 cm from its neighbor or is angulated more than 45 degrees. Nondisplaced fractures or fractures with minimal displacement that do not meet these criteria are considered one-part fractures. A two-part fracture is one in which only a single segment is displaced in relation to the other three; two-part fractures represent approximately 15 per cent of all fractures of the proximal portion of the humerus. A three-part fracture, representing

TABLE 68–2. Fractures of the Humeral Metaphyses and Shaft

Site	Characteristics	Complications
Proximal[92–113]	Middle-aged and elderly adults	Lipohemarthrosis
	Classified as one-part to four-part based on the degree and the location of displacement	Drooping shoulder related to hemarthrosis, capsular tear, muscle or nerve injury
		Osteonecrosis, especially with displaced fractures of humeral neck and four-part fractures
		Osteoarthritis
		Heterotopic ossification
		Rotator cuff tear
		Brachial plexus and, less commonly, axillary artery injury
		Painful arc of motion
Middle[260–268]	Adults > children	Delayed union or nonunion when fracture is transverse or distracted
	Most common at junction of distal and middle thirds	
	Associated fractures in 25 per cent of cases (ulna, clavicle, or humerus)	Radial nerve injury in 5 to 15 per cent of cases
	Characteristic displacements related to sites of muscular attachment	Brachial artery injury
Supracondylar[269–292]	Children >> adults	Brachial artery injury
	Extension (95 per cent) and flexion (5 per cent) types	Median, ulnar, or radial nerve injury
	Paradoxic posterior fat pad sign	Alignment abnormalities
	Supracondylar process may fracture	Heterotopic ossification
		Volkmann's ischemic contracture

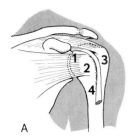

A

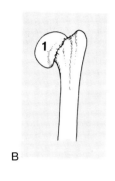

B

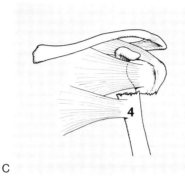

C

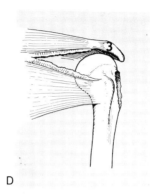

D

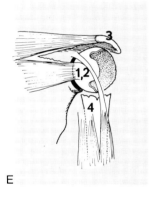

E

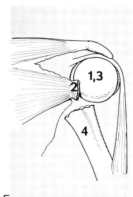

F

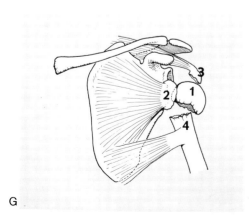

G

FIGURE 68–28. Fractures of the proximal humerus: System of classification.

A Normal situation. Four major segments of the proximal portion of the humerus are identified: 1, humeral head; 2, lesser tuberosity; 3, greater tuberosity; 4, humeral shaft.

B Two-part fracture. In this example, a fracture of the anatomic neck has led to displacement of the humeral head **(1)**. Ischemic necrosis may complicate this rare injury.

C Two-part fracture. In this example, displacement of the humeral shaft **(4)** relates to the pull of the pectoralis major muscle. The rotator cuff is intact and holds the humeral head in a neutral position. Variations of this fracture pattern relate to the extent of impaction, angulation, and comminution.

D Two-part fracture. In this example, displacement of the greater tuberosity **(3)** occurs owing to the forces generated by a portion of the rotator cuff musculature. Retraction of more than 1.0 cm of the entire greater tuberosity or one of its facets is pathognomonic of a longitudinal tear of the rotator cuff. The fragment tends to be large in younger patients and small in older patients. A complication of this injury is impaired motion of the shoulder.

E Three-part fracture. In this injury, the greater tuberosity **(3)** is displaced and the subscapularis muscle rotates the humeral head **(1,2)** so that its articular surface faces posteriorly. The diaphysis **(4)** is displaced relative to the rotated head owing to the action of the pectoralis major muscle.

F Three-part fracture. In this type of injury, the lesser tuberosity **(2)** is detached and displaced by the action of the subscapularis muscle, and the supraspinatus and external rotators cause the articular surface of the humeral head **(1,3)** to face anteriorly. **4,** Humeral shaft.

G Four-part fracture. The articular segment **(1)** is detached from the tuberosities **(2,3)** and from its circulation and is displaced laterally (as shown), anteriorly, or posteriorly, losing contact with the glenoid cavity. The tuberosities usually are retracted by the attached musculature. (From Neer CS II, Rockwood CA Jr: Fractures and dislocations of the shoulder. In CA Rockwood, DP Greene [Eds]: Fractures in Adults. 2nd Ed. Philadelphia, JB Lippincott Co, 1984, p 675.)

approximately 3 or 4 per cent of humeral fractures, occurs when two segments are displaced with relationship to the other two parts, and a four-part fracture, occurring in approximately 3 or 4 per cent of cases, exists when all the humeral segments are displaced. Neer further uses the term fracture-dislocation to indicate that the articular segment of the humerus is displaced beyond the joint space, and he separates this injury from "impression" or "head-splitting" fractures.

The Neer classification system underscores the orthopedic surgeon's concern regarding the degree of displacement of fracture fragments of the proximal portion of the humerus, rather than the specific number of such fragments. As such, it has been used widely to aid in determining the choice of appropriate therapy of these fractures. The application of the Neer classification system is not without difficulties, however, as interpretation of the relationship among the fracture fragments on the basis of routine radiography can be a challenge, and wide interobserver variation regarding the specific type of injury present, even among experienced observers, has been documented.[100, 890–892] CT can be employed as an ancillary technique, allowing more accurate determination of the Neer fracture pattern, particularly in cases of complex humeral fractures.[101, 102]

The classic mechanism of injury is a fall on the outstretched arm in which severe abduction of the shoulder produces a fracture of the humeral neck. A second mechanism of injury is a direct blow on the side of the upper arm. In all types of humeral injury, initial symptoms and signs may be obscured by the thickness of the patient's arm so that accurate diagnosis depends on adequate radiographic examination. In some cases, damage to the axillary vessels or brachial plexus provides additional clues regarding the severity of the injury.

The *one-part (nondisplaced) fracture* is the most frequent pattern of injury. The fracture fragments are closely apposed and are not angulated (Fig. 68–29). Rotation of the humerus usually is followed by movement of all of the fragments as a group.

The *two-part fractures* include isolated displacement of the head with fracture of the anatomic neck, displacement of the shaft with a fracture of the surgical neck, displacement of the greater tuberosity (Fig. 68–30), or displacement of the lesser tuberosity.[99] A two-part fracture with isolated displacement of the humeral head is a rare injury, easily overlooked on initial radiographs, and associated with ischemic necrosis of bone (Fig. 68–28*B*). A two-part fracture with isolated displacement of the shaft owing to a fracture of the surgical neck is a frequent injury; impaction and anterior angulation at the fracture site may be observed (Fig. 68–28*C*). A two-part fracture of the surgical neck also can be associated with anterior and medial displacement of the humeral shaft owing to the pull of the pectoralis major. A third pattern of a two-part surgical neck fracture relates to comminution at the fracture site.

A two-part humeral fracture with displacement of the greater tuberosity is associated with a longitudinal tear of the rotator cuff; the articular segment of the humeral head remains in normal relationship with the shaft (Fig. 68–28*D*). The size of the fracture and the degree of displacement of the greater tuberosity are variable. A two-part humeral fracture with displacement of the lesser tuberosity can occur as an isolated phenomenon[103, 104] or in association

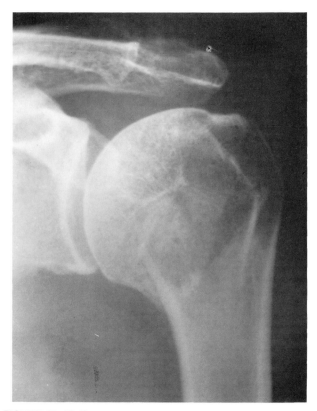

FIGURE 68–29. Fractures of the proximal humerus: One-part (nondisplaced) fracture. Although there are fractures of both the greater tuberosity and the surgical neck of the humerus, no displacement at the sites of fracture is seen.

with a nondisplaced surgical neck fracture. The lesser tuberosity is pulled medially by the subscapularis, but normal alignment between the humeral head and neck is present. Similar fractures of the lesser tuberosity may accompany posterior or anterior dislocations of the glenohumeral joint.

There are two typical patterns of *three-part fractures* of the proximal portion of the humerus; a fracture of the sur-

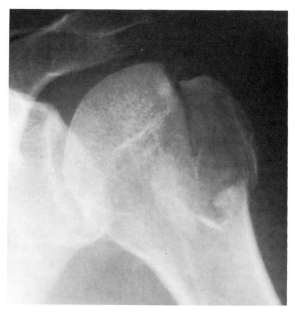

FIGURE 68–30. Fractures of the proximal humerus: Two-part fractures. The greater tuberosity is displaced.

gical neck may be combined with displacement of either the greater tuberosity (Fig. 68–31) or the lesser tuberosity. If the greater tuberosity is avulsed, the subscapularis muscle rotates the humeral head in a posterior direction (Fig. 68–28E); if the lesser tuberosity is avulsed, the supraspinatus, infraspinatus, and teres minor muscles rotate the humeral head in an anterior direction (Fig. 68–28F). The pectoralis major produces anteromedial displacement of the humeral shaft. Open surgical methods are required to reduce these fractures.[105]

The severe *four-part fracture* is characterized by isolation of the humeral articular segment and disruption of its blood supply, rendering it ischemic[106–108] (Fig. 68–28G). Typically, a fracture of the anatomic neck of the humerus is combined with avulsion of the greater and the lesser tuberosities. Displacement of the lesser tuberosity medially related to the pull of the subscapularis; of the greater tuberosity superiorly owing to the pull of the supraspinatus, infraspinatus, and teres minor; and of the shaft medially owing to traction by the pectoralis major is typical. A specific type of four-part fracture of the proximal humerus results in valgus impaction of the articular segment; the frequency of subsequent osteonecrosis of the humeral head is less than that of other displaced four-part fractures.[109]

In association with two-part, three-part, or four-part fractures, the articular surface of the humeral head may be displaced beyond the joint in either an anterior direction (displacement of the greater tuberosity) (Fig. 68–32) or a posterior direction (displacement of the lesser tuberosity).

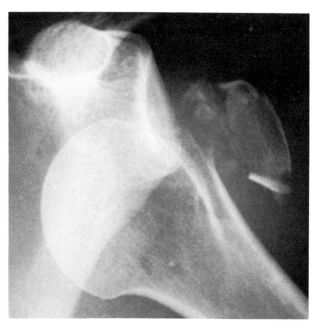

FIGURE 68–32. Fracture-dislocation of the glenohumeral joint. An anterior (subcoracoid) dislocation of the glenohumeral joint is associated with a displaced and comminuted fracture of the greater tuberosity of the humerus.

Pericapsular bone formation is frequent following either type of fracture-dislocation.

Several patterns of intra-articular fracture of the humeral head may be encountered. Impaction of the articular surface against the anterior or posterior rim of the glenoid cavity in cases of anterior or posterior glenohumeral joint dislocation has been considered earlier in this chapter. More severe fragmentation or comminution can accompany central impaction of the humeral head against the glenoid cavity. Complications of fractures of the articular head of the humerus include lipohemarthrosis, production of intra-articular osteocartilaginous fragments, inferior displacement of the humeral head (drooping shoulder), and osteoarthritis.

Lipohemarthrosis, with the release of fat and blood into the articular cavity, can follow intracapsular fractures of the humerus (as well as similar fractures at other sites). The source of the fat within the joint space is assumed to be the bone marrow, so that the detection of radiographic evidence of intra-articular fat should alert the physician that a fracture should be present (see Chapter 67). This rule is not without exception, as it has been proposed that injury to the synovial membrane and surrounding soft tissues also may release fat into the joint. Radiographic demonstration of lipohemarthrosis is facilitated by the inclusion of radiographs obtained with horizontal beam technique. Upright or decubitus films will demonstrate a fat-fluid level with radiolucent fat above and radiodense blood below (Fig. 68–33). CT and MR imaging also allow detection of lipohemarthrosis.

Inferior displacement of the humerus, producing the drooping shoulder, may accompany intra-articular or extra-articular fractures (Fig. 68–20). The findings should not be misinterpreted as a true dislocation of the glenohumeral joint, as the condition is self-limited, the humeral head returning to its normal position with respect to the glenoid cavity over a period of weeks. Its precise pathogenesis is

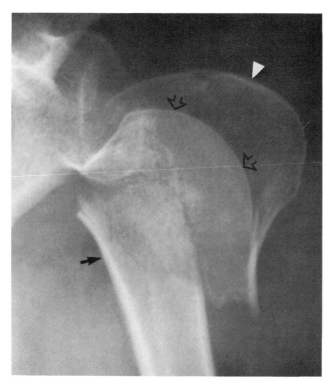

FIGURE 68–31. Fractures of the proximal humerus: Three-part fractures. Fractures involve the surgical neck and greater tuberosity of the humerus. There is medial displacement of the humeral shaft (closed arrow), superior displacement of the greater tuberosity (arrowhead), and rotation of the humeral head with its articular surface facing posteriorly (open arrows). CT confirmed that the lesser tuberosity was intact.

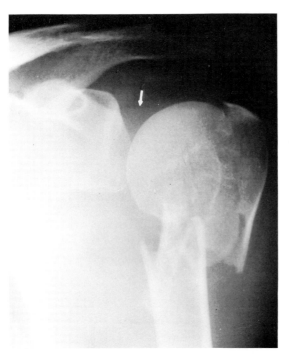

FIGURE 68–33. Lipohemarthrosis: Glenohumeral joint. A two-part fracture of the proximal portion of the humerus (with displacement between the diaphysis and the proximal segment of the bone) is evident. A nondisplaced fracture of the greater tuberosity also is seen. Note the fat-fluid level (arrow) indicating release of fat from the bone marrow. The joint space is widened, with minor inferior displacement of the humeral head (drooping shoulder).

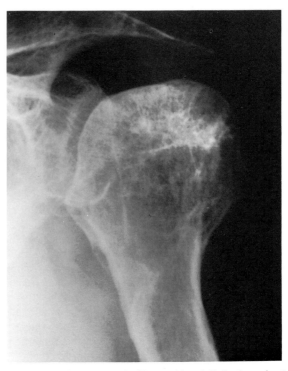

FIGURE 68–34. Osteonecrosis: Humeral head. Following a fracture of the proximal portion of the humerus, ischemic necrosis of the humeral head occurred, manifested radiographically as patchy bone sclerosis and irregularity of the articular surface.

unclear; factors important in its development may include hemarthrosis, detachment of the joint capsule, stretching of the support musculature, or injury to the brachial plexus.[110]

Delayed union or nonunion can accompany any type of fracture of the proximal portion of the humerus and may be accompanied by significant angulation at the site of fracture.[111] *Osteonecrosis* is associated with fractures of the humeral head and neck that lead to loss of the blood supply from both the muscular insertions and the arcuate branch of the internal humeral circumflex artery. This complication, which is reported in 7 to 50 per cent of cases,[112] is most typical of displaced fractures of the anatomic neck of the humerus and a severe fracture or fracture-dislocation of the bone (four-part fracture).[108] The accompanying radiographic features are similar to those that occur in osteonecrosis of the femoral head, including patchy osteolysis and osteosclerosis (Fig. 68–34). Collapse of the articular surface of the humerus following ischemic necrosis is not so marked as in cases of ischemic necrosis of the femoral head owing to the lack of weight-bearing in the upper extremity.

Fractures involving the articular surface of the humeral head may be complicated by *osteoarthritis* with joint space narrowing, sclerosis, and osteophytosis. Fracture-dislocations of the proximal portion of the humerus also can be associated with *heterotopic bone formation* in pericapsular regions (Fig. 68–35). Humeral fractures associated with considerable retraction of the greater tuberosity or the lesser tuberosity are characterized by tears in the *rotator cuff.* Abnormal rotation of the humeral head complicating such severe fractures is related to the unopposed action of intact components of the cuff, and these soft tissue attachments

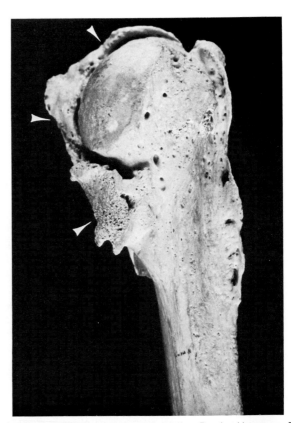

FIGURE 68–35. Heterotopic bone formation: Proximal humerus. Extensive ossification (arrowheads) surrounds the humeral head and neck.

provide an important source of blood supply to the humeral head.

Anterior fracture-dislocation of the proximal portion of the humerus can lead to injury of the nearby *brachial plexus* and, less commonly, the *axillary artery*. The axillary artery lies just anterior and medial to the proximal portion of the humerus; injury of this vessel in cases of humeral fracture is rare and relates to its laceration by fracture fragments or stretching or avulsion when one of its branches (humeral circumflex or subscapular arteries) is entrapped at the fracture site.[113] A brachial plexus injury, which results from contusion or mild traction, may be self-limited.

Fractures of the Clavicle. The clavicle is a horizontally oriented and superficial bone that is anchored at both the acromioclavicular and sternoclavicular articulations. It is the subcutaneous location that is responsible, at least in part, for the high frequency of fractures of this bone. Fractures of the clavicle predominate at the junction of its outer and intermediate thirds, where the two osseous curves are continous. Fracture deformity results from the weight of the arm and the spasm of the musculature crossing from the thorax to the arm.[114] These factors, acting on the coracoclavicular ligament, allow depression of the outer fracture fragment (Fig. 68–36). The proximal fragment is displaced superiorly owing to the action of the sternocleidomastoid muscle. These classic patterns of displacement are modified in the presence of fractures at other clavicular sites.

With regard to the analysis of fractures of the clavicle, it is convenient to divide the bone into three functional segments: a distal or interligamentous segment consisting of the outer 25 to 30 per cent of the bone, the region about and distal to the coracoclavicular ligament; an intermediate segment consisting of the middle 40 to 50 per cent of the bone; and an inner segment consisting of the medial 25 per cent of the bone.[68] Approximately 75 to 80 per cent of clavicular fractures involve the middle segment of the bone, 15 to 20 per cent involve the distal segment, and 5 per cent affect the inner segment.[114] The prognosis of clavicular fractures depends on the precise site of involvement; for example, nonunion is frequent in cases of fracture distal to the coracoclavicular ligament, whereas this complication is rare in cases of fracture of the medial segment of the bone.

The middle segment, located at the junction of the two

curvatures of the clavicle, is the most common site of fracture. In adults and children, the mechanism of injury is usually a fall onto the outstretched hand or a fall on the shoulder.[68] Local pain, swelling, and crepitation are evident at the fracture site. In most cases, the radiographic findings permit prompt and accurate diagnosis[115] (Fig. 68–36), although specialized oblique and angulated projections may be required.[116]

Fractures of the distal portion of the clavicle, related to a force applied on the shoulder driving the humerus and scapula downward, are divided into two types[117]: type I fractures, in which the coracoclavicular ligaments are intact; and type II fractures, in which a portion (conoid portion) of the coracoclavicular ligaments is severed (Fig. 68–37). A characteristic medial flange of bone extending from the distal clavicular fragment may be evident with type II fractures (Fig. 68–38). Type II fractures have a poorer prognosis related to more significant displacement at the fracture site and to nonunion. The degree of osseous displacement may be obscured on routine radiographic examination, requiring stress views (with a weight tied to the ipsilateral wrist) or oblique projections with the patient erect.[117] Four displacement forces exist with regard to type II fractures: the trapezius, attaching to the entire outer third of the clavicle, draws the larger medial fragment posteriorly within its substance; the weight of the arm pulls the outer fragment downward and forward; the trunk muscles attaching to the humerus and scapula displace the outer fragment in a medial direction toward the apex of the thorax; and the scapular ligaments may rotate the outer fragment as much as 40 per cent.[117] Associated fractures of the coracoid process and ribs may be evident (Fig. 68–39). Rarely, a fracture of the distal aspect of the clavicle is accompanied by a longitudinal rupture in the periosteal envelope and a radiographic appearance simulating that of an acromioclavicular joint dislocation (Fig. 68–40) (see Chapter 67).

Direct trauma accounts for the majority of fractures of the medial end of the clavicle (Fig. 68–41). They have been divided into two types: transverse fractures, which do not become displaced because of ligamentous and musculature attachments, and intra-articular fractures. When the costoclavicular ligament remains intact and attached to the outer fragment, displacement does not occur.[68] Intra-articular

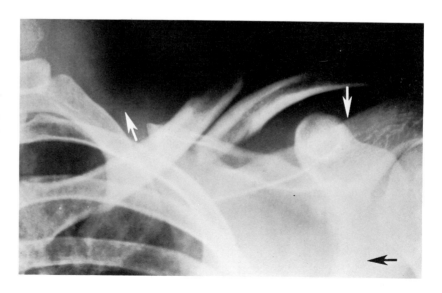

FIGURE 68–36. Clavicular fracture: Intermediate segment. The typical configuration of such a fracture is illustrated. Note that the medial portion of the clavicle is pulled upward by the sternocleidomastoid muscle; the lateral portion is pulled downward by the weight of the arm and inward by the pectoralis major and latissimus dorsi muscles. Arrows indicate the direction of these forces. The result is a bayonet deformity at the fracture site.

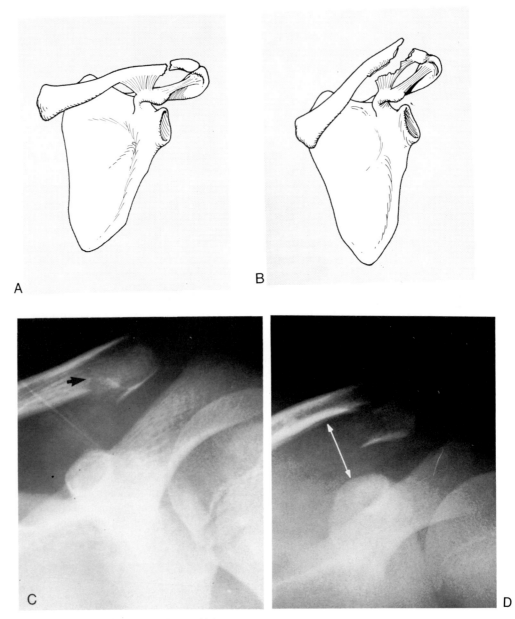

FIGURE 68–37. Clavicular fracture: Distal segment—types of injury.

　A Type I injury. The coracoclavicular ligaments remain intact.

　B Type II injury. The conoid portion of the coracoclavicular ligaments is severed.

　C Type I injury. A subtle fracture (arrow) of the distal clavicle in a child is unassociated with clavicular displacement.

　D Type II injury. Note the widening of the coracoclavicular distance (double-ended arrow), indicating disruption of the coracoclavicular ligaments. This finding may be better evaluated with the patient holding 5 or 10 pounds of weight in the ipsilateral hand or with this weight tied to the ipsilateral wrist.

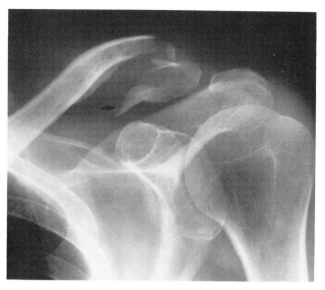

FIGURE 68–38. Clavicular fracture: Distal segment—type II injury. Disruption of the conoid portion of the coracoclavicular ligament has allowed superior migration of the proximal segment of the clavicle. Note the bone flange (arrow) extending from the distal clavicular segment to which the trapezoid portion of the coracoclavicular ligament inserts.

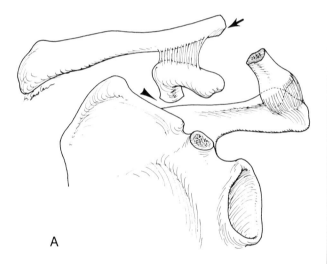

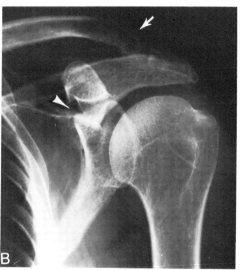

FIGURE 68–39. Clavicular fracture: Associated fracture of the coracoid process. A displaced fracture of the lateral segment of the clavicle (arrows) with intact coracoclavicular ligaments is accompanied by avulsion of the coracoid process (arrowheads).

FIGURE 68–40. Clavicular fracture: Pseudodislocation of the acromioclavicular joint. Following a fracture of the distal portion of the clavicle, the medial aspect of the bone may be displaced through a longitudinal tear in the periosteal envelope (arrowheads). The coracoclavicular ligaments may remain intact. The resulting radiographic appearance resembles that of a dislocation of the acromioclavicular joint when the fracture has occurred close to the lateral end of the clavicle.

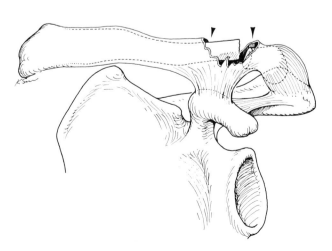

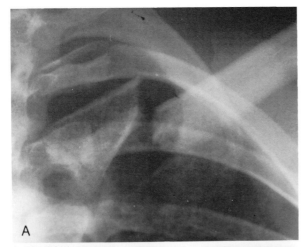

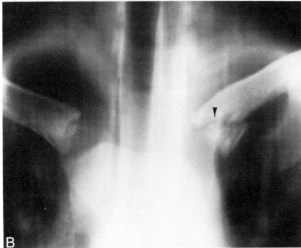

FIGURE 68–41. Clavicular fracture: Inner (proximal or medial) segment.

A An oblique fracture of the clavicle is apparent.

B In this example, an intra-articular fracture is evident (arrowhead).

fractures may be overlooked unless conventional tomography is used. They can result in secondary osteoarthritis with persistent pain.

In children, clavicular fractures heal rapidly without significant sequelae (Fig. 68–42). In adults, resultant deformities secondary to extensive callus formation may be observed. Exuberant callus affecting the middle segment of the clavicle can be associated with persistent neurologic defects and circulatory disturbances owing to compression of the subclavian vessels and brachial plexus against the first rib,[114] and surgical removal of the callus may be required.[118–120] Foreshortening of the clavicle in the form of a bayonet deformity at the site of fracture can occur but it usually is unassociated with significant cosmetic problems.

Fracture of the first rib may accompany fracture of the clavicle (or acromioclavicular joint dislocation).[121] In children, an association of clavicular fracture and atlantoaxial rotary fixation has been noted, consistent with a traumatic insult occurring during a fall onto the shoulder and side of the head.[122] Nonunion of a clavicular fracture is uncommon[123] and, when present, is associated with lack of immobilization. Delayed union or nonunion following fractures of the lateral portions of the clavicle usually is related to

rupture of the coracoclavicular ligament. In the middle portion of the clavicle, delayed union or nonunion may result from local tissue damage, loss of bone stock, stripping or interposition of soft tissues, inadequate fixation of fracture fragments, or infection.[123–125]

A posttraumatic pseudarthrosis of the clavicle must be differentiated from a congenital pseudarthrosis,[126] a distinction that generally is not difficult. Congenital pseudarthrosis of the clavicle usually is manifested as a painless swelling overlying the middle third of the bone, more frequently on the right side. The patients are infants, commonly within the first few weeks of life. On radiographs, the medial segment of the clavicle is elevated and displaced anteriorly and the lateral segment is depressed and displaced posteriorly. Callus and periosteal bone formation are absent.

Fractures of the Scapula. Scapular fractures are infrequent, constituting approximately 1 per cent of all fractures and 5 to 7 per cent of those about the shoulder. Although they may occur as an isolated phenomenon, more commonly and perhaps in as many as 95 per cent of cases,[127] they are associated with additional injuries, including fractures of the ribs, clavicle, and skull. Scapular fractures may involve one or more of the following anatomic regions: glenoid fossa and articular surface, neck, body, spinous process, acromion process, and coracoid process[128, 129] (Fig. 68–43). They are found most frequently in the scapular body, followed by the neck and the other regions of the bone.[127, 129]

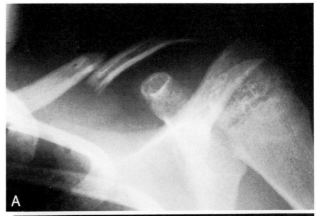

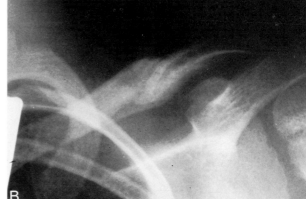

FIGURE 68–42. Clavicular fracture: Rapid healing in children. Observe the solid bone fusion that developed rapidly following a fracture of the intermediate segment of the bone.

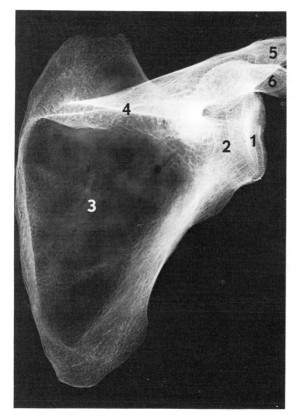

FIGURE 68–43. Scapular fracture: Sites of injury. Fractures of the scapula may involve the glenoid fossa and articular surface (1), the neck (2) or body (3) of the bone, or the spinous (4), acromion (5), or coracoid (6) process. They are most common in the scapular body and neck.

A fracture of the rim of the glenoid cavity occurs in approximately 20 per cent of traumatic glenohumeral joint dislocations. The fracture fragment may be cartilaginous or osteocartilaginous in nature, requiring for diagnosis careful plain film radiography as well as arthrography or arthrotomography in some cases. Either the anterior glenoid rim (in anterior glenohumeral joint dislocations) or the posterior glenoid rim (in posterior glenohumeral joint dislocations) may be affected. Larger portions of the glenoid fossa may be fractured when the humeral head is driven against the glenoid cavity by a direct force.[130, 131] Comminution of the articular surface may require operative intervention.[132] Violent contraction of the triceps muscle, a situation that might occur in an athlete engaged in a throwing sport such as baseball, can lead to avulsion of a portion of the inferior lip of the glenoid cavity.[133]

A fracture in the neck of the scapula typically occurs following a direct blow on the shoulder (Fig. 68–44). When the fracture is complete, the outer fragment is displaced in an inferior direction owing to the effect of gravity on the patient's arm. The fracture line, which may be impacted, extends from the supraclavicular notch above to the coracoid process below. The prognosis is improved if the glenoid cavity is not affected and the coracoclavicular and acromioclavicular ligaments are intact. Combined fractures of the scapular neck and ipsilateral clavicle disrupt the stability of the suspensory structures of the shoulder (i.e., floating shoulder), and muscle forces and the weight of the arm pull the glenoid fragment distally and anteromedially.[134]

Approximately 50 to 70 per cent of scapular fractures involve the body of the bone (Fig. 68–44). The typical mechanism of injury is a direct force of considerable magnitude, which also may result in fractures of neighboring ribs and pneumothorax.[135] Fractures of the body of the scapula owing to indirect forces or to muscular avulsion are less frequent.[136] Radiographs will reveal the vertical or horizontal nature of the fracture line or its comminution. Displacement of the osseous fragment is unusual.

Isolated fractures of the spinous process of the scapula are infrequent and, when present, are the result of direct trauma (Fig. 68–45A). Fractures of the acromion process generally follow direct trauma, although muscular traction can rarely produce a similar lesion.[137] On radiographs, a fracture line is evident, usually adjacent to the acromioclavicular joint, although occasionally at the base of the acromion process (Fig. 68–45B). Significant neurologic injury, although rare in most cases of scapular fracture, is a recognized complication of acromion fractures[129]; depression of the shoulder and contralateral flexion of the neck following these fractures predispose to injuries of the brachial plexus. Of diagnostic importance, the os acromiale, a normal variant of the shoulder, can simulate an acromial fracture. The small osseous density inferior to the acromion that characterizes this extra ossification center is bilateral in approximately 60 per cent of cases.

Fractures of the coracoid process relate to a direct injury from a dislocating humeral head, a direct force on the tip of the coracoid itself, or an avulsion owing to traction on the coracoclavicular ligament (in association with acromioclavicular joint dislocation), the short head of the biceps, or the coracobrachialis.[138, 139] Isolated fractures of the coracoid process are observed in athletes as a result of an avulsion injury or in trapshooters related to repetitive stress from the impact of the recoiling rifle. Anteroposterior radiographs may not demonstrate the coracoid process adequately and must be supplemented with a lateral scapular view or axillary projection, or both (Fig. 68–45C,D). The tip of this process may be displaced in an inferior and medial direction, resembling the appearance of a normal accessory ossification center (infracoracoid bone).

As noted previously, neurologic injuries may be a sequela of a scapular fracture, particularly one that involves the acromion process or leads to avulsion of the coracoid process. Vascular compromise is rare following scapular injuries.[140] Fractures of neighboring bones, including the ribs and clavicle, acromioclavicular joint dislocation, pulmonary involvement, skull fractures, and cerebral contusion may accompany scapular injuries.[141] Considering the great degree of force required to fracture this bone, the high frequency of associated injuries is not unexpected.

An intrathoracic dislocation of the scapula producing a "locked scapula" is a rare injury.[142] Following a direct blow to the scapula or an outward traction force on the arm, the lower margin of the bone becomes locked between adjacent ribs. Fractures of the scapula or ribs may complicate this injury.

Traumatic lateral displacement of the scapula, scapulothoracic dissociation, also is rare and is accompanied by partial or complete amputation through the soft tissue and

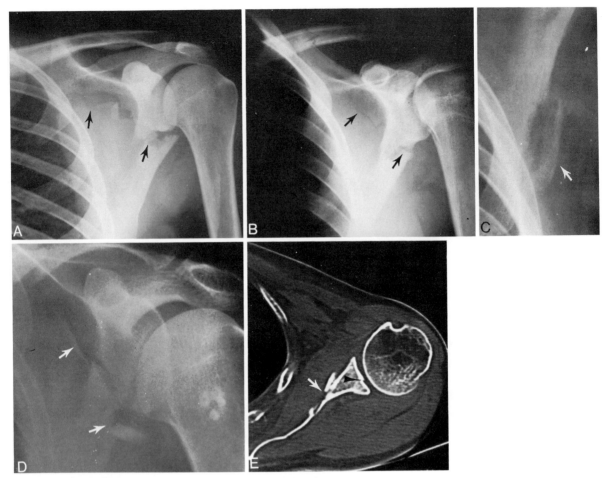

FIGURE 68–44. Scapular fracture: Injuries of the scapular body and neck.

A, B Two examples are shown of horizontal fractures involving the body and neck of the bone (arrows). In **B**, a clavicular fracture also is present.

C A fragment arising from the lateral surface of the bone (arrow) probably represents an avulsion fracture.

D, E The intra-articular extension of a scapular fracture may be difficult to define with routine radiography. In this example, a comminuted fracture of the body and neck of the bone (arrows) extends into the glenohumeral joint, as shown by transaxial CT (arrowhead). A clavicular fracture also was present.

injuries to the brachial plexus and the subclavian artery and vein.[143, 144] In addition to the displacement of the scapula, radiographic findings may include disruption of the acromioclavicular joint and fracture of the clavicle.[145]

Fractures of the First and Second Ribs. Fractures of the first or second rib indicate major trauma to the thorax or shoulder.[146, 147] Associated abnormalities are frequent and potentially serious; these include rupture of the apex of the lung or of the subclavian artery, aneurysm of the aortic arch, tracheoesophageal fistula, pleurisy, hemothorax, cardiac alterations, neurologic injury, and additional fractures. Because of the serious implications of these accompanying abnormalities, the detection of a fracture of the first rib requires a careful evaluation of intrathoracic structures to exclude the presence of additional alterations, although there is no uniform agreement regarding the precise indications for aortography.[148–150]

The first rib is not a superficial structure, being protected by the clavicle; fractures of the first rib related to direct trauma may be combined with disruption of the clavicle. Indirect force owing to a sudden strong contracture of the scalenus anterior muscle combined with traction on the arm and on the serratus anterior muscle can produce a fracture about the subclavian sulcus of the rib.[147] Sudden hyperex-

tension of the neck can produce a similar abnormality. Upper rib fractures are observed following median sternotomy, presumably related to surgical trauma.[151] Stress fractures of these ribs are associated with the lifting of heavy weights or the excessive overhead use of the arms and have been described in hikers carrying heavy backpacks.

Fracture and displacement about the first costovertebral articulations are easily overlooked unless the radiographs are interpreted carefully. Direct or indirect force is implicated. Avulsed fragments at the site of osseous attachment of the adjacent ligaments, such as the radiate or costotransverse ligament, probably indicate severe force and may be combined with pulmonary, pleural, or mediastinal abnormality.

Humeral Diaphysis

The diaphyseal portion, or shaft, of the humerus extends from the upper border of the insertion site of the pectoralis major tendon, close to the surgical neck, in a distal direction to the level of the supracondylar ridge. The diaphysis is cylindrical or tubular in its proximal portion and more triangular, with a flattened anterior surface, in its distal portion. Three surfaces can be identified in the humeral shaft:

the anterior border, extending from the greater tuberosity proximally to the coronoid fossa distally; the medial border, extending from the lesser tuberosity proximally to the medial supracondylar ridge distally; and the lateral border, extending from the posterior aspect of the greater tuberosity proximally to the lateral supracondylar ridge distally.[152] The deltoid tuberosity and the sulcus for the radial nerve and profunda brachii artery are located on the anterolateral surface of the humerus; the anteromedial surface forms the floor of the intertubercular groove; and the posterior surface of the humerus contains the spiral groove for the radial nerve.[152]

Fractures of the humeral diaphysis account for about 3 to 5 per cent of all fractures (see Table 68–2). These humeral fractures may occur as a response to direct trauma (e.g., motor vehicle accidents, blows received during a physical assault, gunshot wounds) or to indirect forces including torsional ones that occur in athletic endeavors, including throwing a ball, shot putting, or arm wrestling.[153–155] Although diaphyseal fractures of the humerus generally heal in a satisfactory fashion, delayed union, nonunion, or malunion of these fractures is well known.[156, 157] An analysis of fractures of the humeral diaphysis reveals the effects of the muscular forces acting on the shaft at varying levels.[152] In fractures occurring above the insertion of the tendon of the pectoralis major muscle, the proximal fragment is displaced into abduction and external rotation, owing to the action of the rotator cuff musculature; fractures occurring in the interval between the insertion of the pectoralis major tendon proximally and the deltoid insertion distally result in adduction of the proximal fragment and lateral displacement of the distal fragment; and fractures occurring distal to the insertion of the deltoid muscle result in abduction of the proximal fragment and proximal displacement of the distal fragment.[152]

The precise fracture configuration depends on the type of

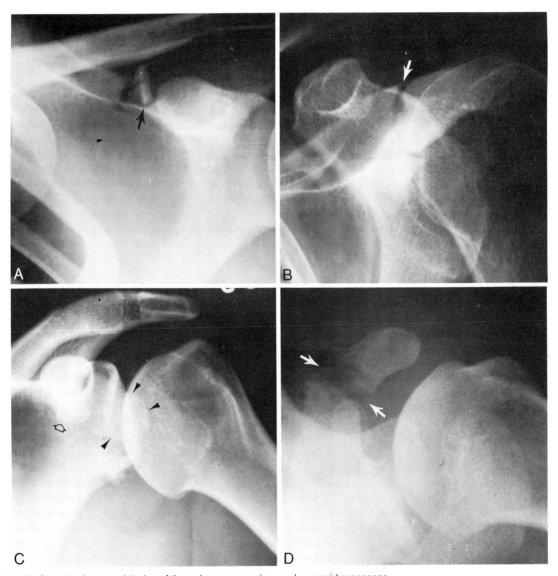

FIGURE 68–45. Scapular fracture: Injuries of the spinous, acromion, and coracoid processes.
  A Spinous process fracture (arrow).
  B Acromion process fracture (arrow).
  C, D Coracoid process fracture (arrows). In this case, observe the position of the displaced coracoid process (arrowheads) on the frontal radiograph **(C)**, the excellent demonstration of the fracture (solid arrows) on the axillary radiograph, and an incidental infracoracoid bone (open arrow).

injury and its force. Transverse fractures of the humeral shaft are most frequent, representing 50 to 70 per cent of all diaphyseal fractures of the humerus; oblique or spiral fractures, each representing about 20 per cent of all humeral diaphyseal fractures, result from torsional forces; and segmental and comminuted fractures constitute the other patterns of humeral shaft fractures[158] (Fig. 68–46). Approximately three fourths of all such fractures involve the middle third of the bone. Routine radiography generally is sufficient for the diagnosis of fractures of the humeral shaft, although two views acquired at approximately 90 degrees to each other are necessary to allow delineation of the patterns of fracture angulation and displacement. Furthermore, views of the adjacent joints (i.e., shoulder and elbow) are necessary in many cases to exclude associated injuries. Ipsilateral fractures of the radius and ulna, resulting in a "floating elbow," are encountered.[159]

Among the complications of fractures of the humeral diaphysis, neurologic injury is most common. Radial nerve palsy occurs in as many as 18 per cent of closed fractures of the humeral shaft.[152] It is associated most often with transverse fractures of the diaphysis, particularly those occurring in the junction of the middle and distal thirds of the bone. In most cases of radial nerve palsy following such fractures, clinical manifestations, which include wrist drop, are transient in nature and complete recovery is expected. In other cases, transection of the radial nerve or its entrapment between the fracture fragments occurs. Routine radiography in cases of radial nerve entrapment may reveal a sharply marginated notch at the periphery of the fracture or a space, or foramen, within the fracture.[160] MR imaging, however, represents a more appropriate technique for the early diagnosis of entrapment of the radial nerve. Injury to the median or ulnar nerve in cases of humeral diaphyseal fracture is rare. The anterior interosseous nerve also may be affected.

Vascular compromise occurring in patients with fracture of the humeral shaft occurs in less than 5 per cent of cases, and such compromise usually is associated with open fractures or those associated with penetrating injury. Transection or an intimal tear of the brachial artery may occur. As routine radiography provides no evidence of vascular injury, arteriography is indicated when diminution or absence of peripheral pulses is detected.

Delayed union or nonunion of humeral shaft fractures is encountered. In general, transverse, segmental, or open fractures unite more slowly than spiral or oblique fractures or comminuted fractures.[152] Separation of fracture fragments related to excessive traction or interposition of soft tissue contributes to improper fracture healing. Malunion accompanied by shortening, angulation, or rotation also is evident in some cases.

Elbow

Although not as frequent as fractures and dislocations about the shoulder, such injuries about the elbow represent 5 to 8 per cent of all fractures and dislocations. Either direct injury, such as the impact of the radius and ulna against the apposing articular surface of the humerus, or indirect injury, such as that resulting from angular forces transmitted through the bones of the forearm, lead to fractures and dislocations about the elbow.[2] Their detection radiographically is made difficult by the complex anatomy of the elbow and, in the child, by the large number and the irregularity of the adjacent ossification centers (see Chapter 67). Diagnostic aid is provided by the presence of intracapsular, extrasynovial fat bodies whose displacement, owing to the occurrence of a traumatic hemarthrosis (or other intra-articular fluid collections and masses) is known as a positive fat pad sign[161–164] (see Chapters 21, 22, and 67). Although not diagnostic of a fracture, the positive fat pad sign should stimulate a careful search for an adjacent fracture in patients with elbow injuries.

Elbow Dislocation. Dislocation of the elbow is a relatively frequent injury, especially in the immature skeleton.[165] The elbow joint ranks third (behind the glenohumeral joint and interphalangeal joints of the fingers) as a site of dislocation, and it is the most common site of dislocation in a child.[2] The usual mechanism of injury is hyperextension (e.g., a fall on the outstretched hand) with the olecranon, driven into the olecranon fossa, serving as a fulcrum to force the elbow apart.[2] The classification of such injuries is based on the direction of displacement and the presence of radial or ulnar dislocation. In cases of dislocation involving both the radius and the ulna, a posterior dislocation (Fig. 68–47) is most frequent (approximately 80 to 90 per cent of all elbow dislocations), as these two bones are displaced in a posterior direction in relation to the distal humerus.[166, 167] In adults, this injury may be complicated by fracture of the coronoid process of the ulna or the radial head, and in children and adolescents, the medial epicondylar ossification center is frequently avulsed and may become entrapped during reduction.[165] Entrapment of the median nerve in the elbow joint after closed reduction of a posterior dislocation of the elbow with fracture of the me-

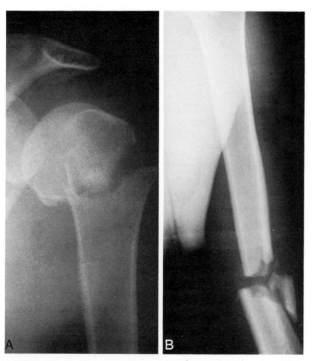

FIGURE 68–46. Humerus: Segmental fracture. The fracture of the surgical neck of the bone **(A)** may be entirely overlooked if attention is directed solely at the diaphyseal fracture **(B)**. A fracture of the scapula also was present in this patient.

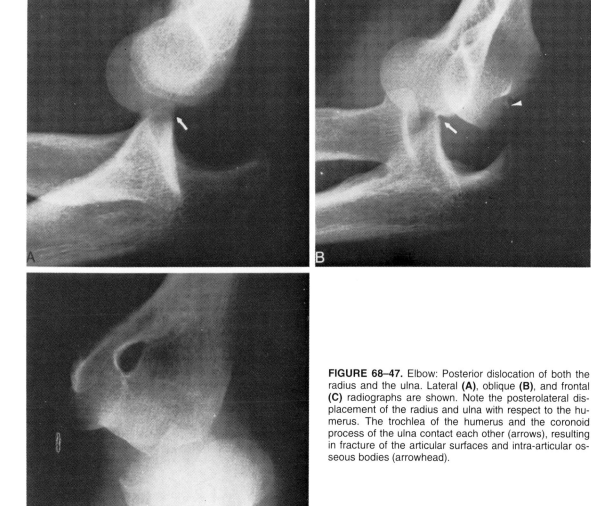

FIGURE 68–47. Elbow: Posterior dislocation of both the radius and the ulna. Lateral **(A)**, oblique **(B)**, and frontal **(C)** radiographs are shown. Note the posterolateral displacement of the radius and ulna with respect to the humerus. The trochlea of the humerus and the coronoid process of the ulna contact each other (arrows), resulting in fracture of the articular surfaces and intra-articular osseous bodies (arrowhead).

dial epicondyle in children can produce a depression in the cortex on the ulnar side of the distal humeral metaphysis.[168–170]

Medial and lateral dislocations of the elbow are not common[171] (Fig. 68–48). Anterior dislocation also is unusual.[172] Rarely, elbow dislocations may be recurrent.[172] The cause of the last injury varies, but a residual defect in the articular surface of the trochlea, attenuation of the collateral ligaments, failure of union of the coronoid process, or anterior capsular stripping may be observed.[174] Indeed, instability of the elbow, particularly medial instability with the elbow extended, is common following a dislocation, related to complete rupture of the medial and sometimes the lateral collateral ligaments, as well as to injury of the anterior capsule and the attachment of the brachialis muscle.[175] Also rare is a divergent dislocation of the elbow in which the radius and ulna move in different directions.[176, 177] This divergent dislocation involves all three joints (i.e., radiocapitellar, ulnotrochlear, and proximal radioulnar) that constitute the elbow. Extensive ligamentous and soft tissue (i.e., annular ligament, interosseous membrane, capsule of the distal radioulnar joint) disruption accompanies this dislocation, and gross instability of the elbow is present.[2] Translocation of the elbow, in which there is reversal of the normal positions of the proximal radius and ulna with the ulna articulating with the capitulum and the radial head articulating with the trochlea, also has been described.[178]

Isolated dislocation of the ulna at the elbow is unusual. Similarly, isolated radial head dislocation without an associated fracture in the ulna is rare in adults. In the child, subluxation of the radial head, which usually but not invariably is transient in nature,[179] is termed nursemaid's elbow or pulled elbow. It is produced by a sudden pull on the child's arm which, when the forearm is in a pronated position, results in slipping of the radial head beneath the annular ligament as it is torn from its attachment to the radial neck.[2, 180] With supination of the forearm, the ligament is restored to its normal position.[2] Routine radiographs, therefore, are normal. Rarely, the annular ligament becomes entrapped in the joint, requiring surgical reduction.[181] Isolated true dislocations of the radial head, without fracture or plastic bowing of the ulna, occasionally are seen in

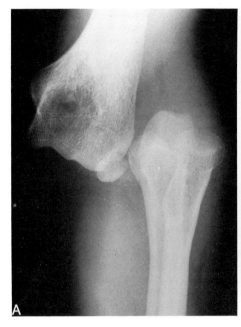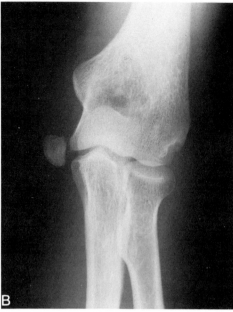

FIGURE 68–48. Elbow: Lateral dislocation of both the radius and the ulna. Prereduction **(A)** and postreduction **(B)** frontal radiographs of a pure lateral dislocation of the elbow are shown. The precise origin of the large osseous fragment is not certain. It could represent an avulsion of the medial epicondyle of the humerus, although the well-corticated margin of the fragment and that of the medial epicondyle itself suggest that if this is the case, a previous injury to the medial epicondyle with nonosseous union may have occurred. That the lateral epicondyle is the source of the osseous fragment is less likely. (Courtesy of A. Polansky, M.D., San Diego, California.)

children.[182] The initial radiographic diagnosis is based on an abnormal position of the radial head, which usually is displaced anteriorly (Fig. 68–49). Within weeks of the injury, curvilinear calcification in the annular ligament may be seen. In the child, traumatic dislocation of the radial head must be differentiated from congenital dislocation of this bone[183, 184] or dislocation associated with osteo-onychodysostosis, or hereditary onycho-osteodysplasia (nail-patella syndrome).[185] Because of the rarity of isolated traumatic dislocation of the radial head,[186] all such cases should be investigated extensively for an associated fracture of the ulna.

The combination of an ulnar fracture and radial head dislocation is termed a Monteggia fracture-dislocation[187–189] (Fig. 68–50). Various types of Monteggia fracture-dislocations are recognized: type I—fracture of the middle or upper third of the ulna with anterior dislocation of the radial head and anterior angulation of the ulna; type II—fracture of the middle or upper third of the ulna with posterior dislocation of the radial head and posterior angulation of the ulna; type III—fracture of the ulna just distal to the coronoid process with lateral dislocation of the radial head; and type IV—fracture of the upper or middle third of the ulna with anterior dislocation of the radial head and fracture of the upper third of the radius below the bicipital tuberosity.[190] Type I injuries are most frequent (approximately 65 per cent), followed by type II (approximately 18 per cent), type III (approximately 16 per cent), and type IV (approximately 1 per cent).[187] These various patterns emphasize the typical occurrence of injuries to more than one structure in the forearm and the rare occurrence of injury isolated to a single bone in the forearm. Although the classic patterns of the Montegia fracture-dislocation include an ulnar fracture, ipsilateral radial shaft fracture and dislocation of the radial head without apparent injury to the ulna have been reported.[191] As the Monteggia fracture-dislocation is a common injury in adults (although rare in children[192–196]) and easily overlooked, multiple views of the elbow should be obtained in all patients who demonstrate fractures of the proximal half of the ulna. A line drawn through the radial

shaft and radial head should align with the capitulum in any projection.[197]

In infants and young children, separation of the entire distal humeral epiphysis may be confused with elbow dislocation.[198, 199] The correct diagnosis of this injury rests on two observations: a normal relationship between the capitulum and radius; and medial displacement of the radius and ulna with respect to the humerus.

Complications of elbow dislocations include heterotopic calcification and ossification[200–202] and neural and vascular injury.[167, 203] Damaged structures include the brachial artery[204, 205] and the median and ulnar nerves.[206] The brachial artery is injured in association with posterior dislocations of the elbow. Such injury is far more common in open rather than closed dislocations; and when there is disruption of the flexor muscles from the medial epicondyle or from a vertical fracture of the medial epicondyle that allows posterior displacement of or traction on the brachial artery.[207]

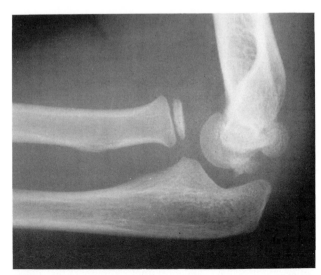

FIGURE 68–49. Elbow: Dislocation of the radial head. Note the anterior position of the radius with respect to the capitulum and abnormal separation of the radius and ulna.

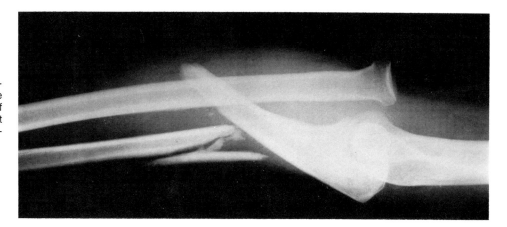

FIGURE 68–50. Monteggia fracture-dislocation (type I). Note the fracture of the upper one third of the ulna with anterior angulation at the fracture site and anterior dislocation of the radial head.

Posttraumatic bone formation occurs as a significant complication in 3 to 5 per cent of elbow injuries, particularly in fracture-dislocations, radial head fractures, and multitrauma patients with head injuries. Calcification or ossification occurs in and around muscles, especially the brachialis muscle, and predominate in the anterior region of the elbow.[2] It usually is visible within 3 to 4 weeks of the injury (see Chapter 95).

Intra-articular Fractures of the Distal Portion of the Humerus. The following discussion pertains principally to injuries in the mature skeleton; those occurring in children and adolescents are discussed in Chapter 67.

Intra-articular fractures of the distal portion of the humerus usually are classified as transcondylar, intercondylar, condylar, epicondylar, transchondral, and miscellaneous in type.[208] *Transcondylar fractures* resemble supracondylar fractures (Fig. 68–51) but are intra-articular in location. The fracture line traverses both condylar surfaces in a horizontal direction. Two types are described: an extension type and a flexion type. The extension variety generally is seen in older patients, particularly those with osteoporosis, and results in a transverse fracture line, which may be subtle, that enters the olecranon and coronoid fossae. Although significant displacement of the fracture fragments generally is not a problem, extensive callus or heterotopic bone formation may be observed and can create mechanical difficulties if it develops in the region of the humeral fossae. The flexion type of transcondylar fracture is associated with significant displacement of the fracture fragments. Typically, the coronoid process of the ulna becomes trapped between the anteriorly displaced condyles and the humeral shaft.

Intercondylar fractures of the distal portion of the humerus (Fig. 68–52) result in comminuted and complex fracture lines that generally include one component that traverses the supracondylar region of the humerus in a transverse or oblique fashion and a second component, vertical or oblique in nature, that enters the articular lumen.[209, 210] The resulting configuration of the fracture is thus T or Y shaped, and the degree of separation between each of the two condylar segments or between both condylar segments and the humeral shaft can be considerable.

These fractures are relatively rare and typically are observed in patients over the age of 50 years.[210, 211] They usually are produced by direct trauma to the elbow in which the ulnar articular surface is driven against the articular surface of the distal portion of the humerus. Indirect forces

can produce similar lesions. The location of the condylar segment in displaced fractures can be anterior or posterior to the humeral shaft, the final position being modified according to the precise mechanism of injury. If the force is applied while the elbow is flexed, the condylar fragments commonly localize anterior to the distal portion of the humerus, whereas if the force is applied during elbow extension, posterior displacement of the condyles frequently is apparent. In some cases, it is the medial condylar fragment that is the larger, whereas in other instances the lateral fragment is larger. Multiple smaller fragments also are common, and, owing to the pull of the attached musculature, they may reveal considerable rotation and displacement.

Complications of intercondylar fractures include soft tissue injury, instability, and loss of elbow function.[212] Other problems, including delay or absence of bone union, injury to nerves (e.g., tardy ulnar palsy) and vessels, and ischemic necrosis of bone, are rare.[213]

The condylar portions of the humerus are separated into medial and lateral structures by the capitulotrochlear sulcus. Each condyle contains an articular and a nonarticular portion. The lateral condyle is composed of the nonarticular lateral epicondyle and the articular capitulum; the medial condyle is composed of the nonarticular medial epicondyle and the trochlea. Condylar fractures imply that the fracture line separates both the articular and the nonarticular portions of one condyle with or without an attached segment of the opposite condyle.[208] These fractures should be distinguished from those involving only an epicondyle (medial or lateral epicondylar fracture) and those affecting the capitulum or the trochlea.

Condylar fractures are relatively uncommon, occurring predominantly in children.[214] Fractures involving the lateral condyle are more frequent than those of the medial condyle (Fig. 68–53). Each can be associated with significant instability and restriction of motion, especially if the fracture fragment is large. In this regard, a classification system has been devised on the basis of the size of the fragment and the presence or absence of disruption of the lateral trochlear ridge.[215] This structure, separating the trochlea and capitulum, is important in providing medial and lateral stability to the elbow. In type I fractures of the condyles, the lateral trochlear ridge is not disrupted, whereas in type II fractures, the larger fracture fragment contains the separated condyle and a portion of this ridge. The latter pattern of injury allows translocation of the radius and the ulna in a medio-

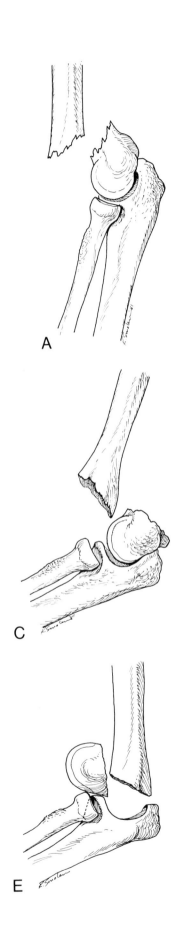

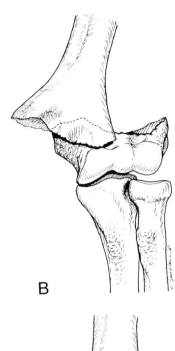

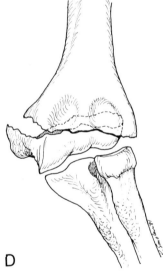

A

B

C

D

E

FIGURE 68–51. Humeral fractures: Supracondylar and transcondylar.

A, B Supracondylar fracture (extension type). A fall on the outstretched hand with the elbow in extension is the probable mechanism of this fracture. On the lateral view **(A)**, the fracture line extends obliquely upward from a more distal point anteriorly to a more proximal point posteriorly. Posterior and proximal displacement of the distal fragment results, in part, from the force of the triceps muscle attaching to the ulna. Observe the sharp margin of the proximal fragment, which projects into the antecubital fossa, accounting for the associated injuries to the brachial artery and median nerve. On the anteroposterior view **(B)** the fracture line generally is transverse in configuration. Displacement and angulation at the fracture site are of variable degree.

C, D Transcondylar fracture (extension type). The fracture line passes through the condyles of the humerus and is intracapsular in location. On the lateral view **(C)**, posterior displacement of the distal fragment predominates. On the frontal view **(D)**, the fracture line commonly is transverse and inferior to that of a supracondylar fracture.

E Transcondylar fracture (Posadas type). Note anterior displacement of the condylar fragment and dislocation of the radius and ulna posteriorly, with the coronoid process wedged between the condyles and the humeral shaft.

(**E**, From DeLee JC, et al: Fractures and dislocations of the elbow. In CA Rockwood Jr, DP Greene [Eds]: Fractures in Adults. 2nd Ed. Philadelphia, JB Lippincott Co, 1984, p 573.)

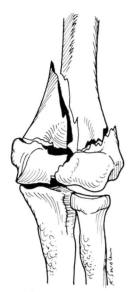

FIGURE 68–52. Humeral fractures: Intercondylar. In this example, a comminuted fracture has led to separation of the trochlear and capitular fragments. Rotation at the fracture site and incongruity of the articular surface are potential complications.

lateral direction and is termed a fracture-dislocation. Because of this instability, type II fractures require more aggressive orthopedic treatment.

A lateral condylar fracture generally appears on radiographs as an oblique radiolucent line extending from a segment of the articular surface of the distal portion of the humerus in a lateral direction, disrupting the supracondylar ridge. If a type II fracture is present, the lateral trochlear ridge is violated, and the ulna may move in a lateral direction with respect to the distal portion of the humerus. A medial condylar fracture usually extends from the trochlear groove in an oblique, upward, and medial direction, terminating at the medial supracondylar ridge (type I injury). If the fracture enters the capitulotrochlear sulcus and disrupts

the lateral trochlear ridge, the less common type II fracture is present.[208] Involvement of the trochlear groove is associated with residual disability owing to incongruity of apposing articular surfaces. Osteoarthritis, delayed union or nonunion, and cubitus varus deformity are recognized complications.

Fractures of the capitulum are rare and involve only the articular surface of the lateral condyle[216–219] (Fig. 68–54). Two types of injury are recognized: type I fractures (Hahn-Steinthal type) are complete in nature and involve a large bony segment of the capitulum; type II fractures (Kocher-Lorenz type) are partial in nature, involving predominantly articular cartilage and producing ''uncapping'' of the condyle.[217] With regard to type I fractures, the fracture line is coronal in configuration, and a fragment of variable size is produced that contains, in addition to the capitulum, a portion of the trochlear lip. The fragment is displaced in an anterior and superior direction, lying in the radial fossa and within the articulation. The lateral humeral condyle is intact.[217] With regard to type II fractures, a small fracture fragment containing cartilage or cartilage and bone is detached and displaced, usually in a posterior direction.

The mechanism of injury is considered to be a direct force, applied through the radial head.[220] The precise position of the elbow at the time of injury is debated; some investigators believe that a direct or indirect force on an elbow that is partially or fully flexed can produce this fracture; others believe that hyperextension of the elbow is required and that the fracture may be accompanied by a tear of the medial collateral ligament.[217] It is even suggested that an anteriorly displaced capitulum fragment indicates an extension injury and a partially displaced fragment indicates a flexion injury.[221] It is the presence of such dislocated pieces of the capitulum that leads to one clinical finding, restricted motion, that may accompany certain of these injuries.

Anteroposterior radiographs may appear surprisingly normal, so that accurate assessment usually depends on the

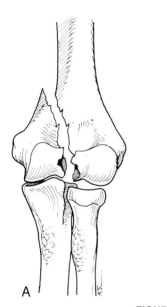
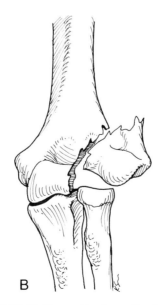
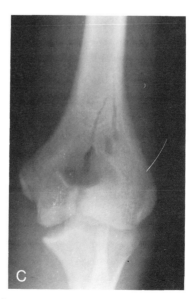

FIGURE 68–53. Humeral fractures: Condylar.
  A Fracture of the medial condyle.
  B Fracture of the lateral condyle.
  C Fracture of the lateral condyle (see text for details).

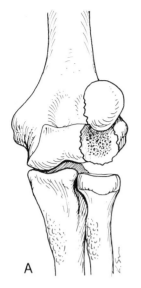

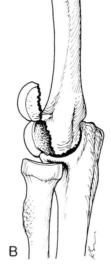

FIGURE 68–54. Humeral fractures: Capitular.

A, B Note the coronal orientation of the fracture line and the characteristic pattern of displacement.

C, D In this example, the capitular fragment (arrow) is seen poorly on the frontal radiograph **(C)**, but its displacement and rotation (arrows) are shown on the lateral radiograph **(D)**.

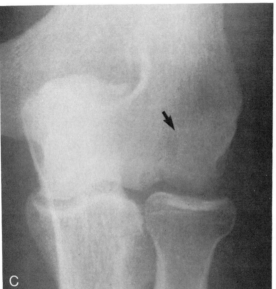

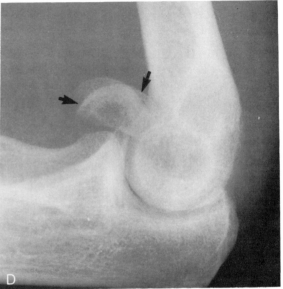

review of optimal lateral radiographs. A semicircular radiopaque shadow representing the displaced capitulum is apparent, usually anterior to the distal portion of the humerus within the radial fossa. Irregularity of the remaining osseous surface of the capitulum may be evident. An associated injury is fragmentation of the radial head. It has been suggested that fragments from a fractured radial head generally do not become located in the proximal portion of the articulation, so that radiographically visible proximal fracture fragments should arouse suspicion of an injury to the capitulum.[217, 221]

The articular surface of the medial condyle, the *trochlea*, rarely is fractured as an isolated event. This structure is well protected owing to its position deep within the elbow.[208] The trochlear fragment with or without a portion of the medial epicondyle is displaced for a variable distance along the medial portion of the articulation (Fig. 68–55).

The *epicondyles*, as well as other osseous structures throughout the elbow, are injured more frequently in the child or adolescent than in the adult (Fig. 68–56). In the mature skeleton, the medial epicondyle is fractured more commonly than the lateral epicondyle, the injury being re-

lated in most cases to a direct force applied to the epicondyle. The fracture may be confined to the medial epicondyle or involve a portion of the adjacent condylar surface. Local pain and tenderness are apparent, and radiographs reveal a fracture fragment that is displaced in a distal or anterior direction by the action of the forearm flexor muscles.[208] In some cases, it may lodge between the apposing articular surfaces of the humerus and ulna. Injury to the adjacent ulnar nerve also may be apparent. Isolated fractures of the lateral epicondyle in the adult are very rare.

Fractures of the Olecranon and Coronoid Processes of the Ulna. Fractures of the olecranon process, representing approximately 20 per cent of all elbow injuries in adults,[2] result from direct injury, indirect injury, or a combination of the two (Fig. 68–57). A transverse or oblique fracture enters the semilunar notch, and the pull of the triceps muscle accounts for displacement of the fragment(s).[208] Significant posterior displacement of the olecranon fragment combined with anterior movement of the remaining portion of the ulna and the radial head is a serious injury that is termed a fracture-dislocation of the elbow.[222]

There is no uniformly accepted classification system for

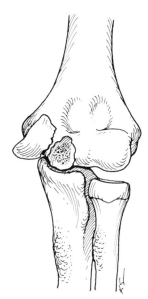

FIGURE 68–55. Humeral fractures: Trochlear. These fractures are rare and of variable configuration, and they may involve portions of the medial epicondyle.

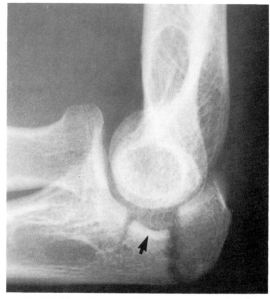

FIGURE 68–57. Ulnar fractures: Olecranon process. A comminuted fracture has led to depression of the articular surface (arrow). A joint effusion is present.

olecranon fractures of the ulna. Some systems use categories of displaced and nondisplaced fractures, others emphasize the configuration of the fracture line, and still others combine these two features.[208, 223, 224] Prognostic factors include the degree of osseous displacement and the ability of the patient to extend the elbow against gravity; the greater the degree of displacement and the more severe the patient's inability to accomplish elbow extension (indicating disruption of the triceps mechanism), the more likely it is that operative intervention is required.

The complications of olecranon fractures include a decreased range of elbow motion, osteoarthritis, and nonunion (the last occurring in approximately 5 per cent of olecranon fractures).[225, 226] Ulnar nerve damage is evident in approximately 10 per cent of patients.

Isolated fractures of the coronoid process of the ulna are rare[227] (Fig. 68–58). More commonly, coronoid fractures are associated with posterior dislocations of the elbow. Isolated fractures of the coronoid process result from either avulsion of the attached brachialis tendon or impaction against the trochlea.[2, 227]

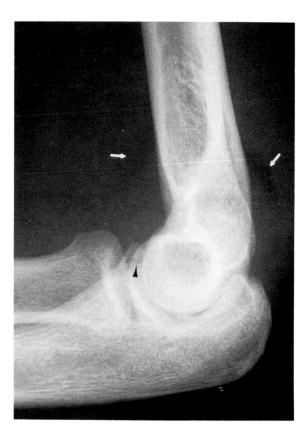

FIGURE 68–58. Ulnar fractures: Coronoid process. A subtle fracture line is evident (arrowhead). Note the positive "fat pad sign" (not well shown in this reproduction) with elevation of both the anterior and the posterior intracapsular fat pads of the elbow (arrows).

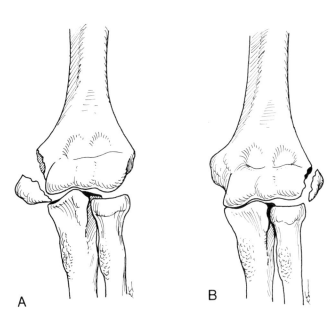

A   B

FIGURE 68–56. Humeral fractures. Epicondylar.
A Fracture of the medial epicondyle.
B Fracture of the lateral epicondyle.

Fractures of the Head and Neck of the Radius. Radial head fractures represent a common injury in adults, resulting principally from indirect trauma. Less frequently, a direct or a violent injury results in a radial head fracture with or without a posterior dislocation of the elbow (in which the head of the radius contacts the capitulum of the humerus).[228] Radial head fractures are classified as undisplaced fractures (Mason type 1), marginal fractures with displacement (e.g., angulation, depression, impaction) (Mason type 2), comminuted fractures (Mason type 3), and, in recognition of their poorer prognosis, fractures associated with elbow dislocation.[208, 229, 230] In addition, an impaction fracture of the radial neck, without involvement of the radial head, is encountered frequently.

The radiographic abnormalities are important in the accurate diagnosis of these injuries, as the physical findings may be relatively minor or nonspecific in nature (Fig. 68–59). The diagnostic importance of a positive "fat pad sign" (see Chapter 22) as well as that of oblique and specialized radiographic projections (see Chapter 1) is well recognized,[231] and the identification of an associated capitulum fracture or intra-articular osseous fragments has been emphasized.

Complications following radial head fractures are infrequent, consisting of a limited range of motion, osteoarthritis, and, in cases of more severe injuries, heterotopic ossification. Such fractures, however, may be part of a more complex or widespread injury, such as an elbow dislocation, a fracture of the the capitulum, subluxation of the distal radioulnar joint (the Essex-Lopresti injury), a Colles' fracture, or a fracture of the scaphoid bone[232] or other carpal bones. The Essex-Lopresti injury consists of a comminuted and displaced radial head fracture and disruption of the distal radioulnar joint (Fig. 68–60). The constant feature of this injury is immediate proximal migration of the radial shaft related to the severity of the radial head fracture.[233] This rare injury results from a longitudinal force applied to the outstretched hand that leads to impaction of the radial head and capitulum. The interosseous membrane is disrupted. Accurate diagnosis requires careful analysis of wrist radiographs. An Essex-Lopresti type injury of the distal radioulnar joint also can result from a fracture-dislocation of the elbow.[234]

Radial and Ulnar Diaphyses

The radius and ulna lie alongside each other, touching at their proximal and distal portions and separated by an interosseous space occupied by the interosseous membrane. This membrane is obliquely oriented, containing fibers that extend from a more proximal position on the radius to a more distal position on the ulna. When a fracture occurs in one

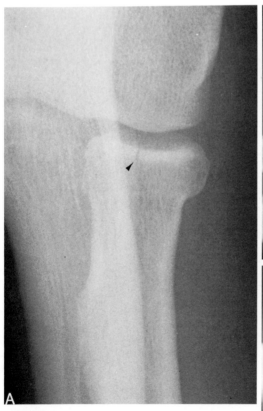

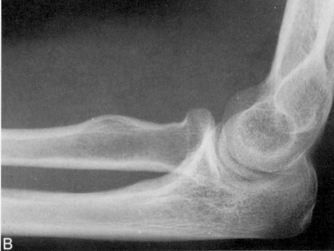

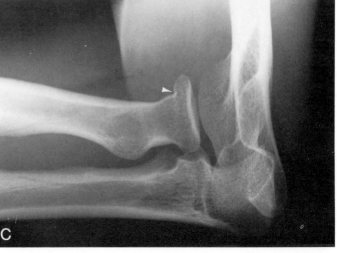

FIGURE 68–59. Radial fractures: Head of the radius.
   A Magnification radiography is used to illustrate a subtle radial head fracture (arrowhead).
   B, C As a supplement to a conventional lateral radiograph **(B)**, a specialized radiographic projection **(C)** is used in the demonstration of a radial head fracture (arrowhead).

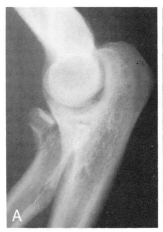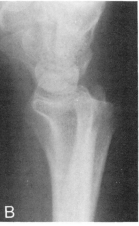

FIGURE 68–60. Essex-Lopresti injury. The components of this injury are a displaced fracture of the radial head **(A)** and disruption of the distal radioulnar joint, with posterior displacement of the distal portion of the ulna in this case **(B)**.

or both bones of the forearm, the muscles that join these bones, the pronator quadratus, pronator teres, and supinator, serve to decrease the interosseous space. The final resting position of the radius following fracture depends on the action of these muscles and others, such as the biceps brachii muscle, and is influenced by the level of the fracture itself. When radial fractures occur in the upper portion of the bone, between the sites of insertion of the supinator above and the pronator teres below, the radius proximal to the fracture is supinated, related to the actions of both the supinator and biceps brachii muscles; when radial fractures occur below the level of attachment of the pronator teres tendon, the proximal fragment assumes a neutral or slightly

supinated attitude. These patterns of rotation of the proximal portion of the radius are important to the orthopedic surgeon who, in reducing the radial fracture, must attempt to eliminate any rotational malalignment. This is accomplished by rotation of the distal radial fragment so it aligns with the proximal fragment. Routine radiography, often supplemented with specialized projections, can be used to judge the degree of supination and pronation of the proximal portion of the radius by analysis of the appearance of the bicipital tuberosity.[235] The bicipital tuberosity of the radius is located medially when the arm is positioned in full supination; laterally when the arm is positioned in full pronation; and posteriorly when the arm is positioned in midpronation.[235, 236] Radiographs of the forearm generally include a frontal anteroposterior projection with the arm supinated. In such a position, the ulnar styloid process is not a border-forming structure on the outer aspect of the distal ulna; on a frontal (posteroanterior) projection of the forearm with the arm pronated, the styloid process is located on the outer margin of the distal ulna.

Injuries involving a single anatomic structure in the forearm are rare (Table 68–3). In common with the pelvis, mandible, and ankle, the forearm can be considered a ring structure owing to the ligamentous and articular connections of the radius and ulna.[237] Disruption of the ring at one site usually is accompanied by disruption at a second (and even third) site. When both injuries are fractures, accurate diagnosis using routine radiography is not difficult. When a fracture and dislocation represent the components of the two injuries (e.g., Monteggia and Galeazzi fracture-dislocations, Essex-Lopresti injury), routine radiographic diagnosis again is straightforward as long as the entire forearm (i.e., elbow to wrist) is surveyed. When a subluxation rep-

TABLE 68–3. Fractures of the Radial and Ulnar Shafts

Site	Characteristics	Complications
Ulna (alone)[293–298]	"Nightstick" fracture: direct blow to forearm, distal ulna > middle ulna > proximal ulna	Displacement at fracture site (uncommon)
	Monteggia injury: Type I: Fracture of middle or upper third of ulna with anterior dislocation of radial head (65 per cent)	Injury to branches of radial nerve (approximately 20 per cent of cases)
	Type II: Fracture of middle or upper third of ulna with posterior dislocation of radial head (18 per cent)	
	Type III: Fracture of ulna just distal to coronoid process with lateral dislocation of radial head (16 per cent)	
	Type IV: Fracture of upper or middle third of ulna with anterior dislocation of radial head and fracture of proximal radius (1 per cent)	
Radius (alone)[299–301]	Proximal and middle segments: Uncommon as usually associated with ulnar fracture	
	Galeazzi's injury: Fracture of the radial shaft with dislocation or subluxation of inferior radioulnar joint, caused by direct blow or fall on the outstretched hand with pronation of forearm, variable degrees of displacement at fracture site	Angulation Entrapment of extensor carpi ulnaris tendon (rare) Delayed union or nonunion
Radius and ulna[302–305]	Closed or open	Delayed union or nonunion (especially of ulna)
	Nondisplaced or displaced (displacement more common in adults than in children)	Infection, especially in open fractures
		Nerve and vascular injuries, especially in open fractures and those with severe displacement
		Compartment syndromes
		Synostosis between radius and ulna (rare)

resents a component of the injury pattern, however, the initial radiographic examination may be interpreted as showing only a single lesion, particularly if the subluxation is transient in nature or appears only in certain positions of the forearm. Scintigraphy, CT, or MR imaging in such instances may provide diagnostic assistance.

Fractures of Both the Radius and the Ulna. Fractures involving both bones of the forearm are common, resulting usually from direct blows sustained during a motor vehicle accident, fall, or fight. The middle segment of the diaphyseal portion of the bones typically is involved, although the peripheral segments may be affected. The sites of fracture in the radius and ulna may occur at approximately the same level or at different levels, and segmental fractures of one of the bones are encountered. Considerable displacement, angulation, and rotation at the fracture sites are common, leading to deformity and loss of function of the forearm (and hand). Analysis of rotational displacement is facilitated by comparison views of the opposite (uninjured) side, by determination of the position of the bicipital tuberosity of the radius (see previous discussion), and by observing an abrupt change in the width of the radius above and below the fracture site. In children, the distal third of the diaphyses of the radius and ulna is involved most commonly, the site of radial fracture generally is more distal than that of the ulnar fracture, and incomplete or bowing fractures of one (or both) bones may be seen.[2]

Complications of these fractures include delayed union or nonunion (especially when infection is present), neurologic and vascular injury (representing an uncommon sequela of such fractures), compartment syndrome, and synostoses.[238, 239]

Fractures of the Ulna. Fractures involving the diaphysis of the ulna may occur as part of a Monteggia fracture-dislocation (see previous discussion) or as an isolated phenomenon. Isolated nondisplaced or minimally displaced fractures of the ulnar shaft are common; typically they result from a direct blow, and are designated nightstick fractures owing to their occurrence during an assault in which the victim raises his or her forearm to protect the head from being struck by a hard object, often a club (Fig. 68–61). Transverse or short oblique fractures, sometimes with a butterfly fragment (see Chapter 67), in the distal or, less commonly, the middle third of the bone are typical. Involvement of the proximal third of the ulna is least common and, in such cases, may be associated with difficulty in maintaining anatomic alignment following fracture reduction. Significantly displaced fractures of the ulnar diaphysis rarely occur as an isolated lesion. Rather, they are associated with dislocations of the proximal or distal radioulnar joint, or both joints.[237]

Fractures of the Radius. Fractures of the diaphysis of the radius occur most commonly as part of the Galeazzi fracture-dislocation (see later discussion) and rarely as an isolated phenomenon. Isolated fractures of the proximal portion of the radial shaft result from a direct blow and are less common than those of the ulna. A fall on the outstretched hand represents a second cause of a fracture of the proximal radial diaphysis, although associated injuries including dislocation of the radial head and capitular fracture usually are evident.[240]

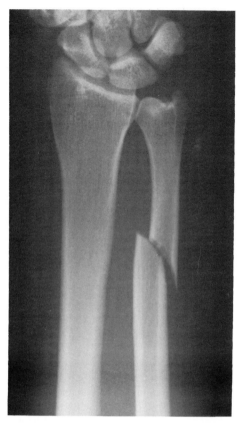

FIGURE 68–61. Fractures of the diaphyses of the radius and ulna: Isolated fracture of the ulna (nightstick fracture). Note the oblique, slightly displaced fracture of the distal portion of the ulna. Radiographically, no lesions of the wrist or elbow were present.

Wrist

Fractures of the Distal Portions of the Radius and Ulna. The most common mechanism of injury to the wrist is a fall on the outstretched hand causing axial compression combined with a bending moment, which leads to dorsiflexion of the joint. Far less frequently, the wrist is in palmar flexion at the time of injury. It is the precise position of the wrist, which also may include varying degrees of radial or ulnar deviation and supination or pronation, combined with other factors, including the age of the patient and the severity of the forces involved, that dictates the type of injury that will occur. With regard to the influence of age alone, metaphyseal fractures of the radius and ulna in young children, physeal separations of the radius in adolescents, scaphoid fractures in young adults, and fractures of the distal portion of the radius or radius and ulna in middle-aged and elderly patients typically follow a fall on the outstretched hand.[2] Fractures of the distal regions of the radius and ulna are approximately 10 times more frequent than those of the carpal bones, and the latter are especially infrequent in children.[4] It generally is believed that the distal portion of the radius yields to a lower level of force and lower angle of dorsiflexion than the carpus.[241]

Many eponyms are used to describe the fractures of the distal ends of the radius and ulna. Examples include Colles' fracture (fracture of the distal portion of the radius with dorsal displacement), Smith's fracture (fracture of the distal

TABLE 68–4. Fractures of the Distal Portions of the Radius and Ulna

Fracture	Mechanism	Characteristics	Complications
Colles'[306, 307] (Pouteau's)	Dorsiflexion	Fracture of distal portion with dorsal displacement	Deformity related to radial shortening and angulation
		Classification system based on extra-articular versus intra-articular location, presence or absence of ulnar fracture	Subluxation or dislocation of inferior radioulnar joint
			Reflex sympathetic dystrophy syndrome
		Varying amounts of radial displacement, angulation, and shortening	Injury to median or, less commonly, radial or ulnar nerve
		Ulnar styloid fracture in about 50 to 60 per cent of cases	Osteoarthritis
			Tendon rupture
		Associated injuries to carpus, elbow, humerus, and femur (in osteoporotic patients), inferior radioulnar joint	
Barton's[308–310]	Dorsiflexion and pronation	Fracture of dorsal rim of radius with intra-articular extension	Similar to those of Colles' fracture
Radiocarpal fracture-dislocation[311, 312]	Dorsiflexion	Uncommon and severe injury	Entrapment of ulnar nerve and artery, tendons
		Associated fractures of dorsal rim and styloid process of radius, ulnar styloid process	
		May be irreducible	
Hutchinson's[241, 308, 313] (chauffeur's)	Avulsion by radial collateral ligament	Fracture of styloid process of radius	Scapholunate dissociation
		Usually nondisplaced	Osteoarthritis
			Ligament damage
Smith's[314] (reverse Colles')	Variable	Fracture of distal portion of radius with palmar displacement	Similar to those of Colles' fracture
		Less common than Colles' fracture	
		Varying amounts of radial comminution, articular involvement	
		Associated fracture of ulnar styloid process	
Ulnar styloid process[2]	Dorsiflexion or avulsion by ulnar collateral or triangular ligament	Usually associated with radial fractures, rarely isolated	Nonunion
		Usually nondisplaced	

portion of the radius with palmar displacement), Barton's fracture (fracture of the dorsal rim of the radius), and Hutchinson's fracture (fracture of the radial styloid process). The major characteristics of these fractures are described in Table 68–4.

The classic Colles' fracture is a transverse fracture, with or without comminution, that extends from the volar to the dorsal surface of the distal radius and is accompanied by impaction and displacement of the dorsal surface of the radius (Fig. 68–62). The typical mechanism, a fall on the

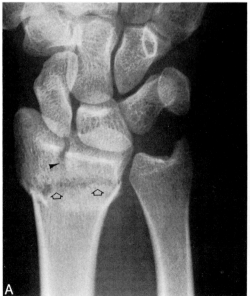 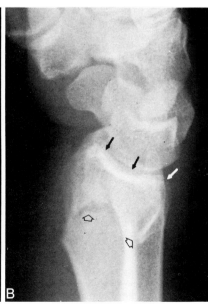

FIGURE 68–62. Wrist fractures: Colles' fracture. Observe the transverse fracture of the distal portion of the radius (open arrows) with extension into the radiocarpal joint (arrowhead). In the lateral projection, dorsal angulation of the articular surface of the radius is apparent (solid arrows) owing to the compaction of bone dorsally. The ulnar styloid process is intact, and there is no evidence of subluxation of the distal portion of the ulna.

outstretched hand, leads to compression of this surface and excess tension (with widening of the fracture line) of the volar surface of the radius. The frequency of Colles' fracture increases with advancing age of the patient, and it is far more frequent in women than in men. A number of classification systems exist for Colles' fractures; many are complex, and some are based upon the number of articulations (i.e., radiocarpal, inferior radioulnar) that are violated and the presence or absence of a fracture of the ulnar styloid process. A fracture of the ulnar styloid process occurs in approximately 50 to 60 per cent of cases, and violation of one or both of these articulations occurs in the majority of cases. Radial shortening and dorsal inclination of the articular surface of the radius (which normally has a 5 to 15 degree volar inclination) are emphasized sequelae of Colles' fractures that, if not corrected, may influence subsequent wrist function.[242, 243] Therefore, precise measurement of such parameters as radial tilt, radial inclination, and ulnar variance on routine radiographs assumes some importance[244] and requires meticulous and sometimes modified radiographic technique.[244, 245] Complications of Colles' fractures are diverse and, unfortunately, common. Such complications include unstable reduction, articular incongruity, subluxation or dislocation of the distal radioulnar joint, median nerve compression resulting in the carpal tunnel syndrome, ulnar nerve injury, entrapment of flexor tendons, the reflex sympathetic dystrophy syndrome, carpal malalignment or fracture, posttraumatic osteolysis of the ulna, and malunion, delayed union, or nonunion.[2, 246–249]

A distal radial fracture similar in position to that of the Colles' fracture but associated with volar (or palmar) angulation or displacement of the distal fragment is known as Smith's fracture (Fig. 68–63). Its mechanism is not clear; it may be related to a fall on the dorsum of the hand or to one on a dorsiflexed wrist with the forearm rotating from a supinated to pronated position. The Smith's fracture is much less common than the Colles' fracture and accurate diagnosis requires careful analysis of the lateral radiograph

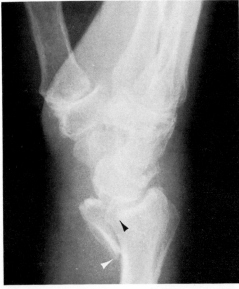

FIGURE 68–63. Wrist fractures: Smith's fracture. A fracture of the distal portion of the radius (arrowheads) involves the volar surface. Note the mild volar and proximal displacement of the fracture fragment and the carpus.

of the wrist. In contrast to Colles' fractures, the distal radial fragment is displaced anteriorly with palmar angulation of the radial articular surface in a Smith's fracture.[2] The Smith's fracture can be extra-articular or intra-articular in nature. Complications of Smith's fractures are similar to those of Colles' fractures and may include injury to the extensor tendons.[250, 251]

A Barton's fracture involves an injury to the dorsal rim of the distal portion of the radius, generally related to dorsiflexion and pronation of the forearm on the fixed wrist and occurring frequently in young patients involved in motorcyle accidents (Fig. 68–64). The size of the fracture fragment is variable, although a large portion of the articular surface of the distal radius may be affected. As this fracture also may occur in the elderly, its differentiation from Colles' fracture becomes important and can be accomplished on the basis of findings on the lateral radiograph of the wrist. Barton's fracture extends in an oblique fashion from the dorsal surface of the radius proximally to the articular surface of the radius distally. It does not classically violate the volar surface of the radius and is accompanied by dorsal displacement of the carpus. A variant of Barton's fracture affects the volar rim of the distal radius, may be more common than its dorsal counterpart, and sometimes is referred to as a reverse Barton's fracture or a type of Smith's fracture. Complications of fractures of the dorsal or volar rim of the distal radius are similar to those of Colles' fracture.

Radiocarpal joint dislocations are rare; they may occur in a dorsal, volar, or radial direction, may appear as an isolated finding or in association with fractures of the dorsal or volar radial rim or radial or ulnar styloid process, and are accompanied by injuries of the radiocarpal ligaments. Very rarely, they are irreducible owing to entrapment of bone fragments within the joint. Neurovascular and tendinous structures also may be compromised.

A fracture of the styloid process of the radius (Fig. 68–65) often is referred to as a Hutchinson's fracture or, owing to its original occurrence when the starting crank of an engine suddenly reversed during an engine backfire, a chauffeur's fracture. It appears to represent an avulsion injury related to the sites of attachment of the radiocarpal ligaments or radial collateral ligament, but such fractures also can occur from a direct blow. The size of the fragment is variable, but its displacement is unusual. In some cases, a fracture of the radial styloid process is a component of a more complex injury of the wrist,[863] including radiocarpal joint dislocations. The fracture is best identified on frontal radiographs of the wrist (although it should not be confused with the irregularity of the lateral surface of the radius that normally may be present at the site of previous physeal closure) and it may not be apparent on lateral radiographs.[2] The fracture line may enter the space between the scaphoid and lunate fossae in the articular surface of the radius and, in such cases, it may be associated with scapholunate dissociation and lesser arc injuries of the wrist[252] (see later discussion).

Although fractures of the styloid process of the ulna usually are a component of a more extensive wrist injury, including a Colles' fracture, an injury isolated to the ulnar styloid process occasionally is observed, perhaps related to an avulsion produced by the ulnar collateral ligament or triangular ligament (Fig. 68–66). The resulting ossific frag-

FIGURE 68–64. Wrist fractures: Barton's fracture. The dorsal rim of the distal portion of the radius is fractured (arrowhead). It is displaced proximally and posteriorly, and there is dorsal subluxation of the carpus (arrows).

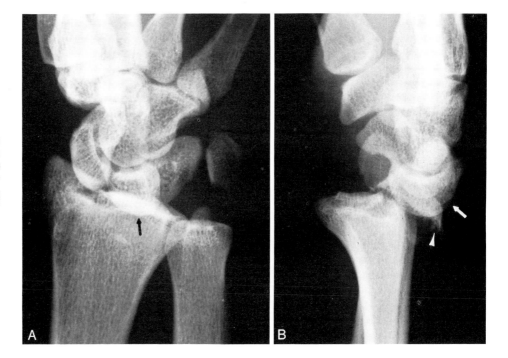

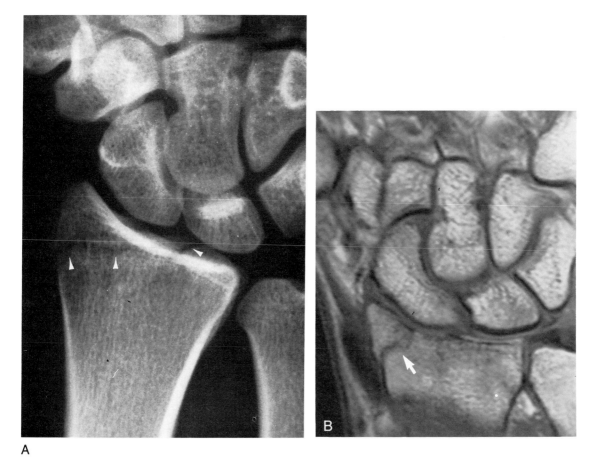

A

FIGURE 68–65. Wrist fractures: Hutchinson's fracture.
   A The fracture line is readily apparent (arrowheads), producing a triangular fragment that is quite large in this case owing to the fact that the fracture line exits ulnarly with respect to the scapholunate space. There is no displacement at the fracture site.
   B A coronal T1-weighted (TR/TE, 733/20) spin echo MR image reveals a fracture (arrows) of the radial styloid process.
   (**B**, Courtesy of S. Eilenberg, M.D., San Diego, California.)

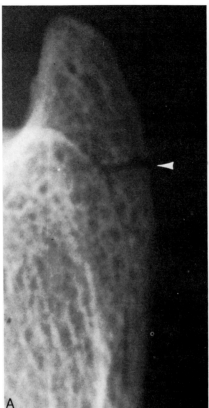

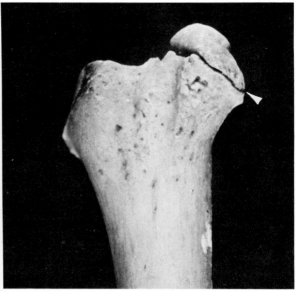

FIGURE 68–66. Wrist fractures: Ulnar styloid process.

A A magnification radiograph reveals a subtle fracture of the styloid process of the ulna (arrowhead).

B An old fracture of the ulnar styloid process is shown (arrowhead). Differentiation of such traumatic changes from developmental alterations of the distal portion of the ulna or from extra centers of ossification (e.g., lunula) can be difficult.

ment resembles the normal area of ossification (lunula) that may appear in the meniscus homologue of the wrist, although its irregular contour as well as the irregularity of the remaining portion of the styloid process generally allows accurate diagnosis of the fracture. Hypertrophy of the fragment with fracture nonunion is encountered infrequently and may be a source of chronic wrist pain.[249]

Dislocation of the Inferior Radioulnar Joint. Although isolated dislocations of the inferior radioulnar joint are seen infrequently,[315–317] dislocation or subluxation of this articulation may occur in association with a fracture of the radius. This combination of findings is termed a Galeazzi fracture-dislocation[315, 318–321] (Fig. 68–67). Classically, the shaft of the radius is fractured in this injury; fractures of the distal end of the radius, which may be associated with dislocation of the ulnar head,[321] and of the radial neck and head, which may be associated with a dislocation of the inferior radioulnar joint, are not regarded as Galeazzi fracture-dislocations unless the radial shaft also is fractured.[322] Comminuted fractures of the radial head combined with dislocations of the distal radioulnar joint are termed Essex-Lopresti injuries (see previous discussion). Most commonly, the fracture accompanying the Galeazzi fracture-dislocation occurs at the junction of the middle and distal thirds of the radius and has a short oblique or transverse configuration. The distal radial fragment is displaced in an ulnar direction. Usually, the dislocation of the ulnar head readily is apparent, although, in some cases, ulnar head subluxation may be more apparent on clinical evaluation. In equivocal cases, arthrography of the radiocarpal joint can be helpful in establishing the existence of an injury to the distal portion of the ulna or surrounding structures.[323] Disruption of the inferior radioulnar joint requires injury to the triangular fibrocartilage,

the major stabilizing structure of the distal portion of the ulna. Thus, contrast opacification of the radiocarpal joint will be associated with filling of the inferior radioulnar joint due to perforation of the intervening triangular fibrocartilage.[320, 324] Fracture of the ulnar head or styloid process also may be identified. Dislocation of the ulna usually occurs in a distal, dorsal, and medial direction; volar dislocation is less frequent.

Owing to the complex anatomy of the distal radioulnar joint, the difficulty in demonstrating this anatomy on routine radiographic examinations, the large number of complex injuries (including the Galeazzi fracture-dislocation and Essex-Lopresti injury) that affect this articulation, and the occurrence of isolated subluxations or dislocations (dorsal or volar) of the distal radioulnar joint,[325–327] a great deal of attention has been given to careful radiographic positioning of the wrist, the application of a number of measurements, and the use of transaxial images provided by CT and MR imaging in the assessment of the position of the distal portion of the ulna with respect to the adjacent radius.[328–330] Compounding the difficulty of diagnosing minor degrees of subluxation of the distal radioulnar joint by routine radiography are problems related to proper positioning of the injured wrist to obtain true lateral views and normal variations in ulnar position related to the degree of pronation or supination of the forearm. CT and MR imaging share diagnostic advantages in the assessment of this joint that include transaxial imaging capabilities, simultaneous visualization of both wrists (allowing comparisons to be made), and delineation of important supporting soft tissue structures (see Chapter 70).

Carpal Injuries. Injuries to the carpus are extremely complex in nature and are well described in a number of review articles to which the interested reader should refer.[244, 331–345] Although the anatomic characteristics of the carpus are well known (see Chapter 22), no uniform description of the functional anatomy of these bones exists. Some investigators regard the wrist as a joint comprising two horizontally arranged rows of bones with the scaphoid serving as a bridge between them. Others employ the vertical approach, identifying three columns of bones: a lateral column consisting of the scaphoid, trapezium, and trapezoid; a central column comprising the lunate and capitate; and a medial column consisting of the triquetrum and hamate (as well as the pisiform). The constituent bones in each of these columns also are not uniformly agreed on. A third concept emphasizes the ringlike nature of the wrist, consisting of a fixed distal half and a mobile proximal half.[333] All agree on the functional importance of the surrounding ligaments, arranged in three layers: the most superficial layer consists of the antebrachial fascia and the transverse carpal ligament; a second layer contains the extrinsic ligaments generally coursing between the carpal bones and the radius, ulna, or metacarpals, including the radial collateral ligament, volar radiocarpal ligaments, meniscus homologue, triangular fibrocartilage, ulnolunate and ulnotriquetral ligaments, ulnar collateral ligament, and dorsal ligaments; and a third or deep layer consisting of intrinsic ligaments, coursing between individual carpal bones in a circular fashion.[333] In general, the extrinsic ligaments are stiffer and less capable of elongation than the intrinsic ligaments,[331] the volar ligaments are stronger and thicker than the dorsal ligaments, and the ligamentous support between the capitate and the lunate may be absent (see Chapter 70).

Two important concepts regarding the radiographic anatomy of the wrist should be emphasized. On the posteroanterior view, three smooth carpal arcs define the normal intercarpal relationships.[342, 343] Arc 1 follows the proximal surfaces of the scaphoid, lunate, and triquetrum; arc 2 is located along the distal surfaces of these same carpal bones; and arc 3 defines the curvature of the proximal surfaces of the capitate and hamate. In the normal situation, these curvilinear arcs roughly are parallel, without disruption, and the interosseous spaces are approximately equal in size. Second, as indicated in Chapter 22, the lateral radiograph of the normal wrist (in neutral position) is characterized by a specific relationship of the longitudinal axes of the radius, scaphoid, lunate, capitate, and third metacarpal. A continuous line can be drawn through these axes of the radius, lunate, and capitate, and this line will intersect a second line through the longitudinal axis of the scaphoid, creating an angle of 30 to 60 degrees. Alterations in these relationships (as well as others) indicate carpal instability, which, in most instances, is related to trauma.

Several characteristic and distinct patterns of carpal instability have been recognized (see Chapter 22). Such patterns sometimes are defined as static when malalignment among

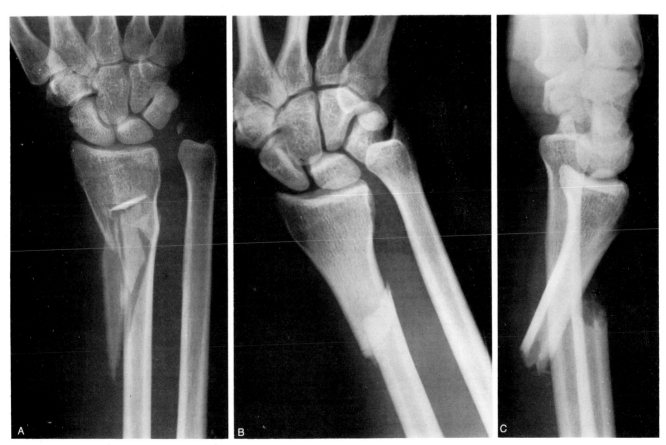

FIGURE 68–67. Galeazzi fracture-dislocation.
   A Observe an oblique fracture of the distal portion of the radial diaphysis, a fracture of the ulnar styloid, and dorsomedial dislocation of the ulna.
   B, C In a different patient, a transverse radial fracture is associated with significant overlapping, shortening, and angulation as well as a volar dislocation of the distal ulna.

the carpal bones is evident on routine radiographs or dynamic when such malalignment requires manipulation of the wrist and is not visible with routine radiography or even specialized views. Anatomically, there are three types of instability: lateral, medial, and proximal.[331] The first pattern relates principally to abnormalities in the central column, consisting of the lunate and the capitate, but affects the lateral carpus as well. Two varieties of this pattern (Fig. 68–68) are emphasized: *dorsal intercalary segment carpal instability* (DICI, DISI, dorsiflexion carpal instability), in which the lunate is tilted dorsally, the scaphoid is flexed, and the scapholunate angle is greater than 70 degrees, is the more common of the two; *volar intercalary segment carpal instability* (VICI, VISI, palmar flexion carpal instability), occurs when the lunate is tilted in a palmar direction and the scapholunate angle is decreased below the normal value of approximately 47 degrees.[341] Although precise analysis of the amount of dorsal or volar lunate tilting requires careful measurements on well-positioned lateral radiographs or tomographic studies, survey of the frontal radiograph alone may allow determination of whether the lunate is tilted in a volar or dorsal direction; with dorsal tilting, the distal contour of the lunate (representing its volar margin) usually is round, and with volar tilting, the distal contour of the lunate (representing its dorsal margin) may be angular.[346] Dorsiflexion instability commonly occurs after scaphoid fractures with scapholunate separation, or dissociation, as well as following fractures of the proximal portion of the radius; palmar flexion instability may be seen after disruption of the lunotriquetral interosseous ligament, excision of the triquetrum, and sprains of the midcarpal joint that attenuate the extrinsic ligaments,[347] as well as in patients using wheelchairs.[348] Similar patterns of instability are seen as a normal variant in persons with ligamentous laxity and in those with various articular disorders, including rheumatoid arthritis and calcium pyrophosphate dihydrate crystal deposition disease.[349]

A second pattern of instability involves the medial aspect of the carpus, one type of which occurs at the articulation between the triquetrum and the hamate and is termed *triquetrohamate dissociation or instability.*[333, 337, 350] It leads to painful clicking on the ulnar aspect of the wrist and is related to traumatically induced pronation and radial flexion.[333] Abnormal motion between the triquetrum and the hamate is observed during fluoroscopy. Another type of medial carpal instability is termed *triquetrolunate dissociation,* indicating abnormal motion at the intervening articulation.[337]

Proximal carpal instability results from disruption of the radiocarpal ligaments or distal radioulnar joint surfaces. Several types exist.[337] *Ulnar translocation* occurs when the carpus shifts in an ulnar direction, which may follow severe capsular injury or articular disorders such as rheumatoid arthritis. An increased space between the scaphoid and the radial styloid process is an important, although not invariable, diagnostic feature. *Dorsal carpal translocation* usually is associated with malunited fractures involving the dorsal rim of the radius and the radial styloid process. *Palmar carpal translocation* accompanies Barton's fractures or disruptions of the volar rim of the radius. *Proximal midcarpal instability,* which may result from malunited fractures of the distal portion of the radius that do not extend into the

radiocarpal joint, leads to disabling pain, tenderness, and, occasionally, a loud snapping sound when the hand is brought voluntarily into ulnar deviation.

The diagnosis of all of these abnormalities requires routine radiography supplemented with special views, including posteroanterior projections in neutral, ulnar, and radial deviation, an anteroposterior projection with tightly clenched fist, and oblique and lateral projections.[342, 351] Fluoroscopic monitoring also can be useful in detecting transient subluxations in the wrist,[352–355] and may be combined with the application of stress.[355]

Dissociated scapholunate movements may accompany tears of the ventral radiocarpal ligaments and scapholunate interosseous ligament complex. This may occur as a complication of lunate or perilunate dislocation, rheumatoid arthritis, and other articular diseases or as an isolated injury. *Scapholunate dissociation* (rotatory subluxation of the scaphoid)[356] is suggested when the distance between the scaphoid and lunate is 2 mm or wider and can be diagnosed almost unequivocally when this distance is 4 mm or wider[342] (Fig. 68–69). Some variability in this width, however, with measurements as great as 5 mm, has been noted in normal persons[357] as well as in those with lunotriquetral coalitions. The finding of a widened scapholunate space implies that an abnormality exists in the scapholunate interosseous ligament,[358] and, perhaps, in the volar or dorsal radiocarpal ligaments as well.[359] When the scaphoid also is tilted in a palmar direction, a ventral radiocarpal ligament tear also is present. Rotatory subluxation of the scaphoid is associated with radiographic findings in addition to widening of the scapholunate space (Terry-Thomas sign) and palmar tilting of the scaphoid.[360–364] These findings include, on the posteroanterior view, a ring produced by the cortex of the distal pole of the scaphoid and a foreshortened scaphoid. Radiographs exposed during radial or ulnar deviation of the wrist or in a posteroanterior position with 10 degrees of tube angulation from the ulna toward the radius may accentuate the gap or space between the scaphoid and the lunate,[360, 365] although a false-positive ring sign also may be seen with wrist deviation in the coronal plane. Wrist arthrography can substantiate the diagnosis of rotatory subluxation of the scaphoid by revealing communication between the radiocarpal and midcarpal compartments. This communication is frequent in older patients, however, owing to small perforations or tears of the interosseous ligaments between the bones of the proximal carpal row, so caution must be applied to the interpretation of the arthrographic findings. Degenerative joint disease of the radiocarpal and midcarpal compartments may complicate this condition.

Virtually any of the carpal bones may be dislocated following an injury; reports describe isolated dislocations of the scaphoid,[366] capitate,[368] triquetrum,[369] trapezium,[370–372] trapezoid,[373–375] and pisiform.[376–378] Furthermore, unusual dislocations or displacements of more than a single carpal bone are encountered,[379] including scaphoid dislocation with axial carpal dislocation,[380] dislocation of the scaphoid and lunate,[381] dislocation of the triquetrum with rotatory subluxation of the scaphoid,[382] dislocation of the lunate and triquetrum,[383] and longitudinal disruption of the ulnar aspect of the carpus.[384] Such injuries are rare, however. Because the lunate and the proximal scaphoid are protected to some

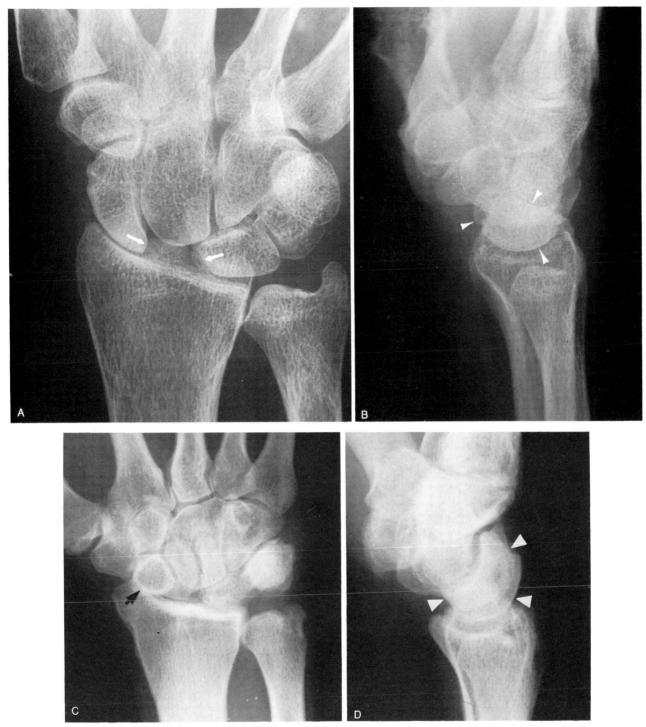

FIGURE 68–68. Lateral (static) carpal instability.

A, B Dorsal intercalary segment instability (DISI). Observe the gap or widening in the scapholunate space (arrows) on the posteroanterior roentgenogram, and dorsiflexion of the lunate (arrowheads) on the lateral radiograph. The radiocarpal and midcarpal joints are narrowed. A small fracture of the volar surface of the lunate is seen.

C, D Volar intercalary segment instability (VISI). Findings include palmar displacement of the distal pole of the scaphoid resulting in a ring-like shadow (arrow) and volar tilting of the lunate (arrowheads).

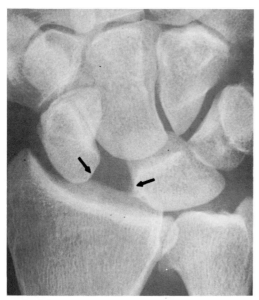

FIGURE 68–69. Scapholunate dissociation (rotatory subluxation of the scaphoid). Findings include widening of the scapholunate distance (arrows) and a foreshortened scaphoid.

extent by the distal radius, a common pattern of injury is a perilunate or transscaphoid perilunate dislocation (Figs. 68–70 and 68–71). In a perilunate dislocation, the lunate remains aligned with the distal radius, and the other carpal bones dislocate, usually dorsally, although on rare occasions in a volar direction.[385, 386] When the wrist is hyperextended, the dorsal cortex of the distal radial articular surface fixes the lunate in place and apposes the scaphoid waist. A fall on the hyperextended hand, creating an abnormal force through the radius, can produce a fracture of the scaphoid,[387] and, with sufficient stress, a dislocation of the carpus occurs. The distal fragment of the scaphoid may move with the distal carpal row, and the proximal fragment may move with the proximal carpal row. With continued hyperextension force, the capitate may force the lunate ventrally, thus converting the perilunate dislocation into a lunate dislocation in which the lunate is displaced in a palmar direction and the capitate appears to be aligned with the distal radius.[388, 389] Variations in the classic patterns of dislocation and associated fractures are common, depending on the exact position of the wrist at the time of injury.[334] Transscaphoid, transcapitate, and transtriquetral fracture-dislocations are encountered, and the radial and ulnar styloid processes also may be affected. Proper radiographic interpretation requires multiple projections, including frontal, lateral, and oblique views. Difficulty in interpretation arises when a fragment is displaced for a considerable distance or when a fracture fragment rotates (e.g., the proximal end of the capitate)[387, 390–392] so that its site of origin is obscure (Fig. 68–72).

Closer inspection of the functional anatomy of the wrist and the patterns of injury has indicated that a predictable sequence of events generally occurs following trauma (Fig. 68–73). The impact and loading conditions in these injuries usually commence about the thenar eminence, initially injuring the radial side of the wrist. Four stages in the resulting abnormalities are defined, with each successive stage indicating increased carpal instability.[338, 393] The stage I injury represents scapholunate dissociation with rotatory sub-

luxation of the scaphoid; the stage II injury is characterized by perilunar instability owing to failure of the radiocapitate ligament or a fracture of the radial styloid process, and leads to a perilunate dislocation; the stage III injury creates ligamentous disruption at the triquetrolunate joint related to partial or complete failure or avulsion of the volar radiotriquetral ligament and dorsal radiocarpal ligaments and may be accompanied by radiographically evident triquetral malrotation, triquetrolunate diastasis, or triquetral fracture; the final stage IV injury is associated with disruption of the dorsal radiocarpal ligaments, freeing the lunate and allowing it to become volarly displaced (lunate dislocation). This series of events affecting ligaments and joint spaces takes place about the circumference of the lunate and is termed a *lesser arc injury. Greater arc injuries* represent fracture-dislocation patterns as this arc passes through the scaphoid, capitate, hamate, and triquetrum. Examples include the relatively common transscaphoid perilunate fracture-dislocation; the transscaphoid, transcapitate, perilunate fracture-dislocation (scaphocapitate syndrome); and the severe and infrequent transscaphoid, transcapitate, transhamate, transtriquetral fracture-dislocation.[338] These injuries also may be divided into various stages based on their severity: stage I: transradial styloid fracture-dislocation; stage II: transscaphoid fracture-dislocation; stage III: transscaphoid, transcapitate fracture-dislocation; stage IV: transscaphoid (or radial styloid), transcapitate, transtriquetral fracture-dislocation; and stage V: complete palmar lunate dislocation associated with carpal fractures.[394]

Dislocations about the common carpometacarpal joint are rare injuries, most typically involving the ulnar aspect of the wrist (Fig. 68–74). They may be isolated to a single metacarpal[395, 396] or, more commonly, involve two or more of the metacarpals.[397–400] Dorsal dislocation predominates. Radiographic abnormalities often are subtle, requiring specialized projections in addition to standard techniques.[401] CT with coronal and sagittal images also is useful. Recognized complications include injuries to the ulnar nerve (in dislocation of the metacarpohamate joint) or median nerve, rupture of extensor tendons, and fractures of one or more metacarpals. Dislocation of the first carpometacarpal articulation also is infrequent and, when present, may be combined with fractures of the base of the first metacarpal (Bennett's fracture-subluxation).[402]

With regard to *fractures of the carpal bones*, they are observed most frequently in the scaphoid (Fig. 68–75). Fractures of the scaphoid are classified principally according to their location (proximal pole, waist, distal body, tuberosity, and distal articular), owing to the influence of the site of involvement on the likelihood of ischemic necrosis and the rate of healing.[241] In general, the prognosis of distal fractures is better than that of proximal fractures because of more rapid osseous healing and less extensive vascular interruption. The most frequent scaphoid fracture occurs in the waist (approximately 70 per cent) or proximal pole (approximately 20 per cent) of the bone, although in children, avulsion fractures of the distal portion of the scaphoid are typical and, with reportable exceptions,[403] generally heal well.[404, 405] Unusual patterns of scaphoid injury include dorsal avulsion fractures[406] and fractures of the osteochondral interface in young children.[407] In any type of fracture, accurate radiographic diagnosis depends on high quality routine and supplementary radiographs[408, 409] and

Text continued on page 2745

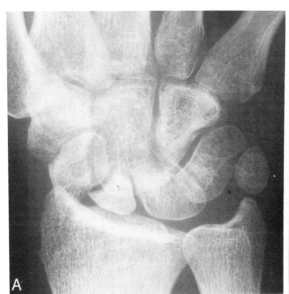
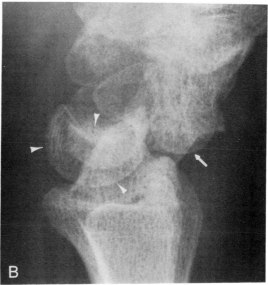
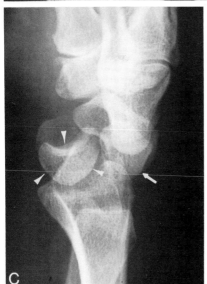

FIGURE 68–70. Perilunate dislocation.

A, B Transscaphoid perilunate dislocation. Findings include a fracture of the scaphoid with osteonecrosis of the proximal pole and a perilunate dislocation characterized by a lunate bone (arrowheads) aligned with the distal radius as well as dorsal displacement of the capitate (arrow) and the rest of the carpus.

C Perilunate dislocation. Observe the alignment of the lunate (arrowheads) with the distal radius and dorsal displacement of the capitate (arrow) and the rest of the carpal bones.

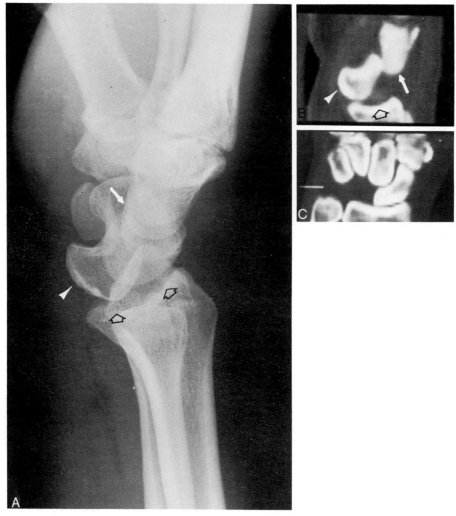

FIGURE 68–71. Lunate dislocation.

A On this lateral radiograph, note volar displacement of the lunate (arrowhead) with the capitate (solid arrow) resting on the dorsal surface of the bone. Neither lunate nor capitate is truly aligned with the distal surface of the radius (open arrows), indicating the difficulty encountered in classifying such lesions as a lunate or perilunate dislocation.

B A sagittally reformatted CT scan shows the relationships among the lunate (arrowhead), capitate (solid arrow), and radius (open arrow).

C A coronally reformatted CT scan reveals that the lunate is absent between the scaphoid and triquetrum owing to its volar displacement. (Courtesy of G. Greenway, M.D., Dallas, Texas.)

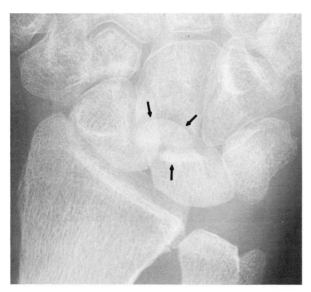

FIGURE 68–72. Scaphocapitate syndrome. Fractures of the scaphoid and capitate resulted from a wrist injury. In this projection, the scaphoid fracture is not well shown. Observe the site of the capitate fracture with 180 degree rotation of the proximal fragment (arrows) so that the proximal articular surface is facing distally. Failure to recognize the abnormal rotation of this fracture fragment will result in improper treatment and therapeutic failure.

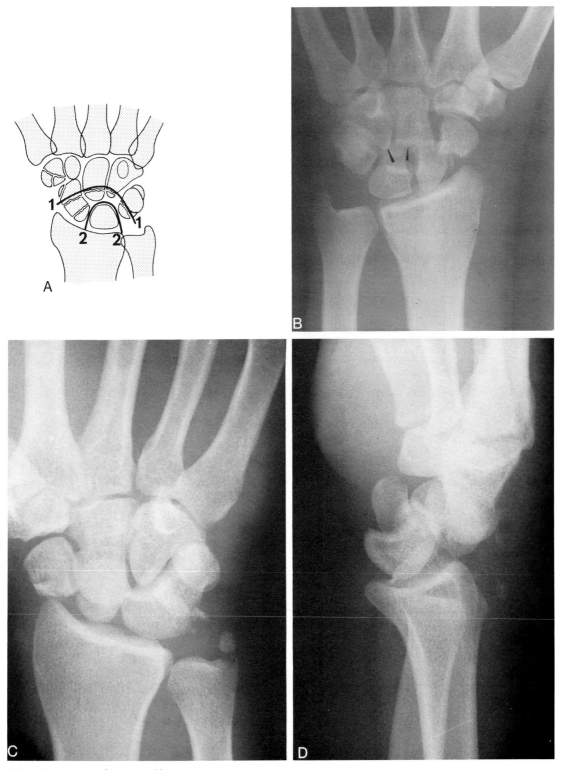

FIGURE 68–73. Wrist injuries: Greater and lesser arcs.

   A The locations of the greater (1) and lesser (2) arcs are shown, as are the common sites of carpal fractures that can be produced experimentally. A pure greater arc injury consists of a transscaphoid, transcapitate, transhamate, transtriquetral fracture-dislocation; a pure lesser arc injury is a perilunate or lunate dislocation. Various combinations of these injury patterns are seen clinically. (From Johnson RP: Clin Orthop Rel Res *149*:33, 1980.)

   B Greater arc injury. Transscaphoid, transcapitate, transtriquetral, perilunate fracture-dislocation with 180 degree rotation of the capitate fragment (arrowheads).

   C, D Greater arc injury. Transscaphoid, transtriquetral, perilunate fracture-dislocation with ulnar styloid fracture.

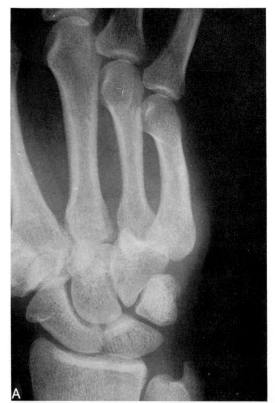

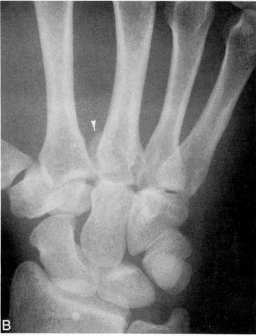

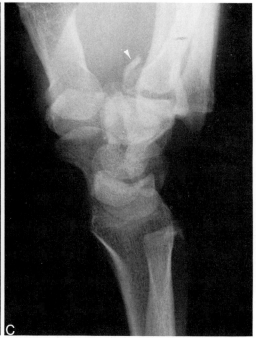

FIGURE 68–74. Dislocations of the common carpometacarpal joint.

A Note the malalignment of the hamate and the bases of the fourth and fifth metacarpal bones related to dorsal dislocation of these metacarpal bones. The joint space is obliterated. Compare with the normal articular space between the third metacarpal bone and capitate.

B, C In this example, a fracture at the base of the third metacarpal bone (arrowheads) is accompanied by dorsal dislocation of the second, third, fourth, and fifth metacarpal bases with respect to the adjacent carpal bones.

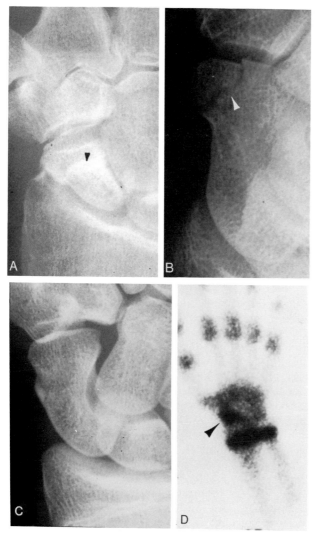

FIGURE 68–75. Carpal scaphoid fractures: Types of fracture.

A Scaphoid waist. A fracture line possessing sclerotic margins is identified (arrowhead).

B Scaphoid tuberosity. An acute fracture is seen (arrowhead).

C, D Scaphoid waist. In this 15 year old boy, the fracture is not evident on initial radiographic examination **(C)**. It is apparent as an area of increased accumulation of the radionuclide (arrowhead) on the bone scan **(D)**.

(**C, D** Courtesy of G. Greenway, M.D., Dallas, Texas.)

even fluoroscopy, magnification radiography, scintigraphy,[410–413] or conventional or computed tomography.[414–417] Diagnostic difficulties arise in the detection of associated fractures or ligamentous instability[418] and in the determination of the age of the fracture when historic data are either lacking or inconclusive.[241] Older scaphoid fractures may possess sclerotic margins with adjacent cysts, although these findings are not present uniformly.

With regard to routine radiography, obliteration, distortion, or displacement of the "scaphoid fat stripe" (which is related to the common tendon sheath of the extensor pollicis brevis and the abductor pollicis longus muscles) may occur in cases of scaphoid fracture, although the diagnostic value of these changes is not clear.[419, 420] Scaphoid fractures, particularly those of the waist, generally are transverse or slightly oblique in orientation and rarely are vertically oriented, and such fractures usually are identified most readily

on posteroanterior radiographs and "scaphoid views."[2, 421] When initial radiographs are not diagnostic, proper management is determined by the results of a careful clinical examination.[422] Dorsal tilting of the lunate simulating that occurring in dorsal segmental instability accompanies displacement of a scaphoid waist fracture[423] (Fig. 68–76).

The time required for healing of a scaphoid fracture varies according to its location. Those in the tuberosity usually heal in 4 to 6 weeks, whereas fractures of the scaphoid waist may require 6 to 8 weeks or longer to heal.[424] The frequency of delayed union or nonunion is greatest in fractures of the proximal pole of the bone and in those associated with displacement of the fragments.[425] Radiographic abnormalities of scaphoid nonunion (Fig. 68–77), which occur in approximately 5 to 15 per cent of cases,[893] include bone sclerosis, cyst formation, widening of the scapholunate space, bone resorption, and, subsequently, osteoarthritis.[426–430] Tendon ruptures may occur as a complication of such nonunion,[431] and CT may reveal hypertrophy of Lister's tubercle on the dorsum of the radius that may predispose to tendon disruption.[432] The frequency of ischemic necrosis following scaphoid fractures is approximately 10 to 15 per cent; this frequency rises to 30 to 40 per cent in case of nonunion. Owing to the vascular anatomy of the scaphoid, the proximal portion of the bone is the site of osteonecrosis, with reportable exceptions.[433]

Patients with scaphoid fractures may have additional wrist injuries, including fractures of the radial styloid process, triquetrum, and capitate, Colles' fractures, and ligamentous disruptions. Careful radiographic assessment of the wrist and, sometimes, the elbow (e.g., to detect an associated radial head fracture) is required.

Isolated fractures of the other carpal bones are less frequent than those of the scaphoid (Fig. 68–78). Triquetral fractures represent 3 to 4 per cent of all carpal fractures.[434] It is the dorsal surface of the triquetrum that typically is fractured, related either to contact with the hamate or ulnar styloid process or to avulsion by the dorsal radiotriquetral ligaments.[435] Such fractures are seen best on lateral and steep oblique projections. Fractures of the body of the triquetrum, which relate to direct blows in most cases, are rare. Isolated fractures of the lunate constitute 2 to 7 per cent of all carpal fractures[434, 436] They may involve the dorsal or volar surfaces of the bone, representing avulsion injuries, or any portion of its body,[437] including the medial facet.[438] Fractures of the hamate represent 2 to 4 per cent of carpal fractures. Fractures of the hamate (Fig. 68–79) may involve any portion of the bone,[439] including the body in which coronal or sagittal fractures occur,[440–442] but those of the hook of the hamate deserve emphasis.[443–445] These latter injuries may result from a fall on the dorsiflexed wrist with a force transmitted through the transverse carpal and pisohamate ligaments or from a direct force, such as occurs in athletes involved in sports that use racquets, bats, or clubs.[446, 894] Accurate clinical and radiographic diagnosis is difficult and specialized techniques, particularly conventional or computed tomography, may be required.[447] Complications of the fractures of the hook of the hamate include nonunion,[448] osteonecrosis,[449] injuries to the ulnar or median nerve,[450] and tendon rupture.[451] Ulnar nerve damage also may follow fractures of the pisiform.[452, 453] Isolated fractures of the capitate,[454] trapezium,[455, 456] and trapezoid are infrequent (Fig. 68–80). Those of the capitate predominate in

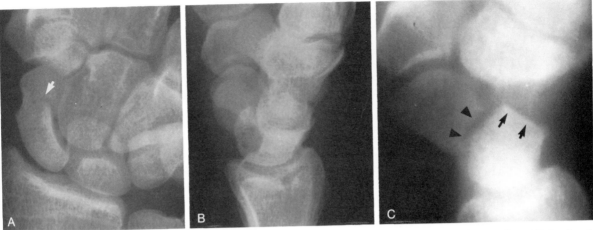

FIGURE 68–76. Carpal scaphoid fractures: Rotation at the fracture site. Frontal **(A)** and lateral **(B)** radiographs reveal a subtle fracture (arrow) of the scaphoid waist with dorsal tilting of the lunate. On a conventional lateral tomogram **(C)**, note that there is no contact of the fracture surfaces of the proximal (arrows) and distal (arrowheads) poles of the bone. (Courtesy of G. Greenway, M.D., Dallas, Texas.)

the neck of the bone, often are combined with metacarpal fractures, and may be associated with scaphoid fractures (scaphocapitate syndrome). Trapezial fractures involve either the body or the palmar ridge of the bone.[457, 458]

Hand

Metacarpophalangeal and Interphalangeal Joint Dislocation. Dislocation of a metacarpophalangeal joint (excluding the thumb) is considerably less frequent than that of a proximal interphalangeal joint of a finger and results from a fall on the outstretched hand that forces the joint into hyperextension (Fig. 68–81A). The index finger is involved most commonly, dislocations of multiple metacarpophalangeal joints are uncommon, and open dislocations of these joints are rare.[459] The volar plate is disrupted, allowing dorsal displacement of the base of the proximal phalanx.[460] Such dislocations are classified as simple (reducible) and complex (potentially irreducible) injuries. In both types, the metacarpal head is displaced into the palm, but with complex dislocations the proximal phalanx is hyperextended only slightly and the metacarpal head is entrapped by the surrounding flexor tendons and lumbrical muscles.[2]

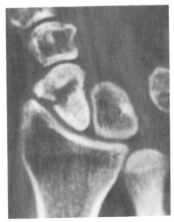

FIGURE 68–77. Carpal scaphoid fractures: Nonunion and osteonecrosis. A direct coronal CT scan shows a large fracture gap with increased density of the proximal portion of the scaphoid bone.

In cases of complex dislocation, radiographs may reveal a widened joint space, indicating interposition of the volar plate within the joint. An adjacent sesamoid also can become displaced into the joint space.[461] Volar dislocation is rare.[462] This, too, may be irreducible.[459] Lateral subluxations, often with spontaneous reduction, are common, are designated strains, are accompanied by injury of the collateral ligament, and generally are characterized by an intact volar plate. Although radiographs commonly are normal in such subluxations, an avulsed fragment of bone from the lateral tubercle of the proximal phalanx may be seen.[459]

Dislocations of the proximal interphalangeal joints are very common, usually involve only one joint, and may occur with or without a major adjacent phalangeal fracture.[463, 464] These dislocations can occur in a posterior or, more rarely, anterior direction (Fig. 68–81B). Posterior dislocation results from a hyperextension injury. Ligamentous and volar plate disruption is a frequent associated finding.[465, 466] Posterior dislocations can occur with only these disruptions (type I), these disruptions and avulsion of a small bone fragment from the volar base of the middle phalanx (type II), or a major fracture fragment (fracture-dislocation) (type III). In the last type, a large volar fragment involving 30 to 50 per cent of the articular surface of the middle phalanx leads to joint instability.[464] Posterior dislocation of a distal interphalangeal joint or the interphalangeal joint of the thumb (Fig. 74–153C) also can be encountered. Such dislocations may be irreducible owing to interposition of the volar plate or flexor tendon.[468, 469] In the interphalangeal joint of the thumb, the sesamoid bones represent an additional structure that can prevent reduction following a dislocation.

A Bennett's fracture-dislocation is a relatively common intra-articular injury that occurs at the base of the first metacarpal[470–473] (Fig. 68–82A). Following an axial blow to a partially flexed first metacarpal, an oblique fracture line separates the major portion of the bone from a small fragment of the volar lip. The base of the metacarpal is pulled dorsally and radially. The Bennett's fracture represents only one of several different fracture patterns that occur at the base of the thumb and should not be confused with a second intra-articular fracture, the Rolando's fracture, in which a Y or T shaped comminuted fracture line is evident (Fig.

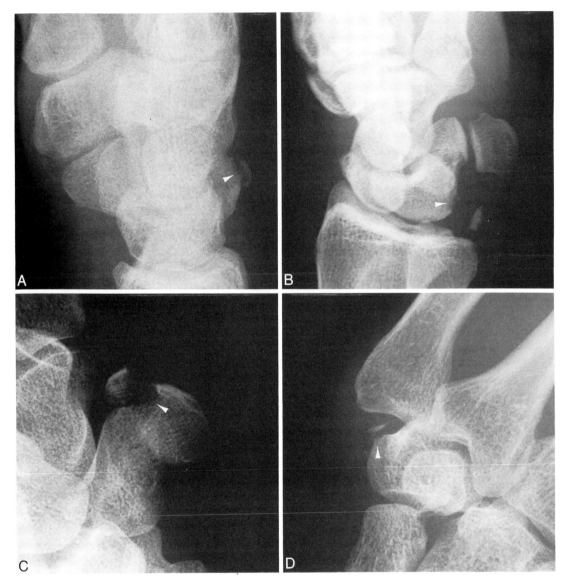

FIGURE 68–78. Carpal fractures.
  A Dorsal surface of triquetrum (arrowhead).
  B Volar surface of lunate (arrowhead) with displaced fragment.
  C Distal surface of pisiform (arrowhead) with displaced fragment.
  D Distal surface of trapezium (arrowhead).

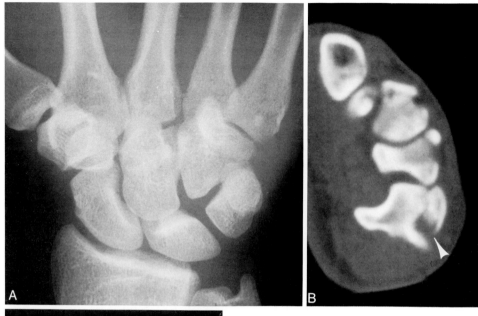

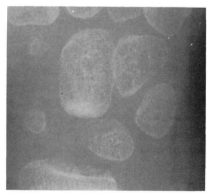

FIGURE 68–79. Carpal fractures: Hamate.

A, B Dorsal surface of the hamate. The frontal radiograph **(A)** reveals widening of the interosseous distance between the hamate and the capitate and subtle loss of parallelism between the hamate and the neighboring bones. A transaxial CT scan **(B)**, accomplished with the ulnar side of the hand against the table, shows the fracture (arrowhead) of the hamate.

C Hook of the hamate. Note the fracture line (arrowhead). Compare with the opposite normal side.

(Courtesy of G. Greenway, M.D., Dallas, Texas.)

68–82*B*). Transverse or oblique extra-articular fractures of the base of the first metacarpal bone also are encountered, as are pure dislocations of the first carpometacarpal joint (Fig. 68–83).

Dislocations and collateral ligament injuries of the first metacarpophalangeal joint are important complications of trauma.[474] Although several types of injuries can be identi-

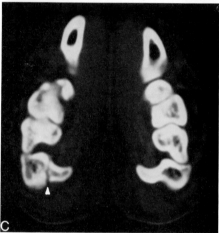

FIGURE 68–80. Carpal fractures: Capitate. Observe compression with bone sclerosis of the proximal portion of the capitate, indicative of a subacute fracture in this child.

fied, that related to a sudden valgus stress applied to the metacarpophalangeal joint of the thumb, the gamekeeper's thumb, has received the most attention.[475–479] Initially described as an occupational hazard in English gamewardens, who, in killing rabbits by twisting their necks, sustained repeated stresses about the first metacarpophalangeal joint, the injury now is recognized to occur in various settings, including skiing[480–482] and breakdancing.[483] Attenuation or disruption of the ligamentous apparatus along the ulnar aspect of the thumb is seen, which may be associated with pain, swelling, tenderness, edema, and pinch instability. Initial radiographs can be negative, although small avulsed fragments from the base of the proximal phalanx can be delineated in some instances (Fig. 68–84). These fragments may be displaced proximally and rotated from 45 degrees to 90 degrees. Radiographs obtained with radial stress applied to the first metacarpophalangeal joint can reveal subluxation[484, 485] (Fig. 68–85), and arthrography may outline leakage of contrast material from the ulnar aspect of the articulation and an abnormal folded position of the ulnar collateral ligament[486, 487] (see Chapter 13). This abnormal position of the collateral ligament, called the Stener lesion,[478] can be identified by MR imaging[488] (see Chapter 70).

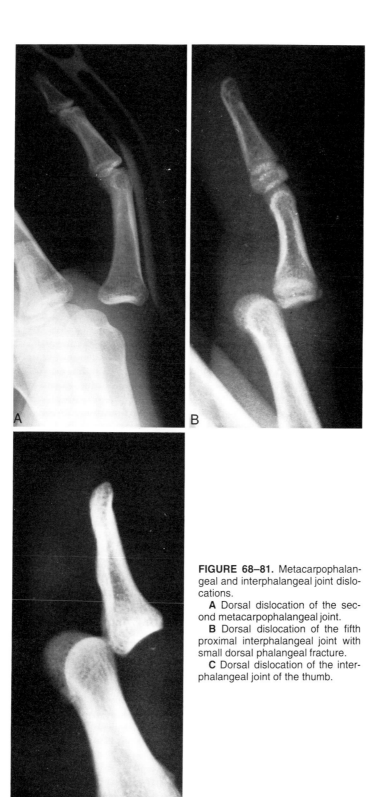

FIGURE 68–81. Metacarpophalangeal and interphalangeal joint dislocations.

A Dorsal dislocation of the second metacarpophalangeal joint.

B Dorsal dislocation of the fifth proximal interphalangeal joint with small dorsal phalangeal fracture.

C Dorsal dislocation of the interphalangeal joint of the thumb.

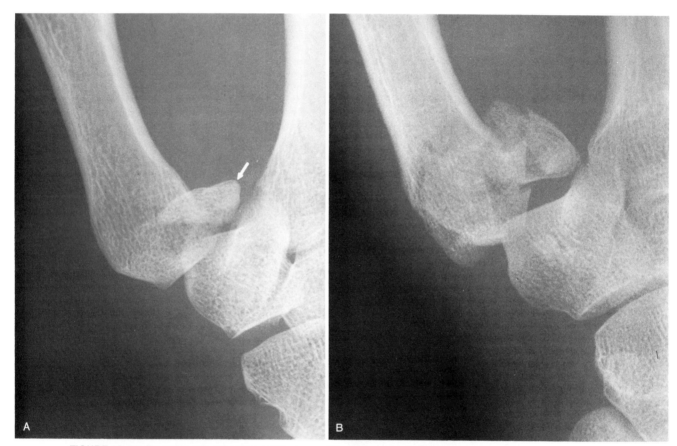

FIGURE 68–82. Fractures and dislocations of the base of the first metacarpal bone.
  A Bennett's fracture-dislocation. Observe the typical oblique fracture of the volar lip of the first metacarpal bone (arrow).
  B Rolando's fracture. A comminuted fracture of the metacarpal base is evident.

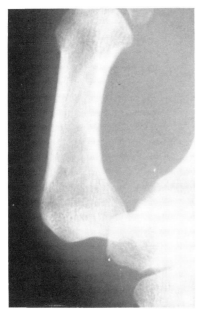

FIGURE 68–83. Dislocation of the first carpometacarpal joint. A dorsal dislocation is evident.

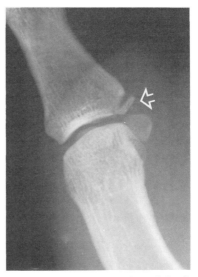

FIGURE 68–84. Gamekeeper's thumb. Note slight displacement of a small fragment (open arrow) arising from the ulnar aspect of the proximal phalanx of the thumb.

Dorsal subluxation or dislocation of the metacarpophalangeal joint of the thumb results from forcible hyperextension. Locking of the joint following this injury may indicate interposition of a sesamoid bone or ligamentous abnormality[474, 489] (Fig. 68–86).

Fractures of the Metacarpal Bones and Phalanges. Fractures of the metacarpal bones, which predominate in the first and fifth digits, generally are classified according to anatomic location: metacarpal head, metacarpal neck, metacarpal shaft, and metacarpal base. Typical locations of fractures include the shaft and neck of the fifth metacarpal (boxer's fracture), the shaft of the third or fourth metacarpal, or both, and the articular surface of the second metacarpal[2, 490, 491] (Fig. 68–87). Displacement, angulation, or rotation commonly is encountered, and the rotation, if not corrected, may lead to serious disability.[492]

Phalangeal fractures are more frequent than those of the metacarpals and most typically involve the distal phalan-

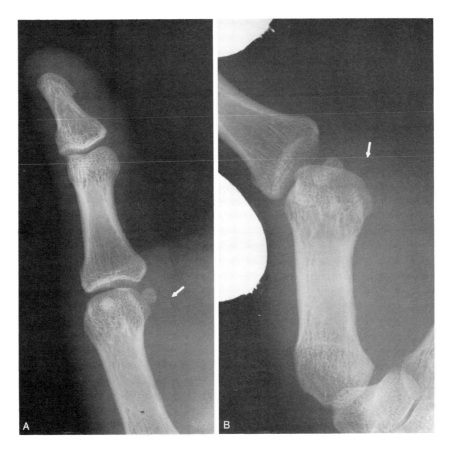

FIGURE 68–85. Gamekeeper's thumb.

A An initial radiograph outlines small osseous fragments adjacent to the first metacarpophalangeal joint (arrow).

B A radiograph obtained during radial stress reveals subluxation of the phalanx on the metacarpal bone. The fracture fragments again are identified (arrow).

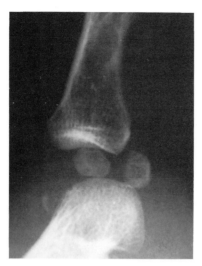

FIGURE 68–86. Dislocation of the first metacarpophalangeal joint: Entrapment of sesamoid bones. Observe the dorsal dislocation, widened joint space, small fracture fragments, and sesamoid bones within the articulation.

ges,[493] followed in order of frequency by the proximal phalanges and the middle phalanges (Fig. 68–88). Important varieties include the mallet fracture (in which an avulsion injury at the base of the dorsal surface of the terminal phalanx is produced by damage to the extensor mechanism),[494, 495] the volar plate fracture (in which a dorsal dislocation of a proximal interphalangeal joint may be associated with an avulsion fracture in the middle phalanx at the site of attachment of the volar plate), any fracture with intra-articular extension or significant rotational deformity, a fracture of the shaft of the proximal or middle phalanx (whose volar surface forms the floor of the flexor tendon sheath so that accurate reduction is desirable), a fracture of the base of the proximal phalanx (in which angulation is easily overlooked owing to superimposition of other bones on the lateral radiograph), and, in the immature skeleton, a physeal separation at the base of the distal phalanx (the nailbed injury, in which an open skin surface leads to secondary infection)[492] (Figs. 68–89 and 68–90). The diagnostic value of multiple radiographic projections, including an internally rotated oblique projection,[496] in the analysis of phalangeal fractures should be recognized.

LOWER EXTREMITY

Hip

Hip Dislocation. Dislocation of the femoral head with or without an acetabular fracture is an injury that usually follows considerable trauma and that may be associated with significant injury elsewhere in the body. Hip dislocations represent approximately 5 per cent of all dislocations.[2] Hip dislocations generally are classified as anterior, posterior, and central in type, although other types such as luxatio erecta (in which the hip is flexed and the leg extends along the torso) are encountered rarely.[497]

Anterior dislocation of the hip is a relatively rare type of dislocation, representing 5 to 10 per cent of all hip dislocations, and it relates to forced abduction and external rotation of the leg.[498, 499] On radiographs, the abnormal position of the femoral head readily is apparent; on frontal radiographs,

an anteriorly displaced femoral head typically moves inferomedially with the femur abducted and externally rotated, and a posteriorly displaced femoral head usually is located superolaterally with the femur adducted and internally rotated, although exceptions to these rules are encountered.[500] Thus, a superior anterior dislocation, sometimes termed a pubic dislocation, may simulate a posterior dislocation of the hip if only the frontal radiograph is analyzed.[2] In anterior hip dislocations, associated fractures of the acetabular rim, greater trochanter, or femoral neck,[501, 502] or, more commonly, femoral head[503, 504] may be observed. A characteristic depression or flattening of the posterosuperior and lateral portion of the femoral head can be seen[505–507] (Fig. 68–91). Rarely, anterior dislocation of the hip may be recurrent.[508–510]

Posterior dislocation of the hip is more common (approximately 80 to 85 per cent of all hip dislocations) and may result from a "dashboard injury" in which the flexed knee strikes the dashboard during a head-on automobile collision.[498, 511–515] Motorcycle accidents provide another important source for this type of hip dislocation.[516] The leg is shortened, internally rotated, and adducted. Associated problems include knee trauma (e.g., patellar, tibial, or fibular fracture, or combinations of these fractures), femoral head or shaft fractures,[517, 518] and sciatic nerve injury. The frequent occurrence of posterior acetabular rim fractures following posterior dislocation of the hip requires careful analysis of routine radiographs and the use of oblique and lateral projections[519–521] (see Chapter 22) (Fig. 68–91). The posteriorly dislocated femoral head usually lies superior to the acetabulum on the frontal radiograph, although it occasionally may lie at the same level as the acetabulum. A persistently widened hip joint may indicate abnormally placed fragments or significant acetabular injury. Conventional or computed tomography (Fig. 68–92) can be used to identify small osseous fragments, deformity of the femoral head, and the extent of damage to the posterior acetabular rim.[522] Two types of the femoral head fractures are seen[2]: shear fractures, which involve principally the inferior and anterior portions of the femoral head, occurring in 7 to 10 per cent of posterior hip dislocations; and compression fractures, which involve mainly the anterior to inferomedial portion of the femoral head, occurring in 13 to 60 per cent of such dislocations and poorly seen on conventional radiographs.[507, 523–525] Additional complications of this injury are periarticular soft tissue calcification and ossification, acetabular labrum tears, acetabular fractures, osteonecrosis of the femoral head, and secondary degenerative joint disease.[526–530] Osteonecrosis may complicate as many as 25 per cent of posterior hip dislocations, especially when the injury is associated with a delay in diagnosis and treatment and a fracture of the posterior acetabular margin. Recurrent posterior dislocations of the hip have been described.[532, 533]

Central acetabular fracture-dislocation usually results from a force applied to the lateral side of the trochanter and pelvis, with the stress applied through the femoral head. Various patterns of acetabular fracture complicate this injury, and hemorrhage into the pelvis also may be observed. Secondary degenerative joint disease is not infrequent.

Traumatic dislocation of the hip usually is encountered in adults, although children and infants also can be affected.[534–539] In the younger age group, dislocation almost always is posterior in type, although anterior dislocations

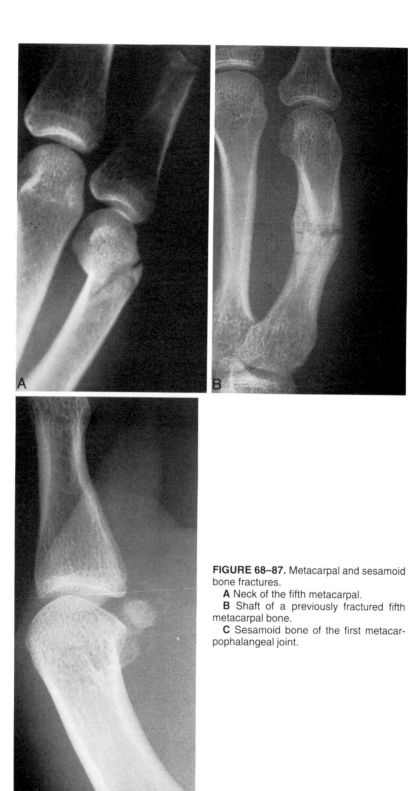

FIGURE 68–87. Metacarpal and sesamoid bone fractures.

A Neck of the fifth metacarpal.

B Shaft of a previously fractured fifth metacarpal bone.

C Sesamoid bone of the first metacarpophalangeal joint.

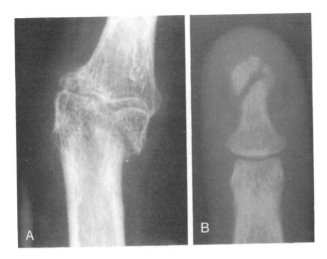

FIGURE 68–88. Phalangeal fractures.

  A A transverse fracture of the distal portion of the proximal phalanx is associated with intra-articular extension.

  B An oblique fracture of the terminal phalanx.

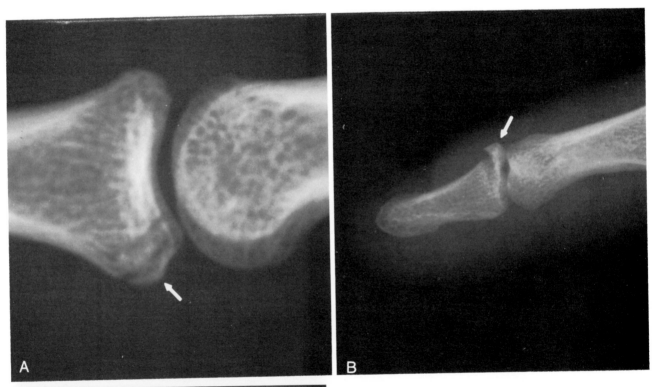

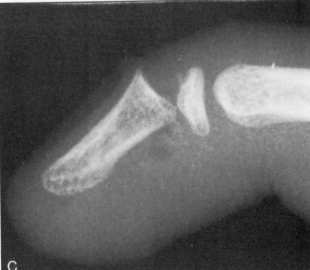

FIGURE 68–89. Phalangeal fractures.

  A, B Avulsion fractures. Small avulsion fractures (arrow) near the proximal interphalangeal or distal interphalangeal joint can result from traction on the volar plate (**A**) or extensor tendons (**B**). Dislocations also may be evident.

  C Nailbed injury. This physeal separation at the base of the distal phalanx, the nailbed injury, is open to the environment with the risk of infection.

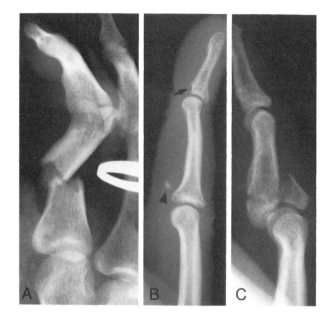

FIGURE 68–90. Phalangeal fractures.
  A Proximal phalanx fracture with displacement. Observe angulation and rotation at the fracture site.
  B Avulsion fracture. An avulsion fracture of the distal phalanx at the site of attachment of the flexor digitorum profundus tendon has led to an osseous defect (arrow) with proximal retraction of the fragment (arrowhead).
  C Fracture-dislocation of the proximal interphalangeal joint. Note the volar dislocation and disruption of the articular surface.

are described.[541, 542] Entrapment of the acetabular labrum[541] or capsule,[542] or osteocartilaginous fragments,[543] may prevent adequate reduction. Such dislocation may be associated with ischemic necrosis of the femoral head[544, 545] or physeal injury,[546] and in the infant, traumatic displacement must be differentiated from developmental dysplasia of the hip.

Fractures of the Proximal Portion of the Femur. The extraordinary amount of attention that has been directed at the diagnosis and treatment of fractures of the femoral neck is indicative of the frequency and the potentially serious nature of these injuries.[900] Although evident as a stress fracture in the young athlete and as a pathologic fracture in patients with skeletal metastasis, Paget's disease, and other disorders, it is the occurrence of fractures of the proximal portion of the femur in elderly persons with osteopenia, particularly women with osteoporosis, that has received the greatest attention.[547–553] In the latter situation, the injuries are similar to insufficiency stress fractures, although a history of minor trauma usually is evident. Two major mechanisms of injury have been proposed in the production of femoral neck fractures: a fall producing a direct blow on the grater trochanter[554]; and lateral rotation of the extremity.[555] Cyclic loading leading to microfractures that become complete following a minor torsional injury and, in young patients, major direct forces along the shaft of the femur with or without a rotational component are additional potential mechanisms of injury.[556] Nondisplaced fractures of the proximal portion of the femur may escape detection on initial routine radiographic examination (Fig. 68–93). Diagnostic help is provided by MR imaging (Fig. 68–94) and bone scintigraphy[895] (also see Chapter 70).

There is no classification system of fractures of the proximal portion of the femur that is accepted uniformly. Anatomic designations, including subcapital, transcervical, basicervical, intertrochanteric, and subtrochanteric, frequently are used to define the location of the fracture and can be modified to include intracapsular fractures (those in the subcapital and transcervical regions) and extracapsular fractures (those in the basicervical and trochanteric regions). Subcapital fractures occur immediately beneath the articular

surface of the femoral head; transcervical fractures pass across the middle of the femoral neck; basicervical fractures occur at the base of the femoral neck; intertrochanteric fractures are located in a line between the greater and lesser trochanters; and subtrochanteric fractures occur subjacent to this.[556] Difficulty in fracture classification based on this anatomic scheme relates to the inability to differentiate clearly between subcapital and transcervical fractures, between basicervical and intertrochanteric fractures, and between intertrochanteric and subtrochanteric fractures in instances in which radiographs are suboptimal, fracture lines are subtle (Fig. 68–95), or marked rotation or angulation occurs at the fracture site.[557, 558]

Intracapsular fractures, which are approximately twice as frequent as those in the trochanteric region,[559] also may be classified according to the direction of the fracture angle or the degree of displacement of the fracture fragments.[560] The former system, which was developed by Pauwels,[561] uses three categories of fracture based on its angle with the horizontal: type I is a fracture that is oriented at 30 degrees from the horizontal; type II is one that is oriented at 50 degrees from the horizontal; and type III is oriented at 70 degrees from the horizontal.[556] The belief that the shearing forces encountered in the more vertical fractures (e.g., type III) led to nonunion was the stimulus for this classification system, but the radiographic accuracy in the detection of the fracture angle subsequently has been challenged.[554, 562] Classification of intracapsular fractures according to the degree of displacement on prereduction radiographs commonly is referred to as the Garden system.[560, 562] Four types of fractures are identified: type I fractures are incomplete or impacted in nature; type II fractures are complete without osseous displacement; type III fractures also are complete with partial displacement of the fracture fragments commonly associated with shortening and external rotation of the distal fragments; and type IV fractures are complete with total displacement of the fracture fragments[556] (Fig. 68–95). It is the type III or IV fracture that is associated with significant complications and technical failures. Difficulty in this latter classification system relates to disagreement regarding the alignment (type IV fracture) or mal-

Text continued on page 2760

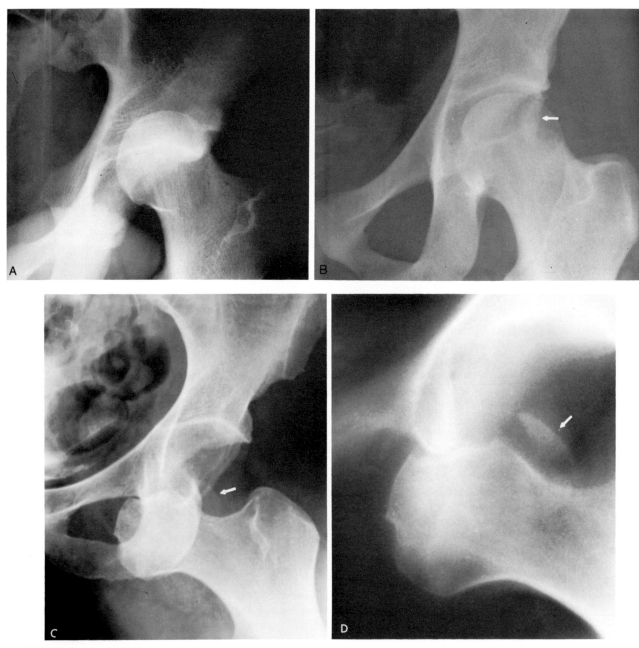

FIGURE 68–91. Hip dislocation.

A, B Posterior dislocation. The initial oblique radiograph reveals a posterosuperior dislocation of the femoral head. Following reduction, note the large osseous fragment of the posterior acetabular rim (arrow).

C, D Anterior dislocation. Plain film and tomogram reveal an inferomedial position of the dislocated femoral head and a fracture fragment of the lateral portion of the head (arrows).

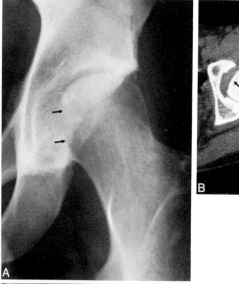

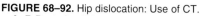

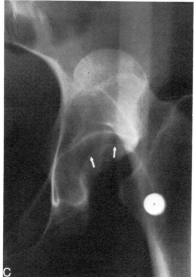

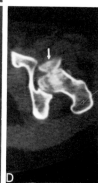

FIGURE 68–92. Hip dislocation: Use of CT.

A, B Posterior dislocation. Following reduction of this injury, the routine radiograph **(A)** reveals a defect in the medial aspect of the femoral head (arrows). This defect (arrow) is well shown with a transaxial CT scan **(B)**.

C, D Posterior dislocation. In this patient, the conventional radiograph **(C)** shows the posterosuperior displacement of the femoral head and a curvilinear bone fragment (arrows) in the joint. Following reduction of the dislocation, a transaxial CT scan **(D)** reveals the fragment (arrow), which represents a portion of the femoral head. This fragment has rotated approximately 180 degrees.

E, F Posterior dislocation. In a third patient, a comminuted fracture of the acetabulum is associated with the dislocation **(E)**. On the transaxial CT image **(F)**, note the fracture of the posterior rim of the acetabulum (arrow), intra-articular fragments, and the displaced femoral head.

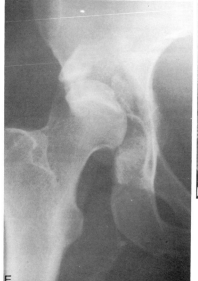

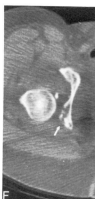

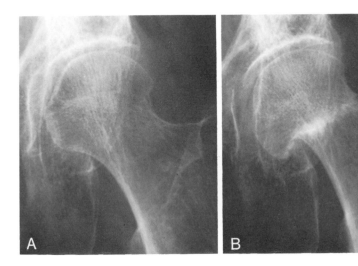

FIGURE 68–93. Fractures of the femoral neck: Difficulties in radiographic diagnosis.

A No obvious abnormalities are evident on the radiograph obtained on the day of injury.

B Six weeks later, a subcapital fracture is evident.

(Courtesy of G. Greenway, M.D., Dallas, Texas.)

FIGURE 68–94. Fractures of the femoral neck: MR imaging.

A, B Subcapital fracture. Although the initial radiograph **(A)** appears normal, a subcapital fracture (arrow) is evident on a coronal T1-weighted (TR/TE, 600/20) spin echo MR image **(B)**.

C, D Intertrochanteric fracture. Although a fracture (arrow) is evident on the initial radiograph **(C)**, it is identified more optimally (arrows) on a coronal T1-weighted (TR/TE, 600/20) spin echo MR image **(D)**.

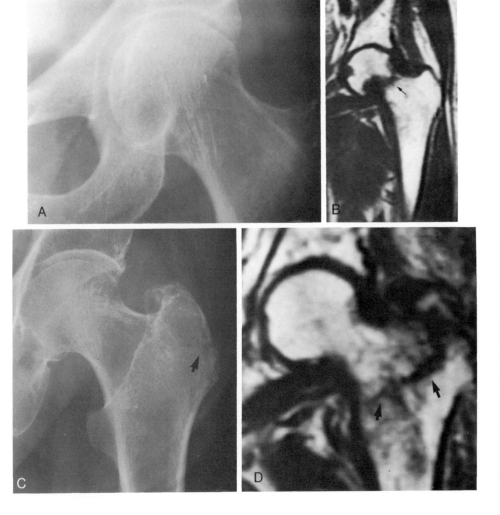

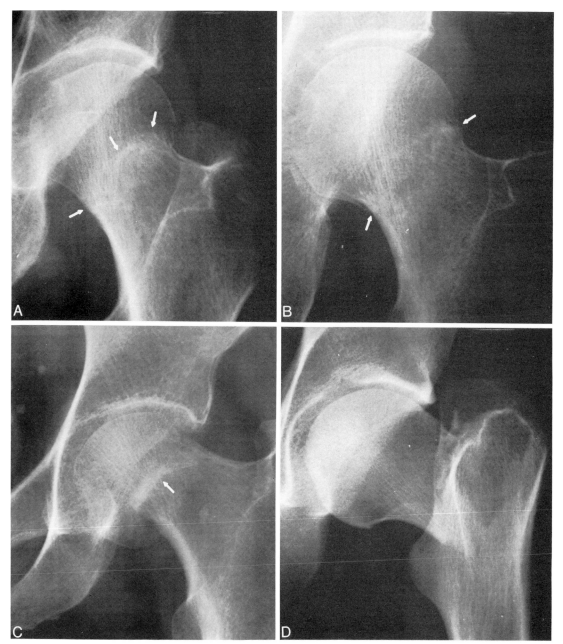

FIGURE 68–95. Fractures of the femoral neck: Intracapsular fractures.

A–C Three examples of intracapsular fractures (arrows) are shown. Observe the bands of increased radiodensity in each case. According to the Garden classification system, these injuries probably represent stage I or II fractures **(A** and **B)** or a stage III fracture **(C)**, but accurate classification requires analysis of lateral radiographs as well. With regard to the anatomic location, these fractures predominantly are subcapital.

D A basicervical fracture of the femoral neck is associated with significant displacement as well as rotation. A lateral radiograph again is required for accurate appraisal.

alignment (type III fracture) of the trabeculae of the femoral head with those of the acetabulum[563] (Fig. 68–96).

Several complications of intracapsular fractures of the femoral neck deserve emphasis. It generally is believed that, under normal circumstances, these fractures will reveal evidence of healing in the first 6 to 12 months. Delayed union and nonunion are not uncommon, and the latter occurs in approximately 5 to 25 per cent of cases.[564–566] Factors predisposing to nonunion include advancing age of the patient, osteoporosis, posterior comminution of the fracture, inadequate reduction, and poor internal fixation technique.[556] The frequency of ischemic necrosis of the femoral head varies from 10 to 30 per cent, increasing in cases with moderate or severe displacement of the fracture fragments or with persistent motion at the fracture site owing to poor stabilization.[567] Measurement of intracapsular pressure in patients with femoral neck fractures reveals elevated values related to hemarthrosis, although the role of the elevated pressure in the pathogenesis of osteonecrosis is not agreed upon.[568–571] Furthermore, it should be noted that the vascular insult to the femoral head may occur not only at the time of fracture but also following attempts at reduction or internal fixation. Bone scintigraphy has been used not only in the initial diagnosis of the fracture but also as a means for detection of osteonecrosis (and other complications) that influences the eventual clinical outcome.[572–577] MR imaging has been employed for these same purposes,[578–580] although routine radiography still remains important in the assessment of posttraumatic osteonecrosis. The resulting radiographic abnormalities are typical, appearing as early as 3

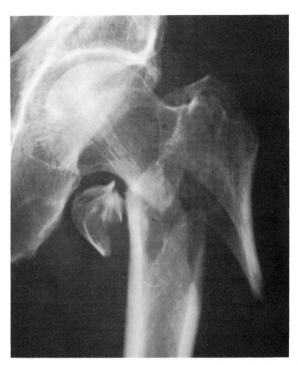

FIGURE 68–97. Fractures of the femoral neck: Intertrochanteric fractures. A comminuted fracture is evident, with displacement of both trochanters.

months and as late as 3 years after the fracture,[2] and consisting primarily of increased radiodensity of the femoral head[581] as well as of irregularity of the articular surface and subchondral radiolucent areas. Late segmental collapse of the necrotic bone is inconstant but, when present, leads to significant clinical manifestations as well as a propensity to develop osteoarthritis.[582, 583]

Additional complications of intracapsular femoral neck fractures include posttraumatic thromboembolic phenomena[556] and postoperative osteomyelitis and septic arthritis.[584]

Intertrochanteric fractures also predominate in elderly patients, with a somewhat higher frequency in women (unlike the overwhelming female predilection observed in intracapsular femoral neck fractures).[2] Osteopenia, usually osteoporosis, is common at the site of fracture, leading to the vulnerability of this femoral region to minor trauma. Direct or indirect force(s) resulting from a fall constitutes the typical mechanism of injury.[585, 586] Fracture comminution is common, leading to multiple fragments of bone, which may include the greater trochanter, the lesser trochanter, or both (Fig. 68–97). The radiographic analysis is complicated by this comminution as well as the typical displacement and rotation that occur.

As in the case of intracapsular fractures of the femoral neck, no uniform classification system exists for intertrochanteric fractures. Available systems are based on stability versus instability or the ease by which fracture reduction can be accomplished[587–590] (Fig. 68–98). As has been emphasized by DeLee,[556] a stable fracture (approximately 50 per cent of cases) is characterized by the absence of comminution of the medial cortices of the proximal and distal fragments and of displacement of the lesser trochanter. Unstable intertrochanteric fractures (approximately 50 per cent of cases) occur in two situations[556]: fractures with reversed

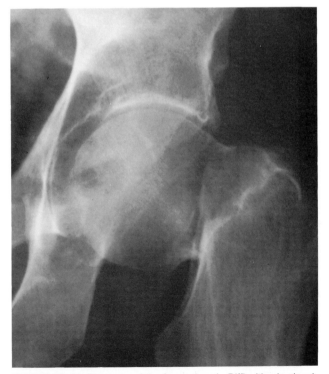

FIGURE 68–96. Fractures of the femoral neck: Difficulties in classification. Although all observers agreed that a displaced fracture of the femoral neck was present in this case, there was disagreement regarding whether it was a type III or type IV fracture in the Garden classification system. Differentiation between these two types requires a decision as to whether the trabeculae of the femoral head and acetabulum are aligned (type IV) or not aligned (type III).

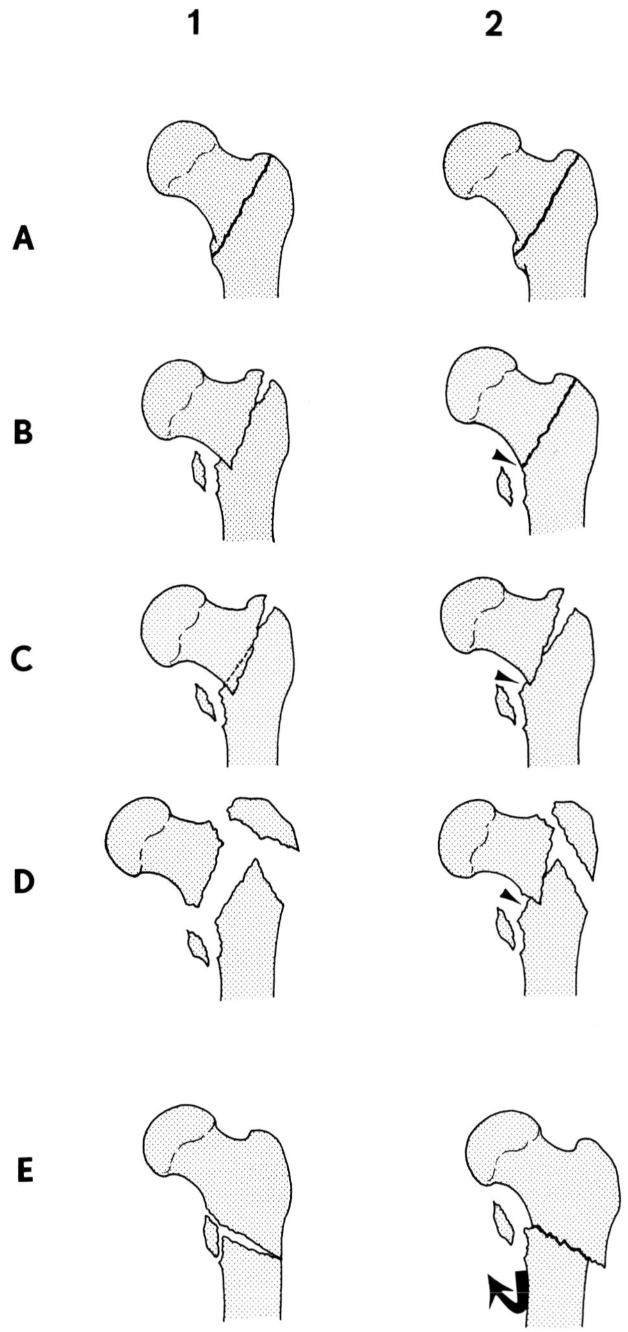

1   **2**

FIGURE 68–98. Fractures of the femoral neck: Intertrochanteric fractures. Evans' classification system. The appearance of the initial radiograph (1) and that following reduction attempts, the postreduction radiograph (2), is shown. Type I fractures are illustrated in **A** through **D**. In each of these instances, the fracture line extends from the region of the lesser trochanter in an upward and outward direction. Type II fractures (**E**) have a reversed obliquity.

A Undisplaced fracture on the initial radiograph; stable on the postreduction radiograph.

B Displaced fracture on the initial radiograph; stable on the postreduction radiograph owing to medial cortical apposition (arrowhead).

C Displaced fracture on the initial radiograph; unstable nonreduced fracture on the postreduction radiograph owing to lack of medial cortical apposition (arrowhead).

D Comminuted fracture on the initial radiograph; unstable nonreduced fracture on the postreduction radiograph owing to lack of medial cortical apposition (arrowhead).

E Fracture with reversed obliquity on the initial radiograph; unstable nonreduced fracture on the postreduction radiograph with a tendency to medial displacement of the femoral shaft owing to the pull of the adductors (curved arrow).

(From De Lee JC: Fractures and dislocations of the hip. In CA Rockwood Jr, DP Greene [Eds]: Fractures in Adults. 2nd Ed. Philadelphia, JB Lippincott Co, 1984, p 1262.)

obliquity in which there is a marked tendency toward medial displacement of the femoral shaft owing to adductor muscle pull or to comminution of the greater trochanter and adjacent posterolateral surface of the shaft; and fractures in which there is absence of contact between the proximal and distal fragments owing to comminution or medial and posterior displacement of fracture fragments.

Complications of intertrochanteric fractures include varus displacement both in nonsurgically treated injuries and in those associated with failure of internal reduction, secondary subcapital fractures (following internal fixation of intertrochanteric fractures), laceration of adjacent vessels (a rare finding), nonunion (which is an uncommon occurrence owing to the fact that these fractures occur in cancellous bone with good blood supply), and ischemic necrosis of the

femoral head (which also is uncommon, appearing in less than 1 per cent of cases).[556, 591, 592]

Isolated fractures of the greater trochanter in adults are infrequent and generally relate to injury (avulsion or direct blow) of the bone following a fall, particularly in elderly persons (Fig. 68–99). Differentiation of a fracture of the greater trochanter from one that also involves the proximal femur (i.e., intertrochanteric fracture) may require tomographic imaging techniques. Furthermore, as fractures of the greater trochanter usually are not significantly displaced, their detection also may necessitate tomography. Similar fractures of the lesser trochanter also are unusual and may represent the initial manifestation of skeletal metastasis. Avulsion injuries of the lesser trochanter are seen more typically in children and adolescents.

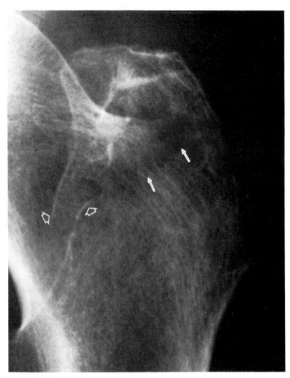

FIGURE 68–99. Fractures of the proximal portion of the femur: Isolated fractures of the greater trochanter. Observe the fracture (solid arrows) with interruption of the intertrochanteric line (open arrows). These injuries should not be misinterpreted as fractures of the femoral neck.

Fractures of the femur that commence immediately below the trochanter are considered subtrochanteric in location, although some of these fractures extend into the trochanteric region, making precise classification difficult. Some classification systems do not separate trochanteric and subtrochanteric fractures, whereas others deal solely with those in the subtrochanteric region[588] or emphasize the configuration of the fracture line[594] (Fig. 68–100). The precise location of the fracture is of more than academic interest, as those that occur more distally are associated with a greater frequency of nonunion or delayed union and implant failure.[556] Problems of fracture union are indicative of the tendency for cortical comminution in cases of subtrochanteric fractures, and surgical failures are reflective of the considerable biomechanical stress in this region of the femur.

Approximately 5 to 30 per cent of fractures of the proximal portion of the femur occur in the subtrochanteric region, the reported frequency varying according to the criteria used to designate a fracture as subtrochanteric in location.[2] These fractures occur in older patients with relatively minor injuries and in younger patients with major trauma. Pathologic fractures also are not infrequent in this region of the femur and are typical of Paget's disease.

Fractures of the Acetabulum. Although the acetabulum represents a portion of the bony pelvis, it also is an essential component of the hip; therefore, a discussion of acetabular fractures is appropriate here owing to their association with hip dislocations as well as their modification of proper function of the joint. The classic description of acetabular fracture belongs to Judet and his colleagues,[595] who devised a classification system based on the specific sites of fracture

and emphasized the need for a complete radiographic examination, including oblique projections. Although these radiographs remain important, more recent modifications in imaging protocols for the injured acetabulum have been proposed in which CT plays an important role.[596–603] With any imaging system, the delineation of four bony landmarks remains fundamental to proper assessment of the extent of injury: the anterior acetabular rim, the posterior acetabular rim, the iliopubic (anterior) column, and the ilioischial (posterior) column (see Chapter 22). Furthermore, with CT, additional features, including the integrity of the acetabular dome and quadrilateral surface as well as the presence of intra-articular osseous fragments and associated fractures of the bony pelvis, readily can be determined (Figs. 68–101 and 68–102).

Although a complete discussion of acetabular fractures is beyond the scope of the current chapter, a few points deserve emphasis. These fractures result from the impact of the femoral head against the central regions of the acetabulum or its rims, especially the posterior rim in association with a posterior dislocation of the hip. Isolated fractures of the anterior or superior portion of the acetabular rim are unusual. The precise location of the force depends on a number of factors, including the degree of flexion or extension, adduction or abduction, and internal or external rotation of the thigh with respect to the bony pelvis, and it accounts for a spectrum of injuries that encompasses pure dislocations of the hip, fractures of the acetabulum, and combinations of the two.[604] The number of categories that have been used to describe the resultant acetabular fractures has varied,[595, 605] although the need to identify the acetabular rims and osseous columns in the assessment of these fractures remains unchallenged. Fractures may involve the anterior or posterior column alone, or a transverse fracture may involve both of these columns. Although displacement of fracture fragments is not uncommon, leading to obvious radiographic abnormalities,[606–610] nondisplaced or occult fractures of the acetabulum present diagnostic difficulties on both the clinical and the radiographic examination,[606] and acetabular fractures in children, although rare, may involve the triradiate cartilage, compounding this difficulty.[611] The complications of acetabular fractures include osteoarthritis of the hip (in cases in which incongruity of the articular surface exists), ischemic necrosis of the femoral head (in cases in which there is an associated posterior dislocation of the hip), heterotopic ossification,[612] and hemorrhage as well as urinary tract, bowel, and peripheral nerve injury (particularly in cases in which there are multiple pelvic fractures).

Femoral Diaphysis

As the femoral shaft represents the strongest portion of the longest and most resilient bone in the human body, it is not surprising that its fracture requires violent force and that associated musculoskeletal injuries, blood loss, and shock are common. Motor vehicle accidents and those involving pedestrians struck by a moving vehicle are frequent causes of such injuries. Simultaneous injury to the head and thoracic or abdominal viscera is of far greater concern in terms of management than that related to fracture healing in the femur. Problems do arise, however, owing to the strong muscle attachments to the greater and lesser trochan-

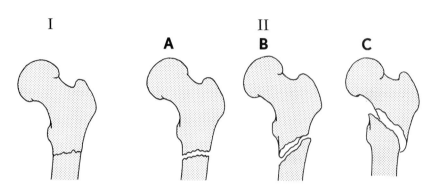

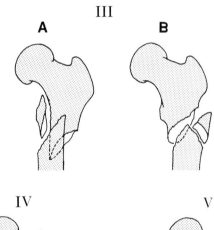

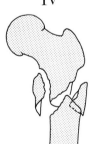

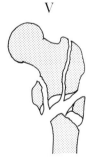

FIGURE 68–100. Fractures of the proximal portion of the femur: Subtrochanteric fractures—Seinsheimer's classification system.

Type I Nondisplaced fractures or those with less than 2 mm of displacement of the fracture fragments.

Type II Two-part fractures.

IIA: Two-part transverse femoral fracture.

IIB: Two-part spiral fracture with the lesser trochanter attached to the proximal fragment.

IIC: Two-part spiral fracture with the lesser trochanter attached to the distal segment.

Type III Three-part fractures.

IIIA: Three-part spiral fracture in which the lesser trochanter is part of the third fragment and in which this fragment has an inferior spike of cortex of variable length.

IIIB: Three-part spiral fracture in which the third fragment is a butterfly type.

Type IV Comminuted fractures with four or more fragments.

Type V Subtrochanteric and intertrochanteric fractures, including those in which the fracture extends through the greater trochanter.

(After Seinsheimer F: J Bone Joint Surg [Am] *60*:300, 1978.)

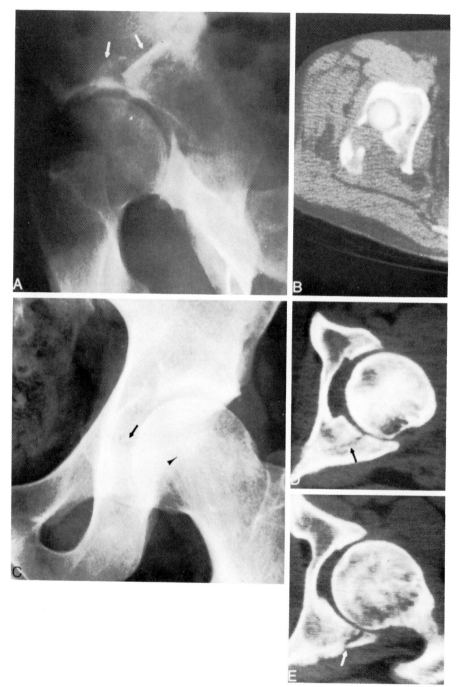

FIGURE 68–101. Acetabular fractures: Use of CT.

A, B An oblique radiograph **(A)** reveals an obvious fracture involving principally the acetabular dome (arrows). A transaxial CT scan **(B)** shows the comminuted nature of the fracture and the extent of involvement of the acetabular roof and posterior rim.

C–E On the frontal radiograph **(C)**, a subtle fracture line is seen (arrow). A fragment of bone also is evident (arrowhead). Two transaxial CT scans **(D, E)** reveal the fracture line affecting mainly the posterior acetabular rim (arrows).

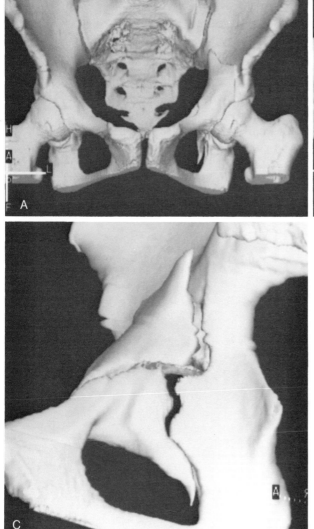

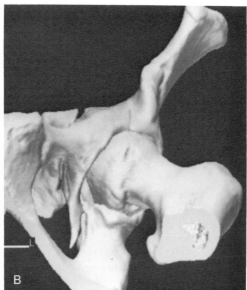

FIGURE 68–102. Acetabular fractures: Use of CT. Three-dimensional images derived from transaxial CT data show, in vivid fashion, a comminuted fracture of the acetabulum with involvement primarily of the iliopubic column.

TABLE 68–5. Fractures of the Femoral Shaft

Site	Characteristics	Complications
Any level[864–872]	Major violence with associated injuries of femur, tibia, patella, acetabulum, hip, and knee	Refracture
		Peroneal nerve injury owing to skeletal traction
	Open or closed	Vascular injury (femoral artery)
	Spiral, oblique, or transverse fracture with possible butterfly fragment and comminution	Thrombophlebitis
		Nonunion (1 per cent of cases), malunion, or delayed union
		Infection
		Fat embolization (approximately 10 per cent of cases)
Proximal	Associated with osteoporosis and Paget's disease	Malalignment
	Less common than midshaft fractures	Nonunion
	Commonly extend into subtrochanteric region	
Middle	Most common site	
	Transverse fracture is most typical	
Distal and supracondylar	Less common than midshaft fractures	Malalignment
		Arterial injury

ters that lead to abduction, flexion, and external rotation of the proximal femoral fragment and to the insertion of the adductor muscles on the medial portion of the distal femoral fragment that lead to its medial angulation. All of these factors contribute to the varus deformity that typifies fractures involving the middle segment of the femoral diaphysis. It is this portion of the shaft that is fractured most commonly. Fractures of the proximal and distal thirds of the femoral diaphysis are less frequent and may extend to the subtrochanteric and supracondylar regions of the femur, respectively.[2]

Classification of femoral shaft fractures can be accomplished in a number of ways, including on the basis of whether they are open or closed, on fracture morphology, or on what portion of the shaft is involved (Table 68–5). Femoral shaft fractures may be classified as simple (with transverse, oblique, or spiral components), segmental, or comminuted.[613, 614] Although transverse or oblique fractures of the femoral diaphysis are very common, comminuted fractures with one or more butterfly fragments also are encountered regularly, as are segmental fractures, leading to therapeutic difficulties.[615–620]

Radiographic diagnosis of femoral shaft fractures usually presents no problems (Fig. 68–103). Diagnostic pitfalls exist in certain situations, however. Fractures and dislocations in the ipsilateral leg occur in 10 to 20 per cent of femoral diaphysis fractures, mandating radiographic examination of the entire extremity. Such injuries include hip dislocations, fractures of the neck or supracondylar region of the femur, tibial or patellar fractures, and ligamentous disruptions of the knee. Occult fractures about the hip (e.g., acetabular fractures), posterior dislocations of the hip, and femoral neck fractures may escape detection on initial radiographs confined to the region of the femoral shaft.[621] As abduction of the proximal femur is typical of an isolated fracture of the femoral diaphysis, an adducted position of the proximal femur that occurs in a patient with a femoral shaft fracture and a posterior dislocation of the ipsilateral hip assumes diagnostic importance.[2] Occult injuries of the knee occur in 5 to 15 per cent of femoral shaft fractures and, in adoles-

cents, may include physeal injuries in the distal femur or proximal tibia that subsequently may lead to physeal growth arrest.[622]

Complications of femoral shaft fractures include arterial injuries (more common in cases of supracondylar fractures of the femur), malunion (rotational or angular deformity and femoral shortening), refracture (occurring in as many

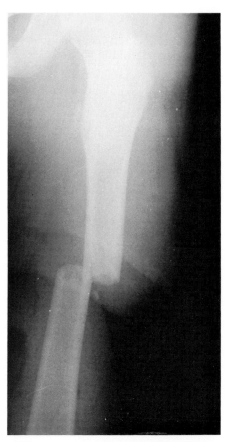

FIGURE 68–103. Femur: Open fracture. Observe the slightly comminuted fracture line and the large soft tissue deficit.

as 9 per cent of cases), fat embolization, and sequelae of associated cranial or visceral injuries.[2]

Knee

Fractures of the Distal Portion of the Femur. These fractures can be classified as supracondylar, intercondylar, or condylar in type. Most of these injuries result from axial loading combined with varus or valgus stress and rotation. They may occur in association with other injuries including ligamentous disruption of the knee, patellar fractures, fracture-dislocations of the hip, and fractures of the tibial shaft.[623] *Supracondylar fractures* (without intra-articular extension) commonly are transverse or slightly oblique in configuration, with varying degrees of displacement and comminution of the fracture fragments.[624, 625] Open or closed fractures are encountered, and injury to the popliteal artery may occur.[626] These supracondylar fractures may be accompanied by a vertical fracture line extending into the knee, leading to *intercondylar fractures* that possess a T or Y configuration,[627] or a vertical fracture alone may be evident.[628, 629] Incongruity of the surface of the femorotibial or patellofemoral compartment, or both, is created by displacement at the fracture site. Oblique radiographs may be required to visualize and categorize these fractures. *Condylar fractures*, in which sagittal or coronal fracture lines are isolated to the region of a single condyle,[630] are more difficult to detect on radiographic examination and may require conventional or computed tomography (Figs. 68–104 and 68–105).

Fractures of the Patella. These fractures result from direct or indirect forces, the latter related to contraction of the quadriceps muscles.[631] Unilateral injuries predominate, although bilateral fractures also are encountered.[632] Transverse fractures are typical, representing approximately 50 to 80 per cent of all patellar fractures, and they generally are the product of indirect force.[633, 634] They may divide the bone into equal-sized components or involve the superior or, more commonly, the inferior pole (Fig. 68–106). Longitudinal (25 per cent) and stellate or comminuted (20 to 35 per cent) fractures are less frequent (Fig. 68–106) and usually result from direct injury, such as striking the dashboard of an automobile (in which case a posterior dislocation of the hip also may be present). Osteochondral fractures occur in combination with patellar dislocation (see later discussion). Displacement of the osseous fragments, particularly in instances of comminuted fractures, can be considerable. Ischemic necrosis is a complication of patellar fractures, involving the proximal fragment and appearing 1 to 3 months after the injury.[635]

Accurate radiographic diagnosis is easy in most patellar fractures, in which comminuted or transverse fracture lines are readily apparent on frontal, oblique, and lateral projections; vertical patellar fractures are best demonstrated on axial radiographic images (''sunrise'' views). Fractures should be differentiated from bipartite patellae, in which separate ossification centers develop in the superolateral aspect of the bone.

Fragmentation and separation of the lower pole of the patella is referred to as Sinding-Larsen-Johanson disease (see Chapter 81), representing a stress-related phenomenon, although the mechanism of injury is debated.[636] Of interest, fracture and dislocation of another sesamoid bone about the knee, the fabella, are reported[637, 638] (68–107).

Fractures of the Proximal Portion of the Tibia. These fractures (Fig. 68–108), which may be extra-articular or intra-articular in nature, commonly are subtle and may be overlooked entirely on routine radiography. Oblique and horizontal-beam projections and conventional or computed tomography (Figs. 68–109 and 68–110) frequently are required for accurate assessment of these injuries, and the tomographic techniques allow further analysis of the extent of displacement and depression of the articular segment.[639–643] MR imaging represents an additional method for diagnosis of occult fractures of the tibial plateau (Fig. 68–111) (see Chapters 67 and 70).[901] Tibial plateau fractures are related to a variety of mechanisms, which include vertical compression, varus or valgus forces, and twisting,[625] and they may be accompanied by injuries to the cruciate or collateral ligaments of the knee[644, 645] which require stress radiography (or MR imaging) for adequate evaluation. Although they may occur in young persons, including those involved in athletics,[646] tibia plateau fractures predominate in middle-aged and elderly persons when the relatively stronger condylar portion of the femur impacts against the plateau. Valgus stress is far more common than varus stress, such that isolated lateral plateau fractures (75 to 80 per cent of all fractures of the tibial plateaus) and combined lateral and medial plateau fractures (10 to 15 per cent of all such fractures) are more frequent than isolated medial plateau fractures (5 to 10 per cent of all plateau fractures)[2] (Fig. 68–112). Fibular head or neck fractures are seen in association with those tibial fractures that involve the lateral plateau. Available classification systems emphasize the location and configuration of the fracture lines.[647–651] Moore[650] has proposed the separation of articular fractures in the proximal tibia into two categories: fractures of the tibial plateau and fracture-dislocations, the latter associated with soft tissue injuries and articular instability (Fig. 68–108).

Important imaging considerations related to tibial frac-

Text continued on page 2773

FIGURE 68–104. Fractures of the distal portion of the femur: Condylar fractures—classification system. Such fractures may be undisplaced **(A)** or displaced **(B–D)**, involve one **(A, B)** or both **(C, D)** condyles, and be oriented principally in the sagittal **(A–C)** or coronal **(D)** plane. (From Hohl M, et al: Fractures and dislocations of the knee. *In* CA Rockwood Jr, DP Greene [Eds]: Fractures in Adults. 2nd Ed. Philadelphia, JB Lippincott Co, 1984, p 1444.)

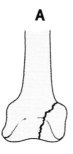 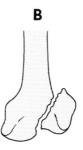 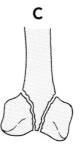 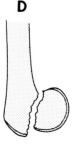

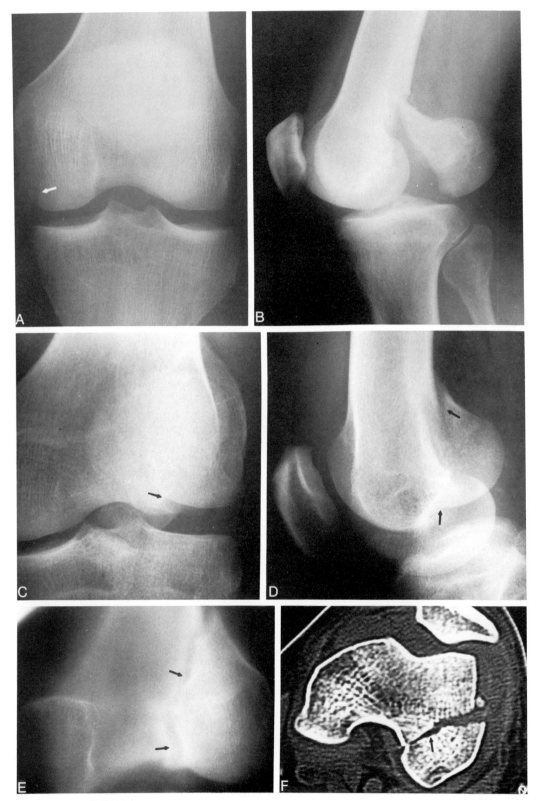

FIGURE 68–105. Fractures of the distal portion of the femur: Condylar fractures.
  A Fracture of the medial condyle (arrow).
  B Fracture of the lateral condyle.
  C–F Fracture of the lateral condyle (arrows).

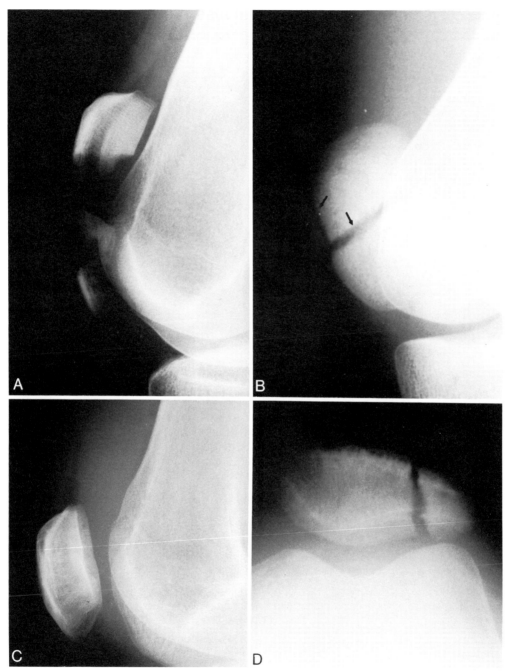

FIGURE 68–106. Patellar fractures.
  A Transverse patellar fracture with comminution and displacement on lateral radiograph.
  B Stellate or comminuted patellar fracture (arrows) on oblique radiograph.
  C, D Longitudinal patellar fracture. The lateral radiograph reveals an effusion, but the axial or tangential projection is required for accurate diagnosis.

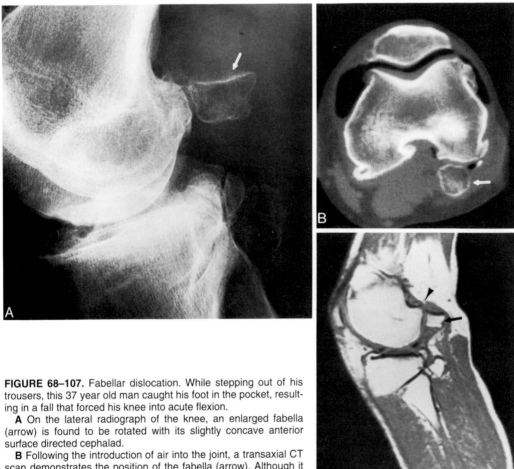

FIGURE 68–107. Fabellar dislocation. While stepping out of his trousers, this 37 year old man caught his foot in the pocket, resulting in a fall that forced his knee into acute flexion.

A On the lateral radiograph of the knee, an enlarged fabella (arrow) is found to be rotated with its slightly concave anterior surface directed cephalad.

B Following the introduction of air into the joint, a transaxial CT scan demonstrates the position of the fabella (arrow). Although it is located behind the lateral condyle, its anterior articular surface is not apposing the femur.

C A sagittal T1-weighted (TR/TE, 600/20) spin echo MR image of the femur, tibia, and fibula demonstrates the rotated fabella (arrow), surrounded by the lateral head of the gastrocnemius muscle, which contains an equivocal tear (arrowhead). The fabella was removed surgically and found to be enlarged; it contained an eburnated articular surface. The tendon of the lateral head of the gastrocnemius muscle was partially ruptured. Postoperatively, the patient recovered completely.

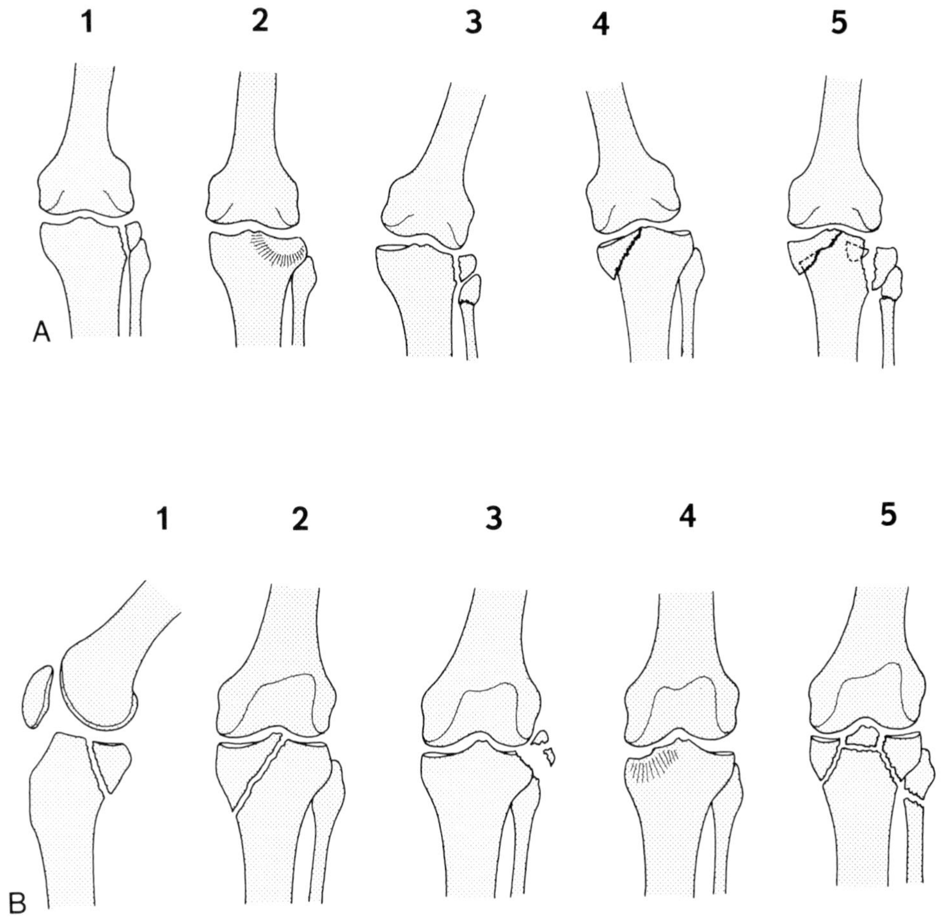

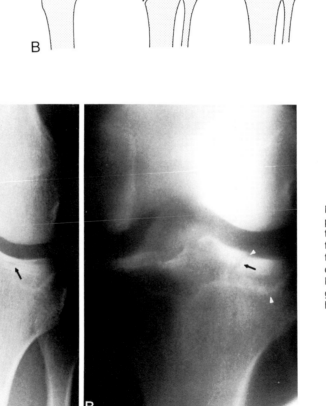

FIGURE 68–108. Fractures of the proximal portion of the tibia: Classification systems.

A Fractures of the tibial plateau. 1, Minimally displaced. 2, Local compression. 3, Split compression. 4, Total condylar depression. 5, Bicondylar.

B Fracture-dislocations of the knee. 1, Split fracture. 2, Entire plateau fracture. 3, Rim avulsion. 4, Rim compression. 5, Four-part fracture.

(**A**, From Hohl M: J Bone Joint Surg [Am] *49*:1456, 1967; **B**, from Hohl M, Moore TM: Articular fractures of the proximal tibia. *In* Evarts CM [Ed]: Surgery of the Musculoskeletal System. New York, Churchill Livingstone, 1983. Used by permission.)

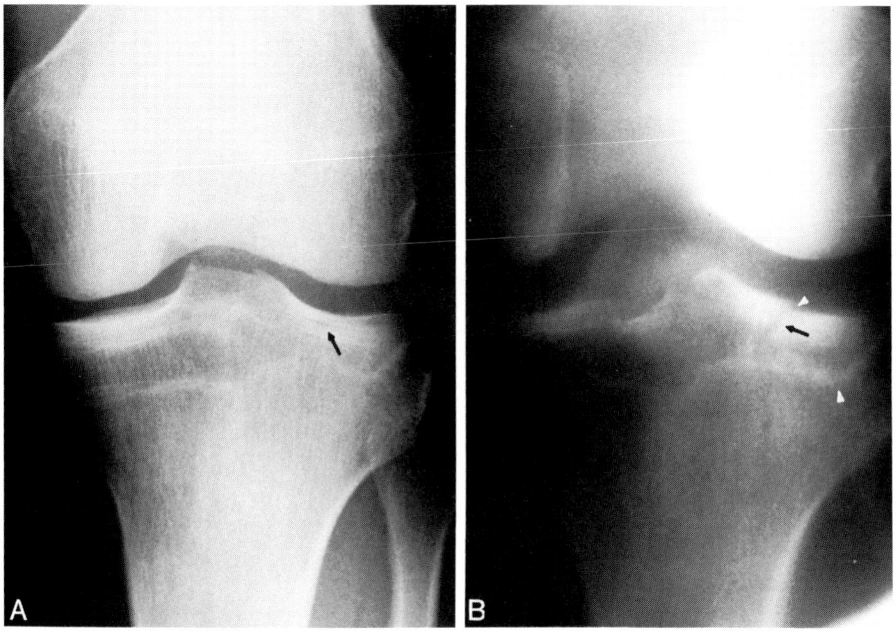

FIGURE 68–109. Fractures of the proximal portion of the tibia: Conventional tomography. Although the fracture line (arrows) is evident on both the routine radiograph **(A)** and the conventional tomogram **(B)**, it is the latter technique that identifies the degree of osseous compression (arrowheads).

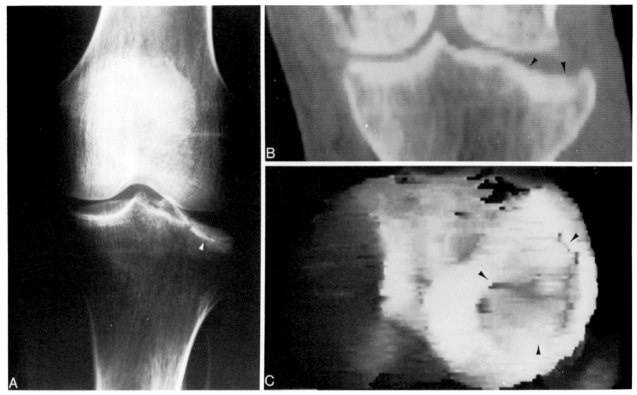

FIGURE 68–110. Fractures of the proximal portion of the tibia: Use of CT.
 A The routine radiograph shows the site of fracture as well as evidence of bone compression (arrowhead).
 B, C A coronal reformatted CT image **(B)** and a three-dimensional CT display **(C)**, in which the tibial plateau is viewed from above, better define the degree of osseous depression (arrowheads).

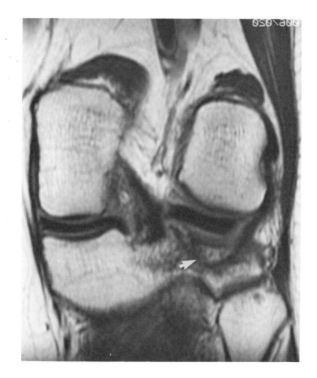

FIGURE 68–111. Fractures of the proximal portion of the tibia: MR imaging. A coronal T1-weighted (TR/TE, 550/20) spin echo MR image reveals a subtle fracture (arrow) of the lateral tibial plateau.

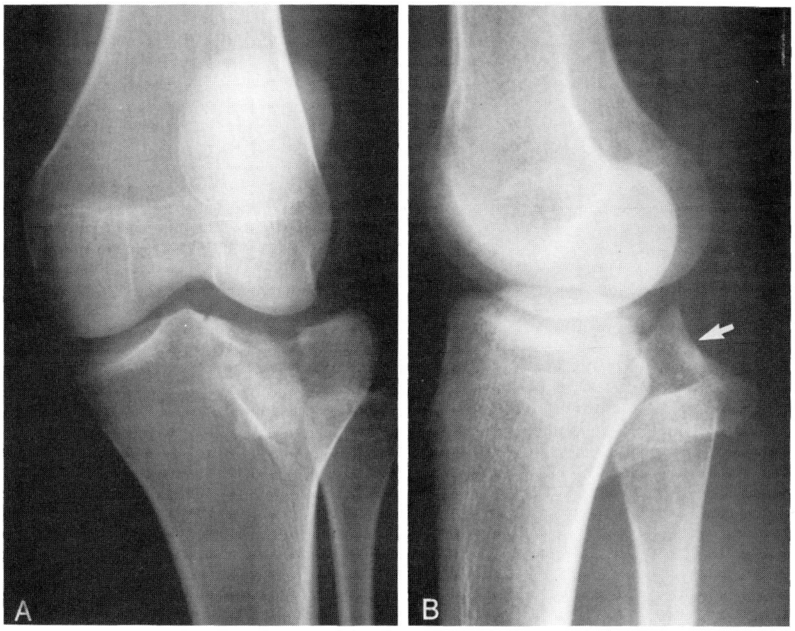

FIGURE 68–112. Fractures of the proximal portion of the tibia: Lateral plateau fractures. Valgus stress has led to a markedly displaced fracture, as shown on a frontal **(A)** and lateral **(B)** radiograph. Note the orientation of the articular surface (arrow) in **B**.

tures include the detection of lipohemarthrosis, avulsion fractures and sites of ligamentous detachment (femoral condyles, fibular head, and intercondylar eminence), meniscal injuries, abnormal widening of the joint space during the application of stress, and disruption of the articular surface. As an approximate guideline, surgical reduction generally is advised for fractures of the tibial plateau that are depressed or displaced by more than 1 cm.[651]

Recognized complications of these injuries include peroneal nerve involvement, ruptures of the popliteal artery, residual varus or valgus angulation, and osteoarthritis.[652, 653]

Fractures of the tibial spine or intercondylar eminence result from violent twisting, abduction-adduction injuries, or direct contact with the adjacent femoral condyle and are indicative of possible damage to the cruciate ligaments of the knee.[625] Varying degrees of osseous displacement are seen.[654] Either the anterior tibial spine (Fig. 68–113) or, less commonly, the posterior tibial spine is affected, and rarely both are involved. Avulsion injuries of the anterior tibial spine occur more commonly in children and in adolescents than in adults and, in children, often result from a fall while bicycling.[655] Such fractures in adults typically are accompanied by ligamentous and meniscal injury, whereas in children they may appear as an isolated phenomenon.[656] Routine radiography supplemented with tunnel projections, radiographs obtained during the application of stress, arthrography, and MR imaging are important in the assessment of these injuries.

Other avulsion fractures may involve the proximal portion of the tibia. Although, rarely, an avulsion injury involves the tibial (or femoral) site of attachment of the medial collateral ligament of the knee, the more common tibial avulsion occurs at the site of insertion of the lateral capsular ligament (see also Chapter 70). This injury, termed a Segond fracture, occurs with the knee in flexion owing to internal rotation of the tibia.[658] The resulting fracture fragment is located laterally, just distal to the joint line. It is elongated in shape and vertically oriented, and is associated with osseous irregularity at the donor site in the tibia. Disruption of the anterior cruciate ligament occurs in 75 to almost 100 per cent of patients with a Segond fracture (although the frequency of Segond fractures in cases of anterior cruciate ligament injury is low), medial ligamentous damage also may be present, and anterolateral rotatory instability of the knee is evident on clinical examination. The fracture fragment eventually may merge with the lateral margin of the tibia, producing an outgrowth that simulates an osteophyte.

Avulsion injuries of Gerdy's tubercle of the tibia relate to the iliotibial band. As opposed to the Segond fracture, the bone fragment arising from Gerdy's tubercle usually is not seen on frontal radiographs of the knee.

Fractures of the Proximal Portion of the Fibula. Isolated fractures of the head or neck of the fibula are distinctly uncommon; the detection of a fracture in these regions should prompt a search for a ligamentous injury or fracture of the knee or ankle. Fibular head or neck fractures result from a direct blow (in which fracture comminution may be identified), a varus force (in which an avulsion fracture of the proximal pole or styloid process of the fibula occurs), a valgus force (which is accompanied by a fracture of the lateral tibial plateau and an injury of the medial collateral ligament), and a twisting force at the ankle (in which pronation and external rotation may lead to a fracture in the fibular neck).[2] The combination of an adduction stress to the knee, rupture of the lateral capsular and ligamentous structures, an injury of the peroneal nerve and, possibly, an avulsion fracture of the fibula is termed the ligamentous peroneal nerve syndrome.[625, 659] Additional complications of fractures of the proximal portion of the fibula include contusion or traction of the biceps tendon, injury to the anterior tibial artery, and avulsion of the fibular head with possible intra-articular entrapment.[625]

Knee Dislocation. This is a rare but serious injury owing to the neurovascular insult that may result from popliteal artery and peroneal nerve damage.[660–664] Dislocations of the knee require major force; typical causes include high-energy trauma resulting from motor vehicle accidents, industrial injury, or falls from a considerable height. Less commonly, these dislocations relate to collisions with a blow to

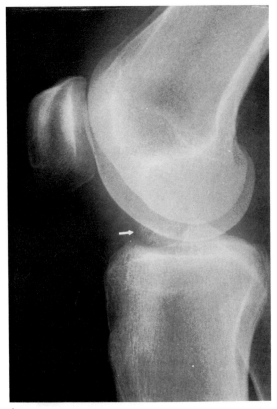

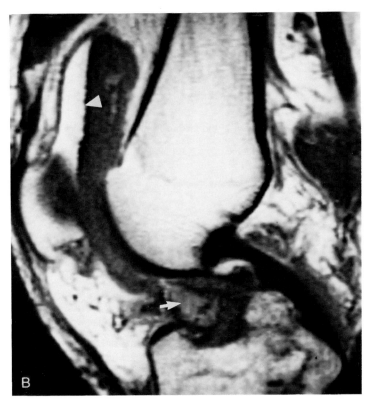

A

FIGURE 68–113. Fractures of the proximal portion of the tibia: Intercondylar eminence fractures.

A Note the osseous fragment (arrow) arising from the anterior aspect of the tibial articular surface. Such injuries generally indicate alteration in the integrity of the cruciate ligaments. The degree of osseous displacement influences the selection of an appropriate therapeutic regimen.

B In a different patient, a sagittal T1-weighted (TR/TE, 886/15) spin echo MR image reveals an avulsion fracture (arrow) of the proximal portion of the tibia and a lipohemarthrosis (arrowhead). In this image, the anterior cruciate ligament cannot be evaluated.

the knee during sporting activities.[665, 666] Closed injuries predominate over open injuries. Associated fractures, although not common, are varied and include tibial and fibular fractures in the injured extremity. Visceral injuries and fractures of the skull and facial bones also are observed, indicating the severity of the trauma. Anterior, posterior, lateral, medial, and rotatory types of dislocation are recognized (Fig. 68–114). Anterior dislocation is the most common type (30 to 50 per cent of all knee dislocations), apparently resulting from hyperextension of the knee with tearing of the posterior capsule and posterior cruciate ligament. The adjacent popliteal artery may be stretched, leading to thrombosis or laceration. Posterior dislocations are next in frequency, although in some reported series they have been more common than anterior dislocations.[666] They may result from crushing blows to the leg[2] with force applied to the anterior surface of the proximal tibia. The extensor mechanism of the knee may be injured at the same time. Medial, lateral, and rotatory (posterolateral) dislocations of the knee are uncommon, but they invariably are associated with damage to the collateral ligaments. Although the precise number of ligaments that are torn, stretched or avulsed during a knee dislocation is variable and dependent on the magnitude of the force and the type of dislocation, injury to both cruciate ligaments is common (although not invariable[667]) as is injury to one or both collateral ligaments. As a general rule, the detection of disruption of four major ligaments of the knee (cruciate ligaments

and collateral ligaments) implies that a dislocation of the joint has occurred.

Rotatory, or posterolateral, dislocation of the knee may be irreducible owing to intra-articular invagination of the medial capsule and medial collateral ligament.[666] Owing to a minor degree of lateral displacement of the tibia, radiographic diagnosis of this injury may be difficult.[2]

Radiographic diagnosis is not difficult in most knee dislocations, however, although multiple views are required to detect associated osteochondral and fibular head fractures as well as avulsion injuries of the tibial spines. Arteriography should be employed to delineate the status of the popliteal artery in patients in whom operative intervention is being contemplated owing to vascular symptoms and signs.[668] Popliteal artery injury occurs in 25 to 50 per cent of knee dislocations, may accompany posterior or anterior knee dislocations, and is encountered in both low- and high-energy injuries.[669, 670] The popliteal vein and tibial and peroneal nerves also may be injured during knee dislocations.

Patellar Dislocation. Traumatic dislocation of the patella can be produced by a direct blow or an exaggerated contraction of the quadriceps mechanism. Abnormalities predisposing to displacement may include an abnormally high patella (patella alta), deficient height of the lateral femoral condyle, shallowness of the patellofemoral groove, genu valgum or recurvatum, lateral insertion of the patellar tendon, muscular weakness, and excessive tibial torsion.[671, 672]

Lateral dislocation predominates, although rare patterns of displacement include vertical (superior) dislocations or rotational dislocations, along either the vertical or the horizontal axis of the bone, the last pattern associated with intercondylar or intra-articular displacement of the patella.[673-681] Medial dislocation of the patella may follow surgical release of the lateral patellar retinaculum.[682] With regard to lateral dislocations of the patella, displacement of the bone may be transient or reduction may be accomplished at the scene of the accident, such that initial radiographs are obtained at a time when the patella no longer is dislocated.[2] Identification of characteristic associated fractures, therefore, assumes diagnostic importance. In particular, osteochondral fractures of the medial patellar facet and lateral femoral condyle are common[683-691] (Fig. 68–115). Axial radiographs are most useful in detecting these fractures.

Recurrent subluxation of the patella is a common problem that may result either from an initial acute traumatic dislocation of the bone or from developmental abnormalities of the femoral condyles, patella, or quadriceps mechanism (e.g., ligament and tendon laxity). It is a problem that requires careful radiographic technique as well as specialized projections (see Chapter 1), supplemented with CT or MR imaging (see Chapters 8 and 70).

Proximal Tibiofibular Joint Dislocation. Although rare, proximal tibiofibular joint dislocation may be seen in parachuting, hang-gliding, sky-diving, and horseback riding injuries. Anterior or, less frequently, posterior dislocation

of the fibular head can be noted.[692-697] Peroneal nerve injury can appear following a posterior dislocation of this joint. Rarely, a superior dislocation can be seen, which is associated with injury to the interosseous membrane and superior dislocation of the lateral malleolus.

Radiographic findings associated with dislocation of the proximal tibiofibular joint may be subtle (Fig. 68–116). As the fibular head is displaced anteriorly, it also moves laterally. This anterolateral movement can be better appreciated when comparison radiographs of the uninvolved side are available or when the relationship of the fibular head to the osseous groove on the posterolateral aspect of the tibia is analyzed carefully (see Chapter 22). Oblique radiographs may reveal complete separation of the tibia and the fibula. In cases of posterior dislocation, the fibular head is displaced medially, overlapped in large part by the tibia on anteroposterior radiographs.

Subluxation of the proximal tibiofibular joint refers to excessive and symptomatic movement without frank dislocation.[698-701] This is a self-limited condition of youth with decreasing symptoms as the patient approaches skeletal maturity, although persistent symptoms and signs may require surgical intervention.

Tibial and Fibular Diaphyses

Of all of the long tubular bones, the tibia is fractured most commonly. Direct or indirect forces applied to the tibia can result in fracture (Table 68–6). Direct forces ac-

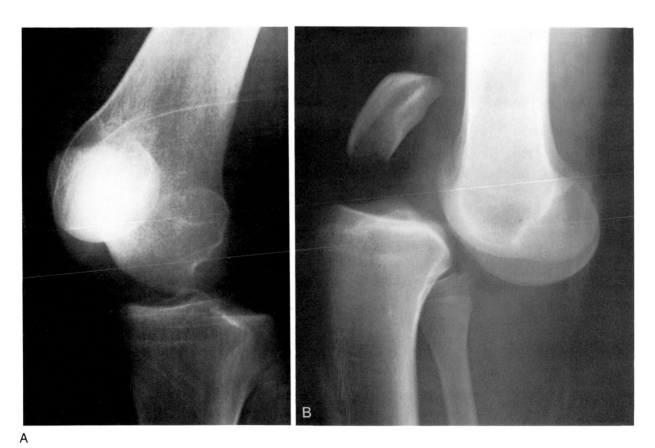

A

FIGURE 68–114. Knee dislocation.
A A lateral dislocation of the tibia with respect to the femur is seen. Abnormal rotation between the two bones also is evident.
B An anterior dislocation of the tibia and fibula is evident.

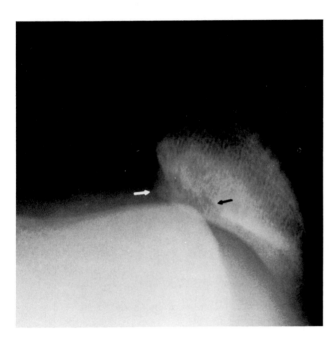

FIGURE 68–115. Patellar dislocation. An axial radiograph reveals lateral dislocation of the patella with fragmentation and erosion of a portion of the patellar articular surface (arrows).

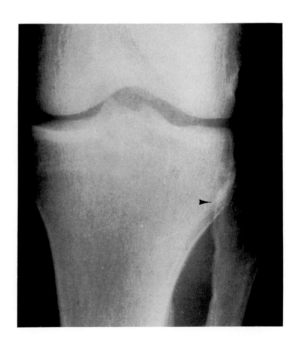

FIGURE 68–116. Proximal tibiofibular joint dislocation. An anterior dislocation is accompanied by anterior and lateral displacement of the fibular head and a reduction in the normal amount of overlap of the tibia and fibula (arrowhead) on the frontal radiograph. Lateral projections, however, also are required for accurate diagnosis.

TABLE 68–6. Fractures of the Tibial and Fibular Shafts

Site	Characteristics	Complications
Tibia[873–887]	Direct or indirect trauma	Delayed union (no osseous union at 20 weeks) in 5 to 15 per cent of cases
	Associated fractures of the fibula especially in direct and severe trauma	Nonunion (no osseous union at 6 months to 1 year) is most common in the distal third of tibia
	Transverse or comminuted fracture in direct trauma; oblique or spiral fracture in indirect trauma; sometimes segmental fractures	Infecton with or without nonunion
	Middle and distal thirds > proximal third	Vascular injury (to anterior tibial artery or, less commonly, posterior tibial artery)
	Minor, moderate, or major categories of injury, the last associated with comminuted and open fractures	Compartment syndrome (anterior > posterior or lateral compartment)
	Prognosis related to amount of displacement, degree of comminution, open or closed fracture, and infection	Nerve injury (uncommon, peroneal and posterior tibial nerves)
	Childhood fractures:	Refracture (especially in athletes)
	Toddler fracture—spiral fracture, undisplaced	Leg shortening
	Proximal metaphyseal fracture—associated with genu valgum deformity	Osteoarthritis (if fracture extends into joint)
		Reflex sympathetic dystrophy syndrome
		Fat embolism
Fibula[888]	Isolated fractures are rare, related to direct injury	Related to those of the associated tibial or ankle injury
	Associated fractures of the tibia and ankle injuries	

counting for tibial shaft fractures are generated during motor vehicle accidents and criminal violence and, when of high energy, lead to skin loss, open and comminuted fractures, and associated fibular fractures (Fig. 68–117). Indirect forces, which may be generated by twisting injuries occurring during sports such as skiing or a fall, lead to spiral or oblique fractures of the tibia (as opposed to the transverse or comminuted fractures associated with direct injury), and the fibula may be left intact. In general, the more severe the force, the more likely that both bones will fracture. Isolated fractures of the shaft of the fibula are uncommon, resulting from a direct blow. More typically, such an apparently isolated fibular fracture in reality is one component of a more complicated injury involving also the ankle (see later discussion). Tibial and fibular fractures occurring together in a single patient may appear at the same level, although it is very common for them to occur at different levels. Because of this, as well as the necessity to determine any rotational component of the fracture or fractures, radiographic evaluation of the entire length of the bones is required.[2] Furthermore, the identification of one fracture in each of these two bones does not exclude the presence of an additional fracture, as segmental fractures of either the tibia or the fibula, or both bones, are encountered regularly. On the basis of clinical manifestations, additional radiographs also may be necessary to identify associated fractures in the ipsilateral femur or acetabulum or even a hip dislocation. As some of these additional injuries may be clinically occult, survey radiographs of the pelvis and ipsilateral femur may be appropriate when a severe injury of the tibia and fibula has occurred.[2] CT may be required in the evaluation of some tibial fractures to assess the relationship of the fracture fragments and the extent of soft tissue injury. In instances of spiral fractures of the tibia, CT provides accurate information regarding the extent of separation of the fragments.[702]

The frequency and rate of union of tibial fractures have varied in reported series, although Sarmiento and

colleagues,[703, 704] using closed reduction and prefabricated bracing of tibial shaft fractures, reported a union rate of 97.5 per cent. The average rate of healing of such fractures in adults is about 16 to 18 weeks in closed injuries and about 4 weeks longer in open injuries. Tibial shaft fractures in children generally heal more quickly. A delayed union of these tibial fractures should be considered present when the fracture line still is readily visible 5 to 6 months after the injury, and a nonunion should be suspected when the fracture line remains apparent more than 6 months after injury.[2] These definitions are not applied rigidly, however; rather, the diagnosis of delayed union or nonunion of a tibial shaft is made on the basis of both clinical and radiologic parameters. The role of scintigraphy and other imaging methods in the assessment of fracture healing is discussed in Chapter 67.

Additional complications of tibial (and fibular) shaft fractures include malunion, infection, neurovascular injury, and compartment syndromes. The most clinically significant malunions of tibial shaft fractures involve angular or rotational deformity, although they are not encountered commonly. The occurrence of osteomyelitis in cases of tibial shaft fractures is not surprising, owing to the superficial location of the bone and the frequency of open fractures. Skin loss at the time of injury may be extensive, particularly when high-energy forces have occurred, and such skin loss contributes to infection at the fracture site. Infected and persistently ununited fractures of the tibial diaphysis are difficult to treat adequately, and amputation of the lower limb eventually may be required. Although vascular injury in cases of tibial shaft fracture is uncommon, fractures involving the proximal portion of the diaphysis may be accompanied by occlusion or laceration of the anterior tibial artery. This artery also may be injured when fractures involving the lower portion of the tibia are displaced posteriorly. Posterior tibial artery involvement is rare in cases of tibial shaft fracture, although such involvement may be apparent when a posterior compartment syndrome is pres-

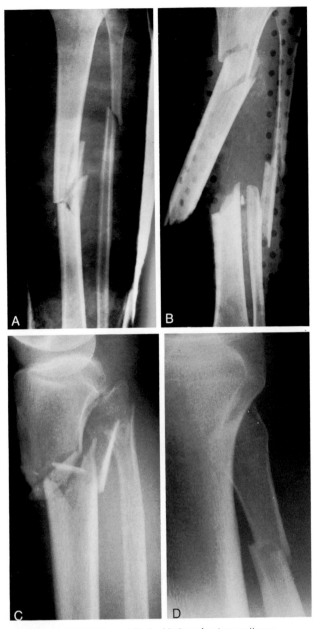

FIGURE 68–117. Tibia and fibula: Various fracture patterns.

A–C Combined injuries of the tibia and fibula usually indicate direct and severe trauma.

D An isolated fracture of the fibula is relatively rare.

ent. The common peroneal nerve is the most commonly injured nerve in patients with a fracture of the diaphysis of the tibia or fibula, although such injury is not frequent. Compartment syndromes, as indicated in Chapter 67, may complicate a variety of musculoskeletal injuries, including fractures of the tibial and fibular shafts. The anterior compartment of the lower leg is involved most commonly in these fractures, particularly in closed but also in open fractures. Its frequency is decreased in fractures that are comminuted or are associated with disruption of the interosseous membrane (or that are open), as spontaneous decompression of the compartment results. Involvement of the posterior or lateral compartment of the lower leg is less frequent.

In children, distinctive fractures of the tibial shaft include a spiral fracture in the first three years of life, designated a toddler's fracture (see Chapter 67), and a fracture involving the proximal metaphysis of the bone.[705–708] Fractures of the proximal metaphyseal region of the tibia, particularly those that are complete or greenstick (not torus) in type and those that occur in children who are 6 years of age or younger, may be associated with a subsequent valgus deformity at the fracture site. The reported frequency of this complication following such fractures has varied from as low as 15 per cent to as high as 75 per cent. The typical age at which this complication occurs is between 3 and 6 years. Although valgus deformity is the expected type of abnormality, varus or recurvatum deformity also has been noted.[707] The fracture configuration usually includes a readily visible gap in the medial side of the tibia with subtle or absent changes laterally. The fibula may or may not be fractured. Valgus displacement at the tibial fracture site typically occurs within the first year following the injury. Such displacement tends to stabilize within a year following its appearance[707] and even may resolve spontaneously.[2] Surgical intervention, including corrective osteotomies, may be followed by recurrence of the deformity. The cause of valgus displacement in these fractures is not clear; it may relate to hyperemia with selective stimulation of the medial portion of the tibial physis or to interposition of the periosteum or a portion of the pes anserinus tissues within the fracture site.[709]

Ankle

Fractures About the Ankle. The treatment of ankle injuries is directed toward restoration of anatomic alignment and reestablishment of normal function (Fig. 68–118). It is important to diagnose both fractures and ligamentous injuries to optimize these therapeutic efforts. Stability of the ankle joint depends on the integrity of a ring formed by the tibia, fibula, and talus, united by surrounding ligaments[710] (Fig. 68–119). A single break in the ring does not allow subluxation of the talus in the mortise, whereas two or more breaks in the ring, whether fractures or a fracture in combination with a ruptured ligament, will allow abnormal talar motion. Displacement of the talus in the ankle joint may be evident on routine radiographs including the mortise view (Fig. 68–120), although the application of stress to the ankle during the radiographic examination can be of considerable diagnostic importance in the detection of instability and of specific sites of ligamentous disruption.[711–713] (Fig. 68–121).

Although ankle fractures may be described using anatomic terminology (e.g., medial or lateral malleolar, bimalleolar or trimalleolar), such a description fails to consider the mechanism of injury and the associated ligamentous disruptions. A comprehensive classification of ankle fractures based on mechanism of injury was first proposed in 1922.[714] Subsequently, Lauge-Hansen derived a more unified and complete classification system that considered both the mechanism of injury and the associated ligamentous abnormalities.[715, 716] Although more complex than other classification systems, the Lauge-Hansen method becomes quite simple to remember and apply once the basic terminology and the association between mechanism and radiographic appearance are understood. This method, however, is not ideal; it is based on the position of the foot relative to the body when, in fact, the foot commonly is fixed to the

FIGURE 68–118. Ankle: Normal anatomy.

A Anteroposterior views show the "mortise and tenon" relationship of the tibia, fibula, and talus.

B This diagram illustrates the cross-sectional appearance of the talar side of the ankle joint. Note that the dorsal narrowing of the talus serves to wedge this bone into the mortise, particularly during weight-bearing and dorsiflexion.

C In this lateral view, the long posterior process of the tibia stabilizes the joint dorsally (solid arrow). The anterior (open arrow) and posterior (arrowhead) colliculi of the medial malleolus also are indicated.

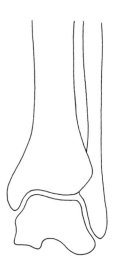
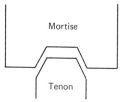
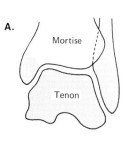
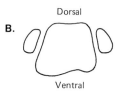
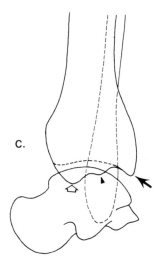

A.

Mortise

Tenon

B.

Dorsal

Ventral

C.

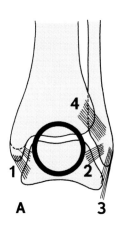
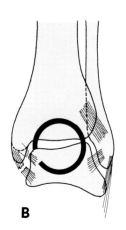
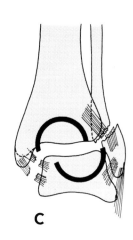

A   B   C

FIGURE 68–119. Ankle: Stable and unstable characteristics.

A The stability of the ankle joint is determined by the status of a ring comprising the mortise and surrounding ligaments. The latter include the deep and superficial deltoid ligaments (1), the anterior (2) and posterior (not shown) talofibular ligaments, the calcaneofibular ligament (3), the anterior (4) and posterior (not shown) tibiofibular ligaments, the inferior transverse ligament (not shown), and the interosseous membrane and ligament (not shown).

B A single break in this ring will not allow displacement.

C Two or more breaks in the ring allow displacement of the mortise.

FIGURE 68–120. Ankle instability: Routine radiography. Direct lateral displacement of the talus with respect to the tibia results in widening of the medial "clear" space (arrowheads) indicative of rupture of the deep deltoid ligament. The superficial deltoid ligament also may be torn. There is a fibular fracture (arrow), which allows the talus to move laterally.

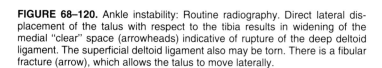
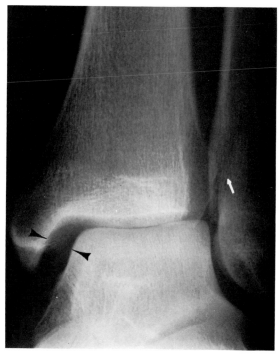

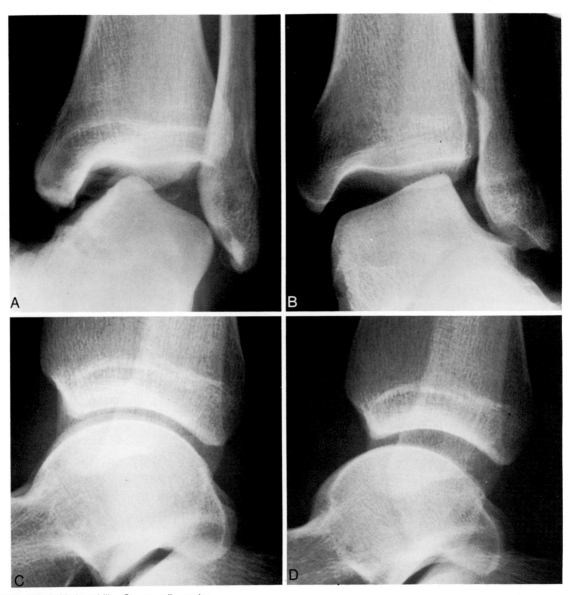

FIGURE 68–121. Ankle instability: Stress radiography.

  A An anteroposterior varus (inversion) stress view (with the foot in neutral position) shows obvious widening of the lateral portion of the joint, indicating some degree of ligamentous disruption. The tibiotalar angle measured 34 degrees. Small fracture fragments are evident.

  B An anteroposterior valgus (eversion) stress view reveals widening of the medial "clear" space indicative of a rupture of the deltoid ligaments.

  C, D Lateral radiographs were obtained without **(C)** and with **(D)** the application of anterior stress (anterior drawer sign). In **D**, note anterior movement of the talus on the tibia.

ground with the body in one of several different positions during a fall. Furthermore, interobserver (and even intraobserver) variation in the application of the Lauge-Hansen classification system appears to be large.[717, 718] Still, this system commonly is employed in the description of ankle injuries. Other classification methods do exist, however, including that of Weber (as a modification of the system of Danis), which is based on the position of fibular fracture with respect to the joint line.[2] Although the Weber system is simple to employ, its lack of descriptive detail and the general absence of reference to injury on the medial side of the ankle may limit its clinical usefulness.[896]

On the basis of experimental results in cadavers, Lauge-Hansen defined five major predictable fracture complexes.[715, 716, 719] Within each grouping are stages of injury, designated by Roman numerals; the higher the number, the greater the applied force and resultant damage. Each of the groups is designated by two characteristic terms. The first term is either *pronation or supination* and refers to the position of the foot at the time of injury. Pronation or supination of the foot tightens various ligamentous and capsular structures of the tibiotalar joint, decreasing flexibility and increasing transmission of forces across the joint to the distal portions of the tibia and fibula. The foot is pronated when there is outward rotation and eversion of the forefoot with abduction of the hindfoot. Supination represents inward rotation and inversion of the forefoot with adduction of the hindfoot.

The second term reflects the direction that the talus is displaced or rotated relative to the mortise formed by the distal regions of the tibia and fibula. There are five possible directions of talar displacement: external rotation (in which the talus is displaced externally or laterally); internal rotation (in which the talus is displaced internally or medially); abduction (in which the talus is displaced laterally without significant rotation; adduction (in which the talus is displaced medially without significant rotation); and dorsiflexion (in which the talus is dorsiflexed on the tibia). Thus, with the foot in either pronation or supination, the talus may be subjected to one of five vectors of force—external rotation, internal rotation, abduction, adduction, or dorsiflexion. It also should be realized that, for example, external rotation of the talus on the tibia and fibula will occur either when the foot is rotated laterally relative to the fixed tibia and fibula or when the body undergoes internal rotation while the foot is fixed. Although these fracture groups result from application of forces with the foot position and direction designated, the end result is classified by the radiographic appearance, specifically, in the first four types, by the configuration of the fibular fracture and not by the mechanism of injury deduced from available clinical information. Indeed, an accurate description of the injury rarely is provided by the patient.

1. *Supination–external rotation fracture* (SER stages I, II, III, and IV). The SER category constitutes almost 60 per cent of all ankle fractures[719] (Figs. 68–122 to 68–125). The fracture complex is caused by external rotation of the supinated foot. In this position, the deltoid ligament is relaxed. External rotation of the foot forces the talus against the fibula, commonly resulting in rupture of the anterior tibiofibular ligament (stage I), although, alternatively, there may be an avulsion fracture arising from the anterior surface of

the fibula or tibia (fracture of Tillaux).[720] Small avulsion fractures usually are not apparent radiographically; furthermore, as most stage I lesions are ligamentous, they too are rarely detected on radiographs. As the mechanism of injury continues, a short oblique fracture of the distal portion of the fibula will occur (stage II). This fracture extends from the anteromedial aspect of the fibula in a dorsal and proximal direction. It usually is evident within 1.5 cm of the tibiotalar joint and rarely is more than 2.5 cm proximal to this joint. The next stage of injury is a fracture of the posterior aspect of the tibia of varying size (stage III). The majority of SER stage III posterior tibial fractures are small and, in some cases, the injury may advance to stage IV without a posterior tibial fracture. The final stage (stage IV) is characterized by a fracture of the medial malleolus or a rupture of the deltoid ligament. Medial malleolar fractures and deltoid ligament ruptures occur with approximately equal frequency in SER injuries.[719] If a typical SER stage II oblique fibular fracture is noted radiographically and there is no evidence of a medial malleolar fracture, a deltoid injury should be suspected when medial soft tissue swelling or widening of the medial aspect of the tibiotalar articulation is apparent.

2. *Supination-adduction fracture* (SAD stages I and II). The SAD category constitutes about 20 per cent of all ankle fractures[719] (Figs. 68–126 and 68–127). These injuries are produced by a medially directed force acting on the supinated foot. Supination causes tension on the lateral ligaments and, with adduction, either a lateral ligament rupture or transverse (traction or avulsion) fracture of the distal portion of the fibula occurs (SAD stage I). The characteristic transverse fibular fracture usually arises just distal to the tibiotalar articulation but, rarely, may be located at the level of or immediately proximal to the joint. Continued pressure from the medially directed talus results in a fracture of the medial malleolus or a rupture of the deltoid ligament (SAD stage II). The malleolar fracture often is oblique or nearly vertical (as is typical of injuries related to compressive forces), but it also may be transverse, a fracture configuration usually attributed to avulsion or traction forces. Thus, the medial malleolar fracture configuration is not significantly distinctive to allow deduction of the mechanism of injury.

The injury to the lateral ligaments, particularly the anterior talofibular ligament, that characterizes the first stage of the SAD complex may represent an avulsion fracture. The fracture fragment often is small and located just distal to the fibular tip, and its identification commonly requires use of a bright light. As a general rule, any small ossicle in this location should be considered evidence of a recent (or remote) injury and not a normal variation of growth.[721]

3 and 4. *Pronation–external rotation fracture* (PER stages I, II, III, and IV); *pronation-abduction fracture* (PAB stages I, II, and III). The PER (Figs. 68–128 and 68–129) and PAB (Fig. 68–130) fractures constitute about 20 per cent of all fractures occurring about the ankle.[719] The two groups commonly are considered together as fractures of the PER stages I and II, and PAB stages I and II cannot be distinguished radiographically. When the foot is pronated, the deltoid ligament is tense. Forceful external rotation or abduction of the talus results in either deltoid ligament rupture (60 per cent) or fracture of the medial malleolus (40 per cent) (PER or PAB stage I). In a PER or PAB stage II

Text continued on page 2787

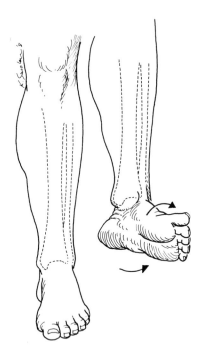

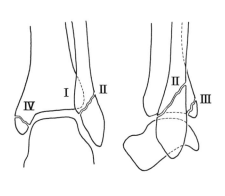

FIGURE 68–122. Ankle injuries: Supination–external rotation fracture. External rotation forces applied to the supinated foot result initially in a rupture of the anterior tibiofibular ligament (stage I). As the forces continue, a short oblique fracture of the distal portion of the fibula occurs (stage II). The next stage of the injury is a fracture of the posterior aspect of the tibia (stage III). The final stage of the injury is a fracture of the medial malleolus (stage IV).

FIGURE 68–123. Ankle injuries: Supination–external rotation fracture—stage II. On anteroposterior **(A)** and lateral **(B)** radiographs, note the typical configuration of the oblique fibular fracture (arrows).

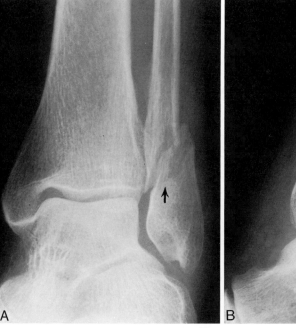

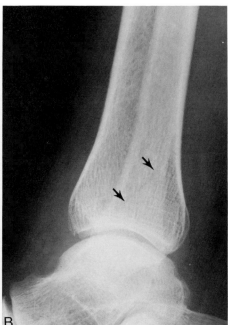

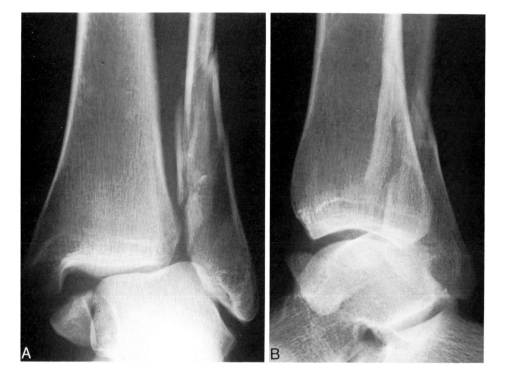

FIGURE 68–124. Ankle injuries: Supination–external rotation fracture—stage IV. Anteroposterior **(A)** and lateral **(B)** radiographs reveal an oblique fibular fracture and a fracture of the medial malleolus.

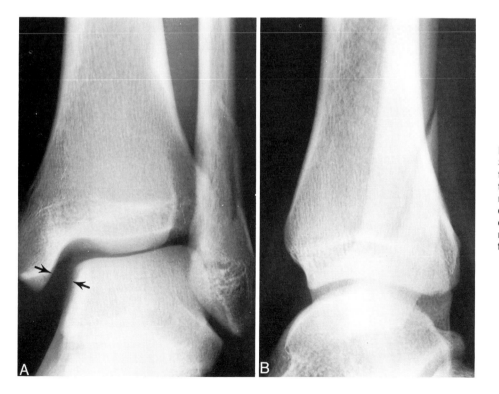

FIGURE 68–125. Ankle injuries: Supination–external rotation fracture—stage IV. In this patient, anteroposterior **(A)** and lateral **(B)** radiographs reveal disruption of the deltoid ligament (manifested by widening of the medial clear space [arrows]) in addition to the fibular fracture.

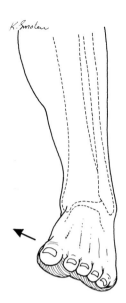

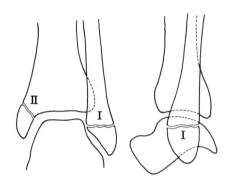

FIGURE 68–126. Ankle injuries: Supination-adduction fracture. Adduction forces applied to the supinated foot initially result in a traction or avulsion fracture of the distal portion of the fibula or rupture of the lateral ligaments (stage I). As forces continue, a fracture of the medial malleolus or a rupture of the deltoid ligament occurs (stage II). The fibular fracture typically is transverse and that of the medial malleolus is oblique or nearly vertical.

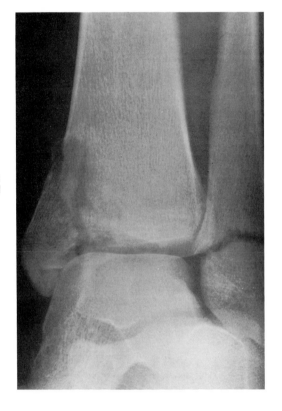

FIGURE 68–127. Ankle injuries: Supination-adduction fracture—stage II. Note the transversely oriented fibular fracture and the nearly vertical fracture of the medial malleolus.

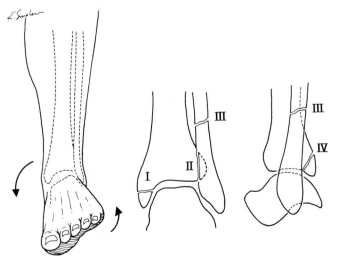

FIGURE 68–128. Ankle injuries: Pronation—external rotation fracture. Forces of external rotation applied to the pronated foot result initially in rupture of the deltoid ligament or a fracture of the medial malleolus (stage I). As forces continue, there is rupture of the anterior tibiofibular ligament (stage II). A high fibular fracture (stage III) and a fracture of the posterior tibial margin (stage IV) are the final stages in this mechanism of injury.

FIGURE 68–129. Ankle injuries: Pronation—external rotation fracture.

A, B Stage III injury. Findings include a fracture of the medial malleolus and an oblique fracture of the fibula (arrowheads), well above the level of the ankle joint.

C, D Stage IV injury. Findings include widening of the medial clear space with an avulsion fracture (arrow), indicating disruption of the deltoid ligament, and a high oblique fibular fracture (arrowheads). The posterior tibial margin also was fractured.

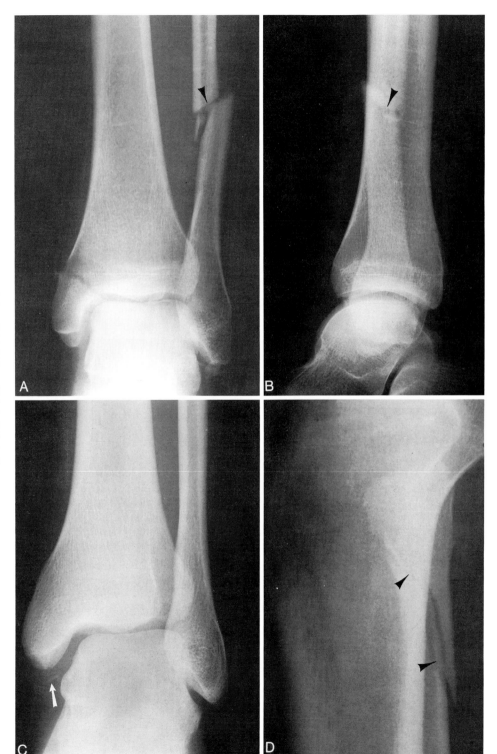

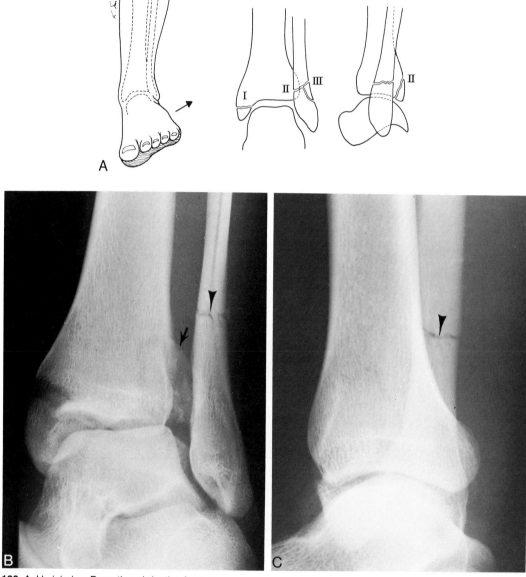

FIGURE 68–130. Ankle injuries: Pronation-abduction fracture.

A The first two stages of this injury are identical to those of the pronation-external rotation fracture complex. Stage III is a transverse supramalleolar fibular fracture that may be comminuted laterally.

B, C Stage III injury. Findings include a transverse supramalleolar fibular fracture (arrowheads) and fractures of the medial malleolus and anterior tibial tubercle (arrow).

lesion, a rupture of the distal tibiofibular syndesmosis also occurs. This latter injury may be purely ligamentous in nature or may be an avulsion fracture arising from either the anterior or the posterior tubercle, or both. PAB stage III fractures include the injuries of the first two stages combined with a transverse supramalleolar fibular fracture. PER stage III injuries include the abnormalities in the first two stages and a short spiral fracture of the fibula more than 2.5 cm above the tibiotalar joint. This latter fibular fracture usually is 6 to 8 cm above the ankle and may even be more proximal in location. Associated rupture of the syndesmosis ligaments and interosseous membrane occurs. PER stage IV fractures include the first three stages in combination with a fracture of the posterior tibial margin. Radiographic detection of the characteristic fibular fracture of either the PAB or PER stage III injury in the absence of a medial malleolar fracture must be associated with a rupture of the deltoid ligament.

Certain diagnostic points regarding these injuries deserve emphasis. A fibular fracture occurring above the joint line and proximal to the distal tibiofibular synostosis may be an important manifestation of an ankle injury. The Dupuytren fracture is one type, occurring in this position and involving the lower portion of the fibular shaft. When it results from a PER injury, the fracture extends from the anterior edge of the fibula in a posteroinferior direction; in a PAB injury the fracture is oblique and extends from the lateral surface of the bone in an inferomedial direction; and in a SER injury, the fibular fracture is oblique, located approximately 4 cm from the distal tip of the fibula, and extends from the anterior edge of the bone in a posterosuperior direction.[2] The Maisonneuve fracture is a second type, involving the proximal portion of the fibular shaft. Although the precise mechanism of this fracture is not agreed upon, it is associated with disruption of the distal tibiofibular syndesmosis and a medial malleolar fracture or tear of the deltoid ligament.[722] It may be overlooked on the basis of clinical findings. Alternatively, when discovered, an evaluation of the ankle is required.[723]

Second, in these pronation injuries, the tibiofibular syndesmosis and interosseous membrane always are disrupted to the level of the most inferior portion of a fibular fracture that involves the distal portion of the diaphysis; with Maisonneuve fractures of the proximal fibula such disruption may or may not be present.[2] Measurement of the syndesmotic region, or lateral clear space, of the ankle therefore becomes important. A width greater than 5.5 mm always is abnormal, indicating syndesmotic rupture. A width of 2 to 5.5 mm is suggestive of such injury and may be an indication for stress radiography of the ankle.

5. *Pronation-dorsiflexion fracture* (PDF stages I, II, III, and IV). The PDF category of ankle fractures was added to the first four categories to provide an explanation for a group of fractures produced by axial loading.[724] These injuries also are designated pilon (pestle) fractures, as the talus is driven into the tibial plafond like a pestle in a mortar.[725–729] Pilon fractures of the tibia constitute less than 0.5 per cent of all ankle fractures.[730] Their mechanism is forced dorsiflexion of the pronated foot, often occurring in a fall from a height, which forces the talus into the ankle mortise (Fig. 68–131). Pilon fractures commonly are associated with additional injuries of the spine, pelvis, and calcaneus, and they may be considered to evolve through several

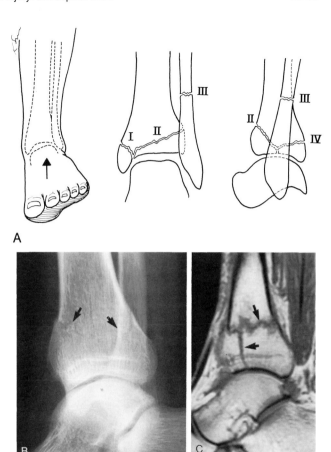

FIGURE 68–131. Ankle injuries: Pronation-dorsiflexion fracture.
A Initially, a fracture of the medial malleolus occurs (stage I). Subsequent injuries include a fracture of the anterior tibial margin (stage II), a supramalleolar fracture of the fibula (stage III), and a transverse fracture of the posterior aspect of the tibia, which connects with the anterior tibial fracture (stage IV).
B, C Stage IV injury. Routine radiography **(B)** and a sagittal T1-weighted (TR/TE, 500/12) spin echo MR image **(C)** show the characteristics of the distal tibial fracture (arrows).

stages. In stage I, a fracture of the medial malleolus is seen. In stage II, a second fracture occurs, arising from the anterior tibial margin. A supramalleolar fracture of the fibula characterizes stage III, and in stage IV it is accompanied by a relatively transverse fracture of the posterior aspect of the tibia, which connects with the anterior tibial fracture. The important radiographic features of PDF fractures are the intra-articular anterior lip fracture of the stage II injury and the comminution of the tibia of the stage IV injury. These features as well as preservation of the normal tibiofibular distance and, in some cases, talar fractures serve to distinguish the pilon injury, which is related to axial compression, from trimalleolar fractures resulting from rotational forces.[729]

An isolated fracture of the posterior tibial margin is a rare lesion that does not fit precisely into the Lauge-Hansen classification system. The mechanism of injury is compression by the talar dome, a situation that might result from kicking an object with the ankle in a neutral position or in plantar flexion. Fractures of the posterior tibial region occur as an isolated lesion or in combination with other injuries. They may be overlooked on the true lateral view of the ankle; their detection is facilitated by the use of an off-lateral projection achieved by slight external rotation of the patient's foot, a maneuver that brings the most prominent portion of the tibia into profile[731] (Fig. 68–132).

An isolated fracture of the anterior margin of the distal portion of the tibia is an uncommon lesion, occurring either as a comminuted injury or as a large fragment involving a significant portion of the joint surface. Comminuted fractures are believed to be related to compression forces resulting from a dorsiflexed talus, whereas larger fragments more often result from a fall on the calcaneus with the talus being forced upward and forward.

In all varieties of ankle fracture, routine radiography represents the primary means of diagnosis and assessment, although it does not diminish the importance of a thorough physical examination.[732] CT remains important in the assessment of complex injuries,[729, 733] and arthrography occasionally is employed in the evaluation of acute ligamentous injuries (see Chapter 13). Bone scintigraphy[734] has limited applications to the analysis of ankle injuries. The role of MR imaging in patients with acute ankle trauma or chronic ankle instability is addressed in Chapter 70.

Ankle Dislocation. Subluxations and dislocations of the ankle, particularly those in a medial or lateral direction, commonly are associated with fracture of the adjacent malleolar surfaces. Displacements owing to extensive ligamentous and capsular injury without fracture can occur in an anterior or posterior direction. Medial dislocation of the talus appears to be the most common type,[2] although lateral, posterior, anterior, posteromedial, superior, and rotatory dislocations also are encountered,[735–737] and any type may be associated with a fracture of the tibial surface (Fig. 68–133). The diagnosis of the specific type of fracture-dislocation usually is accomplished easily by routine radiography; asymmetry of the ankle joint is best delineated on mortise views obtained in 10 degrees of internal rotation.[738] Such assessment is important, as even minor degrees of displace-

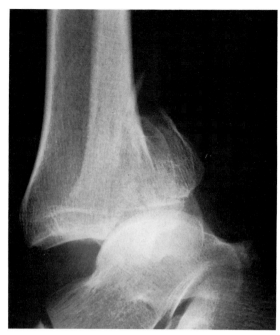

FIGURE 68–133. Ankle injuries: Tibiotalar dislocation. A large posterior tibial fracture is associated with the talar dislocation.

ment of the talus with respect to the tibia can result in secondary degenerative joint disease.[739] Arthrography can be used to demonstrate the presence and site of ligamentous injury, although the examination must be accomplished shortly after the traumatic insult (see Chapter 13).

A peculiar type of ankle injury resulting from severe external rotation of the foot may lead to posterior displacement of the fibula, which becomes locked behind the tibia.[740, 741] This injury, which sometimes is referred to as a Bosworth fracture-dislocation of the ankle,[742] is rare, may be associated with a spiral fracture of the distal fibula, and easily is misdiagnosed on radiographic examination. When both the knee and the ankle are imaged, severe external rotation of the foot readily is apparent, however, and on a true lateral radiograph of the ankle, the fibula courses posterior to the tibia throughout its length.[2] The fibular fracture, if present, must occur within 1 cm of the ankle mortise to ensure that the proximal portion of the fibula is of sufficient length to lodge behind the distal tibia.[740] An anterior variant of this injury also has been described.[743]

Foot

Fractures and Dislocations of the Talus. Of the tarsal bones, injuries of the talus deserve some degree of emphasis, as this bone has functional importance in transmitting the body's weight and allowing motion between the lower leg and foot; it also has unique anatomic characteristics that include a tenuous blood supply (see Chapter 80), which increases its susceptibility to posttraumatic ischemic necrosis, and lack of muscular attachments, which increases the likelihood of dislocation.[744] It is second only to the calcaneus as a site of fracture in the tarsal bones. Such fractures were encountered commonly during World War I, leading to the utilization of the term "aviator's astragalus"[745] and are seen today in a variety of situations in which there occurs sudden hyperextension of the forefoot (e.g., sudden

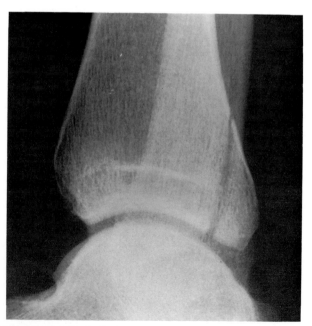

FIGURE 68–132. Ankle injuries: Isolated fracture of the posterior tibial margin. This rare injury may be overlooked on the true lateral projection.

application of the brakes of an automobile to avoid an accident). Avulsion fractures predominate, occurring in the superior surface of the talar neck and the lateral, medial, and posterior aspects of the body[744]; major injuries of the talus also are seen, and these may involve the head, neck, or body, sometimes in association with dislocation of the bone.[746]

With regard to the avulsion fractures, most are produced by a twisting or rotational force combined with flexion or extension stresses (Fig. 68–134). A longitudinal compression force in combination with acute plantar flexion presumably accounts for the avulsion fracture of the anterosuperior surface of the talar neck; eversion stress may lead to osseous avulsion at the site of attachment of the deep fibers of the deltoid ligament to the body of the talus (Fig. 68–135); the posterior process may be fractured during severe plantar flexion of the foot, owing to its compression between the posterior surface of the tibia and the calcaneus; and disruption of the talar body where the bone projects beneath the tip of the lateral malleolus may result from severe dorsiflexion and external rotation.[747] Those fractures involving the posterior process of the talus may be difficult to differentiate from the os trigonum.

Fractures of the head of the talus are rare (Fig. 68–136), may consist of multiple fragments, and probably are related to a longitudinal compression force combined with plantar flexion of the foot.[748] Associated injuries of the tarsal navicular bone and talonavicular joint are encountered.

Fractures of the talar neck are second in frequency to avulsion injuries of the bone (Fig. 68–137). Dorsiflexion related to a force from below or, more rarely, a direct blow to the talus produces this fracture. The extent of the injury varies. Nondisplaced vertical fractures represent the least extensive pattern, whereas displaced fractures combined with subluxation or dislocation of the subtalar joint or both the subtalar and the ankle joints are indicative of considerable injury.[749–751] Complications of talar neck fractures in-

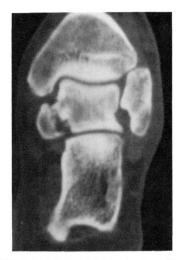

FIGURE 68–135. Talar injuries: Avulsion fracture of talar body. Fractures of the medial portion of the talus may result from avulsion owing to the attachment site of the deep fibers of the deltoid ligament. (Courtesy of G. Greenway, M.D., Dallas, Texas.)

clude delayed union or nonunion, infection, osteoarthritis of adjacent articulations, and ischemic necrosis (Fig. 68–137), the last occurring in a minority of cases of nondisplaced fractures and in as many as 80 to 90 per cent of cases of displaced fractures, particularly those with dislocations.[749, 750, 752, 753] It is the proximal portion of the bone that is affected in ischemic necrosis, with reportable exceptions.[754] The appearance of a linear subchondral lucent area

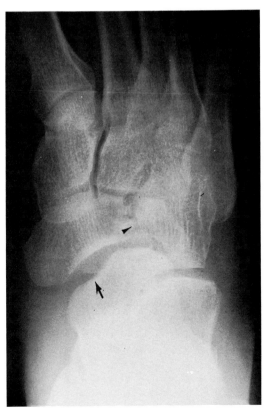

FIGURE 68–136. Talar injuries: Fracture of the head of the talus. In this example, an abnormal depression of the talar head (arrow) is accompanied by a fracture of the tarsal navicular bone (arrowhead) and widening of the talonavicular and calcaneocuboid spaces.

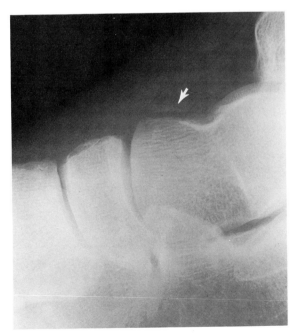

FIGURE 68–134. Talar injuries: Avulsion fracture of talar neck. An example of this relatively common injury is shown (arrow).

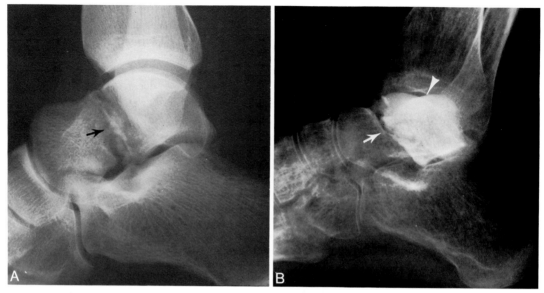

FIGURE 68–137. Talar injuries: Fracture of the talar neck.

A Observe the vertical fracture line (arrow) with slight subluxation leading to widening of the talocalcaneal space in the region of the sustentaculum tali. An acute fracture of the posterior tubercle of the talus also occurred.

B Ischemic necrosis (arrowhead) of the proximal half of the talus, leading to a relative increase in radiodensity of the bone owing to adjacent widespread osteoporosis, is the result of a fracture of the talar neck (arrow).

(the Hawkins sign) in the talar dome on radiographs obtained 1 to 3 months following a talar neck fracture relates to hyperemia and continuity of blood supply and should not be misinterpreted as a crescent sign of osteonecrosis. The absence of such a radiolucent zone is considered a poor prognostic sign, owing to the likelihood of ischemic necrosis of the proximal portion of the talus.

Fractures of the body of the talus are infrequent (Fig. 68–138); they may involve the posterior or lateral process (as discussed previously), the articular surface, or all regions, especially in instances of fracture comminution.[755, 756] Varying amounts of displacement of the fragments and

adjacent articulations (subtalar, ankle) are observed. Complications include ischemic necrosis, osteoarthritis, and delayed union.

Transchondral fractures of the talus (osteochondritis dissecans) are discussed in Chapter 67.

Subluxations or dislocations of the talus generally are accompanied by fractures of the bone, although they may occur as an isolated phenomenon. They usually are classified as subtalar (peritalar) dislocations and total talar dislocations (Fig. 68–139). The first pattern indicates simultaneous disruption of the talocalcaneal and talonavicular articulations.[757–760]

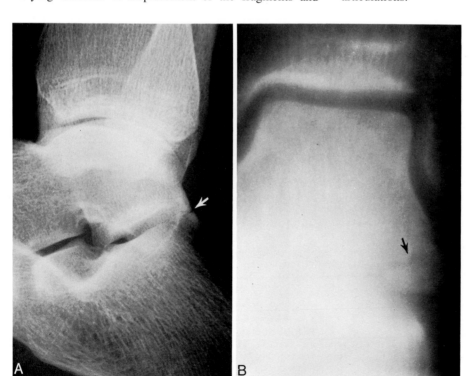

FIGURE 68–138. Talar injuries: Fracture of the body of the talus.

A Fracture (arrow) of the lateral tubercle of the posterior process (Shepherd's fracture).

B Fracture of the lateral process (arrow).

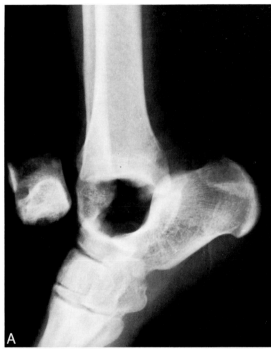

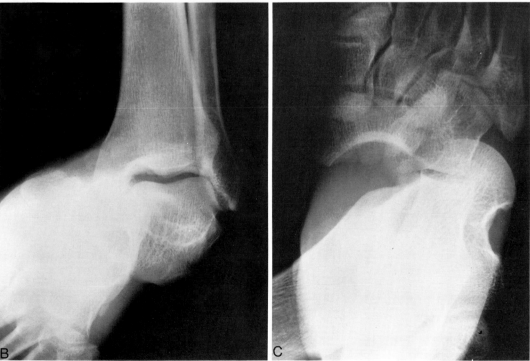

FIGURE 68–139. Talar injuries: Dislocation.
   A Total dislocation of the talus. (Courtesy of J. Hembree, M.D., Palo Alto, California.)
   B, C Medial subtalar dislocation. Note the dislocation of the anterior talocalcaneonavicular and posterior subtalar joints and a relatively normal alignment of the calcaneocuboid joint.

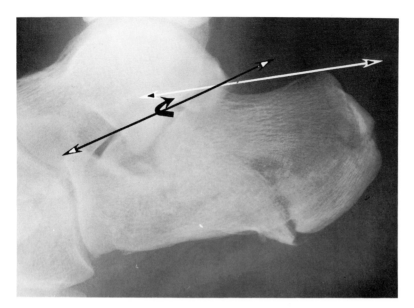

FIGURE 68–140. Calcaneal injuries: Measurement of Böhler's angle. This angle (curved arrow) is formed by the intersection of two lines: The first line is drawn from the highest part of the anterior process of the calcaneus and the highest point of the posterior articular surface; the second line is drawn between the latter point and the most superior part of the calcaneal tuberosity. Böhler's tuber joint angle normally measures between 25 and 40 degrees. In this example it is decreased owing to a complex intra-articular calcaneal fracture.

Medial subtalar dislocations are most frequent, representing approximately 55 to 80 per cent of all such dislocations,[761] and are produced by forceful inversion of the foot with the sustentaculum tali acting as a fulcrum for the posterior portion of the talar body,[762] an injury that occurs most typically in basketball games (basketball foot).[763] Lateral subtalar dislocations are second in frequency, followed by anterior and posterior subtalar dislocations, which are rare. Recurrent dislocations occur but also are rare. Associated fractures are observed in the talus or other bones of the foot and ankle, particularly with medial and lateral subtalar dislocations.

Total dislocation of the talus is an extremely infrequent and serious injury in which the talus generally becomes located medially or laterally.[764] Ischemic necrosis of the talus and infection are two important complications.[765]

Fractures of the Calcaneus. The calcaneus is the most common site of tarsal fracture and, deservingly, such fractures have received a great deal of attention. Although ac-

curate diagnosis commonly is provided by routine and specialized radiographs (see Chapters 1 and 22), especially if attention is directed at Bohler's angle, as depicted on the lateral projection (Fig. 68–140), the complexity of calcaneal anatomy has prompted considerable interest in CT as a technique that ideally displays the extent of injury[766–774] (see Chapter 8). Fractures of the calcaneus can be classified broadly into those that are intra-articular (approximately 75 per cent) and those that are extra-articular (approximately 25 per cent of cases); the former are associated with a poorer prognosis owing to displacement of fragments (typically, varus rotation of the sustentacular fragment, valgus rotation of the lateral fragment, and varus, lateral, and upward displacement of the body fragment) and to disruption of the subtalar articulations.[775, 776] Although further division of these major categories is emphasized in some classification systems, there is no uniformity of opinion regarding the specific fracture designations or the prognostic importance of such subdivisions.[777, 778]

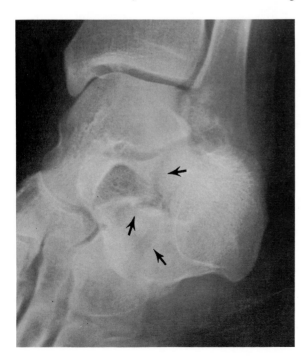

FIGURE 68–141. Calcaneal injuries: Intra-articular fractures. In this oblique radiograph, a comminuted fracture line (arrows) involving the sustentaculum tali extends into the posterior subtalar joint.

Intra-articular fractures (Fig. 68–141) generally occur as a result of a vertical fall in which the talus is driven into the cancellous bone of the calcaneus[779]; this mechanism of injury explains the frequency (10 per cent) of bilateral calcaneal fractures as well as the simultaneous occurrence of spinal injuries. A primary fracture line extends downward toward the plantar surface of the bone (dividing the bone into an anteromedial fragment, including the sustentaculum tali, and a posterior fragment with the posterior facet), and secondary fracture lines extend in two different directions. Those secondary fractures that extend anteriorly may enter the calcaneocuboid joint or exit just proximal to it; those that extend posteriorly may exit just behind the subtalar joint (central depression type) or at the posterior cortex of the tuberosity (tongue type).[780] Comminution and rotation of fragments are common. CT is a useful technique for the delineation of complex intra-articular fractures (Fig. 68–

142). Extra-articular calcaneal fractures (Fig. 68–143) result from several different mechanisms, of which twisting forces are most important. They may localize to the anterior or medial processes, the sustentaculum tali, the body, or the tuberosity. Certain avulsive injuries, such as those affecting the calcaneal tuberosity, are relatively easy to detect on radiographic examination; others, including one that apparently arises at the origin of the extensor digitorum brevis muscle on the lateral surface of the bone, may be somewhat subtle.[780, 781] Fractures of the anterior process of the calcaneus,[782, 783] related to attachment sites of the ligamentum bifurcatum, also may escape detection unless careful analysis of the radiographs is undertaken; acute calcaneal fractures in children, although rare,[784] and stress fractures may be especially difficult to delineate.[785]

The diagnostic problems encountered in intra-articular fractures are of another sort. Fracture comminution and

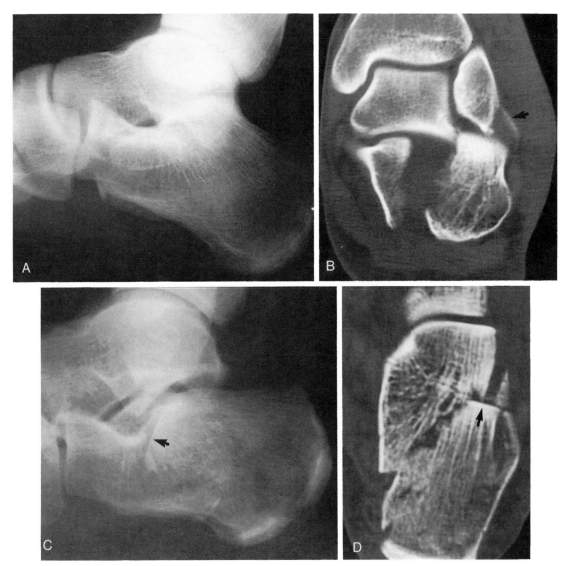

FIGURE 68–142. Calcaneal injuries: Intra-articular fractures. CT.

A, B Although routine radiography **(A)** reveals an intra-articular fracture of the calcaneus, the status of the posterior subtalar joint is difficult to determine. A direct coronal CT scan **(B)** shows marked lateral displacement of the lateral portion of the calcaneus, abutment of this region of the calcaneus and the distal fibula, displacement of the peroneal tendons with a fibular avulsion fracture (arrow), and uncovering of the posterior facet of the talus.

C, D In a second patient, note the depression (arrow) of the posterior facet of the calcaneus on a routine radiograph **(C)**. A comminuted fracture line is seen. A transverse CT scan **(D)** shows the rotated subchondral bone plate (arrow) of this posterior facet and an intact calcaneocuboid joint.

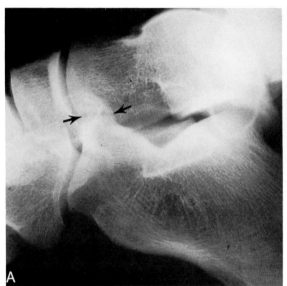

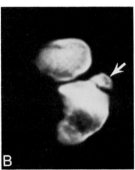

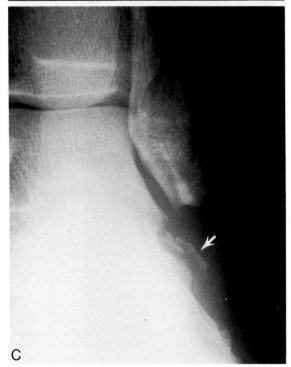

FIGURE 68–143. Calcaneal injuries: Extra-articular fractures.
   A, B Fracture of the anterior process of the calcaneus (arrows). (Courtesy of A. Polansky, M.D., San Diego, California.)
   C Fracture at the origin of the extensor digitorum brevis muscle (arrow).

displacement are common, creating many irregular pieces of bone that are difficult to identify.[786, 787] It is here that conventional[788] or computed[767, 768] tomography is most useful in defining not only the characteristics of the acute injury but also its sequelae, including osteoarthritis of the subtalar joints, malunion, and peroneal tendon dislocation or entrapment between the calcaneus and the fibula.

Fractures of Other Tarsal Bones. Fractures elsewhere in the tarsus are infrequent. Typical sites of injury in the tarsal navicular bone are its dorsal surface near the talonavicular space and the tuberosity and body of the bone.[744] Fractures of the navicular tuberosity may be combined with injuries of the calcaneus and cuboid, whereas isolated fractures of the cuboid and the cuneiforms are rare. In all instances, differentiation between a fracture and the common accessory bones must be accomplished, and the latter themselves may fracture.[789, 790] Fracture of the os peroneum (Fig. 68–144) is rare but may be associated with wide separation of the bone fragments, related to the action of the peroneus longus muscle. It may result from direct trauma or indirect stress that results from violent dorsiflexion of the foot. The latter mechanism of injury also may produce a rupture of the peroneus longus tendon.[791] Such rupture leads to displacement of the os peroneum from its normal position adjacent to the lower border of the cuboid bone or the calcaneocuboid joint.

Tarsal Dislocation. Subluxation, dislocation, and fracture-dislocation are common injuries in the midfoot and hindfoot.[792–795] Of particular interest is the Lisfranc's fracture-dislocation of the tarsometatarsal joints[796–800] (Fig. 68–145). Normally, the heads of the metatarsal bones are joined by transverse ligaments.[798] Similarly, the bases of the metatarsal bones reveal ligamentous connections,[801] except between the base of the first and that of the second metatarsal bone. An oblique ligament extends between the medial cuneiform and the second metatarsal base, anchoring the base of this metatarsal bone, which also is stabilized because of its recessed position between the cuneiforms.

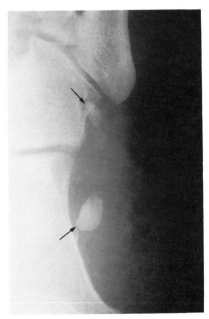

FIGURE 68–144. Fracture of the os peroneum. Note wide separation of the fracture fragments (arrows) and adjacent soft tissue swelling. (Courtesy of M. Pathria, M.D., San Diego, California.)

Injuries of the tarsometatarsal joints can result from direct or, more commonly, indirect trauma (Fig. 68–146). In the latter situation, violent abduction of the forefoot can lead to lateral displacement of the four lateral metatarsal bones with or without a fracture at the base of the second metatarsal bone and the cuboid bone (Fig. 68–145). Accompanying dorsal displacement is more frequent than plantar displacement, a predilection that is explained, at least in part, by the relatively wide configuration of the dorsal surface of the base of the second metatarsal bone. The first metatarsal bone may dislocate in the same direction or in the opposite direction of the other metatarsal bones, depending on the precise vectors of the force.[802, 803]

Radiographic examination usually identifies the dislocation and accompanying fractures, although the findings may be subtle and other techniques, including the application of stress,[800] weight-bearing radiography,[804] and CT,[805] have been emphasized (Fig. 68–147). Proper recognition of abnormal alignment in the tarsometatarsal joints requires knowledge of normal radiographic anatomy.[797] A consistent relationship in the normal foot is the alignment of the medial edge of the base of the second metatarsal bone with the medial edge of the second cuneiform on the frontal and oblique views of the foot. A small space or gap between the bases of the first and second metatarsal bones does not, by itself, represent a definite sign of dislocation; rather, disruption of the alignment of the second metatarsal bone and second cuneiform with a step-off between the bones is more diagnostic of an injury. The normal alignment of the bases of the fourth and fifth metatarsal bones with the cuboid and that of the base of the first metatarsal bone with the medial cuneiform are more variable.

Other varieties of tarsal subluxation and dislocation (Fig. 68–148) have been described, although most are rare.[806–811] These have been well classified by Main and Jowett.[812]

Metatarsophalangeal and Interphalangeal Joint Dislocation. Dislocations at the metatarsophalangeal joints can occur in any direction, related to the mechanism of injury. The first metatarsophalangeal joint commonly is affected.[813] Similarly, patterns of dislocation of interphalangeal joints in the foot are variable (Fig. 68–149). The interphalangeal joint of the hallux most typically is affected. Pseudodislocation of the proximal interphalangeal joint of the fifth toe following trauma has been related to accumulation of joint fluid or soft tissue injury. Sesamoid bone dislocations with or without intra-articular entrapment are rare and usually confined to the first ray.[814–817] Such entrapment, as well as that related to the volar plate,[818] leads to persistent widening of the articulation following attempts at reduction of the dislocation (Fig. 68–150).

Hyperextension of the first metatarsophalangeal joint that occurs in American football, soccer, and basketball players may lead to disruption of the plantar aspect of the joint capsule, which tears away from the metatarsal head, an injury designated turf-toe, owing to its occurrence on playing fields made of artificial turf.[819] Plantar flexion or valgus stress applied to this articulation is a less common mechanism of injury. Rarely, hyperextension of the first metatarsophalangeal joint leads to extensive disruption of the plantar plate with lateral dislocation or proximal or distal migration of the sesamoid bones or sesamoid fracture without joint dislocation[820, 821] (Fig. 68–151). Sequelae of any of these hyperextension injuries include chondromalacia of the

Text continued on page 2800

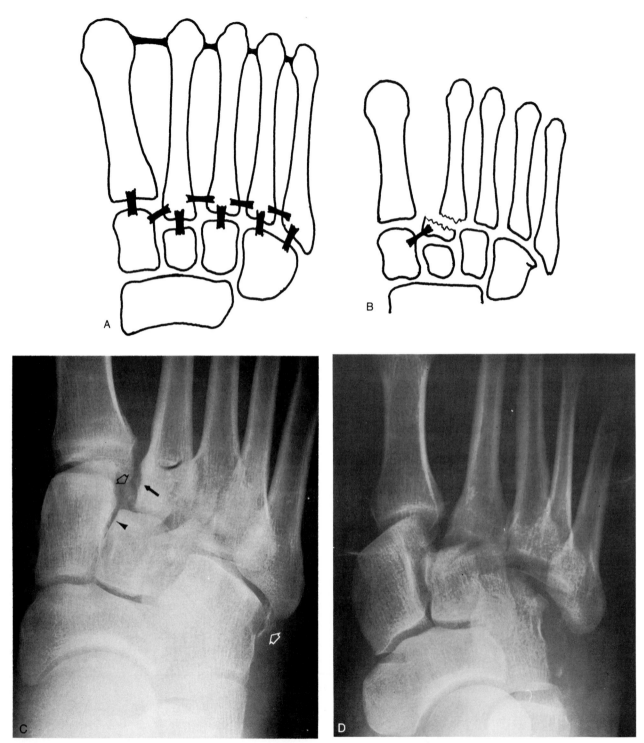

FIGURE 68–145. Lisfranc's fracture-dislocation of tarsometatarsal joints.

A Normal ligamentous anatomy (see text).

B Lateral dislocation of the second through fifth metatarsal bones may be associated with fractures of the base of the second metatarsal bone and cuboid.

C In this patient, note subtle displacement of the second through fifth metatarsal bases. The medial edge of the second metatarsal base (solid arrow) is not aligned with the medial edge of the second cuneiform (arrowhead). Fractures of the base of the second metatarsal bone and cuboid are evident (open arrows).

D One additional example of this injury is shown. Findings include lateral displacement of all of the metatarsal bones and fractures of several of the metatarsal bases and cuboid.

(**A, B,** From Wiley JJ: J Bone Joint Surg [Br] *53*:474, 1971.)

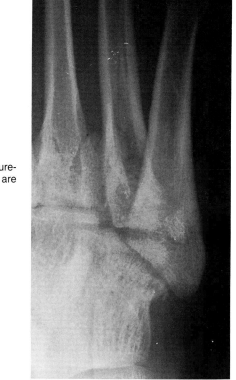

FIGURE 68–146. Injuries of the tarsometatarsal joints. In this example, observe fracture-dislocations at the bases of the fourth and fifth metatarsal bones. Fracture lines also are identified in the diaphysis of the fourth metatarsal bone and the cuboid.

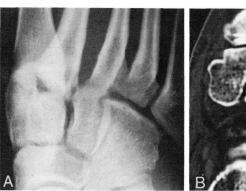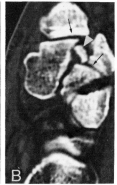

FIGURE 68–147. Injuries of the tarsometatarsal joints: Stress radiography and CT.

A Radiography obtained during the application of valgus stress to the forefoot accentuates the degree of lateral displacement of the metatarsal bases.

B In a second case, a transverse CT scan demonstrates lateral displacement of the bases of the first and second metatarsal bones (arrows) and fractures of the cuneiform bones and second metatarsal base (arrowhead).

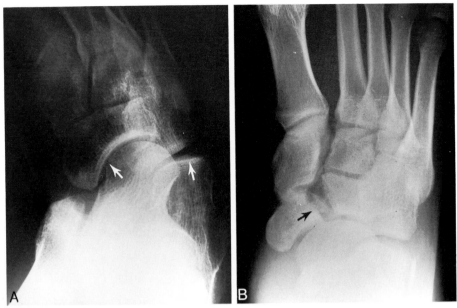

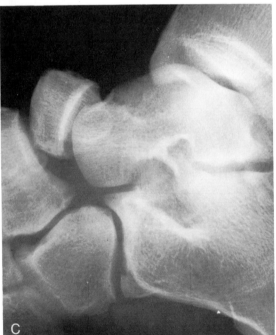

FIGURE 68–148. Tarsal subluxations and dislocations.

A Midtarsal subluxation (subluxation of Chopart's joint). Note medial displacement of the forefoot occurring at the talonavicular and calcaneocuboid spaces (arrows). This has been referred to as a swivel injury. (Courtesy of P. Kaplan, M.D., Charlottesville, Virginia.)

B Tarsal navicular fracture with separation of the first ray. Note the longitudinal fracture of the navicular bone (arrow), which is aligned with the space between the medial and intermediate cuneiforms. This latter space is widened, and adjacent small fracture fragments are seen.

C Tarsal navicular dislocation. A dorsal dislocation of the navicular bone and a calcaneal fracture are seen.

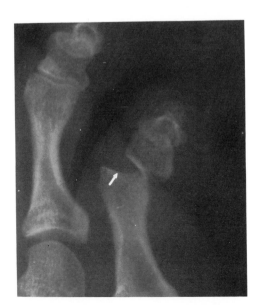

FIGURE 68–149. Dislocation of the interphalangeal joints in the foot. Note the widened proximal interphalangeal joint of the fifth toe (arrow) with lateral displacement of the middle and distal phalanges.

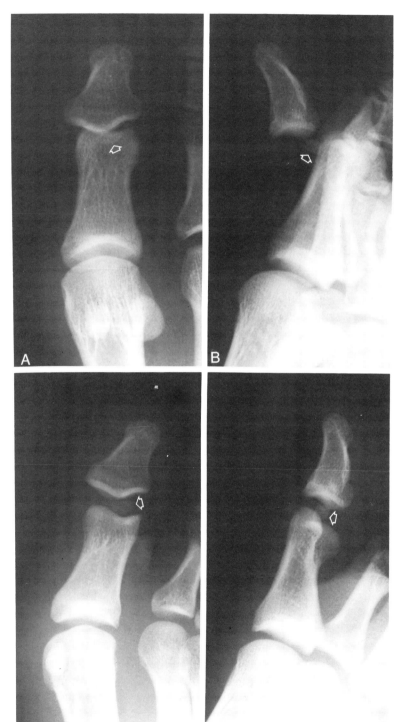

FIGURE 68–150. Dislocation of the interphalangeal joint of the great toe with entrapment of the sesamoid bone.

A, B The initial radiographs reveal dorsal dislocation at the interphalangeal joint of the great toe. Note the position of the sesamoid bone (open arrows).

C, D Following attempts at reduction of the injury, radiographs reveal intra-articular entrapment of the sesamoid bone (open arrows).

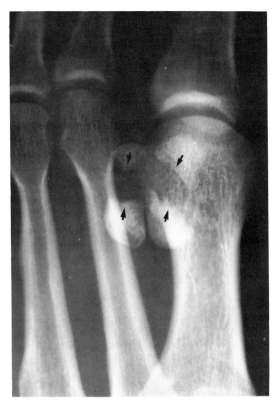

FIGURE 68–151. Disruption of the plantar capsule of the first metatarsophalangeal joint with displaced sesamoid fractures (turf-toe). Note the diastasis between the fracture fragments (arrows). (Courtesy of B. Howard, M.D., Charlotte, North Carolina.)

head of the first metatarsal bone, hallux rigidus or valgus, dorsal osteophytes, and periarticular calcification.[819]

Fractures of the Metatarsal Bones and Phalanges. Metatarsal fractures, which may result from direct or indirect forces or as a response to chronic stress (see Chapter 67) or neuropathic osteoarthropathy (see Chapter 78), may be transverse, oblique, spiral, or comminuted in configuration (Fig. 68–152). Those of the shaft and neck of the bone commonly result from a heavy object falling on the foot; they are relatively infrequent in the first metatarsal bone owing to its larger size and may be associated with significant displacement (which is best observed on the lateral radiographs). Fractures of the metatarsal head are uncommon, result from direct injury, and usually are accompanied by fractures of adjacent metatarsal necks or shafts.

Fractures of the base of the fifth metatarsal bone have received a great deal of attention in the medical literature.[822–825] Two major types exist: an avulsion fracture of the tuberosity and a transverse fracture of the proximal portion of the diaphysis. The latter injury is termed a Jones fracture.[826] Avulsion of a portion of the tuberosity of the fifth metatarsal bone results from an indirect injury associated with sudden inversion of the foot. Its further pathogenesis is debated, with alternative theories implicating the peroneus brevis tendon or the lateral cord of the plantar aponeurosis in the production of the injury.[825] The osseous fragment varies considerably in size as well as degree of displacement, and the fracture line usually is transverse and may enter the cuboid-metatarsal joint space. Differentiation of the fracture from a normal appearing apophysis of the fifth metatarsal bone in children can be difficult; the latter

is oriented in a longitudinal direction and the radiolucent line that exists between it and the parent bone does not enter the cuboid-metatarsal space (Fig. 68–153). Normal sesamoid bones (including the os peroneum and os vesalianum) that occur in this region create further diagnostic difficulty, although they are smooth and round, differing from the appearance of an avulsion fracture.

A fracture in the proximal diaphyseal region of the fifth metatarsal bone, the true Jones fracture, results from either direct or indirect forces and is associated with delayed union or nonunion and refracture.

Fractures of the phalanges of the toes are common and create few diagnostic problems[827] (Fig. 68–154). Of particular importance are displaced intra-articular fractures (which may require surgical reduction) and, in children, physeal injuries of the distal phalanx (the stubbed great toe, which may be open and accompanied by osteomyelitis)[828] (Fig. 68–155). Sesamoid fractures, especially in the first ray, also are encountered (Fig. 68–156).

AXIAL SKELETON

Pelvis

Fractures and Dislocations of the Pelvis. In common with the situation in the skull and in the thoracic cage, the bony pelvis is intimate with vital internal organs and it is the evaluation of these organs that becomes mandatory in cases in which osseous or ligamentous disruption is apparent. Hemorrhage owing to vascular injury of arteries (e.g., hypogastric and superior gluteal arteries and their branches) or veins, injury of the urinary tract (e.g., bladder and urethra), compression of peripheral nerves (e.g., the sacral plexus, sciatic nerve, and lumbosacral nerve roots) and disruption of viscera (e.g., liver and spleen) are among the significant complications of pelvic fractures and dislocations, the frequency of which depends on the site and the magnitude of the abnormal forces. Radiographic examinations directed at the detection of such complications are as fundamental to proper analysis of pelvic fractures and dislocations as are the radiographs of the bones themselves. With regard to the latter radiographs, adequate technique is made difficult owing to patient pain and discomfort and depends on the inclusion of specialized projections (including oblique radiographs and angled views)[829, 830] and CT (with or without three-dimensional display of image data). Accurate interpretation of the radiographs is complicated by the presence of gaseous shadows that obscure osseous and soft tissue detail, yet close inspection is required in the detection of subtle clues that indicate intraperitoneal or retroperitoneal bleeding. Furthermore, as the bony pelvis as a whole is a ringlike structure and, indeed, some of its components also are rings (e.g., pubic rami), it is common to encounter more than a single injury (in the form of a fracture, subluxation, or dislocation), so that the excitement of detecting one abnormal area on the radiograph should not lead to a cursory review of other skeletal parts.

Fractures of the pelvis, which account for approximately 3 per cent of all fractures,[831] have been classified in a number of ways on the basis of such factors as site(s) of involvement, direction of force, and mechanisms of injury.[832–840] No system is ideal, as attention to both biomechanical and anatomic aspects is required. These biome-

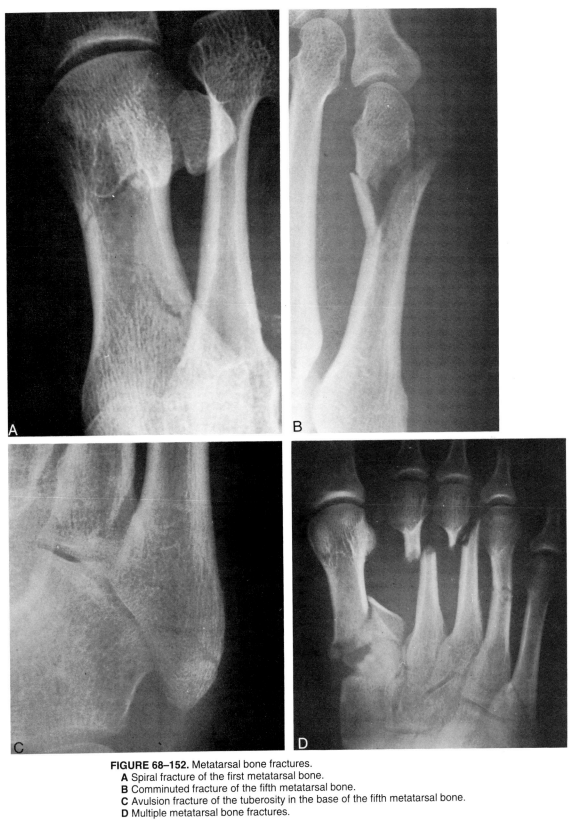

FIGURE 68–152. Metatarsal bone fractures.
A Spiral fracture of the first metatarsal bone.
B Comminuted fracture of the fifth metatarsal bone.
C Avulsion fracture of the tuberosity in the base of the fifth metatarsal bone.
D Multiple metatarsal bone fractures.

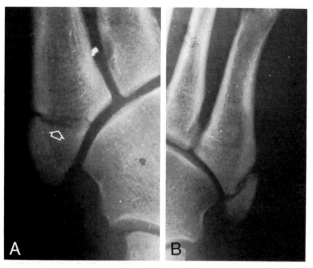

FIGURE 68–153. Metatarsal bone fractures: Fracture at the base of the fifth metatarsal bone.

A The fracture line (open arrow) is identified entering the space between the metatarsal base and the cuboid.

B On the opposite side, a normal apophysis is present. The radiolucent line between it and the metatarsal bone does not enter the joint.

chanics have been well outlined by Tile,[841, 842] whose book should be consulted by the interested reader and whose observations are summarized here.

The major forces acting on the pelvic ring are external rotation, lateral compression (internal rotation), vertical shear, and complex forces (Fig. 68–157).

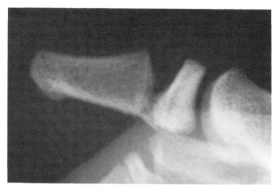

FIGURE 68–155. Physeal injury in the foot: Stubbed great toe. This Salter-Harris type 1 injury of the distal phalanx commonly is associated with violation of the nail bed, creating an open injury.

External Rotation. External rotation may occur when a direct force is applied either to the posterior superior iliac spines (Fig. 68–157*B*) or to the anterior superior iliac spines or the femora (Fig. 68–157*C*). This mechanism of injury relates to disruptive forces in the sagittal plane and, sometimes, is referred to as anteroposterior compression. The pelvis is opened like a book, with diastasis of the symphysis pubis and disruption of the anterior sacroiliac and sacrospinous ligaments. In the absence of a shearing force, the posterior ligaments usually remain intact so that no vertical displacement is seen.

Lateral Compression. A lateral compressive force applied to the iliac crest leads to internal rotation of the hemipelvis with disruption of the anterior portion of the

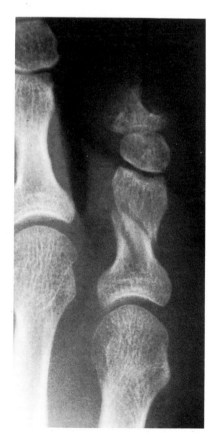

FIGURE 68–154. Phalangeal fractures in the foot. A typical example is shown.

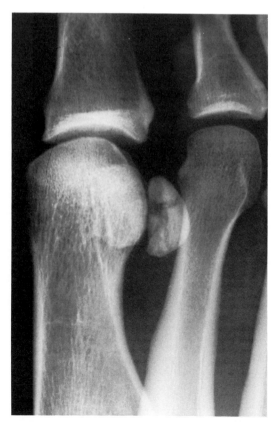

FIGURE 68–156. Sesamoid fractures in the foot. Note a comminuted fracture of the lateral sesamoid bone at the first metatarsophalangeal joint.

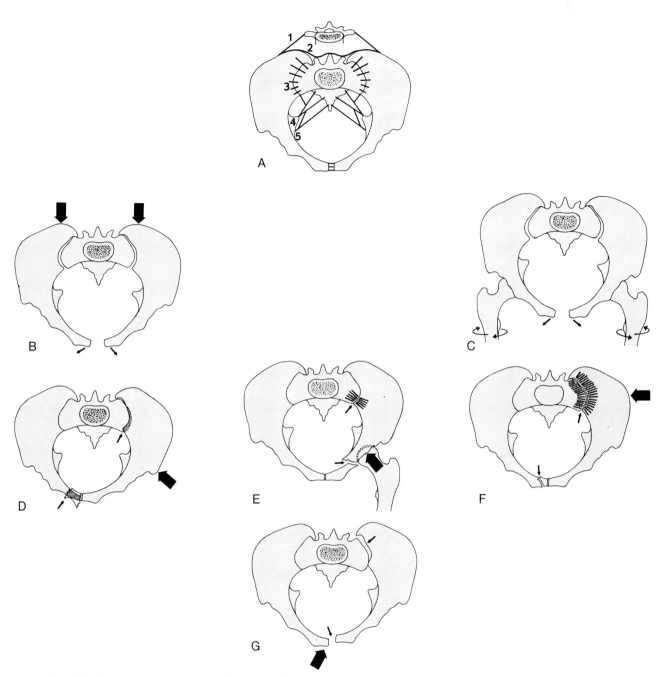

FIGURE 68–157. Fractures and dislocations of the pelvis: Biomechanical principles.

A Normal situation. Schematic representation of the major ligamentous structures is shown. These include the iliolumbar ligaments (1), posterior (2) and anterior (3) sacroiliac ligaments, sacrospinous ligaments (4), and sacrotuberous ligaments (5).

B External rotation forces. A direct blow to the posterior superior iliac spines (large arrows) leads to opening of the symphysis pubis (small arrows). Without the addition of a shearing force, the posterior ligamentous complex remains intact.

C External rotation forces. External rotation of the femora (curved arrows) or direct compression against the anterior superior iliac spines also produces springing of the symphysis pubis (small arrows). Without the addition of a shearing force, the posterior ligamentous complex remains intact.

D Lateral compression forces. A lateral compression force against the iliac crest (large arrow) causes the hemipelvis to rotate internally. The anterior portions of the sacrum and pubic rami (small arrows) are injured.

E Lateral compression forces. A direct force against the greater trochanter (large arrow) leads to similar injuries to the pubic rami and ipsilateral sacroiliac joint ligamentous complex (small arrows).

F Lateral compression forces. A force (large arrow) directed parallel to the trabeculae about the sacroiliac joint may produce impaction of bone posteriorly and disruption of the pubic rami (small arrows).

G Vertical shearing forces. A shearing force (large arrow) crosses perpendicular to the main trabecular pattern, and causes both anterior and posterior injuries (small arrows).

(From Tile M: Fractures of the Pelvis and Acetabulum. Copyright 1984, Williams & Wilkins Co, Baltimore, p 22.)

sacrum and displacement of the anterior pubic rami (Fig. 68–157D). A similar force applied to the greater trochanter will produce disruption of the pubic rami and ipsilateral sacroiliac complex (Fig. 68–157E). A third pattern of lateral compression occurs when the forces are directed parallel to the trabeculae about the sacroiliac joint, causing impaction of bone (Fig. 68–157F). In general, these mechanisms are associated with compression of posterior pelvic structures and the absence of posterior ligamentous disruption.

Vertical Shear. Vertical shearing forces, acting perpendicular to the major trabecular pattern of the posterior pelvic complex, cause displacement of bone and disruption of soft tissues both anteriorly and posteriorly (Fig. 68–157G).

Complex Forces. Complex forces represent the combination of external rotation, lateral compression, and shear.

In this scheme, stability of the pelvic ring is considered to depend primarily on the integrity of its ligamentous structures, especially those located posteriorly. Instability is most characteristic of injuries resulting from vertical shear and complex forces. In severe forms of lateral compression (in which the lateral compressive forces on one side of the pelvis continue to the contralateral side as distracting forces with external rotation of the anterior portion of the pelvis) and of anteroposterior compression (in which all of the sacroiliac ligaments are disrupted), pelvic instability may result.[839] In other classification systems, stable fractures generally are considered to be those that either do not disrupt the osseous ring or disrupt it only in one place, and unstable fractures are those that disrupt the ring in two or more places. This latter approach is well suited to the conventional radiographic examination, which is able to identify directly only osseous elements and to assess indirectly ligamentous structures by delineating sites of diastasis. CT, although possessing superior contrast resolution, allows identification of sites of soft tissue hemorrhage but is unable to define precisely the status of the pelvic ligaments. CT does provide an exquisite cross-sectional display of the bony pelvis[843] and, combined with conventional radiography, can delineate cephalad or posterior displacement of the hemipelvis, which generally is considered a sign of instability.[832] MR imaging eventually may hold the key to the accurate analysis of both the osseous and the ligamentous structures of the pelvis.

In the pages that follow, a summary of injuries of the bony pelvis is organized according to sites of involvement and the presence or absence of disruption of the pelvic ring; this represents a slight modification of the excellent analysis provided by Kane[844] (Table 68–7 and Fig. 68–158).

1. Type I injuries. Type I injuries, which do not lead to disruption of the pelvic ring, constitute approximately 30 per cent of all injuries that involve the bony pelvis. Avulsion fractures, which are considered in Chapter 67, occur at sites of muscular and tendinous insertions, such as the anterior superior iliac spine, anterior inferior iliac spine, ischial tuberosity, symphysis pubis, and iliac crest, particularly in adolescent athletes involved in gymnastics, running, jumping, and hurdling (Fig. 68–158A).

Unilateral fractures of a single ramus are very common (Fig. 68–158B), occur in elderly patients following a fall as well as in the form of a stress fracture in athletes and following hip surgery, and are somewhat more frequent in

TABLE 68–7. Injuries of the Bony Pelvis*

Injuries Without Disruption of the Pelvic Ring
Avulsion fracture
Fracture of the pubis or ischium
Fracture of the iliac wing
Fracture of the sacrum
Fracture or dislocation of the coccyx

Injuries with Single Break in the Pelvic Ring
Fractures of two ipsilateral rami
Fracture near, or subluxation of, the symphysis pubis
Fracture near, or subluxation of, the sacroiliac joint

Injuries with Double Breaks in the Pelvic Ring
Double vertical fractures or dislocations of the pubis (straddle fracture)
Double vertical fractures or dislocations of the pelvis (Malgaigne fracture)
Multiple fractures

Injuries of the Acetabulum
Undisplaced fractures
Displaced fractures

*From Kane WJ: Fractures of the pelvis. *In* CA Rockwood Jr, DP Green (Eds): Fractures in Adults. 2nd Ed. Philadelphia, JB Lippincott Co, 1984, p 1112.

the superior ramus than in the inferior ramus.[845] These fractures, which are encountered about twice as often as those involving two or more rami, may be subtle, requiring for diagnosis oblique radiographic projections, are extremely stable, and yet may be associated with subsequent osteolysis simulating that of a malignant tumor (see Chapter 94).

A fracture of the iliac wing, the Duverney fracture, follows a direct injury and rarely is displaced (Figs. 68–158B and 68–159). An isolated transverse fracture of the sacrum (Figs. 68–158B and 68–160) is rare and easily is overlooked on radiographic examination, necessitating the use of CT in some cases.[846, 847] Isolated fractures of the upper sacral segments may be related to indirect force with the lever arm of the lumbar spine acting on a fixed pelvis; those of the lower segments usually result from a direct blow.[848] Neurologic compromise, related to disruption of higher or lower sacral nerve roots, represents a recognized complication of these fractures. This complication appears to be more frequent in cases of upper sacral (as opposed to lower sacral) fractures, and these injuries of the upper sacrum may be associated with fractures of the lumbar transverse processes and occur predominantly at the S1-S2 level. Transverse fractures of the upper or lower portion of the sacrum should be distinguished from vertical fractures (Fig. 68–161) of the sacrum (which may be associated with additional osseous and ligamentous injuries) and from insufficiency stress fractures (which occur in the osteopenic skeleton and have both a vertical and a horizontal configuration). In all instances of sacral fracture, careful radiographic analysis of the foramina and arcuate lines is required,[849–851] and scintigraphy (with a bone-seeking radiopharmaceutical agent) represents a good screening examination in equivocal cases.[852, 853]

A fracture or dislocation of the coccyx represents an additional example of a type I pelvic injury (Fig. 68–158B). Accurate diagnosis is better accomplished on lateral than on frontal radiographs. These injuries are more common in women than in men and also may occur in persons who ride the rapids sitting in an inflated rubber tube (''tubing'' fractures).

2. Type II injuries. The occurrence of a single break in the pelvic ring may represent an enigma to those who

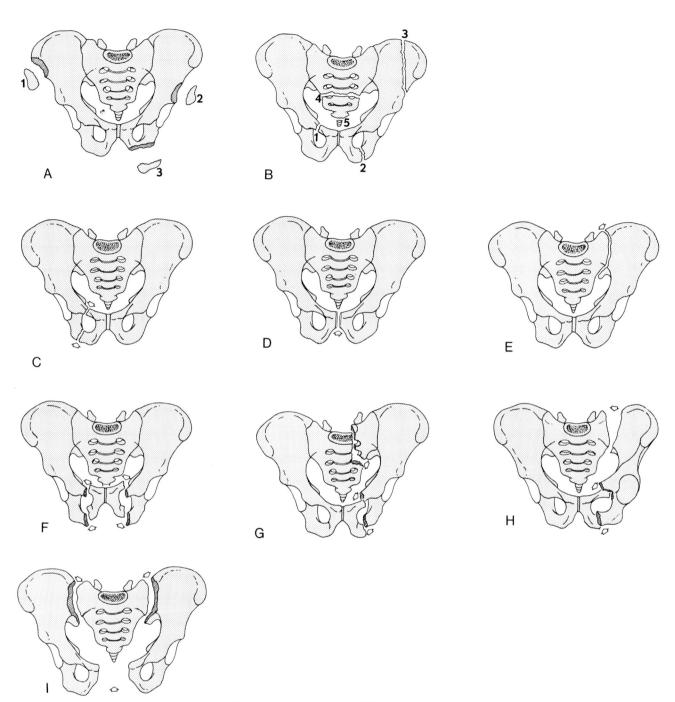

FIGURE 68–158. Fractures and dislocations of the pelvis: Classification system.

A Type I injury: Avulsion fractures. These may involve the anterior superior iliac spine (1), the anterior inferior iliac spine (2), or the ischial tuberosity (3).

B Type I injury: Fractures of a single pubis ramus or iliac wing (Duverney fracture). A single break in the superior or inferior pubic ramus (1, 2), certain fractures of the ilium (3), or some types of fractures of the sacrum (4) or coccyx (5) do not lead to disruption of the pelvic ring.

C Type II injury: Ipsilateral fractures of the pubic rami. Such fractures (open arrows) lead to a single break in the pelvic ring.

D Type II injury: Diastasis of the symphysis pubis. This injury (open arrow), or an isolated fracture of parasymphyseal bone, also leads to a single break in the pelvic ring.

E Type II injury: Subluxation of the sacroiliac joint. This subluxation (open arrow), or an isolated fracture near the sacroiliac joint, is an additional example of a single break in the pelvic ring.

F Type III injury: Straddle fracture. Note disruption of the pelvis in two places owing to bilateral vertical fractures involving both pubic rami (open arrows).

G Type III injury: Malgaigne fracture. Vertical fractures of both pubic rami on one side combined with a sacral fracture (open arrows) lead to disruption of the pelvic ring in two places.

H Type III injury: Malgaigne fracture. Similar vertical fractures of both pubic rami on one side combined with dislocation of the sacroiliac joint (open arrows) again produce disruption of the pelvic ring in two places.

I Complex injury: "Sprung" pelvis. Disruptions of the pelvic ring relate to bilateral dislocations of the sacroiliac joint and diastasis of the symphysis pubis (open arrows).

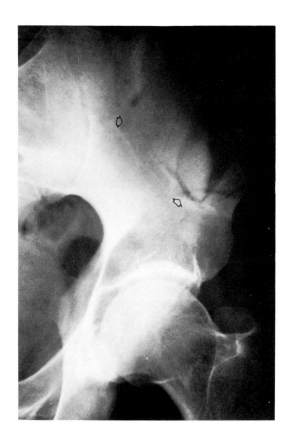

FIGURE 68–159. Fractures and dislocations of the pelvis: Type I fractures of the iliac wing. A comminuted fracture of the ilium (open arrows) does not disrupt the pelvic ring.

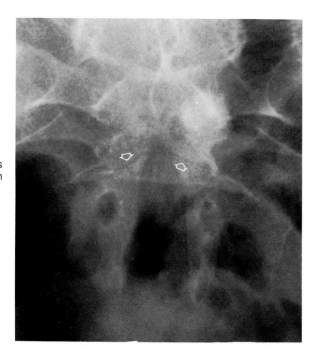

FIGURE 68–160. Fractures and dislocations of the pelvis: Type I fractures of the sacrum. Note the subtle transversely oriented fracture line (open arrows).

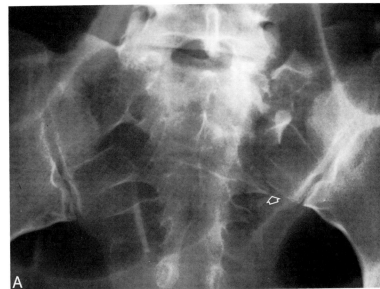

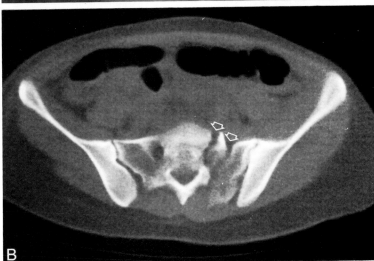

FIGURE 68–161. Fractures and dislocations of the pelvis: Types II and III fractures of the sacrum.

Vertical fractures of the sacrum disrupt the arcuate lines (open arrow), as depicted on frontal radiograph **(A)**. CT **(B)** is better able to define the extent of injury (open arrows).

recognize the difficulty in disrupting a ringlike structure (such as a pretzel) in one place without producing an abnormality somewhere else in the ring. The fact that the bony pelvis is not a rigid structure but one that contains slightly moveable articulations (the symphysis pubis and the sacroiliac joints) explains why its comparison with a pretzel ring is not entirely justified; however, in many instances of an apparently isolated pelvic fracture, bone scintigraphy will indicate that a second region of abnormality truly exists, typically in the form of a subtle diastasis of the sacroiliac articulation.

Ipsilateral fractures of both pubic rami, a fracture of the symphysis itself (Fig. 68–162), subluxation of the sacroiliac joint or symphysis pubis, and a fracture near the sacroiliac articulation are examples of type II pelvic injuries (Fig. 68–158C-E). The conversion of these injuries to a type III pattern represents the next step in a sequence of alterations in which the final result is indicative of the location and extent of the abnormal stresses.[844] The greater the degree of joint diastasis or the more extensive the displacement at the fracture site, the more likely is the occurrence of a second break in the pelvic ring. Diastasis of the symphysis pubis of greater than 15 mm and symphyseal disruption with

overlapping of the pubis represent anterior injuries that should raise the strong possibility of disruption of the posterior aspect of the pelvic ring as well. When symphyseal diastasis is greater than 25 mm, disruption of the sacrospinous and anterior sacroiliac ligaments on one or both sides is highly likely.[842]

An isolated fracture of the symphysis pubis or symphyseal diastasis is a rare injury, and the latter may be difficult to diagnose on the basis of conventional radiographic techniques. Frontal radiographs of the pelvis obtained with the patient standing first on one leg and then on the other may reveal subtle instability of the symphysis pubis, manifested as a changing position of one osseous component with respect to the adjacent one. These injuries, which have been observed in women following pregnancy and in persons who ride real or mechanical horses,[854] may be associated with urethral or bladder disruption, an association that becomes more constant in the presence of greater degrees of symphyseal offset and separation that generally indicate a type III injury pattern.

Similarly, isolated fractures near or separations of the sacroiliac joint are infrequent owing to the likelihood of an accompanying injury to the weaker anterior portion of the

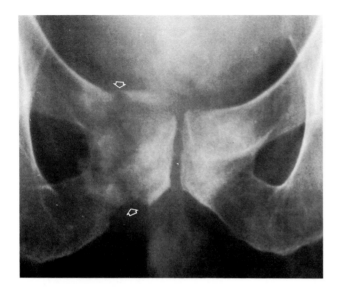

FIGURE 68–162. Fractures and dislocations of the pelvis: Type II parasymphyseal fracture. An insufficiency fracture (open arrows) of parasymphyseal bone in a patient with osteoporosis and rheumatoid arthritis simulates a malignant tumor and disrupts the pelvic ring in one location.

pelvic ring.[844] They usually result from direct trauma to the posterior or posterolateral aspect of the pelvis.

3. Type III injuries. Examples of these injuries, which represent double breaks in the pelvic ring (Fig. 68–163), include straddle fractures (in which there occur vertical fractures of the rami or dislocation of the symphysis pubis) and Malgaigne fractures (in which there is simultaneous disruption of both the anterior and the posterior aspects of the pelvic ring).

Straddle injuries (Figs. 68–158*F* and 68–163) are characterized by disruption of the anterior portion of the pelvis in two places: Bilateral vertical fractures involving both pubic rami or a unilateral fracture of both rami combined with symphyseal diastasis fulfills these criteria.[844] These injuries represent 20 per cent of all pelvic fracture patterns,[835, 855] and are accompanied by urethral or visceral damage in about 30 to 40 per cent of cases.

The term Malgaigne fracture generally is applied to a variety of injuries that have in common disruption of the anterior and posterior regions of the pelvic ring. The forms of this injury include (1) a vertical fracture of both pubic rami combined with either a dislocation of the sacroiliac joint or a fracture of the ilium or sacrum and (2) symphyseal dislocation combined with either a dislocation of the sacroiliac joint or a fracture of the ilium or sacrum[844] (Fig. 68–158*G,H*). With regard to the posterior lesion, sacroiliac joint dislocation is approximately twice as common as a para-articular fracture.[856] The mechanism of Malgaigne fractures, which represent approximately 15 per cent of all injuries of the bony pelvis, is not clear and may involve either direct or indirect forces. The radiographic examination will show sites of osseous disruption, but supplementation with CT is useful in further defining these sites and in delineating subtle articular subluxations.

More extensive disruptions of the pelvis result from massive crushing injuries in which the osseous ring is disrupted in multiple locations or completely shattered (Fig. 68–164).

4. Type IV injuries. Fractures of the acetabulum are considered earlier in this chapter and are illustrated in Figure 68–165.

The mortality associated with all pelvic fractures is about 10 per cent, which in most cases relates to a variety of serious complications.[857] With regard to the complications of pelvic fractures and dislocations, four types deserve emphasis: hemorrhage, urinary tract injury, peripheral nerve injury, and remote injuries.[2] The serious nature of the excessive bleeding that accompanies many of these fractures, particularly type III injuries, is underscored by the necessity for blood transfusions in almost 50 per cent of cases and the significant mortality that follows inadequate blood replacement.[858] Injuries to the urinary tract are associated most typically with symphyseal diastasis or fractures of the pubic rami, or both; urethral damage is somewhat more frequent than that of the bladder, the latter commonly being displaced upward by the accumulating blood. Urethral injuries predominate in men.[859] Microscopic or macroscopic hematuria following a pelvic fracture deserves immediate attention and may require specialized studies, including retrograde urethrography, cystography, or intravenous pyelography, or combinations of the three. Of importance, a catheter should not be placed in the bladder until the extent of urethral damage is known.[2]

Damage to the peripheral nerves occurs in approximately 10 per cent of patients following injuries of the bony pelvis, and this frequency increases in those with sacral fractures.[860] In addition to the bladder, other viscera that are injured in association with fractures and dislocations of the pelvis include the liver, spleen, testes, and bowel as well as the diaphragm.

Thoracic Cage

Fractures and Dislocations of the Sternum. The usual mechanism leading to fractures or dislocations of the sternum is direct trauma, and associated injuries of the anterior portion of the ribs and costocartilages are common.[861] Crushing of the lower anterior aspect of the chest in the region of the mobile portion of the sternum is accompanied by sternal fractures above the site of impact, principally near the junction of the flexible body of the bone and the relatively fixed manubrium; a localized blow to the upper region of the sternum may lead to a transverse fracture at the site of impact.[467] Aortic, other arterial,[897] tracheal, cardiac, and pulmonary injuries represent serious complications of direct sternal trauma. Such injuries may lead to the patient's demise.[898]

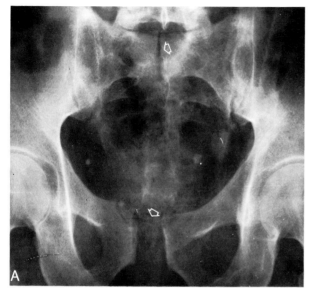

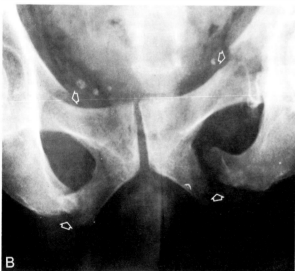

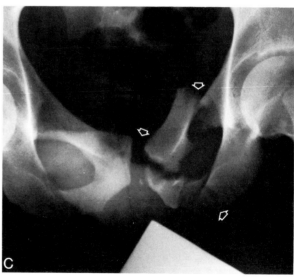

FIGURE 68–163. Fractures and dislocations of the pelvis: Type III injuries.

A In this example, symphyseal diastasis and a vertical fracture of the sacrum (open arrows) have led to disruption of the pelvic ring in two locations.

B A straddle injury with bilateral vertical fractures of both pubic rami (open arrows) is apparent.

C In this variety of a straddle injury, symphyseal diastasis and unilateral vertical fractures of both pubic rami (open arrows) are seen.

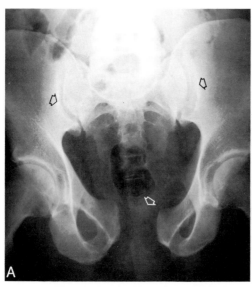

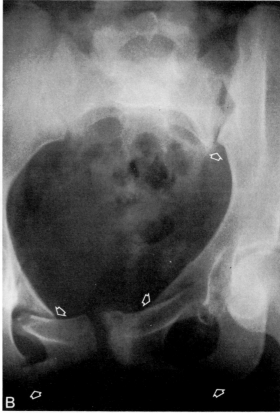

FIGURE 68–164. Fractures and dislocations of the pelvis: Complex injuries.

A A "sprung" pelvis is characterized by subluxations or dislocations of both sacroiliac joints and symphyseal diastasis (open arrows).

B This complex injury includes bilateral vertical fractures of both pubic rami and subluxation of the sacroiliac joint (open arrows).

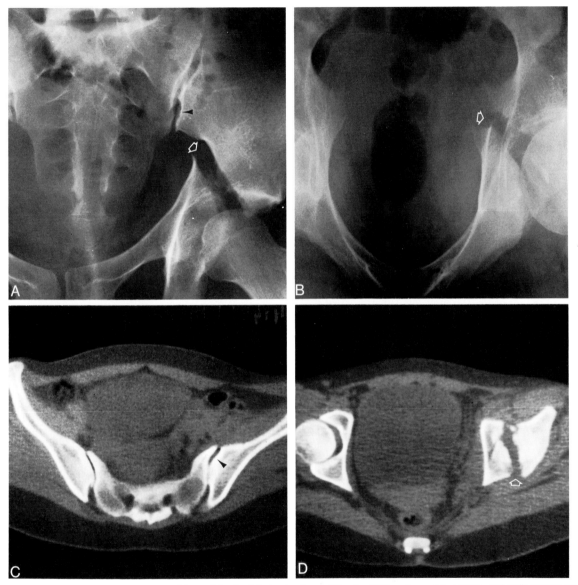

FIGURE 68–165. Fractures and dislocations of the pelvis: Acetabular fractures. Standard **(A)** and angulated **(B)** frontal radiographs reveal the fracture line extending into the hip (open arrows) and subtle subluxation of the left sacroiliac joint (arrowhead). Two transaxial CT scans **(C, D)** confirm the presence of sacroiliac joint subluxation (arrowhead) and a comminuted fracture of the acetabular roof (open arrow).

Indirect mechanisms leading to sternal fractures or dislocations include a blow to the upper thoracic or cervical segment of the spine (which may be fractured) with transmission of the force through the upper ribs or clavicle to the sternum (in which case abnormalities in the form of fractures or dislocations occur in those portions of the bone adjacent to the manubriosternal joint)[467, 862] and stress fractures of the sternum (which are a rare manifestation of chronic progressive kyphosis of the thoracic spine that accompanies osteoporosis, osteomalacia, plasma cell myeloma, and renal osteodystrophy) (Fig. 68–166).

Routine radiography provides important clues regarding the presence of sternal injuries (Fig. 68–167); however, conventional or computed tomography commonly is required for further assessment.

Fractures of the Ribs. Such fractures result from direct injuries owing to blows to the chest or falls[2] and generally are of lesser significance than simultaneous injuries in the nearby lung. Commonly, adjacent areas of multiple ribs are affected. Radiographic detection of these fractures can be difficult, although localized soft tissue swelling represents an important diagnostic clue. Soft tissue emphysema implies that there has been violation of the lung and should prompt a careful search for a pneumothorax.

Certain distinct patterns of rib injuries deserve emphasis. As indicated previously, fractures of the first and second ribs generally imply severe trauma and may be associated with vascular disruptions. Segmental fractures of several ribs, which may occur following a severe crush injury, may be accompanied by separation at their costochondral junctions or by fracture of the sternum; this situation creates a flail chest, in which one portion of the thoracic cage moves

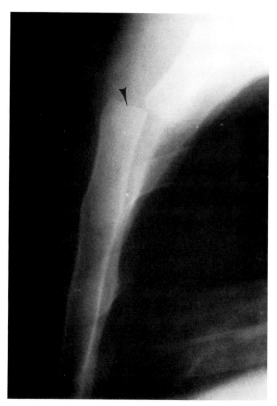

FIGURE 68–167. Dislocations of the sternum. Anterior dislocation (arrowhead) of the body of the bone at the manubriosternal junction is evident.

independently of the remaining portion.[861] Impaired ventilation, pendulum breathing, ineffective cough, hypoxia, and pulmonary edema may occur.[861]

Summary

This chapter provides a summary of many of the sequelae of physical injury to extraspinal sites. Routine radiographic findings are emphasized, although reference is made to the assessment of such injury using other methods such as CT and MR imaging. Both of these techniques as well as arthrography are fundamental to the evaluation of internal derangements of joints, a subject that is addressed in detail in Chapter 70.

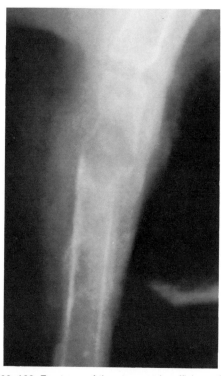

FIGURE 68–166. Fractures of the sternum: Insufficiency fracture in osteomalacia. Note resorption about the fracture site and soft tissue prominence. Biopsy documented the presence of a healing fracture. (Courtesy of J. Schills, M.D., Cleveland, Ohio.)

References

1. Rockwood CA, Green DP: Fractures in Adults. 2nd Ed. Philadelphia, JB Lippincott Co, 1984.
2. Rogers LF: Radiology of Skeletal Trauma. 2nd. Ed. New York, Churchill Livingstone, 1992.
3. Harris JH, Harris WH: The Radiology of Emergency Medicine. Baltimore, Williams & Wilkins Co, 1975.
4. Tachdjian MO: Pediatric Orthopedics. Philadelphia, WB Saunders Co, 1972.
5. Ayella RJ: Radiologic Management of the Massively Traumatized Patient. Baltimore, Williams & Wilkins Co, 1978.
6. Bowerman JW: Radiology and Injury in Sport. New York, Appleton-Century-Crofts, 1977.
7. Saha AK: Dynamic stability of the glenohumeral joint. Acta Orthop Scand 42:491, 1971.
8. Joessel D: Ueber die Recidive der Humerusluxationen. Dtsch Z Chir 13:167, 1880.
9. Hill HA, Sachs MD: The grooved defect of the humeral head. A frequently unrecognized complication of dislocations of the shoulder joint. Radiology 35:690, 1940.
10. Hermodsson I: Röntgenologische Studien über die traumatischen und habituel-

len Schultergelenkverrenkungen nach Vorn und nach Unten. Acta Radiol (Suppl) 20:1, 1934.

11. Symeonides PP: The significance of the subscapularis muscle in the pathogenesis of recurrent anterior dislocation of the shoulder. J Bone Joint Surg [Br] 54:476, 1972.

12. Eyre-Brook AL: Recurrent dislocation of the shoulder. Physiotherapy 57:7, 1971.

13. Rowe CR: Prognosis in dislocations of the shoulder. J Bone Joint Surg [Am] 38:957, 1956.

14. Brav EA: Recurrent dislocation of the shoulder. Ten years' experience with Putti-Platt reconstruction procedure. Am J Surg 100:423, 1960.

15. Palmar I, Widen A: The bone-block method for recurrent dislocation of the shoulder joint. J Bone Joint Surg [Br] 30:53, 1948.

16. Adams JC: Recurrent dislocations of the shoulder. J Bone Joint Surg [Br] 30:26, 1948.

17. Hall RH, Isaac F, Booth CR: Dislocations of the shoulder with special reference to accompanying small fractures. J Bone Joint Surg [Am] 41:489, 1959.

18. Pavlov H, Warren RF, Weiss CB Jr, Dines DM: The roentgenographic evaluation of anterior shoulder instability. Clin Orthop Rel Res 194:153, 1985.

19. Deutsch AL, Resnick D, Mink JH: Computed tomography of the glenohumeral and sternoclavicular joints. Orthop Clin North Am 16:497, 1985.

20. Danzig L, Resnick D, Greenway G: Evaluation of unstable shoulders by computed tomography. A preliminary study. Am J Sports Med 10:138, 1982.

21. Cramer BM, Kramps H-A, Laumann U, Fischedick A-R: CT-Diagnostik bei habitueller Schulterluxation. ROFO 136:440, 1982.

22. Seltzer SE, Weissman BN: CT findings in normal and dislocating shoulders. J Can Assoc Radiol 36:41, 1985.

23. Gould R, Rosenfield AT, Friedlaender GE: Loose body within the glenohumeral joint in recurrent anterior dislocation: CT demonstration. J Comput Assist Tomogr 9:404, 1985.

24. Rafii M, Firooznia H, Bonamo JJ, Minkoff J, Golimbu C: Athlete shoulder injuries: CT arthrographic findings. Radiology 162:559, 1987.

25. Bankart ASB: Recurrent or habitual dislocation of the shoulder joint. Br Med J 2:1132, 1923.

26. Pavlov H, Freiberger RH: Fractures and dislocations about the shoulder. Semin Roentgen 13:85, 1978.

27. Aston JW Jr, Gregory CF: Dislocation of the shoulder with significant fracture of the glenoid. J Bone Joint Surg [Am] 55:1531, 1973.

28. El-Khoury GY, Albright JP, Abu Yousef MM, Montgomery WJ, Tuck SL: Arthrotomography of the glenoid labrum. Radiology 131:333, 1979.

29. Deutsch AL, Resnick D, Mink JH, Berman JL, Cone RO III, Resnick CS, Danzig L, Guerra J Jr: Computed tomography of the glenohumeral joint: Normal anatomy and clinical experience. Radiology 153:603, 1984.

30. Neviaser RJ, Neviaser TJ, Neviaser JS: Concurrent rupture of the rotator cuff and anterior dislocation of the shoulder in the older patient. J Bone Joint Surg [Am] 70:1308, 1988.

31. Gonzalez D, Lopez RA: Concurrent rotator-cuff tear and brachial plexus palsy associated with anterior dislocation of the shoulder. A report of two cases. J Bone Joint Surg [Am] 73:620, 1991.

32. Kirtland S, Resnick D, Sartoris DJ, et al: Chronic unreduced dislocations of the glenohumeral joint: Imaging strategy and pathologic correlation. J Trauma 28:1622, 1988.

33. Hill NA, McLaughlin HL: Locked posterior dislocation simulating a ''frozen shoulder.'' J Trauma 3:225, 1963.

34. McLaughlin HL: Posterior dislocation of the shoulder. J Bone Joint Surg [Am] 34:584, 1952.

35. Shaw JL: Bilateral posterior fracture-dislocation of the shoulder and other trauma caused by convulsive seizures. J Bone Joint Surg [Am] 53:1437, 1971.

36. Vastamaki M, Solenen KA: Posterior dislocation and fracture dislocation of the shoulder. Acta Orthop Scand 51:479, 1980.

37. Din KM: Bilateral four-part fractures with posterior dislocation of the shoulder. A case report. J Bone Joint Surg [Br] 65:176, 1983.

38. Dimon JH III: Posterior dislocation and posterior fracture-dislocation of the shoulder. A report of 25 cases. South Med J 60:661, 1967.

39. Bloom MH, Obata WG: Diagnosis of posterior dislocation of the shoulder with use of Velpeau axillary and angle-up roentgenographic views. J Bone Joint Surg [Am] 49:943, 1967.

40. Arndt JH, Sears AD: Posterior dislocation of the shoulder. Am J Roentgenol 94:639, 1965.

41. Cisternino SJ, Rogers LF, Stufflebam BC, Kruglik GD: The trough line: A radiographic sign of posterior shoulder dislocation. Am J Roentgenol 130:951, 1978.

42. Bernageau J, Patte D: Diagnostic radiologique des luxations postérieures de l'épaule. Rev Chir Orthop 65:101, 1979.

43. Slikva J, Resnick D: An improved radiographic view of the glenohumeral joint. J Can Assoc Radiol 30:83, 1979.

44. Fronek J, Warren RF, Bowen M: Posterior subluxation of the glenohumeral joint. J Bone Joint Surg [Am] 71:205, 1989.

45. Hawkins RJ, Neer CS II, Pianta RM, Mendoza FX: Locked posterior dislocation of the shoulder. J Bone Joint Surg [Am] 69:9, 1987.

46. Samuson RL, Prieto V: Dislocation arthropathy of the shoulder. J Bone Joint Surg [Am] 65:456, 1983.

47. Downey EF Jr, Curtis DJ, Brower AC: Unusual dislocations of the shoulder. Am J Roentgenol 140:1207, 1983.

48. Lynn FS: Erect dislocation of the shoulder. Surg Gynecol Obstet 39:51, 1921.

49. Laskin RS, Sedlin ED: Luxatio erecta in infancy. Clin Orthop Rel Res 80:126, 1971.

50. Kothari K, Bernstein RM, Griffiths HJ, Standertskjold-Nordenstam CG, Choi PK: Luxatio erecta. Skel Radiol 11:47, 1984.

51. Saxena K, Stavas J: Inferior glenohumeral dislocation. Ann Emerg Med 12:718, 1983.

52. Zimmers T: Luxatio erecta: An uncommon shoulder dislocation. Ann Emerg Med 12:716, 1983.

53. Freundlich BD: Luxatio erecta. J Trauma 23:434, 1983.

54. Davids JR, Talbott RD: Luxatio erecta humeri. A case report. Clin Orthop 252:144, 1990.

55. Rowe CR, Pierce DS, Clark JG: Voluntary dislocation of the shoulder. J Bone Joint Surg [Am] 55:445, 1973.

56. Braunstein EM, Martel W: Voluntary glenohumeral dislocation. Am J Roentgenol 129:911, 1977.

57. Howorth MB: Generalized relaxation of the ligaments. Clin Orthop Rel Res 30:133, 1963.

58. Brewer BJ, Wubben RC, Carrera GF: Excessive retroversion of the glenoid cavity. A cause of non-traumatic posterior instability of the shoulder. J Bone Joint Surg [Am] 68:724, 1986.

59. Cotton F: Subluxation of the shoulder downward. Boston Med Surg J 185:405, 1921.

60. Hammond R: Relaxation of the shoulder following bone injury. J Bone Joint Surg 5:712, 1923.

61. Laskin RS, Schreiber S: Inferior subluxation of the humeral head: The drooping shoulder. Radiology 98:585, 1971.

62. Lev-Toaff AS, Karasick D, Rao VM: ''Drooping shoulder''—nontraumatic causes of glenohumeral subluxation. Skel Radiol 12:34, 1984.

63. Uhrist MR: Complete dislocations of the acromioclavicular joint. The nature of the traumatic lesion and effective methods of treatment with an analysis of 41 cases. J Bone Joint Surg 28:813, 1946.

64. Powers JA, Bach PJ: Acromioclavicular separations. Closed or open treatment? Clin Orthop Rel Res 104:213, 1974.

65. Weaver JK, Dunn HK: Treatment of acromioclavicular injuries, especially complete acromioclavicular separation. J Bone Joint Surg [Am] 54:1187, 1972.

66. Eidman DK, Siff SJ, Tullos HS: Acromioclavicular lesions in children. Am J Sports Med 9:150, 1981.

67. Cox JS: The fate of the acromioclavicular joint in athletic injuries. Am J Sports Med 9:50, 1981.

68. Allman FL Jr: Fractures and ligamentous injuries of the clavicle and its articulation. J Bone Joint Surg [Am] 49:774, 1967.

69. Zlotsky NA, Ballard A: Acromioclavicular injuries in athletes. J Bone Joint Surg [Am] 48:1224, 1966.

70. Post M: Current concepts in the diagnosis and management of acromioclavicular dislocations. Clin Orthop Rel Res 200:234, 1985.

71. Montgomery SP, Loyd RD: Avulsion fracture of the coracoid epiphysis with acromioclavicular separation. Report of two cases in adolescents and review of the literature. J Bone Joint Surg [Am] 59:963, 1977.

72. Protass JJ, Stampfli FV, Osmer JC: Coracoid process fracture diagnosis in acromioclavicular separation. Radiology 116:61, 1975.

73. Smith DM: Coracoid fracture associated with acromioclavicular dislocation. A case report. Clin Orthop Rel Res 108:165, 1975.

74. Taga I, Yoneda M, Ono K: Epiphyseal separation of the coracoid process associated with acromioclavicular sprain. A case report and review of the literature. Clin Orthop Rel Res 207:138, 1986.

75. Zanca P: Shoulder pain: Involvement of the acromioclavicular joint. Analysis of 1000 cases. Am J Roentgenol 112:493, 1971.

76. Väätäinen U, Pirinen A, Mäkelä A: Radiological evaluation of the acromioclavicular joint. Skel Radiol 20:115, 1991.

77. Bearden JM, Hughston JC, Whatley GS: Acromioclavicular dislocation: Method of treatment. J Sports Med Phys Fitness 1:5, 1973.

78. Sage J: Recurrent inferior dislocation of the clavicle at the acromioclavicular joint. A case report. Am J Sports Med 10:145, 1982.

79. Leonard MH, Capen DA: Superior entrapment of the clavicle. Am J Sports Med 11:96, 1983.

80. Jain AS: Traumatic floating clavicle. A case report. J Bone Joint Surg [Br] 66:560, 1984.

81. Gearen PF, Petty W: Panclavicular dislocation. Report of a case. J Bone Joint Surg [Am] 64:454, 1982.

82. Cook F, Horowitz M: Bipolar clavicular dislocation. Report of a case. J Bone Joint Surg [Am] 69:145, 1987.

83. Falstie-Jensen S, Mikkelsen P: Pseudodislocation of the acromioclavicular joint. J Bone Joint Surg [Br] 64:368, 1982.

84. Millbourn E: On injuries to the acromioclavicular joint. Treatment and results. Acta Orthop Scand 19:349, 1950.

85. Arner O, Sandahl U, Ohrling H: Dislocation of the acromioclavicular joint—review of the literature and report of 56 cases. Acta Chir Scand 113:140, 1957.

86. Nettles JL, Linscheid R: Sternoclavicular dislocations. J Trauma 8:158, 1968.

87. Tyer HDD, Sturrock WDS, Callow FM: Retrosternal dislocation of the clavicle. J Bone Joint Surg [Br] 45:132, 1963.

88. Selesnick FH, Jablon M, Frank C, Post M: Retrosternal dislocation of the clavicle. Report of four cases. J Bone Joint Surg [Am] 66:287, 1984.

89. Newlin NS: Congenital retrosternal subluxation of the clavicle simulating an intrathoracic mass. Am J Roentgenol 130:1184, 1978.

90. Sadr B, Swann M: Spontaneous dislocation of the sternoclavicular joint. Acta Orthop Scand 50:269, 1979.

91. Levinsohn EM, Bunnell WP, Yuan HA: Computed tomography in the diagnosis of dislocations of the sternoclavicular joint. Clin Orthop Rel Res *140*:12, 1979.

92. Lourie JA: Tomography in the diagnosis of posterior dislocation of the sternoclavicular joint. Acta Orthop Scand *51*:579, 1980.

93. Lee FA, Gwinn JL: Retrosternal dislocation of the clavicle. Radiology *110*:631, 1974.

94. McKenzie JM: Retrosternal dislocation of the clavicle: A report of two cases. J Bone Joint Surg [Br] *45*:138, 1963.

95. Brooks AL, Henning GD: Injury to the proximal clavicular epiphysis. J Bone Joint Surg [Am] *54*:1347, 1972.

96. Lemire L, Rosman M: Sternoclavicular epiphyseal separation with adjacent clavicular fracture. J Pediatr Orthop *4*:118, 1984.

97. Rose SH, Melton J III, Morrey BF, Ilstrup DM, Riggs BL: Epidemiologic features of humeral fractures. Clin Orthop Rel Res *168*:24, 1982.

98. Dehne E: Fractures of the upper end of the humerus: A classification based on the etiology of trauma. Surg Clin North Am 25:28, 1945.

99. Neer CS II: Displaced proximal humeral fractures. Part I. Classification and evaluation. J Bone Joint Surg [Am] *52*:1077, 1970.

100. Kristiansen B, Anderson ULS, Olsen CA, et al: The Neer classification of fractures of the proximal humerus. An assessment of interobserver variation. Skel Radiol *17*:420, 1988.

101. Kilcoyne RF, Shuman WP, Matsen FA III, et al: The Neer classification of displaced proximal humeral fractures: Spectrum of findings on plain radiographs and CT scans. AJR *154*:1029, 1990.

102. Castagno AA, Shuman WP, Kilcoyne RF, et al: Complex fractures of the proximal humerus: Role of CT in treatment. Radiology *165*:759, 1987.

103. Earwaker J: Isolated avulsion fracture of the lesser tuberosity of the humerus. Skel Radiol *19*:121, 1990.

104. LaBriola JH, Mohaghegh HA: Isolated avulsion fracture of the lesser tuberosity of the humerus. A case report and review of the literature. J Bone Joint Surg [Am] *57*:1011, 1975.

105. Hawkins RJ, Bell RH, Gurr K: The three-part fracture of the proximal part of the humerus. Operative treatment. J Bone Joint Surg [Am] *68*:1410, 1986.

106. Neer CS II: Displaced proximal humeral fractures. Part II. Treatment of three-part and four-part displacement. J Bone Joint Surg [Am] *52*:1090, 1970.

107. Stableforth PG: Four-part fractures of the neck of the humerus. J Bone Joint Surg [Br] *66*:104, 1984.

108. Lee DK, Hansen HR: Post-traumatic avascular necrosis of the humeral head in displaced proximal humeral fractures. J Trauma *21*:788, 1984.

109. Jakob RP, Miniaci A, Anson PS, et al: Four-part valgus impacted fractures of the proximal humerus. J Bone Joint Surg [Br] *73*:295, 1991.

110. Ovesen J, Nielsen S: Experimental distal subluxation in the glenohumeral joint. Arch Orthop Trauma Surg *104*:78, 1985.

111. Rooney PJ, Crockshott WP: Pseudarthrosis following proximal humeral fractures. A possible mechanism. Skel Radiol *15*:21, 1986.

112. Kofoed H: Revascularization of the humeral head. A report of two cases of fracture-dislocation of the shoulder. Clin Orthop Rel Res *179*:175, 1983.

113. Zuckerman JD, Flugstad DL, Teitz CC, King HA: Axillary artery injury as a complication of proximal humeral fractures. Two case reports and a review of the literature. Clin Orthop Rel Res *189*:234, 1984.

114. Neer CS II, Rockwood CA Jr: Fractures and dislocations of the shoulder. *In* CA Rockwood Jr, DP Green (Eds): Fractures in Adults. 2nd Ed. Philadelphia, JB Lippincott Co, 1984, p 675.

115. Quesada F: Technique for the roentgen diagnosis of fractures of the clavicle. Surg Gynecol Obstet *42*:424, 1926.

116. Weinberg B, Seife B, Alonso P: The apical oblique view of the clavicle: its usefulness in neonatal and childhood trauma. Skel Radiol 20:201, 1991.

117. Neer CS II: Fracture of the distal clavicle with detachment of the coracoclavicular ligaments in adults. J Trauma *3*:99, 1963.

118. Miller DS, Boswick JA Jr: Lesions of the brachial plexus associated with fractures of the clavicle. Clin Orthop Rel Res *64*:144, 1969.

119. Howard FM, Shafer SJ: Injuries to the clavicle with neurovascular complications. A study of fourteen cases. J Bone Joint Surg [Am] *47*:1335, 1965.

120. Kay SP, Eckardt JJ: Brachial plexus palsy secondary to clavicular nonunion. Case report and literature survey. Clin Orthop Rel Res *207*:219, 1986.

121. Weiner DS, O'Dell HW: Fractures of the first-rib associated with injuries to the clavicle. J Trauma *9*:412, 1969.

122. Goddard NJ, Stabler J, Albert JS: Atlanto-axial rotary fixation and fracture of the clavicle. An association and a classification. J Bone Joint Surg [Br] *72*:72, 1990.

123. Neer CS II: Nonunion of the clavicle. JAMA *96*:1006, 1960.

124. Sakellarides H: Pseudarthrosis of the clavicle. A report of twenty cases. J Bone Joint Surg [Am] *43*:130, 1961.

125. Manske DJ, Szabo RM: The operative treatment of mid-shaft clavicular nonunions. J Bone Joint Surg [Am] *67*:1367, 1985.

126. Owen R: Congenital pseudarthrosis of the clavicle. J Bone Joint Surg [Br] *52*:644, 1970.

127. Ada JR, Miller ME: Scapular fractures. Analysis of 113 cases. Clin Orthop *269*:174, 1991.

128. Imatani RJ: Fractures of the scapula: A review of 53 fractures. J Trauma *15*:473, 1975.

129. McGahan JP, Rab GT, Dublin A: Fractures of the scapula. J Trauma 20:880, 1980.

130. Varriale PL, Adler ML: Occult fracture of the glenoid without dislocation. A case report. J Bone Joint Surg [Am] *65*:688, 1983.

131. Goss TP: Fractures of the glenoid cavity. J Bone Joint Surg [Am] *74*:299, 1992.

132. Hardegger FJ, Simpson LA, Weber BG: The operative treatment of scapular fractures. J Bone Joint Surg [Br] *66*:725, 1984.

133. Heyse-Moore GH, Stoker DJ: Avulsion fractures of the scapula. Skel Radiol *9*:27, 1982.

134. Herscovici D Jr, Fiennes AGTW, Allgöwer M, et al: The floating shoulder: ipsilateral clavicle and scapular neck fractures. J Bone Joint Surg [Br] *74*:362, 1992.

135. McLennan JG, Ungersma J: Pneumothorax complicating fracture of the scapula. J Bone Joint Surg [Am] *64*:598, 1982.

136. Banerjee AK, Field S: An unusual scapular fracture caused by a water skiing accident. Br J Radiol *58*:465, 1985.

137. Rask MR, Steinberg LH: Fracture of the acromion caused by muscle forces. A case report. J Bone Joint Surg [Am] *60*:1146, 1978.

138. Benton J, Nelson C: Avulsion of the coracoid process in an athlete. J Bone Joint Surg [Am] *53*:356, 1971.

139. Froimson AI: Fracture of the coracoid process of the scapula. J Bone Joint Surg [Am] *60*:710, 1978.

140. Stein RE, Bone J, Korn J: Axillary artery injury in closed fracture of the neck of the scapula. A case report. J Trauma *11*:528, 1971.

141. Evans DL: Fatigue fracture of the ulna. J Bone Joint Surg [Br] *37*:618, 1955.

142. Nettrour LF, Krufky EL, Mueller RE, Raycroft JF: Locked scapula: Intrathoracic dislocation of the inferior angle. A case report. J Bone Joint Surg [Am] *54*:413, 1972.

143. Oreck SL, Burgess A, Levine AM: Traumatic lateral displacement of the scapula: A radiographic sign of neurovascular disruption. J Bone Joint Surg [Am] *66*:758, 1984.

144. Rubenstein JD, Ebraheim NA, Kellam JF: Traumatic scapulothoracic dissociation. Radiology *157*:297, 1985.

145. Kelbel JM, Jardon OM, Huurman WW: Scapulothoracic dissociation. A case report. Clin Orthop Rel Res *209*:210, 1986.

146. Richardson JD, McElvein RB, Trinkle JK: First rib fracture: A hallmark of severe trauma. Ann Surg *181*:251, 1975.

147. Lorentzen JE, Movin M: Fracture of the first rib. Acta Orthop Scand *47*:632, 1976.

148. Fisher RG, Ward RE, Ben-Menachem Y, Mattox KL, Flynn TC: Arteriography and the fractured first rib: Too much for too little? Am J Roentgenol *138*:1059, 1982.

149. Woodring JH, Fried AM, Hatfield DR, Stevens FK, Todd EP: Fractures of first and second ribs: Predictive value for arterial and bronchial injury. Am J Roentgenol *138*:211, 1982.

150. Livoni JP, Barcia TC: Fracture of the first and second rib: incidence of vascular injury relative to type of fracture. Radiology *145*:31, 1982.

151. Woodring JH, Royer JM, Todd EP: Upper rib fractures following median sternotomy. Ann Thorac Surg *39*:355, 1985.

152. Ward EF, Savoie FH, Hughes JL: Fractures of the diaphyseal humerus. *In* BD Browner, JB Jupiter, AM Levine, PG Trafton (Eds): Skeletal Trauma. Fractures, Dislocations, Ligamentous Injuries. Philadelphia, WB Saunders, 1992, p. 1177.

153. Garth WP Jr, Leberte MA, Cool TA: Recurrent fractures of the humerus in a baseball pitcher. J Bone Joint Surg [Am] *70*:305, 1988.

154. Heilbronner DM, Manoli A II, Morawa LG: Fractures of the humerus in arm wrestlers. Clin Orthop *149*:169, 1980.

155. Hartonas GD, Verettas DJ: Fracture of the humerus in a shotput athlete. Injury *18*:68, 1987.

156. Healy WL, White GM, Mick CA, et al: Nonunion of the humeral shaft. Clin Orthop *219*:206, 1987.

157. Reginato AJ, Feldman E, Rabinowitz JL: Traumatic chylous knee effusion. Ann Rheum Dis *44*:793, 1985.

158. Mast JW, Spiegel PG, Harvey JP Jr, et al: Fractures of the humeral shaft. A retrospective study of 240 adult fractures. Clin Orthop *112*:254, 1975.

159. Pierce RA Jr, Hodurski DF: Fractures of the humerus, radius and ulna in the same extremity. J Trauma *19*:182, 1979.

160. Duthie HL: Radial nerve in osseous tunnel at humeral fracture site diagnosed radiographically. J Bone Joint Surg [Br] *39*:746, 1957.

161. Norrell HG: Roentgenologic visualization of extracapsular fat: its importance in diagnosis of traumatic injuries to the elbow. Acta Radiol Diagn *42*:205, 1954.

162. Murphy WA, Siegel MJ: Elbow fat pads with new signs and extended differential diagnosis. Radiology *124*:659, 1977.

163. Kohn AM: Soft tissue alterations in elbow trauma. AJR *82*:867, 1959.

164. Quinton DN, Finlay D, Butterworth R: The elbow fat pad sign: Brief report. J Bone Joint Surg [Br] *69*:844, 1987.

165. Rogers LF: Fractures and dislocations of the elbow. Semin Roentgenol *13*:97, 1978.

166. Kini MG: Dislocation of the elbow and its complications. J Bone Joint Surg *22*:107, 1940.

167. Linscheid RL, Wheeler DK: Elbow dislocations. JAMA 194:1171, 1965.

168. Matev I: A radiological sign of entrapment of the median nerve in the elbow joint after posterior dislocation. A report of two cases. J Bone Joint Surg [Br] *58*:353, 1976.

169. Green NE: Entrapment of the median nerve following elbow dislocation. J Pediatr Orthop *3*:384, 1983.

170. Floyd WE III, Gebhardt MC, Emans JB: Intra-articular entrapment of the median nerve after elbow dislocation in children. J Hand Surg [Am] *12*:704, 1987.

171. Exarchou EJ: Lateral dislocation of the elbow. Acta Orthop Scand *48*:161, 1977.

172. Cohn I: Fractures of the elbow. Am J Surg *55*:210, 1942.

173. Symeonides PP, Paschaloglou C, Stavrou Z, Pangalides TH: Recurrent dislocation of the elbow. Report of three cases. J Bone Joint Surg [Am] *57*:1084, 1975.

174. Josefsson PO, Gentz CF, Johnell O, et al: Dislocations of the elbow and intraarticular fractures. Clin Orthop *246*:126, 1989.

175. Josefsson PO, Johnell O, Wendeberg B: Ligamentous injuries in dislocations of the elbow joint. Clin Orthop *221*:221, 1987.

176. Andersen K, Mortensen AC, Gron P: Transverse divergent dislocation of the elbow. A report of two cases. Acta Orthop Scand *56*:442, 1985.

177. Holbrook JL, Green NE: Divergent pediatric elbow dislocation. A case report. Clin Orthop *234*:72, 1988.

178. Eklöf O, Nybonde T, Karlsson G: Luxation of the elbow complicated by proximal radio-ulnar translocation. Acta Radiologica *31*:145, 1990.

179. Frumken K: Nursemaid's elbow: A radiographic demonstration. Ann Emerg Med *14*:690, 1985.

180. Salter RB, Zaltz C: Anatomic investigations of the mechanism of injury and pathologic anatomy of ''pulled elbow'' in young children. Clin Orthop *77*:134, 1971.

181. Triantafyllou SJ, Wilson SC, Rychak JS: Irreducible ''pulled elbow'' in a child. A case report. Clin Orthop *284*:153, 1992.

182. Earwaker J: Posttraumatic calcification of the annular ligament of the radius. Skel Radiol *21*:149, 1992.

183. Caravias D: Some observations on congenital dislocation of the head of the radius. J Bone Joint Surg [Br] *39*:86, 1957.

184. White J: Congenital dislocation of the head of the radius. Br J Surg *30*:377, 1942.

185. Elliott KA, Elliott GB, Kindrachuk WH: The radial subluxation-fingernail defect-absent patella syndrome. Am J Roentgenol *87*:1067, 1962.

186. Wiley JJ, Pegington J, Horwich JP: Traumatic dislocation of the radius at the elbow. J Bone Joint Surg [Br] *56*:501, 1974.

187. Bruce HE, Harvey JP Jr, Wilson JC Jr: Monteggia fractures. J Bone Joint Surg [Am] *56*:1563, 1974.

188. Peiro A, Andres F, Fernandez-Esteve F: Acute Monteggia lesions in children. J Bone Joint Surg [Am] *59*:92, 1977.

189. Giustra PE, Killoran PJ, Furman RS, Root JA: The missed Monteggia fracture. Radiology *110*:45, 1974.

190. Bado JL: The Monteggia Lesion. Springfield, Ill, Charles C Thomas, 1962.

191. Simpson JM, Andreshak TG, Patel A, et al: Ipsilateral radial head dislocation and radial shaft fracture. A case report. Clin Orthop *266*:205, 1991.

192. Wiley JJ, Galey JP: Monteggia injuries in children. J Bone Joint Surg [Br] *67*:728, 1985.

193. Letts M, Locht R, Wiens J: Monteggia fracture-dislocation in children. J Bone Joint Surg [Br] *67*:724, 1985.

194. Kalamchi A: Monteggia fracture-dislocation in children. Late treatment in two cases. J Bone Joint Surg [Am] *68*:615, 1986.

195. Papavasiliou VA, Nenopoulos SP: Monteggia-type elbow fractures in childhood. Clin Orthop *233*:230, 1988.

196. Olney BW, Menelaus MB: Monteggia and equivalent lesions in childhood. J Pediatr Orthop *9*:219, 1989.

197. Storen G: Traumatic dislocation of the radial head as an isolated lesion in children: Report of one case with special regard to roentgen diagnosis. Acta Chir Scand *116*:144, 1959.

198. Rogers LF, Rockwood CA Jr: Separation of the entire distal humeral epiphysis. Radiology *106*:393, 1973.

199. Mizuno K, Hirohata K, Kashiwagi D: Fracture-separation of the distal humeral epiphysis in young children. J Bone Joint Surg [Am] *61*:570, 1979.

200. Loomis LK: Reduction and after-treatment of posterior dislocation of the elbow. Am J Surg *63*:56, 1944.

201. Thompson HC III, Garcia A: Myositis ossificans (aftermath of elbow injuries). Clin Orthop Rel Res *50*:129, 1967.

202. Josefsson PO, Johnell O, Gentz CF: Long-term sequelae of simple dislocation of the elbow. J Bone Joint Surg [Am] *66*:927, 1984.

203. Kerin R: Elbow dislocation and its association with vascular disruption. J Bone Joint Surg [Am] *51*:756, 1969.

204. Hofammann KE III, Moneim MS, Omer GE, Ball WS: Brachial artery disruption following closed posterior elbow dislocation in a child—assessment with intravenous digital angiography. A case report with review of the literature. Clin Orthop Rel Res *184*:145, 1984.

205. Grimer RJ, Brooks S: Brachial artery damage accompanying closed posterior dislocation of the elbow. J Bone Joint Surg [Br] *67*:378, 1985.

206. Malkawi H: Recurrent dislocation of the elbow accompanied by ulnar neuropathy: A case report and review of the literature. Clin Orthop Rel Res *161*:270, 1981.

207. Goldman MH, Kent S, Schaumburg E: Brachial artery injuries associated with posterior elbow dislocation. Surg Gynecol Obstet *164*:95, 1987.

208. DeLee JC, Green DP, Wilkins KE: Fracture and dislocations of the elbow. *In* CA Rockwood Jr, DP Green (Eds): Fractures in Adults. 2nd Ed. Philadelphia, JB Lippincott Co, 1984, p 559.

209. Riseborough EJ, Radin EL: Intercondylar T-fractures of the humerus in the adult (a comparison of operative and non-operative treatment in twenty-nine cases). J Bone Joint Surg [Am] *51*:130, 1969.

210. Miller WA: Comminuted fractures of the distal end of the humerus in the adult. J Bone Joint Surg [Am] *46*:644, 1964.

211. Bickel WH, Perry RE: Comminuted fractures of the distal humerus. JAMA *184*:553, 1963.

212. Gabel GT, Hanson G, Bennett JB, et al: Intraarticular fractures of the distal humerus in the adult. Clin Orthop *216*:99, 1987.

213. Mitsunaga MM, Bryan RS, Linscheid RL: Condylar nonunions of the elbow. J Trauma *22*:787, 1982.

214. Knight RA: Fractures of the humeral condyles in adults. South Med J *48*:1165, 1955.

215. Milch H: Fractures and fracture dislocations of the humeral condyles. J Trauma *4*:592, 1964.

216. Kleiger B, Joseph H: Fractures of the capitellum humeri. Bull Hosp J Dis *25*:64, 1964.

217. Alvarez E, Patel MR, Nimberg G, Pearlman HS: Fracture of the capitellum humeri. J Bone Joint Surg [Am] *57*:1093, 1975.

218. Grantham SA, Norris TR, Bush DC: Isolated fracture of the humeral capitellum. Clin Orthop Rel Res *161*:262, 1981.

219. Schild H, Muller HA, Klose K: The halfmoon sign. Australas Radiol *26*:273, 1982.

220. Keon-Cohen BT: Fractures of the elbow. J Bone Joint Surg [Am] *48*:1623, 1966.

221. Milch H: Unusual fractures of the capitellum humeri and the capitellum radii. J Bone Joint Surg *13*:882, 1931.

222. Stug LH: Anterior dislocation of the elbow with fracture of the olecranon. Am J Surg *75*:700, 1948.

223. Horne JG, Tanzer TL: Olecranon fractures: A review of 100 cases. J Trauma *21*:469, 1981.

224. Colton CL: Fractures of the olecranon in adults: classification and management. Injury *5*:121, 1973–1974.

225. Eriksson E, Sahlen O, Sandahl U: Late results of conservative and surgical treatment of fracture of the olecranon. Acta Chir Scand *113*:153, 1957.

226. Kiviluoto O, Santavirta S: Fractures of the olecranon. Acta Orthop Scand *49*:28, 1978.

227. Regan W, Morrey B: Fractures of the coronoid process of the ulna. J Bone Joint Surg [Am] *71*:1348, 1989.

228. Gaston SR, Smith FM, Baab OD: Adult injuries of the radial head and neck. Importance of time element in treatment. Am J Surg *78*:631, 1949.

229. Mason JA, Shutkin NM: Immediate active treatment of fractures of the head and neck of the radius. Surg Gynecol Obstet *76*:731, 1943.

230. Swanson AB, Jaeger SH, La Rochelle D: Comminuted fractures of the radial head. The role of silicone-implant replacement arthroplasty. J Bone Joint Surg [Am] *63*:1039, 1981.

231. Greenspan A, Norman A: Radial head—capitellum view: An expanded imaging approach to elbow injury. Radiology *164*:272, 1987.

232. Funk DA, Wood MB: Concurrent fractures of the ipsilateral scaphoid and radial head. Report of four cases. J Bone Joint Surg [Am] *70*:134, 1988.

233. Edwards GS Jr, Jupiter JB: Radial head fractures with acute distal radioulnar dislocation. Essex-Lopresti revisited. Clin Orthop *234*:61, 1988.

234. Bock GW, Cohen MS, Resnick D: Fracture-dislocation of the elbow with inferior radioulnar dissociation: a variant of the Essex-Lopresti injury. Skel Radiol *21*:315, 1992.

235. Evans EM: Rotational deformity in the treatment of fractures of both bones of the forearm. J Bone Joint Surg [Am] *27*:373, 1945.

236. Creasman C, Zaleske D, Ehrlich MG: Analyzing forearm fractures in children. The more subtle signs of impending problems. Clin Orthop *188*:40, 1984.

237. Goldberg HD, Young JWR, Reiner BI, et al: Double injuries of the forearm: A common occurrence. Radiology *185*:223, 1992.

238. Vince KG, Miller JE: Cross-union complicating fracture of the forearm. Part I. Adults. J Bone Joint Surg [Am] *69*:640, 1987.

239. Vince KG, Miller JE: Cross-union complicating fracture of the forearm. Part II. Children. J Bone Joint Surg [Am] *69*:654, 1987.

240. Billett DM: An uncommon fracture dislocation of the radius. J Trauma *17*:243, 1977.

241. Dobyns JH, Linscheid RL: Fractures and dislocations of the wrist. *In* CA Rockwood Jr, DP Green (Eds): Fractures in Adults. 2nd Ed. Philadelphia, JB Lippincott Co, 1984, p 411.

242. McQueen M, Caspers J: Colles fracture: Does the anatomical result affect the final function? J Bone Joint Surg [Br] *70*:649, 1988.

243. Porter M, Stockley I: Fractures of the distal radius. Intermediate and end results in relation to radiologic parameters. Clin Orthop *220*:241, 1987.

244. Mann FA, Wilson AJ, Gilula LA: Radiographic evaluation of the wrist: What does the hand surgeon want to know? Radiology *184*:15, 1992.

245. Johnson PG, Szabo RM: Angle measurements of the distal radius: a cadaver study. Skel Radiol *22*:243, 1993.

246. Atkins RM, Duckworth T, Kanis JA: Features of algodystrophy after Colles' fracture. J Bone Joint Surg [Br] *72*:105, 1990.

247. Bickerstaff DR, Bell MJ: Carpal malalignment in Colles' fractures. J Hand Surg [Br] *14*:155, 1989.

248. Paley D, McMurtry RY: Median nerve compression by volarly displaced fragments of the distal radius. Clin Orthop *215*:139, 1987.

249. Burgess RC, Watson HK: Hypertrophic ulnar styloid nonunions. Clin Orthop *228*:215, 1988.

250. Itoh Y, Horiuchi Y, Takahashi M, et al: Extensor tendon involvement in Smith's and Galeazzi's fractures. J Hand Surg [Am] *12*:535, 1987.

251. Thomas WG, Kershaw CJ: Entrapment of extensor tendons in a Smith's fracture: Brief report. J Bone Joint Surg [Br] *70*:491, 1988.

252. Mudgal CS, Jones WA: Scapho-lunate diastasis: A component of fractures of the distal radius. J Hand Surg [Br] 15:503, 1990.

253. Osmond-Clarke H: Recurrent dislocation of the shoulder: The Putti-Platt operation. J Bone Joint Surg [Br] 30:19, 1948.

254. Magnuson PB, Stack JK: Bilateral habitual dislocation of the shoulders in twins, a family tendency. JAMA 144:2103, 1940.

255. Eden R: Zur Operation der habituellen Schulterluxation unter mitteilung eines neuen Verfahrens bei Abris am inneren Plafannenrande. Dtsch Ztschr Chir 144:269, 1918.

256. Hybbinette S: De la transplantation d'un fragment osseux pour remédier aux luxations récidivantes de l'épaule: Constatations et résultats opératoires. Acta Chir Scand 71:411, 1932.

257. Oudard P: La luxation récidivante de l'épaule (variété antero-interne). Procédé opératoire. J Chir 23:13, 1924.

258. Trillat A: Traitement de la luxation récidivante de l'épaule: Considérations techniques. Lyon Chir 49:986, 1954.

259. Helfet AJ: Coracoid transplantation for recurring dislocation of the shoulder. J Bone Joint Surg [Br] 40:198, 1958.

260. Stewart MJ: Fractures of the humeral shaft. Current Pract Orthop Surg 2:140, 1964.

261. Lemperg R, Liliequist B: Dislocation of the upper proximal epiphysis of the humerus in newborns. Acta Paediatr Scand 59:337, 1970.

262. Epps CH Jr: Fractures of the shaft of the humerus. In CA Rockwood Jr, DP Green (Eds): Fractures in Adults. 2nd Ed. Philadelphia, JB Lippincott Co, 1984, p 653.

263. Klenerman L: Fractures of the shaft of the humerus. J Bone Joint Surg [Br] 48:105, 1966.

264. Whitson RO: Relation of the radial nerve to the shaft of the humerus. J Bone Joint Surg [Am] 36:85, 1954.

265. Pollock FH, Drake D, Bovill EG, Day L, Trafton PG: Treatment of radial neuropathy associated with fractures of the humerus. J Bone Joint Surg [Am] 63:239, 1981.

266. Shah JJ, Bhatti NA: Radial nerve paralysis associated with fractures of the humerus. A review of 62 cases. Clin Orthop Rel Res 172:171, 1983.

267. Kaiser TE, Sim FH, Kelly PJ: Radial nerve palsy associated with humeral fractures. Orthopedics 4:1245, 1981.

268. Collins DN, Weber ER: Anterior interosseous nerve avulsion. Clin Orthop Rel Res 181:175, 1983.

269. Eppright RH, Wilkins KE: Fractures and dislocations of the elbow. In CA Rockwood Jr, DP Green (Eds): Fractures in Adults. Philadelphia, JB Lippincott Co, 1975, p 487.

270. DePalma AF: The management of fractures and dislocations. 2nd Ed. Philadelphia, WB Saunders Co, 1970.

271. Hoyer A: Treatment of supracondylar fractures of the humerus by skeletal traction in an abduction splint. J Bone Joint Surg [Am] 34:623, 1952.

272. Murphy WA, Siegel MJ: Elbow fat pads with new signs and extended differential diagnoses. Radiology 124:659, 1977.

273. Kamal AS, Austin RT: Dislocation of the median nerve and brachial artery in supracondylar fractures of the humerus. Injury 12:161, 1980.

274. Symeonides PP, Paschalogluo C, Pagalides T: Radial nerve enclosed in the callus of a supracondylar fracture. J Bone Joint Surg [Br] 57:523, 1975.

275. Tachdjian MO: Pediatric Orthopedics. Philadelphia, WB Saunders Co, 1972.

276. Arnold JA, Nascu RJ, Nelson CL: Supracondylar fractures of the humerus. The role of dynamic fractures in prevention of deformity. J Bone Joint Surg [Am] 59:589, 1977.

277. Norman O: Roentgenological studies on dislocations in supracondylar fractures of the humerus. Ann Radiol 18:395, 1975.

278. Fowles JV, Kassab MT: Displaced supracondylar fractures of the elbow in children. J Bone Joint Surg [Br] 56:490, 1974.

279. Kamal AS, Austin RT: Dislocation of the median nerve and brachial artery in supracondylar fractures of the humerus. Injury 12:161, 1980.

280. Rogers LF: Fractures and dislocations of the elbow. Semin Roentgenol 13:97, 1978.

281. Smith L: Deformity following supracondylar fractures of the humerus. J Bone Joint Surg [Am] 42:235, 1960.

282. D'Ambrosia RD: Supracondylar fractures of the humerus—prevention of cubitus varus. J Bone Joint Surg [Am] 54:60, 1972.

283. Dodge HS: Displaced supracondylar fractures of the humerus in children—treatment by Dunlop's traction. J Bone Joint Surg [Am] 54:1408, 1972.

284. Aitken AP, Smith L, Blackett CW: Supracondylar fractures in children. Am J Surg 59:161, 1943.

285. Blount WP, Schulz I, Cassidy RH: Fractures of the elbow in children. JAMA 146:699, 1951.

286. King D, Secor C: Bow elbow (cubitus varus). J Bone Joint Surg [Am] 33:572, 1951.

287. Parkinson C: The supracondyloid process. Radiology 62:556, 1954.

288. Engber WD, McBeath AA, Cowle AE: The supracondylar process. Clin Orthop Rel Res 104:228, 1974.

289. Barnard LB, McCoy SM: The supracondyloid processes of the humerus. J Bone Joint Surg 28:845, 1946.

290. Thomsen PB: Processus supracondyloidea humeri with concomitant compression of the median nerve and the ulnar nerve. Acta Orthop Scand 48:391, 1977.

291. Kolb LW, Moore RD: Fractures of the supracondylar process of the humerus. J Bone Joint Surg [Am] 49:532, 1967.

292. Symeonides PP: The humerus supracondylar process syndrome. Clin Orthop Rel Res 82:141, 1972.

293. Dymond IWD: The treatment of isolated fractures of the distal ulna. J Bone Joint Surg [Br] 66:408, 1984.

294. Reckling FW: Unstable fracture-dislocations of the forearm (Monteggia and Galeazzi lesions). J Bone Joint Surg [Am] 64:857, 1982.

295. Fowles JV, Sliman N, Kassab MT, Saib K: The Monteggia lesion in children. Fracture of the ulna and dislocation of the radial head. J Bone Joint Surg [Am] 65:1276, 1983.

296. Mullick S: The lateral Monteggia fracture. J Bone Joint Surg [Am] 59:543, 1977.

297. Mullan GB, Franklin A, Thomas NP: Adult Monteggia lesion with ipsilateral wrist injuries. Injury 12:413, 1981.

298. Barquet A, Caresani J: Fracture of the shaft of the ulna and radius with associated dislocation of the radial head. Injury 12:471, 1981.

299. Galeazzi R: Uber ein besonderes Syndrom bei Verlizunger im Bereich der unter Armknochen. Arch Orthop Unfallchir 35:557, 1934.

300. de Carvalho A, Moller JT, Vestergard-Anderson T: Radiological aspects of the Galeazzi lesion. Eur J Radiol 4:169, 1984.

301. Cetti NE: An unusual cause of blocked reduction of the Galeazzi injury. Injury 9:59, 1977.

302. Alpar EK, Thompson K, Owen R, Taylor JF: Midshaft fracture of forearm bones in children. Injury 13:153, 1981.

303. Smith H, Sage FP: Medullary fixation of forearm fractures. J Bone Joint Surg [Am] 39:91, 1957.

304. Knight RA, Purvis GD: Fractures of both bones of the forearm in adults. J Bone Joint Surg [Am] 31:755, 1949.

305. Watson FM, Eaton RG: Post-traumatic radio-ulnar synostosis. J Trauma 18:467, 1978.

306. Colles A: On the fractures of the carpal extremity of the radius. Edinb Med Surg J 10:182, 1814.

307. Frykman G: Fracture of the distal radius, including sequelae—shoulder-hand-finger syndrome, disturbance in the distal radio-ulnar joint, and impairment of nerve function: A clinical and experimental study. Acta Orthop Scand 108(Suppl):1, 1967.

308. Cautilli RA, Joyce MF, Gordon E, Juarez R: Classifications of fractures of the distal radius. Clin Orthop Rel Res 103:163, 1974.

309. Ellis J: Smith's and Barton's fractures. A method of treatment. J Bone Joint Surg [Br] 47:724, 1965.

310. DeOliveira JC: Barton's fractures. J Bone Joint Surg [Am] 55:586, 1973.

311. Bilos ZJ, Pankovich AM, Yelda S: Fracture-dislocation of the radiocarpal joint. J Bone Joint Surg [Am] 59:198, 1977.

312. Fernandez DL: Irreducible radiocarpal fracture-dislocation and radioulnar dissociation with entrapment of the ulnar nerve, artery and flexor profundus II–V. Case report. J Hand Surg 6:456, 1981.

313. Fitzsimons RA: Colles' fracture and chauffeur's fracture. Br Med J 2:357, 1938.

314. Thomas FB: Reduction of Smith's fracture. J Bone Joint Surg [Br] 39:463, 1957.

315. Hughston JC: Fracture of the distal radial shaft. Mistakes in management. J Bone Joint Surg [Am] 39:249, 1957.

316. Heiple KG, Freehafer AA, Van't Hof A: Isolated traumatic dislocation of the distal end of the ulnar or distal radio-ulnar joint. J Bone Joint Surg [Am] 44:1387, 1962.

317. Snook GA, Chrisman D, Wilson TC, Wietsma RD: Subluxation of the distal radio-ulnar joint by hyperpronation. J Bone Joint Surg [Am] 51:1315, 1969.

318. Wong PCN: Galeazzi fracture-dislocations in Singapore 1960–1964. Incidence and results of treatment. Singapore Med J 8:186, 1967.

319. Reckling FW, Cordell LD: Unstable fracture-dislocations of the forearm. The Monteggia and Galeazzi lesions. Arch Surg 96:999, 1968.

320. Mikic ZD: Galeazzi fracture-dislocations. J Bone Joint Surg [Am] 57:1071, 1975.

321. Walsh HPJ, McLaren CAN, Owen R: Galeazzi fractures in children. J Bone Joint Surg [Br] 69:730, 1987.

322. Khurana JS, Kattapuram SV, Becker S, et al: Galeazzi injury with an associated fracture of the radial head. Clin Orthop 234:70, 1988.

323. Rienau G, Gay R, Martinez C, Mansat C, Mansat M: Lésions de l'articulation radio-cubitale inférieure dans les traumatismes de l'avantbras et du poignet. Intérêt de l'arthrographie. Rev Chir Orthop 57(Suppl 1):253, 1971.

324. Resnick D: Arthrography in the evaluation of arthritic disorders of the wrist. Radiology 113:331, 1974.

325. Trousdale RT, Amadio PC, Cooney WP, et al: Radio-ulnar dissociation. A review of twenty cases. J Bone Joint Surg [Am] 74:1486, 1992.

326. Schiller MG, Ekenstarn FA, Kirsch PT: Volar dislocation of the distal radio-ulnar joint. A case report. J Bone Joint Surg [Am] 73:617, 1991.

327. Aulicino PL, Siegel JL: Acute injuries of the distal radioulnar joint. Hand Clin 7:283, 1991.

328. Törnvall AH, Ekenstarn FA, Hagert CG, et al: Radiologic examination and measurement of the wrist and distal radio-ulnar joint. New aspects. Acta Radiol Diagn 27:581, 1986.

329. Olerud C, Kongsholm J, Thuomas K-A: The congruence of the distal radio-ulnar joint. A magnetic resonance imaging study. Acta Orthop Scand 59:183, 1988.

330. King GJ, McMurtry RY, Rubenstein JD, et al: Kinematics of the distal radioulnar joint. J Hand Surg [Am] 11:798, 1986.

331. Taleisnik J: Carpal instability. J Bone Joint Surg [Am] 70:1262, 1988.

332. Wilson AJ, Mann FA, Gilula LA: Imaging of the hand and wrist. J Hand Surg [Br] 15:153, 1990.

333. Fisk GR: The wrist. J Bone Joint Surg [Br] 66:396, 1984.

334. Mayfield JK, Johnson RP, Kilcoyne RK: Carpal dislocations: pathomechanics and progressive perilunar instability. J Hand Surg 5:226, 1980.

335. Mayfield JK: Mechanism of carpal injuries. Clin Orthop Rel Res 149:45, 1980.

336. Taleisnik J: Post-traumatic carpal instability. Clin Orthop Rel Res 149:73, 1980.

337. Taleisnik J: Classification of carpal instability. Bull Hosp J Dis 44:511, 1984.

338. Yeager BA, Dalinka MK: Radiology of trauma to the wrist: dislocations, fracture dislocations, and instability patterns. Skel Radiol 13:120, 1985.

339. Mayfield JK: Patterns of injury to carpal ligaments. A spectrum. Clin Orthop Rel Res 187:36, 1984.

340. Hockley B: Carpal instability and carpal injuries. Australas Radiol 23:158, 1979.

341. Linscheid RL, Dobyns JH, Beabout JW, Bryan RS: Traumatic instability of the wrist. Diagnosis, classification, and pathomechanics. J Bone Joint Surg [Am] 54:1612, 1972.

342. Gilula LA, Weeks PM: Post-traumatic ligamentous instabilities of the wrist. Radiology 129:641, 1978.

343. Gilula LA: Carpal injuries: Analytic approach and case exercises. Am J Roentgenol 133:503, 1979.

344. Meyrueis JP, Cameli M, Jan P: Instabilité du carpe. Diagnostic et formes cliniques. Ann Chir 32:555, 1978.

345. Sebald JR, Dobyns JH, Linscheid RL: The natural history of collapse deformities of the wrist. Clin Orthop Rel Res 104:140, 1974.

346. Cantor RM, Braunstein EM: Diagnosis of dorsal and palmar rotation of the lunate on a frontal radiograph. J Hand Surg 13:187, 1988.

347. Linscheid RL, Dobyns JH, Beckenbaugh RD, Cooney WP III, Wood MB: Instability patterns of the wrist. J Hand Surg 8:682, 1983.

348. Pennes DR, Shirazi KK, Martel W: Bilateral palmar flexion instability: A complication of wheelchair use. Am J Roentgenol 141:1327, 1983.

349. Resnick D, Niwayama G: Carpal instability in rheumatoid arthritis and calcium pyrophosphate deposition disease. Pathogenesis and roentgen appearance. Ann Rheum Dis 36:311–318, 1977.

350. Lichtman DM, Schneider JR, Swafford AR, Mack GR: Ulnar midcarpal instability—clinical and laboratory analysis. J Hand Surg 6:515, 1981.

351. Jones WA: Beware the sprained wrist. The incidence and prognosis of scapholunate instability. J Bone Joint Surg [Br] 70:293, 1988.

352. Braunstein EM, Louis DS, Greene TL, et al: Fluoroscopic and arthrographic evaluation of carpal instability. AJR 144:1259, 1985.

353. Protas JM, Jackson WT: Evaluating carpal instabilities with fluoroscopy. Am J Roentgenol 135:137, 1980.

354. Jackson WT, Protas JM: Snapping scapholunate subluxation. J Hand Surg 6:590, 1981.

355. White SJ, Louis DS, Braunstein EM, Hankin FM, Greene TL: Capitate-lunate instability: Recognition by manipulation under fluoroscopy. Am J Roentgenol 143:361, 1984.

356. Watson H, Ottoni L, Pitts EC, et al: Rotary subluxation of the scaphoid: A spectrum of instability. J Hand Surg [Br] 18:62, 1993.

357. Cautilli GP, Wehbé MA: Scapho-lunate distance and cortical ring sign. J Hand Surg [Am] 16:501, 1991.

358. Ruby LK, An KN, Linscheid RL, et al: The effect of scapholunate ligament section on scapholunate motion. J Hand Surg [Am] 12:767, 1987.

359. Berger RA, Blair WF, Crowninshield RD, et al: The scapholunate ligament. J Hand Surg [Am] 7:87, 1982.

360. Hudson TM, Caragol WJ, Kaye JJ: Isolated rotatory subluxation of the carpal navicular. Am J Roentgenol 126:601, 1976.

361. Boyes JG: Subluxation of the carpal navicular bone. South Med J 69:141, 1976.

362. Frankel VH: The Terry-Thomas sign. Letter to Editor. Clin Orthop Rel Res 129:321, 1977.

363. Howard FM, Fahey T, Wojcik E: Rotatory subluxation of the navicular. Clin Orthop Rel Res 104:134, 1974.

364. Crittenden JJ, Jones DM, Santarelli AG: Bilateral rotational dislocation of the carpal navicular. Case report. Radiology 94:629, 1970.

365. Kindynis P, Resnick D, Kang HS, et al: Demonstration of the scapholunate space with radiography. Radiology 175:278, 1990.

366. Maki NJ, Chuinard RG, D'Ambrosia R: Isolated, complete radial dislocation of the scaphoid. A case report and review of the literature. J Bone Joint Surg [Am] 64:615, 1982.

367. Phillips CD, Keats TE: The development of post-traumatic cyst-like lesions in bone. Skel Radiol 15:631, 1986.

368. Lowrey DG, Moss SH, Wolff TW: Volar dislocation of the capitate. Report of a case. J Bone Joint Surg [Am] 66:611, 1984.

369. Soucacos PN, Hartofilakidis-Garofalidas GC: Dislocation of the triangular bone. Report of a case. J Bone Joint Surg [Am] 63:1012, 1981.

370. Boe S: Dislocation of the trapezium (multangulum majus). A case report. Acta Orthop Scand 50:85, 1979.

371. Holdsworth BJ, Shackleford I: Fracture dislocation of the trapezio-scaphoid joint—the missing link? J Hand Surg [Br] 12:41, 1987.

372. Stevanovic MV, Stark HH, Filler BC: Scaphotrapezial dislocation. A case report. J Bone Joint Surg [Am] 72:449, 1990.

373. Ostrowski DM, Miller ME, Gould JS: Dorsal dislocation of the trapezoid. J Hand Surg [Am] 15:874, 1990.

374. Inoue G, Inagaki Y: Isolated palmar dislocation of the trapezoid associated with attritional rupture of the flexor tendon. A case report. J Bone Joint Surg [Am] 72:446, 1990.

375. Goodman ML, Shankman GB: Palmar dislocation of the trapezoid—a case report. J Hand Surg 8:606, 1983.

376. Sundaram M, Shively R, Patel B, Tayob A: Isolated dislocation of the pisiform. Br J Radiol 53:911, 1980.

377. Minami M, Yamazaki J, Ishii S: Isolated dislocation of the pisiform: A case report and review of the literature. J Hand Surg [Am] 9:125, 1984.

378. McCarron RF, Coleman W: Dislocation of the pisiform treated by primary resection. A case report. Clin Orthop 241:231, 1989.

379. Pai C-H, Wei D-C, Hu S-T: Carpal bone dislocations: An analysis of twenty cases with relative emphasis on the role of crushing mechanisms. J Trauma 35:28, 1993.

380. Richards RS, Bennett JD, Roth JH: Scaphoid dislocation with radial-axial carpal disruption. AJR 160:1075, 1993.

381. Coll GA: Palmar dislocation of the scaphoid and lunate. J Hand Surg [Am] 12:476, 1987.

382. Goldberg B, Heller AP: Dorsal dislocation of the triquetrum with rotary subluxation of the scaphoid. J Hand Surg [Am] 12:119, 1987.

383. Fowler JL: Dislocation of the triquetrum and lunate: Brief report. J Hand Surg [Br] 70:665, 1988.

384. Norbeck DE Jr, Larson B, Blair SJ, et al: Traumatic longitudinal disruption of the carpus. J Hand Surg [Am] 12:509, 1987.

385. Pournaras J, Kappas A: Volar perilunar dislocation. A case report. J Bone Joint Surg [Am] 61:625, 1979.

386. Klein A, Webb LX: The crowded carpal sign in volar perilunar dislocation. J Trauma 27:82, 1987.

387. Stein F, Siegel MW: Naviculocapitate fracture syndrome. A case report—new thoughts on the mechanism of injury. J Bone Joint Surg [Am] 51:391, 1969.

388. MacAusland WR: Perilunar dislocation of the carpal bones and dislocation of the lunate bone. Surg Gynecol Obstet 79:256, 1944.

389. Dunn AW: Fractures and dislocations of the carpus. Surg Clin North Am 52:1513, 1972.

390. El-Khoury GY, Usta HY, Blair WF: Naviculocapitate fracture-dislocation. Am J Roentgenol 139:385, 1982.

391. Resnik CS, Gelberman RH, Resnick D: Transscaphoid, transcapitate, perilunate fracture dislocation (scaphocapitate syndrome). Skel Radiol 9:192, 1983.

392. Brekkan A, Karlsson J, Thorsteinsson T: Case report 252. Skel Radiol 10:291, 1983.

393. Mayfield JK: Patterns of injury to carpal ligaments. A spectrum. Clin Orthop Rel Res 187:36, 1984.

394. Cooney WP, Bussey R, Dobyns JH, et al: Difficult wrist fractures. Perilunate fracture-dislocations of the wrist. Clin Orthop 214:136, 1987.

395. Chen VT: Dislocation of carpometacarpal joint of the little finger. J Hand Surg [Br] 12:260, 1987.

396. Ho PK, Choban SJ, Eshman SJ, et al: Complex dorsal dislocation of the second carpometacarpal joint. J Hand Surg [Am] 12:1074, 1987.

397. Lawlis JF III, Gunther SF: Carpometacarpal dislocations. Long-term follow-up. J Bone Joint Surg [Am] 73:52, 1991.

398. Hazlett JW: Carpometacarpal dislocations other than the thumb: A report of 11 cases. Can J Surg 71:315, 1968.

399. Hsu JD, Curtis RM: Carpometacarpal dislocations on the ulnar side of the hand. J Bone Joint Surg [Am] 52:927, 1970.

400. Joseph RB, Linscheid RL, Dobyns JH, Bryan RS: Chronic sprains of the carpometacarpal joints. J Hand Surg 6:172, 1981.

401. Fisher MR, Rogers LF, Hendrix RW: Systematic approach to identifying fourth and fifth carpometacarpal joint dislocations. Am J Roentgenol 140:319, 1983.

402. Gunther SF: The carpometacarpal joints. Orthop Clin North Am 15:259, 1984.

403. Mody BS, Belliappa PP, Dias JJ, et al: Nonunion of fractures of the scaphoid tuberosity. J Bone Joint Surg [Br] 75:423, 1993.

404. Vahvanen V, Westerlund M: Fracture of the carpal scaphoid in children. A clinical and roentgenological study of 108 cases. Acta Orthop Scand 51:909, 1980.

405. Cockshott WP: Distal avulsion fractures of the scaphoid. Br J Radiol 53:1037, 1980.

406. Compson JP, Waterman JK, Spencer JD: Dorsal avulsion fractures of the scaphoid: Diagnostic implications and applied anatomy. J Hand Surg [Br] 18:58, 1993.

407. Larson B, Light TR, Ogden JA: Fracture and ischemic necrosis of the immature scaphoid. J Hand Surg [Am] 12:122, 1987.

408. Tiel-van Buul MMC, van Beek EJR, Dijkstra PF, et al: Radiography of the carpal scaphoid. Experimental evaluation of ''The Carpal Box'' and first clinical results. Invest Radiol 27:954, 1992.

409. Lindequist S, Larsen CF: Radiography of the carpal scaphoid. An experimental investigation evaluating the use of oblique projections. Acta Radiol (Diagn) 27:97, 1986.

410. Young MRA, Lowry JH, Laird JD, et al: 99Tc-MDP bone scanning of injuries of the carpal scaphoid. Injury 19:14, 1988.

411. Brismar J: Skeletal scintigraphy of the wrist in suggested scaphoid fracture. Acta Radiol Diagn 29:101, 1988.

412. Tiel-van Buul MMC, van Beek EJR, Broekhuizen AH, et al: Radiography and scintigraphy of suspected scaphoid fracture. A long-term study in 160 patients. J Bone Joint Surg [Br] 75:61, 1993.

413. Tiel-van Buul MMC, van Beek EJR, Dijkstra PF, et al: Significance of a hotspot on the bone scan after carpal injury—evaluation by computed tomography. Eur J Nucl Med 20:159, 1993.

414. Smith DK, Linscheid RL, Amadio PC, et al: Scaphoid anatomy: Evaluation with complex motion tomography. Radiology 173:177, 1989.

415. Tehranzadeh J, Davenport J, Pais MJ: Scaphoid fracture: Evaluation with flexion-extension tomography. Radiology 176:167, 1990.

416. Pennes DR, Jonsson K, Buckwalter KA: Direct coronal CT of the scaphoid bone. Radiology 171:870, 1989.

417. Nakamura R, Imaeda T, Horii E, et al: Analysis of scaphoid fracture displacement by three-dimensional computed tomography. J Hand Surg [Am] 16:485, 1991.

418. Cooney WP III, Dobyns JH, Linscheid RL: Fractures of the scaphoid: A rational approach to management. Clin Orthop Rel Res 149:90, 1980.

419. Andersen JL, Grøn P, Langhoff O: The scaphoid fat stripe in the diagnosis of carpal trauma. Acta Radiol Diagn 29:97, 1988.

420. Corfitsen M, Christensen SE, Cetti R: The anatomical fat pad and the radiological "scaphoid fat stripe." J Hand Surg [Br] 14:326, 1989.

421. Brøndum V, Larsen CF, Skov O: Fracture of the carpal scaphoid: Frequency and distribution in a well-defined population. Eur J Radiol 15:118, 1992.

422. Dias JJ, Thompson J, Barton NJ, et al: Suspected scaphoid fractures. The value of radiographs. J Bone Joint Surg [Br] 72:98, 1990.

423. Smith DK, Gilula LA, Amadio PC: Dorsal lunate tilt (DISI configuration): Sign of scaphoid fracture displacement. Radiology 176:497, 1990.

424. Dias JJ, Taylor M, Thompson J, et al: Radiographic signs of union of scaphoid fractures. An analysis of inter-observer agreement and reproducibility. J Bone Joint Surg [Br] 70:299, 1988.

425. Szabo RM, Manske D: Displaced fractures of the scaphoid. Clin Orthop 230:30, 1988.

426. Dias JJ, Brenkel IJ, Finlay DBL: Patterns of union in fractures of the waist of the scaphoid. J Bone Joint Surg [Br] 71:307, 1989.

427. Gelberman RH, Wolock BS, Siegel DB: Fractures and non-unions of the carpal scaphoid. J Bone Joint Surg [Am] 71:1560, 1989.

428. Black DM, Watson HK, Vender MI: Scapholunate gap with scaphoid nonunion. Clin Orthop 224:205, 1987.

429. Mack GR, Bosse MJ, Gelberman RH: The natural history of scaphoid non-union. J Bone Joint Surg [Am] 66:504, 1984.

430. Ruby LK, Stinson J, Belsky MR: The natural history of scaphoid nonunion. A review of fifty-five cases. J Bone Joint Surg [Am] 67:428, 1985.

431. McLain RF, Steyers CM: Tendon ruptures with scaphoid nonunion. A case report. Clin Orthop 255:117, 1990.

432. Quinn SF, Murray W, Watkins T, et al: CT for determining the results of treatment of fractures of the wrist. AJR 149:109, 1987.

433. Sherman SB, Greenspan A, Norman A: Osteonecrosis of the distal pole of the carpal scaphoid following fracture—a rare complication. Skel Radiol 9:189, 1983.

434. Botte MJ, Gelberman RH: Fractures of the carpus, excluding the scaphoid. Hand Clin 3:149, 1987.

435. Levy M, Fischel RE, Stern GM, Goldberg I: Chip fractures of the os triquetrum. The mechanism of injury. J Bone Joint Surg [Br] 61:355, 1979.

436. Cetti R, Christensen S-E, Reuther K: Fracture of the lunate bone. Hand 14:80, 1982.

437. Teisen H, Hjarbaek J: Classification of fresh fractures of the lunate. J Hand Surg [Br] 13:458, 1988.

438. Viegas SF, Wagner K, Patterson R, et al: Medial (hamate) facet of the lunate. J Hand Surg [Am] 15:564, 1990.

439. Ogunro O: Fracture of the body of the hamate bone. J Hand Surg 8:353, 1983.

440. Takami H, Takahashi S, Hiraki S: Coronal fractures of the body of the hamate: Case reports. J Trauma 32:110, 1992.

441. Loth TS, McMillan MD: Coronal dorsal hamate fractures. J Hand Surg [Am] 13:616, 1988.

442. Gillespy T III, Stork JJ, Dell PC: Dorsal fracture of the hamate: Distinctive radiographic appearance. AJR 151:351, 1988.

443. Schlosser H, Murray JF: Fracture of the hook of the hamate. Can J Surg 27:587, 1984.

444. Murray WT, Meuller PR, Rosenthal DI, Jauernek RR: Fracture of the hook of the hamate. Am J Roentgenol 133:899, 1979.

445. Parker RD, Berkowitz MS, Brahms MA, Bohl WR: Hook of the hamate fractures in athletes. Am J Sports Med 14:517, 1986.

446. Stark HH, Chao E-K, Zemel NP, et al: Fracture of the hook of the hamate. J Bone Joint Surg [Am] 71:1202, 1989.

447. Papilion JD, DuPuy TE, Aulicino PL, et al: Radiographic evaluation of the hook of the hamate: A new technique. J Hand Surg [Am] 13:437, 1988.

448. Carter PR, Eaton RG, Littler JW: Ununited fracture of the hook of the hamate. J Bone Joint Surg 59:583, 1977.

449. Failla JM: Osteonecrosis associated with nonunion of the hook of the hamate. Orthopedics 16:217, 1993.

450. Manske PR: Fracture of the hook of the hamate presenting as carpal tunnel syndrome. Hand 10:181, 1978.

451. Minami A, Ogino T, Usui M, Ishii S: Finger tendon rupture secondary to fracture of the hamate. A case report. Acta Orthop Scand 56:96, 1985.

452. Fleege MA, Jebson PJ, Renfrew DL, et al: Pisiform fractures. Skel Radiol 20:169, 1991.

453. Georgoulis A, Hertel P, Lais E: Die Fraktur und die Luxationsfraktur des Os pisiforme. Unfallchirurg 94:182, 1991.

454. Rand JA, Linscheid RL, Dobyns JH: Capitate fractures. A long-term follow-up. Clin Orthop Rel Res 165:209, 1982.

455. Shirazi KK, Agha FP, Amendola MA: Isolated fracture of greater multangular. Br J Radiol 55:923, 1982.

456. Abbitt PL, Riddervold HO: The carpal tunnel view: Helpful adjuvant for unrecognized fractures of the carpus. Skel Radiol 16:45, 1987.

457. Griffen AC, Gilula LA, Young VL, et al: Fracture of the dorsoulnar tubercle of the trapezium. J Hand Surg [Am] 13:622, 1988.

458. Botte MJ, von Schroeder HP, Gellman H, et al: Fracture of the trapezial ridge. Clin Orthop 276:202, 1992.

459. Hubbard LF: Metacarpophalangeal dislocations. Hand Clin 4:39, 1988.

460. Kaplan EB: Dorsal dislocation of the metacarpophalangeal joint of the index finger. J Bone Joint Surg [Am] 39:1081, 1957.

461. Sweterlitsch PR, Torg JS, Pollack H: Entrapment of a sesamoid in the index metacarpophalangeal joint: Report of two cases. J Bone Joint Surg [Am] 51:995, 1969.

462. Khuri SM, Fay JJ: Complete volar metacarpophalangeal joint dislocation of a finger. J Trauma 26:1058, 1986.

463. Vicar AJ: Proximal interphalangeal joint dislocations without fractures. Hand Clin 4:5, 1988.

464. Lubahn JD: Dorsal fracture dislocations of the proximal interphalangeal joint. Hand Clin 4:15, 1988.

465. Moberg E: Fractures and ligamentous injuries of the thumb and fingers. Surg Clin North Am 40:297, 1960.

466. Nance EP Jr, Kaye JJ, Milek MA: Volar plate fractures. Radiology 133:61, 1979.

467. Scher AT: Associated sternal and spinal fractures. Case reports. S Afr Med J 64:98, 1983.

468. Phillips JH: Irreducible dislocation of a distal interphalangeal joint: Case report and review of literature. Clin Orthop Rel Res 154:188, 1981.

469. Rayan GM, Elias LS: Irreducible dislocation of the distal interphalangeal joint caused by long flexor tendon entrapment. Orthopedics 4:35, 1981.

470. Green DP, O'Brien ET: Fractures of the thumb metacarpal. South Med J 65:807, 1972.

471. Griffiths JC: Fractures at the base of the first metacarpal bone. J Bone Joint Surg [Br] 46:712, 1964.

472. Howard FM: Fractures of the basal joint of the thumb. Clin Orthop 220:46, 1987.

473. Pellegrini VD Jr: Fractures at the base of the thumb. Hand Clin 4:87, 1988.

474. Miller RJ: Dislocations and fracture dislocations of the metacarpophalangeal joint of the thumb. Hand Clin 4:45, 1988.

475. Neviaser RJ, Wilson JN, Lievano A: Rupture of the ulnar collateral ligament of the thumb (gamekeeper's thumb). Correction by dynamic repair. J Bone Joint Surg [Am] 53:1357, 1971.

476. Coonrad RW, Goldner JL: A study of the pathological findings and treatment in soft-tissue injury of the thumb metacarpophalangeal joint with a clinical study of the normal range of motion in one thousand thumbs and a study of post mortem findings of ligamentous structures in relation to function. J Bone Joint Surg [Am] 50:439, 1968.

477. Campbell CS: Gamekeeper's thumb. J Bone Joint Surg [Br] 37:148, 1955.

478. Stener B: Displacement of the ruptured ulnar collateral ligament of the metacarpophalangeal joint of the thumb. A clinical and anatomical study. J Bone Joint Surg [Br] 44:869, 1962.

479. Sakellarides HT, DeWeese JW: Instability of the metacarpophalangeal joint of the thumb. Reconstruction of the collateral ligaments using the extensor pollicis brevis tendon. J Bone Joint Surg [Am] 58:106, 1976.

480. Schultz RJ, Fox JM: Gamekeeper's thumb: Result of skiing injuries. NY State J Med 73:2329, 1973.

481. Primiano GA: Skiers' thumb injuries associated with flared ski pole handles. Am J Sports Med 13:425, 1985.

482. van Dommelen BA, Zvirbulis RA: Upper extremity injuries in snow skiers. Amer J Sports Med 17:751, 1989.

483. Winslet MC, Clarke NMP, Mulligan PJ: Breakdancer's thumb—partial rupture of the ulnar collateral ligament with a fracture of the proximal phalanx of the thumb. Injury 17:201, 1986.

484. Downey EF Jr, Curtis DJ: Patient-induced stress test of the first metacarpophalangeal joint: A radiographic assessment of collateral ligament injuries. Radiology 158:679, 1986.

485. Louis DS, Huebner JJ Jr, Hankin FM: Rupture and displacement of the ulnar collateral ligament of the metacarpophalangeal joint of the thumb. Preoperative diagnosis. J Bone Joint Surg [Am] 68:1320, 1986.

486. Linscheid RL: Arthrography of the metacarpophalangeal joint. Clin Orthop Rel Res 103:91, 1974.

487. Resnick D, Danzig LA: Arthrographic evaluation of injuries of the first metacarpophalangeal joint: Gamekeeper's thumb. Am J Roentgenol 126:1046, 1976.

488. Spaeth HJ, Abrams RA, Bock GW, et al: Gamekeeper thumb: Differentiation of nondisplaced and displaced tears of the ulnar collateral ligament with MR imaging. Work in progress. Radiology 188:553, 1993.

489. Yamanaka K, Yoshida K, Inoue H, Inoue A, Miyagi T: Locking of the metacarpophalangeal joint of the thumb. J Bone Joint Surg [Am] 67:782, 1985.

490. Margles SW: Intra-articular fractures of the metacarpophalangeal and proximal interphalangeal joints. Hand Clin 4:67, 1988.

491. McKerrell J, Bowen V, Johnston G, et al: Boxer's fractures—conservative or operative management. J Trauma 27:486, 1987.

492. Barton NJ: Fractures of the hand. J Bone Joint Surg [Br] 66:159, 1984.

493. DaCruz DJ, Slade RJ, Malone W: Fractures of the distal phalanges. J Hand Surg [Br] 13:350, 1988.

494. Stark HH, Gainor BJ, Ashworth CR, et al: Operative treatment of intra-articular fractures of the dorsal aspect of the distal phalanx of digits. J Bone Joint Surg [Am] 69:892, 1987.

495. Wehbe MA, Schneider LH: Mallet fractures. J Bone Joint Surg [Am] 66:658, 1984.

496. Street JM: Radiographs of phalangeal fractures: Importance of the internally rotated oblique projection for diagnosis. AJR *160*:575, 1993.

497. Eddy RJ, Connell DG: Luxatio erecta of the hip. AJR *151*:412, 1988.

498. Epstein HC: Traumatic dislocations of the hip. Clin Orthop Rel Res *92*:116, 1973.

499. Zamani MH, Saltzman DI: Bilateral traumatic anterior dislocation of the hip: Case report. Clin Orthop Rel Res *161*:203, 1981.

500. Bassett LW, Gold RH, Epstein HC: Anterior hip dislocation: Atypical superolateral displacement of the femoral head. Am J Roentgenol *141*:385, 1983.

501. Sadler AH, DiStefano M: Anterior dislocation of the hip with ipsilateral basicervical fracture. A case report. J Bone Joint Surg [Am] *67*:326, 1985.

502. Korovessis P, Droutsas P, Spastris P, et al: Anterior dislocation of the hip associated with fracture of the ipsilateral greater trochanter. A case report. Clin Orthop *253*:164, 1990.

503. Scham SM, Fry LR: Traumatic anterior dislocation of the hip with fracture of the femoral head. Clin Orthop Rel Res *62*:133, 1969.

504. Yandow DR, Austin CW: Femoral defect after anterior dislocation. J Comput Assist Tomogr *7*:1112, 1983.

505. Dussault RG, Beauregard G, Fauteaux P, Laurin C, Boisjoly A: Femoral head defect following anterior hip dislocation. Radiology *135*:627, 1980.

506. DeLee JC, Evans JA, Thomas J: Anterior dislocation of the hip and associated femoral-head fractures. J Bone Joint Surg [Am] *62*:960, 1980.

507. Tehranzadeh J, Vanarthros W, Pais MJ: Osteochondral impaction of the femoral head associated with hip dislocation: CT study in 35 patients. AJR *155*:1049, 1990.

508. Dall D, Macnab I, Gross A: Recurrent anterior dislocation of the hip. J Bone Joint Surg [Am] *52*:574, 1970.

509. Haddad RJ Jr, Drez D: Voluntary recurrent anterior dislocation of the hip. A case report. J Bone Joint Surg [Am] *56*:419, 1974.

510. Guyer B, Levinsohn EM: Recurrent anterior dislocation of the hip: Case report with arthrographic findings. Skel Radiol *10*:262, 1983.

511. Larson CB: Fracture dislocations of the hip. Clin Orthop Rel Res *92*:147, 1973.

512. Whitehouse GH: Radiological aspects of posterior dislocation of the hip. Clin Radiol *29*:431, 1978.

513. Canale ST, Manugian AH: Irreducible traumatic dislocations of the hip. J Bone Joint Surg [Am] *61*:7, 1979.

514. Epstein HC: Posterior fracture-dislocations of the hip; long-term follow-up. J Bone Joint Surg [Am] *56*:1103, 1974.

515. Smith GR, Loop JW: Radiologic classification of posterior dislocations of the hip: Refinement and pitfalls. Radiology *119*:569, 1976.

516. Yang R-S, Tsuang Y-H, Hang Y-S, et al: Traumatic dislocation of the hip. Clin Orthop *265*:218, 1991.

517. Butler JE: Pipkin type-II fractures of the femoral head. J Bone Joint Surg [Am] *63*:1292, 1981.

518. Klasen JH, Binnendik B: Fracture of the neck of the femur associated with posterior dislocation of the hip. J Bone Joint Surg [Br] *66*:45, 1984.

519. Armbuster TG, Guerra J, Resnick D, Goergen TG, Feingold ML, Niwayama G, Danzig LA: The adult hip: An anatomic study. Part I. The bony landmarks. Radiology *128*:1, 1978.

520. Quackenbush D, DiDonato R, Butler D: A modified lateral projection for anterior and posterior lips of the acetabulum. Radiology *125*:536, 1977.

521. Judet R, Judet J, Letournel E: Fracture of the acetabulum: Classification and surgical approaches for open reduction. J Bone Joint Surg [Am] *46*:1615, 1964.

522. Calkins MS, Zych G, Latta L, et al: Computed tomography evaluation of stability in posterior fracture dislocation of the hip. Clin Orthop *227*:152, 1988.

523. Richardson P, Young JWR, Porter D: CT detection of cortical fracture of the femoral head associated with posterior hip dislocation. AJR *155*:93, 1990.

524. Hougaard K, Lindequist S, Nielsen LB: Computerised tomography after posterior dislocation of the hip. J Bone Joint Surg [Br] *69*:556, 1987.

525. Hougaard K, Thomsen PB: Traumatic posterior fracture-dislocation of the hip with fracture of the femoral head or neck, or both. J Bone Joint Surg [Am] *70*:233, 1988.

526. Hougaard K, Thomsen PB: Coxarthrosis following traumatic posterior dislocation of the hip. J Bone Joint Surg [Am] *69*:679, 1987.

527. Proctor H: Dislocations of the hip joint (excluding "central" dislocation) and their complications. Injury *5*:1, 1973.

528. Paterson I: The torn acetabular labrum. A block to reduction of a dislocated hip. J Bone Joint Surg [Br] *39*:306, 1957.

529. Dameron TB Jr: Bucket-handle tear of acetabular labrum accompanying posterior dislocation of the hip. J Bone Joint Surg [Am] *41*:131, 1959.

530. Connolly JF: Acetabular labrum entrapment associated with a femoral-head fracture-dislocation. A case report. J Bone Joint Surg [Am] *56*:1735, 1974.

531. Rashleigh-Belcher HJC, Cannon SR: Recurrent dislocation of the hip with a "Bankart-type" lesion. J Bone Joint Surg [Br] *68*:398, 1986.

532. Graham B, Lapp RA: Recurrent posttraumatic dislocation of the hip. A report of two cases and review of the literature. Clin Orthop *256*:115, 1990.

533. Provenzano MP, Holmes PF, Tullos HS: Atraumatic recurrent dislocation of the hip. A case report. J Bone Joint Surg [Am] *69*:938, 1987.

534. Hovelius L: Traumatic dislocation of the hip in children. Report of two cases. Acta Orthop Scand *45*:746, 1974.

535. Hammelbo T: Traumatic hip dislocation in childhood. A report of three cases. Acta Orthop Scand *47*:546, 1976.

536. Schlonsky J, Miller PR: Traumatic hip dislocations in children. J Bone Joint Surg [Am] *55*:1057, 1973.

537. Gaul RW: Recurrent traumatic dislocation of the hip in children. Clin Orthop Rel Res *90*:107, 1973.

538. Petterson H, Theander G, Danielsson L: Voluntary habitual dislocation of the hip in children. Acta Radiol (Diagn) *21*:303, 1980.

539. Barquet A: Traumatic hip dislocation in childhood. A report of 26 cases and a review of the literature. Acta Orthop Scand *50*:549, 1979.

540. Hougaard K, Thomsen PB: Traumatic hip dislocation in children. Follow up of 13 cases. Orthopedics *12*:375, 1989.

541. Shea KP, Kalamchi A, Thompson GH: Acetabular epiphysis-labrum entrapment following traumatic anterior dislocation of the hip in children. J Pediatr Orthop *6*:215, 1986.

542. Cinats JG, Moreau MJ, Swersky JF: Traumatic dislocation of the hip caused by interposition in a child. A case report. J Bone Joint Surg [Am] *70*:130, 1988.

543. Barrett IR, Goldberg JA: Avulsion fracture of the ligamentum teres in a child. A case report. J Bone Joint Surg [Am] *71*:438, 1989.

544. Barquet A: Avascular necrosis following traumatic hip dislocation in childhood. Factors of influence. Acta Orthop Scand *53*:809, 1982.

545. Barquet A: Natural history of avascular necrosis following traumatic hip dislocation in childhood. A review of 145 cases. Acta Orthop Scand *53*:815, 1982.

546. Fiddian NJ, Grace DL: Traumatic dislocation of the hip in adolescence with separation of the capital epiphysis. Two case reports. J Bone Joint Surg [Br] *65*:148, 1983.

547. Lender M, Makin M, Robin G, Steinberg R, Menczel J: Osteoporosis and fractures of the neck of the femur: Some epidemiologic considerations. Isr J Med Sci *12*:596, 1976.

548. Vose GP, Lockwood RM: Femoral neck fracturing: Its relationship to radiographic bone density. J Gerontol *20*:300, 1965.

549. Stevens J, Freeman PA, Nordin BEC, Barnett E: The incidence of osteoporosis in patients with femoral neck fracture. J Bone Joint Surg [Br] *44*:520, 1962.

550. Lowell JD: Fractures of the hip. N Engl J Med *274*:1418, 1966.

551. Lowell JD: Fractures of the hip. N Engl J Med *274*:1480, 1966.

552. Nilsson BE: Spinal osteoporosis and femoral neck fracture. Clin Orthop Rel Res *68*:93, 1970.

553. Horiuchi T, Tokuyama H, Igarashi M, et al: Spontaneous fractures of the hip in the elderly. Orthopedics *11*:1277, 1988.

554. Linton P: On different types of intracapsular fractures of the femoral neck. Acta Chir Scand *90*(Suppl 86):1, 1944.

555. Backman S: The proximal end of the femur. Acta Radiol *146*(Suppl):1, 1957.

556. DeLee JC: Fractures and dislocations of the hip. *In* CA Rockwood Jr, DP Green (Eds.): Fractures in Adults. 2nd Ed. Philadelphia, JB Lippincott Co, 1984, p 1211.

557. Kenerman L, Marcuson RW: Intracapsular fractures of the neck of the femur. J Bone Joint Surg [Br] *52*:514, 1970.

558. Askin SR, Bryan RS: Femoral neck fractures in young adults. Clin Orthop Rel Res *114*:259, 1976.

559. Alffram PA: An epidemiologic study of cervical and trochanteric fractures of the femur in an urban population. Analysis of 1,664 cases with special reference to etiologic factors. Acta Orthop Scand *65*(Suppl):11, 1964.

560. Garden RS: Stability and union in subcapital fractures of the femur. J Bone Joint Surg [Br] *46*:630, 1964.

561. Pauwels F: Der Schenkenholsbruck, em mechanisches Problem. Grundlagen des Heilungsvorganges. Prognose und kausale Therapie. Stuttgart, Beilageheft zur Zeitschrift fur Orthopaedische Chirurgie, Ferdinand Enke, 1935.

562. Garden RS: Reduction and fixation of subcapital fractures of the femur. Orthop Clin North Am *5*:683, 1974.

563. Fransden PA, Anderson E, Madsen F, et al: Garden's classification of femoral neck fractures. An assessment of inter-observer variation. J Bone Joint Surg [Br] *70*:588, 1988.

564. Barnes R, Brown JT, Garden RS, Nicoll EA: Subcapital fractures of the femur. J Bone Joint Surg [Br] *58*:2, 1976.

565. Barr JS: Experiences with a sliding nail in femoral neck fractures. Clin Orthop Rel Res *92*:63, 1973.

566. Arnold WD, Lyden JP, Minkoff J: Treatment of intracapsular fractures of the femoral neck. J Bone Joint Surg [Am] *56*:254, 1974.

567. Sevitt S: Avascular necrosis and revascularization of the femoral head after intracapsular fractures. J Bone Joint Surg [Br] *46*:270, 1964.

568. Melberg P-E, Körner L, Lansinger O: Hip joint pressure after femoral neck fracture. Acta Orthop Scand *57*:501, 1986.

569. Stromqvist B, Nilsson LT, Egund N, et al: Intracapsular pressures in undisplaced fractures of the femoral neck. J Bone Joint Surg [Br] *70*:192, 1988.

570. Crawford EJP, Emery RJH, Hansell DM, et al: Capsular distension and intracapsular pressure in subcapital fractures of the femur. J Bone Joint Surg [Br] *70*:195, 1988.

571. Holmberg S, Dalen N: Intracapsular pressure and caput circulation in nondisplaced femoral neck fractures. Clin Orthop *219*:124, 1987.

572. Holder LE, Schwarz C, Wernicke PG, et al: Radionuclide bone imaging in the early detection of fractures of the proximal femur (hip): Multifactorial analysis. Radiology *174*:509, 1990.

573. Fairclough J, Colhoun E, Johnston D, et al: Bone scanning for suspected hip fractures. A prospective study in elderly patients. J Bone Joint Surg [Br] *69*:251, 1987.

574. Strömqvist B, Hansson LI, Nilsson LT, et al: Prognostic precision in postoperative 99mTc-MDP scintimetry after femoral neck fracture. Acta Orthop Scand *58*:494, 1987.

575. Alberts KA, Dahlborn M, Ringertz H: Sequential scintimetry after femoral neck fracture. Acta Orthop Scand *58*:217, 1987.

576. Hirano T, Taguchi A, Suzuki R, et al: Correlation of 99mTc-MDP scintimetry and histology in cervical hip fracture. Acta Orthop Scand *58*:33, 1987.

577. Alberts KA: Prognostic accuracy of preoperative and postoperative scintimetry after femoral neck fracture. Clin Orthop 250:221, 1990.

578. Speer KP, Spritzer CE, Harrelson JM, et al: Magnetic resonance imaging of the femoral head after acute intracapsular fracture of the femoral neck. J Bone Joint Surg [Am] 72:98, 1990.

579. Rizzo PF, Gould ES, Lyden JP, et al: Diagnosis of occult fractures about the hip. Magnetic resonance imaging compared with bone-scanning. J Bone Joint Surg [Am] 75:395, 1993.

580. Quinn SF, McCarthy JL: Prospective evaluation of patients with suspected hip fracture and indeterminate radiographs: Use of T1-weighted MR images. Radiology 187:469, 1993.

581. Bayliss AP, Davidson JK: Traumatic osteonecrosis of the femoral head following intracapsular fracture: Incidence and earliest radiological features. Clin Radiol 28:407, 1977.

582. Phemister DB: Fractures of the neck of the femur, dislocation of the hip and obscure vascular disturbances producing aseptic necrosis of the head of the femur. Surg Gynecol Obstet 59:415, 1934.

583. Catto MA: The histological appearances of late segmental collapse of the femoral head after transcervical fracture. J Bone Joint Surg [Br] 47:777, 1965.

584. Barr JS: Diagnosis and treatment of infections following internal fixation of hip fractures. Orthop Clin North Am 5:847, 1974.

585. Cleveland M, Bosworth DM, Thompson FR: Intertrochanteric fractures of the femur. J Bone Joint Surg 29:1049, 1947.

586. Cleveland M, Bosworth DM, Thompson FR, Wilson HJ, Ishizuka T: A ten year analysis of intertrochanteric fractures of the femur. J Bone Joint Surg [Am] 41:1399, 1959.

587. Evans EM: The treatment of trochanteric fractures of the femur. J Bone Joint Surg [Am] 31:190, 1949.

588. Boyd HB, Griffin LL: Classification and treatment of trochanteric fractures. Arch Surg 58:853, 1949.

589. Herrlin K, Strömberg T, Lidgren L, et al: Trochanteric fractures. Classification and mechanical stability in McLaughlin, Ender and Richard osteosynthesis. Acta Radiol Diagn 29:189, 1988.

590. Sernbo I, Johnell O, Gentz C-F, et al: Unstable intertrochanteric fractures of the hip. Treatment with Ender pins compared with a compression hip-screw. J Bone Joint Surg [Am] 70:1297, 1988.

591. Mariani EM, Rand JA: Subcapital fractures after open reduction and internal fixation of intertrochanteric fractures of the hip. Report of three cases. Clin Orthop 245:165, 1989.

592. Søballe K, Christensen F: Laceration of the superficial femoral artery by an intertrochanteric fracture fragment. A case report. J Bone Joint Surg [Am] 69:781, 1987.

593. Fielding JW, Magliata HJ: Subtrochanteric fractures. Surg Gynecol Obstet 122:555, 1966.

594. Seinsheimer F: Subtrochanteric fractures of the femur. J Bone Joint Surg [Am] 60:300, 1978.

595. Judet R, Judet J, Letournel E: Fractures of the acetabulum: Classification and surgical approaches for open reduction. Preliminary report. J Bone Joint Surg [Am] 46:1615, 1964.

596. Sauser DD, Billimoria PE, Rouse GA, Mudge K: CT evaluation of hip trauma. Am J Roentgenol 135:269, 1980.

597. Shirkhoda A, Brashear HR, Staab EV: Computed tomography of acetabular fractures. Radiology 134:683, 1980.

598. Mack LA, Harley JD, Winquist RA: CT of acetabular fractures: Analysis of fracture patterns. Am J Roentgenol 138:407, 1982.

599. Harley JD, Mack LA, Winquist RA: CT of acetabular fractures: Comparison with conventional radiography. Am J Roentgenol 138:413, 1982.

600. Walker RH, Burton DS: Computerized tomography in assessment of acetabular fractures. J Trauma 22:227, 1982.

601. Rafii M, Firooznia H, Golimbu C, Waugh T Jr, Naidich D: The impact of CT in clinical management of pelvic and acetabular fractures. Clin Orthop Rel Res 178:228, 1983.

602. Tillie B, Fontaine Ch, Stahl Ph, et al: The place of computed tomography in the diagnosis and treatment of acetabular fractures. A review of 88 cases. Fr J Orthop Surg 1:13, 1987.

603. Martinez CR, Di Pasquale TG, Helfet DL, et al: Evaluation of acetabular fractures with two- and three-dimensional CT. RadioGraphics 12:227, 1992.

604. Knight RA, Smith H: Central fractures of the acetabulum. J Bone Joint Surg [Am] 40:1, 1958.

605. Letournel E: Acetabulum fractures: Classification and management. Clin Orthop Rel Res 151:81, 1980.

606. Rogers LF, Novy SB, Harris NF: Occult central fractures of the acetabulum. Am J Roentgenol 124:96, 1975.

607. Dunn AW, Russo CL: Central acetabular fractures. J Trauma 13:695, 1973.

608. Nerubay J, Glancz G, Katznelson A: Fractures of the acetabulum. J Trauma 13:1050, 1973.

609. Lansinger O: Fractures of the acetabulum. A clinical, radiological and experimental study. Acta Orthop Scand (Suppl) 165:7, 1977.

610. Lovelock JE, Monaco P: Central acetabular fracture dislocations: An unusual complication of seizures. Skel Radiol 10:91, 1983.

611. Weisel A, Hecht HL: Occult fracture through the triradiate cartilage of the acetabulum. Am J Roentgenol 134:1262, 1980.

612. Bosse MJ, Poka A, Reiner CM, et al: Heterotopic ossification as a complication of acetabular fracture. Prophylaxis with low-dose irradiation. J Bone Joint Surg [Am] 70:1231, 1988.

613. Winquist RA, Hansen ST Jr: Comminuted fractures of the femoral shaft treated by intramedullary nailing. Orthop Clin North Am 11:633, 1980.

614. Winquist RA, Hansen ST Jr, Clawson DK: Closed intramedullary nailing of femoral fractures. J Bone Joint Surg [Am] 66:529, 1984.

615. Hooper GJ, Lyon DW: Closed unlocked nailing for comminuted femoral fractures. J Bone Joint Surg [Br] 70:619, 1988.

616. Brumback RJ, Reilly JP, Poka A, et al: Intramedullary nailing of femoral shaft fractures. Part I. Decision-making errors with interlocking fixation. J Bone Joint Surg [Am] 70:1441, 1988.

617. Brumback RJ, Uwagie-Ero S, Lakatos RP, et al: Intramedullary nailing of femoral shaft fractures. Part II. Fracture-healing with static interlocking fixation. J Bone Joint Surg [Am] 70:1453, 1988.

618. Franklin JL, Winquist RA, Benirschke SK, et al: Broken intramedullary nails. J Bone Joint Surg [Am] 70:1463, 1988.

619. Lhowe DW, Hansen ST: Intramedullary nailing of open fractures of the femoral shaft. J Bone Joint Surg [Am] 70:812, 1988.

620. Christie J, Court-Brown C, Kinninmonth AWG, et al: Intramedullary locking nails in the management of femoral shaft fractures. J Bone Joint Surg [Br] 70:206, 1988.

621. Daffner RH, Riemer BL, Butterfield SL: Ipsilateral femoral neck and shaft fractures: an overlooked association. Skel Radiol 20:251, 1991.

622. Hresko MT, Kasser JR: Physeal arrest about the knee associated with non-physeal fractures in the lower extremity. J Bone Joint Surg [Am] 71:698, 1989.

623. Siliski JM, Mahring M, Hofer HP: Supracondylar-intercondylar fractures of the femur. Treatment by internal fixation. J Bone Joint Surg [Am] 71:95, 1989.

624. Seinsheimer F III: Fractures of the distal femur. Clin Orthop Rel Res 153:169, 1980.

625. Hohl M, Larson RL, Jones DC: Fractures and dislocations of the knee. In CA Rockwood Jr, DP Green (Eds): Fractures in Adults. 2nd Ed. JB Lippincott Co, 1984, p 1429.

626. Klingensmith W, Oles P, Martinez H: Arterial injuries associated with dislocation of the knee or fracture of the lower femur. Surg Gynecol Obstet 120:961, 1965.

627. Neer CS, Grantham SA, Shelton ML: Supracondylar fracture of the adult femur. J Bone Joint Surg 49:591, 1967.

628. Pogrund H, Husseini N, Bloom R, Finsterbush A: The cleavage intercondylar fracture of the femur. Clin Orthop Rel Res 160:74, 1981.

629. Giles JB, DeLee JC, Heckman JD, Keever JE: Supracondylar-intercondylar fractures of the femur treated with a supracondylar plate and lag screw. J Bone Joint Surg [Am] 64:864, 1982.

630. Lewis SL, Pozo JL, Muirhead-Allwood WFG: Coronal fractures of the lateral femoral condyle. J Bone Joint Surg [Br] 71:118, 1989.

631. Carpenter JE, Kasman R, Matthews LS: Fractures of the patella. J Bone Joint Surg [Am] 75:1550, 1993.

632. Hensal F, Nelson T, Pavlov H, Torg JS: Bilateral patellar fractures from indirect trauma. A case report. Clin Orthop Rel Res 178:207, 1983.

633. Lotke PA, Ecker ML: Transverse fractures of the patella. Clin Orthop Rel Res 158:180, 1981.

634. Bostrom A: Fracture of the patella. A study of 422 patellar fractures. Acta Orthop Scand (Suppl)143:5, 1972.

635. Scapinelli R: Blood supply of the human patella. Its relation to ischaemic necrosis after fracture. J Bone Joint Surg [Br] 49:563, 1967.

636. Heckman JD, Alkire CC: Distal patellar pole fractures. A proposed common mechanism of injury. Am J Sports Med 12:424, 1984.

637. Dashefsky JH: Fracture of the fabella. A case report. J Bone Joint Surg [Am] 59:698, 1977.

638. Frey C, Bjorkengren A, Sartoris D, et al: Knee dysfunction secondary to dislocation of the fabella. Clin Orthop 222:223, 1987.

639. Rafii M, Lamont JG, Firoozna H: Tibial plateau fractures: CT evaluation and classification. CRC Crit Rev Diagn Imag 27:91, 1987.

640. Elstrom J, Pankovich AM, Sassoon H, Rodriguez J: The use of tomography in the assessment of fractures of the tibial plateau. J Bone Joint Surg [Am] 58:551, 1976.

641. Raffi M, Firooznia H, Golimbu C, Bonamo J: Computed tomography of tibial plateau fractures. Am J Roentgenol 142:1181, 1984.

642. Newberg AH, Greenstein R: Radiographic evaluation of tibial plateau fractures. Radiology 126:319, 1978.

643. Dias JJ, Stirling AJ, Finlay DBL, Gregg PJ: Computerised axial tomography for tibial plateau fractures. J Bone Joint Surg [Br] 69:84, 1987.

644. Dietz GW, Wilcox DM, Montgomery JB: Segond tibial condyle fracture: Lateral capsular ligament avulsion. Radiology 159:467, 1986.

645. Hastings DE: Knee ligament instability—a rational anatomical classification. Clin Orthop Rel Res 208:104, 1986.

646. McConkey JP, Meeuwisse W: Tibial plateau fractures in alpine skiing. Amer J Sports Med 16:159, 1988.

647. Anglen JO, Healy WL: Tibial plateau fractures. Orthopedics 11:1527, 1988.

648. Honkonen SE, Järvinen MJ: Classification of fractures of the tibial condyles. J Bone Joint Surg [Br] 74:840, 1992.

649. Hohl M: Tibial condylar fractures. J Bone Joint Surg [Am] 49:1455, 1967.

650. Moore TM: Fracture-dislocation of the knee. Clin Orthop Rel Res 156:128, 1981.

651. Waddell JP, Johnston DWC, Neidre A: Fractures of the tibial plateau: A review of ninety-five patients and comparison of treatment methods. J Trauma 21:376, 1981.

652. Ottolenghi CE: Vascular complications in injuries about the knee joint. Clin Orthop Rel Res 165:148, 1982.

653. Jensen DB, Bjerg-Nielsen A, Laursen N: Conventional radiographic examination in the evaluation of sequelae after tibial plateau fractures. Skel Radiol 17:330, 1988.
654. Meyers MH, McKeever FM: Fracture of the intercondylar eminence of the tibia. J Bone Joint Surg [Am] 41:209, 1959.
655. Nichols JN, Tehranzadeh J: A review of tibial spine fractures in bicycle injury. Amer J Sports Med 15:172, 1987.
656. Kendall NS, Hsu SY, Chan K-M: Fracture of the tibial spine in adults and children. A review of 31 cases. J Bone Joint Surg [Br] 74:848, 1992.
657. Dietz GW, Wilcox DM, Montgomery JB: Segond tibial condyle fracture: Lateral capsular ligament avulsion. Radiology 159:467, 1986.
658. Goldman AB, Pavlov H, Rubenstein D: The Segond fracture of the proximal tibia: A small avulsion that reflects major ligamentous damage. AJR 151:1163, 1988.
659. Platt H: On the peripheral nerve complications of certain fractures. J Bone Joint Surg 10:403, 1928.
660. Hill JA, Rana NA: Complications of posterolateral dislocation of the knee. Case report and literature review. Clin Orthop Rel Res 154:212, 1981.
661. Kennedy JC: Complete dislocation of the knee joint. J Bone Joint Surg [Am] 45:889, 1963.
662. Reckling FW, Peltier LF: Acute knee dislocations and their complications. J Trauma 9:181, 1969.
663. Meyers MH, Harvey JR Jr: Traumatic dislocation of the knee joint. A study of eighteen cases. J Bone Joint Surg [Am] 53:16, 1971.
664. Taylor AR, Arden GP, Rainey HA: Traumatic dislocation of the knee. A report of forty-three cases with special reference to conservative treatment. J Bone Joint Surg [Br] 54:96, 1972.
665. Frassica FJ, Sim FH, Staeheli JW, et al: Dislocation of the knee. Clin Ortho 263:200, 1991.
666. Roman PD, Hopson CN, Zenni EJ Jr: Traumatic dislocation of the knee: A report of 30 cases and literature review. Orthop Review 16:917, 1987.
667. Cooper DE, Speer KP, Wickiewicz TL, et al: Complete knee dislocation without posterior cruciate ligament disruption. Clin Orthop 284:228, 1992.
668. Kaufman SL, Martin LG: Arterial injuries associated with complete dislocation of the knee. Radiology 184:153, 1992.
669. Bloom MH: Traumatic knee dislocation and popliteal artery occlusion. Phys Sports Med 15:143, 1987.
670. McCoy GF, Hannon DG, Barr RJ, et al: Vascular injury associated with low-velocity dislocations of the knee. J Bone Joint Surg [Br] 69:285, 1987.
671. Brattstrom H: Shape of the intercondylar groove normally and in recurrent dislocation of the patella. Acta Orthop Scand (Suppl)68:5, 1964.
672. Brattstrom H: Patella alta in non-dislocating knee joints. Acta Orthop Scand 41:578, 1970.
673. Frangakis EK: Intra-articular dislocation of the patella. A case report. J Bone Joint Surg [Am] 56:423, 1974.
674. Allen FJ: Intercondylar dislocation of the patella. S Afr Med J 18:66, 1944.
675. Deaderick C: Case of rupture of quadriceps femoris tendon with dislocation of the patella beneath the intercondyloid groove of the femur. Ann Surg 11:102, 1890.
676. Feneley RCL: Inter-articular dislocation of the patella. Report of a case. J Bone Joint Surg [Br] 50:653, 1968.
677. Murakami Y: Intra-articular dislocation of the patella. A case report. Clin Orthop Rel Res 171:137, 1982.
678. Moed BR, Morawa LG: Acute traumatic lateral dislocation of the patella: An unusual case presentation. J Trauma 22:516, 1982.
679. Hanspal RS: Superior dislocation of the patella. Injury 16:487, 1985.
680. van den Brock TAA, Moll PJ: Horizontal rotation of the patella. Acta Orthop Scand 56:436, 1985.
681. Corso SJ, Thal R, Forman D: Locked patellar dislocation with vertical axis rotation. A case report. Clin Orthop 279:190, 1992.
682. Miller PR, Klein RM, Teitge RA: Medial dislocation of the patella. Skel Radiol 20:429, 1991.
683. Milgram JE: Tangential osteochondral fracture of the patella. J Bone Joint Surg 25:271, 1943.
684. Morscher E: Cartilage-bone lesions of the knee joint following injury. Reconstr Surg Traumatol 12:2, 1971.
685. Ahstrom JP: Osteochondral fracture in the knee joint associated with hypermobility and dislocation of the patella. J Bone Joint Surg [Am] 47:1491, 1965.
686. Frandsen PA, Kristensen H: Osteochondral fracture associated with dislocation of the patella: Another mechanism of injury. J Trauma 19:195, 1979.
687. McDougall A, Brown JD: Radiological sign of recurrent dislocation of the patella. J Bone Joint Surg [Br] 50:841, 1968.
688. Freiberger RH, Kotzen LM: Fracture of the medial margin of the patella, a finding diagnostic of lateral dislocation. Radiology 88:902, 1967.
689. Rorabeck CH, Bobechko WP: Acute dislocation of the patella with osteochondral fracture. A review of eighteen cases. J Bone Joint Surg [Br] 58:237, 1976.
690. Jacobsen K, Metz P: Occult traumatic dislocation of the patella. J Trauma 16:829, 1976.
691. Vainionpää S, Laasonen E, Pätiälä H, Rusanen M, Rokkannen P: Acute dislocation of the patella. Acta Orthop Scand 57:331, 1986.
692. Ogden JA: Dislocation of the proximal fibula. Radiology 105:547, 1972.
693. Parkes JC II, Zelko RR: Isolated acute dislocation of the proximal tibiofibular joint. Case report. J Bone Joint Surg [Am] 55:177, 1973.
694. Conforty B, Tal E, Margulies Y: Anterior dislocation of the head of the fibula. J Trauma 20:902, 1980.
695. Falkenberg P, Nygaard H: Isolated anterior dislocation of the proximal tibiofibular joint. J Bone Joint Surg [Br] 65:310, 1983.
696. Weinert CR Jr, Raczka R: Recurrent dislocation of the superior tibiofibular joint. Surgical stabilization by ligament reconstruction. J Bone Joint Surg [Am] 68:126, 1986.
697. Giachino AA: Recurrent dislocations of the proximal tibiofibular joint. J Bone Joint Surg [Am] 68:1104, 1986.
698. Ogden JA: Subluxation and dislocation of the proximal tibiofibular joint. J Bone Joint Surg [Br] 56:145, 1974.
699. Baciu CC, Tudor A, Olaru I: Recurrent luxation of the superior tibiofibular joint in the adult. Acta Orthop Scand 45:772, 1974.
700. Sijbrandij S: Instability of the proximal tibio-fibular joint. Acta Orthop Scand 49:621, 1978.
701. Sharma P, Daffner RH: Case report 389. Skel Radiol 15:505, 1986.
702. Gershuni DH, Skyhar MJ, Thompson B, et al: A comparison of conventional radiography and computed tomography in the evaluation of spiral fractures of the tibia. J Bone Joint Surg [Am] 67:1388, 1985.
703. Sarmiento A: A functional below-the-knee brace for tibial fractures. J Bone Joint Surg [Am] 52:295, 1970.
704. Sarmuento A, Gersten LM, Sobol PA, et al: Tibial shaft fractures treated with functional brace: Experience with 780 fractures. J Bone Joint Surg [Br] 71:602, 1989.
705. Skak SV, Jensen TT, Poulsen TD: Fracture of the proximal metaphysis of the tibia in children. Injury 18:149, 1987.
706. Zionts LE, Harcke HT, Brooks KM, et al: Posttraumatic tibia valga: A case demonstrating asymmetric activity at the proximal growth plate on technetium bone scan. J Pediatr Orthop 7:458, 1987.
707. Robert M, Khouri N, Carlioz H, et al: Fractures of the proximal tibial metaphysis in children: Review of a series of 25 cases. J Pediatr Orthop 7:444, 1987.
708. Brougham DI, Nicol RO: Valgus deformity after proximal tibial fractures in children. J Bone Joint Surg [Br] 69:482, 1987.
709. Wood KB, Bradley JP, Ward WT: Pes anserinus interposition in a proximal tibial physeal fracture. A case report. Clin Orth￼p 264:239, 1991.
710. Neer CS: Injuries of the ankle joint—evaluation. Conn St Med J 17:580, 1953.
711. Karlsson J, Lansinger O: Lateral instability of the ankle joint. Clin Orthop 276:253, 1992.
712. Rijke AM, Jones B, Vierhout PAM: Stress examination of traumatized lateral ligaments of the ankle. Clin Orthop Rel Res 210:143, 1986.
713. Larsen E: Experimental instability of the ankle. A radiographic investigation. Clin Orthop Rel Res 204:193, 1986.
714. Ashhurst APC, Brumer RS: Classification and mechanism of fractures of the leg bones involving the ankle. Based on a study of three hundred cases from the Episcopal Hospital. Arch Surg 4:51, 1922.
715. Lauge-Hansen N: Fractures of the ankle: Genetic roentgenologic diagnosis of fractures of the ankle. Am J Roentgenol 71:456, 1954.
716. Lauge-Hansen N: Fractures of the ankle: Clinical use of genetic roentgen diagnosis and genetic reduction. Arch Surg 64:488, 1952.
717. Nielsen JØ, Dons-Jenson H, Sørensen HT: Lauge-Hansen classification of malleolar fractures. An assessment of the reproducibility in 118 cases. Acta Orthop Scand 61:385, 1990.
718. Thomsen NOB, Overgaard S, Olsen LH, et al: Observer variation in the radiographic classification of ankle fractures. J Bone Joint Surg [Br] 73:676, 1991.
719. Kristensen TB: Treatment of malleolar fractures according to Lauge-Hansen's method. Acta Chir Scand 97:362, 1949.
720. Protas JM, Kornblatt BA: Fractures of the lateral margin of the distal tibia. The Tillaux fracture. Radiology 138:55, 1981.
721. Berg EE: The symptomatic os subfibulare. Avulsion fracture of the fibula associated with recurrent instability of the ankle. J Bone Joint Surg [Am] 73:1251, 1991.
722. Pankovich AM: Maisonneuve fracture of the fibula. J Bone Joint Surg [Am] 58:337, 1976.
723. Lock TR, Schaffer JJ, Manoli A II: Maisonneuve fracture: Case report of a missed diagnosis. Ann Emerg Med 16:805, 1987.
724. Lauge-Hansen N: Fractures of the ankle. V. Pronation-dorsiflexion fracture. Arch Surg 67:813, 1953.
725. Ayeni JP: Pilon fractures of the tibia: a study based on 19 cases. Injury 19:109, 1988.
726. Bourne RB: Pylon fractures of the distal tibia. Clin Orthop 240:42, 1989.
727. Mast JW, Spiegel PG, Pappas JN: Fractures of the tibial pilon. Clin Orthop 230:68, 1988.
728. Giachino AA, Hammond DI: The relationship between oblique fractures of the medial malleolus and concomitant fractures of the anterolateral aspect of the tibial plafond. J Bone Joint Surg [Am] 69:381, 1987.
729. Mainwaring BL, Daffner RH, Riemer BL: Pylon fractures of the ankle: A distinct clinical and radiologic entity. Radiology 168:215, 1988.
730. Yde J: The Lauge-Hansen classification of malleolar fractures. Acta Orthop Scand 51:181, 1980.
731. Mandell J: Isolated fractures of the posterior tibial lip at the ankle as demonstrated by an additional projection, the ''poor'' lateral view. Radiology 101:319, 1971.
732. Auletta AG, Conway WF, Hayes CW, et al: Indications for radiography in patients with acute ankle injuries: Role of the physical examination. AJR 157:789, 1991.
733. Magid D, Michelson JD, Ney DR, et al: Adult ankle fractures: Comparison of plain films and interactive two- and three-dimensional CT scans. AJR 154:1017, 1990.

734. Maurice H, Watt I: Technetium-99m hydroxymethylene diphosphonate scanning of acute injuries to the lateral ligaments of the ankle. Brit J Radiol 62:31, 1989.

735. Toohey JS, Worsing RA Jr: A long-term follow-up study of tibiotalar dislocations without associated fractures. Clin Orthop 239:207, 1989.

736. Colville MR, Colville JM, Manoli A II: Posteromedial dislocation of the ankle without fracture. J Bone Joint Surg [Am] 69:706, 1987.

737. Segal LS, Lynch CJ, Stauffer ES: Anterior ankle dislocation with associated trigonal process fracture. A case report and literature review. Clin Orthop 278:171, 1992.

738. Goergen TG, Danzig LA, Resnick D, Owen CA: Roentgenographic evaluation of the tibiotalar joint. J Bone Joint Surg [Am] 59:874, 1977.

739. Ramsey PL, Hamilton W: Changes in tibiotalar area of contact caused by lateral talar shift. J Bone Joint Surg [Am] 58:356, 1976.

740. Hoblitzell RM, Ebraheim NA, Merritt T, et al: Bosworth fracture-dislocation of the ankle. A case report and review of the literature. Clin Orthop 255:257, 1990.

741. Molinari M, Bertoldi L, De March L: Fracture dislocation of the ankle with the fibula trapped behind the tibia. A case report. Acta Orthop Scand 61:471, 1990.

742. Bosworth DM: Fracture-dislocation of the ankle with fixed displacement of the fibula behind the tibia. J Bone Joint Surg [Am] 29:130, 1947.

743. Schatzker J, Johnson RG: Fracture dislocation of the ankle with anterior dislocation of the fibula. J Trauma 23:420, 1983.

744. Rogers LF, Campbell RE: Fractures and dislocations of the foot. Semin Roentgenol 13:157, 1978.

745. Anderson HG: The Medical and Surgical Aspects of Aviation. London, Oxford University Press, 1919.

746. Kenwright J, Taylor RG: Major injuries of the talus. J Bone Joint Surg [Br] 52:36, 1970.

747. Dimon JH: Isolated displaced fracture of the posterior facet of the talus. J Bone Joint Surg [Am] 43:275, 1961.

748. Coltart WD: "Aviator's astralagus." J Bone Joint Surg [Br] 34:545, 1952.

749. Hawkins LG: Fractures of the neck of the talus. J Bone Joint Surg [Am] 52:991, 1970.

750. Canale ST, Kelly FB Jr: Fractures of the neck of the talus. Long-term evaluation of seventy-one cases. J Bone Joint Surg [Am] 60:143, 1978.

751. Lorentzen JE, Christensen SB, Krogsoe O, Sneppen O: Fractures of the neck of the talus. Acta Orthop Scand 48:115, 1977.

752. Canale ST: Fractures of the neck of the talus. Orthopedics 13:1105, 1990.

753. Bodamer WJ, Torre RJ, Cotch MT, et al: Avascular necrosis of the talar head. A complication of group 4 fracture of the talar neck. J Amer Podiat Assoc 77:217, 1987.

754. Lieberg OU, Henke JA, Bailey RW: Avascular necrosis of the head of the talus without death of the body: Report of an unusual case. J Trauma 15:926, 1975.

755. Sneppen O, Christensen SB, Krogsoe O, Lorentzen J: Fracture of the body of the talus. Acta Orthop Scand 48:317, 1977.

756. Heckman JD, McLean MR: Fractures of the lateral process of the talus. Clin Orthop Rel Res 199:108, 1985.

757. El-Khoury GY, Yousefzadeh DK, Mulligan GM, Moore TE: Subtalar dislocation. Skel Radiol 8:99, 1982.

758. Monson ST, Ryan JR: Subtalar dislocation. J Bone Joint Surg [Am] 63:1156, 1981.

759. St Pierre RK, Velazco A, Fleming LL, Whitesides T: Medial subtalar dislocation in an athlete. A case report. Am J Sports Med 10:240, 1982.

760. Mattingly DA, Stern PJ: Bilateral subtalar dislocations. A case report. Clin Orthop Rel Res 177:122, 1983.

761. Zimmer TJ, Johnson KA: Subtalar dislocations. Clin Orthop 238:190, 1989.

762. Buckingham WW Jr: Subtalar dislocation of the foot. J Trauma 13:753, 1973.

763. Grantham SA: Medial subtalar dislocation: Five cases with a common etiology. J Trauma 4:845, 1964.

764. Detenbeck LC, Kelly PJ: Total dislocation of the talus. J Bone Joint Surg [Am] 51:283, 1969.

765. Ritsema GH: Total talar dislocation. J Trauma 28:692, 1988.

766. Heger L, Wulff K: Computed tomography of the calcaneus: Normal anatomy. Am J Roentgenol 145:123, 1985.

767. Heger L, Wulff K, Seddiqi MSA: Computed tomography of calcaneal fractures. Am J Roentgenol 145:131, 1985.

768. Pablot SM, Daneman A, Stringer DA, Carroll N: The value of computed tomography in the early assessment of comminuted fractures of the calcaneus: A review of three patients. J Pediatr Orthop 5:435, 1985.

769. Gilmer PW, Herzenberg J, Frank JL, Silverman P, Martinez S, Goldner JL: Computerized tomographic analysis of acute calcaneal fractures. Foot Ankle 6:184, 1986.

770. Crosby LA, Fitzgibbons T: Computerized tomography scanning of acute intra-articular fractures of the calcaneus. A new classification system. J Bone Joint Surg [Am] 72:852, 1990.

771. Rosenberg ZS, Feldman F, Singson RD: Intra-articular calcaneal fractures: computed tomographic analysis. Skel Radiol 16:105, 1987.

772. Bradley SA, Davies AM: Computed tomographic assessment of old calcaneal fractures. Brit J Radiol 63:926, 1990.

773. Janzen DL, Connell DG, Munk PL, et al: Intraarticular fractures of the calcaneus: Value of CT findings in determining prognosis. AJR 158:1271, 1992.

774. Richardson ML, Vu MV, Vincent LM, et al: CT measurement of the calcaneal varus angle in the normal and fractured hindfoot. J Comput Assist Tomogr 16:261, 1992.

775. Eastwood DM, Gregg PJ, Atkins RM: Intra-articular fractures of the calcaneum. Part I: Pathological anatomy and classification. J Bone Joint Surg [Br] 75:183, 1993.

776. Essex-Lopresti P: The mechanism, reduction technique, and results in fractures of the os calcis. Br J Surg 39:395, 1952.

777. Paley D, Hall H: Intra-articular fractures of the calcaneus. A critical analysis of results and prognostic factors. J Bone Joint Surg [Am] 75:342, 1993.

778. Giachino AA, Uhthoff HK: Intra-articular fractures of the calcaneus. J Bone Joint Surg [Am] 71:784, 1989.

779. Palmer I: The mechanism and treatment of fractures of the calcaneus. J Bone Joint Surg [Am] 30:2, 1948.

780. Norfray JF, Rogers LF, Adamo GP, Groves HC, Heiser WJ: Common calcaneal avulsion fracture. Am J Roentgenol 134:119, 1980.

781. Brijs S, Brijs A: Calcaneal avulsion: a frequent traumatic foot lesion. Fortschr Rontgenstr 156:495, 1992.

782. Nielsen S, Agnhold J, Christensen H: Radiologic findings in lesions of the ligamentum bifurcatum of the midfoot. Skel Radiol 16:114, 1987.

783. Renfrew DL, El-Khoury GY: Anterior process fractures of the calcaneus. Skel Radiol 14:121, 1985.

784. Schantz K, Rasmussen F: Calcaneus fracture in the child. Acta Orthop Scand 58:507, 1987.

785. Starshak RJ, Simons GW, Sty JR: Occult fracture of the calcaneus—another toddler's fracture. Pediatr Radiol 14:37, 1984.

786. Soeur R, Remy R: Fractures of the calcaneus with displacement of the thalamic portion. J Bone Joint Surg [Br] 57:413, 1975.

787. Stephenson JR: Displaced fractures of the os calcis involving the subtalar joint: The key role of the superomedial fragment. Foot Ankle 4:91, 1983.

788. Champetier J, Laborde Y, Letoublon Ch, Yver R, Coulomb M, Vincent J: Fractures articulaires du calcanéum. J Radiol 61:269, 1980.

789. Mains DB, Sullivan RC: Fracture of the os peroneum. A case report. J Bone Joint Surg [Am] 55:1529, 1973.

790. Mikami M, Azuma H: Fracture of the os tibiale externum. A case report. J Bone Joint Surg [Am] 60:556, 1978.

791. Thompson FM, Patterson AH: Rupture of the peroneus longus tendon. Report of three cases. J Bone Joint Surg [Am] 71:293, 1989.

792. Main BJ, Jowett RL: Injuries of the midtarsal joint. J Bone Joint Surg [Br] 57:89, 1975.

793. Dewar FP, Evans DC: Occult fracture-subluxation of the midtarsal joint. J Bone Joint Surg [Br] 50:386, 1968.

794. Brantigan JW, Pedegana LR, Lippert FG: Instability of the subtalar joint. Diagnosis by stress tomography in three cases. J Bone Joint Surg [Am] 59:321, 1977.

795. Vuori J-P, Aro HT: Lisfranc joint injuries: Trauma mechanisms and associated injuries. J Trauma 35:40, 1993.

796. Cássebaum WH: Lisfranc-fracture-dislocations. Clin Orthop Rel Res 30:116, G1963.

797. Foster SC, Foster RR: Lisfranc's tarsometatarsal fracture-dislocation. Radiology 120:79, 1976.

798. Wiley JJ: The mechanism of tarso-metatarsal joint injuries. J Bone Joint Surg [Br] 53:474, 1971.

799. Wilson DW: Injuries of the tarso-metatarsal joints. Etiology, classification and results of treatment. J Bone Joint Surg [Br] 54:677, 1972.

800. Goossens M, DeStoop N: Lisfranc's fracture-dislocations: etiology, radiology, and results of treatment. A review of 20 cases. Clin Orthop Rel Res 176:154, 1983.

801. Blouet JM, Rebaud C, Marquer Y, Duval JM, Husson JL, Jourdain R, Masse A: Anatomy of the tarsometatarsal joint and its applications to dislocation of this articular surface. Anat Clin 5:9, 1983.

802. Ashhurst APC: Divergent dislocation of the metatarsus. Ann Surg 83:132, 1926.

803. Aitken AP, Poulson D: Dislocations of the tarsometatarsal joint. J Bone Joint Surg [Am] 45:246, 1963.

804. Faciszewski T, Burks RT, Manaster BJ: Subtle injuries of the Lisfranc joint. J Bone Joint Surg [Am] 72:1519, 1990.

805. Goiney RC, Connell DG, Nichols DM: CT evaluation of tarsometatarsal fracture-dislocation injuries. Am J Roentgenol 144:985, 1985.

806. Fagel VL, Ocon E, Cantarella JC, Feldman F: Case report 183. Skel Radiol 7:287, 1982.

807. Dines DM, Hershon SJ, Smith N, Shelton P: Isolated dorsomedial dislocation of the first ray at the medial cuneonavicular joint of the foot: A rare injury to the tarsus. A case report. Clin Orthop Rel Res 186:162, 1984.

808. Macy NJ, DeBoer P: Mid-tarsal dislocation of the first ray. A case report. J Bone Joint Surg [Am] 65:265, 1983.

809. Tountas AA: Occult fracture-subluxation of the midtarsal joint. Clin Orthop 243:195, 1989.

810. Kollmannsberger A, DeBoer P: Isolated calcaneo-cuboid dislocation: Brief report. J Bone Joint Surg [Br] 71:323, 1989.

811. Yamashita F, Sakakida K, Hara K, et al: Diastasis between the medial and the intermediate cuneiforms. J Bone Joint Surg [Br] 75:156, 1993.

812. Main BJ, Jowett RL: Injuries of the midtarsal joint. J Bone Joint Surg [Br] 57:89, 1975.

813. Salamon PB, Gelberman RH, Huffer JM: Dorsal dislocation of the metatarsophalangeal joint of the great toe. A case report. J Bone Joint Surg [Am] 56:1073, 1974.

814. Barnett JC, Crespo A, Daniels VC: Intra-articular accessory sesamoid dislocation of the great toe. Report of a case. J Fla Med Assoc 66:613, 1979.

815. Szues R, Hurwitz J: Traumatic subluxation of the interphalangeal joint of the hallux with interposition of the sesamoid bone. AJR *152*:652, 1989.

816. Meaney JFM, Desmond JM: Case report 721. Skel Radiol *21*:319, 1992.

817. Miki T, Yamamuro T, Kitai T: An irreducible dislocation of the great toe. Report of two cases and review of the literature. Clin Orthop *230*:200, 1988.

818. Katayama M, Murakami Y, Takahashi H: Irreducible dorsal dislocation of the toe. Report of three cases. J Bone Joint Surg [Am] *70*:769, 1988.

819. Rodeo SA, O'Brien S, Warren RF, et al: Turf-toe: An analysis of metatarsophalangeal joint sprains in professional football players. Amer J Sports Med *18*:280, 1990.

820. Graves SC, Prieskorn D, Mann RA: Posttraumatic proximal migration of the first metatarsophalangeal joint sesamoids: A report of four cases. Foot Ankle *12*:117, 1991.

821. Potter HG, Pavlov H, Abrahams TG: The hallux sesamoids revisited. Skel Radiol *21*:437, 1992.

822. Munro TG: Fractures of the base of the fifth metatarsal. J Canad Assoc Radiol *40*:260, 1989.

823. Dameron TB Jr: Fractures and anatomic variations of the proximal portion of the fifth metatarsal. J Bone Joint Surg [Am] *57*:788, 1975.

824. Torg JS, Balduini FC, Zelko RR, Pavlov H, Peff TC, Das M: Fractures of the base of the fifth metatarsal distal to the tuberosity. Classification and guidelines for non-surgical and surgical management. J Bone Joint Surg [Am] *66*:209, 1984.

825. Richli WR, Rosenthal DI: Avulsion fracture of the fifth metatarsal: Experimental study of pathomechanics. Am J Roentgenol *143*:889, 1984.

826. Jones R: Fractures of the base of the fifth metatarsal bone by indirect violence. Ann Surg *35*:697, 1902.

827. Galant JM, Spinosa FA: Digital fractures. A comprehensive review. J Amer Podiatr Assoc *81*:593, 1991.

828. Pinckney LE, Currarino G, Kennedy LA: The stubbed great toe: A cause of occult compound fracture and infection. Radiology *138*:375, 1981.

829. Resnik CS, Stackhouse DJ, Shanmuganathan K, et al: Diagnosis of pelvic fractures in patients with acute pelvic trauma: Efficiency of plain radiographs. AJR *158*:109, 1992.

830. Edeiken-Monroe BS, Browner BD, Jackson H: The role of standard roentgenograms in the evaluation of instability of pelvic ring disruption. Clin Orthop *240*:63, 1989.

831. Weil GC, Price EM, Rusbridge HW: The diagnosis and treatment of fractures of the pelvis and their complications. Am J Surg *44*:108, 1939.

832. Pennal GF, Tile M, Waddell JP, Garside H: Pelvic disruption: Assessment and classification. Clin Orthop Rel Res *151*:12, 1980.

833. Watson-Jones R: Dislocations and fracture-dislocations of the pelvis. Br J Surg *25*:773, 1938.

834. Huttinen VM, Slatis P: Fractures of the pelvis. Trauma mechanism, types of injury, and principles of treatment. Acta Chir Scand *137*:576, 1971.

835. Conolly WB, Hedberg EA: Observations on fractures of the pelvis. J Trauma *9*:104, 1969.

836. Looser KG, Crombie HD Jr: Pelvic fractures: An anatomic guide to severity of injury. Am J Surg *132*:638, 1976.

837. Trunkey DD, Chapman MW, Lim RC Jr, Dunphy JE: Management of pelvic fractures in blunt trauma injury. J Trauma *14*:912, 1974.

838. Young JWR, Burgess AR, Brumback RJ, Poka A: Pelvic fractures: Value of plain radiography in early assessment and management. Radiology *160*:445, 1986.

839. Young JWR, Resnick CS: Fracture of the pelvis: Current concepts of classification. AJR *155*:1169, 1990.

840. Dalal SA, Burgess AR, Siegel JH, et al: Pelvic fracture in multiple trauma: Classification by mechanism is key to pattern of organ injury, resuscitative requirements, and outcome. J Trauma *29*:981, 1989.

841. Tile M: Fractures of the Pelvis and Acetabulum. Baltimore, Williams & Wilkins Co, 1984.

842. Tile M: Pelvic ring fractures: Should they be fixed? J Bone Joint Surg [Br] *70*:1, 1988.

843. Gill K, Bucholz RW: The role of computerized tomographic scanning in the evaluation of major pelvic fractures. J Bone Joint Surg [Am] *66*:34, 1984.

844. Kane WJ: Fractures of the pelvis. *In* CA Rockwood Jr, DP Green (Eds): Fractures in Adults. 2nd Ed. Philadelphia, JB Lippincott Co, 1984, p 1093.

845. Rankin LM: Fractures of the pelvis. Ann Surg *106*:266, 1937.

846. Fountain SS, Hamilton RM, Jameson RM: Transverse fractures of the sacrum. A report of six cases. J Bone Joint Surg [Am] *59*:486, 1977.

847. Montana MA, Richardson ML, Kilcoyne RF, Harley JD, Shuman WP, Mack LA: CT of sacral injury. Radiology *161*:499, 1986.

848. Sabiston CP, Wing PC: Sacral fractures: Classification and neurologic implications. J Trauma *26*:1113, 1986.

849. Jackson H, Kam J, Harris JH Jr, Harle TS: The sacral arcuate lines in upper sacral fractures. Radiology *145*:35, 1982.

850. Northrop CH, Eto RT, Loop JW: Vertical fracture of the sacral ala. Significance of non-continuity of the anterior superior sacral foraminal line. Am J Roentgenol *124*:102, 1975.

851. Shild H, Muller HA, Klose K, Ahlers J, Huwel N: Anatomie, Rontgenologie und Klinik der Sakrumfrakturen. ROFO *134*:522, 1981.

852. Balseiro J, Brower AC, Ziessman HA: Scintigraphic diagnosis of sacral fractures. Am J Roentgenol *148*:111, 1987.

853. Balseiro J, Brower AC, Ziessman HA: Scintigraphic diagnosis of sacral fractures. AJR *148*:111, 1987.

854. Berg PM: Acute pelvic disruption, the bucking horse injury. Orthop Trans *3*:271, 1979.

855. Peltier LF: Complications associated with fractures of the pelvis. J Bone Joint Surg [Am] *47*:1060, 1965.

856. Holdsworth FW: Dislocations and fracture-dislocations of the pelvis. J Bone Joint Surg [Br] *30*:461, 1948.

857. Failinger MS, McGanity PLJ: Unstable fractures of the pelvic ring. J Bone Joint Surg [Am] *74*:781, 1992.

858. Hauser CW, Perry JF Jr: Massive hemorrhage from pelvic fractures. Minn Med *49*:285, 1966.

859. Colapinto V: Trauma to the pelvis: Urethral injury. Clin Orthop Rel Res *151*:46, 1980.

860. Huittinen VM, Slatis P: Nerve injury in double vertical pelvic fractures. Acta Chir Scand *138*:571, 1972.

861. Kattan KR: Trauma to the bony thorax. Semin Roentgenol *13*:69, 1978.

862. Gopalakrishnan KC, El Masri WS: Fractures of the sternum associated with spinal injury. J Bone Joint Surg [Br] *68*:178, 1986.

863. Helm RH, Tonkin MA: The chauffeur's fracture: simple or complex? J Hand Surg [Br] *17*:156, 1992.

864. Carr CR, Wingo CH: Fractures of the femoral diaphysis. A retrospective study of the results and costs of treatment by intramedullary nailing and by traction and a spica cast. J Bone Joint Surg [Am] *55*:690, 1973.

865. Froimson AI: Treatment of comminuted subtrochanteric fractures of the femur. Surg Gynecol Obstet *131*:465, 1970.

866. Doporto JM, Rafique M: Vascular insufficiency complicating trauma to the lower limb. J Bone Joint Surg [Br] *51*:680, 1969.

867. Zickel RE: Fractures of the adult femur excluding the femoral head and neck: A review and evaluation of current therapy. Clin Orthop Rel Res *147*:93, 1980.

868. Bernstein SM: Fractures of the femoral shaft and associated ipsilateral fractures of the hip. Orthop Clin North Am *5*:799, 1974.

869. Zettas JP, Zettas P: Ipsilateral fractures of the femoral neck and shaft. Clin Orthop Rel Res *160*:63, 1981.

870. Seinsheimer F: Subtrochanteric fractures of the femur. J Bone Joint Surg [Am] *60*:300, 1978.

871. Grosz CR, Shaftan GW, Kottmeier PK, Herbsman H: Volkmann's contracture and femoral shaft fractures. J Trauma *13*:129, 1973.

872. Isaacson J, Louis DS, Costenbader JM: Arterial injury associated with closed femoral-shaft fracture. Report of five cases. J Bone Joint Surg [Am] *57*:1147, 1975.

873. Ellis H: Disabilities after tibial shaft fractures. J Bone Joint Surg [Br] *40*:190, 1958.

874. Ellis H: The speed of healing after fracture of the tibial shaft. J Bone Joint Surg [Br] *40*:42, 1958.

875. Weissman SL, Herold HZ, Engelberg M: Fractures of the middle two-thirds of the tibial shaft. Results of treatment without internal fixation in 140 consecutive cases. J Bone Joint Surg [Br] *48*:257, 1966.

876. Nicoll EA: Fractures of the tibial shaft. A survey of 705 cases. J Bone Joint Surg [Br] *46*:373, 1964.

877. Melis GC, Sotgiu F, Lepori M, Guido P: Intramedullary nailing in segmental tibial fractures. J Bone Joint Surg [Am] *63*:1310, 1981.

878. Brighton CT: Treatment of nonunion of the tibia with constant direct current. J Trauma *21*:189, 1981.

879. Rosenthal RE, MacPhail JA, Ortiz JE: Non-union in open tibial fractures. Analysis of reasons for failure of treatment. J Bone Joint Surg [Am] *59*:244, 1977.

880. Trueta J: Blood supply and the rate of healing of tibial fractures. Clin Orthop Rel Res *105*:11, 1974.

881. Van der Linden W, Sunzel H, Larsson K: Fractures of the tibial shaft after skiing and other accidents. J Bone Joint Surg [Am] *57*:321, 1975.

882. Macnab I, de Haas WG: The role of periosteal blood supply in the healing of fractures of the tibia. Clin Orthop Rel Res *105*:27, 1974.

883. Rhinelander FW: Tibial blood supply in relation to fracture healing. Clin Orthop Rel Res *105*:34, 1974.

884. Jefferys CC: Spasm of the posterial tibial artery after injury. J Bone Joint Surg [Br] *45*:223, 1963.

885. Currarino G, Pinckney LE: Genu valgum after proximal tibial fractures in children. Am J Roentgenol *136*:915, 1981.

886. Skak SV: Valgus deformity following proximal tibial metaphyseal fracture in children. Acta Orthop Scand *53*:141, 1982.

887. Visser JD, Veldhuizen AG: Valgus deformity after fracture of the proximal tibial metaphysis in childhood. Acta Orthop Scand *53*:663, 1982.

888. Pankovich AM: Maisonneuve fracture of the fibula. J Bone Joint Surg [Am] *58*:337, 1976.

889. Huber H, Gerber C: Voluntary subluxation of the shoulder in children. A long-term follow-up study of 36 shoulders. J Bone Joint Surg [Br] *76*:118, 1994.

890. Sidor ML, Zuckerman JD, Lyon T, et al: The Neer classification system for proximal humeral fractures. An assessment of interobserver reliability and intraobserver reproducibility. J Bone Joint Surg [Am] *75*:1745, 1993.

891. Siebenrock KA, Gerber C: The reproducibility of classification of fractures of the proximal end of the humerus. J Bone Joint Surg [Am] *75*:175, 1993.

892. Burstein AH: Fracture classification systems: Do they work and are they useful? J Bone Joint Surg [Am] *75*:1743, 1993.

893. Duppe H, Johnell O, Lundborg G, et al: Long-term results of fracture of the scaphoid. A follow-up study of more than thirty years. J Bone Joint Surg [Am] *76*:249, 1994.

894. Futami T, Aoki H, Tsukamoto Y: Fractures of the hook of the hamate in athletes. Eight cases followed for 6 years. Acta Orthop Scand *64*:469, 1993.

895. Evans PD, Wilson C, Lyons K: Comparison of MRI with bone scanning for suspected hip fracture in elderly patients. J Bone Joint Surg [Br] *76*:158, 1994.

896. Michelson J, Curtis M, Magid D: Controversies in ankle fractures. Foot Ankle *14*:170, 1993.

897. Ben-Menachem Y: Avulsion of the innominate artery associated with fracture of the sternum. AJR *150*:621, 1988.

898. Brookes JG, Dunn RJ, Rogers IR: Sternal fractures: A retrospective analysis of 272 cases. J Trauma *35*:46, 1993.

899. de Laat EAT, Visser CPJ, Coene LNJEM, et al: Nerve lesions in primary shoulder dislocations and humeral neck fractures. J Bone Joint Surg [Br] *76*:381, 1994.

900. Koval KJ, Zuckerman JD: Functional recovery after fracture of the hip. J Bone Joint Surg [Am] *76*:751, 1994.

901. Barrow BA, Fajman WA, Parker LM, et al: Tibial plateau fractures: Evaluation with MR imaging. RadioGraphics *14*:553, 1994.

69

Physical Injury: Spine

Mini Pathria, M.D.

Fractures, dislocations, and soft tissue injuries can involve the spine at any level. In most instances, prominent clinical manifestations and radiologic abnormalities allow prompt and accurate diagnosis. The advent of CT scanning and MR imaging has had a significant impact on the ability to detect and categorize traumatic lesions of the spine. It is beyond the scope of this chapter to discuss all the diagnostic features of the many abnormalities of the spine related to trauma. This chapter presents an overview of some of the more common and important spinal injuries, with an emphasis on conventional radiography, the most widely applied imaging method for studying the injured spine.

BASIC PRINCIPLES

Injuries to the spine may be categorized according to anatomic location, presumed mechanism of injury, and presence or absence of instability. Traditionally, the spine has been subdivided longitudinally into cervical, thoracic, and lumbar anatomic regions. When discussing spinal injuries, however, these anatomic divisions fail to account adequately for the different types of injuries encountered. For this reason, in this chapter the spine is divided into five distinct anatomic and functional segments: occipitoatlantoaxial, lower cervical, upper thoracic, thoracolumbar, and lower lumbar. These five segments undergo distinctly different types of injuries owing to their anatomic differences and different types and ranges of physiologic motion.

Most spinal injuries occur in the lower cervical and thoracolumbar regions, areas of the spine that are capable of voluntary straightening and that normally have a large range of motion[1-4] (Fig. 69–1). The cervicocranium and

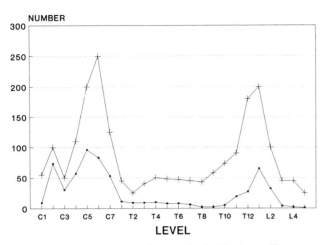

FIGURE 69–1. Anatomic distribution of spinal fractures. The prevalence of spinal fractures is highest in the lower cervical and thoracolumbar regions. (Adapted from Jefferson G: R Soc Med *21*:625, 1927, and Daffner RH, et al: Skel Radiol *15*:518, 1986.)

upper thoracic region also show significant but lower rates of injury, but these regions are at particularly high risk for neurologic damage. In addition to anatomic classification of an injury by longitudinal level, categorization also can be based on its location in the transverse plane. A variety of classification systems based on the level of injury in the sagittal axis of the vertebrae have been developed. Sagittal classification systems divide the spine into either anterior and posterior segments or anterior, middle, and posterior segments to take into account the mechanism and stability of spinal injuries.

Multilevel noncontiguous injuries occur in 4.5 to 7.6 per cent of patients.[5, 6] Unrecognized secondary sites of injury may lead to mechanical or neurologic deficit, pain, or deformity if they are not detected at the time of initial presentation.[6] The relatively high prevalence of noncontiguous

spinal injury has led to protocol imaging of the entire spine in multitrauma patients in whom one injury is detected.[5] Secondary injuries are seen most frequently in patients in whom the primary traumatic lesion is in the upper thoracic region.[5, 6] In Calenoff and associates' series of patients with noncontiguous spinal trauma, upper thoracic fractures accounted for 16 per cent of all primary lesions but represented the primary injury site in 47 per cent of all cases of noncontiguous trauma.[6]

Spinal injuries, particularly in the cervical and thoracolumbar regions, also can be classified on the basis of their presumed mechanism (Table 69–1). A force acting on the spine has both direction and magnitude, and when sufficient force is applied to a given tissue for a significant length of time, the tissue will fail.[7] Flexion, extension, rotation, compression, distraction, or shear forces may produce damage in isolation or in combination.[2, 3, 7–12] Determination of presumptive mechanism solely on the basis of radiographic analysis is largely speculative, and decisions are reached on the basis of the end result of an injury that may have multiple complex forces. Classification systems of injury based on mechanism of spinal trauma are relatively recent; almost all of the in vitro analyses of spinal injury mechanisms date from the past few decades.[7, 13–18] Data generated from biomechanical analyses of isolated cadaveric spinal segments are limited but have led to improved understanding of how spinal injuries are produced.

The basic spinal unit consists of two adjacent vertebrae, their anterior articulation via the intervertebral disc, their posterior facet articulations, and their ligamentous attachments.[7, 13] Experimental work done by Roaf using isolated cadaveric spinal segments has demonstrated that the intervertebral disc and spinal ligaments are highly resistant to compression, distraction, flexion, and extension but are vulnerable to rotary and horizontal shear forces.[7] The disc and ligaments are largely incompressible, whereas bone is less able to resist vertically applied loads. The osseous endplates, rather than the intervertebral soft tissues, fail when

---

TABLE 69–1. Classification of Injuries of the Cervical Spine*

Hyperflexion Injuries
Disruptive hyperflexion
   Hyperflexion sprain (momentary dislocation)
   Hyperflexion-dislocation (locked facets)
     Bilateral
     Unilateral (with associated rotational force)
   Spinous process fracture
Compressive hyperflexion
   Wedgelike compression of vertebral body
   Comminuted (teardrop) fracture of vertebral body
   Hyperflexion fracture-dislocation (type IV)
Hyperflexion or shearing forces
   Anterior atlanto-occipital dislocation (?)
   ''Pure'' anterior atlantoaxial dislocation (without associated fracture)
   Anterior fracture-dislocation of the dens

Hyperextension Injuries
Disruptive hyperextension
   Horizontal fracture of the anterior arch of C1
   Hangman's fracture (traumatic spondylolisthesis of C2)
   Anteroinferior margin of the body of the axis (C2)
   Hyperextension sprain (momentary dislocation)
   Spinous process fracture

Compressive hyperextension
   Posterior arch of the atlas fracture
   Vertebral arch fracture (articular pillar, pedicle, lamina)
   Hyperextension fracture-dislocation (types IV-V)
Hyperextension or shearing forces
   Posterior fracture-dislocation of the dens
   ''Pure'' posterior atlantoaxial dislocation (without associated fracture)

Hyperrotation Injuries
Rotary atlantoaxial dislocation
Anterior and posterior ligament disruption

Lateral Hyperflexion Injuries
Fracture of transverse process
Uncinate process fracture
Lateral fracture-dislocation of the dens
Brachial plexus avulsion associated with cervical fractures or dislocations, or both
Lateral wedgelike compression of vertebral body

Axial Compressive Injuries
Isolated fracture of the lateral mass of the atlas
Burst fracture of Jefferson (C1)
Vertical and oblique fractures of the axis body
Burst fracture of a vertebral body

*From Gehweiler JA Jr, Osborne RL Jr, Becker RF: The Radiology of Vertebral Trauma. Philadelphia, WB Saunders Co, 1980, p 107.

pure compressive or tensile forces are applied to the spine. Axial compression results in vertebral endplate failure, followed by protrusion of nuclear material into cancellous bone.[7] These data suggest that pure compression or distraction produces fractures, whereas rotary or shear forces result in intervertebral dislocations.

Spinal injuries frequently are subdivided further into stable and unstable categories. Instability frequently is mentioned but rarely is defined and remains a controversial concept.[19] In 1949, on the basis of his study of a large number of thoracolumbar fractures, Nicoll suggested a new classification of thoracolumbar fractures that was the first to divide injuries systematically into stable and unstable categories.[9] He believed that all fractures in which the interspinous ligaments were intact should be considered stable, whereas injuries associated with disruption of the interspinous ligaments were unstable.[9] Holdsworth elaborated on Nicoll's classification of thoracolumbar injuries and expanded the classification system to encompass the entire spine.[10] Holdsworth first defined the ''posterior ligament complex'' and suggested that injuries isolated to the posterior ligaments at any spinal level were sufficient to produce instability.[10] The posterior ligament complex consists of the articular capsules, ligamenta flava, interspinous ligament, and supraspinous ligament. Holdsworth considered the posterior ligamentous complex to be the key to maintaining spinal stability and noted that rarely was it injured owing to pure flexion.[10] He suggested that unstable injuries were unusual unless frank dislocation or an associated rotational force also was present.[10] Roaf, using isolated spinal segments, confirmed Holdsworth's observation that pure flexion rarely injured the posterior ligaments unless preceded by vertebral body fracture.[7] Holdsworth noted that the anterior portions of the vertebral bodies were connected by the intervertebral disc, with stability based primarily on the strong anulus fibrosus.[10] Holdsworth attributed little significance to injuries limited to the anterior structures and did not define an equivalent anterior ligamentous complex.[2, 10] Holdsworth considered all hyperextension injuries to be stable in flexion owing to maintenance of the posterior ligament complex.

Whitesides, like Holdsworth, also considered the spine to consist of two columns but thought that both were important in maintaining spinal stability.[20] He defined a stable spine as one that ''can withstand axial compressive forces anteriorly through the vertebral bodies, tension forces posteriorly, and rotational stresses . . . without progressive kyphosis.''[20] Whereas Holdsworth considered any injury isolated to the vertebral body to be a stable one, Whitesides thought that such injuries could be unstable.[10, 20]

Biomechanical analysis has shown that isolated rupture of Holdsworth's posterior complex is insufficient for the development of spinal instability.[8, 11, 21–23] Bedbrook showed that division of the posterior ligament complex alone did not interfere with spinal stability and that potential instability was seen only when the disc was disrupted, with further instability ensuing when the anterior longitudinal ligament was stripped.[21] Bedbrook's work showed the limitations of the two column spinal concept. Denis introduced the concept of the three column spine in 1983, based on a retrospective review of 412 thoracolumbar injuries.[8] Denis' anterior column consists of the anterior longitudinal ligament, anterior portion of the anulus fibrosus, and anterior half of

the vertebral body. The middle column consists of the posterior longitudinal ligament, posterior portion of the anulus fibrosus, and posterior half of the vertebral body. Denis' posterior column is essentially the same as that described by Holdsworth, formed by the posterior osseous arch and the posterior ligaments, consisting of the capsular ligaments, ligamenta flava, interspinous ligament, and supraspinous ligament.[8, 23] This three column classification system is widely used in the assessment of spinal trauma.

Denis also subdivided spinal fractures into minor and major types as a guide to the likelihood of the presence or absence of instability. Minor fractures include isolated fractures of the transverse processes, articular facets, pars interarticularis (i.e., spondylolysis), or spinous process.[8] These injuries all involve the posterior column, are limited to that column, and do not lead to acute instability. Major injuries involve more than one column or result in sufficient deformity to consider them a separate group of injuries. Major spinal injuries were classified into four different categories: compression fractures (48 per cent), burst fractures (14 per cent), fracture-dislocations (16 per cent), and seat-belt type injuries (5 per cent). Denis based his classification on the presence or absence and presumed mode of failure for each of the three spinal columns.[8] According to his complex classification system, which includes over 20 subtypes, the middle column is the most important in determining the potential for instability. Daffner and colleagues have described five radiographic signs that indicate the presence of instability as defined by middle column disruption.[24] These signs are (1) vertebral displacement of greater than 2 mm; (2) widened interlaminar space; (3) widened facet joints; (4) disruption of the posterior margin of the vertebral body; and (5) widened interpediculate distance.[24] Each sign indicates major skeletal, ligamentous, or articular disruption and the presence of any one, according to these authors, is sufficient to establish the diagnosis of spinal instability.[24]

Denis' system subdivides instability into three types. Instability of the first degree (mechanical instability) refers to situations in which the spine is insufficiently constrained against buckling and angulation.[8] This type of instability places the patient at risk for progressive chronic kyphosis.[8] Instability of the second degree (neurologic instability) applies to those injuries at risk for delayed neurologic compromise even if no deficit exists at presentation.[8] Instability of the third degree (mechanical and neurologic instability) includes those injuries in which both progressive osseous displacement and progressive neurologic injury may develop.[8] White and coworkers define clinical instability of the spine as the inability to maintain vertebral relationships in such a way that spinal cord and nerve root damage are avoided, and subsequent deformity and excessive pain do not develop.[13, 14] Their definition is widely used when assessing the potential instability of a traumatic lesion of the spine. Although this definition is somewhat broad, it takes into account both actual and potential instability in both mechanical and neurologic terms.

IMAGING METHODS

Conventional Radiography

The screening examination for the injured spine consists of conventional radiographs, and this method is emphasized in this chapter. Radiography has the advantages of being widely available and rapid; in addition, the radiographic equipment is portable, and the examination can be performed without moving the spine in the acutely injured patient. Its high spatial resolution and excellent ability to allow visualization of osseous structures make radiography the ideal initial examination in patients in whom skeletal injury is suspected. Most fractures can be detected with appropriate projections, and subluxations or malalignments often are easiest to appreciate visually on radiographs.[25] Routine anteroposterior and lateral projections, frequently used ancillary views, and numerous special views have been developed to facilitate visualization of the entire spine. The goal of radiography in the injured patient is to obtain high quality, diagnostic images without moving the patient inappropriately or placing the patient at any neurologic risk.[25] The study can be repeated as often as necessary and can be performed after placement of orthoses or orthopedic hardware. Modifications in film positioning and tube centering and angulation may be necessary after placement of traction or fixation devices.[26] The common routine and ancillary projections for specific anatomic regions are discussed in the sections covering injuries of each anatomic area.

Additional imaging methods for evaluation of the injured spine include conventional tomography, CT scanning, ultrasonography, MR imaging, and myelography (either alone or, more commonly, combined with CT). The use of each of these methods is reviewed briefly in the setting of the spinal injury.

Conventional Tomography

Both conventional tomography and CT scanning are used extensively for the detection and characterization of spinal fractures and malalignments. Considerable evidence exists that both conventional tomography and CT scanning allow the detection of fractures not evident on plain radiographs.[27–30] Conventional tomography has been available for a longer time than CT and its use for detailed evaluation of the osseous components of spinal injury has been described by numerous authors.[27, 30, 31] Conventional tomography can be used for evaluation of spinal regions in which radiographs are inadequate technically, such as the cervicothoracic junction in large patients. In patients with known fractures, conventional tomography can help characterize

the injury and demonstrate additional fractures in the involved or adjacent vertebrae[27] (Fig. 69–2). In patients with normal or equivocal radiographs in whom a spinal injury is suspected on clinical grounds, conventional tomography allows identification of fractures not detected on the screening study.[27, 31, 32] Conventional tomography is particularly helpful when the initial radiographs are equivocal or suggestive of abnormality but not definitive; in this setting, 25 to 65 per cent of patients have fractures detected with conventional tomograms.[27, 30, 32] In comparison to conventional tomograms, routine radiographs reveal fewer fractures, with reported sensitivities of 41 to 93 per cent for the three view study.[30, 31] Conventional tomography is particularly useful for evaluation of the craniocervical junction owing to the complex vertebral anatomy and numerous overlying cranial and facial structures in this region. Its superiority for fracture detection is most pronounced at the anterior and posterior portions of the atlas and axis and at the posterior neural arches of the more caudal vertebrae.[31, 32] Typically, only anteroposterior or both anteroposterior and lateral multidirectional tomograms at 3 to 5 mm intervals are obtained.[27, 30, 31] With most currently used types of x-ray equipment, the lateral views require rolling the patient into the lateral decubitus position; great care must be taken to maintain spinal support and alignment. Some universal tomographic units with tilting tables allow lateral tomography to be performed in the upright or the supine position but these are largely unavailable, particularly with regard to the widespread availability of CT.[25, 33] In the setting of trauma, the anteroposterior study should be obtained first. If this shows a grossly unstable injury, rolling the patient for lateral tomography is not advisable if a CT examination can be performed.

Computed Tomography

Data comparing the accuracies of conventional tomography and CT are limited, and the choice of which of these methods to use depends on availability and physician preference. Currently, CT is used more frequently than conventional tomography because of its more widespread availability, superior contrast resolution, decreased examination time, lower radiation dose, diminished need for patient manipulation, and ability to perform multiplanar reconstruction.[29, 34–36] Malalignment generally is considered easier to detect using conventional tomography, but the routine use

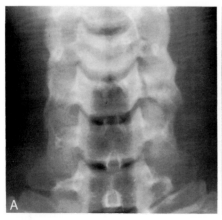
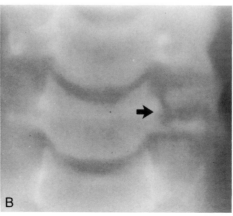

FIGURE 69–2. Spinal fracture: Conventional tomography. An anteroposterior radiograph **(A)** and conventional tomogram **(B)** illustrate a vertical fracture of the left facet of the C5 vertebra, with loss of height of the lateral mass. The fracture is seen more clearly on the conventional tomogram (arrow) owing to lack of superimposition.

of sagittal reconstruction after CT may mitigate this criticism.[12, 19, 34–37] Planar reconstructions often are helpful for understanding complex anatomic regions. Even curved coronal reconstructions can be obtained with software modification to follow the spinal curvatures more closely.[38]

The selection of levels to be studied should be made after a thorough review of the conventional radiographs. Slice selection typically is performed on the basis of lateral scout images in the cervical and lumbar regions and on an anteroposterior scout image of the thoracic spine. The author routinely obtains both an anteroposterior and a lateral scan. In all trauma cases, these images are filmed twice, once alone and once with the slice levels superimposed on the images. In complex injuries, this technique makes it easier to determine the exact orientation and position of the anatomic structures seen in the transaxial plane. Scanning at least one spinal level above and below a recognized fracture is recommended because of the high frequency of contiguous injuries.[29] Osseous anatomy is seen best on CT sections obtained with thin (1.5 to 2 mm) sections, using small body calibration to obtain high spatial resolution.[39]

Dynamic sequential CT scanning with automatic table increments shortens total examination time markedly in comparison to conventional spinal examinations.[40] Multiplanar reformation also is aided by the dynamic imaging technique because motion between slices is minimized, resulting in fewer misregistration artifacts.[40] Spinal immobilization or traction must be maintained throughout the study and dislodgment of any traction equipment as the CT table moves must be avoided.[41] Dedicated CT traction devices constructed of radiolucent plastic have been devised that allow constant, stable traction with minimization of metallic and misregistration artifacts.[41]

Imaging in the transaxial plane makes it difficult to detect those fractures that are parallel to the CT slices. Transaxial images alone may be inadequate for the identification of horizontal fractures, such as those that occur at the base of the odontoid process and at the thoracolumbar level with distraction injuries. Although the transaxial images may fail to demonstrate these transversely oriented fractures, they usually are apparent on good quality reconstructions.[12, 34] The routine use of 1.5 mm CT sections reduces the number of missed fractures and also permits superior reconstruction.[29] Knowledge of the characteristic sites and CT appearance of these injuries, as well as close correlation with conventional radiographs, leads to greater accuracy in the detection of transverse fractures. These fractures characteristically appear as broad bands of low attenuation rather than as a thin lucent line, as is seen typically with vertical fractures.[29] Similar broad bands of low attenuation may be seen in patients with significant kyphosis, lordosis, or scoliosis. The "pseudofractures" produced by these spinal deformities are a partial volume artifact consisting of two adjacent vertebrae and the intervening disc and are particularly evident on thick slices.[42]

CT has higher sensitivity than conventional radiography in the detection of vertebral fractures, particularly those involving the posterior osseous elements. McAfee and colleagues analyzed the use of CT in evaluation of thoracolumbar injuries.[12] They found CT to be more sensitive than radiography for diagnosis of posterior element fractures and for evaluating facet joint malalignment. Acheson and coworkers conducted a study of 49 patients with cervical

fractures detected by CT scanning from among a group of 160 patients examined with this method after suffering blunt trauma.[29] Of the 136 fractures detected in these patients, only 64 (47 per cent) were seen or suspected on the initial radiographic examination.[29] All but one of the fractures found by CT alone occurred in vertebrae already identified as abnormal by plain film (e.g., detection of a second fracture) or at a level above or below a recognized fracture.[29] These data do not imply that the sensitivity of CT for fracture detection is 100 per cent. Pech and collaborators evaluated the sensitivity of CT for fractures of the cervical spine produced in cadavers subjected to experimental trauma.[43] All comminuted vertebral body fractures, including displaced intracanalicular bone fragments, were detected. Despite the use of 1.5 mm slices and sagittal reformation, CT failed to detect seven of nine fractures of the spinous process, five of six superior facet fractures, and three of 14 pedicle or laminar fractures.[43] Other studies also have indicated that CT can lead to missed diagnosis of posterior arch fractures, particularly those that are oriented horizontally.[44]

CT appears to be the optimal method for detection of pneumorrhachis (gas within the spinal canal). Pneumorrhachis most often is iatrogenic, being derived from a lumbar or cervical puncture or due to penetrating wounds to the spinal canal. Unusual causes of pneumorrhachis include extension of pneumocephalus due to cranial fractures, a posttraumatic subarachnoid space–pleural fistula, and rupture of bowel loops entrapped within a fracture-dislocation of the spine.[45–47]

The development of three-dimensional rendering of sequential transaxial CT images has enhanced the ability to visualize musculoskeletal structures.[48–50] The spine lends itself well to such image reformatting to better appreciate its complex anatomic and spatial relationships (Fig. 69–3).

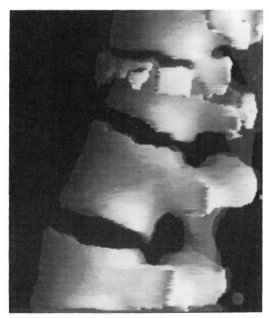

FIGURE 69–3. Fracture-dislocation: Three-dimensional CT scanning. A three-dimensional surface rendering derived from CT data of the spine shows a fracture of the L1 vertebral body with comminution of the superior endplate. The T12 vertebral body is displaced anteriorly.

Wojcik and coworkers first described the use of three-dimensional transaxial CT for the evaluation of acute cervical trauma and noted its superiority over conventional CT in cases of complex cervical injury.[49] Although no new numerical data were created by the three-dimensional rendering, the spatial relationships at the site of trauma were much more obvious and understandable than on the standard transaxial images, according to these authors.[49] Helical CT offers the advantage of greater speed than serial CT; both are able to provide three-dimensional images, but the images from helical CT can be obtained in about one fifth the time it takes for conventional CT.[50]

The role of myelography has diminished greatly since the advent of CT and MR imaging; however, intrathecal administration of contrast medium prior to performing contrast-enhanced CT still is used frequently in complex cases of spinal injury. Conventional myelography necessitates patient motion to optimize layering of the contrast agent against the anterior spinal structures and may be dangerous in the acutely traumatized person. The prone position appears to lead to more osseous displacement than the supine or decubitus position.[51] The addition of water-soluble nonionic intrathecal contrast medium prior to CT is widely employed, particularly for preoperative assessment of the neurologically injured patient. The use of myelography and contrast-enhanced CT probably will decrease as MR imaging becomes more readily available.

Contrast-enhanced CT is particularly helpful when the thecal sac is compressed by soft tissue, such as disc or hematoma, or when a dural tear is suspected.[12, 25, 52–57] Intrathecal enhancement generally is performed via a supine C1-C2 puncture in an attempt to minimize potential injury from patient motion. The advantages of contrast enhancement over conventional CT include better visualization of the spinal cord, improved detection of soft tissue lesions compressing the spinal cord, such as herniated disc or epidural hematoma, and detection of laceration of the spinal cord, nerve roots, and dura.[25, 52, 54, 55, 57] Contrast-enhanced CT is superior to conventional tomography and myelography in localizing the site of neural canal compromise in thoracolumbar fractures.[12] Spinal cord compression can be delineated on the myelogram but is easier to appreciate on the contrast-enhanced CT scan. Intrinsic cord trauma is very difficult to detect in the face of severe compression.[51] Tears, fissures, and disruption of the cord can be differentiated from extradural compression.[54, 55] Severe disruption of the spinal cord can cause an appearance of an absent cord as contrast medium fills the spinal canal completely[53, 54] (Fig. 69–4). Dural tears result in extravasation of contrast agent outside the spinal canal.[52, 57] Identification of dural tears is important despite the fact that most heal spontaneously because of the resultant risk of meningitis, nerve root entrapment, and delayed posttraumatic meningocele formation.[52, 57]

The role of contrast-enhanced CT in the patient with complete spinal cord injury is somewhat controversial. It has been suggested that the remote chance of improvement in these patients does not justify the performance of a myelogram, as little information that would change management would be gained.[25, 54] Allen and coworkers did perform contrast-enhanced CT in 19 patients with complete cord injury, and they noted neurologic improvement in four

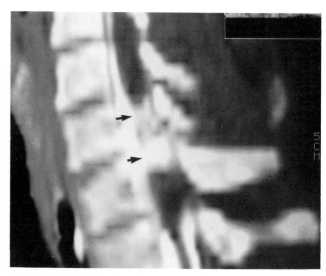

FIGURE 69–4. Spinal cord transection: Contrast-enhanced CT. A sagittal reconstruction of transaxial CT data of the cervical region after intrathecal administration of contrast medium shows discontinuity of the spinal cord with contrast agent filling the defect (arrows). (Courtesy of G. Bock, M.D., Winnipeg, Manitoba, Canada.)

patients, only one of whom was found to have a compressive lesion warranting surgery on contrast-enhanced CT.[55]

Magnetic Resonance Imaging

The role of MR imaging in the evaluation of the acutely traumatized patient currently is evolving. Although this method has been used widely for assessment of the spine and spinal cord, its application to the acutely injured patient has become widespread only recently. The multitrauma patient often is unstable hemodynamically and typically is connected to an array of monitoring and life support systems. The development of ventilation and monitoring devices compatible with MR imaging has greatly increased the physician's ability to examine the severely injured patient acutely.[58, 59] Conventional ventilators are contraindicated because the strong magnetic field adjacent to the MR imaging unit interferes with both the mechanical switches and the microprocessors that control the equipment.[58] Similarly, electrically operated intravenous pumps, used for administration of precise doses of drugs in patients in unstable condition, also are not usable within the area of the MR imager.[60] The conventional halo, vest, and skull pins employed for cervical traction also may be incompatible with MR imaging, and traction equipment replacement or modification of traction equipment typically is necessary to perform the examination safely.[61–64] Several short-term and long-term cervical traction devices compatible with MR imaging now are available commercially.[56, 60, 62, 65] Clayman and associates evaluated nine commonly used nonferrous cervical braces and orthoses for MR imaging compatibility.[62] They found that orthoses containing electrically conductive loops produced eddy currents that resulted in significant image degradation. The best results were obtained with aluminum or graphite-carbon composite components connected by plastic joints.[62] Imaging may be difficult in patients who already have undergone surgical fixation with ferromagnetic materials, such as stainless steel fixation wires, owing to ferromagnetic artifacts from the hardware. Biocompatible titanium wire allows for undistorted imaging of the surgical fixation site.[66] MR imaging of the patient with a penetrating gunshot wound to the spinal canal should be preceded by careful assessment of the position and ferromagnetic properties of any retained projectile. Although patients with nonferromagnetic bullets have been imaged safely, knowledge of the type of bullet is mandatory to predict the risk of movement or deflection.[61, 67] Imaging of the spinal cord in patients after gunshot injuries may be of limited value even if the bullet is nonferromagnetic. Prior studies of gunshot injuries to the spinal cord have found no correlation between the appearance of the spinal cord at surgery and neurologic prognosis, except for cases with frank cord transection.[68]

Despite the difficulties in imaging the traumatized patient, MR imaging clearly is superior to all other imaging methods in the assessment of the spinal cord and is particularly useful in patients with neurologic deficits out of proportion to their bony injury. The ability to survey long segments of the spine and the multiplanar capability afforded by MR imaging offer significant advantages over CT scanning. Perhaps the most advantageous feature of MR imaging is the superb contrast resolution of all the spinal and paraspinal soft tissue structures. Prior to the introduction of MR imaging, the status of the paraspinal musculature, intervertebral disc, spinal ligaments, and spinal cord was difficult to assess noninvasively.[66, 69–71]

Both T1- and T2- or T2*-weighted sequences are essential for adequate detection and characterization of bone and soft tissue injury. Typically, both sagittal and transaxial planes are used in the assessment of the injured spine. Oblique planes of section can be useful for evaluating anatomic structures that are not parallel to the three conventional orthogonal planes, such as the neural foramina and exiting nerve roots.[72, 73] Surface coils typically are used to obtain high resolution images with sufficient signal intensity.[70]

The bone marrow changes associated with acute fractures are best assessed on T1-weighted images. The integrity of the cortex and alterations in the vertebral configuration are well evaluated on T1-weighted or proton density–weighted spin echo MR sequences.[70, 71, 74] Vertebral body fractures are detected readily, although more fractures and a greater number of fragments and their sites of origin can be seen with CT, particularly in cases of comminuted fracture.[67, 70, 71, 74] MR imaging fails to allow identification of a significant number of posterior element fractures detected by CT, particularly in the cervical region.[65, 69–71, 74, 75] MR imaging detects only 25 to 66 per cent of posterior element fractures seen with CT scanning.[65, 67, 71, 74]

T2-weighted spin echo images are essential for assessment of the cord substance and paraspinal soft tissues.[75] Ligamentous injury can be identified by noting alterations in both the morphology and the signal intensity of the spinal ligaments and paraspinal soft tissues. The normal anterior longitudinal ligament, posterior longitudinal ligament, and anulus fibrosus appear as thin linear bands of low signal intensity on all sequences.[53, 69, 72, 76] The interspinous ligaments are less well defined and are of intermediate signal intensity. The supraspinous ligament is well seen on

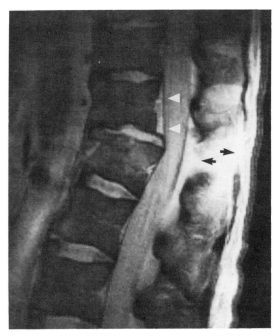

FIGURE 69–5. Ligament disruption: MR imaging. The T12 vertebral body is displaced anteriorly relative to the L1 vertebral body. Sagittal T2-weighted (TR/TE, 2000/80) spin echo MR image shows discontinuity of the supraspinous and interspinous ligaments (arrows). High signal intensity is seen in the T12-L1 interspinous region and in the fractured L1 vertebral body due to hemorrhage or edema, or both. In addition, the posterior longitudinal ligament is stripped from the T12 vertebral body (arrowheads).

the midline sagittal slice as a discrete band of low signal intensity overlying the tips of the spinous processes.[69, 70] The ligaments are best evaluated for tears on the sagittal T2-weighted images.[69, 70, 74] Ligament tears can be seen directly by observing the presence of ligamentous discontinuity or associated soft tissue hemorrhage, or they can be diagnosed by noting indirect criteria, such as kyphosis and malalignment[69, 70, 74, 77, 78] (Fig. 69–5). Supraspinous ligament rupture typically occurs in its midportion, between the osseous elements. Rupture of the anterior longitudinal ligament and posterior longitudinal ligament is easiest to detect in the region at the periphery of the disc, where the ligaments blend with the outermost fibers of the anulus fibrosus.[76] Assessment of the spinal ligaments is hampered significantly by patient scoliosis and obliquity of position.[69] The sensitivity and specificity of MR imaging for ligament evaluation are difficult to establish as not all injured patients undergo surgical exploration of the site of trauma. In one study of 37 patients with spinal injury, correlation with surgical findings and patient follow-up suggested a sensitivity of 90 per cent and specificity of 100 per cent for MR imaging.[69]

The presence and size of traumatic epidural hematomas can be assessed readily on MR images.[70, 71, 79] Massive epidural hematoma is uncommon after trauma, but small to moderate amounts of epidural hemorrhage are frequent in traumatized patients. Bohlman has emphasized the relationship between massive epidural hemorrhage and spinal injuries in patients with ankylosing spondylitis.[80] The epidural space contains loose areolar tissue and has an extensive venous plexus devoid of valves and anastomoses but with

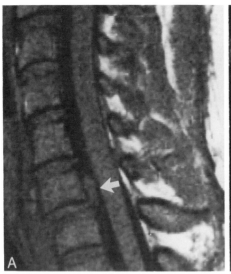 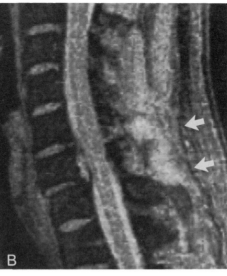

FIGURE 69–6. Traumatic disc herniation: MR imaging. The MR image was obtained after reduction of a unilateral facet lock at the C5-C6 vertebral level.

A T1-weighted (TR/TE, 600/20) spin echo MR image shows a large central disc herniation (arrow) at the C6-C7 level.

B T2*-weighted (TR/TE, 200/13; flip angle, 30 degrees) gradient recalled echo sequence shows the disc herniation as well as edema in the interspinous soft tissues posteriorly (arrows).

tributaries from the vertebral bodies, spinal cord, and extraspinal paravertebral venous plexus.[81] Epidural hematoma is most apparent acutely when the mass of low signal intensity is easily differentiated from epidural fat. At this stage, the epidural hematoma can mimic a disc herniation or disc extrusion although it typically is of higher signal intensity than the normal disc on T2-weighted images.[79, 82] Epidural hematomas, unlike herniated discs, more frequently are located posteriorly and often extend over more than one intervertebral segment.[81] As the hematoma evolves, mass effect persists, but its signal intensity approaches that of fat, which may obscure its margins.[70, 74, 83] The mechanism of T1 shortening in subacute hematomas is mainly due to the presence of methemoglobin. With time, hemoglobin, which contains ferrous iron, is oxidized to methemoglobin, which contains ferric iron and is strongly paramagnetic.[83]

The prevalence of traumatic disc herniation in patients with spinal injury generally is reported to be 3 to 9 per cent. The presenting feature is an acute central or anterior cord syndrome.[84] The true prevalence may be much higher because detection of disc herniation prior to the advent of MR imaging was difficult. In series employing MR imaging, acute disc herniations reportedly are present at the level of injury in 33 to 48 per cent of patients with unstable cervical spine injury.[84, 85] Fifty per cent of these disc herniations occur at the level of injury or at the level above or below the traumatized region.[74] Most frequently the cervical spine is the site of traumatic disc herniation, particularly its lower levels.[80, 86, 87] Traumatic disc herniation appears to be less common at the thoracolumbar region than in the cervical spine.[53, 85] Detection of herniated discs with conventional radiography and CT often is difficult in the presence of a spinal injury owing to the presence of hematoma, edema, and bone fragments at the site of trauma. All 26 traumatic disc herniations reported by Bohlman initially were diagnosed at the time of surgery in patients undergoing laminectomy or anterior fusion for vertebral fracture or subluxation.[80] In 16 patients with traumatic disc herniation detected preoperatively by MR imaging reported in another series, none was diagnosed on plain films or CT scans.[85] MR imaging appears to be more accurate than CT for the detection and assessment of the position of herniated disc

material in the injured spine.[65, 71, 84, 85] The traumatized disc is best seen on the T2- or T2*-weighted images and often has a higher signal intensity than the other, normal discs[74, 85] (Fig. 69–6). The presence of associated osteophytes and spinal stenosis suggest that the disc herniation is chronic.[65, 75] Osteophytes usually can be distinguished from discs, particularly with the use of gradient echo techniques.[60] The frequency of disc herniation appears to be similar in patients with normal, moderate, and severe spinal cord injury.[84, 85]

Ultrasonography

Spinal ultrasonography is not used in the setting of acute trauma but plays a role in the intraoperative assessment of the injured spine, particularly the traumatized spinal cord. Spinal sonography has been facilitated by the development of high frequency transducers and improvements in equipment portability.[88–90] Spinal ultrasonography in the adult requires a defect in the osseous arch to obtain adequate access to the spinal canal. Intraoperative sonography of the spinal canal is possible via a posterior approach following a standard posterior laminectomy or via an anterior approach after corpectomy.[88, 91, 92] To visualize small superficial musculoskeletal structures, use of a 5 MHz or higher frequency transducer is desirable.[89, 90] Visualization is optimized by the use of a saline pool with the scanner head placed 2 to 3 cm away from the first tissue interface.[88, 92, 93]

In 1984, Montalvo and colleagues reported their experience with intraoperative spinal sonography in 39 patients and were the first authors to illustrate the usefulness of this technique in a large group of patients with acute and delayed complications of spinal trauma.[92] Ultrasonography was useful for detection of retropulsed fragments of bone, epidural hematoma, and foreign bodies, allowing direct assessment of spinal cord compression.[92] Real-time ultrasonography also has been utilized to monitor reduction of acute thoracolumbar burst fractures.[93] Restoration of the posterior vertebral body alignment and reduction of retropulsed bone fragments can be visualized directly at the time of placement of distraction rods using this technique.[93]

The major use of ultrasonography is assessment of traumatic lesions of the spinal cord itself. Acute lesions of the parenchymal cord appear as foci of increased echogenicity within the cord substance; the size of the area of abnormal echogenicity correlates with the severity of the patient's neurologic deficit.[91] Chronic abnormalities of the spinal cord, such as intramedullary cysts, subarachnoid cysts, and myelomalacia, can be differentiated accurately. Intraoperative ultrasonography probably is more reliable than MR imaging or contrast-enhanced CT in distinguishing drainable cysts from myelomalacia.[91, 94] Intraoperative sonography also is useful for confirming proper catheter placement and cyst collapse in patients undergoing cyst shunting.[92]

SPINAL CORD TRAUMA

General Considerations

The annual incidence of spinal cord injuries is over 40 injuries per 1 million people in the United States.[95, 96] The highest prevalence is seen in patients aged 20 to 34 years, with men involved more than twice as frequently as women.[96, 97] The case fatality rate between 1970 and 1977 was 11.2 per cent, and the average cost of treating a single patient with spinal cord injury in 1980 was estimated to be a quarter of a million dollars.[96] Motor vehicle accidents and falls account for most of these devastating injuries. Approximately one third of patients with spinal cord damage resulting from trauma develop complete quadriplegia or paraplegia.[97] A disproportionately high rate of quadriplegia is seen in patients suffering from injuries that occurred during sporting activities.[80, 95, 97] Regardless of the form of therapy employed, fewer than 2 to 3 per cent of patients with initially complete spinal cord lesions ever walk again.[20, 80, 98, 99] Presumably most of this small group represents the 2 to 4 per cent of spinal cord injured patients who suffer reversible concussion.[20, 98]

The prevalence of spinal cord injury in patients with vertebral trauma is difficult to estimate because many patients with minor vertebral injuries do not come to medical attention or are not hospitalized, leading to overestimation of the risk of spinal cord injury when only hospitalized patients are included in the survey. Riggins and Kraus, basing their conclusions on a survey of 18 counties in Northern California, estimated the risk of spinal cord injury in a patient with vertebral injury to be 14 per cent.[95] The risk was highest in patients with displaced fractures involving both the vertebral body and the posterior osseous elements in the cervical region.[33, 95] The authors acknowledged that this rate probably is an overestimation owing to the selection bias inherent in the study, as the fracture surveys were limited to patients hospitalized at four major institutions, which would be expected to have as patients the more seriously injured persons.[95]

Classification of Injuries

The prevalence of osseous injury in patients with spinal cord trauma is quite consistent in different series because all patients with neurologic deficit come to medical attention. In studies in which 50, 619, 384, and 123 patients with spinal cord injury were investigated, the rates of fractures or vertebral malalignment were 66, 62, 63, and 64 per cent, respectively.[95, 100, 101]

Acute spinal cord injury may result from irreversible structural lesions, such as laceration, transection, or severe contusion; intrinsic reversible lesions, such as concussion or mild contusion; or extrinsic reversible lesions, such as cord compression.[59] Spinal cord concussion (spinal shock) produces a transient neurologic deficit without any recognizable morphologic or microscopic alterations in the cord.[68, 98] The initial neurologic deficit may be profound and is thought to be due to alterations at a neurochemical or neuroendocrine level.[102, 103] Spinal cord concussion typically is the result of injuries producing a rapid change in cord velocity after trauma and, by definition, resolves completely within 24 to 48 hours.[20, 98] The cervical cord is affected most frequently, perhaps related to preexisting lesions producing spinal canal narrowing or hypermobility.[98]

Spinal cord contusions are intrinsic cord lesions with macroscopic or microscopic alterations (or both) produced by an admixture of necrosis, hemorrhage, and edema. They may produce a reversible or, more commonly, an irreversible neurologic deficit. Early contusions tend to be a few small central hemorrhages, which gradually enlarge and coalesce with variable amounts of surrounding edema.[102, 103] Radiographic and clinical distinction between concussion and contusion may be difficult in mild cases of contusion. Even under ideal imaging circumstances, tiny petechial hemorrhages may be impossible to detect.[100] Numerous types of therapy have been employed to effect more rapid and complete recovery of function in these patients. These therapies, including steroids, cord cooling, fibrinolysis, myelotomy, and neurochemical modification, have been reviewed in detail by de la Torre.[102] In general, only minimal effectiveness has been demonstrated for the various treatments used for cord contusion.

Transection and laceration are irreversible lesions of the spinal cord produced by anatomic discontinuity of the spinal cord nerve tracts.[59, 68] The spinal cord is surprisingly tough and rarely is torn, lacerated, or transected, even in the presence of massive fracture-dislocations.[103, 104] It may be difficult to distinguish transection from massive contusion if the cord is examined more than a few days after the injury. Spinal cord dissolution owing to autodestruction after severe contusive injuries typically develops 24 to 48 hours after the injury and can simulate the appearance of complete cord rupture.[103] Unlike transection, there is a potential for neurologic improvement in patients with contusion.

All forms of intrinsic cord lesions are unlikely to benefit from decompressive surgery.[80, 102, 103] Decompression is indicated when cord compression results in neurologic deficit or places the patient at risk for the development of a deficit. Compression of the intrinsically normal spinal cord generally produces a reversible neurologic defect. Cord edema from compression may develop but no necrosis or hemorrhage is identified in the cord substance.[102] Cord edema due to compressive lesions has a good prognosis and shows rapid resolution clinically and radiographically.

Clinical Assessment

The clinical manifestations of spinal cord injury are variable and depend on the location and extent of the lesion. Schneider and coworkers published their classic review of traumatic spinal cord syndromes in 1973.[105] These authors classified spinal cord injury syndromes into eight major categories: (1) bulbar-cervical dissociation, (2) Dejerine onionskin pattern, (3) anterior spinal cord syndrome, (4) central spinal cord syndrome, (5) conditions simulating central cord syndrome, (6) thoracic spinal artery insufficiency, (7) fluctuating tetraplegia, and (8) immediate complete areflexic tetraplegia syndrome.[105] These eight clinical syndromes have well-defined physical findings and allow prediction of the level and type of cord injury with considerable accuracy. They are mentioned throughout this chapter, and the interested reader is referred to the work of Schneider and colleagues for more detailed information regarding the underlying pathophysiology and management of these lesions.[105]

Bulbar-cervical dissociation refers to interruption of the high cervical cord and results in instant death owing to immediate, complete pulmonary and cardiac arrest.[105] The Dejerine onionskin pattern is due to a lesion at the midcervical level and results in injury to the spinal cord that produces asymmetric facial hypoesthesia as well as medullary dysfunction. The anterior spinal cord injury syndrome is characterized by complete motor paralysis below the level of the lesion and loss of pain, touch, and temperature sensations, but with preservation of the posterior column functions of vibration, motion, and position sensations.[105] This form is one of the commonest patterns of spinal cord injury encountered after severe cervical injury and may result from a fracture-dislocation leading to cord compression, a direct injury to the anterior portion of the cord, or an acutely herniated disc.[105] The central cervical spinal cord syndrome produces disproportionately greater motor loss in the upper extremities as compared to the lower, with variable amounts of sensory loss.[105] Unlike the situation with the anterior cord syndrome, a significant potential exists for neurologic recovery with this lesion.[105] The central cord injury pattern often is present without significant radiographic findings, in which case it characteristically is due to hyperextension, particularly in the spondylitic patient.[105–107] The central cord syndrome may be mimicked by injuries involving the crossing fibers of the pyramidal decussation or trauma causing bilateral injury to the brachial plexus.[105] The syndrome of thoracic anterior spinal insufficiency is produced by a thoracolumbar fracture or dislocation and is characterized by a disproportionately high level of neurologic deficit, occurring many segments cranial to the osseous lesion. It is due to midthoracic vascular insufficiency resulting from arterial injury or occlusion as a result of the trauma.[105] Fluctuating tetraplegia (quadriplegia) with a pattern of vascular recovery is manifested by a gradual recovery of deep pain sensation, followed by a gradual return of temperature and superficial pain sensation. Recovery of both motor and sensory function appears to be due to resolution of hypoxia of the spinal cord owing to reestablishment of circulation via tributaries of the anterior spinal artery.[105] Recovery of somatosensory evoked potentials within 4 hours of spinal cord injury correlates with an improved prognosis in this pattern.[103] The final pattern of spinal cord injury, immediate complete areflexic tetraplegia (quadriplegia) syndrome, usually is irreversible, particularly if it persists for longer than 24 hours.[103, 105]

Clinical assessment, combined with somatosensory evoked potentials and diagnostic imaging, is used to determine the type, severity, and prognosis of acute spinal cord injuries.[102] The most widely used clinical assessment scale for myelopathy is that devised by Frankel and associates.[108] The Frankel scale, which was developed on the basis of clinical examination of 682 patients with closed spinal injuries,[108] has five categories: (1) complete motor and sensory loss (grade A), (2) complete motor loss with complete or partial preserved sensation (grade B), (3) preserved motor power (nonfunctional) (grade C), (4) preserved motor power (functional) (grade D), and (5) no deficit or complete neurologic recovery (grade E).[108] This scale does not distinguish between normal patients and those with only radiculopathy or reflex changes.[84, 108] Distinction between grades C and D often is difficult owing to subjective differences in assessment of the purposefulness of patient movement.[74] The functional status often evolves over time, either worsening or improving over a period of months or years.

Imaging Assessment

Imaging of spinal cord trauma directly is not possible with conventional radiography or conventional tomography. CT affords a crude assessment of the severely injured cord but also is limited in evaluating lesions of the cord other than compression. The use of myelography and intrathecal contrast-enhanced CT is discussed in the previous section. Although myelography and contrast-enhanced CT can provide valuable information about cord compression and can allow identification of complete disruption of the cord substance, they are inadequate for assessment of nondisrupted lesions of the cord substance.

Perhaps the greatest advance made possible by MR imaging in the spinal injury patients is the ability to evaluate intrinsic lesions of the spinal cord noninvasively. Numerous studies have attempted to correlate the MR imaging appearance of the injured cord with the pathologic features of the underlying lesion and its prognosis.[64, 74, 84, 109–112] On MR imaging, spinal cord transection with complete cord discontinuity manifests filling of the defect by cerebrospinal fluid and adhesions.[113] Although MR imaging demonstrates cord transection noninvasively, its advantage over contrast-enhanced CT is much more apparent for milder forms of intrinsic cord pathology.

Several studies have suggested that irreversible damage to the cord secondary to contusion exhibits different MR imaging features from the reversible lesion of concussion. Kulkarni and associates have described three patterns of morphologic and signal intensity alterations on MR imaging and correlated these three types with the potential for neurologic recovery.[64, 111] The poorest prognosis is associated with the type 1 pattern, in which cord hemorrhage results in inhomogeneity of the cord substance on T1-weighted sequences.[64] This pattern develops within hours of the injury and is associated with a very poor prognosis; no improvement in Frankel classification or Trauma Motor Index is noted in many cases.[111, 112] Acutely, within 72 hours of the injury, the hemorrhagic area is hypointense relative to the cord on T2-weighted images, presumably owing to loss of phase coherence created by the magnetic susceptibility of intracellular deoxyhemoglobin.[56, 99, 111] The signal intensity alterations are seen to better advantage on T2-weighted spin echo sequences than on gradient echo studies.[56, 74] These areas of low signal intensity may be difficult to detect when low field systems are used.[114] T2-

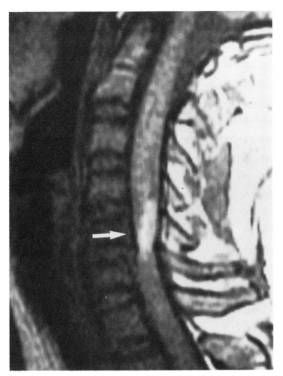

FIGURE 69–7. Spinal cord hemorrhage: MR imaging. T1-weighted (TR/TE, 500/20) spin echo MR image shows an oval region of high signal intensity within the cord (arrow) in a patient who developed a complete neurologic deficit after trauma. This sequence was obtained 9 days after the injury. The high signal intensity is due to methemoglobin in the area of hematomyelia. (Courtesy of A. Flanders, M.D., Philadelphia, Pennsylvania.)

weighted images obtained 3 to 7 days after cord hemorrhage show residual hypointensity in the center of the lesion with a thin rim of peripheral hyperintensity due to extracellular methemoglobin. After a variable period of time (8 days in one study), the hemorrhage becomes evident as an area of high signal intensity on T1-weighted images owing to conversion of the entire region to methemoglobin[74] (Fig. 69–7). In Flanders and coworkers' series of 78 patients with acute cervical trauma, the presence of intramedullary hemorrhage always was predictive of a complete lesion and was present in 91 per cent of patients with a complete neurologic defect.[74] In Silberstein and colleagues' series, all patients with cord transection and hemorrhage as noted on MR images also had complete motor paralysis and a poor prognosis.[115]

The type 2 pattern was the most common pattern encountered in the series of Kulkarni and associates, seen in 18 of 33 patients.[111] This pattern is thought to be due to cord edema and was associated with a good prognosis with improvement of neurologic status in all patients in their series.[64] Although the cord may be enlarged focally, normal signal characteristics are maintained on T1-weighted sequences in this pattern. Acutely, the area of edema is hyperintense relative to the normal spinal cord on T2-weighted sequences.[64, 99, 112] This area of hyperintensity frequently is linear or spindle-shaped, presumably owing to proximal and distal extension of edema around a microscopic area of hemorrhage or necrosis. Similar linear areas of high signal intensity, extending proximally and distally from the site of injury, are noted in mild contusions produced in an animal model.[99, 103] Cord edema can be identified as early as 4 hours after the injury, peaks at 72 hours, and then resolves rapidly, usually over a period of a few days.[56, 64, 102] This time course corresponds to pathologic changes in the cord seen in experimental models of spinal cord injury. Small petechial hemorrhages are noted within 30 min of injury; by 4 hours, extensive coagulation necrosis involving up to 40 per cent of the central gray and subjacent white matter is present.[102, 103] Maximal edema after moderately severe concussion is seen pathologically 2 to 3 days after the injury.[102]

The type 3 pattern was encountered in only two patients in Kulkarni and associates' series[64]; it consisted of cord enlargement and normal signal intensity on T1-weighted images. On T2-weighted images, in the acute situation, a central area of hypointensity was surrounded by a thick rim of hyperintensity.[64] This appeared to be an intermediate pattern with mixed MR imaging features and was associated with an intermediate prognosis.

Schaefer and coworkers have correlated the MR imaging appearance of the acutely injured cervical cord with the admission neurologic examination in 78 patients.[74, 84] Features associated with severe neurologic deficit included intramedullary hematoma and spinal cord edema extending over more than one spinal segment.[74, 84] Findings seen in patients with less severe injuries were a normal cord or a small area of contusion, with edema limited to one spinal segment.[74, 84] All patients with a neurologic deficit manifested some cord abnormality on MR imaging, and no patient with a grossly abnormal cord at MR imaging was normal neurologically.[74] Yamashita and coworkers found that the degree of cord compression, rather than the signal intensity of the cord, was the most accurate prognostic variable for determining clinical prognosis.[110] These authors used a midfield strength magnet, which may not have been as sensitive in detecting signal alterations.[100, 110]

Posttraumatic Progressive Myelopathy

Patients whose conditions previously were stable may develop progression of neurologic deficit long after the time of acute injury. The development of a new neurologic deficit or unexplained progression of previous neurologic deficits requires prompt investigation and intervention when appropriate. Posttraumatic progressive myelopathy is the term applied to a clinical syndrome consisting of the delayed onset of progressive spasticity and of motor and sensory dysfunction after spinal cord injury. Severe pain and autonomic nervous system dysfunction also may be present. This syndrome is estimated to develop in 2 per cent of patients after traumatic spinal cord injury.[116] Posttraumatic progressive myelopathy appears to be independent of the site or severity of the initial injury.[94, 117] The syndrome may develop secondary to a variety of pathologic conditions of the cord. Prior to the introduction of MR imaging, posttraumatic progressive myelopathy was thought to be due to only two pathologically distinct forms of spinal cord damage, noncystic myelomalacia or posttraumatic syringomyelia, also known as posttraumatic cystic myelopathy or posttraumatic spinal cord cyst.[94, 109, 116, 118] The pathogenesis of these lesions may be the breakdown of an area of hematomyelia with cyst development, or the syndrome may result from nonhemorrhagic cord trauma.[118] Nonhemorrhagic trauma can lead to the development of a myelomalacic core of tissue because of ischemia, the action of released enzymes, or vasospasm induced by increased levels of epinephrine.[118] Progressive dilation of the small cystic spaces may be due to the production of cerebrospinal fluid by the gliotic lining tissue or to the presence of cerebrospinal fluid that enters the cyst via enlarged Virchow-Robin spaces or channels.[116, 118] Because only the cystic form of posttraumatic progressive myelopathy is suitable for operative drainage, preoperative distinction between syringomyelia and myelomalacia is essential for selection of appropriate patients for cyst drainage.[94, 116, 119]

It now is recognized that posttraumatic progressive myelopathy may develop in association with cord compression and involves a much wider range of pathologic conditions of the cord. The chronically injured cord can manifest a variety of intrinsic cord lesions, such as atrophy, syringomyelia, myelomalacia, arachnoid cyst, and tethering by adhesions, as well as extrinsic cord compression by mechanical factors, such as malalignment and retropulsed fracture fragments or disc.[60, 109, 110, 119] Yamashita and colleagues evaluated 14 patients with new symptoms after remote spinal cord injury; in their series syringomyelia was the most common MR imaging finding.[110] Silberstein and coworkers described the MR imaging findings in a larger series of 94 patients who developed new symptoms after a previous spinal cord injury.[109] Criteria for inclusion included increasing myelopathy, an ascending neurologic deficit, pain, hyperhidrosis, and increase in muscle spasm. Symptoms developed a mean of 114 months after the original injury.[109] The most frequent findings on MR imaging were atrophy (43 per cent) and syrinx (41 per cent). Other lesions detected included cord compression (24 per cent) and myelomalacia (26 per cent). Conversely, some patients had a completely normal appearing spinal cord (18 per cent).[109] A strong correlation was noted between cord compression and atrophy or myelomalacia; an inverse relationship existed between cord compression and syringomyelia.[109]

Posttraumatic Syringomyelia

Posttraumatic syringomyelia is an important cause of progressive neurologic deterioration. Because syringomyelia can be treated successfully with drainage of the cystic cavity, correct diagnosis is important. The prevalence of this entity is difficult to determine because its diagnosis, prior to the development of contrast-enhanced CT and MR imaging, was difficult to establish. Posttraumatic syringomyelia has been estimated to occur in 0.9 to 2 per cent of patients who have sustained spinal injury.[117, 118] Decades after their initial injury, patients can develop pain, sensory or motor loss, or brain stem involvement.[117]

Myelography shows arachnoiditis and adhesions at the level of injury as well as focal alterations in the size of the spinal cord.[94, 116, 118, 120, 121] The diagnosis of a spinal cord cyst should not be based on detection of focal areas of cord enlargement, because many cysts occur in spinal cords of normal size.[116, 121, 122] The typical spinal cord cyst is seen in a normal-sized or atrophic cord, is located in the dorsal aspect of the cord at or above the level of injury, and is larger than one half the cord diameter, although considerable variability may occur in its size.[116, 118] The average

length of a syrinx is 6.0 cm, although the lesions can be as small as 0.5 cm or occupy the entire length of the spinal canal.[116] Change in the diameter of a normal or atrophic cord in different positions can help in establishing the diagnosis of syringomyelia.[120–122] Up to 50 per cent of patients with syrinx show alterations in cord size with positional changes; decrease in size on moving from the prone to the supine position is most characteristic.[120–122] Positional alterations in cord size may be easier to detect with contrast-enhanced CT than with conventional myelography.[120]

Unenhanced CT and contrast-enhanced CT performed immediately after injection are relatively insensitive unless the cyst is large enough to be appreciated as an area of abnormal attenuation within the cord substance. Seibert and colleagues were the first to note the value of delayed CT for the detection of syringomyelia.[116] The CT examination was performed 3 to 6 hours after the intrathecal instillation of metrizamide, a water-soluble contrast agent. These investigators noted that the contrast agent filled the cyst, rendering it apparent on the delayed CT scans.[116] Subsequent authors have noted that both myelomalacia and posttraumatic syrinx become enhanced with the delayed technique, although myelomalacia tends to involve a shorter segment of the spinal cord and be less dense and less well defined.[119, 120] The major difficulties with delayed contrast-enhanced CT are that the technique is invasive, is time consuming, and generally necessitates hospitalization.[94]

Currently, MR imaging is the imaging method of choice for detection of posttraumatic syringomyelia and myelomalacia.[110, 123] With MR imaging, the cystic cavity in posttraumatic syringomyelia shows signal intensity characteristics similar to those of cerebrospinal fluid on all sequences (Fig. 69–8). Myelomalacia may appear of lower signal intensity than cerebrospinal fluid in T2-weighted images; unlike the cyst, which is hypointense relative to cord in proton density images, myelomalacia appears isointense or hyperintense relative to the spinal cord in proton density images.[119] In many patients, the distinction may not be clear-cut, as myelomalacia probably precedes the development or propagation of cyst formation, and the two lesions frequently coexist.[94, 120]

CERVICAL SPINE: GENERAL CONSIDERATIONS
Protocol Imaging

Recent years have seen a marked increase in requests for cervical radiographs in patients sustaining injury, particularly as a result of the widely taught recommendations of the American College of Surgeons (ACS), the routine application of cervical spine immobilizers, and concerns about potential litigation.[124–127] In 96 per cent of hospitals that deal with acute trauma cervical radiographs are obtained as a routine or protocol examination in all blunt trauma patients.[128] The ACS Committee on Trauma recommends obtaining crosstable lateral views of the cervical spine within 1 hour of presentation in all major trauma victims.[129] According to the ACS, cervical spine fractures should be assumed to be present in any multitrauma patient, particularly if the patient sustains a blunt injury above the clavicle.[129] The ACS states that ''the absence of neurologic deficit or pain does not rule out injury to the cervical spine. Such an

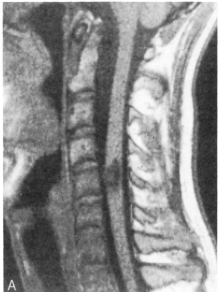
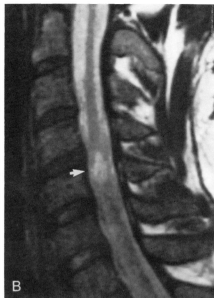

FIGURE 69–8. Posttraumatic syrinx: MR imaging. Two patients with posttraumatic cervical syringomyelia are illustrated.

A T1-weighted (TR/TE, 500/17) spin echo MR image shows an oval area of low signal intensity within the spinal cord posterior to the C5 vertebral body, corresponding to a small syrinx.

B T2-weighted (TR/TE, 2200/78) spin echo MR image in another patient with a posttraumatic syrinx shows high signal intensity in the area of the cyst (arrow).

injury should be presumed present until ruled out by adequate roentgenographic examination."[130] It has been suggested by other physicians that the lateral radiograph of the cervical spine is "more important to the patient's welfare than is any other diagnostic modality—including history and physical examination."[131]

Several authors have questioned these recommendations and the rationale for protocol examination in alert, asymptomatic persons, noting that the benefit of such routine radiographs has yet to be established.[125–128, 132] The prevalence of cervical spine injury in all trauma patients is low and may be as little as 2 per cent at some institutions.[125–127] The low yield from routine protocol examination has led to numerous attempts to identify those risk factors that correlate with cervical spine abnormality.[125–128, 132]

It generally is accepted that early radiographs should be obtained in all patients with pain or neurologic deficit referable to the cervical spine as well as in those patients who are not fully alert and cooperative at the time of their initial evaluation.[125, 126, 129, 131–133] Bohlman reported a delay in diagnosis of cervical injury in 100 of 300 patients with significant spinal trauma.[80] It is unclear from this series how often the delay was due to lack or inadequacy of radiographic evaluation. The major reasons cited for failure to diagnose cervical injury at initial examination in the emergency room included patients' decreased level of consciousness, head injury, alcohol intoxication, and associated fractures or multiple injuries.[80] There is little argument that in patients with concomitant head injury, diminished level of consciousness, alcohol intoxication, or multisystem injury, cervical spine injuries cannot be excluded reliably on the basis of a physical examination.[25, 80, 122, 131–134]

Considerable controversy exists, however, over the prevalence of spinal trauma in alert, asymptomatic persons and over the need to obtain radiographs in all patients who have been injured. Although numerous anecdotal case reports of asymptomatic cervical fractures exist, the thoroughness of the clinical examination has been questioned in these cases.[127, 135] In Williams and coworkers' series, 12 of 50 cases of cervical fracture, which included six multiple trauma patients, were not diagnosed at initial clinical examination.[131] Neck pain was delayed or absent in these patients, although many were not alert at the time of their initial presentation.[131] Walter and colleagues reported that for 12 of 67 patients with cervical fractures no note was present in their medical record documenting symptomatic neck pain, but the majority of these were multitrauma victims; four had altered mental status and four showed tenderness to palpation.[133] It has been suggested that the "asymptomatic" clinical fracture may be a myth and that unnecessary evaluation of patients at no risk should be curtailed.[135]

Virtually all patients with cervical spine injuries and a normal level of consciousness have symptoms or signs referable to the cervical spine.[125–128] Fischer evaluated 333 consecutive patients after head trauma with class 1 level of consciousness (alert, responds immediately to questions, follows complex commands, may be disoriented and confused) and found that all five patients with cervical injury had signs or symptoms, or both, referable to the cervical spine.[125] No correlation was found between the presence of a cervical injury and other major concomitant injuries, skull fractures, or intracranial trauma.[125] Symptoms and signs of cervical injury were present in many patients with normal spines; only five of 42 (11 per cent) of symptomatic patients manifested cervical trauma on their radiographic examination or at follow-up.[125] In the series of Bachulis and associates, all patients with cervical fractures and a normal level of consciousness complained of neck pain or had tenderness to palpation.[126] In another large series of 132 alert, asymptomatic trauma patients who had CT scanning of the lower cervical spine because of inadequate visualization on conventional radiographs, only one insignificant nondisplaced transverse process fracture was identified.[128] The cost of the radiographic and CT examinations in these 132 patients was $59,202.[128]

Screening Examination

The goals of initial radiographic screening of the cervical spine include detection of all injuries, assessment of neural canal or foraminal encroachment, and determination of spinal stability.[33] Considerable controversy exists regarding how many and which radiographic views constitute an adequate examination of the cervical spine.[127, 128, 130, 132, 136] Typically, the initial radiograph obtained is a supine crosstable lateral view centered on C4.[132] Lack of visualization of the lower cervical region on this view is a major cause for missed initial diagnosis.[33, 134] Arm traction may be necessary to obtain adequate visualization of the lower cervical vertebrae and may be used if upper extremity injuries are not present. This position tends to hyperextend the cervical region and is not advisable in patients with neurologic injury.[33] If the C7-T1 junction cannot be visualized with arm traction, an additional swimmer's view is obtained in patients without upper extremity injuries. Patients with a neurologic deficit or those who cannot be examined adequately for such deficits are studied with CT if the lower cervical region is not seen on the supine crosstable lateral view.

The crosstable lateral view of the cervical spine has a maximum sensitivity of only 73 to 86 per cent and should not by itself be considered an adequate screening examination.[29, 30, 125–127] Streitwieser and coworkers evaluated 71 patients with abnormal radiographs, persistent severe cervical pain, or neurologic deficit. Using thin-section conventional tomography as their gold standard, they identified a total of 101 cervical fractures in 44 of these 71 patients.[30] On the basis of the crosstable lateral view alone, 82 per cent of these fractures were detected. The addition of supine anteroposterior and open-mouth odontoid views increased the sensitivity of the plain radiographic examination to 93 per cent.[30] The fractures missed on the three-view examination consisted of one undisplaced odontoid fracture, one fracture of the C2 lateral mass, and one vertebral endplate fracture.[30] Only the odontoid fracture would be considered unstable.[30] Acheson and colleagues, using CT as the gold standard, reported that the sensitivity of the conventional radiographic examination for cervical spine fractures was only 42 per cent.[29] Although CT detected numerous fractures that were not seen on plain radiographs, most of these were second fractures occurring in vertebrae that already had been identified as abnormal. Only one of the 49 patients with cervical spine fractures had a completely normal three-view screening examination.[29]

In the author's experience, the three-view study is an adequate screening examination for most cervical spine injuries. Additional views that have been recommended for the routine workup of trauma patients include standard oblique, supine angulated oblique, pillar (vertebral arch), and flexion-extension views.[132, 136, 137] One author's complete cervical series for suspected cervical trauma consists of 11 projections.[136] Although the addition of multiple projections does increase the detection rate for fractures, particularly undisplaced posterior arch fractures, the clinical utility of these additional views is controversial. Certain injuries, such as undisplaced facet or laminar fractures, are difficult to recognize without these additional projections, but most of the missed injuries are stable.[132] Flexion-extension views may demonstrate ligamentous disruption not evident on conventional radiographs and are discussed in more detail later. Additional projections are most useful when they are tailored to the patient's symptoms or are obtained to clarify suspected abnormalities on the routine series. Equivocal radiographic findings or indirect indicators of trauma, such as soft tissue swelling, warrant further investigation, as does persistent, unexplained pain or a neurologic deficit referable to the cervical region.

Radiologic algorithms devised for use when there is clinical suspicion of cervical injury have been proposed and appear to be a reasonable approach to patient management.[127, 132] Vandemark has proposed a logical approach to the traumatized patient that stratifies patients according to their risk of injury and suggests appropriate radiographs for each category of patient.[127] Patients are assigned to one of four possible risk categories on the basis of their history and clinical features. The category 1 patient, deemed to be at no risk for spinal injury, does not need radiographs. This category includes patients with no historical or physical findings referable to the cervical region. The category 2 patient, considered to be at low risk because the history and mechanism of injury show that the physiologic range of cervical motion is unlikely to have been exceeded, should have an erect three-view series. The category 3 patient is at moderate risk because of the force of injury and should undergo supine lateral, swimmer's, anteroposterior, and odontoid views, followed by upright oblique views after the initial radiographs are approved by the clinician or radiologist. The category 4 patient is at high risk, owing to the force of the injury, altered mental status, abnormal neurologic examination, or prominent cervical symptoms. For these patients all the radiographs are taken in the supine position, with lateral, anteroposterior, odontoid, and shallow oblique films constituting the complete examination.[127] Close communication between the radiologist and emergency personnel is imperative to ensure that the radiographic examination is appropriate for the perceived risk of injury.[33, 25, 127] It likewise is mandatory that both the radiologist and the referring physician understand that significant injury may be present even if the radiographs are completely normal.

Soft Tissue Swelling

Retropharyngeal and retrotracheal soft tissue swelling are important indirect indicators of cervical trauma.[124, 138–143] Other indirect signs suggestive of cervical injury include displacement or obliteration of the prevertebral fat stripe, tracheal displacement or contour abnormalities, laryngeal dislocation, and tracheal laceration with retropharyngeal gas and elevation of the hyoid bone.[1, 124, 144]

Examination of the cervical radiographs should include careful evaluation of the width and contour of the prevertebral soft tissues. Prevertebral soft tissue swelling may not be present acutely, and its absence should not be used to exclude significant injury.[138, 139] Swelling due to edema and hemorrhage is maximal within the first 3 days after the injury.[138] Radiographs obtained more than 2 weeks after the episode may not reveal any abnormalities of the soft tissues, as most hematomas disappear within this period.[138]

Traditionally, 4 to 5 mm or 0.3 times the anteroposterior dimension of the vertebral body width is considered the normal maximum width of the prevertebral soft tissues at

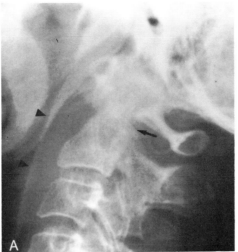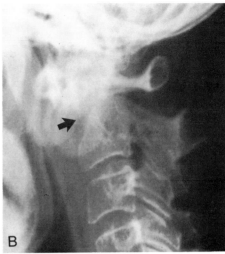

FIGURE 69–9. Soft tissue swelling.

A The neutral view shows abnormal widening of the prevertebral tissues anterior to the C1 and C2 vertebral bodies (arrowheads). A subtle step-off of the posterior margin of the C2 vertebral body is seen in this view (arrow).

B The flexion view shows displacement of the odontoid fracture (arrow), which was responsible for the soft tissue alterations.

the level of the retropharynx, anterior to the upper four cervical vertebrae[4, 139, 145, 146] (Fig. 69–9). Unfortunately, significant overlap is present in the measurements obtained in noninjured and injured patients.[138, 139] Templeton and colleagues noted that in more than 65 per cent of normal patients the traditional 4 to 5 mm upper limit is exceeded and suggested instead the use of 7 to 10 mm as the upper limit of normal.[139] The use of 7 mm as the upper limit of normal has been advocated for both children and adults.[124, 141] The retropharyngeal soft tissues are particularly difficult to assess in the presence of endotracheal, nasogastric, or orogastric tubes. Unsuccessful attempts to pass these tubes or traumatic intubations also produce soft tissue alterations in the absence of cervical trauma.

No significant difference in the width of the retropharyngeal soft tissues is seen with flexion and extension in the adult.[138] Dramatic changes in the retropharyngeal measurement can take place with axial rotation, lateral bending, and swallowing, however.[142] After testing of numerous positions and maneuvers, Martinez and coworkers noted that the action that resulted in the biggest increase in the prevertebral tissues was screaming.[142] Soft tissue thickness also increases with body weight and age in normal persons.[147, 148] Infants have wider retropharyngeal soft tissues, particularly in flexion, that normally may be up to 75 per cent of the vertebral body width.[149] Careful attention to the contour of soft tissues is necessary, particularly in the region of the cervicocranium, which is the most common site of spinal injury in the young child.[149]

The retrotracheal space, the inferior (below C5) continuation of the retropharyngeal space, typically is wider than the retropharyngeal space owing to the presence of the esophagus.[138, 139, 146] The retrotracheal space, measured immediately below the thyroid cartilage, has a mean width of 12.4 mm (range, 8 to 17 mm) in normal persons.[146] The upper limit of normal suggested by other authors has been 22 mm.[124, 141] In the presence of cervical spondylosis, thickening of the retrotracheal space frequently is present, rendering measurement in the presence of prominent anterior osteophytosis unreliable.[146] The wide range of normal values and the large capacity for hemorrhage at this level make evaluation far more difficult than in the retropharyngeal area.[138]

Prevertebral hematoma typically is present in injuries involving the anterior bony and ligamentous structures but is much less common in injuries isolated to the posterior elements.[138–140] In the absence of osseous injury, soft tissue swelling may be the most apparent radiographic finding in patients sustaining anterior ligamentous injuries to the cervical region.[140] Soft tissue swelling is not detected reliably in patients with isolated posterior ligament injury.[140]

The cervical prevertebral fat stripe is a thin radiolucent line located immediately anterior to the vertebrae and represents areolar tissue in the retropharyngeal and retroesophageal spaces.[143] A thin collection of air in the esophagus, a frequent normal finding, should not be confused with this structure. Widening of the prevertebral fat stripe due to obesity may result in an abnormal retropharyngeal and retrotracheal soft tissue thickness.[147] Whalen and Woodruff have suggested that anterior displacement of the prevertebral fat stripe is more accurate than increased width of the prevertebral tissues for detecting fractures.[143] Unfortunately, this structure is not visualized radiographically in all patients. In their review of 318 patients, Templeton and coworkers noted that the prevertebral fat stripe was rarely identified in patients with spinal injuries, suggesting that its presence in a normal location helps exclude injury but that its absence is of limited significance.[139]

Prevertebral hematoma can be visualized readily with cross sectional imaging methods. This finding is particularly helpful in patients with hyperextension sprain injuries when associated spondylosis and the absence of fractures render interpretation of the radiograph difficult.[78] On CT scans, hemorrhage produces thickening of the prevertebral tissues and displacement or obliteration of the prevertebral fat stripe. In MR images, acute prevertebral hemorrhage is isointense with gray matter in T1-weighted images but appears of higher signal intensity in T2-weighted images.[78]

CERVICAL SPINE: OCCIPITOATLANTOAXIAL REGION

General Considerations

The occipitoatlantoaxial region, also known as the cervicocranial junction, differs both anatomically and functionally from the remainder of the cervical spine and serves as the transition between these two regions. Injuries to the occipitoatlantoaxial region typically are the result of direct trauma to the head rather than to the spine. The occipitoatlantoaxial segment is particularly vulnerable in children younger than 12 years and represents the most common site of cervical spine injury in this age group.[80, 149, 150–152] In children, 50 to 83 per cent of traumatic cervical spine lesions involve the cervicocranium, compared with 16 to 24 per cent of all cervical injuries in adults.[80, 147–149, 153]

The osseous anatomy of both the C1 vertebra (atlas) and the C2 vertebra (axis) differs considerably from that of the remaining spinal vertebrae. The occipitoatlantal joint is reinforced by a unique ligamentous arrangement that allows moderate flexion and extension and minimal lateral flexion but restricts other movements markedly. In contradistinction, the primary motion at the C1-C2 joint is rotation rather than flexion or extension, which are the dominant motions in the lower cervical segment. The atlanto-occipital joints are cup-shaped synovium-lined joints located superolateral to the odontoid process. Their anatomic configuration, the capsular ligaments, and the external and internal craniocervical atlanto-occipital ligaments help maintain the stability of the paired atlanto-occipital joints.[154, 155] The external ligaments consist of the anterior and posterior atlanto-occipital membranes, which extend from the anterior and posterior arches of C1, respectively, to the foramen magnum.[154] The atlantoaxial ligament connects C1 to C2 anteriorly.[153, 154] Further reinforcement is provided by the internal ligaments, which consist of the apical ligament, paired alar ligaments, tectorial membrane, and vertical portion of the cruciform ligament. The tectorial ligament is the superior continuation of the posterior longitudinal ligament. It is a broad bilaminar ligament that lies posterior to the odontoid process and its ligaments.[153–155] Anterior to the tectorial membrane is the cruciate ligament, which has a transverse component posterior to the odontoid process (known as the transverse ligament) and a vertical component extending superiorly to the occiput.[153, 156] The alar ligaments extend from the posterolateral aspects of the apex of the dens to the inferomedial aspect of the occipital condyles.[156–158] The apical ligament is a thin midline structure that extends from the tip of the odontoid process to the base of the occiput. The atlas is connected only loosely to the occiput by the two articular capsules and the weak anterior, posterior, and lateral occipitoatlantal membranes.[153, 154, 159, 160] Stability of the occipitoatlantal joint is maintained primarily by the ligamentous attachments between the occiput and the axis.[159] The tectorial membrane and the alar ligaments are the major restrictors to extension at the occipitoatlantal joint.[160, 161] Rupture of both the tectorial and the alar ligaments is necessary for anterior dislocation of the cranium relative to the cervical spine.[162] The cruciate ligament and apical ligament, the only other connections between the axis and the occiput, are weak and do not play a major role in maintaining atlanto-occipital joint stability.

Atlanto-occipital Dislocation

Atlanto-occipital dislocation, subluxation, and instability may be secondary to acute trauma or a variety of nontraumatic conditions. Nontraumatic atlanto-occipital dislocation has been associated with rheumatoid arthritis, congenital skeletal anomalies, Down's syndrome, infection, and calcium pyrophosphate dihydrate crystal deposition at the craniovertebral junction.[155, 163] Nontraumatic atlanto-occipital dislocation has the same radiographic manifestations as traumatic dislocation unless additional features of the underlying disease can be identified. Traumatic atlanto-occipital dislocation is a rare injury that almost always is fatal because of associated transection of the spinomedullary junction.[80, 153, 159, 164]

Bucholz found atlanto-occipital dislocation to be the most common spinal injury resulting in immediate death in 178 victims of multiple trauma.[164] Thirteen of 38 cadaveric radiographs demonstrating cervical injuries showed atlanto-occipital dislocation on the postmortem films.[164] In Davis and coworkers' series of 50 autopsies in deaths due to craniospinal injury, the majority of osseous and ligamentous injuries also involved the cervico-occipital junction.[101]

Although the large majority of cases of atlanto-occipital dislocation result in death, the injury is not invariably fatal or neurologically catastrophic. Most survivors have some neurologic injury, but up to 20 per cent have no deficit at the time of presentation.[161, 162, 165, 166] Cranial nerve dysfunction, most commonly involving the sixth and more caudal cranial nerves, is the most common neurologic abnormality, presumably resulting from avulsion of the nerve roots from the brain stem.[159, 162] Direct trauma to the medulla may be manifested by dyspnea, hypertension, and cardiac arrhythmias.[161] Other neurologic deficits associated with atlanto-occipital dislocation include diffuse spasticity, quadriplegia, quadriparesis, and hemiparesis.

The mechanism of injury is controversial, although most authors believe it results from a combination of hyperextension and distraction.[159, 161, 162, 166] This injury is more common in children than in adults and typically results from motor vehicle accidents to pedestrians.[152, 159, 160, 166] Traumatic atlanto-occipital dislocation also has been documented in postmortem studies of abused children.[151] The relatively small size of the occipital condyles, the ligamentous laxity, the more horizontal plane of the atlanto-occipital joint, the weak cervical musculature, and the greater weight of the cranium place the young child at greater risk.[151, 159, 160, 167]

The conventional lateral radiograph is the initial examination that suggests the presence of this unusual injury. Radiographically, the diagnosis of atlanto-occipital dislocation may be difficult to establish, with up to 40 per cent of cases not being appreciated on the initial examination.[165] The most apparent finding is retropharyngeal soft tissue swelling. Retropharyngeal air may be present if the pharynx also is lacerated.[162] Avulsion fractures of the occipital condyles and clivus are highly suggestive of this injury.[168, 169] Associated fractures of the atlas and axis also have been described.[152, 155, 161, 170] Typically, the cranium is subluxated anteriorly relative to the cervical spine; however, superior displacement or, rarely, posterior subluxation occurs in other cases. Specific signs of anterior or posterior atlanto-occipital dislocation include displacement of the basion (midsagittal point of the anterior lip of the foramen magnum at the lower tip of the clivus) from its normal position superior to the odontoid process, malalignment between the spinolaminar line of C1 and the posterior margin of the foramen magnum, and failure of the clival line to intersect the odontoid process.[145, 153, 162, 166, 445, 446] Longitudinal dis-

POWERS RATIO

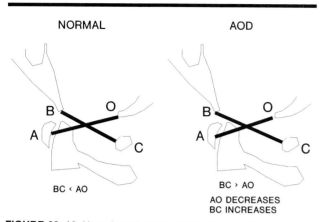

NORMAL   **AOD**

BC ‹ AO   BC › AO

AO DECREASES
BC INCREASES

FIGURE 69–10. Use of the Powers ratio to identify atlanto-occipital dissociation (AOD) is illustrated. See text for details.

traction injuries manifest different radiographic findings, such as increase in the dens-basion distance and widening of the occipitoatlantal joints.[152, 160, 166]

Wholey and coworkers, basing their work on an analysis of lateral cervical radiographs in 480 adults and 120 children, described in detail the normal relationship between the odontoid process and the basion.[141] They noted a remarkably constant relationship between the basion and the odontoid process. The middle of the upper aspect of the odontoid process normally lay directly below the basion at an average distance of 5 mm in the adult.[141] In infants and young children, this distance approached 1 cm.[141] Powers and colleagues noted that the dens-basion measurement in their series of normal subjects exceeded the normative values reported by Wholey and coworkers in up to 85 per cent of examinations.[171] They found a mean dens-basion distance of 9.0 ± 3.6 mm and noted that the value was the same for both children and adults.[171] Bulas and associates confirmed Wholey and colleagues' finding that the normal dens-basion distance in children is less than 1 cm in the majority of cases; they found a mean distance of 8.3 ± 4.2 mm in their review of 156 pediatric radiographs.[160] They noted that the dens-basion distance is affected by magnification and is increased when skeletal traction is applied; therefore, Bulas and coworkers suggested using 12.5 mm as the upper limit of normal.[160]

As an alternative method of evaluating occipitoatlantal alignment, Powers and colleagues described a quantitative technique that is valuable for the radiographic diagnosis of anterior cranial subluxation.[171] This alternative is based on the ratio between two lines rather than absolute measurements, so it is unaffected by variations in patient size or film magnification. The first line (BC) is the distance between the basion (B) and the posterior arch of C1 (C) at the spinolaminar line. The second line (AO) is the measurement between the posterior margin of the anterior arch (A) of C1 and the posterior lip of the foramen magnum, known as the opisthion (O). These anatomic landmarks are not affected significantly during flexion, extension, or rotation of the neck and usually can be identified on the lateral view, although the opisthion frequently is difficult to delineate.[145, 160, 172, 445, 446] Owing mainly to difficulty in identifying the opisthion, the BC/OA ratio could not be measured in 46 per cent of children in one series.[160] In normal persons, the ratio of BC/OA is 0.77 ± 0.09.[171] In the patients with atlanto-occipital dislocation described by Powers and colleagues, all but one had a ratio greater than or equal to 1.15 (Fig. 69–10). The smallest measurement in the atlanto-occipital dislocation group was 1.0. No overlap between normal and abnormal values was present in this series.[171]

The sensitivity of the Powers ratio has been questioned as it relies exclusively on anterior cranial translation.[145, 160, 166] This method is valid only when atlanto-occipital dislocation results in anterior translation of the cranium but is insensitive for longitudinal or posterior displacement (Fig. 69–11). The Powers ratio similarly is not accurate when congenital anomalies are present at the cervicocranium or when the osseous ring of C1 is fractured.[172]

A significant proportion of patients with atlanto-occipital dislocation manifest only longitudinal distraction and have a normal Powers ratio. The lack of significant anterior displacement in this type of injury also may result in a normal sagittal basion-odontoid relationship.[152, 166] Distraction injuries are particularly common in the pediatric population.[152, 160, 166] Only six of 11 children with atlanto-occipital dislocation reported by Bulas and coauthors had an abnormal Powers ratio, whereas the basion-dens distance was greater than 1.4 cm in all cases.[160] Five of 10 children with atlanto-occipital dislocation reported by Maves and collaborators had had a longitudinal traction type of injury.[152] The occipital condyles are displaced from the superior facets of the atlas and the atlanto-occipital joint is widened to more than

FIGURE 69–11. Atlanto-occipital dissociation: Horizontal translation type.
  A The basion (arrow) is displaced anteriorly relative to its normal position above the tip of the odontoid process.
  B Similar malalignment of the basion (arrow) is seen in a different patient with atlanto-occipital dissociation. Note the extensive soft tissue swelling in both examples. The Powers ratio is abnormal in both cases.

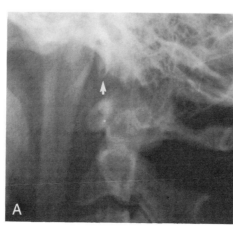

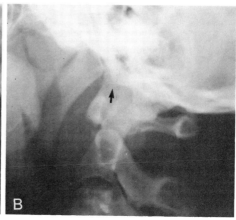

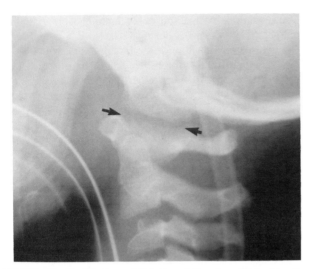

FIGURE 69–12. Atlanto-occipital dissociation: Longitudinal traction type. Longitudinal separation of the atlanto-occipital joints is observed, with more than 5 mm distance between the occipital condyles and the lateral masses of the atlas (arrows). The distance between the basion and the dens also is abnormally increased.

5 mm if the cranium is distracted superiorly[160, 166] (Fig. 69–12). This joint often is difficult to visualize, particularly in the older child and adult, owing to superimposition of the mastoid process.[160]

CT allows assessment of the osseous alignment in this region without moving the patient.[172] Both coronal and sagittal image reconstructions are necessary to comprehend the pattern of displacement fully. On coronal reconstructions, the atlanto-occipital joints slope from superolateral to anteromedial and normally appear about 1 mm thick.[156] Widening of these joints and avulsion fractures may be seen in patients with atlanto-occipital dislocation. The midline sagittal reconstruction can be used to derive the Powers ratio as all the necessary anatomic landmarks are seen well in this reconstruction plane.[172] Associated findings observed in the upper cervical region with CT scanning include hemorrhage around the foramen magnum, thickening of the anterior tectorial membrane, and extradural hemorrhage.[160] MR imaging also has been used to establish the diagnosis of atlanto-occipital dislocation, and some investigators have suggested that MR imaging, owing to its ability to allow visualization of the ligamentous structures directly, is the single best method for evaluation.[165] The sagittal images show the malalignment between the clivus and the dens; edema and hemorrhage in the prevertebral tissues, spinal ligaments, and bone marrow also can be identified.[165, 173] MR imaging similarly allows evaluation of damage to the spinal cord in patients surviving atlanto-occipital dislocation.[173]

Atlantoaxial Subluxation

The dens normally is tightly bound to C1 by the dense inelastic fibers of the transverse ligament, which is attached bilaterally to tubercles on the inner surface of the lateral masses of C2.[17, 156, 157] The transverse ligament lies in a shallow groove on the posterior aspect of the odontoid process and prevents forward subluxation of the atlas on the axis with flexion of the neck. The accessory atlantoaxial ligaments, which extend upward from the tubercles directly to the lateral margins of the odontoid process, reinforce the function of the transverse ligament.[156, 174] The function of this ligament also is augmented minimally by the more flexible alar ligaments, which limit rotation and, to a lesser degree, lateral bending.[17, 170, 175] The horizontal atlantoaxial joints confer minimal stability because both cartilaginous articular surfaces are convex, minimizing contact while affording a large amount of motion.[153, 157]

Isolated posttraumatic atlantoaxial subluxation is a rare injury. Only 1 per cent of 300 cervical injuries reported by Bohlman were of this type.[80] In an autopsy series of 50 patients who died as a result of craniospinal injury, only one case of a traumatic transverse ligament tear was identified.[101] Fielding and colleagues reported 11 cases of posttraumatic atlantoaxial subluxation. All patients in their series were men who had suffered severe trauma to the head.[17] Neck pain was a constant presenting feature, and neurologic deficit was present in three of the 11 injured patients.

Nontraumatic atlantoaxial subluxation is far more frequent, with rheumatoid arthritis probably representing the most common cause of transverse ligament incompetence.[176] Numerous other arthritides and connective tissue disorders, including the seronegative spondyloarthropathies, have an association with atlantoaxial subluxation.[177, 178] A variety of congenital anomalies and disorders also show this association with atlantoaxial subluxation.[175] Five to 30 per cent of patients with Down's syndrome have laxity of the transverse ligament.[179–181] Associated hypoplasia of the posterior arch of C1, present in 26 per cent of children with Down's syndrome, further narrows the spinal canal diameter and places the cord at higher risk.[179, 181] Inflammatory rupture of the transverse ligament likewise can occur owing to a variety of inflammatory processes of the head and neck.[175, 176]

Traumatic tears of the transverse ligament or avulsion fractures at its site of insertion are sufficient to allow displacement of C1 relative to C2 (Fig. 69–13). Almost all cases of atlantoaxial displacement manifest anterior dislocation of the atlas relative to the axis. Isolated cases of posterior atlantoaxial dislocation have been described in the absence of a fracture, but this is an exceedingly rare event[175, 182] (Fig. 69–14). Displacements of up to 5 or even 10 mm can develop after isolated transverse ligament rupture; further displacement requires insufficiency of the alar and other secondary ligaments.[170, 183, 184] In vitro studies suggest that ligamentous failure is a sudden phenomenon and involves the body of the ligament more commonly than the osteoperiosteal portion.[17, 170] The ligament is elastic and retracts once ruptured; consequently, reducing the osseous subluxation does not result in reapposition of the retracted fragments.[170]

The normal distance between the dens and the posterior margin of the anterior arch of C1 is less than 3 mm in adults and 5 mm in children.[170, 185, 186] The normal atlantoaxial distance is maintained in both flexion and extension of the neck. Very young children have substantial amounts of unossified cartilage in the upper portion of the odontoid process; in hyperextension, the anterior arch may not appear to have any bone contact, as it lies above the ossified portion of the odontoid process.[148, 187] Measurements of the atlantoaxial distance are reliable only when the odontoid

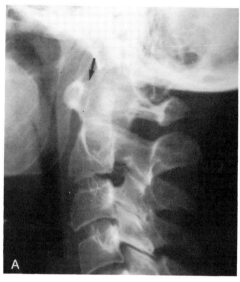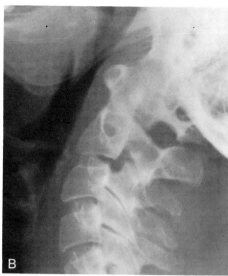

FIGURE 69–13. Atlantoaxial subluxation.

A The flexion view shows abnormal widening of the atlantoaxial space (arrow), which measures 4 mm.

B The subluxation is completely reduced in extension.

process is intact and attached to the C2 body.[175] Spuriously large measurements are obtained when the odontoid process is eroded by infection, pannus, or tumor; widened atlantoaxial distances in these circumstances do not imply transverse ligament rupture. Abnormal widening of this interval because of transverse ligament incompetence is more apparent with flexion of the cervical spine.[17, 136, 153] Concomitant displacement of the C1 spinolaminar line relative to C2 also is seen.[188]

In many normal persons the width of the atlantoaxial interval is uneven, with superior widening resulting in a V-shaped predens space.[176] Nine per cent of adults show this configuration, which is most prominent on radiographs obtained during flexion of the neck.[176] Mild posterior tilting of the dens also is a common normal finding and similarly results in the V-shaped space.[189, 190] Posterior tilting is not associated with any displacement of the odontoid process, as may be seen with an odontoid fracture.[189] The 26 patients reported by Bohrer and colleagues all had an atlantoaxial distance less than 7 mm at the cranial aspect of the joint; the majority of patients with a V-shaped joint had a maximum atlantoaxial distance of 4 mm.[176] A normal atlantoaxial distance is seen in these patients when it is measured at the lower aspect of the anterior arch of C1.

Neurologic deficit is variably present, even in patients with dramatic displacement and atlantoaxial widening. Significant amounts of displacement can be tolerated in this region owing to the large size of the spinal canal. According to Steel's rule of thirds, the spinal cord and odontoid process each occupy a third of the anteroposterior diameter of the ring of C1, leaving the last third as "safe" space.[170] Some of this safe space actually is occupied by the transverse ligament itself, which is 4 to 5 mm wide in its normal state.[175] In patients with rheumatoid arthritis, neurologic symptoms are rare until the atlantoaxial distance approaches 9 mm.[177] The gradual development of subluxation in these patients also may be protective.

The distance between the anterior arch of C1 and the dens can be assessed with CT, but the CT examination typically is performed in the neutral or extended position, limiting its sensitivity for atlantoaxial subluxation. In transaxial CT scans, the normal atlantoaxial space appears to be less than 1 mm wide.[156] The intact transverse ligament often can be seen in CT scans as a curvilinear, enhancing soft tissue structure of variable thickness.[156] A normal CT examination does not exclude atlantoaxial subluxation unless the study is obtained with cervical flexion. MR imaging affords a more sensitive method for the detection of atlantoaxial instability and allows concomitant assessment of the degree of cord compression.[191] Flexion and extension sagittal MR images are necessary for evaluating the craniocervical junction. MR imaging may underestimate the degree of subluxation owing to the small diameter of the head coil, which precludes full flexion and extension of the neck.[191]

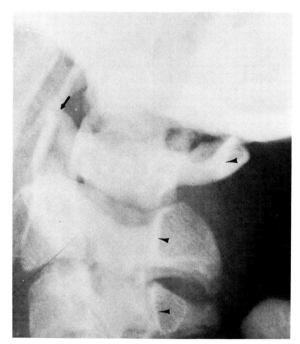

FIGURE 69–14. Posterior atlantoaxial dislocation. In this unusual injury, the atlas is displaced posteriorly with respect to the axis. Note the offset in the spinolaminar lines (arrowheads). The odontoid process (arrow) is intact.

Patients with chronic atlantoaxial subluxation may develop a mass in the craniovertebral junction as a result of repetitive mechanical irritation.[192] These nonmalignant pseudotumors are composed of fibrous and granulation tissue and typically are of low signal intensity in MR images.[192]

Atlantoaxial Rotatory Fixation

Atlantoaxial rotatory fixation is a confusing entity that is difficult to define, diagnose, and manage. The exact pathologic or anatomic basis for this lesion is unclear and probably a variety of mechanisms exist that lead to the same lesion. Atlantoaxial rotatory fixation can be defined as persistent pathologic fixation of the atlantoaxial joints in a rotated position such that the atlas and axis move as a unit, rather than independently as is the normal situation.[183, 193, 194] This form of C1-C2 malalignment often occurs after minor or moderate trauma, but it also may develop spontaneously or after an inflammatory condition involving the pharynx or upper respiratory tract. The first comprehensive review of traumatic atlantoaxial rotatory fixation was published in 1907 by Corner, who described 20 cases of this entity, eight of which were identified in postmortem specimens.[195] He established the diagnosis of atlantoaxial rotatory fixation on the basis of an abnormal rotational malalignment between C1 and C2. The postmortem specimens, unlike the clinical cases he and other subsequent authors have reported, exhibited associated fractures of the odontoid process in six of the eight cases, as well as other fractures of the cervicocranium.[195] This highly select group of postmortem specimens does not correspond well with the patients seen clinically, in whom fractures and a fatal outcome are rare.

The primary function of the C1-C2 joint is rotation. Normally, the atlas rotates 30 to 50 degrees in either direction relative to the axis.[153, 183, 193, 195] Only after a minimum of 20 to 30 degrees of rotation at this level does rotation of the lower cervical spine develop.[137] When the head is rotated to the right, the left articular mass of C1 slides anteriorly while the right articular mass rotates posteromedially.[194, 196] With continued rotation, the left articular mass continues to move anteriorly but also rotates in a medial direction.[194, 196] The movement of the right articular mass is always greater, causing the left alar ligament to become taut and restrict any further motion. Lateral tilting of the head to the left in this situation relaxes the alar ligament, allowing rotation to continue. This relationship explains why rotation is facilitated by a slight tilt of the head to the opposite direction.[157, 158, 194] In atlantoaxial rotatory fixation, the relationship generally is fixed within the range of motion attainable during normal rotation. Fielding and Hawkins developed a four level classification system of atlantoaxial rotatory fixation based on the direction and degree of displacement.[184] Type 1 atlantoaxial rotatory fixation is the most common and consists of fixed rotation within the physiologic range of motion, with an intact transverse ligament and a normal atlantoaxial distance. Type 2 lesions are characterized by deficiency of the transverse ligament with atlantoaxial displacement of 3 to 5 mm. In type 3 atlantoaxial rotatory fixation, atlantoaxial subluxation of more than 5 mm is present owing to deficiency of both the transverse and the secondary (predominantly the alar) ligaments. Atlantoaxial distances as large as 22 mm have been reported in type 3 lesions.[197] The type 4 lesion is extremely rare and occurs when both lateral masses of C2 are displaced posteriorly relative to those of C1.

The patient has a persistent, painful torticollis and the typical ''Cock Robin'' position of the head, consisting of slight flexion, cranial rotation, and tilting of the head contralateral to the direction of rotation.[183, 184, 194, 195, 198] Over 80 causes of torticollis have been reported, and the presence of torticollis is a sign of an underlying disorder, rather than a diagnosis per se.[198] Pain over the occiput is common and may be unilateral and aggravated by motion.[157, 194] The occipital neuralgia may be due to trauma to the second cervical nerve, which runs for a portion of its course in the C1-C2 capsular tissues.[157, 194, 199] Vertebral artery compromise may occur with severe rotation, particularly when combined with anterior subluxation of C1 and C2. Brain stem and cerebellar infarction, and even death, may ensue as a result of vessel damage in cases of severe rotation.[18] With longstanding deformity, facial flattening toward the side of the tilt may develop.[184, 200] Despite the dramatic clinical and radiographic findings, neurologic deficit is seen in only a minority of patients. Unilateral dislocation with rotation of 45 degrees narrows the adult canal to 12 mm without exceeding the critical diameter necessary for the cord.[157] Rotation of 65 degrees is necessary before the critical diameter of the canal is reached. At 65 degrees of rotation, the spinal canal diameter approaches 7 mm.[157]

The most characteristic radiographic abnormality in rotatory fixation is a persistent abnormality in the relationship of the odontoid process to the lateral masses of C2. This abnormal relationship of C1 and C2 is best demonstrated in the anteroposterior open-mouth odontoid view[184, 196, 197] (Fig. 69–15). In this view, the dens is positioned eccentrically between the lateral masses of C1, and the anteriorly displaced lateral mass appears wider, more rectangular, and closer to the midline[196, 200, 201] (Fig. 69–16). This appearance occurs because the long axis of the lateral mass is almost 45 degrees oblique; with rotation, the anterior mass is seen en face whereas the posterior mass appears foreshortened.[183] Asymmetry in the distance between the dens and the C1 lateral masses characteristically is present, with diminution of this distance on the side rotated anteriorly. Unilateral medial offset of the foreshortened posterior facet is a prominent feature.[196] On the side on which the lateral mass has rotated posteriorly, the C1-C2 articulation often is obscured owing to overlapping of the osseous structures as the thick central cartilage contact points no longer are in apposition.[157, 167, 183, 200] Spinous process deviation is not a prominent feature clinically or radiographically unless an associated lateral tilting of the head is present.[195, 200] These same radiographic appearances also can be seen in normal children and adults imaged in a position of voluntary cranial rotation and in patients with reversible torticollis, but in these two groups the positioning abnormality is reversible.[153, 165, 193, 202]

The anteroposterior view of the lower cervical spine may demonstrate a gradual compensatory contralateral rotation but otherwise is unrevealing.[157] The lateral projection often is more confusing than revealing in atlantoaxial rotatory fixation. Because of the rotation and lateral tilt of the atlas, its posterior arches do not overlap. This appearance can mimic occipitalization of the atlas or other congenital craniocervical anomalies.[200] Voluntary lateral bending also is associated with atlantal rotation and can mimic a rotatory

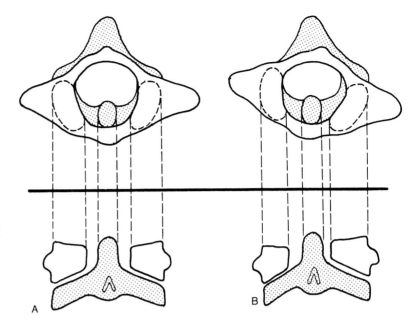

FIGURE 69–15. Atlantoaxial relationships. The atlantoaxial joint is seen in the neutral position **(A)** and on rotation to the right side **(B),** viewed from above (on top) and from the frontal plane (on bottom).

A In the neutral position, the odontoid process is located midway between the lateral masses of the atlas. The lateral atlantoaxial joints are symmetric.

B With rotation, anteromedial rotation and upward shift of the left atlantal articular mass are associated with medial approximation to the odontoid process. The right atlantal articular mass moves inferiorly and posteromedially, and it possesses a narrow profile. The left lateral atlantoaxial joint is widened, and the right is narrowed. Persistence of the findings is consistent with atlantoaxial rotatory fixation.

dislocation.[167] The atlas characteristically is hyperflexed relative to the axis, although this finding is difficult to determine unless a true lateral view of the atlas is obtained.[157] The anteriorly rotated lateral mass tends to overlie the anterior arch of C1, obscuring the region of the atlas and dens. Assessment of the atlantoaxial distance and the integrity of the odontoid process on the lateral view may be difficult or inaccurate when unilateral rotation is present.[195, 200, 203] Compensatory lordosis of the lower cervical vertebrae may be present.[157] Other views rarely are helpful for assessing the C1-C2 relationship. Modified views of the skull base have been advocated for assessment of the atlantoaxial relationship, but these projections require hyperextension of the cervical spine.[136, 167] Modified basilar projections now are rarely obtained in the traumatized patient and have been supplanted by CT.

Rotatory fixation can be diagnosed only when the abnormal relationship between the lateral masses of the atlas and axis is shown to be irreducible. Serial exposures taken with

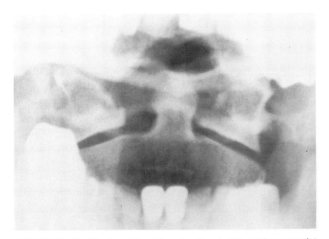

FIGURE 69–16. Atlantoaxial rotatory fixation. In this patient, persistent rotation of the C1-C2 vertebral bodies was present. Note the asymmetry in the shape of the C1 lateral masses and the asymmetric distance between the dens and the lateral masses of the atlas.

different amounts of rotation can be used to evaluate the C1-C2 relationship. Anteroposterior views of the odontoid process obtained with 15 degrees of rotation of the head to both sides and similar views with lateral tilting of the head to both sides have been advocated.[183] In patients without neurologic deficit, in those who have not had an injury, or in those who are not examined soon after the traumatic episode, dynamic fluoroscopy can demonstrate the fixed C1-C2 relationship.[183, 194, 196, 204]

Conventional radiographic examination often is inconclusive and difficult to interpret because of the anatomic distortion and overlap of the craniocervical structures. The interpretation of sequentially rotated radiographs or of findings observed during cineradiography or fluoroscopy often is confusing, and the patient may have difficulty cooperating during the examination. CT scanning both in the resting position and with maximal rotation of the head to the contralateral side now is considered the optimal method for evaluation.[201, 205] Thick slices actually are easier to assess because the axis of a tilted vertebra can be determined from a single slice. The use of static CT examinations for the diagnosis of atlantoaxial rotatory fixation was first described by Fielding and coworkers in 1978.[206] In their case report, the abnormal vertebral relationship was well demonstrated with no patient discomfort and without the need for any patient movement. Rinaldi and colleagues in 1979 used CT scans obtained with cranial rotation to both sides to demonstrate that the abnormal vertebral relationship was fixed, regardless of position.[194] Kowalski and associates obtained functional CT scans in the resting and rotated positions in six patients with atlantoaxial rotatory fixation, as well as in two patients with torticollis and in six normal volunteers.[193] Studies were done in the resting (i.e., rotated) position and with maximal rotation to the contralateral side. The initial static images in all three groups of subjects (normal subjects also were asked to rotate their heads) were identical. In patients with rotatory fixation, no change in the relationship of C1 and C2 was evident when the resting and contralateral rotation studies were compared; in normal

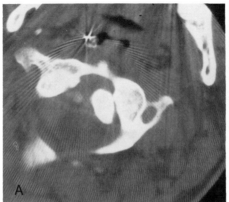
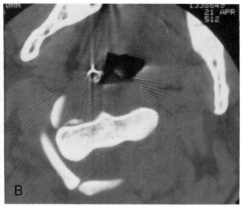

FIGURE 69–17. Atlantoaxial rotatory fixation. Transaxial CT scans at the level of the atlas **(A)** and axis **(B)** show rotatory malalignment between C1 and C2. This abnormal relationship did not change with cranial rotation.

subjects and in patients with torticollis, such comparison revealed reduction or correct of the deformity[193] (Fig. 69–17). It should be noted that patients with atlantoaxial rotatory fixation often can rotate the head further in the direction of their deformity; they are unable to rotate the head to the contralateral side or correct the deformity.[184]

Grisel's syndrome is the term applied to unilateral or bilateral atlantoaxial subluxation in association with an inflammatory condition of the head or neck.[203, 208–210] Unilateral anterior subluxation, producing rotatory malalignment, is most common.[203] Typically, patients are between 5 and 12 years of age; there is no sex predominance.[167, 175, 203, 207–209] Although rotatory displacement is the most typical deformity, the term displacement, rather than fixation, is preferred because many patients have some residual motion present in the upper cervical region[203] (Fig. 69–18).

Infection of the C1-C2 joint itself usually is not present in Grisel's syndrome. Tearing, swelling, and entrapment of the capsular tissues and synovium, combined with muscle spasm, are thought to result in the atlantoaxial subluxation, but the exact pathogenesis is not well understood.[194] Possible causes of malalignment include ligamentous stretching, inflammatory effusion in the anterior median atlantoaxial

joint, muscle spasm, and regional hyperemia leading to osteoporosis at the sites of ligamentous attachment with subsequent ligament dysfunction.[203] The anatomic basis for the inflammatory effusion, which is believed to be the most likely explanation for Grisel's syndrome, has been elucidated by Parke and coworkers.[209] A venous vascular plexus connects the posterosuperior pharynx with the periodontoidal vascular plexus.[209] The absence of lymph nodes about this plexus allows free lymphovenous anastomosis and transfer of septic exudates from the pharynx to the anterior median C1-C2 joint.[203, 209]

Patients typically have neck and throat pain as presenting features, followed by atlantoaxial subluxation and torticollis.[175, 203, 209] Predisposing factors include contiguous infection, typically pharyngitis or tonsillitis, pharyngeal abscess, dental infection, surgical procedures such as mastoidectomy and tonsillectomy, and numerous other inflammatory conditions of the head and neck.[167, 175, 203, 208] The hypertrophic state of the peripharyngeal tissues in children may explain the marked predominance of patients under 15 years of age in reported series of Grisel's syndrome. Neurologic dysfunction in Grisel's syndrome is uncommon, probably owing to the capacious size of the spinal canal at the C1-C2 level. Neurologic complications occur in up to 15 per cent of cases, however, and range from radiculopathy to myelopathy and even death.[175, 203, 208]

Fractures of the Atlas

The atlas differs from all the remaining vertebrae in its anatomy as it lacks both a body and a spinous process.[199, 210] It develops from three ossification centers, one unipartite or multipartite center in the anterior arch and bilateral unipartite centers in each lateral mass.[199, 210] These ossification centers are well formed by the age of 2 years. The two posterior centers fuse by the age of 3 to 5 years, whereas the anterior segment typically does not fuse with the posterior centers until the age of 5 to 9 years.[199] By this age, the spinal canal at the level of C1 has attained its adult size.[141, 211] In young children, the synchondroses represent the points of weakness in the C1 ring.[150]

The ring of C1 can be divided into an anterior arch (20 per cent), paired lateral masses (40 per cent), and a posterior arch (40 per cent).[212, 213] The anterior arch serves as the attachment site for the longus colli muscle and the anterior

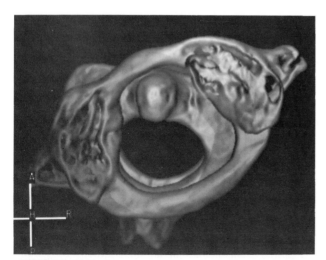

FIGURE 69–18. Grisel's syndrome. This 10 year old girl developed torticollis 6 weeks after an episode of tonsillitis and pharyngitis. Three-dimensional transaxial reconstruction of CT data of the C1-C2 region shows the rotatory malalignment between C1 and C2. (Courtesy of S. Wall, M.D., San Francisco, California.)

longitudinal ligament, and its concave posterior surface articulates with the odontoid process of the axis. A region of weakness exists where the anterior arch joins the lateral mass bilaterally.[214] The lateral masses of C1 are large and articulate superiorly with the occipital condyles and inferiorly with the lateral masses of C2. They are obliquely oriented medially and wedge-shaped on the anteroposterior projection with a narrow medial edge and wider lateral wall. The superior facet is larger and more concave than the inferior facet. The transverse processes of C1 are the longest in the cervical spine and contain a foramen through which the vertebral artery passes.[199, 213] The posterior arches are curved and serve as the attachment site for the ligamentum nuchae and the rectus capitis posterior minor muscle.[213] The weakest part of the posterior arch is at the site of a groove on its cranial surface, the vertebral artery sulcus.[213]

Atlantal fractures constitute 2 to 13 per cent of cervical fractures and between 1 and 2 per cent of all vertebral fractures.[3, 33, 186, 214] In two large series with a total of 1150 patients with cervical injuries, 4.8 per cent of cervical fractures involved the atlas.[213, 214] The clinical findings of an atlantal fracture are nonspecific and consist of suboccipital pain, headaches, and neck stiffness.[186] Compression of the greater occipital sensory nerve producing occipital neuralgia or dysphagia resulting from retropharyngeal hematoma also may be present.[170, 186, 214] Vertebral artery involvement is rare, but arterial ruptures and development of arteriovenous fistulae in association with atlantal fractures have been reported.[186] In general, fractures of C1 are not associated with neurologic deficit.

A variety of fractures of the osseous ring of C1 have been described, but only a few occur with significant frequency. Gehweiler and colleagues classified fractures of C1 into 5 types: (1) the burst Jefferson fracture, (2) posterior arch fractures, (3) horizontal fractures of the anterior arch, (4) lateral mass fractures, and (5) transverse process fractures. The last two types are extremely rare.[213] The most common fracture of C1 is disruption of its posterior arch as it is compressed between the basiocciput and the posterior arch of C2 during hyperextension of the neck[145, 151, 153, 213–215] (Fig. 69–19). Fractures of the posterior arch may be unilateral or bilateral; if bilateral, the dorsal fragment may be angulated cranially owing to traction produced by the rectus capitis muscle.[199] Ten per cent of fractures of the posterior arch of C1 are unilateral.[199] It has been demonstrated in vitro that fractures of the posterior arch develop asynchronously; if the force is arrested after fracture of one side, the contralateral arch may remain intact.[216]

Isolated fractures of the posterior arch are stable and are not associated with significant prevertebral soft tissue swelling. They usually are readily apparent on the lateral view of the cervical spine, particularly when they are bilateral.[186] Unilateral fractures of the posterior arch may be better visualized on lateral radiographs obtained with a few degrees of cranial rotation.[186, 217] Transaxial CT scans obtained along the plane of the posterior arch are recommended when the radiographic findings are equivocal or when there is strong clinical suspicion of an atlas fracture.[28, 214, 218] Fractures must be differentiated from congenital clefts of the posterior arch, which are present in 4 per cent of persons.[219] Fractures can be diagnosed accurately as a consequence of their clinical manifestations and by their characteristic location and configuration as seen on imaging studies. Con-

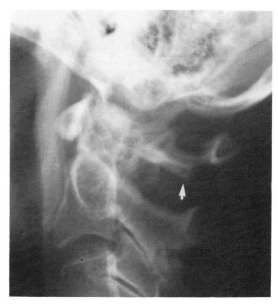

FIGURE 69–19. Fracture of the posterior arch of the atlas. The fracture (arrow) occurred after a hyperextension injury. Note the absence of soft tissue swelling with this isolated posterior injury.

genital clefts typically occur in the region of the synchondroses or in the midline, show no displacement, and characteristically have well-defined, rounded, and sclerotic borders.[186, 213, 219–221] Unlike congenital clefts, fracture margins are sharp and noncorticated, and bone resorption about the fracture site can be identified on follow-up studies. These fractures tend to heal slowly, with minimal or no callus formation; pseudarthrosis is common.[199]

Axial compressive loading of C1 results in the Jefferson fracture, which occurs when the lateral masses of C1 are compressed between the occipital condyles and the articular facets of C2.[1, 145, 213] The wedge-shaped articular masses are driven apart by the compressive force, resulting in fractures of both the anterior and the posterior arches. The classic Jefferson fracture consists of bilateral disruption of both anterior and posterior arches with lateral displacement of both lateral masses. The classic four-part fracture as described by Jefferson appears to be relatively rare, and most cases studied with CT scanning manifest fewer than four fracture lines.[215, 222] It now is recognized that this injury may be unilateral or bilateral and can manifest two, three, or four fracture lines.[222] Hays reported that in vitro attempts to produce the classic four-part fracture are unsuccessful; all 46 cadaveric specimens tested developed two- or three-part fractures with no specimen manifesting more than one fracture of the anterior arch.[222]

The Jefferson fracture is difficult to differentiate from isolated fractures of the posterior arch on the basis of findings in the lateral projection alone. Marked prevertebral edema is suggestive of a Jefferson fracture because posterior arch injuries typically are not associated with significant retropharyngeal edema. Interposition of the basion between the anterior arch of C1 and the dens reflects loss of vertical height of the atlas and is another suggestive finding in the lateral radiograph.[223] The atlantoaxial distance is normal unless a concomitant rupture of the transverse ligament is present. The fracture is characterized more readily on the open-mouth odontoid view owing to the presence of lateral displacement of the lateral masses of the atlas relative to those of the axis.[16, 145] Unilateral offset of the lateral masses or bilateral offset, particularly when the combined displacement is 3 mm or greater, is highly specific for injuries to the atlantoaxial region (Fig. 69–20). No normal persons in Jacobson and Adler's review of the atlantoaxial relationships manifested total offset of the lateral masses of 3 mm or more.[224] The typical amount of total offset of the lateral masses present with Jefferson fractures is 3 to 9 mm.[219]

True offset of the lateral masses must be differentiated from malalignments produced by congenital anomalies, uneven skeletal maturation of C1 and C2, head positioning, and normal variations in the size of the lateral masses.[219, 224–227] In young children between the ages of 3 months and 4 years, ''pseudospread'' of the ring of C1 frequently is present and, indeed, may be evident in over 90 per cent of children in their second year of life.[227] This appearance is due to discrepant growth between the atlas and the axis; the atlas shows a neural growth pattern and matures earlier than the axis, which shows a somatic growth pattern.[225, 227] Total offsets of the lateral masses of 4 to 6 mm are not unusual in normal, young children and should not mistakenly be considered evidence of a Jefferson fracture, which is extremely rare in this age group.[227] Congenital anomalies of the C1 ring also may lead to bilateral offset of the lateral masses in the absence of fracture in both children and adults. Simultaneous anterior and posterior congenital clefts, although rare, can produce displacement of the lateral mass, even though the total displacement tends to be 1 to 2 mm, which is less than the amount that typically is encountered with a Jefferson fracture.[219]

Minimal degrees of displacement of the lateral masses of the atlas and axis may be seen in healthy persons. Offsets of 1 mm are within the normal range and can be discounted safely. An offset of more than 1 mm can be seen in 7.7 per cent of normal persons.[224] Tilting of the head can produce up to 4 mm of lateral translation at the C1-C2 joints. Lateral tilting produces convergent bilateral offset, with medial displacement of one lateral mass and lateral displacement of the opposite lateral mass. Lateral tilting of the head also causes narrowing of the distance between the dens and lateral mass on one side and widening on the contralateral side.[226] Rotation of the head produces foreshortening of the posteriorly rotated lateral mass on the anteroposterior view and leads to medial displacement of the superiorly rotated lateral mass.[224] Minimal degrees of asymmetry of the lateral masses can be seen in normal persons, even with the head in the neutral position.[226]

The fractures of the anterior arch of C1 are difficult to evaluate on lateral and anteroposterior odontoid projections. A modified basal view, obtained with the x-ray beam directed 10 degrees caudal to the orbitomeatal line, may be helpful for detection of undisplaced fractures of the anterior arch.[228] Posteroanterior occlusal views performed with intraoral dental film placed adjacent to the posterior pharyngeal wall have been employed.[199] Currently, CT is used most widely to evaluate the integrity of the anterior arch of the atlas.[229]

In the typical Jefferson fracture, the transverse ligament is intact and no instability is present (see later discussion). The displacement of the bony fragments in a centripetal pattern serves to decompress the spinal canal; therefore, cord damage is uncommon.[214, 215] One review of classic four-part Jefferson fractures revealed no cases with permanent neurologic injury.[215] If the fracture results in comminution in the region of the tubercle to which the transverse ligament attaches, the normal C1-C2 relationship becomes unstable, and a highly dangerous situation results[230] (Fig. 69–21). Transverse ligament damage should be suspected if more than 7 mm of total lateral displacement of the lateral masses is seen on the anteroposterior view.[16, 213, 230] Spence and coworkers demonstrated in a cadaver model that transverse ligament rupture occurred when the mean total lateral displacement measured 6.3 mm (range, 4.8 to 7.6 mm).[16]

The prevalence of instability in Jefferson fractures is difficult to determine. Using Spence and colleagues' criterion of greater than 6.9 mm of lateral offset as an indicator of instability, Landells and Van Peteghem found that six of 13 Jefferson fractures were unstable.[214] Lee and Woodring reported on 72 patients with fractures of the atlas; 60 of these fractures were stable and limited to the posterior arch.[215] Of the remaining 12 fractures, 11 were unstable as a result of anterior arch comminution, rupture of the posterior longitudinal ligament, or both, allowing C1-C2 subluxation to occur.[215] In Lee and Woodring's series, C1 fractures involving the anterior arch were unstable in 11 of 12 patients.[215] Five fractures were associated with a tear of the transverse ligament.[215] These injuries differed from the classic Jefferson fracture in that none of the 12 patients had the classic four breaks in the osseous ring of the atlas but instead showed two or three breaks in this ring.[215]

Horizontal fractures of the anterior arch are less common than fractures of the posterior arch of the atlas or Jefferson fractures. These injuries occur as a result of cervical hyperextension producing avulsion of the tubercle of the anterior arch of the atlas by the superior oblique portion of the longus colli muscle and the anterior longitudinal ligament.[212, 231] Stewart and colleagues reported seven cases of this injury; three were associated with fractures of the odontoid process, and in two additional patients fractures of the posterior elements of the atlas were evident. Isolated fractures of the anterior arch occurred in only two of the seven cases.[212] The fracture is seen on the lateral radiograph as an irregular radiolucent line passing through the middle or inferior part of the anterior arch of C1, associated with prevertebral edema[145, 212] (Fig. 69–22). These fractures may be difficult to distinguish from accessory ossicles, overlapping bony structures, and calcification of the longus colli muscle.[212, 217, 229] Coned lateral views are particularly helpful. Transaxial CT scans alone are not recommended, as the fracture typically is transverse and undisplaced.[231] However, coronal and sagittal reconstructions of transaxial CT data can help in the identification of the fracture line and bone displacement.[229]

Isolated fractures of the lateral mass or transverse process of the atlas are rare.[213, 214] Isolated fractures of the medial aspect of the C1 lateral mass may be related to avulsion by the transverse ligament.[231] Lateral flexion of the head probably is a contributing factor, particularly when the fracture fragment is large.[232] These fractures are seen only on the anteroposterior open-mouth odontoid view. The normal notchlike defect seen in the superior aspect of the medial portion of the articular mass should not be confused with an articular mass fracture.[232]

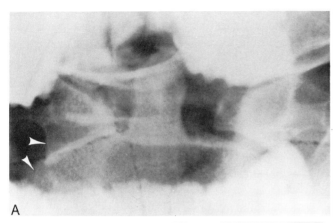
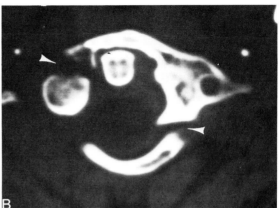
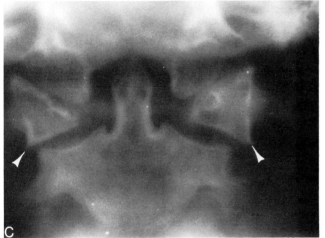
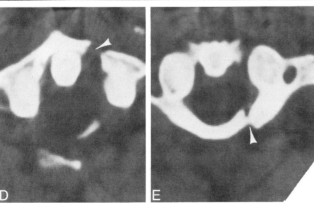

FIGURE 69–20. Jefferson fracture.

A, B In this patient, the initial open-mouth radiograph **(A)** shows an asymmetric position of the odontoid process between the lateral masses of the atlas. The right lateral atlantoaxial joint is obliterated, and offset in the position of the lateral borders of the right lateral masses of the atlas and axis is seen (arrowheads). CT scanning **(B)** reveals two fractures of the atlas (arrowheads). Identification of such fractures requires analysis of multiple contiguous transaxial scans.

C In a different patient, conventional tomography in the frontal projection shows bilateral displacement of the lateral masses of the atlas (arrowheads) with respect to the axis. This implies two or more breaks in the ring of the atlas.

D, E In a third patient, transaxial CT scans allow identification of the fractures (arrowheads) in the anterior and posterior arches of the atlas.

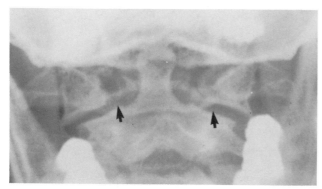

FIGURE 69–21. Unstable Jefferson fracture. Bilateral lateral offset of the lateral masses of the axis is seen. The total offset is greater than 7 mm, which implies transverse ligament incompetence. Avulsion fractures are present at the insertion sites of the transverse ligament (arrows).

Fractures of the Axis

The axis serves as the transitional vertebra between the cervicocranium above and the remaining portion of the cervical spine below.[233, 234] It has unique anatomy and is the largest of the cervical vertebrae. Its most distinctive feature is the presence of the dens, a toothlike projection located above the body. The dens, in conjunction with the anterior arch of C1 and the transverse ligament, prevents anterior and posterior subluxation of C1 on C2.[174] The horizontal inclination of the C1-C2 articular facets confers little stability on this region.[174]

The body of C2 and each posterior neural arch develop from their own primary ossification center.[190] The vertebral body is separated from the ossification centers of the posterior neural arches by the neurocentral synchondroses, which typically fuse between the ages of 4 and 6 years.[188] These three centers are distinct from the ossification centers that form the odontoid process. The odontoid process arises from the sclerotome of C1; it separates from the C1 centrum in fetal life, migrates caudally, and fuses with the axis.[187] At birth, the dens is separated from C2 by a cartilaginous plate, the dentocentral synchondrosis, that is continuous with the neurocentral synchondrosis.[190, 235] This physeal plate is present until the age of 4 to 6 years and can be visualized as a radiolucent area below the level of the C1-C2 articular facets.[187, 190] The extreme cranial tip of the odontoid process develops from a separate ossification center, the ossiculum terminale. This ossicle may be transverse or V-shaped; it enlarges gradually and fuses with the dens by the age of 12 years.[153, 187, 190]

The axis lacks clearly defined pedicles. The pedicle region of C2 is covered cranially by the superior articulating facet and is pierced by the foramina through which the vertebral artery passes.[233, 236] The laminae are thick and broad and fuse with a large bifid spinous process.[237] The superior articular facet lies lateral to the vertebral body whereas the inferior articular facet is located posteriorly. The atlantoaxial joint lies anterior to the facet articulations of the lower cervical vertebrae and corresponds anatomically to the lateral masses of the lower cervical vertebrae. The axis does not have a conventional lateral mass or articular pillar.[237]

Fractures of the Odontoid Process

Fractures of the odontoid process make up 7 to 13 per cent of all cervical spine injuries.[33, 238, 239] They represent the most common fracture of the axis in most series, constituting up to 55 per cent of C2 fractures.[3, 201, 238] The mechanism of injury resulting in fractures of the odontoid process is not well understood, although the pathomechanics probably are determined by the ligamentous attachments.[174] Attempts to reproduce odontoid fractures experimentally have been largely unsuccessful. A review of the literature suggests that the mechanism of injury is complex and that the fracture is a result of a combination of extreme flexion, extension, or rotation, along with a shearing force.[174, 240] Most fractures of the dens are the result of a major force, such as occurs in a motor vehicle accident or in a fall.[240]

The mortality rate of odontoid fractures is difficult to determine because it is unclear how many patients suffering this injury die instantly. Five of 38 cadavers in which cervical spine fractures had caused death prior to hospital admission showed fractures of the odontoid process.[164] The majority of patients with odontoid fractures have no neurologic deficit and manifest posterior upper cervical pain, which often radiates to the occiput, and paravertebral spasm. At the time of presentation 75 to 89 per cent of patients are intact neurologically.[174, 241] Acutely, after an odontoid fracture, the most common neurologic deficits are transient mild upper extremity weakness, lower extremity hyperreflexia, and diminished occipital sensation.[174, 240, 241] Neural deficit may develop weeks or months after the injury due to gradual or delayed atlantoaxial subluxation.[242] In their review of the literature, Anderson and D'Alonzo found 50 reported cases of delayed myelopathy after odon-

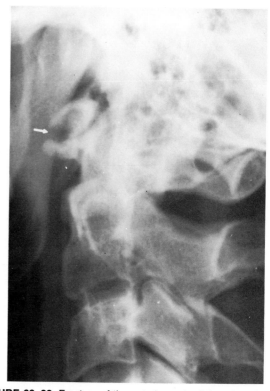

FIGURE 69–22. Fracture of the anterior arch of the atlas. Observe the horizontal configuration of the fracture (arrow).

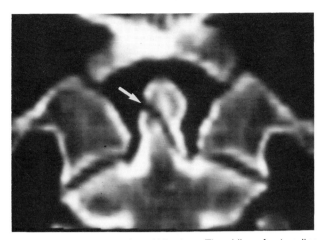

FIGURE 69–23. Type 1 odontoid fracture. The oblique fracture line through the upper portion of the dens (arrow) is easily seen on this coronal reconstruction of transaxial CT data.

toid fractures, with varying degrees of neurologic involvement and with unpredictable neurologic progression.[241] Of those who survive the initial trauma, mortality rates of 5 to 8 per cent typically are reported.[174, 238, 242] The prevalence of nonunion of odontoid fractures varies greatly from series to series, with rates of nonunion ranging from 5 to 63 per cent.[174, 241] Prior to the development of a satisfactory classification system, the risk of nonunion in any given case was difficult to establish. The Schatzker classification system, which uses categories of high or low fractures that are based on the relationship of the fracture line to the insertion of the accessory ligament, did not predict clinical outcome.[174] The widely used classification of odontoid fractures described by Anderson and D'Alonzo[241] is based on fracture location and has both therapeutic and prognostic implications.

Type 1 fractures are the least common variety of odontoid fractures. These are unilateral oblique fractures occurring through the tip of the dens and probably are secondary to an alar ligament avulsion[241] (Fig. 69–23). A review of reported odontoid fractures yielded only five possible examples of this injury, leading some authors to doubt its

existence and to suggest that it be removed from the classification of the dens injuries.[145, 233] Its mechanism justifies its inclusion as a variant of occipitocervical injury rather than as a dens injury.[145] Because this rare injury is located above the transverse ligament, it does not produce instability even if nonunion ensues. The fracture rarely is displaced and heals uneventfully.[241] The injury is best evaluated on the anteroposterior open-mouth odontoid view. The fracture can be differentiated easily from the round, corticated os terminale, a normal ossicle located at the superior tip of the odontoid process.[175]

Type 2 fractures probably are the most common type of odontoid fracture, representing 31 to 65 per cent of dens fractures.[33, 233, 238, 241] This injury occurs at the junction of the dens with the body of C2 and disrupts the blood supply to the odontoid process, which enters adjacent to its base[240] (Fig. 69–24). In children, the fracture occurs through the cartilaginous plate between the body and the dens, preserving its blood supply, and it has a good prognosis.[148, 240–243] Approximately 50 per cent of type 2 fractures are displaced more than 2 mm at the time of presentation.[241] Anterior displacement is more common than posterior displacement. Posterior displacement is believed to be due to cervical hyperextension, whereas anterior displacement is the result of hyperflexion.[244] Displacement is thought to result from the shearing force related to an intact transverse ligament.[174] In Schatzker and associates' series of 37 patients with dens fractures, 14 patients had fractures that were displaced 5 mm or more, but it is unclear how many of these patients had type 2 injuries.[174] A large multicenter study reported a displacement rate of 68 per cent; displacement in half of these fractures was over 5 mm.[240] Displacement of more than 4 mm generally is considered evidence of instability.[238, 240, 242] Angulation of the dens was seen in 28 of 96 cases of odontoid fractures and averaged 13.3 degrees.[238, 240]

The rate of nonunion for type 2 fractures is high, with most large series reporting a nonunion rate of 26 to 36 per cent.[240] Evidence exists that the presence of displacement or angulation, or both, increases the risk of developing nonunion.[174, 238, 240, 242] Schatzker and colleagues suggested that fracture displacement greater than 5 mm, particularly in a posterior direction, has a higher nonunion rate.[174] Clark

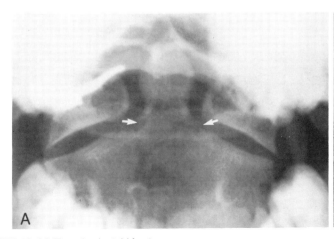
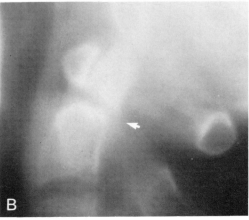

FIGURE 69–24. Type 2 odontoid fracture.
  A The anteroposterior open-mouth view shows a transverse fracture (arrow) across the base of the dens at the same level as the articulations of the C1-C2 lateral masses.
  B The lateral conventional tomogram confirms the presence of a fracture (arrow) at the base of the dens.

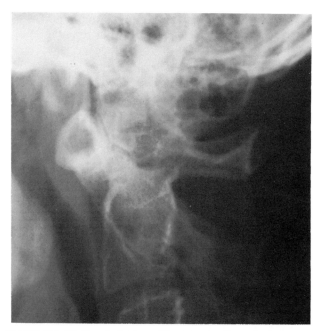

FIGURE 69–25. Os odontoideum. The lateral radiograph shows amputation of the axis, which is without an identifiable odontoid process. A separate ossicle located superiorly represents the os odontoideum. Note the hypertrophied anterior arch of the atlas suggesting chronic altered stresses in this region.

and White also reported that fracture displacement more than 5 mm or angulation greater than 10 degrees is associated with a higher rate of fracture nonunion.[240] Hadley and coworkers noted a nonunion rate of 67 per cent in patients with fracture displacement greater than 5 mm, compared to an overall nonunion rate of 26 per cent in all cases of type 2 fractures.[236]

Considerable controversy has developed over whether the os odontoideum represents a congenital anomaly or is the result of an unrecognized nonunited type 2 odontoid fracture.[187, 245] Most authors believe that an os odontoideum is an acquired posttraumatic abnormality in the majority of cases.[187, 245] This ossicle can be distinguished from an acute odontoid fracture radiographically by noting the presence of a rounded or oval ossified mass possessing smooth, thin cortical borders and being smaller in size than expected for a complete odontoid process, and a wide gap between the ossicle and the body of C2.[187] Hypertrophy of the anterior arch of C1 on the lateral view, indicating a chronic lesion at the atlantoaxial level, helps confirm that an os odontoideum is not an acute fracture[187, 245] (Fig. 69–25).

Type 3 fractures also are relatively common injuries. In these cases, horizontal or oblique fractures adjacent to the base of the dens extend into the cancellous bone of the C2 vertebral body. The fracture line usually extends into the joints between the lateral masses of C1 and C2.[145, 233, 242] Although the fractures frequently are displaced, fracture nonunion is unusual.[241] Nonunion rates of zero to 13 per cent are reported.[240] Anteroposterior displacement at the fracture site is seen in 58 per cent of type 3 fractures.[238] As with type 2 fractures, the displacement typically is anterior. Lateral tilting of the dens greater than 5 degrees was seen in 66 per cent of patients in one series of type 3 odontoid fractures.[246]

The lateral and anteroposterior open-mouth odontoid views are most useful in the assessment of the dens. An anteroposterior view with cranial angulation of the tube (modified Waters view) may be necessary to visualize the upper portion of the odontoid process. The normal dens is recognized easily in the submentovertex view of the skull, but its base is foreshortened in this view, and fractures may be obscured. This radiographic projection requires cervical hyperextension and is not done in the patient with an acutely traumatized cervical spine. Nonvisualization of the dens in this projection is uncommon but suggests an underlying abnormality, such as os odontoideum or bone erosion.[247] Flexion and extension views should be avoided in the patient with a dens fracture as the resultant bone displacement may be fatal.[174] Because many odontoid fractures are horizontal, conventional tomography or reformatted thin section CT scans are preferable to routine transaxial CT images. Transaxial CT scans may fail to detect fractures at the base of the odontoid process.[29, 205]

Fractures of the odontoid process are best demonstrated on the anteroposterior open-mouth view. This view often is difficult to obtain in an unconscious or combative patient. In the setting of severe trauma, the frontal view of the dens often is inadequate as the dens is obscured by overlying endotracheal or nasogastric tubes. Type 1 fractures are seen only on this projection, provided that there is adequate visualization of the tip of the odontoid process. The normal gap between the central incisors and the clefts in the anterior and posterior arches of C1 may mimic the appearance of a type 1 fracture.[248] In types 2 and 3 fractures, the fracture line at the base of the odontoid process or within the C2 centrum can be identified even if the upper part of the odontoid process is obscured. The fracture line may be very subtle in cases of undisplaced fracture. The normal synchondrosis at the base of the odontoid process should not be confused with a fracture. The synchondrosis normally is wide in infants and young children; a persistent faint radiolucent line in this location may be seen in as many as one third of normal persons throughout life.[151, 220] Mach bands produced by the inferior margins of the incisors, the occiput, the posterior arch of C1, and the tongue also should be recognized as normal variants rather than as fractures of the odontoid process.[145] Lateral tilting of the odontoid process of more than 5 degrees likewise has been emphasized as an important indicator of a type 3 odontoid fracture.[246] In nontraumatized persons in one series, the odontoid process never was tilted laterally more than 3 degrees on the anteroposterior open-mouth odontoid projection.[246] Normal lateral tilting of the odontoid process has been described in another series of patients, but no measurements were provided.[183]

Displaced or angulated odontoid fractures usually are apparent on the lateral view (Fig. 69–26). Atlantal displacement is congruent with the degree of odontoid displacement because the integrity of the transverse ligament is maintained. Even if the odontoid step-off is not visualized, malalignment between the spinolaminar lines of C1 and C2 may be apparent.[188] The lateral view may not demonstrate the odontoid fracture in the absence of displacement or angulation, although prevertebral soft tissue swelling typically is present.[145, 158] Coned, tightly collimated views centered on the odontoid process can be extremely helpful in questionable cases and may obviate conventional tomography or CT scanning. Disruption of the anterior or posterior

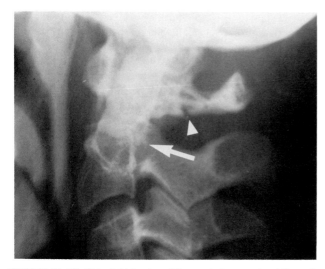

FIGURE 69-26. Odontoid fracture. The posterior margin of the axis is discontinuous owing to an odontoid fracture. Note the posterior displacement and angulation of the dens (arrow). This patient also has fractures of the posterior arch of C1 (arrowhead), consistent with a hyperextension injury.

cortex typically is seen, although subtle disruption may be obscured by overlying osseous structures. Type 2 fractures can be distinguished from type 3 fractures by noting the presence of disruption of the "ring shadow" of the axis, a feature seen only in type 3 injuries[239, 246] (Fig. 69-27). The "ring shadow" is a composite of structures, including the junction of the body of the axis with its lateral masses, the cortex of the facet joints, and the vertebral margin; the dens itself does not form any of the borders of the ring.[239]

Fracture healing typically takes place within 3 to 6 months after the injury. The radiographic signs of fracture nonunion consist of a persistent radiolucent line with sclerotic bone margins, exaggerated bone resorption, and persistent motion at the fracture site.[174] Conventional tomography or CT scanning may be helpful in the diagnosis of fracture nonunion because union often is difficult to assess on conventional radiographs.[240]

Fractures of the Body and Posterior Arch of the Axis

With the exception of odontoid fractures, the most common injury of the axis vertebra is traumatic spondylolisthesis of the pars interarticularis.[237, 238] Traumatic spondylolisthesis of the axis accounts for 4 to 23 per cent of all cervical spine fractures.[238, 244, 249, 250] In 1965, this fracture was first termed the "hangman's fracture" by Schneider and colleagues because of its similarity to the osseous injury produced by judicial hanging.[251] Despite its popular name, the injury typically results from a motor vehicle accident or a fall. Patients of all ages can manifest this injury; traumatic spondylolisthesis has been reported in infants and young children.[238, 243] This injury is defined as bilateral avulsion of the neural arches from the vertebral body, with or without subluxation, with the odontoid process remaining intact.[233, 236, 250-252] The fractures occur through the pars interarticularis of C2 or through the adjacent portion of the articulating facet[233] (Fig. 69-28). Extension into the posterior vertebral cortex is seen in up to 18 per cent of cases and is considered a variant or part of the spectrum of this injury[233, 236, 239, 250] (Fig. 69-29). Extension into one or both vertebral artery foramina also is common.

The hangman's fracture typically is the result of vertical compression and hyperextension, although other mechanisms of injury also can produce similar findings.[250, 252, 253] The frequent association of traumatic spondylolisthesis and facial injury supports hyperextension as the most common mechanism of injury.[234, 238, 249, 252, 253] In one series, 79 per cent of patients had associated wounds to the face or to the frontal and apical regions of the skull.[253] Because the superior facet of the axis is located far anterior to its posterior facet, hyperextension leads to concentration of forces on the region of the pars interarticularis.[233, 236] Radiographically, the only condition that may be confused with this fracture is chronic spondylolysis of the axis, an extremely rare lesion that often is associated with complex congenital anomalies of the cervical spine.[254-256]

Traumatic spondylolisthesis of C2 has been classified by Effendi and associates into three types: Type 1 is a nonangulated, undisplaced or minimally displaced (less than 2 to

FIGURE 69-27. Type 3 odontoid fracture.

A Disruption of the "ring shadow" of the axis is seen on the lateral view (arrows) owing to extension of the fracture lines into the C2 vertebral body.

B The type 3 fracture in a different patient also shows disruption of the C2 ring (arrows).

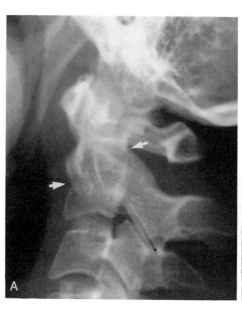
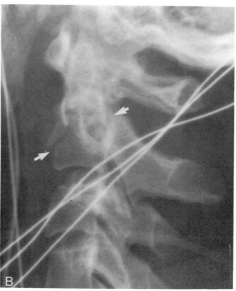

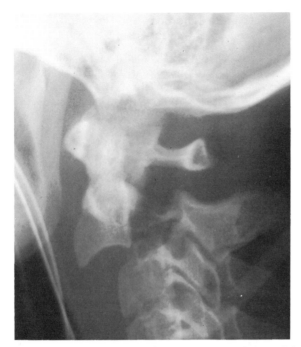

FIGURE 69–28. Hangman's fracture. Fractures through the pedicles on both sides of the axis are present with marked anterior displacement of the C2 vertebral body. Note the lack of concomitant anterior displacement of the spinolaminar line.

3 mm) fracture with a normal disc at C2-C3; type 2 is an anteriorly displaced or angulated fracture of the C2 vertebral body with C2-C3 disc disruption; and type 3 manifests anterior displacement and hyperflexion of the axis in association with unilateral or bilateral C2-C3 facet dislocations.[252] This classification system is not based solely on findings seen in the static lateral radiographs; supervised flexion and extension views in all type 1 injuries are recommended to avoid undergrading the injury.[252] In Effendi and colleagues' series, type 1 injuries were the most common, seen in 65 per cent of patients. The type 1 pattern of injury can be considered stable as long as flexion and extension views show no displacement or angulation.[252, 257] Types 2 and 3, which are considered unstable by Effendi and coworkers, were seen in 28 per cent and 7 per cent of patients, respectively.[252] In other reported series, type 2 fractures have been more common, with most fractures showing anterior displacement of the axis.[249, 250, 257]

Levine and Edwards modified the Effendi classification by subdividing the type 2 injuries into those that were displaced and, using a new designation they named a type 2A injury, those in which significant angulation was present without marked translation.[257] These authors believed the mechanism of injury in patients with the type 2A category was flexion-distraction rather than hyperextension.[257] The type 3 dislocation probably is related to hyperflexion and compression as the accompanying facet dislocations suggest flexion rather than extension.[252, 257] In Levine and Edwards' series, only patients with type 3 fractures did not manifest facial injury, further supporting flexion as the likely mechanism.[257]

The lateral view of the cervical spine demonstrates the fractures in more than 90 per cent of patients.[250] Prevertebral hematoma often is not present in type 1 injuries

because damage to the anterior vertebral column has not occurred.[249] Prevertebral hematoma is found in patients with types 2 and 3 injuries, however, related to the disruption of the disc that occurs in these categories.[249] The fracture lines run obliquely in a superoposterior to an anteroinferior direction and are located immediately anterior to the inferior articular facet.[236] Anterior subluxation of the C2 vertebral body relative to the body of C3 typically is present. In addition, retrolisthesis of the posterior elements of C2 relative to those of C3 may be present. Retrolisthesis may be recognized by noting posterior displacement of the spinolaminar line of C2 relative to C3. Displacement of this line by 2 to 3 mm is a normal variant, seen in both children and adults.[258] Because the dens and transverse ligament are intact, the dens is displaced along with the body of C2.[236] This injury is recognized easily when the fractures are distracted sufficiently to produce these characteristic displacements. CT scanning may be necessary for detection of undisplaced fractures of the pars interarticularis. CT scans demonstrate the fracture lines, their extension into the vertebral foramina, and displaced bony fragments to better advantage than routine radiography.[250, 259]

Although this injury generally is considered unstable, usually little neurologic damage occurs owing to decompression of the spinal canal by the separated fragments.[236, 238, 249–253, 257] Neurologic deficits were present in six of 21 patients in one series; the deficits improved in three of these patients.[250] In Effendi and colleagues' series of 131 hangman's fractures, transient neurologic deficits developed in 13 per cent of patients, but only four of 17 neurologic deficits did not resolve spontaneously.[252] In the series of Francis and associates, 6.5 per cent had neurologic damage.[253] Other series reported no cases of long-term neurologic deficit.[234, 238, 249] The paucity of neurologic injury contrasts with the immediate death produced by judicial hanging with the use of a "long drop" and a submental knot.[251, 260] In hanging, the hyperextension force is sustained

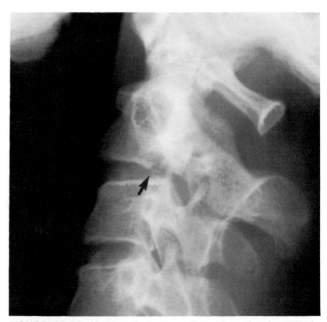

FIGURE 69–29. Hangman's fracture. Extension of a hangman's fracture into the C2 vertebral body at its posteroinferior corner (arrow) is seen. The C2 vertebral body is displaced anteriorly.

and associated with tensile injury to the bone, soft tissues, and spinal cord owing to the gravitational pull of the body across the injury site.[164, 236, 251–253] Hangman's fractures may result in a fatal injury at the time of the trauma, which can lead to underestimation of the true prevalence of severe neurologic deficit. In Bucholz's review of cervical spine radiographs of 178 multiple trauma victims who died at the time of injury, eight had sustained hangman's fractures.[164] This injury was exceeded only by atlanto-occipital dissociation as a cause of sudden death after spinal trauma.[164] Six of eight cadaveric spines exhibiting hangman's fractures were grossly unstable, with complete ligamentous dissociation between the cervicocranium and the remainder of the cervical spine.[164]

Normal pseudosubluxation at the C2-C3 posterior vertebral margins in children should not be confused with a hangman's fracture. The normally greater relative range of motion in the upper cervical spine in children, the horizontal orientation of the facet joints, the displacement of the axis of movement from the disc to the C2 body at this level, and ligamentous laxity all are all responsible for this appearance in the young child.[151, 158, 185, 261] Apparent subluxation in normal children can be dramatic, particularly with flexion of the cervical spine.[158, 261] The pseudosubluxation of childhood can be differentiated from traumatic spondylolisthesis of C2 by assessing the position of the spinolaminar line of the axis. In pseudosubluxation, the spinolaminar line of C2 passes within 1 mm of a tangent connecting the spinolaminar line of C1 with that of C3.[158, 259] The spinolaminar line of C2 is displaced posteriorly, typically by more than 2 mm, in the presence of a hangman's fracture.[261] The spinolaminar line may be difficult to use as an index of displacement if the patient is rotated or if the posterior arch of C1 is hypoplastic or unfused.

Other fractures that frequently involve C2 are the extension teardrop fracture (Fig. 69–30) and avulsion fractures seen in association with hyperextension dislocation. These two injuries accounted for 19 per cent of all C2 injuries in one large series.[233] Both injuries involve the anteroinferior corner of the C2 vertebral body and are related to hyperextension. The extension teardrop fracture characteristically is devoid of any neurologic impairment, whereas the avulsion fracture associated with extension dislocation characteristically is associated with an acute cervical central cord syndrome.[233, 262] Extension teardrop fractures can occur at any cervical level but are most common at C2.[233] The extension teardrop fracture of C2 is more common in older patients with osteoporosis or underlying cervical spondylosis.[145] This fracture results from avulsion of the anteroinferior portion of the vertebral body by the anterior longitudinal ligament, is triangular, and has a vertical height that is equal to or exceeds its horizontal width.[233, 262] The vertebral fragment may be distracted anteriorly or rotated anteroinferiorly.[237] Hyperextension dislocation more typically involves the lower cervical spine but is not rare at the C2-C3 level. The avulsion fracture seen in this severe injury is mediated through Sharpey's fibers and always is wider than it is tall.[233, 262] A less common fracture of the C2 vertebral body is an oblique fracture occurring below the odontoid process and superior articulating facets caused by rotational and lateral bending injuries.[263] Owing to the obliquity of the fracture plane, these injuries are difficult to identify on both frontal and lateral radiographs. Increase in the antero-

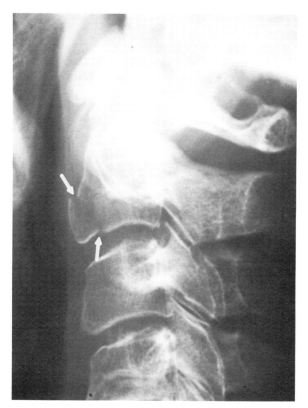

FIGURE 69–30. C2 extension teardrop fracture. A triangular fracture (arrows) is present at the anteroinferior margin of the axis. Note that the height of the fragment exceeds its width.

posterior diameter of the C2 vertebral body, related to displacement of the fracture fragments, produces the "fat C2 sign."[263] The enlargement of C2 can be recognized by the presence of offset at the anterior or posterior vertebral margin relative to that of C3.

Rarely, isolated fractures of the pedicle, lateral mass, lamina, or spinous process of the axis are encountered. These injuries represent 1 to 6 per cent of all C2 fractures.[233, 237, 238] Unilateral pedicle and laminar fractures presumably are related to hyperextension combined with rotation.[237, 264] The fractures of the spinous process occur close to the spinolaminar line and must be differentiated from an unfused apophysis.[237] These injuries may be difficult to detect on conventional radiographs and often require oblique projections, conventional tomography, or CT scanning for adequate delineation.

CERVICAL SPINE: LOWER CERVICAL REGION

General Considerations

The lowest five cervical vertebrae all are similar in their anatomy, articular morphology, and ligamentous attachments. The vertebral bodies are rectangular and have well-defined, straight endplates. Each vertebral body has bilateral superior extensions, known as the uncinate processes, which normally are located posterolaterally and extend forward one half to two thirds of the sagittal diameter of the body.[136] Each transverse process has a perforation that allows passage of the vertebral artery. The cervical pedicles are very short and broad and connect the vertebral body to the lateral masses. The superior and inferior articular facets are flat and inclined approximately 45 degrees in an anterior to posterior direction.[136] The vertebral bodies articulate with each other via the intervertebral disc, uncinate processes, and intervertebral facet joints. The ligamentous attachments consist of the anterior longitudinal ligament, posterior longitudinal ligament, capsular (interfacet) ligaments, ligamenta flava, and interspinous and supraspinous ligaments. The ligaments and intervertebral disc bind the vertebrae. Above the level of C6, the supraspinous ligament is replaced by a thin midline ligamentum nuchae.[265]

The cervical ligaments and facet capsule are relatively lax, allowing a considerable range of motion in flexion and extension.[136] Flexion is limited by the posterior ligaments, the vertebral bodies, and the noncompressible disc. Extension is limited largely by an intact anterior longitudinal ligament, which is a broad band consisting of several layers of fibers and extending across the anterior vertebral margins. The deepest fibers cross only one intervertebral space; others cross two or three adjacent vertebrae; and the most superficial fibers extend over four or five vertebrae.[265]

In flexion, the cervical vertebrae rotate anteriorly, with progressively less forward motion at each successively lower level.[201, 266] The interfacet joints widen posteriorly, and the interspinous distances increase uniformly. Maximal overall range of motion in normal adults is seen between C4 and C6.[136, 158, 267] The mean range of motion at the C4-C5 level and at the C5-C6 level in adults is 20 degrees.[13, 14, 136] The normal range of flexion and extension at C6-C7 is slightly less than at C4-C5 and C5-C6.[158] Some investigators have suggested that extension is more prominent at C6-C7 whereas flexion is the dominant motion at C4-5 and C5-6.[136] The supraspinous and interspinous ligaments and ligamenta flava are composed largely of elastic tissue, thus allowing flexion and extension of the neck without significant folding.[267] The capsular ligaments are weak, are torn easily, and provide little stability.

Fractures of the lower cervical spine are extremely common. It is estimated that 65 to 81 per cent of nonfatal vertebral injuries in adults involve this region.[3, 33, 82] Unlike the situation with fractures of the cervicocranium, radiographic evaluation of injuries in the lower cervical spine often is used to predict the mechanism of injury. Numerous classification systems have been developed to categorize injuries of this region according to their presumed mechanism.[3, 4, 145, 268] Most injuries are due to hyperextension or hyperflexion, either alone or combined with rotation. Axial loading, lateral bending, and shearing account for a much smaller proportion of lower cervical injuries.

Hyperextension Injuries

Hyperextension of the lower cervical spine is a common mechanism of injury, accounting for 25 to 50 per cent of all cervical injuries.[3, 244, 269] As with hyperflexion, this mechanism produces a wide spectrum of osseous and soft tissue spinal injuries. The hyperextension injuries occur as a result of abrupt deceleration, most commonly from a motor vehicle accident or from an impacting force on the face or head.[80, 88, 262] Eight to 20 per cent of motor vehicle accidents are rear-end collisions and characteristically result in deceleration hyperextension or whiplash injuries.[88] The force in hyperextension is maximal in the lower cervical region, at

C5 and C6.[88, 269] Many hyperextension injuries in the lower cervical region reveal few radiographic abnormalities or none at all, even when the injury is unstable or results in severe neurologic damage. In patients with neurologic damage and normal radiographs, hyperextension injury should be suspected, particularly when the patient has had concomitant facial or skull trauma.[106, 269]

Lower cervical injuries associated with hyperextension include avulsion of the ring apophysis, the extension teardrop fracture, hyperextension dislocation, and hyperextension sprain. In the immature spine, hyperextension may produce an avulsion fracture of the inferior ring apophysis.[270, 271] This injury can be conceptualized as the equivalent of a Salter-Harris type 3 fracture of a long bone physis, with separation of a portion of the epiphyseal center from the remainder of the epiphysis.[271] Its appearance is similar to that of the avulsion fracture that occurs with hyperextension in the adult spine. However, unlike its adult counterpart, the apophysis avulsion fracture characteristically is not associated with soft tissue swelling, other osseous injury, or significant neurologic damage.[262, 270] Follow-up examinations show that healing has occurred with the formation of a pronounced bone excrescence in the inferior vertebral margin related to fusion of the avulsed apophysis with the underlying vertebral body.[270, 271] The subsequent fusion implies that discal dispacement into the defect, as is seen in the classic limbus vertebra, does not occur with apophysis avulsion fracture.[272]

The extension teardrop fracture is an avulsion fracture that arises from the anteroinferior corner of a vertebral body. The axis is involved most commonly, and the fracture usually is not associated with any neurologic deficit.[262, 273] Unlike the flexion teardrop fracture, the triangular fracture produced by hyperextension is small and does not exceed in size one quarter of the sagittal diameter of the vertebral body. It similarly is not associated with vertebral body displacement, a feature typically present in flexion teardrop injuries.[87, 273] The most characteristic feature is that the vertical height of this fracture exceeds its horizontal dimension (Fig. 69–30). The extension teardrop fracture should be distinguished from the smaller avulsion fracture of the anteroinferior corner of the vertebral body seen in patients who have sustained a hyperextension dislocation in the lower cervical region.[10, 262]

Hyperextension dislocation occurs when the spine is hyperextended without any associated axial compression.[268] The C5-C6 level is affected most frequently, followed by C4-C5.[106] This injury may produce very subtle radiographic alterations or none at all because the spine characteristically returns to normal or near normal alignment after the injury.[78] A hyperextension dislocation injury is suspected because of the profound neurologic deficit produced, despite the paucity of the radiographic findings. Hyperextension dislocation injuries occur when the traumatic force causes injury to the anterior longitudinal ligament and then either ruptures the disc or produces an avulsion fracture at the site of insertion of the anulus fibrosus.[262] In up to 30 per cent of cases, prevertebral hematoma is the only radiographic finding.[106, 262] Rupture of the anterior longitudinal ligament and the intervertebral disc results in formation of a prominent prevertebral hematoma.[78, 106, 262, 274] Associated injuries to the paracervical musculature, airway, and esophagus may lead to the appearance of prevertebral air and a further

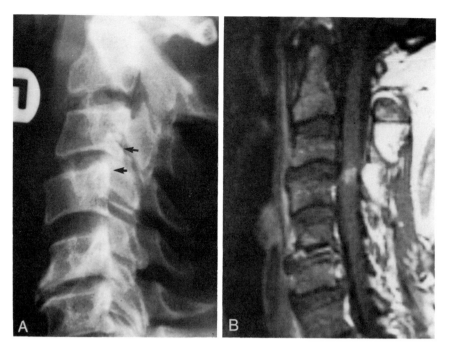

FIGURE 69–31. Hyperextension injury.

A The plain film shows 4 mm of retrolisthesis of the C3 vertebral body relative to that of C4 (arrows) with facet malalignment. Note the presence of spondylotic changes in the lower cervical spine.

B A sagittal T1-weighted (TR/TE, 600/20) spin echo fat-suppressed image obtained after intravenous administration of a gadolinium-based contrast agent shows enhancement in the injured spinal cord at the C3-C4 vertebral level.

increase in the width of the prevertebral soft tissues. Esophageal perforation is a rare but extremely serious complication of hyperextension injuries.[275] Proposed mechanisms include trapping or pinching of the esophagus between the vertebral bodies as a result of rupture of the anterior longitudinal ligament or impingement on the sharp edge of one of the separated vertebral bodies.[275]

Retrolisthesis of the vertebra above the discal injury often is present but may be of minimal degree.[3, 80] Marar noted the presence of obvious retrolisthesis in 20 per cent of his patients with hyperextension-induced cord damage but did not quantitate it.[269] Retrolisthesis of only 2 to 3 mm is seen in some patients with ankylosing spondylitis who develop severe neurologic deficit after injury.[80] These minor degrees of malalignment may occur even with an intact posterior longitudinal ligament if the ligament has been stripped from its normal attachment sites. In elderly patients, underlying spondylosis deformans makes the distinction of acute from chronic retrolisthesis very difficult.[78] In degenerative slippage, anterolisthesis of 5 mm (range, 2 to

9 mm) or retrolisthesis of 2.5 mm (range, 2 to 4 mm) may be seen in the absence of trauma.[276] Anterolisthesis characteristically is associated with osteoarthrosis of the facet joints, whereas retrolisthesis is strongly associated with narrowing of the intervertebral disc and relative preservation of the facet joints.[276] In contradistinction, traumatic slippage characteristically is associated with abnormal widening of the facet joints and facet joint fractures; unlike the situation with degenerative slippage, traumatic slippage may be seen in patients under the age of 40 years[276] (Fig. 69–31). Isolated anterior widening of the disc space may be the only clue to the presence of this subtle injury.[106, 262, 268, 274] Disc space widening may not be apparent on the neutral lateral view but may become obvious only after the patient is placed in skeletal traction.[106] Extension views obtained carefully accentuate this abnormality and confirm the presence of instability.[274] Extension views also may demonstrate small, well-defined, linear, horizontal radiolucent clefts of the anterior portion of the anulus fibrosus[162, 277] (Fig. 69–32). Some authors have suggested that, in patients

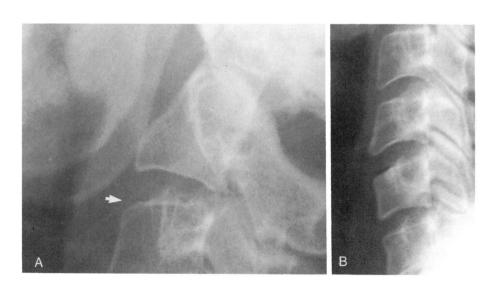

FIGURE 69–32. Hyperextension injury: Annular vacuum.

A Prevertebral soft tissue swelling is present in a patient with facial lacerations from a hyperextension injury. Note the linear gas collection in the anulus at the superior endplate of the C3 vertebral body (arrow), as well as mild widening of the anterior C2-C3 intervertebral disc.

B An annular vacuum is apparent at the C5 level (arrow).

who have suffered trauma, this radiolucent cleft results from nitrogen gas accumulating within a traumatic avulsion of the disc from the anterior cartilaginous endplate.[277] These radiolucent clefts often are difficult to distinguish from the more common linear or irregular lucent areas (vacuum phenomena) seen in the anulus fibrosus or nucleus pulposus in patients with degenerative disc disease. Vacuum phenomena related to discal degeneration typically are associated with other degenerative changes, such as disc space loss, osteophytes, and anular calcification.[278] They also are strongly associated with compressed, deformed anterosuperior vertebral corners, suggesting previous trauma with a prior minimal compressive injury.[278] The presence of anular gas in association with a normal vertebral body or located adjacent to the inferior endplate is more suggestive of an acute extension injury.[278] The gas can persist for up to 5 years after trauma.[278] Such gas must not be confused with the normal radiolucent area produced by a Mach band phenomenon at the superior margin of the disc.[279]

The characteristic avulsion fracture seen in hyperextension dislocation appears as a thin, linear shadow arising from the inferior vertebral endplate. This fracture is produced by avulsion at the site of attachment of Sharpey's fibers and typically is wider than it is tall.[262] In 20 cases of hyperextension dislocation reported by Edeikin-Monroe and colleagues, avulsion fractures were identified in 13 (65 per cent) patients.[262] Other authors state that such avulsion fractures are less common and that the diagnosis of a hyperextension dislocation is established on the basis of the clinical findings and nonspecific radiographic indicators, such as soft tissue swelling.[106, 274] In Regenbogen and co-workers' review of cervical cord injuries in patients with cervical spondylosis, the avulsion fracture was present in only 9 per cent of cases.[106] Because no fracture occurs in a large number of cases, this injury often is difficult to recognize radiographically and probably is underreported.[274] Other fractures resulting from hyperextension dislocation injuries in the lower cervical region are uncommon. On the basis of cadaveric studies, Marar has suggested that transverse fractures develop just inferior to the pedicles after hyperextension and backward displacement of the vertebral body, although he noted that none of these fractures could be seen on conventional radiographs.[269] Horizontal radiolucent regions projecting across the vertebral body related to arthrosis of the uncinate joints may be misinterpreted as fractures in this clinical setting.[248, 280, 281] The "pseudofracture" created at the superior margin of the uncinate process characteristically is horizontal, is associated with disc space narrowing, and occurs most commonly in the lower cervical region.[280, 281]

Hyperextension of the cervical spine in patients with ankylosing spondylitis or in those with spinal stenosis produces a similar clinical syndrome, although the traumatic event may be minor. Taylor and Blackwood, who first described the syndrome of hyperextension dislocation as a cause of neurologic deficit in patients whose radiographs are normal, subsequently reported that significant injury can occur in the spondylitic spine even in the absence of ligament damage or frank vertebral displacement.[107, 282] This injury, often referred to as a hyperextension sprain, does not result in significant disruption of the spinal ligaments, osseous structures, or discs. In a hyperextension sprain, neurologic damage is sustained during the injury, but spinal

stability is maintained. Distinction between a sprain and a reduced dislocation may be impossible on the basis of conventional radiographic findings. In both hyperextension sprain and hyperextension dislocation, severe neurologic damage is thought to occur when the spinal cord is caught between the posterior margin of the vertebral body or posterior osteophytes and the infolded ligamenta flava, particularly in the spondylitic spine.[78, 106, 107, 274] Regenbogen and coworkers reported that spinal cord injury in the absence of radiographic findings was present in 28 per cent of patients over the age of 40 years with traumatic cervical spinal cord lesions.[106] Among the 28 per cent with no fracture or dislocation, 96 per cent had severe cervical spondylosis.[106] An additional 20 per cent of patients showed only minimal evidence of osseous trauma. Conventional tomography and myelography failed to reveal occult fractures or disc herniations in both groups of patients, suggesting that the spinal cord was injured solely by dynamic compression between osteophytes and the ligamenta flava.

The characteristic neurologic defect in hyperextension sprain is the central cord syndrome related to hemorrhage in the central gray matter.[78, 105] The normal cervical canal shortens by 2 to 3 cm in extension, resulting in a slackened cervical cord that can undergo transverse folding by an accordion-like mechanism.[158, 283] Despite the elasticity of the ligamenta flava, these ligaments become infolded by the normal decrease in the interlaminar distances in extension (which may be as much as 55 per cent), and the sagittal width of the thecal sac is narrowed by up to 30 per cent.[107, 158] In the presence of spondylosis, anterior osteophytes act as a counterpoint of compression and lead to even greater narrowing of the spinal canal.[107] In addition, hyperextension causes the posterior longitudinal ligament to thicken and both the dural diameter and spinal cord diameter to increase, leading to even greater stenosis of the spinal canal.[284] Marar has noted that maximum infolding of the ligamenta flava occurs at an angle of 30 degrees prior to full extension of the cervical spine and suggests that infolding of the ligamenta flava may not be responsible for the cord damage.[269] Instead, narrowing of the spinal canal may be most significant between the posteroinferior corner of the vertebral body and the superior aspect of the spinolaminar junction of the vertebral body below, resulting in a "pincers mechanism."[284]

Neurologic deficit resulting from hyperextension sprain is seen not only in patients with cervical spondylosis.[284–286] Transient neuropraxia, typically appearing and disappearing 36 to 48 hours after the injury, also can occur in patients with developmental spinal stenosis, congenital intervertebral fusion, cervical ligamentous laxity, and cervical disc herniation in the absence of osteophyte formation.[284, 285] Congenital spinal stenosis increases the risk of spinal cord injury significantly. The sagittal diameter of the spinal canal traditionally is determined by measuring the distance between the midpoint of the posterior margin of the vertebral body to the nearest point of the spinolaminar line at the same vertebral level.[211, 284, 286] The normal sagittal diameter of C4, C5, and C6 is 17 to 18.5 mm (range, 14 to 23 mm).[286] Alternatively, cervical canal stenosis can be detected by the ratio of the diameter of the spinal canal to the width of the vertebral body. Normally, the width of the vertebral body and the diameter of the spinal canal are approximately the same (ratio of 1). A ratio of the width of the spinal canal to that of the vertebral body below 0.80 indicates a stenotic canal in 96.3 per cent of cases.[284, 286] An advantage of the ratio method is that it does not depend on film magnification or body type.[284, 286]

MR imaging appears to be the optimal method for evaluating the patients with neurologic injuries whose radiographic findings are equivocal. The large prevertebral hematoma characteristically seen with hyperextension ligamentous injuries is well delineated so long as the studies are performed within 1 to 2 weeks after the injury.[78, 86] Acute hematomas are isointense with surrounding soft tissues on T1-weighted spin echo MR images, but the associated edema is of high signal intensity on the proton density– and T2-weighted images.[78] Disruption of the anterior longitudinal ligament, anterior portion of the anulus fibrosus, and intervertebral disc at the level of injury, which previously could be demonstrated only on pathologic specimens, now can be visualized directly with MR imaging.[78, 86] Separation of the disc from the vertebral endplate produces a region of increased intradiscal signal intensity paralleling the vertebral endplate on T2-weighted spin echo MR sequences. This appearance was seen in five of seven patients in one series.[86] Other features identifiable by MR imaging that are very difficult or impossible to detect on routine radiography include multilevel spinal involvement, associated disc herniation, and middle column involvement.[78, 86] MR imaging also allows noninvasive assessment of spinal cord injury in patients with hyperextension sprain of the cervical spine.

Extension Rotation Injuries

A combination of extension, compression, and rotation produces unilateral pillar or facet fractures, which represent 3 to 11 per cent of all cervical spine fractures.[287, 288] Bilateral fractures of the lateral masses resulting from pure hyperextension are much less common than unilateral fractures.[268] Fractures of the lateral masses are more common than generally is appreciated because they are very difficult to detect on conventional radiographs and their true prevalence is underestimated. Facet fractures occur most commonly at C6 and C7 and result in radiculopathy in 6 to 39 per cent of patients.[287] Fractures of the superior facet are associated with persistent radiculopathy more frequently than are fractures of the inferior facet.

Fractures of the articular mass (pillar) often are difficult to visualize on frontal and lateral projections unless they are displaced or severely comminuted. In one study, only two of 16 facet fractures demonstrated by multidirectional conventional tomography were diagnosed on the basis of plain films.[287] The fracture line itself may be visible on either the anteroposterior or the lateral projection. On the anteroposterior view, disruption of the smoothly undulating cortical margin of the lateral mass or rotation of the fracture fragment may be evident.[145] The oblique projection is most useful for detecting fractures of the pillar region. Conventional upright posteroanterior oblique films are contraindicated when a cervical injury is suspected. Supine anteroposterior oblique views obtained by rotating the patient's head also are not preferred in this clinical situation. McCall and associates have described the anteroposterior supine trauma oblique view, obtained by rotating the x-ray tube 45 degrees toward the side being evaluated.[137] This maneuver provides a distorted but adequate oblique projection of the

pedicles, foramina, and lateral masses and is extremely helpful in evaluation of the facet joints and lateral masses.[137] Abel has described an exaggerated supine oblique view obtained with 60 degrees of rotation of the cervical spine that results in increased separation of the anterior and posterior elements, affording excellent visualization of the facet joints.[289] Pillar views also can be used to evaluate the lateral masses. The pillar view is oriented tangentially to the facet joints and shows the lateral masses along their short axis. This view is obtained with the patient in the anteroposterior supine position with the head rotated maximally away from the facet joints that are being evaluated. The central ray is directed caudally at an angle of 35 degrees, entering at the inferior border of the thyroid cartilage.[288] A single pillar view can be obtained by hyperextending the nonrotated head with the central ray directed 20 to 30 degrees caudally.[288]

The pillar fracture that results from extension of the cervical spine usually appears as a simple vertical or oblique radiolucent line, although such fractures may be more severe, accompanied by crushing or comminution of the bone and loss of pillar height[145, 268] (Fig. 69–33). Fractures of the articular process associated with flexion of the cervical spine, such as those occurring in patients with unilateral or bilateral facet subluxation or lock, typically are horizontal and limited to the tip of the superior articulating facet of the lower vertebra.[290] Compressed, distorted lateral masses frequently are identified on cervical radiographs obtained in persons without a history of trauma. The significance of these deformities is controversial. Some authors consider all compressed lateral masses to be due to acute or remote injuries.[136, 291] Other authors have noted the existence of considerable variability in the appearance of the lateral masses and suggest that decrease or asymmetry in height alone is not a reliable feature of an articular process fracture.[145, 288] The normal lateral masses show decreasing height from cranial to caudal, with an average height of 8.6 mm at C3 and 6.2 mm at C7.[288] Two to 3 mm of asymmetry in height of the lateral masses is noted in 46 per cent of normal persons.[288] Apparent unilateral compression of the lateral mass is most common at C6, partly related to the orientation of the facets. Apparent bilateral compression also is seen predominantly in the lower cervical spine, particularly at C6 or C7.[288]

Conventional tomography and CT scanning are more sensitive for detection of fractures of the articular process than are conventional radiographic projections.[43, 44, 287] Because of the small size of the facets, thin sections are necessary with either technique to avoid missing the injury owing to volume averaging artifacts. Fractures of the facets also may be difficult to detect with CT scanning because they frequently are horizontal or displaced minimally.[43, 44] The fracture line may simulate the appearance of a normal or distracted facet joint or of a locked facet joint.[44] Persistent neck pain can result from hypertrophic changes in the previously injured apophyseal joints.[287] CT scanning allows excellent evaluation of the degree of bony proliferation and impingement of soft tissues in such cases.

Hyperflexion Injuries

One of the most common, if not the most common, mechanisms resulting in cervical spine injury is hyperflex-

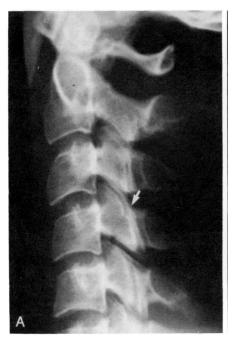
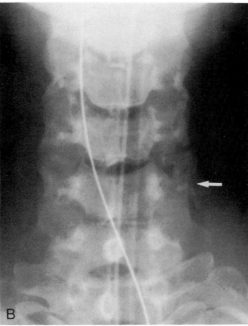

FIGURE 69–33. Extension rotation injury: Facet fractures.

A A vertical fracture of the C4 facet process is apparent (arrow).

B An anteroposterior view in a different patient demonstrates comminution of the articular process (arrow) of the C6 vertebra on the left.

ion of the cervical region.[3, 33, 80] Indeed, 46 to 79 per cent of all cervical injuries are due to hyperflexion.[33] In one radiographic review of 401 cervical injuries, 315 (79 per cent) were thought to be due to hyperflexion.[3] Hyperflexion injuries usually are caused by a blow to the posterior aspect of the cranium, forcing the face toward the chest.[268] This mechanism is responsible for a large variety of bone and soft tissue abnormalities.

The hyperflexion sprain is predominantly a ligamentous injury with disruption of the ligaments of the posterior column and, in severe cases, the posterior longitudinal ligament and posterior portion of the anulus fibrosus in the middle column. The injury typically occurs in the absence of any fracture, although minor wedgelike compressions of the anterior portion of the vertebral body occasionally coexist.[266, 292] The disrupted ligaments, in order of disruption, are the supraspinous ligament, interspinous ligament, ligamenta flava, and capsule of the facet joint; in severe cases, the posterior longitudinal ligament and posterior aspect of the anulus fibrosus also are disrupted. The injury relates to pure flexion without any major axial compressive force; tension in the posterior ligaments results in their rupture.[228, 292] Presenting features can consist of pain, a transient neurologic defect such as paresthesias of the upper or lower extremities, or both, and, rarely, complete tetraplegia.[293] Neurologic defect usually is mild and reversible, with persistent pain and muscle spasm being the dominant clinical features.[292] The spinal level that is injured most commonly in hyperflexion varies with age. In the child and adolescent, the injury typically occurs at the C2-C3 or C3-C4 level, whereas injury of the lower cervical levels usually occurs in adults.[292] These injuries need to be recognized and treated promptly to prevent the delayed development of pain, progressive kyphosis, and eventual neurologic deficit. Approximately 20 to 33 per cent of patients with posterior ligamentous disruption who are treated conservatively develop progressive kyphosis and

delayed spinal instability.[82, 134, 266, 292] Cervical kyphosis of more than 20 degrees in children or 10 degrees in adults has been suggested as a criterion for operative fixation.[292] Partial ligamentous disruptions respond well to conservative therapy but total ruptures typically require anterior or posterior cervical fusion.[292, 293]

Radiographs of the cervical spine frequently are normal despite the presence of a clinically evident cord injury.[293] When radiographs are positive, widening of the interspinous distance or the posterior aspect of the apophyseal joints is evident. Interspinous widening that is more than 2 mm greater than the width at both adjacent levels has been suggested as a sensitive criterion of spinal instability.[24, 267] An interspinous distance that is more than 1.5 times the distance in both adjacent levels definitely is abnormal and indicates the presence of anterior cervical dislocation.[185, 294] In extreme voluntary flexion, the normal interspinous distance may be as much as 1.5 times greater than the interspinous distance in either the level above or the level below, but not in both levels.[185, 294] Localized kyphotic angulation of the cervical spine is highly suggestive of this injury.[266, 293] Focally exaggerated kyphosis is required for diagnosis of the injury, because diffuse kyphosis of the cervical spine may result from voluntary flexion or muscle spasm. Another radiographic feature in patients with hyperflexion injury of the cervical spine is kyphosis at a single spinal level with persistent lordosis in the remaining portions of the cervical spine.[266] Kyphosis at one spinal level that is 11 degrees greater than at adjacent levels in the cervical spine indicates the presence of posterior ligament damage.[14] If the posterior portion of the anulus fibrosus is disrupted as well, anterior narrowing and posterior widening of the disc space and anterior rotation or 1 to 3 mm displacement of the superior vertebrae may be present.[59, 145, 266, 293] Anterior vertebral displacement may be more prominent when it is associated with a compression fracture or a flexion injury.[266] Minor degrees of anterior vertebral displacement resulting from injury are difficult to distinguish from degenerative anterolisthesis. Anterior displacement of the vertebral body of more than 3.5 mm indicates frank dislocation.[13, 14, 266]

If this injury is suspected, supervised flexion and extension views may help to demonstrate these radiographic findings.[293] In flexion injuries, abnormal alignment at the injured level is exaggerated with flexion of the neck and often is corrected with extension of the neck[266, 293] (Fig. 69–34). These views should be obtained only in an alert, cooperative patient who is able to perform these maneuvers actively.

The normal cervical spine typically displays a smooth lordotic curve. Straightening of the cervical spine in the supine position is not a significant finding and does not imply muscle spasm. Even in the erect position, in up to 20 per cent of normal people, the cervical spine is straight or shows a smooth gradual kyphosis with the head held in the neutral position.[266] Complete absence of flexion at all cervical levels is abnormal and indicates either a lack of patient effort or an inability to flex the neck, typically as a result of muscle spasm or soft tissue injury.[267] In normal persons, flexion of at least 3 degrees at three or more consecutive levels in the cervical spine should be present for flexion to be adequate.[267] In patients who show no cervical flexion, the examination must be considered inadequate and a repeat study should be obtained.[267] Seventy to 75 per cent of normal persons are able to reverse the normal cervical lordosis voluntarily; this percentage probably is less in the acutely injured patient.[266, 267, 292] Therefore, an adequate flexion-extension examination may not be possible acutely because of pain and muscle spasm. Delayed flexion and extension views may be more efficacious.[292, 293, 295]

A pure hyperflexion injury of the spine may spare the posterior ligaments and result only in osseous disruption limited to the anterior vertebral column. In the immature cervical spine, flexion may produce an avulsion of the anterior portion of the superior vertebral ring apophysis.[270] This injury characteristically is associated with other vertebral abnormalities, particularly compression fractures of the superior endplate.[270] In adults, simple compression fractures of one or more vertebrae are encountered. The wedge compression fracture consists of comminution of the anterosuperior aspect of the endplate of that vertebral body without concomitant injury to the posterior portion of the vertebral body, posterior bony elements, or spinal ligaments.[145, 201] These simple compression fractures are relatively benign injuries because they do not compromise the neural canal and generally heal uneventfully.[295] The fracture is best seen on the lateral view and is manifested as loss of anterior vertebral height, buckling or step-off of the anterior or superior endplate (or of both), and soft tissue swelling.[145] Although prognosis generally is favorable, delayed spinal instability develops after compression fractures in up to 20 per cent of patients, despite the absence of any indication of spinal instability at the time of initial presentation.[295, 296] Such instability presumably relates to unrecognized posterior ligamentous injury at the time of the flexion force.

The clay-shoveler's fracture is an oblique fracture of the spinous process of the sixth cervical through third thoracic vertebrae that results from avulsion by the supraspinous ligament.[4, 145, 201] The injury derives its name from its common occurrence in Australian clay miners.[201] This injury also is referred to as root-puller's or Schipper's disease; the juvenile form, due to traumatic avulsion of the secondary center of ossification of the spinous process, has been referred to as Schmitt's disease.[297] The fracture may involve a single or multiple spinous processes (Fig. 69–35). The most commonly fractured level is C6 or C7, although the T1 and T2 vertebrae also are injured frequently.[145, 297] Isolated fractures of the spinous process are due to hyperflexion in most cases, but a direct blow to these superficial structures also can result in a fracture. Fractures of the spinous processes related to hyperextension causing crushing of the posterior elements also have been described.[244, 266] These fractures are best seen on the lateral view unless the spinous processes are obscured by overlying soft tissues. The anteroposterior view may show malalignment and displacement of the inferior tip of the involved spinous process. Occasionally, a "double spinous process" shadow related to simultaneous visualization of the fractured base and the caudally displaced tip of the spinous process is evident.[297, 298] Rarely, hyperflexion produces an avulsion fracture of the lamina due to traction at the site of attachment of the ligamentum flavum.[299]

Unstable flexion injuries of the cervical spine include bilateral locking of the facet joints and flexion teardrop fractures. Bilateral facet locks are a consequence of severe flexion forces that cause complete ligamentous disruption of the posterior and middle spinal columns and variable disruption of the anterior spinal column. The horizontal orientation of the cervical facet joints allows dislocation to occur in the absence of bony disruption.[2, 145] Rupture of the posterior portion of the anulus fibrosus, the posterior longitudinal ligament, and the capsular, interspinous, and supraspinous ligaments invariably is present in these cases.[292, 300, 301] In some cases, rupture or stripping of the anterior longitudinal ligament also is present and may produce an avulsion fracture of the anterosuperior corner of the vertebral body.[292] As the facet joints lock, marked narrowing of the spinal canal and intervertebral neural foramina result.[137, 300] Such narrowing leads to a neurologic deficit in up to 75 per cent of patients with this injury.[301] Foraminal or spinal canal narrowing may be aggravated by concomitant soft tissue injury leading to hemorrhage or discal herniation. The prevalence of associated traumatic disc herniation in patients with bilateral facet locks has been estimated to be zero to 50 per cent; in one report, six of 68 patients with malalignment of the facet joints had a concomitant disc herniation.[302] Narrowing of the intervening disc is suggestive of a traumatic disc herniation but is not always present. CT-myelography or MR imaging is necessary to allow accurate assessment of the status of the intervertebral disc. Recognition of this discal herniation is important because reduction of the vertebral subluxation with traction may aggravate the neurologic deficit if the disc is drawn posteriorly into the spinal canal.[302]

Bilateral facet locks are recognized easily on lateral radiographs owing to the severe spinal malalignment (Fig. 69–36). Anterior displacement of the superior vertebra invariably is present and typically is greater than half the width of the vertebral body.[301] The anterolisthesis is increased by flexion of the cervical spine, but even in full extension, a similar degree of anterolisthesis is present.[301] Focal kyphosis also is present characteristically. Associated injuries include avulsion fractures of the spinous process

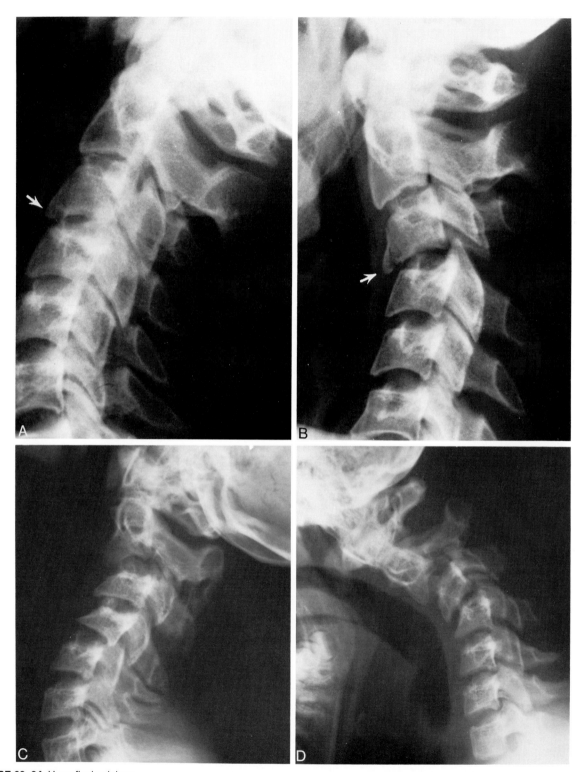

FIGURE 69–34. Hyperflexion injury.

 A, B Lateral radiographs of the cervical spine are obtained with extension **(A)** and flexion **(B)** of the neck. In **A,** vertebral alignment appears normal. A subtle fracture of the third vertebral body is seen (arrow). In **B,** anterior displacement of the C3 vertebral body with respect to C4 is obvious. Note the narrowing of the anterior aspect of the intervening intervertebral disc and widening of the apophyseal joints and interspinous distance at this level. The fracture again is evident (arrow).

 C, D In a different patient, progressive instability of the cervical spine occurred 10 months **(C)** and 1 year **(D)** after an acute, unrecognized hyperflexion injury.

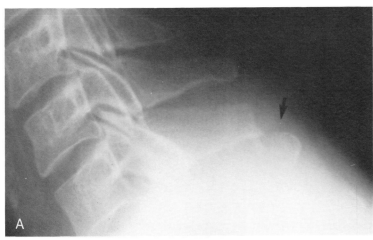

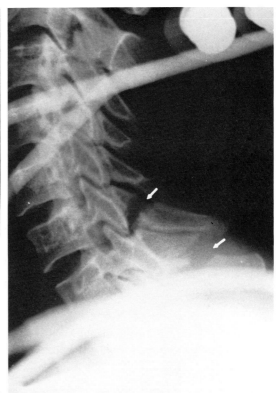

FIGURE 69–35. Fractures of the spinous process.

  A The lateral view shows an isolated fracture of the tip of the spinous process of C6 (arrow) due to hyperflexion (clay-shoveler's fracture).

  B Oblique fractures of the spinous processes of the C6 and C7 vertebrae are present (arrows).

B

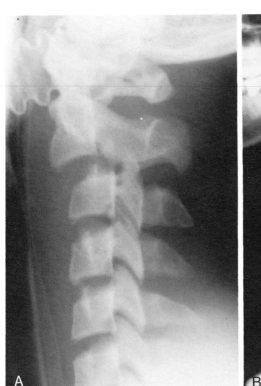

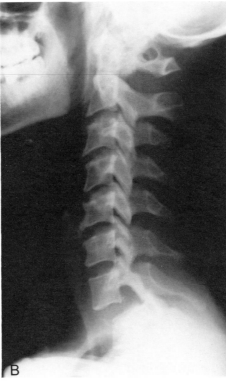

FIGURE 69–36. Bilateral facet locks.

  A Bilateral facet locks are present at the C2-C3 level with anterolisthesis of greater than 50 per cent of the vertebral width.

  B Bilateral facet locks at the C7-T1 vertebral level show marked anterolisthesis and lack of rotation at the injured level.

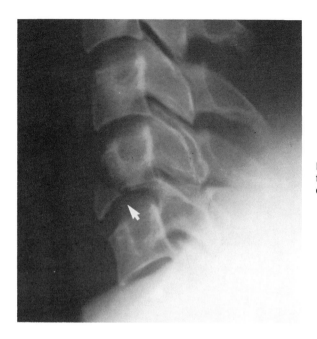

FIGURE 69–37. Flexion teardrop fracture. A triangular fracture (arrow) of the anteroinferior margin of the C5 vertebral body is present. Posterior displacement of this vertebral body is minimal.

above the locked level and triangular fractures of the anterosuperior corner of the inferior vertebral body.[273, 293] The presence of a triangular body fracture suggests incompetence of the anterior longitudinal ligament with the fracture resulting from avulsion.[293] On CT scans, this injury produces the ''naked'' facet sign bilaterally, whereby the articular surfaces of both apophyseal joints at one spinal level no longer are in apposition.[37, 43]

Flexion teardrop fractures, like bilateral facet locks, are highly unstable injuries that characteristically result in severe neurologic deficit.[34, 87, 303, 304] Complete quadriplegia, paraplegia, the Brown-Séquard syndrome, or the anterior cord syndrome develops in 87 per cent of patients with this injury.[273, 303] The characteristic neurologic deficit seen is the anterior cord syndrome, consisting of complete motor paralysis and partial sensory dysfunction with loss of pain, touch, and temperature sensations but preservation of posterior column function.[87, 303, 304] This injury is the result of combined flexion and axial loading with the most common inciting events being diving and motor vehicle accidents.[303] The flexion teardrop injury typically involves the lower cervical spine, with C5 being the most common level of involvement, representing 55 per cent of affected vertebrae in one series.[273, 303]

The vertebral body is divided into a smaller anteroinferior fragment and a larger posterior fragment.[303] Indeed, the name of this injury, proposed by Schneider and Kahn in 1956, was based on the similarity of the anterior fracture fragment to ''a drop of water dripping from the vertebral body'' or a ''teardrop''[87] (Fig. 69–37). The anteroinferior teardrop fragment frequently is large and often involves one third to one half of the vertebral body.[273] Dystrophic calcification of degenerated fibers in the anulus fibrosus, an extremely common finding in adults, should not be confused with a teardrop fracture of the vertebral body.[305] The calcified anulus typically is small, amorphous, and separated from the vertebral body by a well-defined radiolucent band of soft tissue. The teardrop fragment typically remains aligned with the vertebral body below or shows minimal

anterior and downward displacement. The most specific finding in this injury is posterior displacement of the inferior aspect of the larger posterior fragment of the fractured vertebral body relative to the vertebra below (Fig. 69–38). This retrolisthesis is seen in 78 to 89 per cent of cases and results in compression or destruction of the anterior portion of the cervical spinal cord.[87, 273, 303] Retrolisthesis of the posterior portion of the vertebral body and the neural arch results in offset of the spinolaminar line and widening of

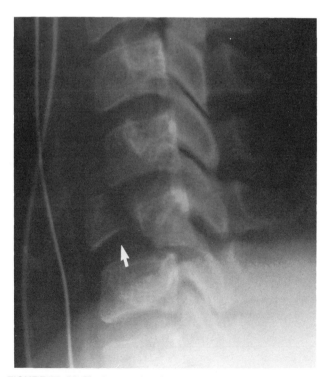

FIGURE 69–38. Flexion teardrop fracture. A fracture of the anteroinferior corner of the C5 vertebral body (arrow) is seen. The posterior portion of the C5 vertebral body is displaced posteriorly, with widening of the C5-C6 facet joints.

the facet joints. The cervical spine superior to the site of the fracture typically remains aligned with the large posteriorly displaced posterior fragment.[273, 303] If anterolisthesis or retrolisthesis is absent, widening of the space between adjacent facet joints and, less commonly, between adjacent laminae and spinous processes suggests the presence of this hyperflexion injury.[303, 304] Sagittal fractures of the vertebral body and laminae, consistent with axial loading, occur in the large majority of patients.[303] The most commonly associated fracture, seen in 67 per cent of cases, is a sagittal vertebral body fracture.[273] Other commonly associated fractures involve the posterior arch in 48 per cent, the articular mass in 20 per cent, and the spinous process in 7 per cent.[273] Associated abnormalities include anterior wedging of the vertebral body in 87 per cent of cases, posterior disc space narrowing, fractures of the lamina, and focal kyphosis.[303]

Flexion Rotation Injuries

Unilateral facet lock is the only common cervical injury produced by the combination of flexion and rotation and represents between 4 and 16 per cent of all cervical spine injuries.[145, 268, 290, 306] Rupture of the interspinous ligament and the capsule of the apophyseal joint allows the ipsilateral inferior facet of one vertebra to pivot, dislocate, and come to rest in the neural foramen anterior to the superior facet of the vertebral body below.[145, 201, 290, 292, 301, 306] The spinal cord is impinged on by the posterosuperior aspect of the body below and by the lamina above.[268] The posterior longitudinal ligament and anulus fibrosus usually are damaged only minimally.[301, 306] More extensive damage to these structures allows increasing anterolisthesis and mechanical instability.[301] The most common levels of involvement are C4-C5 and C5-C6, which are involved in 54 to 79 per cent of cases.[292, 306]

Although this injury is considered mechanically stable, the presence of neurologic damage or an associated facet fracture should suggest potential mechanical and neurologic instability.[14, 132, 145] Neurologic deficit is relatively uncommon; however, spinal cord damage or radiculopathy or both may develop if significant spinal stenosis occurs at the site of subluxation. Unilateral facet lock was responsible for cervical cord damage in 86 of 525 patients (16 per cent) with cervical trauma evaluated by Scher.[306] Early diagnosis, preferably within 2 weeks of the injury, is essential for an easy reduction and for restoration of any nerve root deficit that may be present owing to impingement.[292, 306]

Numerous radiographic manifestations of unilateral facet lock have been described, but the diagnosis may be difficult, with some cases misdiagnosed as cervical subluxation or dislocation secondary to a hyperflexion injury.[292, 306] Unilateral facet lock produces alterations of spinal alignment on the lateral and anteroposterior projections but is easiest to recognize on oblique views. Anterior subluxation of the superior vertebra typically is present, but the degree of subluxation is less than that seen with bilateral facet locks, averaging one quarter of the sagittal diameter of the vertebral body.[145, 301] The magnitude of the anterolisthesis is never greater than half this sagittal diameter; it is exaggerated by flexion of the neck and reduces considerably, although not completely, with hyperextension.[301] Anterior subluxation of 3 to 7 mm was present in 22 of 27 cases

reported by Young and coworkers; in five of 27 patients, vertebral displacement less than 3 mm was identified.[290] Because subluxation may be minimal or even absent, careful attention to the facet joints themselves is essential.[306] The lateral view demonstrates abrupt rotation of the facet joints at the level of the dislocation, with loss of normal superimposition of the paired facets at and superior to the level of injury[4, 145, 292, 306] (Fig. 69–39). The vertebrae above the lock are seen in the oblique projection rather than in the lateral projection as are the caudal vertebrae. Displacement and rotation of the articular facets produces the classic "bow tie" appearance.[145, 290] The bow tie appearance is formed by the anteriorly displaced facet above and the normally positioned facet below.[145] This sign was present in only 33 per cent of patients in one series, however.[290] Abrupt alteration of the laminar space, the distance between the posterior margin of the facet joint and the spinolaminar line, is another sign of rotation that is evident on the lateral radiograph and is present in almost all cases of unilateral facet lock.[290] The laminar space frequently is difficult to measure at C2 and C7; therefore, this sign is less useful in the diagnosis of dislocations at the extreme ends of the cervical spine.[290] Associated findings seen on the lateral view include vertebral fractures and divergence of the spinous processes, the latter finding being seen in 37 per cent of cases and resulting from rupture of the interspinous ligament.[290, 306] The typical associated fractures of the ver-

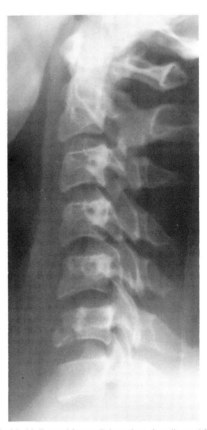

FIGURE 69–39. Unilateral facet dislocation. A unilateral facet lock is present at the C5-C6 spinal level, with a fracture of the anteroinferior margin of the C6 vertebral body. Note the minimal anterolisthesis in this patient. The facet joints at the C6 and C7 levels are superimposed normally, whereas all the facet joints above the level of the lock are rotated.

tebral body are triangular anteroinferior and anterosuperior fractures; less commonly the posteroinferior corner of the vertebral body is disrupted.[273] Associated facet fractures also are common.[273, 287] It is impossible from the lateral view alone to determine which side is involved.

The anteroposterior view demonstrates rotation of the spinous processes at the site of the lock with lateral stepoff of the spinous processes above the site of the injury. This finding is noted in only 33 to 40 per cent of cases.[137, 306] Lateral cervical flexion also may be apparent. Unlike most cervical spine injuries, the abnormality of vertebral alignment is most evident on oblique projections.[137, 145] Oblique radiographs allow identification of the side of injury, show the facet malalignment, demonstrate narrowing of the intervertebral foramen, and may permit detection of associated facet fractures.[137, 306] Associated fractures, typically involving the vertebral bodies and spinous processes, were present in 35 per cent of cases reported by Scher.[306] These fractures are well seen on the lateral projection, whereas oblique views are most helpful for detecting fractures of the articular facets and pedicles.[137, 306]

Despite the numerous radiographic findings, this injury can be extremely difficult to recognize and characterize, particularly on technically inadequate rotated radiographs obtained with portable equipment. This injury is missed on the initial examination in up to one half of patients because the radiographic signs and clinical manifestations are subtle or overlooked.[290, 292] The malalignment, however, is recognized easily using either lateral conventional tomography or CT scanning. The latter method or MR imaging is recommended if associated neurologic injury is present, as it may demonstrate bony fragments impinging on the nerve root (Fig. 69–40). On CT scans, facet subluxation can be recognized by noting the malalignment of the articular processes. The normal facet joints are recognized by their characteristic semilunar configuration, which together form

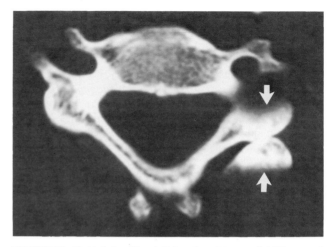

FIGURE 69–41. Unilateral facet dislocation. A transaxial CT scan of a unilateral left-sided facet lock shows that the straight articular surfaces (arrows) no longer are in contact. The curved, nonarticular bony margins are in abnormal contact, denoting a facet lock.

a circular shadow with the two straight adjacent joint surfaces bisecting the circle in a horizontal plane.[44] With facet subluxation and perched facets, the "naked" facet sign is seen, in which a bare articular surface is visualized without its corresponding articular facet.[37] With a frank lock, the convex portions of the joints, rather than the straight portions, are in contact; the flat articular portions of the facets form the anterior and posterior margins of the joint on the side of the lock[44] (Fig. 69–41). Associated uncovertebral joint subluxation at the level of the injury, due to rotation of one vertebral body relative to the other, also is present frequently.[44]

Lateral Hyperflexion Injuries

Lateral hyperflexion injuries are caused by a force delivered directly to the lateral aspect of the skull or cervical spine.[268] The most well known fracture produced by this mechanism is unilateral lateral wedging of the vertebral body and its associated lateral mass.[268] However, a variety of other osseous injuries can result from lateral bending. In a series of 23 patients with lateral hyperflexion injuries reported by Schaaf and coworkers, five types of injuries were recognized. In decreasing order of frequency, these were (1) transverse process fracture; (2) uncinate process fracture; (3) laterally displaced odontoid fracture; (4) brachial plexopathy in association with a cervical fracture or dislocation; and (5) lateral wedge type fracture of a vertebral body.[307] Associated fractures of the neural arches, similar to those occurring in extension, are present in the majority of patients. This association suggests that the laterally flexed spine, when it undergoes compression, tends also to hyperextend.[307] These injuries are uncommon and represent only 6 per cent of all injuries to the cervical spine.[307] They occur most frequently in children, adolescents, and young adults, probably as a result of greater flexibility in these persons.[268] Many of the osseous injuries produced by lateral flexion of the cervical spine characteristically are not apparent on lateral radiographs and require anteroposterior and oblique views for adequate assessment.

Lateral flexion, combined with forceful traction, is thought to be the mechanism underlying cervical fracture-

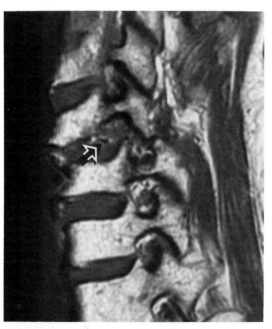

FIGURE 69–40. Unilateral facet dislocation. Oblique T1-weighted (TR/TE, 500/12) spin echo MR image in a cadaver with a surgically created facet lock illustrates narrowing of the neural foramen (arrow) at the injured level.

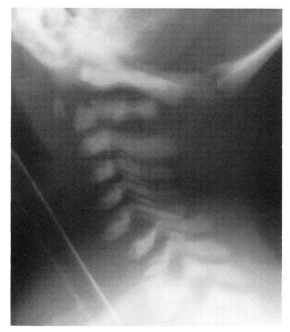

FIGURE 69–42. Cervical dislocation during delivery. A dislocation at the C6-C7 level developed as a result of birth trauma during vaginal delivery of an infant in breech presentation. The infant was quadriplegic at birth as a result of his spinal dislocation.

dislocations occurring during childbirth.[308] Difficult deliveries, particularly in cases of breech presentation with a hyperextended fetal head, can produce severe injury to the spinal cord, nerve roots, meninges, and vessels, in addition to spinal abnormalities[151, 308] (Fig. 69–42). Injury may be limited to the soft tissue structures of the cervical spine or associated with fractures of the superior endplate of the vertebral body below the level of the dislocation. The degree of neurologic deficit varies depending on the level of injury and its severity; death, complete quadriplegia, and minor transient deficits all have been documented.[308]

Axial Loading Injuries

Burst fractures of the cervical vertebrae typically are the result of combined flexion and axial loading.[266] This type of fracture is seen predominantly in areas of the spine capable of voluntary straightening, such as the occipitocervical junction, lower portion of the cervical spine, and thoracolumbar spine. Of these three sites, burst fractures of the lower cervical spine are the least common. Only 36 of 401 cervical spine injuries in one series were of this type.[3] The C5, C6, and C7 levels typically are involved.[3] Neurologic deficit is common as the cord is stretched across the posterior aspect of the vertebral body or compressed by retropulsed bone fragments.[268] Neurologic deficit was present in 85 per cent of patients with burst fractures of the cervical spine reported by Beatson.[301] The true prevalence of neurologic defect probably is lower but is difficult to determine because in some series the authors include flexion teardrop fractures in their definition of a burst fracture.

Burst fractures of the cervical spine characteristically result in retropulsion of the posterosuperior vertebral margin into the spinal canal (Fig. 69–43). The sagittal vertebral widening and presence of retropulsed bone may lead to confusion with a flexion teardrop injury, but the burst fracture lacks the characteristic anteroinferior triangular fragment, is more comminuted, exhibits more loss of vertebral height, and is not associated with cervical kyphosis, interspinous fanning, or subluxation of the facet joints.[145, 201] The flexion teardrop fracture is grossly unstable, whereas burst fractures typically maintain integrity of the ligaments of the posterior spinal column. The discs adjacent to a burst fracture frequently are disrupted, and it is the integrity of the posterior spinal column that maintains stability in these injuries.[301] On the anteroposterior view, burst fractures characteristically are associated with a sagittal fracture line that extends across the entire height of the involved vertebral body.[145] This sagittal fracture line is difficult to appreciate on conventional radiographs but may be recognized on a well-penetrated anteroposterior view.

Axial compression can produce an isolated sagittal fracture of the vertebral body without any comminution or bone retropulsion. This rare injury produces the paradoxic situation of quadriplegia with minimal radiographic abnormality.[309] The radiographic findings of this fracture are subtle, although soft tissue swelling typically is present. Minimal compression of the anterosuperior corner of the vertebral body is seen on the lateral view; the vertical radiolucent shadow representing the fracture occasionally is visualized on the anteroposterior radiograph[309] (Fig. 69–44). A similar vertical radiolucent region may be seen as a result of a thin collection of air in the larynx; this appearance should not be misinterpreted as a sagittal fracture line.[248] Lee and col-

FIGURE 69–43. Cervical burst fracture.

A The lateral radiograph demonstrates loss of height of the C7 vertebral body with retropulsed bone (arrow) within the spinal canal.

B Transaxial CT scan shows the displaced bone (arrowheads) narrowing the spinal canal.

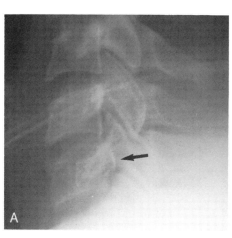
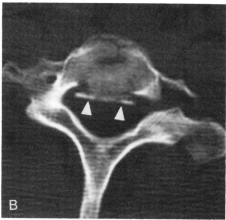

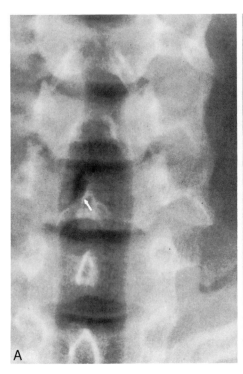
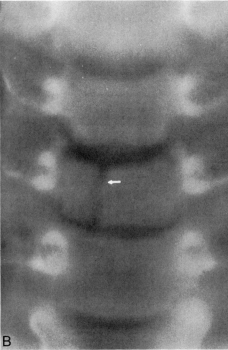

FIGURE 69–44. Axial compression injury.

A The isolated sagittal fracture (arrow) is difficult to identify on the conventional radiograph.

B The fracture line (arrow) is evident on the frontal conventional tomogram.

leagues identified this type of fracture in seven of 270 consecutive patients with cervical fractures. The anteroposterior radiograph allowed identification of the injury in only two patients; two additional patients had suggestive radiographs; in three patients the injury was detected with either conventional tomography or CT scanning.[309] Five of seven patients had multiple sagittal fractures and six of seven patients had associated posterior element fractures.[309]

UPPER THORACIC SPINE

General Considerations

If compression deformities secondary to osteoporosis are excluded, fractures of the thoracic spine above the thoracolumbar junction are uncommon.[310] It has been estimated that only 30 per cent of all traumatic thoracic fractures occur above the T10 level.[311, 312] Although the upper thoracic spine is injured infrequently, these injuries are important clinically because of the relative youth of the injured population, the high rate of permanent neurologic deficit from injuries in this region, and the severity of the injuries occurring in this region.[104, 310, 313, 314] The majority of significant upper thoracic spine injuries are due to motor vehicle accidents or falls, although numerous other mechanisms, including direct trauma to the upper back, athletic injuries, and projectile wounds, also have been implicated.[310, 311, 314, 315] As many as 22 to 56 per cent of patients with upper thoracic injury in some series are injured as a result of a motorcycle accident.[310, 314, 316] The injury occurs when the rider is thrown over the handlebars and lands on the upper thoracic spine, producing forced flexion.[316] A high rate of concomitant fractures in other portions of the spine is seen in these patients.[5, 6, 310] Indeed, as many as 17 per cent of patients with fractures of the upper thoracic spine have another spinal fracture at a noncontiguous level.[310] The

most common associated injuries involve the cervical spine, followed in frequency by the thoracolumbar junction.[5, 310]

A brief review of the pertinent gross anatomy is necessary to understand the characteristic fractures that occur in this region. The thoracic spine is composed of 12 vertebrae, each consisting of a load-bearing vertebral body and a neural arch that resists tension.[20, 312, 317] The vertebral body consists of cancellous bone centrally, surrounded by a thin compact layer of cortical bone. The vertebral strength in compression decreases by up to 50 per cent with the loss of osseous tissue that accompanies aging.[312] The superior and inferior endplates normally are straight, whereas the sides of the vertebral bodies have a mild concavity.[312] The thoracic pedicles are relatively thin and extend posterolaterally to join the large articular facets. In the upper thoracic spine, these large overlapping facets are almost coronal in orientation and play an important role in maintaining stability during spinal flexion and extension.[2, 37, 312] The facet orientation also provides significant resistance to anterior vertebral translation.[312, 317] Posterior to the articular facets lie the paired laminae, which are broad and overlap in the thoracic region. The laminae fuse to form the spinous process, which is long and thin and projects inferiorly.[312]

The unique anatomic feature of the upper thoracic region is the presence of the paired ribs and the costovertebral joints. Throughout the spine, two adjacent vertebrae and connecting soft tissues form the mechanical unit of a motion segment. In the thoracic region, the motion segment is more complex and also encompasses the ribs and their articulations.[15] All the thoracic vertebrae have facets for articulation with the head of the rib; the second through tenth thoracic vertebrae also have facets on their transverse processes, which form a second articulation between the vertebra and the rib.[312] The rib cage restricts motion and increases spinal stiffness, particularly in extension. To a lesser degree, the rib cage also restricts flexion and lateral rotation.[15, 317] The rib cage and intercostal muscles have been estimated to increase the compression tolerance of the spine by a factor of 4.[15, 317] Flexion and extension of the spine are limited to 4 degrees in the upper and 6 degrees in the midthoracic region.[318]

The dominant or primary curve in this area is ventral, with the normal kyphosis developing in utero and persisting throughout life. The thoracic kyphosis is partially explained by a slight discrepancy in the heights of the anterior and posterior portions of the vertebral bodies, the ventral height being 1 to 2 mm less than the dorsal height.[312] Maximal normal wedging is seen at T8, T11, and T12, but mild degrees of anterior wedging are seen at all thoracic levels.[319, 320] Fletcher and Lauridsen and colleagues have developed wedging ratios, derived by comparing the height of the anterior versus the posterior portions of the vertebral body. Wedging ratios of 0.8 in men and 0.87 in women, regardless of age, normally are seen in the lower thoracic spine.[319, 320] The anterior height can be as much as 20 per cent less than the posterior height in a significant number of normal persons.[319, 320] This normal diminution of anterior height and the resultant trapezoidal vertebral configuration should not be misinterpreted as evidence of an acute or chronic fracture.

The unique anatomy of the upper thoracic spine results in fracture patterns that differ from those seen in the more commonly injured cervical and thoracolumbar regions. The magnitude of force necessary to overcome the inherent stability of the upper thoracic spine is greater than that required for the remainder of the spine. The relatively small cross-sectional area of the spinal canal in the upper thoracic region, combined with the high force necessary to create an unstable injury in this region, leads to a high rate of neurologic injury. The spinal canal in the adult is small and circular; the bulk of the canal is occupied by the thoracic cord.[318]

Imaging Assessment

The initial radiographic examination of the traumatized upper thoracic spine consists of supine anteroposterior and lateral radiographs. Adequate visualization of this spinal region frequently is difficult because of overlying soft tissues, particularly on radiographs obtained with portable equipment. The upper four thoracic vertebrae are particularly difficult to see on lateral radiographs. Therefore, close attention must be paid to these vertebrae on the anteroposterior view. A modified swimmer's view can be helpful for evaluating the upper vertebral bodies, but this projection requires arm movement. Despite meticulous positioning, adequate x-ray penetration may be impossible to achieve on the lateral projection of the upper thoracic vertebrae. In some patients, conventional tomography or CT scanning is necessary to allow assessment of suspected injury of the upper thoracic region. Streak artifacts from the soft tissues of the shoulders and the very limited amount of epidural fat in this region make CT scans difficult to evaluate in some patients.[25]

The paravertebral tissues should always be assessed carefully, as osseous disruption from minimal compression fractures often is difficult to appreciate, particularly in the person with osteoporosis. The paraspinal or paravertebral shadow represents the interface between the lung and the paraspinal soft tissues and is well seen on the anteroposterior radiograph, particularly on the left side.[321–323] The right interface is closely applied to the vertebral column, whereas the left interface often shows smooth displacement laterally due to aortic dilation.[321] Osseous alterations that accompany degenerative diseases, infections, tumors, and trauma, as well as a variety of mediastinal disorders, can produce displacement of the paraspinal interface.[321, 322] The majority of acute fractures are associated with the development of a focal paraspinal hematoma that is centered at the level of injury[324] (Fig. 69–45). Gehweiler and colleagues noted paravertebral hematomas in 100 per cent of thoracic fractures between T1 and T11.[324] In upper dorsal fractures, the hematoma may extend over the apex of the lung, forming a pleural cap. Paravertebral hematomas tend to be fusiform or lentiform and resolve gradually within a month of the injury.[322, 323] A hemothorax also is seen commonly in association with severe spinal injury.[310]

The soft tissue changes resulting from an upper thoracic injury, particularly a fracture-dislocation, can mimic those of an aortic transection. Mediastinal widening, paraspinal hematoma, and left apical capping are features that can be seen in both vertebral and vascular injuries.[4, 310, 325–327] Gundry and coworkers have reported that widening of the mediastinum is the most reliable sign of traumatic aortic rupture on conventional radiographs and is seen on the anteroposterior view in 89 per cent of patients with this vascular injury.[327] When soft tissue abnormalities suggestive of aortic injury are present but vascular damage is absent, careful evaluation of the integrity and alignment of the upper thoracic spine is mandatory. Dennis and Rogers studied 54 patients with fractures of the lower cervical or upper thoracic spine (C6-T8) and found a mediastinal width greater than 8 cm in 52 per cent of patients[325] (Fig. 69–46). In all, 69 per cent of patients had either mediastinal widening, left apical pleural fluid, or a widened right paratracheal stripe.[325] In their series, the spinal fracture could be seen on the initial plain film in 51 per cent of patients. Bolesta and Bohlman reported three patients with thoracic fractures who initially were diagnosed as having an aortic rupture on the basis of their admission chest radiographs.[326] All three patients had some neurologic deficit at the time of presentation, but this finding was attributed to cord ischemia resulting from a vascular injury.[326] Aortic trauma reduces the collateral circulation of the spinal arteries, resulting in cord ischemia and necrosis.[326] Aortic and thoracic spinal injury can coexist; Bolesta and Bohlman recommended that an aortogram or other method of aortic evaluation be employed in patients with mediastinal widening, even if an upper thoracic injury is suspected.[326] It has been suggested further that aortic injury itself is due to compression of the vessel between the spine posteriorly and the thoracic cage (manubrium, clavicle, and first rib) anteriorly during chest compression.[328, 329]

Compression Fractures

Compression fractures of the midthoracic spine are common in patients with osteoporosis.[330–332] Eighteen per cent of white women over the age of 50 years demonstrate at least one compression fracture, with prevalence rates approaching 78 per cent among women over 90 years old.[329] Only a small proportion of these patients give a history of

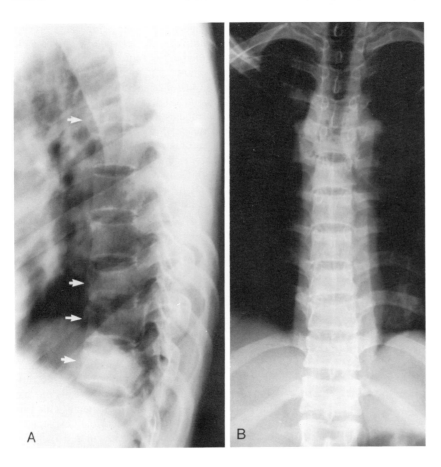

FIGURE 69–45. Thoracic compression fractures with paraspinal hematoma.
A The lateral view shows anterior compression fractures of the T5, T9, T10, and T11 vertebral bodies (arrows). Note the loss of height of the vertebral bodies anteriorly and the presence of angular deformity and cortical disruption of the anterior margins of the fractured vertebrae.
B The anteroposterior view demonstrates widening of both the right and the left paraspinal interfaces due to hematoma.

a specific traumatic event.[332] These fractures typically result from flexion or axial forces, or both, producing compression loading of the vertebral body. The cancellous bone of vertebral body is weaker in compression than in tension.[15] The force required to fracture the vertebral body in an osteoporotic person can be trivial; in younger persons with normal bones, a much greater force is required.[318] With tension loading, failure typically takes place through the disc and endplate rather than through the vertebral body itself.[312]

Denis reported 148 cases of acute traumatic compression fractures in nonosteoporotic persons.[8] The fractures were subclassified as anterior (89 per cent) and lateral (11 per cent) compression injuries. The distribution of acute compression fractures was bimodal, with one peak at the T6-T7 level and the second, larger peak at the thoracolumbar junction. Typical compression fractures cause localized pain and kyphosis but generally do not manifest any acute neurologic deficit. Paraspinal swelling, loss of vertebral height, and cortical disruption typically are apparent (Fig. 69–47). A narrow zone of increased density below the fractured endplate, produced by impacted trabeculae, commonly is present.[333] By Denis' definition of compression fractures, the middle column is intact so there is no loss of height of the posterior vertebral body and no vertebral subluxation.[8] The anteroposterior view may show interspinous widening geometrically in proportion to the degree of anterior vertebral wedging.[23] Many compression fractures are detected as incidental findings on radiographs obtained for some other reason, and their acute or chronic nature cannot be determined.[332]

Typical compression fractures result in failure confined to the anterior column.[8] Because the middle column is normal, this injury generally is considered stable. In severe compression fractures, partial injury to the posterior column may be present, leading to progressive kyphosis with potential mechanical instability.[8] In laboratory studies, vertebral bodies compressed to 50 per cent of their original height show a tendency to return to 70 to 80 per cent of their original height within 72 hours of the injury.[312] Thus, radiographs obtained after a delay may suggest a less significant amount of vertebral compression. The major risk factors for early kyphosis after traumatic compression fractures in nonosteoporotic patients are multiple fractures in the upper thoracic region. Conversely, progressive kyphosis is rare with fractures at the thoracolumbar region.[311] Anterior wedging that is greater than 50 per cent of the height of the vertebral body allows the middle column to act as a fulcrum, potentially leading to damage to the posterior ligamentous complex.[11, 318] Less commonly, nontraumatic compression fractures manifest both anterior and middle column failure, resulting in fractures with a configuration similar to that of burst fractures, with retropulsed fragments of bone and potential neurologic compromise.[330] Careful analysis of the posterior margin of the vertebral body on CT scans is necessary to exclude middle column involvement in any patient with neurologic deficit.[330, 331] Neurologic deficit with an isolated anterior column injury suggests a concomitant disc herniation.[318, 334]

Middle and lower thoracic compression deformities frequently are encountered in elderly patients, even without a history of major trauma. These deformities may be the

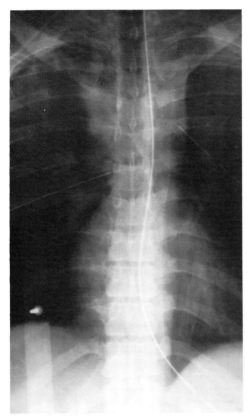

FIGURE 69–46. Mediastinal widening from fracture in the upper thoracic spine. The anteroposterior radiograph shows widening of the mediastinum at the level of the aortic knob and paraspinal hematoma. An aortogram, obtained because of the mediastinal widening, was normal. This patient had a fracture of the T5 vertebral body, which could be detected only by CT scanning. The vertebral fracture and bilateral pneumothoraces were due to a gunshot wound. CT scans revealed no para-aortic hemorrhage; all the soft tissue abnormalities were in the paraspinal region.

"fish vertebra."[335] Fish vertebrae typically are seen at the thoracolumbar or lower lumbar level; the characteristic deformity created by osteoporotic compression fractures in the upper thoracic spine is kyphosis, with anterior collapse or wedging of the vertebral body.[331, 335]

The signal intensity characteristics of an acutely fractured vertebra on MR images are nonspecific, and the compression fracture may be difficult to distinguish from neoplastic tissue. With MR imaging, preservation of normal fatty marrow within the compressed vertebral body is a reliable indicator of a benign fracture that probably is chronic.[337–339] Incomplete replacement of the bone marrow adjacent to the fracture was seen in 14 of 61 vertebral compression fractures, particularly acute fractures.[337] Complete replacement of the bone marrow generally occurs when vertebral compression is related to the presence of skeletal metastasis, although a small proportion of metastases also produce incomplete replacement of the marrow.[337, 338] The distinction between a pathologic and a benign compression fracture is most difficult when the fracture is acute.[337, 339] Traumatic fractures are associated with a higher frequency of disc disruption and fragmentation and a lower frequency of pedicle involvement and large paraspinal masses than are fractures associated with malignant tumors.[337, 338] Both acute benign and pathologic fractures show low signal intensity on T1-weighted MR images and high signal intensity on T2-weighted and short tau (inversion time) inversion recovery (STIR) MR images, but the pattern of increased signal intensity is less homogeneous and less intense in cases of benign fracture[339] (Fig. 69–48). Observing lesions in other, nonfractured vertebrae is the most helpful finding suggesting the presence of underlying neoplastic disease. The marrow signal within the collapsed vertebral body becomes isointense with normal marrow within 1 to 3 months after the injury in the majority of patients.[339] Follow-up MR imaging examinations can be extremely useful in such cases.

Fractures in Children and Adolescents

Upper thoracic fractures in the very young child must be evaluated carefully. This region rarely is traumatized in the young child, so underlying neoplasm, seizures, or child abuse must be considered. Compression fractures of the vertebral bodies, vertebral subluxation, and avulsion fractures of the spinous processes in the thoracic spine are known to occur in abused infants.[340–342] The most common spinal abnormality in the abused child consists of a superior endplate compression fracture, producing notching of the anterior aspect of the vertebral body, associated with mild disc space narrowing.[342] Forceful shaking, resulting in repetitive flexion and extension of the infant's trunk, is the presumed mechanism for the injuries to the vertebral body and spinous process.[341, 342] Other manifestations of child abuse, such as skull and rib fractures, as well as the characteristic metaphyseal fractures, typically are present.[340]

In the older child and adolescent, exaggerated vertebral wedging, vertebral endplate irregularities, Schmorl's nodes, and disc space narrowing are characteristic of Scheuermann's disease. Although numerous theories have been advanced to explain this common condition, the most likely cause of Scheuermann's disease is repetitive traumatic stress to the growing spine.[343, 344] Vertebral wedging in-

consequence of a single fracture due to trivial trauma, multiple separate traumatic events, or slow bone remodeling resulting from ongoing chronic microfractures.[328] Osteoporotic compression fractures are either solitary or disseminated; diffuse deformity involving all the vertebral bodies equally is more common in osteomalacia than in osteoporosis.[335] Solitary compression fractures related to osteoporosis are uncommon above the seventh thoracic vertebra.[331] Identification of an isolated compression fracture in the high thoracic region suggests a cause other than simple osteoporosis.[331] Compression fractures of the upper thoracic spine have been described in nonosteoporotic patients with seizures.[333] These fractures are most common at T4, T5, and T6 and frequently involve multiple vertebral bodies.[333]

Distinction of benign compression fractures from pathologic fractures can be very difficult. Radiographs, CT scans, and MR images all can be used to determine the cause of nontraumatic fractures. The typical deformity of the vertebral endplates in osteoporotic compression fractures consists either of anterior wedging, diffuse compression, or central compression with smooth, diffuse concavity of the upper or lower endplate.[8, 331, 332, 336] The vertebral endplate remains well defined, and the osseous trabeculae are thin, linear, and vertical. Biconcavity caused by depression of both the upper and the lower endplates has been termed

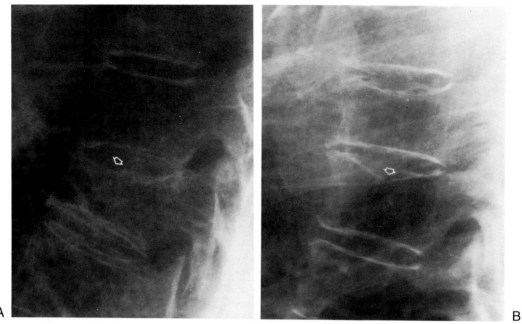

FIGURE 69–47. Compression fractures.

A The lateral radiograph reveals compression of the anterior and middle portions of the superior endplate (open arrow) with loss of height of the vertebral body anteriorly.

B A central compression fracture of the seventh thoracic vertebral body produces a central deformity (open arrow) of the superior endplate with preservation of height of the vertebral body anteriorly and posteriorly.

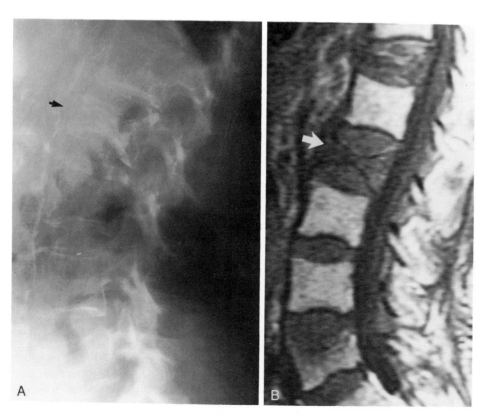

FIGURE 69–48. Osteoporosis with compression fractures.

A The lateral radiograph in this elderly osteoporotic woman demonstrates compression fractures of the L2 vertebral body (arrow) and the superior endplate of L5.

B Sagittal T1-weighted (TR/TE, 600/20) spin echo MR image shows diffuse loss of marrow signal intensity at the T12 and L2 levels (arrow). The L5 vertebral body shows normal fat signal intensity at its inferior aspect. Biopsy of the L2 vertebral body revealed a healing fracture, and the patient had no evidence of malignancy at long-term follow-up.

creases in frequency with duration of competitive waterski jumping, which is one cause of repetitive axial loading, the force implicated most frequently in the development of Scheuermann's spondylodystrophy.[344]

Kümmell's Disease

Kümmell's disease is a form of delayed, posttraumatic collapse of the vertebral body. In 1891, Kümmell reported a delayed posttraumatic vertebral collapse that occurred weeks or even months after an injury.[345] Many underlying mechanisms, including traumatic, nutritional, vasomotor, and neurologic, have been suggested as causative factors.[345] At present, the most widely accepted mechanism for Kümmell's disease is osteonecrosis.[345–347] In 1978, Maldague and coworkers noted the association between vertebral body ischemia and the presence of gas within the vertebral body, also known as the intravertebral vacuum cleft.[346] These authors suggested that the basis for Kümmell's disease may be ischemia associated with the episode of trauma, which leads to osteonecrosis and delayed collapse of the vertebral body. Although Kümmell himself did not note the vacuum cleft sign, evidence exists that osteonecrosis probably is the mechanism accounting for delayed posttraumatic vertebral collapse. Almost all reported cases of intravertebral vacuum clefts occur in noninfectious and non-neoplastic conditions.[347, 348]

The typical vacuum cleft appears as a transverse radiolucent line seen in the centrum of the collapsed vertebral body or adjacent to one of its endplates.[346, 347] The vacuum cleft is exaggerated by spinal extension, particularly in the lateral decubitus position, and diminishes with spinal flexion and prolonged supine positioning.[347] On CT scans, the gas collection may appear more inhomogeneous and irregular than it does on plain films.[347] On MR images, gas is of low signal intensity on all sequences, with magnetic inhomogeneity effects evident on gradient echo images. The typical MR imaging appearance of vertebral osteonecrosis is not that of gas within the cleft, however.[347, 349] Rather, prolonged supine positioning may lead to displacement of the gas by fluid, resulting in high signal intensity within the cleft on T2-weighted images[347, 349] (Fig. 69–49). This thin linear horizontal collection of high signal intensity located centrally within the vertebral body appears to be specific for vertebral osteonecrosis.

Fracture-Dislocations

Complex fracture-dislocations of the upper thoracic spine are more difficult to categorize mechanistically than those of the cervical or thoracolumbar spine because the injuring forces typically are complex. Fracture-dislocation is an unstable injury usually resulting from a combination of hyperflexion and axial loading of the vertebrae, combined with ligamentous disruption by rotatory and shear forces.[8, 310, 318]

Denis described 67 cases of fracture-dislocation involving the thoracic and lumbar spine; of these, 21 (31 per cent) occurred in the upper thoracic region.[8] In comparison to the spinal distribution of compression, burst, and seat-belt injuries, a disproportionate number of fracture-dislocations occur in the high thoracic region.[8, 314] Denis subdivided these injuries into three types according to the predominant mechanism: flexion-rotation, flexion-shear, and flexion-distraction.[8]

These severe injuries are associated with a very high rate of neurologic injury. Most injuries resulting in complete

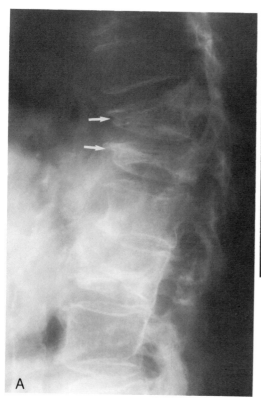
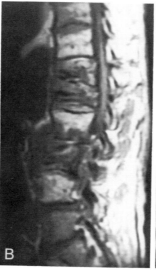
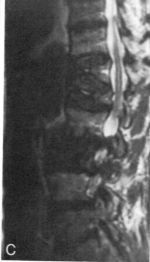

FIGURE 69–49. Kümmell's disease.

A The lateral radiograph illustrates multiple thoracic and lumbar compression fractures. Horizontal collections of gas are present within the T12 and L1 vertebral bodies (arrows), indicating osteonecrosis.

B Sagittal T1-weighted (TR/TE, 500/12) spin echo MR image shows loss of marrow signal intensity in the fractured vertebral bodies.

C Sagittal T2-weighted (TR/TE, 3600/96) fast spin echo MR image shows high signal intensity within the areas of osteonecrosis, presumably due to collection of fluid within the defects.

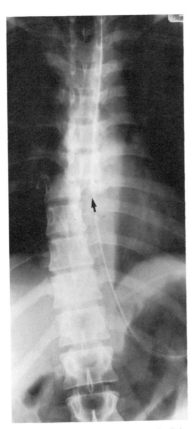

FIGURE 69–50. Thoracic fracture-dislocation. A dislocation is present at the T7-T8 spinal level with lateral displacement and telescoping of the spine at the injured level. The T8 vertebral body has an oblique fracture within its substance. A small portion of the left T8 vertebral centrum (arrow) remains aligned with T7.

paraplegia occur in the middorsal spine, with the majority located at the T3 to T8 levels[310, 316] (Fig. 69–50). The combination of the severe force necessary to cause vertebral injury and the relatively small cross-sectional area of the spinal canal in the upper thoracic spine makes this area particularly vulnerable to spinal cord damage.[317, 318] Approximately 80 per cent of patients with upper thoracic burst fractures, sagittal slice injuries, or anterior dislocations develop paraplegia as a result of their injury.[313] A large proportion, up to 85 per cent, of patients with a neurologic deficit secondary to upper thoracic injury develop complete paraplegia.[313, 315] Irrespective of the type of surgical or nonsurgical treatment, none of the 149 patients reported by Bohlman and coworkers who initially sustained complete paraplegia showed any recovery of neurologic function.[315] Patients who develop an incomplete neurologic lesion may recover function partially, with the best results seen in surgically treated patients with compressive lesions.[315] The most common incomplete cord injury is the anterior cord syndrome; less common incomplete injuries include the central cord syndrome and the Brown-Séquard syndrome of hemiparesis and sensory dissociation.[313] Rarely, thoracic spine translocation occurs without the development of a neurologic deficit.[350–352] It has been suggested that the mechanism of spinal cord sparing in these patients is separation of the vertebral body from the posterior elements. Bilateral fractures through the pedicles at multiple levels allow the vertebral bodies to become displaced while relative integrity is maintained posteriorly.[317, 350, 352] The use of

CT scanning helps to delineate the fracture pattern in such cases, showing bilateral pedicle fractures at the level of the displaced vertebral body, which permits the posterior elements and spinal cord to maintain longitudinal continuity.[351]

Unfortunately, most patients with an upper thoracic fracture-dislocation develop an intrinsic cord lesion or severe cord compression. The typical injury produced by this combination is a fracture-dislocation involving two adjacent vertebrae and all the intervening soft tissues. A predominantly osseous or a mixture of osseous and soft tissue injuries may be evident; pure soft tissue injury disrupting all three columns is rare.[8] The more superior vertebral body may show a variety of fractures, with avulsion fractures of its inferior margin being most common. The superior vertebra is subluxated anteriorly with respect to the inferior vertebra; the average displacement is 8 mm. Facet joint disruption, fractures of the lamina of the superior vertebra, fractures of the superior facet of the inferior vertebra, and a compression fracture of the superior endplate of the inferior vertebra also are present typically.[310] The intervening disc and interspinous ligaments are disrupted, and the disc may be herniated.[318] Rotational deformity, manifested by rotatory malalignment of the pedicles and spinous process above and below the injury, also may be seen[8, 310] (Fig. 69–51). A less common variant of upper thoracic fracture-dislocation, seen in 17 of 218 patients reported by Bohlman and colleagues, is the sagittal slice fracture.[313] This injury

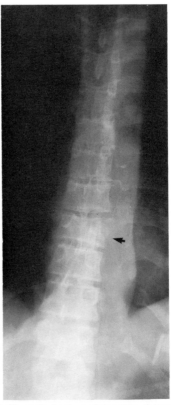

FIGURE 69–51. Thoracic fracture-dislocation. A large paravertebral hematoma is present, and the T9 vertebral body is fractured (arrow). A subtle lateral translocation of the T8 vertebral body to the left relative to T9 is seen. The vertical distance between the pedicles of the eighth and ninth thoracic vertebrae on the left also is increased, indicating disruption of the posterior column. Note the multiple costotransverse dislocations on the left side associated with this rotational injury. The patient was paraplegic immediately after this injury.

occurs when the superior vertebra slices the inferior vertebra in the sagittal plane, with inferior and lateral displacement of the superior vertebral body, resulting in telescoping of the spine.[313, 318] All three columns are disrupted, and the injury is associated with severe neurologic deficit.[318]

Conventional tomography, CT scanning, and MR imaging can be used for additional evaluation of these complex injuries. In the author's experience, the malalignment and degree of displacement are assessed more readily using conventional tomography or MR imaging. CT scanning is superior in the identification of fractures of the posterior elements and in the determination of the extent of encroachment on the spinal canal by displaced bone fragments. Sagittal and coronal reconstructions of the transaxial CT data frequently are necessary for accurate delineation of bone displacement. MR imaging is the method of choice for evaluation of the spinal cord, which frequently is injured in association with upper thoracic injuries.

THORACOLUMBAR SPINE

General Considerations

The thoracolumbar junction is one of the most commonly injured areas of the spine. The region is particularly vulnerable because of its wide range of motion, an orientation of the facet joints that changes from a sagittal to a coronal plane, the absence of significant adjacent supporting structures, such as the rib cage or psoas muscles, and the ability to straighten this spinal segment voluntarily.[52, 353] Unlike the cervical and lumbar regions of the spine, in the thoracolumbar region extension or lordosis is limited; most injuries in this region are secondary to pure flexion or to flexion combined with compression, rotatory, or distraction forces.[2, 3, 8, 20] Spinal flexion results in distraction forces posteriorly and compression forces anteriorly. The pattern of osseous and ligamentous failure depends on the direction and magnitude of the injuring force and the location of its fulcrum of motion.[7, 8, 11, 12, 37]

Numerous classification systems are employed to categorize thoracolumbar injuries; the most widely used are those developed by Denis, Ferguson and Allen, and McAfee and associates.[8, 11, 12] Denis has classified major injuries of the thoracolumbar region into four types[8, 23] (Table 69–2). The first type is the compression fracture, resulting from hyperflexion with compression of only the anterior column and with an intact middle column[8]; the majority of these fractures are associated with a normal posterior column as well. Two subtypes of this injury are described, anterior compression and lateral compression, with the former being eight times more common.[8] In severe anterior compressive injuries, partial failure of the posterior column

related to tension may be present.[8] The second category of major injury, according to Denis, is the burst fracture, characterized by failure of both the anterior and middle columns in compression.[8] The posterior column remains intact functionally, although fractures of the lamina and splaying of the facet joints often are present. Denis' third major category, seat-belt type injuries, represents those injuries in which both the middle and posterior columns fail in tension as a result of spinal flexion and, in some cases, additional distraction.[8] The anterior column may fail partially owing to compression, but the anterior longitudinal ligament maintains its ability to act as a "hinge."[8] The last category in the Denis classification of major injuries is the fracture-dislocation. In this injury, all three columns are disrupted owing to a combination of compression, tension, rotation, and shear.[8] The spine is free to subluxate or dislocate, although radiographs may show little malalignment in the resting position.[8] Most patients with this injury will demonstrate vertebral subluxation or dislocation at the time of their initial presentation. Malalignment in the sagittal, coronal, or transaxial plane may be translational or rotatory.

Ferguson and Allen also developed a classification system for thoracolumbar fractures based on a three column model of the spine.[11] In this classification system, the anterior, middle, and posterior elements (they do not use the term column) are identical to those described as columns by Denis, except that the anterior two thirds of the vertebral body, rather than only the anterior one half, is included in the anterior column.[8, 11] This system also classifies spinal injuries into minor and major groups and then further subdivides major injuries into seven categories on the basis of their presumed mechanism. These classification categories are (1) compressive flexion, (2) distractive flexion, (3) lateral flexion, (4) translation, (5) torsional flexion, (6) vertical compression, and (7) distractive extension.[11] The most common pattern is compressive flexion, which constituted 46 per cent of fractures in Ferguson and Allen's series.[11] This injury can result in three distinctive patterns of abnormality. The first, which is a mild injury, is a compression fracture limited to the anterior column. With more extensive injury, the fracture of the anterior column is associated with ligamentous disruption in the posterior column, producing widening between the spinous processes and facet malalignment. With even greater force, the middle column is disrupted in tension and fragments of bone rotate into the spinal canal.[11] This appearance mimics that associated with middle column failure in compression, but there is no loss of height of the posterior portion of the vertebral body in the compressive flexion injury.[11] Vertical compression produces failure of both the anterior and middle columns and is associated with loss of height of the posterior portion of the vertebral body.[11] The posterior elements may be frac-

TABLE 69–2. Major Fractures and Dislocations of the Thoracolumbar Spine*

Type of Injury	Site of Injury		
	Anterior Column	Middle Column	Posterior Column
Compression fractures	Compression	None	None or distraction
Burst fracture	Compression	Compression	None
Seat-belt injury	None or compression	Distraction	Distraction
Fracture-dislocation	Compression, rotation, shear	Distraction, rotation, shear	Distraction, rotation, shear

*From Denis F: Spine 8:817, 1983.

tured, but there is no ligamentous injury. Although Ferguson and Allen distinguish the type 3 compressive flexion injury from a burst fracture related to compressive loading, the distinction may be difficult radiographically.[11] With CT scanning, retropulsed bone is present in both and often it is difficult to distinguish between these injuries.

The distractive flexion category described by Ferguson and Allen[11] is identical to Denis' seat-belt type injury. Lateral flexion results in compression failure of the vertebral bodies and of the posterior elements on one side. This injury may be limited to the anterior and middle elements or involve all three elements. Lateral bending and unilateral arch fractures suggest this mechanism of injury. Translational injuries produce pure displacement of the vertebral body anteriorly, posteriorly, or laterally.[11] All three spinal elements are disrupted. Torsional flexion produces predominantly ligamentous injury, combined with fractures of the articular processes, vertebral dislocation, and a horizontal slice fracture of the superior vertebral body.[11] Hyperextension injuries of the thoracolumbar region are extremely rare.[11] Denis does not include a comparable category of injury in his classification system.

The classification system developed by McAfee and colleagues was based on the findings in 100 patients with thoracic or thoracolumbar injury.[12] It divides injuries into six categories: (1) wedge compression fracture, (2) stable burst fracture, (3) unstable burst fracture, (4) Chance fracture, (5) flexion distraction injury, and (6) translational injury.[12] As in Denis' and Ferguson and Allen's systems, the McAfee classification is based on a three column spine and divides injuries according to the presence or absence of failure and mechanism of failure of each column. In all three classification systems, the most important feature is the mode of failure, if any, of the middle column. The three classification systems are all comprehensive, and considerable overlap occurs among them in the categories of injury.

Supine anteroposterior and crosstable lateral radiographs constitute an adequate screening examination for the thoracolumbar region in the setting of trauma. Collimated coned views centered on the thoracolumbar region can be very helpful because this area is not well seen in the conventional thoracic and lumbar projections. Most injuries to the thoracolumbar region produce kyphosis, which often is reduced in the supine position. Meticulous attention to osseous alignment is necessary as many unstable injuries of the spine are associated with a nearly normal alignment on supine radiographs. The author does not obtain oblique views of the thoracolumbar region in trauma patients routinely, but these projections may be added for characterization of injuries that are detected on the initial screening views. Radiographs obtained with the patient erect or with flexion of the spine may accentuate the kyphotic deformity and may be obtained when a ligamentous injury is suspected.

Soft tissue alterations due to thoracolumbar injuries, unlike injuries of the upper thoracic spine, characteristically are absent on conventional radiographs. Although displacement of paraspinal soft tissues is present in almost all patients with upper thoracic fractures, fewer than 25 per cent of patients with injuries at the level of T12 or below manifest widening of the paraspinal line.[324] Loss of the fat stripe along the lateral border of the psoas muscle has been advocated as a sensitive indicator of thoracolumbar injury.[324]

In practice, soft tissue alterations are not sufficiently sensitive to be of much assistance in the evaluation of thoracolumbar injuries.

Compression Fractures

The thoracolumbar region is the most common site of traumatic compression fractures, and it also is a major site of fractures resulting from trivial injury in persons with osteoporosis. In large series of traumatic compression fractures, the most common sites of involvement are L1 and L2, followed in frequency by T12, T7, and L3.[8, 311] Between 49 and 65 per cent of traumatic compression fractures occur between T12 and L2.[8, 308] Among osteoporotic compression fractures, a large proportion involve the thoracolumbar region, although the midthoracic region shows a slightly higher prevalence of compression deformities.[331, 332]

These fractures are related to flexion with the fulcrum of flexion located within the vertebral body. The typical thoracolumbar compression fracture results in loss of height of the anterior vertebral body with preservation of the middle and posterior spinal columns.[8, 10] In severe compression fractures, partial or complete posterior ligamentous injury may be present.[8, 11] The usual treatment for these injuries is conservative. Progressive kyphosis is unusual after thoracolumbar compression fractures in the nonosteoporotic person.[20, 311] Vertebral compression that leads to loss of more than 40 per cent of the height of the anterior portion of the vertebral body often requires posterior stabilization, even in the absence of neurologic deficit, to prevent progressive spinal deformity.[313] Compression of 60 to 100 per cent of this vertebral height may require more aggressive management owing to the potential for secondary postural deformity.[20]

Loss of height of the anterior portion of the vertebral body is the most common radiographic finding. In uncomplicated vertebral body fractures, the intervertebral disc remains intact, and no disc space loss is apparent. Isolated central endplate fractures may develop without loss of vertebral height if the force is directed vertically, resulting in displacement of disc material into the vertebral body.[354] These fractures are the equivalent of an acute traumatic Schmorl's node and are manifested as loss of height of the intervertebral disc at the level of the fracture. On CT scans, compression fractures of the thoracolumbar region can be recognized by the presence of an arc of irregular bony fragments displaced circumferentially from the vertebral body.[355, 356] The posterior vertebral wall remains intact, and no retropulsed fragments of bone are present (Fig. 69–52). Fracture lines involving the vertebral body typically involve only its superior aspect, with normal bone seen below the level of the pedicles. The normal vertebral venous channels should not be confused with fracture lines extending into the posterior vertebral margin, which suggest a serious injury.[357]

Burst Fractures

Axial loading or compression of the vertebral body, usually combined with flexion, produces the commonly seen burst fracture.[2, 8, 10, 11, 353, 358] Burst fractures represent 1.5 per cent of all spinal fractures and 14 per cent of thoracolumbar injuries.[8, 353] The peak site of spinal burst fractures is the

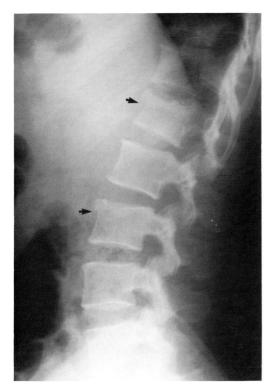

FIGURE 69–52. Compression fractures. Compression fractures are present in the superior endplates of the L1 and L3 vertebral bodies (arrows) with loss of height anteriorly. Note the preservation of height and normal contour of the posterior margins of the vertebral bodies at these levels.

thoracolumbar junction, with T12, L1, and L2 being the most common levels that are involved.[8, 354, 359, 360] The majority of such fractures are associated with neurologic deficit.[359, 360] Neurologic deficit at the time of presentation is seen in 40 to 47.5 per cent of patients with burst fractures.[8, 52] The burst fracture was first named by Holdsworth in 1963, who characterized it as follows: "the body is shattered from within outward."[2, 10] Holdsworth noted that the burst fracture can occur only in the spinal segments with the ability to straighten—namely, the cervical and thoracolumbar regions.[2, 10] Willen and colleagues reported the first experimental production of the burst fracture in 1984[361]; isolated preparations of the vertebral motion segment of L1 that were exposed to an instant dynamic axial force revealed a classic burst fracture, and laxity of the facet joints and an increased range of flexion and extension in the fractured specimens suggested instability.[361]

Characteristic components of this injury are centripetal disruption, increased sagittal diameter, moderate to marked anterior wedging of the vertebral body, unilateral or bilateral laminar fractures, an increased interpediculate distance, involvement of the inferior endplate, and narrowing of the spinal canal related to retropulsion of the posterosuperior portion of the vertebral body.[8, 11, 334, 360, 362] This same pattern of injury has been designated the "crush-cleavage" fracture by other authors.[363] Radiographic and pathologic findings in experimental specimens demonstrate disruption of the intervertebral discs above and below the fracture.[104, 358, 362, 363]

Denis has subclassified burst fractures into five types. Type A fractures result from pure axial load, are manifested by comminution of both the superior and inferior endplates,

and typically occur in the lower lumbar region.[8, 104] This type of fracture is associated with ligamentous preservation, and the extent of retropulsion of bone fragments is less than that in the other types of burst fractures, typically leading to 20 to 50 per cent narrowing of the spinal canal.[104] Type B fractures characteristically occur at the thoracolumbar junction. This subtype of injury is characterized by comminution of only the superior endplate, with frequent coalescence of the fracture lines into a single sagittal fracture that extends into the inferior endplate. Type B injuries are most common, representing 49.2 per cent of all burst fractures in Denis' series.[8] Their mechanism of injury is a combination of axial compression and flexion.[8] Neuropathologic examination of type B injuries demonstrates partial or total rupture of the posterior longitudinal ligament in cases in which large bone fragments are displaced into the spinal canal.[104] Type C (fracture limited to the inferior endplate), type D (burst-rotation injuries), and type E (burst–lateral flexion injuries) patterns of injury are uncommon and together represent only 27 per cent of all burst fractures.[8]

It is essential to differentiate the burst fracture from the more common simple compression fracture because of the potential for spinal instability and compromise of the neural canal in the former. Anterior vertebral wedging can be pronounced in either injury. In burst fractures the average degree of wedging of the anterior portion of the vertebral body is 28 to 47 per cent and does not differ significantly from that seen with compression fractures.[359, 360, 364] Such prominent anterior wedging may lead to a misdiagnosis of an anterior column compression fracture unless careful attention is paid to the integrity of the posterior vertebral margin and posterior elements. Ballock and colleagues have suggested that up to 20 per cent of burst fractures are misdiagnosed as compression fractures on the basis of a review of plain films.[364] It is likely that, prior to the introduction of CT scanning, many burst fractures were misdiagnosed as simple compression fractures that later developed kyphosis and led to neurologic deficit.[365]

Careful evaluation of the posterior margin of the vertebral body usually allows accurate differentiation of these two injuries.[360, 366] The posterior aspect of the normal vertebral body is seen clearly on a well-penetrated, nonrotated lateral view. The posterior cortical line is continuous except in the center of the vertebral body, where it is interrupted by the entry of the nutrient vessels.[366] Disruption, displacement, or rotation of this line indicates disruption of the middle spinal column[366] (Fig. 69–53). All 114 patients with burst fractures reported by Daffner and coworkers had some abnormality of the posterior vertebral margin that was related to the presence of retropulsed bone fragments.[366] Posterior displacement of such fragments is the most common and characteristic finding, occurring in 77 of 114 patients with burst fractures in one series.[366] Loss of height of the posterior aspect of the vertebral body is present in about 60 per cent of patients and allows differentiation of a burst fracture from a compression fracture limited to the anterior column.[8, 23, 364] Ferguson and Allen divide injuries producing retropulsed bone fragments into two major types.[11] One type, identical to that proposed by Denis, is compressive failure of the anterior and middle columns. The other type, the type 3 compressive flexion injury, produces compres-

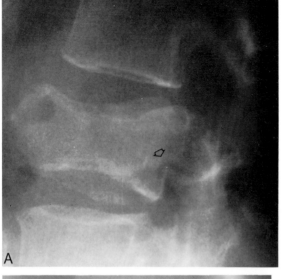

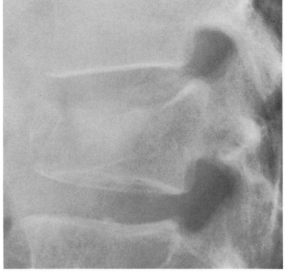

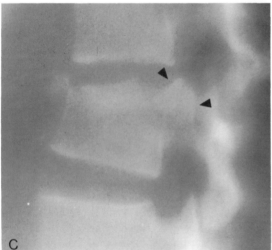

FIGURE 69–53. Thoracolumbar burst fractures.

A The lateral radiograph reveals loss of height of the vertebral body with involvement of the cortex both anteriorly and posteriorly (open arrow).

B A similar fracture pattern in a different patient illustrates loss of height of the vertebral body posteriorly and loss of definition of the posterior margin of the vertebral body due to retropulsed bone.

C A lateral conventional tomogram in a patient with a burst fracture shows the triangular configuration of the retropulsed fragment (arrowheads).

sive failure of the anterior column, tensile failure of the middle column, and tensile failure of the posterior column. Retropulsed bone fragments are seen with both types of major injury, but loss of the posterior height of the vertebral body is seen only when the middle element fails in compression.[11] The retropulsed bone fragment in burst fractures characteristically arises from the posterosuperior corner of the fractured vertebral body superior to the basivertebral foramen.[367, 368] On lateral views, the fragment often is triangular, with its sides formed by the posterior part of the superior endplate, the superior part of the posterior vertebral margin, and the fracture line itself.[367] The retropulsed fragment frequently is comminuted and displaced cranially or caudally by 3 to 8 mm and posteriorly by 2 to 4 mm.[367] Rotation of the fragment may occur such that its superior cortex is facing anteriorly and its posterior cortex is directed superiorly[367–369] (Fig. 69–54). Using CT, Guerra and associates noted rotation of the retropulsed fragment in 30 per cent of patients with burst fractures.[368] This rotation exceeds that produced by endplate depression and angulation and leads to abnormal visualization of a radiodense cortical line at the anterior aspect of the retropulsed fragment.[368, 369]

Posterior element fractures are seen in 50 to 100 per cent of patients with burst fractures.[52, 355, 359, 360, 363] The facet joints normally absorb up to one third of the total force during axial loading, depending on the degree of spinal extension.[361, 370] When the compressive force exceeds the loading capacity of the facet joints, posterior element fractures develop. Typical fractures of the posterior elements associated with burst fractures include vertical fractures of one or both laminae and the spinous process.[8, 52, 360] The laminar fractures may be of the incomplete greenstick variety, with cortical disruption limited to the anterior laminar cortex.[8] Associated dural laceration with entrapment of neural elements within the fracture fragments may develop in patients with laminar fractures.[52, 359] Dural laceration was noted in 11 of 60 patients with burst fractures in one series and was associated with an increased frequency of neurologic deficit.[359]

Posterior element fractures often are difficult to identify on conventional radiographs. A higher rate of posterior element fractures is reported in studies using CT scanning than in those limited to plain film examination. In Willen and associates' series, only 67 per cent of posterior arch fractures seen on CT scans were identified on the radiographs.[104] When the fracture lines are not visible, an abnor-

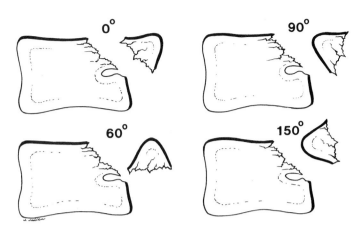

FIGURE 69–54. Burst fracture: Rotation of retropulsed fragment. Diagrammatic representation of how anterior rotation affects the orientation of the bone margins of the retropulsed bone fragment. If the fragment is simply retropulsed without rotating (0 degrees), the transaxial CT scan will demonstrate the posterior cortical margin oriented posteriorly. Rotation of less than 90 degrees results in one bone margin facing anteriorly and one facing posteriorly. Rotation of 90 degrees demonstrates one bone margin directed anteriorly. Greater degrees of rotation are uncommon. (From Guerra J Jr, et al: Radiology *153*:769, 1984.)

mally wide interpediculate distance may be the only indicator of posterior element disruption.[52, 360] This distance is measured as the smallest distance between the inner margins of the two pedicles at a single vertebral level. A retrospective review of 107 fractured thoracic and lumbar vertebrae found that the interpediculate distance could be measured accurately in 96 per cent of patients.[365, 371] Normally, the interpediculate distance increases gradually from the T6 spinal level caudally. In the thoracic region, comparison of measurements made at the injured level with those obtained at both adjacent levels is recommended.[371] As the vertebral foramen is a bony ring and, therefore, at least two fractures are necessary to produce significant widening,[368] an interpediculate distance greater than 2 or 3 mm more than that at the adjacent levels is a highly accurate indicator of a posterior arch fracture.[24, 360, 371] The mean value for interpediculate distance in cases of burst fracture is increased by 25 per cent[359] (Fig. 69–55). However, such widening is not present in all cases; in one series, only 55 per cent of burst fractures had an abnormally wide interpediculate distance.[364]

Some authors suggest that posterior element fractures are correlated with the presence of neurologic compromise.[52, 359] Other investigators have not noted an association between neurologic deficit and posterior element disruption.[367, 370] It likewise is controversial whether the presence of posterior element fractures always implies potential instability. Holdsworth considered all burst fractures to have intact posterior ligaments and to be stable.[10] Whitesides divided burst fractures into stable and unstable categories, based on the presence of failure of osseous or ligamentous elements, or of both, in the posterior complex.[20] Denis considered all burst fractures to be unstable because of the potential for mechanical or neurologic deterioration, even if no neurologic deficit is present at the time of presentation.[8] McAfee and associates considered most burst fractures of the thoracolumbar junction to be stable injuries.[370] McAfee and collaborators outlined five features of burst fractures that indicated instability.[370] These features are (1) progressive neurologic deficit, (2) posterior element disruption, (3) kyphosis that progresses 20 degrees or more in the presence of a neurologic deficit, (4) loss of height of the vertebral body of more than 50 per cent with facet joint subluxation, and (5) retropulsed bone fragments detectable on CT scans in the presence of an incomplete neurologic injury.[370]

CT scanning is the optimal method for identifying the

presence of posterior element fractures and retropulsed bone fragments, features not present in simple compression fractures (Fig. 69–56). The failure of the posterior vertebral wall usually is readily apparent. In some cases, particularly when a small fragment is impacted between the pedicles, the fracture lines may not be apparent, however, and only subtle flattening of the posterior vertebral margin is seen.[355] With CT, the degree of narrowing of the spinal canal produced by retropulsed bone fragments can be quantitated in the preoperative and immediate postoperative periods. In the preoperative patient, narrowing of the spinal canal ranges from 31 to 87 per cent, averaging approximately 55 to 60 per cent.[8, 353, 358, 360] On the basis of autopsy data from patients with burst fractures, Willen and colleagues have noted that when the canal is narrowed by more than 50 per cent, disruption of the posterior longitudinal ligament is present[104] (Fig. 69–57).

Many attempts have been made to correlate the degree of canal narrowing with the extent of neurologic impairment. Some authors have found no such correlation.[52, 353, 356, 363] Other investigators have suggested that a threshold value for the degree of narrowing exists which, if not reached, makes neurologic compromise unlikely.[8] Denis found a higher rate of neurologic compromise in patients in whom the spinal canal was narrowed by more than 50 per cent, but he found no significant correlation between quantitative measurement of narrowing and the extent of neurologic deficit.[8] Fortijne and coworkers found a significant association between the percentage of narrowing of the sagittal diameter of the spinal canal and the presence or absence of a neurologic deficit. The correlation between sagittal stenosis and neurologic deficit was highest for injuries in the thoracolumbar and lumbar levels; only a weak association was seen in cases of injury of upper thoracic vertebrae.[372] At the thoracolumbar level, these investigators found a probability of neurologic deficit of 0.29, 0.51, and 0.71 for cases in which 25 per cent, 50 per cent, and 75 per cent stenosis was evident, respectively.[372] Although the extent of canal stenosis predicted the likelihood of a neurologic deficit, no association of such stenosis was found with the severity of that deficit.[372] This lack of association is not surprising given the potential discrepancy between the position of the bone fragment at the time of maximal impact and its resting position.[12, 14, 353]

A variety of methods of treatment are used for the management of thoracolumbar burst fractures. The primary goal

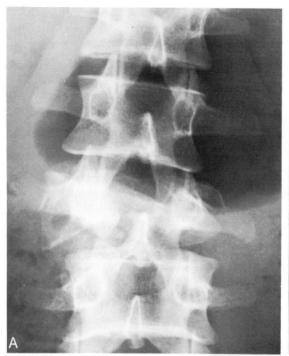

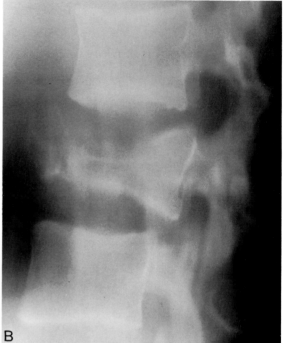

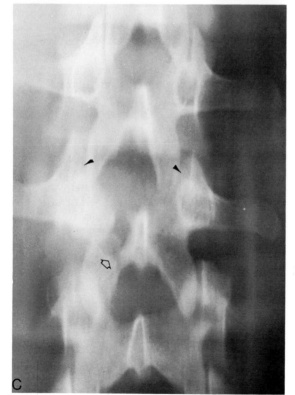

FIGURE 69–55. Burst fracture.

A The frontal radiograph shows loss of height of the vertebral body and widening of the interpediculate distance.

B Conventional tomography in the lateral projection better defines the vertebral deformity and posterior displacement of a portion of the vertebral body into the spinal canal.

C Conventional tomography in the frontal projection confirms widening of the interpediculate distance, splaying of the posterior joints (arrowheads), and a fracture of the lamina (open arrow).

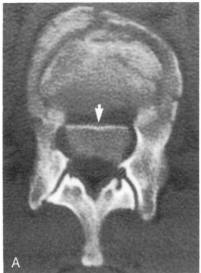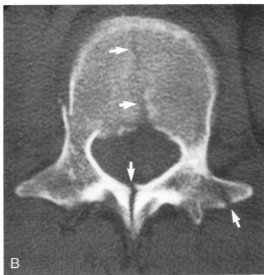

FIGURE 69–56. Burst fracture: CT scanning.

A A transaxial CT scan through the superior aspect of the L3 vertebral body shows comminution of the superior endplate and a large fragment of retropulsed bone within the spinal canal. Note the rotation of the fragment, with the superior cortex (arrow) directed anteriorly.

B A more caudal image shows sagittal fracture lines involving the left transverse process, spinous process, and inferior aspect of the vertebral body (arrows).

of surgery is spinal canal decompression and reduction and stabilization of malaligned vertebrae.[20, 373–375] Conservative therapy with postural reduction and immobilization was the mainstay of therapy prior to the development of distraction rodding.[108, 373, 375] Follow-up CT scans in patients treated conservatively demonstrate spontaneous resolution of spinal stenosis as a consequence of resorption of bone fragments and slowly progressive osseous remodeling in a significant proportion of patients.[376, 377] Laminectomy alone is unsuccessful in decompressing the spinal canal and increases the likelihood of kyphotic instability at the site of injury.[20, 313, 365, 369, 378] Distraction rodding tends to correct vertebral malalignment and improves the degree of posttraumatic defor-

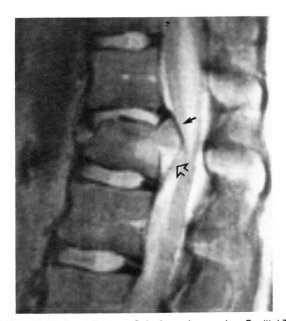

FIGURE 69–57. Burst fracture: Spinal canal narrowing. Sagittal T2-weighted (TR/TE, 1500/60) spin echo MR image shows spinal canal stenosis of more than 50 per cent owing to a large, rotated, retropulsed bone fragment (solid arrow). Note the stripping of the posterior longitudinal ligament from the posterior margin of the vertebral body (open arrow).

mity.[358, 365, 374, 375] After distraction rodding the midsagittal diameter and cross-sectional area of the spinal canal remain diminished by an average of 14 to 29 per cent (range, zero to 55 per cent).[353, 358, 375] Reduction tends to be best with early surgical intervention, preferably within 3 days of the injury.[22, 358] Anterior decompression via a retroperitoneal approach has been advocated as a superior method for decompression.[313, 365, 369, 373] The degree of neurologic recovery in patients with incomplete injuries appears to be improved when this technique was employed; in one report 37 of 42 patients who underwent anterior decompression showed improvement by least one class in motor strength.[373]

Despite image degradation by metal artifact, CT scanning and MR imaging can provide useful information in patients with residual neurologic deficit or pain in the postoperative period. The most common abnormality seen in such patients is the presence of residual bone fragments or exuberant callus indenting the spinal canal.[379] Delayed spinal stenosis with increased cord compression related to fracture healing with hypertrophic callus and ligamentous calcification may develop 1 year or more after trauma.[12, 380] Superimposed degenerative changes of the disc and apophyseal joints, producing further spinal stenosis, can lead to progressive neurologic deficit.[12] Assessment of the posterior osseous arch, the soft tissue structures within the spinal canal, and the integrity of posterior osseous fusion of the postoperative patient often is rendered difficult on CT scans and MR images owing to metal artifact.[379]

Seat-belt Injuries

The term ''seat-belt injury'' or ''lap-belt injury'' is used widely to refer to a class of major injuries of the thoracolumbar region caused by tensile failure of the vertebral column.[8, 20, 23, 381] The term refers to a variety of osseous and ligamentous injuries caused by hyperflexion and, in some cases, superimposed distraction of the spinal column.[8] Not all patients sustaining injuries of this type are wearing seatbelts at the time of the injury, but the term ''seat-belt injury'' or ''seat-belt fracture'' often is used to describe this entire class of injuries. Such injuries occur most frequently at the thoracolumbar and upper lumbar levels, particularly at L1 or L2, which are involved in the majority of adults.[382, 383] In children restrained by lap-belts, the midlumbar level is injured more frequently than the thoracolumbar region.[35, 381] The explanations postulated for this preferential midlumbar involvement include the child's higher center of gravity, larger ratio of head size to body weight, and iliac crests that are incompletely developed, resulting in a poor fit of the lap-belts, which ride up to the midabdominal level.[35, 381] Typically the passenger sustains this injury, not the driver, who probably is protected by contact with the steering wheel.[382, 384]

The fulcrum of flexion in lap-belt injuries is located anterior to the vertebral body, at the level of the anterior abdominal wall where it abuts on the seat-belt.[382, 384] Denis suggested that the flexion fulcrum in many patients who sustain this injury actually is located at the level of the anterior vertebral column, citing to the frequently mild loss of anterior vertebral height.[8] Hyperflexion in this setting subjects the middle and posterior vertebral columns, or all three columns, to distraction forces.[8] The resulting tensile force can lead to purely osseous, purely ligamentous, or combined bony and soft tissue injuries. Because, in general, ligaments withstand tension better than bone, fractures typically are present, particularly in the posterior elements.[7, 20] These injuries, of which the horizontal Chance fracture is the best known subtype, begin posteriorly and propagate anteriorly.[384]

Combination shoulder-lap belts protect the spine against severe flexion. These seat-belts have been reported to be associated with flexion compression injuries of the cervicothoracic junction and anterolateral wedge compression fractures of a thoracolumbar vertebra, with lateral compression occurring on the side opposite the restrained shoulder.[382, 385] The posterior elements are disrupted by distraction contralateral to the site of anterolateral compression of the vertebral body. These injuries have a good prognosis and a low frequency of neurologic deficit. The postulated mechanism is the "roll-out phenomenon," with flexion and rotation occurring about the axis of the shoulder strap as the unrestrained shoulder continues to move forward.[385] The classic seat-belt injury is not seen in persons wearing combination shoulder-lap belts.

Denis believed that this injury is associated with a functional anterior column that prevents frank vertebral subluxation; although compression failure of the anterior osseous column often is present, the anterior longitudinal ligament maintains its ability to act as a "hinge."[8] This preservation of some mechanical constraint probably explains the low rate of neurologic injury in patients with this type of trauma.[8, 382, 384] However, Denis further considered this injury to be mechanically unstable with spinal flexion, which allows excessive buckling about the anterior column.[8]

Denis subdivided seat-belt injuries into four types, depending on whether the injury involves one or two vertebral levels and on whether the middle column fails at the osseous or ligamentous level.[8] The first type, type A, is similar to the horizontal vertebral fracture described by Chance in 1948,[386] which subsequently was referred to as the "Chance fracture" by Smith and Kaufer in their comprehensive review of 24 patients with spinal trauma resulting from the use of lap-type seat-belts.[382] The type A injury is a single level injury with a horizontal fracture extending through all three osseous columns. Chance described three patients with a fracture characterized by "horizontal splitting of the spine and neural arch, ending in an upward curve which usually reaches the upper surface of the body just in front of the neural foramen."[386] The single example that he illustrated showed osseous disruption of the superior vertebral endplate and anterior vertebral column. Chance thought this injury was due to flexion, but he did not know of any anatomic factors that would explain its orientation, nor did he note any association with the use of seat-belts, which were not widely used when he described this fracture.[386] The type B injury is a purely ligamentous injury with rupture of the spinal ligaments, anulus fibrosus, and intervertebral disc. Types C and D injuries are characterized by involvement of the vertebrae and soft tissue at two adjacent spinal levels. Type C injuries reveal osseous failure of the posterior elements, combined with a fracture of the posterior portion of the vertebral body (middle column) with subsequent extension into the disc anteriorly.[8] Type D injuries are associated with osseous failure of the posterior elements and disruption of the posterior longitudinal ligament and posterior portion of the anulus (middle column) and disc.[8] Type A injuries are most common (47.3 per cent), followed in frequency by types C (26.3 per cent) and D (15.8 per cent) injuries.[8] Type B injuries were the least common, seen in only 10.6 per cent of patients.[8]

The radiographic findings of a seat-belt injury depend on whether the injury is predominantly osseous or soft tissue. In general, distraction at the level of the posterior fracture or sites of ligament disruption, relative preservation of or increase in the height of the vertebral body, and mild focal kyphosis are seen[8, 383, 384] (Fig. 69–58). Posterior ligamentous damage results in interspinous widening, increased height of the intervertebral foramina, and either widening, superior subluxation, perching, or locking of the facet joints.[8, 36, 37, 382] Interspinous widening often is difficult to assess in this region owing to the changing orientation of the spinous processes from a nearly vertical to a horizontal slant and to obscuring of the posterior elements on the lateral view as a result of overlying structures and inadequate x-ray penetration.[324] More than 20 degrees of flexion or more than 10 degrees of lateral bending of the upper lumbar levels (in the absence of a fracture) is possible only when the ligamentous disruption extends anteriorly to the level of the facet joints and posterior portion of the anulus fibrosus.[22] Sufficient angulation may be present to give rise to an "empty" or "vacant" appearance to the vertebral body as a result of cephalad displacement of the posterior elements of the cranial vertebra.[380] If the posterior fibers of the anulus fibrosus are disrupted, widening of the posterior portion of the disc space may be apparent. The characteristic injury seen with this mode of failure is a horizontal fracture extending transversely through the vertebral body, pedicles, and other posterior elements[8, 384, 386] (Fig. 69–59). Careful scrutiny of these structures on the anteroposterior view is recommended because the posterior elements often are obscured on the lateral radiograph.[383] Disruption of the ovoid margin of the pedicle and a horizontal fracture through the transverse margin are easiest to see, although the transverse fracture through the lamina and spinous process also may be visualized on well-exposed radiographs.[383] In some cases, the widened interspinous distance is associated with a small avulsion fracture of one of the spinous

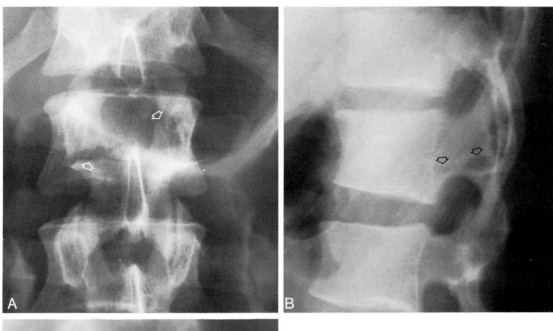

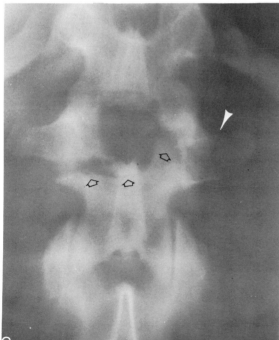

FIGURE 69–58. Seat-belt fracture.

A, B Frontal and lateral radiographs reveal a horizontal fracture (arrows) involving the laminae, articular processes, pedicles, and the posterior portion of the first lumbar vertebral body. Note the widening of the distance between the spinous processes of the T12 and L1 vertebral bodies.

C On a frontal conventional tomogram, the transverse fracture involving the right and left laminae (open arrows) and the left transverse process (arrowhead) is well seen.

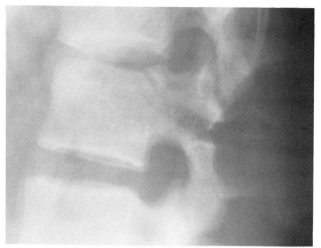

FIGURE 69–59. Seat-belt fracture. A horizontal fracture is seen splitting the pedicle and spinous process of the L2 vertebra. The fracture enters the L1-L2 intervertebral disc space near the posterior margin of the vertebral body.

processes.[23] Similar well-defined avulsion fractures arising from the posteroinferior margin of the vertebral body also may be present.[382] Associated avulsion of the nerve roots related to distraction with subsequent pseudomeningocele formation has been described in association with this injury.[387] The horizontal plane of the fractures often renders them difficult to see with CT scanning, but typically they are evident on good quality sagittal image reconstructions of transaxial CT data.[12] In Taylor and Eggli's review of 365 CT examinations in children assessed for abdominal trauma, all five seat-belt injuries escaped detection on the transaxial CT scans.[381] Indeed, conventional tomography has been recommended for evaluation of these injuries.[8] If concomitant rupture of the anterior spinal ligaments is present, subluxation or dislocation of the vertebral bodies may occur; in this case the injury becomes a fracture-dislocation, rather than a seat-belt injury, and is associated with a much higher rate of neurologic injury.[8, 23, 382] All three patients with neurologic injury as a result of a seat-belt–related spinal injury described by Smith and Kaufer had associated vertebral translation.[382] Both conventional tomography and CT scanning are helpful in the elucidation of the nature of the posterior injury and are essential for the exclusion of posterior element fractures and facet disruption. On CT scans, the normal thoracolumbar facet joints are well visualized. The superior facets are oriented in an anteromedial to posterolateral direction with respect to the vertebral body, are continuous with the pedicles, and have a concave articular surface.[36] The inferior facet normally lies posterior to the superior facet. The inferior facets have a flat or convex articular margin and are continuous with the spinous process.[36] The "naked" facet refers to the appearance of an articular process no longer in contact with its apposing articular facet.[37] This appearance is seen with subluxated and perched facets. Facet malalignment often is easier to appreciate on sagittal and coronal image reconstructions of transaxial CT data.[36, 37, 388]

Fracture-Dislocations

The main characteristic of this severe injury is complete disruption of all three spinal columns, allowing vertebral subluxation and dislocation.[2, 8] Fracture-dislocations account for 10 to 20 per cent of all thoracolumbar injuries; 16 per

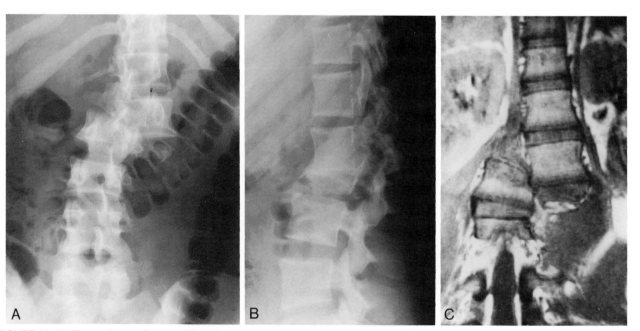

FIGURE 69–60. Thoracolumbar fracture-dislocation.
  A The anteroposterior radiograph demonstrates a fracture-dislocation at the L1-L2 vertebral level. Multiple fractures are present. Severe comminution of the L2 vertebral body and posterior elements on the left is seen. Note the rotational deformity at the level of the dislocation with a change in orientation of the spinous process and pedicle.
  B The lateral view also shows the fractures and rotatory deformity.
  C A coronal T1-weighted (TR/TE, 600/20) spin echo MR image illustrates disruption of the intervening intervertebral disc and shows alteration in signal intensity in the L2 vertebral body as a result of the fractures.

cent of the 412 thoracic and lumbar injuries reported by Denis were of this type.[8, 389] The spinal distribution of fracture-dislocation is bimodal, as with compression fractures, with one peak at the T6-T7 level and a second peak at the thoracolumbar junction.[8] Denis subdivided fracture-dislocations into three types. Type A, which represents the vast majority of these injuries, is caused by a combination of spinal flexion and rotation.[8] The posterior and middle columns fail in tension and rotation, whereas the anterior column fails in compression and rotation. Rotatory stability at the thoracolumbar region is provided largely by the facet joints and ligaments, which are disrupted in this injury.[20] Less common categories of this injury are type B, which is a shearing injury of all three spinal columns, and type C, which is related to severe flexion and distraction, resulting in tensile failure of all three columns.[8] Each of these injuries is associated with a very high rate of neurologic deficit. Indeed, 53 to 93 per cent of patients with vertebral dislocation develop a permanent neurologic deficit, typically complete paraplegia, after their injury.[8, 388, 389]

Many of the radiographic features of fracture-dislocation have been discussed in the section of this chapter dealing with upper thoracic fractures. The major hallmark of these severe injuries is the presence of intervertebral subluxation or dislocation; loss of height of a vertebral body is not a characteristic feature in these injuries.[8, 388] In one series, anterior subluxation averaged one third the width of the vertebral body.[388] Such subluxation is better seen on the lateral view, whereas rotation and lateral translation are seen to better advantage on the anteroposterior projection. Radiographic signs suggestive of rotation injury include slice fractures of the vertebral body, multiple fractures of the ribs or transverse processes, dislocation of the costotransverse joints, unilateral displaced fractures of the articular facets, and rotatory malalignment between the pedicles and spinous processes of vertebrae located above and below the injury[2, 8, 334] (Fig. 69–60). The rotational "slice fracture" is a horizontal fracture involving the superior endplate and a horizontal sliver-like fracture of the vertebral body below the dislocation; the upper vertebra, intervertebral disc, and slice fracture fragment are displaced as a unit, which pivots relative to the caudal vertebra.[2] The interpediculate distance is normal, and the posterior cortex of the vertebral body characteristically remains intact.[388] Radiographic signs suggestive of shear injury include lateral vertebral translation, severely comminuted fractures of the ar-

ticular processes, multiple fractures of the spinous processes, and free-floating laminae.[2, 3, 8]

Vertebral dislocations rarely may be seen in which no fractures of the posterior elements are present.[388] In such cases, the degree of vertebral translation is out of proportion to the extent of disruption of the vertebral body and posterior elements.[388] Rotational malalignment often is seen and may be easier to detect with CT scans than with plain films. In severe dislocations of the spine, two vertebral bodies may be seen in a single CT scan, a finding referred to as the "double vertebrae" sign[388] (Fig. 69–61). Locking of the facet joints due to rotatory or lateral vertebral dislocation can be recognized by careful assessment of the positions of the articulating facets at the injured level on CT scans.[36, 388]

LOWER LUMBAR SPINE

General Considerations

Fractures and dislocations of the lumbar spine below L2 are relatively uncommon. The lower lumbar region is well protected by overlying soft tissues and is relatively immobile. The lumbar vertebrae are bulky and have thicker cortices than the vertebrae in other regions of the spine. Although injuries of the lower lumbar region are less common than those in more mobile spinal regions, fractures, subluxations, and dislocations of the low lumbar region are not uncommon in the setting of severe multisystem trauma. Supine anteroposterior and crosstable lateral radiographs of the lumbar spine usually are obtained in this clinical setting. Coned-down lateral views of the lumbosacral junction can be helpful but usually are not necessary for the assessment of acute trauma. Oblique views also are helpful in the demonstration of the pars interarticularis, but usually they are not obtained in the acutely injured patient.

Fractures and Dislocations

Compression fractures of the lower lumbar spine in patients with osteoporosis are uncommon. When they develop, central endplate compression resembling Schmorl's nodes, rather than anterior vertebral wedging, is seen (Fig. 69–62). Mechanical testing has shown that resistance to collapse is greatest in the lumbar vertebrae owing to the presence of a thick anterior vertebral cortex that resists compression. Preferential central depression of the superior and inferior endplates occurs.[331] Compression fractures involving the anterior column of the lower lumbar spine also are uncommon, representing less than 20 per cent of all acute thoracic and lumbar compression injuries.[8] A disproportionate number of compression injuries in this region are related to lateral, rather than anterior, flexion.[8]

Burst fractures of the lower lumbar vertebrae also are far less common than the same injuries at the thoracolumbar junction. In Denis' series of 59 burst fractures, only 15 occurred below the L2 level.[8] The majority of these were located at L3, with L4 and L5 vertebral bodies rarely manifesting a burst injury. Burst fractures of the L5 vertebral body represented only 1.2 percent of all spinal fractures treated at Southern Illinois University.[390] Three series describing a total of 15 patients with such burst fractures noted deficits of the lumbar motor nerve roots in seven patients and radicular pain or sensory changes with intact

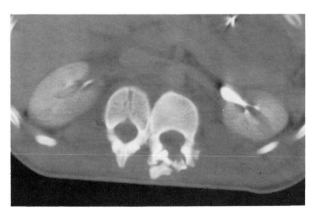

FIGURE 69–61. Thoracolumbar fracture-dislocation. A "double vertebrae" sign is seen on this CT scan.

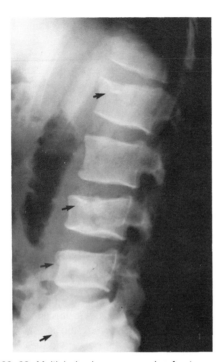

FIGURE 69–62. Multiple lumbar compression fractures. A 23 year old man who had been involved in a motor vehicle accident 1 month previously complained of progressive spinal deformity. The lateral radiograph demonstrates compression deformities of the superior endplate (arrows) of multiple lumbar vertebral bodies. Note the subchondral sclerosis related to partial healing of these subacute injuries. These changes are similar to the deformities seen with Scheuermann's disease.

motor function in three patients; the remaining patients were intact neurologically.[390–392] No relationship was found between the degree of spinal canal compromise and the neurologic status.[390] Unlike the situation with thoracolumbar burst fractures, kyphosis is not seen with low lumbar burst fractures although loss of lordosis may be present.[8, 391] Progressive vertebral collapse and lordosis rarely are seen in patients with low lumbar injury.[390, 392]

Vertebral dislocation is much less common in the lower lumbar spine than in the thoracic region or at the thoracolumbar junction. Only three of 21 lumbar dislocations described by Kaufer and Hayes were below the L1-L2 level.[389] Dislocation of the lumbosacral joint also is a rare injury that frequently is accompanied by fractures of the sacrum or lower lumbar spine.[393, 394] Typically, marked anterior and lateral displacement of the lumbar spine is present, suggesting a complex mechanism that includes compressive hyperflexion as well as rotational or shear forces.[393–395] Associated disruption or interlocking of the facet joints in the lower lumbar spine or lumbosacral junction is easier to recognize on CT scans than on conventional radiographs.[395] Marked anterior vertebral displacement also can be seen in patients with bilateral fractures of the pedicles, which allow vertebral body displacement and maintain posterior element congruity.[396, 397] Significant dislocations mandate surgical stabilization to prevent residual spinal instability.[398]

Fractures of the transverse processes of the vertebrae result from lateral flexion-extension or, less commonly, from a direct blow, or they may be seen in association with a Malgaigne fracture of the pelvis.[6, 399] These fractures tend to occur in the absence of other vertebral fractures, although

multiple transverse processes often are involved.[398] Denis reported on 56 fractures of the transverse process in 28 patients; such represented 13.6 per cent of all thoracolumbar fractures identified in his series.[8] The most commonly involved levels were L3 and L4. Denis considered these fractures to be minor, stable injuries[8]; however, other authors have attributed more clinical significance to them. Indeed, a high frequency of associated abdominal, thoracic, and genitourinary injuries has been reported in patients with fractures of the transverse process.[399] Sturm and colleagues reported associated abdominal visceral injury in 21 per cent of patients with transverse process fractures, but their patients all had multiple injuries and a high mortality rate was seen.[399] The fractures are most evident on the anteroposterior radiograph, in which disruption of the cortex and displacement of the fractured tip of the transverse process can be seen (Fig. 69–63). Isolated fractures of the transverse processes may be difficult to identify owing to the relatively thin bone in this region and overlying bowel gas. Bulging or blurring of the margin of the psoas muscle may be noted but is a very nonspecific finding.[201] Scoliosis convex to the side of a unilateral transverse process fracture occurs in a large proportion of patients, presumably as a result of the unopposed action of the contralateral quadratus lumborum muscle.[396]

Isolated fractures of the pedicles may be related to trauma or represent fatigue fractures caused by repetitive stress.[400–402] When acute trauma is the mechanism of injury, such fractures are extremely rare. Almost all patients with traumatic pedicle fractures have osseous disruption at other sites within the vertebra. Abel has described transverse fractures of the pedicles of L4 and L5, typically associated with vertical fractures of the transverse process at the same level, as a result of extreme torsion.[403] Fatigue fractures of the pedicle have been reported in patients engaged in athletic activities and in patients with contralateral defects of the pars interarticularis.[400–402, 404, 405] Pedicle fractures must be distinguished from the rare retrosomatic clefts, which are congenital abnormalities of the pedicle characterized by unilateral or bilateral coronal osseous defects.[404]

Spondylolisthesis

Spondylolisthesis, with anterior slippage of the superior vertebra on the inferior one, may be due to a variety of osseous lesions, the most common being osteoarthritis of the facet joints and defects of the pars interarticularis. Bilateral pars interarticularis defects effectively divide the vertebra into two segments.[406] The anterosuperior segment consists of the vertebral body, pedicles, transverse processes, and superior facets. The posteroinferior segment consists of the inferior facet, laminae, and spinous process.[406] Acute fractures of the pars interarticularis are far less common than chronic spondylolysis as a cause of traumatic anterior vertebral displacement. The normal pars interarticularis can withstand considerable force; attempts to produce traumatic fractures of this structure in cadaveric specimens have been unsuccessful.[407] Acute fractures of the pars interarticularis are always secondary to severe trauma, usually that related to a hyperextension injury.[407, 408] These acute fractures typically are undisplaced, although frank spondylolisthesis may develop.[396, 407–409] Distinction from a chronic spondylolysis can be made by the history of severe trauma,

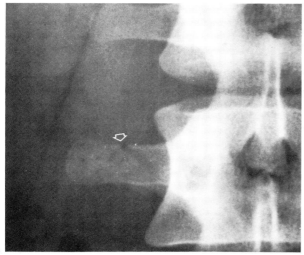

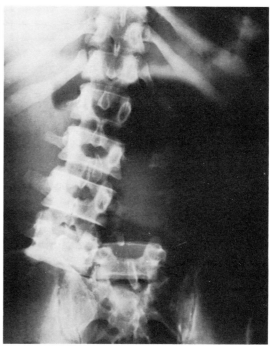

FIGURE 69–63. Fractures of the transverse process.
  A An oblique fracture line is evident (open arrow).
  B Lateral translocation between the fourth and fifth lumbar vertebral bodies is seen. Multiple transverse processes on the left side are fractured.
  (**B**, Courtesy of R. Kilcoyne, M.D., Denver, Colorado.)

the acute appearance of the fracture line, evidence of subsequent callus formation during healing, and increased accumulation of the radionuclide on bone scintigraphy.[407, 410]

Wiltse and coworkers have classified spondylolisthesis into five categories: (1) dysplastic, related to congenital anomalies of the upper portion of the sacrum or neural arch of L5; (2) isthmic, caused by fatigue fractures of the pars interarticularis (type A), elongation of the pars interarticularis (type B), or acute fractures of the pars interarticularis (type C); (3) degenerative, related to intersegmental instability; (4) traumatic, secondary to fractures of the neural arch in regions other than the isthmus; and (5) pathologic, resulting from generalized or localized bone disease.[396] Of these, the most common are the type 2A or 2B isthmic lesions or those related to degenerative causes.[396, 411] The most widely accepted theory regarding type 2A isthmic defects is that they represent fatigue fractures resulting from repeated trauma and stress.[396, 409, 412–414] The type 2B lesion, an elongated pars interarticularis, probably is related to healing of repeated microfractures in the isthmic region.[396] The elongated pars interarticularis frequently is thinned and eventually may separate, at which time the lesion becomes reclassified as a type 2A lesion.

Spondylolysis

The prevalence of pars interarticularis defects has been reported to be between 2.3 and 10 per cent.[413–416] The majority of these defects appear to be asymptomatic.[396, 412] An increased prevalence is seen in male subjects, and a strong hereditary component appears to exist.[413, 417] Many authors have reported a high frequency of pars interarticularis defects among family members, the prevalence being as high as 27 to 69 per cent among close relatives.[412, 417] Definite racial differences in the prevalence of these defects are seen: only 1.95 per cent of blacks have pars interarticularis defects, whereas in certain Eskimo communities the prevalence may be as high as 60 per cent.[414]

Pars interarticularis defects occurring below the age of 5 years are unusual. The prevalence of such defects rises precipitously between the ages of 5.5 and 6.5 years; by the age of 6.5 years, the prevalence of defects of the pars interarticularis is approximately 5 per cent, similar to the 5.8 per cent prevalence rate in adults.[412, 414, 417] Virtually all defects of the pars interarticularis develop by the age of 18 years, but usually before the age 15 years[396] (Fig. 69–64). Patients with such defects have been noted to have a higher frequency of spina bifida occulta at the level of the defect; nine of 11 patients with pars interarticularis defects in one series had a developmental deficiency of the posterior vertebral arch.[411–413, 418] Congenital anomalies of the upper por-

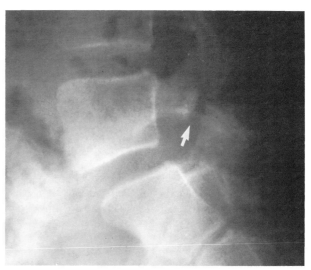

FIGURE 69–64. Spondylolysis of the L5 vertebra. Radiolucent defects (arrow) are seen in the pars interarticularis of the L5 vertebra in this 10 year old child. Spondylolisthesis is minimal, but the vertebral body is normal in morphology.

tion of the sacrum or affected vertebral arch were present in 85 of 253 cases reported by Rothman and Glenn.[419] Perhaps the deficiency of the posterior neural arch results in additional abnormal stresses concentrated on the isthmic region.[393, 413, 419]

Radiographic Abnormalities

Radiographic abnormalities of the pars interarticularis or isthmus, the region of the lamina between the superior and inferior articular facets, parallel those seen with stress fractures in other locations.[420] The earliest radiographic change is osteopenia, followed by the development of endosteal callus. The fracture line itself may not be apparent at this phase. When no discrete fracture line is seen, sclerosis is the dominant finding.[420] With healing, sclerosis, narrowing, and elongation of the pars interarticularis can be seen. The lateral view usually demonstrates the defect, particularly in the presence of spondylolisthesis. The fracture line courses from a posterosuperior to an anteroinferior direction through the pars interarticularis. A pseudospondylolysis or artifactual pars interarticularis defect may be seen in the lateral view at L2 or L3 in normal persons.[421] These apparent defects are created by imperfect superimposition of the transverse processes overlying the posterior vertebral arch. The resulting radiolucent regions tend to have sharp cortical margins and are located slightly more superiorly than the radiolucent areas associated with a true spondylolysis.[421]

The anteroposterior view demonstrates the pars interarticularis defect in only a small proportion of cases, although secondary signs such as laminar thickening, laminar fragmentation, and vertebral malalignment may be recognized. Fragmentation of the lamina is seen in cases in which defects of the pars interarticularis have been present for long periods of time; such fragmentation was apparent in 14.2 per cent of cases in one series.[416] The normal facet joints, which project as a radiolucent region that extends in a caudal and medial direction, should not be confused with pars interarticularis defects, which extend in a caudal and lateral direction on the anteroposterior view.[416] A supine anteroposterior view with 30 degrees of cephalad angulation of the x-ray beam has been suggested to allow visualization of the par interarticularis.[422] This view demonstrates the region of the pars interarticularis at the L4 and L5 levels in the frontal plane, with minimal distortion, foreshortening, and obscuring by overlying bony structures.[416, 422] The 30 degree angled view is more sensitive than the conventional anteroposterior view, demonstrating 55 per cent of pars interarticularis defects compared with 32 per cent of such defects on the conventional anteroposterior radiographs in one series.[416]

Oblique radiographs usually are not necessary but occasionally may be helpful. On oblique radiographs, the isthmic defect appears as a collar around the neck of the so-called "Scottie dog" of Lachapèle.[412] Oblique views do not always show pars interarticularis defects, partly because of the changing obliquity of the isthmic region from a cranial to caudal direction in the spine. Some authors have suggested that multiple oblique views allow adequate visualization of the pars interarticularis at all levels.[416] Collimated lateral views were most sensitive for detection of pars interarticularis defects in one large review that compared lateral, collimated lateral, anteroposterior, cranially angled anteroposterior, and oblique views.[416]

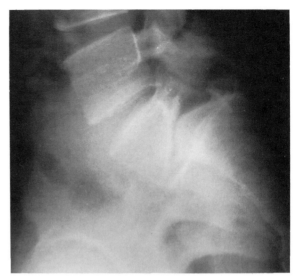

FIGURE 69–65. Spondylolysis and spondylolisthesis. Grade 3 anterolisthesis of the L5 vertebra relative to the sacrum is present. The posterior aspect of the L5 vertebral body is hypoplastic, resulting in a trapezoidal configuration. The sacrum also shows deformity from long-standing spondylolisthesis, with erosion of its anterosuperior margin.

Secondary changes in the morphology of the vertebral body may be evident in cases of pars interarticularis defect.[396] Posterior wedging of greater than 20 per cent and a trapezoid configuration of the fifth lumbar vertebral body is a well-recognized manifestation of bilateral isthmic spondylolysis at that level.[412, 423] Normal mild posterior wedging of the fifth lumbar vertebral body is common, however. A more pronounced trapezoidal shape of this vertebral body in patients with pars interarticularis defects may be related to altered biomechanical stresses.[412, 423] Associated erosion of the anterior and posterior surfaces of the sacrum, producing a domed or beaked appearance, also may be present in such patients[412] (Fig. 69–65).

Approximately one fifth of patients with spondylolysis have a unilateral defect.[418] Whether the defect truly is unilateral or whether the patient had bilateral defects with healing occurring only on one side is not known.[418] Unilateral spondylolysis frequently is associated with reactive sclerosis and hypertrophy of the contralateral pedicle and lamina.[418, 424, 425] This appearance has led to an erroneous diagnosis of an osteoid osteoma, although the absence of a nidus and the presence of dense homogeneous sclerosis favor reactive hypertrophy.[424] An osteoid osteoma and spondylolysis with reactive bone require accurate differentiation, because excision of a hypertrophied arch in cases of contralateral pars interarticularis defects can lead to painful spinal instability.[425] Associated scoliosis, convex toward the side of the pars interarticularis defect, is seen in approximately 75 per cent of cases.[424, 425] Unilateral arch hypertrophy commonly is associated with rotational instability, manifested by tilting of the spinous process toward the side of the isthmic defect.[418] The tilt is seen when the patient is in the upright position, resolves with recumbency, and is related to slippage of the facet joint on the side of the defect.[418] Unilateral hypertrophy presumably represents a physiologic response to excessive stress and an attempt to buttress an unstable posterior arch.[418, 424, 425] When the stress is excessive, fractures of the contralateral pars interarticularis or, less commonly, other portions of the contralateral arch may develop.[405, 418]

Malalignment

Spondylolisthesis associated with bilateral pars interarticularis defects occurs most frequently at the L5-S1 level. Over 90 per cent of pars interarticularis defects that allow slippage occur at this level, with the remainder occurring mainly at L4-L5.[411, 419] By contrast, degenerative spondylolisthesis secondary to facet osteoarthritis occurs at L4-L5 in 90 per cent of cases and is four times more frequent in women.[396, 411] Idiopathic vertebral hypoplasia can mimic a spondylolisthesis because of diminution of the anteroposterior sagittal dimension of the hypoplastic vertebral body. With hypoplasia, the anterior surfaces of the vertebral bodies remain aligned, whereas malalignment of the posterior margins of the vertebral bodies is evident.[423]

Vertebral slippage may be categorized as tangential or angular. Tangential slipping at the L5-S1 level may be classified further into five grades according to the resulting relationship between the fifth lumbar vertebral body and the superior surface of the sacrum.[409] Grade 5, or complete spondyloptosis, is most severe. Angular slipping results in an increase in lumbar lordosis related to diminished contact between the posterior surfaces of the fifth lumbar and first sacral vertebrae as the body of L5 tilts anteriorly on the sacrum.[409]

The definition of instability in spondylolysis is controversial. Hensinger suggested that abnormalities in the shape of the sacrum and fifth lumbar vertebral body denote instability.[412] Wiltse and coworkers, in their classic articles on spondylolysis, did not indicate any radiographic criteria for instability.[396, 414] Some authors consider any spine in which a slip has developed to be unstable; other investigators maintain that changes in vertebral alignment during motion or loading are necessary for spinal instability to occur.[426]

Still other authors define instability as an excessive range of spinal movement.[426] Penning and Blickman reviewed the role of flexion and extension radiographs in the assessment of lumbar spondylolisthesis.[426] They noted local hypermobility at the spondylolisthetic level in as many as 75 per cent of patients but noted that parallel displacement of adjacent vertebral bodies does not occur.[426]

Other Imaging Studies

Transaxial CT scans demonstrate defects of the pars interarticularis, although scans must include the region above the plane of the disc for accurate diagnosis.[427] Careful analysis of the CT scans is necessary to ensure that defects of the pars interarticularis are not misinterpreted as portions of the facet joints.[427] On transaxial images, the CT slice cephalad to the neural foramen is at the top or above the superior aspect of the apophyseal joints. At this level, a normal appearance is that of an intact ring, consisting of the medial walls of the pedicles, the pars interarticularis, the laminae, and the anterior margin of the spinous process.[428] In all cases of spondylolysis, a defect or "incomplete ring" is apparent on the slice above the neural foramen.[411, 428] The presence of a complete ring on CT scans at this level excludes the presence of a pars interarticularis defect.[428] Pars interarticularis defects can be differentiated from facet joints by noting the absence of dense subarticular margins, the presence of irregularity or fragmentation at the edges of the spondylolytic defect, and the absence of normal notches about the facet joint that serve as insertion sites for the joint capsule.[427] A pars interarticularis defect also appears more horizontal than the typical facet joint, which has a smooth oblique orientation[411, 419] (Fig. 69–66). Frequently, the medial aspect of the bone just anterior to the pars interarticularis defect has a small, radiodense, rounded excrescence that extends medially and caudally.[411, 418] Foraminal osteophytes, a normal variant seen in the lumbar spine, may mimic these excrescences.[429] Fractures of the inferior facet

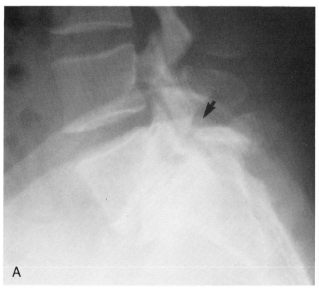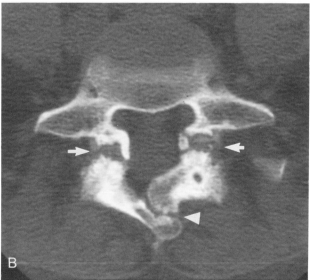

FIGURE 69–66. Spondylolisthesis: CT scanning.
  A The lateral radiograph shows spondylolysis of the L5 vertebra (arrow) with grade 2 anterolisthesis.
  B A transaxial CT scan through the bilateral defects of the pars interarticularis shows irregularity and fragmentation at the margins of the defects (arrows). Note the horizontal inclination of the spondylolytic regions. Spina bifida also is present (arrowhead).

occurring after laminectomy also may simulate a pars inter-articularis defect. These fractures occur below the isthmus, a feature best appreciated on coronal reformations of transaxial CT data.[411, 430]

With severe spondylolisthesis a "double canal" appearance may be seen.[419] In addition, in spondylolisthesis, CT scans may reveal "pseudobulging" of the intervertebral disc in which soft tissue projects posteriorly into the spinal canal.[411] This artifactual appearance is related to projection of a portion of the anulus fibrosus posterior to the slipped vertebra.[411] Pseudobulging of the intervertebral disc appears more extensive with greater degrees of vertebral slippage. Important characteristics of the pseudobulge include irregularity of the posterior margin of the intervertebral disc and an apparent increased transverse diameter of the disc, which extends into the neural foramina.[411] Six per cent of patients with spondylolysis have a true disc herniation, most commonly at the level above the defect.[419] The canal below the defect appears stenotic in the sagittal plane.[411] On MR images, pars interarticularis defects typically are of intermediate signal intensity on all pulse sequences, although their signal intensity is somewhat variable depending on the exact composition of the tissues within the defect.[415] The defects are best seen on sagittal T1-weighted and proton density spin echo MR images, which also are excellent for demonstrating associated spondylolisthesis and disc herniation.[415] Normal variations in marrow signal intensity of the pars interarticularis are common and may make detection of undisplaced pars interarticularis defects difficult.[406] The pars interarticularis is best evaluated in a medial imaging plane that passes through the pedicle; more lateral MR images can result in the appearance of a pseudodefect through the isthmic region.[415]

The central and foraminal stenosis associated with spondylolisthesis also is well depicted on MR images.[406, 415] The foramen assumes a flattened, more horizontal configuration and may have a bilobed appearance.[406] This foraminal deformity can be detected on sagittal reformations of transaxial CT data but is easier to evaluate on sagittal MR images. Using reformatted CT data, flattening of the neural foramen in the sagittal dimension was seen in 84 of 136 patients with spondylolisthesis.[419] Obliteration or nearly complete loss of the fat surrounding the nerve root suggests nerve root entrapment within the foramen.[406] Such entrapment is particularly common when pars interarticularis defects are present at the L5 level. The angulation of the sacrum results in significant stenosis of the superior recess of the L5 neural foramen, even with minimal degrees of vertebral slippage.[406]

Radiography, conventional tomography, CT scanning, and MR imaging all allow recognition of the morphologic abnormalities in established cases of pars interarticularis defects. Bone scintigraphy, in contrast to the former techniques, affords a functional assessment of metabolic activity in the region of the isthmus. Discordance between radiographic and scintigraphic findings in pars interarticularis defects is well recognized.[420, 431–435] Pennell and colleagues developed a radiographic grading system for pars interarticularis defects that correlated with scintigraphic activity.[420] These authors classified the radiographic appearance of the pars interarticularis as follows: type 0, normal; type 1, sclerosis; type 2, an evolving or healed stress fracture; type 3, a nonunited fracture with a well-defined radiolucent defect.[420] Scintigraphy was positive in 73 per cent of patients with type 1 injuries, whereas only 40 per cent of patients with type 2 and 17 per cent of patients with type 3 injuries had abnormal planar bone scans.[420] Thus, it appears that acute stress injuries of the pars interarticularis may not be apparent radiographically and that sites of long-standing spondylolysis may not be active metabolically.[431, 435] Despite such data, whether or not a reliable correlation exists between clinical symptoms and the pattern of radionuclide uptake in patients with spondylolysis is controversial.[433] The scintigraphic appearance of spondylolysis is not specific, and final diagnosis depends on clinical and radiographic evaluation.[435]

Single photon emission computed tomography (SPECT) is more sensitive for detection of stress injuries to the pars interarticularis than is conventional planar imaging.[432, 433] The heightened sensitivity of SPECT over planar images is most evident for lesions involving the posterior neural arch.[434] SPECT allows accurate differentiation between radionuclide accumulation in the neural arch and that in the vertebral body.[433, 434] In one series of 71 patients with abnormal SPECT images, only 32 had findings on planar scintigraphy.[432] Similarly, in a series of 54 abnormal lesions detected on SPECT studies, only 20 (37 per cent) were seen on planar images.[434]

Avulsion of the Ring Apophysis

The ring apophyses are narrow cartilaginous mounds present at both the superior and inferior vertebral endplates, from which they are separated by a thin layer of cartilage.[436] The ring apophyses normally begin to calcify at the age of 6 years; ossification occurs at the beginning of adolescence.[437] The apophyses fuse with the vertebral body by the end of skeletal growth, typically by the age of 18 to 25 years. Their development occurs at different rates at the various spinal levels, with relatively slow progression in the lumbar area.[438] The ring apophyses do not participate in longitudinal vertebral growth but serve as traction apophyses, being closely associated with the attachments of the longitudinal spinal ligaments and the intervertebral Sharpey's fibers.[436–440] Some discrepancy is found in the literature regarding whether the ring is always complete or whether deficiency in its posterior portion exists in some or all normal persons.[437, 441] Posterior ring apophyses are visualized radiographically less frequently than their anterior counterparts.[440]

Avulsions of the posterior apophyseal ring of the lumbar vertebrae, like spondylolysis, are traumatic lesions that develop in children and adolescents. Fractures of the vertebral ring apophysis in the lumbar spine are now a well-documented cause of low back and leg pain.[436, 442–444] Patients typically first come to medical attention in adolescence or young adulthood with back and leg pain, paraspinal spasm, mechanical findings of nerve entrapment, and a relative paucity of focal neurologic findings.[444] Associated disc herniation is present in up to 90 per cent of patients.[436, 438] Whether the disc herniation produces the avulsion fracture or whether the fracture results in anular disruption is unclear.[436] Disc herniation in patients less than 21 years of age is associated with vertebral endplate avulsions in as many as 19 per cent of cases.[439] This injury often is not recog-

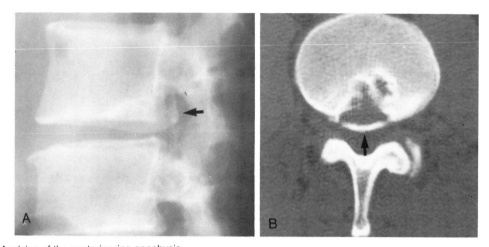

FIGURE 69–67. Avulsion of the posterior ring apophysis.

A The lateral radiograph shows a bone fragment (arrow) located posterior to the L3-L4 intervertebral disc. Note the narrowing of the intervertebral disc space and the irregularity of the posteroinferior margin of the L3 vertebral body, the source of the displaced bone fragment.

B The CT scan demonstrates the characteristic arcuate configuration of the displaced apophyseal fragment (arrow) and the Schmorl's node–like defect at the posteroinferior margin of the vertebral body.

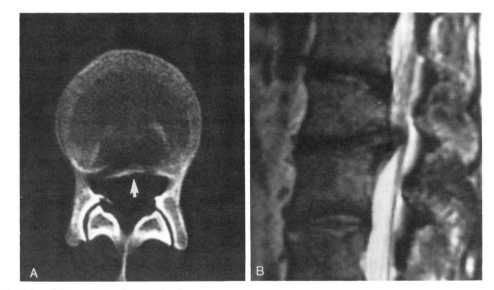

FIGURE 69–68. Avulsion of the posterior ring apophysis.

A A transaxial CT scan through the inferior aspect of the L2 vertebra demonstrates an arcuate bone fragment displaced into the spinal canal (arrow) as well as a defect in the posterior aspect of the vertebral body.

B Sagittal (TR/TE, 3400/96) fast spin echo MR image shows an intervertebral disc herniation at the L2-L3 vertebral level with a "7" configuration, consistent with apophysis avulsion.

nized because of unfamiliarity with the entity and failure to recognize its characteristic radiographic features.

Apophyseal fractures have been recognized throughout the spine, but the most common levels of involvement are the inferior ring apophyses of the lower lumbar vertebrae, particularly the posteroinferior margin of L4.[436, 442, 444] Alternatively, some authors have suggested that the posterior cephalad rim of the sacrum is affected most frequently.[443] This discrepancy can be explained by the imaging method used; rim avulsions of the sacrum are extremely difficult to visualize on conventional radiographs and are diagnosed by CT scanning or MR imaging in most cases.[443]

Takata and associates have classified these fractures into three types on the basis of a review of CT studies in 29 patients with 31 avulsions of the posterior ring apophysis.[443] Type I injuries are simple separations of the posterior osseous vertebral rim and occur in younger children, under the age of 13 years. The underlying vertebral body appears normal and only an arcuate bone fragment is seen displaced into the spinal canal. Ten of 31 fractures in the series reported by Takata and colleagues fit this description.[443] Type II injuries occur in older children and adolescents. In this type, a fragment of the posterior vertebral body and its overlying cartilage are displaced, resulting in a thicker and larger fragment. Nine of 31 fractures in this same series demonstrated this pattern; the avulsed vertebral body fragment was easily recognized on the CT scan.[443] Type III fractures involve a larger amount of the vertebral body such that the resulting fragment is larger than the vertebral rim. A rounded osseous defect is seen in the bone adjoining the fracture site. This pattern was most common and was present in 12 of 31 cases reported by Takata and coworkers.[443] Type IV injuries are an additional category proposed by Epstein and associates.[444] This rare pattern represents a fracture of both the cephalad and the caudad apophyses and spans the full length of the posterior margin of the vertebral body.[444]

Conventional radiographs must be examined carefully because these lesions are difficult to see. Findings seen on the lateral view include mild disc space narrowing, irregularity of the posterior vertebral corner, and an irregular wedge-shaped ossific defect displaced into the spinal canal.[444] On CT scans, the osseous fracture fragment has a characteristic arcuate or semilunar configuration that parallels the posterior border of the vertebral body[439, 442, 443] (Fig. 69–67). The fragment may appear irregular rather than arcuate if it contains a large fragment of the vertebral body.[443] This fragment must be differentiated from osteophytes, calcified disc fragments, and calcification or ossification of the posterior longitudinal ligament.[442] The fragment is more difficult to characterize on MR images because it may be difficult to distinguish the osseous rim from the low signal intensity of the posterior longitudinal ligament.[442] On sagittal MR images, the displaced fracture fragment is seen as a structure that is hypointense or is of mixed signal intensity with a Y or "7" shape, elevating an intact posterior longitudinal ligament[439, 441] (Fig. 69–68). Discontinuity and truncation of the normally convex posteroinferior margin of the vertebral body and disc prolapse adjacent to the fragment also are present.[441] Hypointense signal within the disc on T2-weighted images, consistent with degeneration, also may be recognized.[441]

SUMMARY

Spinal trauma is complex, involving a wide range of soft tissue and osseous injuries in a variety of spinal regions. Knowledge of the anatomic and functional characteristics in the different spinal regions allows the radiologist to understand the injuries that are unique to each area. This review has emphasized the role of diagnostic imaging in evaluating the acutely injured patient with spinal injury.

References

1. Jefferson G: Discussion on spinal injuries. R Soc Med 21:625, 1927.
2. Holdsworth F: Review article: Fractures, dislocations, and fracture-dislocations of the spine. J Bone Joint Surg [Am] 51:1534, 1970.
3. Daffner RH, Deeb ZL, Rothfus WE: "Fingerprints" of vertebral trauma—a unifying concept based on mechanisms. Skel Radiol 15:518, 1986.
4. Rogers LF: The spine. In R Hurley, D Terry (Eds): Radiology of Skeletal Trauma. 2nd Ed. New York, Churchill Livingstone, 1992, p. 000.
5. Gupta A, El Masri WS: Multilevel spinal injuries: Incidence, distribution and neurological patterns. J Bone Joint Surg [Br] 71:692, 1989.
6. Calenoff L, Chessare JW, Rogers LF, et al: Multiple level spinal injuries: Importance of early recognition. AJR 130:665, 1978.
7. Roaf R: A study of the mechanics of spinal injuries. J Bone Joint Surg [Br] 42:810, 1960.
8. Denis F: The three column spine and its significance in the classification of acute thoracolumbar spinal injuries. Spine 8:817, 1983.
9. Nicoll EA: Fractures of the dorso-lumbar spine. J Bone Joint Surg [Br] 31:376, 1949.
10. Holdsworth FW: Fractures, dislocations, and fracture-dislocations of the spine. J Bone Joint Surg [Br] 45:6, 1963.
11. Ferguson RL, Allen BL Jr: A mechanistic classification of thoracolumbar spine fractures. Clin Orthop 189:77, 1984.
12. McAfee PC, Yuan HA, Fredrickson BE, et al: The value of computed tomography in thoracolumbar fractures: An analysis of one hundred consecutive cases and a new classification. J Bone Joint Surg [Am] 65:461, 1983.
13. White AA, Johnson RM, Panjabi MM, et al: Biomechanical analysis of clinical stability in the cervical spine. Clin Orthop 109:85, 1975.
14. White AA, Southwick WO, Panjabi MM: Clinical instability in the lower cervical spine: A review of past and current concepts. Spine 1:15, 1976.
15. Panjabi MM, Brand RA, White AA: Mechanical properties of the human thoracic spine. J Bone Joint Surg [Am] 58:642, 1976.
16. Spence KF, Decker S, Sell KW: Bursting atlantal fracture associated with rupture of the transverse ligament. J Bone Joint Surg [Am] 52:543, 1970.
17. Fielding JW, Cochran GVB, Lawsing JF III, et al: Tears of the transverse ligament of the atlas: A clinical and biomechanical study. J Bone Joint Surg [Am] 56:1683, 1974.
18. Daffner RH, Charlton OP, Gehweiler JA, et al: A model for investigation of mechanisms of cervical spine trauma. Skel Radiol 3:213, 1979.
19. Pathria MN, Petersilge CA: Spinal trauma. Radiol Clin North Am 29:847, 1991.
20. Whitesides TE: Traumatic kyphosis of the thoracolumbar spine. Clin Orthop 128:78, 1977.
21. Bedbrook GM: Stability of spinal fractures and fracture dislocations. Paraplegia 9:23, 1971.
22. Nagel DA, Koogle TA, Piziali RL, et al: Stability of the upper lumbar spine following progressive disruptions and the application of individual internal and external fixation devices. J Bone Joint Surg [Am] 63:62, 1981.
23. Denis F: Spinal instability as defined by the three-column spine concept in acute spinal trauma. Clin Orthop 189:65, 1984.
24. Daffner RH, Deeb ZL, Goldberg AL, et al: The radiologic assessment of post-traumatic vertebral stability. Skel Radiol 19:103, 1990.
25. Kassel EE, Cooper PW, Rubenstein JD: Radiology of spinal trauma: Practical experience in a trauma unit. J Can Assoc Radiol 34:189, 1983.
26. Bank WO, Kerland RK, Kesselring LW: Improved lateral cervical spine radiography through halo traction device. AJR 137:29, 1981.
27. Russin LD, Guinto FC: Multidirectional tomography in cervical spine injury. J Neurosurg 45:9, 1976.
28. Steppe R, Bellemans M, Boven F, et al: The value of computed tomography scanning in elusive fractures of the cervical spine. Skel Radiol 6:175, 1981.
29. Acheson MB, Livingston RR, Richardson ML, et al: High-resolution CT scanning in the evaluation of cervical spine fractures: Comparison with plain film examinations. AJR 148:1179, 1987.
30. Streitwieser DR, Knopp R, Wales LR, et al: Accuracy of standard radiographic views in detecting cervical spine fractures. Ann Emerg Med 12:538, 1983.
31. Maravilla KR, Cooper PR, Sklar FH: The influence of thin-section tomography on the treatment of cervical spine injuries. Radiology 127:131, 1978.
32. Anderson LD, Smith BL, DeTorre J, et al: The role of polytomography in the diagnosis and treatment of cervical spine injuries. Clin Orthop 165:64, 1982.
33. Berquist TH: Imaging of adult cervical spine trauma. RadioGraphics 8:667, 1988.
34. Brant-Zawadzki M, Miller EM, Federle MP: CT in the evaluation of spine trauma. AJR 136:369, 1981.

35. Miller JA, Smith TH: Seatbelt induced Chance fracture in an infant. Pediatr Radiol 21:575, 1991.
36. Manaster BJ, Osborn AG: CT patterns of facet fracture dislocations in the thoracolumbar region. AJR 148:335, 1987.
37. O'Callaghan JP, Ullrich CG, Yuan HA, et al: CT of facet distraction in flexion injuries of the thoracolumbar spine: The "naked" facet. AJR 134:563, 1980.
38. Rothman SLG, Dobben GD, Rhodes ML, et al: Computed tomography of the spine: Curved coronal reformations from serial images. Radiology 150:185, 1984.
39. Orrison WW, Johansen JG, Eldevik OP, et al: Optimal computed-tomographic techniques for cervical spine imaging. Radiology 144:180, 1982.
40. Brown BM, Brant-Zawadzki M, Cann CE: Dynamic CT scanning of spinal column trauma. AJR 139:1177, 1982.
41. Stimac GK, Burch D, Livingston RR, et al: A device for maintaining cervical spine stabilization and traction during CT scanning. AJR 149:345, 1987.
42. Boechat MI: Spinal deformities and pseudofractures. AJR 148:97, 1987.
43. Pech P, Kilgore DP, Pojunas KW, et al: Cervical spinal fractures: CT detection. Radiology 157:117, 1985.
44. Yetkin Z, Osborn AG, Giles DS, et al: Uncovertebral and facet joint dislocations in cervical articular pillar fractures: CT evaluation. AJNR 6:633, 1985.
45. Silver SF, Nadel HR, Flodmark O: Pneumorrhachis after jejunal entrapment caused by a fracture dislocation of the lumbar spine. AJR 150:1129, 1988.
46. Delamarter RB, Heller J, Bohlman HH: Cervical pneumomyelogram secondary to a closed fracture-dislocation of the thoracic spine. Spine 14:1421, 1989.
47. Newbold RG, Wiener MD, Vogler JB III, et al: Traumatic pneumorrhachis. AJR 148:615, 1987.
48. Fishman EK, Magid D, Ney DR, et al: Three-dimensional imaging. Radiology 181:321, 1991.
49. Wojcik WG, Edeiken-Monroe BS, Harris JH: Three-dimensional computed tomography in acute cervical spine trauma: A preliminary report. Skel Radiol 16:261, 1987.
50. Ney DR, Fishman EK, Kawashima A: Comparison of helical and serial CT with regard to three-dimensional imaging of musculoskeletal anatomy. Radiology 185:865, 1992.
51. Pay NT, George AE, Benjamin MV, et al: Positive and negative contrast myelography in spinal trauma. Radiology 123:103, 1977.
52. Brant-Zawadzki M, Jeffrey RB Jr, Minagi H, et al: High resolution CT of thoracolumbar fractures. AJR 138:699, 1982.
53. Goldberg AL, Rothfus WE, Deeb ZL, et al: The impact of magnetic resonance on the diagnostic evaluation of acute cervicothoracic spinal trauma. Skel Radiol 17:89, 1988.
54. Cooper PR, Cohen W: Evaluation of cervical spinal cord injuries with metrizamide myelography–CT scanning. J Neurosurg 61:281, 1984.
55. Allen RL, Perot HL, Gudeman SK: Evaluation of acute nonpenetrating cervical spinal cord injuries with CT metrizamide myelography. J Neurosurg 63:510, 1985.
56. Mirvis SE, Wolf AL: MRI of acute cervical spine trauma. Appl Radiol 12:15, 1992.
57. Morris RE, Hasso AN, Thompson JR, et al: Traumatic dural tears: CT diagnosis using metrizamide. Radiology 152:443, 1984.
58. Mirvis SE, Borg U, Belzberg H: MR imaging of ventilator-dependent patients: Preliminary experience. AJR 149:845, 1987.
59. Beale SM, Pathria MN, Masaryk TJ: Magnetic resonance imaging of spinal trauma. Top Magn Reson Imaging 1:53, 1988.
60. Mirvis SE, Wolf A: Emerging MRI role: Assessing cervical spine trauma. MRI Decisions 1:20, 1990.
61. Shellock FG, Curtis JW: MR imaging and biomedical implants, materials, and devices: An updated review. Radiology 180:541, 1991.
62. Clayman DA, Murakami ME, Vines FS: Compatibility of cervical spine braces with MR imaging: A study of nine nonferrous devices. AJNR 11:385, 1990.
63. McArdle CB, Wright JW, Prevost WJ, et al: MR imaging of the acutely injured patient with cervical traction. Radiology 159:273, 1986.
64. Kulkarni MV, McArdle CB, Kopanicky D, et al: Acute spinal cord injury: MR imaging at 1.5 T. Radiology 164:837, 1987.
65. Mirvis SE: MR provides clues to cervical spine trauma. Diagn Imaging 7:116, 1988.
66. Mirvis SE, Geisler F, Joslyn JN, et al: Use of titanium wire in cervical spine fixation as a means to reduce MR artifacts. AJNR 9:1229, 1988.
67. Tracy PT, Wright RM, Hanigan WC: Magnetic resonance imaging of spinal injury. Spine 14:292, 1989.
68. Yashon D, Jane JA, White RJ: Prognosis and management of spinal cord and cauda equina bullet injuries in sixty-five civilians. J Neurosurg 31:163, 1970.
69. Emery SE, Pathria MN, Wilber RG, et al: Magnetic resonance imaging of posttraumatic spinal ligament injury. J Spinal Disord 2:229, 1989.
70. McArdle CB, Crofford MJ, Mirfakhraee M, et al: Surface coil MR of spinal trauma: Preliminary experience. AJNR 7:885, 1986.
71. Tarr RW, Drolshagen LF, Kerner TC, et al: MR imaging of recent spinal trauma. J Comput Assist Tomogr 11:412, 1987.
72. Peck WW: Current status of MRI of the cervical spine. Appl Radiol 1:17, 1989.
73. Edelman RR, Stark DD, Saini S, et al: Oblique planes of section in MR imaging. Radiology 159:807, 1986.
74. Flanders AE, Schaefer DM, Doan HY, et al: Acute cervical spine trauma: Correlation of MR imaging findings with degree of neurologic deficit. Radiology 177:25, 1990.
75. Mirvis SE, Geisler FH, Jelinek JJ, et al: Acute cervical spine trauma: Evaluation with 1.5-T MR imaging. Radiology 166:807, 1988.
76. Grenier N, Greselle J, Vital J, et al: Normal and disrupted lumbar longitudinal ligaments: Correlative MR and anatomic study. Radiology 171:197, 1989.
77. Harris JH Jr, Yeakley JW: Hyperextension-dislocation of the cervical spine: Ligament injuries demonstrated by magnetic resonance imaging. J Bone Joint Surg [Br] 74:567, 1992.
78. Goldberg AL, Rothfus WE, Deeb ZL, et al: Hyperextension injuries of the cervical spine. Skel Radiol 18:283, 1989.
79. Gundry CR, Heithoff KB: Epidural hematoma of the lumbar spine: 18 surgically confirmed cases. Radiology 187:427, 1993.
80. Bohlman HH: Acute fractures and dislocations of the cervical spine. J Bone Joint Surg [Am] 61:1119, 1979.
81. Pear BL: Spinal epidural hematoma. AJR 115:155, 1972.
82. Garth WP, Van Patten PK: Fractures of the lumbar lamina with epidural hematoma simulating herniation of a disc. J Bone Joint Surg [Am] 71:771, 1989.
83. Unger EC, Glazer HS, Lee JKT, et al: MRI of extracranial hematomas: Preliminary observations. AJR 146:403, 1986.
84. Schaefer DM, Flanders A, Northrup BE, et al: Magnetic resonance imaging of acute cervical spine trauma: Correlation with severity of neurologic injury. Spine 14:1090, 1989.
85. Pratt ES, Green DA, Spengler DM: Herniated intervertebral discs associated with unstable spinal injuries. Spine 15:662, 1990.
86. Davis SJ, Teresi LM, Bradley WG Jr, et al: Cervical spine hyperextension injuries: MR findings. Radiology 180:245, 1991.
87. Schneider RC, Kahn EA: Chronic neurological sequelae of acute trauma to the spine and spinal cord. I. The significance of the acute-flexion or "tear-drop" fracture-dislocation of the cervical spine. J Bone Joint Surg [Am] 38:985, 1956.
88. Knake JE, Gabrielsen TO, Chandler WF, et al: Real-time sonography during spinal surgery. Radiology 151:461, 1984.
89. Harcke HT, Grissom LE, Finkelstein MS: Evaluation of the musculoskeletal system with sonography. AJR 150:1253, 1988.
90. Kaplan PA, Matamoros A, Anderson JC: Sonography of the musculoskeletal system. AJR 155:237, 1990.
91. Mirvis SE, Geisler FH: Intraoperative sonography of cervical spinal cord injury: Results in 30 patients. AJNR 11:755, 1990.
92. Montalvo BM, Quencer RM, Green BA, et al: Intraoperative sonography in spinal trauma. Radiology 153:125, 1984.
93. McGahan JP, Benson D, Chehrazi B, et al: Intraoperative sonographic monitoring of reduction of thoracolumbar burst fractures. AJR 145:1229, 1985.
94. Gebarski SS, Maynard FW, Gabrielsen TO, et al: Posttraumatic progressive myelopathy. Radiology 157:379, 1985.
95. Riggins RS, Kraus JF: The risk of neurologic damage with fractures of the vertebrae. J Trauma 17:126, 1977.
96. Bracken MB, Freeman DH, Hellenbrand K: Incidence of acute traumatic hospitalized spinal cord injury in the United States, 1970-1977. Am J Epidemiol 113:615, 1981.
97. National Spinal Cord Injury Statistical Center: Spinal Cord Injury. Birmingham, University of Alabama, 1991.
98. Del Bigio MR, Johnson GE: Clinical presentation of spinal cord concussion. Spine 14:37, 1989.
99. Hackney DB, Asato R, Joseph PM, et al: Hemorrhage and edema in acute spinal cord compression: Demonstration by MR imaging. Radiology 161:387, 1986.
100. Hackney DB: Denominators of spinal cord injury. Radiology 177:18, 1990.
101. Davis D, Bohlman H, Walker AE, et al: The pathological findings in fatal craniospinal injuries. J Neurosurg 34:603, 1971.
102. de la Torre JC: Spinal cord injury: Review of basic and applied research. Spine 6:315, 1981.
103. Osterholm JL: The pathophysiological response to spinal cord injury. J Neurosurg 40:5, 1974.
104. Willen JAG, Gaekwad UH, Kakulas BA: Burst fractures in the thoracic and lumbar spine: A clinico-neuropathologic analysis. Spine 14:1316, 1989.
105. Schneider RC, Crosby EC, Russo RH, et al: Traumatic spinal cord syndromes and their management. Clin Neurosurg 20:424, 1973.
106. Regenbogen VS, Rogers LF, Atlas SW, et al: Cervical spinal cord injuries in patients with cervical spondylosis. AJR 146:277, 1986.
107. Taylor AR: The mechanism of injury to the spinal cord in the neck without damage to the vertebral column. J Bone Joint Surg [Br] 33:543, 1951.
108. Frankel HL, Hancock DO, Hyslop G, et al: The value of postural reduction in the initial management of closed injuries of the spine with paraplegia and tetraplegia. Paraplegia 7:179, 1969.
109. Silberstein M, Tress BM, Hennessy O: Prediction of neurologic outcome in acute spinal cord injury: The role of CT and MR. AJNR 13:1597, 1992.
110. Yamashita Y, Takahashi M, Matsuno Y, et al: Chronic injuries of the spinal cord: Assessment with MR imaging. Radiology 175:849, 1990.
111. Kulkarni MV, Bondurant FJ, Rose SL, et al: 1.5 tesla magnetic resonance imaging of acute spinal trauma. RadioGraphics 8:1059, 1988.
112. Bondurant FJ, Cotler HB, Kulkarni MV, et al: Acute spinal cord injury: A study using physical examination and magnetic resonance imaging. Spine 15:161, 1990.
113. Mathis JM, Wilson JT, Barnard JW, et al: MR imaging of spinal cord avulsion. AJNR 9:1232, 1988.

114. Yamashita Y, Takahashi M, Matsuno Y, et al: Acute spinal cord injury: Magnetic resonance imaging correlated with myelopathy. Br J Radiol 64:201, 1991.

115. Silberstein M, Tress BM, Hennessy O: Delayed neurologic deterioration in the patient with spinal trauma: Role of MR imaging. AJNR 13:1373, 1992.

116. Seibert CE, Dreisbach JN, Swanson WB, et al: Progressive posttraumatic cystic myelopathy: Neuroradiologic evaluation. AJNR 2:115, 1981.

117. Vernon JD, Silver JR, Ohry A: Post-traumatic syringomyelia. Paraplegia 20:339, 1982.

118. Quencer RM, Green BA, Eismont FJ: Posttraumatic spinal cord cysts: Clinical features and characterization with metrizamide computed tomography. Radiology 146:415, 1983.

119. Quencer RM, Sheldon JJ, Donovan Post MJ, et al: MRI of the chronically injured cervical spinal cord. AJR 147:125, 1986.

120. Stevens JM, Olney JS, Kendall BE: Post-traumatic cystic and non-cystic myelopathy. Neuroradiology 27:48, 1985.

121. Rossier AB, Foo D, Naheedy MH, et al: Radiography of posttraumatic syringomyelia. AJNR 4:637, 1983.

122. Kan S, Fox AJ, Vinuela F, et al: Spinal cord size in syringomyelia: Change with position on metrizamide myelography. Radiology 146:409, 1983.

123. Modic MT, Weinstein MA, Pavlicek W, et al: Nuclear magnetic resonance imaging of the spine. Radiology 148:757, 1983.

124. Clark WM, Gehweiler JA, Laib R: Twelve significant signs of cervical spine trauma. Skel Radiol 3:201, 1979.

125. Fischer RP: Cervical radiographic evaluation of alert patients following blunt trauma. Ann Emerg Med 13:905, 1984.

126. Bachulis BL, Long WB, Hynes GD, et al: Clinical indications for cervical spine radiographs in the traumatized patient. Am J Surg 153:473, 1987.

127. Vandemark RM: Radiology of the cervical spine in trauma patients: Practice pitfalls and recommendations for improving efficiency and communication. AJR 155:465, 1990.

128. Mirvis SE, Diaconis JN, Chirico PA, et al: Protocol-driven radiologic evaluation of suspected cervical spine injury: Efficacy study. Radiology 170:831, 1989.

129. American College of Surgeons: Initial assessment and management. Committee on Trauma: Advanced Trauma Life Support Course. Chicago, American College of Surgeons, 1989.

130. American College of Surgeons: Spine and spinal cord trauma. Committee on Trauma: Advanced Trauma Life Support Course. Chicago, American College of Surgeons, 1989.

131. Williams CF, Bernstein TW, Jelenko C III: Essentiality of the lateral cervical spine radiograph. Ann Emerg Med 10:198, 1981.

132. Wales LR, Knopp RK, Morishima MS: Recommendations for evaluation of the acutely injured cervical spine: A clinical radiologic algorithm. Ann Emerg Med 9:422, 1980.

133. Walter J: Clinical presentation of patients with acute cervical spine injury. Ann Emerg Med 13:512, 1984.

134. Bohlman HH: Complications of treatment of fractures and dislocation of the cervical spine. In CH Epps Jr (Ed): Complications of Orthopedic Surgery. Philadelphia, JB Lippincott, 1978.

135. Gatrell CB: "Asymptomatic" cervical injuries: A myth? Am J Emerg Med 3:263, 1985.

136. Abel MS: Occult traumatic lesions of the cervical vertebrae. CRC Rad Nucl Med 6:469, 1975.

137. McCall IW, Park WM, McSweeney T: The radiological demonstration of acute lower cervical injury. Clin Radiol 24:235, 1973.

138. Penning L: Prevertebral hematoma in cervical spine injury: Incidence and etiologic significance. AJR 136:553, 1981.

139. Templeton PA, Young JWR, Mirvis SE, et al: The value of retropharyngeal soft tissue measurements in trauma of the adult cervical spine. Skel Radiol 16:98, 1987.

140. Miles KA, Maimaris C, Finlay D, et al: The incidence and prognostic significance of radiological abnormalities in soft tissue injuries to the cervical spine. Skel Radiol 17:493, 1988.

141. Wholey MH, Bruwer AJ, Hillier LB: The lateral roentgenogram of the neck. Radiology 71:350, 1958.

142. Martinez JA, Timberlake GA, Jones JC, et al: Factors affecting the cervical prevertebral space in the trauma patient. Am J Emerg Med 6:268, 1988.

143. Whalen JP, Woodruff CL: Radium therapy and nuclear medicine. AJR 109:445, 1970.

144. Polansky A, Resnick D, Sofferman RA, et al: Hyoid bone elevation: A sign of tracheal transection. Radiology 150:117, 1984.

145. Harris JH, Edeiken-Monroe B: The Radiology of Acute Cervical Spine Trauma. 2nd Ed. Baltimore, Williams & Wilkins, 1987.

146. Oon CL: Some sagittal measurements of the neck in normal adults. Br J Radiol 37:674, 1964.

147. Lewis CA, Castillo M, Hudgins PA: Cervical prevertebral fat stripe: A normal variant simulating prevertebral hemorrhage. AJR 155:559, 1990.

148. Sistrom CL, Southall EP, Peddada SD, et al: Factors affecting the thickness of the cervical prevertebral soft tissues. Skel Radiol 22:167, 1993.

149. Apple JS, Kirks DR, Merten DF, et al: Cervical spine fractures and dislocations in children. Pediatr Radiol 17:45, 1987.

150. Ehara S, El-Khoury GY, Sato Y: Cervical spine injury in children: Radiologic manifestations. AJR 151:1175, 1988.

151. Sherk HH, Schut L, Lane JM: Fractures and dislocations of the cervical spine in children. Orthop Clin North Am 7:593, 1976.

152. Maves CK, Souza A, Prenger EC, et al: Traumatic atlanto-occipital disruption in children. Pediatr Radiol 21:504, 1991.

153. Shapiro R, Youngberg AS, Rothman SLG: The differential diagnosis of traumatic lesions of the occipito-atlanto-axial segment. Radiol Clin North Am 11:505, 1973.

154. Schweitzer ME, Hodler J, Cervilla V, et al: Craniovertebral junction: Normal anatomy with MR correlation. AJR 158:1087, 1992.

155. El-Khoury GY, Clark CR, Dietz FR, et al: Posterior atlantooccipital subluxation in Down syndrome. Radiology 159:507, 1986.

156. Daniels DL, Williams AL, Haughton VM: Computed tomography of the articulations and ligaments at the occipito-atlantoaxial region. Radiology 146:709, 1983.

157. Coutts MB: Atlanto-epistropheal subluxations. Arch Surg 29:297, 1934.

158. Penning L: Normal movements of the cervical spine. AJR 130:317, 1978.

159. Pang D, Wilberger JE: Traumatic atlanto-occipital dislocation with survival: Case report and review. Neurosurgery 7:503, 1980.

160. Bulas DI, Fitz CR, Johnson DL: Traumatic atlanto-occipital dislocation in children. Radiology 188:155, 1993.

161. Eismont FJ, Bohlman HH: Posterior atlanto-occipital dislocation with fractures of the atlas and odontoid process. J Bone Joint Surg [Am] 60:397, 1978.

162. Woodring JH, Selke AC, Duff DE: Traumatic atlantooccipital dislocation with survival. AJR 137:21, 1981.

163. Rosenbaum DM, Blumhagen JD, King HA: Atlantooccipital instability in Down syndrome. AJR 146:1269, 1986.

164. Bucholz RW: Unstable hangman's fractures. Clin Orthop 154:119, 1981.

165. Bundschuh CV, Alley JB, Ross M, et al: Magnetic resonance imaging of suspected atlanto-occipital dislocation: Two case reports. Spine 17:245, 1992.

166. Kaufman RA, Dunbar JS, Botsford JA, et al: Traumatic longitudinal atlantooccipital distraction injuries in children. AJNR 3:415, 1982.

167. Englander O: Non-traumatic occipito-atlanto-axial dislocation: A contribution to the radiology of the atlas. Br J Radiol 15:341, 1942.

168. Jones DN, Knox AM, Sage RM: Traumatic avulsion fracture of the occipital condyles and clivus with associated unilateral atlantooccipital distraction. AJNR 11:1181, 1990.

169. Bettini N, Malaguti MC, Sintini M, et al: Fractures of the occipital condyles: Report of four cases and review of the literature. Skel Radiol 22:187, 1993.

170. Steel HH: Anatomical and mechanical considerations of the atlanto-axial articulations. J Bone Joint Surg [Am] 50:1691, 1968.

171. Powers B, Miller MD, Kramer RS, et al: Traumatic anterior atlanto-occipital dislocation. Neurosurgery 4:12, 1979.

172. Gerlock AJ, Mirfakhraee M, Benzel EC: Computed tomography of traumatic atlantooccipital dislocation. Neurosurgery 13:316, 1983.

173. Goldberg AL, Baron B, Daffner RH: Atlantooccipital dislocation: MR demonstration of cord damage. J Comput Assist Tomogr 15:174, 1991.

174. Schatzker J, Rorabeck CH, Waddell JP: Fractures of the dens [odontoid process]: An analysis of thirty-seven cases. J Bone Joint Surg [Br] 53:392, 1971.

175. Greenberg AD: Atlanto-axial dislocations. Brain 91:655, 1968.

176. Bohrer SP, Klein A, Martin W III: "V" shaped predens space. Skel Radiol 14:111, 1985.

177. Weissman BNW, Aliabadi P, Weinfeld MS: Prognostic features of atlantoaxial subluxation in rheumatoid arthritis patients. Radiology 144:745, 1982.

178. Koss JC, Dalinka MK: Atlantoaxial subluxation in Behcet's syndrome. AJR 134:392, 1980.

179. Martich V, Ben-Ami T, Yousefzadeh DK, et al: Hypoplastic posterior arch of C-1 in children with Down syndrome: A double jeopardy. Radiology 128:125, 1992.

180. Singer SJ, Rubin IL, Strauss KJ: Atlantoaxial distance in patients with Down syndrome: Standardization of measurement. Radiology 164:871, 1987.

181. White KS, Ball WS, Prenger EC, et al: Evaluation of the craniocervical junction in Down syndrome: Correlation of measurements obtained with radiography and MR imaging. Radiology 186:377, 1993.

182. Haralson RH, Boyd HB: Posterior dislocation of the atlas on the axis without fracture. J Bone Joint Surg [Am] 51:561, 1969.

183. Wortzman G, Dewar FP: Rotary fixation of the atlantoaxial joint: Rotational atlantoaxial subluxation. Radiology 90:479, 1968.

184. Fielding JW, Hawkins RJ: Atlanto-axial rotatory fixation. J Bone Joint Surg [Am] 59:37, 1977.

185. Penecot GF, Couraud D, Hardy JR, et al: Roentgenographical study of the stability of the cervical spine in children. J Pediatr Orthop 4:346, 1984.

186. Sherk HH, Nicholson JT: Fractures of the atlas. J Bone Joint Surg [Am] 52:1017, 1970.

187. Fielding JW, Hensinger RN, Hawkins RJ: Os odontoideum. J Bone Joint Surg [Am] 62:376, 1980.

188. Scher AT: Displacement of the spinolaminar line—a sign of value in fractures of the upper cervical spine: A report of 2 cases. S Afr Med J 56:58, 1979.

189. Swischuk LE, Hayden CK, Sarwar M: The posteriorly tilted dens. Pediatr Radiol 8:27, 1979.

190. Ogden JA: Radiology of postnatal skeletal development. XII. The second cervical vertebra. Skel Radiol 12:169, 1984.

191. Smoker WRK, Keyes WD, Dunn VD, et al: MRI versus conventional radiologic examinations in the evaluation of the craniovertebral and cervicomedullary junction. RadioGraphics 6:953, 1986.

192. Sze G, Brant-Zawadzki MN, Wilson CR, et al: Pseudotumor of the craniovertebral junction associated with chronic subluxation: MR imaging studies. Radiology 161:391, 1986.

193. Kowalski HM, Cohen WA, Cooper P, et al: Pitfalls in the CT diagnosis of atlantoaxial rotary subluxation. AJNR 8:697, 1987.
194. Rinaldi I, Mullins WJ, Delaney WF, et al: Computerized tomographic demonstration of rotational atlanto-axial fixation: Case report. J Neurosurg 50:115, 1979.
195. Corner EM: Rotary dislocations of the atlas. Ann Surg 45:9, 1907.
196. Jacobson G, Adler DC: Examination of the atlanto-axial joint following injury with particular emphasis on rotational subluxation. AJR 76:1081, 1956.
197. Akbarnia BA, Vafaie M: Atlantoaxial rotary fixation: Report of a case with massive displacement. Spine 8:907, 1983.
198. Kiwak KJ: Establishing an etiology for torticollis. Postgrad Med 75:126, 1984.
199. Plaut HF: Fractures of the atlas resulting from automobile accidents: A survey of the literature and report of six cases. AJR 40:867, 1938.
200. Fielding JW, Hawkins RJ, Hensinger RN, et al: Atlantoaxial rotary deformities. Orthop Clin North Am 9:955, 1978.
201. Harris JH Jr: Acute injuries of the spine. Semin Roentgenol 13:53, 1978.
202. Ogden JA, Murphy MJ, Southwick WO, et al: Radiology of postnatal skeletal development. XIII. C1-C2 interrelationships. Skel Radiol 15:433, 1986.
203. Wetzel FT, La Rocca H: Grisel's syndrome: A review. Clin Orthop 240:141, 1989.
204. Hall FM: CT in atlantoaxial rotatory fixation. AJR 150:947, 1988.
205. Baumgarten M, Mouradian W, Boger D, et al: Computed axial tomography in C1-C2 trauma. Spine 10:187, 1985.
206. Fielding JW, Stillwell WT, Chynn KY, et al: Use of computed tomography for the diagnosis of atlanto-axial rotatory fixation. J Bone Joint Surg [Am] 60:1102, 1978.
207. Grobman LR, Stricker S: Grisel's syndrome. Ear Nose Throat J 69:799, 1990.
208. Mathern GW, Batzdorf U: Grisel's syndrome: Cervical spine clinical, pathologic and neurologic manifestations. Clin Orthop 244:131, 1989.
209. Parke WW, Rothman RH, Brown MD: The pharyngovertebral veins: An anatomical rationale for Grisel's syndrome. J Bone Joint Surg [Am] 66:568, 1984.
210. Ogden JA: Radiology of postnatal skeletal development. XI. The first cervical vertebra. Skel Radiol 12:12, 1984.
211. Yousefzadeh DK, El-Khoury GY, Smith WL: Normal sagittal diameter and variation in the pediatric cervical spine. Radiology 144:319, 1982.
212. Stewart GC, Gehweiler JA Jr, Laib RH, et al: Horizontal fracture of the anterior arch of the atlas. Radiology 122:349, 1977.
213. Gehweiler JA, Duff DE, Martinez S, et al: Fractures of the atlas vertebra. Skel Radiol 1:97, 1976.
214. Landells CD, Van Peteghem PK: Fractures of the atlas: Classification, treatment and morbidity. Spine 13:450, 1988.
215. Lee C, Woodring JH: Unstable Jefferson variant atlas fractures: An unrecognized cervical injury. AJR 158:113, 1992.
216. Suss RA, Bundy KJ: Unilateral posterior arch fractures of the atlas. AJNR 5:783, 1984.
217. Cone RO, Flournoy J, MacPherson RI: The craniocervical junction. RadioGraphics 1:1, 1981.
218. Kershner MS, Goodman GA, Perlmutter GS: Computed tomography in the diagnosis of an atlas fracture. AJR 128:688, 1977.
219. Gehweiler JA, Daffner RH, Roberts L: Malformations of the atlas vertebra simulating the Jefferson fracture. AJR 140:1083, 1983.
220. Wilkinson RH, Strand RD: Congenital anomalies and normal variants. Semin Roentgenol 14:7, 1979.
221. Chambers AA, Gaskill MF: Midline anterior atlas clefts: CT findings. J Comput Assist Tomogr 16:868, 1992.
222. Hays MB, Alker GJ Jr: Fractures of the atlas vertebra: The two-part burst fracture of Jefferson. Spine 13:601, 1988.
223. Flournoy JG, Cone RO, Saldana HA, et al: Jefferson fracture: Presentation of a new diagnostic sign. Radiology 134:88, 1980.
224. Jacobson G, Adler DC: An evaluation of lateral atlantoaxial displacement in injuries of the cervical spine. Radiology 61:355, 1953.
225. Budin E, Sondheimer F: Lateral spread of the atlas without fracture. Radiology 87:1095, 1966.
226. Paul LW, Moir WW: Non-pathologic variations in relationship of the upper cervical vertebrae. AJR 61:519, 1949.
227. Suss RA, Zimmerman RD, Leeds NE: Pseudospread of the atlas: False sign of Jefferson fracture in young children. AJR 140:1079, 1983.
228. England AC, Shippel AH, Ray MJ: A simple view for demonstration of fractures of the anterior arch of C1. AJR 144:763, 1985.
229. Swartz JD, Puleo S: Fractures of the C-1 vertebra: Report of two cases documented with computed tomography. J Comput Assist Tomogr 7:311, 1983.
230. O'Brien JJ, Butterfield WL, Gossling HR: Jefferson fracture with disruption of the transverse ligament: A case report. Clin Orthop 136:135, 1976.
231. Jevtich V: Horizontal fracture of the anterior arch of the atlas. J Bone Joint Surg [Am] 68:1094, 1986.
232. Barker EG Jr, Krumpelman J, Long JM: Isolated fracture of the medial portion of the lateral mass of the atlas: A previously undescribed entity. AJR 126:1053, 1976.
233. Burke JT, Harris JH: Acute injuries of the axis vertebra. Skel Radiol 18:335, 1989.
234. Brashear HR, Venters GC, Preston ET: Fractures of the neural arch of the axis. J Bone Joint Surg [Am] 57:879, 1975.
235. McClellan R, El Gammal T, Willing S, et al: Persistent infantile odontoid process: A variant of abnormal atlantoaxial segmentation. AJR 158:1305, 1992.

236. Elliott JM, Rogers LF, Wissinger JP, et al: The hangman's fracture: Fractures of the neural arch of the axis. Radiology 104:303, 1972.
237. Martinez S, Morgan CL, Gehweiler JA, et al: Unusual fractures and dislocations of the axis vertebra. Skel Radiol 3:206, 1979.
238. Hadley MN, Browner C, Sonntag VKH: Axis fractures: A comprehensive review of management and treatment in 107 cases. Neurosurgery 17:281, 1985.
239. Harris JH Jr, Burke JT, Ray RD, et al: Low (Type III) odontoid fracture: A new radiographic sign. Radiology 153:353, 1984.
240. Clark CR, White AA III: Fractures of the dens: A multicenter study. J Bone Joint Surg [Am] 67:1340, 1985.
241. Anderson LD, D'Alonzo RT: Fractures of the odontoid process of the axis. J Bone Joint Surg [Am] 56:1663, 1974.
242. Southwick WO: Current concepts review: Management of fractures of the dens (odontoid process). J Bone Joint Surg [Am] 62:482, 1980.
243. Ruff SJ, Taylor TKF: Hangman's fracture in an infant. J Bone Joint Surg [Br] 68:702, 1986.
244. Gehweiler JA Jr, Clark WM, Schaaf RE, et al: Cervical spine trauma: The common combined conditions. Radiology 130:77, 1979.
245. Holt RG, Helms CA, Munk PL, et al: Hypertrophy of C-1 anterior arch: Useful sign to distinguish os odontoideum from acute dens fracture. Radiology 173:207, 1989.
246. Thomeier WC, Brown DC, Mirvis SE: The laterally tilted dens: A sign of subtle odontoid fracture on plain radiography. AJNR 11:605, 1990.
247. Gurney JW: Absent dens on submentovertex view of the skull: New sign of an abnormal odontoid. J Can Assoc Radiol 37:38, 1986.
248. Kattan KR, Pais MJ: Some borderlands of the cervical spine. Part I. The normal (and nearly normal) that may appear pathologic. Skel Radiol 8:1, 1982.
249. Pepin JW, Hawkins RJ: Traumatic spondylolisthesis of the axis: Hangman's fracture. Clin Orthop 157:133, 1981.
250. Mirvis SE, Young JWR, Lim C, et al: Hangman's fracture: Radiologic assessment in 27 cases. Radiology 163:713, 1987.
251. Schneider RC, Livingston KE, Cave AJE, et al: "Hangman's fracture" of the cervical spine. J Neurosurg 22:141, 1965.
252. Effendi B, Roy D, Cornish B, et al: Fractures of the ring of the axis: A classification based on the analysis of 131 cases. J Bone Joint Surg [Br] 63:319, 1981.
253. Francis WR, Fielding JW, Hawkins RJ, et al: Traumatic spondylolisthesis of the axis. J Bone Joint Surg [Br] 63:313, 1981.
254. Gehweiler JA, Martinez S, Clark WM, et al: Spondylolisthesis of the axis vertebra. AJR 128:682, 1977.
255. Kish KK, Wilner HI: Spondylolysis of C2: CT and plain film findings. J Comput Assist Tomogr 7:517, 1983.
256. Black KS, Gorey MT, Seideman B, et al: Congenital spondylolisthesis of the 6th cervical vertebra: CT findings. J Comput Assist Tomogr 15:335, 1991.
257. Levine AM, Edwards CC: The management of traumatic spondylolisthesis of the axis. J Bone Joint Surg [Am] 67:217, 1985.
258. Kattan KR: Backward "displacement" of the spinolaminal line at C2: A normal variation. AJR 129:289, 1977.
259. Gerlock AJ, Mirfakhraee M: Computed tomography and hangman's fractures. South Med J 76:727, 1983.
260. Wood-Jones F: The ileal lesion produced by judicial hanging. Lancet 1:53, 1913.
261. Swischuk LE: Anterior displacement of C2 in children: Physiologic or pathologic? A helpful differentiating line. Radiology 122:759, 1977.
262. Edeiken-Monroe B, Wagner LK, Harris JH Jr: Hyperextension dislocation of the cervical spine. AJR 146:803, 1986.
263. Smoker WRK, Dolan KD: The "fat" C2: A sign of fracture. AJR 148:609, 1987.
264. Abel MS, Teague JH: Unilateral lateral mass compression fractures of the axis. Skel Radiol 4:92, 1979.
265. Halliday DR, Sullivan CR, Hollinshead WH, et al: Torn cervical ligaments: Necropsy examination of the normal cervical region of the spinal column. J Trauma 4:219, 1964.
266. Green JD, Harle TS, Harris JH: Anterior subluxation of the cervical spine: Hyperflexion sprain. AJNR 2:243, 1981.
267. Bohrer SP, Chen YM, Sayers DG: Cervical spine flexion patterns. Skel Radiol 19:521, 1990.
268. Whitley JE, Forsyth HF: The classification of cervical spine injuries. AJR 83:633, 1960.
269. Marar BC: Hyperextension injuries of the cervical spine: The pathogenesis of damage to the spinal cord. J Bone Joint Surg [Am] 56:1655, 1974.
270. Jonsson K, Niklasson J, Josefsson PO: Avulsion of the cervical spinal ring apophyses: Acute and chronic appearance. Skel Radiol 20:207, 1991.
271. Lawson JP, Ogden HA, Bucholz RW, et al: Physeal injuries of the cervical spine. J Pediatr Orthop 7:428, 1987.
272. Ghelman B, Freiberger RH: The limbus vertebra: An anterior disc herniation demonstrated by discography. AJR 127:854, 1976.
273. Lee C, Kwang SK, Rogers LF: Triangular cervical vertebral body fractures: Diagnostic significance. AJR 138:1123, 1982.
274. Cintron E, Gilula LA, Murphy WA, et al: The widened disk space: A sign of cervical hyperextension injury. Radiology 141:639, 1981.
275. Agha FP, Raji MR: Oesophageal perforation with fracture dislocation of cervical spine due to hyperextension injury. Br J Radiol 55:369, 1982.
276. Lee C, Woodring JH, Rogers LF, et al: The radiographic distinction of degen-

erative slippage (spondylolisthesis and retrolisthesis) from traumatic slippage of the cervical spine. Skel Radiol 15:439, 1986.

277. Reymond RD, Wheeler PS, Perovic M, et al: The lucent cleft, a new radiographic sign of cervical disc injury or disease. Clin Radiol 23:188, 1972.

278. Bohrer SP, Chen YM: Cervical spine annulus vacuum. Skel Radiol 17:324, 1988.

279. Daffner RH, Gehweiler JA: Pseudovacuum of the cervical intervertebral disc: A normal variant. AJR 137:737, 1981.

280. Daffner RH, Deeb ZL, Rothfus WE: Pseudofractures of the cervical vertebral body. Skel Radiol 15:295, 1986.

281. Goldberg RP, Vine HS, Sacks BA, et al: The cervical split: A pseudofracture. Skel Radiol 7:267, 1982.

282. Taylor AR, Blackwood W: Paraplegia in hyperextension cervical injuries with normal radiographic appearances. J Bone Joint Surg [Br] 30:245, 1948.

283. Pitman MI, Pilman CA, Greenberg IM: Complete dislocation of the cervical spine without neurological deficit. J Bone Joint Surg [Am] 59:134, 1977.

284. Torg JS, Pavlov H, Genuario SE, et al: Neurapraxia of the cervical spinal cord with transient quadriplegia. J Bone Joint Surg [Am] 68:1354, 1986.

285. Ladd AL, Scranton PE: Congenital cervical stenosis presenting as transient quadriplegia in athletes. J Bone Joint Surg [Am] 68:1371, 1986.

286. Pavlov H, Torg JS, Robie B, et al: Cervical spinal stenosis: Determination with vertebral body ratio method. Radiology 164:771, 1987.

287. Woodring JH, Goldstein SJ: Fractures of the articular processes of the cervical spine. AJR 139:341, 1982.

288. Vines FS: The significance of "occult" fractures of the cervical spine. AJR 107:493, 1969.

289. Abel MS: The exaggerated supine oblique view of the cervical spine. Skel Radiol 8:213, 1982.

290. Young JWR, Resnik CS, DeCandido P, et al: The laminar space in the diagnosis of rotational flexion injuries of the cervical spine. AJR 152:103, 1989.

291. Smith GR, Beckly DE, Abel MS: Articular mass fracture: A neglected cause of post-traumatic neck pain? Clin Radiol 27:335, 1976.

292. Braakman M, Braakman R: Hyperflexion sprain of the cervical spine: Follow-up of 45 cases. Acta Orthop Scand 58:388, 1987.

293. Fazl M, LaFebvre J, Willinsky RA, et al: Posttraumatic ligamentous disruption of the cervical spine, an easily overlooked diagnosis: Presentation of three cases. Neurosurgery 26:674, 1990.

294. Naidich JB, Naidich TP, Farfein C, et al: The widened interspinous distance: A useful sign of anterior cervical dislocation in the supine frontal projection. Radiology 123:113, 1977.

295. Mazur JM, Stauffer ES: Unrecognized spinal instability associated with seemingly "simple" cervical compression fractures. Spine 8:687, 1983.

296. Stauffer ES, Kelly EG: Fracture-dislocations of the cervical spine: Instability and recurrent deformity following treatment by anterior interbody fusion. J Bone Joint Surg [Am] 59:45, 1977.

297. Cancelmo JJ Jr: Clay shoveler's fracture: A helpful diagnostic sign. AJR 115:540, 1972.

298. Zanca P, Lodmell EA: Fracture of the spinous processes. Radiology 56:427, 1951.

299. Cimmino CV, Scott DW III: Laminar avulsion in a cervical vertebra. AJR 129:57, 1977.

300. Salomone JA, Steele MT: An unusual presentation of bilateral facet dislocation of the cervical spine. Ann Emerg Med 16:1390, 1987.

301. Beatson TR: Fractures and dislocations of the cervical spine. J Bone Joint Surg [Br] 45:21, 1963.

302. Eismont FJ, Arena MJ, Green BA: Extrusion of an intervertebral disc associated with traumatic subluxation or dislocation of cervical facets. J Bone Joint Surg [Am] 73:1555, 1991.

303. Kim KS, Chen HH, Russell EJ, et al: Flexion teardrop fracture of the cervical spine: Radiographic characteristics. AJR 152:319, 1989.

304. Scher AT: Tear-drop fractures of the cervical spine—radiological features. S Afr Med J 62:355, 1982.

305. Kerns S, Pope TL, de Lange EE, et al: Annulus fibrosus calcification in the cervical spine: Radiologic-pathologic correlation. Skel Radiol 15:605, 1986.

306. Scher AT: Unilateral locked facet in cervical spine injuries. AJR 129:45, 1977.

307. Schaaf RE, Gehweiler JA, Miller MD, et al: Lateral hyperflexion injuries of the cervical spine. Skel Radiol 3:73, 1978.

308. Stanley P, Duncan AW, Isaacson J, et al: Radiology of fracture-dislocation of the cervical spine during delivery. AJR 145:621, 1985.

309. Lee C, Kwang SK, Rogers LR: Sagittal fracture of the cervical vertebral body. AJR 139:55, 1982.

310. Rogers LF, Thayer C, Weinberg PE, et al: Acute injuries of the upper thoracic spine associated with paraplegia. AJR 134:67, 1980.

311. Sutherland CJ, Miller F, Wang GJ: Early progressive kyphosis following compression fractures. Clin Orthop 173:216, 1983.

312. Maiman DJ, Pintar FA: Anatomy and clinical biomechanics of the thoracic spine. Clin Neurosurg 38:296, 1992.

313. Bohlman HH: Current concepts review: Treatment of fractures and dislocations of the thoracic and lumbar spine. J Bone Joint Surg [Am] 67:165, 1985.

314. Griffith HB, Gleave JRW, Taylor RG: Changing patterns of fracture in the dorsal and lumbar spine. Br Med J 1:891, 1966.

315. Bohlman HH, Freehafer A, Dejak J: The results of treatment of acute injuries of the upper thoracic spine with paralysis. J Bone Joint Surg [Am] 67:360, 1985.

316. Daffner RH, Deeb ZL, Rothfus WE: Thoracic fractures and dislocations in motorcyclists. Skel Radiol 16:280, 1987.

317. El-Khoury GY, Whitten CG: Trauma to the upper thoracic spine: Anatomy, biomechanics, and unique imaging features. AJR 160:95, 1993.

318. Bolesta MJ, Bohlman HH: Injuries of the thoracic spine. In HL Frankel (Ed): Spinal Cord Trauma. Amsterdam, Elsevier Science, 1992.

319. Fletcher GH: Anterior vertebral wedging—frequency and significance. AJR 57:232, 1947.

320. Lauridsen KN, De Carvalho A, Andersen AH: Degree of vertebral wedging of the dorso-lumbar spine. Acta Radiol 25:29, 1984.

321. Dalton CJ, Schwartz SS: Evaluation of the paraspinal line in roentgen examination of the thorax. Radiology 66:195, 1956.

322. Lien HH, Kolbenstvedt A, Lund G: The thoracic paraspinal shadow: A review of the appearances in pathological conditions. Clin Radiol 35:215, 1984.

323. Norman A: Segmental bulge of the linear thoracic paraspinal shadow (paravertebral line). J Bone Joint Surg [Am] 44:352, 1962.

324. Gehweiler JA, Daffner RH, Osborne RL: Relevant signs of stable and unstable thoracolumbar vertebral column trauma. Skel Radiol 7:179, 1981.

325. Dennis LN, Rogers LF: Superior mediastinal widening from spine fractures mimicking aortic rupture on chest radiographs. AJR 152:27, 1989.

326. Bolesta MJ, Bohlman HH: Mediastinal widening associated with fractures of the upper thoracic spine. J Bone Joint Surg [Am] 73:447, 1991.

327. Gundry SR, Burney RE, Mackenzie JR, et al: Assessment of mediastinal widening associated with traumatic rupture of the aorta. J Trauma 23:293, 1983.

328. Crass JR, Cohen AM, Motta AO, et al: A proposed new mechanism of traumatic aortic rupture: The osseous pinch. Radiology 176:645, 1990.

329. Cohen AM, Crass JR, Thomas HA, et al: CT evidence for the osseous pinch mechanism of traumatic aortic injury. AJR 159:271, 1992.

330. Kaplan PA, Orton DF, Asleson RJ: Osteoporosis with vertebral compression fractures, retropulsed fragments, and neurologic compromise. Radiology 165:533, 1987.

331. DeSmet AA, Robinson RG, Johnson BE, et al: Spinal compression fractures in osteoporotic women: Patterns and relationship to hyperkyphosis. Radiology 166:497, 1988.

332. Melton LJ, Kan SH, Frye MA, et al: Epidemiology of vertebral fractures in women. Am J Epidemiol 129:1000, 1989.

333. Isard HJ: A roentgen evaluation of vertebral fractures resulting from convulsive shock therapy. AJR 68:247, 1952.

334. Roberts JB, Curtiss PH: Stability of the thoracic and lumbar spine in traumatic paraplegia following fracture of fracture-dislocation. J Bone Joint Surg [Am] 52:1115, 1970.

335. Resnick DL: Fish vertebrae. Arthritis Rheum 25:1073, 1982.

336. Sartoris DJ, Clopton P, Nemcek A, et al: Vertebral-body collapse in focal and diffuse disease: Patterns of pathologic processes. Radiology 160:479, 1986.

337. Yuh WT, Zachar CK, Barloon TJ, et al: Vertebral compression fractures: Distinction between benign and malignant causes with MR imaging. Radiology 172:215, 1989.

338. Hayes CW, Jensen ME, Conway WF: Non-neoplastic lesions of vertebral bodies: Findings in magnetic resonance imaging. RadioGraphics 9:883, 1989.

339. Baker LL, Goodman SB, Perkash I, et al: Benign versus pathologic compression fractures of vertebral bodies: Assessment with conventional spin-echo, chemical-shift, and STIR MR imaging. Radiology 174:495, 1990.

340. Cullen JC: Spinal lesions in battered babies. J Bone Joint Surg [Am] 57:364, 1975.

341. Kleinman PK, Zito JL: Avulsion of the spinous processes caused by infant abuse. Radiology 151:389, 1984.

342. Swischuk LE: Spine and spinal cord trauma in the battered child syndrome. Radiology 92:733, 1969.

343. Alexander CJ: Scheuermann's disease: A traumatic spondylodystrophy? Skel Radiol 1:209, 1977.

344. Horne J, Cockshott WP, Shannon HS: Spinal column damage from water ski jumping. Skel Radiol 16:612, 1987.

345. Brower AC, Downey E Jr: Kummell disease: Report of a case with serial radiographs. Radiology 141:363, 1981.

346. Maldague BE, Noel HM, Malghem JJ: The intravertebral vacuum cleft: A sign of ischemic vertebral collapse. Radiology 129:23, 1978.

347. Malghem J, Maldague B, Labaisse M: Intravertebral vacuum cleft: Changes in content after supine positioning. Radiology 187:483, 1993.

348. Resnick D, Niwayama G, Guerra J Jr, et al: Spinal vacuum phenomena: Anatomical study and review. Radiology 139:341, 1981.

349. Naul LG, Peet GJ, Maupin WB: Avascular necrosis of the vertebral body: MR imaging. Radiology 172:219, 1989.

350. Gertzbein SD, Offierski C: Complete fracture-dislocation of the thoracic spine without spinal cord injury: A case report. J Bone Joint Surg [Am] 61:449, 1979.

351. Sasson A, Mozes G: Briefly noted: Complete fracture-dislocation of the thoracic spine without neurologic deficit, a case report. Spine 12:67, 1987.

352. Simpson AHRW, Williamson DM, Golding SJ, et al: Thoracic spine translocation without cord injury. J Bone Joint Surg [Br] 72:80, 1990.

353. Shuman WP, Rogers JV, Sickler ME, et al: Thoracolumbar burst fractures: CT dimensions of the spinal canal relative to postsurgical improvement. AJR 145:337, 1985.

354. Smith GR, Curtis HN, Loop JW: Jumpers' fractures: Patterns of thoracolumbar spine injuries associated with vertical plunges. Radiology 122:657, 1977.

355. Wilson BPM, Finlay D: Computerized tomography of injury to the thoracolumbar spine. Injury 18:185, 1987.

356. Kilcoyne RF, Mack LA, King HA, et al: Thoracolumbar spine injuries associated with vertical plunges: Reappraisal with computed tomography. Radiology 146:137, 1983.

357. Sartoris DJ, Resnick D, Guerra J: Vertebral venous channels: CT appearance and differential considerations. Radiology 155:745, 1985.

358. Willen J, Lindahl S, Irstam L, et al: Unstable thoracolumbar fractures: A study by CT and conventional roentgenology of the reduction effect of Harrington instrumentation. Spine 9:214, 1984.

359. Cammisa FP, Eismont FJ, Green BA: Dural laceration occurring with burst fractures and associated laminar fractures. J Bone Joint Surg [Am] 71:1044, 1989.

360. Atlas SW, Regenbogen V, Rogers LF, et al: The radiographic characterization of burst fractures of the spine. AJR 147:575, 1986.

361. Willen J, Lindahl S, Irstam L, et al: The thoracolumbar crush fracture. An experimental study on instant axial dynamic loading: The resulting fracture type and its stability. Spine 9:624, 1984.

362. Fredrickson BE, Edwards WT, Rauschning W: Vertebral burst fractures: An experimental, morphologic, and radiographic study. Spine 17:1012, 1992.

363. Lindahl S, Willen J, Nordwall A, et al: The crush-cleavage fracture: A ''new'' thoracolumbar unstable fracture. Spine 8:559, 1983.

364. Ballock RT, MacKersie R, Abitbol J, et al: Can burst fractures be predicted from plain radiographs? J Bone Joint Surg [Br] 74:147, 1992.

365. DeWald RL: Burst fractures of the thoracic and lumbar spine. Clin Orthop 189:150, 1984.

366. Daffner RH, Deeb ZL, Rothfus WE: The posterior vertebral body line: Importance in the detection of burst fractures. AJR 148:93, 1987.

367. Jelsma RK, Kirsch PT, Rice JF, et al: The radiographic description of thoracolumbar fractures. Surg Neurol 18:230, 1982.

368. Guerra J Jr, Garfin SR, Resnick D: Vertebral burst fractures: CT analysis of the retropulsed fragment. Radiology 153:769, 1984.

369. Laasonen EM, Riska EB: Preoperative radiological assessment of fractures of the thoracolumbar spine causing traumatic paraplegia. Skel Radiol 1:231, 1977.

370. McAfee PC, Hansen AY, Lasda NA: The unstable burst fracture. Spine 7:365, 1982.

371. Martijn A, Veldhuis EFM: The diagnostic value of interpediculate distance assessment on plain films in thoracic and lumbar spine injuries. J Trauma 31:1393, 1991.

372. Fontijne WPJ, deKlerk LWL, Braakman R, et al: CT scan prediction of neurological deficit in thoracolumbar burst fractures. J Bone Joint Surg [Br] 74:683, 1992.

373. McAfee PC, Bohlman HH, Yuan HA: Anterior decompression of traumatic thoracolumbar fractures with incomplete neurological deficit using a retroperitoneal approach. J Bone Joint Surg [Am] 67:89, 1985.

374. Rubenstein JD, Gertzbein S: Radiographic assessment of Harrington rod instrumentation for spinal fractures. J Can Assoc Radiol 35:159, 1984.

375. Benson DR: Unstable thoracolumbar fractures, with emphasis on the burst fracture. Clin Orthop 230:14, 1988.

376. Fidler MW: Remodelling of the spinal canal after burst fracture: A prospective study of two cases. J Bone Joint Surg [Br] 70:730, 1988.

377. Chakera TMH, Bedbrook G, Bradley CM: Spontaneous resolution of spinal canal deformity after burst-dispersion fracture. AJNR 9:779, 1988.

378. Malcolm BW, Bradford DS, Winter RB, et al: Post-traumatic kyphosis: A review of forty-eight surgically treated patients. J Bone Joint Surg [Am] 63:891, 1981.

379. Golimbu C, Firooznia H, Rafii M, et al: Computed tomography of thoracic and lumbar spine fractures that have been treated with Harrington instrumentation. Radiology 151:731, 1984.

380. Weisz GM: Post-traumatic spinal stenosis. Arch Orthop Trauma Surg 106:57, 1986.

381. Taylor GA, Eggli KD: Lap-belt injuries of the lumbar spine in children: A pitfall in CT diagnosis. AJR 150:1355, 1988.

382. Smith WS, Kaufer H: Patterns and mechanisms of lumbar injuries associated with lap seat belts. J Bone Joint Surg [Am] 51:239, 1969.

383. Rogers LF: The roentgenographic appearance of transverse or Chance fractures of the spine: The seat belt fracture. AJR 111:844, 1971.

384. Dehner JR: Seatbelt injuries of the spine and abdomen. AJR 111:833, 1971.

385. Miniaci A, McLaren AC: Anterolateral compression fracture of the thoracolumbar spine: A seat belt injury. Clin Orthop 240:153, 1989.

386. Chance GQ: Note on a type of flexion fracture of the spine. Br J Radiol 21:452, 1948.

387. Kachooie A, Bloch R, Banna M: Post-traumatic dorsal pseudomeningocele. J Can Assoc Radiol 36:262, 1985.

388. Gellad FE, Levine AM, Joslyn JN, et al: Pure thoracolumbar facet dislocation: Clinical features and CT appearance. Radiology 161:505, 1986.

389. Kaufer H, Hayes JT: Lumbar fracture-dislocation. J Bone Joint Surg [Am] 48:712, 1966.

390. Finn GA, Stauffer ES: Burst fracture of the fifth lumbar vertebra. J Bone Joint Surg [Am] 74:398, 1992.

391. Court-Brown CM, Gertzbein SD: The management of burst fractures of the fifth lumbar vertebra. Spine 12:308, 1987.

392. Fredrickson BE, Hansen AY, Miller H: Burst fractures of the fifth lumbar vertebra. J Bone Joint Surg [Am] 64:1088, 1982.

393. Das De S, McCreath SW: Lumbosacral fracture-dislocations. J Bone Joint Surg [Br] 63:58, 1881.

394. Resnik CS, Scheer CE, Adelaar RS: Lumbosacral dislocation. J Can Assoc Radiol 36:259, 1985.

395. Graves VB, Keene JS, Strother CM, et al: CT of bilateral lumbosacral facet dislocation. AJNR 9:809, 1988.

396. Wiltse LL, Newman PH, Macnab I: Classification of spondylolysis and spondylolisthesis. Clin Orthop 117:23, 1976.

397. Jacobs RR: Bilateral fracture of the pedicles through the fourth and fifth lumbar vertebrae with anterior displacement of the vertebral bodies. J Bone Joint Surg [Am] 59:409, 1977.

398. Gilsanz V, Miranda J, Cleveland R, et al: Scoliosis secondary to fractures of the transverse processes of lumbar vertebrae. Radiology 134:627, 1980.

399. Sturm JT, Perry JF: Injuries associated with fractures of the transverse processes of the thoracic and lumbar vertebrae. J Trauma 24:597, 1984.

400. Abel MS: Jogger's fracture and other stress fractures of the lumbo-sacral spine. Skel Radiol 13:221, 1985.

401. Traughber PD, Havlina JM Jr: Bilateral pedicle stress fractures: SPECT and CT features. J Comput Assist Tomogr 15:338, 1991.

402. Ireland ML, Micheli LJ: Bilateral stress fracture of the lumbar pedicles in a ballet dancer. J Bone Joint Surg [Am] 69:140, 1987.

403. Abel MS: Transverse posterior element fractures associated with torsion. Skel Radiol 17:556, 1989.

404. Johansen JG, McCarty DJ, Haughton VM: Retrosomatic clefts: Computed tomographic appearance. Radiology 148:447, 1983.

405. Aland C, Rineberg BA, Malberg M, et al: Fracture of the pedicle of the fourth lumbar vertebra associated with contralateral spondylolysis. J Bone Joint Surg [Am] 68:1454, 1986.

406. Jinkins JR, Matthes JC, Sener RN, et al: Spondylolysis, spondylolisthesis, and associated nerve root entrapment in the lumbosacral spine: MR evaluation. AJR 159:799, 1992.

407. Cope R: Acute traumatic spondylolysis: Report of a case and review of the literature. Clin Orthop 230:162, 1988.

408. Roche MB: Bilateral fracture of the pars interarticularis of a lumbar neural arch. J Bone Joint Surg [Am] 30:1005, 1948.

409. Fullenlove TM, Wilson JG: Traumatic defects of the pars interarticularis of the lumbar vertebrae. AJR 122:634, 1974.

410. Melamed A: Fracture of pars interarticularis of lumbar vertebra. AJR 94:584, 1965.

411. Teplick GJ, Laffey PA, Berman A, et al: Diagnosis and evaluation of spondylolisthesis and/or spondylolysis on axial CT. AJNR 7:479, 1986.

412. Hensinger RN: Current concepts review: Spondylolysis and spondylolisthesis in children and adolescents. J Bone Joint Surg [Am] 71:1098, 1989.

413. Jackson DW, Wiltse LL, Cirincione RJ: Spondylolysis in the female gymnast. Clin Orthop 117:68, 1976.

414. Wiltse LL, Widell EH, Jackson DW: Fatigue fracture: The basic lesion in isthmic spondylolysis. J Bone Joint Surg [Am] 57:17, 1975.

415. Grenier N, Kressel HY, Schiebler ML, et al: Isthmic spondylolysis of the lumbar spine: MR imaging at 1.5T. Radiology 170:489, 1989.

416. Amato M, Totty WG, Gilula LA: Spondylolysis of the lumbar spine: Demonstration of defects and laminal fragmentation. Radiology 153:627, 1984.

417. Baker DR, McHollick W: Spondyloschisis and spondylolisthesis in children. J Bone Joint Surg [Am] 38:933, 1956.

418. Maldague BE, Malghem JJ: Unilateral arch hypertrophy with spinous process tilt: A sign of arch deficiency. Radiology 121:567, 1976.

419. Rothman SLG, Glenn WV Jr: CT multiplanar reconstruction in 253 cases of lumbar spondylolysis. AJNR 5:81, 1984.

420. Pennell RG, Maurer AH, Bonakdarpour A: Stress injuries of the pars interarticularis: Radiologic classification and indications for scintigraphy. AJR 145:763, 1985.

421. El-Khoury GY, Yousefzadeh DK, Kathol MH, et al: Pseudospondylolysis. Radiology 139:71, 1981.

422. Libson E, Bloom RA: Anteroposterior angulated view: A new radiographic technique for the evaluation of spondylolysis. Radiology 149:315, 1983.

423. Frank DF, Miller JE: Hypoplasia of the lumbar vertebral body simulating spondylolisthesis. Radiology 133:59, 1979.

424. Wilkinson RH, Hall JE: The sclerotic pedicle: Tumor or pseudotumor? Radiology 111:683, 1974.

425. Sherman FC, Wilkinson RH, Hall JE, et al: Reactive sclerosis of a pedicle and spondylolysis in the lumbar spine. J Bone Joint Surg [Am] 59:49, 1977.

426. Penning L, Blickman JR: Instability in lumbar spondylolisthesis: A radiologic study of several concepts. AJR 134:293, 1980.

427. Grogan JP, Hemminghytt S, Williams AL, et al: Spondylolysis studied with computed tomography. Radiology 145:737, 1982.

428. Langston JW, Gavant ML: Incomplete ring sign: A simple method for CT detection of spondylolysis. J Comput Assist Tomogr 9:728, 1985.

429. Helms CA, Sims R: Foraminal spurs: A normal variant in the lumbar spine. Radiology 160:153, 1986.

430. Rothman SLG, Glenn WV Jr, Kerber CW: Postoperative fractures of lumbar articular facets: Occult cause of radiculopathy. AJR 145:779, 1985.

431. Papanicolaou N, Wilkinson RH, Emans JB, et al: Bone scintigraphy and radiography in young athletes with low back pain. AJR 145:1039, 1985.

432. Bellah RD, Summerville DA, Treves ST, et al: Low-back pain in adolescent athletes: Detection of stress injury to the pars interarticularis with SPECT. Radiology 180:509, 1991.

433. Collier BD, Johnson RP, Carrera GF, et al: Painful spondylolysis or spondylo-

listhesis studied by radiography and single-photon emission computed tomography. Radiology *154*:207, 1985.

434. Ryan PJ, Evans PA, Gibson T, et al: Chronic low back pain: Comparison of bone SPECT with radiography and CT. Radiology *182*:849, 1992.

435. Gelfand MH, Strife JL, Kereiakes JG: Radionuclide bone imaging in spondylolysis of the lumbar spine in children. Radiology *140*:191, 1981.

436. Handel SF, Twiford TW, Reigel DH, et al: Posterior lumbar apophyseal fractures. Radiology *130*:629, 1979.

437. Bick EM, Copel JW: The ring apophysis of the human vertebra: Contribution to human osteogeny. II. J Bone Joint Surg [Am] *33*:783, 1951.

438. Keller RH: Traumatic displacement of the cartilaginous vertebral rim: A sign of intervertebral disc prolapse. Radiology *110*:21, 1974.

439. Banerian KG, Wang AM, Samberg LC, et al: Association of vertebral end plate fracture with pediatric lumbar intervertebral disk herniation: Value of CT and MR imaging. Radiology *177*:763, 1990.

440. Nanni G, Hudson RM: Posterior ring apophyses of the cervical spine. AJR *139*:383, 1982.

441. Rothfus WE, Goldberg AL, Deeb ZL, et al: MR recognition of posterior lumbar vertebral ring fracture. J Comput Assist Tomogr *14*:790, 1990.

442. Wagner A, Albeck MJ, Madsen FF: Diagnostic imaging in fracture of lumbar vertebral ring apophyses. Acta Radiol *33*:72, 1992.

443. Takata K, Inoue S, Takahashi K, et al: Fracture of the posterior margin of a lumbar vertebral body. J Bone Joint Surg [Am] *70*:589, 1988.

444. Epstein NE, Epstein JA, Mauri T: Treatment of fractures of the vertebral limbus and spinal stenosis in five adolescents and five adults. Neurosurgery *24*:595, 1989.

445. Harris JH, Carson GC, Wagner LK: Radiologic diagnosis of traumatic occipitovertebral dissociation: 1. Normal occipitovertebral relationships on lateral radiographs of supine subjects. AJR *162*:881, 1994.

446. Harris JH, Carson GC, Wagner LK, et al: Radiologic diagnosis of traumatic occipitovertebral dissociation: 2. Comparison of three methods of detecting occipitovertebral relationships on lateral radiographs of supine subjects. AJR *162*:887, 1994.

70

Internal Derangements of Joints

Donald Resnick, M.D.

To derange is to disturb the condition, action, and function of, and derangement is the act of deranging.[1] The term internal derangement of a joint, therefore, is applied appropriately to any condition that leads to joint dysfunction. Internal derangements of joints have been the subject of renewed interest and intense investigation by a number of medical specialists, including sports medicine physicians, orthopedic surgeons, and radiologists. In large part, such interest and investigation have related to the increased number of persons involved in recreational sports, the development and refinement of diagnostic and therapeutic arthroscopy, and the introduction of MR imaging as a diagnostic technique. Although other imaging methods, such as arthrography, computed arthrotomography and ultrasonography, can be employed for the assessment of internal derangements of joints, MR imaging has unique advantages, which have been well-documented, that ensure its prominent role in this assessment.

In this chapter, diagnostic imaging of internal derangements of joints is reviewed. To focus the discussion of this broad topic, only the more important derangements in six anatomic regions are analyzed. These regions are the wrist, elbow, shoulder, hip, knee, and ankle and foot. Furthermore, although competing techniques such as arthrography and computed arthrotomography are addressed, their coverage is brief as emphasis is placed on the prominent role of MR imaging in the assessment of internal derangements of joints. The interested reader should refer to sections of this book that deal with these additional imaging methods (see Chapters 8, 11, and 13). Some anatomic information essential to the interpretation of the MR imaging abnormalities is included, although further discussion of such anatomy is contained in Chapter 22. Finally, a number of conditions occurring around these anatomic regions also are included, although these conditions do not fall precisely into the category of internal derangements of joints.

WRIST

Osseous Anatomy

The distal aspects of the radius and ulna articulate with the proximal row of carpal bones. On the lateral surface of the radius is the radial styloid process, which extends more distally than the remainder of the bone, and from which arises the radial collateral ligament of the wrist joint. The articular surface of the radius is divided into an ulnar and a radial portion by a faint central ridge of bone. The ulnar portion articulates with the lunate and the radial portion articulates with the scaphoid. The articular surface is continuous medially with that of the triangular fibrocartilage. The medial surface of the distal radius contains the concave ulnar notch, which articulates with the distal ulna. The posterior surface of the distal radius is convex and grooved or irregular in outline to allow passage of tendons and tendon sheaths. A prominent ridge in the middle of this surface is the dorsal tubercle of the radius. The anterior surface of the distal radius allows attachment of the palmar radiocarpal ligament.

The distal end of the ulna contains a small round head and a styloid process. The lateral aspect contains an articular surface for contact with the ulnar notch of the radius. The ulna also has a distal articular surface, which is intimate with the triangular fibrocartilage. The ulnar styloid process, which extends distally from the posteromedial aspect of the bone, gives rise to the ulnar collateral ligament. Between the styloid process and inferior articular surface, the ulna has an area for attachment of the triangular fibrocartilage and a dorsal groove for the extensor carpi ulnaris tendon and sheath.

The proximal row of carpal bones consists of the scaphoid, lunate, and triquetrum, as well as the pisiform bone within the tendon of the flexor carpi ulnaris. The distal row of carpal bones contains the trapezium, trapezoid, capitate, and hamate bones. The dorsal surface of the carpus is convex from side to side, and the palmar surface presents a deep concavity, termed the carpal groove or canal. The medial border of this palmar carpal groove contains the pisiform and hook of the hamate. The lateral border of the carpal groove contains the tubercles of the scaphoid and the trapezium. A strong fibrous retinaculum attaches to the palmar surface of the carpus, converting the groove into a carpal tunnel, through which pass the median nerve and flexor tendons.

The distal row of carpal bones articulates with the bases of the metacarpals. The trapezium has a saddle-shaped articular surface for the first metacarpal. The trapezoid fits into a deep notch in the second metacarpal. The capitate articulates mainly with the third metacarpal, but also with the second and fourth metacarpals. The hamate articulates with the fourth and fifth metacarpals. The bases of the metacarpals articulate not only with the distal row of carpal bones but also with each other.

Articular Anatomy

The wrist consists of a series of articulations or compartments (Fig. 70–1):

1. Radiocarpal compartment.
2. Distal (inferior) radioulnar compartment.
3. Midcarpal compartment.
4. Pisiform-triquetral compartment.
5. Common carpometacarpal compartment.
6. First carpometacarpal compartment.
7. Intermetacarpal compartments.

Radiocarpal Compartment. The radiocarpal compartment (Fig. 70–2) is formed proximally by the distal surface of the radius and the triangular fibrocartilage and distally by the proximal row of carpal bones exclusive of the pisiform. In the coronal plane, the radiocarpal compartment is a C-shaped cavity with a smooth, shallow curve, which is concave distally. In the sagittal plane, this compartment also is C-shaped, but the curve is more acute. Interosseous ligaments extend between the carpal bones of the proximal row and prevent communication of this compartment with the midcarpal compartment (see later discussion). A triangular fibrocartilage prevents communication of the radiocarpal and inferior radioulnar compartments, whereas a meniscus may attach to the triquetrum, preventing communication of the radiocarpal and pisiform-triquetral compartments.

The radial collateral ligament is located at the radial limit

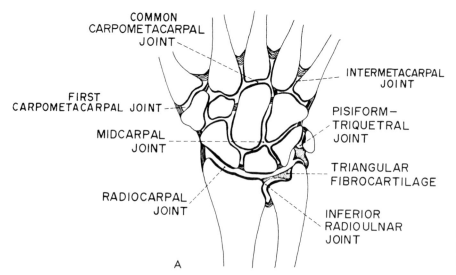

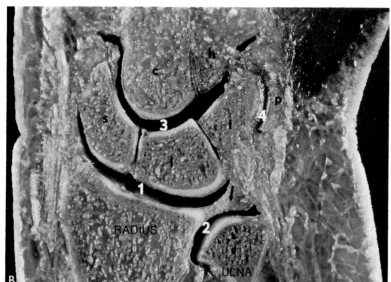

FIGURE 70–1. Articulations of the wrist: General anatomy. Observe the various wrist compartments on a schematic drawing (A) and photograph (B) of a coronal section. These include the radiocarpal (1), inferior radioulnar (2), midcarpal (3), and pisiform-triquetral (4) compartments. Note the triangular fibrocartilage (arrow). s, Scaphoid; l, lunate; t, triquetrum; p, pisiform; h, hamate; c, capitate.

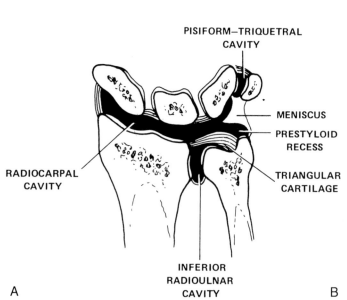

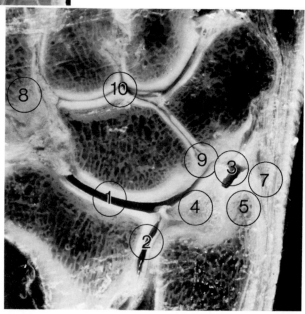

FIGURE 70–2. Radiocarpal compartment.

A Detailed drawing of the radiocarpal compartment. Note its C shape, with a Y-shaped ulnar limit produced by the meniscus. The proximal limb or diverticulum at the ulnar limit of the radiocarpal compartment is the prestyloid recess, which is intimate with the ulnar styloid. The distal limb extends along the triquetrum and may, in some instances, communicate with the pisiform-triquetral compartment.

B Coronal section of cadaveric wrist. Identified structures are the radiocarpal compartment (1), inferior radioulnar compartment (2), prestyloid recess (3), triangular fibrocartilage (4), ulnar styloid (5), ulnar collateral ligament (7), scaphoid (8), interosseous ligament between lunate and triquetrum (9), and midcarpal compartment (10).

(From Resnick D: Radiology 113:331, 1974.)

of the radiocarpal compartment, whereas the ulnar limit of this compartment is the point at which the meniscus is firmly attached to the triquetrum. This ulnar area is Y-shaped; a proximal limb or diverticulum, termed the prestyloid recess, approaches the ulnar styloid and a distal limb is intimate with two thirds of the proximal aspect of the triquetrum.

Palmar radial recesses extend proximally from the radiocarpal compartment beneath the distal articulating surface of the radius. These recesses vary in number and size.

Distal (Inferior) Radioulnar Compartment. The inferior radioulnar compartment (Figs. 70–1 and 70–2) is an L-shaped articulation whose proximal border is the cartilage-covered head of the ulna and ulnar notch of the radius. Its limit is the triangular fibrocartilage. This latter ligament is a band of tough fibrous tissue that extends from the ulnar aspect of the distal radius to the base of the ulnar styloid (see later discussion).

Midcarpal Compartment. The midcarpal compartment (Figs. 70–1 and 70–3) extends between the proximal and distal carpal rows. On the ulnar aspect of this compartment, the head of the capitate and the hamate articulate with a concavity produced by the scaphoid, lunate, and triquetrum. This ulnar side widens between the triquetrum and hamate. On the radial aspect of the midcarpal compartment, the trapezium and trapezoid articulate with the distal aspect of the scaphoid. The radial side of this compartment is termed the trapezioscaphoid space.

Pisiform-Triquetral Compartment. The pisiform-triquetral compartment (Figs. 70–1 and 70–3) exists between the palmar surface of the triquetrum and the dorsal surface of the pisiform. A large proximal synovial recess can be noted. The pisiform-triquetral compartment is surrounded by a loose fibrous articular capsule.

Common Carpometacarpal Compartment. The common carpometacarpal compartment exists between the base of each of the four medial metacarpals and the distal row of carpal bones. This synovial cavity extends proximally between the distal portion of the carpal bones, and distally between the bases of the metacarpals, to form three small intermetacarpal joints. Occasionally, the articulation between the hamate and the fourth and fifth metacarpals is a separate synovial cavity, produced by a ligamentous attachment between the hamate and fourth metacarpal (Fig. 70–1).

First Carpometacarpal Compartment. The carpometacarpal compartment of the thumb is a separate saddle-shaped cavity between the trapezium and base of the first metacarpal (Fig. 70–1). It possesses a loose, fibrous capsule, which is thickest laterally and dorsally.

Intermetacarpal Compartments. Three intermetacarpal compartments extend between the bases of the second and third, the third and fourth, and the fourth and fifth metacarpals (Fig. 70–1). These compartments usually communicate with each other and with the common carpometacarpal compartment.

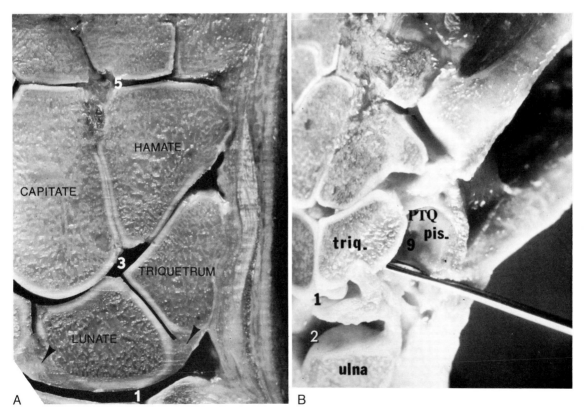

FIGURE 70–3. Midcarpal and pisiform-triquetral compartments.
  A Midcarpal compartment (coronal section). The ulnar side of the midcarpal compartment (3) is well shown. This compartment is separated from the radiocarpal compartment (1) by interosseous ligaments (arrowheads) extending between bones of the proximal carpal row. Observe the common carpometacarpal compartment (5) between the distal carpal row and the bases of the four ulnar metacarpals.
  B Pisiform-triquetral compartment (coronal section). This compartment (PTQ-9) exists between the triquetrum (triq.) and pisiform (pis.). The radiocarpal (1) and inferior radioulnar (2) compartments also are indicated.

Anatomy of the Triangular Fibrocartilage Complex

The distal radioulnar joint is stabilized primarily by the triangular fibrocartilage complex (TFCC) of the wrist.[2, 3] The components of the TFCC are not agreed upon but include the triangular fibrocartilage (TFC) itself, the dorsal and volar radioulnar ligaments, the ulnomeniscal homologue, the ulnar collateral ligament, and the sheath of the extensor carpi ulnaris tendon. The TFC is thicker peripherally than centrally and may be fenestrated centrally, especially in middle-aged and elderly persons (Fig. 70–4A). The thick and strong marginal portions of the TFC, composed of lamellar collagen, often are referred to as the dorsal and volar radioulnar ligaments. The TFCC arises from the ulnar aspect of the lunate fossa of the radius, courses toward the ulna, and inserts in the fovea at the base of the ulnar styloid process.[4] As it extends distally, it is joined by fibers of the ulnar collateral ligament, becomes thickened in the form of the meniscus homologue, and inserts distally into the lunate, triquetrum, hamate, and base of the fifth metacarpal bone.[4] On its volar aspect, the TFCC is attached strongly to the triquetrum (the ulnotriquetral ligament) and to the lunotriquetral interosseous ligament and less strongly to the lunate bone (the ulnolunate ligament); on its dorsolateral aspect, the TFCC is incorporated into the floor of the sheath of the extensor carpi ulnaris tendon.[4]

When the radius and ulna are of equal length, a situation designated neutral ulnar variance, the distal portion of the radius transmits approximately 80 per cent of the axial load across the wrist, and the distal portion of the ulna transmits approximately 20 per cent.[5, 6] Surgical removal of the TFCC decreases the load borne by the distal portion of the ulna by approximately 12 per cent, and removal of the distal portion of the ulna eliminates the load borne across the ulnar aspect of the wrist. When the ulna is short relative to

the radius, a situation designated minus ulnar variance and seen in association with Kienböck's disease, a diminution in the force borne by the distal portion of the ulna is evident. When the ulna is long relative to the radius, a situation designated positive ulnar variance and seen in association with disruption of the TFCC, lunotriquetral interosseous ligament tears, and the ulnar impaction syndrome, an increase in the force borne by the distal portion of the ulna is apparent.[4]

Ligamentous Anatomy

A number of ligaments about the distal portions of the radius and ulna and the carpal bones have been described. Some of these are considered intrinsic ligaments, arising and inserting on carpal bones, and others are considered extrinsic ligaments, joining the distal portion of the radius and the carpal bones (Fig. 70–5).

Interosseous Ligaments. The bones of the proximal carpal row are joined by two interosseous (or intrinsic) ligaments, the scapholunate interosseous ligament (joining the proximal surfaces of the scaphoid and lunate) and the lunotriquetral interosseous ligament (joining the proximal surfaces of the lunate and triquetrum). These ligaments connect the corresponding bones from their palmar to dorsal surfaces. They may have a triangular configuration when sectioned in the coronal plane, they are reinforced by fibers derived from the extrinsic radiocarpal ligaments (see later discussion) and, when intact, they separate the radiocarpal and midcarpal compartments of the wrist. Disruption of these proximal intercarpal ligaments allows communication of the radiocarpal and midcarpal compartments of the wrist (Fig. 70–4B). Disruption of the scapholunate interosseous ligament, when combined with disruption of one or more of the volar extrinsic radiocarpal ligaments, allows

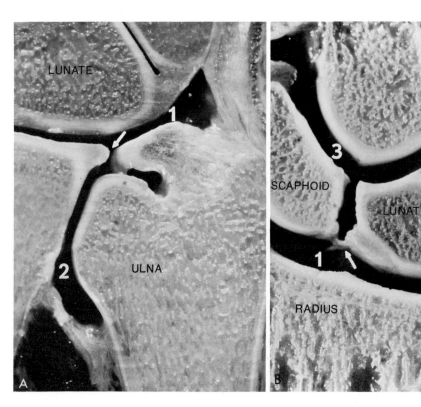

FIGURE 70–4. Age-related fenestrations of the triangular fibrocartilage and interosseous ligaments.

A In elderly persons, fenestrations (arrow) may develop in the triangular fibrocartilage, allowing communication of the radiocarpal (1) and inferior radioulnar (2) compartments.

B In elderly persons, progressive deterioration of the scapholunate interosseous ligament (arrow) eventually may allow communication of the radiocarpal (1) and midcarpal (3) compartments.

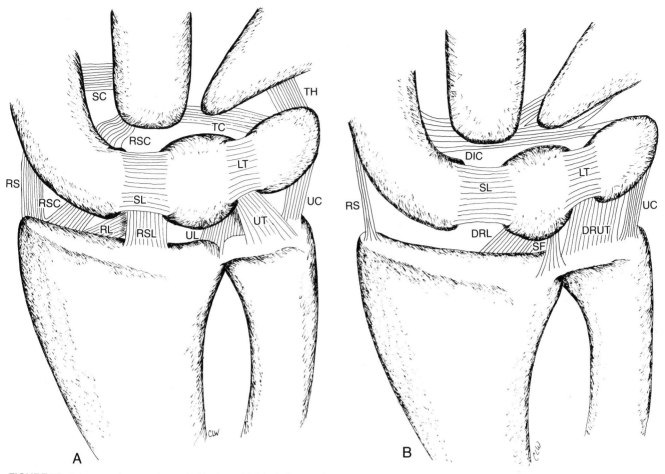

FIGURE 70–5. Ligamentous anatomy: Extrinsic and intrinsic ligaments.

A Palmar aspect of the wrist. Illustrated structures include the radioscaphoid (RS) portion of the radial collateral ligament, radioscaphocapitate ligament (RSC), radiolunotriquetral ligament (RL), radioscapholunate ligament (RSL), scaphocapitate ligament (SC), triquetrocapitate ligament (TC), triquetrohamate ligament (TH), ulnar collateral ligament (UC), ulnolunate ligament (UL), ulnotriquetral ligament (UT), and scapholunate (SL) and lunotriquetral (LT) interosseous ligaments.

B Dorsal aspect of the wrist. Illustrated structures include the radioscaphoid (RS) portion of the radial collateral ligament, scapholunate (SL) and lunotriquetral (LT) interosseous ligaments, dorsal intercarpal ligament (DIC), dorsal radiolunate ligament (DRL), dorsal radioulnotriquetral ligament (DRUT), ulnar collateral ligament (UC), and a prominent synovial fold (SF).

(From North ER, Thomas S: J Hand Surg [Am] *13:*815, 1988. © 1988, Churchill Livingstone, on behalf of the Journal of Hand Surgery, New York.)

separation of the scaphoid and lunate bones, designated scapholunate dissociation.[7]

Three additional interosseous ligaments are found in the distal carpal row. These unite the trapezium and the trapezoid bones, the trapezoid and the capitate bones, and the capitate and the hamate bones. These distal interosseous ligaments do not extend from the volar to the dorsal portions of the wrist capsule, explaining the communication of the midcarpal and common carpometacarpal compartments of the wrist.[3]

Palmar Radiocarpal Ligaments. Radiocarpal (extrinsic) ligaments of the wrist commonly are considered in two groups: palmar radiocarpal ligaments and dorsal radiocarpal ligaments. The former are more important to wrist function than the latter, representing significant stabilizers of wrist motion.[8–11] The terminology applied to these ligaments is not constant, and only one system of nomenclature is emphasized here (Fig. 70–5).

There are three volar (or palmar) radiocarpal ligaments: the radioscaphocapitate (radiocapitate) ligament, the radiolunotriquetral (radiotriquetral) ligament, and the radioscapholunate (radioscaphoid and radiolunate) ligament. The

strong radioscaphocapitate ligament arises from the volar and radial aspects of the radial styloid process and extends in a distal and ulnar direction. It traverses a groove in the waist of the scaphoid bone, to which it may attach, and terminates in the center of the volar aspect of the capitate.[3] Some fibers of the radioscaphocapitate ligament may extend to the triquetrum, although other fibers connecting the scaphoid to the triquetrum sometimes are referred to as the palmar scaphotriquetral ligament.[1371] The large radiolunotriquetral ligament arises from the volar lip and styloid process of the radius adjacent to the radioscaphocapitate ligament, and it is directed distally in an ulnarward direction across the volar aspect of the lunate bone to attach to the palmar aspect of the triquetrum.[3] This ligament serves as volar sling for the lunate. The radioscapholunate ligament is located more medially and deeper than the other two volar ligaments. It arises from the volar aspect of the distal portion of the radius and inserts into the proximal and volar surface of the scapholunate space. This ligament reinforces the scapholunate interosseous ligament, and its disruption, along with that of the scapholunate interosseous ligament, leads to scapholunate dissociation.[3] Separate bundles of fibers in the region of the scapholunate interosseous ligament sometimes are referred to as radiolunate and radioscaphoid ligaments.[12]

Volar Ulnocarpal Ligaments. Two bands of ligamentous tissue arise from the anterior margin of the TFC and the base of the ulnar styloid process and extend distally, downward, and laterally to the lunate and triquetral bones, respectively.[3] The band inserting on the lunate is designated the ulnolunate ligament, and that inserting on the triquetrum is designated the ulnotriquetral ligament (Fig. 70–6); a distal portion of the ulnotriquetral ligament extends onto the volar aspect of the capitate and hamate.[3]

Other Volar Carpal Ligaments. Ligamentous tissue connects the volar aspects of the capitate and triquetral bones. This tissue sometimes is designated the capitotriquetral (intrinsic) ligament. In other instances, ligamentous tissue arising from the volar aspect of the capitate is described as having a V-shape, representing a deltoid or arcuate ligament, whose ulnar arm extends to the triquetrum and whose radial arm extends to the scaphoid bone. Disruption of the ulnar arm of the arcuate ligament may be responsible for volar intercalated carpal instability, or VISI (see Chapter 68). Furthermore, the space of Poirier, representing an area of normal weakness in the volar aspect of the capsule just proximal to the deltoid ligament, is the site through which volar dislocation of the lunate occurs.

Dorsal Radiocarpal Ligaments. The dorsal capsule of the wrist contains an area of thickening that extends from the articular surface of the radius toward the lunate and triquetral bones. This area sometimes is viewed as a single structure or as several separate structures, leading to such designations as the radioscapholunotriquetral ligament, the radioscaphoid ligament, the radiolunate ligament, and the radiotriquetral ligament (Fig. 70–5). The radiotriquetral component of these ligaments appears to be the most consistent of the structures, although its site of origin may be Lister's tubercle of the radius, the radial styloid process, or both structures.[13, 14] Although variation in the terminology applied to the dorsal radiocarpal ligaments exists, they generally are regarded as functionally less important than the volar radiocarpal ligaments.

Other Dorsal Carpal Ligaments. Several intrinsic dorsal ligaments bind together the carpal bones. Among these, the dorsal intercarpal ligament, consisting of the triquetroscaphoid and triquetrotrapezial fascicles, appears most prominent.[14]

Collateral Ligaments. The collateral ligaments of the wrist, the radial collateral ligament and the ulnar collateral ligament (Fig. 70–5), represent thickenings of the fibrous capsule and functionally are less important than the collateral ligaments in other joints such as the knee and elbow. The radial collateral ligament extends from the tip of the styloid process of the radius to attach to the waist of the scaphoid bone, with fibers continuing to the trapezium and blending with the transverse carpal ligament and the dorsal capsular ligament. The ulnar collateral ligament is attached proximally to the base and body of the styloid process of the ulna with an extension into the TFC; distally, it attaches

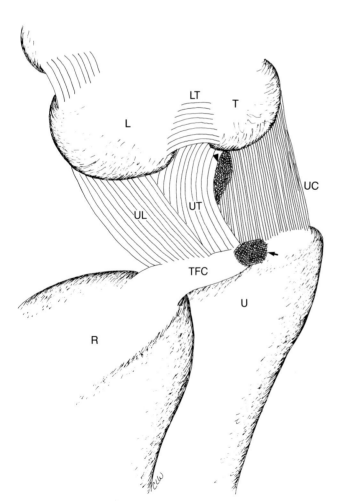

FIGURE 70–6. Ligamentous anatomy: Volar ulnocarpal ligaments. The lunate (L), triquetrum (T), radius (R), and ulna (U) are indicated. Illustrated structures include the ulnolunate (UL) and ulnotriquetral (UT) ligaments, triangular fibrocartilage (TFC), lunotriquetral interosseous (LT) and ulnar collateral (UC) ligaments. The two shaded areas represent the prestyloid recess (arrow) and entrance site to the pisiform-triquetral joint (arrowhead). (From North ER, Thomas S: J Hand Surg [Am] *13*:815, 1988. © 1988, Churchill Livingstone, on behalf of the Journal of Hand Surgery, New York.)

to the triquetrum, pisiform, hamate, and fifth metacarpal bone and the transverse carpal ligament.[3]

Soft Tissue Anatomy

Flexor Retinaculum. On the volar aspect of the wrist, a strong broad ligament, the flexor retinaculum or transverse carpal ligament, extends from its lateral attachment to the tuberosities of the trapezium and scaphoid to its medial attachment to the pisiform bone and hook of the hamate bone (Fig. 70–7). Its functions may include maintenance of the contour of the carpus and fixation of the flexor tendons during flexion of the wrist, preventing the loss of power that would occur with bowstringing of the tendons.[3]

Carpal Tunnel. Beneath the carpus on the palmar aspect of the wrist, the carpal tunnel is a confined soft tissue compartment that is bounded volarly by the flexor retinaculum and dorsally, medially, and laterally by the carpal bones (Fig. 70–7). Coursing through the carpal tunnel are a number of structures that include the median nerve, the eight deep and superficial flexor tendons and tenosynovial sheaths, the tendon and synovial sheath of the flexor pollicis longus muscle, the radial and ulnar bursae, and fat. The precise relationship among the structures varies according to the specific level within the canal (i.e., proximal, intermediate, and distal portions) and the position of the wrist (i.e., neutral, flexion, and extension).[15, 16] At the level of the proximal portion of the carpal tunnel, its walls include the trapezium and scaphoid bones laterally, the capitate, hamate, and triquetrum bones dorsally, the pisiform bone medially, and the flexor retinaculum superficially.[15] At this proximal level, the median nerve is just deep to the flexor retinaculum and palmaris longus tendon and is located between the flexor pollicis longus deeply and laterally and the flexor digitorum superficialis tendons deeply and medially. The median nerve is slightly flattened by the adjacent tendons. At the level of the intermediate portion, or midportion, of the carpal tunnel, the relationships of the median

nerve are similar to those evident in the proximal portion, although the nerve may be located more deeply.[15] At this level, the hook of the hamate bone forms the ulnar wall of the carpal tunnel. At the distal portion of the carpal tunnel, the flexor retinaculum attaches to the hook of the hamate, and the median nerve still maintains a flattened appearance.[15] With the wrist in neutral position, the median nerve within the carpal tunnel is found either anterior to the superficial flexor tendon of the index finger or interposed more posterolaterally between this tendon and the flexor pollicis longus tendon.[16] With wrist extension, the median nerve assumes (or maintains) an anterior position between the superficial index finger flexor tendon and the flexor retinaculum, while the flexor tendons move posteriorly; with wrist flexion, the flexor tendons shift anteriorly toward the retinaculum and the position of the median nerve is more variable.[16]

Ulnar Tunnel (Guyon's Canal). The ulnar nerve passes through a fibro-osseous tunnel known as Guyon's canal, in the anteromedial portion of the wrist (see Chapter 77). The tunnel is approximately 4 cm in length, extending from the proximal edge of the pisiform bone to the origin of the hypothenar muscles at the level of the hamulus.[17, 18] The volar margin of the tunnel is the pisohamate interosseous ligament. The ulnar artery and, occasionally, communicating veins accompany the ulnar nerve through the canal.[17]

Digital Flexor Tendon Sheaths and Synovial Sacs of the Palm. The flexor tendons of the fingers, the sublimis digitorum and profundus digitorum, are enveloped by digital sheaths from a line of insertion of the flexor profundus to a line 1 cm proximal to the proximal border of the deep transverse ligament[19] (Fig. 70–8). This arrangement, which is not constant, is most frequent in the index, middle, and ring fingers.[20] Any of these three sheaths may extend to the wrist.[21] The flexor sheath of the thumb extends from the terminal phalanx to a point 2 to 3 cm proximal to the proximal volar crease of the wrist, although on occasion a septum separates proximal and distal halves of the sheath.[20]

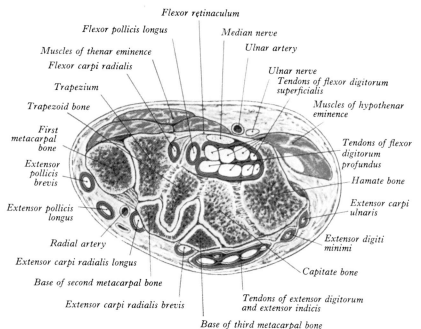

FIGURE 70–7. Flexor retinaculum and carpal tunnel. A transverse section through the wrist shows the tendons and their synovial sheaths passing beneath the flexor retinaculum. The section is slightly oblique and divides the distal row of the carpus and the bases of the first, second, and third metacarpal bones. (From Williams PL, Warwick R [Eds]: Gray's Anatomy. 36th British edition. Edinburgh, Churchill Livingstone, 1980, p 583.)

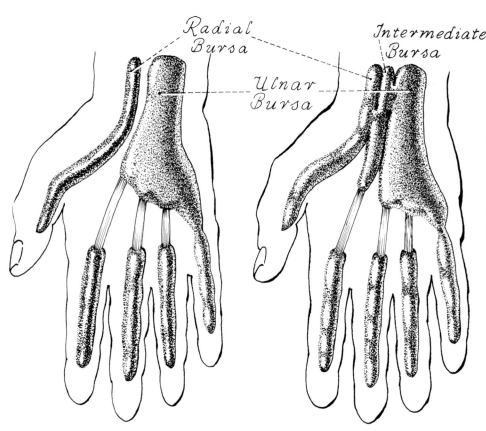

FIGURE 70–8. Digital flexor tendon sheaths and synovial sacs of the palm. The radial and ulnar bursae may be separate, distinct cavities or may communicate via an intermediate bursa. Note the flexor tendon sheaths which, in the second, third, and fourth fingers, usually terminate just proximal to the metacarpophalangeal joints. The tendon sheaths in the first and fifth fingers usually communicate with the bursae in the wrist. (From Resnick D: AJR *124:* 14, 1975. Copyright 1975 American Roentgen Ray Society.)

The synovial sheath of the little finger also commences at its terminal phalanx. It may end near the deep transverse ligament or continue into the palm, expanding to envelop the adjacent tendons of the second, third, and fourth fingers.[19, 20] The digital sheath of the thumb lies distally near the proximal phalanx, but as it ascends toward the palm it separates from the metacarpal head.

Communication between the individual digital tendon sheaths and synovial sacs or bursae in the palm is not constant[21]; most frequently, such continuation is noted involving the first digit (Fig. 70–8). Not uncommonly the digital sheath of the fifth finger also continues into the palm.[20] Such communication is uncommon in the second, third, and fourth fingers.

The ulnar bursa on the medial aspect of the palm comprises three communicating invaginations[19, 20]; a superficial extension lies in front of the flexor sublimis, a middle one lies between the tendons of the sublimis and the profundus, and a deep extension is found behind the flexor profundus. The bursa, beginning at the proximal end of the digital sheaths, spreads out proximally, overlying the third, fourth, and fifth metacarpals. A statistical analysis of the tendon sheath patterns in the hand using air insufflation techniques in 367 cases demonstrated that the ulnar bursa communicated with the sheaths of the little finger in 81 per cent, of the index finger in 5.1 per cent, of the middle finger in 4.0 per cent, and of the ring finger in 3.5 per cent of cases.[21]

The radial bursa is the expanded proximal continuation of the digital sheath of the flexor pollicis longus. It is found on the radial aspect of the palm overlying the second metacarpal. It continues proximally along the volar radial aspect of the wrist, terminating about 2 cm above the transverse carpal ligament.[19]

Intercommunications between the ulnar and radial bursae may be noted in 50 per cent of cases (Fig. 70–8). Such connection is made via intermediate bursae. These accessory synovial sacs may be posterior in location, between the carpal canal and flexor profundus digitorum of the index finger, or, less commonly, anterior in location, between the superficial and deep tendons of the index finger. A separate carpal sheath that does not communicate with either radial or ulnar bursa may be found enveloping the index flexor tendons.[19] Additionally, a small synovial sac may enclose the tendon of the flexor carpi radialis as it passes under the crest of the trapezium.[19]

Extensor Tendon Sheaths. Several synovial sheaths are located in the dorsum of the wrist beneath the dorsal carpal ligament; they extend for a short distance proximal and distal to that ligament (Fig. 70–9). By insular attachments of the dorsal carpal ligament on the posterior and lateral surfaces of the radius and ulna, six distinct avenues are created for transport of ligamentous structures. The most medial compartment (sixth compartment) contains the extensor carpi ulnaris tendon and sheath (4 to 5 cm in length), lying at the dorsomedial aspect of the distal ulna. In the fifth compartment, a long sheath (6 to 7 cm in length) covers the extensor digiti quinti proprius, which lies in close proximity to and may communicate with the inferior radioulnar joint. The fourth compartment on the posteromedial aspect of the radius contains a large sheath (5 to 6 cm in length) enclosing the tendons of the extensor digitorum communis and the extensor indicis proprius. In the third compartment are the sheath (6 to 7 cm in length) and tendon of the extensor pollicis longus. The sheath may extend as far distally as the trapezium or first metacarpal bone. Lateral to this in the second compartment are sheaths

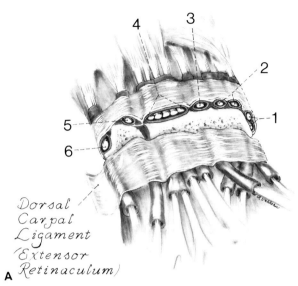
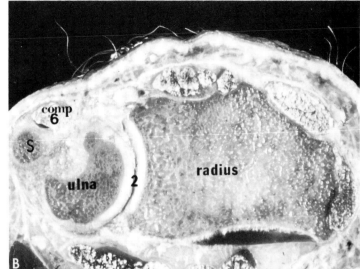

FIGURE 70–9. Extensor tendons and tendon sheaths.

A Drawing showing dorsal carpal ligament and extensor tendons surrounded by synovial sheaths traversing dorsum of wrist within six separate compartments. These compartments are created by the insular attachment of the dorsal carpal ligament on the posterior and lateral surfaces of the radius and ulna. The extensor carpi ulnaris tendon and its sheath are in the medial compartment (6) and are closely applied to the posterior surface of the ulna.

B Cross section through distal end of radius and distal ulna reveals relationship of the extensor carpi ulnaris tendon and tendon sheath (comp 6) and ulnar styloid (S). The inferior radioulnar compartment (2) also is shown.

(From Resnick D: Med Radiogr Photogr *52*:50, 1976.)

(5 to 6 cm in length) covering the extensor carpi radialis longus and extensor carpi radialis brevis, which may communicate with the sheath of the extensor pollicis longus. Finally, a compartment along the lateral aspect of the radius (first compartment) contains a common synovial sheath (5 to 6 cm in length) enclosing the abductor pollicis longus and extensor pollicis brevis.

Distal Radioulnar Joint Abnormalities

Functional Anatomy. The functional anatomy and pathomechanics of the distal radioulnar joint have received a great deal of emphasis.[22–25] Nathan and Schneider[25] have emphasized those features that are fundamental to optimal function of this joint:

1. The articulating surface between the ulnar head and the sigmoid notch of the radius must be intact. The sigmoid notch and two thirds of the ulnar head are covered with articular cartilage. The ulnar head has two surfaces that articulate with the TFC and sigmoid notch of the radius, respectively.[24] The articulation of the ulnar head with the concave sigmoid notch is not congruous; the radius of curvature of the concave surface of the notch is larger than that of the corresponding convex articular surface of the ulna. This situation implies limited joint congruency, and it enables simultaneous sliding and rotation when the forearm is pronated and supinated. As the forearm moves from supination to pronation, the ulnar head rotates up to 150 degrees and also glides several millimeters in a proximal-to-distal direction within the sigmoid notch.[25] The radius translates on the seat of the ulnar head; in full supination, the ulnar head rests on the palmar aspect of the notch, and in full pronation it rests against the dorsal lip of the notch.[24]

2. The soft tissue and ligamentous support system of the distal radioulnar joint must be intact. The precise structures providing stability to this joint are not agreed upon entirely, although recent evidence has implicated various components of the TFCC (consisting of the TFC or articular disc, the dorsal and volar radioulnar ligaments, the ulnar collateral ligament, the meniscus homologue, and the sheath of the extensor carpi ulnaris tendon) in this regard.[26] Ekenstam and Hagert[27] and Nathan and Schneider[25] considered the TFCC to consist of three parts: a cartilaginous central portion (the disc or TFC) and surrounding thick dorsal and volar radioulnar ligaments. These authors emphasized that the central portion serves as a cushion for the ulnar head and ulnar-sided carpal bones and as the load-bearing component of the TFCC and that the dorsal and volar radioulnar ligaments primarily are responsible for stabilization of the distal radioulnar joint. This hypothesis is consistent with the occurrence of defects of the articular disc itself that may exist without joint instability. In addition to the TFCC, the annular ligament and interosseous membrane of the forearm constrain the radius and the ulna.[23]

3. A proper relationship between the lengths of the radius and ulna must exist (Fig. 70–10). As indicated earlier, changes in the length of the ulna relative to that of the radius, designated positive and negative ulnar variance, alter the distribution of compressive forces across the wrist. Consequences of a short ulna, or minus ulnar variance, include increased force applied to the radial side of the wrist and to the lunate bone, which may explain the association of negative ulnar variance and Kienböck's disease. With such variance, the TFC is thicker, and abnormalities of the TFCC are uncommon.[26] A consequence of a long ulna, a positive ulnar variance, is the ulnar impaction or ulnar abutment syndrome (see later discussion), with resulting limitation of rotation and subsequent relaxation of the ligamentous fixation of the wrist.[18] The TFC is thinner in instances of positive ulnar variance, and degenerative perforation of this structure (as well as disruption of the lunotriquetral interosseous ligament) may be observed.

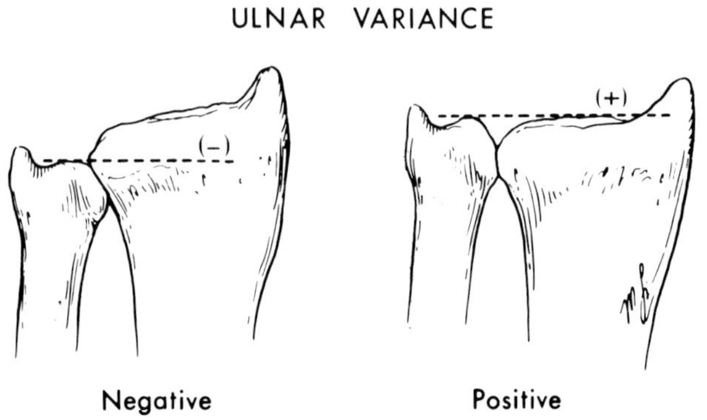

ULNAR VARIANCE

FIGURE 70–10. Ulnar variance. Diagrams of negative and positive ulnar variance are shown.

Pathologic Anatomy. A variety of systems have been used to classify disorders of the distal radioulnar joint.[25, 26, 28–30] Palmer[26] used two major categories, traumatic lesions and degenerative lesions, to describe such disorders, indicating the relative infrequency of the traumatic lesions (Fig. 70–11). Traumatic abnormalities (Class 1) were subdivided further according to their precise anatomic location. A Class 1A lesion represented a tear or perforation of the horizontal portion of the TFCC, usually occurring as a 1 to 2 mm slit located 2 to 3 mm medial to the radial attachment of the TFCC. A Class 1B lesion represented a traumatic avulsion of the TFCC from its insertion site in the distal portion of the ulna that could be associated with a fracture of the base of the styloid process of the ulna. This type of lesion was considered evidence of instability of the distal

radioulnar joint. A Class 1C lesion represented a distal avulsion of the TFCC at its site of attachment to the lunate bone (ulnolunate ligament) or triquetrum (ulnotriquetral ligament). Once again, such a lesion implied instability of the distal radioulnar joint. A Class 1D lesion represented an avulsion of the TFCC from its attachment to the radius at the distal aspect of the sigmoid notch that could be associated with an avulsion fracture.

Degenerative abnormalities (Class 2) also were subdivided according to their extent and location. Five types of degenerative lesions were detailed: wear of the central region of the horizontal portion of the TFCC without perforation (Class 2A lesion); similar wear with evidence of chondromalacia of the ulnar aspect of the lunate bone or the radial aspect of the ulnar head, or both areas (Class 2B lesion); perforation of the horizontal portion of the TFCC, occurring in a more ulnar location than a traumatic perforation (Class 2C lesion); such perforation combined with degenerative changes of the articular surfaces of the lunate bone and ulnar head and disruption of the lunotriquetral interosseous ligament (Class 2D lesion); and the ulnar impaction syndrome with complete absence of the horizontal portion of the TFCC, disruption of the lunotriquetral interosseous ligament, osteoarthritis of the distal radioulnar joint, and degenerative changes about the ulnocarpal space (Class 2E lesion).

The anatomic basis of this classification system is valuable, but this system is very extensive and may be difficult to apply clinically. A simpler method has been described by Nathan and Schneider,[25] in which four possible categories of pathologic lesions are considered: (1) instability of the distal radioulnar joint (including traumatic disruption

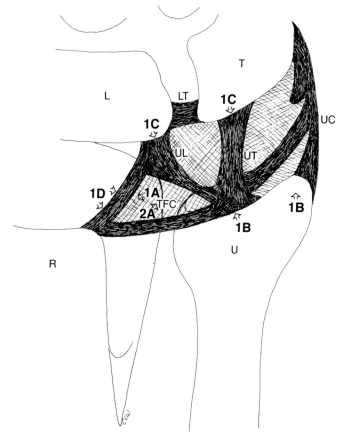

FIGURE 70–11. Pathologic anatomy of the distal radioulnar joint. Illustrated structures are the radius (R), ulna (U), lunate (L), triquetrum (T), triangular fibrocartilage (TFC), ulnolunate (UL) and ulnotriquetral (UT) ligaments, ulnar collateral ligament (UC), and lunotriquetral interosseous ligament (LT). The sites of the lesions mentioned in the text under the categories of 1A, 1B, 1C, 1D, and 2A are indicated. (Modified from Palmer AK: J Hand Surg [Am] *14*:594, 1989. © 1989, Churchill Livingstone, on behalf of the Journal of Hand Surgery, New York.)

of the TFCC with or without dislocation of the joint or fracture of the radius or ulna, or both bones; disruption of the TFCC associated with inflammatory diseases such as rheumatoid arthritis; and ulnar head excision); (2) impingement of the ulna on the carpus; (3) incongruity of the distal radioulnar joint (including that related to traumatic or inflammatory disorders); and (4) isolated lesions of the articular disc (which occur without instability of the distal radioulnar joint). This system, with some modifications, is used in the following discussion.

Lesions of the Triangular Fibrocartilage Complex (TFCC). Lesions of the TFCC are variable in extent; they may be confined to the horizontal or flat portion of the TFCC (referred to as the TFC or articular disc) or involve one or more components of the TFCC with or without instability of the distal radioulnar joint. Those lesions confined to the TFC, a load-bearing structure only, may or may not be symptomatic (manifest as ulnar-sided wrist pain and tenderness and, in some instances, a palpable or audible click during rotation of the forearm) and are not associated with instability of the distal radioulnar joint.[25] Such isolated lesions of the articular disc generally are related to degeneration or trauma, although a congenital basis also has been suggested.[31] An increased frequency of degenerative lesions with advancing age of the patient has been documented arthrographically (see Chapter 13), and similar data have been derived from cadaveric studies. More extensive lesions of the TFCC, including avulsions from its proximal, distal, or radial sites of attachment, as indicated earlier, usually are regarded as traumatic in pathogenesis.[26]

Degenerative lesions of the TFC are more common than traumatic lesions. Either type may result in full-thickness defects, as can be documented with arthrography and MR imaging. Although such full-thickness defects commonly are referred to as tears, Gilula and Palmer[32] have objected to the use of this word, indicating that it implies that a structure has been torn, as commonly is seen with trauma, and that most of these defects relate to progressive wear. The terms communicating (or full-thickness) and noncommunicating (or partial-thickness) defects are used in the following discussion, although the term defect also is not an ideal designation for a finding that may be a normal variation and clinically insignificant.[1372]

The role of arthrography in the diagnosis of defects of the articular disc is well established although, as indicated in Chapter 13, disagreement exists regarding the optimal arthrographic technique and, more specifically, the need for injection of contrast material into more than one wrist compartment (i.e., radiocarpal and distal radioulnar joints). The presence of contrast material in the inferior radioulnar compartment following radiocarpal compartmental opacification (Fig. 70–12) or in the radiocarpal compartment following inferior radioulnar compartmental injection is the sine qua non of a communicating, or complete, defect in the TFC. Partial, or noncommunicating, defects involving the proximal aspect of the TFC can be opacified with injection of contrast material into the inferior radioulnar joint, and those involving the distal aspect of the TFC can be opacified with injection of contrast material into the radiocarpal joint. Intrasubstance degeneration, or tears within the TFC, are invisible to the arthrographer. Other traumatic abnormalities of the TFCC, as described by Palmer,[26] may be associated with distinctive arthrographic findings. Traumatic avulsion of the TFCC from its insertion into the distal ulna (Class 1B lesion) is not visualized during arthrography when the radiocarpal joint is injected but may be seen as extravasation of contrast material when arthrography is performed using an injection into the distal radioulnar joint; traumatic avulsion of the TFCC from its distal attachment to the lunate or the triquetrum (Class 1C lesion) will not lead to a communicating defect of the TFC itself but may be accompanied by capsular leakage of contrast material when either

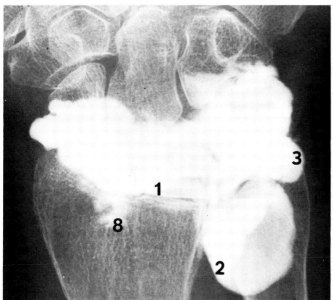 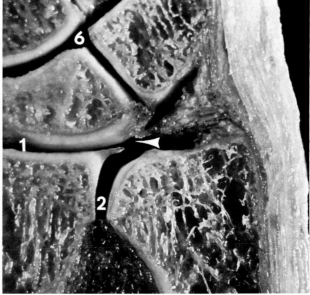

A   B

FIGURE 70–12. Communicating defects of the triangular fibrocartilage: Radiocarpal joint arthrography. A frontal radiograph **(A)** following opacification of the radiocarpal compartment (1) reveals its communication with the inferior radioulnar compartment (2). This communication is possible when a defect exists in the triangular fibrocartilage. Such a defect (arrowhead) is illustrated on a photograph of a coronal section of the wrist **(B)**. Other indicated structures are the midcarpal compartment (6), volar radial recesses (8), and prestyloid recess (3).

the radiocarpal or the midcarpal compartment is injected; and traumatic avulsion of the TFCC from its attachment to the radius at the distal aspect of the sigmoid notch generally is seen as a communicating defect at the site of disruption when either the radiocarpal or the distal radioulnar joint is opacified.[26]

The role of MR imaging in the evaluation of lesions of the TFCC has received increased attention.[33–42, 1372, 1373] In young persons, the normal TFC is characterized by homogeneously low signal intensity on virtually all MR pulse sequences and in the coronal, sagittal, and transverse planes. In the coronal plane, the normal TFC usually appears as an elongated triangle with its apex attaching to the articular cartilage of the radius (Fig. 70–13). The triangle may be thinner in persons with positive ulnar variance and thicker in those with negative ulnar variance. The ulnar attachment of the TFC may appear bifurcated, with two bands of low signal intensity separated by a region of higher signal intensity. The prestyloid recess of the radiocarpal joint, which extends toward the tip of the styloid process of the ulna, also may reveal higher signal intensity. Adjacent structures of the TFCC including the meniscus homologue are identifiable.

Although low signal intensity characterizes the MR imaging appearance of the normal TFC, two regions of higher signal intensity that are encountered normally may simulate the appearance of a lesion (Fig. 70–14): (1) The articular cartilage of the distal portion of the radius separates the apex of the TFC from the adjacent bone. The linear configuration of this region of articular cartilage is similar to that of a tear, but its signal intensity characteristics are those of cartilage and not those of fluid. A radial avulsion of the TFCC is associated with fluid accumulation in this same region, an appearance not evident in the normal situation.

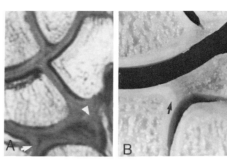

FIGURE 70–14. Triangular fibrocartilage complex: MR imaging. Normal appearance.

A Coronal T1-weighted (TR/TE, 800/20) spin echo MR image shows inhomogeneous low signal intensity in the triangular fibrocartilage. Note intermediate signal intensity in the region of the articular cartilage (arrow) of the radius and at the ulnar limit of the triangular fibrocartilage complex (arrowhead).

B In a coronal section of the ulnar side of the wrist, observe the articular cartilage (arrow) of the radius and fibrofatty tissues (arrowhead) in the ulnar aspect of the triangular fibrocartilage complex.

(2) The ulnar limit of the TFC is of higher signal intensity than that of the flat portion of the TFC. The signal intensity characteristics of this area usually are not those of fluid. Differentiation of this normal appearance from an avulsion of the proximal attachment site of the TFCC may prove difficult.

On sagittal images, the normal TFC is of low signal intensity and reveals a discoid shape lying adjacent to the articular cartilage of the distal end of the ulna. Its central portion may appear thinner than its volar and dorsal portions. On transaxial images, a triangular region of low signal intensity characterizes the normal TFC.

Although the previous description of the MR imaging characteristics of the normal TFC has emphasized its low signal intensity, regions of higher signal intensity within the TFC on T1-weighted spin echo MR images are encountered regularly[39, 42] (Fig. 70–15). The basis for this hyperintensity is the presence of histologic changes (including mucinous and myxoid alterations) related to the age of the person and typically considered degenerative in nature.[43, 44] In one cadaveric study, no degenerative lesions or communicating defects of the TFC were detected in the first two decades of life, whereas after the fifth decade of life, 100 per cent of wrists had degenerative lesions in the TFC and more than 40 per cent of the wrists had communicating defects of the TFC.[43] Degeneration of the TFC invariably is situated in the thinner central portion and initially occurs and is much more severe on the ulnar, or proximal, surface of the TFC, owing to more intensive biomechanical forces in this region.[39] The rotational movements that occur during pronation and supination of the hand produce a drilling effect on the ulnar surface of the TFC that is much more stressful than the gliding movements of the carpal condyle on the carpal surface of the TFC. Progression of degeneration on the surface of the TFC leads to erosion, thinning, and finally perforation of this structure. There is a close correlation between the changes in the TFC and those in the articular cartilage of the lunate and distal portion of the ulna.[43]

The increased signal intensity in the degenerative TFC on T1-weighted spin echo MR images can simulate the appearance of traumatic lesions of the TFC, and in extreme cases, the MR imaging findings may be falsely attributed to

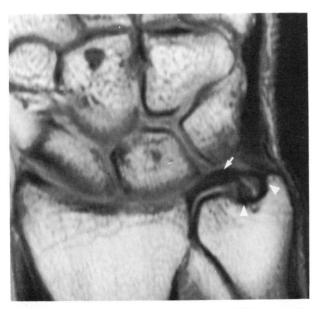

FIGURE 70–13. Triangular fibrocartilage complex: MR imaging. Normal appearance. In a coronal proton density–weighted (TR/TE, 2000/20) spin echo MR image, observe the low signal intensity of the triangular fibrocartilage (arrow), with bifurcated bands of low signal intensity (arrowheads) attaching to the styloid process of the ulna. The scapholunate and lunotriquetral interosseous ligaments are not well seen in this image. Note two bone islands, appearing as foci of low signal intensity, in the lunate and capitate. (Courtesy of A. G. Bergman, M.D., Stanford, California.)

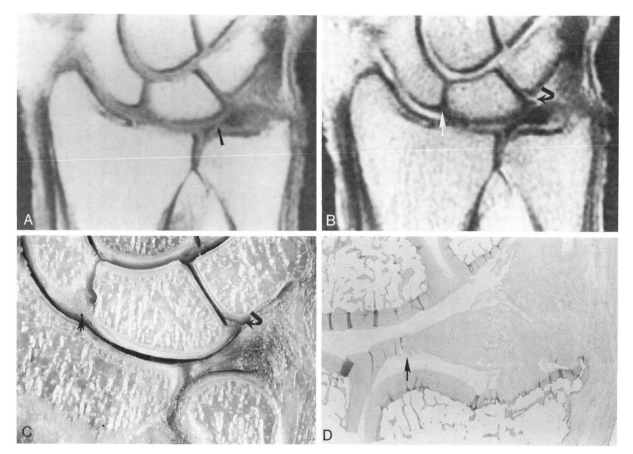

FIGURE 70–15. Triangular fibrocartilage complex: MR imaging. Degenerative changes.

A Coronal T1-weighted (TR/TE, 600/20) spin echo MR image. The triangular fibrocartilage shows bandlike low signal intensity except for its radial and ulnar attachment sites. Apparent discontinuity of the triangular fibrocartilage (arrow) is seen near its radial attachment. The scapholunate and lunotriquetral ligaments are not well shown.

B Coronal T2-weighted (TR/TE, 2000/60) spin echo MR image at the same level as **A**. The triangular fibrocartilage is of low signal intensity and appears to be intact. Perforated lunotriquetral (curved arrow) and intact scapholunate (straight arrow) interosseous ligaments are depicted clearly.

C Coronal section of the specimen. The triangular fibrocartilage and scapholunate interosseous ligament (arrow) are not perforated. The lunotriquetral interosseous ligament (curved arrow) is perforated.

D Histologic preparation of a coronal section of the specimen. The portion of the triangular fibrocartilage that showed discontinuity on the T1-weighted spin echo MR image is not perforated, but it is degenerated (arrow). Mucoid degeneration and surface fibrillation are more severe on the ulnar surface of the triangular fibrocartilage. The articular cartilage is seen at the radial attachment of the triangular fibrocartilage. (From Kang HS, et al: Radiology 181:401, 1991.)

a traumatically induced communicating defect. The detection of less high signal intensity in the TFC on T2-weighted spin echo MR images is useful in differentiating TFC degeneration from TFC perforation in which high signal intensity on T2-weighted spin echo MR images is evident.[39] These data support the concept that reliance on T1-weighted spin echo MR images alone in the analysis of lesions of the TFC creates diagnostic difficulty, as such images, in instances of severe degeneration of the TFC, often reveal alterations in signal intensity and morphology of the TFC that simulate those of perforation. The situation encountered in the analysis of the TFC with MR imaging is similar to that resulting from mucinous change within the menisci of the knee and the glenoid labrum (see later discussion).

Although it is difficult to differentiate between a traumatically induced communicating defect of the TFC and one related to degeneration using MR imaging (or standard arthrography), characteristic MR imaging features frequently allow an accurate diagnosis of some type of com-

municating defect or perforation of the structure. Linear regions of high signal intensity, identical to that of fluid, traversing the entire thickness of the TFC on T1-weighted and T2-weighted spin echo MR images (or gradient echo images) are strong evidence that a communicating defect is present (Figs. 70–16 and 70–17). Although similar regions of high signal intensity extending partially through the thickness of the TFC are compatible with the diagnosis of a noncommunicating defect (Fig. 70–18), the accuracy of this finding is not established. The presence of fluid in the distal radioulnar joint represents a secondary MR imaging finding of perforation of the TFCC[41] but, as an isolated abnormality, this finding is not diagnostic of such a perforation.

Most previous investigations of the value of MR imaging in the assessment of the TFC have relied upon findings derived from spin echo sequences. Gradient echo imaging sequences also may be valuable, however. On multiplanar gradient recalled (MPGR) MR images in which a low flip angle is used, fluid accumulating within communicating

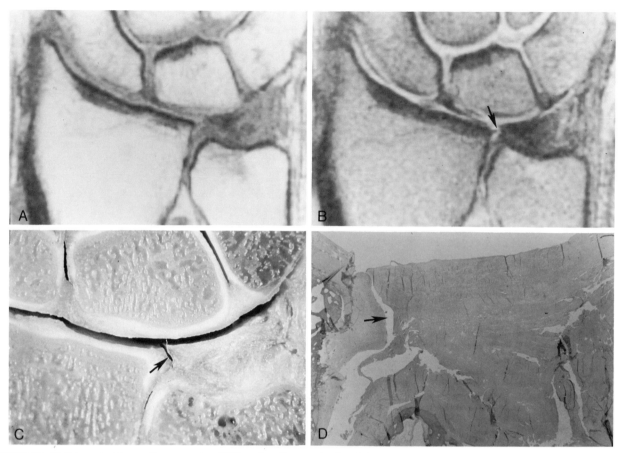

FIGURE 70–16. Triangular fibrocartilage complex: MR imaging. Communicating defect.

A Coronal T1-weighted (TR/TE, 600/20) spin echo MR image. The signal intensity of the triangular fibrocartilage and scapholunate and lunotriquetral interosseous ligaments is diffusely increased.

B T2-weighted (TR/TE, 2000/60) spin echo MR image. The signal intensity of the triangular fibrocartilage and the scapholunate and lunotriquetral interosseous ligaments is lower than in the T1-weighted spin echo MR image. Focal high signal intensity (arrow) near the radial attachment of the triangular fibrocartilage is consistent with the presence of a communicating defect.

C Coronal section of the specimen. The triangular fibrocartilage is perforated (arrow) near its radial attachment. The scapholunate and lunotriquetral interosseous ligaments are not perforated.

D Histologic section. The triangular fibrocartilage is perforated near its radial attachment (arrow). Degeneration of the triangular fibrocartilage is more severe on its ulnar surface and adjacent to the edge of the perforation.

(From Kang HS, et al: Radiology *181*:401, 1991.)

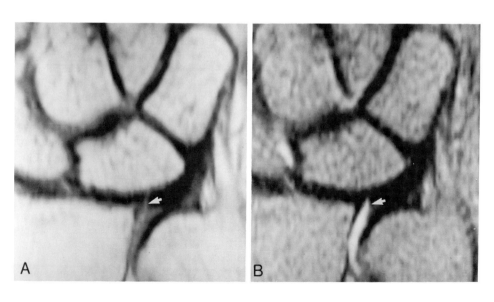

FIGURE 70–17. Triangular fibrocartilage complex: MR imaging. Communicating defect.

A Coronal proton density (TR/TE, 2500/20) spin echo MR image. Note the linear region of increased signal intensity (arrow) in the triangular fibrocartilage.

B T2-weighted (TR/TE, 2500/80) spin echo MR image. Fluid of high signal intensity is present in the defect (arrow) within the triangular fibrocartilage and in the distal radioulnar joint. Fluid also is present in the midcarpal joint.

(Courtesy of M. Zlatkin, M.D., Hollywood, Florida.)

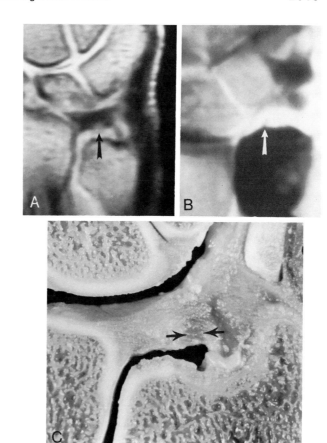

FIGURE 70–18. Triangular fibrocartilage complex: MR imaging. Noncommunicating defect.

A Coronal T2-weighted (TR/TE, 2000/80) spin echo MR image. Note a region of abnormal signal intensity *(arrow)* in the proximal surface of the triangular fibrocartilage.

B Digital arthrogram with injection of the distal radioulnar joint. This is the third part of a three-part wrist arthrogram in which the inferior radioulnar joint was opacified. Observe a linear collection of contrast material *(arrow)* consistent with a partial tear of the proximal surface of the triangular fibrocartilage.

C Coronal section of the wrist. The region of the noncommunicating defect of the triangular fibrocartilage *(arrows)* is evident.

defects in the TFC is of high signal intensity (Fig. 70–19). When gradient recalled imaging is combined with volumetric acquisition, thin sections of the TFC may be obtained, which may accentuate the abnormalities associated with such defects. With volumetric acquisition of image data, radial reconstructions of the TFC also are possible.[1372] In one study, short tau inversion recovery (STIR) MR imaging was found to be more useful than spin echo MR imaging in the assessment of the TFCC[41] (Fig. 70–20). The role of MR arthrography in this assessment is not clear; however, this procedure requires at least one injection into the radiocarpal or distal radioulnar joint and perhaps two separate injections into the radiocarpal and distal radioulnar joints and, therefore, is more complicated and time-consuming than standard MR imaging (Figs. 70–21 and 70–22).

The relative diagnostic value of MR imaging and standard arthrography in the detection of defects of the TFC has been studied.[37, 41] The lack of a standard of reference in the diagnosis of TFC defects makes such comparisons difficult, however, as even arthroscopy performed by expert orthopedic surgeons is not without diagnostic error. For example, surface irregularities of the TFC may be interpreted as communicating defects by some arthroscopists. Close agreement appears to exist in the results of MR imaging and arthrography in the assessment of defects of the TFC.[41] At this time, state-of-the-art MR imaging and arthrography can be considered equally accurate in this assessment. With either technique, however, the presence of degenerative communicating or noncommunicating defects of the TFC in middle-aged and elderly persons who are asymptomatic, and of degenerative or traumatically induced communicating or noncommunicating defects of the

TFC in patients without ulnar-sided wrist pain, makes assessment of the clinical relevance of the findings more difficult.[45, 46]

Despite the widespread availability of wrist arthrography and the increasing availability of MR imaging as a means to study the TFCC, there are those who maintain steadfastly

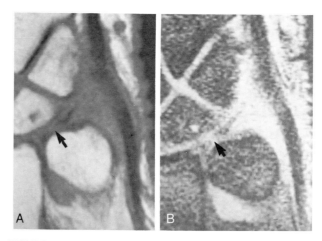

FIGURE 70–19. Triangular fibrocartilage complex: MR imaging. Communicating defect. Spin echo versus multiplanar gradient recalled (MPGR) MR imaging.

A Coronal T1-weighted (TR/TE, 600/20) spin echo MR image. Discontinuity (arrow) in the low signal intensity of the triangular fibrocartilage is seen. Note fluid of intermediate signal intensity about the distal portion of the ulna.

B Coronal MPGR (TR/TE, 500/15; flip angle, 20 degrees) MR image. Fluid of high signal intensity is seen in the defect (arrow) in the triangular fibrocartilage and about the distal portion of the ulna.

(Courtesy of C. Sebrechts, M.D., San Diego, California.)

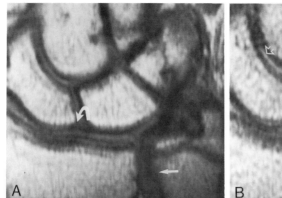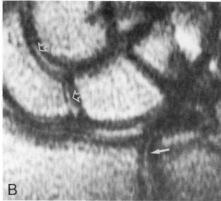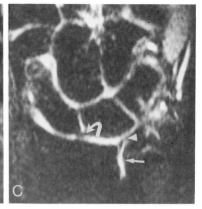

FIGURE 70–20. Triangular fibrocartilage complex: MR imaging. Communicating defect. Spin echo versus short tau inversion recovery (STIR) MR images.

A Coronal proton density–weighted (TR/TE, 1700/20) spin echo MR image. The triangular fibrocartilage is of low signal intensity and appears normal. Fluid is seen in the distal radioulnar joint (straight arrow), and the scapholunate interosseous ligament (curved arrow) is normal.

B Coronal T2-weighted (TR/TE, 1700/70) spin echo MR image. Fluid in the distal radioulnar joint (straight arrow) is of high signal intensity. There is questionable extension of this fluid into the substance of the triangular fibrocartilage. Note the fluid in the midcarpal joint, including the space between the scaphoid and the lunate (open arrows).

C STIR (TR/TE, 1650/25; inversion time, 160 msec) MR image. Fluid of high signal intensity in the distal radioulnar joint (straight arrow) extends into a defect (arrowhead) in the triangular fibrocartilage. The scapholunate ligament (curved arrow) appears normal.

(From Schweitzer ME, et al: Radiology *182*:205, 1992.)

that the advantages of wrist arthroscopy outweigh those of either imaging method, and that arthroscopy, even when used alone (without other diagnostic methods), is effective in the assessment of the TFCC.[1343] Recent technical advances have led to more reliable arthroscopic examinations of the wrist, in which the TFCC (as well as other intra-articular structures) can be inspected directly.[1344] When compared with conventional open procedures of the wrist, arthroscopy is associated with reduced morbidity; when compared with arthrography and MR imaging, arthroscopy provides a truer three-dimensional display of the TFCC.[1343] Instrumentation introduced through one or more portals can be used to allow arthroscopic treatment of lesions of the TFCC, particularly Class 1A and 2C lesions. Reports have indicated therapeutic success following excision of unstable tissue fragments in the central portion of the TFCC and following repair with sutures of peripheral separations, or

detachments, of the TFCC.[1343] Complications of such arthroscopy include infection, painful incisions, injury to cutaneous nerves, and reflex sympathy dystrophy, but they are infrequent. Further investigation is required to determine the benefits of arthrography or MR imaging vis-à-vis those of arthroscopy in the analysis of various abnormalities of the TFCC.

Ulnar Impaction Syndrome. The ulnar impaction syndrome, also termed ulnocarpal abutment, ulnolunate impaction syndrome, and ulnar abutment syndrome, is defined as a degenerative condition characterized by ulnar-sided wrist pain, swelling, and limitation of motion related to excessive load bearing across the ulnar aspect of the wrist.[47, 48] Chronic impaction of the ulnar head against the TFCC and ulnar-sided carpal bones results in progressive deterioration of the TFCC, chondromalacia of the lunate and head of the ulna, and attrition of the lunotriquetral interosseous liga-

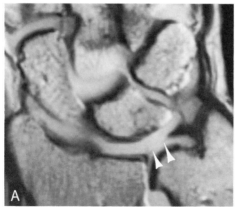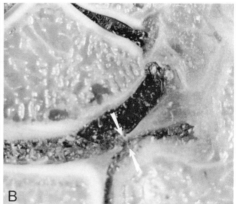

FIGURE 70–21. Triangular fibrocartilage complex: MR imaging. Communicating defect. MR arthrography.

A Coronal T1-weighted (TR/TE, 800/20) MR image following intra-articular injection of a copper sulfate solution into the radiocarpal compartment of a cadaveric wrist. Note the communicating defect (arrowheads) in the triangular fibrocartilage. The lunotriquetral interosseous ligament also is disrupted, allowing filling of the midcarpal joint.

B Coronal section of the wrist. The defect (arrows) in the triangular fibrocartilage is evident. The abnormality of the lunotriquetral interosseous ligament is not seen well in this section.

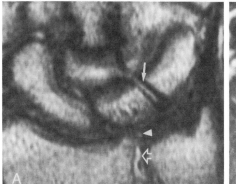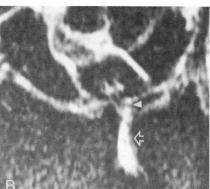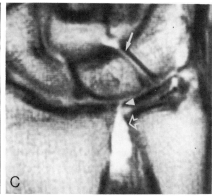

FIGURE 70–22. Triangular fibrocartilage complex: MR imaging. Communicating defect. Spin echo and STIR MR images and MR arthrography.

A Coronal T2-weighted (TR/TE, 1700/70) spin echo MR image. Note fluid of high signal intensity (open arrow) in the distal radioulnar joint and the increased signal intensity (arrowhead) in the triangular fibrocartilage, consistent with a defect. Fluid also is present in the midcarpal joint between the lunate and the triquetrum (solid arrow), although the lunotriquetral and scapholunate interosseous ligaments appear intact.

B Coronal STIR MR image. Fluid of high signal intensity is seen in the distal radioulnar joint (open arrow) and in the defect (arrowhead) in the triangular fibrocartilage. The lunotriquetral and scapholunate interosseous ligaments appear intact.

C MR arthrography with radiocarpal compartment injection of gadolinium compound. A coronal T1-weighted (TR/TE, 200/20) spin echo MR image shows that the injected material extends through a defect (arrowhead) in the triangular fibrocartilage into the distal radioulnar joint (open arrow), and through a defect in the lunotriquetral interosseous ligament into the space between the lunate and the triquetrum (solid arrow) and other portions of the midcarpal joint.

(From Schweitzer ME, et al: Radiology *182*:205, 1992.)

ment.[47] The ulnar impaction syndrome almost always is associated with a positive ulnar variance severe enough to allow transfer of excessive compressive forces from the ulna to the triquetrum and the lunate via the TFCC.[48] This syndrome is distinguished from a second condition, the ulnar impingement syndrome which, as classically described, consists of a short ulna impinging on the distal portion of the radius, causing a painful, disabling pseudarthrosis.[49] Although the ulnar impaction syndrome has been identified in patients with a neutral or a positive ulnar variance, it is not associated with a negative ulnar variance.[47] Causes of this syndrome include developmental alterations in ulnar length, malunion of a fracture of the distal portion of the radius, premature growth arrest of the distal radial physis, an Essex-Lopresti fracture-dislocation, and radial head resection.

Routine radiographs in patients with the ulnar impaction

syndrome may reveal alterations in the ulnar side of the proximal portion of the lunate, the radial side of the proximal portion of the triquetrum, and the ulnar head. Findings include bone sclerosis, cysts, and osteophytes.[48] Arthrography often demonstrates communicating defects of the TFC and disruption of the lunotriquetral interosseous ligament. MR imaging also documents these abnormalities of the TFC and lunotriquetral interosseous ligament, and chondromalacia and alterations in the subchondral bone of the proximal surfaces of the lunate and triquetrum may be evident (Figs. 70–23 and 70–24).

Partial excision of the TFC accomplished arthroscopically commonly is not successful in patients with a positive ulnar variance and the ulnar impaction syndrome. More extensive procedures, such as shortening of the ulna or resection of the ulnar head, in these patients appear to be more beneficial.

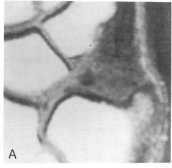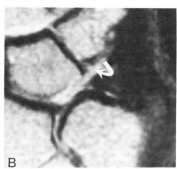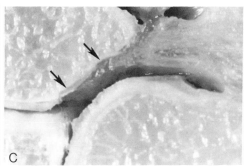

FIGURE 70–23. Ulnar impaction syndrome: MR imaging.

A Coronal T1-weighted (TR/TE, 600/20) spin echo MR image. There is a large communicating defect of the triangular fibrocartilage and a mild positive ulnar variance. The lunotriquetral interosseous ligament is not well seen. Note the irregularity of the ulnar aspect of the proximal portion of the lunate.

B Coronal T2-weighted (TR/TE, 2000/60) spin echo MR image. Fluid of high signal intensity in the radiocarpal and distal radioulnar joint outlines the large communicating defect in the triangular fibrocartilage. Note a defect (curved arrow) of the lunotriquetral interosseous ligament and irregularity of the proximal articular surface of the lunate.

C Coronal section of the wrist. Defects are seen in the triangular fibrocartilage and lunotriquetral interosseous ligament. The articular cartilage and subchondral bone of the lunate are eroded (straight arrows).

(From Kang HS, et al: Radiology *181*:401, 1991.)

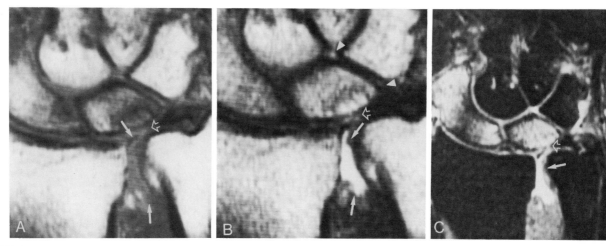

FIGURE 70–24. Ulnar impaction syndrome: MR imaging.

A Coronal proton density–weighted (TR/TE, 1700/20) spin echo MR image. A large communicating defect (open arrow) in the triangular fibrocartilage is evident. Fluid (solid arrows) is apparent in the distal radioulnar joint. The lunotriquetral interosseous ligament is not well seen. Note abnormal regions of low signal intensity in the lunate and scaphoid, consistent with marrow edema. The lunate changes have occurred as a consequence of the ulnar impaction syndrome.

B Coronal T2-weighted (TR/TE, 1700/70) spin echo MR image. The communicating defect (open arrow) of the triangular fibrocartilage again is evident. Fluid fills the distal radioulnar joint (solid arrows). Fluid (arrowheads) is seen in the midcarpal joint, including the space between the lunate and triquetrum. High signal intensity in the proximal portion of the lunate is indicative of marrow edema.

C Coronal STIR MR image (TR/TE, 1650/25; inversion time, 160 msec). Defects are seen in the triangular fibrocartilage (open arrow) and lunotriquetral interosseous ligament. Fluid fills the distal radioulnar joint (solid arrow) and portions of the radiocarpal and midcarpal joints. Marrow edema in the scaphoid and lunate is manifest as regions of increased signal intensity.

(From Schweitzer ME, et al: Radiology *182:*205, 1992.)

Ulnar Impingement Syndrome. The ulnar impingement syndrome is associated with clinical manifestations that are similar to but often more disabling than those accompanying the ulnar impaction syndrome. Pain may be aggravated during pronation and supination of the forearm.[47] Three radiographic features are characteristic of the ulnar impingement syndrome: a minus ulnar variance such that the ulna does not articulate with the sigmoid notch of the radius; a scalloped concavity of the distal portion of the radius; and convergence of the ulna to the distal portion of the radius.[49] Causes of this syndrome include resection of the distal portion of the ulna (Darrach procedure) and growth arrest of the ulna. The latter condition may occur secondary to trauma or a developmental abnormality (e.g., multiple hereditary exostoses).

Instability of the Distal Radioulnar Joint. The distal radioulnar joint is involved in pronation and supination of the forearm, during which the radius moves with respect to a relatively fixed ulna. Although, by convention, subluxation or dislocation of the distal radioulnar joint is described as that of the ulna subluxing or dislocating relative to the radius, in actuality, it is the radiocarpal mass that subluxes or dislocates in relation to the relatively stationary ulnar head.[50] Conventional terminology, however, is used in the following discussion.

Although there is general agreement that the stability of the distal radioulnar joint depends on a number of structures, including the dorsal and volar radioulnar ligaments, (volar) ulnocarpal ligaments, ulnar collateral ligament, extensor carpi ulnaris tendon, and the pronator quadratus and flexor carpi ulnaris muscles, the contributions of each to such stability in attitudes of pronation and supination of the forearm are controversial.[22–25, 27, 51] The importance of the dorsal and volar radioulnar ligaments as a stabilizing factor, preventing subluxations and dislocations of the distal ra-

dioulnar joint, appears certain, but their precise role in this respect is not clear. Linscheid,[24] in a discussion of stability of the distal radioulnar joint, indicated that the dorsal radioulnar ligament is under tension, or is taut, in pronation, and the volar radioulnar ligament is under tension in supination; Ekenstam[22] reported the opposite. Nathan and Schneider[25] emphasized the popularly held opinion that distal radioulnar joint instability is caused by a deficiency or disruption of various components of the TFCC. Such disruption may appear as an isolated phenomenon related to injury, as a finding accompanied by a fracture (e.g., Colles' fracture, fracture of the styloid process of the ulna), or as a consequence of inflammatory diseases such as rheumatoid arthritis. Clinical manifestations include pain, weakness, loss of forearm rotation, and snapping. Dorsal instability predominates, and physical examination confirms a dorsal prominence of the ulnar head, especially in a position of forearm pronation.

The detection of subluxation of the distal portion of the ulna by routine radiography may be quite difficult, as slight variations in wrist position alter the relationship of the radius and ulna. Although a number of radiographic measurements can be employed to more accurately assess the positions of the distal portions of the radius and ulna,[52] they are time-consuming and difficult to apply clinically. Tomographic techniques, such as CT scanning and MR imaging, which provide transverse or cross-sectional data, may be advantageous in the diagnosis of distal radioulnar joint instability[53–55]; evaluation of the wrist in the neutral position and with pronation and supination of the forearm, and comparison of the injured and opposite wrists commonly are required. Even with these techniques, accurate appraisal of the relative position of the ulna with respect to the radius requires construction of a number of lines, typically drawn (1) along the dorsal surface of the radius from Lister's tubercle to the dorsal ulnar border of the bone, (2) as a perpendicular to this line through the dorsal ulnar border of the radius, and (3) as a perpendicular to the second line through the palmar border of the ulnar head.[56] In the normal situation, the bulk of the ulnar head is located between lines 1 and 3, slight changes in its position are detected when volar or dorsal stress is applied to the wrist, and little difference in the position of the ulnar heads (with respect to the distal portion of the radii) in the two extremities is evident. Furthermore, the anatomic landmarks required for construction of these lines are constant and usually identified easily. As subtle displacements may characterize minor degrees of distal radioulnar joint instability, however, a comparison of findings in the injured and noninjured wrist is essential. Although both CT and MR imaging allow such comparison, the advantages of MR imaging include direct multiplanar analysis of the distal radioulnar joint, visualization of the dorsal and volar radioulnar ligaments, and assessment of nearby structures such as the extensor carpi ulnaris tendon and other components of the TFCC that also may be affected.

Carpal Abnormalities

Carpal Instability. As indicated in Chapter 68, since the landmark publications by Linscheid and coworkers[57] and Dobyns and collaborators,[58] the subject of carpal instability has received a great deal of attention. Both the extrinsic and the intrinsic ligaments of the wrist contribute to carpal stability, whereas the role of the collateral ligament system in this function is limited. Biomechanically, the extrinsic ligaments are stiffer than the intrinsic ligaments, and the intrinsic ligaments are capable of greater elongation before permanent deformity occurs.[59] The volar radiocarpal and intercarpal ligaments generally are regarded as the most important structures stabilizing the carpus.

The patterns of carpal instability commonly are divided into dissociated and nondissociated types. The dissociated instability patterns usually indicate more extensive ligamentous damage than the nondissociated instability patterns. The former patterns may be recognized on routine radiographic analysis owing to disruptions in the normal relationships among the carpal bones.[48] Dissociative instability patterns include transscaphoid fractures and complete tears of the scapholunate or lunotriquetral interosseous ligament, or both ligaments, which may occur in association with attenuation or disruption of the palmar or dorsal extrinsic ligaments, or both types of extrinsic ligaments. Nondissociative instability patterns represent abnormalities of alignment or relationship of the carpal bones with intact interosseous ligaments.[48] Nondissociative instability patterns are less common than dissociative instability patterns and may result from attenuation of the palmar or dorsal radiocarpal or ulnocarpal ligaments in the presence of intact scapholunate and lunotriquetral interosseous ligaments. Such intact interosseous ligaments are suggested by routine posteroanterior radiographs of the wrist in which carpal alignment appears normal.[48] Therefore, a normal radiographic appearance does not exclude the presence of carpal instability. Indeed, carpal instability patterns sometimes are classified as static or dynamic, based upon the presence (i.e., static instability) or absence (i.e., dynamic instability) of radiographically detectable carpal abnormalities.[60] Patients with

dynamic instability of the carpal bones may be able voluntarily to change the carpal alignment from normal to abnormal during certain movements of the wrist, or such abnormal carpal alignment may be elicited during manipulation of the wrist during physical examination.

Anatomically, there are three types of carpal instability: lateral instability, which usually occurs between the scaphoid and the lunate; medial instability, which occurs between the triquetrum and the lunate or between the triquetrum and the hamate; and proximal instability, which occurs when the abnormal carpal alignment is secondary to an injury of the radius or to massive radiocarpal disruption.[60] The patterns of instability that result from ligamentous disruption in the proximal carpal row (i.e., between the scaphoid and lunate or between the lunate and triquetrum) include scapholunate dissociation, which produces dorsal intercalated segmental instability (DISI), and lunotriquetral dissociation, which leads to volar intercalated segmental instability (VISI) (Fig. 70–25).

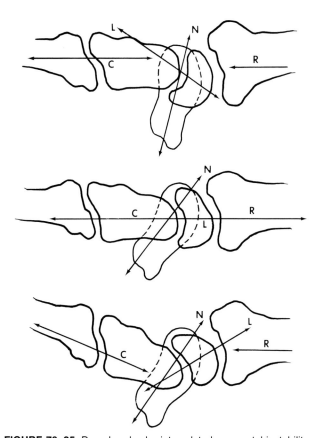

FIGURE 70–25. Dorsal and volar intercalated segmental instability. Lateral projection. Line drawings of longitudinal axes of third metacarpal, navicular (N) or scaphoid, lunate (L), capitate (C), and radius (R) in dorsal intercalated segmental instability (DISI) (upper drawing), in normal situation (middle drawing), and in volar intercalated segmental instability (VISI) (lower drawing). When the wrist is normal, a continuous line can be drawn through the longitudinal axes of the capitate, the lunate, and the radius, and this line will intersect a second line through the longitudinal axis of the scaphoid, creating an angle of 30 degrees to 60 degrees. In DISI, the lunate is flexed toward the back of the hand and the scaphoid is displaced vertically. The angle of intersection between the two longitudinal axes is greater than 60 degrees. In VISI, the lunate is flexed toward the palm and the angle between the two longitudinal axes is less than 30 degrees. (From Linscheid RL, et al: J Bone Joint Surg [Am] *54*:1612, 1972.)

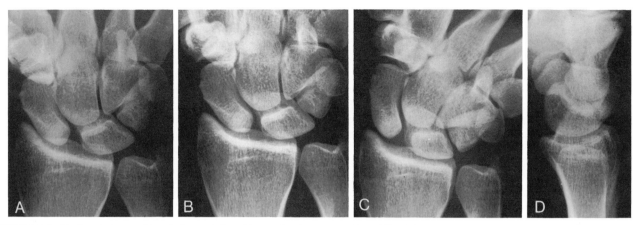

FIGURE 70–26. Scapholunate dissociation and dorsal intercalated segmental instability (DISI): Routine radiography with specialized projections. Routine posteroanterior (PA) radiograph **(A)**, PA radiograph with the patient clenching his fist **(B)**, and PA radiograph with ulnar deviation of the wrist **(C)** show widening of the scapholunate interosseous space and a rounded distal border of the lunate, indicative of dorsal tilting of the lunate with visualization of its volar surface. The lateral radiograph **(D)** confirms DISI. (Courtesy of G. Greenway, M.D., Dallas, Texas.)

Diagnosis of many of the static patterns of carpal instability, such as scapholunate dissociation (Fig. 70–26), triquetrolunate dissociation, scapholunate advanced collapse (SLAC), and ulnar translocation of the carpus, can be established on the basis of findings on routine radiographs, particularly if the observer has knowledge of the standard measurements used to analyze the relationships among the carpal bones[48] (see Chapter 68). Dynamic patterns of carpal instability, however, may escape detection when routine radiographs alone are evaluated. Although bone scintigraphy can be used as a diagnostic screening method, assessment of soft tissue abnormalities, particularly those of the ligaments, is best accomplished with arthrography or MR imaging.

As indicated in Chapter 13, arthrography can be used for the diagnosis of communicating defects of the scapholunate and lunotriquetral interosseous ligaments (Fig. 70–27). Such defects, however, may relate not to injury but to progressive deterioration, a process that increases in frequency with advancing age (see Chapter 22). Indeed, when bilateral arthrography is employed, patterns of communication between the radiocarpal and midcarpal joints in the injured and symptomatic side also may be observed in the uninjured and asymptomatic side.[61] Furthermore, the identification of all full-thickness defects of the scapholunate and lunotriquetral ligaments, in the opinion of some experts, requires sequential opacification of the radiocarpal and midcarpal compartments, owing to the presence of some defects that allow flow of contrast material in only one direction (see Chapter 13). The demonstration of com-

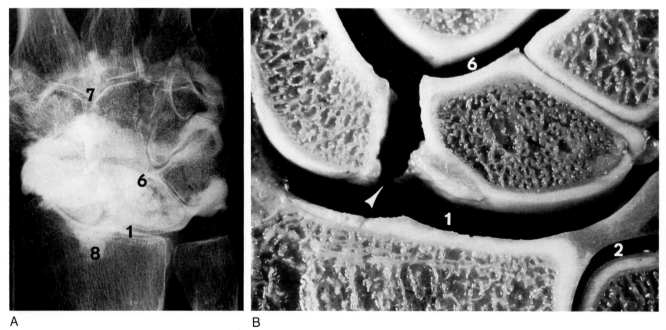

FIGURE 70–27. Intercarpal ligaments: Routine arthrography. Communicating defect of scapholunate interosseous ligament. A frontal radiograph **(A)** following opacification of the radiocarpal compartment (1) reveals its communication with the midcarpal (6) and common carpometacarpal (7) compartments. This communication is possible when a defect exists in the interosseous ligaments extending between bones of the proximal carpal row. On a photograph **(B)** of a coronal section of the cadaveric wrist, observe disruption of the scapholunate ligament (arrowhead). The inferior radioulnar compartment (2) and volar radial recesses (8) also are indicated.

munications between the radiocarpal and midcarpal compartments may depend not only on which compartment is injected but also on which joint is injected first, the amount of contrast material introduced, and the delay between injections.[62] Accurate analysis of arthrographic findings also requires careful monitoring during the injection process; such monitoring can be accomplished with fluoroscopy, videorecording, or digital technique[63–65] (Fig. 70–28).

Although MR imaging does not resolve the question of the clinical significance of the ligamentous abnormalities, the technique has been found useful for the identification of defects of the scapholunate and lunotriquetral interosseous ligaments[33, 36, 38, 40, 41] and, in a preliminary fashion, for the assessment of the dorsal and volar radiocarpal and carpal ligaments.[12, 14, 1345] The coronal plane is most useful for delineation of the interosseous ligaments, although the

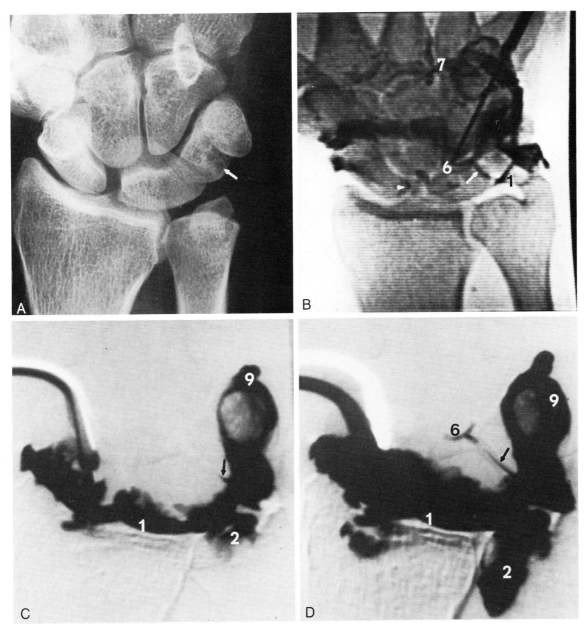

FIGURE 70–28. Intercarpal ligaments: Digital arthrography. Communicating defect of lunotriquetral interosseous ligament (and triangular fibrocartilage).

A, B In this patient, the initial radiograph **(A)** reveals subtle loss of parallelism between the apposing surfaces of the lunate and the triquetrum and cystic changes in the triquetrum (arrow). The scapholunate space is abnormally wide. In **B**, a midcarpal compartment (6) injection of contrast material shows communication with the radiocarpal compartment (1) via the space between the lunate and the triquetrum (arrow). Although the contrast agent flows normally between the distal portions of the scaphoid and the lunate (arrowhead), it did not reach the radiocarpal compartment in this area. The common carpometacarpal (7) compartment also is opacified.

C, D In a cadaver, subtraction images are provided following the injection of 1.0 ml **(C)** and 2.0 ml **(D)** of contrast material into the radiocarpal compartment (1). In **C**, opacification of this compartment, the inferior radioulnar compartment (2) (indicating a tear of the triangular fibrocartilage), and the pisiform-triquetral compartment (9) is seen. A small amount of contrast agent is present in the space between the lunate and triquetrum (arrow). In **D**, opacification of the midcarpal compartment (6) has begun through a tear in the lunotriquetral interosseous ligament (arrow).

(C, D, From Resnick D, et al: AJR *142*:1187, 1984. Copyright 1984, American Roentgen Ray Society.)

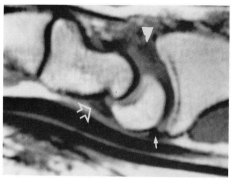

FIGURE 70–29. Dorsal intercalated segmental instability (DISI): MR imaging. Sagittal MPGR MR image (TR/TE, 533/15; flip angle, 35 degrees). Note dorsal tilting of the lunate with respect to the radius and capitate. Parts of the dorsal radiocarpal ligament (arrowhead), volar radioscaphocapitate ligament (open arrow), and volar radioscapholunate ligament (solid arrow) are seen. (Courtesy of S. Eilenberg, M.D., San Diego, California.)

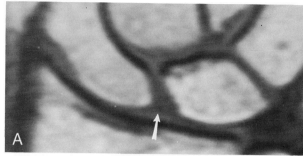

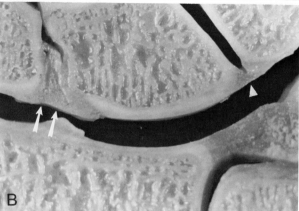

FIGURE 70–30. Intercarpal ligaments: MR imaging. Normal scapholunate interosseous ligament.

A Coronal T1-weighted (TR/TE, 800/20) spin echo MR image. Note the linear region of low signal intensity (arrow) representing the normal scapholunate interosseous ligament. The lunotriquetral interosseous ligament is not well seen.

B Coronal section of the wrist. The normal scapholunate interosseous ligament (arrows) is evident. The lunotriquetral interosseous ligament (arrowhead) also is normal.

transaxial plane also demonstrates these ligaments, and the sagittal plane provides additional information regarding the relationship among the carpal bones and, hence, may be valuable in the identification of dorsal or palmar tilting of the lunate (Fig. 70–29). Of the two interosseous ligaments, the scapholunate interosseous ligament is visualized more consistently, although some investigators have indicated that the lunotriquetral ligament also can be identified regularly.[1374] On coronal spin echo or gradient echo images, the normal scapholunate interosseous ligament typically is seen as a thin or triangular (delta-shaped) structure of low signal intensity traversing the space between the scaphoid and the lunate (Fig. 70–30). When visualized, the normal lunotriquetral interosseous ligament has a similar appearance, extending between the lunate and the triquetrum. An abnormality of the scapholunate interosseous ligament is suggested when it is elongated, incomplete, courses other than in a horizontal direction, or is not seen at all (Figs.

70–31 and 70–32). An abnormality of the lunotriquetral interosseous ligament is suggested when it is elongated, incomplete, or extends in a direction other than horizontal. Although the successful visualization of a lunotriquetral

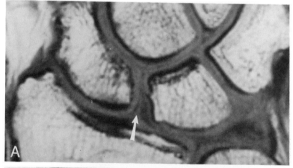

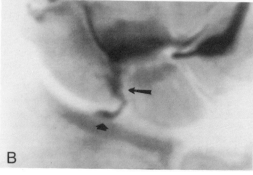

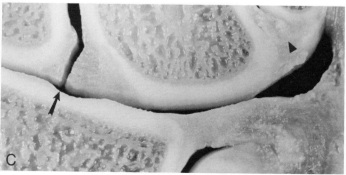

FIGURE 70–31. Intercarpal ligaments: MR imaging and digital arthrography. Communicating defect of the scapholunate interosseous ligament.

A Coronal T1-weighted (TR/TE, 800/20) spin echo MR image shows discontinuity of the scapholunate interosseous ligament (arrow). The lunotriquetral interosseous ligament is not seen.

B Digital arthrographic image following a midcarpal injection shows leakage of contrast material through the scapholunate interosseous space (upper arrow) with opacification of the radiocarpal compartment (lower arrow).

C Coronal section reveals the defect (arrow) in the scapholunate interosseous ligament. The lunotriquetral interosseous ligament (arrowhead) and triangular fibrocartilage are intact.

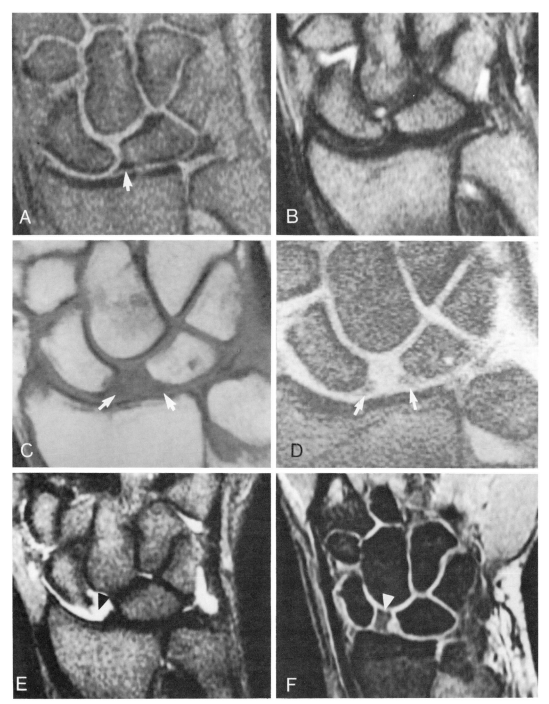

FIGURE 70–32. Intercarpal ligaments: MR imaging. Communicating defect of the scapholunate interosseous ligament.

A, B Coronal T1-weighted (TR/TE, 600/20) spin echo MR image obtained with chemical presaturation of fat (ChemSat) **(A)** and coronal T2-weighted (TR/TE, 2000/80) spin echo MR image **(B)**. In **A**, altered morphology of the scapholunate interosseous ligament (arrow) is seen. The triangular fibrocartilage is normal. In **B**, the scapholunate ligament is not well seen. Note fluid of high signal intensity in the midcarpal joint, including the region of the scapholunate interosseous space.

C, D Coronal T1-weighted (TR/TE, 600/20) spin echo MR image **(C)** and MPGR MR image (TR/TE, 500/15; flip angle, 20 degrees) **(D)** in a second patient. Note the altered morphology of the scapholunate interosseous ligament (arrows) with scapholunate widening or dissociation. The triangular fibrocartilage also is disrupted. (Courtesy of C. Sebrechts, M.D., San Diego, CA.)

E, F Coronal T2-weighted (TR/TE, 3600/105) fast spin echo MR image **(E)** and coronal spoiled gradient recalled (SPGR) MR image (TR/TE, 58/10; flip angle, 60 degrees) obtained with three-dimensional Fourier transform (3DFT) and chemical presaturation of fat (ChemSat) **(F)** in a third patient. Fluid (arrowheads) of high signal intensity in **E** and of low signal intensity in **F** in the scapholunate interosseous space is evident.

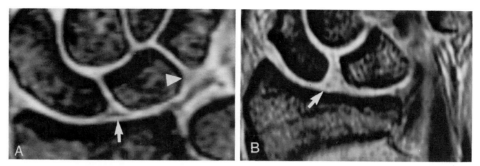

FIGURE 70–33. Intercarpal ligaments: MR imaging. Three-dimensional Fourier transform (3DFT) gradient recalled MR imaging. Normal and abnormal scapholunate interosseous ligament.

   A Normal scapholunate interosseous ligament. A coronal 3DFT (TR/TE, 60/11; flip angle, 10 degrees) MR image shows the low signal intensity and linear morphology that characterize the normal scapholunate (arrow) and lunotriquetral (arrowhead) interosseous ligaments. The triangular fibrocartilage also is normal. (Courtesy of S. K. Brahme, M.D., La Jolla, California.)

   B Communicating defect of the scapholunate interosseous ligament. A coronal oblique 3DFT (TR/TE, 60/10; flip angle, 30 degrees) MR image shows altered morphology (arrow) of the scapholunate interosseous ligament.

interosseous ligament is dependent on the specific imaging parameters employed, its nonvisualization on MR images, often has not been a reliable indicator of abnormality.[39, 41] A secondary (although nonspecific) finding associated with a defect of the scapholunate or lunotriquetral interosseous ligament is the presence of fluid in the adjacent portions of the midcarpal joint and in the scapholunate or lunotriquetral interosseous space, respectively.

   Volumetric gradient echo imaging provides thin contiguous sections of the wrist (Fig. 70–33). With this method, the scapholunate and lunotriquetral interosseous ligaments generally are delineated well. Nonvisualization of either ligament, but particularly the scapholunate interosseous ligament, with volumetric imaging is strong evidence that an abnormality exists.

   Schweitzer and coworkers,[41] in a study of the value of MR imaging of patients with chronic wrist pain, employed routine spin echo images, STIR images, and MR arthrography (with injection of gadolinium compound into the

radiocarpal joint) (Fig. 70–34). The results of the MR examinations were tabulated using conventional arthrography and arthroscopy as two standards of reference. These investigators found failure to visualize the scapholunate interosseous ligament on technically optimal MR images to be moderately helpful as a sign of a defect. Abnormal morphology of this ligament resulted in decreased sensitivity but markedly increased specificity in cases of ligamentous disruption. The standard T1-weighted spin echo MR sequence proved the most accurate, and this accuracy was better than that of conventional arthrography. When conventional arthrography was the standard, the MR arthrography images were slightly more accurate than the other sequences. The presence of fluid in the midcarpal compartment had a high sensitivity for scapholunate interosseous ligament abnormality. For analysis of the lunotriquetral interosseous ligament, failure of its visualization with MR imaging was not a useful sign of abnormality; however, when the morphology of the lunotriquetral interosseous lig-

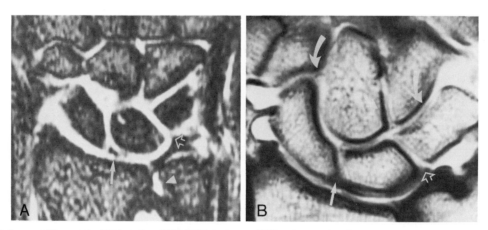

FIGURE 70–34. Intercarpal ligaments: MR imaging. STIR MR imaging and MR arthrography. Communicating defects of the scapholunate and lunotriquetral interosseous ligaments and the triangular fibrocartilage.

   A Coronal STIR (TR/TE, 1650/25; inversion time, 160 msec) MR image. Observe fluid in the distal radioulnar joint (arrowhead), altered morphology in the radial aspect of the triangular fibrocartilage and the scapholunate interosseous ligament (solid arrow), and nonvisualization of the lunotriquetral interosseous ligament (open arrow).

   B MR arthrography following injection of gadolinium compound into the radiocarpal compartment. A coronal T1-weighted (TR/TE, 500/20) spin echo MR image shows the communicating defect in the lunotriquetral interosseous ligament (open arrow) with opacification of the midcarpal compartment (curved arrows). The scapholunate interosseous ligament (straight arrow) and triangular fibrocartilage appear intact. Standard arthrography and arthroscopy confirmed communicating defects of the triangular fibrocartilage and scapholunate and lunotriquetral interosseous ligaments.

   (From Schweitzer ME, et al: Radiology *182*:205, 1992.)

ament was assessed, the specificity of the MR observations was high. The presence of fluid in the midcarpal joint also was a helpful indicator of a lunotriquetral interosseous ligament tear and had high sensitivity, similar to that noted for the scapholunate interosseous ligament. With conventional arthrography as the standard, all of the MR imaging sequences showed similar accuracy with regard to assessment of the lunotriquetral interosseous ligament; with arthroscopy as the standard, conventional T1-weighted spin echo MR images and MR arthrography were most accurate. Arthrography alone showed similar accuracy to MR imaging in the evaluation of the lunotriquetral interosseous ligament.

These results suggest that although MR arthrography may improve accuracy in the assessment of the interosseous ligaments (and the TFCC), its invasive and time-consuming nature does not appear to justify the procedure; that the presence of fluid in the midcarpal joint is an important secondary indicator of abnormality in the scapholunate or lunotriquetral interosseous ligament and, because of this, T2-weighted spin echo MR images are required; and that conventional arthrography and standard MR imaging generally provide similar information in the assessment of these interosseous ligaments.

Evaluation of the dorsal and volar extrinsic radiocarpal ligaments and many intrinsic carpal ligaments with MR imaging is best accomplished with volumetric gradient echo MR sequences (Fig. 70–35). The oblique orientation of many of these ligaments makes analysis of sequential images mandatory, and reformatted images in these oblique planes may be required.[12, 14] The clinical usefulness of such MR imaging in the detection of alterations in these ligaments is not established yet[33] and, ultimately, comparison of findings in the injured and noninjured wrist may be required. The role of MR arthrography in this regard also is not clear (Fig. 70–35C,D).

Osteonecrosis. Osteonecrosis of the carpal bones affects three principal sites: the lunate bone (i.e., Kienböck's disease), the scaphoid bone (particularly its proximal portion following a fracture of the waist of the bone), and less commonly, the capitate bone (typically its proximal portion either on an idiopathic basis or following an injury) (Fig. 70–36). Rarely, other carpal bones such as the hamate are sites of ischemic necrosis. The features of osteonecrosis at these sites are discussed in Chapters 79, 80, and 81, and only the MR imaging aspects of these conditions are discussed here.

MR imaging currently is regarded as the most sensitive and specific imaging method for the detection of osteonecrosis.[66-68] Although much of the reported data concerning this sensitivity of MR imaging relates to osteonecrosis of the femoral head, similar sensitivity certainly is expected regarding the diagnosis of ischemic necrosis in other bones, including the carpus.[36, 38, 40] Bone scintigraphy, particularly single photon emission computed tomography (SPECT), possesses similar diagnostic sensitivity in cases of osteonecrosis; however, advantages of MR imaging, which include anatomic and diagnostic specificity, tomographic display allowing analysis of the integrity of the articular surfaces, and simultaneous delineation of soft tissues, ensure its general superiority in the evaluation of osteonecrosis. The signal intensity characteristics of the infarcted zone that have been used to judge the severity and ultimate prognosis of

osteonecrosis of the femoral head (see Chapter 80) have not been tested yet in instances of carpal osteonecrosis.

MR imaging in cases of Kienböck's disease indicates its superior diagnostic sensitivity when compared with routine radiography and, in some cases, bone scintigraphy.[69-71] The diagnostic specificity of MR imaging in Kienböck's disease is high. In instances in which the entire lunate is affected with or without bone collapse, the imaging pattern almost is specific, particularly when adjacent bones, including the distal portion of the radius, are not affected and a negative (minus) ulnar variance also is observed. MR imaging is less specific when only a portion of the lunate is involved, as other conditions such as an intraosseous ganglion may lead to similar alterations. A radiocarpal joint effusion and adjacent synovial inflammation may accompany Kienböck's disease and, in such cases, the improper diagnosis of a systemic articular disease such as rheumatoid arthritis may be offered. On T1-weighted spin echo MR images, the typical appearance of Kienböck's disease is that of diffuse or focal regions of low signal intensity; on T2-weighted spin echo MR images, low signal or high signal intensity regions within portions of the lunate are seen (Fig. 70–37). These regions may correspond not only to sites of bone necrosis and reactive granulation tissue but also to areas of surrounding marrow edema. Therefore, an overestimation of the extent of bone necrosis is possible based on the distribution of marrow abnormalities delineated with MR imaging. This overestimation of the disease process may be accentuated on STIR MR images. The extent of collapse of the lunate bone in Kienböck's disease is variable and can be precisely defined by conventional tomography, CT, or MR imaging. The sagittal plane is especially valuable in delineating the degree of bone collapse and, with MR imaging, sagittal sections also can reveal the relationship of the elongated and fragmented lunate bone to the flexor tendons. The extent of bone collapse, when combined with other factors such as rotation of the scaphoid bone, proximal migration of the capitate bone, and osteoarthritis of the radiocarpal joint, has been used to stage the disease and influences the choice of a therapeutic option. These options include immobilization alone, radial shortening or lunate revascularization procedures, scaphocapitate or triscaphe fusion, wrist arthrodesis, and proximal row carpectomy.

Osteonecrosis of the scaphoid bone is an important complication of its fracture (see Chapter 68). Almost universally, posttraumatic osteonecrosis involves the proximal portion of the scaphoid, and this finding is observed most commonly following fractures of the waist or proximal pole of the bone. Routine radiography eventually will reveal regions of increased density and cyst formation within the necrotic zone, but scintigraphic and MR imaging abnormalities will antedate the radiographic findings. Both of these last two imaging methods are sensitive to the diagnosis of scaphoid osteonecrosis, although the specificity of MR imaging is greater (Figs. 70–38 and 70–39). Osteonecrosis of the scaphoid bone also may occur secondary to corticosteroid medication and, rarely, on an idiopathic basis.

Improper Fracture Healing. Although fractures may involve any of the carpal bones (see Chapter 68), those of the scaphoid are most common and may be followed by improper fracture healing (i.e., delayed union and nonunion). Causes of improper fracture healing of the scaphoid bone include a delay in initial diagnosis of the fracture,

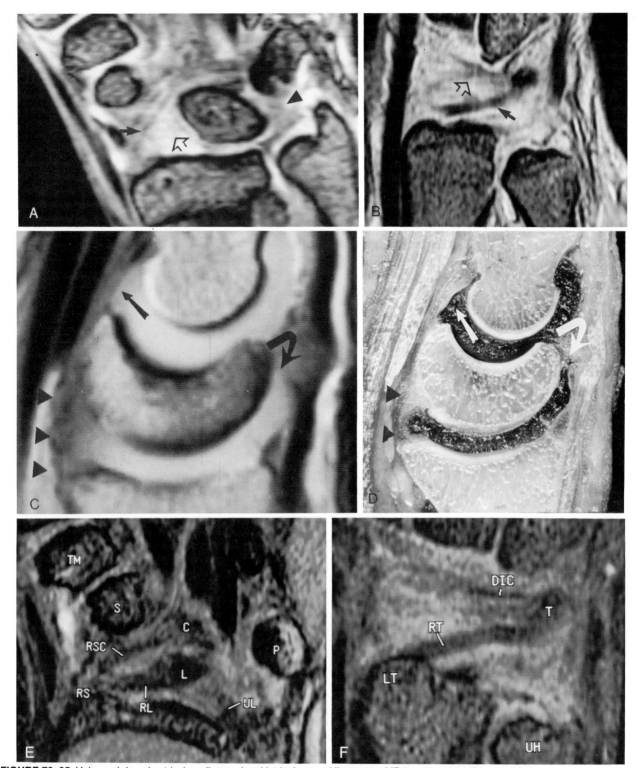

FIGURE 70–35. Volar and dorsal extrinsic radiocarpal and intrinsic carpal ligaments: MR imaging and MR arthrography.

A Normal volar ligaments. Coronal oblique 3DFT gradient recalled MR image (TR/TE, 60/10; flip angle, 30 degrees). Illustrated structures include radioscaphocapitate ligament (solid arrow), radiolunate segment of the radiolunotriquetral ligament (open arrow), and possibly, a portion of the ulnotriquetral ligament (arrowhead).

B Normal dorsal ligaments. Coronal oblique 3DFT gradient recalled MR image (TR/TE, 60/10; flip angle, 30 degrees). Illustrated structures include radiotriquetral ligament (closed arrow) and dorsal intercarpal ligament (open arrow).

C, D Normal and abnormal dorsal and volar ligaments. Sagittal T1-weighted (TR/TE, 800/20) spin echo MR image following injection of copper sulfate solution into the radiocarpal compartment of a cadaveric wrist **(C)**, and a sagittal section of the wrist **(D)**. Note the normal appearance of the radiolunate portion of the volar radioscapholunate ligament (arrowheads) and volar radioscaphocapitate ligament (solid arrows), and a tear (curved arrows) of the dorsal radiocarpal ligament.

E Normal volar ligaments. Paracoronal 3DFT gradient recalled MR image (TR/TE, 37/8; flip angle, 12 degrees). Illustrated structures include radioscaphocapitate ligament (RSC), radiolunate segment (RL) of radiolunotriquetral ligament, and a portion of the ulnolunate ligament (UL). Also identified are the radial styloid process (RS), lunate bone (L), distal pole of scaphoid bone (S), capitate wrist (C), trapezium bone (TM), and pisiform bone (P).

F Normal dorsal ligaments. Identical MR imaging sequence as in **E**. Note Lister's tubercle (LT), ulnar head (UH), and dorsal tubercle of triquetral bone (T). Identified structures are the dorsal intercarpal ligament (DIC) and, in this case, a single radiotriquetral ligament (RT).

(**E, F,** Courtesy of D. K. Smith, M.D., San Antonio, Texas; from Smith DK: AJR *161:*119–125, 352–357, 1993.)

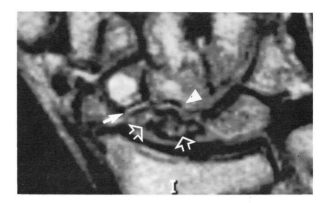

FIGURE 70–36. Scaphocapitate syndrome: MR imaging. This patient had a fracture of the midportion of the scaphoid bone and of the proximal portion of the capitate bone (scaphocapitate syndrome) that was followed by osteonecrosis at both sites. A coronal proton density–weighted (TR/TE, 2000/35) MR image reveals nonunion of the scaphoid fracture (solid arrow) with osteonecrosis of its proximal pole (open arrows) manifest as decreased size, an irregular contour, and low signal intensity. The proximal pole of the capitate bone (arrowhead) also is irregular, and cystic lesions in the capitate bone and distal portion of the scaphoid are manifest as regions of high signal intensity.

rotation or displacement at the fracture site, inadequate immobilization, interposition of soft tissue in the fracture gap, and a tenuous blood supply.[72–75] Routine radiography provides some information regarding the diagnosis of delayed union or nonunion, although interobserver disagreement in the interpretation of the radiographs is encountered.[76] Uncertainty regarding the presence or absence of trabeculae traversing the fracture line is common when conventional radiographs alone are analyzed. CT provides more definitive evidence of a persistent fracture line, especially if direct coronal or sagittal images, or both, are included.

MR imaging, representing a tomographic technique, shares many of the advantages of CT in the diagnosis of delayed union or nonunion of scaphoid fractures. The fracture site can be identified readily, and the degree of displacement or angulation of the fracture fragments can be determined if coronal, sagittal, and transaxial images are obtained. High signal intensity in the fracture defect on T2-weighted spin echo and certain gradient echo MR images is consistent with the presence of fluid, a certain sign of fracture nonunion (see Fig. 70–37). Persistent low signal intensity on T1-weighted and T2-weighted spin echo MR

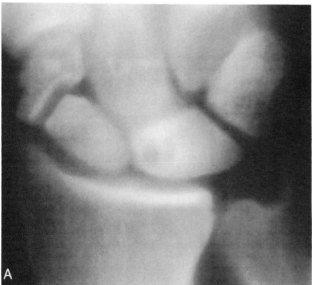

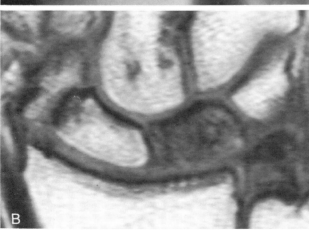

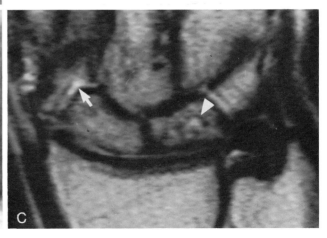

FIGURE 70–37. Kienböck's disease and nonunion of a scaphoid fracture: MR imaging.

A Conventional tomography shows cystic changes and sclerosis in the lunate bone and an ununited fracture of the midportion of the scaphoid bone. The fracture lines are smooth with sclerotic margins. A mild negative ulnar variance is seen.

B A coronal T1-weighted (TR/TE, 800/20) spin echo MR image reveals low signal intensity throughout the lunate bone and in the fracture gap of the scaphoid bone.

C A coronal T2-weighted (TR/TE, 2500/60) spin echo MR image shows foci of high signal intensity (arrowhead) in the lunate bone. Fluid of high signal intensity (arrow) is evident in a portion of the fracture gap in the scaphoid bone.

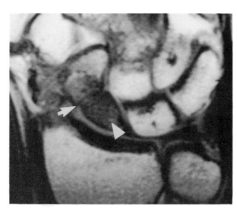

FIGURE 70–38. Osteonecrosis of the scaphoid bone following a fracture. A coronal T1-weighted (TR/TE, 583/20) spin echo MR image shows the site (arrow) of a previous fracture of the midportion of the scaphoid bone. Note the low signal intensity in the proximal pole of the scaphoid bone (arrowhead). (Courtesy of S. Eilenberg, M.D., San Diego, California.)

images may indicate the presence of fibrosis at the fracture site. Marrow continuity across the fracture line represents strong evidence that fracture healing has occurred. Furthermore, with MR imaging, additional bone, ligament, and tendon injuries can be detected.

Carpal Tunnel Abnormalities

Carpal Tunnel Syndrome. As indicated in Chapter 77, the carpal tunnel syndrome is a relatively common entrapment neuropathy affecting the median nerve within the carpal tunnel in the palmar aspect of the wrist (Fig. 70–40). Clinical findings include paresthesias of the fingers in the distribution of the median nerve and weakness and atrophy of the thenar muscles. The carpal tunnel syndrome is more frequent in women than in men, and affected patients usually are in the fourth to sixth decades of life. Unilateral involvement predominates with increased frequency of involvement in the dominant hand, although bilateral involvement is noted in 10 to 40 per cent of cases. Physical examination relies, in part, on reproduction of the symptoms by gentle percussion on the median nerve at the level of the

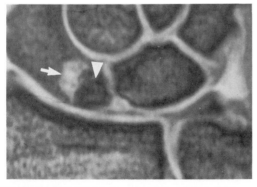

FIGURE 70–39. Osteonecrosis and cyst formation of the scaphoid bone following fracture. A coronal MPGR MR image (TR/TE, 200/15; flip angle, 25 degrees) shows a cyst (arrow) occurring adjacent to a fracture line in the scaphoid bone, with altered signal intensity in the proximal pole of the scaphoid bone (arrowhead) secondary to osteonecrosis. Note the normal appearance of the triangular fibrocartilage and the scapholunate and lunotriquetral interosseous ligaments.

wrist (i.e., Tinel's sign). In most cases, accurate diagnosis based on clinical history and the results of physical examination and electromyographic studies is straightforward. The list of potential causes of the carpal tunnel syndrome is impressive, including a variety of systemic diseases (e.g., acromegaly, thyroid disorders, plasma cell myeloma, amyloidosis, diabetes mellitus, hemophilia), masses, anatomic anomalies (e.g., persistent median artery), occupational or accidental trauma, and inflammatory processes, although this syndrome commonly occurs on an idiopathic basis (see Chapter 77).

Diagnostic imaging plays a minor role in the assessment of the carpal tunnel syndrome. Ultrasonography, CT, and MR imaging have been used for this purpose.[36, 38, 40, 77–80] The MR imaging findings of the carpal tunnel syndrome have been delineated in detail by Mesgarzadeh and coworkers,[81] who emphasize four consistent findings: swelling of the median nerve, best evaluated at the level of the pisiform bone; flattening of the median nerve, best evaluated at the level of the hamate bone; palmar bowing of the flexor retinaculum, best evaluated at the level of the hamate bone; and increased signal intensity of the median nerve on T2-weighted spin echo images (Fig. 70–41). The pattern of enlargement of the median nerve is variable, however; the nerve may be diffusely enlarged or focally enlarged, especially at the level of the pisiform bone.[80] Focal enlargement of the median nerve at this latter level may result in a nerve that is two to three times larger than at the level of the distal portion of the radius. Thus, careful assessment of the size of the median nerve on transaxial images, extending from the region of the distal radius to that of the pisiform bone, is required for accurate diagnosis and, indeed, the use of ratios of nerve size at various levels of the wrist may aid in this diagnosis.[15, 81] The ratio of the cross-sectional area of the median nerve at the pisiform level divided by that at the level of the distal radius is approximately 1 in normal persons, whereas in those with the carpal tunnel syndrome, this ratio may be greater than 2. As the median nerve may appear flattened at the level of the hamate bone in patients with the carpal tunnel syndrome, using this region as a site for measuring the cross-sectional area of the median nerve in ratio calculations may be diagnostically misleading. Although quantitative analysis of the size of the median nerve on MR images at various levels of the wrist is a complicated process and one not commonly employed in clinical practice, swelling of the median nerve at the level of the pisiform bone and compression of the median nerve at the level of the hamate bone can be judged qualitatively, and these remain important observations in diagnosis of the carpal tunnel syndrome. Similarly, increased signal intensity in the medial nerve on T2-weighted spin echo and gradient echo MR images is a valuable diagnostic sign which may be apparent at multiple levels of the wrist. Although such increased signal intensity may extend as far distally as the bases of the metacarpal bones, it rarely extends proximal to the distal radioulnar joint.[81]

Vascular events may be important in the pathogenesis of the carpal tunnel syndrome, suggesting a potential role for gadolinium-enhanced MR imaging in its diagnosis in some patients. In one study, intravenous administration of a gadolinium compound and positioning the wrist in neutral, flexed, and extended positions were employed during MR imaging of patients with the carpal tunnel syndrome.[1375]

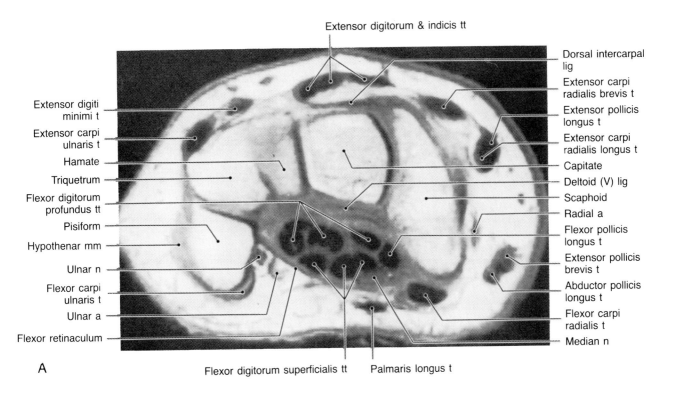

Extensor digitorum & indicis tt

Dorsal intercarpal lig

Extensor carpi radialis brevis t

Extensor pollicis longus t

Extensor carpi radialis longus t

Capitate

Deltoid (V) lig

Scaphoid

Radial a

Flexor pollicis longus t

Extensor pollicis brevis t

Abductor pollicis longus t

Flexor carpi radialis t

Median n

Extensor digiti minimi t

Extensor carpi ulnaris t

Hamate

Triquetrum

Flexor digitorum profundus tt

Pisiform

Hypothenar mm

Ulnar n

Flexor carpi ulnaris t

Ulnar a

Flexor retinaculum

A

Flexor digitorum superficialis tt Palmaris longus t

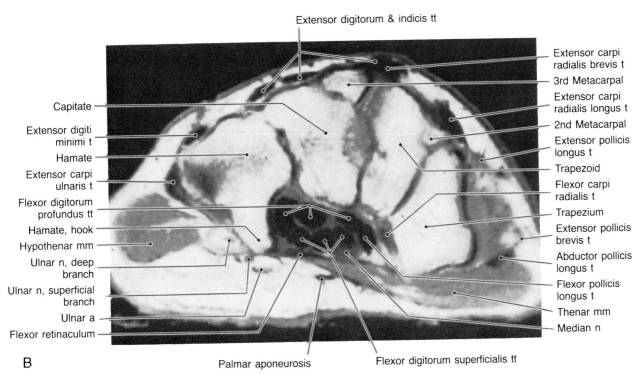

Extensor digitorum & indicis tt

Extensor carpi radialis brevis t

3rd Metacarpal

Extensor carpi radialis longus t

2nd Metacarpal

Extensor pollicis longus t

Trapezoid

Flexor carpi radialis t

Trapezium

Extensor pollicis brevis t

Abductor pollicis longus t

Flexor pollicis longus t

Thenar mm

Median n

Capitate

Extensor digiti minimi t

Hamate

Extensor carpi ulnaris t

Flexor digitorum profundus tt

Hamate, hook

Hypothenar mm

Ulnar n, deep branch

Ulnar n, superficial branch

Ulnar a

Flexor retinaculum

B

Palmar aponeurosis Flexor digitorum superficialis tt

FIGURE 70–40. Normal carpal tunnel: MR imaging.
A Transaxial T1-weighted (TR/TE, 600/20) MR image of the wrist at the level of the pisiform bone.
B Transaxial T1-weighted (TR/TE, 600/20) MR image of the wrist at the level of the hook of the hamate bone.
(From Kang HS, Resnick D: MRI of the Extremities: An Anatomic Atlas. Philadelphia, WB Saunders Co, 1991.)

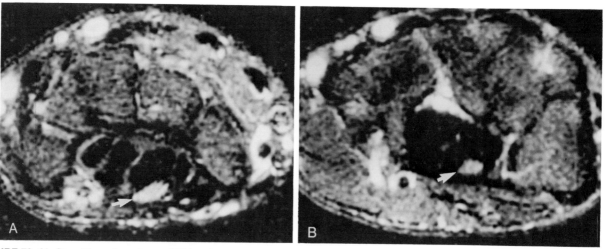

FIGURE 70–41. Carpal tunnel syndrome: MR imaging.
  A Transaxial T2-weighted (TR/TE, 3000/66) fat-suppressed fast spin echo MR image of the wrist at the level of the pisiform bone. Note the diffuse enlargement of and increased signal intensity in the median nerve (arrow).
  B Transaxial T2-weighted (TR/TE, 3000/66) fat-suppressed fast spin echo MR image of the wrist at the level of the hook of the hamate bone. Although the signal intensity in the median nerve (arrow) is increased, the nerve is smaller at this level than at the level of the pisiform bone.
  (Courtesy of M. Schweitzer, M.D., Philadelphia, Pennsylvania.)

Two distinctly abnormal patterns of enhancement of signal intensity in the median nerve were observed: marked enhancement attributed to nerve edema; and no enhancement attributed to nerve ischemia. The diagnostic value of these supplementary MR techniques requires further analysis.

Inflammation of the flexor tendon sheaths is considered an important and, perhaps, the most common cause of the carpal tunnel syndrome, based mainly on surgical findings. The MR imaging abnormalities of such tenosynovitis include enlargement of individual tendon sheaths owing to effusions and increased separation between adjacent tendons in the carpal tunnel, increased signal intensity resulting from fluid in the enlarged tendon sheaths, and volar bowing, or convexity, of the flexor retinaculum. The findings may be subtle, however, requiring comparison with the opposite uninvolved wrist and, in some cases, the intravenous administration of gadolinium compounds. Tenosynovitis resulting from rheumatoid arthritis, gout, calcium pyrophosphate dihydrate crystal deposition disease, and other systemic articular disorders generally leads to similar MR imaging findings, although additional bone and joint alterations may be evident. Regions of persistent low signal intensity within the carpal tunnel on T2-weighted spin echo and gradient echo MR images may be encountered in patients with gout or amyloidosis (primary or secondary to long-term hemodialysis). MR imaging findings accompanying some tumors in the carpal tunnel are diagnostic (Fig. 70–42).

The role of MR imaging in the evaluation of persistent or recurrent carpal tunnel syndrome following carpal tunnel release is not clear yet. Typically, such release, which may be done operatively or endoscopically, is accomplished by dividing the transverse carpal ligament (flexor retinaculum) near its ulnar insertion on the hook of the hamate. Following such surgery, incomplete visualization or palmar displacement of the transverse carpal ligament is evident, and the contents of the carpal tunnel also are displaced volarly.[81] Potential MR imaging findings associated with persistent or recurrent carpal tunnel syndrome following such surgery

are incomplete resection of the transverse carpal ligament, scar formation associated with low signal intensity about the incised flexor retinaculum, and persistent or recurrent flexor tenosynovitis.

As in other regions of the body, the differentiation of fluid, which may indicate significant inflammatory disease, and fat within the carpal tunnel on the basis of findings on standard MR imaging sequences may be difficult. Chemical presaturation of fat with or without prior intravenous injection of gadolinium compounds or STIR MR sequences may be useful in this differentiation.

Ulnar Tunnel Syndrome. Compression of the ulnar nerve as it traverses through the ulnar tunnel, or Guyon's canal, in the volar aspect of the wrist is well recognized (see Chapter 77). Causes of such entrapment include

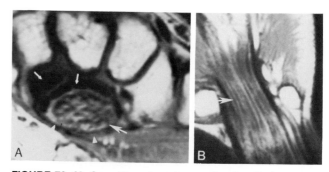

FIGURE 70–42. Carpal tunnel syndrome related to fibrolipomatous hamartoma of the median nerve: MR imaging.
  A Transaxial T1-weighted (TR/TE, 500/15) spin echo MR image of the wrist at the level of the base of the first metacarpal bone shows a large mass (large arrow) of the median nerve that has led to dorsal displacement of the flexor tendons (small arrows) and volar bowing of the flexor retinaculum (arrowheads). Note the inhomogeneous signal intensity of the tumor, resulting from its fibrous and fatty components.
  B Coronal T1-weighted (TR/TE, 500/15) spin echo MR image of the volar aspect of the wrist shows a mass (arrow) composed of longitudinally oriented cylindrical regions of low and high signal intensity.

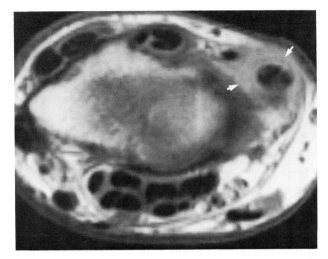

FIGURE 70–43. Tenosynovitis of the extensor carpi ulnaris tendon sheath: MR imaging. Transaxial T1-weighted (TR/TE, 600/20) MR image of the wrist at the level of the radiocarpal joint shows fluid of intermediate signal intensity (arrows) about the extensor carpi ulnaris tendon in the sixth extensor compartment. (Courtesy of S. K. Brahme, M.D., La Jolla, California.)

masses (e.g., tumors and ganglion cysts), vascular injury (e.g., aneurysms or thrombosis of the ulnar artery), anatomic variations (e.g., presence of abductor digiti minimi muscles within the canal), muscle hypertrophy (e.g., enlargement of the palmaris brevis muscle), fractures (e.g., fractures of the hook of the hamate bone or the pisiform bone), and hypertrophy of the transverse carpal ligament.[17] Although the MR imaging abnormalities associated with the ulnar tunnel syndrome are not well documented, findings similar to those of the carpal tunnel syndrome are likely.

Abnormalities of the Extensor and Flexor Tendons and Tendon Sheaths

Tendinitis and Tenosynovitis. Inflammation may affect either the extensor tendons and sheaths or the flexor tendons and sheaths, or both. De Quervain's syndrome relates to tendinitis and tenosynovitis affecting the abductor pollicis longus and extensor brevis tendons and sheaths in the first extensor compartment. Involvement occurs at the level

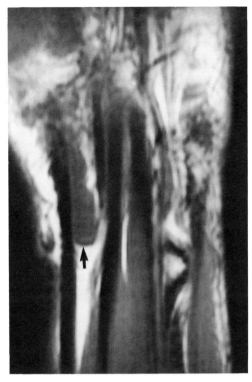

FIGURE 70–44. Tenosynovitis of the flexor carpi radialis tendon sheath: MR imaging. A coronal T1-weighted (TR/TE, 600/14) spin echo MR image of the volar aspect of the wrist shows the enlarged tendon sheath (arrow) containing fluid or inflammatory tissue.

of or just proximal to the styloid process of the radius. Similarly, involvement of the extensor carpi ulnaris tendon and sheath in the sixth extensor compartment at the level of the distal portion and styloid process of the ulna may be evident (Fig. 70–43). Inflammatory changes in the flexor tendons and sheaths in (or about) the carpal tunnel already have been noted (Fig. 70–44).

The MR imaging abnormalities of tendinitis and tenosynovitis include enlargement and increased signal intensity of the affected tendon and enlargement of its sheath owing to the accumulation of fluid (Fig. 70–45). Although the findings usually are quite apparent, misdiagnosis is possible owing to the magic angle phenomenon.[83, 84] This phenomenon results from variations in the T2 times of poorly hy-

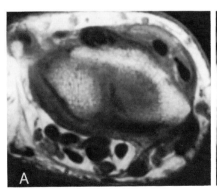
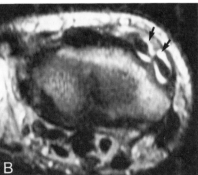
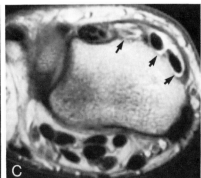

FIGURE 70–45. Tenosynovitis of the tendon sheaths of the extensor pollicis longus and the extensor carpi radialis brevis and longus tendons: MR imaging. Transaxial T1-weighted (TR/TE, 700/17) **(A)** and T2-weighted (TR/TE, 2000/80) **(B)** spin echo MR images and a transaxial T1-weighted (TR/TE, 650/20) spin echo MR image following the intravenous administration of gadolinium compound **(C)** show the enlarged tendon sheaths. The high signal intensity (arrows) in **B** and **C** is consistent with the presence of synovial inflammatory tissue.

drated tissues such as tendons related to their orientation with the magnetic field. T2 augmentation of tendons (and other structures) is maximum at the magic angle, in which the tendon orientation is 55 degrees with respect to the orientation of the main magnetic field, and such augmentation decreases proportionately with orientation angles that are greater or less than 55 degrees. The resulting increased signal intensity within the tendon is evident only when short (e.g., 10 to 25 msec) echo times (TE) are employed, and it is not apparent when the tendon is parallel to the main magnetic field. Portions of the extensor tendons of the wrist (as well as the tendons about the shoulder and ankle) are oriented at or close to the magic angle.[84] Thus, increased signal intensity within such tendons on short TE MR imaging sequences (i.e., routine T1-weighted and proton density spin echo sequences) should not be misinterpreted as evidence of tendinitis or tendon degeneration. The magic angle effect disappears on long TE MR imaging sequences (i.e., T2-weighted spin echo sequences).

Tendon Rupture. Any of the extensor or flexor tendons of the wrist, as well as those of the fingers, can rupture as a response to an acute injury or chronic inflammation as in rheumatoid arthritis. Interruption of the tendon and surrounding fluid or inflammatory tissue are the findings noted on MR images.

Giant Cell Tumor of Tendon Sheath. As indicated in Chapter 95, giant cell tumors of soft tissue may arise from tendon sheaths (as well as joint capsules and ligamentous tissue). Although they may be observed about the wrist, they are far more frequent in the fingers. Soft tissue swelling or a mass with or without erosion of the subjacent bone and without calcification is evident. The relationship of giant cell tumors of the tendon sheath to diffuse or localized (pigmented) villonodular or nodular synovitis is not clear (see Chapter 95), although they may contain hemosiderin deposits. Owing to the presence of hemosiderin deposition or dense acellular fibrous tissue, low signal intensity within the lesion on both T1- and T2-weighted spin echo MR images may be seen (Fig. 70–46). This pattern, however, is not invariable, and regions of high signal intensity on T2-weighted spin echo MR images are encountered.[1376]

Abnormalities of the Joint Synovium and Capsule

Ganglion Cysts. Ganglion cysts about the wrist are common, although their precise cause is debated (see Chapter 95). Most commonly, ganglion cysts appear on the dorsum of the wrist, although they also occur volarly and in other locations. The site of origin may be the joint capsule, tendon, or tendon sheath. Ganglion cysts contain fluid that may be slightly more viscous than joint fluid. They rarely calcify. A soft tissue mass is evident on radiographic examination. Anechoic oval, round, or lobulated cystic masses are seen with ultrasonography.[1377] Arthrography (see Chapter 13) occasionally reveals communication between the opacified joint and the cyst (Fig. 70–47). Similarly, tenography may reveal communication between the opacified tendon sheath and the ganglion cyst. Low to intermediate signal intensity on T1-weighted spin echo MR images and high signal intensity on T2-weighted spin echo MR images within the ganglion cyst are typical (Fig. 70–48).

Adhesive Capsulitis. Adhesive capsulitis is encountered most frequently in the shoulder, although involvement of the ankle, hip, and wrist also is seen (see Chapter 13). Physical or neurologic injury are two potential causes of this condition. Restricted joint capacity with extravasation of contrast material is evident during arthrography (Fig. 70–49). MR imaging of adhesive capsulitis is not rewarding unless intra-articular administration of gadolinium (MR arthrography) is employed.

Articular Diseases. MR imaging has been used to assess the extent of rheumatoid arthritis and other synovial inflammatory diseases in the wrist (and in other locations) (see Chapters 25 and 26). Its advantages when compared with routine radiography include more accurate assessment of cartilage and bone destruction, the extent of synovial inflammation, and the activity of the disease process (Fig. 70–50). Marginal and central bone erosions and subchondral cystic lesions can be identified, owing to the tomographic nature of the study and to the high signal intensity of synovial fluid and inflammatory tissue on the T2-

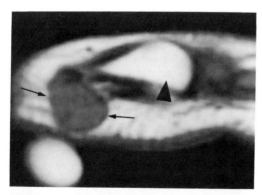

FIGURE 70–46. Giant cell tumor of a tendon sheath: MR imaging. A sagittal T1-weighted (TR/TE, 500/14) spin echo MR image of the fifth finger reveals a mass (arrows) of low signal intensity in the volar soft tissues beneath the diaphysis of the proximal phalanx (arrowhead). It remained of low signal intensity in T2-weighted spin echo MR images and at surgery represented a giant cell tumor of the tendon sheath. (Courtesy of G. Greenway, M.D., Dallas, Texas.)

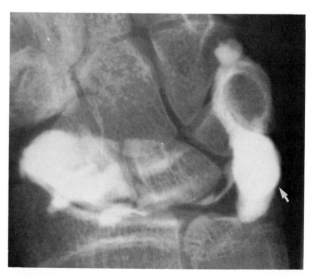

FIGURE 70–47. Ganglion cysts: Arthrography. A radiocarpal joint arthrogram reveals normal opacification of the pisiform-triquetral joint and filling of a proximal ganglion cyst (arrow).

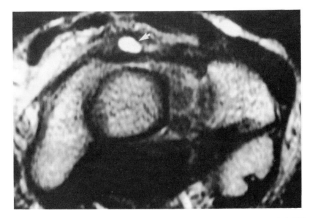

FIGURE 70–48. Ganglion cysts: MR imaging. A transaxial T2-weighted (TR/TE, 2000/80) spin echo MR image of the wrist at the level of the midcarpal joint shows a small ganglion cyst (arrow) just superficial to the dorsal intercarpal ligament and deep to the extensor tendons. (Courtesy of A. G. Bergman, M.D., Stanford, California.)

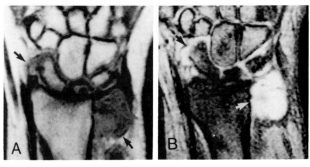

FIGURE 70–50. Rheumatoid arthritis: MR imaging.

A A coronal T1-weighted (TR/TE, 600/25) spin echo MR image shows abnormal synovial tissue and fluid in the distal radioulnar joint and radial aspect of the radiocarpal joint (arrows). Note erosions of the scaphoid, lunate, and triquetral bones.

B A coronal MPGR MR image (TR/TE, 500/15; flip angle, 30 degrees) shows regions (arrows) of high signal intensity, corresponding to sites of abnormal synovial tissue and fluid, and changes in signal intensity in the lunate and triquetrum.

(Courtesy of W. Glenn, M.D., Long Beach, California.)

weighted spin echo and gradient echo MR images. Differentiation between such fluid and synovial pannus is difficult on the basis of findings derived from standard MR imaging sequences. The use of intravenously injected gadolinium compounds has been emphasized; enhancement of signal intensity within inflamed synovial tissue allows its differentiation from joint fluid (which does not show such enhancement) on T1-weighted spin echo MR images obtained immediately after the injection of gadolinium (see Chapter 25). Owing to leakage of gadolinium into the joint fluid, delayed MR images following intravenous administration

of gadolinium are not useful in this differentiation. In a similar fashion, routine or gadolinium-enhanced MR imaging can be used to evaluate the extent of tendon sheath involvement in rheumatoid arthritis and other synovial inflammatory diseases. As enhancement of signal intensity in synovial tissue following the intravenous administration of gadolinium generally implies active inflammation, this technique may be beneficial in monitoring the therapeutic response of the disease.

The diagnosis of pigmented villonodular synovitis and idiopathic synovial (osteo)chondromatosis (Fig. 70–51) can be established effectively with MR imaging (see Chapter 95).

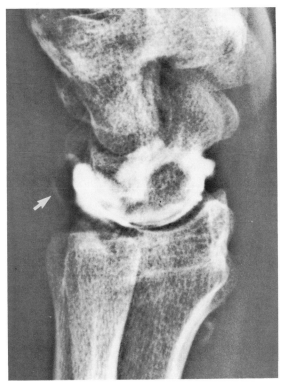

FIGURE 70–49. Adhesive capsulitis: Arthrography. Note the restricted capacity of the opacified radiocarpal joint and the visualization of periarticular lymphatic channels (arrow). (Courtesy of E. C. Hanson, M.D., Loma Linda, California.)

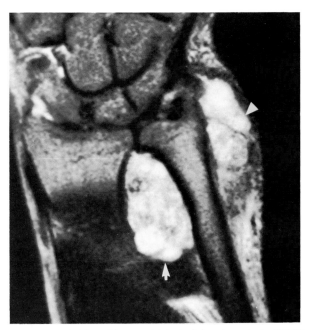

FIGURE 70–51. Idiopathic synovial (osteo)chondromatosis: MR imaging. A coronal T2-weighted (TR/TE, 1800/80) spin echo MR image reveals cartilage nodules of high signal intensity in the distal radioulnar joint (arrow) and about the outer surface of the ulna (arrowhead). Regions of low signal intensity represent foci of calcification or ossification.

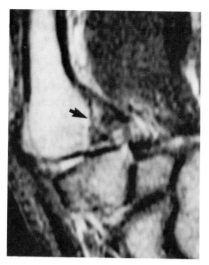

FIGURE 70–52. Bennett's fracture of the first metacarpal bone: MR imaging. A coronal T2-weighted (TR/TE, 2000/80) spin echo MR image shows a fracture (arrow) in the ulnar portion of the base of the first metacarpal bone, associated with radial displacement of the remaining portion of the bone and an effusion in the first carpometacarpal joint.

Other Abnormalities

Occult Bone Injuries. The utilization of MR imaging to evaluate occult bone injuries is discussed in Chapter 67. Such injuries include acute infractions and chronic stress fractures. Although most reported data related to this use of MR imaging are based on studies of occult bone injuries about the knee and hip, a similar role exists for MR imaging in cases of wrist and hand fractures (Fig. 70–52). Occult fractures of the distal portion of the radius in elderly persons and of scaphoid fractures in young adults are two examples of injuries that can be detected with MR imaging. The sensitivity of the MR imaging examination in this regard is at least equal and probably superior to that of bone scintigraphy, and a negative MR imaging examination virtually excludes the presence of a fracture. Bone scintigraphy, however, still represents an effective sensitive

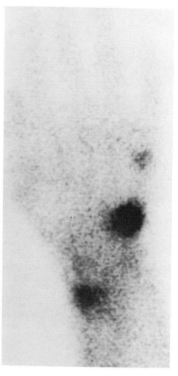

FIGURE 70–53. Occult fractures of the hand and wrist: Bone scintigraphy. In this elderly patient who had fallen, note increased accumulation of the radionuclide at sites of fracture in the distal radius, hamate bone, and fifth metacarpal bone.

method for the diagnosis of occult bone injuries (Fig. 70–53), and CT is both sensitive and specific (Fig. 70–54).

Gamekeeper's Thumb. Owing to the importance of injury to the ulnar collateral ligament of the metacarpophalangeal joint of the thumb and to the potential role of MR imaging in its diagnosis, a short discussion of this condition is included here (also see Chapter 68). Classically described in English game wardens and hence known as gamekeeper's thumb, tears of the ulnar collateral ligament of the first metacarpophalangeal joint remain common, accounting for

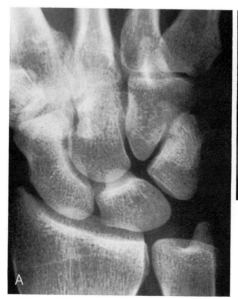

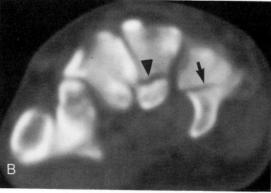

FIGURE 70–54. Occult fractures of the hand and wrist: CT scanning. In this 39 year old woman who fell from a horse, routine radiographs **(A)** were interpreted as normal. A transaxial CT scan **(B)** shows a fracture of the hook of the hamate bone (arrow) and the volar surface of the capitate bone (arrowhead). (Courtesy of G. Greenway, M.D., Dallas, Texas.)

approximately 6 per cent of all skiing injuries.[85] The injury results from violent abduction of the thumb. When disrupted, the torn end of the ulnar collateral ligament can become displaced superficial to the adductor pollicis aponeurosis, a finding known as the Stener lesion[86] (Fig. 70–55). The interposed aponeourosis interferes with healing, and surgery has been advocated for the treatment of displaced tears of the ulnar collateral ligament. Occasionally, displacement of this ligament can be inferred from the presence of an avulsed bone fragment. The absence of bone avulsion, however, does not eliminate the possibility of a Stener lesion.

Arthrography of the first metacarpophalangeal joint has been employed in the assessment of gamekeeper's thumb.[87–89] Arthrographic findings of this injury include extravasation of contrast material along the ulnar aspect of the joint. A filling defect has been described, representing the Stener lesion, produced by interposition of the dorsal

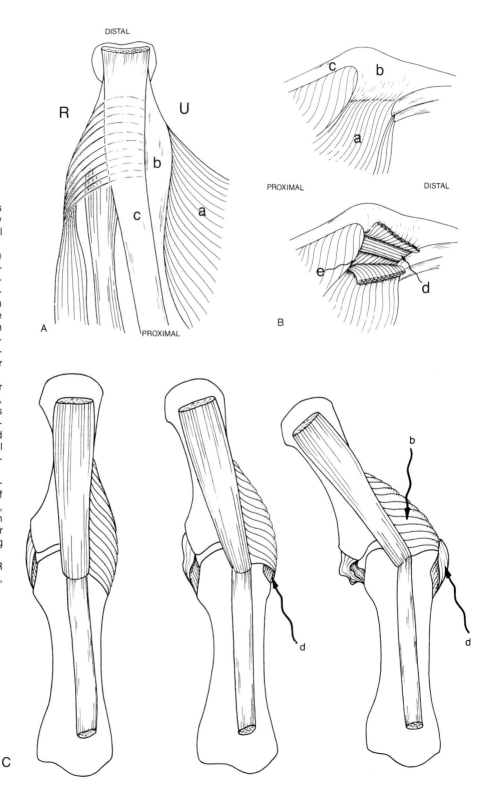

FIGURE 70–55. Gamekeeper's thumb: Mechanism of injury. Anatomy of ligaments of metacarpophalangeal joint of thumb.

A Dorsal aspect showing radial (R) and ulnar (U) sides of metacarpophalangeal joint. Tendon of extensor pollicis longus (c) passes over the metacarpophalangeal joint, running from proximal to distal aspect of digit. The adductor pollicis (a) inserts in part on the proximal phalanx, some of its fibers fusing with a portion of the dorsal aponeurosis, termed the adductor aponeurosis (b).

B Ulnar aspect showing adductor pollicis (a), adductor aponeurosis (b), and tendon of the extensor pollicis longus (c). In lower drawing, the adductor pollicis has been incised and opened, exposing the ulnar collateral (d) and accessory collateral (e) ligaments.

C Dorsal aspect of first metacarpophalangeal joint following rupture of ulnar collateral ligament. With time, torn ligament (d) can protrude from the proximal edge of the adductor aponeurosis (b), the latter preventing its return.

(From Resnick D, Danzig LA: AJR 126:1046, 1976. Copyright 1976, American Roentgen Ray Society.)

aponeurosis between the torn ligament and its phalangeal attachment, although the sensitivity of this arthrographic finding is not clear.

MR imaging can be employed successfully for the identification of the Stener lesion.[90] On coronal MR images of the first metacarpophalangeal joint, the normal ulnar collateral ligament appears as a band of low signal intensity medial to the joint (Fig. 70–56A). The adductor aponeurosis often is visible as a paper-thin band of low signal intensity superficial to the ulnar collateral ligament and extending from the distal half of the ulnar collateral ligament over the base of the proximal phalanx. A nondisplaced tear of the ulnar collateral ligament appears as discontinuity of the ligament distally, without ligamentous retraction and with the adductor aponeurosis covering the distal end of the ulnar collateral ligament (Fig. 70–56B). Displacement of the ulnar collateral ligament, or the Stener lesion, is associated with proximal retraction or folding of the ligament. The proximal margin of the adductor aponeurosis may be seen to abut the folded ulnar collateral ligament, creating a rounded region of low signal intensity designated a "yo-yo on a string" appearance (Fig. 70–56C).[90]

ELBOW

The articulation about the elbow has three constituents: (1) humeroradial—the area between the capitulum of the humerus and the facet on the radial head; (2) humeroulnar—the area between the trochlea of the humerus and the trochlear notch of the ulna; and (3) superior (proximal) radioulnar—the area between the head of the radius and radial notch of the ulna and the annular ligament.

Although the superior or proximal radioulnar area generally is considered a separate articulation, it is convenient to discuss all three areas of the elbow region together.

Osseous Anatomy

The osseous structures about the elbow include the proximal end of the ulna and radius and the distal end of the humerus (Figs. 70–57 and 70–58).

The proximal end of the ulna contains two processes, the olecranon and the coronoid. The olecranon process is smooth posteriorly at the site of attachment of the triceps tendon. Its anterior surface provides the site of attachment of the capsule of the elbow joint. The coronoid process contains the radial notch, below which is the ulnar tuberosity.

The proximal end of the radius consists of head, neck, and tuberosity. The radial head is disc-shaped, containing a shallow, cupped articular surface, which is intimate with the capitulum of the humerus. The articular circumference of the head is largest medially, where it articulates with the radial notch of the ulna. The radial neck is the smooth, constricted part of the bone below the radial head. The radial tuberosity is located beneath the medial aspect of the neck.

The distal aspect of the humerus is a wide, flattened structure. The medial third of its articular surface, termed the trochlea, is intimate with the ulna. Lateral to the trochlea is the capitulum, which articulates with the radius. The sulcus is between the trochlea and the capitulum. A hollow area is found on the posterior surface of the humerus above the trochlea, termed the olecranon fossa; the posterior capsular attachment of the humerus is located above this fossa. A smaller fossa, the coronoid fossa, lies above the trochlea on the anterior surface of the humerus, and a radial fossa lies adjacent to it, above the capitulum. The anterior capsular attachment to the humerus is located above these fossae. When the elbow is fully extended, the tip of the olecranon process is located in the olecranon fossa, and when the elbow is flexed, the coronoid process of the ulna is found in the coronoid fossa and the margin of the radial head is located in the radial fossa.

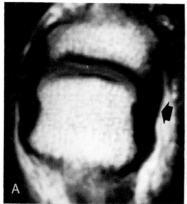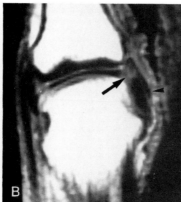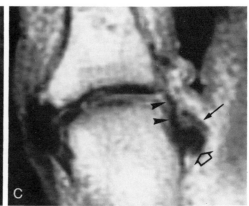

FIGURE 70–56. Gamekeeper's thumb: MR imaging.

  A Normal appearance of the ulnar collateral ligament. A coronal T1-weighted (TR/TE, 500/20) spin echo MR image of the first metacarpophalangeal joint shows the normal ulnar collateral ligament (arrow) as a band of low signal intensity. The adductor aponeurosis is not visible.

  B Nondisplaced tear of the ulnar collateral ligament. A coronal T1-weighted (TR/TE, 500/20) spin echo MR image of the first metacarpophalangeal joint shows disruption of the ulnar collateral ligament (arrow) and a superficial curvilinear structure of low signal intensity (arrowhead), representing the adductor aponeurosis.

  C Displaced tear of the ulnar collateral ligament (Stener lesion). A coronal T1-weighted (TR/TE, 500/20) spin echo MR image of the first metacarpophalangeal joint reveals a yo-yo appearance. The adductor pollicis aponeurosis (arrowheads) looks like a string holding a yo-yo, the balled up, displaced ulnar collateral ligament (open arrow). The thin region of low signal intensity (solid arrow) represents an avulsed bone fragment.

  (From Spaeth HJ, et al: Radiology 188:553, 1993.)

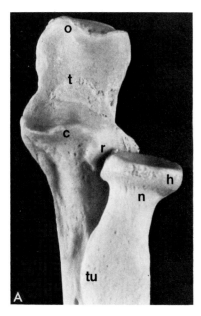

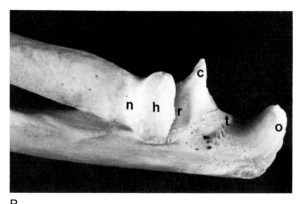

FIGURE 70–57. Elbow joint: Osseous anatomy. Radius and ulna.
A Radius and ulna, anterior aspect. Note the olecranon (o), coronoid process (c), trochlear notch (t), radial notch (r), radial head (h), radial neck (n), and radial tuberosity (tu).
B Radius and ulna, lateral aspect.

The medial epicondyle is a blunt osseous projection of the distal humerus. The posterior smooth surface of this epicondyle is crossed by the ulnar nerve. The anterior surface of the medial epicondyle is the site of attachment of superficial flexor muscles of the forearm. The lateral epicondyle is located on the lateral surface of the distal humerus. Its lateral and anterior surface represents the site of origin of the superficial group of extensor muscles of the forearm.

The degree of congruity of apposing articulating surfaces of radius, ulna, and humerus varies in different positions of the elbow joint; the greatest congruity exists when the forearm is in a position midway between full supination and full pronation and the elbow is flexed to a right angle. When the elbow is extended, the inferior and posterior aspects of the trochlea contact the ulna; when the elbow is flexed, the trochlear notch slides forward on the anterior aspect of the ulna, exposing the posterior aspect of that bone. The capitulum and the radial head are reciprocally curved; in a midprone position, extensive contact occurs between radius and capitulum.

Articular Anatomy

The articular surface of the humerus consists of a grooved trochlea, the spheroidal capitulum, and a sulcus between them (Fig. 70–59). It is covered with a continuous layer of articular cartilage. The ulnar articulating surface is the trochlear notch. This notch is covered with cartilage, which is interrupted in a transverse fashion across its deepest aspect. The trochlear notch of the ulna and the trochlea of the humerus articulate. The radial articulating area is the radial head, which is covered with articular cartilage. This cartilage is continuous with that along the sides of the radial head including an area in the superior radioulnar articulation. The radial head articulates with the capitulum and the capitulotrochlear groove.

A fibrous capsule completely invests the elbow. The attachments of its broad, thin, and weak anterior part are the anterior humerus along the medial epicondyle and above the coronoid and radial fossae, the anterior surface of the

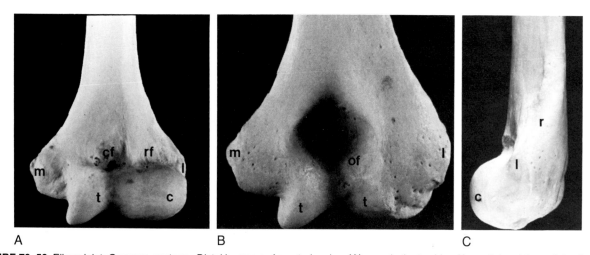

FIGURE 70–58. Elbow joint: Osseous anatomy. Distal humerus. An anterior view **(A)** reveals the trochlea (t), capitulum (c), medial epicondyle (m), lateral epicondyle (l), coronoid fossa (cf), and radial fossa (rf). A posterior view **(B)**, oriented in the same fashion, outlines some of the same structures and, in addition, the olecranon fossa (of). In a view of the lateral surface of the humerus **(C)**, observe the capitulum (c), lateral epicondyle (l), and lateral supracondylar ridge (r).

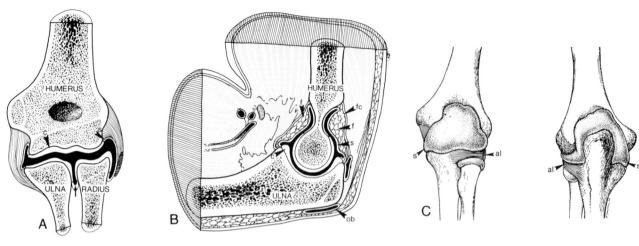

FIGURE 70–59. Elbow joint: Articular anatomy.

A, B Drawings of coronal **(A)** and sagittal **(B)** sections. Observe synovium (s), articular cartilage (c), fibrous capsule (fc), anterior and posterior fat pads (f), and olecranon bursa (ob). Note the extension of the elbow joint between radius and ulna as the superior radioulnar joint (arrow).

C A drawing of the anterior (left) and posterior (right) aspects of the distended elbow joint with the fibrous capsule removed. Observe the synovial membrane (s) and the annular ligament (al) extending around the proximal radius, constricting the joint cavity.

(From Warwick R, Williams P [Eds]. Gray's Anatomy. 15th British edition. Philadelphia, WB Saunders Co, 1973.)

ulnar coronoid process, and the annular ligament. The superior attachments of its thin, weak posterior part are the posterior surface of the humerus behind the capitulum, the olecranon fossa, and the medial epicondyle. Inferomedially the capsule is attached to the upper and lateral margins of the olecranon. Laterally the capsule is continuous with that about the superior radioulnar joint. The fibrous capsule is strengthened at the sides of the articulation by the radial and ulnar collateral ligaments.

The synovial membrane of the elbow lines the deep surface of the fibrous capsule and annular ligament. It extends from the articular surface of the humerus and contacts the olecranon, radial, and coronoid fossae and the medial surface of the trochlea. A synovial fold projects into the joint between the radius and ulna, partially dividing the articulation into humeroulnar and humeroradial portions.

There are several fat pads located between fibrous capsule and synovial membrane (Fig. 70–60). Fat pads are located near the synovial fold between the radius and ulna, and over the olecranon, coronoid, and radial fossae. These fat pads are extrasynovial but intracapsular. On lateral radiographs, an anterior radiolucent area represents the summation of radial and coronoid fossae fat pads. These fat pads are pressed into their respective fossae by the brachialis muscle during extension of the elbow. A posterior radiolucent region represents the olecranon fossa fat pad. It is pressed into this fossa by the triceps muscle during flexion of the elbow. The anterior fat pad normally assumes a teardrop configuration anterior to the distal humerus on lateral radiographs of the elbow exposed in approximately 90 degrees of joint flexion. The posterior fat pad normally is not visible in radiographs of the elbow exposed in flexion. Its occasional appearance on such radiographs may reflect unusually large fat pads or slightly oblique projections. Any intra-articular process that is associated with a mass or fluid may produce a ''positive fat-pad sign'' characterized by elevation and displacement of anterior and posterior fat pads.

The superior radioulnar joint exists between the radial

head and the osseous-fibrous ring formed by the annular ligament and the radial notch of the ulna. This notch is lined with articular cartilage that is continuous with that on the lower part of the trochlear notch. The radial head also is covered with cartilage. The annular ligament is attached anteriorly to the anterior margin of the radial notch. It encircles the head of the radius, and posteriorly it contains several bands that attach to the ulna near the posterior

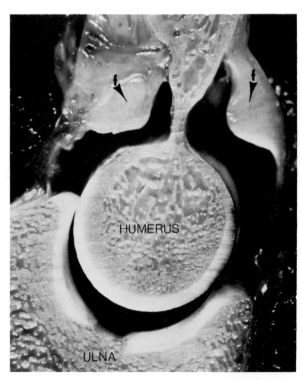

FIGURE 70–60. Elbow joint: Anatomy of intracapsular fat pads. A sagittal section of the elbow in a cadaver after distention of the joint with air reveals the elevated anterior and posterior fat pads (f).

margin of the radial notch. The superior portion of the annular ligament is lined with fibrocartilage where it apposes the circumference of the radial head. The inferior portion of the annular ligament is covered with synovial membrane, which extends downward onto the radial neck. The quadrate ligament, a thin, fibrous layer, covers the synovial membrane.

Along the posterior aspect of the elbow, a subcutaneous bursa, the olecranon bursa, separates the skin from the ulnar olecranon (Fig. 70–61). It is situated like a cap on the olecranon process.

Ligamentous Anatomy

Radial and ulnar collateral ligaments reinforce the fibrous capsule of the elbow[91] (Fig. 70–62). The radial collateral ligament is a thick, roughly triangular band of fibrous tissue that attaches superiorly to the lateral epicondyle of the humerus, beneath the common origin of the extensor muscles, and inferiorly to the radial notch of the ulna and the annular ligament. The ulnar collateral ligament is composed of three distinct bands that are continuous with each other. The anterior band extends from the anterior aspect of the medial epicondyle of the humerus to the medial edge of the coronoid process; a posterior band passes from the posterior aspect of the medial epicondyle to the medial edge of the olecranon; a thin intermediate band extends from the medial epicondyle to merge via a transverse or oblique band (the ligament of Cooper) with the anterior and posterior bands on the coronoid process and the olecranon.

As noted earlier, the annular ligament is a thick band of fibrous tissue that attaches to the anterior and posterior

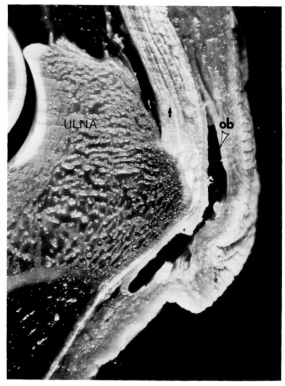

FIGURE 70–61. Olecranon bursa. A sagittal section through the ulna demonstrates the synovium-lined olecranon bursa (ob) between the skin and ulnar olecranon. Note the triceps tendon (t).

margins of the radial notch of the ulna. It serves as a restraining ligament, preventing withdrawal or inferior displacement of the head of the radius from its socket.

Anatomy of Muscles and Tendons

It is convenient to divide the many muscles about the elbow into four groups: posterior group, anterior group, lateral group, and medial group.[92, 93] (Fig. 70–63). The muscles of the posterior group are the triceps and the anconeus. The triceps consists of three muscle bellies: the long head of the triceps muscle arises by a strong tendon from the infraglenoid tubercle of the scapula near the inferior margin of the glenoid cavity, and it descends into the arm between the teres major and teres minor muscles; the lateral head of the triceps muscle originates from the posterior and lateral surfaces of the humerus and from the lateral intermuscular septum; and the medial head of the triceps muscle arises from the posterior surface of the humerus, medial and below the radial groove, and from the medial and lower part of the lateral intermuscular septum. After receiving the muscular fibers, the tendon of the triceps muscle descends to attach to the upper surface of the olecranon process of the ulna and to the antebrachial fascia near the anconeus muscle and tendon. The anconeus muscle is small and triangular, arising from a tendon on the posterior surface of the lateral epicondyle of the humerus. It descends toward the ulna, covering the posterior aspect of the annular ligament and attaching to the lateral surface of the olecranon process and upper posterior surface of the shaft of the ulna.

The muscles of the anterior group are the biceps brachii and brachialis. The biceps brachii muscle typically consists of two heads, the short head and the long head, although in approximately 10 per cent of persons an additional head or multiple additional heads also are evident. The short head of the biceps brachii muscle arises from the tip of the coracoid process, in common with the coracobrachialis, and the long head of the biceps brachii muscle arises from the supraglenoid tubercle of the scapula and extends through the glenohumeral joint into the intertubercular groove of the humerus (see later discussion). The two major muscle bellies of the biceps join to form a common tendon approximately 6 or 7 cm above the elbow, which attaches to the posterior aspect of the radial tuberosity. An aponeurosis (i.e., bicipital aponeurosis) arises from the tendon, passes across the brachial artery, and terminates in the fascia that overlies the origin of the flexor muscles of the forearm. The brachialis muscle originates mainly from the anterior aspect of the lower portion of the humerus, descends across the elbow joint, and inserts as a tendon into the tuberosity and anterior surface of the coronoid process of the ulna.

The lateral group of muscles includes the supinator and brachioradialis muscles and the extensor muscles of the wrist and hand (i.e., extensor carpi radialis longus, extensor carpi radialis brevis, extensor digitorum, extensor digiti minimi, and extensor carpi ulnaris muscles). The brachioradialis muscle is superficially located, arising from the lateral supracondylar ridge of the humerus and the anterior surface of the lateral intermuscular septum. After extending below the elbow, this muscle ends as a tendon that is attached to the lateral aspect of the distal portion of the radius, just above the styloid process. The extensor carpi radialis longus muscle is deep to the brachioradialis muscle,

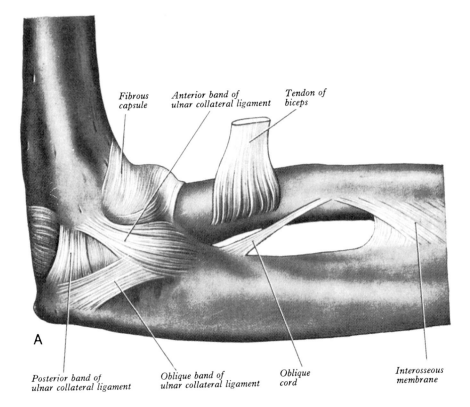

A

Fibrous capsule

Anterior band of ulnar collateral ligament

Tendon of biceps

Posterior band of ulnar collateral ligament

Oblique band of ulnar collateral ligament

Oblique cord

Interosseous membrane

FIGURE 70–62. Elbow joint: Ligamentous anatomy.
  A Medial aspect of the elbow.
  B Lateral aspect of the elbow.
  (From Williams PL, Warwick R [Eds]: Gray's Anatomy. 36th British edition. Edinburgh, Churchill Livingstone, 1980, p 431.)

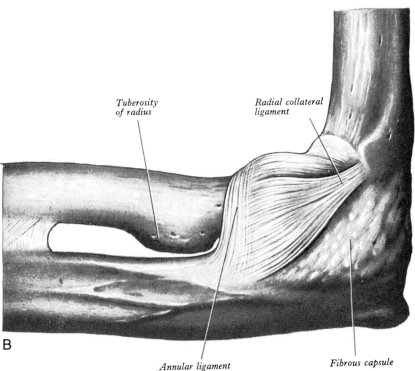

B

Tuberosity of radius

Radial collateral ligament

Annular ligament

Fibrous capsule

also arising from the lateral supracondylar ridge of the humerus and lateral intermuscular septum. Its tendon commences at the distal one third of the shaft of the radius where it is located laterally, passes beneath the extensor retinaculum, and terminates by attaching to the dorsoradial surface of the base of the second metacarpal bone. At the level of the elbow, the extensor carpi radialis brevis, extensor digitorum, extensor digiti minimi, and extensor carpi ulnaris muscles all appear as a single mass. The supinator is the deepest muscle in the lateral group, originating from the lateral epicondyle of the humerus, from the supinator crest of the ulna, and from the radial collateral and annular ligaments of the elbow and superior radioulnar joint. It courses inferiorly, wrapping about the proximal portion of the radius and inserting on the proximal aspect of the diaphysis of the radius.

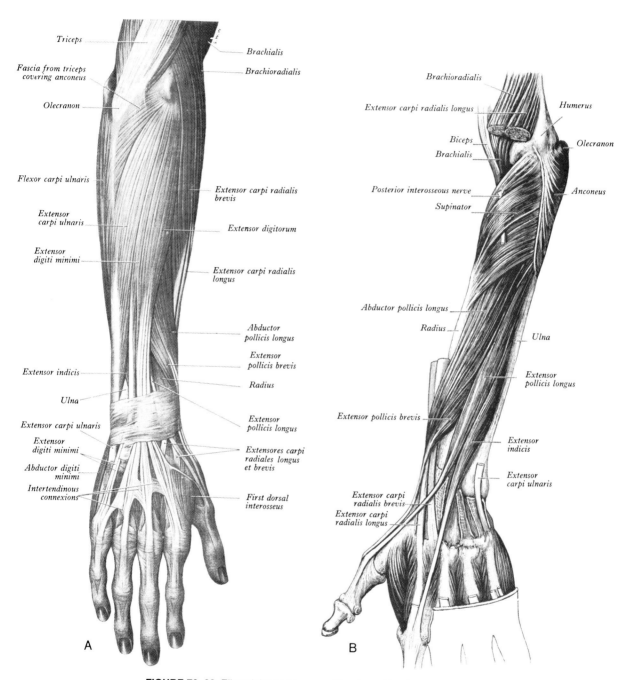

FIGURE 70–63. Elbow joint and forearm: Muscle and tendon anatomy.
A Superficial muscles of the extensor aspect of the forearm.
B Deep muscles of the extensor aspect of the forearm.

Illustration continued on following page

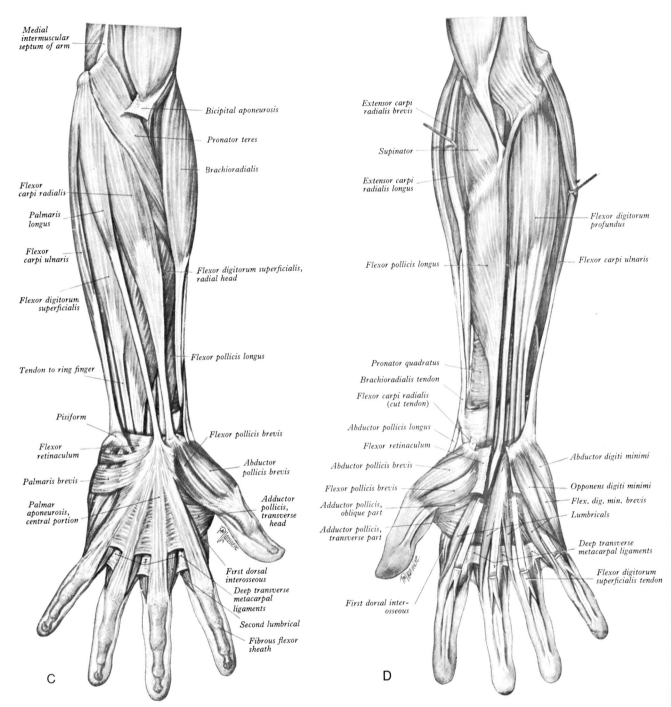

FIGURE 70–63 *Continued*
C Superficial muscles of the flexor aspect of the forearm.
D Deep muscles of the flexor aspect of the forearm.
(From Williams PL, Warwick R [Eds]: Gray's Anatomy. 36th British edition. Edinburgh, Churchill Livingstone, 1980, pp 574, 576, 580, 581.)

The medial group of muscles includes the pronator teres, the palmaris longus, and the flexors of the hand and wrist (flexor carpi radialis, flexor digitorum superficialis, flexor carpi ulnaris, flexor digitorum profundus, and flexor pollicis longus). The most superficial of these muscles is the pronator teres. It has origins from the humerus just above the medial epicondyle (the humeral head) and the medial side of the coronoid process (the ulnar head). The median nerve enters the forearm between these two parts of the muscle and is separated from the ulnar artery by the ulnar head of the muscle. After passing across the forearm, the muscle ends in a tendon that is attached to the lateral aspect of the radial shaft. The other muscles all arise from the common flexor tendon, which also gives rise to a portion of the humeral head of the pronator teres muscle, and these other muscles are arranged from anterior to posterior as the flexor carpi radialis, the palmaris longus, the flexor carpi ulnaris, and the flexor digitorum superficialis. They extend distally, attaching as tendons to various bones in the wrist (i.e., carpus) and hand. The flexor digitorum profundus muscle arises from the upper portion of the anterior and medial surfaces of the ulna, the coronoid process, and the interosseous membrane, and it ends as four tendons that attach to the index, third, fourth, and fifth fingers. The flexor pollicis longus muscle arises from the anterior surface of the radius, near its tuberosity, and the interosseous membrane and, after passing distally, attaches to the palmar surface of the base of the distal phalanx of the thumb.

Anatomy of Vessels and Nerves

The major artery about the elbow is the brachial artery, which extends superficial to the brachialis muscle and medial to the biceps muscle and tendon. Approximately 1 to 2 cm distal to the elbow joint, it divides into the radial and ulnar arteries. The radial artery descends further between the brachioradialis and pronator teres muscles, and the larger ulnar artery crosses obliquely below the cubital fossa under the pronator teres and flexor muscles. Recurrent branches of the radial and ulnar arteries form a network of vessels about the elbow joint.

Three major nerves exist in the elbow region. The median nerve parallels the course of the brachial artery, courses anterior to it in the cubital area, and descends further between the superficial and deep heads of the pronator teres muscle. The ulnar nerve is present on the posteromedial side of the elbow and passes in a groove between the olecranon process of the ulna and the medial epicondyle of the humerus. The radial nerve descends above the elbow between the brachialis and the brachioradialis muscles and divides near the elbow into deep and superficial branches.

Tendinous, Ligamentous, and Muscle Abnormalities

Although uncommon, avulsions (and tears) of tendons about the elbow are encountered. Avulsion at sites of tendinous attachment may occur as a complication of systemic diseases such as primary and secondary hyperparathyroidism, systemic lupus erythematosus, rheumatoid arthritis, and osteogenesis imperfecta,[93, 94] or as a consequence of physical injury.[95–98] The tendons of the biceps brachii and the triceps are involved most commonly. Routine radiographic features of such avulsions include a joint effusion and bone fragmentation and displacement (see Chapter 68). Although other imaging methods such as CT and ultrasonography may be used to delineate tendinous injuries,[99] MR imaging appears most suitable to this task.[100]

Normal tendons about the elbow (and elsewhere) appear as smooth, linear structures of low signal intensity on MR imaging sequences. A magic angle phenomenon, however, occasionally leads to regions of intermediate signal intensity within the tendons when MR sequences using short echo times (TE) are employed (see previous discussion). Tendinous tears and avulsion are associated with irregular and frayed contours and alterations in signal intensity of the tendons (Figs. 70–64 to 70–66). The extent of abnormality relates to the severity of the injury (i.e., complete or partial tears). Complete tears are accompanied by discontinuity and retraction of the tendon, and partial tears are accompanied by some remaining intact tendinous fibers. Alterations in signal intensity depend on the age of the injury, although high signal intensity within the tendon itself and the adjacent soft tissues and bone commonly is present on T2-weighted spin echo MR images. Obliteration of nearby fat planes and local hematomas also are seen. With healing, scar formation develops in the injured tendon that may lead to regions of low to intermediate signal intensity, even on T2-weighted spin echo images.

Although rupture of the distal portion of the tendon of the biceps brachii muscle is rare, constituting less than 5 per cent of all biceps tendon injuries, it represents an important injury about the elbow. The typical mechanism of injury relates to forceful hyperextension applied to a flexed and supinated forearm. Complete rupture, with avulsion of the tendinous attachment to the radial tuberosity, generally occurs in men after 40 years of age and in the dominant extremity. Local pain and swelling, a palpable defect about the elbow, and a proximal lump related to the retracted muscle allow accurate clinical diagnosis. Accurate diagnosis is more difficult in cases of complete tears without such retraction and of partial tears of the tendon. In these cases, MR imaging may be useful for diagnosis.[1378, 1379] The transaxial plane is particularly important in this diagnosis. Findings include absence of the tendon distally, a fluid-filled tendon sheath, a mass in the antecubital fossa, and muscle edema or atrophy in cases of complete rupture; and high signal intensity within the tendon, fluid in the tendon sheath, and thinning or thickening of the distal tendon in cases of partial tears.[1379]

Chronic overuse syndromes such as tennis elbow also can lead to tendinous alterations. Clinical and imaging abnormalities predominate on the lateral side of the joint, in the region of the humeral epicondyle and capitulum. Rarely, similar abnormalities are detected in the medial side of the elbow joint (Fig. 70–67). Although the type of pathologic lesion associated with chronic overuse syndromes of the elbow varies, partial tearing of fibers within the extensor tendons (and, less commonly, the flexor tendons) from their epicondylar attachments is typical. Periostitis and soft tissue edema are associated findings. Regions of high signal intensity on T2-weighted spin echo images in the tendon, the soft tissue, and the bone may be evident. Increased signal intensity in the anconeous muscle also has been seen in association with tennis elbow, affecting the lateral epicondyle of the humerus.[1366]

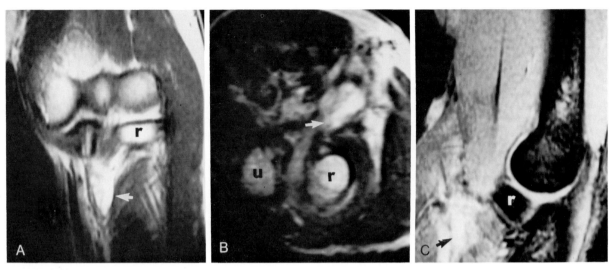

FIGURE 70–64. Biceps brachii tendon: Tears.

A, B Acute partial avulsive injury in a 78 year old man. Coronal T2-weighted (TR/TE, 2000/70) spin echo MR image **(A)** shows fluid of high signal intensity (arrow) adjacent to the radial tuberosity. The head of the radius (r) is indicated. A transaxial T2-weighted (TR/TE, 2000/80) spin echo MR image **(B)** shows a region of high signal intensity (arrow) anterior to the neck of the radius (r). The ulna (u) also is indicated.

C Acute complete avulsive injury in a 48 year old man. A sagittal MPGR MR image (TR/TE, 500/15; flip angle, 30 degrees) shows regions of high signal intensity (arrow) anterior to the notch of the radius (r). The tendon is retracted, and a prominence of the biceps muscle in the anterior portion of the upper arm is seen. (**C** Courtesy of S. K. Brahme, M.D., La Jolla, California.)

Ligament disruptions about the elbow can accompany severe physical trauma (e.g., elbow dislocation) or occur as a response to less extensive acute trauma (e.g., valgus injury) or chronic stress (e.g., pitching a baseball). Injuries to the ulnar (or medial) collateral ligament predominate.[101] The ulnar collateral ligament is the primary structure in the maintenance of elbow stability in the presence of valgus stress, although other structures such as the adjacent flexor musculature, joint capsule, and articular surfaces contribute to this stability. The anterior band of the ulnar collateral ligament is functionally the most important.[102] Experimental transection of the ulnar collateral ligament results in severe

instability when valgus stress is applied to the elbow.[102, 103] In the athlete involved in throwing a ball or javelin, valgus stress applied to the partially flexed elbow can lead to microtears of fibers, hemorrhage and edema in the ulnar collateral ligament, and eventually, to ligamentous disruption and detachment.[104] Associated injuries in these athletes are abnormalities of the annular ligament and triceps tendon which, in combination with the alterations of the ulnar collateral ligament, are evident only in the dominant extremity. Clinical findings include pain and tenderness in the medial aspect of the elbow, symptoms of ulnar nerve compression, and increased valgus angulation at the elbow elic-

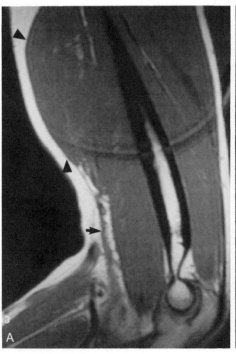

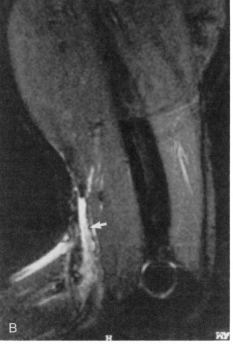

FIGURE 70–65. Biceps brachii tendon: Tears. Complete rupture in a 41 year old man who noted a popping sensation while lifting a heavy weight.

A A sagittal T1-weighted (TR/TE, 570/15) spin echo MR image shows a corkscrew-like appearance of the biceps brachii tendon (arrow). Note the retracted muscle (arrowheads). A wraparound artifact relates to patient positioning for the MR imaging examination.

B A sagittal STIR MR image (TR/TE, 6200/22; inversion time, 150 msec) shows the abnormal biceps brachii tendon (arrow).

(Courtesy of C. Wakeley, M.D., Bristol, England.)

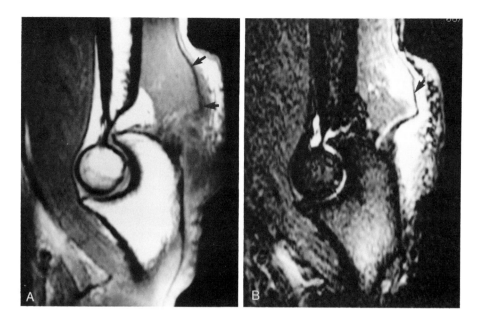

FIGURE 70–66. Triceps tendon: Tears. Acute complete avulsive injury in a 51 year old man. Sagittal T1-weighted (TR/TE, 800/20) **(A)** and T2-weighted (TR/TE, 2500/80) **(B)** MR images show tendon laxity (arrows), disorganization at the ulnar site of attachment, and muscle retraction. Note regions of high signal intensity in **B**.

ited with valgus stress exerted on a partially flexed joint.[105] Additional diagnostic information is provided by radiography obtained during application of stress to the elbow (i.e., increased valgus displacement)[1380] (Fig. 70–68), arthrography (i.e., medial extravasation after intra-articular injection of contrast material),[106] and MR imaging.[100, 104] The MR imaging abnormalities of an acutely or chronically injured ulnar collateral ligament (or other ligaments about the elbow) are laxity, irregularity, poor definition, and increased signal intensity within and around the ligament.[104] The regions of increased signal intensity, which are most prominent on T2-weighted spin echo and gradient echo coronal MR images, reflect the presence of hemorrhage and edema (Fig. 70–69).

Complications of ligamentous disruptions about the elbow depend on their cause. In cases of elbow dislocation, such complications include chronic instability with recurrent dislocations, associated fractures, intra-articular bodies, stretching of the annular ligament, and entrapment of the brachial artery and median nerve. In children, entrapment of the medial epicondyle of the humerus may result from an elbow dislocation.

Muscle injuries about the elbow are seen (Fig. 70–70),

especially in professional athletes. These are discussed in Chapter 67.

Nerve Abnormalities

Entrapment and compression neuropathies about the elbow may involve the ulnar, radial, or median nerve, as discussed in Chapter 77. Those involving the ulnar nerve are the most common. Entrapment of the ulnar nerve in the fibro-osseous tunnel posterior to the medial epicondyle of the humerus results in the cubital tunnel syndrome. Typical causes of this syndrome are injury and progressive cubitus valgus deformity (tardy ulnar nerve palsy), although additional causes include osteoarthritis, rheumatoid arthritis, nerve subluxation, prolonged bedrest, anomalous muscles, masses, and trochlear hypoplasia.[107–110] Clinical manifestations include weakness of the flexor carpi ulnaris muscle, flexor digitorum profundus muscle of the fourth and fifth fingers, and intrinsic hand muscles. The nerve may be enlarged and tender to palpatation.

Although axial radiographs may reveal narrowing of the cubital tunnel related, in part, to osteophytosis,[111] MR imaging represents a far more elegant means to evaluate this

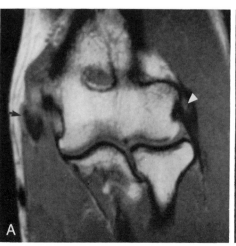
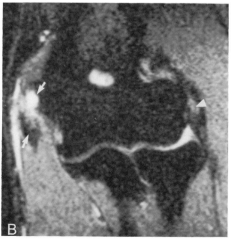

FIGURE 70–67. Flexor tendons: Tears. Acute avulsive injury of the common flexor tendons. A coronal T1-weighted (TR/TE, 600/30) spin echo MR image **(A)** shows avulsion of the flexor tendons (arrow) from the medial epicondyle of the humerus. Abnormal signal intensity also is evident in the common extensor tendons (arrowhead). A coronal STIR MR image **(B)** reveals high signal intensity at the site of flexor tendon avulsion (arrows), altered signal intensity in the common extensor tendons (arrowhead), and a joint effusion. (Courtesy of C. Ho, M.D., Palo Alto, California.)

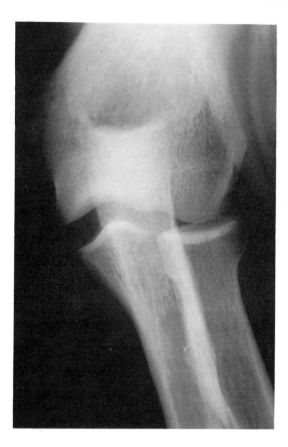

FIGURE 70–68. Ulnar collateral ligament: Tears. Radiograph obtained during the application of valgus stress to a partially flexed elbow reveals widening of the medial side of the joint, indicative of injury to the ulnar collateral ligament.

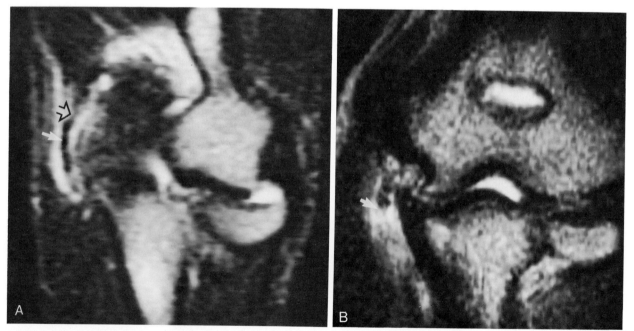

FIGURE 70–69. Ulnar collateral ligament: Tears.
 A In a baseball pitcher with an ulnar collateral ligament injury, a coronal T2-weighted (TR/TE, 2500/80) spin echo MR image shows an ill-defined ulnar collateral ligament, with increased signal intensity, indicating fluid surrounding its margins, particularly medially (solid arrow). In addition, a focus of abnormal increased signal intensity is present within the substance of the proximal portion of the ligament (open arrow).
 B In a second patient, a complete rupture of the ulnar collateral ligament is manifest in a coronal T2-weighted (TR/TE, 2250/80) spin echo MR image as thickening and proximal retraction of the ligament (arrow). Increased signal intensity surrounding the ulnar collateral ligament is indicative of hemorrhage and edema.
 (From Mirowitz SA, et al: Radiology *185:*573, 1992.)

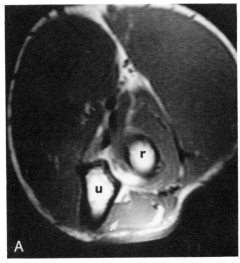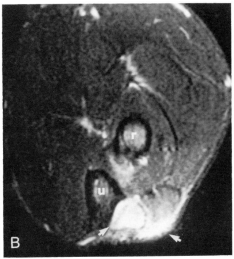

FIGURE 70–70. Muscle injury: Tear with edema of the anconeus muscle in a 30 year old male body builder who developed acute pain during weightlifting. Transaxial T1-weighted (TR/TE, 500/12) **(A)** and T2-weighted (TR/TE, 4000/68) **(B)** spin echo MR images, the latter obtained with chemical presaturation of fat (ChemSat), show altered morphology, and in **B**, increased signal intensity in the anconeus muscle and surrounding tissues (arrows). Inflammatory changes in the biceps tendon also are evident. The radius (r) and ulna (u) are indicated. (Courtesy of C. Sebrechts, M.D., San Diego, California.)

syndrome.[112] MR imaging abnormalities include displacement or shift of the ulnar nerve, a soft tissue mass, and enlargement and increased signal intensity in the compressed nerve (Fig. 70–71). Ulnar nerve enlargement may be focal, occurring at the level of the cubital tunnel, with a normal girth noted proximal and distal to the tunnel.[112]

Entrapment of a portion of the radial nerve may occur just distal to the elbow where the posterior interosseous, or deep, branch passes into the supinator muscle. Causes of this syndrome (supinator syndrome) include elbow dislocations, fractures, rheumatoid arthritis, soft tissue tumors, and traumatic or developmental fibrous bands.[113, 114] The affected patient may be unable to partially or completely extend the fingers at the metacarpophalangeal joints. Deep pain in the posterior portion or dorsum of the forearm, gradual fist weakness, and local pain on compression distal to the lateral humeral epicondyle may simulate the clinical

manifestations of tennis elbow.[112] Median nerve entrapment near the elbow may result from compression by the ligament of Struthers, extending distally from a supracondylar process; hypertrophy of the pronator teres muscle or fibrous bands leading to compression of the nerve in the antecubital area where the nerve passes between the two heads of the pronator teres muscle and then under the edge of the flexor digitorum sublimis muscle (pronator syndrome); and compression of the anterior interosseous nerve (Kiloh-Nevin syndrome), the motor branch of the ulnar nerve (see Chapter 77). MR imaging in cases of radial or median nerve compression may reveal a mass (e.g., lipoma or ganglion cyst), and displacement and abnormal signal intensity within the affected nerve.[112]

Bone Abnormalities

Osteochondral Fractures and Osteochondritis Dissecans. As indicated in Chapter 67, the development and refinement of MR imaging have led to the identification of a number of occult injuries of subchondral bone and cartilage that may escape detection on routine radiographic analysis. Such injuries, which have been investigated most completely about the knee, include trabecular microfractures (bone bruises) and osteochondral fractures. They result from impaction and shearing forces applied to the articular surfaces, and they are manifest on MR images as irregularity of the chondral coat, fracture lines, and marrow edema. The last of these findings results in increased signal intensity on T2-weighted spin echo, gradient echo, and STIR imaging sequences.

Osteochondritis dissecans about the elbow usually affects the capitulum (see Chapter 67). This disorder differs from a developmental alteration of the capitular ossification center known as Panner's disease (see Chapter 81). The precise relationship of osteochondritis dissecans of the capitulum and an osteochondral fracture is not clear, but most investigators regard the former condition as a posttraumatic abnormality that may lead to osteonecrosis. In common with osteochondritis dissecans at other sites, such as the femoral condyles, MR imaging of osteochondritis dissecans of the capitulum (Fig. 70–72) may be used to gain information regarding the integrity of the adjacent articular cartilage,

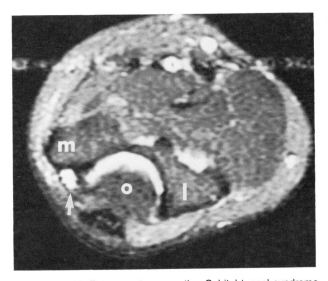

FIGURE 70–71. Entrapment neuropathy: Cubital tunnel syndrome. A transaxial T2-weighted (TR/TE, 2000/70) spin echo MR image, accomplished with chemical presaturation of fat (ChemSat) shows increased signal intensity in the ulnar nerve (arrow) within the cubital tunnel. The medial (m) and lateral (l) epicondyles of the humerus and the olecranon process (o) of the ulna are indicated. A joint effusion is present. (Courtesy of S. K. Brahme, M.D., La Jolla, California.)

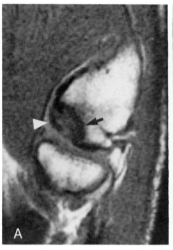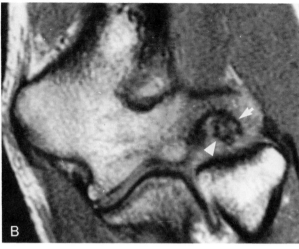

FIGURE 70–72. Osteochondritis dissecans: Capitulum of the humerus in a 16 year old boy.

A A sagittal T1-weighted (TR/TE, 600/20) spin echo MR image shows the concave defect (arrow) of the capitulum containing an ossified body (arrowhead).

B A coronal proton density–weighted (TR/TE, 2000/20) spin echo MR image shows the osseous defect (arrow) containing an ossified body (arrowhead). The integrity of the adjacent articular cartilage cannot be determined.

(Courtesy of M. Schweitzer, M.D., Philadelphia, Pennsylvania.)

the viability of the separated fragment, and the presence or absence of associated intra-articular osseous and cartilaginous bodies.[100] The presence of joint fluid or granulation tissue at the interface between the fragment and the parent bone, manifest as increased signal intensity on T2-weighted spin echo MR images, generally indicates an unstable lesion. Direct visualization of the articular cartilage with standard MR imaging sequences, however, remains problematic, and MR arthrography employing the intra-articular injection of gadolinium compounds may be advantageous (see later discussion). Injected gadolinium is of increased signal intensity on T1-weighted spin echo MR images and may be identified on the surface of the articular cartilage, within defects in the articular cartilage, and in the interface between the osteochondral fragment and subjacent bone. Conventional and computed arthrotomography both provide similar information. With these tomographic techniques, as well as with MR imaging, the extent of bone involvement becomes apparent. Sagittal, coronal, and transaxial images, readily obtained with MR imaging, allow full assessment of the osseous abnormalities.

Chondroepiphyseal Injuries. Accurate radiographic diagnosis of injuries of the elbow in young children is difficult, owing to the large number of developing ossification centers, the normal irregularities of bone in these centers, and the cartilaginous components of these centers that are not visible on routine radiographs. Differentiation among the many types of Salter-Harris type lesions of the growth plate (e.g., type II and type IV injuries of the distal portion of the humerus) may be impossible when standard radiography alone is employed (see Chapter 67). As such differentiation has prognostic implications and may guide the orthopedic surgeon in his or her choice of therapy (i.e., closed reduction versus open reduction and fixation), a diagnostic role for other imaging methods such as arthrography and MR may exist.[115–117] Arthrography using radiopaque contrast material, perhaps combined with conventional tomography or CT, results in coating of the articular surfaces of the distal portion of the humerus and proximal portions of the radius and ulna. Interruption of the articular surface and opacification of fracture lines in the chondroepiphysis are important arthrographic findings, allowing accurate assessment of the extent of injury. Spin echo or gradient echo MR images provide direct visualization of the cartilaginous and osseous components of the chondroepiphyses about the elbow. Physeal separation and violation, fractures, and edema readily are detectable on such images (see Chapter 67).[1423]

Synovial Abnormalities

Synovial Proliferation. Synovial proliferation in the elbow may accompany a variety of disease processes, including rheumatoid arthritis, septic arthritis, crystal deposition disorders, pigmented villonodular synovitis, and idiopathic synovial osteochondromatosis. The accumulation of joint fluid leads to characteristic displacements of the anterior and posterior intracapsular, extrasynovial fat pads of the elbow, which can be recognized with routine radiography, CT, and MR imaging (Fig. 70–73). The finding lacks specificity, indicating only the presence of an effusion, synovial inflammation, or an intra-articular mass, or a combination of these findings. With MR imaging, a joint effusion, best seen in the sagittal plane, is of high signal intensity on T2-weighted spin echo and certain gradient echo MR images.

Rheumatoid arthritis and other synovial inflammatory disorders affecting the elbow lead to proliferation of the synovial membrane and accumulation of joint fluid. The signal intensity characteristics of the abnormal synovium and fluid are similar on standard MR imaging sequences. Intravenous administration of gadolinium compounds leads to enhancement of the signal intensity of the inflammatory tissue and it does not affect the signal intensity of fluid on MR images obtained immediately after the injection.

Pigmented villonodular synovitis may involve the elbow, leading initially to an effusion and subsequently to osteoporosis and even joint space loss and bone erosions. Although the diagnosis may be suggested on the basis of appropriate clinical history and typical radiographic abnormalities, the deposition of hemosiderin in the affected synovial tissue produces regions of persistent low signal intensity on spin echo and, especially, gradient echo MR images. This finding also may be observed in cases of chronic hemarthrosis, hemophilia, synovial hemangioma, and other conditions.

Idiopathic synovial osteochondromatosis, related to metaplasia of the synovial lining, is accompanied by syno-

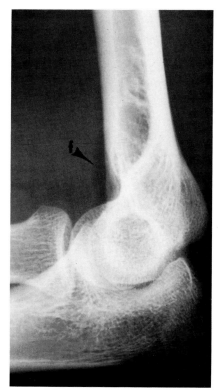
A

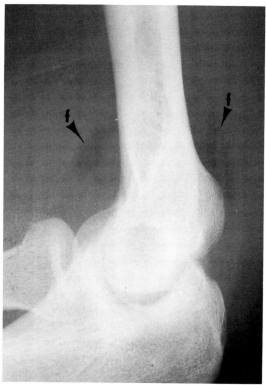
B

FIGURE 70–73. Joint effusion: Routine radiograph and MR imaging.

A On a radiograph of the normal elbow flexed to approximately 90 degrees, the anterior fat pad (f) assumes a teardrop configuration and the posterior fat pad is not visible.

B With a joint effusion, both fat pads (f) are elevated. The anterior fat pad assumes a "sail" configuration, whereas the posterior fat pad becomes visible.

C A sagittal T2-weighted (TR/TE, 2000/80) spin echo MR image shows fluid in the anterior and posterior portions of the joint.

(**C**, Courtesy of S. Fernandez, M.D., Mexico City, Mexico.)

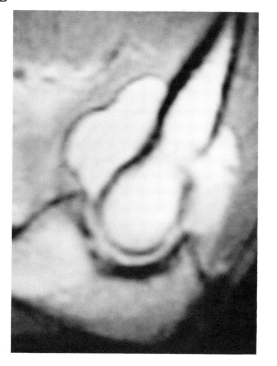
C

vial proliferation and the formation of intrasynovial nodules of cartilage. The fate of these nodules is variable, although they may calcify or ossify, or they may become free within the joint cavity and later become embedded in a distant synovial site. Routine radiography is sensitive to the detection of calcified and ossified intra-articular bodies but insensitive to the detection of nonossified bodies. Arthrography, in which the bodies appear as multiple filling defects within the opacified joint (Fig. 70–74), and MR imaging can be helpful diagnostically. The appearance of idiopathic synovial osteochondromatosis on MR images is dependent on the composition of the cartilage nodules and, specifically, the degree of calcification and ossification. In the absence of such calcification or ossification, the nodules have signal intensity similar to that of fluid; when calcified or ossified, the nodules reveal regions of low signal intensity.

Bursitis. Synovial inflammation and fluid accumulation in the olecranon bursa are seen in rheumatoid arthritis, septic bursitis, and gout and other crystal deposition diseases, and following injury. The diagnosis of olecranon bursitis generally is apparent on physical examination. Imaging methods such as ultrasonography, bursography, and

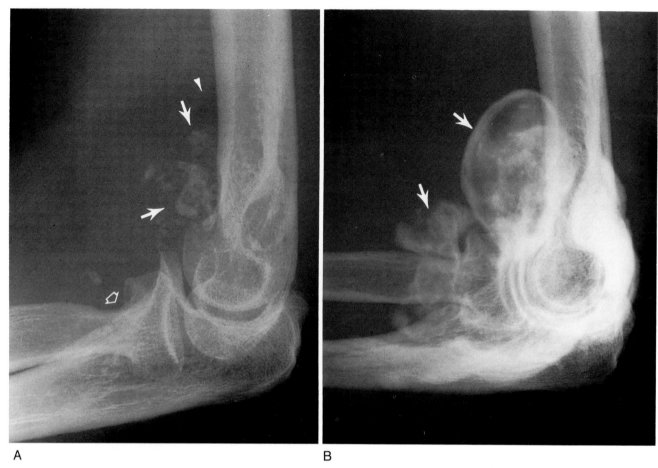

A   B

FIGURE 70–74. Idiopathic synovial osteochondromatosis. This 67 year old woman developed progressive pain and swelling in the elbow over a 6 month period. The radiograph **(A)** outlines irregular ossification in the joint (solid arrows) with displacement of the anterior fat pad (arrowhead) and minor osseous erosion (open arrow) and osteophytes. The arthrogram **(B)** allows identification of multiple radiolucent filling defects (arrows). The diagnosis was confirmed histologically.

MR imaging can be employed in patients with olecranon bursitis but rarely are necessary. A sympathetic effusion in the elbow joint may accompany this condition. In rheumatoid arthritis, subcutaneous nodules may simulate the appearance of olecranon bursitis.

Synovial Cysts. Para-articular synovial cysts that communicate with the elbow joint are a recognized manifestation of rheumatoid arthritis,[118–121] but theoretically, they could occur with any process leading to elevation of intra-articular pressure in the elbow. As in the knee (see later discussion), a valvelike mechanism may exist between the synovial cyst and the elbow joint. Such cysts predominate in the antecubital region,[119] although synovial cysts posterior to the joint also may be evident.[121] Arthrography, cystography, ultrasonography, CT, and MR imaging are all effective in establishing the diagnosis and determining if there is rupture of the contents of the cyst.

Intra-Articular Osteocartilaginous Bodies. Any process leading to disintegration of the articular surface of the elbow joint may be responsible for intra-articular osteocartilaginous bodies, although trauma remains the most important cause. In common with intra-articular bodies in other locations, bodies originating from the joint surface may be composed of cartilage alone, cartilage and bone together, or rarely bone alone, and they may remain at their site of origin, become partially detached or completely free and, if

free, migrate about the joint to become embedded in a distant synovial site. Free bodies in the elbow joint commonly migrate to dependent portions of the joint and to sites of normal depressions in bone, particularly the olecranon fossa. In this last location, intra-articular bodies may prevent full extension of the joint. Once detected, they may be removed arthroscopically.[122, 123]

Calcified bodies in the elbow joint can be detected by routine radiography; however, those that lodge in the olecranon fossa may be overlooked unless conventional tomography or CT is employed. Noncalcified bodies are more difficult to detect. Such detection requires arthrography, conventional arthrotomography, computed arthrotomography (Fig. 70–75), or MR imaging. Of these techniques, computed arthrotomography often is preferred. With computed arthrotomography, purely cartilaginous bodies are manifest as radiodense regions that simulate hypertrophied synovial tissue, creating some diagnostic difficulty. MR imaging is relatively insensitive to the diagnosis of small calcified bodies, as the signal void of these bodies is overlooked easily. Furthermore, small noncalcified cartilaginous bodies are characterized by high signal intensity on T2-weighted spin echo images similar to the signal intensity of joint fluid. MR arthrography (Fig. 70–76) may be useful in the detection of small calcified or noncalcified bodies. Large calcified bodies, owing to the presence of prominent

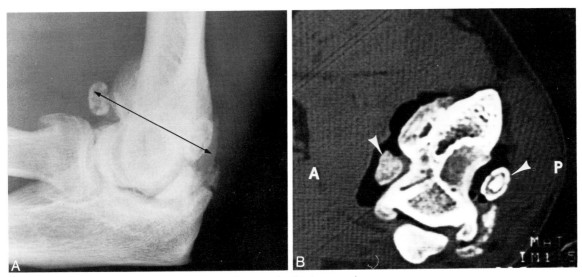

FIGURE 70–75. Intra-articular osteocartilaginous bodies: Computed arthrotomography.
 A The initial radiograph reveals multiple osseous bodies both in front of and behind the distal portion of the humerus.
 B Following the introduction of 10 ml of air, a transaxial CT scan at the approximate level indicated in **A** confirms the intra-articular location of several of the bodies (arrowheads). A, Anterior, P, posterior.

foci of low signal intensity, and large ossified bodies, owing to the presence of bone marrow within them, are detected more easily with MR imaging. Whatever technique is employed, careful inspection of the coronoid, radial, and olecranon fossae of the distal portion of the humerus often is fruitful in the search for intra-articular bodies. In such cases, an inspection of other joint surfaces occasionally will uncover a likely site of origin of these bodies.

SHOULDER

Osseous Anatomy

Glenohumeral Joint. The glenohumeral joint lies between the roughly hemispheric head of the humerus and the

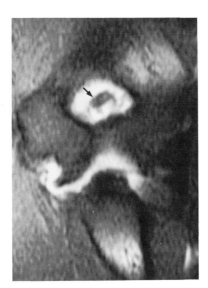

FIGURE 70–76. Intra-articular osteocartilaginous bodies: MR arthrography. A coronal T1-weighted (TR/TE, 950/13) spin echo MR image, obtained following the intra-articular injection of a gadolinium compound and with chemical presaturation of fat (ChemSat), shows a body (arrow) in the olecranon fossa.

shallow cavity of the glenoid region of the scapula. Stability of this articulation is limited, for two reasons: the scapular "socket" is small compared to the size of the adjacent humeral head, so that apposing osseous surfaces provide little inherent stability; the joint capsule is quite redundant, providing little additional support. Stability of the glenohumeral joint is supplied by surrounding structures (see later discussion).

The upper end of the humerus consists of the head and the greater and lesser tuberosities (tubercles) (Fig. 70–77). With the arm at the side of the body, the humeral head is directed medially, upward, and slightly backward to contact the glenoid cavity of the scapula. The head is inclined 130 to 150 degrees with respect to the humeral shaft and has an average retrotorsion angle of 20 to 30 degrees.[124] Beneath the head is the anatomic neck of the humerus, a slightly constricted area that encircles the bone, separating the head from the tuberosities. The anatomic neck is the site of attachment of the capsular ligament of the glenohumeral joint. The greater tuberosity is located on the lateral aspect of the proximal humerus. The tendons of the supraspinatus and infraspinatus muscles insert on its superior portion, whereas the tendon of the teres minor muscle inserts on its posterior aspect. The lesser tuberosity is located on the anterior portion of the proximal humerus, immediately below the anatomic neck. The subscapularis tendon attaches to the medial aspect of this structure. Between the greater and lesser tuberosities is located the intertubercular sulcus or groove (bicipital groove) through which passes the tendon of the long head of the biceps brachii muscle, surrounded by a synovial sheath and fixed by a transverse ligament extending between the tuberosities.[125] The bicipital groove is 30 degrees medial to a line passing from the shaft through the center of the humeral head.[124] The rough lateral lip of the groove is the site of attachment of the tendon of the pectoralis major muscle; the floor of the groove gives rise to the attachment of the tendon of the latissimus dorsi muscle; the medial lip of the groove is the site of attachment of the tendon of the teres major muscle.

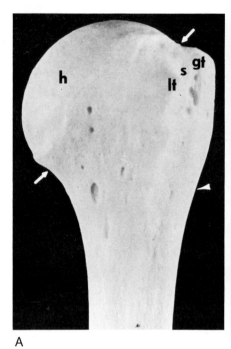

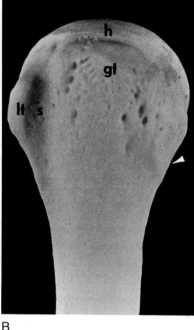

A   B

FIGURE 70–77. Proximal portion of the humerus: Osseous anatomy.

A Anterior aspect, external rotation. Observe the articular surface of the humeral head (h), greater tuberosity (gt), lesser tuberosity (lt), intertubercular sulcus (s), anatomic neck (arrows), and surgical neck (arrowhead).

B Anterior aspect, internal rotation. The same structures as in **A** are indicated. The lesser tuberosity is seen in profile on the medial aspect of the humeral head and the greater tuberosity is seen en face.

The shallow glenoid cavity is located on the lateral margin of the scapula (Fig. 70–78). Although there is variation in the osseous depth of the glenoid region,[126] a fibrocartilaginous labrum encircles and slightly deepens the glenoid cavity.[127] The glenoid contour may be almost flat or slightly curved, or it may possess a deep, socket-like appearance. The average vertical dimension of the glenoid cavity is 35 mm, and the transverse diameter is 25 mm.[124] The glenoid cavity may be either anteverted or retroverted with respect to the plane of the scapula; retroversion (which averages about 7 degrees) is more common than anteversion (which varies from 2 to 10 degrees).[126, 128] Retroversion of the glenoid cavity has been associated with osteoarthritis of the glenohumeral joint.[129] The curvature of the glenoid cavity may be smaller or larger than or identical to the curvature of the humeral head.[124] A supraglenoid tubercle is located above the glenoid cavity, to which is attached the tendon of the long head of the biceps brachii muscle. Below the cavity is a thickened ridge of bone, the infraglenoid tubercle, which is a site of attachment for the tendon of the long head of the triceps muscle.

The width of the glenohumeral joint surface at the central portion of the glenoid, as defined on radiographs, generally is less than 6 mm.[130] The subacromial space, defined as the distance between the head of the humerus and the inferior aspect of the acromion, in adults is approximately 9 or 10 mm; a measurement less than 6 mm in a middle-aged person suggests rotator cuff atrophy or tear.[131]

Acromioclavicular Joint. The lateral or acromial end of the clavicle is a flattened structure with a small, oval articular facet that faces laterally and slightly downward (Fig. 70–79). This facet articulates with the acromial facet of the scapula and is the site of attachment of the joint capsule of the acromioclavicular joint. The inferior surface of the acromial end of the clavicle possesses a rough osseous ridge, termed the trapezoid line. A conoid tubercle is located at the posterior aspect of the lateral clavicle. The trapezoid line and conoid tubercle are the sites of attachment of the trapezoid and conoid parts of the coracoclavicular ligament.

The acromion is a forward protuberance of the lateral aspect of the scapula (Fig. 70–80). An articular facet, the acromial facet, is located on the medial border of the acromion and is small and oval in size and configuration, directed medially and superiorly.

A joint may be noted between the clavicle and coracoid process in 0.1 to 1.2 per cent of people.[132–135] In these cases, a triangular outgrowth from the undersurface of the clavicle approaches the dorsomedial surface of the coracoid process. On dissection, the articulation may be found to contain a capsule and synovial membrane as well as a cartilaginous disc.[136]

FIGURE 70–78. Lateral portion of the scapula: Osseous anatomy. Note the glenoid cavity (g), coracoid process (c), acromion process (a), clavicular facet (cf), and infraglenoid tubercle (t). Also note the anterior (arrow) and posterior (arrowhead) rims of the glenoid region.

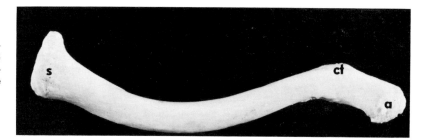

FIGURE 70–79. Clavicle: Osseous anatomy. Superior aspect. A photograph delineates sternal (s) and acromial (a) ends of the clavicle. Note the conoid tubercle (ct) on the posterior surface of the distal clavicle.

Articular Anatomy

Glenohumeral Joint. The articular surfaces of the glenoid and the humerus are covered with hyaline cartilage (Fig. 70–81). The cartilage on the humeral head is thickest at its center and thinner peripherally, whereas the reverse is true on the glenoid portion of the joint. A fibrocartilaginous structure, the labrum, attaches to the glenoid rim and adds an element of stability to the glenohumeral articulation (see later discussion).

A loose fibrous capsule arises medially from the circumference of the glenoid labrum or, anteriorly, the neck of the scapula.[137] It inserts distally into the anatomic neck of the humerus and periosteum of the humeral diaphysis. In certain areas the fibrous capsule is strengthened by its intimate association with surrounding ligaments and tendons; with regard to tendons, the capsule is reinforced above by the supraspinatus, below by the long head of the triceps, anteriorly by the subscapularis, and posteriorly by the infraspinatus and teres minor. The tendons of the supraspinatus, infraspinatus, teres minor, and subscapularis form a cuff—the rotator cuff—which blends with and reinforces the fibrous capsule (see later discussion). The coracohumeral ligament strengthens the upper part of the capsule. It arises from the lateral edge of the coracoid process, extends over the humeral head, and attaches to the greater tuberosity. Anteriorly, the capsule may thicken to form the superior, middle, and inferior glenohumeral ligaments. These ligaments and the recesses formed between them are variable in configuration (see later discussion). The fibrous capsule is strengthened additionally by extensions from the tendons of the pectoralis major and teres major muscles.

Three openings may be found in the fibrous capsule (Fig. 70–82). An anterior perforation below the coracoid process establishes joint communication with the bursa behind the subscapularis tendon, the subscapular "recess." A second opening between the greater and lesser tuberosities allows passage of the tendon and synovial sheath of the long head of the biceps brachii muscle. A third, inconstant perforation may exist posteriorly, allowing communication of the articular cavity and a bursa under the infraspinatus tendon.

A synovial membrane lines the inner aspect of the fibrous capsule. It covers the anatomic neck of the humerus and extends to the articular cartilage on the humeral head. The synovium passes distally to line the bicipital groove and is reflected over the biceps tendon.

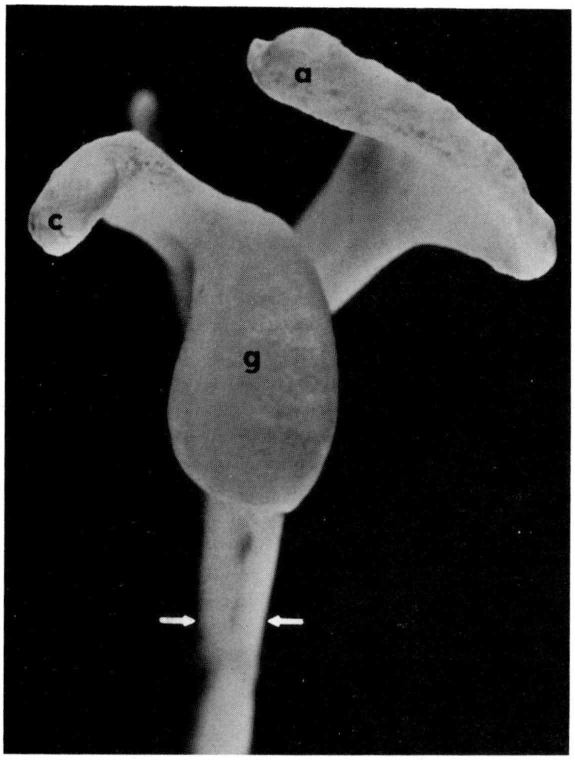

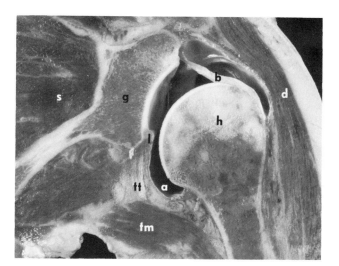

FIGURE 70–81. Glenohumeral joint: Articular anatomy. A coronal section of an air-distended articular cavity reveals the glenoid region (g) of the scapula, humeral head (h), axillary pouch (a), inferior portion of the labrum (l), tendon (b) of the long head of the biceps brachii muscle, portions of the subscapularis (s), deltoid (d), and teres major (tm) muscles, and the tendon (tt) of the long head of the triceps muscle. Note the hyaline cartilage covering both the glenoid cavity and the humeral head. The size of the articular surface of the humerus is much larger than that of the glenoid cavity.

FIGURE 70–80. Lateral aspect of the scapula: Osseous anatomy. The scapular "Y" is well shown, consisting of its lateral border (arrows), glenoid cavity (g), coracoid process (c), and acromion (a).

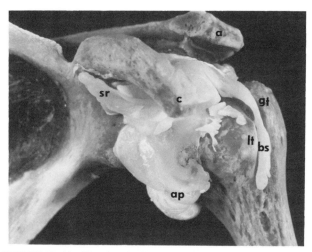

FIGURE 70–82. Glenohumeral joint: Normal articular extensions. A photograph of the anterior portion of a joint that has been distended with methylmethacrylate reveals the acromion (a), coracoid process (c), and greater tuberosity (gt) and lesser tuberosity (lt) of the humerus. Note the finger-like medial extension of the joint, designated the subscapular recess (sr), the axillary pouch (ap), and the synovial sheath (bs) about the tendon of the long head of the biceps brachii muscle. This sheath is located within the intertubercular sulcus.

There are several bursae about the glenohumeral joint:

1. Subscapular bursa. This bursa lies between the subscapularis tendon and the scapula, communicating with the joint via an opening between the superior and middle glenohumeral ligaments or between the middle and inferior glenohumeral ligaments, or in both locations. This bursa is readily apparent on arthrograms of the glenohumeral joint as a tongue-shaped collection of contrast material extending medially from the glenohumeral space underneath the coracoid process.[138] It is prominent in internal rotation but is less obvious in external rotation, as the taut subscapularis muscle compresses the bursa.

2. Bursa about the infraspinatus tendon. This inconstant bursa separates the infraspinatus tendon and joint capsule and may communicate with the joint cavity.

3. Subacromial (subdeltoid) bursa. This important bursa lies between the deltoid muscle and joint capsule[139] (Fig. 70–83). It extends underneath the acromion and the coracoacromial ligament. The subacromial (subdeltoid) bursa is separated from the articular cavity by the rotator cuff and does not communicate with the joint unless there has been a perforation of the cuff. Layers of fat tissue about this bursa have been identified on radiographs of the normal shoulder[140]; a thin, crescentic radiolucent area passes from the inferior aspect of the acromion process and distal clavicle along the outer margin of the upper humerus. Obliteration of the peribursal fat plane is an important sign of shoulder disease and can be recognized not only on routine radiographs[141] but on CT and MR images as well (see later discussion).

4. Bursa above the acromion. This bursa is located on the superior surface of the acromion process of the scapula.

5. Additional bursae. Additional bursae may be found between the coracoid process and the capsule, behind the coracobrachialis, between the teres major and the long head of the triceps, and about the latissimus dorsi.

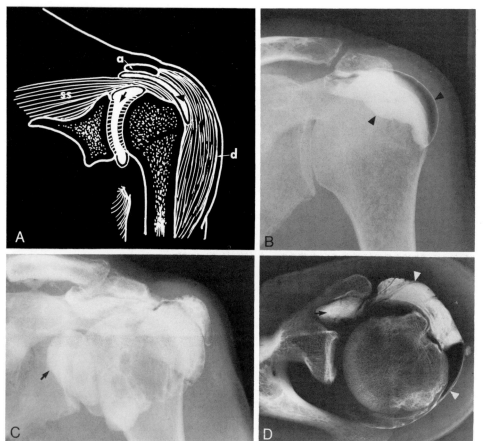

FIGURE 70–83. Subacromial (subdeltoid) bursa: Normal anatomy.

A A diagram of a coronal section of the shoulder shows the glenohumeral joint (arrow) and subacromial (subdeltoid) bursa (arrowhead), separated by a portion of the rotator cuff (i.e., supraspinatus tendon). The supraspinatus (ss) and deltoid (d) muscles and the acromion (a) are indicated.

B A subdeltoid-subacromial bursogram, accomplished with the injection of both radiopaque contrast material and air, shows the bursa (arrowheads) sitting like a cap on the humeral head and greater tuberosity of the humerus. Note that the joint is not opacified, indicating an intact rotator cuff.

C In a different cadaver, a subacromial-subdeltoid bursogram shows a much more extensive structure owing to opacification of the subacromial, subdeltoid, and subcoracoid (arrow) portions of the bursa.

D A radiograph of a transverse section of the specimen illustrated in **C** shows both the subdeltoid (arrowheads) and subcoracoid (arrow) portions of the bursa. The glenohumeral joint is not opacified.

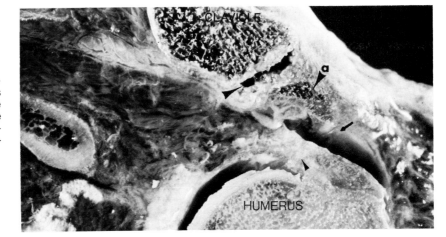

FIGURE 70–84. Acromioclavicular joint: Normal articular anatomy. Visualized structures on this coronal section are the articular space (large arrowheads) between the distal clavicle and acromion (a) (an articular disc is not visible), rotator cuff (small arrowhead), and subacromial (subdeltoid) bursa (arrow).

Acromioclavicular Joint. The articular surfaces about the acromioclavicular joint are covered with fibrocartilage (Fig. 70–84). In the central portion of the articulation is an articular disc[142] that partially or, more rarely, completely divides the joint cavity. The fibrous capsule surrounds the articular margin and is reinforced on its superior and inferior surfaces. Surrounding ligaments include the acromioclavicular and coracoclavicular ligaments (Fig. 70–85). The former ligament, which is located at the superior portion of the joint, extends between the clavicle and acromion. The coracoclavicular ligament, which attaches to the coracoid process of the scapula and clavicle, is composed of a trapezoid part and a conoid part. The trapezoid portion extends from the upper surface of the coracoid process to the trapezoid line on the inferior aspect of the clavicle; the conoid portion extends from the coracoid process to the conoid tubercle on the inferior clavicular surface. The trapezoid and conoid parts of the coracoclavicular ligament may be separated by fat or a bursa.

Normal anteroposterior radiographs of the acromioclavicular joint may reveal a soft tissue plane about the articulation related to the aponeurosis associated with the trapezius and deltoid muscles. Contrast opacification of the joint reveals an L-shaped articular cavity with a horizontal limb extending under the inferior surface of the distal clavicle.[143]

The acromioclavicular joint allows the acromion to glide in a forward and backward direction and to rotate on the clavicle. These movements depend upon additional movements at the sternoclavicular joint.

Soft Tissue Anatomy

Glenohumeral Ligaments. The glenohumeral ligaments represent thickenings, or reinforcements, of the joint capsule (Fig. 70–86). They are not visible on the external surface of the glenohumeral joint but are identifiable from within the glenohumeral joint, as can be appreciated during arthroscopy. Their function is dependent on (1) their collagenous integrity, (2) their sites of attachment, and (3) the position of the arm.[124] There are three glenohumeral ligaments: the superior glenohumeral ligament, the middle glenohumeral ligament, and the inferior glenohumeral ligament. In any person, the number of ligaments present is variable and, even when present, the glenohumeral ligaments vary considerably in size. Anatomic studies have indicated the presence of a superior glenohumeral ligament in 90 to 97 per cent of cases, of a middle glenohumeral ligament in 73 to 92 per cent of cases, and of an inferior glenohumeral ligament in almost 100 per cent of cases.[124, 144, 145] Each extends from the anterior aspect of the glenoid cavity, near the glenoid labrum, to the proximal portion of the humerus. Apertures between these ligaments provide areas of communication between the glenohumeral joint and the subscapular bursa; some variability exists in the size of these apertures as well as that of the bursa itself.[146] The bursa extends medially from the joint, along the superior tendinous border of the subscapularis muscle, toward the inferior surface of the coracoid process.[146]

The detailed anatomy of the glenohumeral ligaments has been summarized by O'Brien and coworkers,[124] whose observations are included here. When present, the superior glenohumeral ligament varies in size from a thin wisp of capsular tissue to a prominent bandlike region within the joint capsule. It arises either from a common origin with the tendon of the long head of the biceps brachii muscle, from the anterior portion of the labrum just anterior to this tendon, or from the middle glenohumeral ligament.[144] It inserts into the fovea capitis just superior to the lesser

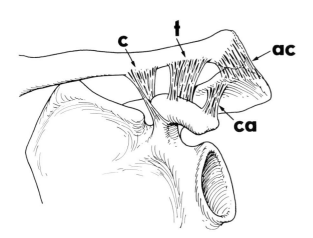

FIGURE 70–85. Acromioclavicular joint: Normal ligamentous anatomy. Important structures are the fibrous capsule of the joint, which is strengthened by the acromioclavicular ligament (ac), the coracoacromial ligament (ca), and the conoid (c) and trapezoid (t) portions of the coracoclavicular ligament.

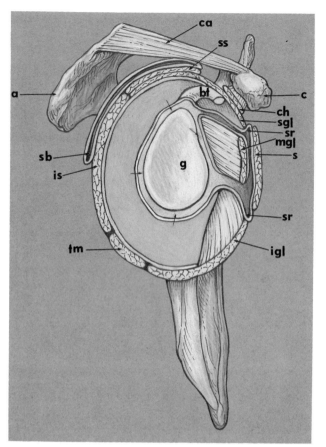

FIGURE 70–86. Glenohumeral joint: Ligamentous and capsular anatomy. A lateral view of an opened glenohumeral joint is shown in which the humeral head has been removed. Identified structures (beginning superiorly and continuing in a clockwise direction) are the coracoacromial ligament (ca), the supraspinatus tendon (ss), the tendon of the long head of the biceps brachii muscle (bt), the coracoid process (c), the coracohumeral ligament (ch), the superior glenohumeral ligament (sgl), an opening into the subscapular recess (sr), the middle glenohumeral ligament (mgl), the subscapularis tendon (s), a second opening into the subscapular recess (sr), the inferior glenohumeral ligament (igl), the teres minor tendon (tm), the infraspinatus tendon (is), the subacromial-subdeltoid bursa (sb), and the acromion (a). Also identified is the cartilage-covered glenoid cavity (g) surrounded by the glenoid labrum (arrows).

tuberosity.[147] In this latter region, it is intimate with the coracohumeral ligament.[146] The functional importance of the superior glenohumeral ligament is debated; however, owing to its small size in some persons, its vulnerability for tearing during forceful abduction of the glenohumeral joint, and its protection from excessive tension by the other glenohumeral ligaments, the superior glenohumeral ligament probably contributes very little to static stability of the glenohumeral joint.[124, 146, 148]

The middle glenohumeral ligament is the least constant of the glenohumeral ligaments and shows the most variability in size. It usually arises from the anterior portion of the labrum below the superior glenohumeral ligament or from the adjacent neck of the glenoid region, and it inserts just medial to the lesser tuberosity of the humerus, under the tendon of the subscapularis muscle, to which it attaches.[124, 147] When thick, the middle glenohumeral ligament can act as an important secondary restraint to anterior translation of the humeral head if the anterior portion of the inferior glenohumeral ligament is damaged.[124]

The inferior glenohumeral ligament is the main stabilizer of the abducted glenohumeral joint. Turkel and colleagues[147] described three portions of this ligament: the superior band of the inferior glenohumeral ligament, representing the thick anterosuperior edge of the ligament; the anterior axillary pouch, representing the region between the superior band and the middle glenohumeral ligament; and the axillary pouch, representing the remainder of the capsule posterior to the superior band. O'Brien and collaborators[124, 145] introduced the term inferior glenohumeral ligament complex, consisting of an anterior band, a posterior band, and an intervening axillary pouch. This complex is a hammock-like structure originating from the glenoid region and inserting into the anatomic neck of the humerus.[124] Its components change in configuration with changes in position of the arm: with abduction and external rotation of the arm, the anterior band fans out to support the humeral head, and the posterior band becomes cordlike; with internal rotation of the arm, the opposite occurs.[124] The anterior and posterior bands often are of equal thickness, although occasionally the posterior band is thicker than the anterior band.[124]

Coracohumeral Ligament. The coracohumeral ligament is the most constant area of thickening of the capsule of the glenohumeral joint (Fig. 70–86). Edelson and colleagues[149] found a coracohumeral ligament in 100 per cent of 20 cadaveric shoulders, and Neer and coworkers[150] detected this ligament in 94 per cent of 63 cadaveric shoulders. The coracohumeral ligament is of variable thickness and generally is trapezoidal in shape. It arises from the lateral aspect of the coracoid process, either at its base[150] or over much of its surface.[149] The coracohumeral ligament then passes over the top of the glenohumeral joint, joining the capsule, and inserts into the greater and lesser tuberosities of the humerus, on either side of the bicipital groove.[149] It is intimate with the rotator interval between the subscapularis and supraspinatus tendons (see later discussion) and with the tendon of the long head of the biceps brachii muscle.

The function of the coracohumeral ligament is not clear. It has been regarded as a central element in the suspension of the humerus, a stabilizer of the tendon of the long head of the biceps brachii muscle, and a structure restraining external rotation of the arm (especially with the arm at the side of the torso).[149, 150] The coracohumeral ligament may prevent inferior displacement of the humeral head,[151, 152] and shortening of this ligament has been noted in cases of adhesive capsulitis of the shoulder (see later discussion).[150]

Glenoid Labrum. The glenoid labrum is a cuff of fibrous and fibrocartilaginous tissue that surrounds the glenoid cavity, serving to deepen the glenoid fossa and to allow attachment of the tendon of the long head of the biceps brachii muscle and the glenohumeral ligaments (Figs. 70–86 and 70–87). According to some investigators, most of the labrum consists of fibrous tissue with fibrocartilage present only in a small and narrow transitional zone where the capsule, the periosteum of the scapular neck, and the hyaline articular cartilage of the glenoid fossa meet.[146, 153] Other investigators, however, have emphasized the fibrocartilaginous nature of the labrum, indicating that the structure modulates from undifferentiated mesenchymal tissue to fibrocartilage during postnatal development in the first decade of life.[154]

The morphology and the capsular relationships of the

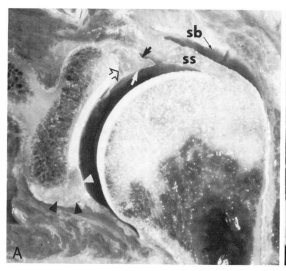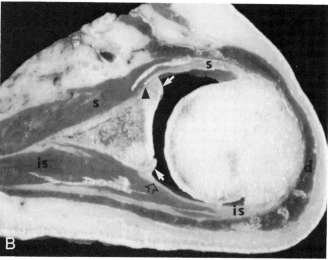

FIGURE 70–87. Glenohumeral joint: Labral anatomy. Coronal **(A)** and transverse **(B)** sections of an air-distended glenohumeral joint show portions of the glenoid labrum. In **A**, note the meniscus-like shape of the superior portion of the labrum (solid arrows) and the rounded appearance of the lower portion of the labrum (arrowheads). The superior portion of the labrum is separated from the adjacent articular cartilage of the glenoid cavity by a small joint recess (open arrow). No such recess is identified inferiorly. Other indicated structures in **A** are the supraspinatus tendon (ss) and a portion of the subacromial-subdeltoid bursa (sb). In **B**, the anterior and posterior portions of the labrum are seen (solid arrows). The posterior part of the joint capsule (open arrow) attaches to the labrum. Anteriorly, a type 1 capsular insertion (arrowhead) is evident (see text for details). In this midglenoid level, other indicated structures are the subscapularis muscle and tendon (s), infraspinatus muscle and tendon (is), and deltoid muscle (d).

glenoid labrum vary according to which portion of the structure is being studied. The inferior part of the labrum generally appears as a rounded and elevated structure that is continuous with the articular cartilage; loosening of the inferior half of the labrum is considered an abnormal finding.[153] In contrast, the superior part of the labrum tends to be meniscal in appearance and normally is more loosely attached and more mobile.[153] This normal laxity leads to diagnostic difficulty in the identification of superior labrum, anterior and posterior (SLAP) lesions (see later discussion). Posteriorly, the capsule of the glenohumeral joint is intimately related to the glenoid labrum along the entire posterior margin of the glenoid cavity. Anteriorly, however, variations in the relationship of the joint capsule and glenoid labrum are encountered. The anterior capsular insertions have been classified into two or three types based upon the proximity of the insertion site to the anterior portion of the labrum.[137, 155] In the three-part classification system, which is used throughout this chapter, a type I capsular insertion occurs close to or into the labrum, a type II capsular insertion occurs more medially, and a type III capsular insertion occurs into the scapular neck; in the two-part classification system, a type I capsular insertion occurs into the labrum, and a type II capsular insertion occurs into the scapular neck. Medial insertions of the anterior portion of the capsule (i.e., type III in the first classification system and type II in the second classification system) generally are considered less stable, perhaps causing or resulting from anterior glenohumeral joint instability. A type I capsular insertion in either classification system usually is considered more stable. The documentation of anterior capsular redundancy as a common finding in fetal glenohumeral joints, however, raises the possibility that such redundancy is a developmental variation rather than a consequence of trauma.[137] Nonetheless, categorizing the type of anterior capsular insertion on the basis of transaxial data supplied by CT and MR imaging remains popular (see later discussion).

The assessment of glenohumeral joint instability using CT and MR imaging requires analysis of the shape of the glenoid labrum in transverse sections. Complicating this assessment is the documented variability of the labral-capsular complex in the presumed normal shoulders of asymptomatic persons. Although a triangular shape of the anterior and posterior portions of the labrum often is considered evidence of a normal structure, imaging studies have confirmed normal variations in labral shape.[156, 157] In one very detailed study employing MR images of 52 shoulders in 30 asymptomatic volunteers, the anterior and posterior parts of the labra varied in shape but showed several dominant features: the anterior part of the labrum was triangular (45 per cent), round (19 per cent), cleaved (15 per cent), notched (8 per cent), flat (7 per cent), or absent (6 per cent); and the posterior part of the labrum was triangular (73 per cent), round (12 per cent), flat (6 per cent), or absent (8 per cent).[157] These findings suggest far more variability in the anterior rather than the posterior portion of the glenoid labrum. Further complicating the imaging analysis of the glenoid labrum are known variations in its shape that relate to rotation of the humeral head[146] and variability in its histologic composition[154] that may lead to modifications in its signal intensity (as seen with MR imaging).

The precise role of the glenoid labrum in providing stability to the glenohumeral joint is not clear. Although a portion of the labrum frequently is detached in cases of anterior glenohumeral joint instability, leading to the designation of a detached glenoid labrum as the essential lesion responsible for the high incidence of recurrent glenohumeral joint dislocations,[158, 159] the labrum is intimately associated with other soft tissue structures that appear to influence the degree of stability of the glenohumeral joint. As it is difficult to define the role of each of these structures in this regard, the designation of the anterior and posterior soft tissue structures of the glenohumeral joint as pillars, supports, or capsular mechanisms seems wise.[146, 160] The anterior capsular mechanism of the glenohumeral joint comprises the synovial membrane, anterior portion of the joint capsule including the glenohumeral ligaments, anterior portion of the glenoid labrum, scapular periosteum, subscapular recess, and subscapularis muscle and tendon; the posterior capsular mechanism consists of the posterior portion of the joint capsule, synovial membrane, posterior portion of the glenoid labrum, scapular periosteum, and posterosuperior structures of the rotator cuff (supraspinatus, infraspinatus, and teres minor muscles and tendons).[146] The anterior and posterior capsular mechanisms are separated superiorly by the coracohumeral ligament and the tendon of the long head of the biceps brachii muscle and inferiorly by the long head of the triceps muscle. A further discussion of these mechanisms is presented later in this chapter.

Rotator Cuff. The tendons of four muscles contribute to the rotator cuff of the shoulder: the supraspinatus muscle, the infraspinatus muscle, the teres minor muscle, and the subscapularis muscle (Fig. 70–88).

The supraspinatus muscle arises from the supraspinatus fossa (i.e., above the spine of the scapula) and overlying fascia, and it extends laterally over the humeral head. It ends as a tendon that inserts into the uppermost facet in the greater tuberosity in common with the infraspinatus tendon posteriorly and the coracohumeral ligament anteriorly.[161]

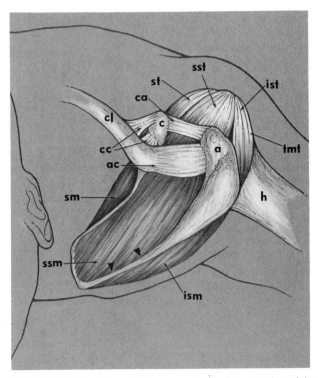

FIGURE 70–88. Rotator cuff: Normal anatomy. Superior view of the rotator cuff and related structures. Identified structures (beginning at the top and continuing in a clockwise direction) are the supraspinatus tendon (sst), infraspinatus tendon (ist), teres minor tendon (tmt), infraspinatus muscle (ism), supraspinatus muscle (ssm), subscapularis muscle (sm), acromioclavicular ligament (ac), coracoclavicular ligament (cc), coracoacromial ligament (ca), and subscapularis tendon (st). Also identified are the clavicle (cl), coracoid process (c), acromion (a), humerus (h), and spine of the scapula (arrowheads).

The tendon forms centrally within the muscle belly and, as it extends laterally, assumes a more anterior position with respect to the muscle fibers (see later discussion). The thick, triangular infraspinatus muscle originates from the infraspinatus fossa (i.e., below the spine of the scapula), overlying fascia, and spine of the scapula. The muscle fibers converge to form a single tendon or multiple tendons, which pass across the posterior aspect of the capsule of the glenohumeral joint to insert on the middle facet in the greater tuberosity of the humerus. A bursa may exist between the tendon and the joint capsule. The teres minor muscle is narrow and elongated, and it arises from the middle portion of the lateral border of the scapula and the dense fascia of the infraspinatus muscle. Its tendon is united with the inferior, posterior surface of the capsule of the glenohumeral joint, and it inserts into the lowest of the three facets in the greater tuberosity of the humerus and directly into the humerus just below this facet. More medially, the quadrilateral space is evident between the teres minor and teres major muscles; the posterior humeral circumflex artery and axillary nerve pass through this space. The subscapularis muscle is large and triangular, and it arises from the medial portion of the subscapular fossa on the anterior surface of the scapula. The subscapularis muscle extends laterally, and its muscle fibers are converted into a tendon that attaches to the lesser tuberosity of the humerus. Close to this site of attachment, the transverse humeral ligament extends between the greater and lesser tuberosities of the humerus. The tendon of the subscapularis muscle is separated from the neck of the scapula by the large subscapular bursa, which communicates with the glenohumeral joint through apertures in the joint capsule (see previous discussion).

These four components of the rotator cuff, the supraspinatus, the infraspinatus, the teres minor, and the subscapularis muscles, are important stabilizers of the glenohumeral joint, channeling the motion of the articulation and preventing excessive sliding at the joint. These muscles are involved in the initial phases of abduction of the arm.[1424] When intact, these rotator cuff muscles also counteract the superior translational force produced by the action of the deltoid muscle. Furthermore, these muscles reinforce the superior (supraspinatus and infraspinatus muscles), posterior (infraspinatus and teres minor muscles), and anterior (subscapularis muscle) portions of the capsule of the glenohumeral joint. The infraspinatus muscle prevents posterior subluxation of the humeral head with internal rotation of the arm, and anterior subluxation of the humeral head with external rotation and abduction of the arm; the teres minor muscle is an external rotator of the humerus and is important in controlling glenohumeral joint stability in an anterior direction; and the subscapularis muscle functions as an internal rotator of the humerus, as a stabilizer preventing anterior subluxation of the humeral head, and as a depressor of the humeral head.[161]

Although the rotator cuff consists of four muscles and their tendons with individual functions, the coordinated action of these structures is required to maintain joint stability. Electromyographic studies have documented that all four muscles of the rotator cuff are active during movement of the glenohumeral joint but with varying force.[162] One cadaveric investigation has shown that, of the four, the subscapularis muscle is the most powerful, followed, in order of decreasing strength, by the infraspinatus, supraspinatus, and teres minor muscles.[163] Although results from other studies have provided similar data,[164] information derived from a limited number of cadaveric specimens may not be applicable to living patients. Furthermore, age-dependent changes in tendons, including those of the rotator cuff, which include mucoid degeneration tendolipomatosis, hypoxic tendinopathy, and even calcification,[165, 166] may alter the relative strengths of the rotator cuff muscles. These changes may predispose the tendon to tear and, furthermore, as described later, alter the signal intensity characteristics of the tendon when examined with MR imaging.

Although the tendons of the rotator cuff pass in front of, over, and behind the humeral head, a normal space in the cuff exists anterosuperiorly where the cuff is perforated by the coracoid process. This space has been designated the rotator interval or rotator interval capsule.[167, 168] It is triangular in shape and located between the anterior border of the supraspinatus tendon and the superior border of the subscapularis tendon. The base of the interval is the coracoid process, and the apex of the interval is the transverse humeral ligament at the intertubercular sulcus of the humerus.[168] Capsular tissue bridges this space. The coracohumeral and superior glenohumeral ligaments are important structures within the rotator interval. The fibers of the joint capsule and superior glenohumeral ligament blend together and insert into the borders of the supraspinatus and subscapularis tendons, the transverse humeral ligament, and the greater and lesser tuberosities of the humerus.[168] The tendon of the long head of the biceps brachii muscle also is intimate with this interval. The rotator interval, with its supporting structures, appears to play an important role in providing stability to and channeling the motion in the glenohumeral joint.[167, 168]

Six arteries contribute regularly to the vascular supply of the tendons of the rotator cuff: the suprascapular, anterior circumflex humeral, posterior circumflex humeral, thoracoacromial, suprahumeral, and subscapular arteries.[124, 169] Approximately two thirds of shoulders reveal a hypovascular zone in the supraspinatus tendon just proximal to its insertion (Fig. 70–89); less commonly, the infraspinatus and the subscapularis tendons reveal similar zones of hypovascularity.[124] A deficiency of blood flow to the supraspinatus tendon has commonly but not uniformly[170] been regarded as important in the pathogenesis of its rupture.

Coracoacromial Arch. The coracoacromial arch is intimate with portions of the rotator cuff, with the tendon of the long head of the biceps brachii muscle, and with the subacromial bursa. It consists of the coracoacromial ligament, the coracoid process, and the acromion (Fig. 70–90). Abnormalities of any of the structures of the arch and of the acromioclavicular joint can lead to impingement on the adjacent soft tissue structures, particularly the rotator cuff, a situation designated the shoulder impingement syndrome.

The coracoacromial ligament is a strong and triangular band that forms part of the roof of the glenohumeral joint. It extends from the edge of the acromion, anterior to the articular surface of the acromioclavicular joint, to the lateral border of the coracoid process of the scapula. The coracoacromial ligament may be uniform in composition or consist of two marginal bands and less dense intervening tissue. A tendon of the pectoralis minor muscle occasionally may pass between the marginal bands of this ligament. The coracoacromial ligament is firm and unyielding,[171] and it generally is regarded as an important cause of the shoulder impingement syndrome (see later discussion).

The coracoid process of the scapula projects from the head of the scapula, in an anterior and lateral direction. It serves as a site of origin of the tendons of the short head of the biceps brachii muscle and of the coracobrachialis muscle and the site of insertion of the tendon of the pectoralis minor muscle and the coracoacromial and coracoclavicular ligaments. The space between the coracoid process and the humeral head varies somewhat in size, although the coracohumeral interval is smallest in internal rotation and for-

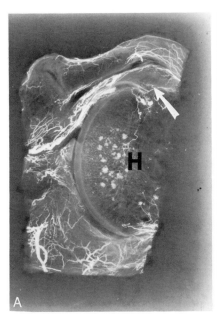
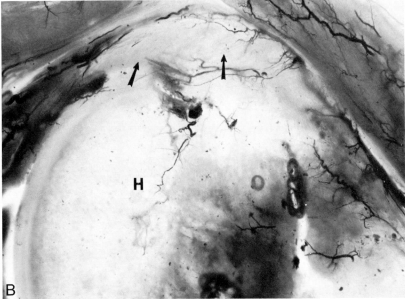

FIGURE 70–89. Rotator cuff: Normal hypovascular zone of the supraspinatus tendon. A radiograph **(A)** and photograph **(B)** of a coronal section of a cadaveric shoulder, following the use of a modified Spalteholz technique to delineate the blood supply of the rotator cuff, reveal a critical zone of relative avascularity in the outer portion of the supraspinatus tendon (arrows) in which tears usually occur. H, Humeral head.

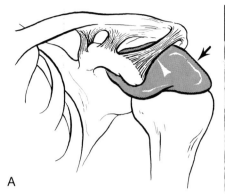

A

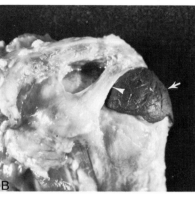

B

FIGURE 70–90. Coracoacromial arch: Normal anatomy.

A Drawing shows the coracoacromial arch, consisting of the coracoid process anteriorly, the acromion posteriorly, and the intervening coracoacromial ligament (arrowhead). Note the intimate relationship between this arch and the subacromial-subdeltoid bursa (arrow).

B An anterior view of a dissected shoulder reveals the coracoacromial ligament (arrowhead) and a latex-filled subacromial-subdeltoid bursa (arrow).

ward flexion of the arm.[161] One form of the shoulder impingement syndrome appears to relate to encroachment of the lesser tuberosity of the humerus on the coracoid process, a situation that can be aggravated by developmental or acquired conditions (e.g., coracoid fractures, fractures of the lesser tuberosity of the humerus, calcification within the subscapularis tendon, glenoid osteotomy, and surgical procedures in which transfer of the coracoid process is accomplished).[172] Transaxial CT has been employed as a means of measurement of the lateral extent of the coracoid process and may be a useful technique in the assessment of coracohumeral impingement.[172]

The acromion projects forward from the lateral end of the scapular spine. The lateral border and tip of the acromion are the sites of origin of the middle fibers of the deltoid muscle; the acromial tip also serves as the attachment site of the coracoacromial ligament. Behind the clavicular facet of the acromion, horizontal fibers of the tendon of the trapezius muscle arise. An accessory bone, the os acromiale, may be apparent at the tip of the acromion in 1 to 15 per cent of shoulders.[173] Its relationship to the shoulder impingement syndrome and disruption of the rotator cuff is not clear.

Variations in the morphology of the acromion have received a great deal of attention owing to their possible association with rotator cuff pathology.[174, 175] Bigliani and coworkers[176] divided the profile shape of the acromion into three types; the undersurface of the bone was categorized as flat (type I), curved (type II), or hooked (type III) (Fig. 70–91). Reported data regarding these shapes have indicated a flat undersurface in 17 to 22 per cent of shoulders, a curved undersurface in 43 to 62 per cent of shoulders, and a hooked undersurface in 16 to 40 per cent of shoulders.[175, 176] This variation in the reported data may relate to changes in the shape of the undersurface of the acromion in its medial and lateral portions or mislabeling of acromial shape when osteophytes or enthesophytes are present.[1425] Type I acromions appear to have the lowest association with the impingement syndrome, and type III acromions appear to have the highest association with this syndrome.[176] The slope of the acromion, a different parameter, relates to its inclination as determined by an angle related to the intersection of two lines, one constructed along the inferior portion of the very anterior and posterior parts of the acromion, and the second line representing the horizontal. The importance of the slope of the acromion, as distinct from a hooked undersurface, in the pathogenesis of the shoulder impingement syndrome has been empha-

sized.[175] A horizontal acromion (i.e., one with a decreased slope) together with an increased length of the acromion, as well as a diminished height of the arch of the bone, leads to increased cover of the humeral head and a diminished space between the humeral head and acromion.

This interest in acromial morphology has led to the definition of the supraspinatus outlet space between the acromion and the humerus.[177] Frontal radiographs of the shoulder provide some information regarding the capaciousness of this outlet; calculations of the space between the humeral head and acromion indicate an average measurement of 9 or 10 mm (6.6 to 13.8 mm in men and 7.1 to 11.9 mm in women).[130] An anteroposterior radiograph of the shoulder made with the patient erect and with a 30 degree caudal tilt of the x-ray beam has been found helpful in assessment of the supraspinatus outlet.[178, 179] Lateral radiographs of the scapula obtained with approximately 10 degrees of caudal

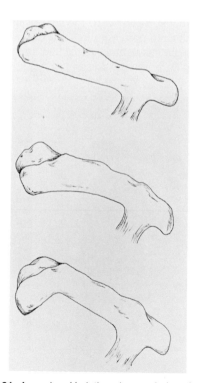

FIGURE 70–91. Acromion: Variations in morphology in the sagittal plane. Three variations in acromial shape are illustrated. The upper drawing depicts a flat undersurface of the acromion; the middle drawing depicts a curved undersurface of the acromion; and the lower drawing depicts a hooked undersurface of the acromion.

angulation of the x-ray tube in a medial to lateral direction, the supraspinatus outlet view, also are useful in the analysis of this space.[176, 177]

Muscles. The muscles about the shoulder are numerous and complex, and their anatomy has been well described by Jobe.[161] A brief summary of this anatomy follows. These muscles can be divided into scapulothoracic muscles, glenohumeral (or scapulohumeral) muscles, and multiple joint muscles[161] (Figs. 70–92 and 70–93).

The scapulothoracic muscles include the trapezius, the rhomboideus major and minor, the levator scapulae, the serratus anterior, the pectoralis minor, and the subclavius. The trapezius muscle is superficial and large. It arises from the spinous processes of the seventh cervical through twelfth thoracic vertebrae (with some anatomic variations) and from the ligamentum nuchae and the external occipital protuberance, and this muscle inserts in the clavicle and acromion and spine of the scapula.[180] In combination with

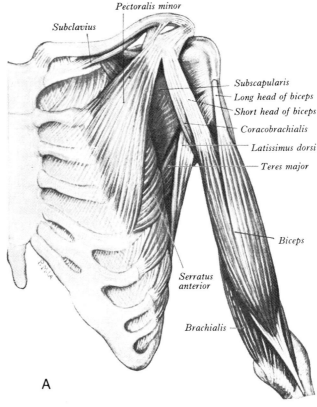

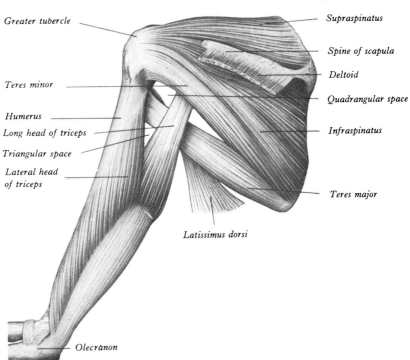

FIGURE 70–92. Deep muscles of the shoulder and upper arm: Normal anatomy.
A Anterior aspect of the shoulder.
B Posterior aspect of the shoulder.
(From Williams PL, Warwick R [Eds]: Gray's Anatomy. 36th British edition. Edinburgh, Churchill Livingstone, 1980, pp 537, 539.)

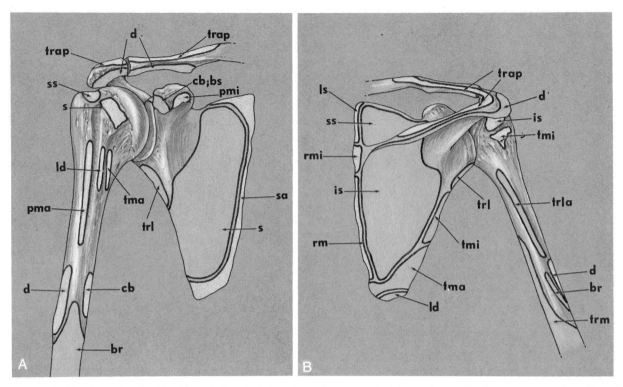

FIGURE 70–93. Muscles of the shoulder: Normal sites of origin and insertion. Sites of origin are depicted in darker gray, and sites of insertion in lighter gray.

A Anterior aspect of the shoulder. Identified structures (starting at the top and proceeding in a clockwise direction) are the deltoid muscle (d), trapezius muscle (trap), coracobrachialis (cb), short head of the biceps brachii muscle (bs), pectoralis minor muscle (pmi), serratus anterior muscle (sa), subscapularis muscle (s), long head of the triceps muscle (trl), teres major muscle (tma), coracobrachialis muscle (cb), brachialis muscle (br), deltoid muscle (d), pectoralis major muscle (pma), latissimus dorsi muscle (ld), subscapularis muscle (s), supraspinatus muscle (ss), and trapezius muscle (trap).

B Posterior aspect of the shoulder. Identified structures (starting at the top and proceeding in a clockwise direction) are the trapezius muscle (trap), deltoid muscle (d), infraspinatus muscle (is), teres minor muscle (tmi), lateral head of the triceps muscle (trla), deltoid muscle (d), brachialis muscle (br), medial head of the triceps muscle (trm), long head of the triceps muscle (trl), teres minor muscle (tmi), teres major muscle (tma), latissimus dorsi muscle (ld), rhomboideus major muscle (rm), infraspinatus muscle (is), rhomboideus minor muscle (rmi), supraspinatus muscle (ss), and levator scapulae muscle (ls).

other muscles attaching to the scapula, the trapezius muscle elevates the lateral angle of the scapula. The rhomboid muscles arise from the spines of the second, third, fourth, and fifth thoracic vertebrae (rhomboideus major) and those of the seventh cervical and first thoracic vertebrae (rhomboideus minor). They insert on the medial border of the scapula. The levator scapulae arises from the posterior tubercles of the transverse processes of the third and fourth cervical vertebrae and from the transverse processes of the atlas and axis. It inserts distally in the upper medial border of the scapula. Either alone or in combination with other scapular muscles, the rhomboids and the levator scapulae muscles control the position of the scapula during active movements of the arm. The serratus anterior muscle takes origin from the upper eight or nine ribs and passes laterally to attach to the superior and inferior angles and medial border of the scapula. The serratus anterior muscle protracts the scapula and participates in upward rotation of this bone.[161] The pectoralis minor muscle arises from the anterior surface of the second through fifth ribs (with some anatomic variations), and it inserts into the base of the coracoid process of the scapula. Aberrant slips of this muscle also may attach to the clavicle, humerus, and glenoid cavity and other portions of the scapula. Working with other scapular muscles, the pectoralis minor aids in forward

movement and rotation of this bone. Finally, the subclavius muscle usually does not attach to the scapula but is involved indirectly in assisting scapulothoracic motion.[161] It arises from the first rib and its costal cartilage and attaches to the inferior surface of the medial third of the clavicle. Rarely, an attachment of this muscle to the coracoid process of the scapula is evident. The subclavius muscle stabilizes the sternoclavicular joint.

The glenohumeral (or scapulohumeral) muscles are the deltoid, teres major, coracobrachialis, and the components of the rotator cuff (supraspinatus, infraspinatus, teres minor, and subscapularis) described earlier in this chapter. The deltoid muscle is large and consists of three major portions: the anterior portion arises from the lateral third of the clavicle; the middle portion arises from the acromion; and the posterior portion arises from the spine of the scapula.[161] All portions of the deltoid muscle insert as a prominent tendon in the deltoid tuberosity on the lateral surface of the humerus. Individual portions of the deltoid muscle or the entire muscle are involved in most movements of the arm with the exception, perhaps, of medial and lateral rotation. The deltoid muscle accounts for 60 per cent of strength in horizontal abduction of the arm, but this muscle has limited leverage in the first 30 degrees of abduction,[161] during which its action mainly is one of upward traction (which is counteracted by various components of the rotator cuff). The teres major muscle arises from the posterolateral surface of the scapula, and it inserts along with the tendon of the latissimus dorsi muscle adjacent to the medial margin of the intertubercular sulcus of the humerus. The function of this muscle is to internally rotate, adduct, and extend the arm. The coracobrachialis muscle arises from the apex of the coracoid process, in common with the origin of the short head of the biceps brachii muscle, and it inserts on the anteromedial surface of the midportion of the humerus. The coracobrachialis muscle is involved in flexion and adduction of the arm.

The last category of muscles, multiple joint muscles, perform action on the glenohumeral joint and one other joint, most commonly the scapulothoracic joint.[161] The pectoralis major, latissimus dorsi, biceps brachii, and triceps (brachii) muscles fall in this category. The pectoralis major muscle arises from the anterior surface of the medial margin of the clavicle, and the anterior surface of the sternum, the upper costal cartilages, and the aponeurosis of the obliquus externus abdominis muscle. The pectoralis major muscle attaches to the lateral edge of the intertubercular groove of the humerus. Its various components, or the muscle as a whole, are involved in adduction and internal rotation of the humerus. The latissimus dorsi muscle originates from the dorsal spines of the seventh thoracic through fifth lumbar vertebrae, iliac crest, and sacrum. It inserts into the medial margin and floor of the intertubercular sulcus. Actions of this muscle are internal rotation and adduction of the humerus and extension of the shoulder. As discussed previously, the biceps brachii muscle is actively involved in elbow motion. Its long head arises from the supraglenoid tubercle atop the glenoid cavity where it is continuous with the superior portion of the glenoid labrum; its short head arises from the tip of the coracoid process of the scapula. The tendon of the long head of the biceps brachii muscle extends laterally above the head of the humerus, enclosed in a synovial sheath, passes behind the transverse humeral ligament, and exits the joint in the intertubercular sulcus. The bicipital tendon is kept within this sulcus by the transverse humeral ligament. The distal attachment sites of the biceps brachii muscle are discussed earlier in this chapter. This muscle is involved in flexion and supination at the elbow. The long head of the triceps muscle originates from the infraglenoid tubercle of the scapula, where it is intimately related to the inferior portion of the glenoid labrum and the joint capsule, and the lateral and medial heads of the triceps muscle arise from the posterior surface of the humeral shaft. The distal attachment site and action at the elbow of the triceps muscle are discussed earlier in this chapter.

Shoulder Impingement Syndrome

Although he was not the first to suggest a relationship between subacromial impingement and chronic shoulder disability, Neer clarified and popularized the concept of the shoulder impingement syndrome in 1972 and is recognized as its main advocate.[181] Based on observations in scapular specimens, Neer described a characteristic bone excrescence that arose from the undersurface of the anterior portion of the acromion that he believed was caused by repeated impingement of the rotator cuff and the humeral head with traction of the coracoacromial ligament. He emphasized the dynamic relationship between (1) the intertubercular sulcus (bicipital groove) and the insertion site of the supraspinatus tendon in the greater tuberosity, and (2) the coracoacromial arch. Neer noted that although the bicipital groove and supraspinatus tendon were located anterior to the coracoacromial arch when the arm was in the neutral position, these structures passed beneath this arch during forward flexion of the arm (Fig. 70–94). He believed that this dynamic relationship explained the occurrence of impingement of portions of the rotator cuff during movements of the arm that eventually could result in complete disruption of the rotator cuff as well as of rupture of the tendon of the long head of the biceps brachii muscle.[181–184] Three progressive stages of the shoulder impingement syndrome were described by Neer[184]: stage 1, consisting of reversible edema and hemorrhage about the rotator cuff, typically seen in patients below the age of 25 years; stage 2, consisting of fibrosis and tendinitis in the rotator cuff, usually seen in patients between the ages of 25 and 40 years; and stage 3, consisting of tendon rupture and subacromial spurs (enthesophytes), generally evident in patients over the age of 40 years.

The basis of the shoulder impingement syndrome is the restricted space that exists between the coracohumeral arch above and the humeral head and tuberosities below. Through this space pass the tendons of the rotator cuff and, within the rotator interval, the tendon of the long head of the biceps brachii muscle and the coracohumeral ligament. The subacromial-subdeltoid bursa, consisting of two serosal surfaces lubricated by synovial fluid and surrounded by a layer of fat (peribursal fat), aids in the passage of these structures.[185] Compression of these structures also is minimized by a normal acromioclavicular joint, a shape of the coracoacromial arch that allows free passage of the subjacent cuff mechanism, and normal capsular laxity.[185] Contributing to the vulnerability of the supraspinatus tendon are the following:

1. A relatively avascular critical zone near the site of attachment of the tendon to the greater tuberosity. Compromise of blood flow to the tendon has been shown experimentally with adduction[186] and flexion[187] at the glenohumeral joint.

2. Anatomic variations in the anterior excursion and slope of the acromion and the shape of its inferior margin (see previous discussion).

3. Abnormal laxity of the capsule of the glenohumeral joint.

The large number of factors that potentially could cause shoulder impingement syndrome have led to several attempts at classification. As one example, Matsen and Arntz[185] divided the causative factors into two groups: structural factors and functional factors. Structural factors relate to the acromioclavicular joint (congenital anomalies or osteophytes), acromion (alterations in shape, fractures with malunion or nonunion, os acromiale, or osteophytes), coracoid process (congenital anomalies or posttraumatic or postsurgical changes), subacromial-subdeltoid bursa (inflammation, thickening, or surgical or nonsurgical foreign bodies), rotator cuff (calcification, thickening, or irregularity related to tendon tears, or postoperative or posttraumatic scars), or humerus (congenital anomalies, fractures with

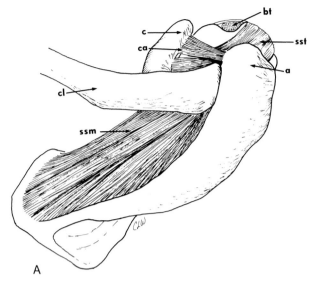

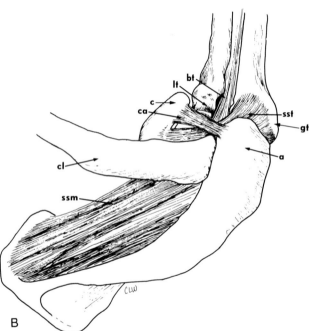

FIGURE 70–94. Shoulder impingement syndrome: Pathogenesis.
  A Superior view of the shoulder with the arm in a neutral position. The supraspinatus tendon (sst) and the tendon of the long head of the biceps brachii muscle (bt) lie anterior to the acromion (a), acromioclavicular joint, and coracoacromial ligament (ca). The supraspinatus muscle (ssm), clavicle (cl), and coracoid process (c) also are indicated.
  B Superior view of the shoulder with forward flexion of the arm. The supraspinatus tendon (sst), greater tuberosity of the humerus (gt), and tendon of the long head of the biceps brachii muscle (bt) become more intimate with the acromion (a), the acromioclavicular joint, and the coracoacromial ligament (ca). The supraspinatus muscle (ssm), coracoid process (c), clavicle (cl), and lesser tuberosity of the humerus (lt) also are indicated.
  (Modified from Rockwood CA Jr: J Bone Joint Surg [Am] 75:409, 1993.)

malunions, or altered position of a humeral head prosthesis). Fu and associates[188] divided impingement syndromes into two major categories: primary impingement occurring mainly in nonathletic persons and related to alterations in the coracoacromial arch; and secondary impinge-

ment occurring mainly in athletes involved in sports requiring overhead movement of the arm, and related to either glenohumeral or scapular instability. The relationship of anterior instability of the glenohumeral joint and rotator cuff impingement has been emphasized repeatedly.[189–191] Such instability results in fatigue of the components of the rotator cuff, allowing the humeral head to translate anteriorly, and mechanical impingement of the supraspinatus tendon on the coracoacromial arch may be seen. As the occurrence of the shoulder impingement syndrome implies a diminution of the space between the coracohumeral arch and the humeral head and its tuberosities, its causes are predictable, related to alterations in any of the components of the arch or humerus that serve to narrow this space; or to transient malposition of the humeral head and glenoid cavity that also leads to diminution of this space. Additional factors intrinsic to the rotator cuff such as ischemia and inflammation make it more vulnerable to the impingement syndrome.

The clinical manifestations of this syndrome are well documented and vary with the severity of the process. Certain occupations such as tree pruning, fruit picking, grocery clerking, longshoring, carpentry, and painting or certain types of athletic activity such as throwing a ball, swimming, tennis, and skiing are common among affected patients.[185] Such patients complain of chronic shoulder pain, stiffness, and weakness, and the findings may be accentuated when the arm is flexed or internally rotated. A limited range of motion usually restricts internal rotation and adduction of the arm. Pain may be provoked by elevation of the shoulder. Matsen and Arntz[185] emphasized the clinical importance of differentiation among signs of subacromial impingement (subacromial crepitus on flexion and rotation), signs of tightness (limited range of motion), and signs of tendon involvement (atrophy, weakness, and pain or restricted motion of the shoulder). Clinical tests for mechanical impingement of the shoulder have been described.[181, 190, 192] Most of these relate to the occurrence of pain during forward flexion and internal rotation of the arm. A painful arc exists between 60 degrees and 120 degrees of shoulder abduction. In general, these various clinical manifestations increase as the stage of the process increases.[192]

Routine radiography plays a minor diagnostic role in the evaluation of patients with early clinical stages of shoulder impingement. Nonspecific sclerosis and cyst formation in the greater tuberosity or osteoarthritis of the acromioclavicular joint may be seen. This last finding, although of value in defining a possible cause of the shoulder impingement syndrome, is not diagnostic of this syndrome. Similarly, evidence of calcific tendinitis and loss of the peribursal fat plane does not allow a specific diagnosis of the shoulder impingement syndrome. Evaluation of the subacromial space may require angulated frontal and lateral radiographs of the shoulder (see earlier discussion).

A specific but late radiographic manifestation of the shoulder impingement syndrome is an anterior acromial enthesophyte.[193, 194, 1346] This enthesophyte may be apparent on routine anteroposterior radiographs of the shoulder (Fig. 70–95) or on those obtained with 30 degrees of caudal angulation of the x-ray beam.[179] Lateral radiographs of the scapula (scapular ''Y'' view) and fluoroscopy represent additional useful techniques for its identification. The enthesophyte extends from the anteroinferior surface of the

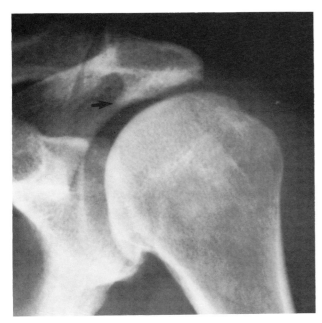

FIGURE 70–95. Shoulder impingement syndrome: Routine radiographic abnormalities. A frontal radiograph of the shoulder shows a large enthesophyte (arrow) extending from the anteroinferior portion of the acromion, associated with osteophytes at the acromioclavicular joint and in the inferior portion of the humeral head.

acromion in a medial and slightly inferior direction toward the coracoid process. It arises at the acromial attachment site of the coracoacromial ligament and differs in location and morphology from a ''pseudospur'' associated with prominence of the acromial angle (see Chapter 39). In some instances, the tip of the acromion simulates the radiographic appearance of a subacromial enthesophyte.

More advanced imaging methods, such as standard arthrography, computed arthrotomography, ultrasonography, and MR imaging, may be employed in patients with the shoulder impingement syndrome, but their role primarily is one of defining the extent and precise cause of the shoulder impingement syndrome and not one of establishing the diagnosis. Each of these techniques can be used to determine the status of the rotator cuff, which may be disrupted in persons with the shoulder impingement syndrome (see later discussion).

The value of MR imaging in the assessment of the shoulder impingement syndrome has been the subject of a number of investigations.[195–197, 1426] Without question, this imaging method allows detection of abnormalities of the rotator cuff (such as changes in its signal intensity or frank disruption), the acromioclavicular joint (such as osteoarthritis with inferiorly protruding osteophytes or capsular hypertrophy), and the subacromial bursa (such as bursitis with the accumulation of bursal fluid). None of these findings, however, is specific for the shoulder impingement syndrome, being seen in asymptomatic persons[198] and in those with other causes of shoulder pain. Part of the difficulty in using MR imaging as a means to diagnose the shoulder impingement syndrome relates to the fact that, owing to constraints on patient positioning mandated by the configuration of the MR gantry, the patient typically is examined with the arm at his or her side and not in the position of impingement. The relationships of the coracoacromial arch and the components of the rotator cuff change during movement of the arm; the absence of depression of the supraspinatus tendon by the coracoacromial arch when the arm is alongside the torso does not exclude the diagnosis of shoulder impingement and, conversely, the presence of such depression with the arm in this position may occur in patients who do not have symptoms and signs of shoulder impingement. Although MR imaging may provide information regarding anatomic features such as acromial morphology that have been associated with shoulder impingement and rotator cuff abnormalities,[199] these features are not diagnostic of the shoulder impingement syndrome. Rather, as with routine radiography, the only MR imaging finding that is specific for this syndrome is a subacromial enthesophyte (Fig. 70–96). Such enthesophytes are observed on coronal oblique and sagittal MR images as bone outgrowths, often containing marrow, extending from the anteroinferior portion of the acromion. When a region of persistently low signal intensity is detected at the tip of the acromion, caution must be exercised in the interpretation of this MR imaging finding, as this appearance may relate to the normal inferior tendon slip of the deltoid muscle rather than to a subacromial enthesophyte.[200]

The severity of the shoulder impingement syndrome guides the orthopedic surgeon with regard to the choice of appropriate therapy. Most patients with stages I and II impingement respond well to conservative care (rest, avoidance of activities requiring overhead movements of the arm, and physical therapy), whereas some with stage II impingement and many with stages III and IV impingement do not respond to such conservative measures and become candidates for surgery. Some form of anterior acromioplasty generally is employed.[179, 181] This can be accomplished arthroscopically or with an open surgical procedure.[201, 202] Acromioplasty usually involves the resection of the anterior third of the undersurface of the acromion and the coracoacromial ligament, although the amount of bone removed may vary. Surprisingly, routine radiographs may reveal little evidence that an acromioplasty has been performed, although the radiodense line normally seen along the undersurface of the acromion and the distal portion of the clavicle may be absent. MR images commonly reveal artifacts, especially with gradient echo sequences, presumably related to small metal fragments that break off from the burring implements used during surgery.[203] The signal intensity within the remaining portions of the acromion may be altered, with regions of decreased signal intensity in both T1- and T2-weighted spin echo images.[203] MR findings related to surgical repairs of the rotator cuff also may be evident (see later discussion).

Rotator Cuff Tears

Classification. A variety of methods have been used to classify failure of the rotator cuff. One simple method is to divide tears of the rotator cuff into those that are acute and those that are chronic. Acute tears occur suddenly or as a result of a definite injury; chronic tears have existed for a long time, generally measured in months or even years.[204] Acute tears have been reported to represent less than 10 per cent of all tears of the rotator cuff.[205] A chronic tear is at risk for acute extension, with the sudden failure of additional fibers and the onset of new clinical manifestations.[204]

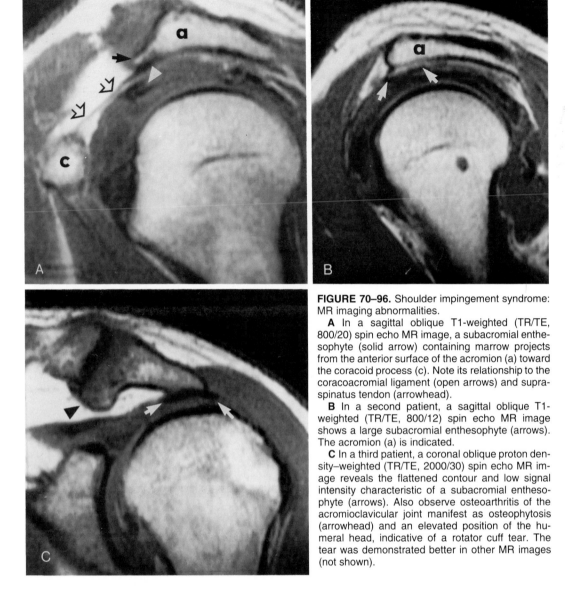

FIGURE 70–96. Shoulder impingement syndrome: MR imaging abnormalities.

A In a sagittal oblique T1-weighted (TR/TE, 800/20) spin echo MR image, a subacromial enthesophyte (solid arrow) containing marrow projects from the anterior surface of the acromion (a) toward the coracoid process (c). Note its relationship to the coracoacromial ligament (open arrows) and supraspinatus tendon (arrowhead).

B In a second patient, a sagittal oblique T1-weighted (TR/TE, 800/12) spin echo MR image shows a large subacromial enthesophyte (arrows). The acromion (a) is indicated.

C In a third patient, a coronal oblique proton density–weighted (TR/TE, 2000/30) spin echo MR image reveals the flattened contour and low signal intensity characteristic of a subacromial enthesophyte (arrows). Also observe osteoarthritis of the acromioclavicular joint manifest as osteophytosis (arrowhead) and an elevated position of the humeral head, indicative of a rotator cuff tear. The tear was demonstrated better in other MR images (not shown).

A second method of classification relates to the depth of the rotator cuff tear (Fig. 70–97). Full-thickness (or complete) tears extend from the articular surface to the bursal surface of the cuff, and partial-thickness (or incomplete) tears involve only the articular surface or the bursal surface of the cuff. A tear within the substance of the rotator cuff (intrasubstance tear) represents a special type of incomplete tear.

Patte[206] has provided an extensive classification system in which lesions are divided according to their extent, their topography in the sagittal and coronal planes, the quality of the involved muscle, and the status of the tendon of the long head of the biceps brachii muscle. In this system, the extent of the lesion is measured in centimeters at the level of the bone insertion and is judged as grade I (partial-thickness and full-thickness tears measuring less than 1 cm in their sagittal diameter), grade II (full-thickness tears that measure approximately 2 cm in their sagittal diameter and that usually are confined to the supraspinatus tendon), grade III (full-thickness tears that measure 4 cm or more in their sagittal diameter and that involve not only the supraspinatus

tendon but also other tendons such as the infraspinatus and subscapularis tendons), and grade IV (massive full-thickness tears with secondary osteoarthritis of the glenohumeral joint). The topography of the tears in the sagittal plane relates to their extent with respect to specific components of the rotator cuff which, from anterior to posterior, are: subscapularis tendon, coracohumeral ligament, supraspinatus tendon, and infraspinatus (as well as teres minor) tendon. Segment 1 lesions are isolated to the subscapularis tendon, usually resulting from a traumatic evolution rather than a degenerative lesion. Segment 2 lesions are isolated to the coracohumeral ligament and, again, typically are traumatic in nature. Segment 3 lesions generally are isolated to the supraspinatus tendon, although additional involvement of other segments also may be seen. Segments 4 and 5 lesions involve the supraspinatus tendon and the superior half (segment 4) or all (segment 5) of the infraspinatus tendon. Segment 6 lesions involve all the components of the rotator cuff. Anterosuperior lesions of the rotator cuff involve segments 1, 2, and 3; superior lesions of the cuff involve segments 2 and 3; and posterosuperior lesions of

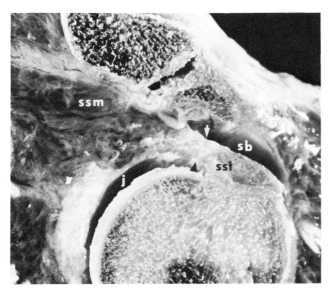

FIGURE 70–97. Rotator cuff tears: Classification system based on depth of the tear. A coronal section of the glenohumeral joint shows portions of the supraspinatus muscle (ssm) and tendon (sst), subacromial bursa (sb), and glenohumeral joint (j). Partial-thickness tears of the rotator cuff may involve either the bursal (arrow) or articular (arrowhead) side of the cuff, or they may occur within its substance. Those on the bursal side of the cuff may be detected by subacromial-subdeltoid bursography, but they are invisible on glenohumeral joint arthrograms. Partial-thickness tears involving the articular side of the cuff may be detected by glenohumeral joint arthrography but not by subacromial-subdeltoid bursography. Intrasubstance tears are not detected with either glenohumeral joint arthrography or subacromial-subdeltoid bursography. Full-thickness tears allow communication of the glenohumeral joint and the subacromial-subdeltoid bursa and may be detected with injection of contrast material into either structure.

the cuff involve segments 4 and 5. This classification system also considers the topography of the tear in the coronal plane. Three stages are described related to the degree of retraction of the tendon proximal to the tear. Finally, the system also is based on the extent of fatty degeneration of the involved muscle (as determined by CT) and on the status of the tendon of the long head of the biceps brachii muscle (i.e., normal, displaced, or torn).

The value of this comprehensive classification system is not proved, but it does emphasize the importance of determining not only the depth of the lesion (i.e., partial-thickness versus full-thickness) but also its coronal and sagittal extent. Although lesions of the rotator cuff generally begin in the supraspinatus tendon, their extension into other components of the rotator cuff is well established, and such extension influences the therapeutic options available and, ultimately, the likelihood of partial or complete recovery of shoulder function.

Incidence. Much of the data regarding the incidence of rotator cuff tears are based upon studies of cadaveric shoulders. In these shoulders, derived mainly from persons who were elderly at the time of death, the reported incidence of full-thickness tears of the rotator cuff has varied from about 5 to 25 per cent,[181, 182, 207–209] and that of partial-thickness tears of the rotator cuff has varied from about 12 to 35 per cent.[204, 205, 207, 209, 210] Data regarding the incidence of rotator cuff tears in living patients are more limited. Such tears

appear to be common in patients who have sustained one or more dislocations of the glenohumeral joint, particularly those older than 50 years of age. In one study, Pettersson[211] noted arthrographic evidence of a partial-thickness or full-thickness tear of the rotator cuff in 30 per cent of patients in the fourth decade of life who had had an anteroinferior dislocation of the glenohumeral joint and in 60 per cent of patients in the sixth decade of life who had had such a dislocation.[204]

The general consensus indicates that partial-thickness tears of the rotator cuff are more common than full-thickness tears and that those of the articular side of the rotator cuff probably are slightly more common than those of the bursal side of the rotator cuff. Intratendinous tears appear to be less frequent than those involving the articular or bursal portion of the rotator cuff. As no standard exists that allows detection of all intrasubstance tears, their true incidence is difficult to ascertain.

The incidence of rotator cuff disruption increases in the later decades of life. The discovery of chronic tears of the rotator cuff as incidental findings on chest radiographs obtained for unrelated reasons is well known. The strength of human tendons decreases in older persons; as an example, it has been shown that the strength of the anterior cruciate ligament in a person in the eighth decade of life is only about 25 per cent of that in a person in the third decade of life.[204]

Etiology and Pathogenesis. Proposed causes of rotator cuff failure have included trauma, attrition, ischemia, and impingement.[204] An association of rotator cuff tears and acute traumatic episodes is well known. One example of this is an isolated rupture of the subscapularis tendon that may result from an anterior dislocation of the glenohumeral joint.[212, 213] This type of rupture predominates in men and in persons over the age of 40 years. It differs from an avulsion fracture of the lesser tuberosity at the site of insertion of the subscapularis tendon, which occurs in elderly women and men,[214] and from tears of the subscapularis tendon that accompany disruptions of most or all of the components of the rotator cuff. Superior dislocations of the glenohumeral joint also are accompanied by disruption of the rotator cuff, as the humeral head is driven upward acutely through the cuff.

Most rotator cuff tears are unrelated to an acute injury. Rather, rupture of the rotator cuff occurs during movements and activities that should not—and usually do not—damage the involved musculotendinous units.[165] This occurrence can be designated a spontaneous rupture. Furthermore, the general consensus is that normal tendons do not rupture spontaneously. Although evidence to the contrary may be provided by arthroscopic evidence corroborating partial-thickness tears of the rotator cuff tendons in the "normal" shoulders of athletes,[204] these lesions may represent minor tendinous avulsion injuries rather than intratendinous tears. Most full-thickness tears of the rotator cuff appear to occur in a tendon that is weakened by some combination of age, repetitive stress, corticosteroid injection, hypovascularity, or damage produced by impingement.[204] A variety of histopathologic changes are observed in tendons prior to their rupture; these include hypoxic tendinopathy, mucinous change, tendolipomatosis, and calcifying tendinopathy, occurring either alone or in combination.[165] The manner in which these histologic abnormalities are interpreted has led to the concepts of an ischemic, degenerative, and mechanical (i.e., impingement) cause for rotator cuff disruption.

The school that emphasizes the importance of ischemic events in failure of the rotator cuff is based, in part, on anatomic studies that confirm the presence of a critical zone of hypovascularity in the distal portion of the supraspinatus tendon.[186, 215] As the supraspinatus tendon is the component of the rotator cuff that tears most often, and its site of failure corresponds closely to the location of this critical zone, hypovascularity has been implicated in the pathogenesis of rotator cuff failure. Brooks and coworkers,[170] however, did not support this concept, indicating that results of perfusion studies (in which the critical zone has been identified) do not represent proof of hypovascularity, and showing that the vascular patterns of the distal portions of both the supraspinatus and infraspinatus tendons are similar.

A second school emphasizes the importance of age-related degeneration of the tendon manifest by changes in cell arrangement, calcium deposition, fibrinoid thickening, fatty infiltration, necrosis, and rents, in the pathogenesis of failure of the rotator cuff.[204, 211, 216] The changes usually are apparent histologically in the tendons of persons in the third or fourth decade of life, and they increase in frequency and severity in the later decades.[165] The alterations may be prominent at the site of attachment of the cuff tendons to the tuberosities of the humerus, leading to tearing away of the tendinous fibers from the bone.[211, 217] The relationship of such degenerative alterations to clinical manifestations that may be interpreted as evidence of tendinitis or to complete failure of the tendon is not clear.[204] These degenerative abnormalities, however, can lead to alterations of the signal intensity in the rotator cuff on MR images that may simulate the signal intensity changes of a tendon tear (see later discussion).

A third theory regarding the pathogenesis of rotator cuff disruption emphasizes extrinsic factors rather than intrinsic factors (i.e., ischemia, degeneration). It is this school that holds to the belief that cuff impingement related to the coracoacromial arch is the most important cause of rotator cuff tears. Although, as indicated earlier, data exist that support this theory, other data tend to refute it. A relationship exists between morphologic changes in the anterior portion of the undersurface of the acromion and in the rotator cuff, supporting the concept that shoulder impingement produces cuff tears, but this relationship is not constant, and partial-thickness (or even complete) tears of the rotator cuff occur in the absence of morphologic abnormalities of the acromion.[218] Furthermore, although results of cadaveric studies, including those using scanning electron microscopy, support the detrimental effects of friction and rubbing (related to the adjacent coracoacromial arch) on the surface of the cuff, these results also confirm the occurrence of intrinsic degeneration of the cuff at a time when the coracoacromial arch is normal.[219, 220] Cadaveric studies also document isolated histologic abnormalities on the articular side of the rotator cuff, whereas the bursal side of the cuff would be expected to be more severely affected in instances of shoulder impingement.[221]

It appears likely that no single factor is responsible for most failures of the rotator cuff and that several working in concert are important in causing rotator cuff tears. Abnormalities intrinsic to the cuff, such as ischemia, contusion, and degeneration, place its fibers at risk. With the application of loads (whether repetitive or abrupt, compressive or tensile), each fiber fails when the applied force exceeds its strength.[204] This may occur a few fibers at a time or en masse (an acute tear or an acute extension of a chronic tear).[204] Once ruptured, the tendons of the cuff show little evidence of healing, perhaps related to their being bathed by the synovial fluid of the glenohumeral joint and subacromial-subdeltoid bursa. With loss of function of the rotator cuff, progressive elevation of the humeral head occurs, leading to deterioration of the glenohumeral joint, contact of the humeral head and acromion, and subacromial enthesophytes, and eventually to disorganization designated cuff arthropathy or the Milwaukee shoulder syndrome (see Chapter 45).

Clinical Abnormalities. Tears of the rotator cuff predominate in patients over the age of 40 years, in men, and in the dominant arm. Shoulder pain, stiffness, and weakening are common clinical manifestations, although patients may be entirely asymptomatic. On physical examination, shoulder crepitus may be elicited when the arm is internally rotated, abducted, and flexed. Weakness of flexion, abduction, and external rotation of the arm may be apparent. Such weakness is greater in patients with large tears and, in such patients, a defect in the rotator cuff may be palpable.

The clinical manifestations of rotator cuff disease may allow accurate diagnosis; however, in some cases, they simulate the findings of other disorders of the shoulder, such as adhesive capsulitis and calcific or noncalcific tendinitis. When the clinical diagnosis is not clear, imaging studies may provide diagnostic help.

Routine Radiographic Abnormalities. No routine radiographic findings are diagnostic of an acute rotator cuff tear that has occurred in the absence of glenohumeral joint dislocation. The peribursal fat plane, which normally is seen as a curvilinear radiolucent region about the lateral margin of the humerus on internal rotation views of the shoulder, may be obliterated in patients with acute tears of the rotator cuff, but such loss also is evident in inflammatory processes of adjacent tissues, including rheumatoid arthritis and calcific tendinitis.[141] The presence of calcification in the tendon of the supraspinatus muscle has been regarded as a finding that rarely coexists with rotator cuff disruption, although a recent arthrographic study in patients with calcific tendinitis has indicated the frequent occurrence of incomplete or complete tears of the rotator cuff.[222] Radiographs obtained during active abduction of the shoulder to 90 degrees from the horizontal or to the maximum extent that is possible may reveal narrowing of the coracoacromial distance in patients with rotator cuff disruption[223, 1367] (Fig. 70–98).

With chronic tears of the rotator cuff, a number of radiographic abnormalities may become apparent[224, 225] (Fig. 70–99):

1. *Narrowing of the acromiohumeral space.* This interosseous space may measure less than the lower limit of normal, 0.6 to 0.7 cm. The narrowing should be evident in both internal and external rotation radiographs, as some diminution of the acromiohumeral space can be seen in external rotation projections in normal persons.

2. *Reversal of the normal inferior acromial convexity.* Elevation of the humeral head leads to closer apposition of the humerus and the acromion and repeated traumatic insult

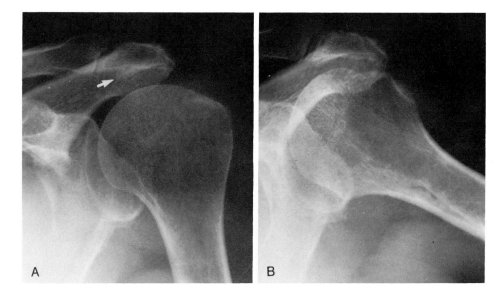

FIGURE 70–98. Rotator cuff tears: Routine radiographic abnormalities. In a 70 year old man with clinical manifestations of the shoulder impingement syndrome and a recent fall with acute exacerbation of shoulder pain, an initial anteroposterior radiograph of the shoulder **(A)** shows mild elevation of the humeral head with respect to the glenoid cavity, leading to narrowing of the acromiohumeral space, and a subacromial enthesophyte (arrow). With abduction of the arm **(B)**, note further narrowing of the acromiohumeral space.

to the acromion. Straightening and concavity of the undersurface of the acromion may then become evident. This finding must be evident on both internal rotation and external rotation projections, as a pseudoconcavity can be seen in normal persons on a single view owing to the anatomic characteristics of the acromion process.

   3. *Cystic lesions and sclerosis of the acromion and humeral head.* Small cystic lesions surrounded by a thin rim of sclerosis can be noted along the inferior aspect of the acromion. Similarly, cysts appear within the greater tuberosity in areas of bony sclerosis and contour irregularity. These latter cystic lesions may develop by the process of synovial intrusion, in which synovial fluid is forced into the

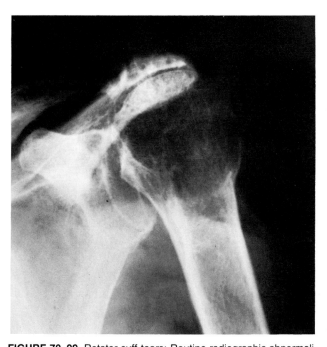

FIGURE 70–99. Rotator cuff tears: Routine radiographic abnormalities. This patient with a chronic rotator cuff tear reveals elevation of the humeral head with respect to the glenoid, contact of the humeral head and the acromion, concavity of the inferior surface of the acromion, and sclerosis and cyst formation on apposing surfaces of acromion and humeral head.

subchondral bone because of repeated stress.[226] The loss of soft tissue and the elevation of the humeral head may allow abutment of the acromion and greater tuberosity in full abduction. Notching of the superior aspect of the humeral neck also may be seen.[226]

   Several limitations of these radiographic findings as diagnostic aids in rotator cuff tears must be noted. First, apparent elevation of the humeral head with malalignment of the humerus and glenoid and narrowing of the acromiohumeral space can be an artifact of the x-ray technique related to incident beam angulation. Second, severe degeneration and atrophy of the rotator cuff without tear can lead to many of the same abnormalities that are noted in association with chronic tears of the rotator cuff. Finally, many of the radiographic changes also can appear in patients with other disorders, particularly those with ''frozen'' shoulders.

   Rotator cuff atrophy and tear can complicate a variety of articular diseases, such as rheumatoid arthritis (Fig. 70–100), ankylosing spondylitis, and septic arthritis. In these processes, synovial inflammation may lead to erosion of the undersurface of the cuff and subsequent disruption. Radiographs reveal the typical signs that are listed above and, additionally, changes of the glenohumeral joint consistent with the underlying disease (e.g., joint space narrowing, osseous erosion). In rotator cuff disruption uncomplicated by the presence of an underlying disorder, the glenohumeral joint may appear surprisingly normal, although secondary degenerative joint disease (cuff arthropathy) can develop later.

   Arthrographic Abnormalities. Standard arthrography remains a popular technique in the diagnosis of some tears of the rotator cuff. In one recent study of full-thickness tears of the rotator cuff, glenohumeral joint arthrography revealed a sensitivity of 93 per cent, an accuracy of 94 per cent, a positive predictive value of 96 per cent, and a negative predictive value of 91 per cent.[1381] Double contrast shoulder arthrography is the preferred technique. Suggested arthrographic modifications include the application of stress,[227] the supplementary use of conventional or computed tomography,[228–230] the use of digital radiographic technique,[231] and the monitoring of intra-articular pressure.[232, 233] As indicated in Chapter 13, complete tears

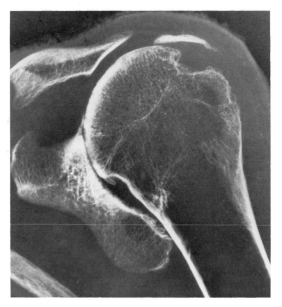

FIGURE 70–100. Rotator cuff tears: Rheumatoid arthritis. A radiograph of a coronal section of the shoulder in a cadaver with rheumatoid arthritis shows marked elevation of the humeral head with resorption of the acromion and distal portion of the clavicle, severe loss of the glenohumeral joint space, and marginal erosions of the humeral head.

of the rotator cuff are associated with abnormal communication between the glenohumeral joint cavity and the subacromial (subdeltoid) bursa (Figs. 70–101 and 70–102). Contrast material can be identified within the bursa as a large collection superior and lateral to the greater tuberosity and adjacent to the undersurface of the acromion. The contrast material in the bursa is separated from the articular cavity by a lucent area of varying size, representing the rotator cuff itself. If the musculature is thick, this lucent region is quite large, whereas if the musculature is atrophic, it is small or even absent. In the presence of a complete rotator cuff tear, contrast material is identified as a "saddle-bag" radiodense area across the surgical neck of the humerus on the axillary view. In some patients with complete tears, the contrast material will pass from the subacromial bursa into the acromioclavicular joint.[234, 235]

Using double contrast shoulder arthrography, the degree of degeneration of the torn rotator cuff can be recognized.[236, 237] Furthermore, the width of the tear itself is identified. The location of the disrupted tendons is apparent as the tendinous ends are coated by positive contrast material. In some patients, the torn rotator cuff tendons are either absent or consist of only a few small pieces.

Killoran and associates[238] have emphasized three potential sources of error in the diagnosis of a complete rotator cuff tear: Inadequate distribution of opaque material within the joint may prevent adequate visualization of the subacromial bursa; the contrast-filled sheath of the biceps tendon may project slightly lateral to the greater tuberosity on external rotation, simulating filling of the subacromial bursa; and inadvertent bursal injection may simulate a complete tear unless it is recognized that the articular cavity is not opacified.

Tears within the substance of the cuff generally will escape arthrographic detection. Tears involving the superior surface of the cuff also will not be demonstrated on gleno-

humeral joint arthrography, although they rarely may be seen with direct subacromial bursography[239] (Fig. 70–103). Tears on the inferior surface of the rotator cuff can be diagnosed on arthrography (Fig. 70–104). In these cases, an irregular circular or linear collection of contrast material may be identified above the opacified joint cavity, near the anatomic neck of the humerus[238] (Fig. 70–103). The intact superficial fibers of the rotator cuff prevent opacification of the subacromial bursa.[240] A false-negative arthrogram in the presence of a partial tear of the rotator cuff can indicate that the tear is too small for recognition or that a fibrous nodule has occluded the defect.

Ultrasonographic Abnormalities. The value of ultrasonography in the assessment of the rotator cuff is discussed in Chapter 11.

Magnetic Resonance Imaging Abnormalities

General Considerations. MR imaging has been applied to the analysis of shoulder disorders, including tears of the rotator cuff, for approximately 10 years. Although the sensitivity and specificity of MR imaging in such analysis still are debated, it is clear that technical advances such as those related to the design of surface coils have led to a gradual improvement in the quality and diagnostic accuracy of MR examinations of the shoulder. Currently, MR imaging generally is considered superior to ultrasonography and conventional arthrography in the assessment of the rotator cuff. Most MR imaging protocols used for this purpose rely heavily on standard spin echo sequences, although additional methods such as routine and volumetric gradient echo sequences, short tau inversion recovery (STIR) imaging, fat

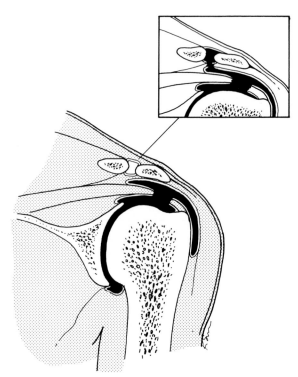

FIGURE 70–101. Full-thickness rotator cuff tears: Glenohumeral joint arthrography. Contrast material extends from the glenohumeral joint through the rotator cuff into the subacromial (subdeltoid) bursa. The inset reveals contrast material extending from the glenohumeral joint through the rotator cuff into the subacromial bursa, and from there into the acromioclavicular joint.

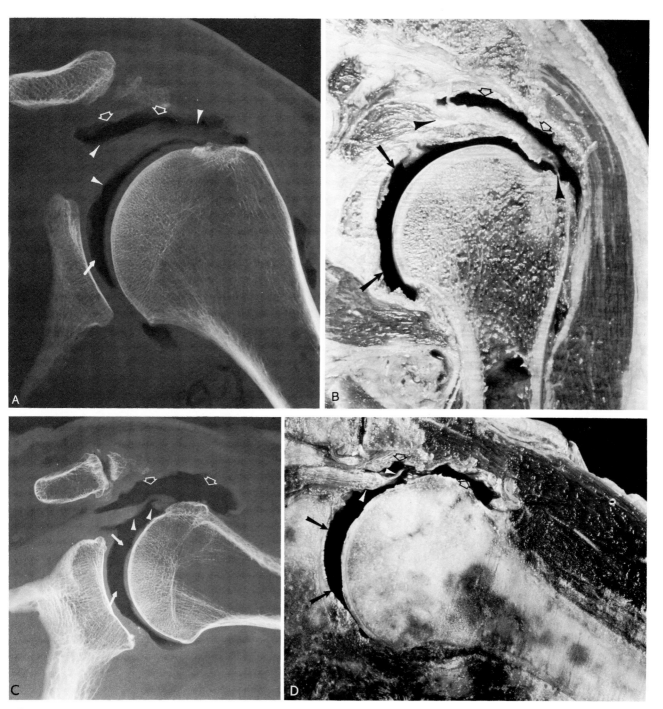

FIGURE 70–102. Full-thickness rotator cuff tears: Glenohumeral joint arthrography. These coronal sections were prepared following air arthrography of the glenohumeral joint in cadavers of elderly persons.

A, B On a corresponding sectional radiograph and photograph, note the irregular and torn rotator cuff (arrowheads), allowing communication of the glenohumeral joint (solid arrows) and subacromial (subdeltoid) bursa (open arrows).

C, D In a different cadaver, note the irregular rotator cuff (arrowheads) with communication of the glenohumeral joint (solid arrows) and subacromial (subdeltoid) bursa (open arrows). The articular cartilage is eroded.

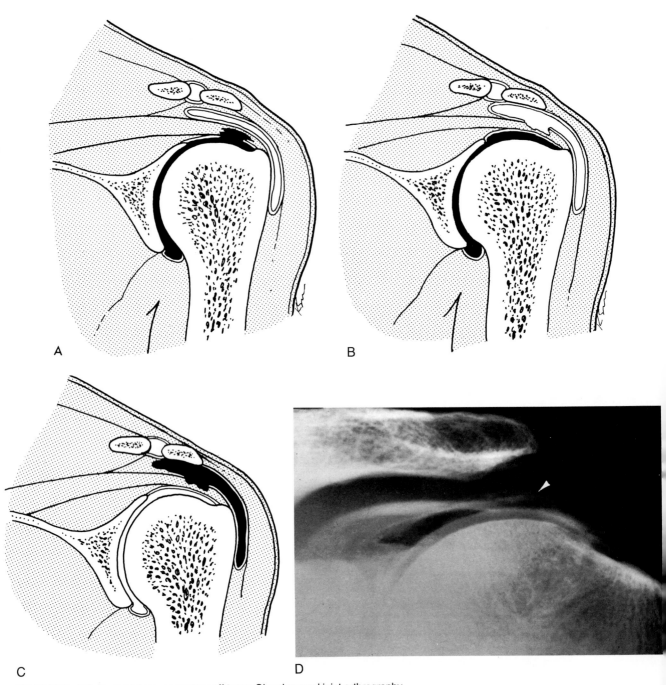

A

B

C   D

FIGURE 70–103. Partial-thickness rotator cuff tears: Glenohumeral joint arthrography.

A Diagram illustrating that a tear on the undersurface of the rotator cuff can produce an irregular collection of contrast material following opacification of the glenohumeral joint.

B, C In the presence of a partial tear on the superior surface of the rotator cuff, glenohumeral joint arthrography is unrewarding. Subacromial bursography may demonstrate an irregular collection of contrast material.

D A double contrast arthrogram reveals a partial tear (arrowhead) on the undersurface of the rotator cuff.

(Courtesy of J. Mink, M.D., Los Angeles, California.)

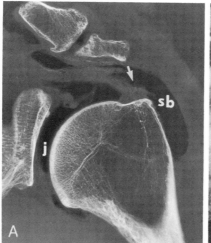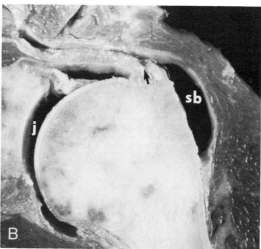

FIGURE 70–104. Partial-thickness rotator cuff tears: Glenohumeral joint arthrography and subacromial (subdeltoid) bursography. A radiograph **(A)** and photograph **(B)** of a coronal section of the shoulder made following separate injections of air into the glenohumeral joint (j) and subacromial (subdeltoid) bursa (sb) reveal degeneration with partial tearing of the superior portion (arrows) of the supraspinatus tendon.

suppression techniques, and MR arthrography may be useful (see later discussion).

The MR imaging examination of the shoulder generally emphasizes three imaging planes: a coronal oblique plane that is parallel to the long axis of the scapula and roughly parallel to the long axis of the supraspinatus tendon; a sagittal oblique plane that is perpendicular to the long axis of the scapula and roughly tangent to the glenoid cavity; and a transaxial plane (Fig. 70–105). For rotator cuff disorders, both the coronal oblique and sagittal oblique planes are useful (Figs. 70–106 and 70–107), although whether both are required for accurate diagnosis is debated.[1382] The coronal oblique plane displays much of the entire length of the supraspinatus tendon, and the sagittal oblique plane displays the coracoacromial arch (including the acromion, coracoid process, and coracoacromial ligament) and all of the components of the rotator cuff. In the transaxial plane, the subscapularis muscle and tendon are well seen, and the location of the tendon of the long head of the biceps brachii muscle can be defined.

The position of the arm during the MR imaging examination is critical to the assessment of the rotator cuff.[1368] Generally, the patient is in a supine position with the arm placed alongside his or her body. A neutral position of the arm (i.e., with the thumb up) is preferred.[241] Although some investigators favor a position of internal rotation of the arm,[196] internal rotation produces overlap of the supraspinatus and infraspinatus tendons and apparent tendon discontinuities, factors that make analysis of the rotator cuff more difficult.[242] With exaggerated external rotation of the shoulder, the tendon of the long head of the biceps brachii muscle is projected close to the critical area of the supraspinatus tendon, and fluid within the bicipital tendon sheath may simulate the appearance of a cuff tear.[242] Therefore, the neutral position of the arm is optimal.

Normal Rotator Cuff. The normal tendons of the supraspinatus, infraspinatus, teres minor, and subscapularis muscles usually have been reported as regions of low signal intensity on all MR imaging sequences, contrasting with areas of high signal intensity in these tendons on some MR imaging sequences that are characteristic of tears.[243–249] Although these differences in signal intensity in the normal and torn tendons of the rotator cuff are fundamental to the diagnosis of cuff disruption, regions of intermediate signal

intensity and inhomogeneity of signal intensity in intact tendons of the rotator cuff are encountered regularly,[250] creating some diagnostic difficulty. Specifically, regions of intermediate and, sometimes, high signal intensity within

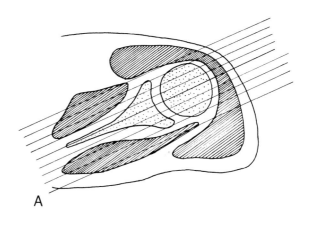

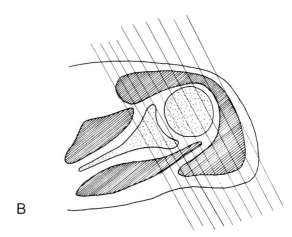

FIGURE 70–105. Rotator cuff tears: MR imaging. Imaging planes. Three MR imaging planes usually are used to study the rotator cuff. The first plane is the transaxial plane from which the orientations of the coronal oblique plane **(A)** and the sagittal oblique plane **(B)** are determined. The coronal oblique plane is parallel to the long axis of the scapula and, with the arm in a neutral position, is approximately parallel to the long axis of the supraspinatus tendon. The sagittal oblique plane is perpendicular to the long axis of the scapula.

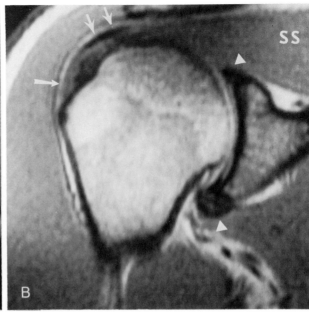

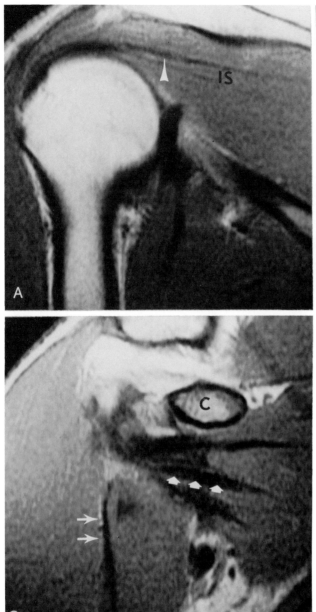

FIGURE 70–106. Normal rotator cuff: MR imaging. Coronal oblique plane. T1-weighted (TR/TE, 800/20) spin echo MR images.

A Posterior MR image. Note the infraspinatus muscle (IS) and its tendon (arrowhead). In this image, the infraspinatus tendon passes over the humeral head.

B Middle MR image. The supraspinatus muscle (SS) and its tendon (upper arrows) are evident. The tendon is inhomogeneous in signal intensity but contains regions of very low signal intensity. The peribursal fat plane (lower arrow) is of high signal intensity, located beneath the deltoid muscle. Superior and inferior portions of the glenoid labrum (arrowheads) are seen as triangular structures of low signal intensity.

C Anterior MR image. Note the subscapularis muscle and its tendinous fibers (short arrows) attaching to the lesser tuberosity of the humerus. A portion of the tendon of the long head of the biceps brachii muscle (long arrows) and the coracoid process (c) are seen.

(From Kursunoglu-Brahme S, et al: Radiol Clin North Am 28: 941, 1990.)

the outer portion of the supraspinatus tendon on T1-weighted and proton density spin echo MR images have been documented both in cadavers with grossly intact tendons and in asymptomatic living persons.[221, 251] These regions may be more conspicuous and more clearly defined with fat suppression MR imaging.[252] The pathogenesis of such regions of intermediate or high signal intensity is not agreed upon, resulting in the emergence of several different theories.

1. *Magic angle phenomenon.* As indicated earlier in this chapter, the spin-spin relaxation for poorly hydrated tissues such as tendons depends on the orientation of the tissues in the magnetic field because of the effects of anisotropy of water molecule motion.[83, 84, 253] Higher signal intensity within normal tendons oriented obliquely to the direction of the main magnetic field, rather than parallel or perpendicular to it, may occur and could account for the regions

of intermediate and high signal intensity in the supraspinatus tendon that are seen on MR images employing short echo times (TE).

2. *Partial volume averaging.* As the distal portion of the supraspinatus tendon may contain fat and muscle fibers in addition to tendinous fibers, averaging of signal intensity of these various components theoretically could occur if the imaging plane were not strictly parallel to the supraspinatus tendon.[250] The persistence of regions of intermediate signal intensity within the supraspinatus tendon on fat-suppressed MR images[252, 253] does not support the importance of volume averaging as a causative factor, however. Furthermore, inability to detect TE-dependent signal oscillation (i.e., in phase and opposed phases of protons of different bindings) typical of fat within these regions on gradient echo images also suggests that partial volume averaging with peritendinous adipose tissue is not a likely cause of areas of increased signal intensity.

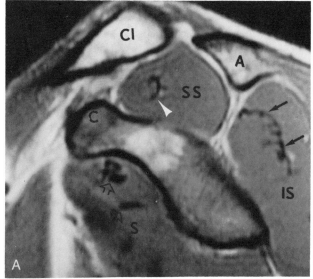

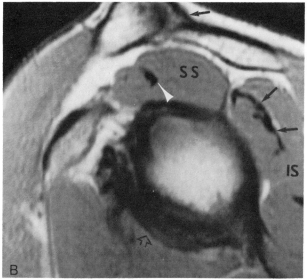

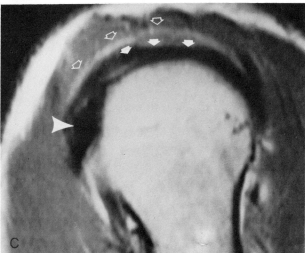

FIGURE 70–107. Normal rotator cuff: MR imaging. Sagittal oblique plane. T1-weighted (TR/TE, 800/20) spin echo MR images.

A Medial MR image. Note the acromion (A), clavicle (Cl), and coracoid process (C). The supraspinatus muscle (SS) and its tendon (arrowhead), the infraspinatus muscle (IS) and its tendon (solid arrows), and the subscapularis muscle (S) and its tendon (open arrows) are shown.

B Middle MR image. Note the region of the acromioclavicular joint (solid arrow), the supraspinatus muscle (SS) and its tendon (arrowhead), the infraspinatus muscle (IS) and its tendon (solid arrows), and the subscapularis tendon (open arrow). A fat plane is seen above and in front of the supraspinatus muscle.

C Lateral MR image. The tendons of the supraspinatus and infraspinatus muscles are seen as a curvilinear region of low signal intensity (solid arrows). The subscapularis tendon (arrowhead) at its site of insertion in the lesser tuberosity is identified. The peribursal fat plane (open arrows) can be seen.

(From Kursunoglu-Brahme S, et al: Radiol Clin North Am *28:* 941, 1990.)

3. *Tendon and muscle anatomy.* The supraspinatus muscle has been reported to consist of two distinct portions: A fusiform portion originates from the anterior supraspinous fossa and inserts via a dominant tendon anteriorly on the greater tuberosity; a second portion of the supraspinatus muscle is located posteriorly with muscle fibers originating from the posterior aspect of the supraspinous fossa and the scapular spine.[253] Several distinct tendinous slips originate from this second portion of the supraspinatus muscle and attach to the greater tuberosity. The orientation of the dominant tendon differs from that of the main muscle by approximately 10 degrees.[253] This anatomic complexity of the distal few centimeters of the supraspinatus tendon may explain its inhomogeneous signal intensity.

4. *Histologic changes in the tendon.* The occurrence of eosinophilic, fibrillar, and mucoid changes in the tendinous fibers of the supraspinatus muscle, which has been confirmed in cadavers,[221] may account for the regions of inhomogeneous and intermediate signal intensity. Such changes, interpreted as evidence of tendon degeneration (i.e., tendinosis, tendinopathy), are discussed later in this chapter.

Although the cause of altered signal intensity within the supraspinatus tendon remains unclear, these changes should not be interpreted as evidence of tendon disruption.[200, 254]

As a general rule, the signal intensity of nondisrupted tendons of the rotator cuff, including the supraspinatus tendon, on T2-weighted spin echo MR images is equal to or less than that on T1-weighted and proton density spin echo MR images. When the signal intensity of the rotator cuff tendons on T2-weighted spin echo images is higher than that on T1-weighted and proton density spin echo MR images, a tendon disruption usually is present. Unfortunately, however, there are exceptions to this rule (see later discussion).

The musculotendinous junction of the supraspinatus muscle generally is apparent over the center of the humeral head (i.e., at the 12 o'clock position) on coronal oblique MR images with the arm held in neutral position. Some variation in this position can be normal, however. Neumann and coworkers,[251] in a study of 55 shoulders in 32 asymptomatic volunteers, observed that the musculotendinous junction was located 15 degrees lateral to the 12 o'clock position in 18 shoulders (33 per cent), 30 degrees lateral to the 12 o'clock position in 4 shoulders (7 per cent), and 15 degrees medial to this 12 o'clock position in 3 shoulders (6 per cent). Some 93 per cent of all musculotendinous junctions in these volunteers were found in a 30 degree radius (i.e., 15 degrees medial to 15 degrees lateral to the 12 o'clock position).

The fat that surrounds the subacromial-subdeltoid bursa generally can be identified on MR images. Although failure to visualize this fat plane has been emphasized as a finding consistent with rotator cuff disruption (see later discussion), portions of it, particularly the subacromial portion, may not be visualized on MR images of asymptomatic persons.[200, 251, 252, 254] Furthermore, small amounts of fluid normally may be present in the subacromial-subdeltoid bursa or in the glenohumeral joint, or in both locations; the detection of such fluid collections during MR imaging of the shoulder is not diagnostic of a tear of the rotator cuff.

Full-Thickness Tears of the Rotator Cuff. The MR imaging features of full-thickness tears of the rotator cuff have been detailed in a number of publications.[241, 244, 246–248, 255–262] The most definite and direct feature of such tears is a tendinous defect that is filled with fluid or granulation tissue, or both (Figs. 70–108 to 70–111). A second direct feature is retraction of the musculotendinous junction beyond the limits of normal (see previous discussion). When the first of these two signs is present alone or when both the first and the second of these signs are present together, the diagnosis of a full-thickness tear of the rotator cuff can be made confidently. When the second finding alone is present, such a tear is likely, although as previously indicated, there is variability in the location of the musculotendinous junction of the supraspinatus muscle in asympto-

matic persons, and this location is influenced by the precise position of the arm during the MR imaging examination. The absence of either of these two direct signs does not exclude the presence of a tear. Small full-thickness tears or those accompanied by scar formation may not reveal obvious regions of tendinous discontinuity on MR images (Fig. 70–112). In these cases, morphologic alterations (e.g., ill-definition, attenuation, or thickening) of the involved segment of the tendon may be evident. Furthermore, small full-thickness tears of the rotator cuff may not be associated with retraction of the musculotendinous junction.

A number of secondary signs of a full-thickness tear of the rotator cuff have been described (Fig. 70–112), but none of these occurring in isolation is diagnostic of such a tear. These signs include: fluid in the subacromial-subdeltoid bursa; fluid in the glenohumeral joint; loss of the peribursal fat plane; and muscle atrophy. The first of these findings, fluid in the subacromial-subdeltoid bursa, may occur in asymptomatic persons or in those with bursitis. Similarly, fluid in the glenohumeral joint also is encountered in asymptomatic persons and may occur in association with arthritis. Although fluid in both the bursa and the joint may be more specific for the diagnosis of rotator cuff disruption than fluid in either one of these locations, this pattern, too, is not diagnostic of a tendon tear and may be evident in patients with inflammatory articular and bursal

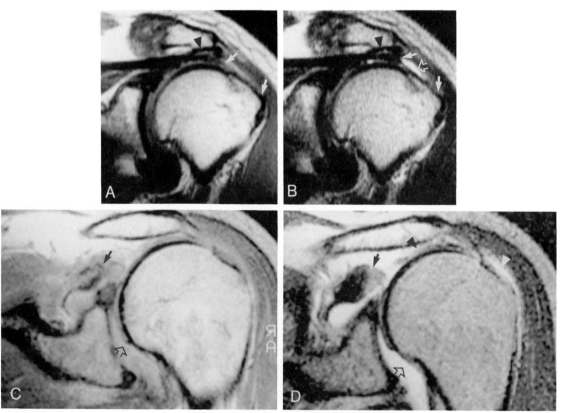

FIGURE 70–108. Full-thickness rotator cuff tears: MR imaging.
  A, B Coronal oblique proton density–weighted (TR/TE, 2000/30) **(A)** and T2-weighted (TR/TE, 2000/80) **(B)** spin echo MR images show discontinuity of the supraspinatus tendon. The tendinous gaps (between solid arrows) are filled with fluid, which is of high signal intensity (open arrow) in **B**. A subacromial enthesophyte (arrowheads) is evident.
  C, D In a second patient, coronal oblique proton density–weighted (TR/TE, 2000/20) **(C)** and T2-weighted (TR/TE, 2000/80) **(D)** spin echo MR images show evidence of a chronic full-thickness tear of the rotator cuff. The supraspinatus tendon is retracted (solid arrows), the humeral head is elevated, and there is fluid in the glenohumeral joint (open arrows) and subacromial-subdeltoid bursa (arrowheads).
  (Courtesy of T. Broderick, M.D., Orange, California.)

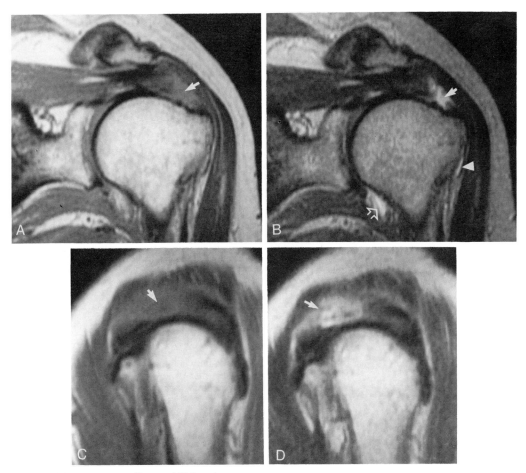

FIGURE 70–109. Full-thickness rotator cuff tears: MR imaging.
A, B In the coronal oblique plane, proton density–weighted (TR/TE, 2000/20) **(A)** and T2-weighted (TR/TE, 2000/60) **(B)** spin echo MR images show fluid in a gap (solid arrows) in the supraspinatus tendon, the fluid being of increased signal intensity in **B.** Also in **B**, note increased signal intensity related to fluid in the glenohumeral joint (open arrow) and subdeltoid bursa (arrowhead). Osteoarthritis of the acromioclavicular joint is evident.
C, D In the same patient, sagittal oblique proton density–weighted (TR/TE, 2000/20) **(C)** and T2-weighted (TR/TE, 2000/60) **(D)** spin echo MR images show the site (arrows) of disruption of the supraspinatus tendon, which is of high signal intensity in **D.**

processes (e.g., rheumatoid arthritis). The loss of the peribursal fat plane is a documented feature of rotator cuff disruption, related to bursal fluid, granulation tissue or scar formation, but it also is a finding seen in asymptomatic persons. Chronic rotator cuff tears are associated with muscle atrophy, but such atrophy also is apparent in patients with neurologic compromise, adhesive capsulitis, and other conditions in which shoulder movement is restricted or absent.

The accumulation of fluid or granulation tissue, or both, in a site of tendon discontinuity leads to a characteristic change in signal intensity evident in about 80 per cent of rotator cuff tears: high signal intensity on T2-weighted spin echo MR images.[257] In about 20 per cent of rotator cuff tears, no such increased signal intensity is evident. In these cases, the diagnosis of a tear is based upon other MR imaging findings related to altered tendon morphology (Fig. 70–113). Extreme caution should be exercised, however, in diagnosing a rotator cuff tear based solely on morphologic alterations, as similar alterations of the tendon may be observed in patients with degenerative abnormalities (tendinosis or tendinopathy) or calcific tendinitis. Analysis of coronal oblique and sagittal oblique images provides information regarding the extent of the full-thickness rotator cuff

tear. As indicated earlier, initial tears in the supraspinatus tendon may extend anteriorly to involve the coracohumeral ligament and subscapularis tendon or posteriorly to involve the infraspinatus tendon and, rarely, the teres minor tendon, or anteriorly and posteriorly to involve the entire cuff. The width of the tendon gap also can be gauged by the size of the high signal intensity region and the presence of tendon retraction. The retracted margin may be of normal size or thickened, the latter related to hemorrhage, edema, fibrosis, or reparative tissue. With massive tears that extend anteriorly to involve the subscapularis tendon or in those that are isolated to the subscapularis tendon,[1383] the bicipital tendon may dislocate medially and, in some cases, may become entrapped within the joint (see later discussion).

The published accuracy of MR imaging in the diagnosis of rotator cuff tears has varied. Zlatkin and collaborators[255] were able to diagnose all 17 surgically confirmed full-thickness tears on the basis of MR imaging abnormalities. These authors diagnosed small full-thickness tears of the rotator cuff following analysis of MR images in two patients who had partial-thickness tears confirmed at surgery. Rafii and colleagues,[257] using MR imaging in the assessment of 31 full-thickness tears that subsequently were confirmed surgically, reported a sensitivity of 0.97, a specificity of 0.94,

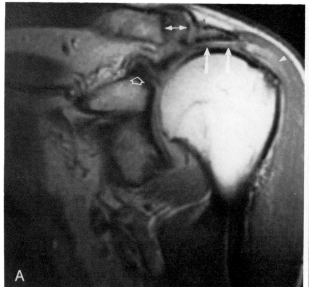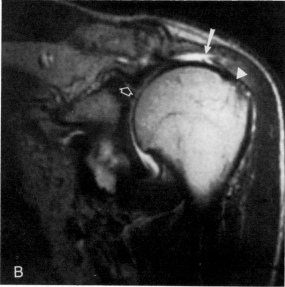

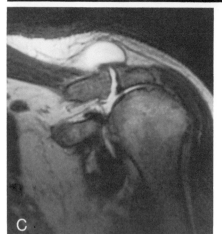

FIGURE 70–110. Full-thickness rotator cuff tears: MR imaging.

A A coronal oblique proton density-weighted (TR/TE, 2000/20) spin echo MR image reveals discontinuity of the supraspinatus tendon (solid arrows), an elevated humeral head with narrowing of the acromiohumeral space, obliteration of the peribursal fat plane (arrowhead), osteoarthritis of the acromioclavicular joint (double-headed arrow), and an ovoid region of low signal intensity (open arrow) which, at arthroscopy, proved to be an intra-articular body.

B A coronal oblique T2-weighted (TR/TE, 2000/70) spin echo MR image reveals fluid within the subacromial bursa (closed arrow) and within a full-thickness tear of the supraspinatus tendon, the intra-articular body (open arrow), and irregularity of the greater tuberosity of the humerus (arrowhead) related to the shoulder impingement syndrome.

(**A, B** From Kursunoglu-Brahme S, et al: Radiol Clin North Am *28:*941, 1990.)

C In a different patient, a coronal oblique T2-weighted (TR/TE, 4100/96) fast spin echo MR image reveals a chronic and massive tear of the rotator cuff. The humeral head contacts the acromion. Fluid of high signal intensity is seen in the glenohumeral and acromioclavicular joints and in a mass (synovial cyst) above the acromioclavicular joint.

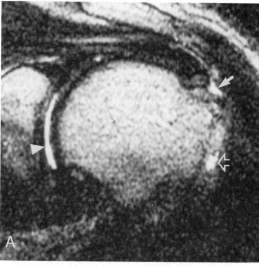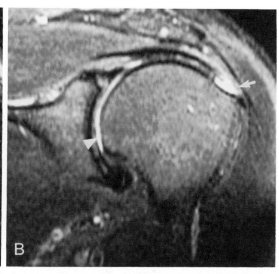

FIGURE 70–111. Full-thickness rotator cuff tears: MR imaging.

A A coronal oblique T2-weighted (TR/TE, 4000/92) fast spin echo MR image shows fluid of high signal intensity in the glenohumeral joint (arrowhead), in a small gap in the supraspinatus tendon (solid arrow), and in the subdeltoid bursa (open arrow). The findings suggest the presence of a partial-thickness bursal-sided tear of the tendon.

B In the same patient, a coronal oblique T2-weighted (TR/TE, 5000/76) fast spin echo MR image obtained with chemical presaturation of fat (ChemSat) better defines the extent of this full-thickness tear of the supraspinatus tendon. Note fluid of high signal intensity in the joint (arrowhead) and in the tendinous gap (solid arrow).

(Courtesy of S. K. Brahme, M.D., La Jolla, California.)

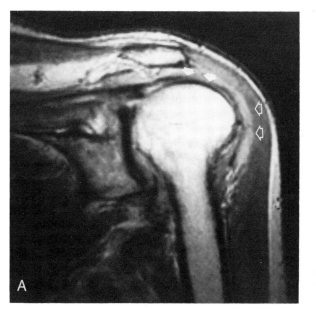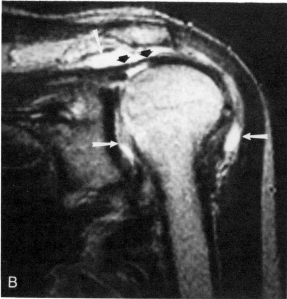

FIGURE 70–112. Full-thickness rotator cuff tears: MR imaging.

A A coronal oblique proton density-weighted (TR/TE, 2000/20) spin echo MR image, obtained with the arm in internal rotation, shows diffuse thinning of the supraspinatus tendon (solid arrows), atrophy of the supraspinatus muscle, and distention of the subdeltoid bursa (open arrows).

B A coronal oblique T2-weighted (TR/TE, 2000/70) spin echo MR image confirms the presence of an attenuated supraspinatus tendon (small arrows) and reveals fluid of increased signal intensity in the glenohumeral joint and subacromial-subdeltoid bursa (large arrows).

(From Kursunoglu-Brahme S, et al: Radiol Clin North Am 28:941, 1990.)

and accuracy of 0.95, a positive predictive value of 0.94, and a negative predictive value of 0.97. Iannotti and co-workers,[259] in an analysis of MR imaging in 33 surgically confirmed full-thickness tears of the rotator cuff, indicated 100 per cent sensitivity and 95 per cent specificity in the assessment of these tears with MR imaging. Nelson and collaborators[260] also reported high accuracy regarding the diagnosis of full-thickness tears of the rotator cuff using MR imaging. Based on these results, it appears that experienced observers interpreting carefully performed MR imaging examinations will provide an accurate diagnosis of a full-thickness rotator cuff tear in more than 90 per cent of patients with such tears, although occasionally they will provide an incorrect diagnosis of a full-thickness tear when a partial-thickness tear or degenerative tendinopathy is present. Less experienced observers, obviously, will not do as well, and both experienced and inexperienced observers will be less successful in correctly diagnosing partial-thickness tears of the rotator cuff.

In an attempt to improve diagnostic accuracy in cases of full-thickness (and partial-thickness) rotator cuff tears, some investigators have employed MR arthrography, accomplished by the injection of gadolinium compounds (or saline) into the glenohumeral joint.[263, 264] This technique combines the advantages of both MR imaging and standard arthrography. The injection of gadolinium compounds

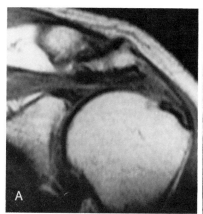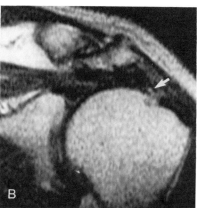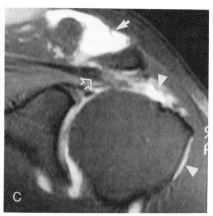

FIGURE 70–113. Full-thickness rotator cuff tears: MR imaging and MR arthrography. Coronal oblique proton density (TR/TE, 2000/20) **(A)** and T2-weighted (TR/TE, 2000/80) **(B)** spin echo MR images show osteoarthritis of the acromioclavicular joint and an enlarged and irregular distal portion of the supraspinatus tendon. Only one region of the tendon, however, reveals increased signal intensity in **B** (arrow). A coronal oblique T1-weighted (TR/TE, 650/20) spin echo MR image obtained with chemical presaturation of fat (ChemSat) following the intra-articular administration of a gadolinium compound **(C)** reveals the high signal intensity of the contrast agent in the glenohumeral joint, subacromial-subdeltoid bursa (arrowheads), and acromioclavicular joint (solid arrow). Note the completely torn and retracted supraspinatus tendon (open arrow).

rather than saline allows the use of T1-weighted spin echo MR images in which the gadolinium compounds have high signal intensity (Fig. 70–114). The main advantage of MR arthrography is direct opacification of full-thickness rotator cuff tears and partial-thickness tears involving the articular side of the cuff (see later discussion). Its disadvantages include a longer examination time, its cost, and its invasiveness. Furthermore, the technique is not useful in the assessment of partial-thickness tears confined to the bursal side of the cuff or intratendinous tears. Hodler and coworkers[263] reported no added accuracy in the diagnosis of full-thickness tears when results of MR arthrography were compared with those of standard MR imaging. These investigators emphasized the value of MR arthrography in the assessment of partial-thickness tears of the rotator cuff, however. One diagnostic pitfall encountered with MR arthrography that may lead to a false-positive diagnosis of a full-thickness tear relates to misinterpretation of the peribursal fat plane as evidence of contrast medium that has leaked into the subacromial-subdeltoid bursa. This pitfall can be eliminated if fat-suppression methods are used in combination with the MR arthrogram.[265, 266] The resulting suppression of the signal intensity from the peribursal fat allows detection of even small amounts of contrast material within the subacromial-subdeltoid bursa (see Fig. 70–113). The main value of MR arthrography of the shoulder performed with or without fat suppression is related to the detection of partial-thickness tears involving the articular side of the rotator cuff and to the differentiation of partial-thickness and small full-thickness tears of the rotator cuff.

The intravenous administration of gadolinium compounds has also been used to investigate rotator cuff disease, including tears (Fig. 70–115). Enhancement of signal intensity in the synovial membrane and in the rotator cuff is a constant finding, but preliminary data have indicated that patterns of enhancement of signal intensity in the rotator cuff do not allow reliable differentiation of rotator cuff tears and degenerative disease (tendinopathy or tendinosis).

Partial-Thickness Tears of the Rotator Cuff. Recent years have witnessed an increased interest in the occurrence of partial-thickness tears of the rotator cuff. In large part, this has related to the increased popularity of shoulder arthroscopy that may be used to diagnose and, in some cases, treat these tears.[267] Minor lesions of the rotator cuff may be decompressed and debrided successfully using arthroscopy, whereas incomplete tears that extend into or exist within the substance of the cuff generally are treated by open surgical technique.[268] Among partial-thickness tears, deep (articular-sided) tears appear to be most frequent, followed by superficial (bursal-sided) tears and those occurring within the substance of the tendon.[268] Incomplete tears of the rotator cuff may be twice as common as full-thickness tears. The detection of partial-thickness tears of the rotator cuff with imaging methods is more difficult than that of full-thickness tears. Arthrography, bursography, and MR imaging are techniques that have diagnostic potential in the assessment of partial-thickness tears of the rotator cuff. Arthrography is useful only in instances of articular-sided defects, and accurate detection of these defects may require filming following exercise of the patient's shoulder or arthrotomographic methods. Bursography, with opacification of the subacromial-subdeltoid bursa, is technically difficult and time-consuming, and it, too, may necessitate tomographic techniques.

MR imaging in cases of partial-thickness tears of the rotator cuff requires careful analysis of patterns of signal intensity and of morphologic alterations in the distal portion of the tendons, particularly the supraspinatus tendon. The value of secondary MR imaging signs of cuff abnormalities in these cases has been emphasized,[255] but these signs lack specificity. Even with such analysis, the results of the MR imaging examinations are not as good diagnostically as in cases of full-thickness tears of the rotator cuff. In five cases of surgically confirmed partial-thickness tears of the rotator cuff, Zlatkin and coworkers,[255] on the basis of MR imaging abnormalities, reported an accurate interpretation in one patient and inaccurate interpretations in four patients (two partial-thickness tears of the inferior surface of the cuff were interpreted as small full-thickness tears and two such tears were interpreted as abnormal but intact tendons). Rafii and collaborators[257] indicated that in only 7 of 16 patients with surgically confirmed partial-thickness tears was the tendinous abnormality manifest as intense increased signal intensity on the T2-weighted spin echo MR images. In the remaining nine patients, focal areas of tendon interruption or depression, marked by regions of moderate to marked increased signal intensity on proton density and T2-weighted spin echo MR images, were seen. Nelson and colleagues[260] were successful in identifying partial-thickness tears of the rotator cuff with MR imaging in 5 of 7

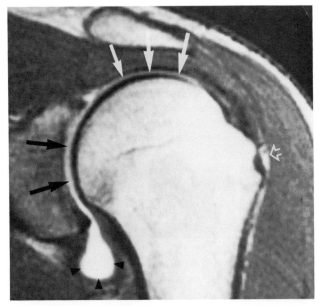

FIGURE 70–114. Normal rotator cuff: MR arthrography. A coronal oblique T1-weighted (TR/TE, 600/20) spin echo MR image following the intra-articular injection of a gadolinium compound reveals that all the contrast material remains in the glenohumeral joint. The high signal intensity fluid coats the undersurface of the supraspinatus tendon (white arrows), fills the space between the humeral head and glenoid cavity (black arrows), and distends the axillary recess (arrowheads). A source of diagnostic error with MR arthrography relates to the high signal intensity of peribursal fat (open arrow) that may be misinterpreted as evidence of fluid escaping from the joint through a full-thickness tear of the rotator cuff. (From Hodler J, et al: Radiology *182*:431, 1992.)

FIGURE 70–115. Full-thickness rotator cuff tears: MR imaging with and without intravenous gadolinium administration and MR arthrography. Coronal oblique proton density (TR/TE, 2000/20) **(A)** and T2-weighted (TR/TE, 2000/80) **(B)** spin echo MR images reveal altered signal intensity in the distal portion of the supraspinatus tendon with high signal intensity in this region in **B** (arrow). The findings are consistent with a small full-thickness tendon tear. A coronal oblique T1-weighted (TR/TE, 600/20) spin echo MR image obtained with chemical presaturation of fat (ChemSat) and immediately following intravenous administration of a gadolinium compound **(C)** shows enhancement of signal intensity in the region of the tendon tear (arrow) and in several areas of the glenohumeral joint itself. A coronal oblique T1-weighted (TR/TE, 600/15) spin echo MR image obtained with chemical presaturation of fat (ChemSat) and following intra-articular injection of a gadolinium compound **(D)** confirms a full-thickness tear of the supraspinatus tendon with the contrast agent of high signal intensity located in the tendinous gap (arrow) and in the subacromial bursa (arrowhead), as well as within the joint.

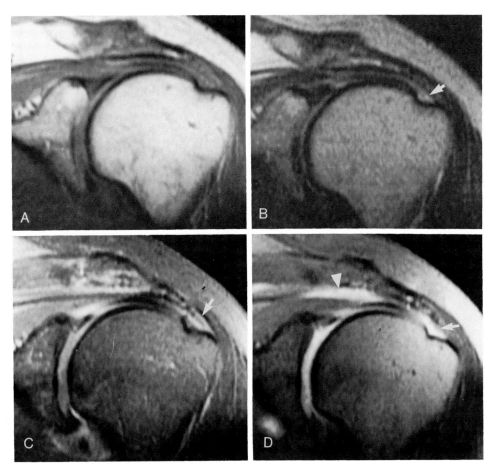

patients who had such tears confirmed surgically. Traughber and Goodwin[269] were unable to detect 4 of 9 partial-thickness tears of the rotator cuff (confirmed with arthroscopy and bursography) using MR imaging.

Careful evaluation of the pattern of increased signal intensity within the rotator cuff on T2-weighted spin echo MR images provides important information regarding the presence and the type of tear of the rotator cuff (Fig. 70–116). A region of increased signal intensity in the superficial portion of the tendon, perpendicular to the long axis of

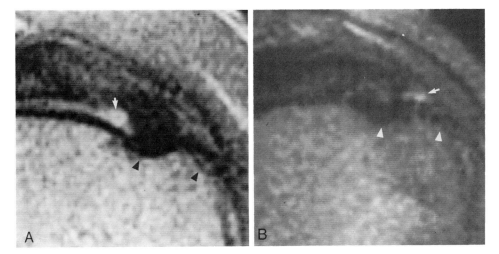

FIGURE 70–116. Partial-thickness rotator cuff tears: MR imaging.

A Partial-thickness tear of the articular side of the supraspinatus tendon. A coronal oblique T2-weighted (TR/TE, 2000/75) spin echo MR image shows a region of high signal intensity (arrow) involving the inferior or articular surface of the supraspinatus tendon. The supraspinatus tendon attaches to the flat portion of the greater tuberosity of the humerus (between arrowheads), allowing one to judge which portion of the tendon is abnormal.

B Partial-thickness tear of the bursal side of the supraspinatus tendon. A coronal oblique T2-weighted (TR/TE, 2000/75) spin echo MR image shows a linear region of high signal intensity (arrow), extending in a horizontal fashion and located in the superior or bursal portion of the tendon. The site of attachment of the supraspinatus tendon to the greater tuberosity of the humerus again is indicated (between arrowheads).

the tendon, on coronal oblique T2-weighted spin echo images is most consistent with the diagnosis of a partial-thickness tear involving the bursal side of the tendon; a similar region in the deep portion of the tendon, again perpendicular to the long axis of the tendon, on these images is most consistent with the diagnosis of a partial-thickness tear involving the articular side of the tendon; a region of increased signal intensity on T2-weighted spin echo MR images that extends in a linear fashion through the entire cuff, without retraction of the tendon, is most consistent with the diagnosis of a small full-thickness tear of the tendon; and a region of increased signal intensity on these images that is parallel to the long axis of the tendon is most consistent with the diagnosis of an intrasubstance

tear of the tendon or, perhaps, acute tendinitis. These patterns of altered signal intensity are helpful clues to correct diagnosis (Figs. 70–117 and 70–118), but they are not foolproof. Partial-thickness tears of the rotator cuff may be associated with changes in tendon morphology (attenuated or thickened tendon) and unassociated with changes in signal intensity.

Some reported studies have indicated that standard spin echo images are not sufficient for the diagnosis of partial-thickness tears of the rotator cuff.[269, 270] STIR imaging sequences may lead to increased diagnostic accuracy in such cases[269] (Fig. 70–119). Studies employing chemical presaturation of fat also may improve diagnostic accuracy,[269] but increased signal intensity in the distal portion of the tendons

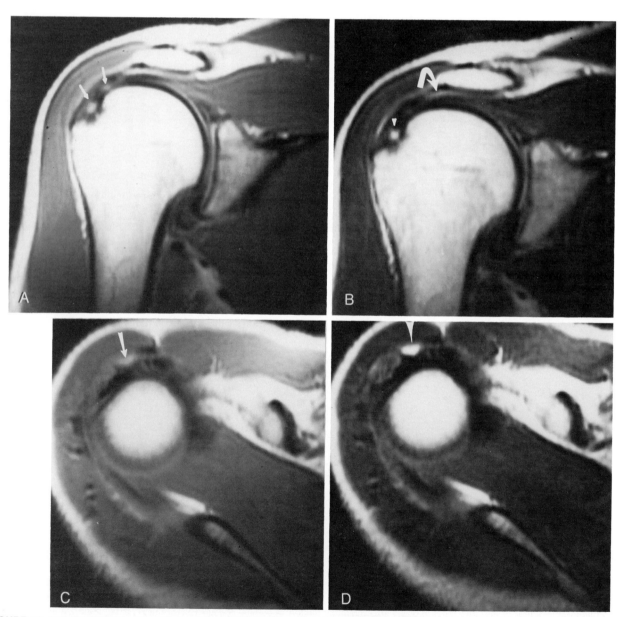

FIGURE 70–117. Partial-thickness rotator cuff tears: MR imaging. Partial-thickness tear of the articular side of the supraspinatus tendon. Coronal oblique proton density (TR/TE, 2000/20) **(A)** and T2-weighted (TR/TE, 2000/70) **(B)** spin echo MR images show two small regions of altered signal intensity (arrows in **A**) in the distal portion of the supraspinatus tendon. One of these regions shows a further increase in signal intensity (arrowhead) in **B**. There is no fluid in the subacromial-subdeltoid bursa (curved arrow in **B**). Transaxial proton density (TR/TE, 2000/20) **(C)** and T2-weighted (TR/TE, 2000/60) **(D)** spin echo MR images confirm a region of altered signal intensity in the leading edge of the supraspinatus tendon which is of intermediate signal intensity (arrow) in **C** and of high signal intensity (arrowhead) in **D**. (From Kursunoglu-Brahme S, et al: Radiol Clin North Am 28:941, 1990.)

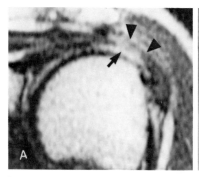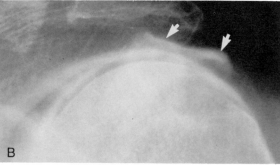

FIGURE 70–118. Partial-thickness rotator cuff tears: MR imaging and arthrography. Partial-thickness tear of the articular side of the supraspinatus tendon. A coronal oblique T2-weighted (TR/TE, 2500/60) spin echo MR image **(A)** shows a region of high signal intensity (arrow) involving the articular portion of the supraspinatus tendon. Some intact tendinous fibers (arrowheads) appear to extend over the region of high signal intensity. Glenohumeral joint arthrography **(B)** confirms a partial-thickness tear (arrows) of the supraspinatus tendon.

of the rotator cuff, even in normal tendons, is encountered with this method.[252] MR arthrography, employing the intra-articular administration of gadolinium compounds, represents an ancillary method that may increase diagnostic accuracy in patients with articular-sided partial-thickness tears of the rotator cuff[263, 264] (Fig. 70–120). Hodler and collaborators,[263] using MR arthrography, were able to correctly diagnose 6 of 13 arthroscopically proven partial-thickness tears of the articular side of the cuff. In 5 of these 13 cases, the results of the MR arthrographic study were interpreted as normal and in two, they were interpreted as evidence of a full-thickness tear.

Surgically Repaired Rotator Cuff Tears. Full-thickness and partial-thickness rotator cuff tears may be entirely asymptomatic and require no therapy. Symptomatic tears of the rotator cuff can be treated conservatively or surgically. Nonoperative methods of treatment include rest, physical therapy, anti-inflammatory medications, and corticosteroid injections. In cases of full-thickness tears that do not respond to these conservative measures, some type of operative repair, which may include tendon-to-tendon repair or tendon advancement to bone with or without an anterior acromioplasty, may be required.[271, 272] Release of the coracoacromial ligament and resection of the outer end of the clavicle also may be done.[273] Occasionally, biologic and

prosthetic grafts are used to repair large cuff defects.[204] Partial-thickness tears of the rotator cuff also may be treated surgically by principles identical to those used in the treatment of full-thickness tears. Arthroscopic management of incomplete tears with debridement, acromioplasty, and even suture placement also is possible, and an approach combining arthroscopic and open techniques can be employed.[274, 1347] Clinical manifestations following any type of surgical repair may relate to persistent or recurrent rotator cuff tear, persistent shoulder impingement, tendinitis, deltoid muscle detachment, and nerve injury.[205]

Imaging of the postoperative shoulder presents a diagnostic challenge. Even after a clinically adequate repair, glenohumeral joint arthrography may reveal communication of the joint and the subacromial-subdeltoid bursa.[275] Furthermore, owing to the presence of adhesions at the site of repair, failure to reveal such communication during arthrography does not eliminate the possibility of a persistent or recurrent rotator cuff tear. At ultrasound examination, defects in the rotator cuff may be detected,[276] although anatomic landmarks are distorted, making sonography less useful here. MR imaging also may be used to evaluate the surgically repaired rotator cuff. As reported by Owen and coworkers,[203] acromioplasty frequently results in alteration of the normal signal intensity of the fatty marrow within

FIGURE 70–119. Partial-thickness rotator cuff tears: MR imaging including STIR images. Partial-thickness tear of the articular side of the supraspinatus tendon. A coronal oblique T2-weighted (TR/TE, 2000/80) spin echo MR image **(A)** reveals a region of high signal intensity (solid arrow) involving the articular side of the supraspinatus tendon, with overlying intact tendinous fibers (arrowhead). Note the presence of a fracture (open arrow) of the greater tuberosity of the humerus and a joint effusion. A coronal oblique STIR (TR/TE, 2000/20; inversion time, 160 msec) MR image **(B)** confirms the partial-thickness tear of the tendon (solid arrow), overlying intact tendinous fibers (arrowhead), and the fracture (open arrows) of the greater tuberosity of the humerus.

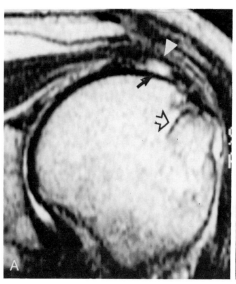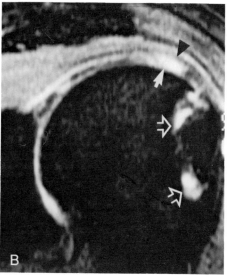

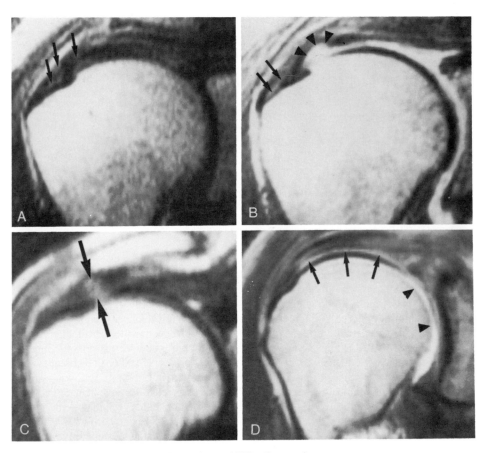

FIGURE 70–120. Partial-thickness rotator cuff tears: MR imaging and MR arthrography.

A, B Partial-thickness tears of the articular and bursal sides of the supraspinatus tendon. A coronal oblique T2-weighted (TR/TE, 2000/80) spin echo MR image **(A)** reveals minor irregularities of signal intensity (arrows) in the supraspinatus tendon, although regions of high signal intensity are not evident. A coronal oblique T1-weighted (TR/TE, 600/20) spin echo MR image following the intra-articular injection of a gadolinium compound **(B)** reveals a partial-thickness tear (arrowheads) of the articular side of the supraspinatus tendon and additional sites (arrows) of intermediate signal intensity of questionable significance. The diagnosis of a partial-thickness tear of the bursal side of the supraspinatus tendon, which was confirmed during bursoscopy, is not possible on the basis of the MR arthrographic findings.

C, D Partial-thickness tear of the bursal side of the supraspinatus tendon. A coronal oblique T2-weighted (TR/TE, 2000/80) spin echo MR image **(C)** shows a region of high signal intensity (arrows) in the supraspinatus tendon, although it is not clear if this indicates a partial-thickness or full-thickness tear. A coronal oblique T1-weighted (TR/TE, 600/20) spin echo MR image following the intra-articular administration of a gadolinium compound **(D)** confirms that the articular side of the supraspinatus tendon is normal (arrows). Note the contrast material within the joint (arrowheads). No information is provided regarding the integrity of the bursal side of the tendon, which was found to be torn during bursoscopy.

(From Hodler J, et al: Radiology *182*:431, 1992.)

the remaining portion of the acromion with persistently decreased signal intensity on both T1-weighted and T2-weighted spin echo MR images. The MR criteria for full-thickness rotator cuff tears in the shoulder after surgery are the presence of fluid-like signal intensity on T2-weighted spin echo MR images that extends through an area of the rotator cuff and the nonvisualization of a portion of the rotator cuff.[203] Although accurate in the identification of 90 per cent of such tears, Owen and collaborators[203] were unable to differentiate partial-thickness cuff tears and repaired tendons. A potential diagnostic role may exist for MR arthrography in the evaluation of complete and incomplete tears following shoulder surgery (Fig. 70–121).

Rotator Cuff Tendinitis, Tendinosis, and Tendinopathy

The designation of tendinitis often is applied loosely to a variety of shoulder problems that lead to focal pain and tenderness and subacromial crepitation. These complaints are common in persons involved in occupations requiring heavy manual labor, frequent arm elevation, and the use of hand tools.[277] Similar symptoms and signs are encountered in persons involved in sporting activities that require considerable shoulder movement. As histologic data supporting the occurrence of true tendon inflammation generally are lacking in these persons, it appears likely that a number of different disorders, such as avulsion or disruption of rotator cuff tendons and shoulder impingement, are responsible for these clinical manifestations. The vulnerability of components of the rotator cuff to ischemia and extrinsic compression during arm elevation has been addressed earlier.

Histologic abnormalities similar to those observed in ligamentous tissue about the elbow in cases of overuse syndrome[278] have been documented in some instances of rotator cuff tendinitis. Initial alterations include fibroblastic invasion and vascular granulation-like tissue that has been described as angiofibroblastic hyperplasia.[278] Subsequent alterations include similar hyperplasia, fibrosis, and vacuolar, mucoid, eosinophilic, and fibrillary degeneration with or

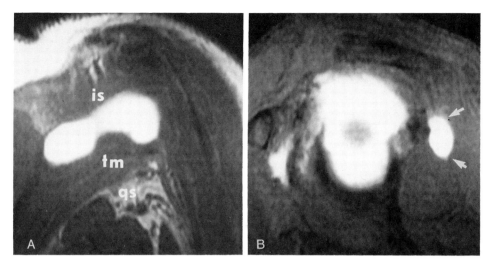

FIGURE 70-121. Full-thickness rotator cuff tears following surgical repair of the rotator cuff: MR arthrography. This patient had had tendon-to-tendon repair of a full-thickness tear of the supraspinatus and infraspinatus tendons, prior to developing recurrent shoulder pain and limitation of motion.

A A coronal oblique proton density (TR/TE, 2200/30) spin echo MR image following the intra-articular injection of a gadolinium compound shows the contrast material of high signal intensity, extending posteriorly, between the infraspinatus muscle (is) and teres minor muscle (tm). Note the quadrilateral space (qs).

B A sagittal oblique T1-weighted (TR/TE, 900/20) spin echo MR image obtained with chemical presaturation of fat (ChemSat) following the intra-articular injection of a gadolinium compound confirms the posterior leakage of contrast material (arrows).

without calcification.[221] In neither the acute nor chronic stages, however, are abundant inflammatory cells evident. When chronic inflammatory cells are detected, they are seen more commonly in the supporting tissues and not in the tendon. The histologic findings are more compatible with an ischemic or degenerative process than an inflammatory one. A more appropriate term for this process is tendinosis or tendinopathy rather than tendinitis.

The reported MR imaging characteristics of rotator cuff tendinosis or tendinopathy (i.e., tendinitis) have included increased signal intensity in a tendon with normal or abnormal morphology and an intact peribursal fat plane.[255] The increase in signal intensity generally is moderate and not extreme, creating an inhomogeneous appearance to the tendon (Fig. 70–122). It is apparent on T1-weighted and proton density spin echo MR images and is less evident on T2-weighted spin echo MR images.[257] Regions of intense signal intensity within the cuff tendons on T2-weighted spin echo MR images that is similar to the signal intensity of fluid are not compatible with the diagnosis of tendinosis or tendinopathy. Such regions suggest the presence of a full-thickness or partial-thickness tear of the rotator cuff. The MR imaging findings of tendinosis or tendinopathy can be identified in asymptomatic persons, suggesting that in most cases they lack clinical importance. Similar MR imaging findings are associated with tendon scars, perhaps related to healing of a previous tendon tear (Fig. 70–123).

Histopathologic observations using cadaveric shoulders have confirmed the presence of tendon degeneration in regions of increased signal intensity on the T1-weighted and proton density spin echo MR images[221, 257] (Fig. 70–122). Increased internal signal intensity has been shown to have

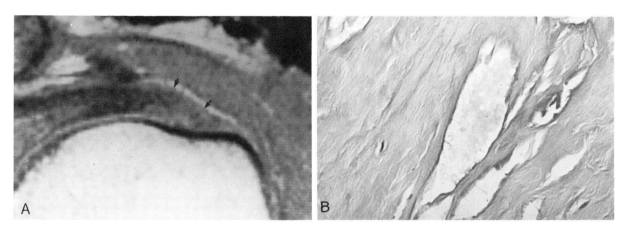

FIGURE 70-122. Tendinosis or tendinopathy of the rotator cuff: MR imaging and histopathology. A coronal oblique proton density–weighted (TR/TE, 2000/25) spin echo MR image **(A)** reveals increased signal intensity in the distal part of the supraspinatus tendon (arrows). There was no further increase in signal intensity in T2-weighted spin echo MR images. The peribursal fat plane is intact. A photomicrograph (hemtoxylin and eosin, x100) **(B)** reveals mucoid and vacuolar degeneration in the affected portion of the supraspinatus tendon. No inflammatory cells are evident. (From Kjellin I, et al: Radiology *181:*837, 1991.)

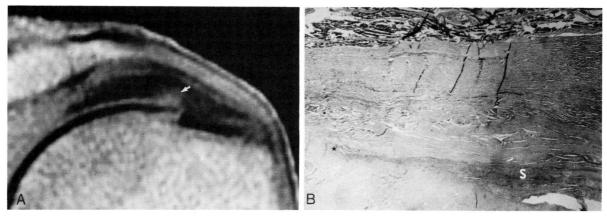

FIGURE 70–123. Tendon scar of the rotator cuff: MR imaging and histopathology. A coronal oblique proton density–weighted (TR/TE, 2000/25) spin echo MR image **(A)** shows increased signal intensity in the articular side of the distal portion of the supraspinatus tendon (arrow). There was no further increase in signal intensity in the T2-weighted spin echo MR images. A photomicrograph (hematoxylin and eosin, × 16) **(B)** demonstrates a linear scar (s) in the articular side of the supraspinatus tendon. The lateral end of the scar is indicated by an asterisk. (From Kjellin I, et al: Radiology 181:837, 1991.)

several different distributions; in general, these reflect the extent of the eosinophilic, fibrillary, and mucoid changes.[221]

Calcific tendinitis of the shoulder and other sites is discussed in Chapter 45. Calcific tendinitis is diagnosed far more easily on plain films than on MR images (Fig. 70–124). Regions of low signal intensity on all imaging sequences are typical of intratendinous (and intrabursal) calcification, but these regions may be difficult to differentiate from a thickened tendon without calcification.[279]

Adhesive Capsulitis

Adhesive capsulitis is one of several terms applied to a clinical condition in which there is severe restriction of active and passive motion of the glenohumeral joint and in which no other cause can be documented. Additional designations for this disorder are capsulitis, periarthritis, and frozen shoulder. Although some investigators prefer the term frozen shoulder to describe this disorder,[280] abnormalities in the capsule of the glenohumeral joint generally are considered fundamental to its pathogenesis, such that the designation adhesive capsulitis is preferred by this author. A similar condition may involve the ankle, wrist, and hip.

Several different systems have been introduced to classify adhesive capsulitis of the shoulder. Lundberg[281] divided the condition into two categories: primary disease, in which no predisposing cause or event can be documented; and secondary disease, in which a traumatic injury has occurred previously. Other investigators use classification systems based on the degree of restriction of the joint capsule,[282] the results of physical examination done with the patient under anesthesia,[283] or the arthrographic findings.[284]

Most patients with adhesive capsulitis are between the ages of 40 and 70 years. Predisposing factors include trauma (Fig. 70–125), hemiplegia, cerebral hemorrhage, diabetes mellitus, hyperthyroidism, and cervical disc disease. Many patients report a period during which the shoulder has been immobile related to pain, injury, cervical spondylosis, or other causes.[280] Unilateral involvement of the shoulder predominates, although subsequent involvement of the opposite shoulder may occur in as many as 20 per cent of patients. Three stages, or phases, of the disease are

recognized[280]: the painful phase, characterized by progressive pain, usually worse at night, over a period of weeks to months; the stiffening phase, 4 to 12 months in length, characterized by slowly progressive loss of shoulder motion; and the thawing phase, usually weeks to months in duration, during which shoulder motion is regained gradually. Although adhesive capsulitis commonly is a self-limited condition that lasts about 12 to 18 months, its outcome is variable and, in some cases, full recovery of shoulder motion never occurs.

The pathogenesis and gross morphologic abnormalities of adhesive capsulitis have been investigated extensively. These investigations have been summarized by Murnaghan.[280] Fifty years ago, Neviaser[285] described the capsular changes that characterize this condition, which consisted of thickening and contraction, and he introduced the term adhesive capsulitis. Approximately 6 years later, McLaughlin[286] confirmed the capsular alterations and indicated also that a proliferative synovitis was evident and that the tendon sheath of the long head of the biceps brachii muscle was involved frequently. At about the same time, Simmonds[287] implicated a chronic inflammatory process of the supraspinatus tendon in the pathogenesis of adhesive capsulitis, and Macnab[288] expanded on this theory, suggesting that an autoimmune response to alterations of the supraspinatus tendon resulted in this condition. Although capsular thickening[285] and adhesions either between the capsule and bicipital tendon[289] or in the subacromial-subdeltoid bursa and beneath the coracoid process[290] have been emphasized in many reports of adhesive capsulitis, they are not confirmed uniformly.[281] The answers to questions regarding the pathogenesis of adhesive capsulitis await further investigations.

Routine radiography rarely contributes to the diagnosis of adhesive capsulitis. Rather, it serves mainly to eliminate other conditions, such as a chronic rotator cuff tear or calcific tendinitis, that may lead to similar clinical manifestations. In adhesive capsulitis, nonspecific periarticular osteoporosis and sclerotic and cystic changes in the greater tuberosity of the humerus are encountered. Rarely, thickening or buttressing of the cortex of the proximal and medial portion of the humeral neck is apparent.

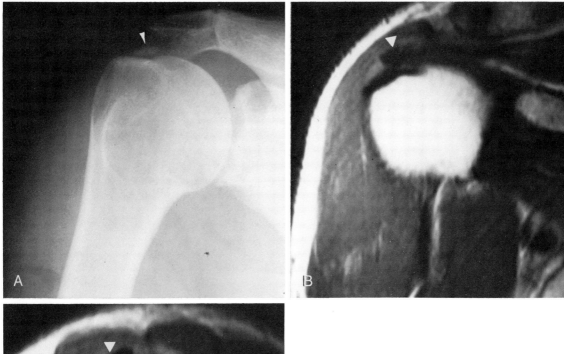

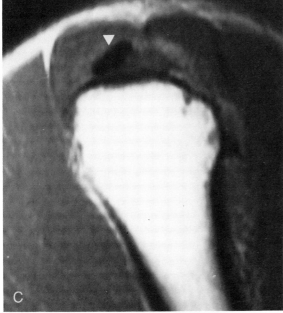

FIGURE 70–124. Calcific tendinitis: Routine radiography and MR imaging. Frontal radiograph **(A)** reveals amorphous calcification in the supraspinatus tendon (arrowhead). Coronal oblique **(B)** and sagittal oblique **(C)** T1-weighted (TR/TE, 700/20) spin echo MR images reveal a region (arrowheads) of low signal intensity indicative of calcification. (From Kursunoglu-Brahme S, et al: Radiol Clin North Am *28:*941, 1990.)

Glenohumeral joint arthrography has been used in the diagnosis and treatment of adhesive capsulitis.[291, 292] Indeed, arthrography is considered by most investigators, although not all,[293] as a reliable means of detecting adhesive capsulitis. Single contrast (radiopaque contrast agent) technique is preferable,[294] and simultaneous determination of the intra-articular pressure has been described.[295] The main arthrographic abnormality in adhesive capsulitis of the glenohumeral articulation is a joint of low capacity evidenced by increased resistance to injection and a ''tight'' feel (Fig. 70–126). Only a small amount of fluid (5 to 8 ml) may be injected successfully, and when the hand is released from the plunger, the fluid may quickly return to the syringe. The subscapular and axillary recesses are small or absent. Filling of the bicipital tendon sheath is variable; in some cases it appears normal, whereas in others it fills poorly or not at all, or contrast may leak from the sheath. Contrast also commonly leaks elsewhere in the joint, particularly from the subscapular recess. An additional finding is irregularity of the capsular insertion.

Joint distention during arthrography, the ''brisement'' procedure,[292] may aid in treatment of this condition.[296] This technique requires slow, intermittent injection of larger and larger volumes of contrast material (mixed with saline solution and lidocaine), allowing some of the fluid to return into the syringe after each injection. The patient is instructed to move the arm carefully during the procedure. In some patients, 100 ml of fluid eventually may be injected, although free extravasation, particularly at the subscapular recess or the bicipital tendon sheath, frequently occurs with extensive distention, and the procedure is halted. Postprocedural physical therapy is advised. With severe capsular restriction, the brisement procedure is less beneficial, and in all patients, symptoms may return, requiring repeated

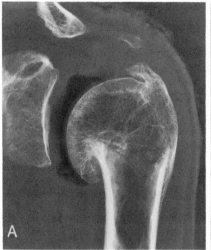 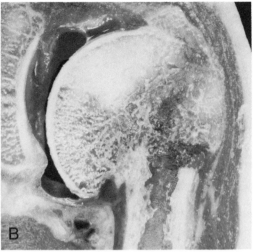

FIGURE 70–125. Adhesive capsulitis: Association with previous trauma. A radiograph **(A)** and a photograph **(B)** of a coronal section of an air-distended glenohumeral joint in a cadaver with a previous fracture of the surgical neck of the humerus show a reduced size of the articular cavity.

examinations. The technique also has been applied to the treatment of adhesive capsulitis in other locations, such as the hip, with inconstant therapeutic results.

There is yet no proven diagnostic role for MR imaging in the assessment of adhesive capsulitis of the shoulder. MR arthrography, however, probably can be used as an alternative to standard arthrography in the diagnosis of this condition, although it is more expensive. The role of ultrasonography as a diagnostic technique in cases of adhesive capsulitis is not clear[1369] but probably is limited.

Bone scintigraphy in patients with adhesive capsulitis of the shoulder reveals nonspecific uptake of the radiophar-

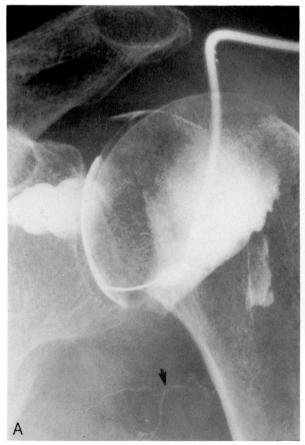 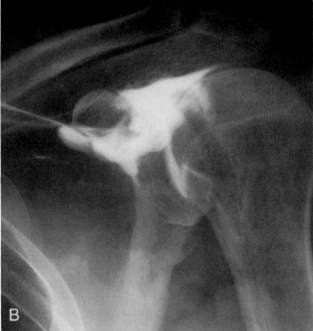

FIGURE 70–126. Adhesive capsulitis: Arthrography.
  A A frontal radiograph obtained following the injection of 5 ml of radiopaque contrast material into the glenohumeral joint reveals a tight-appearing articulation with lymphatic filling (arrow). No axillary pouch is seen.
  B In a second patient, incomplete opacification of the glenohumeral joint is indicative of adhesive capsulitis.

maceutical agent.[293, 297] In general, no association exists between the abnormalities depicted on bone scans and the severity or prognosis of the disease or the arthrographic findings.[293] Arthroscopy has been used to define the extent of synovial and capsular abnormalities in adhesive capsulitis, both before and after manipulation of the shoulder under anesthesia, but the role of shoulder arthroscopy in the diagnosis and treatment of adhesive capsulitis is not established.[280, 298, 299]

Glenohumeral Joint Instability

Classification. Glenohumeral joint instability generally is considered a symptomatic clinical situation in which altered movement of the humeral head with respect to the glenoid cavity occurs. Such instability, in its classic forms, differs from glenohumeral joint laxity in which asymptomatic passive translation of the humeral head on the glenoid fossa is observed.[1384] Glenohumeral joint instability and laxity may coexist. Furthermore, the extent of humeral head translation in patients with glenohumeral joint laxity often is substantial and nearly on a par with that observed in patients with glenohumeral joint instability.[1384] Methods of classification of glenohumeral joint instability are based upon the degree and direction of instability, its chronology, and its pathogenesis. With regard to the degree of instability, dislocations or subluxations of the joint may be encountered. In the former category, no contact remains between the apposing surfaces of the glenoid cavity and the humeral head. With subluxation, abnormal translation of the humeral head in relation to the glenoid cavity is evident, it is not accompanied by complete separation of the apposing articular surfaces, and it usually is greater than the small amount of translation of the humeral head that is a manifestation of the normal range of motion.[300] Subluxation of the glenohumeral joint is transient and often momentary; the humeral head spontaneously returns to its normal position in the glenoid fossa, and the event may be unrecognized by the patient.[301] In one series of patients with anterior subluxation of the glenohumeral joint, a traumatic cause was identified in approximately 90 per cent of cases, and 50 per cent of affected patients were not aware of the problem.[302] Dislocation and subluxation of the glenohumeral joint may occur in several different directions: anterior, posterior, superior, and inferior (Fig. 70–127). With anterior or posterior dislocations, the displaced humeral head may become located in a subcoracoid, subglenoid, subclavicular, or intrathoracic location (anterior dislocations), or in a subacromial, subglenoid, or subspinous location (posterior dislocations), as described in Chapter 68. Subluxations and dislocations of the glenohumeral joint may occur at different times in a single patient, and multidirectional instability may lead to different patterns of displacement of the humeral head in a single shoulder.

With regard to the chronology of instability, acute dislocations are defined as those seen within the first 24 or 48 hours, and chronic dislocations are defined as those evaluated after this time.[301] In common with subluxations of the glenohumeral joint, dislocations of this joint may be transient, with spontaneous reduction of the humeral head. With dislocations of the glenohumeral joint, the humeral head also may be fixed, or locked, in the abnormal position.

Dislocations and subluxations of the glenohumeral joint also may be categorized according to their pathogenesis. They may be traumatic or atraumatic, congenital or acquired, and voluntary or involuntary.

Incidence. Owing to a number of reasons, including its propensity for injury and its inherent instability, the glenohumeral joint is the most common site of dislocation and subluxation in the human body. In one study, approximately 45 per cent of more than 8000 dislocations involved the glenohumeral joint.[303] Approximately 85 per cent of all dislocations about the shoulder affect the glenohumeral joint (as opposed to the acromioclavicular or sternoclavicular joint), and the vast majority of glenohumeral joint dislocations are anterior in nature (see Chapter 68).

Etiology and Pathogenesis. Although developmental factors may lead to congenital instability of the glenohumeral joint and such factors combined with emotional and psychiatric problems may promote voluntary subluxations and dislocations of this joint, trauma is the leading cause of subluxations and dislocations of the glenohumeral joint. Indirect forces are more common than direct forces as causes of glenohumeral joint instability. The combination of abduction, extension, and external rotation forces applied to the arm may result in an anterior dislocation of the glenohumeral joint; axial loading of an adducted, internally rotated arm may produce a posterior dislocation.[301]

Although many structures, such as the components of the rotator cuff, the glenoid labrum, the glenohumeral ligaments, the joint capsule and supporting musculature, and the coracoacromial arch, contribute to glenohumeral joint stability (Fig. 70–128), the contributions of each are not agreed upon. Both static (passive) and dynamic (active) constraints are believed to contribute to shoulder stability.[304] Static constraints include the bone configuration of the glenohumeral joint, and the capsule and ligamentous complex that surrounds the shoulder; dynamic constraints include the muscle and tendon units that surround the glenohumeral joint, particularly the muscles and tendons of the rotator cuff.[305] Matsen and collaborators[301] have provided an excellent summary of the passive and active constraints, and some of their observations are included here.

With regard to passive mechanisms, the stability of the glenohumeral joint is affected by the size, shape, and tilt of the glenoid fossa. Studies have indicated that the glenoid fossa and its contact area may be smaller in shoulders affected by recurrent glenohumeral joint dislocations than in normal shoulders,[306] and that retroversion of the glenoid cavity may be excessive in shoulders demonstrating posterior glenohumeral joint instability.[307] Whether the reported changes are the cause or the effect of glenohumeral joint instability is not clear, however. The glenoid labrum serves to deepen the glenoid cavity, perhaps providing some element of increased stability, but its size is highly variable and often small, such that the contribution of the glenoid labrum to glenohumeral joint stability remains speculative.

The capsule of the glenohumeral joint is large, loose, and redundant, allowing for a great range of motion.[301] Reinforcing the capsule of this joint are the coracohumeral ligament and the three glenohumeral ligaments (Fig. 70–129), whose anatomy has been discussed earlier in this chapter. Although the glenohumeral ligaments are inconstant and variable in size, their importance in providing stability to the glenohumeral joint has been emphasized repeatedly. In combination with the anterior and posterior

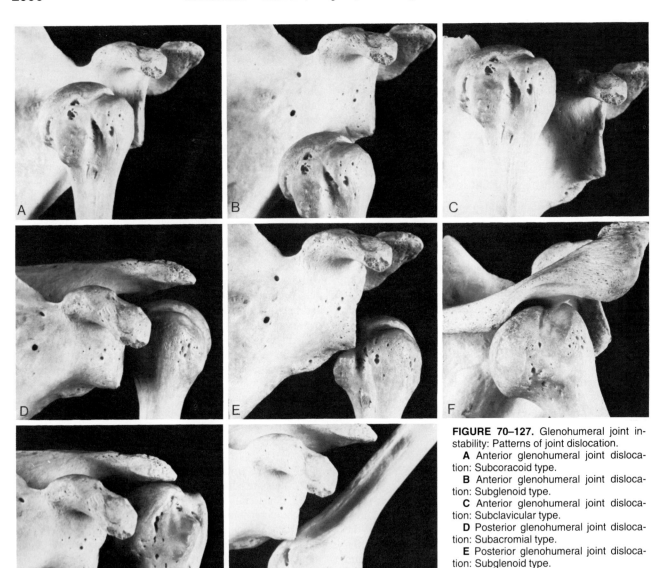

FIGURE 70–127. Glenohumeral joint instability: Patterns of joint dislocation.

A Anterior glenohumeral joint dislocation: Subcoracoid type.

B Anterior glenohumeral joint dislocation: Subglenoid type.

C Anterior glenohumeral joint dislocation: Subclavicular type.

D Posterior glenohumeral joint dislocation: Subacromial type.

E Posterior glenohumeral joint dislocation: Subglenoid type.

F Posterior glenohumeral joint dislocation: Subspinous type.

G Superior glenohumeral joint dislocation.

H Inferior glenohumeral joint dislocation (Luxatio erecta).

portions of the joint capsule, the glenohumeral ligaments appear to limit the translation and rotation of the humerus and, therefore, may serve as the last guardian of shoulder stability after all other passive and dynamic mechanisms have been overwhelmed.[301] The role of the joint capsule and glenohumeral ligaments in this regard has been confirmed in a number of cadaveric studies, the results of which have been summarized by Matsen and coworkers[301]:

1. The anteroinferior capsule restrains anterior subluxation of the abducted arm.

2. The middle glenohumeral ligament limits external rotation at 45 degrees of abduction of the arm.

3. The inferior glenohumeral ligament limits external rotation at 45 to 90 degrees of abduction of the arm.

4. The posterior portion of the capsule and the teres minor muscle and tendon restrain internal rotation of the arm.

5. The lower two thirds of the anterior capsule and the lower portion of the subscapularis muscle and tendon restrain abduction and external rotation of the arm.

Active mechanisms of glenohumeral joint stability include the long head of the biceps brachii muscle and its tendon and the components of the rotator cuff (supraspinatus, infraspinatus, subscapularis, and teres minor muscles and their tendons). The rotator cuff surrounds the humeral head, blending with the capsule of the glenohumeral joint and the capsular ligaments. The components of the rotator cuff can act independently or as a unit, pressing the humeral head into the glenoid fossa and resisting displacing forces resulting from contraction of the major muscles of the shoulder (e.g., deltoid and pectoralis major muscles).[301]

These observations confirm the complexity of the issue of glenohumeral joint stability. Many different structures working independently or in concert provide such stability, and the structures that are operational at any given time depend upon the position of the arm and the type of shoul-

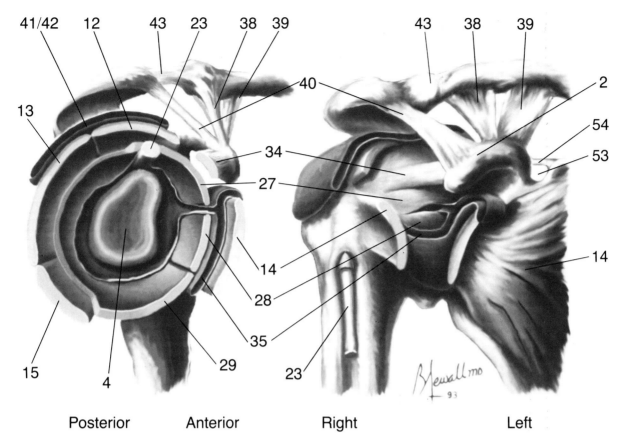

FIGURE 70–128. Capsular complex of the glenohumeral joint, rotator cuff, and supraspinatus outlet: Normal anatomy. On the right, a right shoulder is sketched as if all of the muscles have been dissected away to reveal the glenohumeral, coracohumeral, coracoacromial, and coracoclavicular ligaments. The tendons of the long head of the biceps brachii muscle, the subacromial-subdeltoid bursa, and the subscapularis bursa also are depicted. On the left, the relationships of these structures in the sagittal plane are emphasized. In numerical order, the structures that are illustrated are the following:

  2. Coracoid process
  4. Glenoid cavity
 12. Supraspinatus muscle and tendon
 13. Infraspinatus muscle and tendon
 14. Subscapularis muscle and tendon
 15. Teres minor muscle
 23. Tendon of the long head of the biceps brachii muscle
 27. Superior glenohumeral ligament
 28. Middle glenohumeral ligament
 29. Inferior glenohumeral ligament
 34. Coracohumeral ligament
 35. Subscapularis bursa
 38. Trapezoid ligament
 39. Conoid ligament
 40. Coracoacromial ligament
 41. Subacromial bursa
 42. Subdeltoid bursa
 43. Acromioclavicular joint and ligaments
 53. Suprascapular notch
 54. Superior transverse scapular ligament
(Drawings courtesy of B. O. Sewell, M.D., San Diego, California; From Petersilge CA, et al: MRI Clin North Am *1*:1, 1993.)

der movement taking place. Additional factors related to the presence and amount of joint fluid and cohesive and adhesive mechanisms provided by this fluid also have been identified.[301] Anterior and posterior capsular mechanisms have been defined, underscoring the importance of the coordinated activities of different anatomic structures performing as a functional unit. Instability of the glenohumeral joint occurs when the integrity and coordinated activity of the supporting mechanisms are disrupted. No single or essential lesion appears to form the basis of anterior or posterior instability of the joint. Identification of a detached

portion of the glenoid labrum (Bankart lesion), a compression fracture of the posterolateral surface of the humeral head (Hill-Sachs lesion), a deficiency of one or more of the glenohumeral ligaments, capsular laxity, or detachment or lengthening of the subscapularis muscle as the primary cause of shoulder instability is an oversimplification of a process that is far more complex.

Clinical Abnormalities. The clinical abnormalities related to instability of the glenohumeral joint are variable, being influenced by its atraumatic or traumatic pathogenesis and by its acute or chronic nature. Many patients recall an

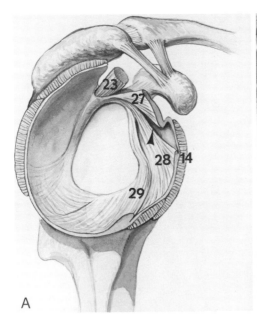
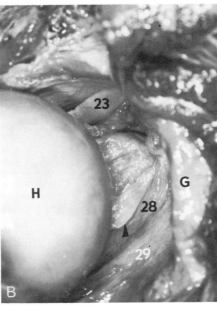

FIGURE 70–129. Capsular complex of the glenohumeral joint: Normal anatomy. The diagram **(A)** provides a simplified depiction of the anterior capsular complex of the glenohumeral joint; a photograph of a dissected shoulder **(B)** also shows this mechanism. The indicated structures are:

14. Subscapularis muscle and tendon

23. Tendon of the long head of the biceps brachii muscle

27. Superior glenohumeral ligament

28. Middle glenohumeral ligament

29. Inferior glenohumeral ligament

G. Glenoid cavity

H. Humeral head

Arrowheads. Opening into the subscapularis bursa

(From Zlatkin M, et al: AJR *150:*151, 1988.)

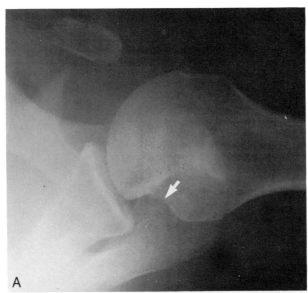

FIGURE 70–130. Anterior glenohumeral joint dislocation: Hill-Sachs and Bankart-type lesions.

A An axillary radiograph of an abducted shoulder reveals a Hill-Sachs lesion (arrow) in the posterolateral aspect of the humeral head, as well as an avulsion fracture of the coracoid process, in a patient with a seizure-induced anterior dislocation of the glenohumeral joint. At the time of this radiograph, the humeral head is not dislocated.

B, C Photographs of macerated humeral **(B)** and scapular **(C)** specimens indicate a Hill-Sachs lesion (arrows) of the humerus and a Bankart-like fracture deformity (arrowheads) of the anterior glenoid rim and anterior surface of the scapula that resulted from a chronic unreduced anterior glenohumeral joint dislocation. The size of these lesions is far greater than that typically seen in clinical practice.

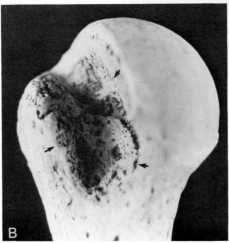
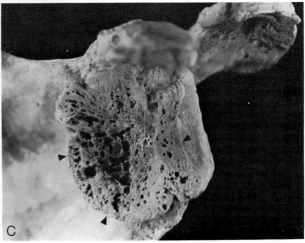

experience in which the humeral head was felt to have been displaced, whether initiated by trauma or not.[1384] Fixed dislocations of the glenohumeral joint usually are identifiable during physical examination of the patient, particularly with anterior dislocation of the glenohumeral joint. Posterior dislocations of this joint are associated with more subtle but definite clinical manifestations, including fixed internal rotation of the affected arm, with limited external rotation and elevation of the arm. The clinical diagnosis of recurrent glenohumeral joint subluxation is more challenging. A history of a minor injury or shoulder discomfort during sporting activities that require movement of the shoulder and physical findings indicative of generalized ligamentous laxity are helpful clues. Manipulative techniques meticulously attempt to document the specific arcs, angles, and directions at which instability is experienced by the patient or examiner, or both.[1384] Although these provocative tests accomplished during physical examination are used to establish the occurrence of subluxation of the glenohumeral joint, imaging examinations are fundamental to accurate diagnosis.

Routine Radiographic Abnormalities. The routine radiographic abnormalities associated with dislocations of the glenohumeral joint are discussed in Chapter 68. In addition to confirming an abnormal position of the humeral head with respect to the glenoid cavity, conventional radiographs are useful in the identification of bone injuries that may occur during the dislocation (Fig. 70–130). Foremost among these injuries are the Hill-Sachs lesion of the humerus and a Bankart-type lesion of the anterior portion of the glenoid rim that may occur during anterior dislocation of the glenohumeral joint, and the trough fracture line of the humerus and an impaction fracture of the posterior

portion of the glenoid rim (reverse Bankart-type lesion) that may occur during posterior dislocation of the glenohumeral joint. Specialized projections may increase the sensitivity of conventional radiographs to the detection of these associated osseous abnormalities (see Chapter 68).[308]

The radiographic assessment of recurrent glenohumeral joint instability includes several views obtained during the application of stress to the shoulder.[301] Small amounts of translational movement of the humeral head with respect to the glenoid cavity may be identified, although similar or perhaps superior data are provided by CT.

Arthrographic Abnormalities. Standard arthrography has a limited role in the assessment of glenohumeral joint instability. Anterior dislocations of the glenohumeral joint are associated with soft tissue damage. As the dislocating humeral head moves anteriorly, it tears the articular capsule or it detaches or lifts the articular capsule from the glenoid and neck of the scapula, producing an abnormal recess of variable size between the subscapular and axillary recesses (Fig. 70–131). On arthrography, the abnormal recess fills with contrast material, obscuring the indentation that normally is present between the subscapular and axillary recesses. This finding is more evident on radiographs taken in internal rotation.

Additional findings related to anterior dislocation are injuries of cartilage and bone. The Bankart deformity involves an avulsion or compression defect of the anteroinferior rim of the glenoid and may be purely cartilaginous in nature. The arthrogram, particularly when performed with double contrast technique, may outline the cartilaginous abnormalities about the glenoid labrum. The second defect associated with previous anterior dislocation is a Hill-Sachs compression deformity on the posterolateral aspect of the

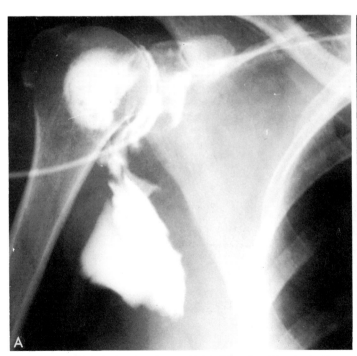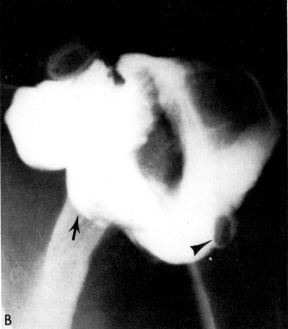

FIGURE 70–131. Anterior glenohumeral joint dislocation: Standard arthrography.

A Following an acute anterior dislocation of the glenohumeral joint with an associated fracture of the greater tuberosity, arthrography outlines an anterior capsular tear with soft tissue extension of contrast material. (Courtesy of J. Mink, M.D., Los Angeles, California.)

B In a patient with previous anterior dislocations of the glenohumeral joint, arthrography demonstrates an abnormal recess (arrow) between the axillary pouch and subscapular recess and an intra-articular body (arrowhead).

humeral head. This finding generally is evident on plain films but may require arthrography for demonstration if the defect is small or involves only cartilage.

Conventional and Computed Arthrotomographic Abnormalities. As the importance of capsular, ligamentous, and labral abnormalities in cases of glenohumeral joint instability became known, tomographic modifications of standard arthrography were applied. Two techniques became popular—conventional arthrotomography and computed arthrotomography.

Conventional arthrotomography was the first of the two techniques to be developed,[309–314] although it rarely is employed today. Thin-section conventional arthrotomography can be accomplished in two ways (prone oblique or supine oblique patient position), each giving a different perspective of the labrum and both requiring considerable experience and expertise on the part of the examiner and meticulous positioning of the patient. Such patients may be positioned in a prone oblique manner, with the affected shoulder facing downward and the neck flexed, with the opposite shoulder moved slightly forward to avoid overlap with the side of interest and the scapula on the involved side directed perpendicular to the table top. Alternatively, a supine oblique position can be used, with the injured shoulder closest to the table. The described techniques of conventional arthrotomography also differ somewhat with regard to the amount of contrast agent that is advocated. In general, 1 or 2 ml of radiopaque contrast material and 10 to 15 ml of air are instilled into the joint.

Computed arthrotomography was the second of these techniques to be developed,[315–322] and it remains popular today. Computed arthrotomography is accomplished following the injection of 10 to 15 ml of air with or without 1 ml of radiopaque contrast material. The patients are examined in the supine position with their arms positioned by their sides and their shoulders in a neutral attitude or in slight internal rotation; to optimally distend the posterior capsule with air, external rotation of the shoulder can be used. Continuous 3 mm sections usually are used, and an average of 15 scans is sufficient. Reformatted coronal or sagittal images rarely are required.

The interpretation of the images obtained with either conventional or computed arthrotomography requires knowledge of the cross-sectional appearance of the normal humeral head and glenoid region of the scapula and of

normal soft tissue structures (Figs. 70–132 to 70–136). The head of the humerus is essentially round and smooth on superior sections taken at the level of the coracoid process, which is the appropriate level for evaluation of a Hill-Sachs lesion; the smooth appearance changes to an irregular one at the level of the cartilage-bone junction in the neck of the humerus, where a constant constriction or concavity is evident between the greater tuberosity and the humeral head itself.[1385] The bicipital groove, located between the greater and lesser tuberosities of the humerus, varies considerably in both depth and configuration.

The articular surface of the glenoid fossa is gently concave and covered by hyaline cartilage, which is normally thinner at the center than at the periphery. On cross section, the posterior margin of the fossa appears larger and more rounded than the more pointed anterior margin. The inclination of the fossa is characterized by mild retroversion superiorly, changing to slight anteversion on progressively caudal sections. The glenoid labrum is a fibrous structure that is firmly attached to the edge of the fossa. In cross section, the labrum appears essentially triangular (Fig. 70–137). On conventional arthrotomography, the anterior portion often is longer and more pointed than the posterior portion, which frequently appears slightly larger, more rounded, and smoother. On computed arthrotomography, the anterior portion most commonly has a smoothly rounded apex, although on occasion the apex is pointed and closely resembles the appearance on conventional arthrotomography. The base of the labrum abuts the articular cartilage of the glenoid, somewhat analogous to the meniscus in the knee. Air or contrast material normally may track between the base of the labrum and the cartilage and should not be mistaken for evidence of partial detachment.

Distention of the glenohumeral joint during conventional or computed arthrotomography (or during MR arthrography) allows identification of the glenohumeral ligaments and sites of capsular insertion. There is variability in the size of the glenohumeral ligaments, however, such that it is not possible to visualize all three ligaments in every case. The anterior capsular insertion is somewhat variable in appearance; the capsule may insert in or near the labrum (type 1) or more medially along the scapular neck (types 2 and 3) (Fig. 70–138). The importance of a type 3 capsular insertion, representing the most medial type of insertion, as a cause or result of anterior instability of the glenohumeral

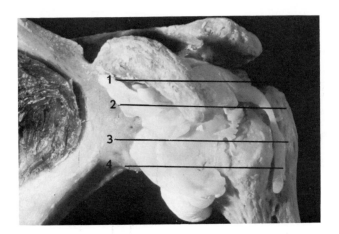

FIGURE 70–132. Cross-sectional appearance of the glenohumeral joint: Normal anatomy. Four anatomic levels of analysis. As demonstrated in this anatomic specimen, in which the glenohumeral joint has been distended with methylmethacrylate, a simplified approach to the assessment of transaxial images provided by conventional or computed arthrotomography (or MR imaging or MR arthrography) emphasizes findings at four specific levels: the superior aspect of the joint (level 1); the region of the subscapularis recess or bursa (level 2); the midglenoid level (level 3); and the inferior glenoid level (level 4). (From Zlatkin M, et al: AJR *150*:151, 1988.)

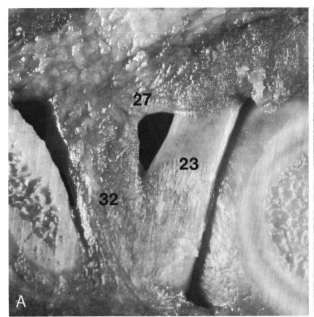 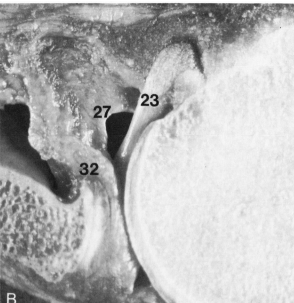

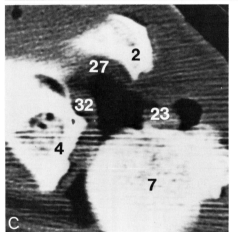

FIGURE 70–133. Cross-sectional appearance of the glenohumeral joint: Normal anatomy. Level 1—superior aspect of the joint.

A, B Two sections, **A** slightly above **B,** show the superior portion of the glenoid labrum (32), the capsule and superior glenohumeral ligament (27), and the tendon of the long head of the biceps brachii muscle (23).

C CT arthrography of the air-distended joint also allows identification of these same structures. The humerus (7), glenoid cavity (4), and coracoid process (2) also are indicated.

(From Zlatkin M, et al: AJR *150:*151, 1988.)

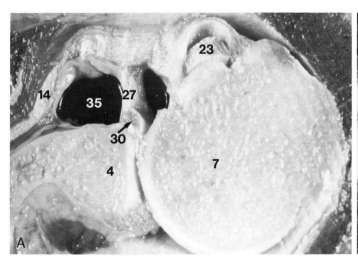 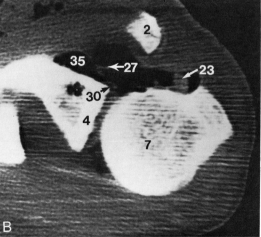

FIGURE 70–134. Cross-sectional appearance of the glenohumeral joint: Normal anatomy. Level 2—the region of the subscapularis recess or bursa. At this level, the lower portion of the superior glenohumeral ligament (27), opening into the subscapularis bursa (35), anterior portion of the glenoid labrum (30), tendon of the long head of the biceps brachii muscle (23), subscapularis tendon (14), coracoid process (2), glenoid cavity (4), and humerus (7) are identified in the anatomic section **(A)** and CT arthrogram **(B).**

(From Zlatkin M, et al: AJR *150:*151, 1988.)

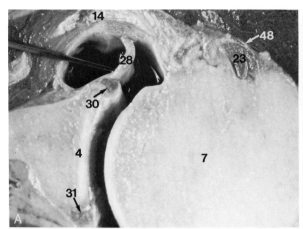
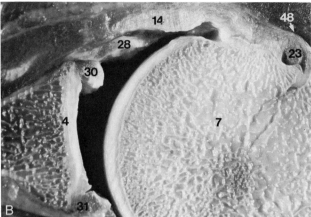

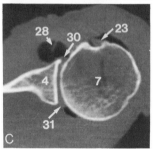

FIGURE 70–135. Cross-sectional appearance of the glenohumeral joint: Normal anatomy. Level 3—midglenoid level.

A, B Two anatomic sections show variations in the appearance of the middle glenohumeral ligament (28). Also note the subscapularis tendon (14), anterior portion of the glenoid labrum (30), posterior portion of the glenoid labrum (31), tendon of the long head of the biceps brachii muscle (23) within the bicipital groove, transverse humeral ligament (48), glenoid cavity (4), and humeral head (7).

C CT arthrography allows identification of some of these same structures.

(From Zlatkin M, et al: AJR *150:*151, 1988.)

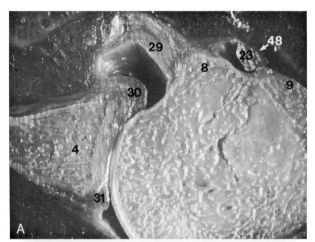

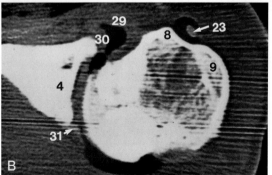

FIGURE 70–136. Cross-sectional appearance of the glenohumeral joint: Normal anatomy. Level 4—inferior glenoid level.

A An anatomic section shows the prominent inferior glenohumeral ligament (29). Also note the anterior portion of the glenoid labrum (30), posterior portion of the glenoid labrum (31), tendon of the long head of the biceps brachii muscle (23), transverse humeral ligament (48), lesser (8) and greater (9) tuberosities of the humerus, and glenoid cavity (4).

B Some of the same structures can be identified in the CT arthrogram.

(From Zlatkin M, et al: AJR *150:*151, 1988.)

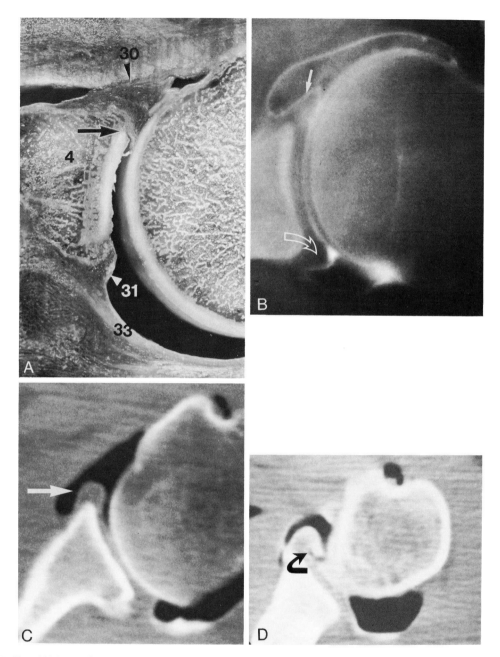

FIGURE 70–137. Glenoid labrum: Conventional and computed arthrotomography. Normal appearance.

A A transverse anatomic section through the lower third of the glenoid cavity shows the anterior (30) and posterior (31) portions of the labrum. The anterior labrum has a triangular configuration, with a cleft or potential space at its base (arrow) where it abuts the articular cartilage of the glenoid cavity (4). The posterior portion of the glenoid labrum appears smaller and more rounded, and the posterior capsule (33) of the joint attaches directly to it.

B With conventional arthrotomography, the apex of the anterior portion of the labrum (solid arrow) is sharp, in comparison with the rounded appearance of the posterior portion of the labrum (open arrow).

C With CT arthrography, the apex of the anterior portion of the labrum (arrow) commonly appears more rounded than with conventional arthrotomography.

D Air or radiopaque contrast material (curved arrow) normally may be seen between the base of the anterior portion of the labrum and articular cartilage of the glenoid cavity.

(From Deutsch AL, et al: Radiology *153:*603, 1984.)

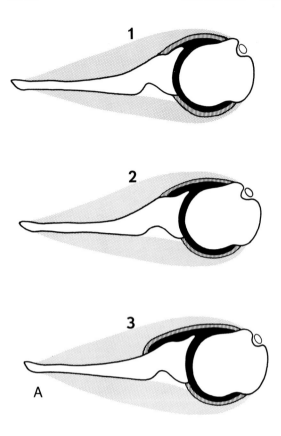

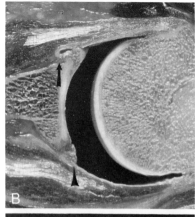

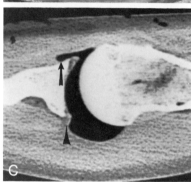

FIGURE 70–138. Cross-sectional appearance of the glenohumeral joint: Normal anatomy. Types of anterior and posterior capsular insertion.

A The three types of anterior capsular insertion are indicated (see text for details). Note that the posterior portion of the capsule attaches directly to the labrum.

B, C A photograph of a transverse anatomic section **(B)** and CT arthrographic image **(C)**, both at the midglenoid level, reveal a type 1 capsular insertion (arrows) and a posterior capsular attachment to the posterior portion of the labrum (arrowheads).

(From Zlatkin M, et al: AJR *150*:151, 1988.)

joint is not clear (Fig. 70–139). The type 1 capsular insertion is the most commonly encountered pattern. The posterior capsule, when normal, invariably inserts in the labrum.

Abnormalities of the glenoid labrum depicted on conventional or computed arthrotomography include foreshortening or thinning or contrast imbibition along its free margin (Fig. 70–140). The labrum also may be completely detached (the true Bankart lesion). An osseous Bankart-type lesion typically is visualized as an elevation of a small sliver of bone and irregularity of the adjacent glenoid rim. A depression along the posterolateral aspect of the humeral head is indicative of a Hill-Sachs lesion.

Both conventional and computed arthrotomographic studies were reported to be highly accurate in the analysis

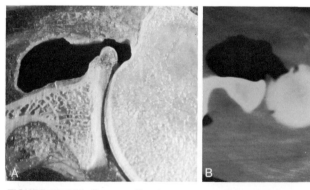

FIGURE 70–139. Cross-sectional appearance of the glenohumeral joint: Pathologic anatomy. Type 3 insertion of the anterior capsule. An anatomic section **(A)** and a corresponding CT arthrographic image **(B)** reveal a large anterior pouch related to a type 3 capsular insertion. The clinical significance of this finding is not clear. (From Zlatkin M, et al: AJR *150*:151, 1988.)

of the glenoid labrum. With regard to the reported series using conventional arthrotomography, Braunstein and O'Connor[310] accurately characterized the anterior labral abnormality seen in all nine of their patients; however, no patients with normal arthrograms were explored, and thus no data on false-negatives are available. Of the 21 patients with surgical confirmation reported by McGlynn and coworkers,[312] the labrum was accurately characterized as normal or abnormal in all cases, and there were no false-positives or false-negatives. Pappas and collaborators[323] examined 46 patients with prone oblique conventional arthrotomography; 18 patients with positive findings and 3 normal subjects had operative intervention in which the accuracy of the interpretations was confirmed. In an analysis of 55 patients undergoing conventional arthrotomography, Deutsch and coworkers[317] found that the technique classified the status of the labrum in 13 of the 16 patients who had surgery or arthroscopy (sensitivity, 86 per cent; accuracy, 81 per cent).

Reported studies also have underscored the accuracy of computed arthrotomography in the assessment of the glenoid labrum. In an investigation of 10 patients, Shuman and others[316] observed that, on the basis of surgical confirmation of the findings, computed arthrotomography correctly characterized the labrum as abnormal in five persons and normal in one. Kinnard and collaborators[315] reported that of 10 patients undergoing computed arthrotomography for evaluation of shoulder instability, three had labral abnormalities confirmed at surgery. Deutsch and colleagues,[317] in an investigation of 81 patients using computed arthrotomography, found that the examination accurately characterized the glenoid labrum as normal, abnormal, or detached in 38 of the 44 patients who had surgery or arthroscopy (sensitivity, 96 per cent; accuracy, 86 per cent). Hill-Sachs defects

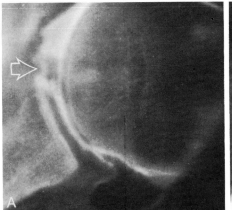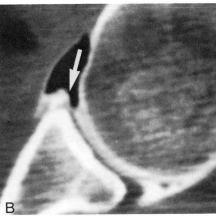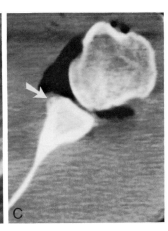

FIGURE 70–140. Glenoid labrum: Conventional and computed arthrotomography. Abnormal appearance.
  A A conventional arthrotomographic image demonstrates irregularity and foreshortening of the anterior portion of the labrum (arrow).
  B With CT arthrography, the anterior portion of the labrum is foreshortened and imbibes contrast material (arrow).
  C With CT arthrography, a scan through the lower portion of the joint shows avulsion of the anterior portion of the labrum with a small fracture (arrow) of the glenoid rim.
  (From Deutsch AL, et al: Radiology *153:*603, 1984.)

were seen in 20 of 29 patients with anterior labral abnormalities, and bicipital tendon abnormalities were evident in six patients.

The reliability of arthrotomographic methods to define clinically significant labral abnormalities, however, may be questioned on the basis of an investigation in 1987 by McNiesh and Callaghan.[324] In this investigation, as well as a subsequent one in which MR imaging was assessed,[157] variations in the normal appearance of the glenoid labrum were described. From material derived from computed arthrotomograms of 72 shoulders in which the labrum had been considered normal at the time of arthroscopy, McNiesh and Callaghan[324] emphasized the occurrence of a notched or cleaved appearance of the anterior labrum, as well as a small labrum, in some cases. Neumann and coworkers,[157] studying the MR images of 50 shoulders in 30 asymptomatic volunteers, expanded on this concept, indicating the presence of many normal variations in labral morphology (see previous discussion). Although these morphologic variations may result from glenohumeral ligamentous attachments to the labrum or from labral degeneration in older persons,[325] ultimately they lead to diagnostic uncertainty with regard to labral integrity in any patient. This diagnostic problem is common to both arthrotomography and MR imaging. Because of this, interpretation of either type of examination commonly relies on the presence or absence of additional abnormalities, such as those of the humeral head (i.e., Hill-Sachs lesion) or glenohumeral capsule or ligaments.

The investigation of Rafii and coworkers[319] in 1986 was the first to provide a detailed analysis of the computed arthrotomographic appearance of the capsular structures of the shoulder. Distention of the glenohumeral joint accomplished during computed arthrotomography (and during MR arthrography) allows visualization of the anterior and posterior capsular insertions of the glenohumeral ligaments, and the coracohumeral ligament. In cases of anterior glenohumeral joint instability, the capsular reflections may appear lax or distorted with either loss or thickening of the anterior subscapular soft tissues (Figs. 70–141 to 70–143). Although isolated tears of the labrum may be detected, these tears frequently are associated with varying degrees of capsular abnormality and, in some cases, with periostitis involving the anterior portion of the scapula. Detachment of the labrum along with one or more of the glenohumeral ligaments may be apparent. With posterior instability of the

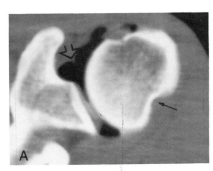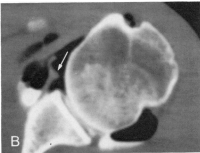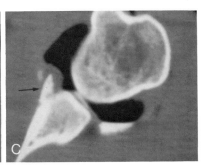

FIGURE 70–141. Glenohumeral joint instability: Computed arthrotomography. Capsular, ligamentous, and labral abnormalities. Three transaxial CT arthrographic images obtained at the level of the superior aspect of the joint (level 1) **(A)**, the midglenoid level (level 3) **(B)**, and the inferior glenoid level (level 4) **(C)**, show a number of abnormalities indicative of previous anterior glenohumeral joint dislocation. In **A**, observe a Hill-Sachs lesion (arrow), irregularity of the superior glenohumeral ligament (open arrow), and nonvisualization of the superoanterior portion of the labrum. In **B**, findings include avulsion of the anterior portion of the labrum at the site of attachment of the middle glenohumeral ligament (arrow) and a redundant anterior capsule. In **C**, observe a fracture (arrow) of the anterior surface of the glenoid rim.

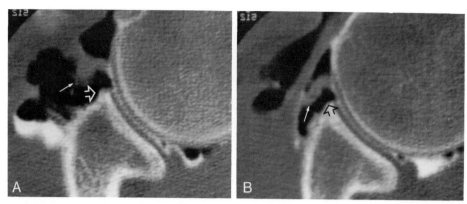

FIGURE 70–142. Glenohumeral joint instability: Computed arthrotomography. Capsular, ligamentous, and labral abnormalities. Two transaxial CT arthrographic images obtained at the level of the subscapularis bursa (level 2) **(A)** and midglenoid level (level 3) **(B)** show abnormality indicative of anterior instability of the glenohumeral joint. In **A**, note irregularity of the inferior portion of the superior glenohumeral ligament (solid arrow) and absence of the anterior portion of the labrum (open arrow). In **B**, note absence of the anterior portion of the labrum (open arrow) at the site of attachment of the middle glenohumeral ligament (solid arrow).

glenohumeral joint, the posterior portion of the glenoid labrum may be torn, shredded, or detached, and capsular laxity may be apparent. Both anterior and posterior abnormalities may be seen with computed arthrotomography in patients with multidirectional instability.

Magnetic Resonance Imaging Abnormalities. Numerous publications have examined the value of MR imaging in the analysis of glenohumeral joint instability.[326–334] Most studies have relied upon standard spin echo MR images, although a few have employed gradient echo images,[334] sometimes combined with additional methods such as radial sectioning of the labrum.[328] Little data exist regarding the value of volumetric gradient echo MR imaging in the assessment of the glenoid labrum, although the ability to obtain thin (1 mm or less), contiguous slices with this technique may prove important. MR arthrography, accomplished with the intra-articular injection of gadolinium compounds or saline, also appears to have diagnostic potential,[270, 335, 1348, 1386–1388] although it is invasive and time-consuming, and the added benefits of this technique are not known yet. With standard MR imaging or MR arthrography, the glenoid labrum is best demonstrated in the transaxial plane (Figs. 70–144 and 70–145), although coronal

oblique (Fig. 70–146) and sagittal oblique (Fig. 70–147) images provide additional information.

Initial investigations dealing with MR imaging of glenohumeral joint instability described the generally low signal intensity and smooth, wedge-shaped appearance of the normal anterior and posterior portions of the labrum, the irregularity of contour and intermediate or high signal intensity of the torn labrum (Figs. 70–148 to 70–150), and slight superiority of this technique when compared with computed arthrotomography in the analysis of labral lesions.[326, 327, 329] In 1991, Legan and associates[330] reported that MR imaging enabled prediction of anterior labral tears with a sensitivity of 95 per cent, a specificity of 86 per cent, and an accuracy of 92 per cent in a series of 88 patients in whom results of arthroscopy were used as the standard. These authors also indicated that MR imaging was less effective in the prediction of tears of the superior portion of the labrum (sensitivity of 75 per cent, specificity of 99 per cent, and accuracy of 95 per cent), and it was unreliable in the prediction of less common, posterior, or inferior labral tears. In this investigation, labral tears were considered to involve the anterior or posterior portion of the labrum if seen on transaxial images and the superior or inferior portion of the labrum if

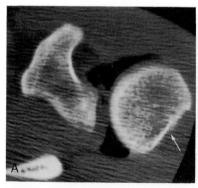 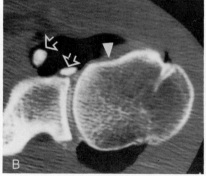 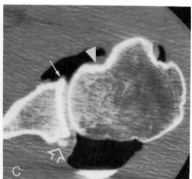

FIGURE 70–143. Glenohumeral joint instability: Computed arthrotomography. Capsular, ligamentous, and labral abnormalities. Three transaxial CT arthrographic images obtained at the level of the superior aspect of the joint (level 1) **(A)**, the midglenoid level (level 3) **(B)**, and the inferior glenoid level (level 4) **(C)**, show abnormalities indicative of multidirectional instability. In **A**, observe a Hill-Sachs lesion (solid arrow). In **B**, note intra-articular bodies (open arrows) and a trough fracture (arrowhead) in the anterior surface of the humeral head. In **C**, the trough fracture (arrowhead) is more apparent. Additional findings include absence of the anterior portion of the labrum (solid arrow) and a fracture (open arrow) of the posterior glenoid rim.

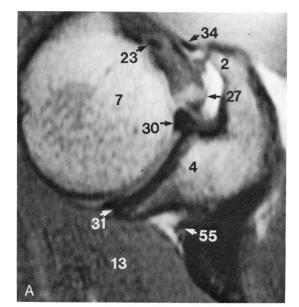

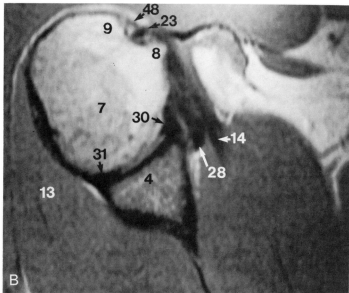

FIGURE 70–144. Cross-sectional appearance of the gleno-humeral joint: Normal anatomy. MR imaging. Transaxial T1-weighted (TR/TE, 600/20) spin echo MR images.

A Level 1—superior aspect of the joint. Note the coracoid process (2), glenoid cavity (4), and smooth humeral head (7). The anterior (30) and posterior (31) portions of the glenoid labrum are of low signal intensity. Portions of the superior glenohumeral ligament (27) and coracohumeral (34) ligament and the tendon of the long head of the biceps brachii muscle (23) are seen. Also labeled are the suprascapular neurovascular bundle (55) and infraspinatus muscle (13).

B Level 3—midglenoid level. Note the glenoid cavity (4), humeral head (7), greater (9) and lesser (8) tuberosities of the humerus, tendon of the long head of the biceps brachii muscle (23), transverse humeral ligament (48), anterior (30) and posterior (31) portions of the glenoid labrum, middle glenohumeral ligament (28), subscapular tendon (14), and infraspinatus muscle (13).

seen on coronal oblique images. The diagnostic criteria for a labral tear included a visibly torn labrum or one that was truncated or absent. A visibly torn labrum was seen as a high signal intensity region traversing the signal void of the normal labrum. The diagnostic value of one additional finding, a glenoid labrum ovoid mass (GLOM), consisting of a rounded, often expanded labral mass of low signal intensity on proton density and T2-weighted spin echo images as a sign of a torn labrum also was emphasized (Fig. 70–150). Inherent bias was introduced in this study, however, owing to the high prevalence of labral abnormalities in the predominately young, athletic patients and to the inclusion of a significant number of patients with recurrent glenohumeral joint subluxations in whom labral abnormalities occur with high frequency. Other investigators[331] were unable to confirm the high sensitivity and specificity of MR imaging in the diagnosis of labral abnormalities that were reported by Legan and collaborators.[330]

The criteria used to diagnose an abnormality of the glenoid labrum with MR imaging include alterations in its morphology and signal intensity. Diagnostic pitfalls exist

with regard to the application of either of these criteria, however (Fig. 70–151). As with computed arthrotomography, MR imaging displays the many variations of labral shape that are evident in asymptomatic persons.[157, 254] A triangular shape of the anterior and posterior portions of the labrum, believed to represent the classic appearance of a normal labrum, has been reported to be evident anteriorly in only 45 per cent of asymptomatic persons and posteriorly in only 73 per cent of asymptomatic persons.[157] The attachment sites of the glenohumeral ligaments and, superiorly, of the tendon of the long head of the biceps brachii muscle may alter the apparent shape of a normal labrum.[200, 254] The signal intensity of the normal anterior portion of the labrum may appear abnormal, owing to the presence of the subjacent articular cartilage of the glenoid cavity, a structure of higher signal intensity.[200] Histologic findings, consisting of mucinous and myxoid changes, within the labrum occur with increased frequency with advancing patient age and can produce regions of intermediate signal intensity, particularly on gradient echo MR images.[334]

As in the case of computed arthrotomography, standard

Text continued on page 3008

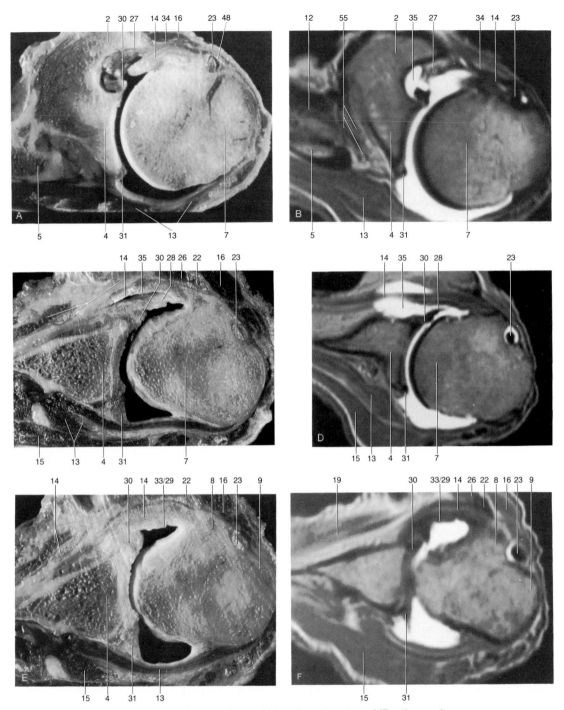

FIGURE 70–145. Cross-sectional appearance of the glenohumeral joint: Normal anatomy. MR arthrography.

A, B Level 1—superior aspect of the joint. Labeled structures are the coracoid process (2), glenoid cavity (4), scapular spine (5), humeral head (7), supraspinatus muscle (12), infraspinatus muscle (13), subscapularis tendon (14), deltoid muscle (16), tendon of the long head of the biceps brachii muscle (23), superior glenohumeral ligament (27), anterior portion of the glenoid labrum (30), posterior portion of the glenoid labrum (31), coracohumeral ligament (34), subscapularis bursa (35), transverse humeral ligament (48), and suprascapular neurovascular bundle (55).

C, D Level 3—midglenoid level. Labeled structures are the glenoid cavity (4), humeral head (7), infraspinatus muscle and tendon (13), subscapularis tendon (14), teres minor muscle (15), deltoid muscle (16), tendon of the short head of the biceps brachii muscle (22), tendon of the long head of the biceps brachii muscle (23), coracobrachialis muscle (26), middle glenohumeral ligament (28), anterior portion of the glenoid labrum (30), posterior portion of the glenoid labrum (31), and subscapularis bursa (35).

E, F Level 4—inferior glenoid level. Labeled structures are the glenoid cavity (4), lesser tuberosity of the humerus (8), greater tuberosity of the humerus (9), infraspinatus tendon (13), subscapularis tendon (14), teres minor muscle (15), deltoid muscle (16), pectoralis major muscle (19), tendon of the short head of the biceps brachii muscle (22), tendon of the long head of the biceps brachii muscle (23), coracobrachialis muscle (26), inferior glenohumeral ligament (29), anterior portion of the glenoid labrum (30), posterior portion of the glenoid labrum (31), and the joint capsule (33).

(From Petersilge CA, et al: MRI Clin North Am *1:*1, 1993.)

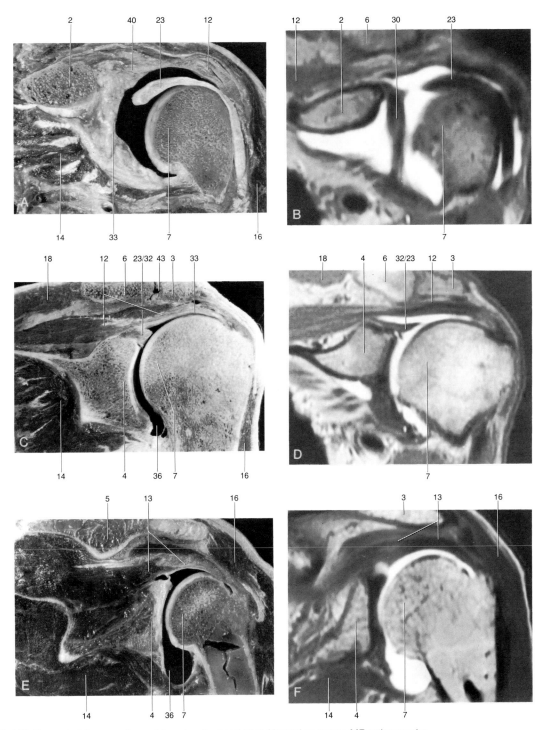

FIGURE 70–146. Coronal oblique sections of the glenohumeral joint: Normal anatomy. MR arthrography.

A, B Anterior aspect of the joint. Labeled structures are the coracoid process (2), clavicle (6), humeral head (7), supraspinatus tendon (12), subscapularis muscle and tendon (14), deltoid muscle (16), tendon of the long head of the biceps brachii muscle (23), anterior labrum (30), anterior capsule (33), and coracoacromial ligament (40).

C, D Middle aspect of the joint. Labeled structures are the acromion (3), glenoid cavity (4), clavicle (6), humeral head (7), supraspinatus muscle and tendon (12), subscapularis muscle (14), deltoid muscle (16), trapezius muscle (18), tendon of the long head of the biceps brachii muscle (23), superior portion of the glenoid labrum (32), joint capsule (33), axillary recess (36), and acromioclavicular joint and ligaments (43).

E, F Posterior aspect of the joint. Labeled structures are the acromion (3), glenoid cavity (4), scapular spine (5), humeral head (7), infraspinatus muscle and tendon (13), subscapularis muscle (14), deltoid muscle (16), and axillary recess (36).

(From Petersilge CA, et al: MRI Clin North Am *1*:1, 1993.)

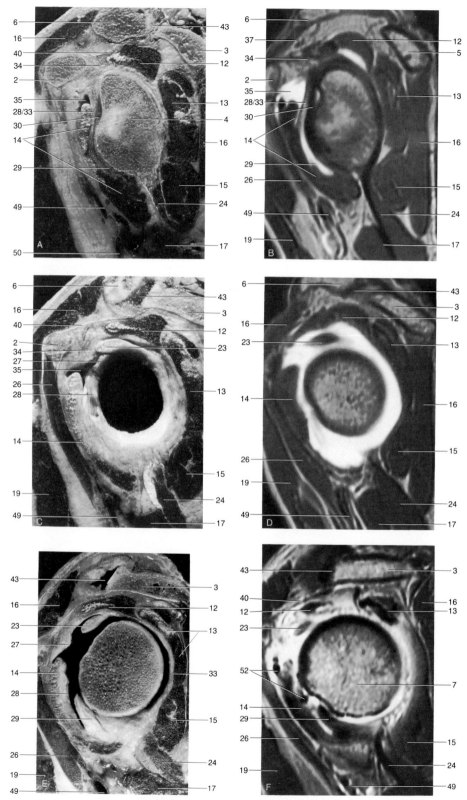

FIGURE 70–147 *See legend on opposite page*

FIGURE 70–148. Glenoid labrum: MR arthrography. Abnormal appearance. A transaxial T1-weighted (TR/TE, 600/20) spin echo MR image obtained following the intra-articular injection of a gadolinium compound **(A)** reveals a linear region (arrow) of high signal intensity in the anterior portion of the labrum. An anatomic section at the same level **(B)** reveals a subtle, undisplaced tear (arrow) in the anterior portion of the labrum. (From Zlatkin M, et al: AJR *150*:151, 1988.)

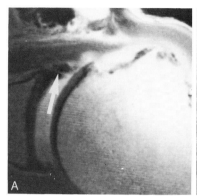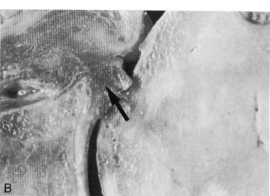

FIGURE 70–149. Glenoid labrum: MR imaging. Abnormal appearance. Labral tear and detachment. Two transaxial proton density–weighted (TR/TE, 2116/30) spin echo MR images at the midglenoid **(A)** and lower glenoid **(B)** levels show detachment (arrow) of the anterior portion of the labrum and an intrasubstance labral tear (arrowhead). (Courtesy of M. Rafii, M.D., New York, New York.)

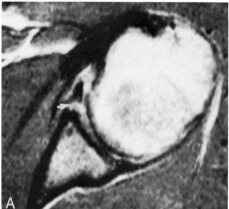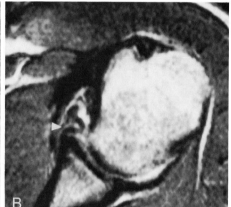

FIGURE 70–147. Sagittal oblique sections of the glenohumeral joint: Normal anatomy. MR arthrography.

A, B Medial aspect at the level of the glenoid cavity. Labeled structures are the coracoid process (2), acromion (3), glenoid cavity (4), scapular spine (5), clavicle (6), supraspinatus muscle (12), infraspinatus muscle (13), subscapularis muscle and tendon (14), teres minor muscle (15), deltoid muscle (16), teres major muscle (17), pectoralis major muscle (19), tendon of the long head of the triceps muscle (24), coracobrachialis muscle (26), middle glenohumeral ligament (28), inferior glenohumeral ligament (29), anterior portion of the glenoid labrum (30), joint capsule (33), coracohumeral ligament (34), subscapularis bursa (35), coracoclavicular ligaments (37), coracoacromial ligament (40), acromioclavicular joint and ligaments (43), axillary artery and brachial plexus (49), and axillary vein (50).

C, D Middle aspect at the level of the medial aspect of the humeral head. Labeled structures are the coracoid process (2), acromion (3), clavicle (6), supraspinatus tendon (12), infraspinatus muscle and tendon (13), subscapularis tendon (14), teres minor muscle (15), deltoid muscle (16), teres major muscle (17), pectoralis major muscle (19), tendon of the long head of the biceps brachii muscle (23), long head of the triceps muscle and its tendon (24), coracobrachialis muscle (26), superior glenohumeral ligament (27), middle glenohumeral ligament (28), coracohumeral ligament (34), subscapularis bursa (35), coracoacromial ligament (40), acromioclavicular joint and ligaments (43), and axillary artery and brachial plexus (49).

E, F Lateral aspect at the level of the midportion of the humeral head. Labeled structures are the acromion (3), humeral head (7), supraspinatus tendon (12), infraspinatus muscle and tendon (13), subscapularis tendon (14), teres minor muscle (15), deltoid muscle (16), teres major muscle (17), pectoralis major muscle (19), tendon of the long head of the biceps brachii muscle (23), long head of the triceps muscle and its tendon (24), coracobrachialis muscle (26), superior glenohumeral ligament (27), middle glenohumeral ligament (28), inferior glenohumeral ligament (29), joint capsule (33), coracoacromial ligament (40), acromioclavicular joint and ligaments (43), axillary artery and brachial plexus (49), and air bubbles (52).

(From Petersilge CA, et al: MRI Clin North Am *1*:1, 1993.)

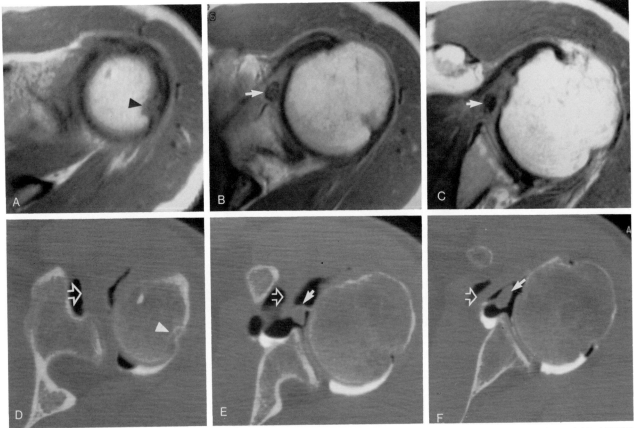

FIGURE 70–150. Glenoid labrum: MR imaging and CT arthrography. Abnormal appearance. Three transaxial proton density–weighted (TR/TE, 2000/19) spin echo MR images **(A–C)** and three transaxial CT arthrographic scans **(D–F)** demonstrate an abnormal anterior portion of the labrum, including a glenoid labrum ovoid mass (GLOM).

 A At the level of the base of the coracoid process, note a Hill-Sachs lesion (arrowhead) of the humeral head.

 B Slightly below the level of **A**, observe the GLOM (closed arrow) of low signal intensity, diagnostic of a labral tear.

 C Slightly below the level of **B**, in the midglenoid region, the GLOM (closed arrow) again is evident.

 D At the level of the base of the coracoid process, note the Hill-Sachs lesion (arrowhead) and a thick superior glenohumeral ligament (open arrow).

 E Slightly below the level of **D**, note the GLOM (closed arrow) adjacent to the inferior portion of the superior glenohumeral ligament (open arrow).

 F Slightly below the level of **E**, in the midglenoid region, the GLOM (closed arrow) is contiguous with the middle glenohumeral ligament (open arrow).

 (Courtesy of J. Quale, M.D., Englewood, Colorado.)

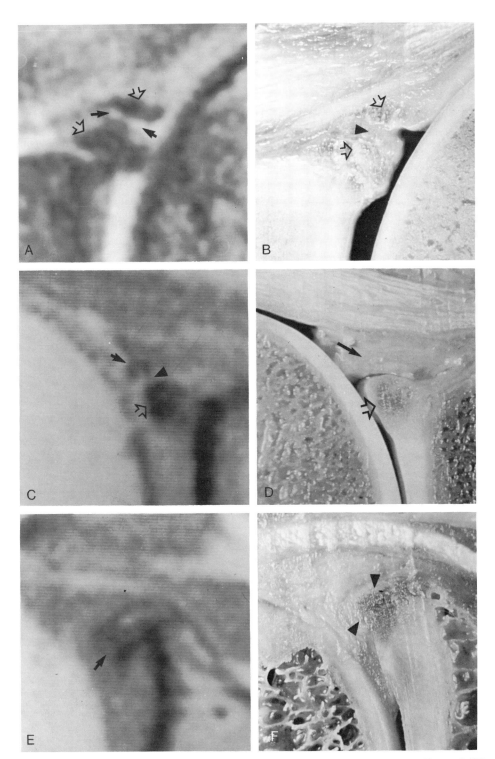

FIGURE 70–151. Glenoid labrum: MR imaging. Tears and pseudotears of the anterior portion of the labrum. Transaxial T1-weighted (TR/TE, 600/20) spin echo MR images **(A, C, E)** and corresponding anatomic sections **(B, D, F)**.

A, B Labral tear. Note the region of high signal intensity (solid arrows) representing a true tear (arrowhead), dividing the labrum into two parts (open arrows).

C, D Normal labrum. Note the normal labrum (open arrows) and adjacent joint capsule, synovium, and middle glenohumeral ligament (solid arrows), producing a pseudotear (arrowhead) in the MR image.

E, F Labral degeneration. Irregular signal intensity in the labrum (solid arrow), simulating the appearance of a labral tear, corresponded to sites of mucinous and myxoid degeneration of a labrum that was grossly intact (arrowheads).

(Courtesy of I. Kjellin, M.D., Loma Linda, California.)

MR imaging or MR arthrography allows detection of capsular and ligamentous abnormalities that may be combined with labral alterations in patients with glenohumeral joint instability. The diagnosis of capsular and ligamentous changes is facilitated by the presence of joint fluid, related either to a native effusion or to the intra-articular injection of a saline solution or gadolinium compound (Figs. 70–152 and 70–153). In MR images, the capsule may appear lax, with an undulating contour, or it may be stripped from the adjacent bone. In elderly persons, disruption of the subscapularis tendon may accompany an anterior glenohumeral joint dislocation. The soft tissue (i.e., ligamentous, capsular, and tendinous) changes may include findings of edema or hemorrhage in the acute stage, appearing as regions of high signal intensity in T2-weighted spin echo and certain gradient echo MR images. Distribution of the soft tissue abnormalities, including those of the labrum, depends on the direction of glenohumeral joint instability (i.e., anterior, posterior, or multidirectional) (Fig. 70–154).

A variety of osseous injuries accompanies glenohumeral joint instability and may be detected with MR imaging. These include fractures of the anterior or posterior portion of the glenoid rim, Hill-Sachs and trough lesions, and avulsion fractures of the lesser or greater tuberosity of the humerus (Figs. 70–155 and 70–156).

The Hill-Sachs lesion is a specific indicator of a prior anterior glenohumeral joint dislocation (Fig. 70–157A). Its radiographic detection is improved when specialized views are used as a supplement to standard methodology. Notch,

or Stryker, views, modified Didiee projections, frontal radiographs obtained with varying degrees of internal rotation of the humerus, and fluoroscopy improve the sensitivity of conventional radiography in the identification of this compression fracture.[336] Transaxial images provided by CT and MR imaging (Fig. 70–157B) provide further diagnostic sensitivity. In one study, in which agreement of findings in two of three different methods (routine radiography, MR imaging and arthroscopy) was used as the standard, MR imaging resulted in a sensitivity of 97 per cent, a specificity of 91 per cent, and an accuracy of 94 per cent in the detection of a Hill-Sachs lesion.[337] The presence of a normal groove in the posterolateral aspect of the proximal humeral metaphysis can lead to difficulty in the diagnosis of the Hill-Sachs lesion on transaxial CT and MR images. This groove, however, is located lower than a Hill-Sachs lesion (Fig. 70–158). The latter is apparent almost universally in the first two or three transaxial images through the superior portion of the humeral head (with 3 mm or 5 mm slice thickness).

Other Labral Abnormalities. In athletes involved in sports requiring repetitive overhead use of the arm, such as in baseball, volleyball, and tennis, an injury of the superior portion of the glenoid labrum may occur, resulting from sudden forced abduction of the arm.[338–341] This injury, which also occurs occasionally in middle-aged persons, may be related to excessive traction, owing to a sudden pull of the tendon of the long head of the biceps brachii muscle, and frequently is referred to as a superior labral, anterior

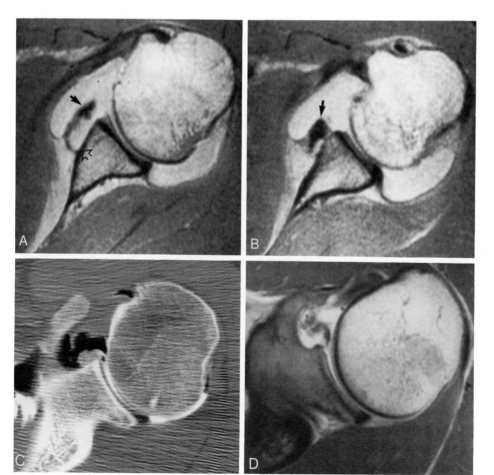

FIGURE 70–152. Anterior glenohumeral joint instability: MR imaging, MR arthrography, and CT arthrography.

A, B Labral detachment and capsular stripping. Two transaxial proton density–weighted (TR/TE, 1800/30) spin echo MR images, **A** being located at a slightly higher level than **B**, show a large joint effusion, detachment of the anterior portion of the labrum (closed arrows), capsular stripping (open arrow), and extra-articular fluid extravasation. (Courtesy of C. Ho, M.D., Stanford, California.)

C, D Labral tear. A transaxial CT arthrogram **(C)** and a transaxial T1-weighted (TR/TE, 850/16) spin echo MR image obtained after the intra-articular administration of a gadolinium compound **(D)** both reveal irregularity of the anterosuperior portion of the labrum. In **D**, high signal intensity is observed at the base of the labrum. (Courtesy of V. Chandnani, M.D., Honolulu, Hawaii.)

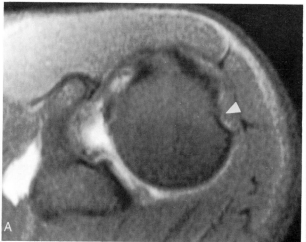
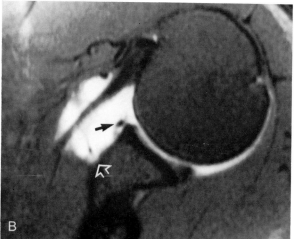
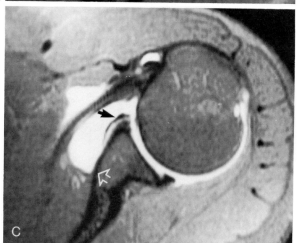

FIGURE 70–153. Anterior glenohumeral joint instability: MR arthrography. Labral tear and detachment, capsular stripping, and Hill-Sachs lesion.

A, B Two transaxial T1-weighted (TR/TE, 600/13) spin echo MR images obtained with chemical presaturation of fat (ChemSat) following the intra-articular injection of a gadolinium compound show, at the higher level **(A)**, a Hill-Sachs lesion (arrowhead) and, at the lower level **(B)**, labral detachment (solid arrow) and capsular stripping (open arrow).

C In a second patient, a transaxial T1-weighted (TR/TE, 750/20) spin echo MR image obtained with chemical presaturation of fat (ChemSat) following the intra-articular injection of a gadolinium compound shows labral detachment and a tear (solid arrow) and capsular stripping (open arrow).

FIGURE 70–154. Posterior and multidirectional glenohumeral joint instability: MR imaging.

A Posterior glenohumeral joint instability. A transaxial proton density–weighted (TR/TE, 2000/30) spin echo MR image shows a tear of the posterior portion of the labrum (solid arrow), a region of low signal intensity (open arrow) that corresponded to a site of calcification evident in the routine radiographs, capsular stripping, and extra-articular fluid.

B Multidirectional glenohumeral joint instability. A transaxial proton density–weighted (TR/TE, 2116/30) spin echo MR image shows abnormalities of both the anterior (open arrow) and posterior (solid arrow) portion of the labrum. (Courtesy of M. Rafii, M.D., New York, New York.)

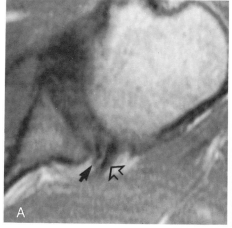
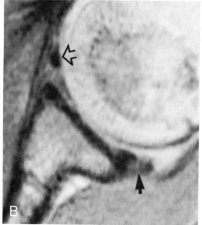

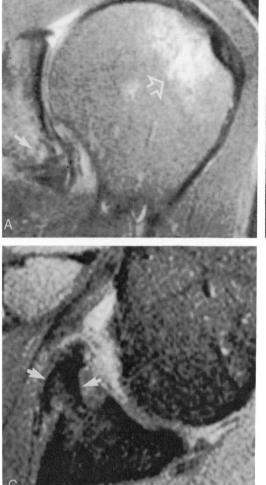

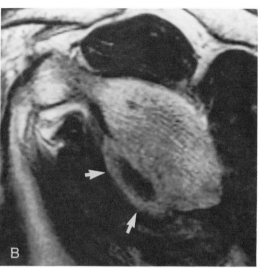

FIGURE 70–155. Anterior glenohumeral joint instability: MR imaging. Acute dislocation in a 50 year old man.

A A coronal oblique fast spin echo MR image (TR/TE, 2650/48) obtained with chemical presaturation of fat (ChemSat) reveals a fracture of the anterior glenoid rim (solid arrow) and high signal intensity in the humeral head (open arrow) consistent with marrow edema secondary to impaction against the glenoid rim during the dislocation.

B A sagittal oblique fast spin echo MR image (TR/TE, 2300/96) shows the fracture of the glenoid rim (arrows).

C A transaxial MPGR MR image (TR/TE, 633/10; flip angle, 35 degrees) reveals the anterior glenoid fracture fragment (arrows).

(Courtesy of S. Eilenberg, M.D., San Diego, California.)

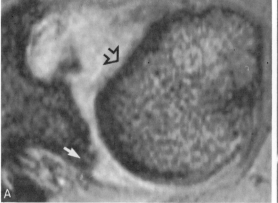

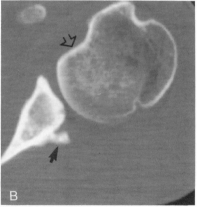

FIGURE 70–156. Posterior glenohumeral joint instability: MR imaging and CT scanning.

A A transaxial spoiled gradient recalled (SPGR) MR image in the steady state (TR/TE, 45/15; flip angle, 20 degrees) shows posterior subluxation of the humeral head, irregularity of the posterior glenoid rim (solid arrow), and a trough fracture (open arrow) involving the anterior surface of the humeral head.

B A transaxial CT scan at a slightly lower level in the same patient confirms posterior displacement of the humeral head, a fracture of the posterior glenoid region (solid arrow), and a trough fracture (open arrow) of the humeral head.

(Courtesy of M. Schweitzer, M.D., Philadelphia, Pennsylvania.)

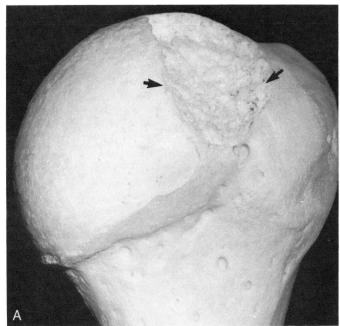
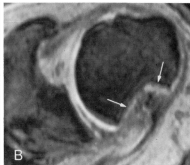

FIGURE 70–157. Anterior glenohumeral joint instability: Hill-Sachs lesion.
   A A photograph of the posterior surface of the humeral head shows the typical location of the Hill-Sachs lesion (arrows).
   B A transaxial 3DFT spoiled gradient recalled acquisition in the steady state MR image (TR/TE, 63/10; flip angle, 60 degrees) obtained with chemical presaturation of fat (ChemSat) shows a large Hill-Sachs lesion (arrows) appearing as a depression in the posterolateral surface of the humeral head at the level of the coracoid process.

and posterior tear (SLAP lesion). The lesion appears to begin posteriorly and to extend anteriorly, it terminates prior to or at the midglenoid notch, and it includes the anchor of the biceps tendon to the glenoid labrum. A fall on the outstretched arm with the shoulder positioned in abduction and slight forward flexion at the time of impact also is a typical mechanism of injury.

The SLAP lesion has been divided into four types: type I lesions, representing approximately 10 per cent of all SLAP lesions, are associated with degenerative fraying of the superior portion of the labrum, but the labrum remains firmly attached to the glenoid rim; type II lesions, representing approximately 40 per cent of all SLAP lesions, are characterized by separation of the superior portion of the glenoid labrum and the tendon of the long head of the biceps brachii muscle from the glenoid rim; type III lesions, representing approximately 30 per cent of all SLAP lesions, are bucket-handle tears of the superior portion of the la-

brum without involvement of the attachment site of the tendon of the long head of the biceps brachii muscle; and type IV lesions, representing approximately 15 per cent of all SLAP lesions, are characterized by a bucket-handle tear of the superior portion of the labrum that extends into the biceps tendon. Clinical findings of SLAP lesions include painful motion of the shoulder and, at times, audible clicking noises.

Both computed arthrotomography[342] (Fig. 70–159) and MR imaging[343, 344, 1370] (Fig. 70–160) have been used to detect SLAP lesions of the glenoid labrum-capsular-bicipital tendon complex, with variable success. In a retrospective analysis of computed arthrotomographic images in 17 patients with surgically proved SLAP lesions, Hunter and coworkers[342] indicated that this imaging method showed abnormalities in 16 of the patients and that in 15 the type of labral tear could be determined. Shoulders with type I lesions revealed superior labral irregularities, those with

FIGURE 70–158. Normal groove in the proximal metaphysis of the humerus.
   A Humeral head. A radiograph of a transverse section at the level of the humeral head reveals a smooth posterior surface. The intertubercular sulcus is seen anteriorly (arrow).
   B Humeral metaphysis. A radiograph of transverse section at the level of the proximal humeral metaphysis shows the normal posterior groove (arrowhead) as well as the intertubercular sulcus anteriorly (arrow).

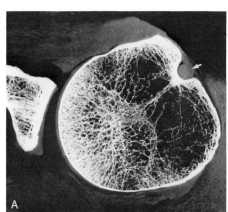
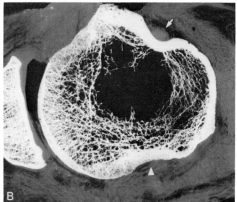

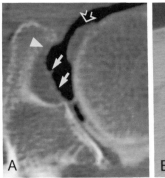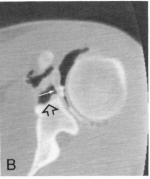

FIGURE 70–159. Superior labral anterior and posterior tear (SLAP lesion): CT arthrography.

A Type I SLAP lesion. A transaxial CT arthrographic image obtained 4 mm below the scapular insertion of the tendon of the long head of the biceps brachii muscle shows subtle fraying (solid arrows) of the anterosuperior portion of the labrum. The bicipital tendon (open arrow) and superior glenohumeral ligament (arrowhead) are indicated.

B Type II SLAP lesion. A transaxial CT arthrographic image reveals labral-capsular separation (open arrow) and marked irregularity of the free edge of the anterosuperior portion of the labrum (solid arrow). (Courtesy of J. Quale, M.D., Englewood, Colorado.)

type II lesions showed labral tears with capsular injury or laxity, those with type III lesions showed a rounded core of soft tissue surrounded by a rim of contrast material and air adjacent to the anterior portion of the labrum (a finding that was designated the Cheerio sign), and shoulders with type IV lesions revealed evidence of a rupture of the tendon of the long head of the biceps brachii muscle. Hodler and associates[343] reviewed MR images and arthroscopic reports in nine patients in whom SLAP lesions were present (using arthroscopic findings as the standard). MR imaging did not allow recognition of simple fraying of the superior portion of the labrum, and the differentiation between complete and partial labral detachments of this portion of the labrum was difficult using MR imaging or even MR arthrography (Fig. 70–161). Detection of abnormalities required analysis of both coronal oblique and transaxial MR images. These authors emphasized the difficulty encountered in the differentiation of significant labral detachment from normal or age-related separation of the labrum.[345, 346] Cartland and

colleagues,[344] in a retrospective analysis of MR images in 10 patients with surgically proved SLAP injuries, indicated the usefulness of this imaging method in the detection and classification of these injuries. Type I lesions were characterized by irregularity of labral contour and a slight increase in its signal intensity, type II lesions were associated with a globular region of high signal intensity interposed between the superior part of the glenoid labrum and the superior portion of the glenoid fossa, type III lesions were accompanied by superior labral tears, and type IV lesions were associated with diffuse high signal intensity in the superior portion of the labrum and in the proximal part of the biceps tendon.

The treatment of SLAP lesions may involve excision of part of the glenoid labrum.[339, 347] The results of such therapy have been inconsistent, however. Indeed, Cooper and co-workers[153] have emphasized the normal laxity of the attachment sites of the superior and anterosuperior portions of the labrum to the glenoid rim that may be difficult to distinguish from a SLAP lesion.

Another specific type of labral lesion has been identified arthroscopically, consisting of a superficial tear of the anteroinferior portion of the labrum.[348] The lesion always is associated with an inferior flap tear with no demonstrable anterior glenohumeral joint instability, and the deep fibers of the inferior glenohumeral ligament remain strongly attached to the labrum and glenoid rim. This lesion has been designated glenolabral articular disruption (GLAD lesion),[348] and it is accompanied by fibrillation and erosion of the articular cartilage in the anteroinferior quadrant of the glenoid fossa. Arthrography of the glenohumeral joint is normal in these cases, and the MR imaging findings have not been studied.

Recurrent unidirectional anterior instability of the glenohumeral joint may be associated not only with a classic Bankart lesion (an avulsion of the anterior labroligamentous structures from the anterior glenoid rim) but also with an avulsion of the periosteal sleeve of the anterior portion of the scapula.[349] This lesion differs from a Bankart lesion because the anterior scapular periosteum does not rupture, thereby allowing the labroligamentous structures to displace medially and rotate inferiorly on the scapular neck. The anterior labroligamentous periosteal sleeve avulsion (ALPSA lesion) is associated with recurrent anterior dislocation of the glenohumeral joint because of the subsequent

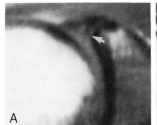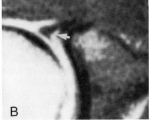

FIGURE 70–160. Superior labral anterior and posterior tear (SLAP lesion): MR imaging. Type II SLAP lesion. Coronal oblique proton density–weighted (TR/TE, 1881/30) **(A)** and T2-weighted (TR/TE, 1881/80) **(B)** spin echo MR images reveal separation (arrows) of the superior portion of the glenoid labrum and the tendon of the long head of the biceps brachii muscle from the superior portion of the glenoid fossa. (Courtesy of P. Fenton, M.D., Toronto, Ontario, Canada.)

FIGURE 70–161. Superior labral anterior and posterior tear (SLAP lesion): MR imaging and MR arthrography. Type II SLAP lesion. A coronal oblique proton density–weighted (TR/TE, 2000/20) spin echo MR image **(A)** and a T1-weighted (TR/TE, 600/20) spin echo MR image following the intra-articular administration of a gadolinium compound **(B)** show disruption (arrows) of the superior portion of the glenoid labrum at its site of attachment. The findings are more obvious in **B**. (From Hodler J, et al: AJR *159*:565, 1992.)

incompetence of the anterior portion of the inferior glenohumeral ligament.

Certain tears of the anterior or posterior portion of the labrum are accompanied by the development of perilabral cysts or ganglia.[1390] The pathogenesis of the cystic lesions is not certain, although similar lesions have been described in association with meniscal tears of the knee (where they are designated meniscal cysts) and with tears or degeneration of the acetabular labrum (in which case they are termed ganglion cysts). In each of these locations, fluid derived from the joint might extend through the tear of the labrum or meniscus into the surrounding soft tissues, leading to cyst formation. In the shoulder, such perilabral cysts or ganglia may extend into the spinoglenoid notch or the suprascapular notch of the scapula, or both notches, and produce an entrapment neuropathy (see later discussion).

Postsurgical Imaging Abnormalities. Numerous operative techniques are used to correct glenohumeral joint instability (see Chapter 68). Recurrent glenohumeral joint instability may occur following any of these techniques, however, related to such factors as persistent abnormalities of the glenoid labrum, joint capsule, or glenohumeral ligaments, compromise of the rotator cuff, or reinjury.[350, 351] Assessment of the postoperative shoulder with advanced imaging methods such as computed arthrotomography and MR imaging is made difficult owing to surgical distortion of normal soft tissue landmarks, incomplete information regarding the nature of the previous surgery, and unavailability of postoperative baseline studies. In one investigation, computed arthrotomography proved useful in confirming the presence of capsular laxity, subscapularis muscle and tendon abnormalities, and Bankart lesions that were either recurrent or not identified during previous shoulder operations.[352] The precise role of imaging examinations in the assessment of the postoperative shoulder, however, requires further analysis.

Biceps Tendon Abnormalities

Anatomic Considerations. The tendon of the long head of the biceps brachii muscle arises from the supraglenoid tubercle or the superior portion of the glenoid labrum, or both structures, and it extends obliquely across the top of the humeral head into the intertubercular sulcus or groove (Fig. 70–162). This groove is bounded by the tuberosities of the humerus. The tendon emerges from the joint at the lower portion of the groove, surrounded by a sheath that communicates directly with the joint. The main arterial supply to the intertubercular portion of the biceps tendon is the anterior circumflex humeral artery.

The tendon of the long head of the biceps brachii muscle is restrained at several levels along its course.[35] The intra-articular portion of this tendon lies beneath the coracohumeral ligament in the rotator interval. The primary restraint of the tendon in this area is the thickened joint capsule about the coracohumeral ligament and edges of the subscapularis and supraspinatus tendons. This restraint is believed to be the major obstacle to medial dislocation of the tendon.[354, 355] Within the intertubercular groove, the biceps tendon is held in place by the tendinous expansion from the insertion of the sternocostal portion of the pectoralis major muscle, the falciform ligament.[356] The relative lack of importance of the transverse humeral ligament in keeping the biceps tendon aligned in the groove has been stressed constantly since an early study by Meyer in 1926.[354] Another key structure in this region is the subscapularis muscle and tendon. The subscapularis tendon inserts into the lesser tuberosity of the humerus. Disruption of the subscapularis tendon leaves the biceps tendon unhindered to slip medially over the lesser tuberosity into the glenohumeral joint. Similar intra-articular displacement of the biceps tendon may occur if the subscapularis tendon is detached from the lesser tuberosity; in this case, although the subscapularis mechanism may remain intact owing to continuity of its fibers with those of the transverse humeral ligament, the biceps tendon may slip medially, by passing over the lesser tuberosity and underneath the subscapularis tendon.

The osseous anatomy of the bicipital groove has been outlined by Cone and coworkers.[357] In their investigation, the average value for the medial wall angle was 56 degrees and the average depth of the groove was 4.3 mm. Although no correlation between the incidence of subluxation and low medial wall angle was found in this study, such a correlation has been noted in other investigations.[358, 359]

Tendinitis. Burkhead[353] has divided tendinitis of the long head of the biceps brachii muscle into two categories: impingement tendinitis and attrition tendinitis. The first and more common of these two types of tendinitis occurs in association with the shoulder impingement syndrome and disruption of the rotator cuff. In this situation, the biceps tendon is impinged between the humeral head, the acromion, and the coracoacromial ligament during elevation and rotation of the arm. Synovial inflammation is not present.[353] Attrition tendinitis is accompanied by peritendinous synovitis and affects the intertubercular portion of the tendon. Stenosis of the bicipital groove related to periostitis leads to tendon attrition and, in some cases, tendon rupture.

The frequency of bicipital tendinitis and tenosynovitis (with or without tendon subluxation) is not clear. Its association with anterior shoulder pain in athletes involved in sports requiring throwing of a ball or in golf or swimming has been noted.[360] The pain may extend down the arm or radiate to the humeral insertion site of the deltoid muscle.[353] The findings usually are unilateral but may be bilateral and are most frequent in the fifth or sixth decade of life. Tenderness with palpation of the bicipital groove may be apparent.

Routine radiography generally is nondiagnostic in cases of bicipital tendinitis and tenosynovitis. A specialized view of the bicipital groove may reveal degenerative changes including bone outgrowths.[357] Glenohumeral joint arthrography may reveal a corrugated pattern of the contrast material that surrounds the tendon, although the finding is infrequent and of questionable significance. The extent of filling of the sheath about the tendon of the long head of the biceps brachii muscle generally is not useful in the diagnosis of bicipital tendinitis or tenosynovitis. Ultrasonography may be valuable in the assessment of the bicipital tendon; in cases of tenosynovitis, fluid in the tendon sheath or an enlarged tendon may be evident.[361]

The diagnostic role of MR imaging in cases of bicipital tendinitis and tenosynovitis is not clear. Evidence of fluid in the sheath of the tendon of the long head of the biceps brachii muscle has been regarded either as a normal finding[252] or as indicative of inflammation, particularly if there

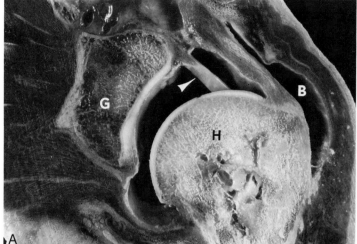

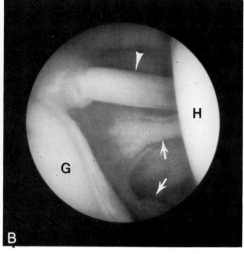

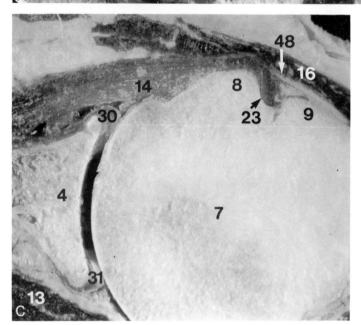

FIGURE 70–162. Tendon of the long head of the biceps brachii muscle: Normal anatomy.

A A coronal section of a cadaveric shoulder following the introduction of air into the glenohumeral joint shows the articular cartilage of the glenoid cavity (G) and humeral head (H). Note the long head of the bicipital tendon (arrowhead) arising from the supraglenoid tubercle. The subacromial (subdeltoid) bursa is identified (B).

B Arthroscopy reveals the long head of the bicipital tendon (arrowhead) attaching to the supraglenoid tubercle. The superior and middle glenohumeral ligaments are indicated (arrows). G, Glenoid cavity; H, humeral head.

C Transverse section at the midglenoid level reveals the following structures: glenoid cavity (4), humeral head (7), lesser (8) and greater (9) tuberosities of the humerus, infraspinatus muscle (13), subscapularis tendon (14), deltoid muscle (16), tendon of the long head of the biceps brachii muscle (23), anterior (30) and posterior (31) portions of the glenoid labrum, and transverse humeral ligament (48).

is no associated effusion in the glenohumeral joint.[252, 256] Kaplan and coworkers,[200] in an MR imaging study of 30 shoulders in asymptomatic volunteers, concluded that fluid in the tendon sheath of the long head of the biceps tendon should be considered abnormal only if it completely surrounds the tendon and a sizable joint effusion is not present. These investigators also indicated that slow blood flow in the anterior circumflex humeral vein may lead to an area of increased signal intensity within the bicipital groove that can be misinterpreted as evidence of tenosynovitis.

Tendon Subluxation and Dislocation. Medial subluxation or dislocation of the tendon of the long head of the biceps brachii muscle may occur as an isolated lesion but generally is observed in association with massive tears of the rotator cuff. Medial displacement of the biceps tendon also may accompany isolated tears or avulsion of the subscapularis muscle or tendon.[362] Once dislocated, the tendon may relocate spontaneously, but more commonly, owing to the development of scar tissue within the sulcus, the tendon remains in a medially displaced position.[353] Factors predisposing to dislocation of the biceps tendon include anomalies and dysplastic changes of the intertubercular groove,[363]

degenerative and attritional changes in the tendon itself, and capsular and ligamentous (i.e., coracohumeral ligament) abnormalities.[364] Even in normal persons, the biceps tendon is pressed against the medial wall of the intertubercular sulcus; hypoplasia of the medial wall of this groove may allow medial subluxation or dislocation of the tendon. Rupture of the coracohumeral ligament may further promote such displacement. Lateral displacement of the tendon of the long head of the biceps brachii muscle does not occur. Posterior dislocation of the tendon may result from a fracture of the greater tuberosity that allows the tendon to slip behind the humerus. It also may occur in association with glenohumeral joint dislocation (Fig. 70–163).

Clinically, there is no pathognomonic finding of a medially dislocated biceps tendon.[364] A snapping sensation as the tendon moves in and out of the bicipital groove may be experienced by the patient. Abbott and Saunders[356] described a provocative diagnostic test that is accomplished during the physical examination: with the arm fully abducted, externally rotated and elevated, it is slowly lowered to the side of the patient during which a palpable or audible click is demonstrated as the tendon slips from its groove. A

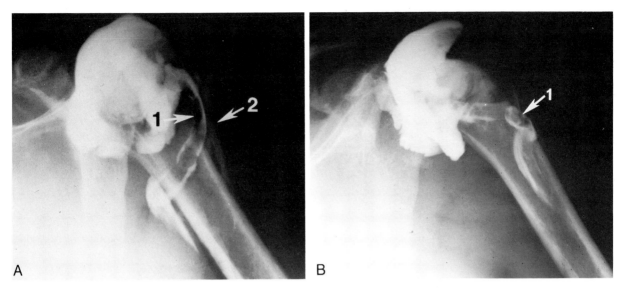

FIGURE 70–163. Tendon of the long head of the biceps brachii muscle: Posterior displacement. Glenohumeral joint arthrography. This 41 year old man sustained an anterior dislocation of the glenohumeral joint that was manipulated and "reduced." Three months later, he had marked restriction of both active and passive motion of the shoulder. An arthrogram of the glenohumeral joint was performed.

A In internal rotation of the humerus, the dislocated long head of the bicipital tendon is seen in an unusual position (1). A bone fragment is also evident (2).

B In external rotation of the humerus, motion is restricted by the posteriorly displaced long head of the bicipital tendon (1). At surgery, the latter was released from its origin and tenodesis in the bicipital groove was performed, reestablishing full shoulder motion.

(From Freeland AE, Higgins RW: Orthopedics 8:468, 1985.)

number of other provocative tests also have been described and are summarized by Burkhead.[353]

Ultrasonography, arthrography, and MR imaging may be used in the assessment of medial dislocation of the biceps tendon. The arthrographic diagnosis of this condition is established by direct visualization of a bicipital tendon within its opacified sheath that is not located in the intertubercular groove (Fig. 70–164) and typically is located medial to the lesser tuberosity. A bicipital groove projection accomplished during arthrography may improve the visualization of the tendon and aid in establishing the diagnosis of tendon dislocation. MR imaging also allows this diagnosis.[365, 366, 1389] The dislocated tendon is seen medial to the bicipital groove, particularly on transaxial (Fig. 70–165) and coronal oblique (Fig. 70–166) MR images. The tendon may appear thickened and may contain abnormal increased signal intensity, and fluid may be seen in the surrounding tendon sheath.[365] Disruption of one or more components of the rotator cuff and the coracohumeral ligament also may be evident. Intra-articular entrapment of the tendon of the long head of the biceps brachii muscle may be documented;

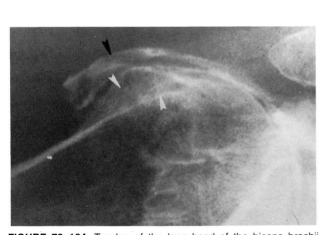

FIGURE 70–164. Tendon of the long head of the biceps brachii muscle: Anterior displacement. Glenohumeral joint arthrography. On a modified axillary view of the shoulder, the contrast-filled tendon sheath and tendon (black arrowhead) is displaced from the intertubercular sulcus (white arrowheads). (Courtesy of A. B. Goldman, M.D., New York, New York.)

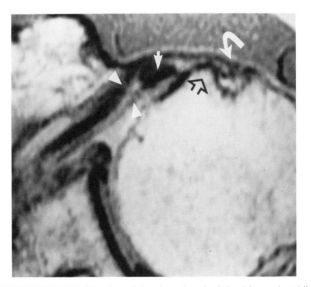

FIGURE 70–165. Tendon of the long head of the biceps brachii muscle: Medial displacement. MR imaging. A 54 year old man fell on his shoulder while skiing and subsequently was unable to abduct his arm. A transaxial proton density–weighted (TR/TE, 2000/30) spin echo MR image shows that the biceps tendon (solid straight arrow) has slipped medially over the lesser tuberosity (open arrow) and appears to be lying between the partially displaced fibers (arrowheads) of the subscapularis tendon. The transverse humeral ligament (curved arrow) appears intact.

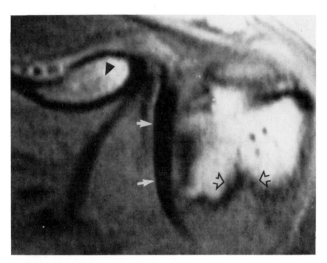

FIGURE 70–166. Tendon of the long head of the biceps brachii muscle: Medial displacement. MR imaging. A coronal oblique proton density–weighted (TR/TE, 2500/20) spin echo MR image at the level of the base of the coracoid process (arrowhead) shows a medially located biceps tendon (solid straight arrows) displaced from the bicipital groove (between open arrows).

access to the joint is provided by disruption of the subscapularis tendon or by detachment of this tendon from the lesser tuberosity of the humerus[366] (Fig. 70–167).

Tendon Rupture. Complete rupture of the tendon of the long head of the biceps brachii muscle may occur proximally, related to impingement or tendon degeneration, or rarely distally, usually resulting from injury (see previous discussion of tendon injuries about the elbow). The weakest portion of the tendon is the segment just distal to its exit from the joint cavity (extracapsular portion), although intracapsular tears of the bicipital tendon also are encountered.[1389] Complete disruption of the bicipital tendon may

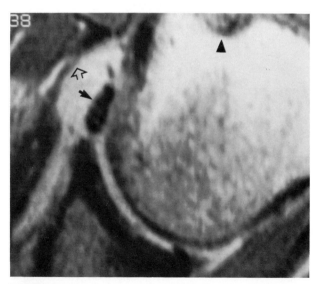

FIGURE 70–167. Tendon of the long head of the biceps brachii muscle: Medial displacement with intra-articular entrapment. MR imaging. A transaxial proton density–weighted (TR/TE, 2000/30) spin echo MR image at the midglenoid level reveals an empty intertubercular sulcus (arrowhead) and intra-articular displacement of the biceps tendon (solid arrow). The subscapularis tendon is torn (open arrow).

be accompanied by an audible pop and, later, by ecchymoses and a change in contour of the soft tissues of the arm. The diagnosis usually is obvious on clinical examination and requires no further diagnostic tests. Partial tears of the biceps tendon, however, may be more subtle and, in these cases, ultrasonography, arthrography, and MR imaging again may be useful. The value of MR imaging relates to direct visualization of the entire length of the tendon of the long head of the biceps brachii muscle when images at appropriate levels of the arm are available. The value of arthrography in this clinical setting, however, is less clear. In the normal glenohumeral joint arthrogram, visualization of the tendon sheath and tendon of the long head of the biceps is not constant. Therefore, although the absence of visualization may indeed represent a tear of the biceps, it is not a reliable sign. Occasionally, following exercise, the tendon sheath will be seen when it was not apparent on preexercise films. Furthermore, leakage of contrast material from the biceps sleeve can be seen in normal persons,[238] although some investigators regard it as a sign of disruption of the transverse bicipital ligament,[367, 368] rupture of the bicipital tendon itself,[369] or overdistention of the articular cavity.

Considering the wide variation in the arthrographic appearance of the bicipital tendon and sheath in normal persons, the radiologist must not rely too heavily on the arthrogram in establishing the existence of a significant abnormality. Still, when a complete bicipital tendon rupture is apparent clinically, arthrography may confirm the diagnosis, demonstrating distortion of the synovial sheath and failing to identify the tendon within the opacified sheath (Figs. 70–168 and 70–169). The arthrographic diagnosis of complete rupture is more accurate in cases of acute tears; with less acute ruptures, shrinkage of adjacent tissues may obscure the abnormal findings. Incomplete tears of the bicipital tendon produce increased width of the tendon and distortion of the synovial sheath.

Rupture of the tendon of the short head of the biceps brachii muscle is extremely rare. The mechanism of injury appears to relate to rapid flexion and adduction of the arm with the elbow extended.[1389]

Entrapment Neuropathies

Several entrapment neuropathies occurring about the shoulder are discussed in Chapter 77, and only two of them are briefly summarized here owing to the importance of MR imaging in their diagnosis.

Suprascapular Nerve Entrapment. The suprascapular nerve is a mixed motor and sensory nerve that carries pain fibers from the glenohumeral and acromioclavicular joints and provides motor supply to the supraspinatus and infraspinatus muscles.[370] It is derived from the upper trunk of the brachial plexus, originating from the fourth, fifth, and sixth cervical nerve roots. The suprascapular nerve passes deep to the trapezius and omohyoid muscles to enter the supraspinatus fossa, passing beneath the superior transverse scapular ligament; it then runs deep to the supraspinatus muscle to enter the infraspinatus fossa through the spinoglenoid notch, passing beneath the inferior transverse scapular ligament at the lateral margin of the spine of the scapula[370] (Fig. 70–170). Two motor branches supplying the supraspinatus muscle are derived from that portion of the supra-

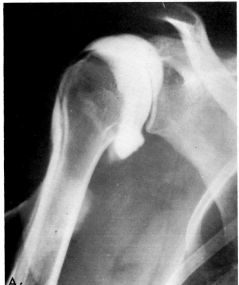
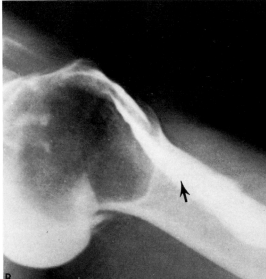
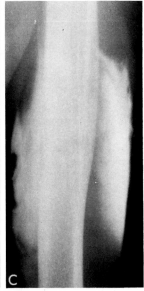

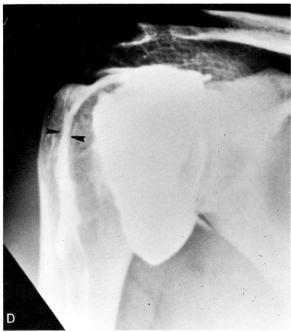

FIGURE 70–168. Tendon of the long head of the biceps brachii muscle: Rupture. Glenohumeral joint arthrography.

A Tear of the transverse bicipital ligament. Note contrast extension for a considerable distance along the course of the bicipital tendon with soft tissue extravasation. (Courtesy of J. Mink, M.D., Los Angeles, California.)

B, C Bicipital tendon rupture. Axillary **(B)** and frontal **(C)** views in a patient with known rupture of the bicipital tendon reveal contrast extension along the course of the bicipital tendon and extravasation into the soft tissues of the arm. The normal lucency of the bicipital tendon itself is not seen within the contrast-filled sheath (arrow).

D Bicipital tendon rupture. This view with the humerus in external rotation shows collapse of the bicipital tendon sheath (arrowheads) with absence of the normal radiolucent shadow of the tendon in this region. (Courtesy of A. B. Goldman, M.D., New York, New York.)

scapular nerve that is in the supraspinatus fossa and, similarly, two motor branches supplying the infraspinatus muscle are derived from that portion of the suprascapular nerve that is in the infraspinatus fossa. Therefore, depending upon the precise site of involvement, entrapment of the suprascapular nerve can lead to weakness and atrophy of both the supraspinatus and infraspinatus muscles, or to weakness and atrophy of the infraspinatus muscle alone.

The first pattern, that of proximal involvement, is more frequent in the general population, whereas distal entrapment of the nerve leading to isolated involvement of the infraspinatus muscle often is seen in male athletes, particularly baseball pitchers and weightlifters.[371] Causes of suprascapular nerve entrapment include fractures of the humerus and scapula, anterior dislocations of the glenohumeral joint, penetrating or surgical trauma, anomalies of the transverse scapular ligaments, tumors, and ganglia.[370, 372–376] A delay in diagnosis is frequent, related in part to the patient not seek-

ing medical treatment until significant shoulder weakness is observed.

MR imaging, as well as ultrasonography and CT, has been used to investigate patients with findings of suprascapular nerve entrapment.[370, 377] Although a variety of benign and malignant soft tissue and bone lesions cause this entrapment, the documentation of periarticular ganglion cysts with MR imaging has been emphasized[370] (Fig. 70–171). These ganglia may lead to proximal or distal entrapment of the suprascapular nerve and are seen as well-defined, smooth masses with low signal intensity on T1-weighted spin echo MR images and high signal intensity on T2-weighted spin echo MR images. An associated finding is atrophy of the infraspinatus muscle alone or both the infraspinatus and supraspinatus muscles. Such ganglia may be accompanied by tears in the adjacent portion of the glenoid labrum, which suggests that their pathogenesis may be similar to that of meniscal cysts in the knee.[1390]

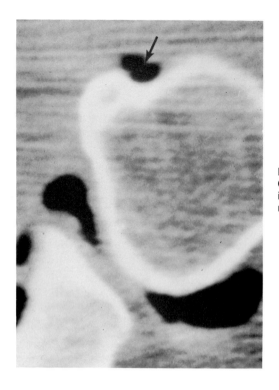

FIGURE 70–169. Tendon of the long head of the biceps brachii muscle: Rupture. Computed arthrotomography. A transaxial CT image following the injection of air into the glenohumeral joint reveals a distended empty bicipital tendon sheath (arrow).

Axillary Nerve Entrapment. The quadrilateral space syndrome represents an entrapment neuropathy of the axillary nerve that occurs within the quadrilateral space of the shoulder. This space is located posteriorly, bounded by the teres minor muscle above, the teres major muscle below, the long head of the triceps muscle medially, and the humeral neck laterally (Figs. 70–170 and 70–172). Passing through this space are the axillary nerve and the posterior humeral circumflex artery.

The quadrilateral space syndrome was described in 1983 by Cahill and Palmer.[378] Clinical findings include skin paresthesias in the distribution of the axillary nerve, weakness of the teres minor muscle or deltoid muscle or both muscles, and tenderness upon palpation of the quadrilateral space. Posterior shoulder pain exacerbated by abduction and external rotation of the arm may be evident. A history of trauma may[379] or may not[379] be present. The dominant arm of athletes involved in sports requiring abduction and external rotation of the arm, as in the cocking motion in throwing, may be affected.[371] One documented cause of this syndrome are fibrous bands in the quadrilateral space; treatment may require surgical lysis of these bands and decompression of the quadrilateral space.[371, 380]

The diagnosis of the quadrilateral space syndrome may be accomplished with arteriography[381] or MR imaging.[382] On subclavian arteriograms, occlusion of the posterior hu-

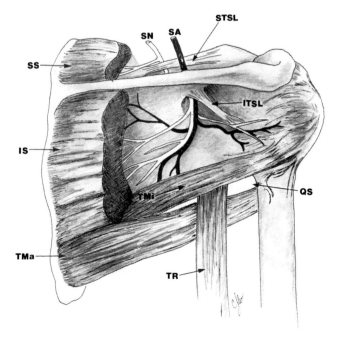

FIGURE 70–170. Suprascapular nerve: Normal anatomy. The suprascapular nerve (SN) adjacent to the suprascapular artery (SA), passes beneath the superior transverse scapular ligament (STSL) in the suprascapular notch, then runs deep to the supraspinatus muscle (SS) and the inferior transverse scapular ligament (ITSL) to pass through the spinoglenoid notch. The infraspinatus muscle (IS), teres minor muscle (TMi), teres major muscle (TMa), and long head of the triceps muscle (TR) also are indicated. The quadrilateral space (QS) is shown. The axillary nerve and the posterior humeral circumflex artery traverse this space. (Modified from Fritz R. C., et al: Radiology *182*:437, 1992.)

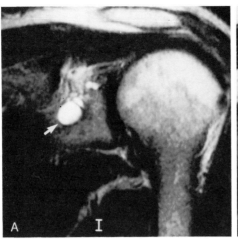 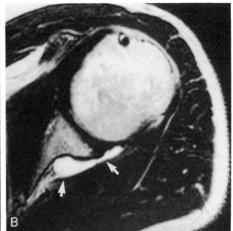

FIGURE 70–171. Suprascapular nerve: Entrapment related to ganglion cysts.

A, B Coronal oblique **(A)** and transaxial **(B)** T2-weighted (TR/TE, 3200/105) fast spin echo MR images reveal a ganglion cyst (arrows) extending medially from the glenohumeral joint to the region of the spinoglenoid notch of the scapula. Although this patient had clinical evidence of entrapment of the suprascapular nerve, no MR imaging findings of muscle atrophy are evident.

C In a second patient, a transaxial MPGR MR image (TR/TE, 383/12; flip angle, 15 degrees) reveals a ganglion cyst of high signal intensity adjacent to the posterior margin of the glenoid cavity. Observe a tear in the adjacent labrum (arrow).

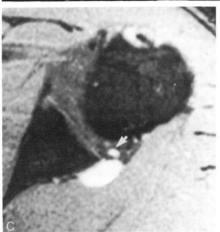

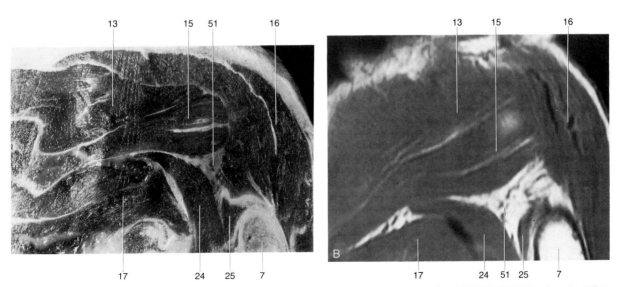

FIGURE 70–172. Quadrilateral space: Normal anatomy. Coronal oblique section **(A)** and T1-weighted (TR/TE, 600/20) spin echo MR image **(B)**. The posterior humeral circumflex artery and the axillary nerve (51) are located in the quadrilateral space. Other identified structures are the humeral diaphysis (7), infraspinatus muscle (13), teres minor muscle (15), deltoid muscle (16), teres major muscle (17), long head of the triceps muscle (24), and lateral head of the triceps muscle (25). (From Petersilge CA, et al: MRI Clin North Am *1:*1, 1993.)

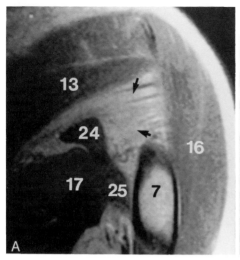
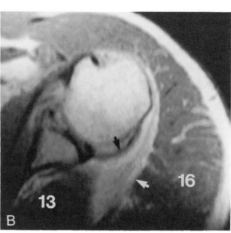

FIGURE 70–173. Quadrilateral space syndrome: MR imaging. Coronal oblique **(A)** and transaxial **(B)** proton density–weighted (TR/TE, 2000/25) MR images show selective atrophy with fatty replacement of the teres minor muscle (arrows). The infraspinatus muscle (13), deltoid muscle (16), teres major muscle (17), and long (24) and lateral (25) heads of the triceps muscle are identified and are not involved. The humeral diaphysis (7) also is seen. Compare **A** with Figure 70–172**B**. (Courtesy of W. Glenn, M.D., Long Beach, California.)

meral circumflex artery can be documented when the arm is abducted and externally rotated, although the artery may be patent when the arm is placed alongside the body. MR imaging reveals atrophy with fatty infiltration of the teres minor muscle or the deltoid muscle, or both muscles (Fig. 70–173).

Synovial Abnormalities

Involvement of the glenohumeral joint in a variety of synovial inflammatory disorders, such as rheumatoid arthritis, the seronegative spondyloarthropathies, crystal deposition diseases, infection, amyloidosis, pigmented villonodular synovitis, and idiopathic synovial (osteo)chondromatosis, is described in appropriate sections of this text. Similar involvement of the subacromial-subdeltoid bursa, either alone or in combination with glenohumeral joint involvement,

also is described in many of these sections. The arthrographic and bursographic findings accompanying these conditions are detailed in Chapter 13. These findings include a corrugated, enlarged synovial space, nodular filling defects, lymphatic filling, adhesive capsulitis with a restricted joint cavity, adhesive bursitis with a contracted bursal cavity, and rotator cuff disruption (Figs. 70–174 and 70–175). In cases of rheumatoid arthritis, para-articular synovial cysts may be encountered, and in cases of septic arthritis, soft tissue abscesses may be evident.

MR imaging in cases of synovitis within the glenohumeral joint or subacromial-subdeltoid bursa shows a variety of findings including an increased amount of synovial fluid, intrasynovial regions of low signal intensity representing fibrous (or rice) bodies, and enhancement of the synovial membrane following the intravenous administration of gadolinium compounds. The extent of cartilaginous and osse-

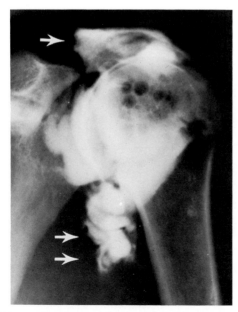

FIGURE 70–174. Septic arthritis: Glenohumeral joint arthrography. Note opacification of a soft tissue abscess (lower arrows) and, owing to a rotator cuff tear, the subacromial-subdeltoid bursa (upper arrow).

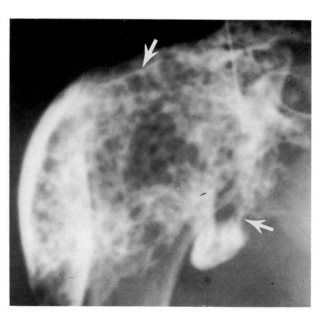

FIGURE 70–175. Rheumatoid arthritis: Subacromial bursography. A frontal radiograph reveals an enlarged subacromial bursa with innumerable nodular filling defects (arrows). (Courtesy of W. J. Weston, M.D., Lower Hutt, New Zealand.)

ous destruction may be identifiable. In cases of pigmented villonodular synovitis or idiopathic synovial (osteo)-chondromatosis, diagnostic MR imaging abnormalities may be seen, owing to the presence of hemosiderin deposition (in pigmented villonodular synovitis) or cartilage nodules (in idiopathic synovial osteochondromatosis) (Fig. 70–176). In amyloidosis, particularly that related to long-term hemodialysis, nodular masses, often with persistent low signal intensity, may be evident (Fig. 70–176).

Bone Abnormalities

A number of radiographically occult bone injuries may lead to significant shoulder disability. These include acute fractures of the tuberosities of the humerus, osteochondritis dissecans of the glenoid cavity or humeral head, stress fractures of the clavicle, scapula, or ribs, and posttraumatic osteolysis of the distal clavicle (see Chapters 67, 68, and 94). When routine radiographs are not rewarding, diagnos-

tic information may be supplied by bone scintigraphy, CT scanning, CT arthrography, or MR imaging (Fig. 70–177).

HIP

Osseous Anatomy

At the hip, the globular head of the femur articulates with the cup-shaped fossa of the acetabulum. This latter structure develops in fetal life from ossification of the ilium, ischium, and pubis. At birth, the acetabulum is cartilaginous, with a triradiate stem extending medially from its deep aspect, producing a Y-shaped physeal plate between ilium, ischium, and pubis. Continued ossification results in eventual fusion of these three bones.

The fully developed acetabular cavity is hemispheric in shape and possesses an elevated bony rim (Fig. 70–178). This rim is absent inferiorly, the defect being termed the acetabular notch. A fibrocartilaginous labrum is attached to

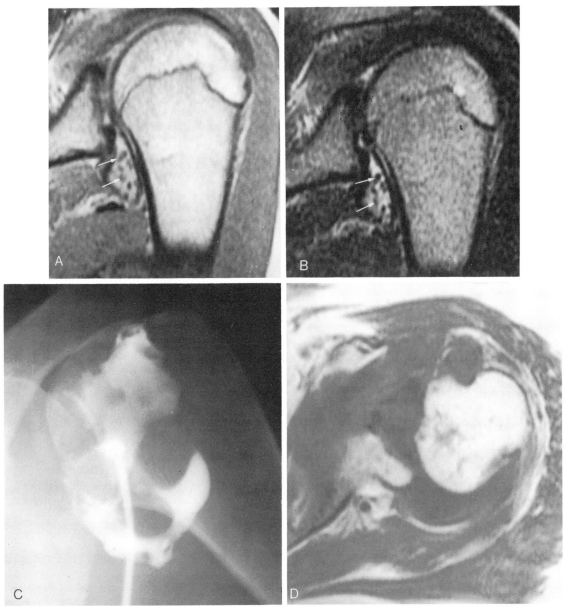

FIGURE 70–176. Idiopathic synovial (osteo)chondromatosis and amyloidosis: MR imaging.
   A, B Idiopathic synovial (osteo)chondromatosis. Coronal oblique proton density–weighted (TR/TE, 2000/30) **(A)** and T2-weighted (TR/TE, 2000/80) **(B)** spin echo MR images show a distended joint containing fluid and multiple calcified bodies (arrows) that are of low signal intensity in both images. (Courtesy of J. Blasingham, M.D., San Diego, California.)
   C, D Amyloidosis. In this patient who had been receiving hemodialysis, glenohumeral joint arthrography **(C)** reveals nodular filling defects. A transaxial T1-weighted (TR/TE, 800/12) spin echo MR image **(D)** shows masses of low signal intensity in the joint. These masses had low signal intensity on T2-weighted images.

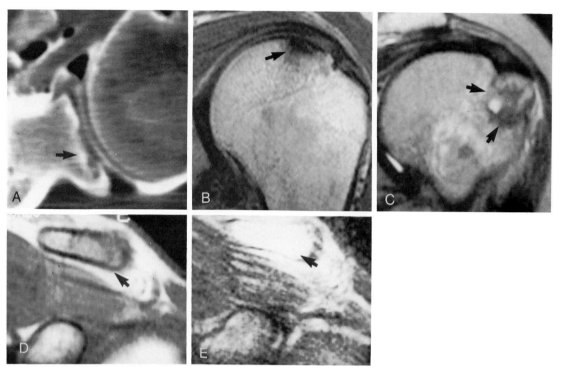

FIGURE 70–177. Occult bone abnormalities: CT arthrography and MR imaging.

A Osteochondritis dissecans of the glenoid cavity. A transaxial CT arthrographic image shows a subtle osseous lesion (arrow) in the posterior region of the glenoid cavity in an 18 year old baseball catcher. Although the overlying cartilage appears normal, a detached chondral fragment was evident at arthroscopy. (Courtesy of G. Greenway, M.D., Dallas, Texas.)

B Osteochondritis dissecans of the humeral head. A coronal oblique T1-weighted (TR/TE, 550/20) spin echo MR image shows a small lesion (arrow) involving the posterior surface of the humeral head. (Courtesy of S. Eilenberg, M.D., San Diego, California.)

C Fracture of the greater tuberosity. A coronal oblique T2-weighted (TR/TE, 3200/104) fast spin echo MR image shows the fracture site (arrows) with areas of high signal intensity extending into the humeral head.

D, E Posttraumatic osteolysis of the clavicle. A coronal oblique T1-weighted (TR/TE, 550/15) spin echo MR image **(D)** and a coronal oblique T2-weighted (TR/TE, 3500/84) fast spin echo MR image obtained with chemical presaturation of fat (ChemSat) **(E)** reveal abnormalities of the distal portion of the clavicle (arrows) in this 30 year old weightlifter. Note the elevated and irregular distal margin of the bone and alterations in the signal intensity of the clavicular marrow, with low signal intensity in **D** and high signal intensity in **E**. (Courtesy of M. Schweitzer, M.D., Philadelphia, Pennsylvania.)

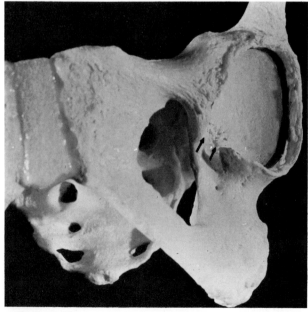

FIGURE 70–178. Acetabular cavity: Osseous anatomy (anterior). A metal marker (black strip) identifies the posterior acetabular rim. This rim is continuous except at the area of the acetabular notch inferiorly (arrows). (From Armbuster TG, et al: Radiology *128:*1, 1978.)

the bony rim, deepening the acetabular cavity. The acetabular floor above the notch, the acetabular fossa, is depressed and irregular. Between the rim and fossa is a smooth horseshoe-shaped articular lunate surface. A discontinuity in the medial aspect of the acetabular roof, termed the superior acetabular notch, appears to represent an accessory fossa in the apex of the acetabulum.[383]

The hemispheric head of the femur extends superiorly, medially, and anteriorly (Fig. 70–179). It is smooth except for a central roughened pit, the fovea, to which is attached the ligament of the head of the femur. The anterior surface of the femoral neck is intracapsular, as the capsular line extends to the intertrochanteric line; only the medial half of the posterior surface of the femoral neck is intracapsular, as the posterior attachment of the hip capsule does not extend to the intertrochanteric crest. The greater trochanter projects from the posterosuperior aspect of the femoral neck–shaft junction and is the site of attachment of numerous muscles, including the gluteus minimus, gluteus medius, and piriformis. The lesser trochanter is located at the posteromedial portion of the femoral neck–shaft junction. The psoas major and iliacus muscles attach to it.

The acetabular angle, iliac angle, and angle of anteversion of the femoral neck are useful radiographic measurements, particularly in the young skeleton. The CE angle of

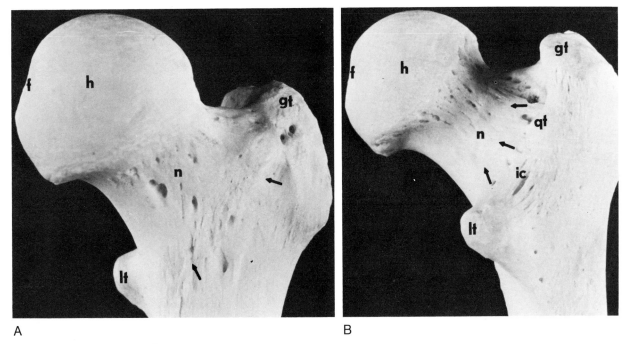

FIGURE 70–179. Proximal femur: Osseous anatomy.
   A Anterior aspect, neutral position. Observe the smooth femoral head (h), fovea (f), neck (n), greater trochanter (gt), and lesser trochanter (lt). The hip capsule attaches anteriorly to the intertrochanteric line (arrows).
   B Posterior aspect, neutral position. The same structures as in **A** are identified. The intertrochanteric crest (ic) and quadrate tubercle (qt) also are indicated. Arrows point to the site of capsular attachment.

Wiberg[384] is an indication of acetabular depth (Fig. 70–180). It is the angle formed by a perpendicular line through the midportion of the femoral head and a line from the femoral head center to the upper outer acetabular margin. The normal CE angle is reported to be 20 to 40 degrees, with an average of 36 degrees.[385] This angle may be slightly larger in women and in older persons. The "teardrop" is a U-shaped shadow medial to the hip joint that has been utilized to detect abnormalities of acetabular depth, thereby establishing a diagnosis of acetabular protrusion (Fig. 70–181). The lateral aspect of the teardrop is the wall of the acetabular fossa, and the medial aspect is the anteroinferior margin of the quadrilateral surface.

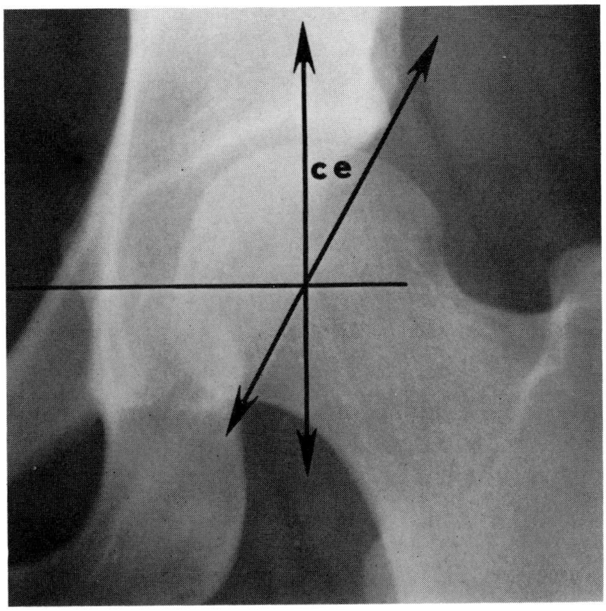

Articular and Soft Tissue Anatomy

The femoral head is covered with articular cartilage, although a small area exists on its surface that is devoid of cartilage, to which attaches the ligament of the head of the femur (Fig. 70–182). The lunate surface is covered with articular cartilage; the floor of the acetabular fossa within this surface does not contain cartilage, but has a fibroelastic fat pad covered with synovial membrane.

A fibrous capsule encircles the joint and much of the femoral neck. The capsule attaches proximally to the acetabulum, labrum, and transverse ligament of the acetabulum. Distally it surrounds the femoral neck; in front, it is attached to the trochanteric line at the junction of the femoral neck and shaft; above and below, it is attached to the femoral neck close to the junction with the trochanters; behind, the capsule extends over the medial two thirds of the neck (Fig. 70–183). Because of these capsular attachments, the physeal plate of the femur is intracapsular and the physeal plates of the trochanters are extracapsular. The fibers of the fibrous capsule, although oriented longitudinally from pelvis to femur, also consist of a deeply situated circular group of fibers termed the zona orbicularis. The fibrous capsule is strengthened by surrounding ligaments, including the iliofemoral, pubofemoral, and ischiofemoral

FIGURE 70–180. CE angle of Wiberg. This is the angle formed by the intersection of a perpendicular line through the midpoint of the femoral head and a line from the femoral head center to the upper outer acetabular margin. The normal value for this angle is reported to be 20 to 40 degrees, with an average of 36 degrees. (From Armbuster TG, et al: Radiology *128*:1, 1978.)

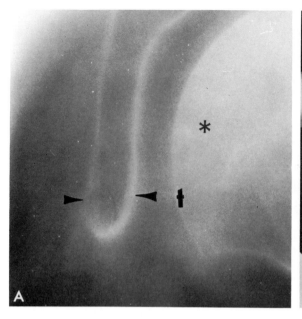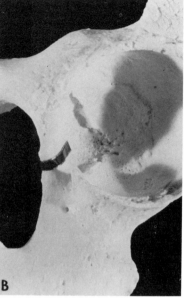

FIGURE 70–181. The "teardrop."

A Anteroposterior tomogram. The "teardrop" (t) and femoral head (asterisk) are seen. The lateral wall of the "teardrop" is the wall of the acetabular fossa. The medial wall is the anteroinferior margin of the quadrilateral surface.

B On a cadaveric specimen, a metal marker has been placed on the teardrop. The quadrilateral surface is not visualized in this projection.

ligaments (Fig. 70–184). The external surface of the capsule is covered by musculature and separated anteriorly from the psoas major and iliacus by a bursa. In this area, the joint may communicate with the subtendinous iliac bursa (iliopsoas bursa) beneath the psoas major tendon through an aperture between the pubofemoral and iliofemoral ligaments.

The extensive synovial membrane of the hip extends from the cartilaginous margins of the femoral head over intracapsular portions of the femoral neck. It is reflected beneath the fibrous capsule and covers the acetabular labrum, the ligament of the head of the femur, and the fat pad in the acetabular fossa.

Important ligaments include the iliofemoral, pubofemoral, and ischiofemoral ligaments, the ligament of the head of the femur, the transverse ligament of the acetabulum, and acetabular labrum. The strong iliofemoral liga-

ment attaches proximally to the anterior inferior iliac spine and the adjoining part of the acetabular rim and distally to the intertrochanteric line on the femur. This ligament becomes taut in full extension of the hip. The pubofemoral ligament extends from the pubic part of the acetabular rim and the superior pubic ramus to the undersurface of the femoral neck, some of its fibers blending with the fibrous capsule. This ligament also becomes taut on hip extension. The ischiofemoral ligament is attached to the ischium below and behind the acetabulum and extends in a superolateral direction across the back of the femoral neck. Its fibers are continuous with those of the zona orbicularis or attach to the greater trochanter. This ligament, as the others, becomes taut in extension of the hip. The ligament of the head of the femur is a weak intra-articular ligament, which is attached to the margin of the acetabular fossa and the transverse ligament of the acetabulum. It extends to a pit

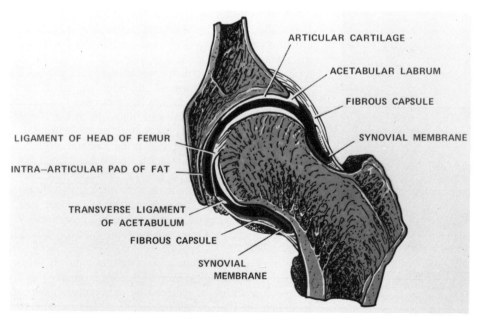

FIGURE 70–182. Hip joint: Normal articular anatomy. Drawing of a coronal section through the hip.

FIGURE 70–183. Hip joint: Normal articular anatomy. Hip arthrogram. The recess capitus (rc) is a thin, smooth collection of contrast medium between apposing articular surfaces and is interrupted only where the ligamentum teres (double arrows) enters the fovea centralis of the femoral head. The ligamentum transversum (lt) is seen as a radiolucent defect adjacent to the inferior rim of the acetabulum. The ligamentum teres bridges the acetabular notch and effectively deepens the acetabulum. The inferior articular recess (iar) forms a pouch at the inferior base of the femoral head below the acetabular notch and ligamentum transversum. The superior articular recess (sar) extends cephalad around the acetabular labrum (lab). The acetabular labrum is seen as a triangular radiolucent area adjacent to the superolateral lip of the acetabulum. The zona orbicularis (zo) is a circumferential lucent band around the femoral neck, which changes configuration with rotation of the femur. The recess colli superior (rcs) and recess colli inferior (rci) are poolings of contrast material at the apex and base of the intertrochanteric line and are the most caudal extensions of the synovial membrane. (From Guerra J Jr, et al: Radiology *128*:11, 1978.)

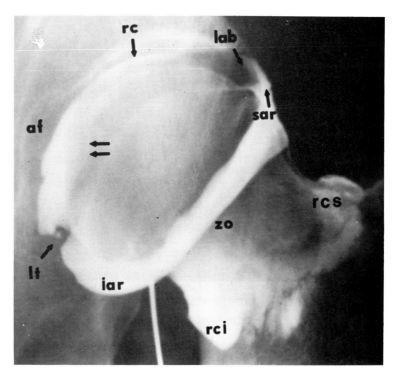

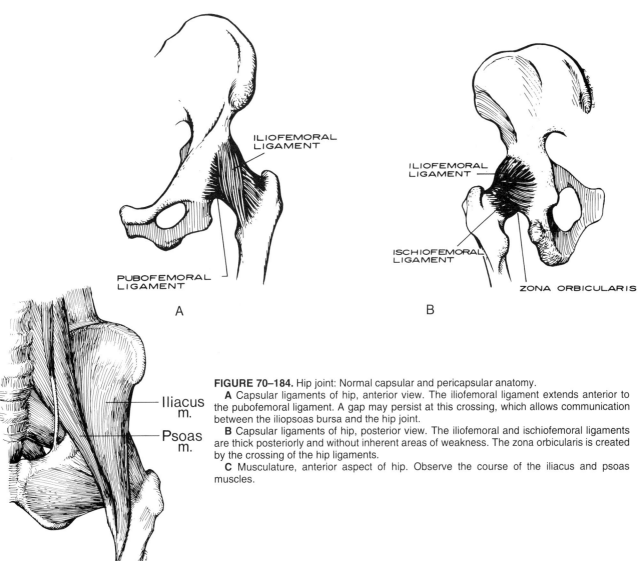

FIGURE 70–184. Hip joint: Normal capsular and pericapsular anatomy.

A Capsular ligaments of hip, anterior view. The iliofemoral ligament extends anterior to the pubofemoral ligament. A gap may persist at this crossing, which allows communication between the iliopsoas bursa and the hip joint.

B Capsular ligaments of hip, posterior view. The iliofemoral and ischiofemoral ligaments are thick posteriorly and without inherent areas of weakness. The zona orbicularis is created by the crossing of the hip ligaments.

C Musculature, anterior aspect of hip. Observe the course of the iliacus and psoas muscles.

on the femoral head. Between these areas of attachment, this ligament is clothed by a synovial sheath. In some persons, the sheath alone is present, without the ligament, and in others, neither sheath nor ligament can be identified. The ligament is stretched when the thigh is flexed, adducted, and laterally rotated. The transverse ligament of the acetabulum is a portion of the acetabular labrum whose fibers extend across the acetabular notch. The acetabular labrum, the fibrocartilaginous rim about the acetabulum, is firmly attached to the bony rim and transverse ligament, is triangular on cross section, and has a free edge or apex that forms a smaller circle that closely embraces the femoral head.

The iliopsoas bursa represents the largest and most important bursa about the hip. It is present in 98 per cent of hips and is located anterior to the joint capsule.[386] It may extend proximally and communicates with the joint space in approximately 15 per cent of normal hips[387, 388] through a gap between the iliofemoral and pubofemoral ligaments. One additional site that represents an inherent weak part of the hip capsule occurs at the crossing of the iliofemoral and iliopubic ligaments. At this site, fluid may extravasate into the fat plane of the obturator externus muscle.[389]

Bursae about the gluteus muscles also may be demonstrated anatomically and radiographically.[390] The bursa deep to the gluteus medius is larger than that deep to the gluteus minimus. Both bursae are intimate with the greater trochanter.

Many muscles are intimate with the hip joint. Some of these are illustrated in Figure 70–185.

Labral Abnormalities

Abnormalities of the acetabular labrum occur both in children and in adults. Those associated with developmental dysplasia of the hip in infants and in young children are discussed in Chapter 86.

Labral Tears. Although tears of the acetabular labrum occurring in association with irreducible traumatic posterior dislocation of the hip in adults were described in 1957 by Paterson[391] and in 1959 by Dameron,[392] and those occurring with falls in elderly patients were described in 1977 by Altenberg,[393] the report in 1986 by Dorrell and Catterall[394] was the first to emphasize the association of acetabular labral tears in adult patients with developmental dysplasia of the hip. In this report, 12 hips in 11 patients ranging in age from 13 to 47 years were affected, and initial clinical manifestations included local pain and aching. In all patients, radiographic evidence of acetabular dysplasia was evident. Additional radiographic findings included subchondral cysts in the acetabulum and a relatively rapid appearance of osteoarthritis of the hip (Fig. 70–186). Standard arthrography revealed evidence of a labral tear in every patient, manifest as an opacified channel extending into the labrum following the introduction of radiopaque contrast material into the hip (Fig. 70–186). The authors concluded that uncovering of the femoral head in patients with developmental dysplasia of the acetabulum leads to mechanical deformation and subsequent degeneration of the labral tissues. In the same year, Suzuki and coworkers,[395] using hip arthroscopy, identified rupture of the posterior or posterosuperior portion of the acetabular labrum in five adolescents and young adults who had hip pain and no evidence of hip dysplasia or arthrographic abnormalities.

In 1988, Ikeda and associates[396] described arthroscopically evident tears involving mainly the posterosuperior portion of the acetabular labrum in seven adolescents or young adults whose routine radiographs were normal. A history of developmental dysplasia of the hip was apparent in only one of these patients. Pain, especially during physical activity and on passive flexion and medial rotation of the hip, was a constant clinical manifestation. Arthrography in some patients showed abnormal shape of the acetabular labrum, characterized by enlargement and a rounded contour, but the actual tears were not opacified. In 1991, Klaue and associates[397] described an acetabular rim syndrome occurring mainly in young adults that was associated with growing pain and locking of the hip. Routine radiography in many cases showed subtle or obvious findings of acetabular dysplasia. In some patients, conventional arthrography or computed arthrotomography revealed hypertrophy, displacement, or truncation of the acetabular labrum but no evidence of labral tears. In 6 of 29 cases, CT showed cysts (or ganglia) in the periacetabular soft tissues or intraosseous cysts (or ganglia) in the acetabular roof. At surgery, in all cases, a tear of the acetabular labrum was apparent, involving the anterosuperior quadrant of the acetabular rim and resembling a bucket-handle tear of a meniscus in the knee. The authors speculated that in cases of acetabular dysplasia, abnormal forces generated in the acetabular rim lead to degenerative abnormalities of the bone, labrum, and adjacent soft tissues. They postulated further that cyst formation within the limbus (i.e., labrum) is analogous to cystic degeneration of a knee meniscus.

Cystic Degeneration of the Labrum and Ganglion Cysts. The concept of cystic deformation of the acetabular labrum, as described by Klaue and collaborators,[397] had been identified earlier in reports by Ueo and Hamabuchi[398] in 1984, and Matsui and colleagues[399] in 1988, and the association of acetabular ganglia and adjacent soft tissue ganglia had been reported by McBeath and Neidhart[400] in 1976 and by Lagier and associates[401] in 1984. Ueo and Hamabuchi[398] reported two adult patients with developmental dysplasia of the acetabulum and chronic hip pain who revealed a deformed cartilaginous labrum due to ganglion cyst formation; and in the report of Matsui and coworkers,[399] a similar lesion was detected in a single young adult. Arthrography in all three patients in these two reports revealed an enlarged and deformed acetabular labrum.

Haller and coworkers[402] and Silver and associates[403] have described seven and three adult patients, respectively, with labral tears, acetabular dysplasia, osteoarthritis of the hip, acetabular ganglion cysts, or para-acetabular soft tissue ganglia, or combinations of these findings. In both reports, gas adjacent to and within the acetabulum represented a diagnostic clue that was evident on routine radiographs and CT. In two patients reported by Haller and collaborators,[402] spin echo MR images showed the soft tissue ganglion cysts adjacent to the labrum; they appeared as well-defined masses of low signal intensity on T1-weighted spin echo MR images and of high signal intensity on T2-weighted spin echo MR images. Haller and associates[402] indicated possible pathogeneses of these ganglia: abnormal pressure on the lateral portion of the acetabulum that leads to the formation of an intraosseous ganglion cyst, which breaks

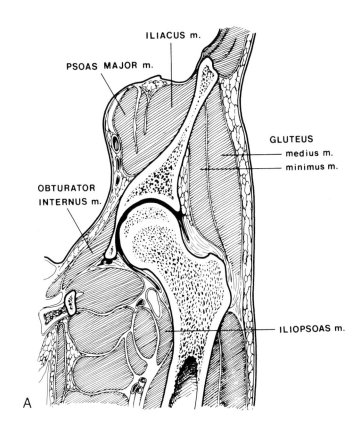

FIGURE 70–185. Hip joint: Normal muscle anatomy.
  A Musculature, coronal section of hip.
  B Musculature, transverse section of hip. Anterior structures are located at the bottom of the drawing.

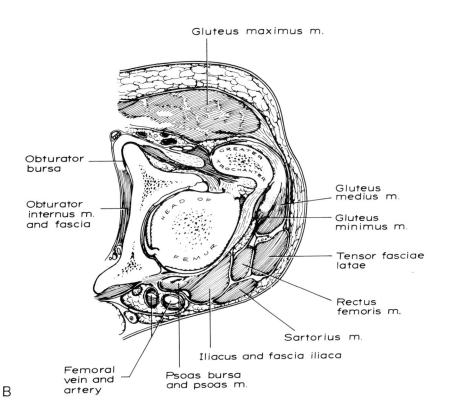

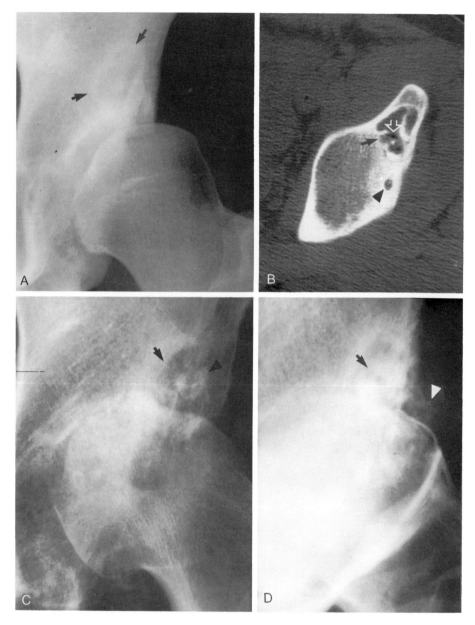

FIGURE 70–186. Acetabulum and acetabular labrum: Developmental dysplasia associated with intraosseous ganglion cysts and labral tears.

A, B In a 27 year old man, routine radiography **(A)** reveals developmental dysplasia of the hip (manifest as a steep, flat acetabular roof and lateral displacement of the femoral head) and a ganglion cyst (arrows) in the acetabulum. A transaxial CT scan **(B)** at the level of the acetabular roof shows the septated intraosseous ganglion cyst (solid arrow) containing gas (open arrow) and a smaller ganglion cyst located posteriorly (arrowhead).

C, D In a second adult patient, routine radiography **(C)** reveals mild developmental dysplasia of the hip associated with severe joint space loss, an acetabular ganglion cyst (arrow), and a bone fragment (arrowhead). Arthrography **(D)** demonstrates contrast opacification of the ganglion cyst (arrow) and a tear of the acetabular labrum manifest as a collection of radiopaque contrast material (arrowhead).

through the outer edge of the bone, creating a soft tissue ganglion; or elevated intra-articular pressure which forces synovial fluid through a labral tear and, subsequently, into the soft tissues, producing a ganglion cyst.

The data in all of these reports of acetabular labral tears and adjacent ganglia generate a number of important observations (Figs. 70–187 to 70–189):

1. Tears of the acetabular labrum occur not only in infants but also in young adults and, rarely, in elderly persons.

2. In adults, these labral tears may or may not be associated with long-standing dysplastic changes of the acetabulum.

3. Ganglion cysts in the acetabulum or adjacent to the acetabular labrum, or in both locations, may be associated with dysplastic acetabuli, with labral tears, or with both findings.

4. Routine radiography may show gas within the osseous and para-articular ganglion cysts.

5. Opacification of the labral tears may be seen during hip arthrography or computed arthrotomography.

6. MR imaging and CT scanning are effective techniques for the detection of the ganglion cysts.

7. The role of MR imaging in the assessment of the torn acetabular labrum is not clear.

Synovial Abnormalities

Synovitis. The involvement of the hip in a variety of articular disorders is well known and is described in appropriate sections of this book. Systemic diseases, such as rheumatoid arthritis and the seronegative spondyloarthropathies, and localized processes, such as septic arthritis, pigmented villonodular synovitis, and idiopathic synovial (osteo)chondromatosis, may affect this articulation. In some cases, routine radiography allows precise diagnosis, although data provided by clinical assessment, other imaging methods, and occasionally, joint aspiration or examination of synovial tissue may be required.

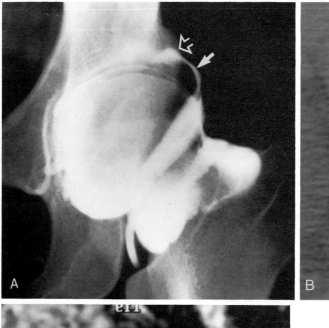

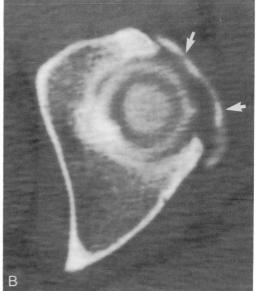

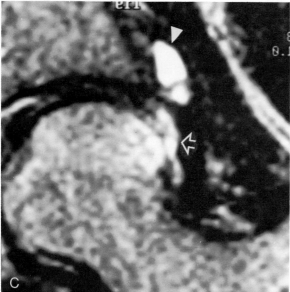

FIGURE 70–187. Acetabular labrum: Tears and cystic degeneration. Standard hip arthrography **(A)** reveals enlargement and rounding of the acetabular labrum (solid arrow) with a cystic collection of contrast material (open arrow). There appears to be mild flattening of the acetabulum consistent with developmental dysplasia. CT arthrography **(B)** confirms a curvilinear collection of contrast material about the enlarged labrum (arrows). A coronal T2-weighted (TR/TE, 3500/102) fast spin echo MR image **(C)** shows fluid of high signal intensity extending from the joint (open arrow) into a cystic mass (arrowhead). (Courtesy of M. Callagher, Sr., M.D., Laguna Niguel, California.)

Contrast opacification of the hip may allow more accurate diagnosis of some of these articular disorders (Fig. 70–190). In idiopathic synovial (osteo)chondromatosis or pigmented villonodular synovitis, the extent of synovial and capsular abnormality can be determined arthrographically.[404] This is important, not only in outlining the severity of the disorder, but also in establishing the correct diagnosis when plain films are not conclusive. In patients with septic arthritis, hip arthrography provides a technique for aspiration and culture and also a means for evaluating cartilaginous, osseous, and synovial abnormalities. Hip arthrography also provides information regarding the origin and nature of intra-articular and para-articular radiodense areas.

As in other regions of the body, bone scintigraphy can be used to assess articular disease in the hip. The examination is sensitive but lacks specificity. Its role includes: confirmation of the presence of an abnormality when results of conventional radiography are negative; demonstration of the anatomic distribution of the disease; and evaluation of the activity of the process.[405] Bone scintigraphy also allows

detection of osseous abnormalities, such as stress fractures and ischemic necrosis, that can produce clinical manifestations simulating those of arthritis.

MR imaging provides information regarding the extent of synovial disease in the hip that is not apparent on routine radiographs (Fig. 70–191). Abnormal collections of joint fluid may be detected.[406] As in other locations, such as the knee, however, the differentiation of synovial inflammatory tissue and a joint effusion using MR imaging may require the intravenous administration of gadolinium compounds. As the assessment of the arthritic hip in the immature skeleton often necessitates analysis of the developing chondroepiphysis, MR imaging is superior to routine radiography.[407]

Synovial Cysts. With any process of the hip that leads to elevation of intra-articular pressure, escape of fluid from the joint through a number of anatomic pathways serves to decompress the articulation. Typically, the fluid passes into a surrounding synovial sac which, with distention, can be seen or palpated. These synovial cysts also can be assessed

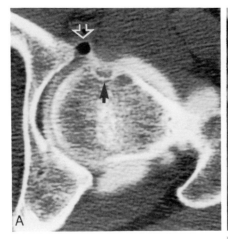

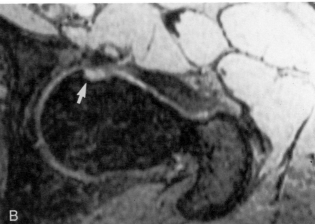

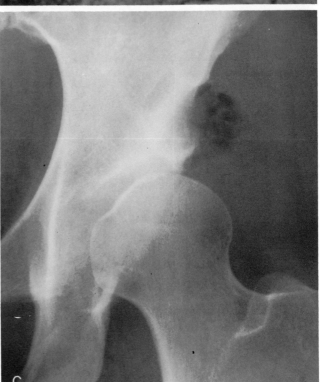

FIGURE 70–188. Acetabular labrum: Tears and cystic degeneration.

A, B In this 23 year old woman, a transaxial CT arthrographic image (obtained by injection of radiopaque contrast material only) **(A)** shows a cystic lesion containing gas (open arrow) and subtle erosion (solid arrow) of the anterior surface of the femoral head. A transaxial 3DFT gradient recalled acquisition in the steady state (GRASS) MR image (TR/TE, 60/11; flip angle, 10 degrees) **(B)** shows the site of bone erosion (solid arrow) with adjacent high signal intensity. (Courtesy of S. K. Brahme, M.D., La Jolla, California.)

C In a second patient, routine radiography shows findings of developmental dysplasia of the hip and gas within a perilabral ganglion cyst. (Courtesy of M. Recht, M.D., Cleveland, Ohio.)

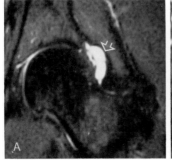

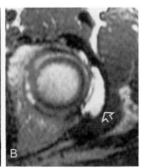

FIGURE 70–189. Acetabular labrum: Tears and cystic degeneration. In a 39 year old woman, a coronal STIR MR image (TR/TE, 4000/17; inversion time, 150 msec) **(A)** shows a cystic collection of high signal intensity (open arrow) within the labrum. A transaxial T2-weighted (TR/TE, 2100/70) spin echo MR image **(B)** reveals the posterolateral location of the cystic lesion (open arrow). (Courtesy of S. K. Brahme, M.D., La Jolla, California.)

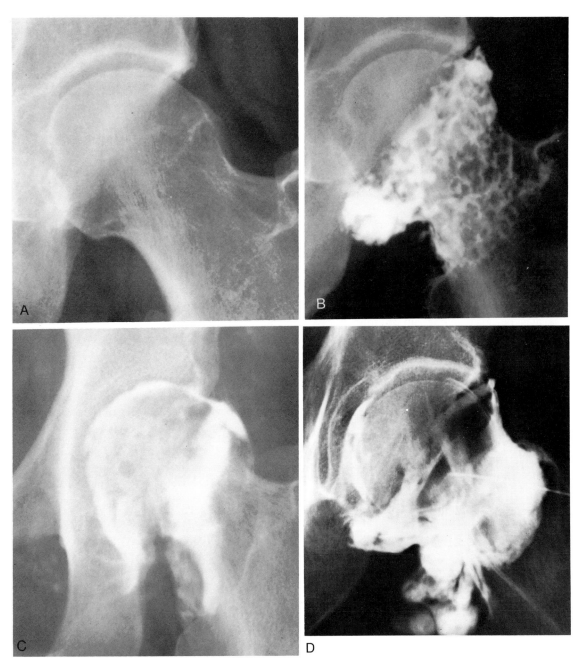

FIGURE 70–190. Synovial disorders: Arthrography.

A, B Idiopathic synovial (osteo)chondromatosis. A routine radiograph **(A)** shows osteophyte formation at the junction of the femoral head and neck, an ossicle adjacent to the lesser trochanter, and a normal joint space. Arthrography **(B)** reveals multiple filling defects within the opacified hip joint that, at surgery, represented noncalcified cartilaginous bodies. (Courtesy of G. Greenway, M.D., Dallas, Texas.)

C Septic arthritis. Arthrography reveals incomplete opacification of the joint, cartilage loss in both the acetabulum and femoral head, and lymphatic filling medially.

D Pigmented villonodular synovitis. Arthrography reveals an enlarged and irregular joint cavity with small, medial collections or pools of contrast material.

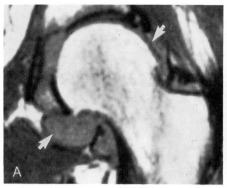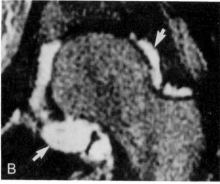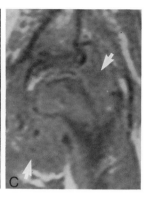

FIGURE 70–191. Synovial disorders: MR imaging.

A, B Idiopathic synovial (osteo)chondromatosis. Coronal proton density–weighted (TR/TE, 2000/20) **(A)** and T2-weighted (TR/TE, 2000/80) **(B)** spin echo MR images show joint distention (arrows) in this 37 year old man with an 8 month history of hip pain. In **A,** the intra-articular process is of low signal intensity; in **B,** it is of high signal intensity. The MR imaging findings simulate those of a joint effusion.

C Septic arthritis. In this child with hematogenous osteomyelitis of the femur and septic arthritis of the hip, a coronal T1-weighted (TR/TE, 500/30) spin echo MR image shows destruction of the femoral capital epiphysis and acetabulum and a mass (arrows) of low signal intensity. (Courtesy of T. Mattsson, M.D., Riyadh, Saudi Arabia.)

with imaging methods, including ultrasonography, CT, arthrography (Fig. 70–192), computed arthrotomography, and MR imaging. Of all the potential locations of synovial cysts about the hip, the iliopsoas bursa deserves special emphasis.

Iliopsoas Bursal Distention. Opacification of the iliopsoas bursa may be noted during hip arthrography. Although this is apparent in 15 per cent of normal hips,[386] communication of the hip and iliopsoas bursa in the presence of intra-articular diseases such as osteoarthritis, rheumatoid arthritis, pigmented villonodular synovitis, infection, calcium pyrophosphate dihydrate crystal deposition disease, and idiopathic synovial (osteo)chondromatosis (Fig. 70–193) may lead to bursal enlargement, producing a mass in the ilioinguinal region that may simulate a hernia and cause obstruction of the femoral vein.[408, 409]

The iliopsoas bursa (also termed the iliopectineal, iliofemoral, iliac, or subpsoas bursa) is the most important of the 15 or more synovium-lined bursae that have been described about the hip. Measuring approximately 3 to 7 cm in length and 2 to 4 cm in width and extending from the inguinal ligament to the lesser trochanter of the femur, the iliopsoas bursa is present in about 98 per cent of adults. It communicates with the hip joint via an aperture ranging in diameter from 1 mm to 3 cm, and enlargement of this channel in the 15 per cent of normal adults who possess this aperture or creation of a communicating pathway in those adults who do not is an expected consequence of virtually any disease process of the hip that leads to an elevation of intra-articular pressure (Fig. 70–194). This phenomenon is somewhat less frequent in children, owing to a decreased prevalence of normal communication between the iliopsoas bursa and the hip.

The iliopsoas bursa is bounded anteriorly by the iliopsoas muscle and posteriorly by the pectineal eminence and the thin portion of the capsule of the hip joint.[410] Its lateral border is the iliofemoral ligament and its medial border is the cotyloid ligament; its superior border is the inguinal ligament and its inferior border is the pubofemoral ligament.[410] When distended, a painless or painful soft tissue mass is created, possibly accompanied by shortening of the stride related to avoidance of hyperextension, flexion of the hip and knee with external rotation of the thigh, weakness of the extremity, and point tenderness inferior to the inguinal ligament and 2 cm lateral to the femoral artery. The mass itself may compress the adjacent neurovascular structures, rarely causing secondary venous obstruction with distal edema, displace pelvic organs, become secondarily infected or traumatized, or induce an abducted gait. In the absence of a clear-cut history of arthritis, the patient with an enlarged iliopsoas bursa initially may be evaluated by a general surgeon, who easily may misinterpret the mass and

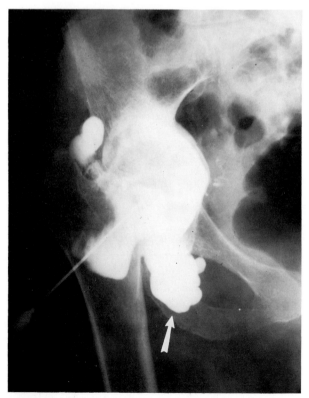

FIGURE 70–192. Synovial cysts: Arthrography. In this 65 year old woman with rheumatoid arthritis and an apparent "femoral hernia," arthrography indicates that the clinically evident soft tissue mass is related to a synovial cyst (arrow). Observe the sacculation of the articular cavity and a protrusio acetabuli defect.

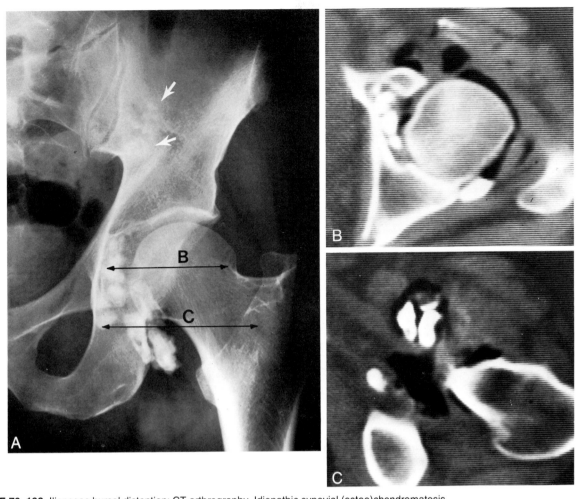

FIGURE 70–193. Iliopsoas bursal distention: CT arthrography. Idiopathic synovial (osteo)chondromatosis.

A An initial radiograph reveals multiple calcified or ossified collections in the acetabular fossa that are extending medially and inferiorly, in the distribution of the iliopsoas bursa. Note the additional subtle calcified collections near the sacroiliac joint (arrows).

B, C Following the introduction of air into the hip, two transaxial CT scans at the levels indicated in **A** document the intra-articular location **(B)** and intrabursal location **(C)** of the bodies. Histologic confirmation of idiopathic synovial (osteo)chondromatosis was obtained.

its associated symptoms and signs as evidence of an inguinal hernia, aneurysm of the femoral artery, undescended testicle, varices, adenopathy, or solid neoplasm. Arteriographic evaluation may lead to inadvertent puncture of the bursa or, at the time of operation, the enlarged synovium-lined structure may present a puzzle to the surgeon, who was anticipating some other disease process.[411] Accurate preoperative diagnosis is provided by arthrography of the hip (which may be combined with CT), direct opacification of the bursa, ultrasonography, MR imaging, or CT alone.[410, 412–415]

With regard to the imaging strategy that is used to evaluate suspected iliopsoas bursal distention or other synovial cysts about the hip, ultrasonography should be performed following conventional radiography in the setting of a probable groin mass or other suggestive clinical manifestations. If a nonpulsatile fluid collection without Doppler evidence of flow is demonstrated, this technique then can be used for diagnostic aspiration of its contents. Fluid analysis should distinguish a synovial cyst or iliopsoas bursitis from a lymphocele, abscess, or hematoma. Subsequent injection of

contrast material into the bursa or cyst may opacify the hip joint, confirming the diagnosis; if not, hip arthrography, CT, or MR imaging may be desirable for delineation of potential articular communication if surgery is being contemplated. The results of conservative management can be followed noninvasively with either ultrasonography or CT. In general, arteriography and lymphangiography have no place in the present-day diagnosis of suspected disease of synovial origin about the hip joint.

Iliopsoas Bursitis. The synovium lining the iliopsoas bursa can be involved in a variety of processes, including rheumatoid arthritis and infection. Typically, such involvement is associated with abnormality in the adjacent hip, particularly when communication between the two structures is evident. As in diseases of the subacromial-subdeltoid, prepatellar, and olecranon bursae, isolated involvement of the iliopsoas bursa may occur, however. CT, MR imaging, and ultrasonography are the best techniques for further evaluation of an inflamed and distended iliopsoas bursa.[416] Afflictions of other bursal cavities about the hip and pelvis can be evaluated similarly (Fig. 70–195).

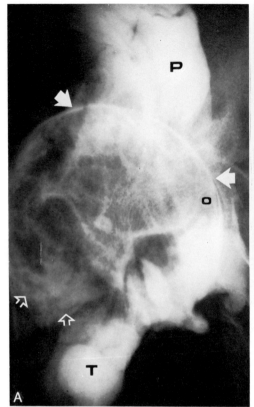

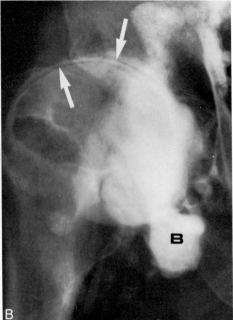

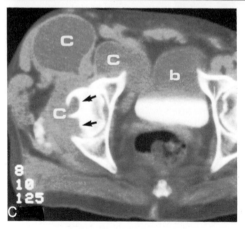

FIGURE 70–194. Iliopsoas bursal distention: Arthrography and CT arthrography.

A Osteoarthritis. This 72 year old woman had a mass in the right groin that was believed to represent an inguinal or femoral hernia. Conventional radiography documented osteoarthritis in the hip. Arthrography demonstrates opacification of a large, multiloculated, communicating iliopsoas bursa with pelvic (P) and thigh (T) extensions. Synovial hypertrophy (open arrows), complete absence of articular cartilage (solid arrows) osteophytosis (o), and flattening of the femoral head indicate advanced degenerative joint disease.

B Legg-Calvé-Perthes disease. In a 71 year old woman with a history of Legg-Calvé-Perthes disease resulting in coxa magna and secondary osteoarthritis, a right inguinal mass suggested a neoplasm. The arthrogram of the hip reveals simultaneous filling of the iliopsoas bursa (B), which lies inferomedial to the articulation. Additional findings are thinning of the femoral and acetabular cartilage (arrows), enlargement and flattening of the femoral head, and nodal opacification from a prior lymphangiogram.

C Rheumatoid arthritis. CT scan was obtained in the evaluation of swelling in the right groin of a middle-aged man with rheumatoid arthritis. The transaxial scan reveals several collections of fluid density (C) around and anterior to the right hip joint, one of which extends into the pelvis with leftward displacement of the urinary bladder (b). Bone erosions also are apparent (arrows). (From Sartoris DJ, et al: Skel Radiol *14:*85, 1985.)

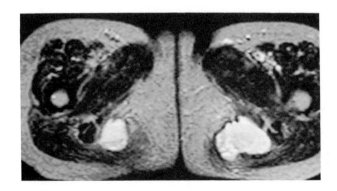

FIGURE 70–195. Trochanteric bursitis: MR imaging. A transaxial T2-weighted (TR/TE, 1500/90) spin echo MR image shows evidence of bilateral trochanteric bursitis. (Courtesy of J. Dillard, M.D., San Diego, California.)

Cartilage Abnormalities

The evaluation of cartilage loss in the hip joint with imaging methods frequently relies upon routine radiography. Although characteristic patterns of such loss allow accurate diagnosis of a number of conditions that affect the hip (see Chapter 50), the detection of small degrees of cartilage destruction in this location is not possible with routine radiography. Indeed, damage to articular cartilage can only be estimated on conventional radiographs related to the presence and distribution of joint space loss and other secondary signs, such as bone sclerosis and osteophytosis. The role of routine radiographs of the hip obtained with the patient standing is not clear, although this technique has been used extensively to evaluate cartilage loss in the knee. Ultrasonography is not effective as a means of detecting cartilage damage in the hip. Arthrotomographic methods may provide some information regarding this detection, but these methods generally are considered insensitive.

Although the value of MR imaging in assessing cartilage lesions in the knee has been investigated thoroughly (see later discussion), the evaluation of similar lesions in the hip using MR imaging has received little attention. Li and co-workers[417] employed standard spin echo MR images in 10 patients with clinically and radiographically documented osteoarthritis of the hip. From data provided by transaxial and coronal images, these investigators developed a grading system based upon the extent of cartilage and bone involvement. Grade 1 abnormalities were characterized by nonhomogeneity of the high signal intensity in the articular cartilage; grade 2 abnormalities were characterized by such nonhomogeneity and discontinuity of the high signal intensity in the articular cartilage, blurring of the adjacent trabeculae, and overall loss of signal intensity in the marrow of the femoral head and neck; grade 3 alterations included those of grade 2 and, in addition, irregularities of the cortical outlines of the femoral head and acetabulum, a zone of intermediate signal intensity between the acetabulum and the femoral head, and regions of intermediate signal intensity surrounded by a rim of low signal intensity in the femoral head; and grade 4 abnormalities represented all of the previous changes plus deformity of the femoral head. These authors concluded that a grading system based on MR imaging findings was more useful than one based on routine radiographic findings in cases of mild to moderate osteoarthritis of the hip.

Although these results suggest a role for MR imaging in the detection of cartilage loss in the hip, the deficiencies of standard MR imaging in the analysis of chondral lesions in the knee has been well documented (see later discussion). Furthermore, the results of an additional study by Hodler and associates[418] emphasized the deficiencies of one particular MR imaging sequence in the detection of cartilage lesions in the acetabulum and femoral head (Fig. 70–196).

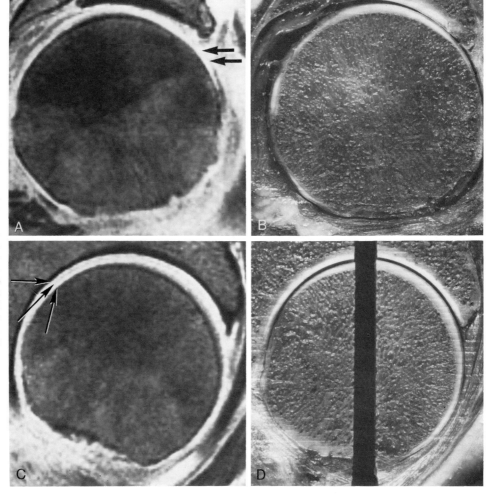

FIGURE 70–196. Cartilage loss: MR imaging. Coronal **(A, B)** and sagittal **(C, D)** T1-weighted (TR/TE, 600/20) spin echo MR images obtained with chemical presaturation of fat (ChemSat) **(A, C)** and corresponding anatomic sections **(B, D)** reveal that although femoral and acetabular cartilage can be differentiated easily in the sagittal MR image **(C,** arrows), this differentiation is difficult in the coronal MR image **(A)**. Femoral cartilage is difficult to differentiate from hyperintense structures within the acetabular fossa and superolaterally (presumably related in part to a joint effusion) **(A,** arrows). (From Hodler J, et al: AJR *159:*351, 1992.)

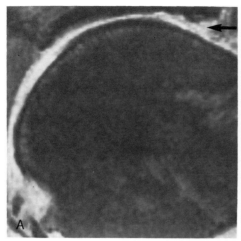
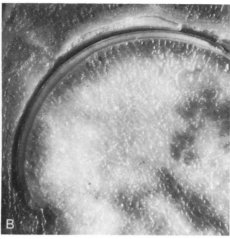

FIGURE 70–197. Cartilage loss: MR imaging. A coronal T1-weighted (TR/TE, 600/20) spin echo MR image obtained with chemical presaturation of fat (ChemSat) **(A)** and a corresponding anatomic section **(B)** reveal difficulty in differentiation between superolateral femoral cartilage and parts of the labrum (arrow), capsule, and surrounding soft tissue. (From Hodler J, et al: AJR *159:*351, 1992.)

In this investigation, femoral heads and acetabula derived from 10 cadavers were imaged with a T1-weighted fat-suppressed (ChemSat) spin echo MR sequence in both the coronal and sagittal planes (using a send-receive extremity coil, a 12 cm field-of-view, and two excitations), and the thickness of the articular cartilage in numerous locations in the femoral head and acetabulum as measured by MR images was compared with that detected on gross inspection of the specimens. The highest correlation between the two measurement methods was found for femoral cartilage, particularly in regions where the femoral cartilage was applied directly to acetabular cartilage. There were significant inconsistencies in the measurements derived from inspection and from MR imaging, however, leading the authors to conclude that fat-suppression spin echo MR images were not sufficiently accurate to be of clinical value (Fig. 70–197).

As is indicated in the section on cartilage lesions in the knee, a number of newer MR imaging sequences and methods may hold more promise for the detection of chondral loss.

Bone Abnormalities

Many localized and generalized diseases of bone may involve the acetabulum or proximal portion of the femur. Classic examples include Paget's disease, fibrous dysplasia, intraosseous lipoma, osteoid osteoma, and Legg-Calvé-Perthes disease. These processes are discussed elsewhere in this book. Three additional conditions are of importance in any discussion of hip disorders: osteonecrosis of the femoral head, transient bone marrow edema (and related disorders), and intracapsular and extracapsular fractures of the femoral neck. Although each of these is considered in detail in other chapters (Chapters 51, 68, 79, and 80), a few additional comments appropriately are placed here.

Osteonecrosis. The causative factors leading to ischemic necrosis of bone are diverse and include trauma, corticosteroid medications, sickle cell anemia and other hemoglobinopathies, Gaucher's disease, alcoholism, pancreatitis, and radiation; furthermore, in many cases, a specific etiologic factor cannot be identified (idiopathic osteonecrosis). Although the site of osteonecrosis in any patient varies according to its precise cause, the femoral head, the femoral condyles, and the humeral head commonly are involved.

The predilection for involvement of the femoral head relates to the vulnerability of a blood supply that includes arteries that extend beneath the capsule of the hip joint.

A desire to identify a sensitive method for detection of osteonecrosis of the femoral head has led to extensive investigation of a number of imaging methods, and the sensitivity of many of these techniques has been found wanting. Routine radiography, conventional tomography, and CT (Fig. 70–198A) are not reliable in the diagnosis of early osteonecrosis of the femoral head, although the two tomographic methods are useful in defining the extent of bone collapse (Fig. 70–198B,C). Scintigraphy using bone-seek-

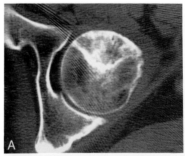
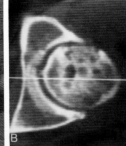
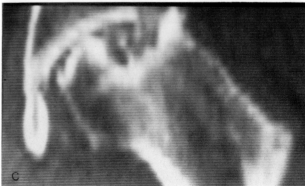

FIGURE 70–198. Osteonecrosis: CT scanning.

A A transaxial CT scan shows features of a segmental region of osteonecrosis involving the anterolateral surface of the femoral head, but the technique generally is not useful in defining early osteonecrosis.

B, C A transaxial CT scan **(B)** and a reformatted coronal CT scan **(C)** at the level indicated in **B** show extensive osteonecrosis of the femoral head manifest as subchondral cysts, bone collapse, and joint space narrowing.

ing radiopharmaceutical agents is sensitive to early changes of osteonecrosis, but the scintigraphic findings lack specificity. Single photon emission computed tomography (SPECT) improves the sensitivity but does not improve the specificity of the radionuclide examination. MR imaging appears best suited to the detection of the early stages of ischemic necrosis of bone.

The MR imaging characteristics of osteonecrosis of the femoral head are variable. Factors that may predispose a femoral head to osteonecrosis and that may be identified on MR images include increased amounts of fatty marrow in the trochanters and the presence of a sealed-off physeal scar.[1391] A diffuse pattern of bone marrow edema, identical to that of transient bone marrow edema (see following discussion), may be identified in the early stages of the process. Subsequently, a more focal process within the femoral head allows a more specific diagnosis (Fig. 70–199). The area of ischemic marrow may be surrounded by a reactive interface that is characterized by low signal intensity on T1-weighted spin echo MR images and an outer margin of low signal intensity and an inner margin of high signal intensity on T2-weighted spin echo MR images. This pattern, often designated a double line sign, is virtually diagnostic of osteonecrosis.[419] The involved segment of the femoral head may extend to the subchondral bone plate or, less commonly, it may occur at a distance from it. The central region within the infarcted area initially may reveal signal characteristics of normal fat but, with chronicity, its signal characteristics may change, resembling those of fluid, hemorrhage, or fibrosis. Staging the ischemic process on the basis of these changing patterns of signal intensity has been attempted, but the prognostic significance of this type of staging system is not clear.[419–421] Modifications of MR imaging methods may be used successfully in the initial diagnosis and subsequent monitoring of osteonecrosis of the femoral head; these modifications include STIR imaging (Fig. 70–200*A*), fat-suppression techniques (Fig. 70–200*B*), and the intravenous administration of gadolinium compounds. Although the last of these may lead to different patterns of enhancement of signal intensity in early and advanced stages of the disease process,[422] the added benefit of contrast administration is not clear and, generally, standard spin echo images are sufficient. Successful application

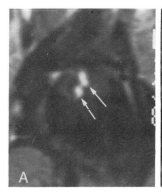
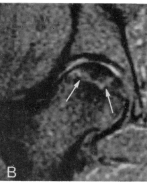

FIGURE 70–200. Osteonecrosis: MR imaging.

A STIR MR imaging. A coronal STIR MR image (TR/TE, 2200/15; inversion time, 160 msec) shows focal regions of high signal intensity (arrows) in the left femoral head, consistent with osteonecrosis.

B Chemical presaturation of fat (ChemSat) MR imaging. A coronal T1-weighted (TR/TE, 650/20) spin echo MR image obtained with ChemSat shows an irregular linear region of high signal intensity (arrows) at the periphery of the zone of osteonecrosis in the right femoral head.

of spin echo images in cases of osteonecrosis of the femoral head usually requires: imaging in more than one plane (coronal, transaxial, or sagittal) and, in some cases, in all three planes; the use of surface coils to allow detection of early disease; and the inclusion of at least one T2-weighted spin echo MR imaging sequence to allow assessment of the healing of the process. Improper diagnosis of osteonecrosis on the basis of MR images may relate to misinterpretation of regions of normal hematopoietic marrow, of normal trabecular groups, or of normal synovial herniation pits in the proximal portion of the femur as abnormal findings.

Transient Bone Marrow Edema. An understanding of this process requires a review of a previously described condition involving the proximal portion of the femur designated transient demineralization (i.e., osteoporosis) of the hip in 1959 by Curtiss and Kincaid[423] (see Chapter 51). Although early reports emphasized the occurrence of this condition in the left femoral head of women in the third trimester of pregnancy, transient osteoporosis about the hip has proven more common in men than women, affecting either the right side or the left side, and occasionally migrating from one side to the other. Early reports also suggested that the diagnosis was based upon the presence of osteopenia of the femoral head, an intact joint space, the absence of bone erosions or collapse, and increased accumulation of bone-seeking radionuclide agents. Although the relationship among transient osteoporosis about the hip, the reflex sympathetic dystrophy syndrome (Sudeck's atrophy), and regional migratory osteoporosis remains controversial, numerous reports have documented the occurrence of pain, restricted motion, and a limp in patients with transient osteoporosis about the hip, leading to its general acceptance as a disease entity.

The application of MR imaging to the assessment of transient osteoporosis about the hip was reported in 1988 by Wilson and collaborators.[424] Their findings, which consisted of altered signal intensity in the marrow of the femoral head and neck, were interpreted as evidence of bone marrow edema (Fig. 70–201*A,B*). Biopsy specimens indicated the presence of normal marrow and bone and the absence of osteonecrosis. Although the histologic data re-

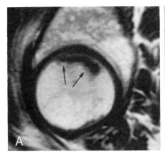
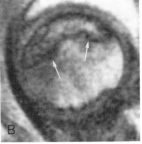

FIGURE 70–199. Osteonecrosis: MR imaging.

A A sagittal T1-weighted (TR/TE, 966/12) spin echo MR image shows a curvilinear region of low signal intensity (arrows) representing osteonecrosis of the femoral head.

B A sagittal T1-weighted (TR/TE, 800/20) spin echo MR image in a second patient reveals a large area of osteonecrosis of the femoral head manifest as a serpentine-like line of low signal intensity (arrows) with a central zone whose signal intensity is similar to that of fat.

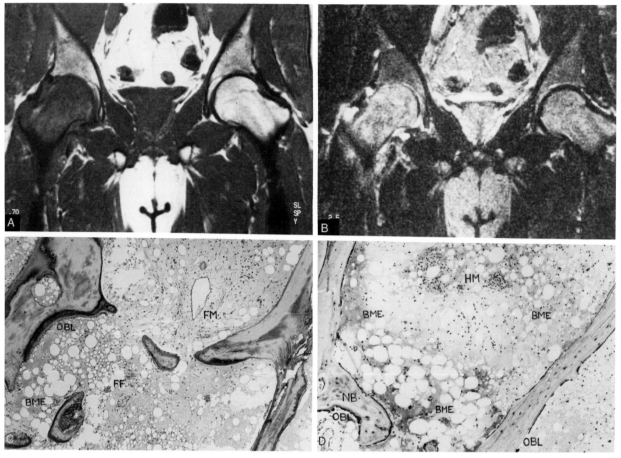

FIGURE 70–201. Transient bone marrow edema: MR imaging and histology.

A, B Coronal T1-weighted (TR/TE, 700/15) **(A)** and T2-weighted (TR/TE, 2500/90) **(B)** spin echo MR images reveal characteristic features of transient bone marrow edema. In **A**, note low signal intensity in the marrow of the right femoral head and neck with normal signal intensity in the adjacent acetabulum. The opposite femur and acetabulum also are normal. In **B**, note high signal intensity in the involved marrow in the right femur and a large joint effusion. The altered signal intensity extends to the base of the femoral neck. Again, the acetabula and left femur appear normal.

C, D Photomicrographs derived from undecalcified sections of material obtained from the affected marrow of the right femur are shown. In **C**, note dark gray osteoid seams with the trabecular surfaces partly covered by active osteoblasts (OBL). Homogeneous material is seen in the marrow cavity, representing marrow edema (BME), fat cell fragmentation (FF), or fibrous marrow regeneration (FM) (trichrome Goldner stain, ×60). In **D**, trabeculae are partly covered by active osteoblasts (OBL), leading to new bone formation (NB). The homogeneous extracellular material now is dark or basophilic, with marrow edema (BME) between fat cells and remnants of hematopoietic marrow (HM) (Giemsa stain, ×60).

(A, B Courtesy of J. Kramer, M.D., Vienna, Austria; **C, D** From Hofmann S, et al: J Bone Joint Surg [Br] *75*:210, 1993.)

ported in this study did not confirm the presence of marrow edema, such histologic confirmation (Fig. 70–201*C,D*) was provided in a study of 10 hips in nine patients reported by Hofman and coworkers[425] in 1993. Furthermore, in this latter study, elevation of the pressure within the involved bone marrow and abnormalities seen during intraosseous venography were documented in five patients, and histologic evidence of bone death was absent.

The association of transient pain and limitation of motion in the hip, radiographically evident osteopenia, and an MR imaging pattern consistent with bone marrow edema appears definite on the basis of results from many reported investigations (see Chapter 51). What also appears definite is the presence of identical marrow findings on MR imaging examinations of painful hips in patients whose routine radiographs do not reveal osteopenia. This is not surprising, owing to the relative insensitivity of conventional radiography in the detection of minor to moderate degrees of bone loss. Therefore, the designation of transient bone marrow edema appears to be more comprehensive than that of transient osteoporosis about the hip.

The relationship between transient bone marrow edema and osteonecrosis of the femoral head, however, is not clear.[1392] Based on their observations, Hofman and coworkers[425] concluded that the bone marrow edema syndrome was an initial phase of nontraumatic ischemic necrosis of the femoral head. Supporters of the idea undoubtedly point to the fact that in cases of proven osteonecrosis, the typical focal changes on MR images sometimes are preceded by diffuse abnormalities characteristic of bone marrow edema; skeptics argue that this is not surprising, because the reparative phase of osteonecrosis is associated with inflammation, hyperemia, marrow congestion, a decrease in fat, and an increase in interstitial fluid.[426] Supporters of the idea call attention to the study by Turner and associates[427] who reported five patients who presented with hip pain and evidence of marrow edema on MR imaging examinations and subsequently developed biopsy-proven marrow and bone necrosis. Skeptics emphasize the characteristic MR imaging findings seen in most patients with osteonecrosis of the femoral head, which allow its differentiation from bone marrow edema.

Vande Berg and collaborators[422] provide further insight into this controversy. These authors emphasized that careful analysis of the diffuse pattern of marrow abnormality that may occur in some patients with osteonecrosis of the femoral head reveals features different from those of bone marrow edema. High spatial resolution T2-weighted spin echo MR images in cases of osteonecrosis showed the lesion to be inhomogeneous and associated with crescent-shaped subchondral marrow areas of low signal intensity. Furthermore, intravenous contrast-enhanced MR images showed intense enhancement within the entire lesion except in the subchondral bone areas, suggesting that the necrotic zone was limited to very small portions of the marrow. These authors concluded that collapse of the subchondral bone in cases of transient bone marrow edema is indicative of epiphyseal fractures rather than osteonecrosis.

As indicated by Solomon,[426] whatever the answer to this puzzle, it is important to recognize the difference between bone marrow edema without osteonecrosis and that with osteonecrosis. The former is a hypervascular, usually self-limiting disorder whereas the latter is unequivocally ischemic in nature.

Femoral Neck Fractures. Fractures of the femoral neck may result from a significant injury, but they also occur spontaneously or following a minor injury in elderly patients, and as a response to the cumulative effects of prolonged stress (i.e., fatigue or insufficiency fractures). Nondisplaced fractures of the femoral neck may be difficult to detect with conventional radiographic techniques, leading to the application of other imaging methods. Of these, bone scintigraphy (Fig. 70–202A) and MR imaging (Figs. 70–202B and 70–203) hold the most promise (see Chapters 67 and 68).

Scintigraphy using bone-seeking radiopharmaceutical agents is useful in the initial diagnosis of the fracture and in the determination of the risk for subsequent osteonecrosis of the femoral head. Bone scintigraphy has proven more sensitive than routine radiography in confirming a femoral neck fracture.[428] Although it has been widely accepted that, in the elderly patient, a traumatic fracture might not be detected with bone scintigraphy for 2 or 3 days after the injury,[429–431] Holder and associates[432] found that patients of all ages, regardless of the time after injury, could undergo bone scintigraphy as soon as they are evaluated. Although their results eliminate one of the deficiencies of radionuclide bone scanning in the assessment of femoral neck fractures, the scintigraphic abnormalities are not specific and they provide little data regarding the morphology of the fracture. The interest in MR imaging in this clinical setting, therefore, is understandable. The MR imaging examination appears to be equally sensitive and far more specific in the detection of fractures of the femoral neck.[433, 1393] This examination may not allow determination of the viability of the femoral head following these fractures[434]; however, it can be tailored in such a fashion that imaging time is limited and costs are competitive with those of other advanced imaging methods.[435] A coronal T1-weighted spin echo MR imaging sequence, requiring approximately 7 min, may be sufficient.[435]

The MR imaging characteristics of a nondisplaced fracture of the femoral neck on T1-weighted spin echo MR sequences are a well-defined linear zone of low signal intensity that may be surrounded by a broader and ill-defined zone of low signal intensity consistent with marrow edema.[436] On T2-weighted spin echo MR images, the fracture line may remain of low signal intensity, but the edematous zone demonstrates high signal intensity. STIR images are very sensitive to the detection of these fractures, which appear as broad bands of high signal intensity within the normal, low signal intensity bone marrow; however, these images are less specific, as the fracture line itself may not be identifiable. The use of fat-suppression in combination with the intravenous administration of gadolinium compounds represents an additional sensitive MR imaging method for the detection of occult fractures of the femoral neck. A variety of MR imaging sequences also can be used to evaluate other subtle fractures, including stress fractures, of the pelvis. CT, however, is a superior method for the assessment of complex fractures and fracture-dislocations about the hip (Fig. 70–204).

Soft Tissue Abnormalities

The many soft tissue abnormalities that can lead to significant clinical manifestations in the hip (and elsewhere) are discussed in Chapter 95. Those related to injury of muscle are described in Chapter 67. Only one condition, which appears to be of soft tissue origin and can lead to hip pain, is discussed here.

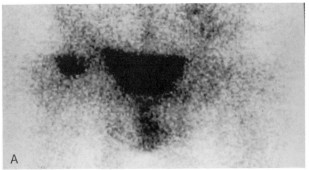
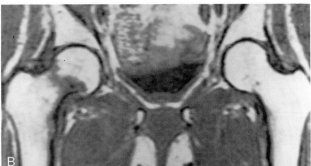

FIGURE 70–202. Femoral neck fractures: Bone scintigraphy and MR imaging. Although initial radiographs were normal in this 75 year old woman who had fallen, bone scintigraphy **(A)** reveals increased accumulation of radionuclide in the right femoral neck. A coronal T1-weighted (TR/TE, 600/20) spin echo MR image **(B)** clearly shows the fracture of the right femoral neck.

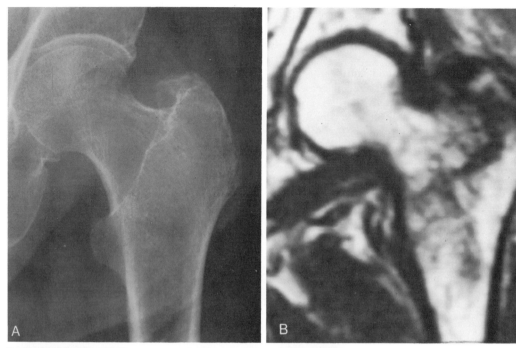

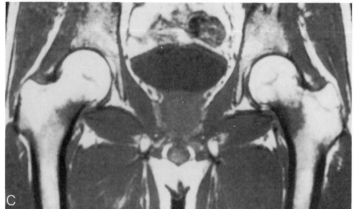

FIGURE 70–203. Femoral neck fractures: MR imaging.

A, B Although the routine radiograph **(A)** was interpreted as normal, the coronal T1-weighted (TR/TE, 600/20) spin echo MR image **(B)** shows a nondisplaced intertrochanteric fracture of the left femur. The fracture is manifest as an irregular line of low signal intensity surrounded by less well defined regions of low signal intensity. (Courtesy of D. Bates, M.D., La Jolla, California.)

C Bilateral fatigue fractures of the medial portion of the femoral necks in a 20 year old military recruit are manifest as zones of low signal intensity in this coronal T1-weighted (TR/TE, 717/20) spin echo MR image. (Courtesy of G. S. Huang, M.D., Taipei, Taiwan.)

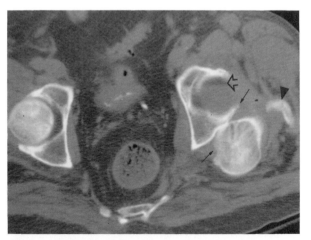

FIGURE 70–204. Complex fracture-dislocation about the hip: CT scanning. A transaxial CT scan reveals evidence of a posterior dislocation of the left hip with fractures (solid arrows) of the femoral head and acetabulum and a lipohemarthrosis with a fat-blood fluid level (open arrow). The top of the greater trochanter of the femur is evident (arrowhead).

A variety of causes have been implicated in the hip pain associated with an audible snapping. Intra-articular abnormalities, including single or multiple osteocartilaginous bodies, typically result in a faint sound associated with true femoral-acetabular motion; extra-articular causes often are characterized by a loud snap and, in some cases, a sudden jump of the fascia lata or gluteus maximus over the greater trochanter as the hip moves in a well-delineated fashion.[437] Other proposed causes have included slipping of the iliopsoas tendon over the iliopectineal eminence[438] and of the iliofemoral ligaments over the anterior portion of the hip capsule.[439]

Several studies[437, 440–442] have confirmed that subluxation of the iliopsoas tendon is one cause of a snapping hip. Iliopsoas bursography,[440, 443] iliopsoas tenography,[441] or hip arthrography in which the iliopsoas bursa also is opacified[437] confirms the changing position of the iliopsoas tendon and its displacement over the iliopectineal line during flexion and extension of the hip. An abrupt change in the position of the tendon coincident with the audible sound and palpable snap is observed.

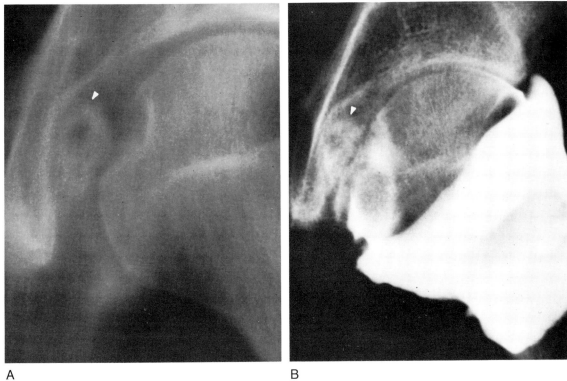

A　　　　　　　　　　　　　　　　　　　　B

FIGURE 70–205. Intra-articular osteochondral bodies: Conventional tomography and arthrography. The conventional tomogram **(A)** reveals an osseous body (arrowhead) in the acetabular fossa. Arthrography **(B)** indicates that contrast material partially surrounds the osseous body (arrowhead). At surgery, an osteochondral body attached to the acetabulum was removed.

Miscellaneous Abnormalities

Although MR imaging is useful in the assessment of many processes involving the hip and adjacent bones and soft tissues, some conditions are better evaluated with other imaging methods. Intra-articular bodies in the hip (and in other joints) may escape detection when MR imaging is used alone. Such bodies, which commonly localize in the region of the acetabular fossa, are detected more easily with routine radiography supplemented with conventional tomography, CT, or arthrography (Fig. 70–205). When combined with routine radiography, MR imaging can be employed effectively in the analysis of osteomyelitis and benign and malignant bone tumors (see Chapters 64, 65,

66, and 83). Osteoid osteomas, however, are better evaluated with CT (Fig. 70–206).

KNEE

The knee joint is the largest and most complicated articulation in the human body. In this articulation, three functional spaces exist: the medial femorotibial space, the lateral femorotibial space, and the patellofemoral space. In the following discussion, general anatomic features of the joint initially are summarized. A more detailed analysis of the anatomy and function of individual structures, such as the menisci and ligaments, is contained in subsequent sections of this chapter that deal with the imaging of each of them.

Osseous, Articular, and Soft Tissue Anatomy

The lower end of the femur contains a medial and lateral condyle, separated posteriorly by an intercondylar fossa or notch (Fig. 70–207). The medial condyle is larger than the lateral condyle and possesses a superior prominence called the adductor tubercle for attachment of the tendon of the adductor magnus muscle. Below this tubercle is a ridge, the medial epicondyle. The lateral condyle possesses a similar protuberance, the lateral epicondyle. The intercondylar fossa, between the condyles, stretches from the intercondylar line posteriorly to the lower border of the patellar surface anteriorly. The patella, the largest sesamoid bone of the body, is embedded within the tendon of the quadriceps femoris. It is oval in outline, with a pointed apex on its inferior surface. The ligamentum patellae (patellar tendon), a continuation of the quadriceps tendon, is attached to the apex and adjacent bone of the patella.

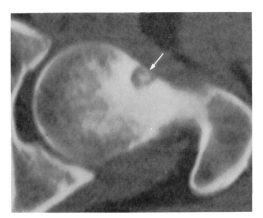

FIGURE 70–206. Osteoid osteoma: CT scanning. The partially calcified nidus (arrow) of an osteoid osteoma and surrounding bone sclerosis are shown effectively in a transaxial CT scan.

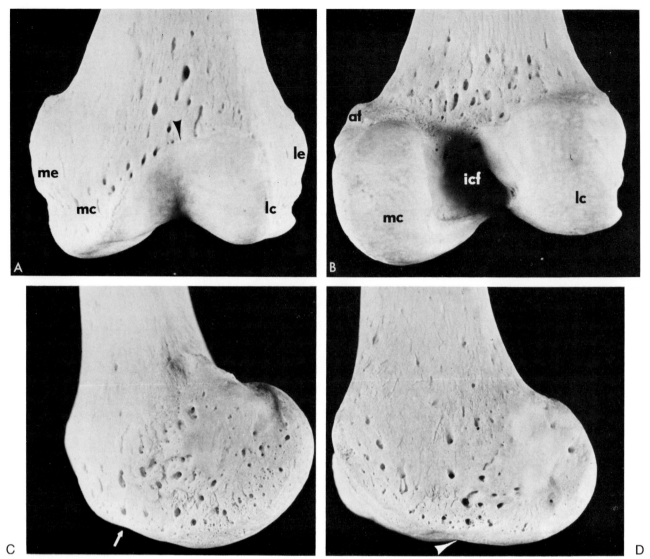

FIGURE 70–207. Distal femur: Osseous anatomy. Anterior **(A)** and posterior **(B)** aspects. Observe the medial (mc) and lateral (lc) condyles, medial (me) and lateral (le) epicondyles, adductor tubercle (at), patellar surface (arrowhead), and intercondylar fossa (icf). Medial **(C)** and lateral **(D)** aspects. On the medial aspect, observe the groove (arrow) that separates the anterior and middle thirds of the distal femur. On the lateral aspect, there is a groove (arrowhead) that divides the femoral surface approximately in half.

Articular surfaces of the femur, tibia, and patella are not congruent. The articular surface of the femur comprises the condylar areas (femorotibial spaces) and the patellar surface (patellofemoral space). A shallow groove is present between each condylar surface and the patellar surface. As viewed from below, the outline of the femoral condylar surfaces generally conforms to that of the tibial articular surfaces. The surface on the lateral femoral condyle appears circular, whereas that on the medial femoral condyle is large and oval, elongated in an anteroposterior direction, with concavity extending laterally.

The tibial articular surfaces are the cartilage-clothed condyles, each with a central hollow and peripheral flattened area (Fig. 70–208). Between the condyles is the intercondylar area. The articular surface of the medial tibial condyle is oval, with its long axis in the sagittal plane, whereas the articular surface of the lateral tibial condyle is circular and smaller in size compared with the medial condyle.

The adjacent articular surfaces of the tibia and femur are more closely fitted together by the presence of the medial and lateral menisci (Fig. 70–209). The medial meniscus is nearly semicircular in shape, with a broadened or widened posterior horn. The anterior end of the medial meniscus is attached to the intercondylar area of the tibia anterior to the attachment of the anterior cruciate ligament. The posterior end of the medial meniscus is attached to the intercondylar area of the tibia between the attachments of the posterior cruciate ligament and lateral meniscus. The peripheral aspect of the medial meniscus is attached to the fibrous capsule and tibial collateral ligament. The lateral meniscus, which is of relatively uniform width throughout, resembles a ring. Its anterior aspect is attached to the intercondylar eminence of the tibia behind and lateral to the anterior cruciate ligament. Its posterior portion is attached to the intercondylar eminence of the tibia just anterior to the attachment of the medial meniscus. The lateral meniscus is grooved posteriorly by the popliteus tendon and its accom-

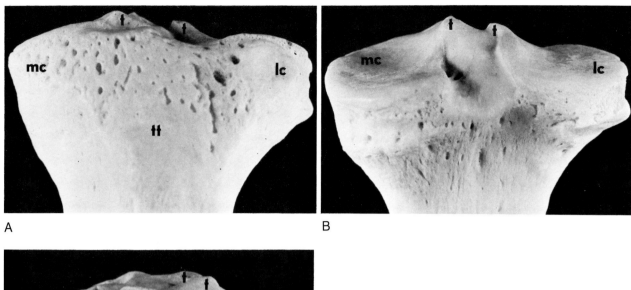

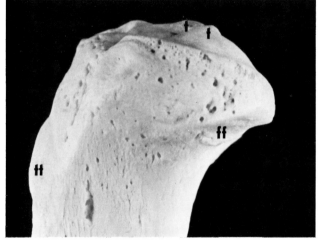

FIGURE 70–208. Proximal tibia: Osseous anatomy. Anterior **(A)** and posterior **(B)** aspects. Structures include the tibial tuberosity (tt), tubercles (t) of intercondylar eminence, medial condyle (mc), and lateral condyle (lc). Lateral aspect **(C)**. Note the tibial tuberosity (tt), tubercles (t) of intercondylar eminence, and fibular facet (ff).

panying tendon sheath. Meniscofemoral ligaments, both anterior and posterior, represent attachments of the posterior horn of the lateral meniscus.

The articular surface of the patella is oval in shape and contains an osseous vertical ridge that divides it into a smaller medial area and a larger lateral area. This patellar ridge fits into a corresponding groove on the anterior surface of the femur. The patellar articulating surface is subdivided still further by two ill-defined horizontal ridges of bone into three facets on either side. One additional vertical ridge of bone separates a narrow elongated facet on the medial border of the articular surface. Contact between these various patellar articular facets and the femur varies, depending on the position of the knee. In full flexion, the most medial facet of the patella contacts the lateral portion of the medial femoral condyle, and the superior aspect of the lateral patellar facet contacts the anterior part of the lateral condyle. With extension of the knee, the middle facet of the patella becomes intimate with the lower portion of the femoral patellar surface, and in full extension, only the lowest patellar articular facets contact the femur. During forced extension of the joint, there is a tendency for the patella to be displaced laterally, a tendency that is prevented by the action of adjacent musculature and the prominence of the lateral patellar surface of the femur.

The fibrous capsule of the knee joint is not a complete structure. Rather, the knee is surrounded by tendinous expansions, which reinforce the capsule. Between the capsule or tendinous expansions and synovial lining are various intra-articular structures, including ligaments and fat pads.

Anteriorly, the fibrous capsule is absent above and over the patellar surface. The ligamentous sheath in this area is composed mainly of a tendinous expansion from the rectus femoris and the vasti musculature, which descends to attach around the superior half of the bone. Superficial fibers continue to descend onto the strong ligamentum patellae. This structure, which represents the continuation of the quadriceps muscle, is attached above to the apex of the patella and below to the tibial tuberosity. Adjacent fibers, the medial and lateral patellar retinacula, pass from the osseous margins of the patella to the tibial condyles. Superficial to these tendinous structures are the expansions of the fascia lata. Above the patella, deficiency of the fibrous capsule creates a suprapatellar bursa, which freely communicates with the articular cavity.

Posteriorly, capsular fibers extend from the femoral surface above the condyles and the intercondylar line to the posterior border of the tibia. This portion of the capsule is strengthened by the oblique popliteal ligament, which is

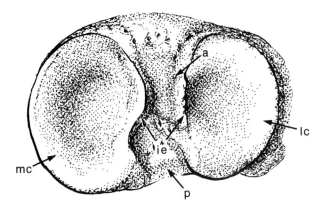

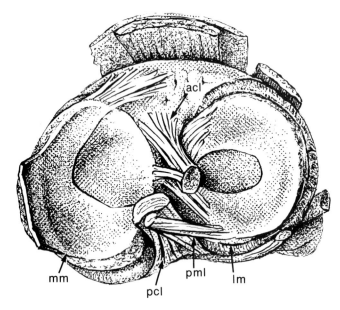

FIGURE 70–209. Knee joint: Normal anatomy. Menisci and cruciate ligaments. Drawings of tibial articular surfaces without (upper) and with (below) the addition of soft tissue structures. Note the medial condyle (mc), lateral condyle (lc), intercondylar eminences (ie), anterior intercondylar area (a), and posterior intercondylar area (p). Soft tissue structures are the medial meniscus (mm), lateral meniscus (lm), posterior cruciate ligament (pcl), posterior meniscofemoral ligament (pml), and anterior cruciate ligament (acl).

derived from the semimembranosus tendon. Additional posterior reinforcement relates to the arcuate popliteal ligament, which emerges from the fibular head to blend with the capsular fibers.

Laterally, capsular fibers run from the femoral to the tibial condyles. In this area, the fibular collateral ligament is found, which is attached above to the lateral epicondyle of the femur and below to the fibular head. There is a space between capsular fibers and the fibular collateral ligament through which extend genicular vessels and nerves.

Medially, the capsule is strengthened by tendinous expansions from sartorius and semimembranosus muscles. These fibers pass upward to the tibial collateral ligament, which is attached above to the medial epicondyle of the femur and below to the medial tibial condyle and shaft. One or more bursae may separate the tibial collateral ligament from the fibrous capsule.[444] On its deep surface, the fibrous capsule connects the menisci and adjacent tibia, a connection termed the coronary ligament.

The tibial and fibular collateral ligaments reinforce the medial and lateral sides of the joint. They are taut in joint extension, and in this position, they prevent rotation of the knee.

The synovial membrane of the knee joint is the most extensive in the body and can be conveniently divided into several parts[445] (Fig. 70–210).

Central Portion. This extends between the patella and the patellar surface of the femur to the cruciate ligaments (Fig. 70–211). This portion lies between femoral and tibial condyles and, in addition, above and below the menisci. An infrapatellar fat pad below the patella, located deep to the patellar ligament, presses the synovial membrane posteriorly. In this area, a vertical infrapatellar synovial fold runs from the synovial surface of the fat pad to the intercondylar fossa. Horizontal alar synovial folds run from each side of the infrapatellar synovial fold.

Suprapatellar Synovial Pouch. This cavity, which develops separately from the knee joint but eventually communicates with it, extends vertically above the patella between the quadriceps muscle anteriorly and the femur posteriorly.

Posterior Femoral Recesses. These recesses lie behind the posterior portion of each femoral condyle, deep to the lateral and medial heads of the gastrocnemius muscle (Fig. 70–212). Single or multiple bursae may be located between the muscular portions and the fibrous capsule and may communicate with the articular cavity.[446–449] The medial and lateral posterior femoral recesses are separated by a thick central septum formed by a broad synovial fold around the cruciate ligaments, which may be continuous with the infrapatellar synovial fold.[450]

Subpopliteal Recess. A small synovial cul-de-sac lies

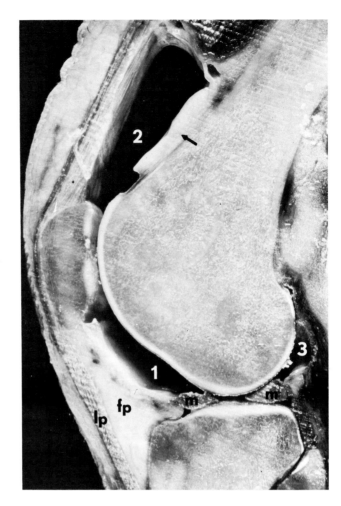

FIGURE 70–210. Knee joint: Normal anatomy: Various parts of the joint. A photograph of an air-distended knee joint outlining ligamentum patellae (lp), infrapatellar fat pad (fp), and menisci (m). The articulation can be divided into a central portion (1), suprapatellar pouch (2), and posterior femoral recesses (3). Note fatty tissue (arrow), which is pressed against the anterior aspect of the femur.

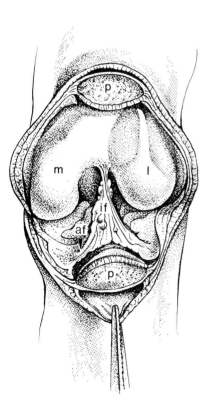

FIGURE 70–211. Knee joint: Normal anatomy. Central portion. The patella (p) has been divided to expose the joint interior. Observe the medial (m) and lateral (l) femoral condyles and alar folds (af) of synovium, which converge to form the infrapatellar fold (if) or ligamentum mucosum.

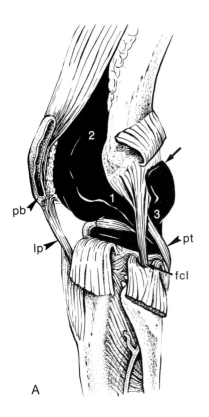

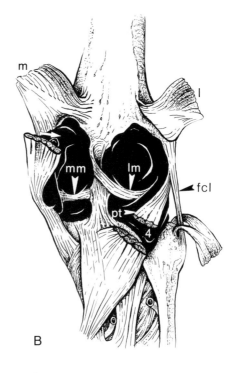

A

B

FIGURE 70–212. Knee joint: Normal anatomy. Suprapatellar synovial pouch and posterior femoral recesses.

A Lateral aspect. Distended joint is indicated in black. Observe the central portion (1), suprapatellar pouch (2), and posterior femoral recesses (3). The prepatellar bursa (pb), ligamentum patellae (lp), fibular collateral ligament (fcl), and popliteus tendon (pt) are indicated. The lateral head of the gastrocnemius muscle has been turned up, exposing a communicating bursa (arrow).

B Posterior aspect. The distended joint is indicated in black. The medial (m) and lateral (l) heads of the gastrocnemius muscle have been sectioned. Note the bursa (arrow) beneath the lifted medial head, medial meniscus (mm), lateral meniscus (lm), popliteus tendon (pt), fibular collateral ligament (fcl), and subpopliteal recess (4).

between the lateral meniscus and the tendon of the popliteus, which may communicate with the superior tibiofibular joint in 10 per cent of adults[451] (Fig. 70–212).

Additional Bursae. Numerous additional bursae may be found about the knee.[445, 447, 452–454] These include the subcutaneous prepatellar and subfascial prepatellar bursae anterior to the patella; deep infrapatellar bursa between the upper tibia and ligamentum patellae; anserine bursa between the tibial collateral ligament and tendons of the sartorius, gracilis, and semitendinosus muscles; and bursae between the semimembranosus tendon and tibial collateral ligament, and between the biceps tendon and fibular collateral ligament.

The anterior and posterior cruciate ligaments extend between the femur and the tibia (Fig. 70–209). The anterior cruciate ligament attaches below to the anterior intercondylar area of the tibia and above to the medial side of the lateral femoral condyle. The posterior cruciate ligament extends from the posterior intercondylar area of the tibia, below the joint line, to the lateral side of the medial femoral condyle. These ligaments prevent excessive posterior displacement (anterior cruciate ligament) or anterior displacement (posterior cruciate ligament) of the femur on the tibia.

A number of normal radiographic landmarks about the knee deserve emphasis. On routine radiographs, the shallow grooves in the distal articular surface of the femur can be recognized.[455–458] The groove on the medial condyle appears as a sulcus at the junction of the anterior and middle thirds of the articular surface on lateral radiographs. In the same projection, the groove on the lateral condyle is located at the center of the articular surface and is generally more prominent. Landmarks allowing identification of each of the tibial condyles on lateral radiographs also have been summarized.[456]

Blumensaat's line is identified as a condensed linear shadow on the lateral radiograph representing tangential bone in the intercondylar fossa.[459, 460] The location and appearance of Blumensaat's line is extremely sensitive to changes in knee position.[456] In the past, Blumensaat's line has been used to provide an indication of the relative position of the patella in lateral projections. Elevation of the distal pole of the patella above this line with the knee flexed 30 degrees has been used as an indicator of patella alta (an elevated position of the patella). More recently, other measurements on lateral radiographs have been suggested as more reliable indicators of patellar position (see later discussion).

The radiographic anatomy of the knee related to soft tissue shadows also has been described. In the lateral projection of a mildly flexed knee, the collapsed suprapatellar pouch creates a sharp vertical radiodense line between an anterior fat pad superior to the patella (anterior suprapatellar fat) and a posterior fat pad in front of the distal supracondylar region of the femur (prefemoral fat pad) (Fig. 70–213). This line generally is less than 5 mm in width, but may be between 5 and 10 mm. Shadows of increased thickness suggest the presence of intra-articular fluid.[461–463] Distortion of soft tissue planes[461, 464] with the production of a piriform mass[465] in this projection and displacement of fat planes about the suprapatellar pouch on frontal projections[466] are additional but less sensitive signs of knee effusions. Axial radiographs reveal abnormal radiodensity in the medial patellofemoral compartment in such cases.[463] Intra-articular fluid in the knee also may cause displacement of the ossified fabella.[467]

In lateral projections, a thin layer of extrasynovial fat hugs the femoral condyles posteriorly.[453] This fat plane extends from the origin of the femoral condyles to the posterior aspect of the lateral tibial condyle, forming a double curve resembling the numeral 3. A fat plane about

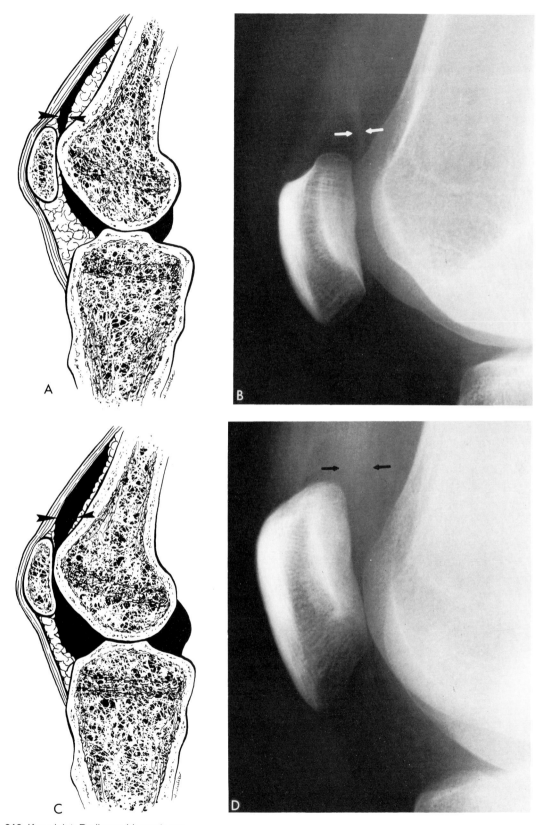

FIGURE 70–213. Knee joint: Radiographic anatomy.

   A, B In normal situations, the collapsed suprapatellar pouch (arrowheads) creates a radiodense area (arrows) that generally is less than 5 mm in width but may be between 5 and 10 mm in width.

   C, D In the presence of intra-articular fluid, distention of the pouch (arrowheads) creates a radiodense region of increased thickness with blurred margins (arrows).

the posterior cruciate ligament also may be visible. These fat planes become distorted in the presence of intra-articular fluid.

Synovial Abnormalities

Joint Effusion. In normal joints, including the knee, fluid is present in small quantities sufficient to coat the numerous folds of the synovial membrane and to pool in one or more joint recesses. In the normal state, there never is sufficient volume of fluid to distend the joint or to separate redundant surfaces of the synovium.[468] The intra-articular pressure within a normal joint may be a negative one compared with ambient atmospheric pressure.[468] The accumulation of abnormal amounts of joint fluid leads to separation of adjacent synovial surfaces, distortion of the joint capsule, and elevation of intra-articular pressure. With large amounts of joint fluid, rupture of the synovial contents or the creation or enlargement of an opening between the joint and a surrounding synovial sac with distention of that sac (i.e., synovial cyst) may occur.

The precise amount of fluid that may be present in a normal knee joint is not clear. What is clear, however, is that such fluid may move from one portion of the joint to another during passive or active movement of the knee, the pattern of flow being guided by the location of intra-articular pressure gradients and physiologic compartmentation.[469] Physiologic compartmentation of a joint is defined as a synovial cavity that is anatomically continuous but is hydraulically divided into separate compartments at physiologic pressures.[470] Pathologic compartmentation of the knee joint may result as a consequence of synovial plicae (see later discussion).

Although abnormal amounts of joint fluid in the knee may be palpated clinically, such fluid also can be detected with several different imaging methods, including routine radiography, ultrasonography, CT, and MR imaging. As indicated earlier, the lateral radiograph of the knee is the most sensitive of all routine radiographic projections in the detection of a joint effusion. Enlargement of the normally collapsed suprapatellar recess is appreciated radiographically on the lateral projection, owing to abnormal separation between a fat body above the patella and the prefemoral fat body (Fig. 70–213). A measurement of 10 mm between these fat bodies is considered definitely abnormal, and a measurement between 5 and 10 mm is considered possibly abnormal. An abnormal measurement can result not only from joint fluid but also from an intra-articular mass or hypertrophy of the synovial membrane. A recent study employing MR imaging has indicated that approximately 4 or 5 ml of fluid in the knee joint is required before an effusion can be detected with conventional radiography.[471]

MR imaging is extremely sensitive to the presence of intra-articular fluid (Fig. 70–214). Such fluid is of low signal intensity on T1-weighted spin echo MR images and of high signal intensity on T2-weighted spin echo MR images and on many gradient echo images. Modifications in these patterns of signal intensity occur in the presence of a hemarthrosis. Furthermore, the differentiation of joint fluid and synovial inflammatory tissue may require additional MR imaging techniques (see later discussion). The precise distribution of joint fluid in the knee as detected with MR imaging depends upon the size of the effusion, the position of the knee during the examination, and anatomic and pathologic factors such as the presence of synovial plicae and synovial cysts. Schweitzer and coworkers,[471] in a study of cadaveric knees, indicated that sagittal MR images allowed detection of as little as 1 ml of fluid, such fluid collecting about the condyles of the femur. Kaneko and collaborators,[472] reviewing MR imaging examinations of 300 traumatized knees, noted the common occurrence of

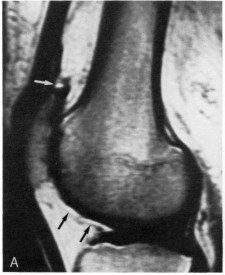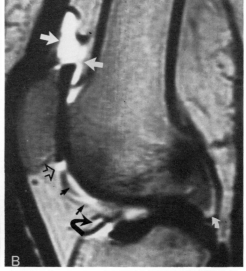

FIGURE 70–214. Joint effusion: MR imaging. Sagittal T1-weighted (TR/TE, 600/20) spin echo MR images obtained after the instillation of 1 ml **(A)** and 15 ml **(B)** of a gadolinium compound show patterns of distribution of fluid in a cadaveric knee joint. In **A**, a small amount of fluid is seen adjacent to the femoral condyle (black arrows) and a tiny amount of fluid is evident in the suprapatellar pouch or recess (white arrow). In **B**, increased fluid is seen in the suprapatellar recess (straight white arrows). Small amounts of fluid are seen distending a superior vertical cleft in Hoffa's infrapatellar fat body (open arrow), filling a horizontally oriented inferior cleft (curved black arrow), extending between the femoral condyle and the infrapatellar fat body (straight solid black arrows), and extending posteriorly about the cruciate ligaments (curved white arrow). (From Schweitzer ME, et al: AJR *159:*361, 1992.)

fluid in the central portion of the joint and in the suprapatellar recess, and the infrequent occurrence of fluid in the posterior femoral or subpopliteal regions of the knee. No reported data currently indicate that the precise patterns of distribution of fluid in the knee are dependent on the specific internal derangements present.

The detection of a knee effusion with MR imaging is aided by differences in the signal intensity of fluid and that of adjacent soft tissue structures. In particular, in the region of the suprapatellar recess and of the anteroinferior portion of the joint, the synovial membrane is intimate with three fat bodies: the anterior and posterior (or prefemoral) suprapatellar fat bodies and the infrapatellar (or Hoffa's) fat body. These fat bodies are intracapsular but extrasynovial in location. The presence of a bland knee effusion (defined as one that results from trauma or an internal derangement) typically does not lead to distortion of the interface between these fat bodies and the adjacent fluid; the presence of a proliferative effusion (defined as one associated with synovial proliferation) may lead to scalloping, truncation, or displacement of these fat bodies and obscuration of the interface between them and the adjacent fluid[473] (Fig. 70–215).

Hemarthrosis and Lipohemarthrosis. A hemarthrosis may result from an injury or a number of articular processes, including pigmented villonodular synovitis, hemophilia and other bleeding disorders, intra-articular tumors (e.g., synovial hemangioma), neuropathic osteoarthropathy, crystal deposition diseases, and renal osteodystrophy. Posttraumatic hemarthrosis of the knee generally is considered a manifestation of serious ligamentous injury, particularly in adults.[474, 475, 1349] A joint effusion appearing within the first few hours following trauma usually is related to a hemarthrosis; nonbloody effusions typically appear 12 to 24 hours after injury.[476, 477] One factor leading to posttraumatic hemarthrosis is a subtle increase in vascular permeability, caused by mechanisms other than gross disruption of vessels.[478]

There are no reliable routine radiographic features of a hemarthrosis. In cases of chronic and recurrent hemarthroses, as in pigmented villonodular synovitis or hemophilia, increased radiodensity of the distended joint owing to intrasynovial hemosiderin deposition occasionally may be evident. In such cases, CT may reveal a thickened synovial membrane and increased attenuation values in the hemosiderin-laden synovial membrane.

MR imaging allows a specific diagnosis in some types of hemarthrosis. Although acute hemorrhagic effusions may have signal intensity characteristics similar to those of normal synovial fluid, subacute and chronic hemarthrosis may reveal high signal intensity on both T1-weighted and T2-weighted spin echo MR images. A fluid level representing a layering phenomenon between serum (above) and sediment (below) also may be seen. In cases of chronic hemarthroses, hemosiderin deposition within the synovial membrane leads to regions of low signal intensity in both T1- and T2-weighted spin echo MR images and, especially, in gradient echo images (Fig. 70–216).

The identification of lipid material in synovial fluid by histochemical and microscopic techniques and by imaging methods has diagnostic utility in the injured patient.[479–482] The discovery of intra-articular fat, when combined with bone marrow spicules, is reliable evidence of an intra-articular fracture, the fat being released from the marrow following cortical violation. Frequently, however, a hemorrhagic effusion containing fat may be observed in patients without fracture, probably related to cartilaginous or ligamentous injury.[483, 484] As fat also is present in the synovium, it is possible that damage to the synovium alone can release fat into the synovial fluid.[484] Other sources of lipids in the synovial fluid include the rich vascular bed between the adjacent cells and the joint and the intra-capsular fat pads. The amount of fat in the synovial fluid is directly proportional to the severity of the joint injury.[483]

The detection of a lipohemarthrosis can be accomplished with several different imaging methods (Fig. 70–217). Routine radiographic examination employing horizontal beam technique allows the demonstration of a fat-blood fluid level following injury to the joint.[482, 486–488] Although this finding is observed most often in the knee (in the region of the suprapatellar recess), it also may be noted in other articulations, such as the elbow, hip, ankle, and glenohumeral joint. In the knee, lipohemarthrosis may accompany fractures of the tibial plateau, proximal portion of the fibula, patella, or distal portion of the femur, as well as soft tissue injury to cartilage, ligaments, fat pads, or synovium.[489] Small amounts of fat and blood in the knee may not be sufficient to produce a fat-blood fluid level on cross-table radiography, however. Occasionally, routine lateral films of the knee taken without horizontal beam technique in patients with significant intra-articular fat allow visualization of the capsule as a water-dense linear structure outlined on both sides by fat.[490]

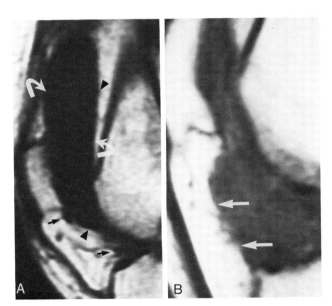

FIGURE 70–215. Bland versus proliferative knee effusion: MR imaging.

A Bland effusion. A sagittal T1-weighted (TR/TE, 600/20) spin echo MR image in a patient with a large, bland effusion (curved arrows) shows fluid extending into the normal recesses (solid straight arrows) in the infrapatellar fat body. The interfaces (arrowheads) between the fluid and the adjacent fat bodies are well defined.

B Proliferative effusion. In a patient with pigmented villonodular synovitis, a sagittal proton density–weighted (TR/TE, 1800/19) spin echo MR image shows distortion and displacement (arrows) of the infrapatellar fat body.

(From Schweitzer ME, et al: AJR *160:*823, 1993.)

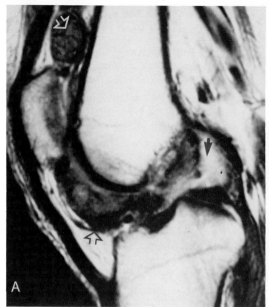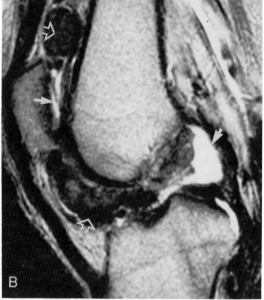

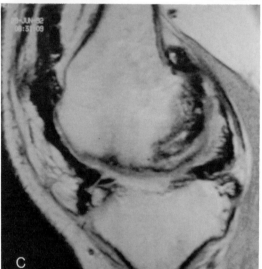

FIGURE 70–216. Chronic hemarthrosis: MR imaging.

A, B Pigmented villonodular synovitis. Sagittal proton density–weighted (TR/TE, 2000/30) **(A)** and T2-weighted (TR/TE, 2000/80) **(B)** spin echo MR images reveal distention of the knee in a patient with pigmented villonodular synovitis. In **A**, note intra-articular fluid of intermediate signal intensity (solid arrow) and intrasynovial hemosiderin deposits of low signal intensity (open arrows). In **B**, the fluid is of high signal intensity (solid arrows), and the hemosiderin reveals low signal intensity (open arrows).

C Hemophilia. Sagittal proton density (TR/TE, 2100/20) spin echo MR image reveals extensive hemosiderin deposition of low signal intensity throughout the joint. Bone erosions, cysts, and osteophytes are evident. (Courtesy of D. Goodwin, M.D., San Diego, California.)

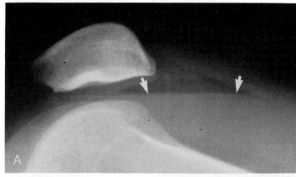

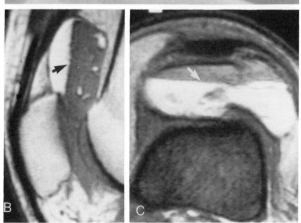

FIGURE 70–217. Lipohemarthrosis: Routine radiography and MR imaging.

A Routine radiography. In a patient with a tibial plateau fracture, a crosstable radiograph (obtained with horizontal beam technique) shows a fluid level (arrows) between fat (above) and blood (below).

B, C MR imaging. In a patient with an avulsion at the tibial site of attachment of the anterior cruciate ligament, a sagittal T1-weighted (TR/TE, 886/15) spin echo MR image **(B)** and a transaxial MPGR MR image (TR/TE, 424/18; flip angle, 20 degrees) show a fluid level (arrows) indicative of a lipohemarthrosis. In **B**, the upper layer, representing fat, is of high signal intensity, and the lower layer, representing blood, is of low signal intensity, although it contains regions of high signal intensity, indicative of fat. In **C**, the upper layer is of intermediate signal intensity, again representing fat, and the lower layer is of high signal intensity and contains regions of intermediate signal intensity representing fat.

Transaxial images provided by CT also demonstrate a lipohemarthrosis as a fat-blood fluid level.[491] This technique appears to be more sensitive than routine radiography, but MR imaging probably is the most sensitive method that allows detection of a lipohemarthrosis. The characteristics of a lipohemarthrosis on MR images are relatively complex.[492] Fat droplets in the knee in the supine patient appear as foci of high signal intensity on T1-weighted coronal spin echo MR images and of intermediate signal intensity on T2-weighted coronal spin echo MR images. In the transaxial and sagittal planes, four distinct signal intensity bands may be evident[492]: a superior band representing floating fat, a central band containing serum, an inferior band of dependent erythrocytes, and a thin band representing chemical shift artifact at the interface of serum and fat. Furthermore, the relative signal intensities of the serum and precipitate vary, depending on the chronicity of the bleed and the specific pulse sequence chosen.

Synovitis. The differentiation of synovial inflammatory tissue and joint fluid is important to the physician who is treating patients with rheumatoid arthritis and related disorders. With most imaging methods, including routine radiography and CT, such differentiation is not possible. MR imaging holds promise in this area (Fig. 70–218).

In 1990, Kursunoglu-Brahme and coworkers[493] reported results in the examination of the knee in 14 patients with classic rheumatoid arthritis, with MR imaging obtained both before and immediately after the intravenous administration of gadopentetate dimeglumine. T1- and T2-weighted spin echo MR images obtained prior to gadolinium administration demonstrated identical signal intensity characteristics in both the effusion and the inflamed synovial membrane. The intravenous administration of the gadolinium compound, however, allowed distinction between effusion and abnormal synovium, with the effusion remaining of low signal intensity and the synovium demonstrating enhancement and increased signal intensity on T1-weighted spin echo MR images. Two years later, Singson and Zalduondo[494] reported that standard spin echo MR images (i.e., those obtained without the intravenous administration of gadolinium compounds) could be used for the same purpose. They indicated that thickened synovium was of intermediate signal intensity on T1-weighted spin echo MR images compared with the lower signal intensity of joint

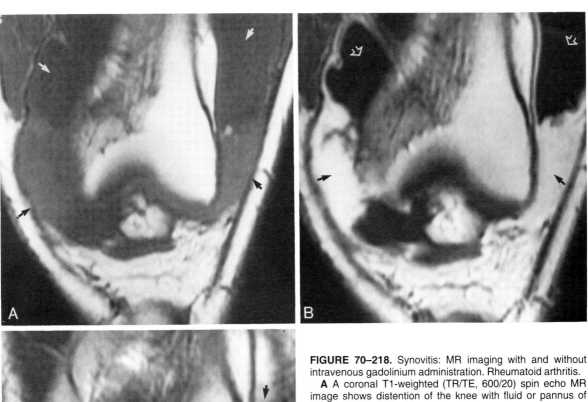

FIGURE 70–218. Synovitis: MR imaging with and without intravenous gadolinium administration. Rheumatoid arthritis.

A A coronal T1-weighted (TR/TE, 600/20) spin echo MR image shows distention of the knee with fluid or pannus of inhomogeneous low signal intensity (arrows).

B An identical T1-weighted (TR/TE, 600/20) spin echo MR image obtained immediately following the intravenous administration of a gadolinium compound reveals pannus of high signal intensity (solid arrows) and joint fluid of low signal intensity (open arrows).

C An identical T1-weighted (TR/TE, 600/20) spin echo MR image obtained in a delayed fashion following the intravenous administration of a gadolinium compound reveals regions of intermediate signal intensity (arrows) throughout the joint.

(Courtesy of S. K. Brahme, M.D., La Jolla, California.)

effusion. In 8 of 12 knees with significant joint effusions and thickened synovium, the abnormal synovium had an intermediate signal intensity on T2-weighted spin echo MR images relative to the high signal intensity of the joint effusion, although in the other four knees, the increased signal intensity of the abnormal synovium was identical to that of the articular fluid.

If intravenous injection of gadolinium compounds is employed as a method of differentiating abnormal synovium and joint fluid, it becomes mandatory to obtain MR images immediately after its injection. The delayed enhancement of joint fluid following intravenous gadolinium administration is well documented.[495, 496] A faster rate and greater degree of enhancement of joint fluid occurs in knees that are exercised compared with those at rest, presumably related to an increased rate of transsynovial flow and more rapid diffusion in the exercised knees.[496] A peripheral rim of enhancing joint fluid in delayed MR images may be misinterpreted as enhanced, thickened synovium; thus, non-inflammatory joint effusions may be mistakenly diagnosed as synovitis.[496] In rheumatoid arthritis, it also is possible that enhancement of the signal intensity of the joint fluid occurs at a more rapid rate, leading to further diagnostic difficulty.

Recent advances related to improved discrimination between synovium and joint fluid (as well as among cartilage, synovium, and joint fluid) have included the application of fat-suppressed imaging and saturation transfer techniques (the latter altering the signal intensity through effects on cross relaxation, or magnetization transfer, between the aqueous and macromolecular components of tissue).[1394] Some of these techniques are addressed later in this chapter in a discussion of cartilage imaging.

Synovial Plicae. The term synovial plicae refers to remnants of synovial tissue that in early development originally divided the joint into three separate compartments, and which may be found normally in the adult knee.[497–506] Usually of no consequence, these structures may become pathologically thickened and lead to symptoms mimicking arthritis, injuries involving the meniscus, and other common internal derangements of the knee. In addition, persistence of these structures in their embryonic form, as complete septa, may cause a variety of intra-articular compartmental syndromes.

The synovial cavity of the adult knee is the most extensive and complex in the body, and it represents in its final form the end result of a sequence of developmental steps that have been studied extensively. In the embryo of 7 weeks' gestation, the tibial and femoral cartilages are separated by unchondrified blastema, which becomes thinned to form a discrete disc or intermediate zone.[507] As the joint continues to grow, and prior to the development of the fibrous joint capsule, adjacent mesenchyme becomes incorporated into an intra-articular position. This embryonic mesenchyme gives rise to the menisci and cruciate ligaments at approximately 8 weeks of development.[507] It generally is agreed that cavities are not seen in the previously solid embryonic synovial mesenchyme until approximately 9 weeks of embryogenesis. Originally, three compartments are partitioned by septa of embryonic synovium: a superior femoropatellar compartment and two inferior femorotibial compartments.[508] These primitive cavities enlarge by proliferation of the lining tissue and extend into the middle por-

tion of the blastemal intermediate zone. At this time, the cavities are irregular in outline and frequently contain strands of tissue, and their lining bears little resemblance to the typical synovial tissue of the adult.[507] Progressive involution of these mesenchymal septa leads to the formation of a single joint space by approximately 12 weeks.[507] Persistence of any portion of these embryonic partitions constitutes a synovial plica. These synovial remnants can be encountered in 18 to 60 per cent of adult knees, a frequency that largely may reflect the diligence and persistence of the examiner.[502, 503]

The three most commonly encountered plicae are classified according to the partitions from which they took origin, as suprapatellar, medial patellar, and infrapatellar (Fig. 70–219). Of these, the infrapatellar plica is most frequent, followed by the suprapatellar plica, and, least commonly, the medial plica.[503] Rarely, a lateral patellar plica is observed.[509] Each of these septa varies widely in size and shape, and various combinations may exist simultaneously. Their identification can be accomplished by arthrography,[500, 510–512] computed arthrotomography,[513, 514] MR imaging, or arthroscopy,[505, 506, 515–518] depending on their location and size.

The suprapatellar plica, or plica synovialis suprapatellaris, represents a remnant of the embryonic septum that divides the suprapatellar cavity from the medial and lateral joint compartments. This synovial fold may vary widely in the adult and most commonly takes one of the following three forms: (1) an intact septum completely dividing the suprapatellar pouch from the remainder of the knee; (2) an intact septum except for a variably sized, centrally placed diaphragm known as the porta; and (3) a variably sized, crescent-shaped fold arising medially from the undersurface of the quadriceps tendon above the level of the patella and extending inferiorly to insert along the medial edge of the knee joint[508] (Fig. 70–220).

On double contrast arthrograms, the suprapatellar plica is best visualized on the lateral view with the knee in full extension. This position allows for complete distention of the suprapatellar pouch. The plica is seen as a thin, delicate fold obliquely crossing the suprapatellar pouch to insert near the patella. On fluoroscopy, it is readily pliable, moving easily with flexion and extension of the knee. With computed arthrotomography, this plica most commonly appears as a fine line parallel to the medial wall of the joint.[513] With MR imaging, it is seen more easily when there is fluid in the joint.

The medial patellar plica has been referred to variously as a wedge, a band, or a shelf.[497] This synovial remnant has its origin on the medial wall of the knee joint, near the suprapatellar plica, and courses obliquely downward relative to the patella, to insert into the synovium, which covers the infrapatellar fat pad (Fig. 70–221). Its inner edge may be rounded, sharp, or smooth, or it may contain small fenestrations.[497] Its configuration varies with knee position, lying transverse to the femur with the knee extended and parallel to the axis of the femur with the joint flexed.

Arthrographic demonstration of the medial patellar plica depends on careful technique and the inclusion of axial views of the patellofemoral compartment.[511, 519, 520] On the axial projections, this plica is seen as a flat, lucent region lying just anterior to the medial femoral condyle in the medial aspect of the patellofemoral joint. In an almost lateral projection, with the knee in slight internal rotation, the

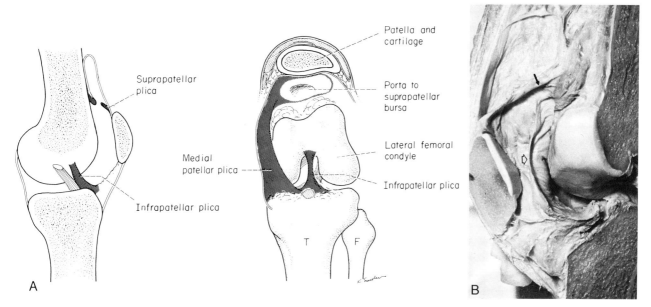

FIGURE 70–219. Synovial plicae: Classification.

A A schematic drawing depicts the three most commonly encountered synovial plicae.

B A sagittal section through the knee demonstrates the suprapatellar plica (solid arrow) and the medial patellar plica (open arrow). (From Deutsch AL, et al: Radiology *141:*627, 1981.)

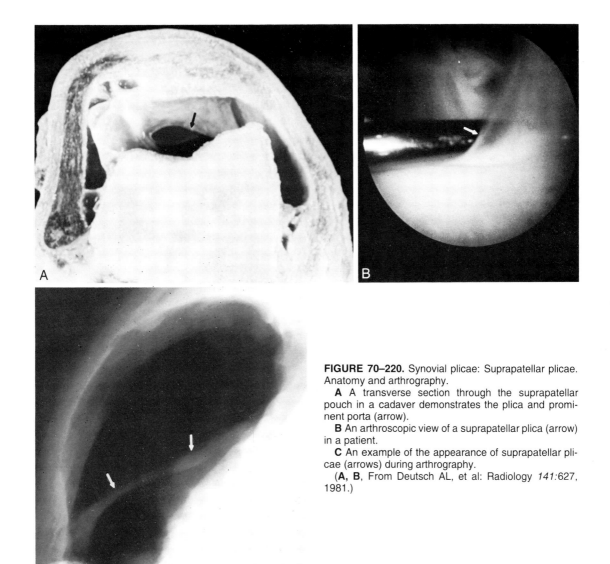

FIGURE 70–220. Synovial plicae: Suprapatellar plicae. Anatomy and arthrography.

A A transverse section through the suprapatellar pouch in a cadaver demonstrates the plica and prominent porta (arrow).

B An arthroscopic view of a suprapatellar plica (arrow) in a patient.

C An example of the appearance of suprapatellar plicae (arrows) during arthrography.

(**A, B,** From Deutsch AL, et al: Radiology *141:*627, 1981.)

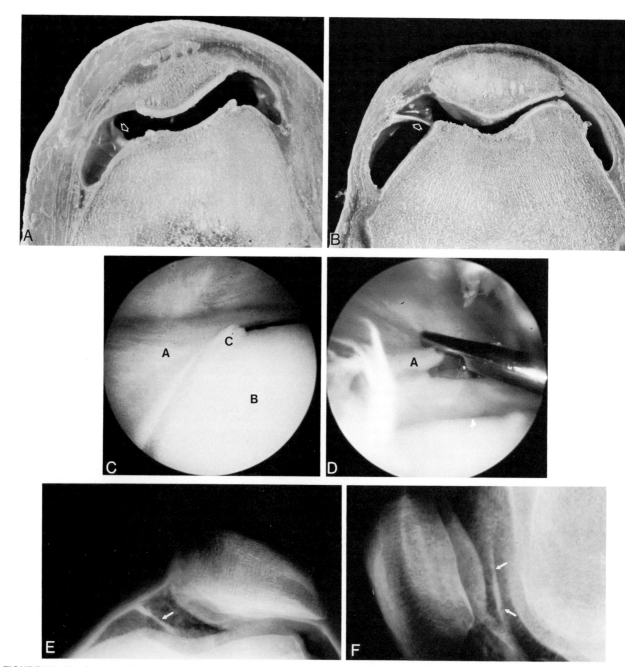

FIGURE 70–221. Synovial plicae: Medial patellar plicae. Anatomy and arthrography.

A, B Transverse sections through cadaveric knee joints at the level of the patella demonstrate medial patellar plicae (arrows). (From Deutsch AL, et al: Radiology *141:*630, 1981.)

C, D Arthroscopy reveals the characteristics of a symptomatic medial patellar plica. In **C**, the plica (A) is "bowstrung" over the femoral condyle (B) in flexion, with localized chondromalacia (C) of the articular surface of the femur. In **D**, the medial patellar plica (A) is resected using basket forceps. (From Richmond JC, McGinty JB: Clin Orthop *178:*185, 1983.)

E, F Arthrographic demonstration of a medial patellar plica (arrows) is provided on axial and near-lateral projections.

medial patellar plica appears as a stringlike radiolucent line superimposed on the superior part of the medial femoral condyle, extending from the suprapatellar bursa to the infrapatellar fat pad.[519] Computed arthrotomography delineates the location and the thickness of this plica.[513, 514] With MR imaging, the medial patellar plica is seen on transaxial and sagittal images when there is fluid in the joint (Fig. 70–222).

The infrapatellar plica, or ligamentum mucosum, represents a vestige of the membranous partition that once separated the medial and lateral embryonic compartments of the knee.[500] It often is fan-shaped, with a narrow femoral margin in the intercondylar notch, widening as it descends through the inferior joint space to attach distally to the inferior and medial aspects of the patellar articular cartilage (Fig. 70–223). From there the plica continues as two fringelike alar folds to cover the infrapatellar fat and separate the synovium from the ligamentum patellae.[521] Its course parallels that of the anterior cruciate ligament, which is located just posterior to it. The course and position of the plica change with increasing flexion of the knee because the site of insertion into the intercondylar fossa is displaced. On

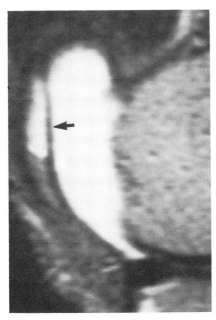

FIGURE 70–222. Synovial plicae: Medial patellar plicae. MR imaging. A sagittal T2-weighted (TR/TE, 1800/60) spin echo MR image through the medial aspect of the joint shows a medial patellar plica (arrow) outlined by fluid of high signal intensity on either side.

rare occasions, the infrapatellar plica may be double, or it may persist into adult life as an intact septum, although it is encountered more commonly as a fenestrated septum or series of fibrous bands in the adult knee.[497, 521]

The infrapatellar plica can be identified on double contrast arthrography both on the lateral and the intercondylar views. Because of their anatomic relationship, the infrapatellar plica easily may be confused with the anterior cruciate ligament, resulting in an incorrect diagnosis in patients with complete disruption of the anterior cruciate ligament.[522]

Symptomatic plicae most commonly are encountered in what has been referred to as the "plica syndrome."[497, 498, 502, 504, 1350] In this syndrome, the medial patellar plica, which

normally exists as a fine, thin, flexible fold of synovium of little clinical significance, becomes pathologically thickened and symptomatic.[515–518, 523–528] Among the postulated factors in the initiation of a traumatic synovitis leading to secondary abnormalities within the plicae are trauma, strenuous exercise, osteochondritis dissecans, injuries to the meniscus, and intra-articular osteocartilaginous bodies. Regardless of the inciting event, when inflammation exists with edema and thickening, fibrous repair may result in increasing collagenization and progressive loss of elasticity.[502] With continued thickening, the plica becomes relatively unpliable and no longer glides normally but snaps against the underlying femoral condyle. Repeated irritation and abrasion result in erosive changes of the articular cartilage of the condyle or even the patella.[514, 523, 524]

The diagnosis may be suspected from the history and physical examination. Classically, the patient relates an episode of blunt or twisting trauma followed by the development of a joint effusion. Excessive stress precipitates a dull, aching pain medial to the patella, which is aggravated by flexion. A clicking sensation without locking or giving way is another common clinical complaint. A palpable or audible snap may occur on knee movement, and a symptomatic plica may be palpated as a tender, bandlike structure parallel to the medial border of the patella. In some cases, a pathologic plica may simulate primary monoarticular arthritis.[526] Alternatively, in rheumatoid arthritis and in other conditions in which a chronic synovial inflammatory process is present, the plicae may become irregularly thickened. The thickened medial plica may be visualized with CT arthrography or MR imaging (Fig. 70–224).

Although much recent attention has focused on the plica syndrome, these embryonic remnants may manifest themselves in another clinically significant manner. Both the suprapatellar and infrapatellar plicae may persist in their entirety and lead to complete compartmentalization of the knee joint. Failure of the suprapatellar partition to involute may produce an entirely separate suprapatellar bursa.[498, 500, 527, 529] Clinically, the bursa may be manifested as a mass in the suprapatellar area, which is cystic or rubbery and firm on palpation.[498, 508] This may be recognized on double contrast arthrography by the appearance of either a small suprapatellar space or an extrinsic compression on the suprapatellar pouch.[500, 529] CT may be of value in further characterizing the nature of the mass and its relation to the

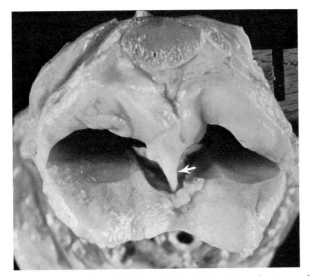

FIGURE 70–223. Synovial plicae: Infrapatellar plicae. Anatomy. A transverse section of a cadaveric knee through the level of the intercondylar notch allows optimal visualization of the course of the infrapatellar plica (arrow) with the patella retracted anteriorly and superiorly. (From Deutsch AL, et al: Radiology *141:*631, 1981.)

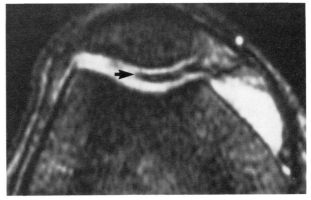

FIGURE 70–224. Synovial plicae: Plica syndrome. A thickened medial patellar plica (arrow) is well shown on a transaxial STIR MR image (TR/TE, 1650/25; inversion time, 160 msec).

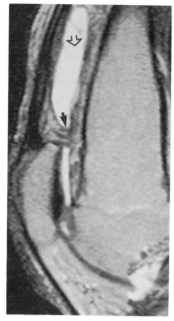

FIGURE 70–225. Synovial plicae: Compartmentalization of the joint. MR imaging. A sagittal T2-weighted (TR/TE, 2100/80) spin echo MR image in a patient who presented with soft tissue fullness in the anterior aspect of the knee shows a distended suprapatellar pouch (open arrow) separated from the knee by a suprapatellar plica (solid arrow).

knee joint. MR imaging also may display the mass[530] (Fig. 70–225). Documentation of a separate bursa is of considerable importance in planning an optimal surgical approach; in this regard, a case has been described in which osteocartilaginous bodies in a separate suprapatellar bursa could not be located by using an infrapatellar surgical incision.[508] Documentation of a separate bursa also is important in the

management of penetrating wounds with acute suppurative bursitis, in which rupture of the partitioning membrane may unnecessarily contaminate the joint.[508]

Persistence of the infrapatellar plica in its entirety will divide the knee joint into separate medial and lateral compartments.[531] This finding may occur in patients who have had a history of previous trauma with healed supracondylar fractures.[500] This fact suggests that trauma may initiate either fibrous thickening and hypertrophy of the infrapatellar plica or intra-articular fibrosis, leading to abnormal compartmentalization of the joint. Similar compartmentalization has been identified in hereditary onycho-osteoarthrodysplasia (the nail-patella syndrome)[500] (Fig. 70–226). The probable relation, however, between anomalies of the patella and aberrations in joint development remains incompletely understood.[532]

Periarticular Synovial and Ganglion Cysts. Minor variations in histologic features and inconsistencies in terminology have led to great confusion regarding the classification of synovial cysts and other periarticular fluid collections. The existence of numerous bursae about the knee[445, 447, 452–454] further complicates the classification of fluid-filled cystic lesions in this location. Although such cysts occurring in the popliteal fossa that communicate with the joint usually are referred to as synovial cysts or Baker's cysts, cysts in this region that do not communicate with the joint and those in other locations about the knee that may or may not communicate with the joint are described using a variety of terms such as noncommunicating synovial cysts, ganglion cysts, meniscal cysts, and juxta-articular myxomas. Subtle differences in the histology of the lesions or in their contents may allow an experienced pathologist to differentiate among these many fluid-filled cysts, although no uniformly accepted classification system exists. In this section, a discussion of some of the more typical synovial and ganglion cysts occurring about the knee is

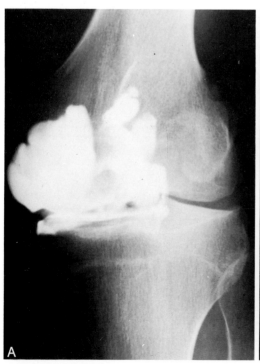
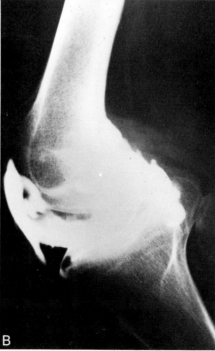

FIGURE 70–226. Synovial plicae: Compartmentalization of the joint. Knee arthrography, in the nail-patella syndrome. Frontal **(A)** and lateral **(B)** views following the initial injection of contrast material into the medial aspect of the joint demonstrate a well-demarcated and independent medial compartment. (From Deutsch AL, et al: Radiology *141*:633, 1981.)

presented. Cystic lesions that generally communicate with an abnormal meniscus (i.e., meniscal cysts) are considered later in this chapter.

Synovial cysts about the knee are most frequent in the popliteal region, where communication between the joint and normal posterior bursae can be identified.[446, 447, 533] The most commonly involved bursa is the gastrocnemiosemimembranosus bursa,[449, 534, 535] located posterior to the medial femoral condyle between the tendons of the gastrocnemius and semimembranosus muscles, with an additional portion anterior to the medial head of the gastrocnemius. The anterior limit of this bursa abuts on the posterior surface of the joint capsule and is relatively thin.[536] Communication between the bursa and the knee joint occurs in 35 to 55 per cent of cadavers[447, 536] and increases in frequency with advancing age. This communication occurs via a transverse slit, usually between 15 to 20 mm in size.[536] The opening may be covered with a fibrous membrane in approximately 70 per cent of cases.[536]

Swelling of this posterior bursa is termed a Baker's cyst.[537, 538] The cause of such cysts is not entirely clear, and various theories have been proposed: (1) Herniation of the synovial membrane of the knee through a weak area in the posterior joint capsule; (2) rupture of the posterior joint capsule with extravasation of fluid into the soft tissues and secondary encapsulation; and (3) rupture of the posterior joint capsule, producing communication with a normally occurring posterior bursa. Of these theories, the third theory seems most probable,[446, 447, 539, 540] as direct observation rarely has documented a synovial herniation from the knee into a normal bursa or a popliteal cyst completely separated from the articular cavity.

The presence of a slit between articular cavity and posterior bursa may be responsible for a ball-valve mechanism that has been noted in conjunction with synovial cysts[541–543]; fluid introduced into a cyst may not enter the joint cavity (Fig. 70–227). Because of this one-way directional flow, arthrography rather than bursography is more accurate in defining the extent of a cyst and its connection with a neighboring joint. This ball-valve mechanism, however, is not present invariably. Rauschning and collaborators[535] have divided popliteal cysts into those with a true one-way valve (approximately 50 per cent of cases) and those in which unimpeded flow of fluid occurs in both directions; a strong positive correlation was found between the presence of a valve mechanism and the absence of articular disorders, and between the absence of a valve mechanism and the presence of joint effusions and disease.

In addition to the gastrocnemiosemimembranosus bursa, a second posterior bursa is located beneath the popliteal

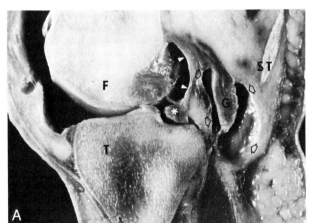
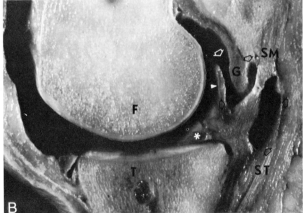
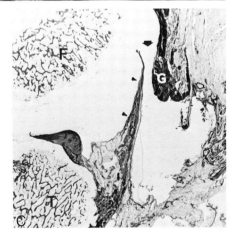

FIGURE 70–227. Synovial cysts: Anatomy of the posterior bursae—photographs and a photomicrograph of sagittal sections through the knee of a cadaveric specimen.

A Sagittal section through the knee at the level of the medial femoral condyle near the intercondylar notch. F, Femur; T, tibia; asterisk, posterior horn of medial meniscus. The anterior margin of the band of tissue directly posterior to the medial femoral condyle is the knee joint capsule (arrowheads). The posterior margin of this same band of tissue is the anterior margin of the gastrocnemiosemimembranosus bursa (arrows), which lies anterior to the medial head of the gastrocnemius muscle (G). The semimembranosus muscle is not seen in this section. The semitendinosus muscle (ST) is seen more posteriorly, with the posterior margin of the bursa (arrows) apposed to it.

B A sagittal section through the medial femoral condyle 1 cm medial to **A**. A transverse slit (white arrow) represents communication between the knee joint and the gastrocnemiosemimembranosus bursa (black arrows). The opening is cranially oriented and arises about 2 cm inferiorly to the most superior aspect of the posterior joint capsule. The semimembranosus muscle (SM) courses obliquely posterior to the medial head of the gastrocnemius muscle (G). The semitendinosus muscle (ST) forms the posterior margin of the gastrocnemiosemimembranosus bursa. Arrowhead, Knee joint capsule; asterisk, posterior horn of medial meniscus.

C Photomicrograph (×1) of a sagittal section at the level of the medial femoral condyle. The transverse slit (solid arrow) is readily apparent. The membranous septum could not be seen. G, Medial head of the gastrocnemius muscle; open arrows, gastrocnemiosemimembranosus bursa; arrowheads, posterior joint capsule. (From Guerra J Jr, et al: AJR *136*:593, 1981. Copyright 1981, American Roentgen Ray Society.)

tendon, which communicates less frequently with the joint. A third posterior bursa exists between the medial head of the gastrocnemius and the distal end of the biceps. A weak point occurs laterally beneath the popliteal tendon, which may represent an extended popliteal tendon sheath. Furthermore, communication may exist between the knee and proximal tibiofibular joint cavity in 10 per cent of adults. Occasionally, anterior, medial, and lateral synovial cysts also may be observed.[544-549] In fact, synovial cysts may extend simultaneously in more than one direction.[550]

Any of these synovial cysts may enlarge, producing a mass with or without pain. Rupture of a cyst is associated with soft tissue extravasation of fluid contents. Ruptures occurring posteriorly can simulate thrombophlebitis,[551] and, in fact, the two conditions can coexist.[552-556] Giant synovial cysts can extend into the calf, ankle, heel, and thigh.[557-561]

Conventional radiography usually provides nonspecific evidence of a synovial cyst. A joint effusion and a soft tissue mass are evident in some cases, although the latter abnormality may be difficult to distinguish from normal soft tissue structures. Occasionally, intrabursal osteocartilaginous bodies or radiolucent collections, calcification in the bursal wall, or bone erosions are seen.[562-567]

Arthrography of the knee is an accurate method of diagnosing synovial cysts,[568-573] although some investigators also recommend ultrasonic[574-586] or isotopic[587-590] examination in this clinical situation. Computed tomography appears of little value in diagnosing these cysts in most cases, although this examination is useful in the evaluation of a suspected synovial cyst when its position is atypical or when it is not opacified on arthrography.[591-594] Imaging of such cysts with MR may provide information regarding the degree of synovial inflammation (see later discussion).

The arthrographic appearance of an abnormal synovial cyst will vary.[595] In most instances, a well-defined, lobulated structure filled with air and radiopaque contrast material will be revealed. It may have an irregular surface related to hypertrophy of its synovial lining (Fig. 70–228) and be associated with adjacent lymphatic filling. Alternatively, the entire cyst or a portion of it may rupture,[596, 597] with extravasation of contrast material into soft tissues posteriorly, or, less commonly, superiorly or anteriorly. Sinus tracts leading from the cyst to the skin surface may be encountered.

MR imaging is effective in the demonstration of intact as well as ruptured popliteal cysts.[598, 599] In one study, however, only a 5 per cent incidence of such cysts was detected in a retrospective analysis of 1000 consecutive MR imaging examinations of the knee performed in patients referred for evaluation of internal derangement, leading the authors to conclude that the reported higher incidence of popliteal cysts detected with arthrography may relate to distention of normal, collapsed bursae.[600] The typical appearance of a popliteal cyst is a well-defined mass of variable size with signal intensity characteristics of fluid, located between the tendons of the medial head of the gastrocnemius muscle and the semimembranosus muscle (Fig. 70–229). Changes in these signal intensity characteristics may indicate hemorrhage[601] or intrabursal osteocartilaginous bodies. The relationship of the cyst to nearby arteries and veins and the documentation of cyst rupture easily are accomplished with MR imaging (Fig. 70–230).

Any inflammatory, degenerative, traumatic, or neoplastic

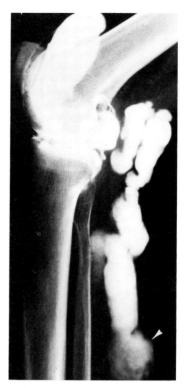

FIGURE 70–228. Synovial cysts: Arthrography. Rheumatoid arthritis. A typical large popliteal cyst extending into the calf is filled with contrast material. It is slightly irregular in contour, particularly inferiorly (arrowhead), which may reflect synovial inflammation. No free extravasation into the soft tissues is seen.

condition that produces a knee effusion can lead to synovial cyst formation. These conditions include rheumatoid arthritis, degenerative joint disease, gout, pigmented villonodular synovitis, and idiopathic synovial (osteo) chondromatosis, as well as other localized or systemic articular conditions. In the absence of any obvious cause, the radiologist must search diligently for meniscal abnormality. Synovial cysts may be noted in children with juvenile chronic polyarthritis[602] or on a familial basis.[603] In children, popliteal cysts appear to have a much better prognosis than in adults, and the frequency of noncommunicating cysts is higher. Surgical removal of synovial cysts without treatment of the underlying articular disease process rarely is successful, as the cyst will recur.[604]

The differential diagnosis of synovial cysts about the knee includes a variety of neoplasms of soft tissue or bone origin,[605-607] thrombophlebitis and hematomas,[608, 609] varicose and focally dilated veins, aneurysms, and other conditions (Fig. 70–231). The simultaneous occurrence of synovial cysts and some of these disorders is well known, especially with regard to venous thrombosis, thrombophlebitis, and cystic degeneration of the popliteal artery.[610-612]

Ganglion cysts classically contain a jelly-like viscous fluid, are loculated or septated, may arise within muscle bundles or be attached to a tendon sheath, and may or may not communicate with a joint. Those occurring about the knee usually are located close to the proximal tibiofibular joint and fibular head (Fig. 70–232), where they may lead to compression of the common peroneal nerve.[613-616] Ganglion cysts in this location (and other locations) may extend into the adjacent bone (Fig. 70–233), contain gas, and mi-

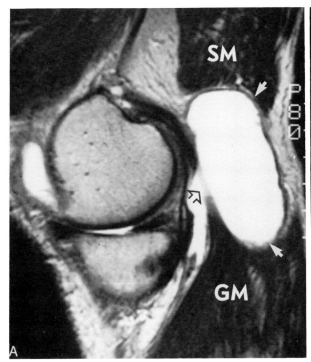

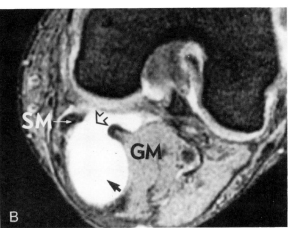

FIGURE 70–229. Synovial cysts: MR imaging.

A A sagittal T2-weighted (TR/TE, 4000/76) fast spin echo MR image shows a channel (open arrow) leading from the joint into a large synovial cyst (solid arrows) located between the semimembranosus muscle (SM) and medial head of the gastrocnemius muscle (GM).

B A transaxial MPGR MR image (TR/TE, 500/11; flip angle, 15 degrees) shows the channel (open arrow) and the synovial cyst (solid arrow) located between the semimembranosus tendon (SM) and the medial head of the gastrocnemius muscle and its tendon (GM).

(Courtesy of S. K. Brahme, M.D., La Jolla, California.)

FIGURE 70–230. Synovial cysts: MR imaging. Cyst dissection.

A A sagittal T1-weighted (TR/TE, 800/20) spin echo MR image shows a large mass (arrows) in the posterior aspect of the knee and calf with low inhomogeneous signal intensity. It begins at the level of the joint.

B A transaxial T2-weighted (TR/TE, 2000/80) spin echo MR image shows the mass (arrows) of inhomogeneous signal intensity superficial to the medial head of the gastrocnemius muscle.

(Courtesy of T. Broderick, M.D., Orange, California.)

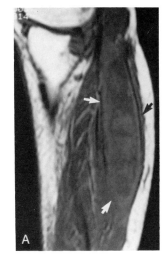

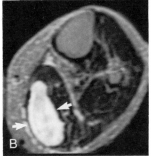

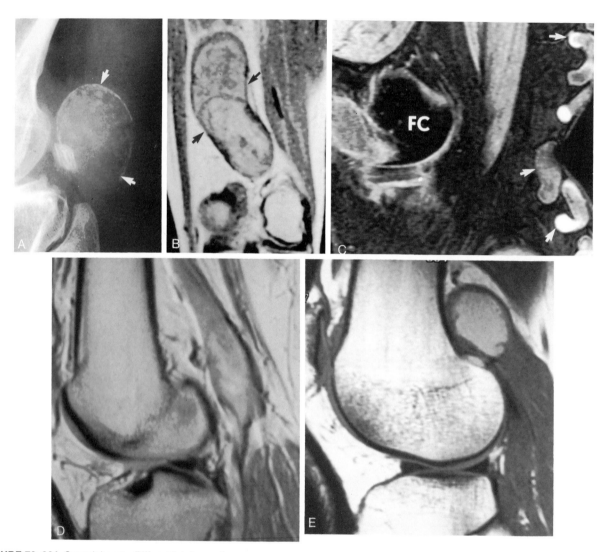

FIGURE 70–231. Synovial cysts: Differential diagnosis.

A Popliteal artery aneurysm. A calcified aneurysm (arrows) is evident behind the knee. (Courtesy of A. Orloff, M.D., San Diego, California.)

B Popliteal artery aneurysm. A coronal proton density–weighted (TR/TE, 1800/20) spin echo MR image shows a large aneurysm (arrows) with inhomogeneous signal intensity behind and just above the knee.

C Varicose veins. A sagittal 3DFT spoiled gradient recalled acquisition in the steady state (SPGR) MR image (TR/TE, 58/10; flip angle, 60 degrees) obtained with chemical presaturation of fat (ChemSat) shows irregular channel-like masses (arrows) of inhomogeneous signal intensity behind the knee. The femoral condyle (FC) is indicated.

D Popliteal vein aneurysm. A sagittal proton density–weighted (TR/TE, 2950/20) spin echo MR image shows the varix of intermediate signal intensity. (Courtesy of J. Spaeth, M.D., Albuquerque, New Mexico.)

E Synovial sarcoma. A sagittal T1-weighted (TR/TE, 500/16) spin echo MR image reveals the tumor of intermediate signal intensity in the lateral head of the gastrocnemius muscle. (Courtesy of D. Witte, M.D., Memphis, Tennessee.)

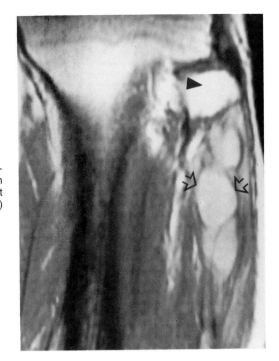

FIGURE 70–232. Periarticular ganglion cysts: MR imaging. A coronal proton density–weighted (TR/TE, 2000/35) spin echo MR image shows a septated ganglion cyst (open arrows) containing fluid of intermediate signal intensity located adjacent to the fibular head (arrowhead). (Courtesy of T. Broderick, M.D., Orange, California.)

grate for considerable distances within the fascial planes. Ultrasonography, CT, and MR imaging can be used in their assessment.[613, 614, 617] Similar lesions may arise close to the tibial insertion site of the pes anserinus tendons, where they have been referred to as ganglion cysts, juxta-articular bone cysts, and pes anserinus bursitis.[618–620] In this location, erosion of the medial tibial margin and periosteal bone proliferation in the form of broad spicules extending perpendicular to the external surface of the cortex may be evident. As in other sites, ganglion cysts near the pes anserinus tendons may be diagnosed using ultrasonography, cystography, CT, or MR imaging (Fig. 70–234). Usually, although not invariably,[620] the signal intensity characteristics of the lesion on various MR imaging sequences are those of fluid.

Intra-Articular Ganglion Cysts. Ganglion cysts arising within the knee joint are encountered infrequently. These cysts arise most typically at two specific sites: the alar folds that cover the infrapatellar fat body; and the cruciate ligaments. Intra-articular ganglion cysts arising from the alar folds were described in 1972 by Muckle and Monahan.[621] These cysts may present as knee pain similar to that of a torn meniscus, joint fullness, or an effusion. They generally are seen as well-defined and smooth masses during conventional arthrography or computed arthrotomography and, with MR images, the signal intensity abnormalities of the lesions are those of fluid (Fig. 70–235). Localized nodular synovitis of the knee may have a similar arthrographic appearance (Fig. 70–236A), although if the nodular lesion contains hemosiderin, it will reveal a different pattern of signal intensity on the MR imaging examination (Fig. 70–236B).

Ganglion cysts arising from the anterior or posterior cruciate ligament were noted during routine necropsy in 1924 by Caan.[622] They were described further in reports by Sjovall[623] in 1942 and Levine[624] in 1948. More modern descriptions belong to Chang and Rose,[625] Yasuda and Majima,[626] and Kaempffe and D'Amato.[627] In 1990, Brown and Dandy,[628] in a retrospective analysis of the results of 6500 arthroscopic examinations of the knee, noted the occurrence

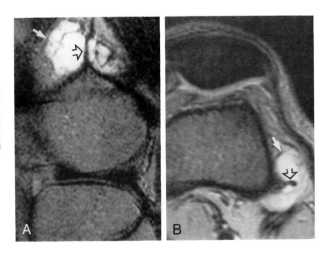

FIGURE 70–233. Subperiosteal ganglion cyst: MR imaging. Ganglion cysts arising close to the surface of a bone can lead to distinctive bone spiculation. This feature is demonstrated (open arrows) in a sagittal T2-weighted (TR/TE, 2200/80) spin echo MR image **(A)** and a transaxial MPGR MR image (TR/TE, 267/15; flip angle, 25 degrees) **(B)** with regard to a ganglion cyst (solid arrows) involving the lateral surface of the distal portion of the femur.

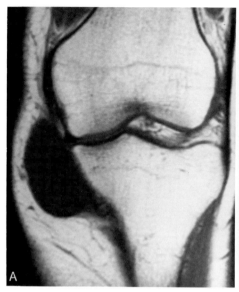 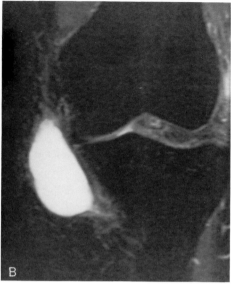

FIGURE 70–234. Pes anserinus ganglion cyst (bursitis): MR imaging. A coronal T1-weighted (TR/TE, 400/20) spin echo MR image **(A)** and a coronal STIR MR image (TR/TE, 2500/40; inversion time, 160 msec) **(B)** show a large, fluid-filled mass adjacent to the anteromedial portion of the tibia.

FIGURE 70–235. Intra-articular ganglion cyst: MR imaging. Alar folds. Sagittal T1-weighted (TR/TE, 500/20) **(A)** and MPGR MR images (TR/TE, 550/25; flip angle, 25 degrees) **(B)** show a septated ganglion cyst located anteriorly and extending into the infrapatellar fat body. (Courtesy of J. Schils, M.D., Cleveland, Ohio.)

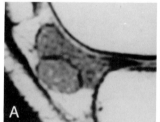 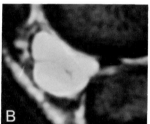

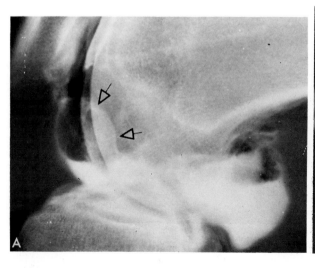 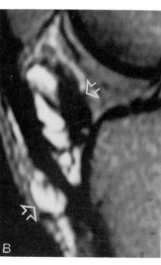

FIGURE 70–236. Localized nodular synovitis: Arthrography and MR imaging.

A Arthrography reveals a nodular mass (arrows) in the region of the infrapatellar fat body that, at surgery, represented localized nodular synovitis.

B In a different patient, a sagittal T2-weighted (TR/TE, 2200/80) spin echo MR image shows a mass (arrows) anterior and posterior to the patellar tendon. It has regions of high and low signal intensity. The low signal intensity is consistent with hemosiderin deposition. Surgical verification of the nature of this lesion was not obtained. (**B**, Courtesy of M. Zlatkin, M.D., Hollywood, Florida.)

FIGURE 70–237. Intra-articular ganglion cysts: CT scanning and MR imaging. Anterior cruciate ligament. A transaxial CT scan **(A)** reveals a well-defined lesion (open arrows) containing fluid (of low attenuation) adjacent to the inner aspect of the lateral femoral condyle close to the site of attachment of the anterior cruciate ligament. A sagittal proton density–weighted (TR/TE, 1200/30) spin echo MR image **(B)** confirms the presence of the mass (open arrow) adjacent to the anterior cruciate ligament (solid arrow).

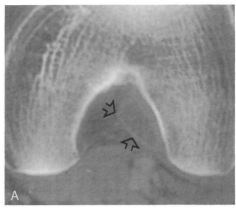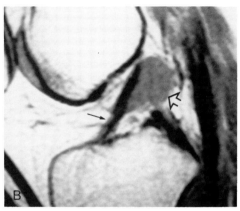

of 38 cases in which an intra-articular ganglion cyst was found. Of these, 28 ganglia arose from the tibial insertion site of the anterior cruciate ligament and one from its femoral insertion site, and six arose from the tibial insertion site of the posterior cruciate ligament. All contained clear fluid, and their average diameter was 5 mm (range: 3 to 8 mm). The clinical manifestations of these ganglion cysts were similar to those of other internal derangements of the knee, and no recurrence of the lesions occurred after arthroscopic excision.[1427]

Routine radiography in such cases may reveal pressure erosion of the femoral condyles, best seen on tunnel views. CT may show an intercondylar soft tissue mass in close proximity to one or both cruciate ligaments (Fig. 70–237A). The MR imaging features consist of a well-defined mass applied to the surface of the anterior cruciate ligament (Fig. 70–237B) or posterior cruciate ligament (Fig. 70–238) with signal intensity characteristics of fluid.[629] These MR imaging findings allow a specific diagnosis in most cases.[1428]

Of related interest, a report by McLaren and coworkers[630] noted the presence of intraosseous cystic lesions at or near the tibial insertion site of the anterior cruciate ligament, posterior cruciate ligament, or both ligaments, in approximately 1 per cent of 1710 knees evaluated with MR imaging. The lesions generally were solitary, and all were spherical and well marginated (Fig. 70–239). The signal intensity characteristics of the intraosseous cysts were typical of a fluid-filled structure surrounded by a rim of sclerotic bone or fibrous tissue. The cruciate ligaments were normal in almost all cases, and no soft tissue masses were evident. Although histologic confirmation of the nature of the lesions was not obtained, the authors speculated that they were in-

traosseous ganglia. The authors further noted the presence of a soft tissue mass adjacent to a similar intraosseous cystic lesion in one additional patient, consistent with the presence of both extraosseous and intraosseous ganglion cysts.

Tumors and Tumor-Like Lesions. A number of tumor and tumor-like lesions may arise from the synovium or capsule of the knee joint or nearby intra-articular tissue. These lesions include pigmented villonodular synovitis and localized nodular synovitis (see Chapters 84 and 95), idiopathic synovial (osteo)chondromatosis (see Chapters 84 and 95), synovial hemangioma (see Chapter 63), intracapsular and capsular chondroma (see Chapter 95), synovial chondrosarcoma (see Chapter 95), synovial lipoma, and lipoma arborescens. In some of these lesions, imaging abnormalities may allow a specific diagnosis.

With pigmented villonodular synovitis, a monoarticular process of the knee in a young adult associated with a radiodense joint effusion, preservation of joint space, and well-defined bone erosions and cysts is typical. The conventional arthrogram in diffuse pigmented villonodular synovitis reveals an enlarged synovial cavity, an irregular synovial outline with pooling of contrast material, and nodular filling defects[631–633] (Fig. 70–240). MR imaging shows synovial proliferation with regions of persistently low signal intensity, consistent with hemosiderin deposition (Fig. 70–241). In idiopathic synovial (osteo)chondromatosis, partially calcified intra-articular and intrasynovial bodies may or may not be evident on routine radiographs (Fig. 70–242). Conventional arthrography shows an enlarged synovial cavity and multiple small, sharply defined filling defects[634, 635] (Fig. 70–243). The nodular lesions in this condition are of variable size but usually are better defined

FIGURE 70–238. Intra-articular ganglion cysts: MR imaging. Posterior cruciate ligament. A coronal T1-weighted (TR/TE, 800/25) spin echo MR image **(A)** and a sagittal T2-weighted (TR/TE, 2000/80) spin echo MR image **(B)** show the large ganglion cyst (open arrows) which arose from the posterior cruciate ligament.

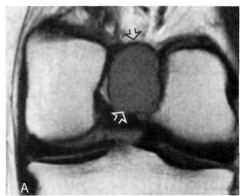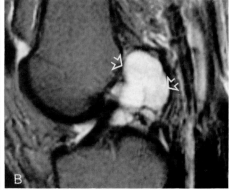

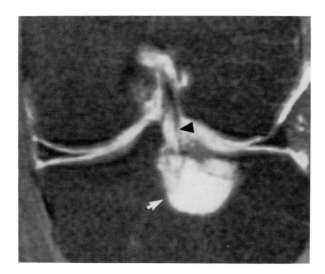

FIGURE 70–239. Intraosseous ganglion cysts: MR imaging. Anterior cruciate ligament. A coronal proton density–weighted (TR/TE, 2850/18) fast spin echo MR image obtained with chemical presaturation of fat (ChemSat) shows a large lesion (arrow) in the tibia close to the site of attachment of the anterior cruciate ligament (arrowhead). Surgical confirmation of the nature of this lesion was not obtained. (Courtesy of G. Applegate, M.D., Van Nuys, California.)

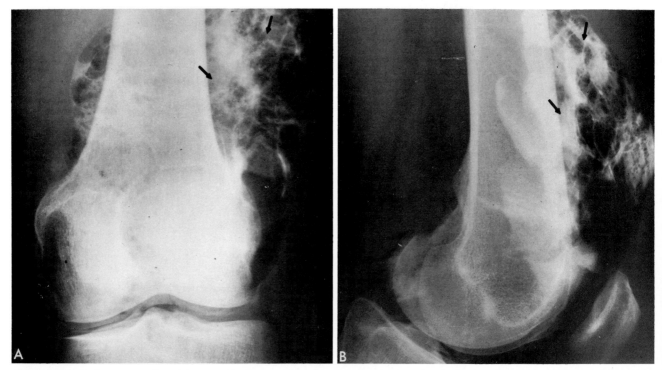

FIGURE 70–240. Pigmented villonodular synovitis: Knee arthrography. Observe the irregular distribution and appearance of contrast material (arrows) in the suprapatellar pouch. (From Dalinka MK, et al: CRC Crit Rev Radiol Sci 5:1, 1973.)

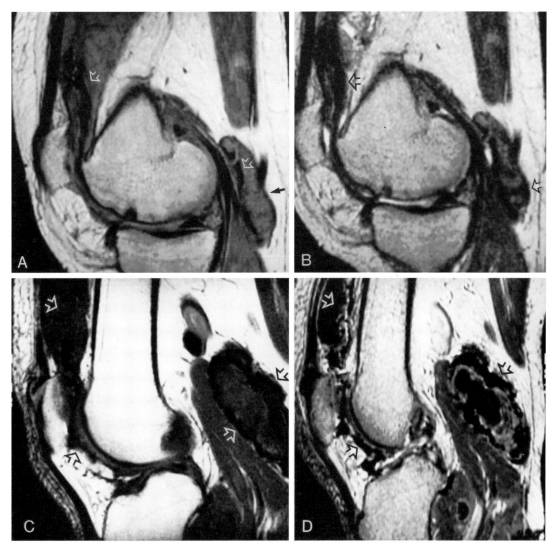

FIGURE 70–241. Pigmented villonodular synovitis: MR imaging.

A, B Sagittal proton density–weighted (TR/TE, 2000/15) **(A)** and T2-weighted (TR/TE, 2000/80) **(B)** spin echo MR images show character-istic features of pigmented villonodular synovitis. In **A**, note involvement of both the joint and a posterior synovial cyst (solid arrow) by a process of inhomogeneous signal intensity. There are regions of very low signal intensity (open arrows) in the joint and synovial cyst. The cartilage is poorly seen and involvement of the femur is evident. In **B**, the regions of very low signal intensity again are evident (open arrows). Small collections of fluid have high signal intensity. (Courtesy of V. Chandnani, M.D., Honolulu, Hawaii.)

C, D A sagittal T1-weighted (TR/TE, 600/12) spin echo MR image **(C)** and a sagittal three-dimensional field echo acquisition with a short repetition time and echo reduction (FASTER) (TR/TE, 18/4.6; flip angle in X axis, 20 degrees, flip angle in Y axis, 25 degrees) obtained following the intravenous administration of a gadolinium compound **(D)** show regions of very low signal intensity (open arrows) in the joint and adjacent synovial cyst that do not enhance following gadolinium administration. A discussion of the FASTER technique is provided by Harms et al: Radiology *173:* 743, 1989. (Courtesy of G. Greenway, M.D., Dallas, Texas.)

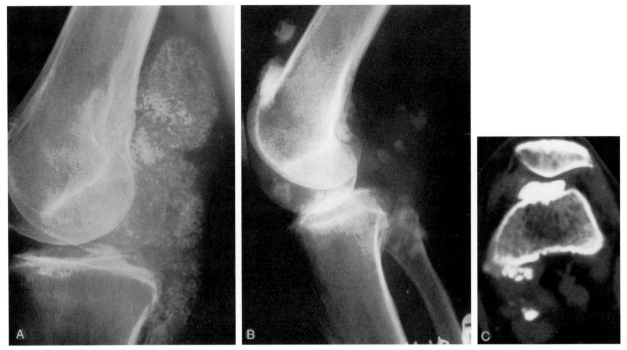

FIGURE 70–242. Idiopathic synovial (osteo)chondromatosis: Routine radiography and CT scanning.

A A lateral radiograph of the knee reveals innumerable small calcific collections scattered throughout the knee and extending posteriorly. (Courtesy of A. G. Bergman, M.D., Stanford, California.)

B, C In a second patient, routine radiography **(B)** shows fewer and larger calcifications in the knee joint with extension into the proximal tibiofibular joint and a posterior synovial cyst. A transaxial CT scan **(C)** confirms the presence of intra-articular and intrabursal calcifications. (Courtesy of G. Greenway, M.D., Dallas, Texas.)

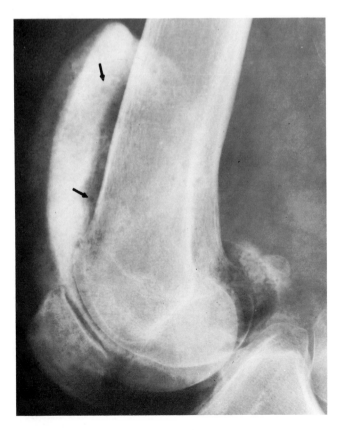

FIGURE 70–243. Idiopathic synovial (osteo)chondromatosis: Arthrography. Observe multiple sharply defined filling defects (arrows) throughout the articular cavity. (From Dalinka MK, et al: CRC Crit Rev Radiol Sci 5:1, 1973.)

arthrographically than those of pigmented villonodular synovitis. MR imaging characteristics of idiopathic synovial (osteo)chondromatosis are variable, depending on the presence or absence of calcification or ossification within the bodies[1395] (Fig. 70–244). Hemangiomas of the synovium occur most frequently in the knee. Initial radiographs may reveal soft tissue masses, calcified phleboliths, and a hemophilia-like arthropathy with osteoporosis and epiphyseal enlargement.[636] Conventional arthrography may reveal single or multiple radiolucent defects, and arteriography will outline hypervascular tumors.[637] MR imaging shows the extent of the lesions, which have variable signal intensity (Fig. 70–245). Intracapsular and capsular chondromas are associated with masses of variable size that may calcify (Fig. 70–246). An infrapatellar location is most typical, and erosion of the lower portion of the patella and displacement of the patellar tendon may be evident. Signal intensity inhomogeneity or homogeneity may be noted on MR imaging examinations (Figs. 70–247 and 70–248). Synovial chondrosarcomas are extremely rare, they occur most often in the knee, they may or may not be related to idiopathic synovial (osteo)chondromatosis, they reveal bizarre calcification, and they are accompanied by inhomogeneity of signal intensity on MR images (Fig. 70–249).

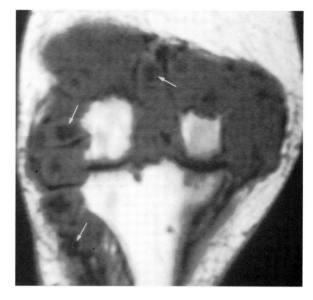

FIGURE 70–244. Idiopathic synovial (osteo)chondromatosis: MR imaging. A coronal T1-weighted (TR/TE, 600/15) spin echo MR image shows fluid of intermediate signal intensity throughout the knee. Note many foci of low signal intensity (arrows), indicative of calcified bodies.

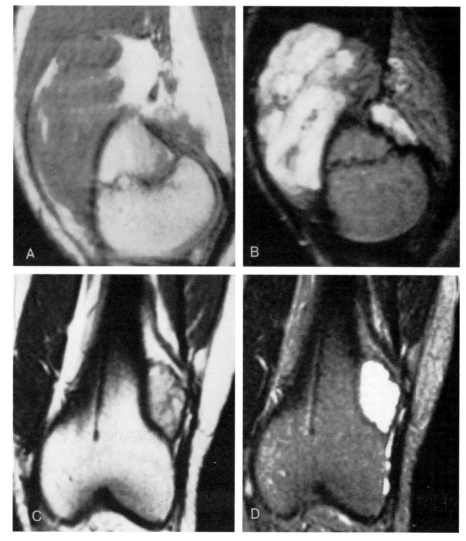

FIGURE 70–245. Synovial hemangioma: MR imaging.

A, B Sagittal T1-weighted (TR/TE, 600/17) **(A)** and T2-weighed (TR/TE, 2000/90) **(B)** spin echo MR images reveal distention of the suprapatellar pouch. The process is of low signal intensity in **A** and inhomogeneous but mainly of high signal intensity in **B**. (Courtesy of M. Pathria, M.D., San Diego, California.)

C, D In a second patient who had a venous hemangioma adjacent to the suprapatellar pouch, coronal proton density–weighted (TR/TE, 2200/20) **(C)** and T2-weighted (TR/TE, 2200/80) **(D)** spin echo MR images reveal the extent of the process, which is of intermediate signal intensity in **C** and of high signal intensity in **D**. (Courtesy of G. Greenway, M.D., Dallas, Texas.)

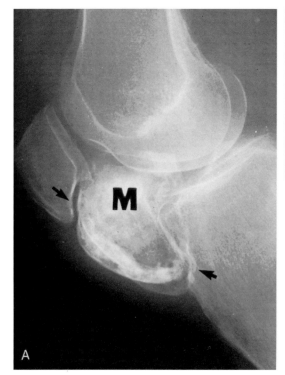

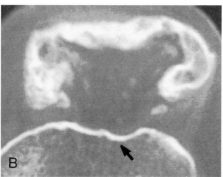

FIGURE 70–246. Intracapsular chondroma: Routine radiography and CT scanning. A frontal radiograph **(A)** reveals the ossified mass (M) that is producing erosion (arrows) of the inferior margin of the patella and the proximal portion of the tibia. A transaxial CT scan **(B)** shows the heavily ossified peripheral portion of the lesion and erosion (arrow) of the metaphysis of the tibia.

FIGURE 70–247. Intracapsular chondroma: MR imaging. A sagittal proton density–weighted (TR/TE, 2500/20) spin echo MR image **(A)** and a sagittal MPGR MR image (TR/TE, 1200/15; flip angle, 70 degrees) **(B)** reveal a large, partly ossified mass in the region of the deep infrapatellar fat body. The mass contains foci whose signal intensity is that of marrow fat. Note erosion of the lower portion of the patella and anterior displacement of the patellar tendon.

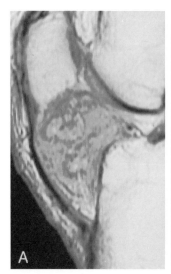
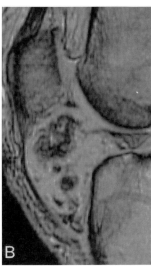

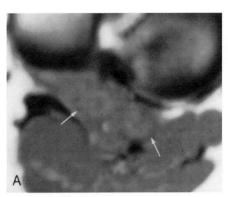
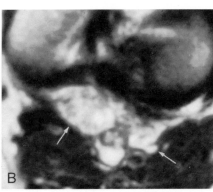

FIGURE 70–248. Capsular chondroma: MR imaging. Transaxial T1-weighted (TR/TE, 600/20) **(A)** and T2-weighted (TR/TE, 2000/80) **(B)** spin echo MR images show the tumor (arrows) arising from the posterior capsule of the knee joint. In **B**, inhomogeneous high signal intensity within the lesion is evident. (Courtesy of S. Montgomery, M.D., Burlington, Vermont.)

FIGURE 70–249. Synovial chondrosarcoma: MR imaging. A sagittal T1-weighted (TR/TE, 867/12) spin echo MR image **(A)** and a STIR MR image (TR/TE, 2500/40; inversion time, 160 msec) **(B)** show the large mass involving the posterior aspect of the knee and posterior soft tissues. The lesion is inhomogeneous but mainly of high signal intensity in **B**. At surgery, the tumor was adherent to the posterior capsule of the knee joint. The final histologic diagnosis was extraskeletal myxoid chondrosarcoma or synovial chondrosarcoma. (Courtesy of G. Greenway, M.D., Dallas, Texas.)

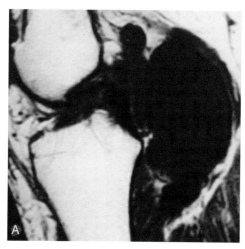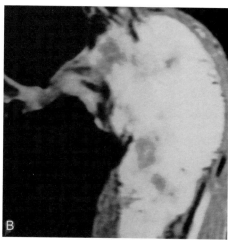

Lipoma arborescens is a rare intra-articular lesion of unknown cause, most commonly located in the knee, consisting of focal deposits of fat beneath the swollen synovial lining.[638] Arthrography reveals numerous moderately well defined defects of variable size.[639, 640] The fatty nature of the process can be determined accurately with CT or MR imaging[641, 642] (Fig. 70–250). Rarely, true lipomas may produce filling defects in the opacified knee during arthrography.[643] Once again, MR imaging provides evidence regarding the fatty nature of the process.

Meniscal Abnormalities

Anatomic Considerations. The menisci of the knee are composed of fibrocartilage and are located between the articular surfaces of the condyles of the femur and the tibial plateaus (Fig. 70–251). They serve to deepen and enlarge the articular surfaces of the proximal portion of the tibia and, thereby, to better accommodate the condyles of the femur. The shapes of the two menisci are not identical. The lateral meniscus appears as a circular structure and, compared with the medial meniscus, covers more of the articular surface of the tibia. Its width is relatively constant from its anterior to posterior portions. The lateral meniscus has a loose peripheral attachment and, posteriorly, is separated from the capsule by the popliteus tendon and its sheath. Therefore, the lateral meniscus normally is more mobile than the medial meniscus. The meniscofemoral ligaments are intimate with the posterior horn of the lateral meniscus (see later discussion). The shape of the medial meniscus is semicircular, and its width is greater posteriorly than anteriorly. The width of its central portion is variable. Peripherally, the medial meniscus is firmly attached to the joint capsule, particularly in its midportion, in the region of the medial (tibial) collateral ligament. The tibial attachment of the meniscus often is referred to as the coronary ligament. The medial meniscus has no direct attachments to any muscle, but indirect capsular connections to the semimembranosus muscle may provide some retraction of its posterior horn.[644]

The posterior fibers of the anterior horn of the medial meniscus are intimate with the transverse (geniculate) ligament of the knee, which connects the anterior horns of both menisci.[645] This ligament is of variable thickness and lies in the frontal plane anterior to the capsule of the knee joint, in the posterior portion of Hoffa's infrapatellar fat body.[646] It can be recognized regularly on MR images (Fig. 70–252) and, occasionally, on lateral radiographs.

The meniscofemoral ligaments are accessory ligaments of the knee that extend from the posterior horn of the lateral meniscus to the lateral aspect of the medial femoral condyle.[645] As they extend across the knee, they are intimate with portions of the posterior cruciate ligament.[647–649] The anterior meniscofemoral ligament, or ligament of Humphrey, passes in front of the posterior cruciate ligament, and the posterior meniscofemoral ligament, or ligament of Wrisberg, passes behind the posterior cruciate ligament. The incidence of these ligaments is not clear, and their size is variable. The reported incidence of one or the other of the two meniscofemoral ligaments in a single knee is 70 to 100 per cent,[647, 649] and the reported incidence of both ligaments in a single knee is 6 to 80 per cent. As a general guide, the ligament of Humphrey probably is present in at least one third of knees, the ligament of Wrisberg probably is present in at least one third of knees, and both ligaments are present in approximately 6 to 10 per cent of knees. The meniscofemoral ligaments are well demonstrated in coronal and sagittal MR images (Figs. 70–252 and 70–253), in which they may lead to an appearance simulating that of a tear of either the posterior cruciate ligament or the posterior horn of the lateral meniscus (see later discussion). The precise function of these ligaments also is not clear. The ligaments become taut when the knee is flexed, and this flexion leads to anterior and medial movement of the posterior horn of the lateral meniscus while the meniscus as a whole rotates backward and outward.[649] These movements appear to provide increased congruity between the meniscotibial socket and the lateral femoral condyle.[645, 647, 648] Shortening of the ligament of Wrisberg in association with absence of a posterior tibial attachment of the lateral meniscus may disturb the meniscal kinetics and may represent one causative factor of a discoid lateral meniscus (see later discussion).

Water represents approximately 75 per cent of the wet content of the meniscus. The dry content of the meniscus is composed of about 75 per cent collagen, 8 to 13 per cent noncollagenous proteins, and 1 per cent hexosamine.[644, 650, 651] The collagen fibers within the meniscus primarily are oriented in a circumferential fashion, thereby resisting the loads applied to them by the femur.[644, 652] Radially oriented

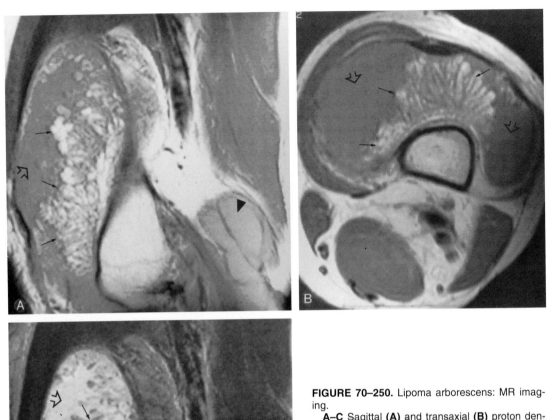

FIGURE 70–250. Lipoma arborescens: MR imaging.

A–C Sagittal **(A)** and transaxial **(B)** proton density–weighted (TR/TE, 2000/20) spin echo MR images and a sagittal T2-weighted (TR/TE, 2000/80) spin echo MR image **(C)** show fatty infiltration of the synovial membrane (solid arrows) associated with a fluid-filled joint (open arrows) and a posterior synovial cyst (arrowheads). Note that the signal intensity of the involved synovium is identical to that of fat. (Courtesy of M. Schweitzer, M.D., Philadelphia, Pennsylvania.)

fibers also are present, however, which may prevent longitudinal splitting of the structure resulting from undue compression.[644] Elastin fibers, accounting for approximately 0.6 per cent of the dry weight of the meniscus, connect the collagen fibers in a bridgelike fashion,[653] and they may contribute to recovery after its deformation.[644]

The vascular supply to the medial and lateral menisci originates predominately from the superior and inferior branches of both the medial and lateral genicular arteries.[645] These vessels give rise to a perimeniscal capillary plexus within the synovial and capsular tissues of the knee that supplies the peripheral border of the meniscus at its attachment to the joint capsule.[645] The central and major portion of the menisci, however, is avascular, deriving its nutrition from the synovial fluid (Fig. 70–254).

The functions of the menisci of the knee have been the subject of intense investigation, the results of which have been summarized by Renström and Johnson.[644] These functions appear to include load transmission, shock absorption, stress reduction, promotion of joint congruity, joint stabili-

zation, limitation of extremes of flexion and extension of the knee, and articular lubrication and nutrition. Investigators have confirmed that the menisci transmit between 30 and 70 per cent of the load applied across the knee, that the lateral meniscus transmits a load equal to or greater than the load transmitted by the medial meniscus, that the posterior horns of the menisci transmit more of the load than the anterior horns, and that the distribution of the load depends on the degree of flexion of the joint.[644] The effects of partial or total meniscectomy on ipsilateral compartmental contact areas and contact pressures and on the transmission of force across the knee may be profound,[1396] although the contribution of such meniscectomy to the development of osteoarthritis of the knee remains controversial (see Chapter 39). The menisci also are important in reducing the shock that is applied to the articular cartilage and subchondral bone of the knee.[654] Meniscectomy reduces the shock absorption capacity of the normal knee by 20 per cent.[644, 655] Similarly, meniscectomy leads to a significant increase in the stress applied to the knee.[656, 657] By filling in the space

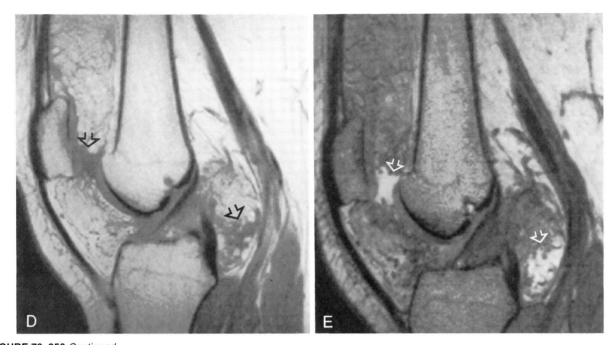

FIGURE 70–250 *Continued*
D, E In a second patient, sagittal proton density–weighted (TR/TE, 1000/15) spin echo **(D)** and 3DFT gradient recalled (TR/TE, 31/10; flip angle, 40 degrees) **(E)** MR images show massive enlargement of the knee joint with a process that is mainly lipomatous in nature. The signal intensity of the infiltrative process primarily is that of fat, although fluid collections (arrows) also are apparent. The popliteal vessels are displaced. (Courtesy of T. Hughes, M.D., San Diego, California.)

between the femur and the tibia, the menisci increase the congruency of the knee joint. By deepening the articular surface of the tibial plateaus, they also stabilize the joint. During the final phases of extension of the knee, the menisci are forced anteriorly, and their anterior position blocks further extension of the joint; conversely, the posterior horns are driven far posteriorly in full flexion of the knee and assist in preventing further flexion.[644] Finally, the menisci may contribute to joint lubrication by reducing the space available for distribution of the fluid that is expressed from the articular cartilage during weight-bearing, and they

may assist in compressing the synovial fluid into the articular cartilage, aiding in joint nutrition.[644]

Pathologic Considerations. Although the vast majority of meniscal lesions are considered traumatic in nature, developmental, inflammatory, infectious, neoplastic, metabolic, and degenerative processes also affect these structures.[658, 659] The discoid-shaped meniscus is the most important of the developmental processes and is discussed later in this chapter. Rheumatoid arthritis, the seronegative spondyloarthropathies, juvenile chronic arthritis, and septic arthritis are among the inflammatory processes that involve

FIGURE 70–251. Menisci of the Knee: Normal anatomy. Coronal section (on left) and view of the upper portion of the tibia (on right). A, anterior; P, posterior. Visualized structures are the medial meniscus (1), lateral meniscus (2), medial collateral ligament (3), fibular collateral ligament (4), anterior cruciate ligament (5), posterior cruciate ligament (6), transverse ligament of the knee (7), and meniscofemoral ligament of Wrisberg (arrow). Observe the relatively large posterior horn of the medial meniscus and its firm attachment to the medial collateral ligament and the more circular configuration of the lateral meniscus, with its relatively uniform size.

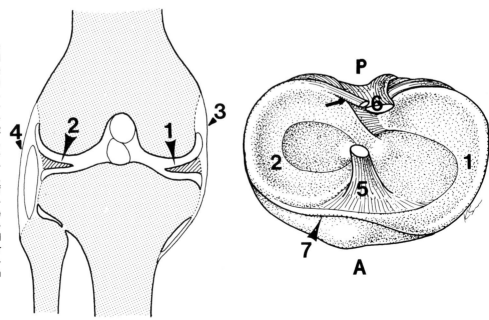

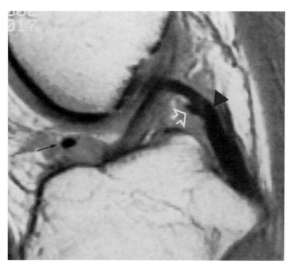

FIGURE 70–252. Transverse (geniculate) ligament of the knee and anterior meniscofemoral ligament (ligament of Humphrey): MR imaging. A sagittal proton density–weighted (TR/TE, 2000/20) spin echo MR image shows the transverse ligament (solid arrow) and anterior meniscofemoral ligament (open arrow) adjacent to the posterior cruciate ligament (arrowhead). The anterior cruciate ligament also is seen. (Courtesy of S. K. Brahme, M.D., La Jolla, California.)

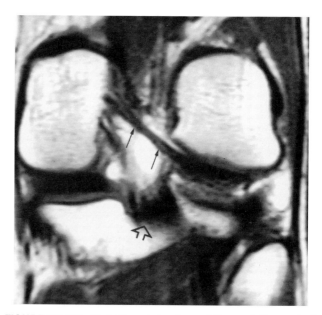

FIGURE 70–253. Posterior meniscofemoral ligament (ligament of Wrisberg): MR imaging. A coronal T1-weighted (TR/TE, 650/20) spin echo MR image shows the posterior meniscofemoral ligament (solid arrows) extending from the region of the posterior horn of the lateral meniscus to the medial femoral condyle. The tibial attachment site of the posterior cruciate ligament is seen (open arrow).

the knee, including the menisci. Generally, owing to their fibrocartilaginous nature, the menisci are more resistant than articular cartilage to the detrimental effects of these processes. Aggressive inflammatory tissue, or pannus, however, can lead to significant changes of the menisci, related to enzymatic destruction and interference with proper nutri-

tion. The peripheral portions of the menisci appear more vulnerable than the central portions,[659] although the entire meniscus may be affected. Pigmented villonodular synovitis and idiopathic synovial (osteo)chondromatosis are addi-

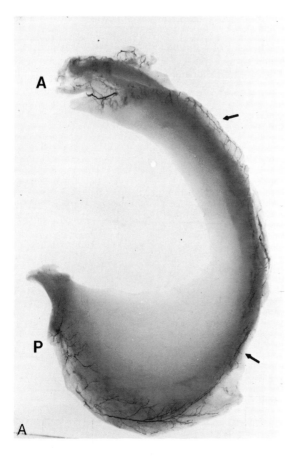

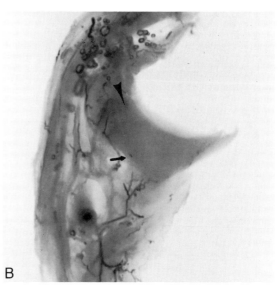

FIGURE 70–254. Menisci of the knee: Normal vascular anatomy.

A Medial meniscus. Note the peripheral arterial blood supply (arrows) and the avascular inner zone. A, Anterior; P, posterior.

B Medial meniscus. A cross section shows a blood vessel in the central zone of the meniscus (arrow) and absence of blood supply in the superior (arrowhead) and inferior surfaces of the meniscus. (From Danzig L, et al: Clin Orthop *172*:271, 1983.)

tional synovial processes that directly or indirectly alter meniscal integrity. All of these processes are discussed elsewhere in this book.

Crystal deposition diseases, particularly those related to calcium pyrophosphate dihydrate (CPPD) and calcium hydroxyapatite (HA) crystal accumulation, affect the menisci. Both of these disorders lead to cartilage calcification (i.e., chondrocalcinosis) that can be detected pathologically and with imaging methods. Diffuse calcification in more than one meniscus and, frequently, in the medial and lateral menisci of both knees in a middle-aged or elderly person is virtually pathognomonic for CPPD crystal deposition. Such deposition and the structural joint changes that may accompany it (i.e., pyrophosphate arthropathy) are discussed in Chapter 44. Alkaptonuria, which is associated with alterations in the metabolism of tyrosine and the accumulation of homogentisic acid and its derivatives in the body's tissues, can lead to abnormal pigmentation of the menisci of the knee and structural joint change (i.e., ochronotic arthropathy). This disease is discussed in Chapter 47.

The association of meniscal abnormalities and degenerative disease is complex. As indicated in Chapter 39, the occurrence of degenerative alterations in the menisci, with or without intrameniscal crystal deposition, and osteoarthritis in the same knee is well recognized.[660, 661] The prominent role played by the menisci in maintaining joint stabilization, promoting joint congruence, stress reduction, and shock absorption suggests that any damage to these structures may be detrimental to the adjacent articular cartilage. Furthermore, the importance of the menisci in promoting joint lubrication and nutrition of the articular cartilage is recognized. Meniscal damage interferes with these functions. Arthroscopic surgery with more limited resection or even repair of meniscal tears is a recent trend that underscores the value of maintaining as much meniscal tissue as possible in an attempt to prevent subsequent deterioration of the articular cartilage and, eventually, osteoarthritis of the knee (see Chapter 39).

Meniscal Degeneration. Changes in the composition of the menisci of the knee have been observed with advancing age, although it is difficult to determine which changes are age-related alone and which occur as a consequence of other age-related phenomena such as osteoarthritis and CPPD crystal deposition disease. In association with osteoarthritis of the knee, the prevalence of horizontal cleavage lesions of the meniscus increases; in one study consisting of 100 random necropsy examinations, the prevalence of such lesions rose from 18.4 per cent in knees without evidence of osteoarthritis to 61.5 per cent in those with severe osteoarthritis.[662] In animal models in which osteoarthritis of the knee was created by ligamentous resection, profound changes in the menisci occur, characterized by initial evidence of small vertical and horizontal tears and by subsequent evidence of extensive disruption.[663] Significant alterations in water content, proteoglycans, and other matrix proteins in the menisci of the knee accompany naturally occurring or experimentally induced osteoarthritis (as well as rheumatoid arthritis).[651] Calcium HA crystal deposition, representing a dystrophic phenomenon, and CPPD crystal accumulation increase with advancing age, and either or both of these crystals can lead to an inflammatory response that, in turn, could evoke or activate proteases and catabolic factors, thus initiating or accelerating meniscal

degeneration.[651] Whatever their cause, degenerative changes in the menisci of the knee are common in middle-aged and elderly persons, especially those with osteoarthritis. Such degenerative changes may predispose to tears of the menisci, owing to a decrease in their elasticity.[662] Whether degenerative meniscal abnormalities are an essential prerequisite for meniscal tears, however, is not clear, as the histologic distinction between acute tears, progressive wear and tear, and degeneration of the meniscus may not be possible.[664]

Degenerative changes of the menisci may lead to imaging abnormalities that often are characteristic and, yet, that occasionally lead to diagnostic problems. On routine radiographs, gas may accumulate within the substance of a chronically fragmented and degenerative meniscus. The gas, representing nitrogen, leads to a thick, radiolucent shadow, often in a compartment of the knee that also reveals evidence of osteoarthritis (joint space narrowing and bone sclerosis). This type of vacuum should be differentiated from a thin, curvilinear collection of gas that may accumulate between the articular surfaces of the femur and the tibia. Gas within the meniscus is a sign of a pathologic process and is reminiscent of the vacuum phenomenon occurring in a degenerative intervertebral disc; gas within the knee joint itself is not a sign of a pathologic process but, rather, its detection generally eliminates the possibility of a large joint effusion. Both types of gas collection may be identified with CT. On MR images of the knee, however, intrameniscal or intra-articular gas produces a signal void that may simulate the appearance of a torn (or calcified) meniscus or other type of intra-articular abnormality[665] (Fig. 70–255).

Meniscal calcification related to calcium HA or CPPD crystal deposition may occur in association with meniscal degeneration. On routine radiographs, the correct diagnosis is made easily and, based upon the pattern and extent of the calcific deposits, a distinction between these two types of crystals often is possible. With MR imaging, however, the meniscal calcification may be overlooked completely, and its signal void may lead to obscuration of other meniscal findings (Fig. 70–256). With any imaging method, meniscal calcification should be differentiated from a discrete focus of ossification within the meniscus, the meniscal ossicle (see later discussion).

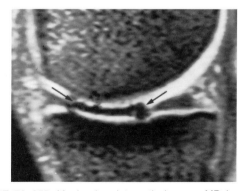

FIGURE 70–255. Meniscal or intra-articular gas: MR imaging. A signal void (arrows) related to gas in the knee joint, as demonstrated in this sagittal MPGR MR image (TR/TE, 500/11; flip angle, 30 degrees), may lead to diagnostic difficulty in the interpretation of meniscal integrity with MR imaging. (Courtesy of C. Hayes, M.D., Richmond, Virginia.)

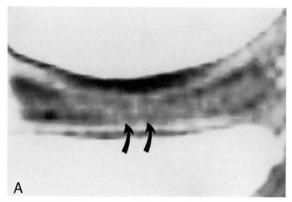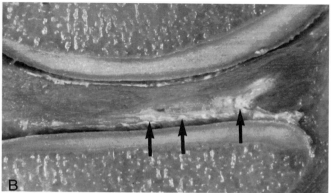

FIGURE 70–256. Meniscal calcification: MR imaging. A sagittal T1-weighted (TR/TE, 500/20) spin echo MR image photographed with meniscal windowing **(A)** reveals inhomogeneities in the signal intensity of the medial meniscus (arrows) that simulate those of a tear. A corresponding anatomic section **(B)** confirms the presence of calcium deposition (arrows) and the absence of a tear. (From Hodler J, et al: *Radiology 184:*221, 1992.)

The presence of mucinous and myxoid degeneration (and other forms of degeneration) in a variety of intra-articular structures, such as the rotator cuff and glenoid labrum of the shoulder and the triangular fibrocartilage complex of the wrist, has received considerable attention, owing to its effect on the signal intensity of those structures during the MR imaging examination. The menisci of the knee participate in these types of degeneration. Thus, in elderly patients, differentiation of clinically significant meniscal tears and clinically insignificant meniscal degeneration with MR imaging may become problematic. The diagnosis of a meniscal tear on the basis of MR imaging is related, in part, on the presence of characteristic changes in signal intensity (see later discussion), but similar changes in signal intensity also are observed with extensive meniscal degeneration (Fig. 70–257). Thus, although the exclusion of a tear of the meniscus in an older person may be accomplished reliably with MR imaging, the documentation of such a tear, as opposed to meniscal degeneration, may not be possible with this imaging method.[666]

Meniscal Tears. Although meniscal tears may be discovered incidentally, they may have a variety of clinical manifestations, foremost of which are knee pain and disability. The nerve supply to the meniscus is similar to the vascular supply, with the peripheral portion of the meniscus being innervated most richly.[667] In adults, invagination of the innervated synovium into the tear, particularly in cases of chronic tear, may generate pain.[662, 665] The pain may lead to a feeling of instability of the joint that often is reported by the patient. Further disability may result from displacement of portions of the torn meniscus, such as occurs with a bucket-handle meniscal tear, because the displaced fragment becomes lodged between the ipsilateral femoral condyle and tibial plateau. Associated injuries, which may include medial collateral and anterior cruciate ligament disruption, amplify the clinical manifestations of meniscal tears.

Pathogenesis. Two categories of meniscal tears commonly are identified: traumatic tears and degenerative tears. Traumatic tears are believed to result from excessive application of force to a normal meniscus. Degenerative tears are believed to result from normal forces acting on a degenerated structure.[659] The former usually are vertical tears that may propagate in a longitudinal or transverse direction and commonly involve the thin edge of the meniscus. Vertical transverse tears appear to be less common than vertical longitudinal tears and characteristically involve the middle third of the lateral meniscus.[659] Degenerative tears are horizontal cleavage lesions that typically occupy the posterior half of the menisci.[659]

In young persons, especially athletes, a single traumatic episode is responsible for the majority of meniscal lesions. The precise mechanisms leading to injury of the meniscus have been well summarized by Crues and Stoller.[669] Meniscal injuries frequently result from twisting strains applied to the knee when it is either slightly flexed or fully extended. In full extension, the stability of the knee joint is increased; therefore, meniscal tears resulting from injury during full extension often are accompanied by ligamentous injuries or fractures of the tibial plateau.[669, 1429] In some instances, the peripheral portion of the meniscus becomes detached from the joint capsule over a variable length. In either situation, displacement of a portion of the meniscus (in cases of meniscal tear) or of the entire meniscus (in cases of meniscal detachment) may occur during subsequent flexion or rotation of the joint.

Degenerative tears occur more commonly in older persons and in association with osteoarthritis of the knee. The degenerative changes in the meniscus include fibrillation, fibrochondrocyte necrosis and proliferation, and loss of normal staining properties of the matrix proteins. These alterations apparently make the meniscus more vulnerable to normal stress, and the cumulative effects of the stress eventually lead to loss of meniscal integrity.

The categorization of a meniscal tear as traumatic or degenerative generally is based on analysis of the clinical history, the age of the patient, and the gross morphology of the meniscus at the time of arthroscopy or open surgery. Imaging abnormalities, particularly those derived from arthrography or MR imaging, provide information regarding the type of meniscal tear. In some instances, however, it is not possible to separate degenerative and traumatic tears of the meniscus on the basis of clinical, imaging, and gross pathologic findings. Even microscopic analysis of the meniscal tissue may not allow such separation.

Classification. There is no uniformly accepted classification system for meniscal tears. Most classification systems emphasize the direction of the tear. Tears can be

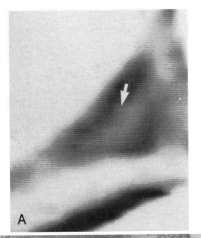

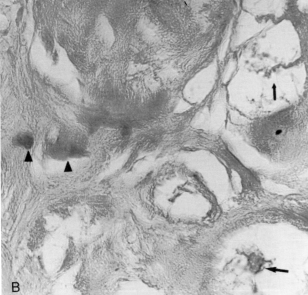

FIGURE 70–257. Meniscal degeneration: MR imaging. A sagittal T1-weighted (TR/TE, 500/20) spin echo MR image photographed with meniscal windowing **(A)** reveals increased signal intensity in the lateral meniscus (arrow), which corresponds to sites of mucoid (arrows) and eosinophilic (arrowheads) degeneration shown histologically (×100) **(B)**. (From Hodler J, et al: Radiology 184:221, 1992.)

the cleavage lesions common in older persons and in degenerated menisci. These tears may extend in a slightly oblique direction, exiting on the superior or inferior surface of the meniscus. Such tears involve either the medial or lateral

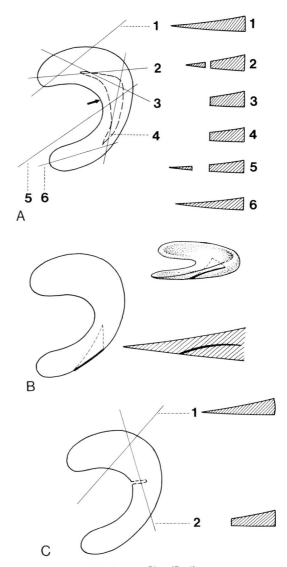

FIGURE 70–258. Meniscal tears: Classification.

A Longitudinal vertical tears (with displacement). The medial meniscus is viewed from above with the posterior horn located superiorly. The longitudinal vertical tear can be seen and the inner fragment is displaced centrally (arrow). The arthrographic appearance as well as the appearance in radial sections obtained with MR imaging will depend on the specific site of the tear. A view of the posterior aspect of the meniscus (1) will be normal. Slightly more anteriorly (2) a vertical tear will be apparent with minimal displacement of the fragment. At positions 3 and 4, an amputated meniscal shadow will be apparent. At position 5, significant displacement of the inner fragment will be observed. The anterior horn of the meniscus (6) will appear normal.

B Longitudinal horizontal tears. The medial meniscus is viewed from above (drawing on left), in front (drawing on top right), and in longitudinal section (drawing on bottom right). The extent and appearance of the tear can be appreciated.

C Radial tear. The medial meniscus is viewed from above, with its posterior horn located superiorly. A radial tear is evident on the inner contour of the meniscus. Some arthrographic views or MR imaging views (with radial sections) (1) will appear normal, whereas others passing through the tear (2) will reveal a blunted, contrast-coated inner meniscal shadow.

described as longitudinal, radial, vertical, or horizontal, and as complete, incomplete, or complex.[658] With most types of tears, the medial meniscus is involved more frequently than the lateral meniscus, and the posterior horn of the medial meniscus and the anterior horn of the lateral meniscus most commonly are affected.

Longitudinal tears are the most frequent type encountered. Such tears may occur in a vertical direction (Fig. 70–258A) dividing the meniscus into inner and outer segments, or in a horizontal direction (Fig. 70–258B), dividing the meniscus into an upper and lower segment, resembling a fish mouth.[658] Vertical longitudinal tears are more common in the medial meniscus than in the lateral meniscus (approximately 3 to 1), and they may involve the peripheral or central portion of the meniscus. They vary in length, being isolated to the posterior horn, midportion, anterior horn, or various combinations of these. When a large part of the meniscus is affected, the inner fragment may be displaced into the central part of the joint, a phenomenon termed a bucket-handle tear. Horizontal longitudinal tears represent meniscus, or both menisci, and they may be accompanied by a meniscal cyst (see later discussion).

A radial tear is a special type of vertical tear that involves the inner margin of the meniscus (Fig. 70–258C). This tear is most frequent in the middle third of the lateral meniscus and, in either meniscus, may extend outwardly for a variable distance in any direction. Such tears sometimes are referred to as parrot beak or flap tears and, when extensive, may divide the meniscus into an anterior and posterior portion.

Although it is optimal to be able to differentiate among these various types of tears on the basis of imaging abnormalities, this commonly is not possible. Many tears are complex in nature, demonstrating features of more than one type of lesion. More significant from an imaging standpoint is the accurate diagnosis of a tear, its proper localization to the medial or lateral meniscus, or both menisci, and documentation of displacement of any meniscal fragments. Differentiation between traumatic and degenerative tears also is not possible on many occasions. Acute traumatic tears in young persons often lead to rounded and smooth margins, and chronic degenerative tears in older persons commonly are associated with frayed, fibrillated, and irregular margins.[658] The localization of a tear to the peripheral portion of the meniscus has therapeutic importance, owing to the possibility of spontaneous healing of this tear (see later discussion). Tears in this region may appear hemorrhagic on gross inspection, an appearance related to the prominent vascular supply to the peripheral portion of the meniscus.

Clinical Abnormalities. The clinical diagnosis of a meniscal tear relies upon careful questioning of the patient and physical examination. A history of pain and a slowly developing joint effusion are helpful clues, but neither finding is diagnostic of a meniscal tear. In cases of a bucket-handle tear of the meniscus, locking of the knee may be reported by the patient, but this, too, is not a pathognomonic finding. Pain and tenderness on palpation of the meniscal margin near the site of tear may be elicited. A positive McMurray test, characterized by an audible snap or pop as an abnormal meniscus extends over a bone protuberance, lends support to the clinical diagnosis of a meniscal tear, but a negative McMurray test does not eliminate the possibility of such a tear.[669]

The reported accuracy in diagnosis of meniscal tears based on results of analysis of the patient's history and physical examination has varied.[670, 671] This accuracy appears to be greater in cases of a medial meniscus tear than in those of a lateral meniscus tear. A diagnostic accuracy of approximately 90 per cent with regard to tears of the medial meniscus and of approximately 70 per cent with regard to tears of the lateral meniscus may be possible when experienced orthopedic surgeons are assessing the knee. In the hands of less experienced physicians, however, a far lower diagnostic accuracy usually is apparent and, independent of the level of experience of the examiner, determination of the precise location, type, and extent of the tear usually is not possible on the basis of the clinical history and physical examination.[669] An interest in the value of imaging studies in the assessment of menisci, therefore, is understandable.

Ultrasonographic Abnormalities. Despite recent interest in the application of ultrasonography to the detection of meniscal tears,[672–674] the technique rarely is employed for this purpose. In one cadaveric study,[672] ultrasonography proved useful in demonstrating even small meniscal tears, and the type of tear could be assessed in some cases. In general, however, it is difficult to study the entire meniscus with ultrasonography, and the results are very dependent upon the experience of the examiner. Although the use of an intra-articular transducer is an interesting extension of sonographic technique,[673] this method requires a skin incision and, therefore, is invasive.

Scintigraphic Abnormalities. Bone scintigraphy has been employed in a limited fashion for the diagnosis of meniscal tears.[675, 676] Even when combined with SPECT, bone scintigraphy is, at best, a moderately sensitive method, and it lacks specificity.

CT Abnormalities. The use of standard CT (i.e., without the introduction of intra-articular contrast material) in the assessment of the menisci of the knee has been studied.[677–682] The reported sensitivity of CT has varied from 63 to 96 per cent, the reported specificity from 81 to 93 per cent, and the reported accuracy from 84 to 91 per cent.[678, 680] In one study, CT was found to be more efficacious than MR imaging (performed with a 0.5 Tesla magnet) in meniscal evaluation,[679] and in another study, CT was found accurate in the diagnosis of a bucket-handle tear of the meniscus (using arthroscopy as the standard) in 49 of 53 patients (92.5 per cent).[681] This method requires thin (2 or 3 mm) contiguous or overlapping transaxial images and angulation of the gantry so that the sections are parallel to the tibial plateau. Diagnostic difficulty arises in cases in which a nondisplaced horizontal tear of the meniscus is oriented parallel to the transaxial imaging plane. When compared with arthrography, CT of the meniscus is noninvasive, can be used to assess both knees, and is not a physician-intensive examination (as the study can be performed within 20 to 25 min by experienced technologists). Disadvantages of the CT examination, when compared with arthrography, are its higher cost, degradation of the images owing to patient movement, poor visualization of the menisci as a result of a hemarthrosis, difficulty in imaging horizontal tears of the meniscus and meniscocapsular separations, and findings related to meniscal degeneration that simulate those of a meniscal tear.[682] Furthermore, modern MR imaging allows more detailed analysis of the knee menisci and other intra-articular and periarticular structures, albeit at a slightly higher cost.

Arthrographic Abnormalities. The use of arthrography in the evaluation of the menisci of the knee is discussed and illustrated in Chapter 13, and only a summary is provided here.

With regard to the normal arthrographic appearance of the menisci, the medial meniscus is identified as a sharply defined, soft tissue triangular shadow (Fig. 70–259). Its posterior horn usually is large, averaging 14 mm in width.[683] Its midportion is somewhat smaller, whereas the anterior horn usually is the smallest portion of the medial meniscus, averaging 6 mm in width.[683] Occasionally, the anterior horn may be larger than the midportion of the medial meniscus. The peripheral surface of the medial meniscus is firmly attached to the medial collateral ligament. Certain normal recesses about the medial meniscus produce focal pouchlike collections of air and contrast material.[684, 685] A superior recess frequently is present above the posterior horn of the medial meniscus. A posterior inferior

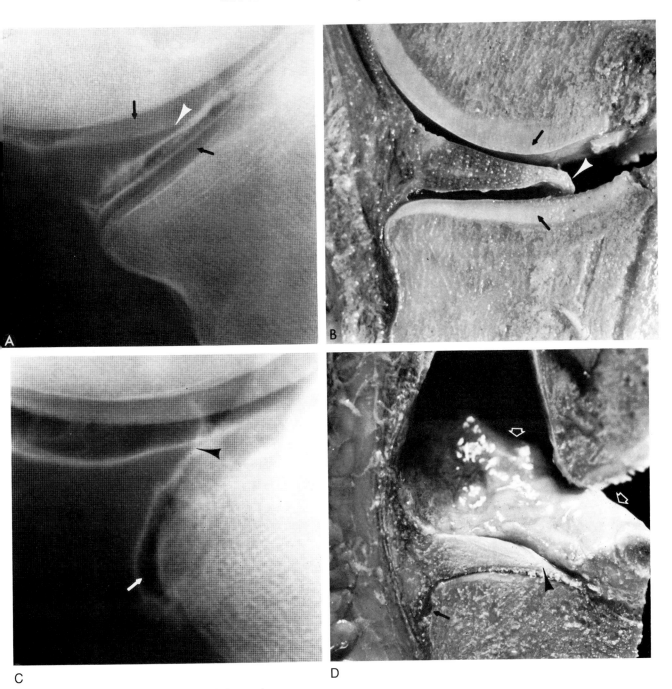

FIGURE 70–259. Normal medial meniscus: Arthrography.
   A, B Posterior horn of the medial meniscus. This segment is relatively large, extending for a considerable distance into the articular cavity (arrowheads). The adjacent articular recesses are small. The articular cartilage (arrows) is smooth.
   C, D Anterior horn of the medial meniscus. The size of this segment is variable (arrowheads). Note the fat pad that overlies the meniscus (open arrows). An inferior recess is visualized (solid arrows).

recess is less common, although the presence of such a recess beneath the anterior horn of the medial meniscus is more frequent. These inferior recesses beneath the medial meniscus generally are small, and some regard recesses that are greater than 2 mm in size as abnormal.[686] The anterior part of the medial meniscus is covered with the base of the infrapatellar fat pad, making evaluation of this region more difficult.

   The lateral meniscus normally is more circular in configuration than the medial meniscus. It too is projected as a sharply defined triangular radiodense area surrounded by air and contrast material (Fig. 70–260). It changes little in size from its anterior to its posterior horn, averaging 10 mm in width.[687] Inferior recesses are frequent beneath both the anterior and the posterior horns of the lateral meniscus. The anterior horn is attached to the lateral ligament, but the posterior horn of the lateral meniscus is separated from this ligament by the synovial sheath of the popliteus tendon. This sheath fills with air and contrast material and overlies the peripheral portion of the posterior horn of the lateral meniscus, producing variable arthrographic findings.[685, 688–691] Two delicate bands of connective tissue,

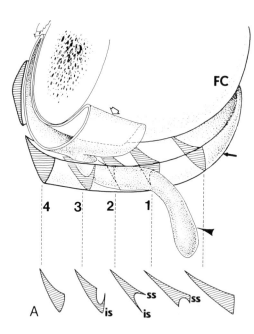

A

FIGURE 70–260. Normal lateral meniscus: Arthrography.

A Diagrammatic representation of the posterolateral aspect of the knee joint demonstrates relationships of the lateral meniscus (solid arrow) and popliteus tendon sheath (arrowhead). The most posterior aspect of the femoral condyle (FC) and synovial reflection (open arrow) are indicated. The popliteus muscle originates posteriorly and inferiorly on the tibia and extends obliquely, anteriorly, and superiorly to insert on the lateral aspect of the femur. The popliteus tendon enters the joint close to the posterior and lateral aspects of the meniscus and passes through an oblique tunnel. Anteroinferior and posterosuperior to the intra-articular portion of the popliteus tendon are recesses, which fill with contrast medium during arthrography. Two bands of connective tissue, termed struts or fascicles, connect the posterior horn of the lateral meniscus to the joint capsule around the popliteal tendon sheath. Classically, (1) the more posterior aspect of the lateral meniscus will reveal an intact superior strut (ss); (2) a slightly more anterior section will reveal both superior strut (ss) and inferior strut (is); (3) a more anterior section will reveal only an inferior strut (is); and (4) a still further anterior section (midportion of the lateral meniscus) will depict an intact meniscus with no visible popliteal tendon sheath.

B, C Posterior aspect of the lateral meniscus (section 2). In this arthrogram and longitudinal section, observe the popliteus tendon sheath (arrowheads), lateral meniscus (arrows), superior strut (ss), and inferior strut (is). The latter strut has been disrupted in the preparation of this section.

D, E Anterior horn of the lateral meniscus. In this arthrogram and longitudinal section, the meniscus (solid arrows) is well shown. Observe the articular cartilage (arrowheads) and prominent recesses (open arrows).

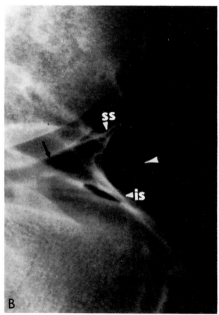

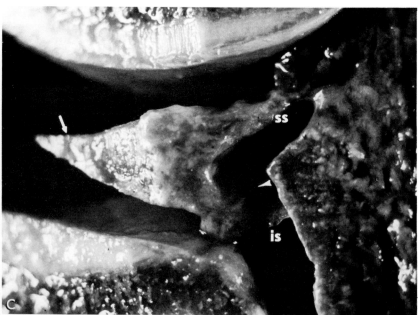

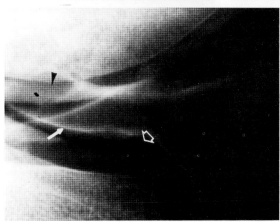

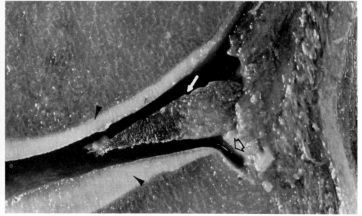

D

E

termed struts or fascicles, connect the posterior horn of the lateral meniscus to the joint capsule around the popliteal tendon sheath. In any one view of this portion of the lateral meniscus, two struts may be observed with the intervening sheath, one strut may be apparent in conjunction with the sheath, or the sheath may be observed without visualization of either strut. Classically, however, arthrography of the most posterior aspect of the lateral meniscus will reveal an intact superior strut; a slightly more anterior view will reveal both struts; and a more anterior projection will reveal an inferior strut. The variability in appearance of the fascicles or struts of the lateral meniscus combined with the presence of an overlying air-filled tendon sheath makes difficult the evaluation of the posterior horn of the lateral meniscus. Narrowing, compression, or absence of the popliteus tendon sheath, however, may indicate tears of the lateral meniscus, discoid menisci, adhesive capsulitis, prior surgery, or a rare congenital abnormality.[692]

Arthrography remains a highly accurate technique for the evaluation of a number of meniscal abnormalities, including tears. The arthrographic appearance of meniscal tears in both adults[693–697] and children[698–700] has been well described. A classification of types of meniscal tears has been used,[693] although specification of a particular type of tear during arthrography often is impossible and, even when possible, may have little clinical significance. The location of the tear in one aspect of the meniscus is of greater significance. In cases of vertical longitudinal (concentric) tears, a vertical radiodense line extending through the meniscus will be observed (Fig. 70–261). The inner fragment may be displaced producing a bucket-handle tear, and may lodge in the central portion of the articulation, where it may or may not be identified during arthrography.[701] A vertical tear along the inner contour of the meniscus (radial tear) will produce a contrast-coated inner meniscal margin and a blunted meniscal shadow (Fig. 70–262). With a horizontal meniscal tear, a radiopaque line of contrast material is apparent overlying the meniscal shadow, extending to the superior or inferior surface (Fig. 70–263). The meniscus may lose its wedge-shaped configuration.

MR Imaging: Historical Review and Perspective. Many of the early descriptions of MR imaging of the knee represented general overviews of the subject. Later, the investigations became more focused, examining various pathologic conditions (e.g., meniscal tears, cruciate ligament disruptions, patellofemoral disorders). Although it is impossible to do justice to all of the investigations that have dealt with MR imaging of the knee, a brief review is required.

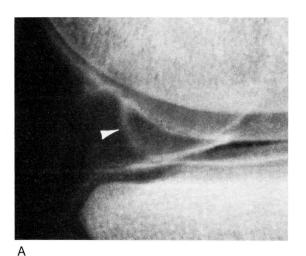

A

FIGURE 70–261. Vertical longitudinal (concentric) meniscal tears: Arthrography. Two examples are shown. In **A**, contrast material coats the tear (arrowhead) in the medial meniscus. In **B**, the tear (arrow) of the medial meniscus is associated with central displacement (arrowhead) of its inner portion.

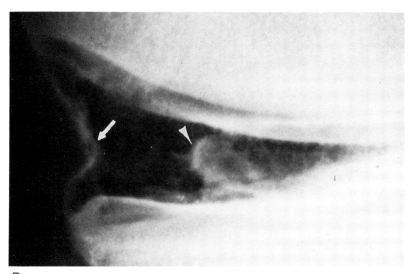

B

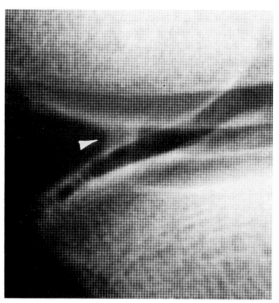

FIGURE 70–262. Vertical radial meniscal tears: Arthrography. Note the radial tear (arrowhead) of the medial meniscus.

The reports in 1983 by Kean and coworkers[702] and Moon and associates,[703] and in 1984 by Li and collaborators[704] were the first to describe the potential of MR imaging in assessing the knee. Although primitive by today's standards, they served as a stimulus for subsequent investigation. In 1985, Reicher and coworkers[705, 706] provided further evidence of this potential, using close imaging-pathologic correlation in cadaveric knees and imaging-arthroscopic correlation in knees of symptomatic patients. The foundation now in place and the potential clearly in sight, the deluge of investigations dealing with MR imaging of the knee began.[707–731] MR imaging was touted early on as a noninvasive diagnostic method that could compete favorably with standard arthrography in the analysis of knee disorders; subsequently, MR imaging became regarded as superior to standard arthrography and as a substitute for or, at the very least, a complement to diagnostic arthroscopy of the knee. With technical advances in the field, MR images of the knee became sharper and the findings more definite. Three-dimensional gradient echo imaging,[732, 733] reformatted or reconstructed multiplanar images,[734] and innovative and

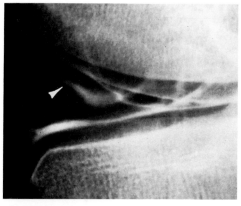

FIGURE 70–263. Horizontal meniscal tears: Arthrography. Note the tear (arrowhead), which is filled with contrast material.

faster MR imaging methods[735] for assessing the knee all were given attention. Furthermore, as many of the MR imaging abnormalities were seen more easily in the presence of a knee effusion, the added benefit of using intra-articular administration of gadolinium was studied. The work of Hajek and coworkers[736, 737] in 1987 gave birth to the concept of gadolinium-enhanced MR arthrography of the knee (and other joints), and the technique remains popular in certain parts of the United States and Europe.[738] MR arthrography, however, is time-consuming and invasive, and it may require access to a fluoroscopic room for injection of contrast material. Furthermore, it sometimes is regarded not as a supplement to standard MR imaging but as a step backward toward conventional arthrography, from which the excitement of MR imaging first took hold.

That MR imaging has invaded the territory once held firm by conventional arthrography is certain. In many institutions in which MR imaging is available, knee arthrography rarely is employed, being reserved for patients who are claustrophobic, who have certain types of metallic implants in whom MR imaging is contraindicated, and who are too large to be placed on the MR imaging table. Is MR imaging needed as a supplement to clinical assessment in an age in which diagnostic and therapeutic arthroscopy is being used increasingly? There are no easy answers to this question. Boden and associates,[739] in an analysis of the financial impact of the diagnostic methods used to evaluate the acutely injured knee, concluded that arthroscopy is more cost-effective than MR imaging if 78 per cent or more of the scanned patients eventually undergo arthroscopy. Ruwe and collaborators,[740] in another study addressing the issue of cost-effectiveness, indicated that the results of MR imaging of the knee in 53 of 103 patients avoided a potentially unnecessary diagnostic arthroscopy, resulting in a net savings of $103,700. As might be expected, the first of these two investigations was accomplished by orthopedic surgeons and published in a journal devoted to arthroscopy, and the second, although resulting from the combined efforts of both orthopedic surgeons and radiologists, was published in a diagnostic radiology journal. Spiers and coworkers,[741] in a study of 58 patients with suspected internal derangements of the knee, indicated the advantages and disadvantages of MR imaging, with the conclusion that MR imaging studies on all patients scheduled for knee arthroscopy would lead to a modest increase in the cost of treatment but one that represented "a small price to pay for a reduction in the morbidity associated with arthroscopy, and the liberation of theatres and surgeons for other work." Noble[742] emphasized the need to avoid unnecessary arthroscopy, indicating that the results of MR imaging of the knee in some patients augment the clinical judgment, "leaving the arthroscope to bring about a practical solution for the patient's demonstrable (and verified) problem."

Few would argue that a diagnostic test, such as MR imaging, is not indicated if the treatment will not be affected by the result, no matter what that result might be.[743] Identification of the correct therapeutic method, however, requires the attention of a highly skilled and often specialized orthopedic surgeon. Such a physician is expected to be able to determine whether or not the results of an MR imaging examination of the knee will affect treatment of the patient. With less skilled physicians, this type of determination may not be possible, and MR imaging may represent an effective means of identifying the problem and, thereby, influencing the decision as to the appropriateness of surgical intervention. Proper interpretation of MR images requires the attention of a highly skilled and often specialized radiologist. Furthermore, owing to the occurrence of positive findings on MR images of the knee in asymptomatic persons,[744] the results of the MR imaging examination must be correlated with those derived from careful clinical assessment and other imaging methods.

MR Imaging: Technical Considerations. Spin echo MR imaging remains the most commonly employed method for assessing disorders of the knee, including those of the menisci. Typically, sagittal and coronal MR images are obtained (Fig. 70–264), the sagittal images often being acquired in the plane of the anterior cruciate ligament (see later discussion). Transaxial MR images also are used, although they have limited value in the diagnosis of meniscal tears. The transaxial images may be acquired with either spin echo or gradient echo methods (Fig. 70–264). There is no uniform agreement regarding the type of spin echo sequences that should be obtained in the coronal and sagittal planes. Typically, in one of these (usually the sagittal plane), proton density and T2-weighted spin echo MR images are acquired, and in the other (usually the coronal

plane), T1-weighted spin echo MR images are obtained. The value of coronal T2-weighted spin echo MR images in the evaluation of the collateral ligaments of the knee is addressed later in this chapter.

The sagittal plane is regarded as most important in assessment of the menisci. Although the menisci also are visualized in the coronal plane, supportive rather than new data regarding the integrity of the menisci usually are derived from the coronal MR images.[1397] In cases of discoid menisci or meniscal cysts, MR images in the coronal plane may provide additional information.[745] High contrast, narrow window width MR images (meniscal windowing) in both the coronal and sagittal planes frequently are employed. These images may be useful in determining the nature and extent of regions of intermediate signal intensity within the menisci, although their usefulness is not agreed upon.[746] In both the coronal and sagittal planes, moderately thin slices (approximately 3 or 4 mm) obtained in a contiguous fashion or with a small interslice gap (approximately 1 mm) are sufficient.

In recent years, two-dimensional fast spin echo sequences, which allow more rapid aquisition of image data, especially for T2-weighted images, than standard spin echo sequences, have been used in many institutions as the pri-

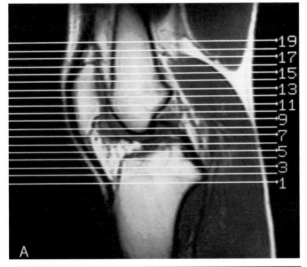

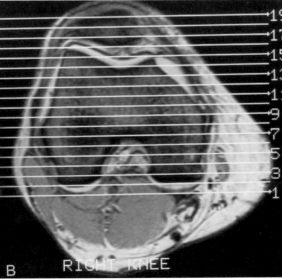

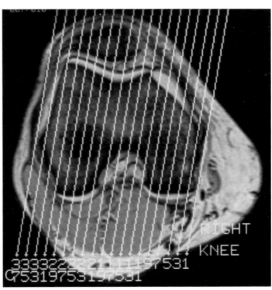

FIGURE 70–264. MR imaging of the knee: Technical considerations. Three MR imaging planes usually are used to evaluate the knee: sagittal (oblique), coronal, and transaxial planes. Various methods may be used to provide the MR images in these three planes. One method is illustrated here. From a sagittal T1-weighted (TR/TE, 400/12) spin echo localizer image **(A)**, transaxial MR images may be programmed. The transaxial images may consist of multiplanar gradient recalled (MPGR) images (TR/TE, 450/15; flip angle, 60 degrees) from which the coronal **(B)** and sagittal oblique **(C)** MR images may be programmed. The sagittal oblique MR images are oriented in an anteromedial to posterolateral direction in order to allow better visualization of the anterior cruciate ligament.

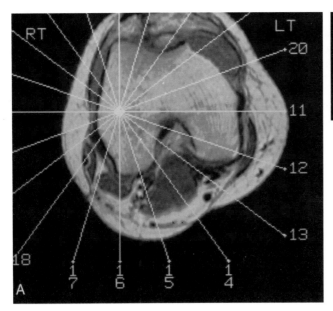

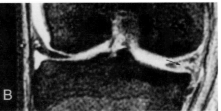

FIGURE 70–265. MR imaging of the knee: Technical considerations. Radial imaging of the menisci. From data supplied from transaxial MR images, radial sections of the menisci (A) can be programmed, which provide an arthrogram-like analysis of the menisci, as shown in a MPGR MR image (TR/TE, 400/12; flip angle, 15 degrees) (B). In this patient, a tear of the medial meniscus (arrow) is present.

mary MR imaging method for the assessment of the menisci (and other structures) in the knee. Although image contrast with this technique is similar to that of standard spin echo images, subtle differences exist (see Chapter 9), including some blurring of normally sharp anatomic margins in the fast spin echo proton density images. In one study, such blurring (as well as other factors) led to decreased sensitivity of fast spin echo sequences (with conventional spin echo sequences used as the gold standard) in the detection of meniscal tears of the knee.[1398]

Gradient recalled MR images also have been used to assess the menisci of the knee. In general, the information displayed is similar to that obtained with spin echo images. Radial imaging can be coupled with gradient recalled MR sequences, providing cross-sectional images perpendicular to the long axis of the meniscus (Fig. 70–265). Radial imaging is best accomplished by programming separately appropriate imaging planes for the medial meniscus and for the lateral meniscus.[745] In one study,[747] the simultaneous analysis of sagittal spin echo MR images and multiplanar gradient recalled (MPGR) radial images led to a slight improvement in sensitivity and specificity in the diagnosis of meniscal tears. Radial MR images increase the conspicuity of meniscal tears but at the expense of anatomic detail.[747] One further problem that arises with radial imaging of the knee is the presence of a signal void in the center of the images, representing the location of the axis of rotation.[745]

Three-dimensional Fourier transformation (3DFT) gradient echo MR imaging of the knee also has been employed in the assessment of the menisci (and other intra-articular structures).[720, 723, 732, 733, 748–750] The advantages of this technique relate to the rapid acquisition of extremely thin (approximately 1 mm) contiguous slices of the knee. Reported data indicate high accuracy in the detection of meniscal tears, although the assessment of the cruciate ligaments and the bone marrow may be less accurate than with standard spin echo images. With three-dimensional MR imaging, meniscal tears may be delineated in the transaxial plane[749, 750] (Fig. 70–266), in addition to the standard coronal and sagittal planes. Furthermore, imaging data acquired

in one plane may be reconstructed in another, and three-dimensional reformatting procedures allow creation of images with apparent depth that then can be rotated in any direction.[745]

MR arthrography has a limited role in the evaluation of the menisci of the knee, although this role may be expanded in instances of persistent or recurrent clinical manifestations following meniscectomy or meniscal repair (see later discussion). Occasionally, when the extent of increased signal intensity within the meniscus is not clear, and specifically, when it is not certain if the altered signal intensity extends to the surface of the meniscus, MR arthrography using gadolinium compounds (or saline) may prove useful (Fig. 70–267). The accumulation of contrast agent within the meniscus is strong evidence that a tear is present, a finding that may be accentuated when fat suppression MR imaging methods also are used.

MR Imaging: Normal Menisci. Two aspects of the MR imaging appearance of the normal meniscus relate to their morphology and their internal signal intensity.

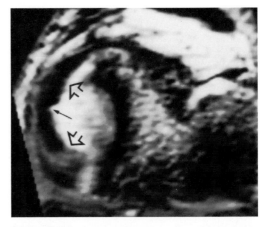

FIGURE 70–266. MR imaging of the knee: Technical considerations. Three-dimensional Fourier transform (3DFT) GRASS MR image (TR/TE, 34/15; flip angle, 60 degrees) of the menisci. In this example, a radial tear (solid arrow) of the medial meniscus (open arrows) is evident. (Courtesy of S. Eilenberg, M.D., San Diego, California.)

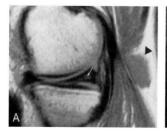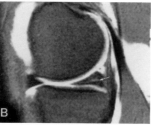

FIGURE 70–267. MR imaging of the knee: Technical considerations. MR arthrography of the menisci. An initial sagittal proton density–weighted (TR/TE, 2200/20) spin echo MR image **(A)** shows altered signal intensity (arrow) in the posterior horn of the medial meniscus. It is not certain if the region of altered signal intensity extends to the inferior surface of the meniscus. A posterior synovial cyst (arrowhead) also is evident. A sagittal T1-weighted (TR/TE, 650/20) spin echo MR image obtained with chemical presaturation of fat (ChemSat) and after the intra-articular administration of a gadolinium compound **(B)** shows fluid of high signal intensity in the joint and in the synovial cyst, but there is no increase in the signal intensity in the meniscus (arrow). The findings suggest that a meniscal tear is not present.

As with arthrography, the normal morphology of the meniscus is characterized by a triangular appearance and a sharp central tip.[731, 1351] This appearance is apparent in both coronal and sagittal planes (Fig. 70–268). In the sagittal plane, in peripheral sections, the anterior and posterior horns of the menisci unite, forming a structure that is shaped like a bow-tie.[712] In central sections, the menisci normally have a rhomboid shape. In the coronal plane, far posterior sections show the menisci as broad and elongated structures extending far into the central portion of the joint. The medial (tibial) collateral ligament is seen adjacent to the midportion of the medial meniscus, with an interface apparent between it and the outer portion of the meniscus. In both the sagittal and coronal images, the course of the popliteus tendon and its sheath and their intimacy with the posterior horn of the lateral meniscus are evident.

Although classic morphologic changes (e.g., blunting of the tip of the meniscus, displacement of a portion of the meniscus, an interrupted appearance of the meniscus, and an abnormality in the size of a segment of the meniscus) occur in the presence of a meniscal tear, there are normal variations in the morphology of the menisci that can lead to diagnostic difficulty. Some of these variations relate to normal anatomic structures, physiologic changes in the

shape of the meniscus, and artifacts of the MR imaging examination itself. The normal anatomic structures that may simulate the appearance of a meniscal tear include the following:

1. *Transverse ligament of the knee.* The transverse ligament of the knee extends between the convex portions of the anterior horns of the medial and lateral menisci. Its size is variable, and it may be absent in some persons. This ligament usually is identified on sagittal MR images of the knee and, occasionally, on coronal images as well. Its course can be traced on sequential sagittal MR images of the central portion of the knee (Fig. 70–269). As it separates from the menisci, particularly the medial meniscus, the space between it and the meniscus may be misinterpreted as evidence of a meniscal tear.

2. *Lateral inferior genicular artery.* The lateral inferior genicular artery is closely applied to the anterior portion of the lateral meniscus.[721] The space between this vessel and the meniscus may be misinterpreted as evidence of a meniscal tear.

3. *Popliteus tendon.* The popliteus tendon and its synovial sheath course between the posterior horn of the lateral meniscus and the joint capsule. An area of intermediate signal intensity between the posterior horn of the lateral meniscus and the popliteus tendon on sagittal MR images may be misinterpreted as evidence of a tear (Fig. 70–269). This area extends in an oblique fashion from posterior above to anterior below and differs in orientation from the usual tear of the posterior horn of the lateral meniscus.

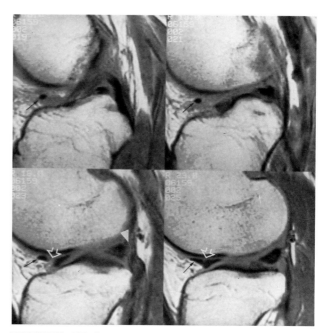

FIGURE 70–269. Pseudotears of the menisci: Transverse ligament of the knee and popliteus tendon. Four sagittal proton density–weighted (TR/TE, 2000/20) spin echo MR images show the course of the transverse ligament of the knee (solid arrows) from its most central position (top left) to its most lateral position (bottom right). As it approaches the anterior horn of the lateral meniscus, a space of intermediate signal intensity (open arrows) between it and the meniscus may be misinterpreted as evidence of a meniscal tear. Posteriorly, the popliteus tendon (arrowhead) separates the posterior horn of the lateral meniscus and the joint capsule. This region also may be misinterpreted as evidence of a meniscal tear.

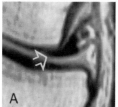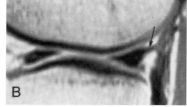

FIGURE 70–268. Normal lateral meniscus of the knee: MR imaging.
A In a coronal proton density–weighted (TR/TE, 2000/20) spin echo MR image, note the normal appearance of the lateral meniscus (open arrow). It is of uniform low signal intensity.

B A sagittal proton density–weighted (TR/TE, 2000/30) spin echo MR image reveals the anterior and posterior horns of the lateral meniscus. The lateral meniscus is of low signal intensity and its morphology is normal. Note the superior fascicle (arrow) of the lateral meniscus.

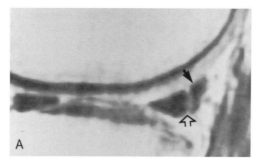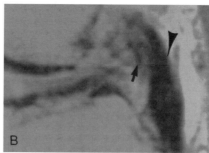

FIGURE 70–270. Pseudotears of the menisci: Anterior meniscofemoral ligament (ligament of Humphrey). Two sagittal proton density–weighted (TR/TE, 2300/30) spin echo MR images photographed with meniscal windowing reveal the course of the anterior meniscofemoral ligament. In **A**, the more lateral image, note the ligament (solid arrow) adjacent to the posterior horn of the lateral meniscus with a space (arrowhead) between them that may be misinterpreted as evidence of a meniscal tear. In **B**, a central image, the anterior meniscofemoral ligament (solid arrow) is located anterior to the posterior cruciate ligament (arrowhead).

4. *Meniscofemoral ligaments.* The meniscofemoral ligaments extend from the posterior horn of the lateral meniscus to the medial condyle of the femur. The anterior branch, or ligament of Humphrey, is directed in an oblique craniomedial orientation, anterior to the posterior cruciate ligament; the posterior branch, or ligament of Wrisberg, has a similar orientation but passes posterior to the posterior cruciate ligament.[751] The relatively high signal intensity related to the loose connective tissue between either one of these ligaments and the most medial part of the posterior horn of the lateral meniscus may be misinterpreted as evidence of a meniscal tear.[751–753] As in most cases of meniscal pseudotears, analysis of sequential MR images allows proper interpretation (Fig. 70–270).

5. *Capsular attachment.* The junctional region between the posterior portion of the medial meniscus and the joint capsule contains peripheral vessels whose signal intensity leads to tissue inhomogeneity that can simulate the appearance of a meniscocapsular detachment.[752] Less conspicuity of this region of increased signal intensity on gradient echo MR images may be useful in differentiating the normal situation from such detachment.[752]

6. *Bursa of the medial collateral ligament.* The bursa of the medial collateral ligament is present in more than 90 per cent of cadaveric knees.[444] This bursa separates the peripheral region of the midportion of the medial meniscus and the medial collateral ligament. Fluid collections accompanying bursitis lead to increased signal intensity in this junctional region that simulates the appearance of meniscocapsular separation.[754]

Physiologic changes in the shape of the meniscus may be observed during the MR imaging examination, and the resulting appearance may simulate those of a meniscal tear. The medial meniscal flounce is one example of these changes.[755] The flounce, which is observed regularly during knee arthrography, relates to traction on the peripheral portion of the medial meniscus that occurs during tibial rotation, leading to waviness or folding of the inner edge of the medial meniscus. A similar phenomenon occurs during MR imaging in the presence of a joint effusion and joint laxity (related to ligamentous injury), when the tibia is rotated for positioning within the magnet.[755] The resulting appearance during the MR imaging examination may resemble that of a meniscal tear.[756]

Certain artifacts produced during the MR imaging examination may lead to findings that simulate those of a meniscal tear.

1. *Volume averaging.* As indicated previously, problems in interpretation of meniscal integrity are encountered at the site of attachment of the meniscus to the capsule. A concavity filled with periarticular fat and neurovascular structures exists in this junctional region.[721, 752] Sagittal images through the periphery of the meniscus often demonstrate a linear artifact of high signal intensity within the normal meniscus (of low signal intensity) due to volume averaging of these junctional tissues and the meniscus. A similar appearance sometimes is seen in the most posterior coronal MR images of the menisci (Fig. 70–271).

2. *Truncation artifact.* Truncation artifacts result from the use of Fourier transform methods to construct MR images of high contrast boundaries, such as between the articular cartilage and the meniscus.[757] Truncation artifacts appear as a series of high and low signal intensity lines, adjacent and parallel to these boundaries. Such a line of high signal intensity within the low signal intensity of the meniscus may simulate the appearance of a meniscal tear. In the knee, truncation artifacts affecting the meniscus have been reported to be most prominent when the acquisition matrix is 128 × 256 and the 128-pixel (phase-encoded) axis is in a superoinferior orientation; acquisition of images using a 192 × 256 or 256 × 256 matrix or with antero-

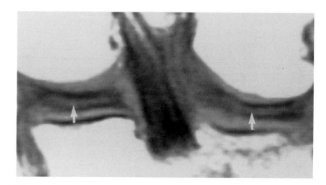

FIGURE 70–271. Pseudotears of the menisci: Volume averaging. Linear regions of intermediate signal intensity (arrows) normally may be evident at the peripheral portions of the medial and lateral menisci. Here they are seen in the posterior portions of both menisci in a coronal T1-weighted (TR/TE, 650/20) spin echo MR image photographed with meniscal windowing.

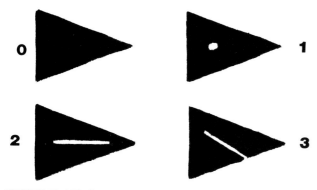

FIGURE 70–272. Grades of intrameniscal signal intensity. The meniscus may appear of uniform low signal intensity (grade 0); it may contain one or several circular foci of intermediate signal intensity (grade 1), or a linear region of intermediate signal intensity that does not extend to an articular surface (grade 2); or it may reveal linear or irregular regions of intermediate signal intensity that extend to the articular surface (grade 3).

posterior orientation of the 128-pixel axis results in a diminution of these artifacts.[757] Truncation artifacts within the meniscus may be accentuated when meniscal windowing is used, and they may be accompanied by similar artifacts within the subchondral bone plate of the tibia. When superimposed on the meniscus, truncation artifacts tend to be subtle, uniform in thickness, and parallel to the surfaces of the menisci, approximately 2 pixels distant from the articular cartilage.[757] They may extend beyond the boundaries of the meniscus.

The second aspect of the MR imaging characteristics of the normal meniscus relates to its internal signal intensity. Although the menisci commonly are described as structures of uniformly low signal intensity, this description is misleading and not accurate. Regions of intermediate signal intensity commonly are encountered within the menisci of asymptomatic persons, and misinterpretation of these regions as tears has led to unnecessary arthroscopy during which the grossly normal appearance of the meniscus has been documented.

In 1987, Stoller and colleagues[717] provided the first full description of the inhomogeneous signal intensity that may be seen in normal menisci. In a cadaver study using close MR imaging–histologic correlation, they developed a grading system based upon the appearance and extent of the areas of higher intrameniscal signal intensity that, with minor modifications, is used today. This grading system recognized three patterns of intrameniscal signal (Fig. 70–272):

Grade 1: One or several punctate regions of intermediate signal intensity not contiguous with an articular surface of the meniscus (the capsular margin of the meniscus is not considered an articular surface).

Grade 2: Linear regions of intermediate signal intensity without extension to the articular surface of the meniscus.

Grade 3: Regions of intermediate signal intensity with extension to an articular surface of the meniscus.

Correlation of the grades of intrameniscal signal intensity and histologic findings confirmed increasing amounts of degenerative changes within those menisci with grades 1 and 2 imaging findings, and evidence of fibrocartilaginous

tears in those menisci with grade 3 imaging findings.[717] The primary pattern of degenerative alteration was mucinous change, appearing as discrete foci in menisci with grade 1 signal intensity and as linear bands in menisci with grade 2 signal intensity. In menisci with grade 3 signal intensity, degenerative alterations were accompanied by distinct cleavage planes with or without macroscopically evident extension to the articular surface of the meniscus.

The occurrence of mucinous and myxoid changes within the meniscus as a consequence of aging is well documented.[666, 758] Thus, intrameniscal regions of intermediate signal intensity detected on MR images of the knee may progress with advancing age of the patient, leading to diagnostic difficulty in the interpretation and clinical significance of grade 3 signal intensity in middle-aged and elderly persons.[666] The appearance of extensive regions of intermediate signal intensity within the menisci of asymptomatic persons in the fourth, fifth, and sixth decades of life and beyond is well recognized. These degenerative abnormalities may predispose the meniscus to structural failure. In one study, patients with documented meniscal tears had evidence of a more advanced degree of meniscal degeneration in the opposite, asymptomatic knee when compared with an age-matched normal control population or patients with nonmeniscal knee disorders.[758] Degenerative changes predominate in the posterior segment of the medial meniscus, the most common site of meniscal tear.

Despite the diagnostic problems encountered caused by age-related meniscal degeneration, the grading system proposed by Stoller and coworkers[717] is useful clinically. This system relies upon the occurrence of grade 3 signal intensity within the meniscus in cases of meniscal tear (Fig. 70–273). Differentiation between grade 2 signal intensity that may extend close to the articular surface of the meniscus and grade 3 signal intensity that violates this surface, obviously, becomes important, as the first pattern generally is regarded as evidence of degenerative changes that cannot be detected at the time of arthroscopy and the second pattern is considered evidence of a meniscal tear that can be found and treated at the time of arthroscopy. In clinical practice, a great deal of time is spent trying to correctly interpret the intrameniscal signal intensity as evidence of a grade 2 or grade 3 pattern. The general consensus emphasizes caution in "overcalling" the extent of intrameniscal signal intensity and in using photographic maneuvers during meniscal windowing to create an illusion of violation of the meniscal surface. The wisdom of this philosophy is underscored by the results of studies by Kaplan and co-

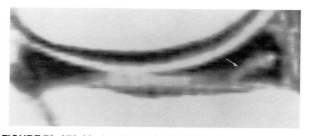

FIGURE 70–273. Meniscal tears: Grade 3 intrameniscal signal intensity. A sagittal proton density–weighted (TR/TE, 2000/20) spin echo MR image photographed with meniscal windowing shows a linear region of intermediate signal intensity (arrow) extending to the inferior surface of the posterior horn of the medial meniscus.

workers[759] and by De Smet and collaborators.[760] In the first of these two investigations, an analysis of MR scans of the knee in 142 consecutive patients revealed 20 patients (14 per cent) in whom it was difficult to decide if the region of intermediate signal intensity extended to the meniscal surface. In 17 of 20 patients, the posterior horn of the lateral meniscus was involved. In 13 of 20 patients who underwent arthroscopy or arthrotomy, no meniscal tears were found. The authors concluded that a meniscal tear is unlikely when the focus of altered intrameniscal signal intensity does not unequivocally involve the meniscal surface. De Smet and associates,[760] in an assessment of MR imaging findings in the knees of 200 consecutive patients, found that more than 90 per cent of menisci with abnormal signal intensity contacting the surface on more than one image were torn, but only 55 per cent of medial menisci and 30 per cent of lateral menisci with such signal intensity patterns on a single MR image were torn. The authors concluded that the presence of regions of intermediate signal intensity within the meniscus that contact the surface of the meniscus on only one image should lead to the diagnosis of a possible tear rather than a definite tear.

In order to determine the prognosis in patients with grade 2 intrameniscal signal intensity, Dillon and collaborators[761] performed a prospective study of this pattern of signal intensity in patients with intact anterior cruciate ligaments. In 27 menisci in 22 patients in whom the initial MR imaging examination showed evidence of grade 2 changes in one or both menisci that had been proven at arthroscopy not to be torn, subsequent evaluation using MR imaging after a period of 11 to 41 months showed an unchanged pattern of signal intensity in 18 of 27 menisci, decreased intrameniscal signal intensity in six menisci, and increased intrameniscal signal intensity in only three menisci. These data support the conclusion that grade 2 patterns of signal intensity within the meniscus generally are stable for at least one to several years.

The effects of physiologic exercise on the patterns of intrameniscal signal intensity have been studied with inconsistent results. Kursunoglu-Brahme and coworkers,[762] evaluating MR images of the knee in 10 healthy subjects before and immediately after 30 min of continuous jogging, found subtle increases in intrameniscal signal intensity (as well as joint effusions) in five of their subjects. It was suggested that the changes in signal intensity occurred as a result of imbibition of water by meniscal proteoglycans in association with the presence of joint fluid. Shellock and collaborators[763, 764] performed MR imaging examinations of the knee in healthy long distance runners and found that there was no increased prevalence of meniscal degeneration or tears in these persons and that none demonstrated an increase in intrameniscal signal intensity or an increase in joint fluid when comparison was made between MR imaging studies obtained before and after competition. MR imaging examinations of the knee in asymptomatic collegiate and professional (American) football and basketball players have shown a high prevalence of signal intensity patterns consistent with meniscal degeneration or tear[765] and a progression of these patterns on sequential examinations.[766]

An expanded classification system of intrameniscal signal intensity was described by Mesgarzadeh and colleagues[752] (Fig. 70–274). Although these authors included the categories of grade 1 and grade 2 signal intensity as

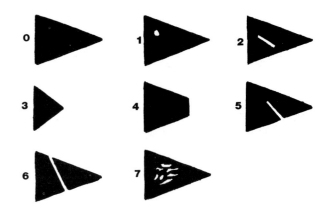

FIGURE 70–274. Grading of intrameniscal signal intensity and meniscal morphology: Expanded classification system. A grade 0 pattern consists of a meniscus that is of homogeneous low signal intensity. Grades 1 and 2 patterns are similar to those previously illustrated. Additional grades (3, 4, 5, 6, and 7) are described in the text. (Modified from Mesgarzadeh M, et al: RadioGraphics 13:489, 1993.)

described by Stoller and coworkers,[717] they classified short and truncated menisci as grade 3 and grade 4 abnormalities, respectively. They further divided the previously described category of grade 3 signal intensity into three new grades: intermediate signal intensity extending to only one surface of the meniscus (grade 5), signal intensity extending to both meniscal surfaces (grade 6), and an irregular pattern of intermediate signal intensity within the meniscus that may or may not extend to the meniscal surface (grade 7). Arthroscopically proven meniscal tears occurred in 2 per cent of menisci with grade 1 signal intensity, 5 per cent of menisci with grade 2 signal intensity, 23 per cent of menisci with grade 3 signal intensity, 71 per cent of menisci with grade 4 signal intensity, 85 per cent of menisci with grade 5 signal intensity, 95 per cent of menisci with grade 6 signal intensity, and 82 per cent of menisci with grade 7 signal intensity. These results indicate that reliance on the presence of violation of the meniscal surface in the diagnosis of meniscal tears will result in a definite but small percentage of false-negative MR imaging examinations, that violation of both meniscal surfaces as opposed to one is a more definite sign of a meniscal tear, and that correct interpretation of the significance of a short and truncated meniscus as seen on MR images is difficult, particularly in patients who have had previous meniscal surgery. The assessment of the significance of grade 7 signal intensity also is difficult (Fig. 70–275). When the altered signal intensity reaches the surface of the meniscus, the diagnosis of a tear in menisci with grade 7 signal intensity becomes more definite; when it does not reach the meniscal surface, there appears to be a high likelihood of prominent meniscal degeneration, particularly in older persons. Such meniscal degeneration may be interpreted as evidence of a meniscal tear during arthroscopy if the meniscus is probed vigorously.

Although most patients who reveal altered signal intensity within the meniscus that does not extend to the meniscal surface do not have a torn meniscus, one exception to this rule deserves emphasis. Prominent areas of intermediate signal intensity confined to the substance of a discoid meniscus may indicate extensive cavitation of that meniscus, which often is regarded as evidence of an intrameniscal tear at the time of arthroscopy (see later discussion).

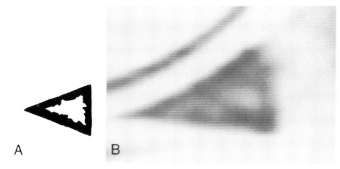

FIGURE 70–275. Intrameniscal signal intensity: Diagnostic difficulty. The presence of extensive regions of intermediate signal intensity within a meniscus that do not extend to the articular surface, as demonstrated diagrammatically **(A)** and in a sagittal proton density–weighted (TR/TE, 2000/20) spin echo MR image photographed with meniscal windowing **(B)**, creates some diagnostic difficulty. A significant percentage of patients with such intrameniscal signal intensity are found to have a meniscal tear at the time of arthroscopic surgery.

MR Imaging: Torn Menisci. Once the many variations of signal intensity that characterize the grossly intact meniscus are mastered, diagnosis of meniscal tears on MR images becomes straightforward. Most reports have indicated that the sensitivity, specificity, and accuracy of MR imaging in the detection of meniscal tears is close to or even greater than 85 to 90 per cent.[714, 716, 725, 767, 768, 1399] Much lower values of the sensitivity, specificity, and accuracy of MR imaging in such detection have been reported, however, which may reflect variations in sample size.[769] Other factors that potentially may explain discrepancies in reported results of MR imaging of the menisci include differences in study populations, technical variations, and observer performance. Furthermore, there is no true standard by which to measure the accuracy of the MR imaging findings. Arthroscopy, which has been used as the standard in most reports dealing with noninvasive imaging studies of the knee, is not without limitations.[770] Not all segments of the posterior horn of the menisci can be visualized directly with arthroscopy, probing of the meniscus rather than direct visualization is used as an arthroscopic test for some tears of the inferior (tibial) surface of the meniscus, and the level of expertise varies among orthopedic surgeons performing arthroscopy (just as it varies among radiologists interpreting MR imaging examinations of the knee).

Assessment of certain parts of the menisci with MR imaging may be difficult. One such region is the free, or inner, edge of each meniscus, where small tears may be obscured by volume-averaging artifacts, leading to a false-negative MR imaging examination. Similarly, meniscal tears may be overlooked during MR imaging in trouble spots such as the posterior horn of the lateral meniscus where normal structures obscure meniscal detail. Tears in this location are not uncommon in patients with associated injuries of the anterior cruciate ligament.[1400] The chance of missing a large (and potentially unstable) meniscal tear in any location is unlikely if the MR images are interpreted by an experienced observer. False-positive results on MR images of the menisci often relate to some of the normal anatomic variations described earlier.

The two MR imaging criteria for diagnosis of the meniscal tear are intrameniscal signal intensity that extends to a meniscal surface and abnormal meniscal morphology (Fig. 70–276). The sagittal plane and T1-weighted and proton density spin echo MR images are more valuable in this diagnosis than the coronal and transaxial planes and T2-weighted spin echo MR images. Although some meniscal tears will fill with fluid and appear as regions of high signal intensity on T2-weighted spin echo images (Fig. 70–277), most do not.

Alterations in morphology of torn menisci take several

FIGURE 70–276. Meniscal tears: Abnormalities of intrameniscal signal intensity and meniscal morphology. Sagittal proton density–weighted (TR/TE, 2000/20) spin echo MR images.

A Posterior horn of the medial meniscus. A grade 3 pattern of intrameniscal signal intensity (arrow) is evident.

B Posterior horn of the medial meniscus. A grade 3 pattern of intrameniscal signal intensity (arrow) and irregularity of the inferior meniscal surface are seen.

C Posterior horn of the medial meniscus. A grade 3 pattern of intrameniscal signal intensity (arrow) and altered meniscal morphology are evident.

D Posterior horn of the lateral meniscus. A grade 3 pattern of intrameniscal signal intensity (arrow) and an irregular inferior and inner meniscal surface are seen.

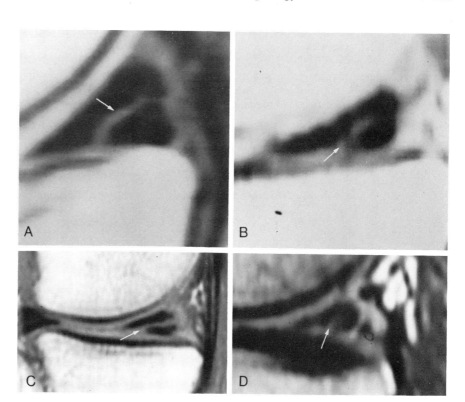

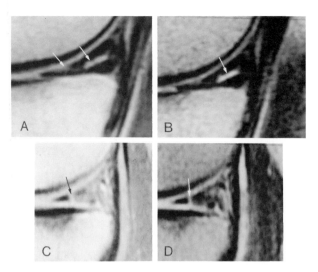

FIGURE 70–277. Meniscal tears: Abnormalities of intrameniscal signal intensity and meniscal morphology. Sagittal proton density–weighted (TR/TE, 2200/20) spin echo MR images **(A, C)** and sagittal T2-weighted (TR/TE, 2200/60) spin echo MR images **(B, D)**.

    A, B Posterior horn of the medial meniscus. Note the grade 3 pattern of intrameniscal signal intensity (arrows) that increases further in signal intensity in **B**. The superior portion of the meniscus is irregular.

    C, D Posterior horn of the medial meniscus. Note the grade 3 pattern of intrameniscal signal intensity (arrows) that reveals a further increase in signal intensity in **D**.

forms. The inner portion of the meniscus may appear blunted on coronal or sagittal MR images. The meniscus may have a normal triangular shape but appear too small (Fig. 70–278). As an example of this, the width of the posterior horn of the medial meniscus normally is greater than the width of the anterior horn of the medial meniscus; when sagittal MR images display a posterior horn of the medial meniscus that is equal in size to or smaller than its anterior horn, a tear should be suspected even if the meniscal contour appears normal. Diagnosis of tears of the free edge of the meniscus often requires careful analysis of both the sagittal and coronal MR images so that subtle blunting or poor definition of the involved portion of the meniscus is recognized. An abrupt change of contour or focal deformity of the meniscus (Fig. 70–279), designated the notch sign,[756] is an important indicator of a meniscal tear, but it can be simulated by the normal meniscal flounce (see previous discussion). The notch sign is a more definite indica-

tor of meniscal tear when it is accompanied by abnormalities of intrameniscal signal intensity.

    Bucket-handle tears of the meniscus are associated with characteristic MR imaging abnormalities (Fig. 70–280). This term is derived from the appearance of the tear, in which the inner displaced meniscal fragment resembles a handle, and the peripheral nondisplaced portion of the meniscus has the appearance of a bucket.[771] Bucket-handle tears usually are observed in young adults and in the medial meniscus, and they may be associated with a history of locking of the knee joint. MR imaging findings include a foreshortened and blunted meniscus with central displacement of its inner fragment.[771, 772] As the peripheral nondisplaced component of the meniscus also may appear relatively normal, recognition of the displaced inner portion of the meniscus is important.[771] In cases of bucket-handle tears of the medial meniscus, the displaced fragment typically appears as a band of low signal intensity extending across

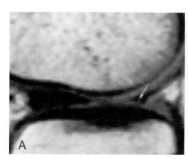
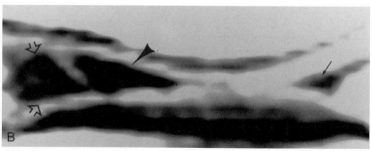

FIGURE 70–278. Meniscal tears: Abnormalities of meniscal morphology. Posterior horn of the lateral meniscus. Sagittal proton density–weighted (TR/TE, 1000/20) spin echo MR images obtained without **(A)** and with **(B)** meniscal windowing show an abnormally small posterior horn of the lateral meniscus (solid arrows). A bucket-handle tear of the posterior portion of the lateral meniscus is present, with a more central fragment displaced anteriorly (open arrows), lying in front of the anterior horn of the lateral meniscus (arrowhead). (Courtesy of A. Nemcek, M.D., Chicago, Illinois.)

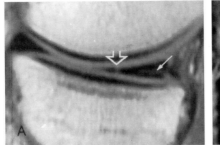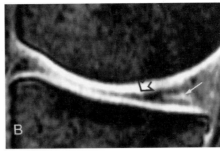

FIGURE 70–279. Meniscal tears: Abnormalities of intrameniscal signal intensity and meniscal morphology. Posterior horn of the medial meniscus. A sagittal proton density–weighted (TR/TE, 2200/20) spin echo MR image **(A)** and a sagittal 3DFT spoiled gradient recalled acquisition in the steady state (SPGR) MR image (TR/TE, 58/10; flip angle, 60 degrees) obtained with chemical presaturation of fat (ChemSat) **(B)** show altered intrameniscal signal intensity (solid arrows) with a further increase in signal intensity in **B** and an irregular notch (open arrows) in the superior surface of the meniscus.

the joint and projecting over the medial tibial eminence.[771] On sagittal MR images, the displaced fragment often lies in front of, below, and parallel to the posterior cruciate ligament. The resulting appearance may simulate that of the normal meniscofemoral ligament of Humphrey or a tear of the anterior cruciate ligament.

Bucket-handle tears involving the lateral meniscus (and, perhaps, a few involving the medial meniscus) may have a different appearance on MR images. This appearance, designated the flipped meniscus sign,[773] relates to displacement of a posteriorly located fragment of the meniscus that still is attached to the central portion of the meniscus (Fig. 70–281). The fragment may flip, or invert, and become located

on top of the anterior horn of the involved meniscus. On sagittal images, the flipped meniscal fragment may be located anterior to the anterior horn of the meniscus with a cleavage plane between the two.[1352] In such cases, a tear or nonvisualization of the posterior horn of the meniscus and an increase in height of the anterior meniscal contour are helpful diagnostic clues.[773] The predilection for the lateral meniscus may relate to its greater mobility.

Meniscocapsular Separation. Meniscocapsular separation refers to disruption of the meniscal attachment to the joint capsule. The posterior horn of the medial meniscus is involved most frequently, perhaps related to its solid adherence to the capsule. Once separated, the mobility of the

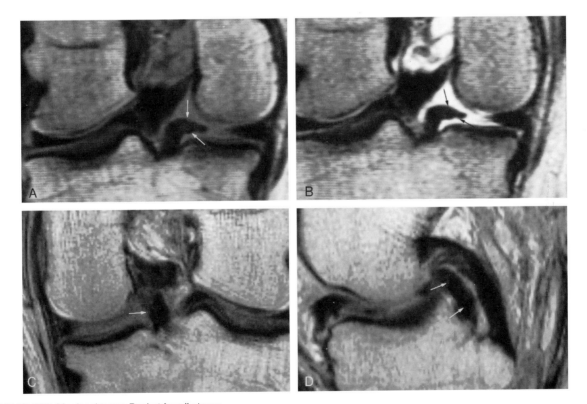

FIGURE 70–280. Meniscal tears: Bucket-handle tears.
  A, B Medial meniscus. Coronal proton density–weighted (TR/TE, 2500/20) **(A)** and T2-weighted (TR/TE, 2500/60) **(B)** spin echo MR images reveal a bucket-handle tear of the medial meniscus with central displacement (arrows) of the inner portion of the meniscus.
  C, D Medial meniscus. Coronal proton density–weighted (TR/TE, 1750/20) **(C)** and sagittal proton density–weighted (TR/TE, 3000/20) **(D)** spin echo MR images reveal a bucket-handle tear of the medial meniscus with central displacement (arrows) of the inner portion of the meniscus. In **D**, the meniscal fragment is located in front of the posterior cruciate ligament. (Courtesy of R. Stiles, M.D., Atlanta, Georgia.)

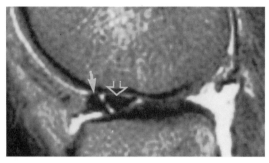

FIGURE 70–281. Meniscal tears: Flipped meniscus sign. Lateral meniscus. A sagittal T2-weighted (TR/TE, 2000/70) spin echo MR image reveals that the posterior horn of the lateral meniscus is not visualized posteriorly but rather is seen anteriorly (solid arrow), located in front of the anterior horn of the lateral meniscus (open arrow). (Courtesy of J. Kirkham, M.D., Minneapolis, Minnesota.)

medial meniscus is increased, and subsequent tears of this structure probably are uncommon. Surgical repair of meniscocapsular separations is a therapeutic option,[774] underscoring the importance of correct diagnosis.

The principles related to the diagnosis of meniscocapsular separation are the same whether the lesion is detected arthrographically or with MR imaging. The presence of fluid between the peripheral portion of the posterior horn of the medial meniscus and the joint capsule is the most important finding on either type of examination. With arthrography, the fluid represents a portion of the injected contrast material; with MR imaging, the fluid is derived from a portion of a joint effusion, and it is observed best in sagittal T2-weighted spin echo images or gradient echo images (in the steady state) employing small to moderate flip angles. The fluid may collect in the entire interface between the meniscus and capsule or in a portion of this interface, particularly its inferior portion (Fig. 70–282). Uncovering of the tibial articular cartilage, owing to central displacement of the medial meniscus, does not appear to be a reliable sign of meniscocapsular separation. The role of MR imaging using intra-articular or intravenous administration of gadolinium compounds in establishing this diagnosis is not clear. At present, arthrography appears to be equally sensitive or more sensitive when compared to MR imaging in establishing a diagnosis of a meniscocapsular separation. Another type of lesion occurring at the periphery of the medial meniscus, disruption of the meniscotibial (coronary) ligament that normally connects the meniscus to the tibia, also can be established with arthrography.[775]

The differential diagnosis of a meniscocapsular separation includes normal recesses that may appear above or below the peripheral portion of the meniscus, a large joint effusion displacing the meniscus, a longitudinal vertical tear through the periphery of the meniscus, and bursitis beneath the tibial collateral ligament.[755]

Meniscal Cysts. Meniscal cysts are multiloculated collections of mucinous material of unknown cause that occur at the periphery of the meniscus and, therefore, appear as a focal mass or swelling at the joint line. These cysts also are referred to as ganglion cysts or juxta-articular myxomas. They appear to be uncommon lesions, observed in approximately 1 per cent of meniscectomies.[776] Although reports have indicated that meniscal cysts on the lateral side of the knee are three to seven times more frequent than those on the medial side,[777–784] meniscal cysts on the medial side are being reported frequently,[785, 786] particularly on MR imaging examinations.[617] Medial meniscal cysts tend to be larger than those on the lateral side,[778] and they are more often asymptomatic.[787] The most common location of meniscal cysts is adjacent to the middle third of the lateral meniscus.[778] Meniscal cysts usually occur in young adult men with an average age of 30 years, but they have been reported in patients as young as 5 years and as old as 80 years.[778]

The precise cause of meniscal cysts is not clear. They have been reported in association with other disorders, such as calcium pyrophosphate dihydrate crystal deposition disease and rheumatoid arthritis.[788] Most observers believe that these cysts are traumatic in nature, although degenerative or congenital factors also may be important. Many, if not most, meniscal cysts are associated with myxoid degeneration and horizontal cleavage tears of the adjacent meniscus that extend into the parameniscal region.[778–780, 787, 789] Fluid from the joint extending into a horizontal tear of the meniscus and subsequently into the cystic lesion is one explanation for their occurrence. Pathologically, cysts are septated lesions containing clear, bloody, or gelatinous fluid that has a high protein content and histochemically is similar if not identical to synovial fluid.[778, 788]

In addition to swelling at the joint line, patients with meniscal cysts may experience pain and limitation of motion, perhaps related to the presence of an underlying meniscal tear. Irritation of the common peroneal nerve in cases of lateral meniscal cysts may be noted.[778] On physical examination, a soft tissue mass is palpable. Meniscal cysts on the lateral side of the knee often are smaller, and they may be located anterior or posterior to the fibular collateral ligament. Such cysts may be palpated posteriorly adjacent to the tendons of the popliteus muscle and the biceps femoris muscle, or anteriorly near the iliotibial band.[778] On the medial side of the knee, meniscal cysts may dissect through the joint capsule and even the medial collateral ligament and, in such cases, may enlarge, appear mobile, and dissect into the soft tissues for considerable distances.[778]

Although the diagnosis of a meniscal cyst often is made clinically, imaging studies may be used to further evaluate the lesion. On routine radiography, gas formation or erosion of bone, in addition to a mass, may be observed.[790, 791] CT typically reveals a well-defined mass containing fluid that often communicates with the adjacent meniscus.[792] Ultrasonography confirms the cystic nature of the lesion and, in some cases, cystic degeneration of the adjacent meniscus.[793]

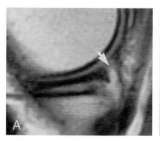
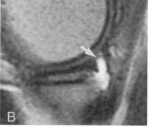

FIGURE 70–282. Meniscocapsular separation: MR imaging. Medial meniscus. Sagittal proton density–weighted (TR/TE, 2000/30) **(A)** and T2-weighted (TR/TE, 2000/80) **(B)** spin echo MR images reveal fluid (arrows) between the posterior portion of the medial meniscus and the joint capsule.

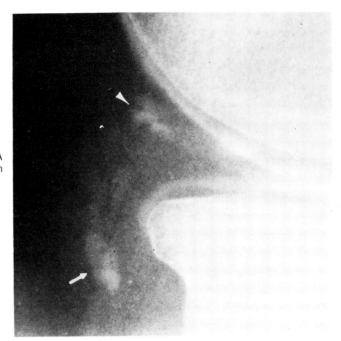

FIGURE 70–283. Meniscal cysts: Arthrography. Medial meniscus. A cyst of the medial meniscus is opacified (arrow) and associated with a horizontal tear of the meniscus (arrowhead).

Standard arthrography may reveal contrast material extending from the joint into a horizontal tear of the meniscus and, from there, pooling in a cystic mass at the periphery of the torn meniscus (Fig. 70–283). Such communication may be more apparent on delayed radiographs following arthrography.[794] Meniscal cysts also may lead to distortion

of the adjacent meniscus on arthrographic examination.[795] On MR images, an ovoid mass of variable size containing fluid is seen[617, 778] (Figs. 70–284 and 70–285). The cyst may extend either anteriorly or posteriorly, and an associated meniscal tear may be evident. Meniscal cysts also may be diagnosed and treated arthroscopically.[778–780, 786]

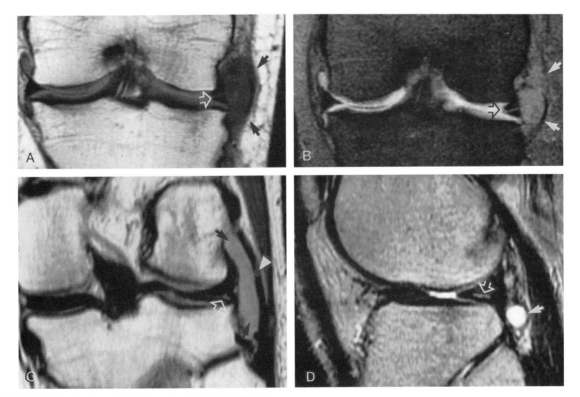

FIGURE 70–284. Meniscal cysts: MR imaging. Lateral meniscus.
   A, B A coronal T1-weighted (TR/TE, 800/12) spin echo MR image **(A)** and a coronal T1-weighted (TR/TE, 750/20) spin echo MR image obtained with chemical presaturation of fat (ChemSat) **(B)** show a mass (solid arrows) adjacent to the midportion of the lateral meniscus. Note a grade 3 pattern of signal intensity (open arrows) in the meniscus, consistent with a horizontally oriented meniscal tear.
   C, D In a second patient, a coronal proton density–weighted (TR/TE, 2200/20) spin echo MR image **(C)** and a sagittal T2-weighted (TR/TE, 2200/80) spin echo MR image **(D)** show a meniscal cyst (solid arrows) associated with a horizontal tear of the lateral meniscus (open arrows). Note that the cyst displaces the lateral (fibular) collateral ligament (arrowhead).

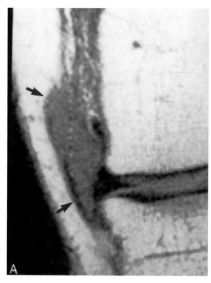
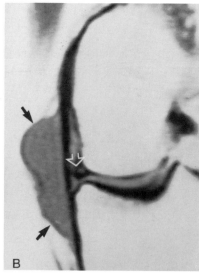
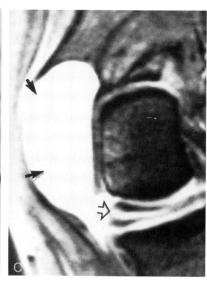

FIGURE 70–285. Meniscal cysts: MR imaging. Medial meniscus.

A A coronal proton density–weighted (TR/TE, 1000/20) spin echo MR image shows the cyst (arrows) adjacent to the midportion of the medial meniscus. Although the meniscus itself looks normal in this scan, a tear of the medial meniscus was evident at arthroscopy. (Courtesy of G. Greenway, M.D., Dallas, Texas.)

B A lobulated meniscal cyst (solid arrows) superficial to the medial (tibial) collateral ligament and a medial meniscal tear (open arrow) are evident in this T1-weighted (TR/TE, 800/25) spin echo MR image that is photographed with meniscal windowing.

C A coronal MPGR MR image (TR/TE, 450/12; flip angle, 15 degrees) shows a large meniscal cyst (solid arrows) and a horizontally oriented tear (open arrow) in the medial meniscus. (Courtesy of H. S. Kang, M.D., Seoul, Korea.)

Discoid Menisci. A discoid meniscus has an altered shape. It is broad and dislike in appearance rather than semilunar in configuration, although intermediate varieties of discoid menisci have been described.[796] These include the slab type (flat, circular meniscus), biconcave type (biconcave disc, thinner in its central portion), wedge type (large but normally tapered meniscus), anterior type (enlarged anterior horn), forme fruste (slightly enlarged meniscus), and grossly torn type (too deformed for accurate classification). A discoid lateral meniscus[797–803] is much more common than a discoid medial meniscus.[801–813]

The reported frequency of discoid lateral menisci varies from 0 to 2.7 per cent,[796, 814] although occasionally a higher frequency, determined by arthrography in children[815] or by direct inspection during meniscectomy,[798, 801, 816] is cited. The usual age of patients at the time of clinical presentation is between 15 and 35 years, and men are affected more frequently. These patients commonly have symptoms of a torn cartilage. Bilateral discoid menisci[817] and a familial occurrence of an abnormal meniscal shape[818] also have been noted.

Three basic theories have been set forth to explain the occurrence of a discoid lateral meniscus: embryologic, developmental, and congenital. An embryologic explanation for discoid menisci has not been determined yet. During development, undifferentiated mesenchymal tissue exists between the cartilaginous precursors of bone.[819] This tissue subsequently cavitates, producing an articular cavity. In some articulations, a portion of the mesenchyme exists as fibrocartilaginous discs or menisci. In knee development, under normal circumstances, undifferentiated mesenchyme evolves into fetal cartilage, which by the 10th week is semilunar in shape, closely resembling the adult meniscus. This normal sequence of embryologic development, therefore, does not contain a stage in which either the medial or

the lateral meniscus is discoid in shape; the appearance of such a meniscus in a child or adult cannot occur through persistence of a fetal stage. Of interest, however, is the demonstration of discoid menisci as normal findings in various vertebrates.

Kaplan[799] has postulated that the discoid lateral meniscus is acquired after birth as a result of an abnormal attachment of its posterior horn to the tibial plateau. He suggested that a primary abnormality of the inferior strut or fascicle will leave a lateral meniscus attached posteriorly only by the meniscofemoral ligament (ligament of Wrisberg) and eventually will produce a discoid meniscus because of repetitive abnormal mediolateral and anteroposterior movement of the meniscus, with subsequent enlargement and thickening of meniscal tissue. Other investigators have noted that this strut frequently is poorly visualized or definitely abnormal in many patients with discoid lateral menisci, observations that lend support to Kaplan's theory. Investigations have documented that a complete type of discoid lateral meniscus with intact ligamentous attachments, which generally is asymptomatic, also exists.

The third theory indicates the importance of congenital factors and is supported by the occurrence of discoid menisci in several members of a single family, and in twins, fetuses, and neonates.[820]

No single classification system exists for discoid menisci. Some systems divide these menisci into complete and incomplete forms (referring to the degree of meniscal interposition between the tibial plateau and femoral condyle in the presence of intact meniscal attachments) and the Wrisberg ligament type, in which the posterior attachment site of the lateral meniscus is altered. Evidence suggests that incomplete and complete discoid menisci are symptomatic only when torn and that the Wrisberg ligament type is associated with a snapping knee.[803] Many authors believe that a discoid lateral meniscus with normal posterior attachments does not require surgical treatment unless it is torn.[803, 820] Some believe that all discoid menisci undergo cystic mucoid degeneration,[821] although this is not accepted uniformly.[820] The Wrisberg ligament type discoid meniscus is believed to be associated with meniscal hypermobility, although the precise movement of such a meniscus during flexion and extension of the knee is not agreed upon. Furthermore, some view the hypermobile meniscus as one in which a posterior capsular tear has occurred and not one related to a developmental alteration in the capsular attachment of the lateral meniscus.[820]

Discoid menisci may be discovered incidentally or associated with clinical manifestations that include pain and a snapping knee. Torn discoid menisci lead to pain, swelling, and locking of the knee, findings in common with all meniscal tears. The classic clinical finding, the snapping knee, may be absent in cases in which the discoid meniscus possesses normal capsular attachments. Accurate diagnosis depends on the results of arthroscopic examination, arthrography, or MR imaging.

Initial plain films in patients with discoid menisci generally are unrewarding, although widening of the articular space in the ipsilateral compartment of the knee documented by weight-bearing radiography, a high fibular head, a "cupped" tibial plateau,[822] and an abnormally shaped lateral malleolus have been observed in patients with discoid lateral menisci. A discoid medial meniscus may be associated with irregularity of the medial margin of the proximal tibial epiphysis.[823] An association of discoid lateral menisci and osteochondritis dissecans of the lateral femoral condyle also has been noted.[824] Arthrography reveals the abnormally large and elongated meniscus, frequently extending to the intercondylar notch (Fig. 70–286). The margins of the body of the meniscus are relatively parallel rather than converging in configuration. An associated meniscal tear frequently is observed.[825]

MR imaging has been used to confirm either an intact or a torn discoid meniscus.[826–828] This can be accomplished by analysis of both sagittal and coronal MR images (Fig. 70–287). Observations based on sagittal images relate to the number of consecutive scans that reveal a bow-tie appearance of the meniscus, in which the anterior and posterior horns of the meniscus still are connected, or continuous. This number is directly related to the width of the meniscus; an enlarged meniscus is compatible with the diagnosis of a discoid meniscus, although no precise dimensions are available for normal menisci. The average transverse diameter of the lateral meniscus appears to be approximately 11 or 12 mm; the visualization of a bow-tie appearance on three or more contiguous sagittal sections that are 5 mm in thickness, or an abnormally thickened bow-tie, or both, are evidence of a discoid lateral meniscus.[827] Similarly, the presence of two adjacent peripheral 5 mm thick sagittal sections demonstrating equal or nearly equal meniscal height is suggestive of this diagnosis.[827] Similar diagnostic rules apply to the analysis of the sagittal MR images in cases of discoid medial meniscus. In the coronal plane, the abnormal shape of the meniscus, involving the entire meniscus or a portion of it, is identified more readily.

The MR imaging criteria for diagnosing a tear of a discoid meniscus are similar to those used to diagnose a tear in a meniscus that is not discoid in shape. The presence of extensive, intermediate signal intensity within a discoid meniscus, however, should be interpreted cautiously. Such a finding in a nondiscoid meniscus usually is considered evidence of mucinous or myxoid change without a tear, unless the region of altered signal intensity extends to the surface of the meniscus. In a discoid meniscus, cavitation or intrasubstance tears may present as areas of intermediate signal intensity that do not violate the meniscal surface (Fig. 70–287).

MR imaging allows analysis of the capsular attachments of the posterior horn of the lateral meniscus. As alterations in the morphology of the meniscofemoral ligament of Wrisberg and similar alterations or absence of other capsular structures, such as the posterior coronary ligament,[829] may be responsible for discoid menisci or altered movement of

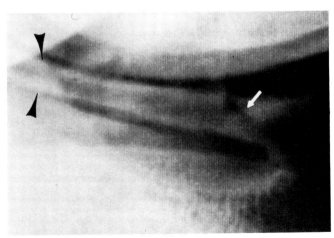

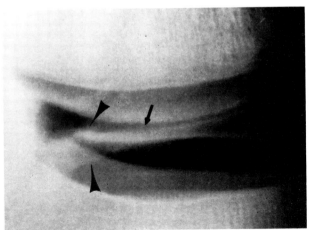

A   **B**

FIGURE 70–286. Discoid menisci: Arthrography.
   A Discoid lateral meniscus (slab type) with tear. Observe that the meniscus extends far into the joint cavity (arrowheads). A vertical tear is evident (arrow).
   B Discoid lateral meniscus (biconcave type). The central extension (arrowheads) and the thinner central portion (arrow) of the meniscus are observed.

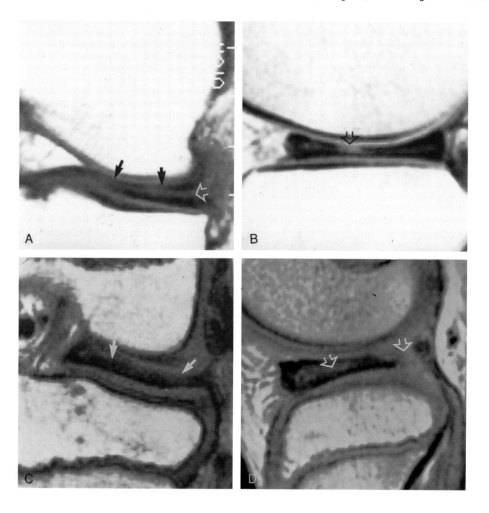

FIGURE 70–287. Discoid menisci: MR imaging. Lateral meniscus.

A, B A coronal T1-weighted (TR/TE, 750/20) spin echo MR image photographed with meniscal windowing (**A**) and a sagittal proton density–weighted (TR/TE, 2300/30) spin echo MR image also photographed with meniscal windowing (**B**) show the enlarged meniscus (solid arrows) and the meniscal tear (open arrows). The presence of large regions of intermediate signal intensity within a discoid meniscus generally is indicative of a tear.

C, D In a second patient, a coronal T1-weighted (TR/TE, 800/20) spin echo MR image (**C**) and a sagittal proton density–weighted (TR/TE, 2000/20) spin echo MR image (**D**) reveal the enlarged meniscus (solid arrows) and a meniscal tear (open arrows). Surgical confirmation of the findings was not obtained. (Courtesy of G. Greenway, M.D., Dallas, Texas.)

the lateral meniscus, analysis of these structures should be accomplished on MR images. One case of a discoid lateral meniscus associated with an abnormally short and thick ligament of Wrisberg has been described in which the MR images allowed a correct diagnosis.[649]

Meniscal Ossicles. Meniscal ossicles represent foci of ossification within the menisci. They rarely are observed in the human knee,[830–835] although they are a normal finding in the knees of certain rodents,[836] as well as of several types of small and large animals.[1401] Ossicles represent hyaline cartilage enclosing lamellar and cancellous bone and marrow. They should be differentiated from meniscal calcifications, which are frequent and relate to calcium pyrophosphate dihydrate crystal deposition in many cases.[837] The origin of meniscal ossicles in humans is controversial; some investigators believe they are vestigial structures,[832, 836] whereas others suggest they are acquired following trauma.[830, 835, 1402] Reports have indicated an association of meniscal ossicles with longitudinal tears of the medial meniscus in which the origin of the ossicles appeared to be an avulsion at the tibial site of attachment of the posterior horn of the medial meniscus.[838, 839] Patients with knee ossicles may be asymptomatic or have local pain and swelling.

Initial films reveal ossification of variable shape in the anterior or posterior portion of either the medial or the lateral meniscus (Fig. 70–288). The most common site is the posterior horn of the medial meniscus. Thus, the radiodense region generally is centrally located within the artic-

ular space. Arthrography confirms the location of the ossification within the meniscus[834] (Fig. 70–289). The meniscus itself may be normal, contain associated tears,[830–832, 838] or be discoid in type.[839]

MR imaging also may be used to diagnose or confirm a meniscal ossicle. As the ossicle may contain bone marrow, the signal intensity characteristics of fat may be seen within the ossicle (Fig. 70–290). The ossicle also may reveal low signal intensity on all MR imaging sequences. MR imaging allows precise localization of the ossicle to the meniscus and provides evidence of any associated meniscal tear.

Meniscal ossicles must be differentiated from other causes of articular radiodensities, particularly intra-articular osteochondral fragments. These latter fragments are not central in location, may move in location from one examination to another, or may appear in the joint recesses. If a meniscal ossicle produces considerable symptoms, requiring meniscectomy, radiography of the removed meniscus will document the intrameniscal location of the ossification.

Postoperative Menisci. Significant changes in the surgical management of meniscal abnormalities in the knee are the consequence of two major factors: the increasing awareness that the menisci have weight-bearing capacity and transmit an important component of the load during daily physical activities[840, 841]; and the current popularity of arthroscopic surgery. Meniscectomy is no longer considered a harmless operation, because of the documentation of progressive damage of the articular cartilage following re-

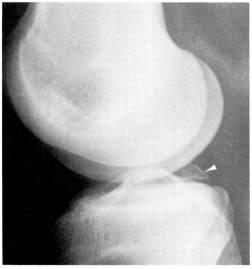

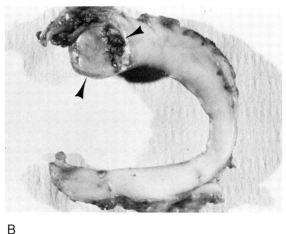

B

A

FIGURE 70–288. Meniscal ossicles: Routine radiography. This 20 year old man injured his knee playing basketball and, during the next year, noted pain, clicking, and popping.
  A The lateral radiograph reveals a bone fragment (arrowhead) in the distribution of the posterior horn of the medial meniscus.
  B In a different patient, an ossicle (arrowheads) in the posterior horn of the medial meniscus is evident. (Courtesy of G. Greenway, M.D., Dallas, Texas.)

moval of the meniscus,[842–846] although similar degenerative changes are encountered when a severely torn meniscus is left in place.[847] The advocacy of partial rather than total meniscectomy appeared to represent a philosophy midway between one that recommended complete removal of all damaged menisci and one that suggested a conservative approach to all meniscal injuries. Although partial and even total meniscectomies still are performed, the development and refinement of arthroscopic techniques have led to the

choice of meniscal repair rather than meniscal resection as a more ideal means to maintain meniscal function and, ultimately, to preserve the integrity of the knee joint. To understand the philosophy behind this choice, one needs to review the details of meniscal healing, regeneration, and remodeling. These are well summarized by Arnoczky,[645] some of whose observations are repeated here.

Meniscal Healing, Regeneration, and Remodeling. The peripheral portion of the meniscus possesses a vascular zone that supports a reparative response to injury similar to that observed in other connective tissues.[848] Inflammatory cell infiltration within a fibrin clot follows an injury to the peripheral portion of the meniscus. Subsequently, fibrovascular scar tissue appears in the injured region, becoming continuous with the adjacent normal meniscal fibrocartilage.[645] In experimental situations, peripheral meniscal tears that also involve the adjacent synovial tissue heal through the development of this scar tissue within 10 weeks of the

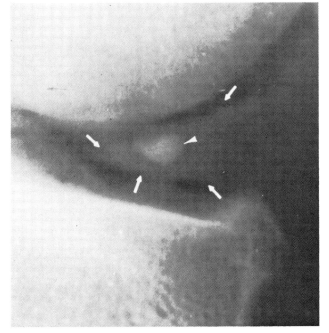

FIGURE 70–289. Meniscal ossicles: Arthrography. In this patient, an arthrogram using air alone confirms that an ossicle (arrowhead) is located in the anterior horn of the lateral meniscus (arrows).

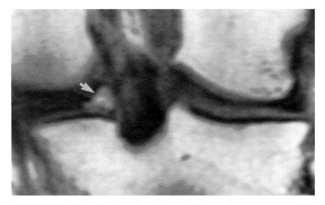

FIGURE 70–290. Meniscal ossicles: MR imaging. A coronal T1-weighted (TR/TE, 600/15) spin echo MR image shows an ossicle containing fat (arrow) within the posterior horn of the medial meniscus. (Courtesy of A. Deutsch, M.D., Los Angeles, California.)

injury.[848] This tissue may be weaker than the normal meniscus, however. Conversion of the scar tissue to normal-appearing fibrocartilage may require months. These results explain the current rationale regarding surgical repair of peripheral meniscal injuries.[645, 849, 850] The success of these repairs relates to the vascular nature of the meniscus on either side or both sides of the tear. Tears involving the central, avascular portion of the meniscus are incapable of repair unless modifications of surgical technique, such as vascular access channels, synovial pedicle flaps, and synovial abrasion, are employed.[645, 848, 851] In general, tears known to be definitely capable of repair are traumatic, are within the vascular zone of the meniscus, and have caused minimum damage to the meniscal body fragment; such tears most commonly are longitudinal and vertical, are peripheral or nearly peripheral, and are 1 cm in length or longer.[1403] Tears that may be suitable for repair are those in the avascular zone or in an area where the vascularity is in doubt; repair of these tears requires healing-enhancement techniques such as rasping of the superior and inferior fringes and the insertion of a fibrin clot.[1403] Tears that are not suitable for repair include those with moderate or severe damage of the meniscus and complete radial tears; partial or complete meniscectomy is required for treatment in such cases.

In experimental studies in animals, regeneration of a meniscus-like structure following total meniscectomy has been observed.[852, 853] Such regeneration may depend upon bleeding from incised perimeniscal vessels that results in an organized clot, cellular proliferation within the clot, and synthesis of a fibrous connective tissue.[645] Owing to the presence of joint motion, a transformation of this fibrous tissue to fibrocartilage may occur over a period of months.[645] The vascular synovial tissue in cases of total meniscectomy and the vascular peripheral meniscal tissue in cases of partial meniscectomy appear to be instrumental in the process of meniscal regeneration.[853] Whether a similar process of meniscal regeneration occurs in humans is a controversial matter, although regeneration of a meniscus-like structure, considerably smaller than a normal meniscus, has been demonstrated in long-term follow-up evaluations in some patients undergoing total meniscectomies.[854] Thus, following total (rather than partial) meniscectomies in humans, regeneration of the peripheral portion of the meniscus appears possible. Despite this evidence, most orthopedic surgeons believe partial meniscectomy is the preferred operation if meniscal removal is considered.[645] Remodeling (rather than regeneration) in the avascular zone of the meniscus may occur after partial meniscectomy, probably related to extrameniscal accretion of new tissue adjacent to the meniscectomy site.[855] The ability of the human meniscus to regenerate or remodel has led to attempts to identify implant material, such as collagen-based scaffolds, that will accelerate the processes.

Partial Meniscectomy and Total Meniscectomy. Despite recent interest in meniscal repair, partial and total meniscectomies still are employed in the treatment of some meniscal tears. Results following partial meniscectomy accomplished by open or arthroscopic surgery have been promising[856-858] and are dependent on the type and location of the meniscal tear and the integrity of the remaining portions of the joint. Retention of the peripheral one third of the meniscus provides stress protection to the outer and middle regions of the ipsilateral compartment of the knee, and its salvage then appears to be physiologically sensible. Spontaneous healing of a tear in the peripheral (or central) portion of the meniscus[859, 860] occurs from an ingrowth of connective tissue and is consistent with anatomic studies indicating a relatively abundant vascular supply to the outer meniscal substance.[861] A peripheral vascular synovial fringe extends a short distance over both the femoral and the tibial surfaces of the menisci, except in the posterolateral region of the lateral meniscus, but it does not contribute any vessels to the meniscal stroma[848]; a vascular response originating from the perimeniscal vessels and peripheral synovial fringe is fundamental to the production of a fibrovascular scar at the site of a torn meniscus, emphasizing that the outer blood supply to the meniscus is sufficient to effect a reparative process in those meniscal lesions with which it communicates.[848]

A total meniscectomy involves the removal of the entire meniscus from its capsular attachment. A partial meniscectomy may involve the removal of the anterior two thirds of the abnormal meniscus, deliberately leaving the posterior horn in place; or, alternatively, the torn portion of the meniscus may be removed, leaving the remainder of the meniscus intact. Following complete meniscectomy, fibrous regeneration of the meniscus occurs within 6 weeks to 3 months.[862] The regenerated meniscus is thinner and narrower than a normal meniscus, with a decreased surface area and diminished mobility. Tears through regenerated menisci, although reported,[863, 864] are rare.

Routine Radiography and Arthrography. Plain film radiographic findings following meniscectomy may include flattening of the ipsilateral femoral condyle, a bone outgrowth projecting inferiorly from the margin of the femoral condyle at the meniscectomy site, and joint space narrowing. Arthrographic evaluation following complete or partial meniscectomy may reveal a retained fragment, a regenerated meniscus, or a tear of the opposite meniscus.[865-868]

During arthrography, the retained posterior horn following incomplete meniscectomy resembles a normal posterior horn (Fig. 70–291), although it may be irregular or contain an obvious tear. Following removal of the inner fragment of a bucket-handle tear, the retained peripheral fragment appears as a truncated shadow with rough, irregular surfaces.[866] With regeneration of the meniscus, a small triangular shadow resembling an equilateral or isosceles triangle is observed, varying from 2 to 7 mm in width.[866] It possesses smooth, well-defined margins but is not associated with adjacent normal recesses at the meniscocapsular junction. Arthrographic findings in cases of tears of the opposite meniscus are no different from those associated with meniscal tears in patients who have not undergone meniscectomy. The torn meniscus may have been overlooked on preoperative imaging examinations or may have occurred following surgery.

MR Imaging. Despite considerable interest in the role of MR imaging in the assessment of the menisci following partial meniscectomy or meniscal repair, the value of this technique remains unclear, and its diagnostic superiority when compared with standard arthrography remains unproved.[1430] A spectrum of MR imaging findings consisting of altered intrameniscal signal intensity and contour alterations is seen following partial meniscectomy or surgical repair of a torn meniscus, and sorting out what is clinically

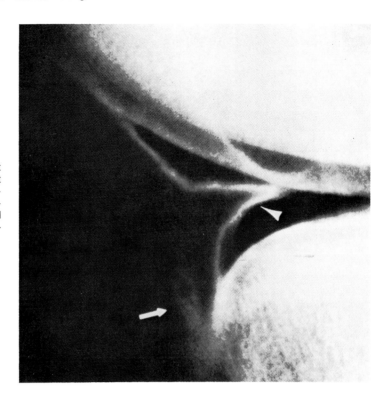

FIGURE 70–291. Postoperative menisci: Retained fragment following meniscectomy. This patient described recurrent symptoms following a partial medial meniscectomy. A retained posterior horn is apparent (arrowhead). A small collection of contrast material (arrow) may represent a partial separation of the meniscus from the medial collateral ligament.

significant from what is not is difficult.[869] Smith and Totty[870] used MR imaging to evaluate 40 patients who had had partial meniscectomies and correlated the appearance of the menisci on MR images with arthroscopic findings which were available for 23 menisci. They emphasized the spectrum of MR appearances of the meniscal remnants and cautioned against applying the classic diagnostic criteria of meniscal tears in the assessment of the postoperative knee. The authors concluded that although standard MR criteria can be used to diagnose tears in postoperative menisci that do not reveal marked contour irregularity (Fig. 70–292), the diagnosis of tears in meniscal segments revealing marked contour irregularity is far more difficult, as such irregularity can be a normal postoperative finding. They further indicated that tears occurring through meniscal remnants with severe contour irregularity may not be detectable

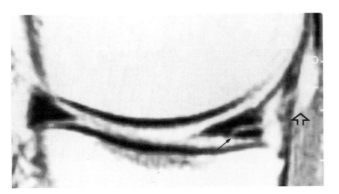

FIGURE 70–292. Postoperative menisci: Meniscal tear following partial meniscectomy. This patient developed recurrent symptoms following a partial meniscectomy for a torn medial meniscus. A sagittal T1-weighted (TR/TE, 800/20) spin echo MR image photographed with meniscal windowing shows a pattern of grade 3 intrameniscal signal intensity (solid arrow) as well as a meniscal cyst (open arrow). Both were confirmed at arthroscopy.

with MR imaging unless displacement of the fragment is evident.

Kent and coworkers[871] emphasized the slow healing response that may follow meniscal surgery and indicated that regions of altered signal intensity within the meniscal remnant on MR images can lead to diagnostic problems, particularly if a history of previous meniscal surgery is not known at the time of image interpretation. The persistence of altered signal intensity within meniscal remnants (as well as within torn menisci that are treated conservatively) also was emphasized by Deutsch and colleagues.[872] In this study, MR imaging examinations were obtained before and after therapy in 17 patients with arthroscopically confirmed meniscal tears who were treated either conservatively or operatively (meniscal repair). Follow-up MR imaging examinations, obtained 3 to 27 months after the initial studies, revealed persistent intrameniscal signal intensity (grade 3) that was unchanged from that on the initial examinations. In three patients, second-look arthroscopy was employed, and these procedures confirmed that grade 3 intrameniscal signal intensity can be observed in repaired menisci that appear intact (i.e., no new or recurrent tear) at the time of subsequent arthroscopic examination. The authors concluded that such intrameniscal signal intensity is not diagnostic of a meniscal retear. Farley and collaborators[873] arrived at conclusions similar to those of Deutsch and colleagues[872] with regard to the lack of clinical significance of grade 3 intrameniscal signal intensity in T1-weighted and proton density spin echo images in previously repaired menisci. These investigators noted, however, that a further increase in the intrameniscal signal intensity on T2-weighted spin echo images, with a resultant signal intensity identical to that of fluid, might be helpful in the diagnosis of a retorn meniscus. The specificity of this finding was 92 per cent, but its sensitivity was only 60 per cent. Although these authors indicated that a fluid-filled meniscal remnant,

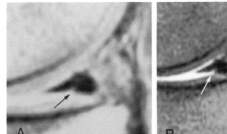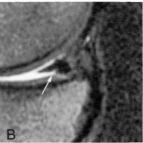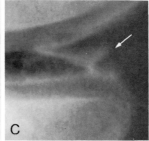

FIGURE 70–293. Postoperative menisci: Meniscal tear following partial meniscectomy. A sagittal proton density–weighted (TR/TE, 2000/30) spin echo MR image photographed with meniscal windowing **(A)** and a sagittal T2-weighted (TR/TE, 2000/80) spin echo MR image **(B)** reveal findings suggesting a tear in the posterior horn of the medial meniscus. In **A**, note irregularity (arrow) of the inferior margin of the meniscus. In **B**, a small amount of fluid (arrow) is present at the site of meniscal tear. Arthrography **(C)** confirms the presence of such a tear (arrow).

a tear at a location other than that of the repair site, and a displaced meniscal fragment all might be used to diagnose a tear in a meniscus that previously had been repaired, they concluded that standard arthrography might be a better procedure for the assessment of the symptomatic, previously repaired meniscus.

Although the previously cited studies differed in their methodology, they all indicate the difficulty encountered in the MR imaging analysis of the repaired or partially resected meniscus. In the absence of a displaced tear, the presence of fluid collections within the meniscus appears to represent the most reliable MR imaging finding of a retear (Fig. 70–293). The fluid is derived from the joint space and, therefore, the finding would be expected to be more common in patients who have sizeable joint effusions. The diagnostic value of standard arthrography in this clinical setting is based primarily on the intrameniscal extension of fluid following an iatrogenic effusion produced by the injection of contrast material into the joint. MR arthrography using gadolinium compounds[1353] or saline shares many of the advantages of standard arthrography in the diagnosis (or exclusion) of a retorn meniscus (Fig. 70–294). Whether the added expense of this procedure, when compared with standard arthrography, is warranted in this clinical situation remains unproved.

MR imaging examinations, as well as quantitative bone mineral analysis,[874] reveal changes in the subchondral bone in the proximal portion of the tibia and in the distal portion of the femur in patients undergoing partial or complete meniscectomies. These changes may reflect the effects of redistribution of stress, osteoarthritis, or even osteonecrosis (Fig. 70–295).

Abnormalities of the Medial Supporting Structures

Anatomic Considerations. The gross anatomy of the supporting structures on the medial side of the knee (Fig. 70–296) often is discussed according to the depth of the tissue, in the form of layers.[875, 876] The most superficial of three layers is represented by fascia that covers the quadriceps mechanism, invests the sartorius tendon, and continues on as the deep fascia of the leg. It rarely is torn with injury. The second layer is the superficial portion of the medial collateral ligament (also called the tibial collateral ligament or superficial medial ligament), which is separated from the first layer at the tibial tuberosity by the gracilis and semitendinosus tendons. The superficial portion of the medial collateral ligament is approximately 10 to 11 cm in length. It is composed of two bundles of fibers, one vertical and one oblique. The vertical fibers originate from the femoral epicondyle and insert in the proximal portion of the tibia, posterior to the pes anserinus tendons. The oblique fibers, often designated the posterior oblique ligament, also originate in the femoral epicondyle and insert in the posteromedial aspect of the proximal portion of the tibia, inferior to the articular surface. The superficial portion of the medial collateral ligament has no meniscal attachment and is able

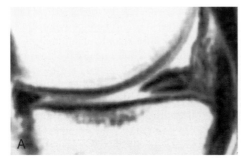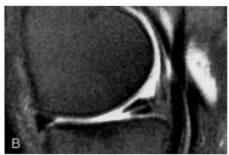

FIGURE 70–294. Postoperative menisci: Meniscal tear following partial meniscectomy. A sagittal T1-weighted (TR/TE, 500/20) spin echo MR image photographed with meniscal windowing **(A)** shows a grade 3 pattern of intrameniscal signal intensity in the posterior horn of the medial meniscus. The meniscus also appears blunted. A sagittal T1-weighted (TR/TE, 733/20) spin echo MR image obtained with chemical presaturation of fat (ChemSat) following the intra-articular administration of a gadolinium compound **(B)** reveals a slight increase in signal intensity in the inferior margin of the resected meniscus, consistent with a tear. A synovial cyst also is seen. The meniscal tear was confirmed arthroscopically.

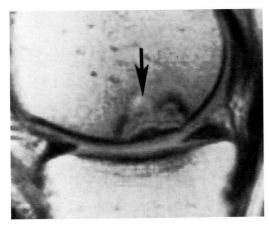

FIGURE 70–295. Postoperative menisci: Osteonecrosis. Following repair of a tear of the posterior horn of the medial meniscus, this patient developed osteonecrosis in the medial femoral condyle. A sagittal proton density–weighted (TR/TE, 2000/20) spin echo MR image shows alterations in signal intensity in the subchondral bone (arrow) of the medial femoral condyle. The meniscus appears normal. (Courtesy of S. K. Brahme, M.D., La Jolla, California.)

the coronary ligament) and, to a lesser extent, to the femur; and it thickens beneath the superficial portion of the medial collateral ligament to form the deep portion of this ligament (also designated the deep medial ligament, deep collateral ligament, or middle capsular ligament).[875] The superficial and deep portions of the medial collateral ligament are separated by a bursa that allows movement between the two. The deep portion of the medial collateral ligament is divided into meniscofemoral and meniscotibial ligaments, which extend from the medial meniscus to the femur and tibia, respectively.

Although this description is useful, the three layers of tissue on the medial side of the knee usually are not identified together at any one anatomic site (with the exception of the region of the superficial portion of the medial collateral ligament). Furthermore, some of these layers may appear to merge in certain anatomic regions. One such region is the posteromedial corner of the knee, in which the second and third layers merge. In this region, an oblique oriented band of fibers, often designated the posterior oblique ligament or the oblique portion of the tibial collateral ligament,[875, 877] extends to the tibia, the fibers being reinforced by the semimembranosus muscle and its tendon.[876–878]

The supporting structures in the medial side of the knee also can be divided into three segments, based on their position in an anteroposterior plane: anterior third, middle third, and posterior third. The anterior third of these sup-

to slide posteriorly over the proximal portion of the tibia during flexion of the knee.[875] The third layer is the capsule of the knee joint, which attaches to the margins of the joint.[876] The capsule is thin anteriorly, providing little stability to the joint; it holds the meniscal rim to the tibia (i.e.,

FIGURE 70–296. Medial supporting structures: Anatomic considerations. (From Williams PL, Warwick R [Eds]: Gray's Anatomy. 35th British edition. Philadelphia, WB Saunders Co, 1973, p 453.)

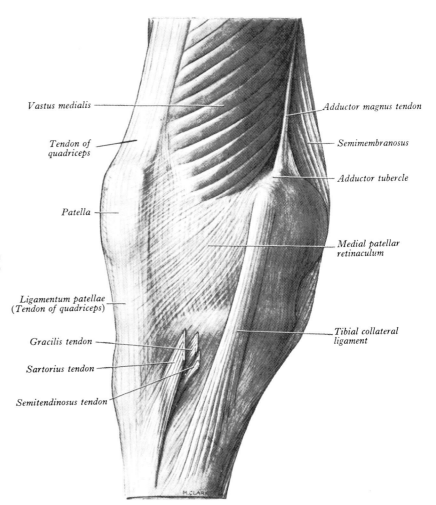

Vastus medialis

Tendon of quadriceps

Patella

Ligamentum patellae (Tendon of quadriceps)

Gracilis tendon

Sartorius tendon

Semitendinosus tendon

Adductor magnus tendon

Semimembranosus

Adductor tubercle

Medial patellar retinaculum

Tibial collateral ligament

porting structures includes the anterior portion of the joint capsule with its reinforcement from the retinaculum of the vastus medialis muscle. The middle third consists of the superficial portion of the medial collateral ligament (i.e., tibial collateral ligament) and the deep portion of the medial collateral ligament (i.e., meniscofemoral and meniscotibial ligaments). The posterior third consists of the posterior oblique ligament with contributing fibers from the vastus medialis, adductor magnus, and semimembranosus muscles.

Pathologic Considerations. The medial supporting structures of the knee, particularly the superficial portion of the medial collateral ligament, act as the primary restraint to limit valgus angulation at the knee.[879–881] Medial structures also serve as the primary restraints to internal rotation of the tibia; if the superficial and deep portions of the medial collateral ligament are sectioned, increased tibial rotation occurs with the knee in either flexion or extension.[880, 881] The medial supporting structures are major secondary restraints to anterior displacement of the tibia.[880, 882] Although deficiencies confined to the medial supporting structures may lead to pure (straight) lateral instability of the knee, such deficiencies commonly are combined with deficiencies of the cruciate ligaments that allow a rotational component, as well.[883–885] Thus, deficiencies in various components of the medial supporting structures, either alone or in combination with deficiencies in other supporting structures, may lead to straight medial, straight anterior, straight posterior, anteromedial, and combined patterns of knee instability (see later discussion).

The medial supporting structures of the knee are injured more frequently than the lateral supporting structures. Most of the major injuries to the medial capsuloligamentous complex are the result of a valgus stress, often produced by a blow to the lateral aspect of the lower portion of the thigh or the leg near the knee (e.g., clipping injury in American football players). The extent of the injury is dependent on whether the valgus forces occur alone or in combination with rotational forces. Pure valgus injuries lead to damage of the tibial collateral ligament with or without damage to the posterior oblique ligament; valgus injuries combined with rotational forces lead initially to damage to the posterior oblique ligament and, possibly, the anterior cruciate ligament and subsequently to damage to the tibial collateral ligament.[886] Rotational forces also may lead to injury of the medial meniscus. O'Donoghue's triad of injury consists of tears of the anterior cruciate ligament, medial collateral ligament, and the medial meniscus,[887] an injury that is particularly frequent in American football players.[1431]

Medial Collateral Ligament Injuries. Tears of the medial collateral ligament may be classified as acute, subacute, or chronic; or according to their severity, varying from a ligament strain (grade I) to partial (grade II) or complete (grade III) ruptures.

Clinical Abnormalities. Although the pattern and distribution of injury to the knee may be defined by a carefully obtained history, physical examination is fundamental to accurate diagnosis of an injury to the medial collateral ligament. A rapidly (less than 2 hours) developing joint effusion following an injury to the knee usually indicates a hemarthrosis, which typically relates to a collateral ligament strain, a tear of the anterior cruciate ligament, a tear of the peripheral portion of a meniscus, or an osteochondral fracture; absence of joint swelling may indicate capsular

disruption of such a degree that the fluid extravasates into the soft tissues surrounding the knee.[883] Localized edema and tenderness are good indicators of the site of disruption of the medial collateral ligament, although complete disruption of the medial ligaments of the knee may occur without significant pain, effusion, or difficulty walking.[883] One important physical finding relates to the response of the knee to the application of valgus stress. Valgus stress testing is performed with the knee in full extension and in 30 degrees of flexion. The extent of opening of the medial side of the injured knee, when compared with the opposite (uninjured) side, is used as a measure of damage to the medial collateral ligament. When such opening occurs during the application of valgus stress to the fully extended knee, damage involving the deep and superficial portions of the medial collateral ligament, including the posterior oblique ligament, is likely; if severe instability is demonstrated during this stress test, damage to the cruciate ligaments also is probable.[886] If the knee is stable in full extension, the semimembranosus corner of the knee is not damaged significantly. If positive results are obtained when valgus stress is applied to the slightly flexed knee, damage to the deep and superficial portions of the medial collateral ligament and, possibly, to the anterior fibers of the posterior oblique ligament has occurred.[886] As subtle widening of the medial side of the knee during valgus stress testing is based on comparison with the contralateral uninjured knee, evidence of abnormality of the contralateral medial collateral ligament in animals sustaining unilateral injuries, an effect that is largely unexplained, may have clinical relevance to humans.[1404]

Routine Radiographic Abnormalities. Routine radiographic abnormalities associated with acute injuries to the medial collateral ligament of the knee include medial soft tissue swelling with or without a joint effusion, rarely an avulsion fracture at the sites of insertion of the ligament, and evidence of associated injuries, such as a fracture of the lateral tibial plateau that may be comminuted, displaced, or depressed. An avulsion of the intercondylar eminence of the tibia indicates an accompanying injury to the anterior cruciate ligament. In cases of chronic injury to the medial collateral ligament, ligamentous calcification or ossification may occur (i.e., Pellegrini-Stieda syndrome).

Arthrographic Abnormalities. Recent tears of the medial collateral ligament may be documented by conventional arthrography. Contrast material introduced into the joint space will extravasate into the adjacent soft tissues. A linear radiodense region may indicate a contrast-coated outer margin of the medial collateral ligament (Fig. 70–297). An elevated meniscus and an enlarged synovial fold between the tibial margin and meniscus may indicate a tear of the coronary ligament.[775]

Two limitations are related to the arthrographic assessment of injuries to the medial collateral ligament. The examination must be performed within the first 24 to 48 hours following injury, because sealing of the synovial membrane after this time may prevent extravasation of contrast material. Furthermore, injuries involving only the superficial portion of the medial collateral ligament (with sparing of the deep portion of this ligament) are not demonstrated on the arthrographic examination.

MR Imaging: Normal Medial Collateral Ligament. Although parts of the medial collateral ligament can be seen

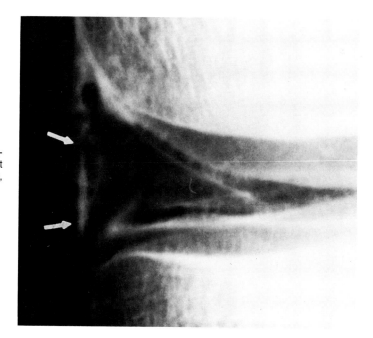

FIGURE 70–297. Medial collateral ligament injuries: Arthrography. A tear of the medial collateral ligament allows contrast material to pass from the articular cavity into the soft tissues, outlining the outer aspect of the ligament (arrows).

in MR images in the transaxial and sagittal planes, the coronal plane best displays this ligament (Fig. 70–298). In the coronal plane, the medial collateral ligament appears as a smooth structure of low signal intensity that extends from the medial epicondyle of the femur above, to the proximal metaphysis of the tibia below. In its lowest portion, the ligament may be separated from the tibial cortex by medial inferior genicular vessels. At the level of the joint line, the medial collateral ligament is separated from the periphery of the medial meniscus by a bursa and surrounding fat. This

junctional tissue should not be misinterpreted as evidence of a meniscocapsular separation. The normal junctional tissue frequently reveals signal intensity characteristics that are indicative of fat and, in such cases, misinterpretation of the normal appearance is not likely. In other instances, however, fluid within the bursa is identified between the medial collateral ligament and the medial meniscus. This may be a normal finding or represent bursitis.[755] Although similar fluid collections may occur with capsular and ligamentous injuries in the medial side of the knee, other findings indicative of trauma, including distortion of the signal intensity characteristics of the adjacent subcutaneous fat, also will be evident. Furthermore, large joint effusions resulting from any cause can lead to bowing or even displacement of the medial supporting structures of the knee.

MR Imaging: Abnormal Medial Collateral Ligament. Injuries of the medial collateral ligament vary in severity and include strains, partial tears, and complete tears. The MR imaging characteristics are dependent on the severity of the injury and its acute or chronic nature.[888–890] With acute injuries, subcutaneous edema or hemorrhage and, in some cases, a joint effusion are evident; with chronic injuries, such edema and hemorrhage are not apparent.

Strains of the medial collateral ligament may lead to slight contour irregularity or thickening of the ligament, but there is no discontinuity of its fibers. In acute strains, subcutaneous edema is an associated finding, but the signal intensity of the ligament usually is normal. Partial tears of the medial collateral ligament lead to discontinuity of some of its fibers which, in acute injuries, is associated with increased signal intensity (particularly in T2-weighted spin echo and gradient echo MR images) within the substance of the ligament (Fig. 70–299) and in the subcutaneous tissues. Complete tears of the medial collateral ligament are associated with frank discontinuity of all of its fibers. In the acute stage, hemorrhage and edema within the ligament and subcutaneous tissues also are evident (Fig. 70–300).

Although the main diagnostic criteria of an injury to the medial collateral ligament are based on its appearance in the MR images, a spectrum of associated abnormalities

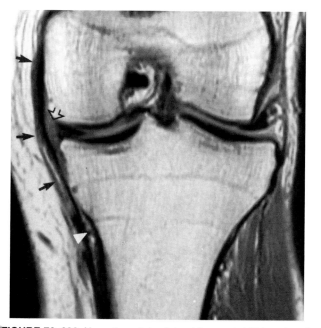

FIGURE 70–298. Normal medial collateral ligament: MR imaging. A coronal T1-weighted (TR/TE, 800/20) spin echo MR image shows the course of the vertical fibers of the superficial portion of the medial collateral ligament (solid arrows). Note that this portion of the ligament is separated (open arrow) from the medial meniscus. The medial inferior genicular vessels are seen (arrowhead).

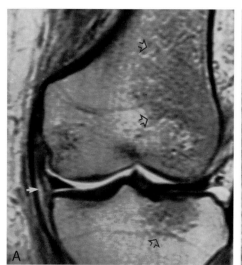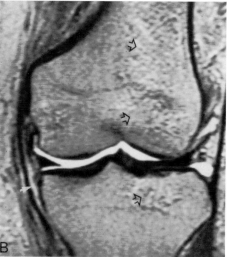

FIGURE 70–299. Injuries of the medial collateral ligament: MR imaging. Partial tear. Coronal proton density–weighted (TR/TE, 2500/20) **(A)** and T2-weighted (TR/TE, 2500/60) **(B)** spin echo MR images show altered signal intensity superficial to and within the substance of the medial collateral ligament (solid arrows), with a higher signal intensity in **B**. Marrow edema (open arrows) in the lateral portions of the femur and tibia indicates the presence of bone bruises. A joint effusion is present.

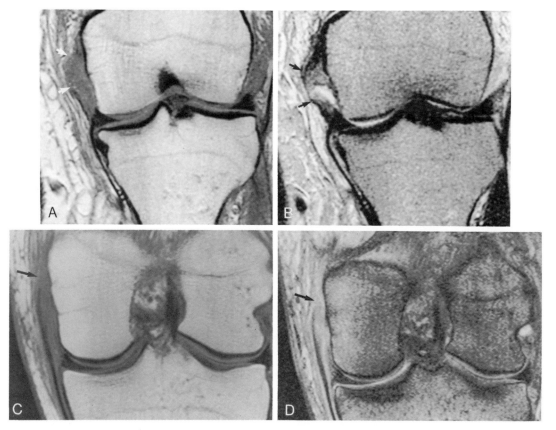

FIGURE 70–300. Injuries of the medial collateral ligament: MR imaging. Complete tear.

   A, B Coronal proton density–weighted (TR/TE, 1500/12) **(A)** and T2-weighted (TR/TE, 1500/80) **(B)** spin echo MR images show complete disruption (arrows) of the fibers of the medial collateral ligament. Note the increase in signal intensity in the ligament and soft tissues in **B**. A joint effusion is present. Additional injuries in this patient included tears of the lateral meniscus and anterior cruciate ligament. (Courtesy of V. Chandnani, M.D., Honolulu, Hawaii.)

   C, D In a second patient, coronal T1-weighted (TR/TE, 550/20) **(C)** and MPGR (TR/TE, 600/15; flip angle, 40 degrees) **(D)** MR images reveal complete disruption (arrows) of the fibers of the medial collateral ligament. The menisci and anterior cruciate ligament appear normal. Fluid and edema are evident about the torn ligament.

produce additional MR imaging changes that can be diagnostically helpful.[890] Bone infractions in the lateral femoral condyle, lateral tibial plateau, or both locations, may be observed, appearing as regions of low signal intensity on T1-weighted spin echo MR images and of high signal intensity on T2-weighted MR images. Associated tears of one or both cruciate ligaments and, less commonly, of the fibular collateral ligament also may be evident, and the lateral meniscus or medial meniscus may be injured.

Semimembranosus Tendon Abnormalities. The posteromedial corner of the knee is anatomically complex and functionally important. Portions of the joint capsule and semimembranosus tendon are intimate in this area, and the region sometimes is designated the semimembranosus corner of the knee.[886] The capsular attachments of the semimembranosus tendon merge with the oblique fibers of the superficial portion of the medial collateral ligament and, as indicated previously, sometimes are designated the posterior oblique ligament of the knee. The semimembranosus tendon is regarded as having five arms of insertion[875]: a direct attachment to the posteromedial portion of the tibia just below the joint line; a slightly anterior attachment to the tibia, just beneath the superficial fibers of the medial collateral ligament; an attachment of its sheath to the posteromedial portion of the capsule; an attachment to the oblique popliteal ligament; and a distal attachment to the superficial fibers of the medial collateral ligament. The semimembranosus corner of the knee, or posterior oblique ligament, may be important in abolishing any valgus laxity in the extended knee.[886] The semimembranosus tendon also may contribute to activation of the posterior oblique ligament.

Many injuries of the posteromedial corner of the knee also involve other medial supporting structures, as well as the medial meniscus, and any peripheral tear of the posterior horn of the medial meniscus usually includes a tear of the posterior oblique ligament.[886] Isolated avulsion injuries involving this corner of the knee, presumably, are rare. Identification of a small bone fragment adjacent to the posteromedial portion of the tibia is consistent with an avulsion injury, but its site of origin usually is not clear. One report has indicated the MR imaging findings of apparent avulsion injuries at or near the tibial sites of attachment of the semimembranosus tendon in two patients who also had tears of the anterior cruciate ligament and posterior horn of the medial meniscus.[891] Surgical findings in these two cases were not described. A case with similar MR imaging finding was reported by Vanek.[1405] Associated injuries again included a tear of the medial meniscus and a rupture of the anterior cruciate ligament. Based on additional cadaveric data, Vanek proposed that the injury was not an avulsion fracture at the site of attachment of the semimembranosus tendon but was produced by varus and external rotation forces on a flexed knee. As such, it was evidence of anterior subluxation of the medial tibial plateau occurring as a result of rupture of the anterior cruciate ligament.

Abnormalities of the Lateral Supporting Structures

Anatomic Considerations. As on the medial side of the knee, the anatomy of lateral supporting structures can be considered in the form of layers (according to the depth of the tissues)[875, 892] or in terms of their position in an anteroposterior plane.[884] Three layers of tissue can be defined[875]: superficial layer, intermediate layer, and deep layer. The superficial layer is composed of the deep fascia of the thigh and calf, including the condensed portion known as the iliotibial tract. The iliotibial tract extends along the lateral portion of the knee and inserts in the proximal, anterolateral surface of the tibia at Gerdy's tubercle. This tract has functionally important capsular and bone attachments that have been referred to as the anterolateral ligament of the knee; some fibers of the iliotibial tract are continuous with those of the vastus lateralis tendon and aponeurosis, forming the lateral patellar retinaculum.[875, 893, 894] The biceps femoris tendon lies just deep to the superficial layer; its main distal attachment is to the head and styloid process of the fibula, although some of its fibers attach to Gerdy's tubercle, blend with the crural fascia of the leg, and extend around the lateral (fibular) collateral ligament.[875]

The second layer consists of the retinaculum of the patella and the patellofemoral ligaments (see later discussion).[892] The third and deepest layer is composed of the capsule of the knee joint and the lateral (fibular) collateral ligament.[875] The lateral collateral ligament extends from the lateral epicondyle of the femur to the proximal lateral surface of the fibular head. It is taut when the knee is extended and loose when the knee is flexed, and it serves as the primary restraint to varus stress at the knee.[879] The deepest layer passes along the posterior portion of the lateral meniscus, comprising the coronary ligament (which is longer than the coronary ligament of the medial meniscus, accounting for the increased mobility of the lateral meniscus), and terminates as the arcuate ligament. The arcuate ligament extends from the styloid process of the fibular head to the posterior portion of the joint capsule (near the termination of the oblique popliteal ligament), and it is intimate with the junction of the popliteus muscle and its tendon.[875] A portion of the joint capsule forms the fabellofibular ligament (in cases in which a fabella is present). The popliteus muscle originates in the posterior surface of the proximal portion of the tibia, attaches to the posterior horn of the lateral meniscus and to the arcuate ligament, and terminates in the lateral femoral condyle, distal and posterior to the attachment site of the lateral collateral ligament.[875, 895, 896] The anatomy of the posterolateral corner of the knee (Fig. 70–301) is complex and not agreed upon.[1406] Some refer to this region simply as the arcuate complex (composed of the arcuate ligament, the lateral collateral ligament, the popliteus muscle and tendon, and the tendon of the lateral head of the gastrocnemius muscle).[884, 897]

Hughston and coworkers[884] divide the lateral supporting structures into the anterior third, middle third, and posterior third of the knee. The structures in the anterior third include the capsular ligament, extending posteriorly from the lateral borders of the patella and patellar tendon to the anterior border of the iliotibial tract, reinforced by the lateral retinaculum of the quadriceps tendon. The structures in the middle third are the iliotibial tract and the capsular ligament deep to it, and this segment extends posteriorly as far as the lateral collateral ligament. Structures in the posterior third, including both capsular and noncapsular ligaments, are designated the arcuate complex of the knee (see previous discussion), and are reinforced by the lateral head of the gas-

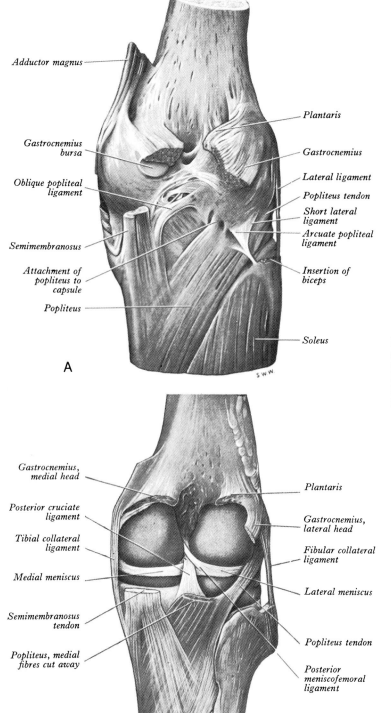

FIGURE 70–301. Posterolateral corner of the knee: Anatomic considerations. Drawings of the superficial **(A)** and deep **(B)** structures in the posterior aspect of the knee are shown. See text for details. (From Williams PL, Warwick R [Eds]: Gray's Anatomy. 36th British edition. Edinburgh, Churchill Livingstone, 1980, pp 452, 453.)

trocnemius muscle and the biceps femoris and popliteus muscles.

Pathologic Considerations. The lateral supporting structures restrain varus angulation at the knee and external rotation of the tibia. The relative contributions of each of these supporting structures in these functions is not clear. The lateral collateral ligament acts as a primary restraint to limit such varus angulation, although deep posterolateral structures provide considerable restraint as a secondary stabilizer. Injuries involving both the lateral collateral liga-

ment and these deep posterolateral structures are associated with greater varus instability than those confined to the lateral collateral ligament.[898] No individual lateral supporting structure appears to act as the primary restraint to external rotation of the tibia; rather, the components of the posterolateral corner of the knee (consisting of the lateral collateral ligament, arcuate ligament, posterior portion of the lateral capsule, and popliteus tendon) function in concert as a complex to limit such external rotation.[898] The lateral supporting structures also act as secondary restraints to limit anterior and posterior motion at the knee. The effect of any one structure in this regard appears to be small, but together the lateral collateral ligament and deep posterolateral structures serve as a major secondary restraint to posterior displacement at the knee from full extension to 30 degrees of flexion.[898]

Injuries to the lateral supporting structures of the knee may be combined with other injuries such as those to the cruciate ligaments. The effects of deficiency of various combinations of knee ligaments and other supporting structures have been studied in vitro, and the data are summarized by Shoemaker and Daniel.[898] Disruptions of both the lateral collateral ligament and deep posterolateral structures yield increases in varus angulation at the knee and external rotation of the tibia and, in addition, minor anteroposterior instability. Combined disruption of the anterior cruciate ligament and deep posterolateral structures without injury to the lateral collateral ligament leads to an increase in anterior movement at the knee without evidence of accentuated external rotation of the tibia or varus angulation of the knee (owing to the restraint provided by the intact lateral collateral ligament). When the anterior cruciate ligament, lateral collateral ligament, and deep posterolateral structures all are incompetent, anterior and varus instability at the knee and exaggerated external rotation of the tibia are seen. Combined injury to the posterior cruciate ligament, lateral collateral ligament, and deep posterolateral structures allows increases in posterior movement, varus angulation, and external rotation of the tibia.

Hughston and collaborators[884] identified six types of lateral instability patterns of the knee encountered in clinical practice: (1) anterolateral rotatory instability caused by disruption of the middle third of the lateral capsular ligament and accentuated by other tears, particularly a tear of the anterior cruciate ligament; (2) posterolateral rotatory instability caused by a tear of the arcuate complex; (3) combined anterolateral and posterolateral rotatory instability caused by disruption of all the lateral capsular ligaments with or without a tear of the iliotibial tract, with an intact posterior cruciate ligament; (4) combined anterolateral and anteromedial rotatory instability caused by tears of the middle thirds of the medial and lateral capsular ligaments with an intact posterior cruciate ligament; (5) combined posterolateral, anterolateral, and anteromedial rotatory instability caused by tears of both the lateral and the medial ligaments; and (6) straight lateral instability caused by tears of the lateral ligaments and the posterior cruciate ligament.

The lateral instability patterns are less frequent than those on the medial side of the knee, although they eventually may be more disabling. Initially, however, clinical findings associated with injuries to the supporting structures in the lateral side of the knee may be subtle and often unrecognized.[884] Acutely, pain and swelling may be evident, the severity of the findings being influenced by the location and extent of the injury. With time, instability of the knee may prevent the patient from participating in sports or even walking. A number of tests administered during physical examination can be employed to check the integrity of the lateral supporting structures as well as of the cruciate ligaments, which also may be injured. Many of these tests rely on the presence or absence, as well as the pattern, of motion that occurs when stress is applied to the injured knee. These tests, which include the anterior and posterior drawer tests

and the adduction and abduction stress tests, are accomplished with varying degrees of flexion or extension of the knee. The results of such testing often allow an accurate diagnosis as to which specific ligaments are injured.[884]

Lateral Collateral Ligament Injuries. Routine radiography in cases of injury to the lateral collateral ligament of the knee generally does not reveal specific findings. Focal soft tissue swelling may be evident in some cases. Furthermore, as the lateral collateral ligament along with the tendon of the biceps femoris muscle attaches to the fibular head and styloid process, avulsion fractures of this portion of the fibula may be seen. The fragment is of variable size and may be large, although it usually is displaced only minimally. Rarely, significant proximal migration, or even entrapment, of the fragment in the lateral compartment of the knee is present. Standard arthrography is not useful in the diagnosis of injuries to the lateral collateral ligament, and the value of CT is restricted to detection of avulsion fractures of the proximal portion of the fibula.

MR imaging represents an effective technique for assessment of the integrity of the lateral collateral ligament and the adjacent tendon of the biceps femoris muscle (Fig. 70–302). These structures can be identified on sagittal, coronal, and transaxial MR images. In posterior MR images in the coronal plane, the normal biceps femoris muscle is seen in the lateral aspect of the leg, above the knee. Its tendon is straight, is of low signal intensity, and attaches to the head and styloid process of the fibula. In coronal images just anterior to those that display the biceps femoris muscle and tendon, the lateral collateral ligament is seen arising from the fibula and extending superiorly and anteriorly to attach to the epicondyle in the distal portion of the femur. It, too, is of low signal intensity. In far lateral MR images in the sagittal plane, a V-shaped region of low signal intensity can be identified. The anterior limb of this region is the lateral collateral ligament, and the posterior limb is the tendon of the biceps femoris muscle. They join in the region of the proximal portion of the fibula. Because of the oblique course of the normal lateral collateral ligament, it may not be seen in its entirety in any single coronal or sagittal MR image.

Disruption of the lateral collateral ligament, the tendon of the biceps femoris muscle, or both structures, is recognized on MR images as an interruption or waviness of these tendons or regions of high signal intensity on T2-weighted spin echo MR images within or adjacent to these tendons[890, 899] (Fig. 70–303). Associated injuries of other lateral supporting structures or the cruciate ligaments also may be evident. In dislocations of the knee, injuries of lateral, medial, and cruciate ligaments are encountered (Fig. 70–304).

Popliteus Muscle and Tendon Injuries. As indicated earlier, the popliteus muscle and tendon contribute significantly to the integrity of the posterolateral region of the knee. The precise role of the popliteus muscle and tendon is not certain, but these structures may initiate and maintain internal rotation of the tibia with respect to the femur, and contribute to prevention of forward displacement of the femur in relation to the tibia during the initial stages of knee flexion.[900] It also has been suggested that the popliteus muscle acts to withdraw, and thereby protect, the lateral meniscus during flexion and rotation of the knee,[900] although some anatomic studies have failed to document a major attachment of the popliteus tendon to the lateral me-

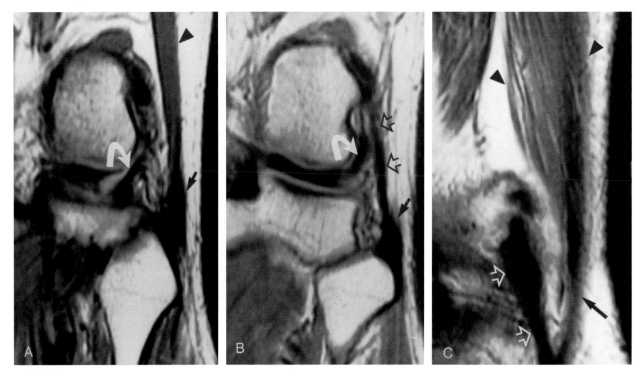

FIGURE 70–302. Normal lateral collateral ligament and biceps femoris muscle and tendon: MR imaging.

A, B Two consecutive coronal proton density–weighted (TR/TE, 2200/20) spin echo MR images show the normal appearance of the biceps femoris muscle (arrowhead) and its tendon (solid straight arrows), and the lateral collateral ligament (open arrows). In **A**, the more posterior scan, the biceps femoris muscle and tendon are seen extending lateral to the joint and inserting into the proximal portion of the fibula. In **B**, the lateral collateral ligament extends from the fibula superiorly to insert into the femur. The popliteus tendon (curved arrows) is identified.

C A sagittal proton density–weighted (TR/TE, 2200/20) spin echo MR image of the lateral aspect of the knee shows the biceps femoris muscle (arrowheads) and its tendon (solid arrow) and the lateral collateral ligament (open arrows). Note the V-like pattern created at the junction of the biceps femoris tendon and lateral collateral ligament.

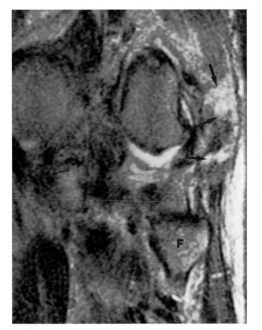

FIGURE 70–303. Injuries of the lateral collateral ligament and biceps femoris muscle and tendon: MR imaging. A coronal T2-weighted (TR/TE, 2500/80) spin echo MR image reveals complete disorganization in the posterolateral region of the knee. Although the fibular head (F) is seen, the tendon of the biceps femoris muscle and the lateral collateral ligament are not identifiable. A joint effusion is seen. Note high signal intensity within the biceps femoris muscle (arrows). An injury of the anterior cruciate ligament also was present in this patient.

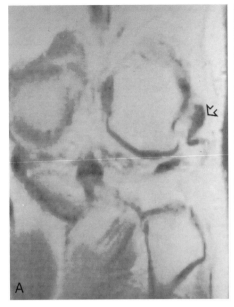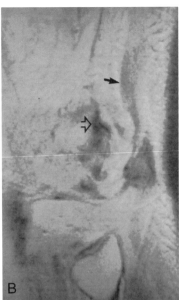

FIGURE 70–304. Injuries of the lateral collateral ligament and biceps femoris muscle and tendon. Coronal **(A)** and sagittal **(B)** proton density–weighted (TR/TE, 1500/40) spin echo MR images reveal interruption and waviness of the lateral collateral ligament (open arrows). The biceps femoris muscle (arrow) is seen, and its tendon is retracted. The anterior and posterior cruciate ligaments also were disrupted in this patient whose knee was dislocated. (Courtesy of A. Newberg, M.D., Boston, Massachusetts.)

niscus.[901] Injuries to the popliteus muscle and tendon may occur in association with injuries to other lateral supporting structures of the knee or, rarely, as an isolated phenomenon.[900, 902, 903] Such isolated injuries may involve sudden external rotation of the tibia when the knee is partially flexed and bearing weight.[902] Clinical findings include an acute hemarthrosis, lateral tenderness, and rarely, injury to the posterior tibial nerve.[902] Avulsion fracture of the femur may be seen with routine radiography, and an abnormal course of or signal intensity within the popliteus tendon or hemorrhage in the popliteus muscle may be seen with MR imaging (Fig. 70–305).

Iliotibial Tract Abnormalities. Injuries to the iliotibial tract usually are combined with injuries to other lateral supporting structures of the knee. Rarely, they may occur as an isolated phenomenon. Avulsion injuries occur at the tibial insertion site of the iliotibial tract (i.e., Gerdy's tubercle), resulting in a small fragment of bone that is difficult

to detect in standard frontal and lateral projections of the knee but that may be seen in oblique projections. As the iliotibial tract can be well evaluated on coronal MR images of the knee, MR imaging can be employed to detect traumatic abnormalities involving this structure. The normal iliotibial tract is observed on coronal MR images as a structure of low signal intensity traversing the lateral portion of the thigh, extending across the lateral aspect of the knee, and inserting in Gerdy's tubercle in the tibia (Fig. 70–306). Discontinuity of this structure and edema in the tibia adjacent to the site of its attachment may be observed when this tract is injured.

The iliotibial tract friction syndrome is related to intense physical activity, as occurs in American football players or long distance runners, that leads to abnormal contact at the iliotibial tract and the lateral femoral epicondyle.[904–906] Pain occurs in the lateral aspect of the thigh and knee, particularly with 30 degrees of flexion of the knee.[906] Although the

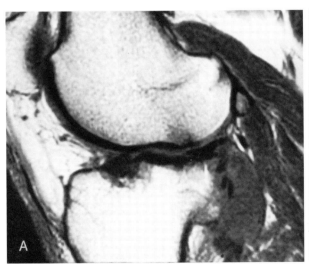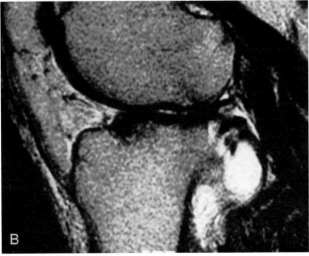

FIGURE 70–305. Injuries of the popliteus muscle: MR imaging. Coronal proton density–weighted (TR/TE, 2000/20) **(A)** and T2-weighted (TR/TE, 2000/80) **(B)** spin echo MR images show an enlarged popliteus muscle with high signal intensity in **B**. The findings are consistent with an intramuscular hematoma. Note anterior translation of the tibia with respect to the femur, indicating a tear of the anterior cruciate ligament. (Courtesy of M. Schweitzer, M.D., Philadelphia, Pennsylvania.)

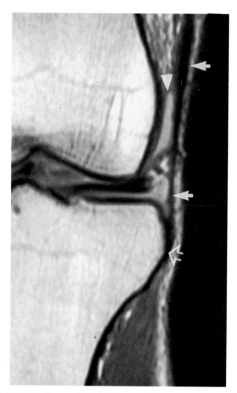

FIGURE 70–306. Normal iliotibial tract: MR imaging. A coronal proton density–weighted (TR/TE, 2000/20) spin echo MR image shows the iliotibial tract (solid arrows) attaching to Gerdy's tubercle (open arrow) in the tibia. A small joint effusion is evident, just medial to the iliotibial tract (arrowhead).

diagnosis of this syndrome can be established on the basis of clinical findings, similar clinical manifestations occur in association with injuries to the lateral ligaments of the knee or lateral meniscus. In one report, MR imaging produced evidence of the iliotibial tract friction syndrome owing to the presence of fluid collections or edema adjacent to the iliotibial tract.[907] The MR imaging findings, however, resemble those of a joint effusion with fluid accumulating in the suprapatellar bursa.

Other Lateral Capsular Ligament Injuries. A characteristic and important injury involves an avulsion fracture of the tibial rim that occurs at the site of attachment of the lateral capsular ligament of the knee. Described in 1879 (before the discovery of x-rays) by Segond,[908] this fracture results from forces of internal rotation and varus stress at the knee and is known simply as the Segond fracture. The resulting bone fragment easily is overlooked unless the lateral margin of the tibia is carefully analyzed on the anteroposterior and tunnel radiographic views of the knee (Fig. 70–307A). An elliptically shaped piece of bone, measuring up to 10 mm in length, occurs at the joint line or just proximal to it, and the donor site in the tibia reveals an irregular surface. The location of the Segond fracture is posterior and slightly proximal to Gerdy's tubercle, the insertion site of the iliotibial tract and, therefore, the fracture should not be misinterpreted as evidence of an injury to the iliotibial tract. With healing, the avulsed fragment may unite with the lateral tibial margin, creating a bone excrescence below the joint line that simulates the appearance of an osteophyte (Fig. 70–307B,C).

Although subtle and seemingly innocent, this lateral tibial rim fracture is indicative of anterolateral instability of the knee, which may become chronic and disabling if the fracture is not recognized and appropriately treated in the acute stage. There is a high association of the Segond fracture with injuries to the anterior cruciate ligament (75 to 100 per cent of cases) and tears of the menisci (60 to 70 per cent of cases).[892, 909]

The MR imaging findings of the Segond fracture also are characteristic.[910] The dominant finding is marrow edema adjacent to the site of fracture (Fig. 70–308). The fracture fragment itself often is not visible, owing to its small size. Associated injuries to the cruciate ligaments and menisci often are visible, and some of these may be accompanied by additional bone injuries with resulting marrow edema.

Abnormalities of the Anterior Supporting Structures

Anatomic Considerations. In the anterior aspect of the knee, ligaments, muscles, aponeuroses, and joint capsule

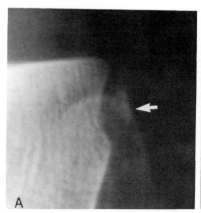
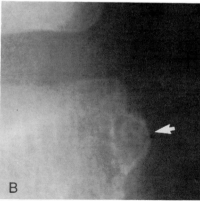
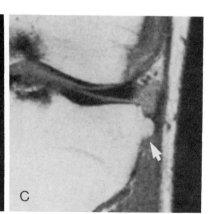

FIGURE 70–307. Injuries of the lateral capsular ligament (Segond fracture): Routine radiography and MR imaging.
  A The typical appearance of the Segond fracture fragment (arrow) is evident.
  B The bone excrescence on the lateral surface of the tibia (arrow) indicates a healed Segond fracture.
  C A coronal T1-weighted (TR/TE, 650/20) spin echo MR image shows the bone prominence (arrow) in the tibia indicative of a previous healed Segond fracture.
  (Courtesy of G. Bock, M.D., Winnipeg, Manitoba, Canada.)

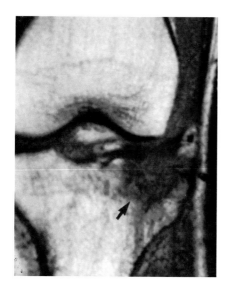

FIGURE 70–308. Injuries of the lateral capsular ligament (Segond fracture): MR imaging. A coronal T1-weighted (TR/TE, 800/25) spin echo MR image shows low signal intensity (arrow) in the lateral aspect of the proximal portion of the tibia, indicating marrow edema. A large joint effusion is evident. The fracture fragment is not well seen. A tear of the anterior cruciate ligament also was present.

converge to surround the centrally located patella, providing an adequate stabilizing system[911] (Fig. 70–309). These structures, individually or in small groups, lead to forces on the patella that are oriented superiorly (quadriceps muscles), inferiorly (patellar tendon), medially (medial patellar retinaculum and vastus medialis muscle), or laterally (lateral patellar retinaculum, vastus lateralis muscle, and iliotibial tract). Together they stabilize the patella, owing to both passive and active elements.

Passive soft tissue stabilizers are the patellar tendon, medial and lateral patellofemoral ligaments, medial and lateral meniscopatellar ligaments, and portions of the fascia lata. The major passive stabilizer of the patella is the patellar tendon (also referred to as the patellar ligament), extending from the inferior pole of the patella to the tibial tuberosity. This is a broad, flat structure 4 to 6 cm in length and approximately 7 mm in thickness, that diminishes in width from top to bottom. The patellar tendon is approximately 3 cm wide superiorly and 2.5 cm wide inferiorly at its insertion site in the tibial tuberosity.[912] The course of the patellar tendon almost is parallel to the long axis of the lower extremity, although it commonly reveals a slight oblique lateral orientation from proximal to distal, which contributes to a tendency toward lateral displacement of the pa-

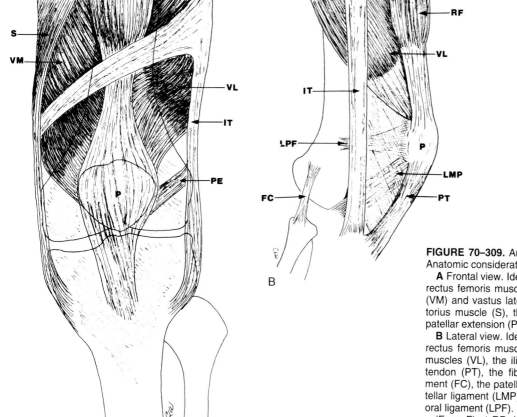

FIGURE 70–309. Anterior supporting structures: Anatomic considerations.

A Frontal view. Identified structures include the rectus femoris muscle (RF), the vastus medialis (VM) and vastus lateralis (VL) muscles, the sartorius muscle (S), the iliotibial tract (IT) and its patellar extension (PE), and the patella (P).

B Lateral view. Identified structures include the rectus femoris muscle (RF), the vastus lateralis muscles (VL), the iliotibial tract (IT), the patellar tendon (PT), the fibular (lateral) collateral ligament (FC), the patella (P), the lateral meniscopatellar ligament (LMP), and the lateral patellofemoral ligament (LPF).

(From Ficat RP, Hungerford DS: Disorders of the Patello-Femoral Joint. Baltimore, Williams and Wilkins, 1977, pp 16, 17.)

tella.[911] Capsular condensations or retinacula link the patella to both medial and lateral epicondyles of the femur and to the anterior portions of the medial and lateral menisci. Medially, these condensations include the medial patellofemoral ligament above and the medial meniscopatellar ligament below; laterally, these condensations include the lateral patellofemoral ligament above and the lateral meniscopatellar ligament below.[911] Further lateral reinforcement is provided by the patellar expansion of the fascia lata. As a group, the lateral soft tissue stabilizers are stronger than the medial soft tissue stabilizers.

The four components of the quadriceps muscle represent the active elements of the soft tissue stabilizers. These components are the rectus femoris, vastus lateralis, vastus medialis, and vastus intermedius muscles, which terminate as four tendons that merge several centimeters above the patella, forming the quadriceps tendon, and subsequently attach to the patella. Three layers of the quadriceps tendon can be identified. The tendon of the rectus femoris muscle is located in the superficial layer. As it descends, its tendinous fibers become deeper in location, situated beneath the fleshy muscle fibers. This tendon attaches to the anterior surface of the patella, with a distal extension that continues on to attach to the superficial part of the patellar tendon. The intermediate or middle layer of the quadriceps tendon results from the fusion of the tendons of the vastus lateralis and vastus medialis muscles. Together, the fused tendons of these two muscles attach to the base of the patella, just posterior to the insertion site of the rectus femoris fibers; individually, they extend over the lateral and medial borders of the patella.[911] The tendon of the vastus intermedius muscle occupies the third, and deepest, layer of the quadriceps tendon, inserting into the base of the patella.

Several bursae exist superficial and deep to these anterior supporting structures. The deep infrapatellar, or pretibial, bursa is situated at the base of the infrapatellar fat body, between the patellar tendon in front and the anterosuperior portion of the tibia behind. Prepatellar bursae exist in front of the patella itself. They may be situated in the subcutaneous tissue, in the aponeurosis, or in the tendinous fibers.

Variations in the shape of the patella, as well as of the patellar surface of the femur, are well recognized,[913–916] and some of these may be causative factors of patellar instability and retropatellar pain. Several classification systems exist for patellar shape (Fig. 70–310), that of Wiberg[913] being cited most often. The Wiberg classification system includes three types of patellar configuration: type 1 patellae have medial and lateral patellar facets, approximately equal in size, both with a concave appearance; type 2 patellae (the most common type) also have concave articular surfaces, with the medial facet being slightly smaller than the lateral facet; and type 3 patellae possess a small medial facet with a convex articular surface. The value of this and other classification systems of patellar (and distal femoral) shape in predicting the likelihood of patellofemoral instability has yet to be proved, and the precision of detecting patellar shape on the basis of axial radiographs of the knee (or transaxial sections provided by CT or MR imaging) requires further study.

The patella has several functions, the most important of which is strengthening the force of knee extension by providing a more anterior fulcrum for this movement. The relationship of the patella and the femur is dependent upon

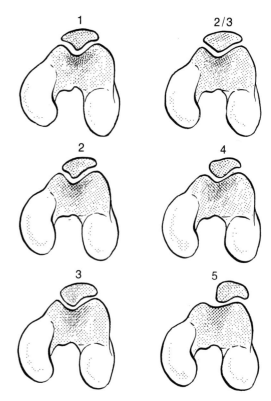

FIGURE 70–310. Patella: Anatomic variations in shape. Patellar configurations have been delineated by Wiberg, Baumgarten, and other investigators and are summarized in this drawing. For each image, the medial condyle is depicted on the left and the lateral condyle is depicted on the right. Type 1 patellae have equal facets, which are slightly concave. Type 2 patellae are similar, with concave surfaces and a smaller medial facet. Type 3 patellae possess a small medial facet with a convex surface. Type 2/3 patellae have a flat medial facet. Type 4 patellae possess a small or absent medial facet. Type 5 (Jagerhut) patellae demonstrate no medial facet, no central ridge, and lateral subluxation.

the degree of flexion or extension of the knee. In the fully extended position, the patella lies above the trochlear surface of the femur, and it rests on a layer of subsynovial fat.[913] Its precise position in a medial-lateral direction in the extended knee depends on the degree of contraction of the quadriceps mechanism.[911] Furthermore, the ''screw home'' mechanism of the femorotibial joint that occurs in the final degrees of extension, in which the tibia rotates externally with respect to the femur, lateralizes the tibial tubercle.[911] This external rotation produces a valgus vector between the line of pull of the quadriceps tendon and that of the patellar tendon, designated the Q-angle. This vector is resisted by the passive and active medial stabilizers of the knee. As the knee is flexed, the tibia internally rotates, decreasing the Q-angle and the lateral vector, and contact of the patella and the trochlea increases, initially involving the lower pole of the patella, and later more and more of the patellar surface. Increasing stability is afforded by the trochlea as it embraces the patella.[911] The point at which the patella becomes centered in the trochlea varies, although at 90 degrees of knee flexion, centering of the patella in the trochlea almost is a universal finding.[917] At this degree of flexion, or with further flexion of the knee beyond 90 degrees, the quadriceps tendon and, eventually, the odd facet of the patella articulate with portions of the femur.[915, 918] The size of the contact area between femur and patella varies according to the position of the knee. In general, the contact area is greater with increasing degrees of knee flexion.[918]

Pathologic Considerations. Abnormalities of the anterior supporting structures of the knee are related to alterations in the anatomy of the patella and adjacent patellar articular surface of the femur and the constantly changing compressive and tensile forces generated during the complex movement of this joint. The syndromes and disorders related to disuse, overuse, misuse, or injuries of various anterior supporting structures include chondromalacia patellae, patellar tendinitis, disruption of the quadriceps musculature and tendon and the patellar tendon, osteochondritis dissecans of the patella, osteochondral fractures of the patella and femur, patellar instability with subluxation or dislocation, Osgood-Schlatter disease, and deep infrapatellar and prepatellar bursitis. A review of some of these entities is provided in the following sections of this chapter, but the interested reader also should refer to other chapters of this book dealing with patellar instability (Chapter 68), chondromalacia and patellofemoral osteoarthritis (Chapter 39), Osgood-Schlatter and Sinding-Larsen–Johansson disease (Chapter 81), and osteochondritis dissecans and osteochondral fractures of the patella (Chapter 67). Furthermore, a review of standard radiographic techniques applied to the patellofemoral joint is contained in Chapter 1, and radiographic measurements used to determine patellar position are contained in Chapter 22. Consideration of chondromalacia patellae also is included in the discussion of the assessment of articular cartilage later in this chapter.

Patellar Tendinitis. Patellar tendinitis appears to represent an overuse syndrome related to sudden and repetitive extension of the knee that may occur in persons, particularly athletes, involved in such activities as kicking, jumping, and running.[919–921] This syndrome, often referred to as jumper's knee, leads to local pain, swelling, and tenderness that ultimately may result in disruption of the patellar tendon. As the major histologic findings associated with patellar tendinitis are not those of inflammation but rather those of fiber failure, mucoid degeneration, and fibrinoid necrosis,[919, 922] the term tendinitis may be inappropriate, as inflammatory changes may represent the response to the injury rather than the primary event.[923] Clinical manifestations include activity-related pain below the patella that initially is intermittent but may become persistent.[920] Men are involved more commonly than women.

Routine radiographs usually do not provide diagnostic information in cases of patellar tendinitis. Soft tissue swelling, thickening of the patellar tendon, and obscuration of portions of the infrapatellar fat body may be evident, but these findings are depicted more easily on CT and MR images. Bone scintigraphy shows nonspecific accumulation of the radionuclide in the infrapatellar soft tissues or patella.[924] Ultrasonography reveals an enlarged and hypoechoic tendon, particularly in its proximal portion.[925–927] With CT, the enlarged tendon with central expansion near the inferior pole of the patella and with decreased attenuation values is evident.[926]

MR images in the sagittal plane display the entire length of the patellar tendon (Fig. 70–311). In an analysis of such images in asymptomatic persons, Schweitzer and associates[1354] noted that the mean thickness of the patellar tendon was 5.2 mm, being slightly thicker in men. The mean

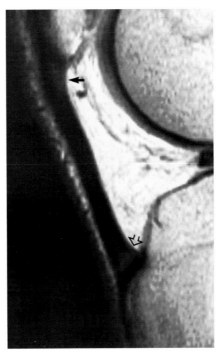

FIGURE 70–311. Normal patellar tendon: MR imaging. As shown in this sagittal proton density–weighted (TR/TE, 3000/20) spin echo MR image, the patellar tendon typically has low signal intensity throughout its length, although intermediate signal intensity in the posterior margin of the proximal portion of the tendon (solid arrow) and in a triangular area near its distal insertion (open arrow) may be evident. (Courtesy of J. Yu, M.D., Columbus, Ohio.)

of the thickness of the patellar tendon to the thickness of the quadriceps tendon in this study was 0.72. Focal regions of increased signal intensity within the patellar tendon in T1-weighted spin echo MR images were frequent, particularly proximally, and the signal intensity did not increase in T2-weighted spin echo MR images. Schweitzer and coworkers[1354] also observed subtle buckling of the patellar tendon in these asymptomatic persons, a finding that was more prominent in those with joint effusions.

MR imaging in patients with patellar tendinitis shows an enlarged sagittal diameter of the tendon, with a mean value of 10.9 mm in one series[923] (Fig. 70–312). The proximal portion of the patellar tendon usually is thickened more than its distal portion, but in severe cases both portions may be involved.[923, 926] An indistinct margin to the posterior aspect of the tendon may be combined with regions of increased intratendinous signal intensity.[922, 923] The increased signal intensity may be more evident on STIR images.

As indicated previously, in certain MR imaging sequences, such as spoiled gradient recalled images in the steady state (spoiled GRASS), foci of increased signal intensity may be seen in tendons that are not enlarged. The cause of these foci is not clear. Regions of cartilage metaplasia or mucoid degeneration may be responsible for these changes. Mucoid degeneration has been documented as a histologic occurrence in patellar tendons, sometimes in association with cystic enlargement (mucoid cysts) of the tendon.[928]

Tears of the Patellar and Quadriceps Tendons. Indirect forces applied to the extensor mechanism of the knee can lead to failure of one or more of its components, includ-

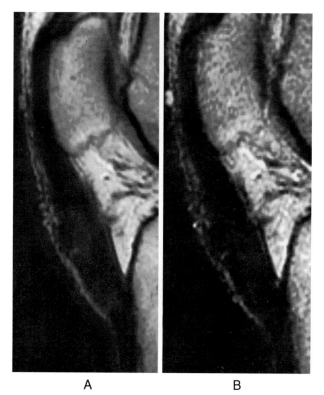

A   B

FIGURE 70–312. Chronic patellar tendinitis: MR imaging. Sagittal proton density–weighted (TR/TE, 2200/30) **(A)** and T2-weighted (TR/TE, 2200/80) **(B)** spin echo MR images show marked thickening of the entire patellar tendon, more pronounced in the middle and distal segments, and indistinctness of the anterior margin of the tendon. No increase in signal intensity within the patellar tendon is seen in **B**. (Courtesy of J. Yu, M.D., Columbus, Ohio.)

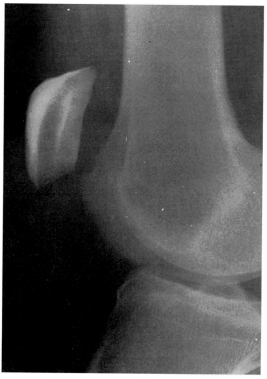

FIGURE 70–313. Complete tears of the patellar tendon: Routine radiography. A complete tear of the patellar tendon is associated with a high position of the patella, designated patella alta.

ing the patella, quadriceps tendon, or patellar tendon.[929] Failure of the patella, resulting in fracture, is common, especially in adults (see Chapter 68). Systemic disorders, such as rheumatoid arthritis, chronic renal disease, and systemic lupus erythematosus, contribute to failure of the quadriceps and patellar tendons (see Chapters 25, 26, 33, and 57), although such failure, particularly of the patellar tendon, may occur in the absence of these causative factors. Patellar tendon ruptures are not uncommon in persons with chronic patellar tendinitis, and they may occur spontaneously or after vigorous physical exercise. Failure of the patellar tendon usually occurs at its junction with the inferior pole of the patella or, less commonly, with the tibial tuberosity, although intrasubstance disruption of the patellar tendon also may occur. Complete tears of the patellar tendon are associated with a high position of the patella, designated patella alta (Fig. 70–313). Incomplete tears are unassociated with this change in patellar position. Although CT and ultrasonography can be used to verify complete or incomplete tears of the patellar tendon, MR imaging displays these tears most vividly (Figs. 70–314 and 70–315). Typically, the tendon is thickened, and complete or incomplete disruption of its fibers is evident. In recent tears, foci of increased signal intensity are observed in the patellar tendon and adjacent soft tissues on T2-weighted spin echo, certain gradient echo, and STIR images.

Partial or complete tears of the quadriceps tendon may result from an injury involving a direct blow to the tendon or forceful flexion of the knee[930]; or they may occur spon-

taneously in association with such chronic diseases as systemic lupus erythematosus, rheumatoid arthritis, gout, or renal failure, or following corticosteroid therapy.[931–934] Rarely, spontaneous rupture of the quadriceps tendon oc-

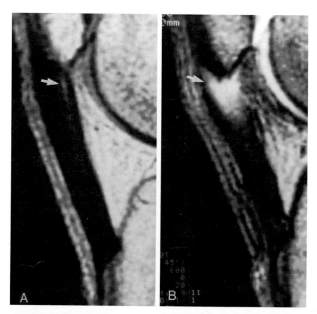

FIGURE 70–314. Partial tears of the patellar tendon: MR imaging. A sagittal T1-weighted (TR/TE, 850/25) spin echo MR image **(A)** and a sagittal MPGR MR image (TR/TE, 600/20; flip angle, 45 degrees) **(B)** reveal a partial tear (arrows) involving the proximal portion of the patellar tendon and thickening of the entire tendon, indicating chronic patellar tendinitis. The findings of partial patellar tendon rupture are much more pronounced in **B**. (Courtesy of S. Fernandez, M.D., Mexico City, Mexico.)

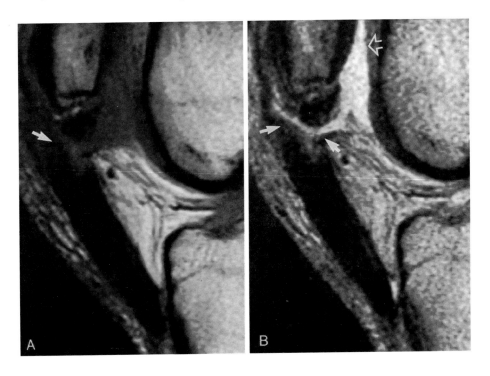

FIGURE 70–315. Complete tears of the patellar tendon: MR imaging. Sagittal proton density–weighted (TR/TE, 2000/20) **(A)** and T2-weighted (TR/TE, 2000/80) **(B)** spin echo MR images reveal complete disruption (solid arrows) of the patellar tendon at its proximal insertion site. The tendon is thickened, fragmentation of the lower pole of the patella is seen, soft tissue edema is present, and a lipohemarthrosis with a fat-blood fluid level (open arrow) is evident. (Courtesy of J. Lyons, M.D., San Diego, California.)

curs in healthy persons.[935] Unilateral or bilateral tendon disruptions have been described. The clinical diagnosis of a complete tear of the quadriceps tendon usually is obvious, based on the patient's history, his or her inability to extend the knee, a hemarthrosis or soft tissue hematoma, and a palpable or visible gap in the soft tissues above the patella.[923, 936–938] Delays in such diagnosis are encountered, however, which in one report ranged from 14 days to 1 year after the injury.[936]

Routine radiographic findings associated with complete tears of the quadriceps tendon include soft tissue swelling, distortion of soft tissue planes above the patella, an inferior position of the patella (patella infera or baja), calcification or ossification within portions of an avulsed patellar fragment, and an undulating patellar tendon[934] (Fig. 70–316A). Similar but less dramatic findings accompany partial tears of the quadriceps tendon. Standard arthrography in cases of partial[939] or complete[940] disruptions of the quadriceps tendon may be diagnostic (Fig. 70–316B). Contrast material introduced into the knee joint will extend outside the quadriceps tendon[941] and, in some cases, will extend into the deep infrapatellar or prepatellar bursa. Owing to the superficial location of the quadriceps tendon, ultrasonography also may be used in its assessment.[942, 1407]

Sagittal MR images display the quadriceps tendon in exquisite detail (Fig. 70–317). A laminated appearance with two, three, or four layers of tissue characterizes the MR imaging appearance of the normal quadriceps tendon.[943] This laminated structure is more evident in the medial aspect of the tendon, and its lateral portion may appear as a single thick band of low signal intensity. Transaxial MR images confirm that the superficial layer of the quadriceps tendon originates from the rectus femoris muscle, the deep layer originates from the vastus intermedius muscle, and the middle layer (or layers) is composed of fibers derived from the vastus medialis and vastus lateralis muscles.[943] The average thickness (anteroposterior plane) of the quadriceps tendon, defined in MR images, is approximately 8 mm, and

its average width (medial-lateral plane) is approximately 35 mm.

With the knee in full extension, the normal quadriceps tendon appears as a relatively straight band of tissue of low signal intensity in sagittal MR images, and in these images the patellar tendon also is straight and of low signal intensity. Tears of the quadriceps tendon lead to partial or complete interruption of its fibers (Fig. 70–318), displayed in all three imaging planes.[937, 938, 943] An undulating, corrugated, or wrinkled appearance to the patellar tendon in the sagittal MR images is secondary evidence of disruption of

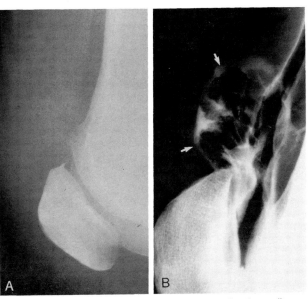

FIGURE 70–316. Tears of the quadriceps tendon: Routine radiography and arthrography.

A Routine radiographic findings include obliteration of normal soft tissue planes above the patella, a joint effusion, and an inferior position of the patella (patella infera or baja).

B Arthrography in a different patient shows anterior extravasation (arrows) of air and radiopaque contrast material above the patella.

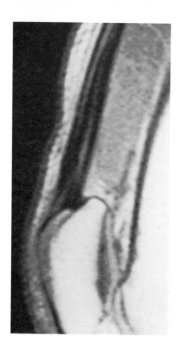

FIGURE 70–317. Normal quadriceps tendon: MR imaging. A sagittal proton density–weighted (TR/TE, 3000/20) spin echo MR image shows a trilaminar appearance of the quadriceps tendon. The superficial layer relates to the tendon of the rectus femoris muscle, the middle layer relates to the tendons of the vastus medialis and vastus lateralis muscles, and the deep layer relates to the tendon of the vastus intermedius muscle. (Courtesy of J. Yu, M.D., Columbus, Ohio.)

FIGURE 70–318. Partial and complete tears of the quadriceps tendon: MR imaging.

A, B Partial tear. Sagittal proton density–weighted (TR/TE, 2500/20) **(A)** and T2-weighted (TR/TE, 2500/80) **(B)** spin echo MR images show disruption of the normal trilaminar appearance of the quadriceps tendon. The tendon (solid arrows) of the vastus intermedius muscle appears intact. The other tendons have retracted (open arrows). Note the high signal intensity at the site of the tear (arrowhead) and in the soft tissues and muscles in **B**.

C, D Complete tear. Sagittal proton density–weighted (TR/TE, 2500/30) **(C)** and T2-weighted (TR/TE, 2500/80) **(D)** spin echo MR images show a complete tear (arrows) of the quadriceps tendon at the tendo-osseous junction. Note the high signal intensity at the site of the tear in **D**. The patella is displaced inferiorly.

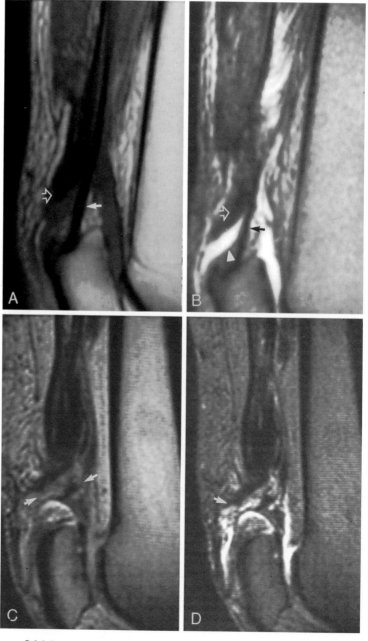

the quadriceps tendon or some other portion of the extensor mechanism[937] (Fig. 70–319). In cases of partial tears of the quadriceps tendon, the alterations in its morphology, as depicted by MR imaging, are more subtle, although careful assessment of serial transaxial images usually allows a correct diagnosis.[943] With either partial or complete tears of this tendon, hemorrhage and edema lead to an increase in signal intensity on T2-weighted spin echo and some gradient echo MR images in the acute stage.

Patellofemoral Instability. Patellofemoral instability is a frequent and complex problem that has been studied extensively. The clinical diagnosis of such instability often is difficult, as the resulting symptoms and signs may simulate those of other disorders of the knee. Although observation of the manner in which the patella moves with respect to the femur during flexion and extension of the knee can be accomplished during physical examination, alterations in such movement may be subtle and, further, disagreement exists regarding the precise normal position of the patella during various degrees of flexion and extension of the knee.[917, 944] It is not surprising, therefore, that clinicians have turned to other diagnostic techniques in an effort to provide verification of patellofemoral tracking abnormalities.

Routine radiography, employing standard radiographic projections, has been used to define the position of the patella, particularly in the vertical plane. On the basis of the lateral projection, the position of the patella relative to the joint line can be ascertained. A high-riding patella, or patella alta, has been associated with recurrent lateral patellar subluxations or dislocations, chondromalacia patellae, Sinding-Larsen–Johansson disease, and joint effusions.[911, 945–947] A low-riding patella, or patella baja, has been identified in neuromuscular disorders, in achondroplasia, and following certain surgical procedures involving transfer of the

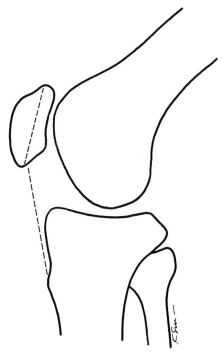

FIGURE 70–320. Patellar position: Insall-Salvati method. The ratio of patellar tendon length to the greatest diagonal length of the patella may be used to diagnose patella alta.

tibial tuberosity.[911] A number of different methods based upon the patellar position in the lateral radiograph have been described to confirm the presence of patella alta or baja; the Insall-Salvati ratio[946] and methods described by Blumensaat,[948] Brattstrom,[949] and Labelle and Laurin[950] are most popular. The advantage of the Insall-Salvati method relates to its nondependency on the degree of flexion of the knee joint. This technique requires determination of the length of the patellar tendon and that of the patella (Fig. 70–320). The normal ratio of the first measurement to the second is approximately 1. Drawbacks to this method, including inability to identify precisely the insertion site of the patellar tendon, and more importantly, variations in patellar shape, have led to interest in a modified Insall-Salvati ratio, in which the length or location of the articular surface of the patella is determined and compared with the position of the joint line or the length of the patellar tendon.[951–953]

Axial radiographic views used to access the configuration of the trochlea, the patellar shape, and the relationship of the patella to the femur also have been employed.[911] A variety of different techniques, described in Chapter 1, are available, but all emphasize the inadequacy of the standard ''skyline'' view in assessing the patellar position. As this view is obtained with knee flexion beyond 90 degrees, it does not allow examination of the patellofemoral relationships in lesser degrees of knee flexion, during which patellar instability is a greater problem. Thus, axial radiographic projections obtained with 20, 30, or 45 degrees of knee flexion have advantages when compared with the skyline view,[911, 954, 955] and many allow detection not only of patellar displacement but also of patellar tilt when a number of lines are constructed and angles measured (Fig. 70–321).

Transaxial images provided by CT and MR imaging (Fig. 70–322) allow assessment of patellar position with the knee

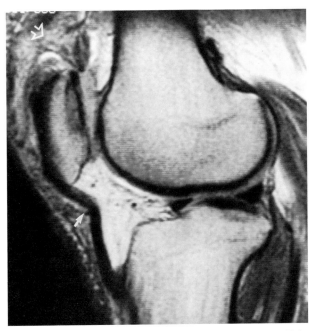

FIGURE 70–319. Complete tear of the quadriceps tendon: MR imaging. A sagittal proton density–weighted (TR/TE, 2000/20) MR image demonstrates an abnormal contour of the patellar tendon (solid arrow) related to a complete tear (open arrow) of the quadriceps tendon.

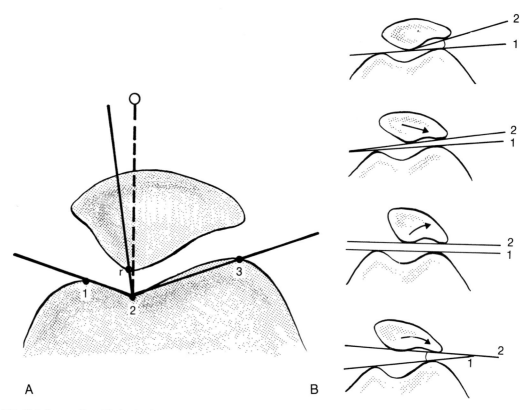

FIGURE 70–321. Patellar position: Methods of measurement of lateral patellar displacement and patellar tilt.
A Merchant and coworkers (Merchant AC, et al: J Bone Joint Surg [Am] *56:*1391, 1974) have suggested that on an axial radiograph, the line connecting the median ridge of the patella (r) and trochlear depth (2) should fall medial to or slightly lateral to a line (O) bisecting angle 1-2-3. Here the first line lies medial to line O, a normal finding.
B Laurin and coworkers have indicated other measurements that might be appropriate. The upper two diagrams reveal the normal situation; the lower two diagrams indicate the abnormal situation. On axial radiographs, normally an angle formed between a line connecting the anterior aspect of the femoral condyles (1) and a second line along the lateral facet of the patella (2) opens laterally. In patients with subluxation of the patella, these lines are parallel or the angle of intersection opens medially.
(**B**, From Laurin CA, et al: J Bone Joint Surg [Am] *60:*55, 1978.)

extended and with minor degrees of knee flexion (with and without contraction of the quadriceps mechanism).[917, 944, 956–958, 1355] Both imaging techniques also allow investigation of patellofemoral relationships during various stages of flexion and extension of the knee, usually accomplished by obtaining multiple static images that are viewed in a movie format.[959] Kinematic MR imaging of the patellofemoral joint has been studied extensively by Shellock and col-

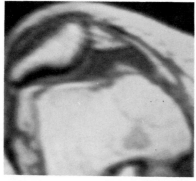

FIGURE 70–322. Patellofemoral instability: MR imaging. A transaxial T1-weighted (TR/TE, 600/20) spin echo MR image obtained with 10 degrees of flexion of the knee shows lateral displacement of the patella.

leagues,[960–964] Brossman and coworkers,[965, 1408] and Niitsu and colleagues.[966] Newer modifications of these techniques allow active movement by the patient, loading the knee to better simulate walking or other physical activities, rapid scanning with a variety of gradient recalled imaging methods, and motion-triggered cine MR imaging. These methods have provided information regarding patterns of lateral subluxation of the patella, the excessive lateral pressure syndrome associated with tilting of the patella (with little or no associated lateral displacement) that increases with flexion of the knee, and medial displacement of the patella that may occur as a complication of arthroscopic lateral retinacular release.[961, 967]

Lateral dislocation (or subluxation) of the patella often is a transient phenomenon, with spontaneous reduction.[968] Diagnosis based upon results of physical examination and clinical history may be difficult, and identification of characteristic osteochondral and avulsion fractures on routine radiography provides important information in many cases (see Chapter 68). Patellar dislocations usually result from a twisting injury with the knee in flexion and the femur rotated internally on a fixed foot. The patella is pulled laterally from the trochlea and across the lateral femoral condyle, leading to osteochondral injuries of the medial patellar facet, lateral femoral condyle, or both structures[969] (Fig. 70–323). The medial retinaculum is injured as a result of dis-

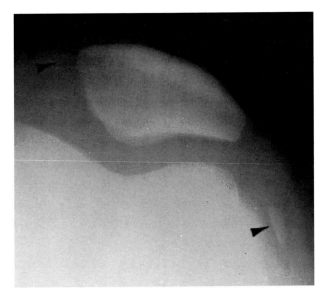

FIGURE 70–323. Patellofemoral instability: Routine radiography. An axial radiograph reveals the characteristic fractures of the lateral femoral condyle and medial aspect of the patella (arrowheads) that may accompany lateral dislocation of the patella.

traction, or a small avulsion fracture at the patellar site of attachment of the medial retinaculum occurs. These pathologic findings can be observed directly on MR images of the knee obtained shortly after the injury[969, 970] (Fig. 70–324). Bone contusions lead to signal intensity changes in the marrow that reflect edema.[1356, 1357] The location of the marrow edema in the lateral femoral condyle following a patellar dislocation may be more lateral and superior to that seen with anterior cruciate ligament injuries.[969] A sprain of the medial retinaculum is characterized by thickening and increased signal intensity in T2-weighted spin echo MR images, related to edema and hemorrhage; disruption and avulsion of the retinaculum are associated with loss of integrity of its fibers, with similar changes in signal intensity.[969] Defects in the articular cartilage of the patella also may be evident, but their detection with MR imaging often requires specialized sequences (see later discussion). Fol-

lowing a lateral patellar dislocation, the patella may assume a more lateral position or may be tilted abnormally, owing to loss of integrity of the medial retinaculum.

Excessive Lateral Pressure Syndrome. Although, traditionally, axial radiographs of the knee have been used to diagnose lateral subluxation of the patella with respect to the femur, they occasionally demonstrate a normally located patella that is abnormally tilted to the lateral side. This finding led to the concept of an excessive lateral pressure syndrome affecting the articular surface of the lateral facet of the patella and that of the adjacent articular portion of the femur. The clinical manifestations of this syndrome have been well summarized by Ficat and Hungerford.[911] Adults or adolescents are affected, and patellofemoral pain, sometimes precipitated by an injury, is evident. Manual subluxation of the patella while the patient flexes the knee may initiate or aggravate the pain. Loss of articular cartilage in the lateral facet of the patella and adjacent articular portion of the femur, and sclerosis and cyst formation in the subchondral bone of the patella and femur may be observed. The cartilage loss is believed to be more extensive and different in location than that seen in classic chondromalacia patellae.[911] Causes of the excessive lateral pressure syndrome are not clear, but they may relate to breakdown in one or more of the structures that contribute to medial stability of the patella (e.g., medial retinaculum and vastus medialis muscle) or to alterations in the shape of the lateral trochlea or lateral articular facet of the patella.[911]

Chondromalacia Patellae. As discussed in Chapter 39, chondromalacia patellae is a term applied to cartilage loss involving one or more portions of the patella that leads to patellofemoral pain. Initially described in 1924 by Aleman[971] as a cause of crepitus and synovitis of the knee, the term has been applied loosely to a host of different disorders leading to patellofemoral pain, in which loss of patellar cartilage either is not documented, is not present, or occurs in combination with other morphologic changes. This has led to the designation patellofemoral pain syndrome as a more appropriate description of those diseases associated with retropatellar pain.[911, 915, 972] Such disorders include (but are not limited to) prepatellar bursitis, deep infrapatellar

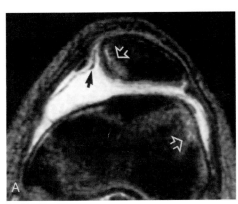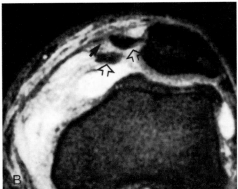

FIGURE 70–324. Patellofemoral instability: MR imaging.
  A A transaxial MPGR MR image (TR/TE, 500/11; flip angle, 15 degrees) shows disruption of the medial patellar retinaculum (solid arrow) and marrow edema with increased signal intensity (open arrows) in the medial aspect of the patella and the lateral femoral condyle. A large joint effusion is present.
  B A transaxial MPGR MR image (TR/TE, 500/11; flip angle, 15 degrees) in a second patient shows disruption of the medial patellar retinaculum (solid arrow) and two bone fragments (open arrows) that originated from the medial aspect of the patella. Note the large joint effusion and soft tissue edema. (Courtesy of S. K. Brahme, M.D., La Jolla, California.)

bursitis, pes anserinus bursitis, the plica syndrome, the excessive lateral pressure syndrome, osteoarthritis, and even meniscal tears.

Fundamental to the diagnosis of chondromalacia patellae is the presence of histologic abnormalities affecting the articular cartilage of the patella. Whether specific histologic findings in the articular cartilage allow separation of chondromalacia from other processes that involve the patellar cartilage is not clear. Goodfellow and colleagues[915] defined two separate processes, basal degeneration and surface degeneration, that affected the patellar cartilage: basal degeneration was defined as fasciculation of collagen in the middle and deep zones of cartilage (that later might affect the chondral surface), and was believed to occur in the ridge separating the medial and odd facets of the patella in young persons, perhaps related to excessive pressure. Surface degeneration was thought to begin in the young and progress throughout life, perhaps culminating in osteoarthritis of the patellofemoral joint.

Numerous classification systems for chondromalacia patellae have been proposed, generally based upon the anatomic extent or the severity of the articular cartilage loss in the patella. As assessment of patellar articular cartilage on the basis of routine and advanced imaging methods is difficult and often inadequate, accurate classification of chondromalacia patellae requires direct observation, and even probing of the articular surface of the patella, which can be accomplished arthroscopically. Arthroscopically evident grades of chondromalacia have been described[973]: (1) fibrillation or softening of articular cartilage involving one or more facets of the patella, without involvement of the femur; (2) erosion or fragmentation of the articular surface that is limited to the patella; and (3) changes in the articular cartilage in both the patella and the femur. Another classification system is based on the anatomic distribution of the changes in the patellar articular cartilage[972]: (1) involving the lateral facet, usually just lateral to the median ridge; (2) involving the medial facets, particularly the odd facet; (3) affecting the median ridge and extending into the medial and lateral facets; (4) involving the central portion of the medial and lateral facets with sparing of the median ridge; and (5) affecting the entire articular cartilage (global chondromalacia). In one further classification system, the extent and depth of the articular cartilage alterations are emphasized[974]: (1) softening and swelling of the cartilage; (2) fissuring and fragmentation of the cartilage in an area 1 cm or less in diameter; (3) fissuring and fragmentation of the cartilage in an area greater than 1 cm in diameter; and (4) erosion of the entire cartilage coat with exposure of subchondral bone. Classification of cartilage changes in the patella also has been based on MR imaging characteristics (see later discussion).[956]

As there is no universally agreed upon definition of chondromalacia patellae, its cause also is not clear. Potential factors include single or recurrent acute episodes of trauma, chronic stress (as in the excessive lateral pressure syndrome), patellofemoral instability, and anatomic or developmental variations in bone morphology.

Assessment of cartilage loss involving the patella using imaging techniques generally is inadequate. Positive findings on routine radiographs require significant and often severe loss of articular cartilage, manifest as joint space narrowing, and secondary changes in the subchondral bone,

evident as sclerosis, cyst formation, and osteophytosis. Standard arthrography and arthrography coupled with conventional tomography or CT also are deficient in the diagnosis of early or mild loss of articular cartilage. Imbibition of contrast material in areas of abnormal cartilage may be observed (Fig. 70–325), but this finding is not sensitive nor specific, as it may occur when arthrographic images are not obtained immediately after injection of the contrast material. Positive results with bone scintigraphy usually indicate more advanced disease with involvement of the subchondral bone. The patellar cartilage is not accessible to investigation with ultrasonography. MR imaging appears to represent the best of an otherwise mediocre group of noninvasive diagnostic techniques for the assessment of patellar cartilage, but it too has many deficiencies. As these deficiencies are not limited to evaluation of the patellar cartilage but apply also to analysis of other articular surfaces in the knee, they are discussed later in this chapter.

Abnormalities of Central Supporting Structures

Anatomic Considerations. The anterior and posterior cruciate ligaments are intracapsular, extrasynovial structures[875, 975, 976] (Fig. 70–326). These bands of dense tissue connect the femur and tibia and are enveloped by a mesentery-like fold of synovium that originates from the posterior intercondylar region of the knee. In one cadaveric study, the mean length of the anterior cruciate ligament was approximately 3.5 cm, and its central portion had a mean width of approximately 1 cm; the mean length of the posterior cruciate ligament was approximately 3.8 cm, and its central portion had a mean width of approximately 1.3 cm.[977] Although not all investigators agree that the posterior

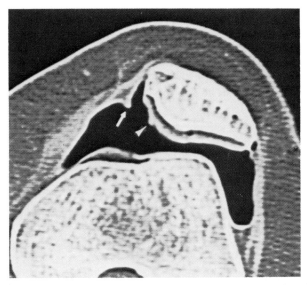

FIGURE 70–325. Chondromalacia patellae: CT arthrography. A transaxial image during computed arthrotomography using air and a small amount of radiopaque contrast material shows cartilage fibrillation (arrowhead) and imbibition of contrast material, especially at the junction of the medial and most medial (odd) facets of the patella, consistent with chondromalacia patellae. A small medial plica (arrow) also is evident. As it is difficult to judge patellar position when large amounts of air or contrast material are placed in the joint, the diagnosis of patellar subluxation is better accomplished with CT alone.

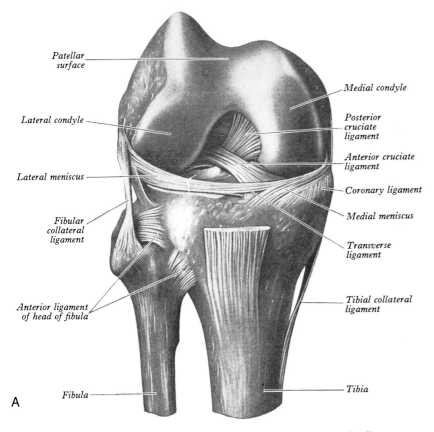

Patellar surface

Lateral condyle

Lateral meniscus

Fibular collateral ligament

Anterior ligament of head of fibula

Medial condyle

Posterior cruciate ligament

Anterior cruciate ligament

Coronary ligament

Medial meniscus

Transverse ligament

Tibial collateral ligament

Fibula

Tibia

A

FIGURE 70–326. Central supporting structures of the knee: Anatomic considerations.

A Anterior aspect of the knee showing the cruciate ligaments and nearby structures.

B, C Superior aspect of the tibia showing the menisci and the tibial attachments of the cruciate ligaments.

(From Williams PL, Warwick R [Eds]: Gray's Anatomy. 36th British edition. Edinburgh, Churchill Livingstone, 1980, pp 400, 485, 486.)

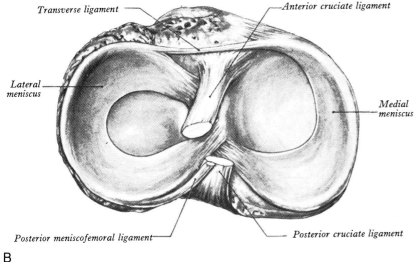

Transverse ligament

Anterior cruciate ligament

Lateral meniscus

Medial meniscus

Posterior meniscofemoral ligament

Posterior cruciate ligament

B

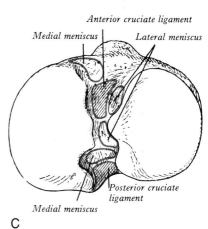

Anterior cruciate ligament

Medial meniscus

Lateral meniscus

Posterior cruciate ligament

Medial meniscus

C

cruciate ligament is longer than the anterior cruciate ligament, the general consensus is that the posterior cruciate ligament is stronger than the anterior cruciate ligament.[978]

The anterior cruciate ligament is attached proximally to a fossa on the posterior aspect of the medial surface of the lateral femoral condyle.[975] Distally, the anterior cruciate ligament is attached to a fossa in front of and lateral to the tibial spines. This attachment site fans out like a foot, allowing the anterior cruciate ligament to tuck under the roof of the intercondylar notch.[875] A few fascicles of the anterior cruciate ligament may blend with the anterior attachment of the lateral meniscus, and the anterior cruciate ligament passes beneath the transverse (geniculate) ligament.[975] The tibial attachment of the anterior cruciate ligament is

stronger and wider than the femoral attachment.[977, 979] The proximal attachment of the anterior cruciate ligament is oriented primarily in the longitudinal axis of the femur, and its distal attachment is in the anteroposterior axis of the tibia.[875] Because of this anatomic arrangement, a twist of the anterior cruciate ligament fibers occurs when the knee moves from extension to flexion. A twist of the anterior cruciate ligament also is evident in the coronal plane, with external rotation of the fibers by approximately 90 degrees as they approach the tibial surface.[875, 977, 980]

The posterior cruciate ligament attaches inferiorly to the tibia in a depression just posterior to and below its articular surface.[975] This attachment site is intracapsular, however. It is rectangular in shape[875] and quite thin.[975] Some fibers of the posterior cruciate ligament extend laterally, to blend with the attachment site of the posterior horn of the lateral meniscus. The proximal, and functionally more important, attachment site of the posterior cruciate ligament is the posterior aspect of the lateral surface of the medial femoral condyle. The femoral attachment is shaped like a half-moon[977] and extends into the intercondylar notch. The longitudinal axis of this femoral attachment is described as more horizontal than that of the anterior cruciate ligament[975] or as in the anteroposterior plane of the femur.[875] The meniscofemoral ligaments of Humphrey and Wrisberg are intimate with the femoral attachment site of the posterior cruciate ligament (see previous discussion).

The spatial orientation of the anterior and posterior cruciate ligaments has been summarized by Arnoczky and Warren.[975] These ligaments cross each other as they extend through the joint. The anterior cruciate ligament courses anteriorly, medially, and distally as it passes from the femur to the tibia, and it turns on itself in a lateral or outward spiral. The posterior cruciate ligament passes posteriorly, laterally, and distally as it extends from the femur to the tibia, and it is narrowest in its midportion. The cruciate ligaments attach to the femur and tibia, not as a single cord, but as a collection of individual fascicles.[975] Although there is some disagreement regarding the presence and number of distinct fascicular bundles,[976] a consensus indicates that two groups of fascicles are evident in the anterior cruciate ligament, and two groups of fascicles are evident in the posterior cruciate ligament. In the anterior cruciate ligament, these two groups are designated the anteromedial bundle or band (arising from the proximal aspect of the femoral attachment and inserting in the anteromedial aspect of the tibial attachment), and the larger posterolateral bundle or bulk (representing the remaining bulk of fascicles that are inserted in the posterolateral aspect of the tibial attachment).[975, 976] As the knee moves from flexion to extension, the anterior cruciate ligament twists on itself, and the functional bundles become manifest. When the knee is extended, the posterolateral bundle is tight, whereas the anteromedial bundle is moderately lax; as the knee is flexed, the anteromedial bundle is tight and the posterolateral bundle is lax.[975] The fascicles in the anteromedial bundle are believed to be longest in flexion, and they may be the primary component that resists anterior displacement of the tibia in flexion; the fascicles in the posterolateral bundle are believed to be longest in extension and may be the primary component that resists hyperextension.[976, 981] In the posterior cruciate ligament, the fascicles are divided into a larger anterior (or anterolateral) portion and a posterior (or posteromedial) portion. The anterior fascicles tighten in flexion of the knee, and the posterior fascicles tighten in extension.[975] Together, portions of the anterior cruciate ligament and the posterior cruciate ligament are taut throughout the range of motion of the knee.

Histologically, the anterior and posterior cruciate ligaments consist mainly of dense fibrous tissue, which, with age, may reveal foci of eosinophilic or mucoid degeneration, or both types of degeneration.[982] The ligaments are composed of collagen fibrils and, at their site of attachment to bone, in common with all ligaments, transitional zones of fibrocartilage and mineralized cartilage are evident.[983, 984] The predominant source of blood supply to the cruciate ligaments is the middle geniculate artery that pierces the

posterior capsule of the knee joint, although an additional blood supply is derived from the inferior medial and lateral geniculate arteries.[875] Nerve fibers are derived from terminal branches of the tibial nerve.[985]

Pathologic Considerations. The anterior cruciate ligament functions as the primary restraint to anterior displacement of the tibia at the knee, and it offers no restraint to posterior displacement of the tibia. Experimental sectioning of the anterior cruciate ligament leads to greater anterior movement of the tibia in 30 degrees of knee flexion than in 90 degrees of flexion.[898] In one study, such sectioning increased anterior tibial displacement from 2.8 mm to 13.0 mm, with a mean value of 6.7 mm.[898] The anterior cruciate ligament also functions as a secondary restraint to tibial rotation, particularly internal rotation of the tibia and with full extension of the knee.[986] Increased tibial rotation is greater when both the anterior cruciate ligament and medial collateral ligament are sectioned than when either structure is sectioned alone.[878] The anterior cruciate ligament also serves as a minor secondary restraint to varus-valgus angulation at full extension of the knee, although the anterior cruciate ligament appears to offer little additional restraint to such angulation beyond that afforded by the medial collateral ligament and lateral collateral ligament.[898]

The posterior cruciate ligament is the primary restraint to posterior displacement of the tibia at the knee.[898] An increase in such displacement following sectioning of the posterior cruciate ligament is greater at 90 degrees of knee flexion than at 30 degrees of knee flexion.[986, 987] The posterior cruciate ligament acts as a major secondary restraint to external tibial rotation, particularly at 90 degrees of flexion, but does not appear to limit internal rotation of the tibia.[898, 986] The posterior cruciate ligament serves as a minor secondary restraint to varus-valgus angulation.[898]

Experimental data provide the following conclusions.[898] Isolated disruption of the anterior cruciate ligament increases anterior movement of the tibia, most evident at 30 degrees of knee flexion, providing the basis for the Lachman test (see later discussion). Isolated disruption of the posterior cruciate ligament increases posterior movement of the tibia, particularly at 75 to 90 degrees of knee flexion, forming the basis for the posterior sag sign (see later discussion). Disruptions of the anterior cruciate ligament, medial collateral ligament, and midportion of the medial aspect of the joint capsule result in large increases in anterior displacement, varus angulation, and internal rotation of the tibia. Disruptions of the anterior cruciate ligament, lateral collateral ligament, and deep posterolateral structures dramatically increase anterior displacement, varus angulation, and external rotation of the tibia. Combined injury of the posterior cruciate ligament, lateral collateral ligament, and deep posterolateral structures results in large increases in posterior displacement of the tibia, varus angulation from full extension to 90 degrees of flexion, and external rotation from 30 degrees to 90 degrees of flexion.

Hughston and coworkers[883] divided the instability patterns into two types: straight instabilities (without a rotatory component) and rotatory instabilities (either simple or combined). By definition, straight instabilities exhibit abnormal motion at the knee without rotation, opening in a manner similar to a book or a door.[885] The common factor exhibited by all straight instability patterns is that, in forced hyperextension, the deficient posterior cruciate ligament is unable to prevent opening of the knee joint and translation of the tibia.[885] Four patterns of straight instability may accompany injuries to the posterior cruciate ligament.[883]

1. Straight medial instability represents instability in hyperextension and is caused by a tear of the posterior cruciate ligament combined with a tear of the medial ligaments of the knee.[883] A positive abduction stress test with the knee in full extension is observed. If the anterior cruciate ligament also is torn, a minimal rotational wobble is evident.[885]

2. Straight lateral instability represents lateral opening of the joint without rotation. It results from tears of the lateral ligaments and the posterior cruciate ligament.[883] It is confirmed by a positive adduction test, accomplished with the knee in full extension. If the anterior cruciate ligament also is torn, a minor rotational wobble again is seen.[885]

3. Straight posterior instability relates to a tear of the posterior cruciate ligament, which may occur as an isolated phenomenon (caused by a force that displaces the tibia posteriorly while the knee is in 90 degrees of flexion) or in combination with injury to the posterior oblique ligament and the arcuate complex of the knee.[883] The large posterior bulk of the posterior cruciate ligament is the site of disruption. This form of instability is manifest by a positive posterior drawer test.

4. Straight anterior instability results from disruption of the posterior cruciate ligament, which may occur in isolation or in combination with tears of the anterior cruciate ligament and the medial and lateral capsular ligaments. It is demonstrated by positive results on several different types of anterior drawer testing, dependent upon which specific structures are torn. If there is no rotational component, the positive anterior drawer sign persists in internal rotation and external rotation of the knee, as well as in the neutral position.[885]

There are three types of simple rotatory instabilities.[883]

1. Anteromedial rotatory instability relates to momentary subluxation of the medial tibial plateau anteriorly and externally on the femur.[885] When mild, this pattern of instability relates to tears of the medial capsule, posterior oblique ligament, and medial collateral ligament; when severe, the anterior cruciate ligament also is injured. Results of an anterior drawer sign with the tibia in external rotation and an abduction stress test with the knee in 30 degrees of flexion are positive.

2. Anterolateral rotatory instability is associated with anterior translation and internal rotation of the lateral plateau of the tibia on the femur. Tears of the anterior cruciate ligament and, in some cases, of the lateral capsular ligament and iliotibial tract are present.[883, 885] The results of adduction stress testing are mildly positive, and jerk and pivot shift testing may be required for diagnosis.[885]

3. Posterolateral rotatory instability usually relates to a direct blow that creates varus angulation and hyperextension of the knee, producing posterolateral subluxation of the tibia on the femur. The sites of injury do not include the cruciate ligaments, but rather are the lateral collateral ligament, arcuate ligament, popliteus tendon, and lateral head of the gastrocnemius muscle.[885] A positive posterolateral drawer sign results.

The instability patterns of the knee are complex, and various combinations of these classic types may be encountered. Proper identification of the type of injury requires careful physical examination, with reliance on the results of many different tests accomplished during application of stress to the injured knee. These tests are described in great detail by Hughston and coworkers.[883] Daniel and Stone[988] have provided a short summary of these tests. Two important tests for anterior cruciate ligament integrity are the Lachman test and pivot shift test. The Lachman test assesses anterior knee laxity and stiffness, accomplished in about 20 degrees of knee flexion. An increase in joint laxity and a decrease in end-point stiffness are signs of injury to the anterior cruciate ligament. A number of different pivot shift tests are described, usually leading to anterior subluxation and subsequent reduction of the tibia, with knee flexion and extension from 10 to 40 degrees as a sequela of anterior cruciate ligament disruption.[988] Two fundamental tests are used to evaluate the integrity of the posterior cruciate ligament.[988] The 90 degree quadriceps active test is performed with the patient in a supine position, with the hip flexed 45 degrees, the knee flexed 90 degrees, and the foot on the table. With contraction of the quadriceps musculature, exaggerated posterior movement of the tibia occurs (positive sag sign). The patient then is asked to slide the foot along the tabletop. Anterior translation of the tibia occurs when the tibia is posteriorly subluxed secondary to disruption of the posterior cruciate ligament.[988] The second test for posterior cruciate ligament integrity is the posterior drawer test, which documents posterior subluxation of the tibia. The test is more useful in acute (rather than chronic) injuries of the posterior cruciate ligament. A posteromedial pivot shift of the knee also has been described, in which positive results relate to injuries not only of the posterior cruciate ligament but also of the medial and posterior collateral ligaments and the posterior oblique ligament.[1409]

Physical examination provides important information regarding which ligament or ligaments are torn. In the acute stage, however, difficulty arises, owing to pain, muscle spasm, and guarding.[994] The results of carefully performed stress testing may allow precise determination of sites of injury. In some instances, physical examination performed with the patient under general anesthesia is required. Noyes and Grood[995] have outlined four concepts that must be understood in order to properly diagnose injuries of the ligaments of the knee: (1) diagnosis of a ligament injury must be expressed as a specific anatomic defect; (2) physical examination must be interpreted using knowledge of three-dimensional motions of the knee; (3) patterns of rotary instability can be characterized by separate subluxations that occur to the medial and lateral tibial plateaus; and (4) diagnosis of ligament and capsular defects requires the use of selected laxity tests for which the primary and secondary restraints have been determined experimentally. These authors also indicated that terms must be precisely defined. They suggested that the term instability should be used only in a general sense to indicate excessive motion of the knee joint, that the term laxity should be used only in a general sense to indicate slackness or loosening of a ligament, that the term instability refers to the condition of increased mobility of the knee joint, and that the term subluxation represents incomplete or partial displacement at the knee, and it requires further descriptive terms to indicate precisely which portions of the joint are malaligned.

Anterior Cruciate Ligament Injuries. Injuries to the

anterior cruciate ligament are among the most frequent sequelae of knee trauma. In one series, almost 40 per cent of ligamentous injuries of the knee involved the anterior cruciate alone and, in an additional 35 per cent of cases, the anterior cruciate ligament was injured in combination with other ligamentous disruptions, particularly those of the medial collateral ligament.[989] Approximately 60 to 75 per cent of acute traumatic hemarthroses are associated with anterior cruciate ligament injury. The classic mechanism of injury to the anterior cruciate ligament (which frequently is evident in skiers and American football players) is indirect trauma leading to decelerating, hyperextension, or twisting forces, often accompanied by an audible pop and the rapid onset of pain, soft tissue swelling, and disability. The combination of external rotation of the tibia with respect to the femur, knee flexion, and valgus stress may produce an anterior cruciate ligament injury, often combined with additional injuries to the medial collateral ligament and the medial meniscus.[990–994] O'Donoghue's triad of injury consists of a tear of the anterior cruciate ligament, complete disruption of the medial collateral ligament, and a tear of the peripheral portion of the medial meniscus. Even when initial injuries are isolated to the anterior cruciate ligament, chronic instability in the anterior cruciate ligament–deficient knee subsequently can lead to additional injuries, such as meniscal tears. The midsubstance of the anterior cruciate ligament is injured most commonly (approximately 70 per cent of cases), followed in frequency by its proximal portion (approximately 20 per cent of cases), and its distal portion (approximately 10 per cent of cases).

Clinical assessment of the knee in patients with anterior cruciate ligament injuries includes physical examination with stress testing. Instillation of a local anesthetic agent into the joint or, in some cases, the use of general anesthesia may be required, particularly when muscle spasm or patient apprehension precludes adequate evaluation. The correct assessment of the severity of knee instability and its type requires the attention of an experienced orthopedic surgeon, and results of stress tests, which may be accomplished with instrumented ligament-testing devices, should be compared with those of the opposite (uninjured) knee. One instrument used for measuring instability of the knee is a KT1000 arthrometer. This instrument allows quantitative analysis of tibial displacement in relation to the femur by tracking the distance between one sensor pad in contact with the tibial tubercle and a second in contact with the patella.[996, 997] The role of arthroscopy in the diagnosis and management of acute knee injuries, including partial and complete tears of the anterior cruciate ligament, is well established. Precise diagnosis requires arthroscopic assessment of the menisci and chondral surfaces as well as the anterior cruciate ligament.[998–1000] Arthroscopy also can be used to evaluate knees with chronically deficient anterior cruciate ligaments. In either acute or chronic tears of the anterior cruciate ligament, arthroscopic difficulty may arise if the synovial membrane overlying the torn ligament is intact.

Routine Radiography. In patients with acute tears of the anterior cruciate ligament, nonspecific soft tissue swelling and a joint effusion may be evident. Several fractures of the proximal portion of the tibia and distal portion of the femur, however, are specific for or imply the likelihood of an injury to the anterior cruciate ligament.

1. *Avulsion fracture of the anterior tibial eminence.* These avulsion fractures (Fig. 70–327) occur at the site of attachment of the anterior cruciate ligament and are more frequent in children and young adolescents than in older adolescents and adults (in whom injuries of the cruciate ligament itself occur). Avulsion fractures of the anterior tibial eminence, especially in adults, may be associated with additional fractures and other injuries such as medial ligamentous and meniscal tears. Undisplaced fractures appear as a horizontal fracture line at the base of the anterior portion of the tibial spine; displaced fractures are accompanied by upward movement of the anterior portion of the fragment, which may become completely detached or even inverted.[1001] Avulsion fractures involving the femoral site of attachment of the anterior cruciate ligament are rare.[1002]

2. *Lateral tibial rim fracture (Segond fracture).* As indicated earlier, a fracture fragment arising at the site of tibial attachment of the lateral capsular ligament reveals a high association with anterior cruciate ligament instability. The fragment usually is located lateral and just inferior to the joint line on the anteroposterior and tunnel radiographic projections (see Fig. 70–307).

3. *Posterior fracture of the lateral tibial plateau.* A subtle fracture of the posterior part of the lateral tibial plateau, visible on the lateral radiograph of the knee, may relate to an avulsion injury at the insertion site of the posterior portion of the joint capsule.[1003] In one study, 11 of 25 patients with tears of the anterior cruciate ligament documented by MR imaging revealed this fracture pattern.[1003] These posterior tibial fractures may be associated with fractures of the lateral tibial rim (Segond fracture). Compression fractures of the posterior portion of the lateral tibial plateau or fractures at the site of attachment of the semimembranosus tendon also may be observed in patients with anterior cruciate ligament tears. These fractures lead to an irregular contour of the plateau on lateral radiographs of the knee.[1003]

4. *Osteochondral fracture of the lateral femoral condyle.* A constant localized chondral or transchondral lesion occurring in the region of the condylopatellar sulcus of the lateral femoral condyle has been observed at the time of surgical reconstruction of anterior cruciate ligament–deficient knees.[1004, 1005] During surgery in some patients it was possible to pull the lateral or posterolateral margin of the

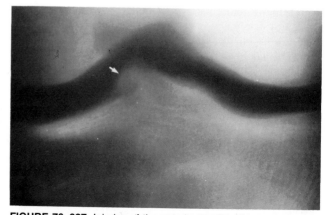

FIGURE 70–327. Injuries of the anterior cruciate ligament: Routine radiography. Avulsion fracture of the anterior tibial eminence. Note the subtle fracture fragment (arrow), which is minimally displaced in an upward direction.

tibia into the sulcus, suggesting that the lesion was the result of an impaction fracture similar to the Hill-Sachs lesion that accompanies an anterior dislocation of the glenohumeral joint. Retrospectively, the sulcus was shown to be abnormal on the lateral radiograph of the knee in many patients.[1006] In one study, only 1 of 47 patients with clinically intact anterior cruciate ligaments had a condylopatellar sulcus greater than 1 mm in depth (as measured on the lateral radiograph), whereas 2 of 52 patients with acute tears of the anterior cruciate ligament and 13 of 70 patients with chronic tears of the anterior cruciate ligament had a sulcus equal to or greater than 1.5 mm in depth.[1007] The significance of this finding, which has been designated the lateral notch sign,[1007] is supported by histologic data that document the presence of focal areas of degenerated cartilage with localized invagination of cartilage into subchondral bone of the condylopatellar sulcus in patients with chronic anterior cruciate ligament tears[1006]; and by MR imaging findings in patients with acute tears of the anterior cruciate ligament that include marrow edema (presumably resulting from injury) in the region of the sulcus (see later discussion). The lateral notch sign is considered present when the depth of the sulcus is greater than 1.5 to 2 mm (Fig. 70–328). The sign appears to be a specific indicator of an anterior cruciate ligament–deficient knee, but it is insensitive, probably occurring in less than 5 per cent of patients with torn anterior cruciate ligaments. It is not clear, however, if the deepening of the sulcus represents an osteochondral fracture or a developmental abnormality that predisposes to, rather than results from, the injury mechanism that causes an anterior cruciate ligament tear.

Arthrography. Several arthrographic techniques have been employed for the evaluation of cruciate ligament injuries, with varying degrees of success. Initial techniques using double contrast arthrography were accurate in less than 50 per cent of cases, stimulating investigation with modified methods of examination. Some investigations report success using a lateral view of the knee, flexed to 90 degrees over the edge of the table[1008] or elevated above the table,[1009] or employing single positive contrast examinations.[1010] Others indicate approximately 75 to 90 per cent accuracy in diagnosing anterior cruciate ligament tears using conventional tomography.[1011] This technique is improved if tomographic exposures are obtained immediately following injection, although this is time-consuming, delaying the meniscal examination.

In a series of articles, Pavlov and collaborators[1012–1016] emphasized the role of double contrast arthrography in the evaluation of the cruciate ligaments. Although the study of the cruciate ligaments can be accomplished following the investigation of the menisci, it is better employed before the menisci are studied, immediately after the introduction of radiopaque contrast material, air, and epinephrine. The knee is passively flexed and extended several times with the patient in the supine, sitting, and prone positions, and attention then is directed to the anterior cruciate ligament. Two techniques are used: a horizontal cross-table lateral radiograph and fluoroscopic spot films. In both instances, the anterior cruciate ligament is examined while being tensed with a simulated "anterior drawer" maneuver. For the horizontal cross-table lateral radiograph, the patient sits with the legs flexed between 45 and 75 degrees over the side of the table, and the proximal end of the tibia is pushed anteriorly with respect to the femoral condyles by a firm pillow located behind the calf. An overpenetrated cross-table lateral radiograph is exposed while the patient holds a grid cassette adjacent to the medial aspect of the knee. Following this, the patient lies on his or her side, with the affected knee dependent and flexed 45 to 75 degrees. A stress band extends around the calf from the side of the table in front of the knee, and the examiner pulls the distal

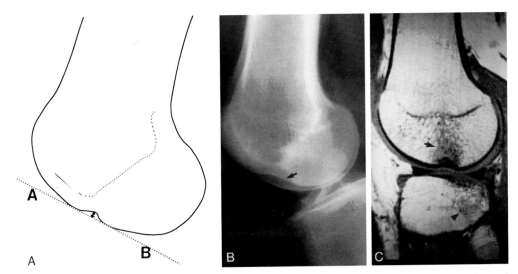

FIGURE 70–328. Injuries of the anterior cruciate ligament: Routine radiography. Osteochondral fracture of the lateral femoral condyle.

A Method of measuring the depth of the lateral condylopatellar sulcus. A line (AB) drawn tangentially across the lower articular surface of the lateral femur forms the reference line. The depth of the sulcus is measured perpendicular to this line at the deepest point (arrowheads). (From Cobby MJ, et al: Radiology *184:* 855, 1992.)

B In a patient with a chronic tear of the anterior cruciate ligament, note the prominent condylopatellar sulcus (arrow).

C In a different patient with a torn anterior cruciate ligament and a deep lateral condylopatellar sulcus, a T1-weighted (TR/TE, 800/30) spin echo MR image shows alterations in marrow signal intensity in the midportion of the lateral femoral condyle (arrow) and in the posterolateral portion of the tibia (arrowhead). These findings are consistent with marrow edema related to impaction fractures. (Courtesy of M. Pathria, M.D., San Diego, California.)

part of the leg posteriorly against the stress band. Although a properly performed cruciate ligament examination takes only 1 or 2 min and is not incompatible with subsequent and adequate investigation of the menisci, it must be carefully and meticulously done. When accomplished by an experienced arthrographer, the accuracy of the technique surpasses 90 per cent,[1014] although similar accuracy has been reported from clinical examination alone.[1017] Of course, arthrography also allows identification of meniscal lesions that commonly accompany injuries of the anterior cruciate ligament.

The fundamental arthrographic criterion of a normal anterior cruciate ligament is an anterior synovial surface that is "ruler-straight" on one or both of these radiographs[1014] (Fig. 70–329). This ligament is considered to be lax but intact if the anterior synovial surface is bowed and concave anteriorly. The arthrographic abnormalities associated with disruption of the anterior cruciate ligament (Fig. 70–329) are more definite when simultaneous visualization of the posterior cruciate ligament is accomplished (decreasing the likelihood of technical inadequacies) and include nonvisualization, a wavy, lumpy, or acutely angulated anterior surface, irregularity of the inferior attachment of the ligament, pooling of the contrast medium in the usual location of the ligament, and visualization of the plica synovialis infrapatellaris (the infrapatellar synovial fold, which otherwise is easily misinterpreted as evidence of a normal anterior cruciate ligament).[1012–1015] It should be emphasized that the abnormal findings frequently are subtle, requiring of the examiner a good deal of experience and knowledge.

An alternative approach to the diagnosis of tears of cruciate ligaments is provided by CT alone or combined with arthrography of the knee[324, 523–527] (Fig. 70–330). Prior descriptions of the CT technique that is required to evaluate the cruciate ligaments have been conflicting not only with respect to the need for intra-articular contrast material but also with respect to whether the contrast material should be radiopaque material, air, or both. There is no uniform agreement regarding the position of the knee in the CT gantry, the necessity for angulation of the gantry, or the benefit of reformatted or even three-dimensional images.

MR Imaging: Technical Considerations. As with the menisci of the knee, spin echo MR imaging is the most popular method used to assess the anterior cruciate ligament (as well as the posterior cruciate ligament). The best plane for analysis of either cruciate ligament is the sagittal plane, but supplementary data supplied by coronal and transaxial MR images are important. In one study, combined analysis of MR images in all three planes led to an improvement in the sensitivity (98 per cent) and specificity (93 per cent) for determining the status of the anterior cruciate ligament when compared with the sensitivity (94 per cent) and specificity (84 per cent) derived from analysis of the sagittal images alone.[1018] The sagittal images commonly are obtained with the leg externally rotated 15 to 30 degrees, and therefore represent sagittal oblique images; or they are obtained by determining the orientation of the anterior cruciate ligament from initial transaxial (or coronal) MR images and using a sagittal oblique imaging plane parallel to this orientation (i.e., a 15 to 30 degree internally rotated imaging plane).[1019–1022] The use of T1- and T2-weighted spin echo MR images or proton density and T2-weighted spin echo MR images in the sagittal plane is helpful for determining changes in signal intensity in the anterior cru-

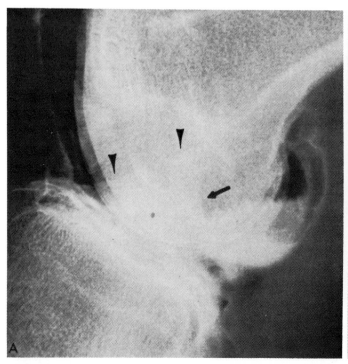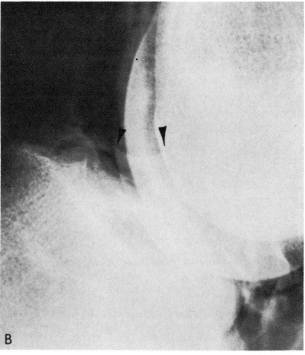

FIGURE 70–329. Injuries of the anterior cruciate ligament: Arthrography.

A On this lateral view, the anterior cruciate (arrowheads) and posterior cruciate (arrow) ligaments are seen. Note their normal appearance and smooth contour.

B A torn anterior cruciate ligament is evident (arrowheads). Note the irregular coating and bowed appearance of the torn ligament.

(**B**, From Dalinka MK, et al: CRC Crit Rev Radiol Sci *5:*1, 1973.)

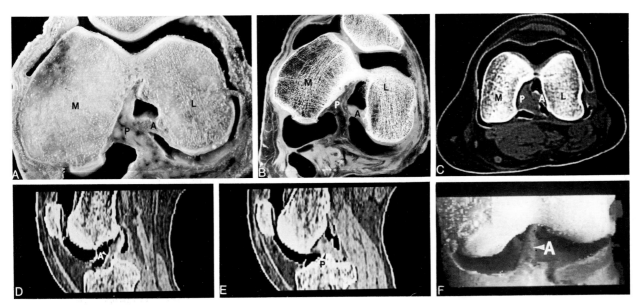

FIGURE 70–330. Normal anterior cruciate ligament: CT arthrography.

 A–C A photograph **(A)** and radiograph **(B)** of a transverse section of a cadaveric knee following the instillation of intra-articular air and a transaxial CT scan **(C)** of the intact specimen show the normal anterior (A) and posterior (P) cruciate ligaments. M, medial femoral condyle; L, lateral femoral condyle.

 D, E Reconstructed sagittal CT images of the normal anterior cruciate ligament (A) and normal posterior cruciate ligament (P) are shown.

 F A three-dimensional CT image displays the normal anterior cruciate ligament (A).

ciate ligament that may accompany acute or subacute injuries. T2-weighted images also improve the contrast between the anterior cruciate ligament and a surrounding joint effusion. The sagittal images usually are 3 or 4 mm in thickness. The use of volumetric (3-dimensional Fourier transform) gradient echo MR images of approximately 1 mm in thickness also may be useful. Gradient echo MR imaging may be coupled with cine technique to provide dynamic, rather than static, data.[1023] The leg is extended during the acquisition of the MR images.[1022]

MR Imaging: Normal Anterior Cruciate Ligament. Identification of the normal anterior cruciate ligament begins with analysis of the sagittal MR images (Fig. 70–331). In choosing a proper sagittal section in which the normal anterior cruciate ligament should be visualized, it often is helpful to find one that displays the intercondylar roof of the femur as a straight line of low signal intensity. Typically, in this section (or sections), the anterior cruciate ligament appears as a straight band of low signal intensity whose course parallels that of the intercondylar line. The anterior cruciate ligament may not be seen in its entirety in this image (or images), but the course of the visible portion of the anterior cruciate ligament still should be parallel to this line of low signal intensity. The anterior cruciate ligament may be seen as a uniform structure of low signal intensity or as one composed of individual fibers of low signal intensity. The individual fibers are identified most frequently at the tibial attachment site of the anterior cruciate ligament. Sometimes, two bands (anterior and posterior) of fibers are seen within the anterior cruciate ligament. The posterior band may reveal increased signal intensity when compared with the anterior band. Indeed, even the anterior band may show regions of increased signal intensity, particularly near its attachment to the tibia, presumably representing regions of fat. With gradient echo MR images, the anterior band is seen regularly, but it may be difficult to see the fibers of the posterior portion of the anterior cruciate ligament. The femoral insertion site of the anterior cruciate ligament may look bulbous, probably related to partial volume artifacts produced by the thickness of the sagittal images and resulting in visualization of a portion of the lateral femoral condyle.

In coronal (Fig. 70–331) and transaxial MR images, the normal anterior cruciate ligament again can be identified. It may not be seen in its entirety in these images, but portions of it are visible and, in the coronal plane, individual fibers may be visualized.

The dominant pattern of signal intensity in the normal anterior cruciate ligament is low, although it is not as low as the signal intensity in the posterior cruciate ligament. The cause for the relative increased signal intensity in the anterior cruciate ligament (Fig. 70–332), particularly in elderly persons, is not clear.[982] Ligament architecture may be a causative factor, leading to increased signal intensity in the anterior cruciate ligament. The obliquely oriented fibers of the anterior cruciate ligament may result in more pronounced volume averaging artifacts during the MR imaging examination. Fat localized between the distal, diverging fascicles of the anterior cruciate ligament also represents a potential source for its increased signal intensity. Furthermore, in older persons, regions of mucoid or myxoid changes within the anterior cruciate ligament may be responsible for changes in its signal intensity.[982]

MR Imaging: Anterior Cruciate Ligament Tears. MR imaging represents a sensitive (90 to 98 per cent), specific (90 to 100 per cent), and accurate (90 to 95 per cent) method for identifying tears of the anterior cruciate ligament.[1018, 1019, 1022, 1024] In one study, its sensitivity to the analysis of the anterior cruciate ligament was superior to that provided by clinical tests such as the Lachman test and the anterior drawer sign.[1024] MR imaging also appeared to be more specific and, possibly, more sensitive than arthrog-

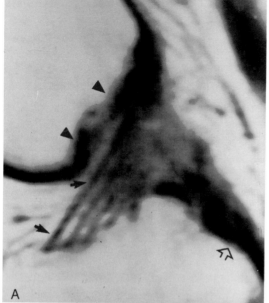
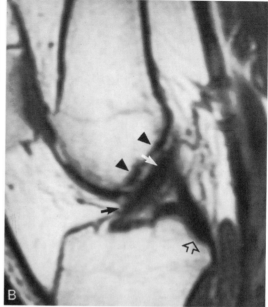
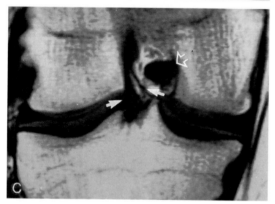

FIGURE 70–331. Normal anterior cruciate ligament: MR imaging.

A Sagittal proton density–weighted (TR/TE, 2000/20) spin echo MR image. The intercondylar roof (arrowheads) is seen as a straight line of low signal intensity. The anterior cruciate ligament (solid arrows) is seen as individual fibers whose course is straight and parallel to the course of the intercondylar roof. The tibial insertion site of the posterior cruciate ligament (open arrow) also is apparent.

B Sagittal proton density–weighted (TR/TE, 2000/20) spin echo MR image. In this example, the intercondylar roof (arrowheads) again is visualized as a straight line of low signal intensity. Although individual fibers of the anterior cruciate ligament are not seen, the ligament (solid arrows) is of low signal intensity and has a course that is parallel to the course of the intercondylar roof. The tibial insertion site of the posterior cruciate ligament (open arrow) is evident.

C Coronal proton density–weighted (TR/TE, 2000/20) spin echo MR image. Fibers of the anterior cruciate ligament (solid arrows) are seen coursing from the lateral femoral condyle to the anterior portion of the tibia. The femoral insertion site of the posterior cruciate ligament (open arrow) is evident.

raphy in demonstrating tears of the anterior cruciate ligament.[1024] The ability of MR imaging to allow differentiation between acute and chronic tears of the anterior cruciate ligament and to enable identification of partial tears of this ligament remains unclear.[1025] The MR imaging diagnosis of injuries to the anterior cruciate ligament relates to the documentation of: (1) abnormalities in the anterior cruciate ligament itself; (2) alterations in the appearance of other structures (e.g., posterior cruciate ligament and patellar tendon) related to the abnormal alignment of the tibia and femur that results from an anterior cruciate ligament tear; and (3) abnormalities that result from bone impaction forces that occur in the course of the injury itself or from the resultant anterolateral instability that accompanies the injury to the anterior cruciate ligament.[1026] Of these three types of abnormalities, those occurring in the anterior cruciate ligament itself are direct evidence of its injury; those reflecting altered alignment of the tibia and femur are indirect but strong evidence of anterior cruciate ligament injury; and those occurring in the adjacent bone are supportive of the diagnosis of an injury to the anterior cruciate ligament and mandate critical assessment (or reassessment) of the

ligament. Furthermore, MR imaging allows confirmation of additional soft tissue damage, such as a tear of the medial meniscus (40 to 80 per cent of cases of acute or chronic tears of the anterior cruciate ligament)[1400] or disruption of the medial supporting structures, or both, that is known to be associated with anterior cruciate ligament injury.

1. Abnormalities of the anterior cruciate ligament itself. The two major alterations occurring within the ligament itself are changes in its morphology or course and changes in its signal intensity.[1018, 1019, 1022, 1024, 1027] A complete tear of the anterior cruciate ligament is accompanied by disruption of all of its fibers and an irregular or wavy contour. These findings are more evident in the sagittal than the coronal MR images, although an indistinct anterior cruciate ligament in coronal MR images through the intercondylar notch, referred to as the empty notch sign, is an important finding of a complete tear of the anterior cruciate ligament, having been noted in 92 per cent of such tears in one study.[1027] In sagittal MR images, the course of the completely torn anterior cruciate ligament may appear depressed (Fig. 70–333), with a decreased slope of residual fibers extending almost parallel to the tibial surface rather

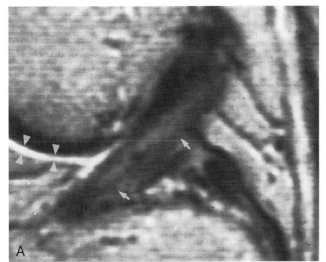
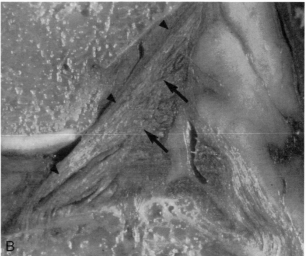

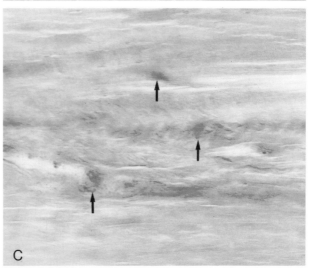

FIGURE 70–332. Normal anterior cruciate ligament: MR imaging. Variations in signal intensity related to eosinophilic degeneration.

A A sagittal T2-weighted (TR/TE, 2000/70) spin echo MR image shows regions of intermediate signal intensity (arrows) in the anterior cruciate ligament. The increased signal intensity is not as great as that of the adjacent joint fluid (arrowheads).

B A corresponding sagittal anatomic section shows that the anterior fibers (arrowheads) of the anterior cruciate ligament are parallel to the imaging plane, whereas the posterior fibers (arrows) of the anterior cruciate ligament have a less steep course and are oriented more obliquely with regard to the sagittal plane.

C A photomicrograph shows extensive eosinophilic degeneration (arrows) in the anterior cruciate ligament.

(From Hodler J, et al: AJR *159:* 357, 1992.)

FIGURE 70–333. Injuries of the anterior cruciate ligament: MR imaging. Chronic complete anterior cruciate ligament tears with alterations in ligament morphology and course.

A A sagittal proton density–weighted (TR/TE, 2150/30) spin echo MR image shows a depressed anterior cruciate ligament (arrow) whose course no longer parallels that of the intercondylar roof.

B A sagittal proton density–weighted (TR/TE, 2000/30) spin echo MR image shows a similar finding (arrow) in a second patient with a chronically torn anterior cruciate ligament.

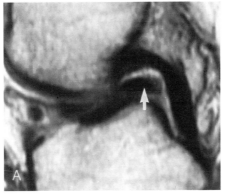
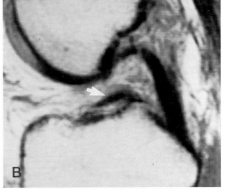

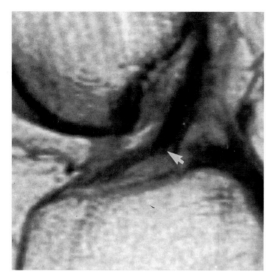

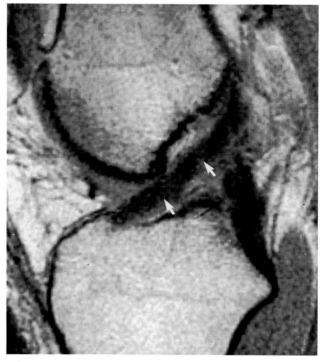

FIGURE 70–334. Injuries of the anterior cruciate ligament: MR imaging. Chronic complete anterior cruciate ligament tears with scar tissue. A sagittal proton density–weighted (TR/TE, 2000/20) spin echo MR image shows a focally angular (arrow) but intact band with low signal intensity that represents a combination of anterior cruciate ligament fragments and associated bridging fibrous scar. (From Vahey TN, et al: Radiology *181:* 251, 1991.)

FIGURE 70–335. Injuries of the anterior cruciate ligament: MR imaging. Chronic complete anterior cruciate ligament tears with scar tissue. A sagittal proton density–weighted (TR/TE, 2000/20) spin echo MR image shows a relatively straight band (arrows) with low signal intensity that bridges the expected origin and insertion of the anterior cruciate ligament. The appearance simulates that of a normal anterior cruciate ligament. At arthroscopy, a chronically torn anterior cruciate ligament that was scarred to the posterior cruciate ligament was found. (From Vahey TN, et al: Radiology *181:* 251, 1991.)

than at an angle to this surface and parallel to the intercondylar roof (as is characteristic of the normal anterior cruciate ligament). In some chronic complete tears of the anterior cruciate ligament, the development of scar tissue results in an angulated appearance of the ligament (Fig. 70–334) or, in some cases, a continuous band of low signal intensity that simulates the appearance of a normal anterior cruciate ligament[1410] (Fig. 70–335). A focal angulation in this band may allow a correct diagnosis of a torn anterior cruciate ligament even in these cases.[1025] With acute or chronic tears of some but not all the fibers of the anterior cruciate ligament, the ligament may appear attenuated, or small, and its course may or may not be altered (Fig. 70–336). Rarely, developmental hypoplasia of the cruciate ligaments produces a similar appearance (Fig. 70–337).

The presence of increased signal intensity within the anterior cruciate ligament on proton density and T2-weighted spin echo MR images usually indicates an acute or subacute injury resulting in complete or partial disruption of the ligament (Fig. 70–338). This pattern of increased signal intensity appears to reflect edematous soft tissues, not joint fluid, in the intercondylar notch.[1025] A cloudlike or amorphous mass of increased signal intensity, with well-defined margins, may be evident. Although such edema is indicative of a recent tear of the anterior cruciate ligament,

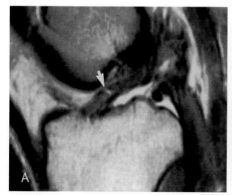
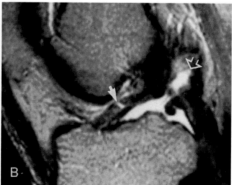
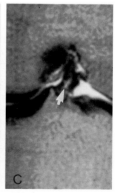

FIGURE 70–336. Injuries of the anterior cruciate ligament: MR imaging. Acute partial anterior cruciate ligament tears with alterations in ligament morphology and signal intensity. Sagittal proton density–weighted (TR/TE, 4000/21) **(A)** and T2-weighted (TR/TE, 4000/105) **(B)** fast spin echo MR images and a coronal T2-weighted (TR/TE, 3200/108) fast spin echo MR image **(C)** show an attenuated appearance of the anterior cruciate ligament with intraligamentous regions (solid arrows) of high signal intensity. Note the joint fluid that is collecting between the anterior cruciate ligament and posterior cruciate ligament (open arrow), consistent with a tear of the synovial lining that surrounds the cruciate ligaments.

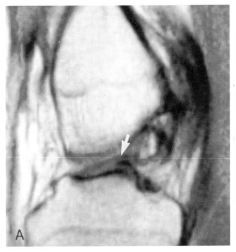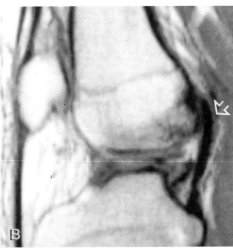

FIGURE 70–337. Hypoplasia of the cruciate ligaments: MR imaging. In this 19 year old man with hypoplasia of the femur, tibia, and patella, the anterior cruciate ligament (solid arrow) and the posterior cruciate ligament (open arrow) also are hypoplastic, as seen in sagittal proton density–weighted (TR/TE, 2200/15) spin echo MR images **(A, B)**. Also note the hypoplastic quadriceps and patellar tendons and anterior translation of the tibia with respect to the femur. (Courtesy of J. Hodler, M.D., Zurich, Switzerland.)

its absence does not exclude the presence of a recent tear.[1025] With chronic tears of the anterior cruciate ligament, edema usually is not evident. The presence of joint fluid about the chronically torn ligament, however, may simulate the appearance of edema in the MR images.[1025]

Although, as indicated in the following discussion, additional soft tissue and bone abnormalities seen with MR imaging may serve as clues to the presence of an anterior cruciate ligament tear, the alterations in the ligament itself represent the most important findings of such a tear, allowing correct diagnosis in more than 90 per cent of cases.[1027] False-positive diagnoses may occur, however, owing to the presence of foci of mucinous or myxoid change within the ligament,[982] partial volume averaging of the anterior cruciate ligament with the lateral femoral condyle or with periligamentous fat, and suboptimal selection of the sagittal imaging plane to view the ligament.[1027] False-negative diagnoses may result from the formation of scar tissue with adherence of the anterior cruciate ligament to the posterior cruciate ligament (simulating a normal course and signal intensity of the anterior cruciate ligament) or from partial tears in which residual intact fibers lead to an appearance of a normal anterior cruciate ligament.[1410] Assessment of all three imaging planes is required to minimize these diagnostic errors. Furthermore, attention should be paid to any additional soft tissue or bone abnormalities that may accompany disruptions of the anterior cruciate ligament.

2. Alterations in other structures related to abnormal alignment of the tibia and femur. Anterior cruciate ligament injuries are associated with anterolateral instability that may be manifest as a forward shift of the tibia with respect to the femur.[1411] This shift, if severe, can be recognized easily, owing to the position of the two bones (Fig. 70–339). If the shift is subtle, its recognition depends upon minor alterations in the configuration of or relationship among other structures in the knee. Examples of these alterations include a relative posterior displacement of the lateral meniscus compared with the posterior margin of the lateral tibial plateau (''uncovered lateral meniscus'' sign), a change in the curvature of the posterior cruciate ligament, and undulation of the patellar tendon.[1412]

The uncovered lateral meniscus sign is positive if a vertical line drawn tangent to the posteriormost cortical margin of the lateral tibial plateau on sagittal MR images intersects any part of the posterior horn of the lateral meniscus; this sign is negative if the vertical line does not intersect the lateral meniscus, but rather, is posterior to the meniscus.[1027] In one study, the uncovered lateral meniscus sign was positive in 18 per cent of cases in which an anterior cruciate ligament tear was present and was negative in all cases in which the anterior cruciate ligament was normal.[1027]

Changes in the curvature of the posterior cruciate ligament in cases of tears of the anterior cruciate ligament have been emphasized in some reports.[1027–1029] A forward shift in

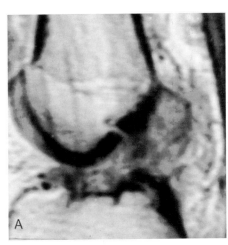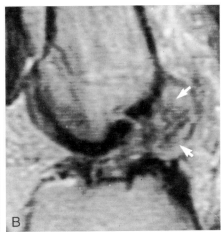

FIGURE 70–338. Injuries of the anterior cruciate ligament: MR imaging. Acute complete anterior cruciate ligament tears with alterations in intraligamentous signal intensity. In sagittal proton density–weighted (TR/TE, 2500/20) **(A)** and T2-weighted (TR/TE, 2500/60) **(B)** spin echo MR images, the anterior cruciate ligament is not visualized. In **B**, note a generalized increase in signal intensity (arrows) in an amorphous mass near the femoral site of insertion of the anterior cruciate ligament.

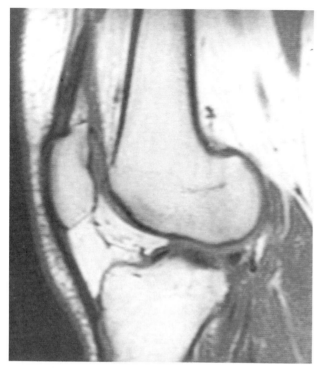

FIGURE 70–339. Injuries of the anterior cruciate ligament: MR imaging. Chronic complete anterior cruciate ligament tears with anterior translation of the tibia. A sagittal T1-weighted (TR/TE, 600/20) spin echo MR image shows obvious forward movement of the tibia with respect to the lateral femoral condyle. Note uncovering of the posterior horn of the lateral meniscus (see text).

the position of the tibia with respect to the femur occurs in patients with anterior cruciate ligament–deficient knees, and this shift may alter the appearance of the smooth curve of the posterior cruciate ligament (Fig. 70–340). A line drawn along the inferior portion of the posterior cruciate ligament and extended superiorly on sagittal MR images normally intersects the medullary cavity of the femur; when this line does not intersect the femur but extends parallel to it, a positive posterior cruciate sign is present.[1029] Alternatively, quantifying the curvature of the posterior cruciate ligament on the basis of the sagittal MR images may be accomplished.[1027] In common with the uncovered lateral meniscus

sign, altered curvature of the posterior cruciate ligament appears to be a specific but insensitive indicator of a tear of the anterior cruciate ligament.[1027, 1030]

Undulation and redundancy of the patellar tendon may result from forward movement of the tibia with respect to the femur (Fig. 70–341), but a similar appearance relates to hyperextension of the knee at the time of the MR imaging examination and a tear of the quadriceps tendon. The patellar tendon sign of a tear of the anterior cruciate ligament appears to be both insensitive and nonspecific.[1354]

3. Abnormalities related to bone impaction forces. Impaction of portions of the femur and tibia may occur acutely in patients with anterolateral instability of the knee. Subcortical infraction and medullary edema and hemorrhage lead to changes in signal intensity of the affected bone marrow, a finding designated a bone bruise (see Chapter 67). Typically, bone bruises lead to geographic or reticular areas of decreased signal intensity on T1-weighted spin echo MR images and increased signal intensity on T2-weighted spin echo MR images obtained soon after the injury. Their conspicuity is increased in short tau inversion recovery (STIR) MR images and those obtained with fat suppression techniques.[1358]

In patients with acute tears of the anterior cruciate ligament, bone bruises have been observed most often in the midportion of the lateral femoral condyle (near the condylopatellar sulcus) and in the posterior portion of the lateral tibial plateau[1006, 1031, 1032, 1413] (Figs. 70–341 and 70–342). Using MR imaging, Murphy and coworkers[1031] detected bone impaction sites involving the posterolateral portion of the tibial plateau in 94 per cent and the lateral femoral condyle in 91 per cent of 32 patients with surgically confirmed acute complete tears of the anterior cruciate ligament. Only 1 of 6 patients with a partial tear of the anterior cruciate ligament displayed similar findings. Kaplan and collaborators[1032] detected 89 occult fractures in MR imaging examinations of 56 knees in patients with acute complete tears of the anterior cruciate ligament. The posterior aspect of the lateral tibial plateau was involved in every case, either as an isolated finding or associated with additional lesions, especially in the midportion of the lateral femoral condyle. Tung and associates[1027] detected MR imaging findings compatible with a bone bruise in 44 per cent of pa-

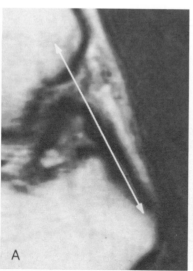
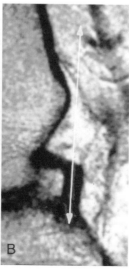

A   B

FIGURE 70–340. Injuries of the anterior cruciate ligament: MR imaging. Normal and abnormal configuration of the posterior cruciate ligament.

A Normal appearance. As shown in this T1-weighted (TR/TE, 600/20) spin echo MR image, a line drawn along the course of the lower portion of the posterior cruciate ligament, when extended superiorly, intersects the femur.

B Acute complete anterior cruciate ligament tear. As shown in a sagittal T2-weighted (TR/TE, 2000/70) spin echo MR image, the appearance of the posterior cruciate ligament may be altered in association with a complete tear of the anterior cruciate ligament. In this case, acute angulation of the posterior cruciate ligament is evident. A line drawn along the course of the lower portion of the posterior cruciate ligament, when extended superiorly, does not intersect the femur. (Courtesy of S. K. Brahme, M.D., La Jolla, California.)

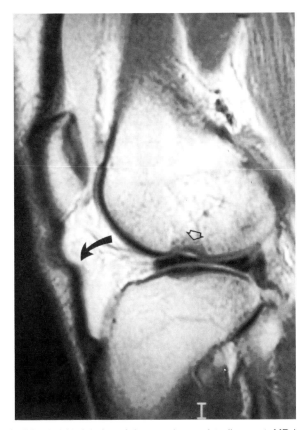

FIGURE 70–341. Injuries of the anterior cruciate ligament: MR imaging. Acute complete anterior cruciate ligament tears with redundancy of the patellar tendon and osteochondral impaction fractures. A sagittal proton density–weighted (TR/TE, 2000/30) spin echo MR image shows buckling of the patellar tendon (curved solid arrow) and an alteration in signal intensity (open arrow) in the lateral condylopatellar sulcus related to an impaction injury. A large joint effusion is present. (From Cobby MJ, et al: Radiology *184:* 855, 1992.)

tients with a complete tear of the anterior cruciate ligament and in 9 per cent of patients who had a normal anterior cruciate ligament at the time of arthroscopy. In patients with a torn anterior cruciate ligament and one or more bone bruises, these bruises were seen in the posterior aspect of the lateral tibial plateau in 32 per cent of cases, in this tibial region and the middle aspect of the lateral femoral condyle in 36 per cent of cases, and in the lateral femoral condyle and medial femoral condyle in 23 per cent of cases. These last investigators emphasized the time-dependent nature of the bone bruises, indicating that they rarely were seen when the MR imaging examination was performed nine or more weeks after the injury. Results of this study indicated a 73

per cent prevalence of bone bruise in patients with anterior cruciate ligament tear who underwent MR imaging within 9 weeks of injury and, in 91 per cent of cases, the lateral compartment of the knee was involved. The authors concluded that the pattern of bone bruise involving the posterior compartment of the lateral tibial plateau, alone or together with that of the middle aspect of the lateral femoral condyle, occurs predominantly but not exclusively in association with acute complete anterior cruciate ligament tear. Such bruises usually are not evident when the patient is examined 9 or more weeks after the knee injury.

Other patterns of bone contusion occurring in patients with anterior cruciate ligament tears relate to avulsion fractures. These occur in the lateral tibial rim (Segond fracture) and posterior margin of the lateral tibial plateau, related to capsular avulsions of the tibia (Fig. 70–343). Marrow edema is evident on the MR imaging examinations, but the fracture fragments may not be appreciated. Anterior cruciate ligament deficiency also may relate to avulsion fractures at its sites of insertion (Fig. 70–344).

Postoperative Anterior Cruciate Ligament. As disruption of the anterior cruciate ligament represents the most frequent of all the ligamentous injuries of the knee, a great deal of thought and study has been directed at its treatment. Left untreated, progressive deterioration of the knee joint, manifest as meniscal tears, further ligamentous damage, and cartilage loss, may occur. Radiographic evidence of osteoarthritis has been reported in approximately one third of patients with anterior cruciate ligament disruption who have been studied serially over a period of years.[1033, 1034] Many variables, however, enter into the decision regarding the need for surgical intervention and the precise type of procedure required. Whether the anterior cruciate ligament is completely or partially torn and the presence or absence of meniscal and other ligamentous damage influence this decision. Furthermore, lifestyle of the patient also plays a significant role in the decision-making process. Persons who are athletic (i.e., high risk lifestyle) are more likely candidates for surgery than those who are sedentary or who are involved in only modest amounts of physical activity. In patients in whom a conservative therapeutic approach is chosen, functional bracing and modifications in lifestyle may represent a sufficient treatment protocol, particularly in instances of isolated or partial tears of the anterior cruciate ligament.

Principles of Ligament Reconstruction. Operative procedures employed for the treatment of the torn anterior cruciate ligament include primary repair of the ligament, ligament repair plus augmentation using various autogenous grafts, and ligament reconstruction using autogenous

FIGURE 70–342. Injuries of the anterior cruciate ligament: MR imaging. Acute complete anterior cruciate ligament tears with osteochondral impaction fractures. Sagittal **(A)** and coronal **(B)** T2-weighted (TR/TE, 2000/80) spin echo MR images in a patient with an acute tear of the anterior cruciate ligament reveal one typical site of bone injury, appearing as a region of high signal intensity (arrows) in the posterolateral aspect of the proximal portion of the tibia.

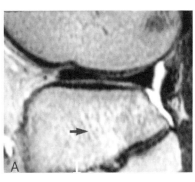
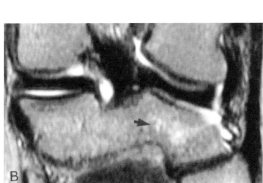

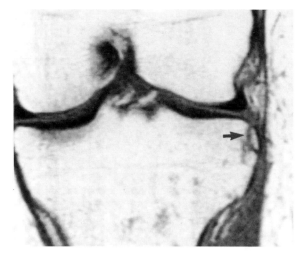

FIGURE 70–343. Injuries of the anterior cruciate ligament: MR imaging. Subacute complete anterior cruciate ligament tears with lateral capsular avulsion fracture (Segond fracture). A coronal T1-weighted (TR/TE, 400/20) spin echo MR image shows a small fracture fragment (arrow) without displacement.

materials, allografts, or prosthetic devices.[1035, 1036] Of the autogenous intra-articular reconstructions, the bone–patellar tendon–bone graft has become the anterior cruciate ligament substitute to which all others are being compared.[1035] The success of this procedure, or other similar ones in which the iliotibial tract, semitendinosus tendon, or gracilis tendon is used as the graft material, depends upon a number of factors, including the structural and material properties of the graft, the intra-articular positioning of the graft, initial tensioning of the graft during implantation, fixation of the graft, and the postoperative rehabilitation regimen.[1035]

Theoretical advantages relate to the choice of the patellar tendon graft. In experimental situations, preparations using

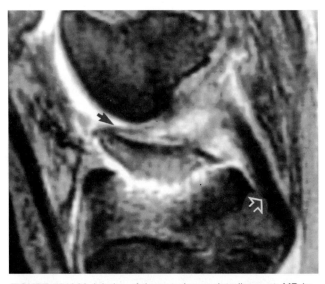

FIGURE 70–344. Injuries of the anterior cruciate ligament: MR imaging. Acute avulsion of the anterior tibial eminence. A sagittal MPGR MR image (TR/TE, 600/20; flip angle, 45 degrees) shows a displaced avulsion fracture of the tibial eminence. Note the insertion of the anterior cruciate ligament (solid arrow) into the fracture fragment. The site of attachment of the posterior cruciate ligament (open arrow) is not involved. (Courtesy of S. Fernandez, M.D., Mexico City, Mexico.)

bone–patellar tendon–bone graft material have been stronger than those using the semitendinosus or gracilis tendon.[1037, 1038] Furthermore, the bone-to-bone apposition used with this graft procedure provides immediate and secure fixation, enabling joint motion soon after surgery. The structural properties of the bone–patellar tendon–bone graft change with time following the surgical procedure. Experimentally, stiffness and ultimate failure of the strength of this preparation decrease over a period of months following surgery, related to increased water content in the graft and, perhaps, to changes in the profile of the collagen fiber and rearrangement of its ultrastructural morphometry.[1039] In animals and in humans, the remodeling process occurring in the graft has been documented repeatedly and is believed to be consistent with synovial revascularization.[1040]

The middle third of the patellar tendon with its accompanying bone plugs or blocks is used.[1041] The femoral insertion site chosen generally is close to or at the normal insertion site of the anterior cruciate ligament. Similarly, the tibial insertion site of the graft usually corresponds closely to that of the anterior cruciate ligament itself. The principle guiding the selection of appropriate femoral and tibial insertion sites is based upon isometry. Isometric points are those regions of ligamentous attachment to the femur and the tibia that allow the graft to undergo minimal (if any) change in its length and associated load during flexion and extension of the knee.[1042] Identification of such isometric points is complicated by the fact that the graft has material and geometric properties different from those of the normal anterior cruciate ligament.[1035] Furthermore, the anterior cruciate ligament is composed of bands of fibers, each with different morphologic characteristics. As the anteromedial band of the anterior cruciate ligament demonstrates the least amount of change in length during knee movement, autogenous graft procedures probably should reproduce the function of this band of the ligament by assuming its sites of femoral and tibial attachment.[1035, 1036] In replacements of the anterior cruciate ligament, isometry is less sensitive to the site of tibial attachment of the graft than to the site of femoral attachment. Accurate positioning of the femoral tunnel through which the graft passes appears to be critical.[1036] If this tunnel is placed too far anteriorly with respect to the normal anatomic insertion site of the anterior cruciate ligament, high strain along the graft occurs as the knee is flexed; in such cases, knee flexion may be restricted, or over a period of time, the graft may elongate.[1035, 1036] Graft placement posterior or distal to the normal site of femoral attachment of the anterior cruciate ligament leads to similar problems during knee extension. Although the position of the tibial tunnel (through which the graft passes) is less critical to the success of the surgery, this tunnel should be positioned so that the graft does not impinge against the roof of the intercondylar notch when the knee is fully extended.[1035, 1043, 1044]

After proper positioning of the graft is achieved, an appropriate graft tension is chosen based upon the desire to restore normal joint kinematics.[1035] This choice is difficult, owing to a viscoelastic response that occurs in all grafts that may lead to stress relaxation. Secure fixation of the graft to the host bone also is essential to surgical success. For bone–patellar tendon–bone grafts, large diameter interference-fit screws often are used to fix the bone plugs to the walls of the femoral and tibial tunnels. These screws serve to press the bone plug against the side of the drill hole, and they may be combined with additional screws or staples used to secure the adjacent soft tissue. Finally, rehabilitation of the knee following surgery is essential, but the need for immobilization or early mobilization of the knee is not agreed upon, resulting in different rehabilitation protocols.[1035]

A variety of prosthetic devices and other means have been used to serve as artificial substitutes for the torn anterior cruciate ligament. Three general types of artificial ligaments exist: prostheses (which are designed to replace the ligament permanently); scaffolds (which produce support for ingrowing tissue by possibly inducing orientated ingrowth of collagen); and stents (which temporarily protect an autogenous graft from excessive strain during the period of its revascularization and collagen maturation).[1414] Such artificial ligaments have considerable appeal owing to the theoretical advantage of immediate strength and therefore a rapid return to full function. In practice, however, numerous complications are seen with many of the ligament substitutes, leading to the current popularity of the bone–patellar tendon–bone graft procedure.

The success of surgical repair of the torn anterior cruciate ligament is influenced by the procedure chosen, the skill of the orthopedic surgeon, and the resolve of the patient during the many months of rehabilitation. Postoperative stiffness of the knee represents a frequent and disabling problem. Failure to regain full extension of the knee after anterior cruciate ligament reconstruction procedures may relate to graft impingement (see later discussion), fat pad fibrosis, the reflex sympathetic dystrophy syndrome, and intra-articular adhesions. The patellar entrapment syndrome results in a loss of knee extension or knee flexion, with reduced patellar mobility.[1045] It may relate to adherence of the patella to the adjacent infrapatellar fat body, leading to contracture of the patellar tendon, a low-lying patella (patella baja or infera), and loss of patellar cartilage. The cyclops lesion is a fibrous nodule that develops anterior to the tibial insertion site of the graft, within the intercondylar notch, and that may lead to loss of knee extension[1046] (Fig. 70–345).

Routine Radiography. The normal radiographic appearance of the knee following reconstruction of the anterior cruciate ligament has been summarized by Manaster and coworkers.[1047] Both frontal and lateral radiographs provide indirect information regarding the placement of the graft material, based upon the position of the tunnels in the femur and the tibia. As indicated previously, these tunnels should exit at the level of the joint in regions close to or at the normal sites of attachment of the anterior cruciate ligament. In the lateral projection, the tibial osseous tunnel begins distally near the tibial tuberosity, courses posteriorly, and exits the tibial articular surface immediately anterior to the anterior tibial spine; in the frontal projection, this tunnel begins in the medial side of the tibia, courses laterally, and exits the tibial articular surface at the intercondylar eminence of the tibial plateau.[1047] In the lateral projection, the intra-articular point of entrance of the femoral tunnel is at the intersection of two lines representing the posterior femoral cortex and the intercondylar shelf; in the frontal projection, the femoral osseous tunnel begins laterally, just superior to the lateral femoral condyle, and emerges on the superolateral aspect of the intercondylar notch.[1047]

Radiographic findings associated with improper placement of the anterior cruciate ligament graft material (i.e., nonisometric attachment) relate to the identification of osseous tunnels in the femur and tibia that vary from the normal landmarks noted previously. The construction of a number of lines on lateral radiographs of the maximally extended knee has been used to identify improperly oriented tibial tunnels.[1048] The location of a tibial tunnel that is completely anterior to the line of the intercondylar roof (Blumensaat's line), as seen in these radiographs, is consistent with impingement on the anterior portion of the graft by the intercondylar roof.[1048] Additional radiographic abnormalities relate to breakage of the screws or staples, fracture of the bone plugs, fracture of the patella (related to the donor sites of the bone blocks), patella baja (related to the patellar entrapment syndrome), and patella alta (related to avulsion or rupture of the patellar tendon).[1045, 1047, 1049–1051]

MR Imaging. Postoperative impingement of the anterior cruciate ligament graft may occur in the intercondylar notch, blocking full extension of the knee and causing erosion and possible disruption of the graft. Although routine radiography may provide indirect evidence of such impingement,[1048] MR imaging allows direct visualization of the graft itself (Fig. 70–345) and potentially is a superior imaging method in establishing the diagnosis of graft impingement. Although an initial report indicated a limited role for MR imaging in the assessment of reconstructed anterior cruciate ligaments,[1052] some of the subsequent investigations of the diagnostic role of MR imaging in this assessment have led to more promising results. Rak and associates[1053] emphasized a poorly delineated graft and buckling of the posterior cruciate ligament as MR imaging findings consistent with graft inadequacy. The low signal intensity of the normal graft material has been emphasized,[1054, 1055] and an increase in signal intensity in the graft, particularly in the distal two thirds of its intra-articular portion, has been attributed to impingement of the graft by the intercondylar roof.[1048, 1056] The results of some studies suggest that persistent low signal intensity in the graft is an indicator of the absence of roof impingement, but the presence of increased signal intensity, although suggesting roof impingement, may occur with or without clinical evidence of knee instability.[1056] Further diagnostic difficulty regarding the interpretation and clinical significance of regions of increased signal intensity within the graft relates to the known occurrence of remodeling of the graft (with revascularization and cellular ingrowth) in the early postoperative period. Such remodeling may lead to some variability in the appearance of the graft on MR imaging studies. In one study, only 2 of 15 autografts (bone–patellar tendon–bone grafts) in clinically stable knees appeared as bands of low signal intensity in the MR images.[1057]

At this time, MR imaging appears to represent an effective technique for assessing the precise position of the intraosseous tunnels,[1058] but its value in allowing detection of clinically significant graft impingement is not clear. MR imaging also reveals time-dependent changes in configuration and signal intensity within the patellar tendon when a portion of it has been used for the anterior cruciate ligament reconstructive procedure.[1059]

Posterior Cruciate Ligament Injuries. Injuries to the posterior cruciate ligament are less frequent than those to the anterior cruciate ligament, they require greater force,

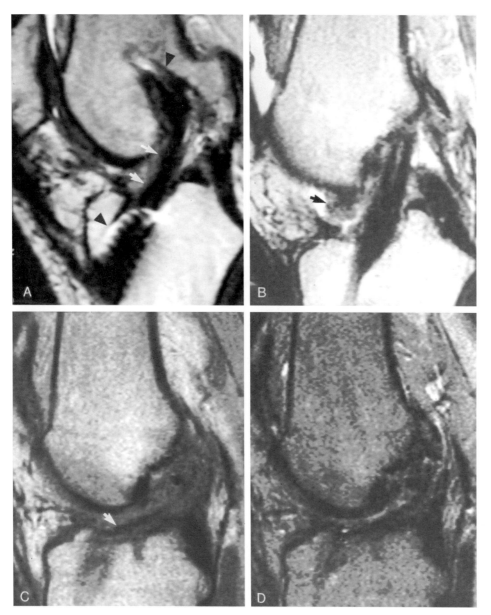

FIGURE 70–345. Postoperative anterior cruciate ligament: MR imaging.

A Normal appearance. A sagittal T2-weighted (TR/TE, 3800/100) spin echo MR image in an asymptomatic patient with a bone–patellar tendon–bone autograft shows the sites of the intraosseous tunnels (arrowheads) and a graft (arrows) that is straight in contour and of low signal intensity. A slight increase in signal intensity in the distal portion of the patellar tendon is evident.

B Cyclops lesion. A sagittal T2-weighted (TR/TE, 8000/135) spin echo MR image shows a nodular region (arrow) of low signal intensity anterior to the reconstructed anterior cruciate ligament. At surgery, a fibrous nodule, or cyclops lesion, was found.

C, D Autograft rupture. Sagittal proton density–weighted (TR/TE, 2400/20) **(C)** and T2-weighted (TR/TE, 2400/80) **(D)** spin echo MR images reveal only a portion of the autograft (arrow) and, in **D**, adjacent high signal intensity.

(B–D, Courtesy of M. Recht, M.D., Cleveland, Ohio.)

and they initially may be unrecognized, leading to a delay in diagnosis.[1359] Injuries to this ligament represent approximately 5 to 20 per cent of all knee injuries. The usual mechanism of injury producing a tear of the posterior cruciate ligament is a force applied to the anterior aspect of the proximal portion of the tibia with the knee flexed. This mechanism occurs from a fall or when the knee of a passenger in a car strikes the dashboard. Posterior cruciate ligament injuries also may result from extreme hyperextension or hyperflexion of the knee or from rotational or valgus forces applied to the knee.[1060–1062] They may occur as an isolated phenomenon (30 per cent of cases) or in association with other capsular, ligamentous, or meniscal injuries (70 per cent of cases).

Although the reported prevalence of posterior cruciate ligament injuries is low (less than 20 per cent of all ligamentous injuries of the knee), subtle clinical findings in some cases of isolated injury to the posterior cruciate ligament may lead to missed diagnoses. Pain, swelling, and a hemarthrosis[1063] may be evident; however, the frequent lack

of soft tissue swelling or ecchymosis in these cases may result in a diagnosis of a knee sprain with conservative (and often inadequate) therapy.[1064] The posterior drawer test, in which stress is applied to the anterior surface of the tibia in an attempt to produce posterior translation of the tibia with respect to the femur, is positive in 30 to 75 per cent of cases of posterior cruciate ligament tears, and a posterior sag sign represents additional evidence of such a tear.[988] Although arthroscopy can provide direct evidence of a tear of the posterior cruciate ligament, diagnostic problems arise owing to incomplete visualization of this ligament at arthroscopy when the anterior cruciate ligament is intact or misinterpretation of a normal meniscofemoral ligament of Humphrey as an intact posterior cruciate ligament. Imaging studies can be used to supplement the clinical assessment.

Routine Radiography. In cases of injury to the posterior cruciate ligament, routine radiography may reveal avulsion fractures at the tibial site of insertion of the ligament. This may occur in adults or in children. A joint effusion may be present. Owing to the nonspecific nature of a joint effusion

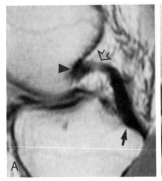
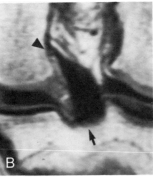

FIGURE 70–346. Normal posterior cruciate ligament: MR imaging.

A Sagittal proton density–weighted (TR/TE, 2000/20) spin echo MR image. Note the femoral (arrowhead) and tibial (solid arrow) insertion sites of the posterior cruciate ligament. It has an arcuate course and is of low signal intensity except for its proximal portion (open arrow), where intermediate signal intensity may relate to the magic angle phenomenon.

B Coronal proton density–weighted (TR/TE, 2000/20) spin echo MR image. The femoral (arrowhead) and tibial (solid arrow) insertion sites of the posterior cruciate ligament again are identified. The ligament is of low signal intensity and has a smooth contour.

and to the infrequent occurrence of an avulsion fracture, however, routine radiography rarely contributes to the diagnosis of a posterior cruciate ligament injury.

MR Imaging: Normal Posterior Cruciate Ligament. The posterior cruciate ligament normally appears as a band-like structure of low signal intensity on sagittal, coronal, and transaxial MR images (Fig. 70–346). In sagittal MR images, it is arcuate in shape when the knee is in a neutral position or mildly flexed. With increasing flexion, the ligament becomes taut and, with hyperextension, it appears lax.[1065] The posterior cruciate ligament is seen in its entirety in a single MR image or possibly two contiguous MR images in the sagittal plane. The meniscofemoral ligament, consisting of the anterior (ligament of Humphrey) and posterior (ligament of Wrisberg) branches, leads to ovoid regions of low signal intensity, either applied to the surface of the posterior cruciate ligament or adjacent to it.[726] In the coronal plane, the posterior cruciate ligament again is identified in a single MR image or perhaps two contiguous MR images. It possesses a gentle curve. Occasionally, in elderly persons, mucoid or eosinophilic degeneration in the poste-

rior cruciate ligament may lead to regions of intermediate signal intensity (Fig. 70–347).

MR Imaging: Posterior Cruciate Ligament Tears. Tears of the posterior cruciate ligament usually occur in its midsubstance, or less commonly, at its femoral or tibial insertion site.[1065] Disruption of all or a portion of its fibers is evident on the MR imaging examination, especially in sagittal images (Figs. 70–348 to 70–350). Regions of high signal intensity within the ligament may be evident on T2-weighted spin echo MR images in cases of acute or subacute tears of the posterior cruciate ligament (Figs. 70–348 and 70–349). These regions may relate to hemorrhage or joint fluid collecting within the torn ligament. The diagnosis of avulsion fractures of the tibia at the site of insertion of the posterior cruciate ligament is possible with MR imaging (Fig. 70–351), although correlation with routine radiography is required.

Sonin and associates[1415] reported the MR imaging findings in 47 patients with injury to the posterior cruciate ligament, the diagnosis being confirmed arthroscopically in 24 patients. Complete tears (45 per cent), partial tears (47 per cent), and bone avulsions (8 per cent) were seen. Associated ligamentous (38 per cent) or meniscal (47 per cent) injuries were frequent. Regions of altered signal intensity in the bone marrow, compatible with contusions or fractures, also were common (36 per cent). Localization of such regions to the anterior portion of the tibial articular surface is particularly characteristic.

Tears of the posterior cruciate ligament are treated by primary repair, involving suturing of the ligament, that may be combined with graft augmentation.[1065, 1360] The role of MR imaging in the assessment of the repaired posterior cruciate ligament is not documented.

Cartilage Abnormalities

Anatomic Considerations. Articular hyaline cartilage is a complex structure whose integrity is fundamental to proper joint function. Covering the articulating ends of bones in synovial joints, articular cartilage has unique structural characteristics that provide an extremely smooth and resilient surface that can withstand the high pressure and rapid velocity generated during normal articular movement. Articular cartilage is composed primarily of collagen and proteoglycans, as detailed in Chapter 23.

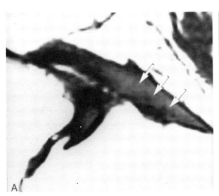
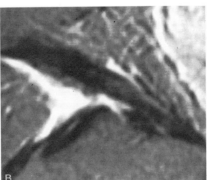
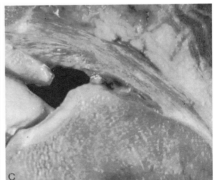

FIGURE 70–347. Normal posterior cruciate ligament: MR imaging. Variations in signal intensity related to eosinophilic degeneration. Sagittal T1-weighted (TR/TE, 500/20) **(A)** and T2-weighted (TR/TE, 2000/70) **(B)** spin echo MR images show regions of intermediate signal intensity (arrows) that are much more prominent in **A** than in **B**. A corresponding anatomic section **(C)** shows that the posterior cruciate ligament is grossly normal and its fibers are parallel to the sagittal plane. (From Hodler J, et al: AJR *159:* 357, 1992.)

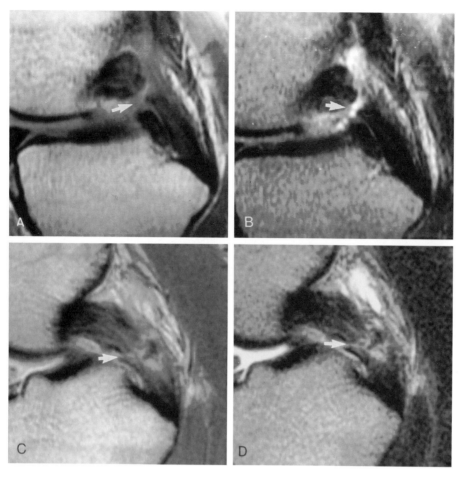

FIGURE 70–348. Injuries of the posterior cruciate ligament: MR imaging. Acute complete posterior cruciate ligament tears with alterations in ligament morphology and signal intensity.

A, B Sagittal proton density–weighted (TR/TE, 2000/30) **(A)** and T2-weighted (TR/TE, 2000/80) **(B)** spin echo MR images reveal complete disruption (arrows) of the posterior cruciate ligament, with an increase in signal intensity in **B**.

C, D Sagittal proton density–weighted (TR/TE, 2200/20) **(C)** and T2-weighted (TR/TE, 2200/80) **(D)** spin echo MR images in a second patient again show complete disruption (arrows) of the posterior cruciate ligament, with an increase in signal intensity in **D**.

Macroscopic and microscopic analysis of articular cartilage indicates a structure whose composition changes throughout its substance (Fig. 70–352). Its superficial, or tangential, zone, representing approximately 5 to 10 per cent of its total thickness, is composed of flattened and elongated cells oriented parallel to the surface of the joint. The collagen fibers are horizontally disposed, and the ma-

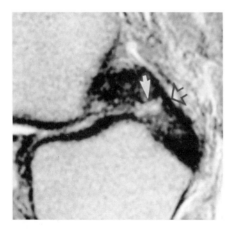

FIGURE 70–349. Injuries of the posterior cruciate ligament: MR imaging. Acute partial posterior cruciate ligament tears with alterations in ligament morphology and signal intensity. A sagittal T2-weighted (TR/TE, 2000/80) spin echo MR image shows that the posterior cruciate ligament has an irregular contour and contains a region (solid arrow) of high signal intensity. Some of the fibers of the posterior cruciate ligament are intact (open arrow).

trix contains less proteoglycan than that present in other zones. The second zone, located deep to the superficial zone and designated the transitional or intermediate stratum, contains chondrocytes that are larger and appear singly or in groups. The third zone, designated the radiate stratum, contains columns of large cells that are oriented perpendicular to the surface, following the pattern of collagen deposition. This is the largest layer of articular cartilage, representing 70 to 80 per cent of its total thickness. The fourth and deepest zone is designated the calcified stratum, composed of nonviable cells and heavily calcified matrix. The inferior surface of the calcified zone of cartilage is irregular or undulating, with tongues of tissue that extend into and interdigitate with the subchondral bone. The tidemark represents a basophilic line, recognized on histologic analysis, that marks the junction between the calcified and noncalcified cartilage. The subchondral bone contains a thin plate that overlies the cancellous trabeculae that surround the marrow elements.

Nourishment of articular cartilage is derived from three sources: the synovial fluid, through a process of intrusion and extrusion of fluid that occurs with normal movement; the vessels of the synovial membrane; and the vessels of the underlying marrow cavity, which may penetrate or extend completely through the calcified layer of cartilage.

Pathologic Considerations. Healing of articular cartilage following an acute injury or a chronic insult is marginal at best, owing to its relative avascularity and its sparse cellularity. Healing of a cartilage defect that does not involve the subchondral bone plate relies entirely on chondro-

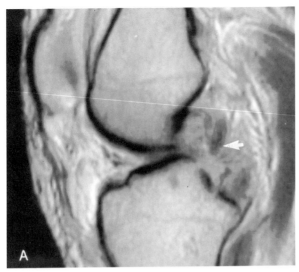
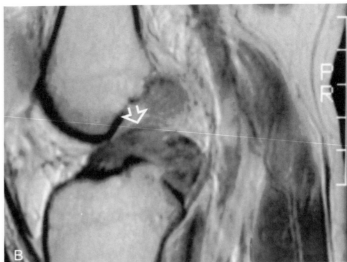

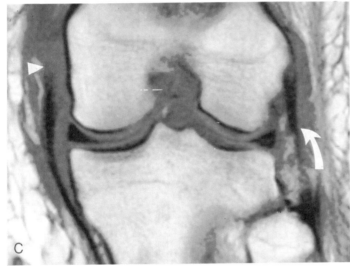

FIGURE 70–350. Injuries of the posterior cruciate ligament, anterior cruciate ligament, lateral collateral ligament, and medial collateral ligament: MR imaging. Acute tears of all ligaments following knee dislocation. Sagittal **(A, B)** and coronal **(C)** proton density–weighted (TR/TE, 4000/21) fast spin echo MR images in this patient reveal disruption of the posterior cruciate ligament (solid straight arrow), anterior cruciate ligament (open arrow), medial collateral ligament (arrowhead), and lateral collateral ligament (curved solid arrow). Disruption of three or more of the major ligaments of the knee generally suggests a dislocation of the joint.

FIGURE 70–351. Injuries of the posterior cruciate ligament: MR imaging. Acute avulsion of the posterior tibial eminence. A sagittal T1-weighted (TR/TE, 600/20) spin echo MR image shows a large, slightly displaced bone fragment (solid arrows) to which the posterior cruciate ligament (open arrow) attaches.

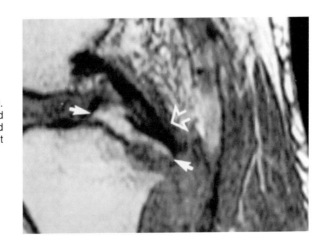

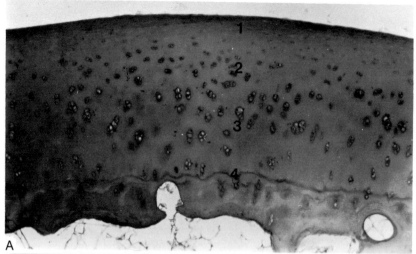

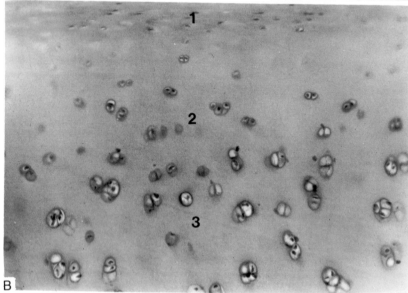

FIGURE 70–352. Cartilage abnormalities: Anatomic considerations. Photomicrographs (×80, ×200) reveal the superficial or tangential zone of cartilage (1) with flattened cartilage cells, the transitional zone (2) with numerous irregularly distributed cells, the radiate stratus (radial zone) (3) with a columnar arrangement of cells, and the calcified stratum (4) adjacent to the osseous surface.

cyte proliferation at the margins of the injured area. Although chondrocytes can proliferate, the response generally is inadequate to lead to complete healing of the lesion. With cartilage injuries that extend to the subchondral bone plate, a healing response characterized by granulation tissue and fibroblastic proliferation is evident.[1066, 1067] The resulting fibrocartilaginous scar tissue differs morphologically from normal hyaline cartilage.

The overall cellularity, fluid content, and collagen and glycosaminoglycan composition of articular cartilage does not change significantly with age.[1068] Although aging articular cartilage appears yellow, there is no evidence to suggest that this pigment has any functional significance.[1068] Cartilage fibrillation, however, is an age-dependent process, occurring initially at the periphery of the joint surfaces and in the superficial layers.[1069, 1070] Splitting, fraying, and pitting of the articular surface characterize this fibrillation, which on chemical analysis is associated with depletion of glycosaminoglycans and with normal collagen concentration.[1068] Such cartilage fibrillation is not regarded as synonymous with osteoarthritis, although it may progress to involve the deeper layers of cartilage. The initial stages of osteoarthritis are characterized by softening of the articular cartilage, with disruption occurring along the planes of the collagen fibrils. This process may extend vertically, involv-

ing deeper layers of the cartilage, progressing to reach the tidemark and, with abrasion of the abnormal cartilage, exposing the subchondral bone. The changes of osteoarthritis resemble those of aging but, in loaded (i.e., weight-bearing) portions of a joint, are more extensive. The morphologic changes of osteoarthritis, however, certainly resemble those of aging, differing primarily in extent. The relationships of those changes in articular cartilage that relate to aging, those that relate to osteoarthritis, and those that are designated as chondromalacia are not clear.

Cartilage Degeneration. Owing to the difficulty in distinguishing among the cartilage alterations of aging and those occurring in chondromalacia and osteoarthritis, all of these findings are considered together here. From an imaging standpoint, many of the standard methods (e.g., conventional radiography, arthrographic and tomoarthrographic techniques, and ultrasonography) used to evaluate cartilage degeneration relate to the assessment of chondral loss. None of these is ideal. Some, such as standard radiography, require the use of films obtained during weight-bearing or application of stress, and others, such as arthrographic methods, require the injection of contrast material. Ultrasonography is applicable only when the articular surfaces can be positioned in such a manner as to allow their assessment with probes placed on the skin surface. Scintigraphy generally requires the presence of changes in the subchondral bone. MR imaging, however, appears unique in its ability to demonstrate not only cartilage loss but internal chondral derangement as well.

Routine Radiography. As indicated in Chapter 39, routine radiographic assessment of cartilage loss, particularly in weight-bearing joints such as the knee, includes standard radiographic projections and those obtained with weight-bearing, varus or valgus stress, knee flexion, or combinations of these techniques. Most of these methods are adequate for the determination of cartilage loss in the more involved weight-bearing compartment (i.e., medial femorotibial or lateral femorotibial compartment) and inadequate for the assessment of such lesions in the less involved weight-bearing compartment. Tunnel views, accomplished with knee flexion in the supine or standing position, may be more valuable than standard radiographic projections, based on the more extensive cartilage loss evident in the posterior portion of the femoral condyles. Radiographs obtained with the application of varus or valgus stress to the knee also may allow a better assessment of the extent of cartilage loss in the more involved weight-bearing compartment but do not improve the analysis of chondral deterioration in the less involved weight-bearing compartment.

Arthrography. Contrast material injected into the joint cavity allows visualization of portions of articular cartilage. Because of the differences in shape of the articular surfaces of the femur and tibia, the tibial cartilage is more completely evaluated than the femoral cartilage. Knee arthrography with conventional tomography may improve visualization of cartilaginous surfaces.[1071]

The role of arthrography in the diagnosis of chondromalacia of the patella has been the subject of debate. Most observers regard its role as minor or nonexistent,[1072, 1073] although others are more optimistic.[1074, 1075] The posterior surface of the patella is V-shaped, with medial and lateral facets separated by an osseous ridge. Routine lateral projections during arthrography demonstrate only a small amount of the patellar cartilaginous surface, that near the apex of the ridge. Axial projections increase the cartilaginous area that can be visualized, and oblique projections that are tangential to the medial and lateral facets may further improve this visualization.[1076] If overhead and fluoroscopic filming is accomplished using lateral, oblique, and axial positions supplemented with conventional or computed tomography, the diagnosis of chondromalacia indeed may be substantiated by arthrography in some patients.[1077–1080] On arthrography, chondromalacia produces absorption or imbibition of contrast material by the patellar cartilage. Nodular elevation, fissuring, or diminution of the cartilaginous surface may be apparent.

Contrast examination of the knee in patients with degenerative joint disease delineates abnormalities of the articular cartilage and menisci and the presence of intra-articular osseous bodies and popliteal cysts.[1072] Arthrography in these persons does have certain limitations: Proper positioning during arthrography in the elderly patient with degenerative disease can be extremely difficult and time-consuming; tangential portions of the cartilaginous surface are the only areas that are visualized adequately; and evaluation of femoropatellar disease is difficult, as the patellar cartilage is not well shown. Despite these shortcomings, arthrography may delineate generalized cartilaginous thinning or localized cartilaginous defects. A rough, irregular surface with imbibition of contrast material may be apparent.

Compared with routine and weight-bearing radiographic films, arthrography adds little additional information regarding alterations in the more involved femorotibial compartment.[1072] In the less involved (contralateral) compartment, arthrography may reveal information regarding cartilaginous integrity not obtainable by these other examinations (Fig. 70–353).

Meniscal alterations in patients with degenerative joint disease can include acute tears, similar in appearance to those occurring in patients without degenerative joint disease, or degenerative tears. These latter tears appear as swollen, irregular meniscal surfaces with fragmented inner contours and imbibition of contrast material. Horizontal

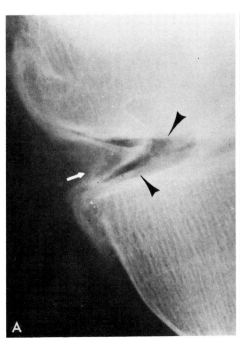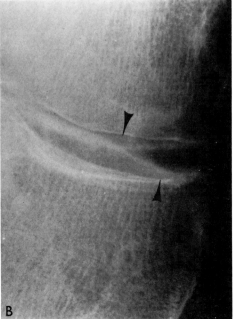

FIGURE 70–353. Cartilage abnormalities: Arthrography. In a patient with osteoarthritis of the knee, arthrography reveals severe denudation of articular cartilage in both the femur and the tibia (arrowheads) in the medial femorotibial compartment **(A)**. The medial meniscus is swollen, with an incomplete vertical tear (arrow) and an irregular inner contour. In the lateral femorotibial compartment **(B)** thinning of the articular cartilage can be seen (arrowheads), although the lateral meniscus appears normal.

collections of contrast material within the involved meniscus represent degenerative crevices.

Ultrasonography. As indicated in Chapter 39, the role of ultrasonography in the assessment of the articular cartilage is limited by the necessity of positioning the joint in such a manner as to provide proximity to the articular surface for a probe placed on the skin. Although acute flexion of the knee allows sonographic analysis of portions of the articular cartilage in the femoral condyles, the cartilage in the proximal portion of the tibia and the posterior surface of the patella is not evaluated. Information derived from this procedure, therefore, is incomplete.

MR Imaging: Normal Articular Cartilage. The application of MR imaging to the assessment of articular cartilage, particularly that of the knee, has been the subject of numerous investigations. Owing to its excellent contrast resolution, its ever-increasing spatial resolution, and the ability to obtain images in any plane, the superiority of MR imaging, when compared with other imaging methods, in this assessment seems guaranteed. In practice, however, the usefulness of this technique in providing clinically important information regarding the integrity of the articular cartilage is not certain. Although severe chondral abnormalities, including full-thickness defects and denudation of the articular surface, are delineated with MR imaging, the detection of more superficial cartilage lesions with this imaging method is far more challenging. Despite the application of modified MR imaging sequences and newer MR imaging methods, the results of prior investigations have been inconsistent and often have not withstood critical analysis. A multitude of MR pulse sequences have been advocated, including T1-weighted,[1081–1083] proton density–weighted,[1084] and T2-weighted[1084–1086] standard spin echo sequences; fast spin echo sequences[1416]; T1-weighted inversion recovery sequences[1087]; magnetization transfer contrast sequences[1088, 1394]; fat-suppressed sequences[1089, 1090]; and both two- and three-dimensional gradient recalled echo sequences.[1091–1095] The reported sensitivity and specificity for detecting cartilage lesions with these sequences have ranged from a low of 31 per cent[1092] and 50 per cent,[1085] respectively, to a high of 100 per cent[1085, 1094] for each. Recently, MR arthrography enhanced with intra-articular administration of gadolinium compounds has been shown to be effective in the detection of cartilage abnormalities,[1096, 1097] but this method is time-consuming and invasive.

In addition to the uncertainty regarding the efficacy of these sequences in enabling the depiction of cartilage lesions, the appearance of normal cartilage with the various sequences also is unclear. The majority of descriptions of cartilage in spin echo and gradient echo images has indicated a homogeneous signal intensity or a subtle bilaminar appearance[1081, 1092, 1093] (Fig. 70–354). A study using high-resolution spin echo imaging found a trilaminar appearance of normal cartilage.[1098] The cause of the different signal intensities in the three layers is uncertain, but it was postulated that the different layers corresponded to the different histologic zones of cartilage.[1098] The thin surface layer was believed to represent the histologically superficial zone, with the middle layer representing the transitional zone, and the deep layer representing a combination of the deep radiate zone, the calcified cartilage zone, and the subchondral bone.

Recht and collaborators,[1099] in a study of cadaveric knees

in which multiple MR imaging methods were employed, found that a bilaminar or trilaminar appearance of articular cartilage occasionally was present with spin echo and certain gradient echo sequences, but this was not a consistent finding. The reason for the variability in the appearance of cartilage with these sequences was uncertain. With fat-suppressed spoiled gradient recalled acquisition in the steady state (SPGR) sequences, cartilage appeared to have a trilaminar appearance, consisting of a superficial region of high signal intensity, an intermediate region of low signal intensity, and a deep region of high signal intensity (Fig. 70–355). Determination of the cause of the different signal intensities in the three layers and their histologic correlation was not possible in this study. The superficial location of the outer region of high intensity suggested the possibility that this region corresponded to the histologically apparent superficial zone of cartilage.

Rubenstein and collaborators,[1100] using spin echo MR imaging sequences in the analysis of bovine articular cartilage, also detected a trilaminar appearance of normal cartilage (with signal intensity characteristics corresponding closely to those reported by Recht and coworkers[1099]). Results of polarized light microscopy of histologic specimens confirmed the three zones, and transmission electron microscopy showed different collagen arrangements in the zones. With rotation of the specimens with respect to the main magnetic field, an isotropic effect on signal intensity was noted, especially in the hypointense second lamina. Because of the preferential alignment of water molecules associated with collagen, angular rotation of the cartilage in the direction of minimum dipolar coupling (55 degrees to the magnetic field, i.e., the magic angle) caused the cartilage to have a homogeneous appearance. Rubenstein and colleagues[1100] concluded that the MR imaging appearance of the three layers of articular cartilage is strongly influenced by an isotropic arrangement of the collagen and by the alignment of the specimen relative to the magnetic field, and that similar principles can be expected to apply to MR imaging characteristics of normal human articular cartilage.

The results of available studies underscore the complexity of the issue of MR imaging of articular cartilage. As the MR imaging appearance of normal articular cartilage is not agreed upon and certainly is influenced by the precise imaging method or sequence employed, disagreement regarding the value of MR imaging in assessing abnormal cartilage is to be expected (see following discussion). Ultimately, the role of MR imaging in this regard may relate, not to the analysis of the morphology of articular cartilage, but rather to its physiology. Specifically, the integrity of articular cartilage relates to proper nutrition in which nutrients and waste products are moved in and out of the cartilage matrix, mainly as a result of diffusion of synovial fluid.[1101–1103] Although the most widely used technique for the in vitro evaluation of diffusive transport in cartilaginous tissues is the radioactive tracer method[1104, 1105] (in which measurements are made of the intrachondral flux of a radioisotope contained in a bath to which the cartilage is exposed), MR imaging also may be employed for this purpose.[1106]

MR Imaging: Abnormal Articular Cartilage. The use of MR imaging in the study of abnormal cartilage has been investigated extensively. Although MR imaging sequences and techniques have varied, analysis of the knee, particu-

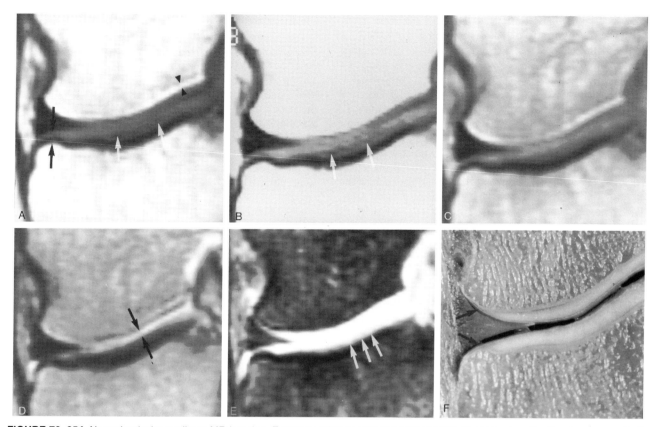

FIGURE 70–354. Normal articular cartilage: MR imaging. Femoral and tibial articular cartilage (lateral compartment) without macroscopically visible focal defects examined with spin echo and gradient echo sequences.

A Coronal T1-weighted (TR/TE, 600/20) spin echo MR image. Cartilage is represented by a superficial layer of intermediate signal intensity and a deep layer of low signal intensity (black arrows). The presence of a chemical shift artifact is suggested, which may explain the difference in thickness of the deep hypointense layer between the tibial and femoral sides. A hyperintense line at the periphery of the femoral fat marrow is consistent with this suggestion (arrowheads). The normal articular cartilage shows slight irregularity (white arrows).

B Coronal T1-weighted (TR/TE, 600/20) spin echo MR image photographed with meniscal windowing. Slight cartilage irregularity is more pronounced (arrows).

C Coronal proton density–weighted (TR/TE, 2000/20) spin echo MR image. There is reduced contrast. The cartilage appears to be more homogeneous.

D Coronal T2-weighted (TR/TE, 2000/70) spin echo MR image. The superficial layer of cartilage is narrower. The differentiation between the cartilage surface and the joint fluid is difficult (arrows).

E Coronal MPGR MR image (TR/TE, 450/15; flip angle, 15 degrees). The superficial layer of cartilage demonstrates high signal intensity. Differentiation between the fluid and the surface of the articular cartilage is difficult. Cartilage irregularities potentially simulate fluid-filled ulcerations (arrows).

F Corresponding anatomic section. The cartilage is grossly normal. Note that its thickness is significantly less at the periphery of the joint.

(From Hodler J, et al: J Comput Assist Tomogr *16:*597, 1992.)

FIGURE 70–355. Normal articular cartilage: MR imaging. Patellofemoral articular cartilage. Transaxial 3DFT SPGR acquisition in the steady state MR image (TR/TE, 52/10; flip angle, 60 degrees) obtained with chemical presaturation of fat (ChemSat). The articular cartilage is of high signal intensity, and the bone and synovial fluid (arrowhead) are of low signal intensity. The articular cartilage possesses a trilaminar appearance, best appreciated in the lateral patellar facet and the lateral femoral condyle; the superficial portion of articular cartilage is of high signal intensity, a thin intermediate region shows low signal intensity, and the deep portion of the articular cartilage is of high signal intensity.

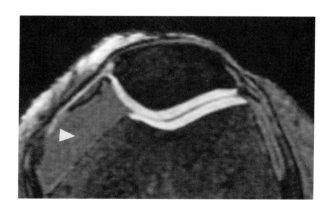

larly the patellofemoral joint, has received the most attention. The choice of the patellofemoral joint is a wise one, owing to the thickness of the normal articular cartilage of the patella, the frequent occurrence of chondromalacia patellae and osteoarthritis of the patellofemoral compartment, and the adequate display of this compartment provided by transaxial MR images. Numerous MR imaging sequences have been employed in the study of the patellar articular cartilage, some more successfully than others. As a general rule, any MR imaging sequence that is insensitive to the detection of abnormal patellar cartilage will be even less sensitive to cartilage changes in other locations, such as the femorotibial compartments and hip, owing to more complex regional anatomy. In fact, in any site, angular or curved articular surfaces can lead to diagnostic difficulty during MR imaging, owing to partial volume artifacts that lead to superimposition of subchondral bone and articular cartilage. Thin section imaging displays that can be accomplished with the use of volumetric gradient echo MR sequences may diminish these artifacts but not eliminate them.

The choice of a standard by which the results of MR imaging of articular cartilage can be assessed creates added difficulty. Although gross morphologic and histologic analysis can be used as a standard in cadaveric studies, arthroscopy generally is chosen as the standard in patient studies. Differences in examiner expertise, terminology, sites of analysis, and techniques of measurement (landmarks may be better defined on cross-sectional images than during arthroscopy) are encountered that make arthroscopy a less than ideal standard by which to judge the sensitivity and specificity of MR imaging abnormalities.

With MR imaging, two fundamental findings of abnormal articular cartilage are sought: altered thickness and modified signal intensity. With regard to the first, detection of decreased thickness of articular cartilage as the sine qua non for cartilage abnormality is an oversimplification. Diminution in cartilage thickness is a well-known manifestation of moderate to advanced osteoarthritis; however, thickening of cartilage may occur following its injury, a finding documented repeatedly in animal models in which the knee has been rendered unstable with surgical techniques.[1107–1109] Cartilage, like other connective tissues, swells when injured, a finding that is well documented during arthroscopic assessment of chondromalacia. The cause of posttraumatic cartilage thickening is not clear; an increase in proteoglycan content, of water, or of both, may be important in the pathogenesis of cartilage thickening.[1109, 1110] Thus, this increase in cartilage thickness may represent hypertrophy secondary to repair or edema, owing to recurrent injury in the experimentally produced unstable knee.[1111] Long-term studies in such knees have indicated that cartilage breakdown and loss may follow the stage of cartilage thickening.[1112] Similarly, thickening of articular cartilage may represent an early manifestation of osteoarthritis in humans, and progressive loss of articular cartilage may indicate more advanced disease.

The accurate determination of increased or decreased cartilage thickness with MR imaging requires identification of its most superficial and deepest layers on sequential images in any plane. An ideal MR imaging sequence used to assess articular cartilage is one that, among other attributes, allows precise definition of the interfaces between the surface of the cartilage and the joint space and between the deepest layer of cartilage and the subchondral bone. The interface between the deepest layer of cartilage and the subchondral bone is anatomically complex, however, consisting of a layer of calcified cartilage, a subchondral bone plate, and the adjacent spongy trabeculae and marrow of the subchondral bone. Furthermore, the interface between the superficial layer of cartilage and the joint space changes according to the congruency of the apposing articular surfaces, the presence of any gap or tissue void between these surfaces, and the presence, amount, and composition of joint fluid. Thus, identification of a specific MR imaging sequence that provides good delineation of these two interfaces in one particular clinical situation and in one anatomic location does not necessarily indicate that this same sequence is useful in other situations and in different anatomic locations. The presence of a joint effusion generally is regarded as an advantage in delineation with MR imaging of superficial changes in the articular cartilage, as long as an imaging sequence is chosen that accentuates the differences in signal intensity of the fluid and the articular cartilage. This principle forms the basis for the use of MR arthrography (with intra-articular instillation of saline or gadolinium compounds) in the assessment of articular cartilage, especially in patients in whom native joint fluid is either absent or minimal (see later discussion). With spin echo MR imaging, T2-weighted sequences lead to an arthrogram-like effect in patients with joint effusions, with synovial fluid hyperintense relative to hyaline cartilage. Multislice gradient echo MR sequences (employing a longer echo time and low flip angle) also lead to this arthrogram-like effect[1113] (Fig. 70–356). Alternatively, if a single-slice or volumetric positive-contrast technique is desired, a minimal repetition time (TR), minimal echo time (TE), intermediate flip angle GRASS sequence may be used.[1113] Evaluation of intrinsic cartilage lesions is facilitated by optimizing contrast-to-noise ratios between synovial fluid and hyaline cartilage. A multiplanar sequence for this purpose would have a minimal TE and a large flip angle, leading to a T1-weighted appearance with synovial fluid hypointense relative to hyaline cartilage.[1113] If a single-scan or three-dimensional technique is desired, a GRASS sequence at minimal TR and TE and intermediate flip angle may be used.

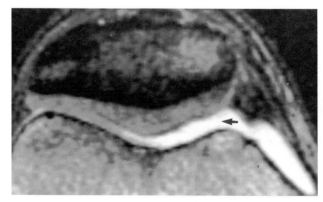

FIGURE 70–356. Normal articular cartilage: MR imaging. Patellofemoral articular cartilage. Transaxial MPGR MR image (TR/TE, 450/20; flip angle, 15 degrees). The presence of joint fluid (arrow) of high signal intensity allows improved visualization of the surface of the articular cartilage.

The second fundamental finding of cartilage abnormality is altered signal intensity. The clinical significance of this finding, however, in the absence of alterations in cartilage thickness or surface irregularities of cartilage is not entirely clear, as correlative histologic and histochemical data generally are lacking. Some previous MR imaging studies of patellofemoral cartilage have employed grading systems in which the lowest grade has consisted of intrachondral alterations of signal intensity (hypointensity or hyperintensity) occurring in the absence of chondral surface irregularities or alterations of cartilage thickness,[956, 1099] but the reported data do not allow assessment of the clinical significance of this grade of abnormality.

Complicating the MR imaging analysis of abnormal articular cartilage are technical and anatomic pitfalls. The chemical shift artifact is the spatial misrepresentation of predominantly water-containing tissue versus fat-containing tissue that occurs along the frequency-encoding axis.[1114] The articular cartilage whose surface is perpendicular to this axis appears thicker or thinner than it is actually, leading to diagnostic error. Rotation of the frequency- and phase-encoding gradients allows more accurate appraisal of the true thickness of this articular cartilage. As indicated previously, partial volume-averaging artifacts also can lead to improper analysis of cartilage integrity.

A description of the most frequently employed MR imaging techniques for cartilage assessment follows.

1. Standard spin echo sequences. Standard T1-weighted and T2-weighted spin echo images have been used to analyze hyaline cartilage (Figs. 70–357 and 70–358). The T1-weighted spin echo MR images provide good anatomic detail and high contrast between cartilage and subchondral bone, but they are associated with poor contrast between cartilage and joint fluid. The advantages of T2-weighted spin echo MR images include an arthrogram-like effect when a joint effusion is present and the ability to delineate signal intensity changes within the articular cartilage; their disadvantages include poor contrast between articular cartilage and subchondral bone and insufficient resolution to allow detection of contour abnormalities in the absence of a joint effusion. Hayes and collaborators,[1081] in a cadaveric study of the patellar cartilage, found T1-weighted spin echo MR images to be satisfactory for defining cartilage morphology, allowing detection of focal cartilage lesions (as small as 3 or 4 mm in diameter) and diffuse chondral thinning. With these images, contrast between joint fluid and cartilage was found to be less than that provided by T2-weighted spin echo MR images, but adequate to permit visualization of more advanced cartilage lesions. These investigators indicated that T2-weighted spin echo MR images were less useful, owing to decreased spatial resolution, poor contrast between subchondral bone and cartilage, and poor delineation of changes in signal intensity within the cartilage. Speer and coworkers[1092] noted the value of an arthrogram-like effect on T2-weighted spin echo MR images provided by a joint effusion in the detection of partial-thickness and full-thickness cartilage lesions of the knee. De Smet and co-investigators[1115] noted distinctive defects or fissures of high signal intensity in the patellar articular cartilage on sagittal T2-weighted spin echo MR images that corresponded to arthroscopically proven sites of chondromalacia. McCauley and associates[1084] also emphasized the importance of T2-weighted, as well as proton density, spin echo MR images in the diagnosis of cartilage lesions. In their study of chondromalacia patellae, focal cartilage abnormalities in signal intensity or contour on one or both of these MR images yielded the highest correlation with the arthroscopic diagnosis of chondromalacia. In a commentary on this investigation, Hodler and Resnick[1083] indicated that they had confirmed several of these findings, mainly: (1) the importance of focal changes in signal intensity in the diagnosis of localized cartilage defects; (2) the infrequency of direct depiction of chondral contour abnormalities; (3) the relative insensitivity of proton density–weighted images alone; and (4) the value of the combined analysis of different MR imaging sequences. These last investigators also indicated that MR imaging is better suited for visualization of cartilaginous defects that do not contain any tissue, rather than those containing residual fibrillated cartilage or granulation tissue. Hodler and collaborators[1116] subsequently reported an MR imaging investigation of femorotibial articular cartilage in cadavers in which they concluded that the

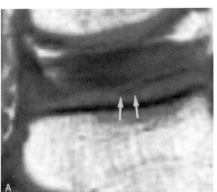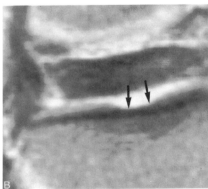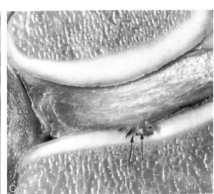

FIGURE 70–357. Articular cartilage abnormalities: MR imaging. Femorotibial articular cartilage (lateral compartment). Standard spin echo MR images. Focal defect in the tibial articular cartilage.

A Coronal oblique T1-weighted (TR/TE, 600/20) spin echo MR image. The tibial cartilage is focally thinned (arrows). The depth of the articular cartilage defect is underestimated.

B Coronal oblique T2-weighted (TR/TE, 2000/70) spin echo MR image. The defect is filled with hyperintense joint fluid that depicts the extent of the defect more exactly but not its precise form (arrows).

C Corresponding anatomic section. A deep focal defect nearly extends to the subchondral bone. Fibrillation within the defect may explain part of the fact that the T1-weighted MR images led to an underestimation of the size of the defect (arrows).

(From Hodler J, et al: J Comput Assist Tomogr *16:*597, 1992.)

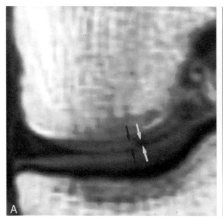
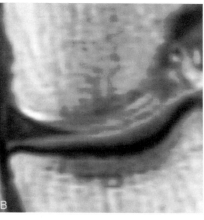
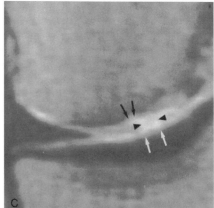
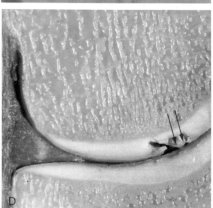

FIGURE 70–358. Articular cartilage abnormalities: MR imaging. Femorotibial articular cartilage (medial compartment). Standard spin echo MR images. Focal defect in the femoral articular cartilage.

A Coronal T1-weighted (TR/TE, 600/20) spin echo MR image. The lateral (more central) part of the defect is hypointense (white arrows). Medially (more peripherally), minimally increased signal intensity is seen within the deep hypointense cartilage layer (black arrows).

B Coronal proton density–weighted (TR/TE, 2000/20) spin echo MR image. The lateral part of the defect is less obvious, while hyperintensity is more marked than on the T1-weighted spin echo MR image in the medial part of the defect.

C Coronal T2-weighted (TR/TE, 2000/70) spin echo MR image. The medial part of the defect is well demarcated (black arrows), while differentiation between the lateral part of the lesion and the joint fluid is difficult (arrowheads). The presence of joint fluid simulates cartilage irregularity on the tibial surface (white arrows).

D Corresponding anatomic section. A gross cartilage defect with some tissue within the lateral (central) part (arrows) is evident.

(From Hodler J, et al: J Comput Assist Tomogr *16*:597, 1992.)

value of those MR imaging sequences (i.e., T1-weighted, proton density, and T2-weighted spin echo sequences, as well as multiplanar gradient recalled sequences) used routinely in the analysis of internal derangements of the knee in the detection of focal defects of the hyaline cartilage is limited. Brown and Quinn,[1117] using proton density and T2-weighted spin echo MR images, concluded that such images were valuable only in the diagnosis of advanced lesions of chondromalacia patellae.

2. Standard spin echo sequences combined with fat-suppression techniques. Although many fat-suppression techniques are available, most are based on four methods or their modifications[1118]: Dixon and chopper methods, the hybrid method, frequency-selection presaturation (ChemSat), and short tau inversion recovery (STIR). The Dixon and chopper methods are based on the production of separate water- and fat-based MR images, and the hybrid method in the spin echo mode of data acquisition uses a single two-excitation MR sequence.[1118] The ChemSat technique initially involves the selective excitation of fat (as compared with water) with a narrow-band pulse in the absence of any gradients, and subsequently dephases the signal of fat with added gradients and then immediately continues with the choice of a specific imaging sequence.[1118] The ChemSat technique is most effective when high field strength magnets are used. Inhomogeneities in the magnetic field lead to inconsistent fat suppression in some cases, an artifact that can be minimized through the use of a smaller field of view.

The assessment of articular cartilage using fat-suppression methods combined with standard spin echo technique has received limited attention (Fig. 70–359). In one study,

Chandnani and coworkers[1089] used both standard and hybrid suppression methods with and without the intra-articular injection of saline solution and gadopentetate dimeglumine in the analysis of femorotibial cartilage in cadaveric knees. These investigators found the hybrid fat suppression technique combined with T1-weighted spin echo MR imaging sequences with or without saline injection to be superior to standard spin echo MR images alone in the visualization of the articular cartilage. With this method, intra-articular fluid is of low signal intensity compared with the high signal intensity of the articular cartilage. Thus, the interfaces between the chondral surface (of high signal intensity) and the joint fluid (of low signal intensity), and between the chondral surface (of high signal intensity) and the subchondral bone (of low signal intensity) are well seen. Koskinen and collaborators,[1119] in a study of cadaveric patellae with a low field strength magnet, arrived at similar conclusions. König and associates[1091] also found chemical shift (and gradient refocused) images to be more useful than standard spin echo MR sequences in the detection of early osteoarthritis, although they indicated that the presence of a joint effusion led to some diagnostic difficulty in the assessment of articular cartilage. The results of most of these investigations reinforce the concept that fat-suppression imaging methods combined with standard spin echo MR imaging, by changing the dynamic range of the images, afford excellent contrast between articular cartilage and surrounding structures in both the presence and absence of a joint effusion, but its effectiveness in delineating intrachondral abnormalities is not proved.

3. STIR sequences. Although STIR sequences are used extensively for the analysis of infections, tumors, and trau-

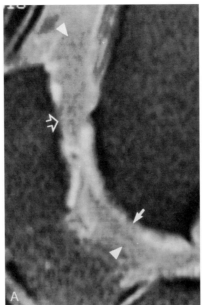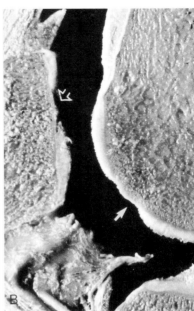

FIGURE 70–359. Articular cartilage abnormalities: MR imaging. Patellofemoral articular cartilage. T1-weighted spin echo MR images with hybrid method of fat suppression. Cartilage fibrillation and erosion. A sagittal T1-weighted (TR/TE, 500/20) spin echo MR image following the intra-articular injection of saline **(A)** shows cartilage thinning in the femoral condyle (solid arrow) and erosion of cartilage (open arrow) in the patella. Note the low signal intensity of the saline (arrowheads). The cartilage findings (solid and open arrows) are corroborated in the corresponding anatomic section **(B)**.

(From Chandnani V, et al: Radiology *178:*557, 1991.)

matic disorders of bone and soft tissue, their application to the assessment of articular cartilage lesions has received little attention. STIR imaging sequences are effective in depressing the signal intensity in the bone marrow and, therefore, may allow clear separation between the articular cartilage and subchondral bone. The interface between cartilage and joint fluid generally is poorly delineated with such sequences, however, as both fluid and cartilage reveal high (fluid) or moderately high (cartilage) signal intensity. STIR imaging is extremely sensitive to the detection of joint fluid, subchondral cystic lesions containing such fluid, and marrow alterations in regions of subchondral bone sclerosis.[1122]

4. Fast spin echo sequences. Fast spin echo MR imaging sequences are used increasingly to provide images with the desired type of contrast in a shorter acquisition time. For example, heavily T2-weighted images can be obtained far more rapidly with fast spin echo rather than standard spin echo techniques. The disadvantages of the fast spin echo method include a loss of spatial resolution along the phase-encoded axis that is exaggerated on images obtained with short echo times and that leads to image blurring and to a decrease in the number of images that can be obtained at any given repetition time (when compared with standard spin echo methods). Furthermore, as fat reveals a relatively high signal intensity even in heavily T2-weighted fast spin echo images, the combination of fast spin echo imaging and fat-suppression techniques has become popular.

The application of fast spin echo MR imaging sequences to cartilage analysis has not been studied extensively. In common with T2-weighted standard spin echo methods, an arthrogram-like effect provided by joint fluid on fast spin echo images obtained with long repetition times may prove useful in delineating the chondral surface. Such was the case in one study by Broderick and coworkers[1416] who used a dual fast spin echo pulse sequence combined with fat suppression to evaluate the knees in patients with osteoarthritis and in normal persons. These investigators indicated that cartilage and adjacent fluid could be easily differentiated in short TE and long TR images. In almost all cases,

contrast resolution allowed detection of inhomogeneity of signal intensity in diseased cartilage, and correlation of MR imaging findings and those at arthroscopy was high. A tendency of cartilage abnormalities to be underestimated with this fast spin echo technique also was noted, however.

5. Gradient recalled echo sequences. Both two- and three-dimensional gradient recalled echo (GRE) sequences have been used to study articular cartilage.[1091–1095, 1099, 1113, 1120, 1121] Many of these sequences provide high contrast between articular cartilage, synovial fluid, and subchondral bone; some allow the acquisition of radial sections that are perpendicular to the articular surface (Fig. 70–360), and those using volumetric acquisition allow thin contiguous scans and reformatting of image data in any plane that is desired (Fig. 70–360). Disagreement exists regarding the selection of specific GRE scanning parameters that are optimal for analysis of articular cartilage, however. As examples, fast imaging with steady precession (FISP) with a flip angle of 70 degrees and a short repetition time (TR) has been advocated for the assessment of degenerative changes in hyaline cartilage[1123]; and short TR fast low-angle shot (FLASH) sequences with a flip angle of 12 degrees have been considered appropriate for the general evaluation of articular cartilage.[1091] In a detailed analysis of various GRE techniques that were used to assess the patellofemoral joint in normal volunteers, Yao and coworkers[1113] arrived at the following conclusions:

1. For optimal contrast-to-noise ratios (synovial fluid–cartilage), the best multiplanar sequence (for TE less than 23 msec) is with a short TE and a large flip angle (e.g., TR/TE, 400/9; flip angle, 73 degrees).

2. If a single scan or three-dimensional technique providing optimal contrast-to-noise ratios is desired, a GRASS sequence at minimal TR and TE and intermediate flip angle (e.g., TR/TE, 18/9; flip angle, 32 degrees) is best.

3. For optimal signal-to-noise ratios (for both synovial fluid and hyaline cartilage), the best multiplanar sequence employs a short TE and an intermediate flip angle (e.g., TR/TE, 400/9; flip angle, 30 degrees).

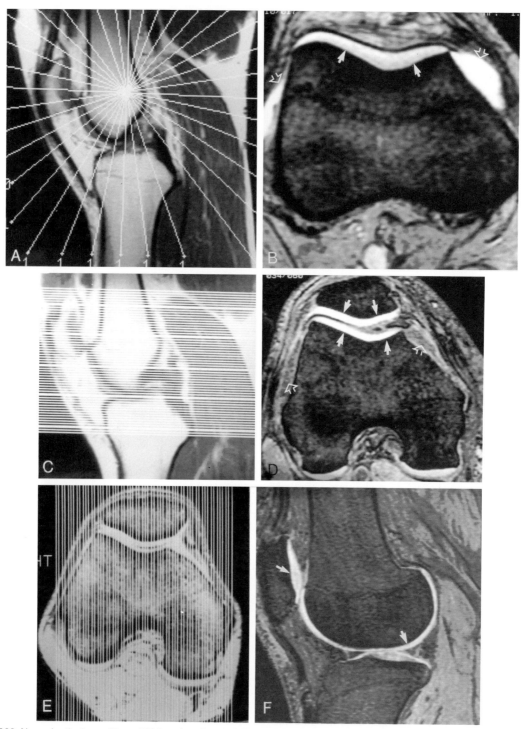

FIGURE 70–360. Normal articular cartilage: MR imaging. Femoral, tibial, and patellar articular cartilage. Gradient recalled echo sequences.

A, B Multiplanar gradient recalled (MPGR) MR images with radial sections to assess femoral cartilage. From a sagittal T1-weighted (TR/TE, 450/20) spin echo MR localizer image **(A)**, radial sections can be programmed such that the plane of individual images is perpendicular to the articular surface of the distal portion of the femur. One such MPGR MR image (TR/TE, 450/15; flip angle, 20 degrees) is shown **(B)**. Note the high signal intensity of articular cartilage (solid arrows) with a trilaminar appearance and the high signal intensity of joint fluid (open arrows).

C, D Three-dimensional Fourier transform (3DFT) SPGR acquisition in the steady state with assessment of patellar and femoral cartilage. From a similar sagittal T1-weighted (TR/TE, 450/20) spin echo MR localizer image **(C)**, transaxial SPGR MR images (TR/TE, 52/10; flip angle, 60 degrees) obtained with chemical presaturation of fat (ChemSat) **(D)** can be obtained. Note the high signal intensity of articular cartilage (solid arrows) and the low signal intensity of joint fluid (open arrows).

E, F Three-dimensional Fourier transform (3DFT) SPGR acquisition in the steady state with assessment of femoral and tibial cartilage. From a transaxial MPGR MR image (TR/TE, 450/15; flip angle, 20 degrees) **(E)**, sagittal SPGR MR images (TR/TE, 52/10; flip angle, 60 degrees) obtained with chemical presaturation of fat (ChemSat) **(F)** can be obtained. Note the high signal intensity and trilaminar appearance of articular cartilage (solid arrows).

4. If a short TR, high signal-to-noise technique is desired, GRASS (e.g., TR/TE, 18/9; flip angle, 13 degrees) is superior to FLASH.

Recht and colleagues[1099] assessed the patellofemoral articular cartilage in cadavers using the intra-articular administration of saline and a number of GRE sequences and standard spin echo sequences including: two fat-suppressed three-dimensional spoiled GRASS (SPGR) sequences; a nonfat-suppressed three-dimensional SPGR sequence; a three-dimensional GRASS sequence; and T1-weighted, proton density–weighted, and T2-weighted spin echo sequences (Fig. 70–361). Using grading systems for the severity of the cartilage as seen in the various MR images, and for the confidence level of the observer, and employing close MR imaging–pathologic correlation, these investigators found that the fat-suppressed three-dimensional SPGR sequences provided the most accurate results, with a sensitivity of 96 per cent, a specificity of 95 per cent, and an accuracy of 95 per cent. The two SPGR sequences (TR/TE, 52/5; flip angle, 30 degrees; and TR/TE, 52/10; flip angle, 60 degrees) revealed a trilaminar appearance in regions of normal articular cartilage. With these sequences, regions of abnormal cartilage were characterized by loss of the surface layer and sometimes of the deeper layers of cartilage (Fig. 70–362). Abnormal low signal intensity frequently was seen in the articular cartilage adjacent to the area of cartilage loss. No statistically significant difference was identified between the two fat-suppressed SPGR sequences in the detection of lesions. The sequence with flip angle of 60 degrees and echo time of 10 msec was slightly superior for allowing correct staging of the cartilage lesions; in this sequence, 24 of 25 lesions were graded within one grade of the corresponding macroscopic grade. Although these results are promising, the SPGR sequences are time-consuming, and their effectiveness in displaying cartilage abnormalities in regions other than the patellofemoral joint (Fig. 70–363) is not proved.

6. MR arthrography. As indicated earlier, MR arthrography has been used in the evaluation of many articulations, including the knee. The rationale for its application to the assessment of articular cartilage is based upon the improved visualization of the chondral surface that results when joint fluid is present. MR arthrography can be accomplished with the intra-articular injection of saline or gadolinium compounds; the advantages of gadolinium administration in-

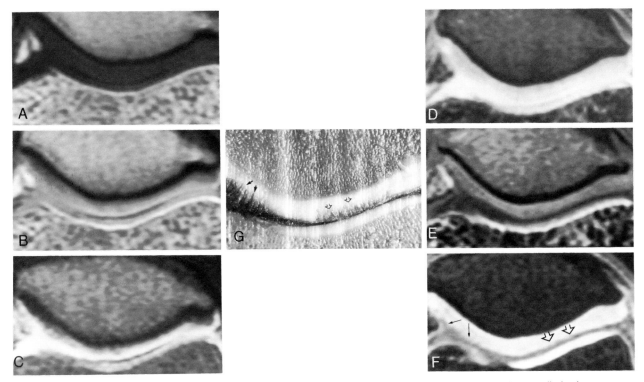

FIGURE 70–361. Articular cartilage abnormalities: MR imaging. Patellar articular cartilage. Spin echo and gradient recalled echo sequences. A variety of transaxial MR imaging sequences are used to analyze a grade 2 cartilage lesion (minor surface fibrillation or loss of less than 50 per cent of the cartilage thickness) of the lateral patellar facet and a grade 3 cartilage lesion (severe surface fibrillation or loss of more than 50 per cent of the cartilage thickness but without exposure of subchondral bone) of the medial patellar facet.
    A T1-weighted (TR/TE, 500/14) spin echo MR image.
    B Proton density–weighted (TR/TE, 2000/20) spin echo MR image.
    C T2-weighted (TR/TE, 2000/70) spin echo MR image.
    D Three-dimensional Fourier transform (3DFT) GRASS MR image (TR/TE, 40/10; flip angle, 30 degrees).
    E 3DFT spoiled GRASS MR image (TR/TE, 40/5; flip angle, 30 degrees).
    F 3DFT fat-suppressed (ChemSat) spoiled GRASS MR image (TR/TE, 52/10; flip angle, 60 degrees).
    The medial (solid arrows) and lateral (open arrows) patellar facet lesions are indicated in the corresponding transverse anatomic section **(G)**.
    The patellar cartilage abnormalities are seen best in **F** (solid arrows and open arrows). The absence of cartilage in the medial femoral condyle is secondary to the plane of sectioning and is not a true cartilage lesion.
    (From Recht MT, et al: *Radiology 187:*473, 1993.)

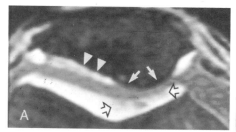

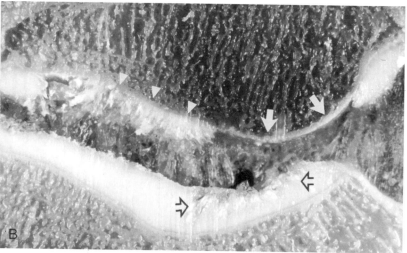

FIGURE 70–362. Articular cartilage abnormalities: MR imaging. Patellar and femoral articular cartilage. A transaxial 3DFT SPGR acquisition in the steady state MR image (TR/TE, 60/10; flip angle, 60 degrees) obtained with chemical presaturation of fat (ChemSat) **(A)** and a corresponding transverse anatomic section **(B)** are shown. In **A**, the articular cartilage of the patella is focally absent (solid arrows) or severely thinned (arrowheads), and that of the femur reveals surface irregularity and altered signal intensity (between open arrows). The corresponding cartilage regions are indicated (closed and open arrows and arrowheads) in **B**. (From Recht MT, et al: Radiology *187*:473, 1993.)

clude its high signal intensity on T1-weighted spin echo MR images that allows for high spatial resolution and shorter examination time (Fig. 70–364). As MR arthrography can be coupled with other MR imaging techniques, including various gradient recalled sequences, saline injection also may be employed. In one study in which focal defects were created in the articular cartilage in cadaveric knees, MR arthrography using gadolinium compounds, as compared with saline, enabled detection of smaller chondral lesions.[1096]

Some disadvantages exist to the use of MR arthrography. As with standard arthrography, a needle puncture and proper localization of the needle in the joint are required, lengthening examination time. An underestimation of cartilage thickness, particularly with gradient echo imaging, may occur. In part, this may result from a delay in examination time, allowing imbibition of the gadolinium compound (or saline) into the superficial layers of cartilage. Overestimation of cartilage thickness, particularly with T1-weighted spin echo imaging, also may be encountered. Furthermore, the long-term effects of gadolinium compounds on the articular cartilage and synovial membrane are not known.

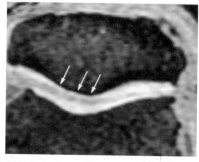

FIGURE 70–363. Articular cartilage abnormalities: MR imaging. Patellar articular cartilage. A transaxial 3DFT SPGR acquisition in the steady state MR image (TR/TE, 58/10; flip angle, 60 degrees) obtained with chemical presaturation of fat (ChemSat) shows diffuse cartilage thinning (arrows) involving mainly the medial portion of the patella. Fluid of low signal intensity is seen between the femoral and patellar cartilage.

7. Magnetization transfer contrast. Magnetization transfer contrast (MTC), or saturation transfer imaging, is a newer MR imaging method that improves contrast in gradient recalled sequences and that is sensitive to the interaction between water and macromolecules.[1124] With MTC, low-power radiofrequency irradiation is applied off resonance to selectively saturate H-1 nuclei with a short T2, as part of a conventional gradient recalled echo MR imaging sequence. The saturation of the short T2 component then is transferred to the bulk water protons via a magnetization exchange process, which is highly selective for water protons.[1124, 1125] MTC, therefore, provides unique information regarding the interaction between water and macromolecules.[1125] Compared with standard gradient recalled echo MR images, MTC images demonstrate increased contrast between many tissue pairs.[1125] When applied to the analysis of the knee, MTC has been shown to improve contrast in standard single-section gradient recalled echo images with regard to fat-muscle, muscle–flowing blood, and cartilage–synovial fluid interfaces[1126] (Fig. 70–365). The improvement of contrast between the articular cartilage and synovial fluid also is apparent on three-dimensional images,[1126] images that otherwise are associated with decreased contrast. Although contrast generation with MTC is complex, MTC images and T2-weighted images generally reveal increased signal intensity in similar regions.[1124] Thus, synovial fluid is of high signal intensity on MTC images. The sharp contrast generated between the cartilage and the synovial fluid with MTC suggests that the cartilage contains macromolecules that strongly interact with water protons.[1126] With MTC, hypertrophic synovial tissue also reveals increased signal intensity, underscoring the potential of saturation transfer imaging to allow discrimination among cartilage, joint fluid, and pannus.[1394]

Chondral and Osteochondral Injury. Two types of fractures involve articular cartilage: shearing fractures that produce chondral or osteochondral lesions confined to the superficial surfaces of the joint; and fractures in periarticular bone that also pass through the articular cartilage of the joint.[1127] These latter fractures often extend perpendicularly through the cartilage as a direct extension of the fracture line within the bone. Resulting incongruity of the joint

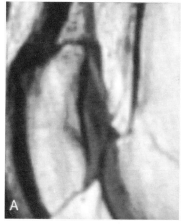 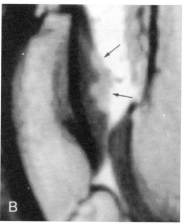 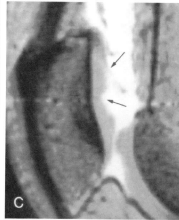

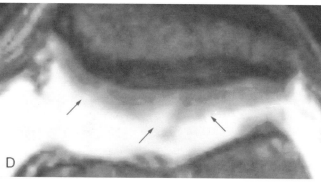

FIGURE 70–364. Articular cartilage abnormalities: MR arthrography. Patellar articular cartilage.

A A sagittal T1-weighted (TR/TE, 700/15) spin echo MR image shows subtle alterations in signal intensity in the patellar articular cartilage.

B In the same patient, a sagittal T1-weighted (TR/TE, 700/15) spin echo MR image obtained following the intra-articular injection of a gadolinium compound shows surface irregularity of the patellar articular cartilage (arrows) with imbibition of fluid.

C In the same patient, a sagittal three-dimensional MR image using fast imaging with steady-state precession (FISP) (TR/TE, 30/10; flip angle, 35 degrees) obtained following the intra-articular administration of a gadolinium compound better defines the surface irregularity of the patellar articular cartilage (arrows).

D In the same patient, a transaxial three-dimensional MR image using FISP (TR/TE, 30/10; flip angle, 35 degrees) obtained following the intra-articular administration of a gadolinium compound dramatically displays the extent of articular cartilage abnormalities in the patella (arrows).

(Courtesy of J. Kramer, M.D., Vienna, Austria.)

surface often is underestimated with routine radiography and is assessed more actively with imaging methods that allow indirect (e.g., arthrography) or direct (e.g., MR imaging) visualization of the chondral surface.

Chondral and osteochondral lesions, as well as osteochondritis dissecans, are discussed in detail in Chapter 67. As many of these lesions involve the articular surfaces of the knee (e.g., femoral condyles, patella), a few additional comments are appropriately placed here. Rotatory or shearing forces generated by acute trauma or impaction forces occurring during a joint dislocation can lead to injury of the articular surface, in which a portion of the surface is avulsed. The injuries may be purely chondral, may include a tiny or large fragment of bone and the entire overlying cartilage, or rarely, may involve bone alone if the overlying cartilage already has been eroded by an unrelated joint process.[1127] The resulting fragment may remain in situ or it may be partially or completely detached. If completely detached, it may become a free body in the joint, sometimes lodging and becoming embedded in a distant portion of the synovial membrane.

The pathologic characteristics of chondral and osteochondral fractures have been described in detail by Milgram.[1127–1130] The cartilage injury often is more complex than a simple fracture line, consisting of comminution and crushing of cartilage tissue. Beneath the disrupted chondral fragment, the remaining cartilage may appear relatively normal or may demonstrate a blister-like effect. Acutely,

any bone that has been separated along with the overlying cartilage appears normal histologically and, at its base, local hemorrhage and crushing of exposed trabeculae may be observed. In more chronic cases, the osteochondral fragment may be attached by a soft tissue pedicle to its site of origin. The composition of this pedicle varies: it may be secure or loose, cartilaginous or fibrous, long or short, and avascular or vascular.[1127] In the knee, osteochondral fractures of the femoral condyles commonly result in a mobile lesion containing considerable portions of overlying, intact cartilage and fibrous and cartilaginous pedicles. At any site, repair at the base of an osteochondral lesion is associated with fibrocartilaginous proliferative tissue derived from subchondral bone. Even empty craters may contain such tissue.

The detection of an osteochondral fragment containing a sizeable piece of bone that is located in its original osseous bed, is free in the joint cavity, or is embedded in the synovial membrane, can be accomplished reasonably well with routine radiography, conventional tomography, or CT. The detection of an osteochondral fragment containing a small piece of bone or a purely chondral fragment located in any of these sites frequently requires additional imaging methods, such as standard arthrography (Fig. 70–366), conventional arthrotomography, computed arthrotomography, or MR imaging, that provide indirect or direct evidence that such a fragment is present.

Evaluation of chondral and osteochondral fractures and

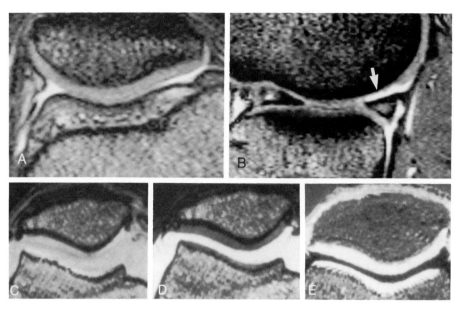

FIGURE 70–365. Normal and abnormal articular cartilage: MR imaging with magnetization transfer contrast (MTC) or saturation transfer (ST) imaging. Patellar and femoral articular cartilage.

A Normal patellar articular cartilage. A transaxial single section gradient recalled echo MR image (TR/TE, 650/15; flip angle, 40 degrees) obtained with MTC reveals the smooth patellar articular cartilage, which is of low signal intensity when compared with the joint fluid.

B Abnormal femoral articular cartilage. In a sagittal single section gradient recalled echo MR image obtained with MTC, a chondral defect (arrow) of the lateral femoral condyle is apparent. Note fluid of high signal intensity within the cartilage defect.

C–E Normal patellar and femoral articular cartilage. Transaxial images in an unfrozen cadaveric knee after the intra-articular injection of 55 ml of saline to simulate a joint effusion. Conventional 3DFT GRASS MR image (TR/TE, 60/7; flip angle, 20 degrees) **(C)**; addition of on-resonance pulsed ST to the sequence in **C (D)**; and ST subtraction image, obtained by subtracting image **D** from image **C (E)**. Note the decreased signal intensity of articular cartilage in **D** compared to **C.** This leads to an improvement in contrast between cartilage and fluid, but it decreases the contrast at the cartilage-bone interface. In **E,** ST subtraction provides high contrast at both the cartilage-fluid and cartilage-bone interfaces.

(A, B Courtesy of M. Solomon, M.D., San Jose, California; **C–E,** courtesy of C. Peterfy, M.D., and H. Genant, M.D., San Francisco, California.)

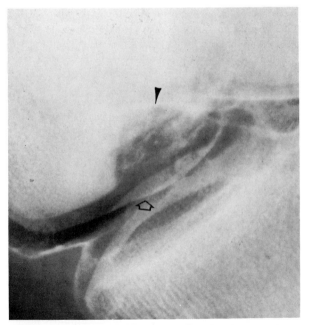

FIGURE 70–366. Osteochondritis dissecans: Arthrography. This lesion in the medial femoral condyle (arrowhead) is well shown with conventional arthrography. Note the swollen articular cartilage (open arrow) over the lesion. (From Wershba M, et al: Clin Orthop 107:81, 1975.)

osteochondritis dissecans with MR imaging has received considerable attention.[1131–1136, 1417] Such evaluation includes analysis of the site and size of the lesion, the integrity of the overlying cartilage, and in the case of osteochondritis dissecans, the stability of the lesion. When a lesion is associated with intact cartilage and is not ballottable at the time of arthroscopy (or open surgery), it is regarded as stable. A lesion that is loose in situ is ballottable, although the overlying cartilage is normal.[1135] Grossly loose lesions are associated with a disrupted chondral surface and partial or complete separation of the fragment. The MR imaging criteria used to judge stability generally are based on the appearance of the junctional zone between the fragment and the parent bone (Figs. 70–367 and 70–368). The absence of high signal intensity in this zone on T2-weighted spin echo and certain gradient echo sequences usually indicates a stable lesion.[1134, 1135] The presence of such high signal intensity in the junctional zone is a strong (although not infallible) indicator of an unstable lesion. High signal intensity may result from granulation tissue at the base of the lesion or it may relate to fluid that extends from the joint cavity through cartilage defects. Although the presence of joint fluid in the base of the lesion clearly indicates cartilage violation, differentiation between this fluid and granulation tissue with MR imaging is difficult in some cases. MR arthrography, in which gadolinium compounds injected in-

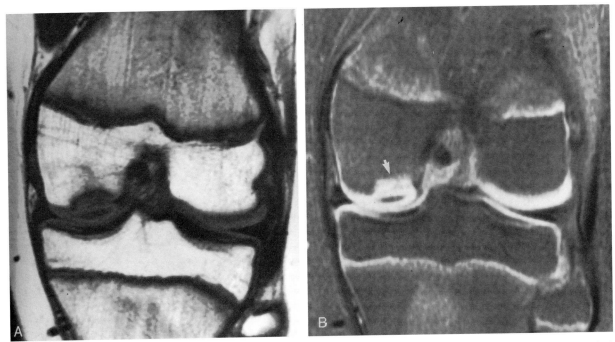

FIGURE 70–367. Osteochondritis dissecans: MR imaging. Coronal T1-weighted (TR/TE, 600/20) **(A)** and T1-weighted (TR/TE, 800/20) **(B)** spin echo MR images, the latter image obtained with fat suppression, show the typical location of osteochondritis dissecans in the inner aspect of the medial femoral condyle. In **B**, note the high signal intensity at the base of the lesion (arrow), a poor prognostic sign. (From Bosch E, et al: Physician Sportsmed *21*:116, 1993.)

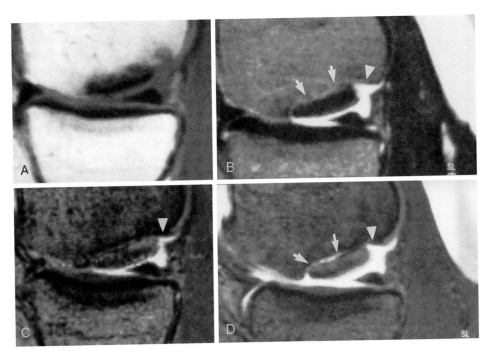

FIGURE 70–368. Osteochondritis dissecans: MR imaging and MR arthrography.
  A, B Sagittal T1-weighted (TR/TE, 700/15) **(A)** and T2-weighted (TR/TE, 2500/90) **(B)** spin echo MR images show a large osteochondral lesion in the medial femoral condyle. In **B**, note a slight increase in signal intensity at the base of the lesion (arrows), which represents either fluid or granulation tissue. Also in **B**, because of the high signal intensity of the joint fluid, a posterior defect in the articular cartilage is apparent (arrowhead). Note the large synovial cyst.
  C In the same patient, a sagittal three-dimensional MR image using FISP shows the posterior disruption of the articular cartilage (arrowhead) but fails to reveal increased signal intensity at the base of the lesion.
  D In the same patient, a sagittal three-dimensional FISP MR image obtained following the intra-articular administration of a gadolinium compound reveals definite fluid (arrows) at the base of the lesion, indicating a poor prognosis. The posterior cartilaginous defect again is seen (arrowhead).
  (Courtesy of J. Kramer, M.D., Vienna, Austria.)

tra-articularly can be detected at the interface of the fragment and parent bone, can confirm disruption of the articular cartilage. MR imaging following the intravenous administration of gadolinium compounds, in which accentuation of signal intensity occurs in the junctional zone, provides strong evidence that granulation tissue is present. These supplementary methods improve the accuracy of MR imaging in defining stability in cases of osteochondritis dissecans, although large lesions (equal to or greater than 0.8 cm²) and those with thick (equal to or greater than 3 mm) sclerotic margins as defined by routine radiography generally are unstable.[1135] Furthermore, bone scintigraphy can be used to judge lesion stability, as unstable lesions usually reveal accumulation of the radionuclide in flow, blood pool, and delayed phases of the examination.[1135] Thus, the relative value of MR imaging in the analysis of lesion stability is not clear.

The role of MR imaging in allowing direct assessment of the cartilage surface in cases of osteochondritis dissecans or chondral or osteochondral fractures is limited by the inadequacies of many standard sequences in accurately delineating articular cartilage (see previous discussion). The role of MR imaging in determining the presence of necrosis in fragments containing considerable quantities of bone also is not clear. Finally, the relative value of MR imaging, when compared with other imaging methods, in the detection of free bodies within the joint or those embedded in the synovial membrane, is questionable (see later discussion). MR imaging, however, is sensitive to the diagnosis of occult subcortical femoral and tibial fractures that, with time, may progress to osteochondral sequelae.[1136]

Abnormalities of Subchondral Bone

Occult Injuries. The detection of occult injuries in the distal portion of the femur and the proximal portion of the tibia with MR imaging has been emphasized repeatedly[1019, 1027, 1031, 1032, 1136–1139] and is discussed in Chapter 67. Many of these injuries result from forces that lead to impaction of one articular surface against another, and they frequently are accompanied by additional insults to the menisci and to intra-articular (i.e., cruciate) and periarticular ligaments. Experimentally, transarticular loading has led to fractures through the zone of calcified cartilage and subchondral bone, frequently with step-off displacement and little or no change in the gross appearance of the articular cartilage; MR imaging has documented soft tissue swelling, joint effusions, and alterations of signal intensity in the bone marrow as transient accompanying phenomena.[1140] Such alterations in signal intensity within subchondral marrow following injury to the knee (or to other joints) have led to the introduction of the term "bone bruise."[1139] The precise histologic correlates of a bone bruise are not clear, although microfractures of trabeculae and hyperemia, edema, and hemorrhage in adjacent marrow probably contribute to the changes in signal intensity. Reticulated regions of low signal intensity are apparent in T1-weighted spin echo MR images, and similar regions of inhomogeneous high signal intensity are observed in T2-weighted spin echo MR images (Fig. 70–369). STIR imaging sequences dramatically display these lesions as areas of high signal intensity within involved marrow. The MR imaging characteristics of bone

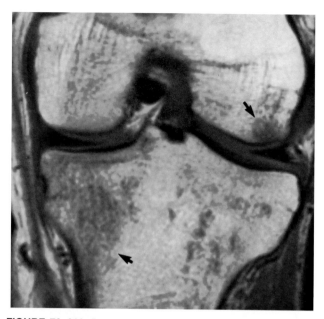

FIGURE 70–369. Bone bruises: MR imaging. In a patient with an anterior cruciate ligament tear, a coronal T1-weighted (TR/TE, 600/20) spin echo MR image shows the typical reticulated regions of low signal intensity (arrows) involving principally the medial tibial plateau and the lateral femoral condyle. These regions revealed increased signal intensity in the T2-weighted spin echo MR images (not shown). (From Bosch E, et al: Physician Sportsmed *21*:116, 1993.)

bruises are similar to those noted in cases of transient painful bone marrow edema (see Chapter 51).

Additional occult cartilage and bone injuries about the knee include stress fractures (insufficiency and fatigue fractures) (Fig. 70–370), osteochondral fractures, and acute fractures of the femoral condyles and tibial plateaus (Fig. 70–371) that generally extend into the chondral surfaces.[1139] Although differentiation among these injuries generally is possible on the basis of MR imaging findings coupled with information derived from the patient's history, clinical examination, and results of other imaging studies, this is not always possible. A constant component of all types of occult injury is a poorly defined area of decreased signal intensity in T1-weighted spin echo MR images, and of increased signal intensity in T2-weighted spin echo MR images, within the bone marrow, presumably related to edema, hemorrhage, hyperemia, or even osteonecrosis, or combinations of these findings.[1139] This may be the only component of a bone bruise, whereas with osteochondral fractures, stress fractures, and acute fractures, additional MR imaging features may be evident (see Chapter 67). These occult injuries may occur together or in isolation, and one type of injury, such as a bone bruise, later may develop into another.[1136] The sensitivity of the MR imaging examination in detection of any of these occult injuries is equal to and probably better than bone scintigraphy, even single photon emission computed tomography (SPECT). The specificity of the MR imaging examination surely is superior to bone scintigraphy and, by modifying and shortening the MR imaging examination, its cost may not differ significantly from that of bone scintigraphy. In all cases, when an occult injury to cartilage and subchondral bone is detected with MR imaging, attention must be directed to

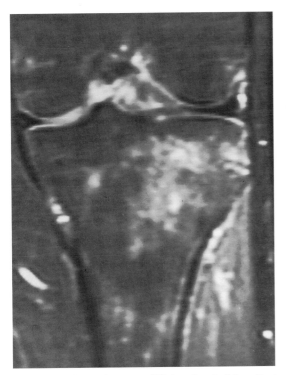

FIGURE 70–370. Stress fractures: MR imaging. In this patient who developed knee pain after starting a new jogging program, a coronal T1-weighted (TR/TE, 750/20) spin echo MR image obtained with chemical presaturation of fat (ChemSat) and after the intravenous injection of a gadolinium compound reveals areas of increased signal intensity in the lateral tibial plateau. (From Bosch E, et al: Physician Sportsmed *21*:116, 1993.)

other structures, such as the menisci and the collateral and cruciate ligaments, that also may be injured.

Hematopoietic Hyperplasia. A report in 1989 by Deutsch and coworkers[1141] was the first to emphasize the occurrence of islands of hypercellular but otherwise normal-appearing hematopoietic marrow in the metaphysis of

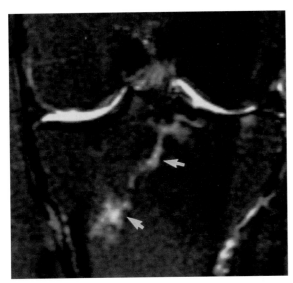

FIGURE 70–371. Occult acute fractures: MR imaging. Although routine radiographs were normal in this patient who had sustained an injury to the knee, a coronal T2-weighted (TR/TE, 4000/102) fast spin echo MR image obtained with chemical presaturation of fat (ChemSat) reveals the fracture line (arrows) in the tibial plateau.

the distal femur in asymptomatic persons, particularly obese women of menstruating age who also are cigarette smokers. These islands demonstrated low signal intensity on both T1-weighted and T2-weighted spin echo images, prompting initial concern about the possibility of occult myeloproliferative neoplasms. A similar alteration of marrow signal intensity about the knee in an obese woman subsequently was reported by Schuck and Czarnecki,[1142] and in this patient, marrow alterations were noted not only in the distal portion of the femur but in the proximal portion of the tibia, proximal aspect of the femora, and iliac crest. Shellock and collaborators[1143] observed a high prevalence (43 per cent) of hematopoietic bone marrow hyperplasia in the distal femoral metaphysis of marathon runners when compared with healthy volunteers (3 per cent) and with patients with symptoms of knee disorders (15 per cent). The femoral epiphysis and the proximal portion of the tibia were not affected. These authors postulated that the prevalence of such marrow hyperplasia in marathon runners may indicate a response to the anemia encountered in highly conditioned aerobically trained athletes. Other investigators also have confirmed the presence of hematopoietic bone marrow about the knee, emphasizing its localization to the femoral metaphysis, some variability in the pattern of decreased marrow signal intensity, and accentuated changes in signal intensity when opposed-phase gradient echo MR sequences are employed.[1144, 1145, 1361]

The major differential diagnostic considerations of MR imaging findings are lymphoma or other myeloproliferative disorders and sickle cell anemia or other hemoglobinopathies. Although benign hematopoietic hyperplasia may not be confined to the distal femoral metaphysis in all cases, this distribution provides the most important clue to correct diagnosis. Furthermore, the absence of increased signal intensity on T2-weighted spin echo MR images favors a diagnosis of benign hematopoietic hyperplasia over that of most primary and secondary bone tumors and osteomyelitis.

Osteonecrosis. Ischemic necrosis involving the bones about the knee is second in frequency only to that of the femoral head (see Chapters 79 and 80). Typical sites of involvement are the femoral condyles and proximal portion of the tibia, although involvement of the diaphyseal and metaphyseal regions of the femur and tibia is encountered. Ischemic necrosis of the patella is rare and usually is associated with a patellar fracture, previous surgery, or the administration of corticosteroid medications. Osteonecrosis of the fibula is extremely rare.

As discussed in detail in Chapters 79 and 80, the causes of osteonecrosis are diverse and, in some cases, no causative factors can be identified, a situation designated primary (or spontaneous) osteonecrosis. Primary osteonecrosis about the knee is a condition of middle-aged and elderly men and women who present with the spontaneous onset of knee pain. The weight-bearing portion of the medial femoral condyle is affected most frequently, although involvement of the lateral femoral condyle or the medial or lateral regions of the proximal portion of the tibia, or combinations of these sites, is encountered. One or both knees may be affected, and an association of this condition with meniscal tears and, later, with osteoarthritis is recognized. Furthermore, as indicated in Chapters 79 and 80, a variety of imaging methods may be used to diagnose osteonecrosis

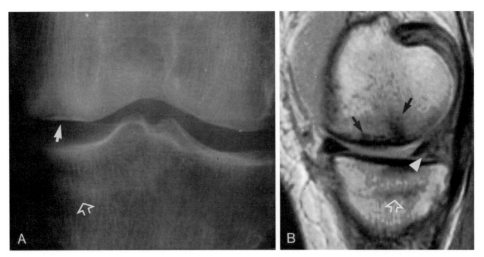

FIGURE 70–372. Primary (spontaneous) osteonecrosis about the knee: Routine radiography and MR imaging. The routine radiograph **(A)** reveals flattening of the medial femoral condyle (solid arrow) and a subchondral radiolucent region surrounded by bone sclerosis. A linear area of bone sclerosis in the tibia (open arrow) represents a stress fracture. A sagittal proton density–weighted (TR/TE, 2000/30) spin echo MR image **(B)** reveals regions of low signal intensity (solid arrows) in the subchondral bone of the femur (reflecting bone sclerosis and edema) and a tear of the posterior horn of the medial meniscus (arrowhead). Note the linear area of low signal intensity in the tibia (open arrow), representing the stress fracture. A joint effusion is present.

about the knee, of which bone scintigraphy and MR imaging are most sensitive, and to define its distribution and extent. The classic feature of bone necrosis as displayed by bone scintigraphy is the increased accumulation of the radiopharmaceutical agent at or near the site of involvement, although decreased accumulation or no accumulation (i.e., cold lesion) of the radionuclide may be found in the acute stages of the process. The MR imaging features of osteonecrosis are more variable, influenced by the stage of the process. Decreased signal intensity in the involved bone marrow in T1-weighted spin echo MR images and increased signal intensity in this region in T2-weighted spin echo MR images usually are evident, even in early stages of osteonecrosis. Later findings in cases of osteonecrosis involving the femoral condyles or subchondral bone of the tibia include flattening of the articular surface and areas of persistent low signal intensity that reflect the presence of bone sclerosis (Fig. 70–372). Similar findings are displayed by more conventional techniques, such as routine radiography and conventional tomography (Fig. 70–372).

Widespread infarcts in the diaphyseal and metaphyseal regions of the femur and tibia lead to serpentine-like areas about the lesions whose signal intensity characteristics relate to the presence of sclerotic bone and granulation tissue (Fig. 70–373).

Miscellaneous Abnormalities

Intra-Articular Bodies. Although intra-articular bodies composed of cartilage alone or cartilage and bone together may be evident in virtually any joint, those of the knee are encountered most frequently. Any process that leads to acute disruption or chronic disintegration of the articular surface can give rise to one or more free or synovial-embedded intra-articular bodies. Examples of such processes include chondral and osteochondral fractures, osteochondritis dissecans, osteoarthritis, neuropathic osteoarthropathy, rheumatoid arthritis, gout, calcium pyrophosphate dihydrate crystal deposition disease, calcium

hydroxyapatite crystal deposition disease, osteonecrosis, and rheumatoid arthritis. Furthermore, primary synovial (osteo)chondromatosis, a rare disorder of unknown cause, leads to metaplasia of the synovial lining with the formation of cartilage nodules that may calcify or ossify and become free within the joint cavity.

Regardless of their source of origin, intra-articular bodies all demonstrate similar histopathologic alterations once they are free in the joint space.[1127] They receive their nutrition from the synovial fluid and may contain any or all of the principal cells of bone tissue (i.e., osteoblasts, osteocytes,

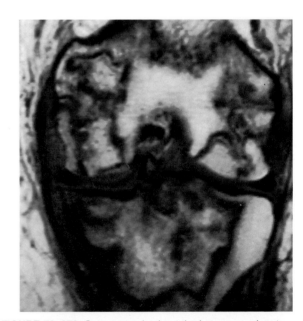

FIGURE 70–373. Osteonecrosis about the knee secondary to corticosteroid medications: MR imaging. A coronal T1-weighted (TR/TE, 632/17) spin echo MR image shows widespread regions of osteonecrosis in both femoral condyles and the proximal portion of the tibia characterized by serpentine-like areas of low signal intensity. (Courtesy of J. Goobar, M.D., Ostersund, Sweden.)

chondroblasts, chondrocytes, fibroblasts, osteoclasts, and their precursor cells). The osteoblasts and osteoclasts can differentiate and perform their functions without the presence of any blood supply.[1127] The origin of these cells may be the nidi of the free bodies themselves or, more likely, the synovial membrane. The surface cells of free bodies form more cartilaginous layers than osseous layers; as these layers are formed, the deeper cells are deprived of their nutrition, die, and calcify.[1127]

Calcified free or embedded intra-articular bodies that are large usually are identified easily with routine radiography. Classically, they appear layered, without recognizable trabeculae. Occasionally, irregular radiodense nodules at the periphery of the bodies create a mulberry-like appearance.[1146] Smaller bodies, unless heavily calcified, are more difficult to detect with routine radiography or, sometimes, even with conventional tomography or CT. With any of these imaging methods, the search for intra-articular bodies is more rewarding if normal recesses and dependent portions of the knee (or other joint) are analyzed carefully. Common locations for intra-articular bodies in the knee are the suprapatellar recess (particularly in instances in which a suprapatellar plica is present), popliteus tunnel, recesses beneath the menisci, and the intercondylar notch.[1147] Free bodies within the knee may pass into an adjacent synovial cyst. Multiple intra-articular bodies in the knee are present in approximately 30 per cent of cases.[1147] A calcified area localized to the region of the posterior horn of the medial meniscus may represent a meniscal ossicle rather than an intra-articular body (see previous discussion).

The detection of small calcified or noncalcified bodies in the knee may require the combination of arthrography and either conventional tomography or CT (Fig. 70–374). Large amounts of air with or without a small amount of radiopaque contrast material are injected in the joint. Transaxial CT images may be employed with the patient supine or prone, depending on the suspected location of the fragment. Care must be exercised so that the tibial spines are not misinterpreted as evidence of intra-articular osseous bodies.

Small calcified or noncalcified bodies in the knee may escape detection with MR imaging, especially if a joint

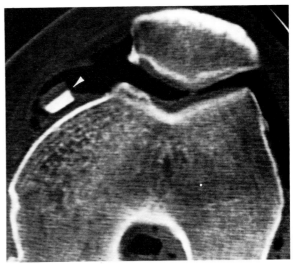

FIGURE 70–374. Intra-articular bodies: CT arthrography. Following the introduction of air into the knee joint, a transaxial CT scan reveals the fragment (arrowhead), consisting of cartilage and bone in the medial aspect of the articulation.

effusion is not present. A joint effusion makes their detection easier (Fig. 70–375). In the absence of a knee effusion, MR arthrography may represent an effective technique for demonstrating such bodies. In general, however, the diagnosis of free or embedded bodies in the knee is better accomplished with computed arthrotomography than with MR imaging.

Bursitis. Any of the bursae about the knee may become inflamed, leading to the accumulation of bursal fluid. Prepatellar bursitis (''housemaid's'' knee), deep infrapatellar bursitis, anserinus bursitis, and bursitis involving a suprapatellar recess that is isolated from the remaining portion of the knee by a suprapatellar plica are typical examples. Ultrasonography[1362] and MR imaging represent the two most effective imaging methods for diagnosis of these conditions. With MR imaging, bursal fluid is of high signal intensity on T2-weighted spin echo images (Fig. 70–376) as well as on STIR images. Prepatellar bursitis may result

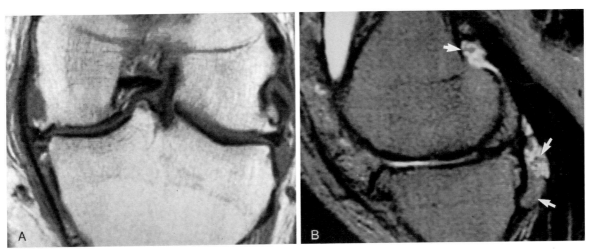

FIGURE 70–375. Intra-articular bodies: MR imaging. In this patient with severe osteoarthritis of the knee, a coronal T1-weighted (TR/TE, 800/25) spin echo MR image **(A)** shows loss of the medial femorotibial joint space and osteophytes in the marginal regions of the femur and tibia. A sagittal T2-weighted (TR/TE, 2000/80) spin echo MR image **(B)** reveals multiple intra-articular bodies (arrows) appearing as foci of low signal intensity surrounded by joint fluid of high signal intensity.

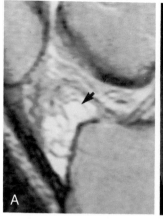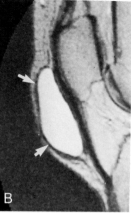

FIGURE 70–376. Bursitis: MR imaging.
A Deep infrapatellar bursitis. A sagittal T2-weighted (TR/TE, 2300/70) spin echo MR image shows fluid of high signal intensity (arrow) in the deep infrapatellar bursa. (Courtesy of M. Zlatkin, M.D., Hollywood, Florida.)
B Prepatellar bursitis. A sagittal T2-weighted (TR/TE, 2000/80) spin echo MR image shows fluid of high signal intensity (arrows) in the prepatellar bursa. (Courtesy of E. M. Bellon, M.D., Cleveland, Ohio.)

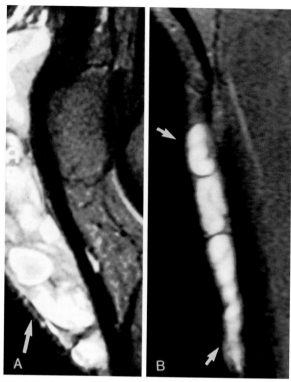

FIGURE 70–377. Prepatellar and anterior soft tissue masses.
A Prepatellar hematoma. A sagittal T2-weighted (TR/TE, 2433/80) spin echo MR image shows a large, septated mass of high signal intensity, representing a hematoma, anterior to the patella (arrow). (Courtesy of S. Eilenberg, M.D., San Diego, California.)
B Varicosities. A sagittal T1-weighted (TR/TE, 600/20) spin echo MR image obtained with chemical presaturation of fat (ChemSat) shows a septated mass of high signal intensity (arrows), which corresponded to clinically evident varicose veins.

from chronic stress, as may occur with prolonged kneeling, or synovial inflammatory diseases such as rheumatoid arthritis or gout. Rheumatoid nodules and gouty tophi may lead to a prepatellar soft tissue mass, although the imaging characteristics of these lesions usually differ from those of fluid. The differential diagnosis of prepatellar and anterior soft tissue masses also includes hematomas and varicosities (Fig. 70–377).

A bursa may be present at the tibial insertion site of the pes anserinus tendons (see Fig. 70–234). Inflammation of this bursa may occur, leading to a large fluid-filled mass. Erosion or proliferation of the subjacent bone may be evident in these cases. The histologic findings associated with this condition may lead to a diagnosis of a ganglion, rather than bursitis, in some cases.

Hoffa's Disease. Hoffa's disease is a term that has been applied to traumatic and inflammatory changes occurring in the infrapatellar fat body. This rare condition is seen in young, athletic persons in whom pain, swelling, and limitation of joint motion may occur. The fat body hypertrophies and may become entrapped between the femur and the tibia when the flexed knee is extended suddenly. MR imaging reveals alterations in signal intensity in the infrapatellar fat body (Fig. 70–378), which resemble those related to scarring after knee arthroscopy.

ANKLE AND FOOT

Osseous Anatomy

The distal end of the tibia contains the medial malleolus and articular surface (Fig. 70–379). The broad malleolus has an articular facet on its lateral surface, which is comma-shaped in configuration. On the posterior surface of the distal tibia is a groove, just lateral to the medial malleolus, related to the tendon of the tibialis posterior. The inferior surface of the tibia represents the articular area for the talus. It is smooth, wider anteriorly than posteriorly, concave an-

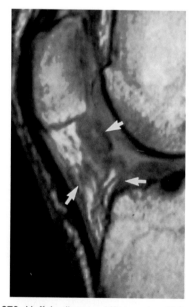

FIGURE 70–378. Hoffa's disease: MR imaging. This male adolescent had undergone several arthroscopic procedures in which resection of a medial patellar plica and an enlarged and inflamed infrapatellar fat body had been accomplished. He presented with recurrent anterior knee pain. A sagittal proton density–weighted (TR/TE, 2700/20) spin echo MR image shows serpentine-like and irregular areas of low signal intensity (arrows) in the deep infrapatellar fat body. Repeat arthroscopy confirmed inflammation of the fat pad and adjacent synovial membrane. (Courtesy of G. Bock, M.D., and P. Major, M.D., Winnipeg, Manitoba, Canada.)

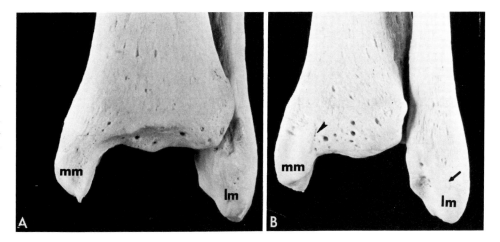

FIGURE 70–379. Distal tibia and fibula: Osseous anatomy. Anterior **(A)** and posterior **(B)** aspects. Observe the medial malleolus (mm), lateral malleolus (lm), groove for the tendon of the tibialis posterior muscle (arrowhead), and groove for the peroneal tendons (arrow).

teriorly to posteriorly, and minimally convex medially to laterally. The articular surface on the inferior tibia is continuous with that on the medial malleolus. The triangular fibular notch is on the lateral side of the tibia. This notch represents the site of attachment of various ligaments that connect the distal tibia and fibula.

The distal end of the fibula contains the lateral malleolus (Fig. 70–379). This structure projects more inferiorly than the medial malleolus and contains a triangular facet on its medial surface for articulation with the talus, and an irregular surface above this facet for the interosseous ligament. Posterior to the convex articular facet is a depression, the malleolar fossa.

The dorsal surface of the talus contains the trochlear articular surface (Fig. 70–380). This surface is convex anteriorly to posteriorly and concave from side to side. The medial surface of the talar body possesses a facet that articulates with the medial malleolus. The lateral surface of the body contains a triangular articular facet that is intimate with the lateral malleolus.

Assessment of alignment of the ankle on radiographs is important in the evaluation of this joint following trauma. Small degrees of lateral displacement of the talus on the tibia may result in the rapid development of secondary degenerative arthritis. It has been shown that even 1 mm of lateral displacement of the talus reduces the tibiotalar contact areas by 42 per cent.[1148] Incomplete ligament tears may result in relatively small amounts of displacement, which may be difficult to detect radiographically. This has stimulated investigators to propose radiographic criteria for assessment of tibiotalar alignment.[1149]

A short, concave cortical line representing the posteromedial surface of the talus was used by some investigators to determine tibiotalar displacement.[1150] This line actually delineates the insertion of the deep deltoid fibers, however, and does not represent the true medial articular surface. In addition, this line cannot be accurately identified with moderate internal or external rotation of the talus, precluding accurate measurements on rotation radiographs. The main pitfalls of previously reported measurement techniques include (1) inability to accurately identify the posteromedial border of the talus with extreme degrees of rotation, (2) lack of an identifiable posterolateral talar landmark, and (3) variations in the weight-bearing line of the tibia with rotation, because this bone is not a true cylinder even above the metaphysis.

In the adult, the coronal plane of the ankle is oriented in about 15 to 20 degrees of external rotation with reference to the coronal plane of the knee[1151] and therefore the lateral malleolus is slightly posterior to the medial malleolus. To obtain a true anteroposterior radiograph of the tibiotalar articulation, the ankle must be positioned with the medial and lateral malleoli parallel to the tabletop; that is, in about 15 to 20 degrees of internal rotation, or the mortise view.[1152] This positioning places the medial articular surface tangent to the x-ray beam, and the short concave line representing the posteromedial surface of the talus falls slightly lateral to the medial articular surface. With this view, the radiographic medial clear space represents the actual width of the medial joint space. In adults, the normal interosseous space is about 2.5 to 3.5 mm.[1153]

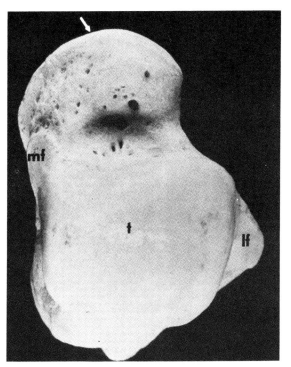

FIGURE 70–380. Talus: Osseous anatomy. Dorsal aspect. Structures include the trochlear surface (t), medial facet (mf) for articulation with the medial malleolus, and lateral facet (lf) for articulation with the lateral malleolus. The distal surface (arrow) of the talus articulates with the tarsal navicular surface.

Articular Anatomy

Talocrural (Ankle) Joint. The articular surfaces are cartilage-covered and the bones are connected by a fibrous capsule and by the deltoid, the anterior and posterior talofibular, and the calcaneofibular ligaments (Fig. 70–381). The fibrous capsule is attached superiorly to the medial and lateral malleoli and tibia and inferiorly to the talus. The talar attachment of the capsule is close to the margins of the trochlear surface except anteriorly, where the attachment to the neck of the talus is located at some distance from the articular margin. The capsule is weak both anteriorly and posteriorly, but it is reinforced medially and laterally by various ligaments. A synovial membrane lines

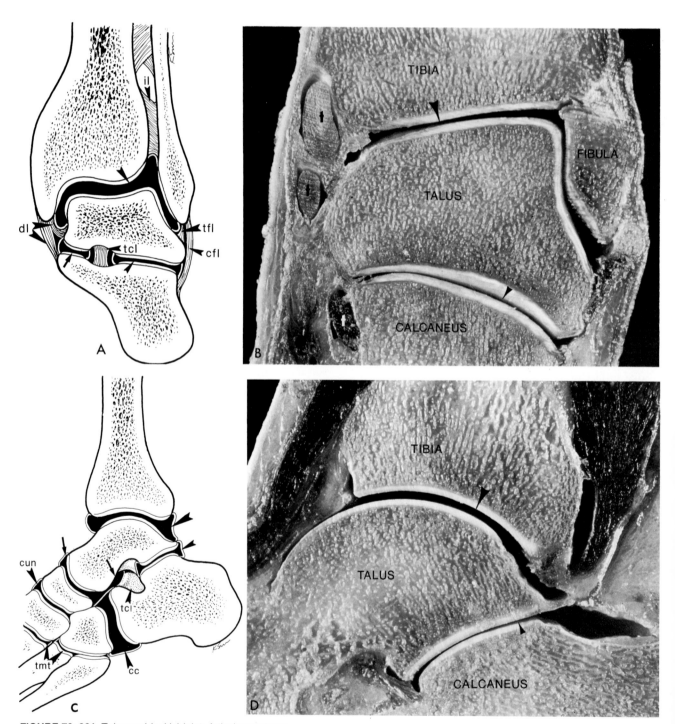

FIGURE 70–381. Talocrural (ankle) joint: Articular anatomy.
   A, B A drawing and photograph of a coronal section through the distal tibia, fibula, and talus, outlining the ankle joint (large arrowheads), interosseous ligament (il) of tibiofibular syndesmosis, interosseous talocalaneal ligament (tcl), portions of the deltoid ligament (dl), posterior talofibular ligament (tfl), calcaneofibular ligament (cfl), surrounding tendons (t), subtalar joint (small arrowheads), and talocalcaneonavicular joint (arrow).
   C, D Some of the same structures as in **A** and **B** can be identified in a drawing and photograph of a sagittal section of the ankle. Additional articulations that can be seen are the calcaneocuboid (cc), cuneonavicular (cun), and tarsometatarsal (tmt) joints.

the inner aspect of the capsule and extends for a short vertical distance between the tibia and fibula. In this latter area, cartilage may be found on the osseous surfaces, continuous with that in the ankle joint.

Surrounding ligaments[1154] include the deltoid, anterior and posterior talofibular, and calcaneofibular ligaments:

1. *Deltoid ligament.* This medial ligament is triangular in shape and is attached above to the apex and the posterior and anterior borders of the medial malleolus. It contains superficial, middle, and deep fibers. Superficial fibers run anteriorly to the tuberosity of the tarsal navicular bone and blend with the plantar calcaneonavicular ligament. Middle fibers attach to the sustentaculum tali of the calcaneus, and posterior fibers pass to the medial talar surface, including its tubercle.

2. *Anterior talofibular ligament.* This ligament extends from the anterior margin of the lateral malleolus to the lateral articular facet on the neck of the talus.

3. *Posterior talofibular ligament.* This ligament attaches to the lateral malleolar fossa and extends horizontally to the lateral tubercle of the talus and medial malleolus.

4. *Calcaneofibular ligament.* This structure extends from the lateral malleolus to the lateral surface of the calcaneus. It is crossed by the peroneus longus and peroneus brevis tendons. These last three ligaments constitute the lateral ligamentous complex of the ankle.

The soft tissue anatomy of the talocrural joint governs the radiographic manifestations of an articular effusion. On lateral radiographs, an ankle effusion produces a teardrop-shaped dense shadow anterior to the joint, extending along the neck of the talus,[1155] a finding that is accentuated when the ankle is dorsiflexed.[1156] A similar radiodense area in the posterior aspect of the joint or a lobulated mass (indicative of articular communication with the posterior subtalar joint) in this region is an additional, although less reliable, sign of an ankle effusion.

Distal Tibiofibular Joint. This fibrous joint consists of a strong interosseous ligament that unites the convex sur-face of the medial distal fibula and the concave surface of the adjacent fibular notch of the tibia. Additionally, the anterior and posterior tibiofibular ligaments reinforce this articulation. Below this ligamentous joint, an upward prolongation of the synovial membrane of the ankle (talocrural joint) can extend 3 to 5 mm. This synovial recess may be associated with cartilaginous surfaces on tibia and fibula.

Talocalcaneal Joints (Figs. 70–382 to 70–384).[1157, 1158] The talocalcaneal joints are two in number: the subtalar (posterior talocalcaneal or posterior subtalar) joint and the talocalcaneonavicular (anterior subtalar) joint. These articulations are separated by the tarsal canal and sinus and their contents.

The subtalar joint exists between the posterior talar facet of the calcaneus and the posterior calcaneal facet of the talus. The talar facet is oval and concave and extends distally and laterally at an angle of approximately 45 degrees with the sagittal plane. The posterior calcaneal facet is oval and convex anteroposteriorly. This synovium-lined joint, which may communicate with the talocrural or ankle joint in approximately 10 to 20 per cent of persons,[1157–1160] contains a capsule that contributes to the interosseous talocalcaneal ligament, the major bond between talus and calcaneus. Additional structures binding talus and calcaneus are the anterior talocalcaneal ligament (extending from the lateral talar tubercle to the proximal medial calcaneus), the medial talocalcaneal ligament (extending from the medial talar tubercle to the sustentaculum tali), and the lateral talocalcaneal ligament (extending from the lateral surface of the talus to that of the calcaneus).

The talocalcaneonavicular joint also is a synovium-lined articulation, which exists between the head of the talus, the posterior surface of the navicular bone, the anterior articular surface of the calcaneus, and the proximal surface of the plantar calcaneonavicular ligament or "spring" ligament. The distal surface of the head of the talus is oval and convex, directed inferiorly and medially to articulate with the oval, concave proximal surface of the navicular bone. The plantar surface of the talar head has three articular

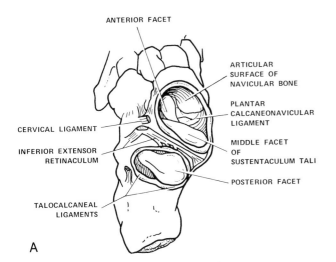
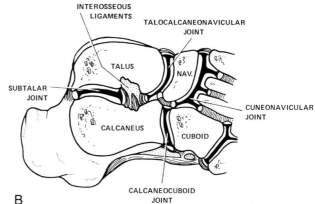

FIGURE 70–382. Talocalcaneal joints: Articular anatomy.

A Superior surface of calcaneus. Note the broad convex posterior talar facet separated from the anterior and middle talar facets by the tarsal canal and its ligamentous structures. Two completely independent synovium-lined articulations are formed.

B Oblique section of the foot. The interosseous ligaments between the talus and calcaneus are well shown, and the two separate talocalcaneal articulations are indicated. Note the independent calcaneocuboid and cuneonavicular joint cavities.

(**A, B** From Resnick D: Radiology *111:*581, 1974.)

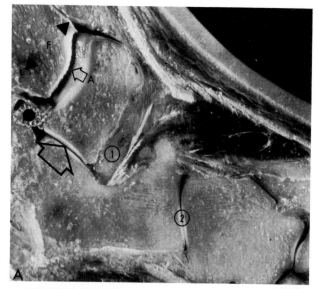

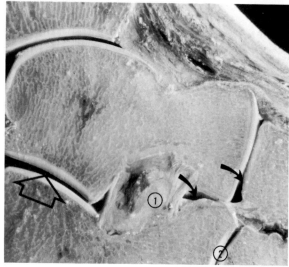

FIGURE 70–383. Talocalcaneal joints: Sagittal cross-sectional anatomy.

A A lateral sagittal section through the fibula (F) and ankle (A) demonstrates the subtalar articulation (open arrow) between the posterior facets of the talus and calcaneus. The tarsal sinus (1) and posterior talofibular ligament (black dot) are indicated. A separate calcaneocuboid joint (2) is evident.

B A more medial sagittal section outlines the talocalcaneonavicular (curved arrows) and subtalar (open arrow) joint cavities completely separated by the contents of the tarsal sinus (1). The calcaneocuboid articulation (2) again is indicated.

(From Resnick D: Radiology *111*:581, 1974.)

areas separated by indistinct osseous ridges: the posterior area is large and oval, is convex in shape, and articulates with the sustentaculum tali of the calcaneus; the second area, anterolateral to the posterior area, is flattened, articulating with the superior surface of the calcaneus; and the navicular area, directed distally, is oval and convex, articulating with the tarsal navicular bone. The anterior articular surface of the talus also contacts the plantar calcaneonavicular ligament. This ligament has a central area that consists of fibrocartilage and bridges the triangular space between the anterior and middle talar facets of the calcaneus and navicular bone. The posterior surface of the joint capsule

contributes to the interosseous ligament. On its medial side, this articulation is enlarged or deepened by a portion of the deltoid ligament, which is attached to the plantar calcaneonavicular ligament. Movements are coordinated between the talocalcaneonavicular and subtalar articulations and include inversion and eversion of the foot.

Calcaneocuboid Joint (Fig. 70–385). This joint is formed between apposing quadrilateral facets on the calcaneus and cuboid bones, and its capsule is reinforced by surrounding ligaments, including the long plantar ligament (extending from the plantar surface of the calcaneus to the cuboid and third through fifth metatarsals) and the plantar calcaneocuboid ligament (extending from calcaneus to cuboid). The calcaneocuboid and talocalcaneonavicular joints often are referred to collectively as the transverse tarsal joint. Movements at the calcaneocuboid articulation are limited to gliding and rotation.

Cuneonavicular, Intercuneiform, Cuneocuboid, and Cuboideonavicular Joints (Fig. 70–385). The cuneonavicular joint is formed between the concave articular surfaces of the posterior portion of the three cuneiforms and the convex distal surface of the navicular. The articular capsule of this joint is continuous with two intercuneiform joints (small joint cavities between the proximal portions of the cuneiform bones), cuneocuboid joint (articulation between apposing facets on the cuboid bone and lateral cuneiform), and cuboideonavicular joint (inconstant cavity between cuboid and navicular bones). Movements at all of these joints occur simultaneously and include slight amounts of gliding and rotation of one bone on another.

Tarsometatarsal and Intermetatarsal Joints. The medial cuneiform and first metatarsal bones possess an independent medial tarsometatarsal articulation (Fig. 70–385). The intermediate tarsometatarsal joint is located between the second and third metatarsal bones and the intermediate and lateral cuneiforms. This joint may communicate with the intercuneiform and cuneonavicular joints. The lateral tarsometatarsal joint exists between the distal aspect of the cuboid and the base of the fourth and fifth metatarsal bones. A limited amount of gliding motion may occur between tarsals and metatarsal bones, the motion being accentuated at the medial tarsometatarsal joint. The tarsometatarsal joints extend distally between the metatarsal bases as intermetatarsal joints. Slight gliding motion can occur at these latter articulations.[1161]

Tendon Sheath and Bursal Anatomy

Tendons with accompanying tendon sheaths are intimate with the ankle joint[1162–1165] (Fig. 70–386). Anteriorly, there are sheaths about the tendons of the tibialis anterior, extensor hallucis longus, extensor digitorum longus, and peroneus tertius muscles. Medially, sheaths are present about the tendons of the tibialis posterior, flexor digitorum longus, and flexor hallucis longus muscles. Laterally, the common sheath of the tendons of the peroneus longus and peroneus brevis muscles may be appreciated.[1166]

Important tendons, aponeuroses, and bursae are located about the calcaneus. The plantar aponeurosis contains strong fibers that adhere to the posteroinferior surface of the bone. The Achilles tendon, which is the thickest and strongest human tendon, attaches to the posterior surface of the calcaneus approximately 2 cm below the upper surface

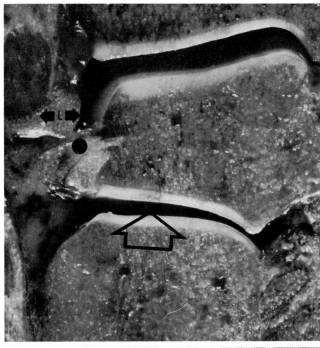

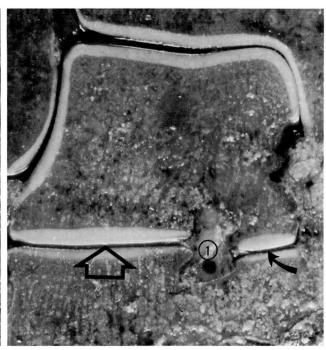

B

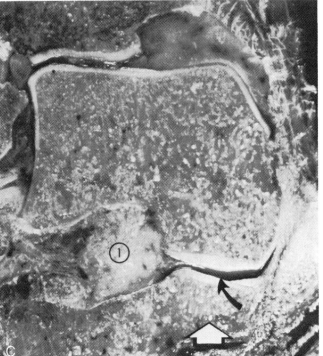

FIGURE 70–384. Talocalcaneal joints: Coronal cross-sectional anatomy.

A A section through the subtalar articulation (open arrow) is shown. The lateral (L) malleolus and posterior talofibular ligament (black dot) are indicated.

B A more anterior section outlines separate subtalar (open arrow) and talocalcaneonavicular (curved arrow) joints. The interosseous ligaments (1) are labeled.

C This most anterior section is through the sustentaculum tali (heavy arrow) and talocalcaneonavicular joint (curved arrow). The tarsal sinus (1) is well shown as it expands on the anterolateral aspect of the foot.

(From Resnick D: Radiology *111:*581, 1974.)

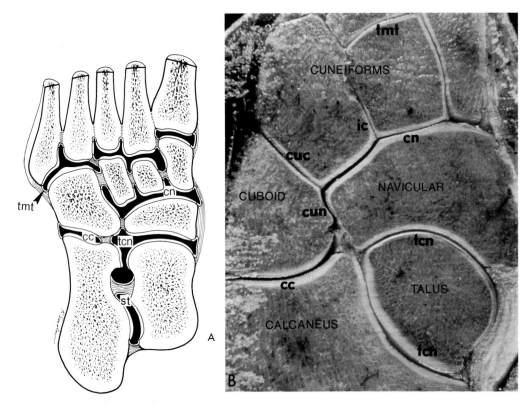

FIGURE 70–385. Joints of the midfoot: Articular anatomy.
  A, B Drawing and photograph of an oblique transverse section through the midfoot, outlining the following articulations: subtalar (st), talocalcaneonavicular (tcn), cuneonavicular (cn), calcaneocuboid (cc), cuboideonavicular (cun), cuneocuboid (cuc), intercuneiform (ic), and tarsometatarsal (tmt) joints.

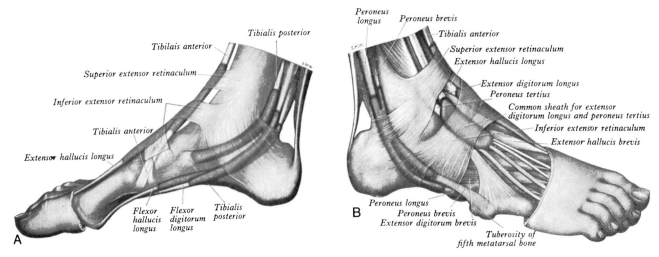

FIGURE 70–386. Tendon sheaths about the ankle: Normal anatomy.
  A Medial aspect of the ankle.
  B Lateral aspect of the ankle.
  (From Williams PL, Warwick R [Eds]: Gray's Anatomy. 36th British edition. Edinburgh, Churchill Livingstone, 1980, pp 611, 612.)

of the bone. The retrocalcaneal bursa exists between the Achilles tendon and the posterosuperior surface of the calcaneus[1167, 1168] (Fig. 70–387). This bursal space is lined with synovium, which extends over both the Achilles tendon and the inferior limit of the preachilles fat pad. The posterior surface of the calcaneus is covered with cartilage.

A triangular radiolucent area, the posterior triangle or preachilles fat pad, is normally observed on lateral radiographs of the ankle. The posterior margin of the triangle is the Achilles tendon and the anterior border is the flexor hallucis longus.[1169] Obscuration of portions of the preachilles fat pad occurs in instances of tendinous rupture,[1170] but similar findings may indicate accessory or anomalous muscles of the lower calf.

Soft Tissue Anatomy

Crural Interosseous Membrane. This membrane is tightly stretched between the interosseous borders of tibia and fibula.[1171] Its upper limit is just inferior to the proximal tibiofibular joint, and its lower limit contains fibers that blend with those about the distal tibiofibular joint. The oblique fibers in the crural interosseous membrane extend inferiorly and laterally from tibia to fibula. A large oval opening in the superior aspect of the membrane allows passage of the anterior tibial vessels; a smaller distal opening allows passage of the perforating branch of the peroneal artery.

Retinacula and Aponeurosis. Owing to the change in orientation of the tendons from a vertical attitude in the lower leg to a horizontal attitude in the foot, five retinacula act to maintain close approximation of the tendons to the bones about the ankle and thereby prevent bowstringing of these tendons[1172, 1173] (Fig. 70–386):

1. *Superior extensor retinaculum.* The superior extensor retinaculum is attached to the anterior surface of the lateral

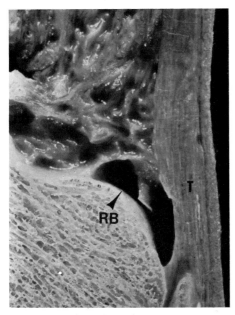

FIGURE 70–387. Retrocalcaneal bursa: Normal anatomy. In this sagittal section, observe the retrocalcaneal bursa (RB), which is located between the Achilles tendon (T) and upper border of the calcaneus. Above the bursa, the preachilles fat pad can be identified. (From Resnick D, et al: Radiology *125:*355, 1977.)

malleolus and to the anterior surface of the medial portion of the tibia, and it is continuous with the deep fascia of the lower leg. This structure serves to reinforce the crural fascia and to contain the tendons of the tibialis anterior, extensor hallucis longus, extensor digitorum longus, and peroneus tertius muscles on the dorsal surface of the ankle.

2. *Inferior extensor retinaculum.* The inferior extensor retinaculum is a Y-shaped structure whose base is attached laterally to the calcaneus. Two limbs or bands are evident medially: An upper limb is located at the level of the ankle and attaches to the medial malleolus; a lower limb attaches to the plantar aponeurosis. This retinaculum serves to prevent bowstringing of the dorsal tendons.

3. *Flexor retinaculum.* The flexor retinaculum is located medially, enclosing the tarsal tunnel. It extends between the medial malleolus and the calcaneus. Three septae divide the tarsal tunnel into four compartments: The first compartment encloses the tendon of the tibialis posterior muscle; the second compartment encloses the tendon of the flexor digitorum longus muscle; the third compartment encloses the neurovascular bundle (i.e., posterior tibial vessels and the tibial nerve); and the fourth compartment encloses the tendon of the flexor hallucis longus muscle.

4 and 5. *Superior and inferior peroneal retinacula.* The two peroneal retinacula are laterally located fascial thickenings that extend from the lateral malleolus to the calcaneus. These retinacula serve to hold the tendons of the peroneus longus and brevis muscles firmly in place behind the fibula.

The plantar aponeurosis is a longitudinally oriented, strong fibrous structure located in the plantar aspect of the foot.[1173] The central portion is the thickest part of this aponeurosis; this portion arises on the calcaneal tuberosity, initially broadens, and subsequently thins distally before dividing into five separate structures that each extend to one of the toes. The medial and lateral portions of the plantar aponeurosis are thinner and smaller than the central portion. Two vertical intermuscular septa arise from the junction of the central portion of the plantar aponeurosis with the medial and lateral portions, dividing the plantar muscles into medial, lateral, and intermediate groups.[1173]

Muscles and Tendons. The anatomy of the musculature of the lower portion of the leg and the foot has been detailed by Jaffe and coworkers.[1173] A summary of this anatomy is provided by Schweitzer and Resnick.[1172] The musculature of the lower portion of the leg is divided into three compartments: posterior, lateral, and anterior (Fig. 70–388).

1. *Posterior compartment.* The muscles of the posterior compartment are separated into a superficial layer (consisting of the gastrocnemius, soleus, and plantaris muscles) and a deep layer (consisting of the popliteus, tibialis posterior, flexor hallucis longus, and flexor digitorum longus muscles). The two heads of the gastrocnemius muscle arise from the medial (medial head) and lateral (lateral head) femoral condyles. These two heads combine in the midcalf to form a single muscle belly that ends in a large, flat tendon, the Achilles tendon. Deep to the gastrocnemius muscle lies the soleus muscle. This muscle originates as two heads: one head originates from the superior portion of the fibula and the other originates from the posterior and medial aspects of the tibia and the popliteal line. The usual insertion site of the soleus muscle is in the midportion of

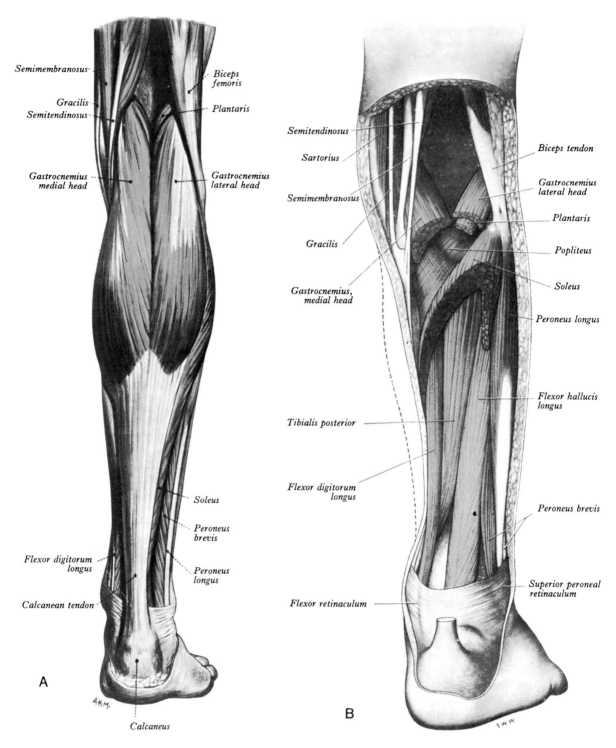

FIGURE 70–388. Musculature of the lower portion of the leg: Normal anatomy.
A Posterior aspect, superficial layer of muscles.
B Posterior aspect, deep layer of muscles.

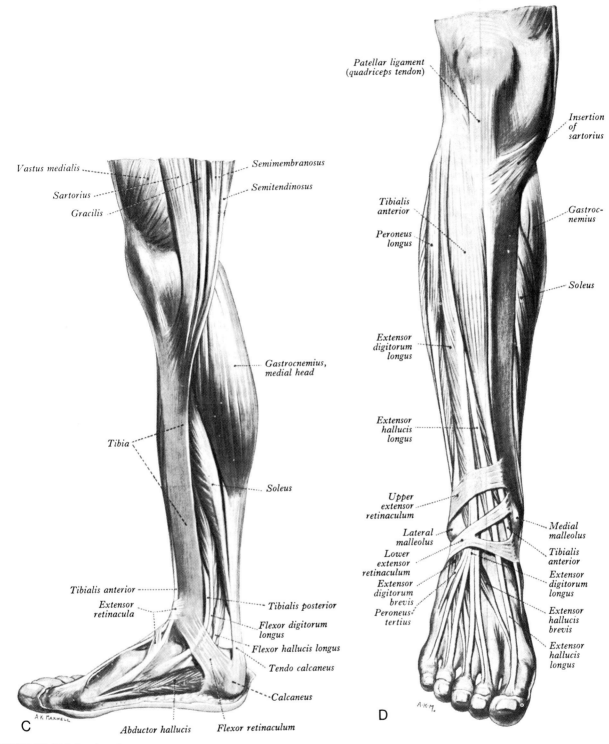

FIGURE 70–388 *Continued*
C Medial aspect.
D Anterior aspect.
(From Williams PL, Warwick R [Eds]: Gray's Anatomy. 36th British edition. Edinburgh, Churchill Livingstone, 1980, pp 606–609.)

the Achilles tendon. The small plantaris muscle originates from the lateral femoral condyle. It forms a tendon in the proximal portion of the leg, and it extends distally to insert in the Achilles tendon.

The most lateral structure in the deep posterior compartment is the flexor hallucis longus muscle. This muscle originates in the posterior aspect of the middle portion of the fibula, and it extends distally to insert in the distal phalanx of the great toe. The flexor digitorum longus muscle originates from the posterior aspect of the tibia and inserts distally in the form of four slips that pass to the distal phalanges of the second, third, fourth, and fifth toes. The tibialis posterior muscle arises from the posterior aspects of the tibia and fibula and the interosseous membrane. This muscle represents the deepest and most central structure of the posterior compartment. Its distal insertion is in the navicular, cuneiforms, calcaneus, and metatarsals of the second, third, and fourth toes.

The tendons of the flexor hallucis longus, flexor digitorum longus, and tibialis posterior muscles are intimately related at the level of the medial malleolus. In this region, the tendons lie in a groove, the tendon of the tibialis posterior muscle being most anterior, the tendon of the flexor digitorum longus muscle being in the intermediate position, and the tendon of the flexor hallucis longus muscle being located posteriorly. A mnemonic device, "Tom, Dick, and Harry," indicates the anterior-to-posterior relationships of these three tendons: "T" for the tibialis posterior tendon, "D" for the flexor digitorum longus tendon, and "H" for the flexor hallucis longus tendon.

2. *Lateral compartment.* The peroneus longus and peroneus brevis muscles lie in the lateral compartment of the lower leg. Both originate from the lateral aspect of the fibula, the origin of the peroneus longus muscle being more superior than that of the peroneus brevis muscle. The myotendinous junction of the peroneus longus occurs above the ankle, at the level of the soleal insertion in the Achilles tendon. The myotendinous junction of the peroneus brevis is located slightly more distally. Both tendons pass lateral to the ankle; the peroneus longus tendon extends medially across the foot to insert in the first metatarsal bone and medial cuneiform; the tendon of the peroneus brevis muscle inserts in the base of the fifth metatarsal bone.

The peroneus brevis and peroneus longus tendons are intimately related at the level of the lateral malleolus. In this location, the peroneus longus tendon is located posterior to the tendon of the peroneus brevis muscle. Above this level, the muscle belly of the peroneus brevis is located posterior to the tendon of the peroneus longus muscle. Below and anterior to the level of the lateral malleolus, the peroneus longus tendon is located inferior and posterior to the peroneus brevis tendon.

3. *Anterior compartment.* The muscles of the anterior compartment are the extensor digitorum longus, peroneus tertius, extensor hallucis longus, and tibialis anterior.

The extensor digitorum longus is the most lateral muscle in this compartment. It originates from the upper aspect of the tibia and the fibula and the intervening interosseous membrane. Distally, it divides into four slips, which run forward on the dorsum of the foot and extend into the second, third, fourth, and fifth toes. The tendon of the extensor digitorum longus muscle begins at the approximate level of the lateral malleolus.

The peroneus tertius muscle is intimately related to the extensor digitorum longus muscle. It arises from the lower third of the medial surface of the fibula, the adjoining anterior surface of the interosseous membrane, and the anterior crural intermuscular septum. The tendon of the peroneus tertius muscle inserts in the base of the fifth metatarsal bone.

The extensor hallucis longus muscle arises from the middle and distal portions of the fibula and the anterior surface of the interosseous membrane. Its distal attachment is to the dorsal aspect of the base of the distal phalanx of the great toe. The tibialis anterior muscle originates from the lateral aspect of the tibia, from the anterior surface of the interosseous membrane, and from the deep surface of the fascia cruris. The insertion of the tibialis anterior muscle is to the medial and inferior surfaces of the medial cuneiform bone and the adjacent portion of the base of the first metatarsal bone.

The tendons of the tibialis anterior, extensor hallucis longus, and extensor digitorum longus muscles lie alongside each other in the anterior portion of the lower leg. The most medial of these structures is the tibialis anterior tendon and the most lateral of these structures is the extensor digitorum longus tendon, with the tendon of the extensor hallucis longus muscle lying in an intermediate position. The mnemonic device, "Tom, Harry, and Dick," can be used to define the medial to lateral relationships of these three tendons (i.e., "T" for the tibialis anterior, "H" for the extensor hallucis longus, and "D" for the extensor digitorum longus).

The muscles of the foot commonly are described according to layers rather than compartments (Fig. 70–389). The plantar muscles are arranged in four different layers. The muscles in the superficial layer include the abductor hallucis, flexor digitorum brevis, and abductor digiti minimi. These three muscles extend from the tuberosity of the calcaneus to the toes. The abductor hallucis muscle is located medially, arising from the medial aspect of the calcaneal tuberosity, the plantar aponeurosis, and the flexor retinaculum. The fibers of this muscle terminate as a tendon that inserts in the proximal phalanx of the great toe. The medial and lateral plantar vessels and nerve pass deep to the proximal portion of the abductor hallucis muscle.

The flexor digitorum brevis muscle arises by a narrow tendon from the medial aspect of the calcaneal tuberosity and from the plantar aponeurosis. It inserts distally in the middle phalanges of the second, third, fourth, and fifth toes. The abductor digiti minimi muscle is located laterally. It arises in large part from the lateral portion of the calcaneal tuberosity. Distally, its tendon extends over a groove in the plantar surface of the fifth metatarsal bone and attaches to the lateral side of the proximal phalanx of the fifth digit.

The second layer of plantar muscles consists of the quadratus plantae and lumbrical muscles as well as the tendons of the flexor hallucis longus and flexor digitorum longus muscles. The quadratus plantae muscle also is known as the flexor digitorum accessorius muscle. It arises from the medial and lateral portions of the calcaneal tuberosity, and it terminates in tendinous slips that join the long flexor tendons to the second, third, and fourth toes. The lumbricales consist of four small muscles extending in a medial-to-lateral direction. These muscles arise from the tendons of

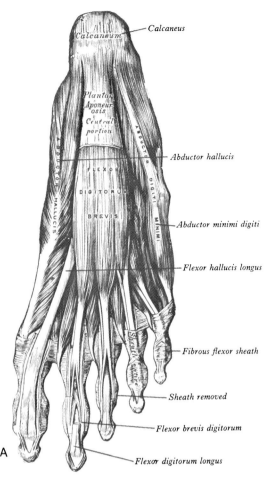

A

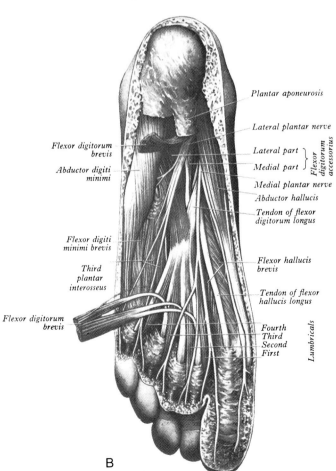

B

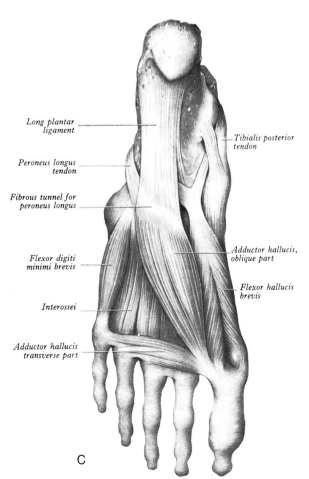

C

FIGURE 70–389. Musculature of the foot: Normal anatomy.
  A Superficial muscles.
  B Intermediate muscles.
  C Deep muscles.
(From Williams PL, Warwick R [Eds]: Gray's Anatomy. 36th British edition. Edinburgh, Churchill Livingstone, 1980, pp 614, 616.)

the flexor digitorum longus muscle, and they insert in the dorsal digital expansions in the proximal phalanges.

The third layer of plantar muscles consists of the flexor hallucis brevis, adductor hallucis, and flexor digiti minimi brevis muscles. The flexor hallucis brevis muscle is located medially, originating from the cuboid and lateral cuneiform bones. Distally, this muscle divides into medial and lateral parts, each terminating as a tendon that inserts in the base of the proximal phalanx of the great toe. Each tendon contains a sesamoid bone beneath the first metatarsophalangeal joint. The adductor hallucis muscle arises as two heads. The oblique head originates from the second, third, and fourth metatarsal bases and the long plantar ligament. The transverse head arises from the capsules of the third, fourth, and fifth metatarsophalangeal joints and the deep transverse ligament. The two heads of this muscle join and insert in the lateral sesamoid bone of the great toe and the base of the first phalanx of the hallux. The flexor digiti minimi brevis muscle originates from the medial aspect of the plantar surface of the base of the fifth metatarsal bone, from the cuboid bone, and from the sheath of the peroneus longus tendon. The tendon of the flexor digiti minimi brevis muscle inserts in the base of the proximal phalanx of the fifth toe.

The fourth layer of plantar muscles is the deepest, and it consists of the seven interosseous muscles. These muscles, which originate from the metatarsal bases, are further divided into four dorsal and three plantar muscles. The dorsal interossei muscles insert laterally in the proximal phalanges; the plantar interossei muscles insert medially.

The extensor digitorum brevis muscle represents the only intrinsic muscle in the dorsal aspect of the foot. It arises from the superolateral portion of the calcaneus, anterior to the groove for the peroneus brevis tendon, from the interosseous talocalcaneal ligament, and from the inferior extensor retinaculum. This muscle inserts in the lateral aspect of the proximal phalanges of the first, second, third, and fourth toes.

Tendon Abnormalities

Anatomic Considerations. Numerous tendons extend from the lower portion of the leg into the foot, across the ankle. These include the peroneus longus and peroneus brevis tendons laterally; the Achilles tendon posteriorly; the posterior tibialis, flexor hallucis longus, and flexor digitorum longus tendons medially; and the anterior tibialis, extensor hallucis longus, extensor digitorum longus, and peroneus tertius tendons anteriorly. With the exception of the Achilles tendon, all of these tendons change from a vertical orientation in the lower leg to a horizontal orientation in the foot at or near the level of the ankle, a modification in direction that is accomplished by means of a pulley system consisting either of bone (i.e., the malleoli) or of retinacula.[1174] To promote smooth movement at their sites of angulation, tendons are surrounded by either: (1) a sheath of parietal synovium and tenosynovial fluid in fibro-osseous tunnels (e.g., flexor hallucis longus tendon), under a bone pulley (e.g., peroneal tendons under the lateral malleolus), or under a fascial sling (e.g., anterior tibialis tendon under the extensor retinaculum); or (2) loose connective tissue, termed a peritenon (e.g., Achilles tendon).[1174] Where tendons are applied to the surface of a bone, a groove or sulcus

is present to promote angular deviations in their course that occur about the ankle. Examples include a groove in the posterior portion of the tibia for the tibialis posterior and flexor digitorum longus tendons, grooves in the posterior surface of the tibia and the talus and the inferior surface of the sustentaculum tali of the calcaneus for the flexor hallucis longus tendon, and a groove in the posterior surface of the fibula that houses the peroneus brevis tendon (and, to a lesser extent, the peroneus longus tendon). These grooves vary in size and in depth. The groove behind the fibula, through which pass the tendons of the peroneus brevis and peroneus longus muscles, is the smallest and most shallow, perhaps explaining the occurrence of subluxation of these tendons (see later discussion).

The movements of the ankle and foot are intimately related and complex. These movements lead to the development of dynamic forces in the many regional tendons whose magnitude is related to the osseous anatomy that varies somewhat from one person to another, the volume of the contracting muscles, and the rapidity and type of movement. As the tendons of the ankle and foot are subjected to tremendous functional demands, not only during physical exertion but also as a response to routine activities such as walking, it is not surprising that a variety of tendon and tendon sheath abnormalities are encountered.

Pathologic Considerations. Jahss[1175] has classified disorders of the tendons about the ankle and in the foot according to the following general categories: tenosynovitis, tethering, tears, dislocations, tumors and pseudotumors, ossification, congenital anomalies, contractures, and iatrogenic injuries. Inflammatory changes in or about a tendon, often designated tenosynovitis, can be more precisely defined according to which type of tissue is affected. Such inflammation can affect a tendon sheath, the surrounding tissues, the region between the sheath and the tendon, or the tendon substance. If the tendon sheath itself is involved, the term tenosynovitis is most appropriate. Paratenosynovitis refers to inflammation of tissues about a tendon sheath, and paratendinitis refers to inflammation about a tendon that has no sheath. Peritendinitis is defined as inflammation of a peritenon. Tendinitis indicates inflammation within the substance of the tendon. Although such terminology is anatomically correct, inflammation commonly involves more than one of these structures, such that paratenosynovitis, tenosynovitis, and tendinitis can occur simultaneously. Inflammation of any or all of these structures may relate to direct or indirect injury, occupational stress and overuse syndromes, misuse syndromes related to anomalies of the foot or other structures, and local or systemic rheumatic diseases.[1164] Although paratenosynovitis, paratendinitis, peritendinitis, tenosynovitis, and tendinitis occur in many different anatomic sites, inflammation leads to increased regional vascularity and cellular infiltration. When synovitis is a component of the inflammatory process, an increase in synovial fluid is apparent. Adhesions may develop between the sheath and the tendon (i.e., stenosing or constrictive tenosynovitis), leading to altered or restricted movement in a tendon sheath–tendon unit that normally requires smooth, almost frictionless function. The wall of the sheath may thicken and become irregular, producing narrowing of the avenue through which the tendon or tendons pass. The pathologic findings that produce narrowing or constriction of the tendon sheath appear to be more common in locations, such as the sheath that surrounds the peroneus longus and peroneus brevis tendons, in which more than one tendon occupies a single sheath.[1174]

Tenosynovitis in the ankle and foot relates primarily to either a systemic rheumatic disease, an infection, or local mechanical factors. Rheumatoid arthritis, the seronegative spondyloarthropathies, and gout are among the rheumatic diseases that lead to such tenosynovitis. Infective tenosynovitis can relate to a variety of microorganisms, although gonococcal or atypical mycobacterial infections deserve emphasis. Mechanical tenosynovitis is the most common type of disease, however. Causes of mechanical tenosynovitis include overuse syndromes in athletes, improper footwear, and bone anomalies (such as pes planus, an accessory navicular bone, and an enlarged peroneal tubercle).[1175]

Paratenosynovitis may result from any inflammatory process that originates in the soft tissues and extends to the vicinity of a tendon sheath. Tendinitis, or inflammation in the substance of the tendon itself, may relate to an injury leading to disruption of some of the tendinous fibers, xanthomatosis, gouty or rheumatoid involvement of the tendon, or irritation by enlargement or irregularity of an adjacent bone (e.g., flexor hallucis longus tendinitis produced by an enlarged os trigonum).[1175] Peritendinitis also may occur secondary to a systemic process, such as rheumatoid arthritis, or spontaneously, particularly in the Achilles tendon and the tendon of the tibialis posterior muscle. Relative avascularity of these two tendons may make them more susceptible to this condition, which can lead to their attrition and eventual rupture.

By definition, a tethered tendon is one whose range of movement is limited, owing to its abnormal fixation to an adjacent structure. Causes of such tethering include anatomic anomalies (such as a single tendon sheath surrounding two tendons that normally have separate sheaths, or an accessory tendon that increases the volume of tissue within a single sheath), fractures with resulting deformities that lead to abnormal fixation or displacement of the tendon or its sheath (e.g., tethering of the peroneal tendons as a result of lateral extrusion of fragments of the calcaneus), a hypertrophied os trigonum that leads to constriction and displacement of the flexor hallucis longus tendon within its sheath, fracture-dislocations of the ankle that may lead to tethering or even incarceration of one or more regional tendons, and checkrein deformities resulting from abnormal fixation of the flexor hallucis longus tendon under or just proximal to the flexor retinaculum (usually related to a fracture of the lower portion of the tibia) or under the annular ligament (which may occur secondary to a fracture, infection, or tumor).[1175]

Partial or complete tears of the tendons of the foot and ankle may relate to a laceration, especially in the sole of the foot or, more commonly, they may occur spontaneously. Spontaneous ruptures of these tendons (as well as those at other sites) usually imply some type of intrinsic pathologic process, as normal tendons rarely rupture in this fashion. Tendon degeneration in older persons or chronic inflammation in younger persons, particularly athletes, may predispose to spontaneous rupture. Although virtually any tendon of the foot or ankle may be affected, spontaneous disruptions of the tibialis posterior tendon and the Achilles tendon are encountered most frequently. Those of the tibialis anterior tendon, flexor hallucis longus tendon, and ten-

dons of the peroneus longus and peroneus brevis muscles are far less common.

Additional lesions of tendons and their sheaths in the foot and ankle include tumors and tumor-like disorders (e.g., lipomas, xanthomas, gouty tophi, rheumatoid nodules, chondromas, pigmented villonodular tenosynovitis, idiopathic tenosynovial osteochondromatosis), anomalies (e.g., accessory or duplicated tendons and aberrant tendon insertions), contractures related to neuromuscular disease, infections, and ossification (e.g., ossification of the Achilles tendon). Many of these conditions are discussed elsewhere in this book (see Chapters 64, 67, 77, 84, and 95).

Imaging Considerations. The assessment of tendon and tendon sheath abnormalities can be accomplished with a number of different imaging techniques. Routine radiography and bone scintigraphy lack sensitivity, ultrasonography is applicable to analysis of only those tendons accessible to a probe placed on the skin, and tenography provides indirect evidence of tendon abnormality and requires a needle puncture. CT and MR imaging are the two most commonly employed techniques for evaluation of the tendons of the foot and ankle. At this time, MR imaging generally is considered the best available imaging method in the detection of tendinitis, tenosynovitis, and partial and complete tendon ruptures; CT is superior to MR imaging in the delineation of tendon calcification and retinacular avulsions of bone; and CT and MR imaging are of approximately equal value when applied to the analysis of tendon dislocations.[1176]

Routine Radiography. Routine radiographic findings associated with abnormalities of the tendons and tendon sheaths of the foot and ankle include: soft tissue swelling, a change in contour, calcification, or ossification of a tendon, bone proliferation, fracture fragments, and sesamoid displacement. Soft tissue swelling or fullness may accompany tenosynovitis, but the finding is not specific. A change in contour of an inflamed or torn tendon is best appreciated in locations where the tendon is surrounded by abundant fat (e.g., Achilles tendon), but the finding may be subtle unless low kilovolt radiography (see Chapter 5) or xeroradiography (see Chapter 6) is employed. Achilles tendinitis or a rupture of the Achilles tendon may be accompanied by edema or hemorrhage, with obscuration of portions of the preachilles fat body, and associated retrocalcaneal bursitis (which may occur in systemic rheumatic disorders and in Haglund's syndrome) leads to obliteration of the normal radiolucent retrocalcaneal recess between the Achilles tendon and the posterosuperior portion of the calcaneus (Fig. 70–390). Calcific tendinitis in the foot is rare; ossification of the Achilles tendon is seen, however, and is detected readily by routine radiography (see later discussion and Chapter 95).

Osseous proliferation or erosion is a recognized manifestation of inflammation of tendons and tendon sheaths that are located close or applied directly to the surface of a bone (Fig. 70–391). In the foot and ankle, this finding most commonly is observed in the posteromedial portion of the tibia in patients with rheumatoid arthritis or a seronegative spondyloarthropathy who have involvement of the tibialis posterior tendon and sheath. Infections of tendons and tendon sheaths also can lead to infective or reactive periostitis in the subjacent bone (see Chapter 64).

Avulsion fractures related to sites of retinacular attach-

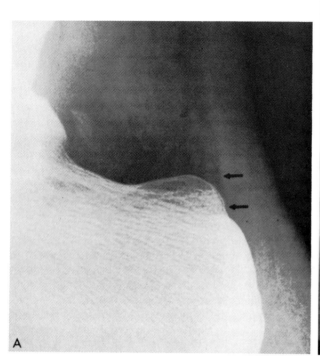
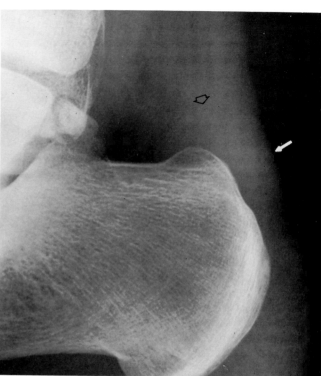

FIGURE 70–390. Retrocalcaneal bursa: Routine radiography. Normal appearance and retrocalcaneal bursitis.

A Normal appearance. Normally, with the foot in a neutral position, fat about the retrocalcaneal bursa produces a triangular radiolucent area (arrows), designated the retrocalcaneal recess, between the Achilles tendon and the calcaneus in lateral radiographs of the ankle.

B Retrocalcaneal bursitis. Inflammation, synovial hypertrophy, and effusion result in an enlarged fluid-filled retrocalcaneal bursa, which extends above the calcaneus as a radiodense area (open arrow). The Achilles tendon and surrounding tissue also are thickened (solid arrow).

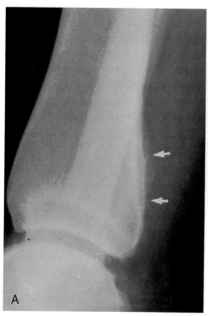
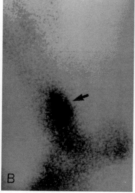
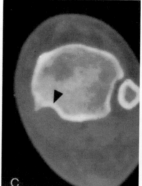
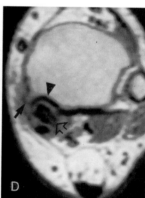

FIGURE 70–391. Tibialis posterior tendinitis and tenosynovitis: Bone proliferation and erosion displayed by routine radiography, bone scintigraphy, CT scanning, and MR imaging.

A A lateral radiograph shows soft tissue swelling and bone proliferation involving the posterior surface of the tibia (arrows).

B Bone scintigraphy shows increased accumulation (arrow) of the radiopharmaceutical agent in the distal portion of the tibia.

C A transaxial CT scan reveals bone erosion (arrowhead) of the tibia subjacent to the tibialis posterior tendon.

D A transaxial T1-weighted (TR/TE, 900/20) spin echo MR image confirms the presence of tibial erosion (arrowhead) and bone proliferation (solid arrow) adjacent to the tibialis posterior tendon (open arrow).

(Courtesy of T. Broderick, M.D., Orange, California.)

ment may occur as a response to tendon subluxation or dislocation. An elongated bone fragment located lateral to the distal portion of the fibula is characteristic of a dislocation of the peroneal tendons (see later discussion) and may be seen as an isolated finding or in association with complex fracture-dislocations about the ankle.[1177, 1178] Displacement of the os peroneum may occur in patients with rupture of the tendon of the peroneus longus muscle.[1179] This sesamoid bone ossifies in approximately 5 to 20 per cent of persons, and normally is located adjacent to the lower border of the cuboid bone or at the level of the calcaneocuboid joint. Proximal migration with or without fragmentation of the os peroneum is consistent with attrition and rupture of the peroneus longus tendon just distal to the location of the sesamoid bone.

Ultrasonography. High resolution ultrasonography is an inexpensive and noninvasive technique that can be applied to the assessment of tendon abnormalities[1176] (see Chapter 11). In the foot and ankle, the Achilles tendon is evaluated most easily and accurately with ultrasonography. The normal Achilles tendon shows an internal network of fine parallel and linear fibrillar echoes that become more numerous and thinner as the ultrasonic frequency is increased.[1180] Sonographic abnormalities of the Achilles tendon include increased thickness, interruption, fragmentation, or disappearance of the tendon fibrils.[1180] With ultrasonography, complete tears of the tendon are accompanied by retraction of the fragments and a tendinous gap that may be filled with a hematoma.[1176] Ultrasound examinations that are performed meticulously and interpreted by experienced observers are most likely to be beneficial in the evaluation of the Achilles tendon and other tendons in the foot and ankle.

Computed Tomography. CT can be used effectively to study the tendons of the foot and ankle.[1176, 1181–1184] Transaxial CT images are the easiest to acquire and provide the most useful information, although reformatted transaxial data in the coronal or sagittal plane occasionally are required. The CT features of a normal tendon include a smooth contour, a size similar to that on the opposite side, a well-defined margin, and attenuation values (75 to 115 Hounsfield units) higher than those of the respective muscles.[1176] Tenosynovitis is manifest as an enlarged tendon with an inhomogeneous appearance. The surrounding swollen, fluid-containing tendon sheath has a lower attenuation value than the tendon itself.[1184] Tendon displacement, tethering, or rupture may be evident, and the relationship of the tendon to the adjacent bone is identified readily. Tendon ruptures are associated with partial or complete discontinuity of the fibers and a decrease in attenuation values (30 to 50 Hounsfield units). Diagnostic difficulties are encountered with CT, owing to beam-hardening artifacts that cause inaccurate assessment of attenuation values and to the presence of surrounding inflammation that obscures the contour of the tendon and the tendon sheath. MR imaging is superior to CT in delineating small amounts of fluid around the tendon and allowing differentiation of scar tissue from edema and fluid.[1176] CT is superior to MR imaging in demonstrating regions of tendon calcification and avulsion fractures related to the retinacula.

Tenography. Tenography is a procedure in which tendon sheaths are opacified directly with contrast medium. Initially used as a diagnostic method, tenography now is performed less commonly for this purpose because CT and

MR imaging seem more efficient in the assessment of tendon disorders. Tenography still can be employed for therapeutic purposes, however.[1185]

The peroneal tendon sheath was the first to be studied with tenography.[1166, 1186–1188] The normal peroneal tenogram outlines the common sheath of the peroneus longus and peroneus brevis muscles and the point of bifurcation of this sheath into separate sheaths enclosing either tendon (Fig. 70–392). These sheaths can be traced for variable distances in the foot, appearing smooth in outline and containing a radiolucent tendon without displacement. The peroneal tenogram may be abnormal following calcaneal fractures (see later discussion). Abnormal findings include extrinsic compression and irregularity of the sheath, lateral or anterior displacement of the tendons and sheath, complete obstruction of contrast flow, and tendon rupture. Peroneal tenography (and subtalar arthrography) also can be accompanied by lidocaine injection to localize the source of obscure pain in patients with previous calcaneal fractures.[1166]

Contrast opacification of additional tendon sheaths about the ankle has been accomplished.[1164, 1176, 1189, 1190] Irregularity or nonvisualization of the injected tendon sheath is consistent with the diagnosis of stenosing tenosynovitis. More important, proper placement of the needle within the tendon sheath can be confirmed during the tenographic procedure, allowing accurate intrasynovial instillation of local anesthetic agents or corticosteroid preparations.

MR Imaging. MR imaging has been applied to the assessment of the tendons and other structures in the ankle and foot.[1176, 1191–1199] The tibialis posterior tendon[1200, 1201] and

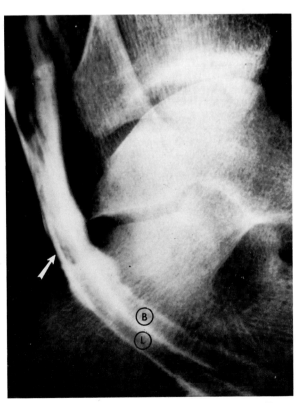

FIGURE 70–392. Peroneal tenography: Normal tenogram. The normal peroneal tenogram reveals a smooth synovial sheath (arrow) separating into sheaths enclosing the peroneus brevis (B) and peroneus longus (L) tendons. No impingement or deviation of the contrast-filled sheaths can be seen.

(From Resnick D, Goergen TG: Radiology *115*:211, 1975.)

the Achilles tendon[1202–1204] have received the greatest attention. The most commonly employed MR imaging sequences used in the ankle and foot are standard spin echo, multiplanar gradient recalled echo, and short tau inversion recovery (STIR) sequences. The use of three-dimensional Fourier transform (3DFT) gradient recalled images allows the rapid acquisition of thin, contiguous sections of the foot and ankle and reformatting of image data in oblique planes parallel to the long axis of the tendons,[1198] although this method is not used routinely. MR images can be obtained in the sagittal, coronal, or transaxial (plantar) plane, or combinations of these planes. The specific planes selected depend upon the particular anatomic regions and structures to be evaluated and the clinical questions involved. Similarly, the position of the patient (supine versus prone), the inclusion of one foot and ankle or both feet and ankles, and the need for flexion of the knee or flexion, extension, or a neutral position of the foot are influenced by the specific indications for the MR imaging examination.[1174] With regard to the assessment of the tendons of the ankle and foot, at least two different imaging planes are required, T2-weighted spin echo (or some type of gradient recalled echo) images should be obtained in at least one plane, and both feet and ankles should be included in at least one plane, providing a means to compare the findings in the symptomatic side with those in the asymptomatic side. Standard T1-weighted spin echo MR images are useful for anatomic delineation of the tendons, and T2-weighted spin echo MR images are valuable for the detection of fluid, edema, hemorrhage, or scar formation in or about the tendons.[1176] The presence of adjacent fat, as occurs about the Achilles tendon, aids in the MR imaging assessment of some tendons.

With minor exceptions, the normal tendons in the ankle and foot are homogeneous and of low signal intensity with all MR imaging sequences. They generally are equal in size in the two sides of the body and have a smooth contour. There are some exceptions to these general rules, however.

1. Magic angle effect. As indicated earlier, an increased signal intensity may be seen in normal tendons oriented obliquely with respect to the main magnetic field, an effect that is greatest when this orientation is at 55 degrees to that of the magnetic field (Fig. 70–393). This effect is greater when the MR imaging examination employs spin echo techniques with short echo times or gradient echo techniques. The tibialis posterior tendon approximates this orientation at its site of attachment to the navicular bone, resulting in a normal appearance of increased signal intensity or heterogeneous signal intensity in this area. This alteration in signal intensity may be accentuated by volume averaging of different signal intensities derived from the joint capsule and fat in this region.[1195] Although the change in signal intensity has a typical appearance that allows distinction from a tear, the absence of abnormal findings on T2-weighted spin echo images is useful in eliminating the diagnosis of tendon pathology.[1199] Furthermore, repeating the MR imaging examination with a foot in plantar flexion will diminish or eliminate this magic angle phenomenon.[1198]

2. Tenosynovial fluid. The differentiation of a thickened tendon from one surrounded by a fluid-filled synovial sheath is difficult on T1-weighted spin echo MR images. Furthermore, the presence of small or even moderate amounts of fluid within a tendon sheath, by itself, is not diagnostic of an abnormality, as such fluid is seen in asymptomatic persons.[1199] Tenosynovial fluid is more frequent in flexor tendons (as compared to extensor tendons) and may be particularly prominent about the flexor hallucis longus tendon.[1418] The precise amount of fluid that defines an abnormality of the tendon or tendon sheath has not been determined.

3. Bulbous tendon insertion sites. Insertion sites of tendons may appear bulbous (Fig. 70–394), perhaps related to volume averaging of their signal intensity with that of adjacent cortical bone. This appearance can simulate that of a tendon disruption, particularly of the tibialis posterior tendon.[1201]

4. Tendon striations. When three-dimensional gradient recalled MR images are obtained, longitudinal lines of intermediate signal intensity in the distal portion of the tibialis posterior tendon may be noted.[1198] These lines probably

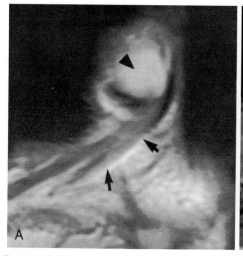
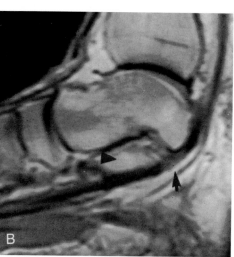

FIGURE 70–393. Tendons about the ankle: MR imaging. Normal variations—magic angle phenomenon.

A Peroneus longus and brevis tendons. A sagittal T1-weighted (TR/TE, 600/20) spin echo MR image reveals a slight increase in signal intensity (arrows) of the peroneus tendons as they course about the distal portion of the fibula (arrowhead). This alteration in signal intensity relates to the magic angle phenomenon.

B Flexor hallucis longus tendon. A sagittal T1-weighted (TR/TE, 600/20) spin echo MR image shows a slight increase in signal intensity (arrow) in the flexor hallucis longus tendon near the sustentaculum tali (arrowhead) related to the magic angle phenomenon.

(Courtesy of D. Goodwin, M.D., and D. Salonen, M.D., San Diego, California.)

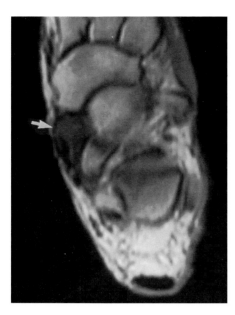

FIGURE 70–394. Tendons about the ankle: MR imaging. Normal variations—bulbous tendon insertion sites. As shown in this trans-axial T1-weighted (TR/TE, 600/20) spin echo MR image, the navicular insertion site (arrow) of the tibialis posterior tendon normally may appear bulbous and of increased signal intensity.
(Courtesy of D. Goodwin, M.D., and D. Salonen, M.D., San Diego, California.)

represent branches of the tendon, although their appearance may simulate that of a tendon tear.

In common with the findings derived by ultrasonography and CT, the major MR imaging finding of tenosynovitis is abnormal accumulation of fluid within the tendon sheath. This fluid is of low signal intensity on T1-weighted spin echo MR images and of high signal intensity on T2-weighted spin echo images. Pannus and scar formation about a tendon are characterized by intermediate signal intensity on T1-weighted spin echo MR images and intermediate to high signal intensity on T2-weighted spin echo MR images. Tendinitis is accompanied by focal areas of high signal intensity within the substance of the tendon on proton density and T2-weighted spin echo MR images.[1176] With chronic tendinitis, the tendon is enlarged and of low signal intensity in both T1-weighted and T2-weighted spin echo MR images.[1176]

Tendon ruptures may be acute or chronic, and partial or complete. With MR imaging, recent tendon tears frequently reveal regions of increased signal intensity in T2-weighted spin echo MR images and in certain gradient echo images, owing to the presence of edema and hemorrhage. Remote tendon tears generally do not have these high signal intensity characteristics, owing to the presence of scar tissue. With regard to the extent of the tendon tear, three MR imaging patterns have been described[1176, 1200] (Fig. 70–395):

Type 1. Partial tendon rupture with tendon hypertrophy. The involved tendon appears hypertrophied or bulbous, and it reveals heterogeneous signal intensity. Focal areas of increased signal intensity are noted within its substance. The MR imaging pattern corresponds to a surgically evident, partially torn tendon possessing vertical splits and defects.

Type 2. Partial tendon rupture with tendon attenuation. The involved tendon is stretched and attenuated in size, MR imaging findings that correspond to those found at surgery.

Type 3. Complete tendon rupture with tendon retraction. The involved tendon is discontinuous and, in some cases, a gap is evident that is filled with fluid, fat, or scar tissue depending upon the age of the tear. The size of the gap, reflecting the degree of tendon retraction, is variable, both with MR imaging and at surgery.

The extent of the tendon tear, as well as its location, influences the type of surgical repair that may be attempted.[1200] A small focal area of tendon rupture may be treated with surgical resection and end-to-end tendon anastomosis; a large area of tendon rupture may require side-to-side tendon anastomosis; and a large tendon rupture with tendon retraction may preclude direct anastomosis of the torn ends of the tendon, requiring arthrodesis in some cases in order to prevent further foot deformities.[1205–1207]

Tendon subluxation or dislocation is detected easily with MR imaging, as with CT, owing to an abnormal relationship of the tendon with the adjacent tissues. The tendon itself may be enlarged or partially torn, and associated soft tissue and bone injury may be evident.

Abnormalities of the Achilles Tendon. The Achilles tendon, which serves to plantar flex the foot at the ankle, is the longest and strongest tendon in the lower leg and, along with the tibialis posterior tendon, is one of the most commonly injured tendons in the foot.

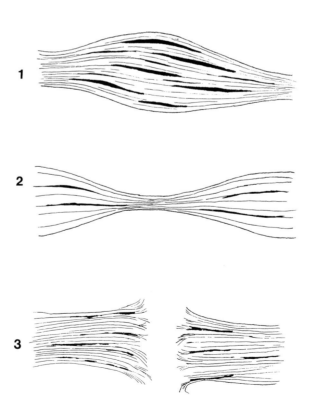

FIGURE 70–395. Tendons about the ankle: MR imaging. Types of tendon tears. Type 1 tears are characterized by partial disruption of the tendon with vertical splits and a bulbous or hypertrophied appearance. Type 2 tears are characterized by partial disruption of the tendon, which appears attenuated. Type 3 tears are characterized by complete disruption of the tendon and retraction of the torn ends.
(Modified from Rosenberg ZS, et al: Radiology *169:*229, 1988.)

Anatomy. The Achilles tendon is formed by the confluence of the gastrocnemius and soleus tendons, and courses along the posterior surface of the ankle, separated from the ankle joint by the preachilles fat body (Fig. 70–388). The precise contributions of the gastrocnemius and soleus tendons to the Achilles tendon is variable; the gastrocnemius tendon usually contributes more tendinous fibers to the Achilles tendon than does the soleus tendon.[1174] In adults, the Achilles tendon is about 10 to 15 cm in length.[1208] Superiorly, the Achilles tendon is a flattened band of tissue. As it descends, it becomes rounded, assuming a cordlike shape.[1208] It then fans out, as it approaches the tubercle of the calcaneus. Close to the point of attachment of the tendinous fibers to the calcaneus, the fibers take a spiral twist; the posterior strands swing from the medial to the lateral side and capture the outer rim of the posterior surface of the calcaneus, while the anterior fibers run from the lateral to the medial side and insert into the inner border of these same structures.[1208] The vulnerable region of the Achilles tendon is just proximal to the inception of this spiral twist, involving a segment between 2 and 6 cm from its insertion into the calcaneus.[1208] The normal blood supply in this region is tenuous,[1209] a situation reminiscent of that in the distal portion of the supraspinatus tendon and one that may be responsible for tendinous disruption. Some studies have indicated, however, that another area of diminished blood supply in the Achilles tendon occurs just above its bone insertion,[1432] a site that rarely ruptures, suggesting that factors other than vascular supply are important in the pathogenesis of Achilles tendon disruption.[1210] The Achilles tendon does not possess a tendon sheath. Rather, it is covered by a peritenon whose system of vessels extends within and outside the Achilles tendon.

The distal portion of the Achilles tendon is approximately 4 to 7 mm in thickness. It has a flat to slightly concave anterior margin and rounded medial, posterior, and lateral aspects that give the tendon a crescent shape.[1174] Just prior to its insertion into the calcaneus, the Achilles tendon assumes a more ovoid shape with a flattened anterior margin.[1174] These features are best displayed in sagittal and transaxial MR images (Fig. 70–396).

Tendinitis, Paratendinitis, and Peritendinitis. As the Achilles tendon does not possess a tendon sheath, inflammatory disorders are best classified as tendinitis (inflammation of the Achilles tendon itself), paratendinitis (inflammation about the Achilles tendon), and peritendinitis (inflammation of its peritenon). Any of the inflammatory processes may be acute or chronic in nature, and acute episodes of inflammation may occur in or about a tendon that reveals chronic inflammatory changes as well. Inflammatory disease of the Achilles tendon may result from a systemic rheumatic disorder (such as rheumatoid arthritis) or relate to a local response to overuse or misuse of the foot and ankle. Older, sedentary people or young athletes may be affected. An increase in the level of training or a change in training protocol (e.g., running on hills as opposed to flat terrain), tibia vara, excessive pronation of the foot, or a cavus foot may cause acute and chronic tendinitis, paratendinitis, or peritendinitis.[1174]

Chronic tendinitis leads to thickening of the Achilles tendon. One or both feet may be involved. The tendon is enlarged and slightly tender, and crepitation may be palpated when the foot is flexed and extended repeatedly.

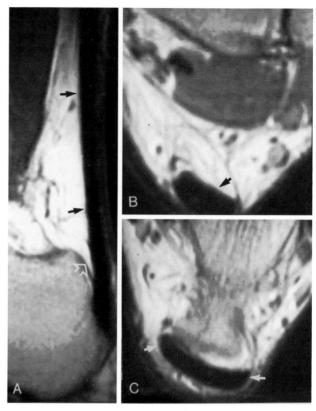

FIGURE 70–396. Normal Achilles tendon: MR imaging.
A A sagittal T1-weighted (TR/TE, 650/20) spin echo MR image shows the smooth straight contour of the Achilles tendon (solid arrows) and its sharp interface with the preachilles fat pad. Note the triangular region of fat (open arrow) that separates the Achilles tendon and the posterosuperior portion of the calcaneus.
B, C Transaxial T1-weighted (TR/TE, 650/20) spin echo MR images at the level of the ankle joint **(B)** and just above the calcaneal attachment of the Achilles tendon **(C)** show the changing shape of the Achilles tendon (arrows). In **B**, the anterior margin of the Achilles tendon is flat or slightly concave; in **C**, a wider structure with a flat anterior margin is evident.

Chronic peritendinitis is associated with adhesions between the peritenon and adjacent Achilles tendon. The involved tendon feels thickened, fibrotic, and nodular on physical examination, and it may be tender to palpation.

The classic MR imaging feature of chronic Achilles tendinitis with or without surrounding peritendinitis and paratendinitis is a diffusely or focally enlarged or thickened tendon[1202, 1203, 1211] (Fig. 70–397). The signal intensity in the involved portion of the Achilles tendon generally is low; when intratendinous foci of increased signal intensity are observed in T2-weighted spin echo MR images, an accompanying partial tear of the Achilles tendon is likely. Peritendinitis or paratendinitis alone may lead to changes in the preachilles fat body with a normal-appearing Achilles tendon (Fig. 70–398).

Partial and Complete Tendon Ruptures. Complete disruption of the Achilles tendon by indirect violence is 5 to 6 times more common in men than in women, and the left side is affected more often than the right.[1208] Although athletes of any age may develop Achilles tendon disruption, complete rupture of this tendon usually occurs in persons between the ages of 30 and 50 years. The typical patient is a middle-aged sedentary man who partakes in strenuous

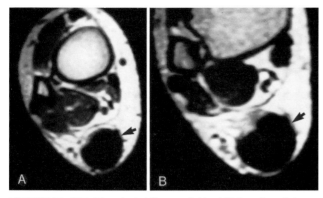

FIGURE 70–397. Chronic Achilles tendinitis: MR imaging. A transaxial proton density–weighted (TR/TE, 2500/20) spin echo MR image at the level of the distal portions of the tibia and fibula **(A)** and a transaxial T2-weighted (TR/TE, 2500/70) spin echo MR image at a slightly lower level **(B)** show a markedly enlarged Achilles tendon (arrows), which is of low signal intensity in both images.

activity requiring sudden or forceful dorsiflexion or pushoff of the foot.[1175] Clinical findings include severe pain, local soft tissue swelling and hemorrhage, and a positive Thompson test, in which the patient is unable to stand tiptoe on the affected leg.[1175] Predisposing factors include chronic tendinitis, partial tears of the Achilles tendon, tendon ossification or calcification, rheumatoid arthritis, systemic lupus erythematosus, and local injection or systemic administration of corticosteroid preparations. Local causative factors also may include tendon ischemia and anatomic variations. It has been proposed that inadequately interwoven collagen bundles of the soleus and the gastrocnemius muscles lead to asynchronous rubbing of tendinous fibers at the vulnerable level of the Achilles tendon, 2 to 6 cm proximal to the calcaneus.[1212] Ruptures also may occur due to incongruity

between the tones of muscle and tendon fibers, alignment abnormalities such as exaggerated pronation of the foot, or ineffective or poorly designed footwear.[1203]

The MR imaging findings of a partial or complete tear of the Achilles tendon (Figs. 70–399 and 70–400) include discontinuity of some or all of its fibers, intratendinous regions of increased signal intensity in T2-weighted spin echo MR images and STIR images, and in the case of total disruption of the Achilles tendon, a tendinous gap that is filled with blood and edema of increased signal intensity in these images. The tendon often is enlarged, sometimes grossly enlarged. Diagnostic difficulty arises in the differentiation of partial tears and those complete tears in which tendon retraction is not a prominent feature. Diagnostic difficulty also arises in differentiating chronic tendinitis without tendon disruption from such tendinitis accompanied by a partial tear of the Achilles tendon. In general, however, MR imaging appears more accurate (when compared with CT and ultrasonography) (Fig. 70–401) in allowing identification of partial and complete tears of the Achilles tendon.[1202, 1213–1215]

Although conservative treatment (i.e., casting of the leg) of Achilles tendon ruptures may be sufficient in older and sedentary patients, surgical repair often is required, particularly in athletes who wish to resume their previous level of physical activity. Suturing alone, suturing reinforced with tendinous or fascial grafts (e.g., flexor hallucis or plantaris tendon or the fascia lata), or synthetic materials may be used.[1204, 1216–1218] The role of MR imaging in the selection of patients who will derive the greatest benefit from surgery involves identification of the site and extent of the tendon

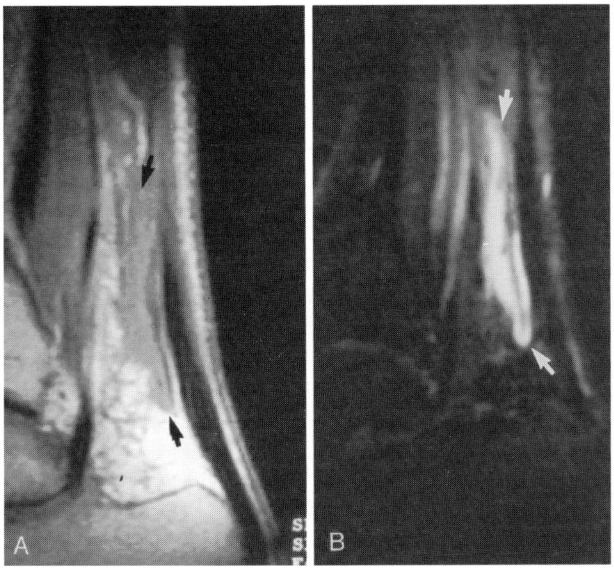

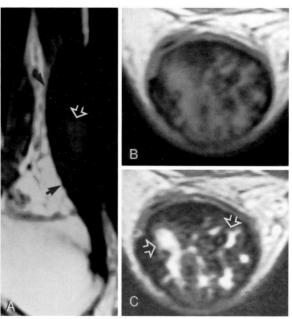

FIGURE 70–399. Chronic Achilles tendinitis with partial tear: MR imaging.

A A sagittal T1-weighted (TR/TE, 600/25) spin echo MR image shows a massively enlarged Achilles tendon (solid arrows) containing a region of intermediate signal intensity (open arrow).

B, C Transaxial proton density–weighted (TR/TE, 2000/20) **(B)** and T2-weighted (TR/TE, 2000/80) **(C)** spin echo MR images through the enlarged segment of the Achilles tendon show its inhomogeneous signal intensity, with regions of high signal intensity (open arrows) in **C**.

FIGURE 70–398. Achilles peritendinitis and paratendinitis: MR imaging. In a soccer player, a sagittal T1-weighted (TR/TE, 700/15) spin echo MR image **(A)** shows an irregular region of intermediate signal intensity (arrows) within the preachilles fat body. A sagittal STIR MR image (TR/TE, 5000/22; inversion time, 150 msec) shows high signal intensity (arrows) anterior to the Achilles tendon. (Courtesy of C. Wakeley, M.D., Bristol, England.)

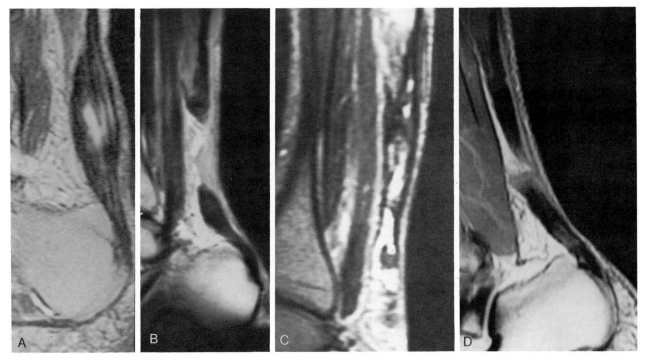

FIGURE 70–400. Chronic Achilles tendinitis with partial or complete tear: MR imaging.

A Partial tear. A sagittal T2-weighted (TR/TE, 2000/70) spin echo MR image shows an enlarged Achilles tendon containing irregular regions of high signal intensity.

B Complete tear. A sagittal proton density–weighted (TR/TE, 3000/30) spin echo MR image shows complete disruption of the Achilles tendon and a proximal segment that is inhomogeneous in signal intensity. Note edema and hemorrhage of high signal intensity about the acutely torn tendon.

C Complete tear. A sagittal T2-weighted (TR/TE, 1800/80) fat-suppressed spin echo MR image reveals an acute and complete tear of the Achilles tendon with multiple regions of high signal intensity. (Courtesy of D. Levey, M.D., Corpus Christi, Texas.)

D Complete tear. A sagittal proton density–weighted (TR/TE, 2000/20) spin echo MR image reveals a chronic tear characterized by complete disruption of the Achilles tendon.

rupture and the degree of separation of the torn ends of the tendon.[1174] Assessment of the position of the tendon fragments in MR images performed with the foot in a plantar flexed position may have some value.[1214] Following surgical repair, MR imaging can be used to evaluate the healing response of the Achilles tendon.[1174] A decrease in signal intensity within the Achilles tendon and an increase in its

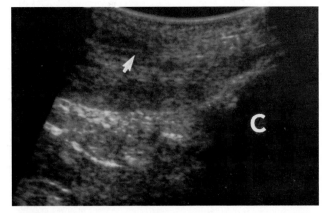

FIGURE 70–401. Chronic Achilles tendinitis with partial tear: Ultrasonography. A longitudinal scan of the ankle (with the cephalad aspect to the reader's left and the posterior aspect at the top of the image) shows a thickened Achilles tendon with coarse sonographic features (arrow) consistent with a partial tear (C = calcaneus). (Courtesy of T. Broderick, M.D., Orange, California.)

size, owing to the formation of scar tissue, are observed, although these findings occur gradually over a period of months or even a year. Similarly, MR imaging can be used to monitor the healing response within torn Achilles tendons that are treated conservatively.[1211, 1213, 1215] Preliminary data also suggest that this method allows assessment of the Achilles tendon following its repair with prosthetic implants.[1204]

Recurrent rupture of the Achilles tendon may occur following conservative or surgical treatment of the initial tendinous tear. These retears may appear weeks or even months after the initiation of therapy.[1175]

Calcification and Ossification. Calcification within the substance of the Achilles tendon relates to calcium hydroxyapatite or calcium pyrophosphate dihydrate crystal deposition (see Chapters 44 and 45). The calcific deposits are linear, occurring close to the tendinous insertion into bone, and they are well shown with routine radiography. Indeed, such calcification may be overlooked during evaluation of MR images. The relationship of calcification in the Achilles tendon to chronic tendinitis and to clinical manifestations is not clear.

Ossification in the Achilles tendon takes two forms. More commonly, an enthesophyte develops at the calcaneal site of insertion of the tendon, and it appears to have little clinical significance (Fig. 70–402). Less commonly, a discrete ossicle of variable size or diffuse ossification occurs within the tendon several centimeters from its calcaneal

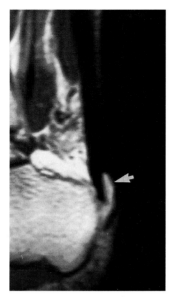

FIGURE 70–402. Calcaneal enthesophyte: MR imaging. A sagittal T1-weighted (TR/TE, 800/12) spin echo MR image shows a large calcaneal enthesophyte (arrow) containing marrow that arises at the site of insertion of the Achilles tendon.

attachment site (see Chapter 95). The process may be unilateral or bilateral, is often associated with a history of injury, and frequently is accompanied by evidence of tendon thickening (Fig. 70–403).

Urate Tophi, Rheumatoid Nodules, and Xanthomas. Involvement of the Achilles tendon in gout, rheumatoid arthritis, and various hypercholesterolemic conditions may lead to intratendinous nodules or diffuse thickening of the tendon (see Chapters 25, 26, 43, and 61). On palpation, the Achilles tendon may be nodular and enlarged. Ultrasonography, CT, and MR imaging (Fig. 70–404) represent effective methods for evaluation of these tendinous changes.[1419, 1420]

Abnormalities of the Tibialis Posterior Tendon

Anatomy. The tibialis posterior muscle plays a critical role in stabilizing the hindfoot, including the talus and subtalar joints, preventing valgus deformity of the hindfoot and excessive pronation of the forefoot. This muscle is involved in inversion and plantar flexion of the foot. As the flexor digitorum longus muscle acts in a fashion similar to that of the tibialis posterior muscle, incompetence of the latter muscle related to inflammation or rupture may be occult clinically.

The tibialis posterior muscle is the deepest of the flexor muscles of the foot. Its origin commonly is divided into two parts: the medial part of the muscle originates from the posterior surface of the interosseous membrane and from the posterior surface of the tibia; the lateral part of the muscle arises mainly from the posterior surface of the fibula. As it descends in the lower portion of the leg, the tendon of the tibialis posterior muscle is deep to that of the flexor digitorum longus muscle and lies within a groove behind the medial malleolus of the tibia (Figs. 70–405 to 70–407). From here, the tendon of the tibialis posterior muscle enters the foot by passing deep to the flexor retinaculum and superficial to the deltoid ligament. Distally, the tendon inserts via a superficial branch into the tuberosity of the navicular bone and into the medial cuneiform bone. A

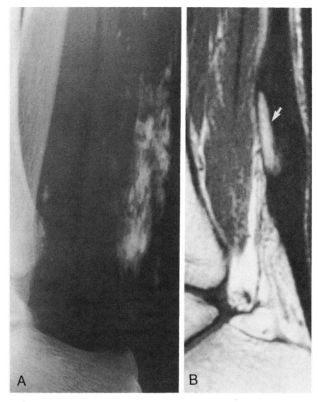

FIGURE 70–403. Achilles tendon ossification: Routine radiography and MR imaging.

A Note diffuse plaquelike ossification in the Achilles tendon.

B In a second patient, an elongated ossicle (arrow) containing marrow is located in a thickened portion of the Achilles tendon, as shown in a sagittal T1-weighted (TR/TE, 800/20) spin echo MR image.

(Courtesy of J. Yu, M.D., Columbus, Ohio.)

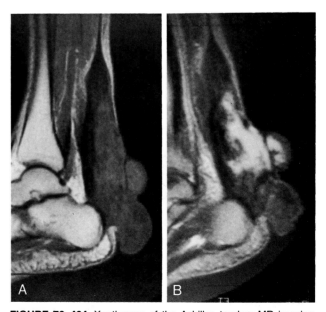

FIGURE 70–404. Xanthomas of the Achilles tendon: MR imaging. Sagittal T1-weighted (TR/TE, 800/30) **(A)** and T2-weighted (TR/TE, 2000/80) **(B)** spin echo MR images show a large mass infiltrating the Achilles tendon. Note the high signal intensity within the mass in **B**. The Achilles tendon is partially torn. The opposite side was involved similarly. (From Tehranzadeh J, et al: Skel Radiol *21*:79, 1992.)

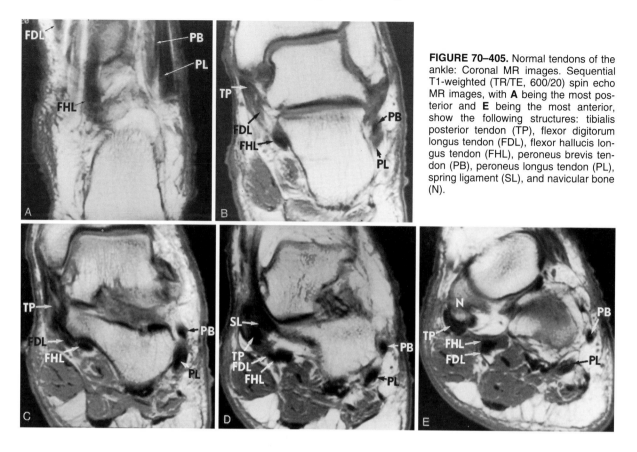

FIGURE 70–405. Normal tendons of the ankle: Coronal MR images. Sequential T1-weighted (TR/TE, 600/20) spin echo MR images, with **A** being the most posterior and **E** being the most anterior, show the following structures: tibialis posterior tendon (TP), flexor digitorum longus tendon (FDL), flexor hallucis longus tendon (FHL), peroneus brevis tendon (PB), peroneus longus tendon (PL), spring ligament (SL), and navicular bone (N).

lateral branch contributes to the tendon of the flexor hallucis brevis muscle and inserts into the intermediate cuneiform bone and the bases of the second, third, and fourth metatarsal bones. These insertion sites in the cuneiform and metatarsal bones underscore the contribution of the muscle to maintenance of the longitudinal arch of the foot. Disruption of the tibialis posterior tendon, which is being recognized increasingly, is associated with inability to supinate and invert the foot while the toes are being wiggled, and with progressive and painful planovalgus deformity of the foot.[1219]

Tendinitis, Tenosynovitis, and Rupture. Inflammatory changes in the tendon and tendon sheath of the tibialis posterior muscle are encountered as a result of altered mechanics of the foot or as a response to a systemic articular disease such as rheumatoid arthritis or a seronegative spondyloarthropathy. Spontaneous rupture of the tibialis posterior tendon (i.e., occurring in the absence of a systemic rheumatic disease) classically is seen in patients in the fifth and sixth decades of life (average age, 55 years), with two thirds of cases occurring in women.[1175, 1206, 1207, 1220, 1221] Unilateral involvement occurs in approximately 90 per cent of cases, with a left-sided predominance. Bilateral abnormalities of the tibialis posterior tendon are more frequent in cases associated with an underlying rheumatic disease. A spectrum of clinical alterations is encountered, depending

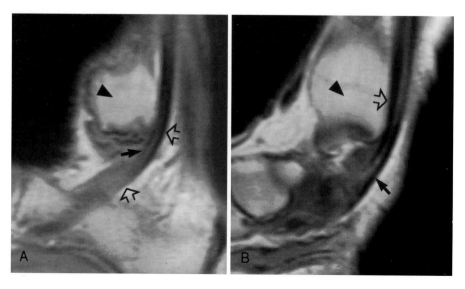

FIGURE 70–406. Normal tendons of the ankle: Sagittal MR images.

A A sagittal T1-weighted (TR/TE, 600/20) spin echo MR image through the lateral malleolus (arrowhead) shows portions of the peroneus longus (open arrows) and peroneus brevis (solid arrow) tendons.

B A sagittal T1-weighted (TR/TE, 600/20) spin echo MR image through the medial malleolus (arrowhead) reveals the tibialis posterior (open arrow) and flexor digitorum longus (solid arrow) tendons.

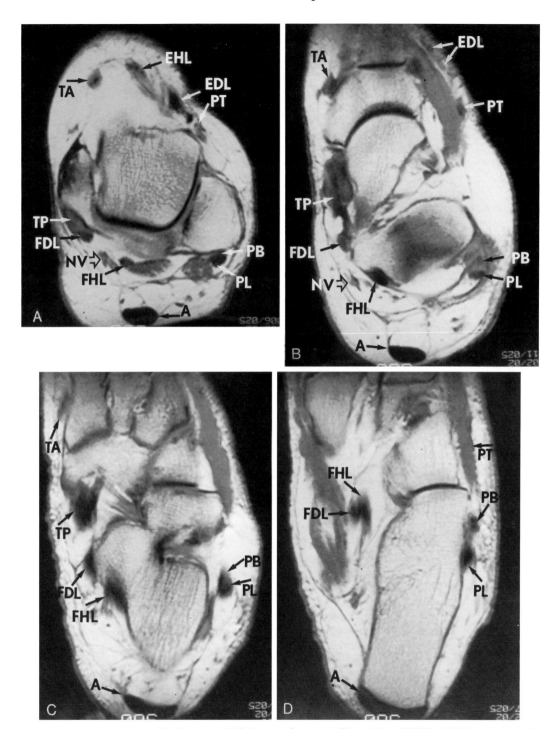

FIGURE 70–407. Normal tendons of the ankle: Transaxial MR images. Sequential T1-weighted (TR/TE, 600/20) spin echo MR images, with **A** being the most superior (at the level of the ankle joint) and **D** being the most inferior, show the following structures: tibialis posterior tendon (TP), flexor digitorum longus tendon (FDL), flexor hallucis longus tendon (FHL), posterior tibial artery and tibial nerve (NV), Achilles tendon (A), tibialis anterior tendon (TA), extensor hallucis longus tendon (EHL), extensor digitorum longus tendon (EDL), peroneus tertius tendon (PT), peroneus longus tendon (PL), and peroneus brevis tendon (PB).

upon the extent and chronicity of the changes. Initial manifestations include pain, swelling, and tenderness to palpation of the affected tendon. Progressive involvement results in weakness of inversion of the foot and flattening of the medial longitudinal arch of the foot, with the eventual appearance of severe pes planus deformity. Similar abnormalities also are identified in young athletic persons involved in tennis, soccer, ice hockey, basketball, and ballet dancing,[1174, 1222] and in children.[1433]

The cause of spontaneous rupture of the tibialis posterior tendon unrelated to a systemic rheumatic disease appears to result from local mechanical factors. The tibialis posterior tendon is the thickest of the medial group of tendons in the foot and resists the considerable weight-bearing forces that otherwise would lead to collapse of the longitudinal arch. Acute angulation of the tendon behind the medial malleolus and, perhaps, a vulnerable blood supply make it susceptible to injury.[1175, 1223] Pes planovalgus occurring as a developmental abnormality or as a result of initial weakening of the tibialis posterior tendon accentuates the forces placed on this tendon, leading to progressive tendinous alterations and eventual tendon rupture. Acute fractures about the ankle may be responsible for some cases of rupture of the tibialis posterior tendon.[1224] Furthermore, an accessory ossicle of the navicular bone may provide the site of attachment of some of the fibers of the tibialis posterior tendon (see Chapter 90), also predisposing to tendon failure.

Jahss has classified abnormalities (i.e., degeneration) within the tibialis posterior tendon and surrounding structures according to the severity of involvement (Fig. 70–408). Stage IA disease, representing approximately 13 per cent of all such abnormalities, is mild or clinically occult. Manifestations, which usually have been present for approximately 4 to 12 months, include minimal swelling, mild tenderness, slight weakness during inversion of the foot, and minimal valgus deformity of the hindfoot during weight-bearing. Pathologic findings include longitudinal splits in the deep surface of the tendon with a normal outer surface and sheath. Stage IB disease, representing approximately 44 per cent of cases of tendon degeneration, is moderate in extent. Clinical abnormalities usually have been manifest for a period of 12 to 18 months and are associated with CT and MR imaging findings (see later discussion). Pathologic alterations include more extensive deep splitting of the tibialis posterior tendon, intramural degeneration, tendon laxity, and irregularity of the external surface of the tendon and adhesions among it, the sheath, and the flexor retinaculum. Stage II or advanced disease represents 17 per cent of all cases of tibialis posterior tendon degeneration. Symptoms have been present for a period of approximately 18 to 30 months, and pes planus and heel valgus deformities and medial prominence of the head of the talus are observed. Pathologic findings include an elongated and fibrotic tendon, which is adherent to the medial malleolus. Bone proliferation in the medial malleolus is observed. The tendon is significantly degenerated, and its sheath is atrophic with scar formation. Multiple longitudinal tears of the tendon may be evident, and migration of the flexor digitorum longus tendon into the space previously occupied by the tibialis posterior tendon is seen, accounting for the failure to opacify the latter during tenography. Stage IIIA disease, present in approximately 15 per cent of patients with degeneration of the tibialis posterior tendon, represents complete rupture of the tendon. Symptoms usually have been present for 30 months to 4 years, and increasing peritalar subluxation, particularly during weight-bearing, is evident. In addition to tendon rupture, pathologic findings include separation of the scarred and frayed proximal and distal portions of the tendon with adherence of these portions to subjacent bone. The final stage, stage IIIB, is associated with complete tendon rupture and peritalar dislocation. It represents approximately 11 per cent of cases of degeneration of the tibialis posterior tendon. This stage occurs in patients who have had clinical manifestations for many years. Severe valgus deformity and medial dislocation of the talar head are observed on radiographic examination. The superior portion of the calcaneus abuts the undersurface of the talar neck in the sinus tarsi. With weight-bearing, valgus rotation and superior displacement of the calcaneus obliterate the sinus tarsi. Secondary osteoarthritis in the subtalar joints is evident. The pathologic

findings are similar to but more severe than those occurring in stage IIIA disease. The value of this staging system relates to the choice of appropriate therapy. Although conservative treatment, including orthoses, casting, and anti-inflammatory medications, may be an option in lesser degrees of degeneration of the tibialis posterior tendon,[1174] surgery often is required. Jahss[1175] recommends repair of tendon tears and plication of the tendon (if it is elongated) in stages IA and IB disease. More extensive surgical procedures, including triple arthrodesis, may be necessary for more severe involvement.

Although routine radiographs and those obtained during weight-bearing allow the diagnosis of long-standing disruption of the tibialis posterior tendon (Fig. 70–409), owing to the presence of a number of deformities (e.g., an increase in the angle between the long axis of the talus and that of the calcaneus, a sag at the calcaneonavicular and naviculo-cuneiform articulations, and lateral subluxation of the navicular bone with respect to the talus),[1363] these methods are less useful in the early diagnosis of such disruption. CT and MR imaging appear to be more valuable than ultrasonography and tenography in the evaluation of degeneration, inflammation, and disruption of the tibialis posterior tendon. Rosenberg and coworkers[1200] used a classification system of tibialis posterior tendon rupture in which three categories based upon surgical findings were defined: type 1 lesions represented partially torn, bulbous, or hypertrophied tendons with vertical splits and defects; type 2 tears represented partially torn, attenuated tendons; and type 3 tears represented complete tendinous disruption with an intratendinous gap. In the evaluation of 32 cases of clinically suspected chronic tears of the tibialis posterior tendon, these investigators found CT to be sensitive and specific in 90 per cent and 100 per cent of cases, respectively, and MR imaging to be sensitive and specific in 95 per cent and 100 per cent of cases, respectively. The accuracy in detecting rupture of this tendon was found to be 91 per cent for CT and 96 per cent for MR imaging. The overall accuracy, which reflected the percentage of cases correctly diagnosed as well as those that were correctly classified, was 59 per cent for CT and 73 per cent for MR imaging. These investigators concluded that MR imaging was superior to CT in providing greater definition of tendon outline, vertical splits, synovial fluid, edema, and tissue degeneration; they concluded that CT was superior to MR imaging in showing associated bone abnormalities such as periostitis, subtalar osteoarthritis, and subtalar dislocation.

With both CT and MR imaging, type 1 partial tears are associated with tendon hypertrophy and, when longitudinal splitting is prominent, tendon division into two parts. With MR imaging, an abnormal increase in signal intensity may be seen within the enlarged or bifurcated tibialis posterior tendon, especially in proton density–weighted spin echo MR images, but occasionally also in T2-weighted spin echo and STIR images.[1174] Type 2 partial tears lead to a diminution in the size of the tibialis posterior tendon, especially its width. Complete tears of the tibialis posterior tendon are associated with tendon retraction and a gap[1174] (Fig. 70–410).

Schweizer and coworkers[1201] compared the MR imaging findings in patients with clinically suspected or surgically confirmed complete tears of the tibialis posterior tendon with those in normal persons. These investigators found

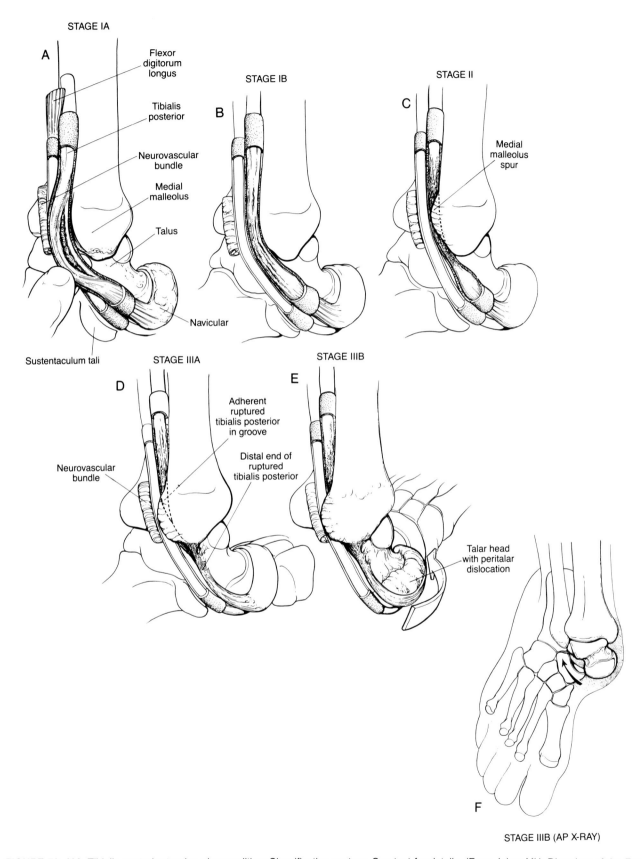

FIGURE 70–408. Tibialis posterior tendon abnormalities: Classification system. See text for details. (From Jahss MH: Disorders of the Foot and Ankle. 2nd Ed. Philadelphia, WB Saunders Co, 1991, p 1485.)

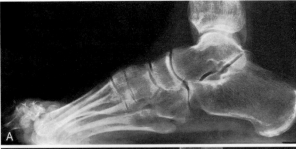

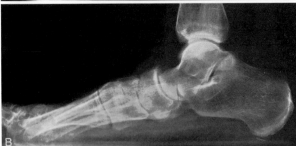

FIGURE 70–409. Injuries of the tibialis posterior tendon: Routine and weight-bearing radiography. Complete tears. Although a lateral radiograph obtained without weight-bearing (A) appears normal, a lateral radiograph obtained with weight-bearing (B) shows plantar flexion of the distal portion of the talus with malalignment at the talonavicular joint. (From Myerson M, et al: Foot and Ankle 9:219, 1989.)

that there was overlap in the size of the distal portion of the tibialis posterior tendon in patients with tears and in normal persons, and that such overlap also was evident with regard to alterations in intratendinous signal intensity (i.e., increased signal intensity in T1-weighted and, to a lesser extent, T2-weighted spin echo MR images). They found that abnormalities such as changes in the alignment of the talus and navicular bone, prominence of the medial tubercle of the navicular bone, and an accessory ossicle in the navicular bone were useful MR imaging findings in predicting a tear of the tibialis posterior tendon. These latter abnormalities, however, also can be seen on routine radiographs, conventional tomograms, and CT scans.

The value of MR imaging in the assessment of the degenerated or torn tibialis posterior tendon requires further analysis. Similarly, any role for MR imaging in the evaluation of this tendon following surgical repair awaits the

results of additional studies.[1174] The application of reformatted three-dimensional Fourier transform gradient recalled MR imaging to the analysis of this and other tendons in the foot and ankle may lead to more accurate diagnosis of tendon injury,[1198] although this too is not yet proved.

Abnormalities of the Flexor Hallucis Longus Tendon. Abnormalities of the flexor hallucis longus tendon are encountered less commonly than those of the Achilles and tibialis posterior tendons. Such abnormalities include tendinitis and partial or complete disruption, partial tethering (i.e., os trigonum syndrome), and complete tethering (i.e., checkrein deformity).[1175]

Injuries of the tendon of the flexor hallucis longus muscle at the level of the medial malleolus are observed in athletes, particularly dancers, who actively plantar flex their feet. Indeed, this tendon often is considered the Achilles tendon of the foot in dancers, and inflammation of the flexor hallucis longus tendon in dancers frequently is referred to as dancer's tendinitis.[1225] The flexor hallucis longus tendon extends through a fibro-osseous tunnel from the posterior aspect of the talus to the level of the sustentaculum tali, much like a rope through a pulley.[1225] Irritation and swelling of the tendon in this area may lead to triggering of the great toe,[1175] a condition known as hallux saltans.[1225] Such inflammation may result not only from the trauma associated with ballet dancing or other sports requiring repetitive pushoff maneuvers from the forefoot, but also from systemic rheumatic diseases (such as rheumatoid arthritis) or acute trauma (e.g., comminuted calcaneal fractures).[1174] The tendon eventually may rupture with loss of plantar flexion of the interphalangeal joint of the hallux.[1226, 1227]

Flexor hallucis longus tendinitis usually occurs behind the medial malleolus but it occasionally can be found at Henry's knot, under the base of the first metatarsal bone, where the flexor digitorum longus tendon crosses over the flexor hallucis longus tendon or at the level of the head of the first metatarsal bone where the tendon of the flexor hallucis longus muscle passes between the sesamoid bones.[1225]

MR imaging can be used to assess inflammation or rupture of the flexor hallucis longus tendon (Fig. 70–411), although fluid in the sheath of this tendon may be a normal finding in patients with large ankle effusions, owing to communication of the sheath with the ankle in approximately 20 per cent of normal persons.[1174]

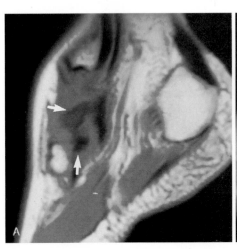

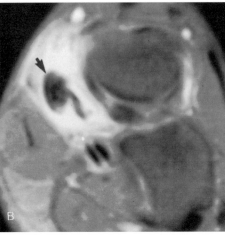

FIGURE 70–410. Injuries of the tibialis posterior tendon: MR imaging. Acute complete tear.

A A sagittal T1-weighted (TR/TE, 800/12) spin echo MR image shows disorganization of the tibialis posterior tendon (arrows) near its navicular site of insertion. Note a mass of intermediate signal intensity about the tendon.

B A coronal T1-weighted (TR/TE, 650/20) spin echo MR image obtained with chemical presaturation of fat (ChemSat) following the intravenous administration of a gadolinium compound reveals the torn tibialis posterior tendon (arrow). Note enhancement of signal intensity about the torn tendon.

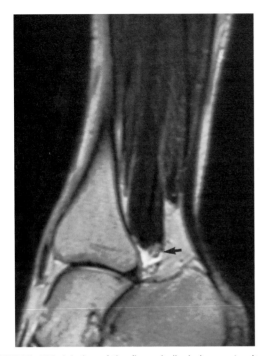

FIGURE 70–411. Injuries of the flexor hallucis longus tendon: MR imaging. Acute partial tear. This 43 year old man heard a pop while running, which was followed immediately by severe pain. A sagittal T2-weighted (TR/TE, 3500/102) fast spin echo MR image shows the site of tendon tear (arrow), which is associated with high signal intensity. Other images showed that some of the tendinous fibers were intact.

Partial tethering of the tendon of the flexor hallucis longus muscle may result from hypertrophy of the os trigonum, a condition designated the os trigonum syndrome. The posterior aspect of the talus normally has two tubercles, the medial tubercle and the lateral tubercle, between which is found the fibro-osseous tunnel of the flexor hallucis longus tendon.[1225] The os trigonum is the ununited lateral tubercle of the talus, is present in approximately 10 per cent of persons, and is bilateral in 50 per cent of persons. The medial edge of the os trigonum (or trigonal process of the talus) lies under the flexor hallucis longus tendon, on the lateral side of the flexor hallucis longus tunnel, and it may lead to compression of the tendon in this area. Resulting symptoms often are designated the talar compression syndrome or posterior impingement syndrome of the ankle,[1228, 1229] and they are common in activities such as those occurring during ballet dancing (e.g., demi-pointe, full pointe, tendu, the frappé, the relevé, or leaving the ground in a jump), in which full weight-bearing occurs with maximum plantar flexion at the ankle.[1225] These maneuvers decrease the space between the superior border of the os calcis and the posterior lip of the tibia, in which the os trigonum (or trigonal process) is found. Laxity of the lateral ligaments of the ankle may predispose to or accentuate this syndrome. Pain and tenderness are apparent in the postero-lateral region of the ankle, findings that may simulate those of peroneal or Achilles tendinitis.[1225] Although radiographs will reveal an os trigonum in many patients with a posterior impingement syndrome, the size of the os is a poor indicator of the severity of the clinical manifestations. Furthermore, this syndrome may occur in the absence of an os trigonum, and a prominent os trigonum can occur in the

absence of this syndrome. Soft tissue entrapment between the calcaneus and talus or a plica in the posterior region of the ankle (with or without an os trigonum) also may lead to the posterior impingement syndrome.[1225, 1230] CT or MR imaging is useful in defining the relationship between the os trigonum and flexor hallucis longus tendon in some patients with this syndrome.[1175]

The checkrein deformity consists of a fixed tethering of the flexor hallucis longus tendon under, or just proximal to, the flexor retinaculum (internal annular ligament) of the ankle, which leads to unexplained flexion contracture of the interphalangeal joint of the hallux with a mild extension contracture of the first metatarsophalangeal joint (claw hallux).[1175] A healing fracture of the lower portion of the tibia may lead to this deformity, related to posttraumatic adhesions.

Abnormalities of the Tibialis Anterior Tendon. The tendon of the tibialis anterior muscle is invested by a synovial sheath and traverses three retinacular tunnels. This tendon begins near the junction of the lower and middle thirds of the tibia and slightly below this level acquires a tendon sheath with which it descends further into the ankle and foot.[1208] The three retinacular tunnels are contributed to by the superior extensor retinaculum and the bifurcating limbs of the inferior extensor retinaculum.[1208]

Spontaneous rupture of the tibialis anterior tendon is rare.[1231–1233] Ruptures may occur at various levels of the tendon, although those appearing between the superior and inferior extensor retinacula are most common.[1208] Rupture also may occur at the level of the medial tarsometatarsal joint, perhaps related to a dorsal osteophyte.[1175] Spontaneous ruptures appear most typically in patients over the age of 45 or 50 years, and they may be complete or partial in extent. Athletes, such as runners, soccer players, and hikers, also may develop ruptures of the tibialis anterior tendon.[1174] Injuries relate to forced plantar flexion of the foot and eversion of the ankle.[1208] Footdrop results from these injuries, which create difficulty in walking, although women who wear high-heeled shoes may experience only minor difficulty during walking.[1208] Thus, accurate diagnosis may be delayed. On clinical examination, a mass related to protrusion of the proximal portion of the torn tendon above the inferior retinaculum may be noted.[1175] Retraction of the torn end beneath the superior retinaculum also may be seen. Inflammation of the adjacent tendon sheaths frequently is apparent. MR imaging (Fig. 70–412), and CT allow accurate diagnosis in most cases.

Abnormalities of the Peroneal Tendons

Anatomy. The peroneus longus and brevis muscles are important lateral stabilizers of the ankle joint (see Figs. 70–386, 70–388, 70–405 to 70–407). The peroneus longus muscle serves to evert and dorsiflex the foot, the contribution to eversion being far more apparent when the foot is off the ground. Along with the peroneus brevis muscle, the peroneus longus muscle acts to maintain the concavity of the foot in takeoff of the foot from the ground during walking and in tiptoeing. The peroneus brevis muscle contributes to eversion of the foot.

In their course from the ankle to the foot, the tendons of these two muscles come to lie together behind the lateral malleolus in a common synovial sheath (Fig. 70–413). Here, the tendon of the peroneus longus muscle lies in a retrofibular groove that is shared by the tendon of the pe-

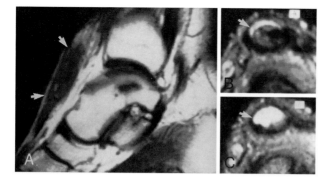

FIGURE 70–412. Injuries of the tibialis anterior tendon: MR imaging. Acute complete tear. This 22 year old man twisted his ankle while running and developed pain and swelling in front of the ankle.

A A sagittal T1-weighted (TR/TE, 450/15) spin echo MR image shows an enlarged tibialis anterior tendon and sheath (arrows) containing foci of increased signal intensity.

B, C Two transaxial T2-weighted (TR/TE, 1800/90) spin echo MR images obtained near the ankle joint are shown. At the higher level **(B)**, fluid of high signal intensity (arrow) is evident within the sheath and surrounds the tendon. At the lower level **(C)**, the fluid-filled sheath (arrow) is seen, but the tibialis anterior tendon is not visible.

roneus brevis muscle. Indeed, the peroneus brevis tendon lies more securely within this groove than the posteriorly located peroneus longus tendon.[1208] The tendons and their sheath are kept in place and supported within the groove by the superior peroneal retinaculum, a structure that inserts into the medial and lateral ridges of the sulcus, converting the groove into a tunnel. More distally, the peroneus longus tendon is applied to the lateral surface of the calcaneus, inferior to the tendon of the peroneus brevis muscle and the peroneal trochlea (a depression in the lateral surface of the calcaneus), and above the calcaneal tubercle that serves as the insertion site for the calcaneofibular ligament. In this

area, the peroneus longus tendon passes beneath a tunnel created by the inferior peroneal retinaculum. Further distally, the tendon of the peroneus longus muscle is intimate, first with the lateral side, and then with the inferior surface of the cuboid bone. Beneath the cuboid bone, this tendon lies within a groove that is converted to a tunnel by the long plantar ligament. The tendon of the peroneus brevis muscle, after passing behind the fibula, runs forward on the lateral surface of the calcaneus, above the peroneus longus tendon. Here, it lies close to but above the peroneal trochlea in an osteoaponeurotic canal created by the inferior peroneal retinaculum. Two distal extensions of the common

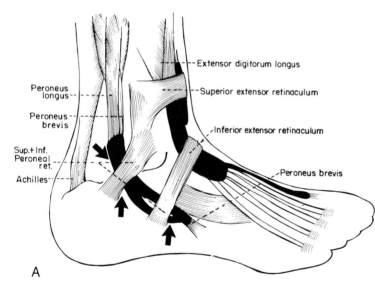

FIGURE 70–413. Peroneal tendons and tendon sheath: Normal anatomy.

A A drawing depicts the peroneus longus and brevis tendons and their sheath. (From Gilula LA, et al: Radiology *151*:581, 1984.)

B A lateral sagittal section of the foot and ankle demonstrates the peroneus brevis (B) and peroneus longus (L) tendons passing around the lateral malleolus (arrowhead). The peroneus brevis can be followed close to the base of the fifth metatarsal bone (M).

C A slightly more medial sagittal section through the calcaneus (CAL) and cuboid (CUB) bone outlines the peroneus longus (L) tendon as it crosses underneath the foot.

(**B, C** From Resnick D, Goergen TG: Radiology *115*: 211, 1975.)

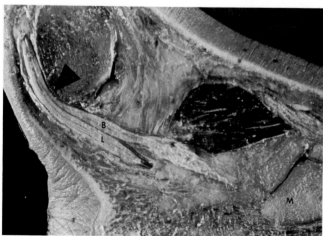

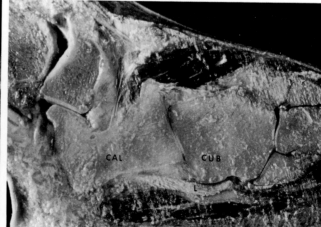

synovial sheath individually surround the peroneus longus and peroneus brevis tendons. The intimate relationship of the common peroneal tendon sheath and the calcaneofibular ligament explains the arthrographic finding of opacification of the sheath following injuries to the ankle joint. Tears of the calcaneofibular ligament allow the synovial sheath to become apposed to the ankle joint, explaining its opacification during arthrography. Isolated tears of the anterior talofibular ligament are not associated with this pattern of communication.

Subluxation and Dislocation. Subluxation and dislocation of the peroneal tendons often are classified as habitual (i.e., voluntary) and traumatic.[1208, 1234–1237] Habitual subluxations commonly are bilateral and are reproduced by voluntary maneuvers involving the ankle and foot, often leading to a snapping sensation or sound. Such snapping relates to anterior movement of the peroneus brevis tendon, which carries with it the tendon of the peroneus longus muscle, enclosed within the common tendon sheath, although the two never lie in front of the lateral malleolus.[1208]

Traumatic dislocations of the peroneal tendons are associated with disruption of the superior retinaculum or stripping of the periosteal membrane in the distal portion of the fibula at the sites of attachment of this retinaculum. In either situation, the retinaculum becomes functionally deficient, allowing the peroneal tendons to subluxate in a lateral or forward direction. Rarely do they assume a position anterior to the fibula, however. These injuries are common in athletes, particularly those involved in hockey, soccer, and basketball. The mechanism of injury appears to be inversion at the ankle with the foot in a position of plantar flexion, a mechanism that also can lead to injury to the lateral ligaments of the ankle. Congenital variations of the shape of the retrofibular groove or the strength of the superior peroneal retinaculum can predispose to subluxation or dislocation of the peroneal tendons. Routine radiography may disclose a small avulsion fracture adjacent to the lateral surface of the lateral malleolus, an important and often diagnostic observation (Fig. 70–414). Identification of subluxation or dislocation of the peroneal tendons also can be accomplished with peroneal tenography, ultrasonography, CT (Fig. 70–414), and MR imaging.[1174, 1237, 1239] Accurate diagnosis is important as, if left untreated, chronic recurrent subluxation, tendon tears, and stenosing tenosynovitis may develop.[1238]

Entrapment or Impingement. Fractures of the calcaneus may be associated with lateral displacement of the lateral wall of the bone, resulting in narrowing of the fibulocalcaneal space. Entrapment of the peroneal tendons between the fibula, calcaneus, and talus or subluxation or dislocation of the peroneal tendons, or a combination of the two, may result.[1240] Clinical manifestations of peroneal tendon entrapment include findings of tenosynovitis, limited subtalar motion, local tenderness, and an antalgic gait. Once again, diagnostic information is provided by routine radiography, supplemented with ultrasonography, peroneal tenography (Fig. 70–415), or MR imaging.

Tendinitis and Tenosynovitis. Inflammatory changes in the peroneal tendons or their sheath usually result from acute injury or chronic stress. Typical causes include calcaneal fractures with peroneal tendon entrapment, systemic rheumatic disorders, tarsal coalition, congenital or acquired hypertrophy of the peroneal tubercle, altered foot mechanics, and improper footwear.[1164, 1237] Pain, tenderness, and swelling are common clinical manifestations.

Ultrasonography, tenography (Fig. 70–416), and MR imaging (Fig. 70–417), can be applied to the diagnosis of inflammation of the peroneal tendons and sheath. MR imaging reveals significant fluid within the sheath of the peroneal tendons and, possibly, altered tendon size and intratendinous signal intensity.[1174] Differentiation of physiologic versus pathologic collections of fluid in the peroneal tendon sheath, however, is difficult. Furthermore, tears of the calcaneofibular ligament allow communication of the ankle and the peroneal tendon sheath, accounting for fluid in the sheath in some patients who have had ankle trauma.

Rupture. Partial or complete disruption of one or both peroneal tendons can accompany an acute injury (e.g., calcaneal fracture) or occur spontaneously.[1241–1243] Spontaneous ruptures of these tendons are rare, usually occurring in young adults and involving the peroneus brevis tendon.[1175] Partial tears are more common than complete disruptions of

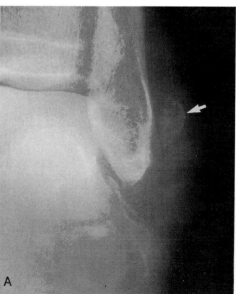
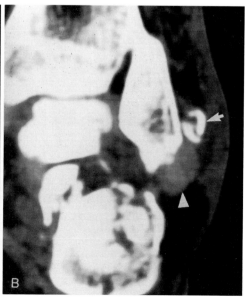

FIGURE 70–414. Injuries of the peroneal tendons and sheath: Routine radiography and CT scanning. Peroneal tendon dislocation. In this patient with a comminuted calcaneal fracture, a routine radiograph **(A)** reveals the avulsed fibular bone fragment (arrow) that is characteristic of a peroneal tendon dislocation. A coronal CT scan **(B)** confirms the bone avulsion (arrow). Note its relationship to the peroneal tendons (arrowhead) and the fracture of the calcaneus.

A

B

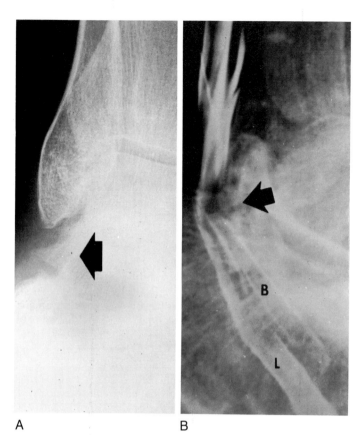

A   B

FIGURE 70–415. Injuries of the peroneal tendons and sheath: Routine radiography and peroneal tenography. Entrapment or impingement. In a patient with a previous calcaneal fracture, the routine radiograph **(A)** reveals a lateral calcaneal spicule (arrow) beneath the fibula. The peroneal tenogram **(B)** outlines impingement and compression of the sheath as it passes around the lateral malleolus (arrow) associated with incomplete filling of the peroneus brevis (B) and peroneus longus (L) sheaths. (**B** From Resnick D, Goergen TG: Radiology *115:*211, 1975.)

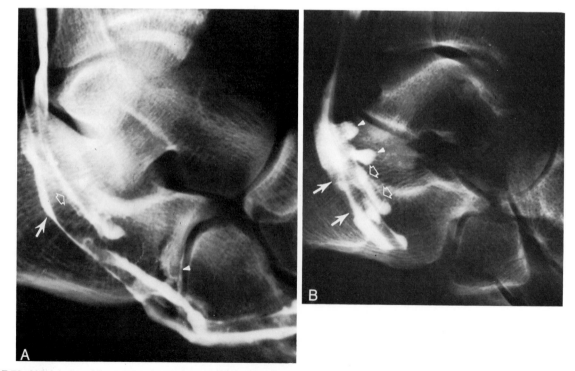

FIGURE 70–416. Injuries of the peroneal tendons and sheath: Peroneal tenography. Stenosing and nodular tenosynovitis.
 A A lateral view following injection of the peroneal tendon sheaths shows filling of the peroneus longus (solid arrow) and peroneus brevis (open arrow) sheaths. Contrast material enters the calcaneocuboid joint (arrowhead), indicative of a capsular tear or defect in the tendon sheath. There is nonfilling of the superior margin of the peroneus brevis, consistent with fibrosis.
 B In a second patient, the margins of the peroneus longus (solid arrows) and peroneus brevis (open arrows) tendon sheaths are markedly irregular, with pseudodiverticula (arrowheads) of the peroneus brevis tendon sheath.
 (From Gilula LA, et al: Radiology *151:*581, 1984.)

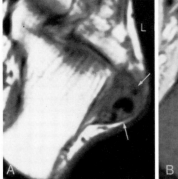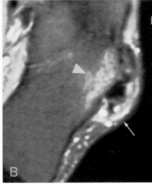

FIGURE 70–417. Injuries of the peroneal tendons and sheath: MR imaging. Peroneal tendinitis and tenosynovitis. A transaxial T1-weighted (TR/TE, 400/17) spin echo MR image (**A**) and a transaxial T2-weighted (TR/TE, 3300/100) fast spin echo fat-suppressed MR image (**B**) obtained at a slightly more inferior level than **A** show a fluid-filled mass (arrows) about the peroneus longus and peroneus brevis tendons. Note the reactive edema of the marrow of the calcaneus (arrowhead) in **B**. (Courtesy of S. Eilenberg, M.D., San Diego, California.)

the peroneal tendons. The occurrence of ruptures of the peroneus longus tendon may lead to a fracture or a change in position of the os peroneum (Fig. 70–418), which may be retracted proximally, even as far as the level of the lateral malleolus (see previous discussion).

In the usual situation, longitudinal splits and hypertrophy of the peroneus brevis tendon are evident pathologically. MR imaging allows identification of abnormal signal intensity or size of the tendon (Fig. 70–419). A diagnostic pitfall is the occurrence of a normal variation leading to bifurcated insertions of this tendon.[1174] In cases of complete disruption of either the peroneus longus or peroneus brevis tendon, analysis of serial MR images in one or more imaging planes will document the absence of a normal tendon structure.

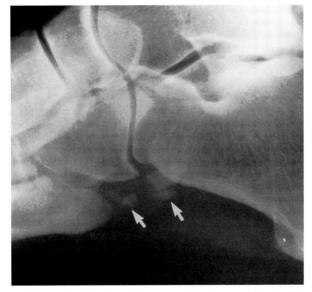

FIGURE 70–418. Injuries of the peroneal tendons and sheath: Routine radiography. Complete tear of the peroneus longus tendon with fracture of the os peroneum. A lateral radiograph reveals fragmentation of the os peroneum (arrows), indicative of a rupture of the peroneus longus tendon.

Retraction of the torn tendon is less common in cases of peroneal tendon disruption than in those of disruption of the Achilles tendon.[1174]

Ligament Abnormalities

Anatomic Considerations. The primary function of the ankle joint is to provide stability during locomotion. Such stability relates not only to the configuration of the three principal bones, the tibia, fibula, and talus, that form the ankle, but also to the surrounding soft tissue structures, particularly the ligaments, that bind the bones together and the muscles and tendons that regulate ankle movement. Spanning the ankle joint are more than 10 ligaments as well as four retinacula, numerous tendons (some with sheaths), and no muscles save for the occasional fibers of the peroneus tertius muscle.[1244] A thick fibrous membrane holds the shafts of the tibia and fibula together, four syndesmotic ligaments bind the lower ends of the bones, and two sets of collateral ligaments connect the malleoli to the talus, calcaneus, and tarsal navicular bone.[1208] Despite this extensive arrangement, composed of bones, ligaments, retinacula, tendons, and a fibrous membrane, acute or chronic ankle instability is one of the most important and common problems encountered in clinical practice. Indirect or direct violence can disrupt one or more of these structures, as well as nearby vessels and nerves. Although many types of fractures about the ankle represent direct evidence of this violence (see Chapter 68), injury to nearby ligaments ultimately may be responsible for chronic disability.

Anatomically, the ligaments of the ankle are grouped according to their location into three complexes: the tibiofibular complex, the medial complex, and the lateral complex. The ligaments in the lateral complex are injured most commonly, usually related to an inversion stress; the ligaments in the medial complex are injured less frequently, generally related to an eversion stress and often in association with a fibular fracture; and the ligaments of the tibiofibular complex may be injured owing to external rotation at the ankle or forced dorsiflexion of the foot, often in combination with a fracture of the fibula.

Tibiofibular Complex. The interlacing fibers of the crural interosseous membrane pass obliquely downward from the interosseous ridge of the tibia to that of the fibula. Descent of the fibula, which occurs during the pushoff phase of gait, leads to more acute angulation of these fibers. Just above the inferior tibiofibular syndesmosis, the lower of two apertures in the crural interosseous membrane provides a passageway for the perforating branch of the peroneal artery. In instances of total tibiofibular diastasis in which the syndesmotic ligaments and the distal fibers of the crural interosseous membrane are torn, this artery may be injured.[1208]

Four ligaments, collectively designated the syndesmotic ligaments, bind together the apposing portions of the tibia and fibula (Fig. 70–420). From above downward, they are the interosseous ligament, the anterior tibiofibular ligament, the posterior tibiofibular ligament, and the transverse tibiofibular ligament. The anatomy of these ligaments has been well defined by Kelikian.[1208] The interosseous ligament represents the lowermost portion of the crural interosseous membrane and consists of short, thick fibers that join the concave surface of the peroneal groove of the tibia to the convex surface of the fibula. It is triangular in configura-

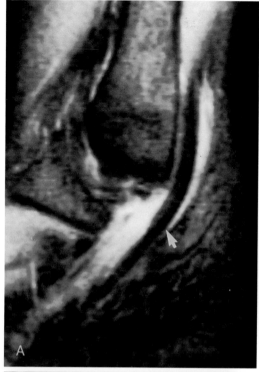
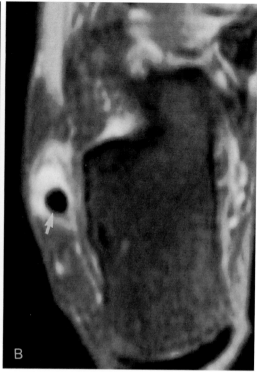

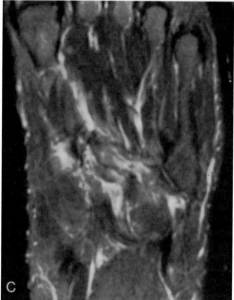

FIGURE 70–419. Injuries of the peroneal tendons and sheath: MR imaging.

A Complete tear of the peroneus brevis tendon. A sagittal MPGR MR image (TR/TE, 500/11; flip angle, 25 degrees) shows the peroneus longus tendon (arrow) with a fluid-filled sheath. The peroneus brevis is not visualized. (Courtesy of C. Sebrechts, M.D., San Diego, California.)

B Complete tear of the peroneus brevis tendon. In a second patient, a transaxial proton density–weighted (TR/TE, 2000/20) spin echo MR image obtained with chemical presaturation of fat (ChemSat) shows fluid of high signal intensity about the peroneus longus tendon (arrow) with nonvisualization of the peroneus brevis tendon. (Courtesy of C. Sebrechts, M.D., San Diego, California.)

C Complete tear of the peroneus longus tendon. A transaxial T2-weighted (TR/TE, 3000/80) fat-suppressed fast spin echo MR image shows nonvisualization of the distal portion of the peroneus longus tendon, with high signal intensity in the plantar soft tissues. (Courtesy of S. Eilenberg, M.D., San Diego, California.)

tion, with a broad base distally and a pointed apex proximally. In combination with injuries of the crural interosseous membrane, disruption of the interosseous ligament occurs when forces lead to diastasis of the distal portions of the tibia and fibula. In injuries that involve external rotation of the talus with lateral displacement and external rotation of the fibula, an open-book type of disruption of the interosseous ligament occurs in combination with disruption of the anterior tibiofibular ligament.[1208]

The anterior tibiofibular ligament extends between the anterolateral surface of the tibia (including the anterior tubercle) to the adjacent anterior surface of the fibula. This ligament is the weakest of the four syndesmotic ligaments and the first to yield with injuries that produce external

rotation of the fibula. In association with oblique fractures of the lateral malleolus, occurring with supination and external rotation at the ankle, an avulsion fracture of the anterior tubercle of the tibia at the site of insertion of the anterior tibiofibular ligament, rather than disruption of the ligament itself, may occur.[1208]

The posterior tibiofibular ligament is the posterior counterpart of the anterior tibiofibular ligament, extending from the posterolateral surface of the tibia (including the posterior tubercle) to the adjacent posterior surface of the fibula. External rotation and posterior displacement of the fibula lead to disruption of this ligament or an avulsion fracture of the posterior tibial tubercle.

The transverse tibiofibular ligament represents the low-

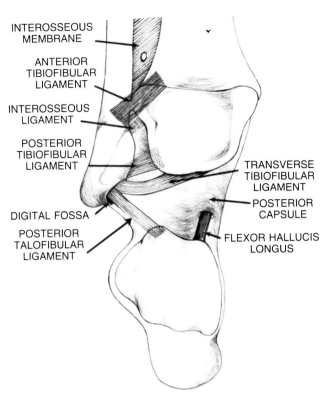

INTEROSSEOUS
MEMBRANE

ANTERIOR
TIBIOFIBULAR
LIGAMENT

INTEROSSEOUS
LIGAMENT

POSTERIOR
TIBIOFIBULAR
LIGAMENT

TRANSVERSE
TIBIOFIBULAR
LIGAMENT

POSTERIOR
CAPSULE

DIGITAL FOSSA

POSTERIOR
TALOFIBULAR
LIGAMENT

FLEXOR HALLUCIS
LONGUS

FIGURE 70–420. Syndesmotic ligaments and related structures: Normal anatomy. See text for details. (From Kelikian H, and Kelikian AS: Disorders of the Ankle. Philadelphia, WB Saunders Co, 1985, p 5.)

ermost portion of the posterior tibiofibular ligament, although it often is considered to be a distinct structure.[1208] In common with the remaining portions of the posterior tibiofibular ligament, the transverse tibiofibular ligament inserts into the posterior surface of the tibia. Laterally, however, the transverse tibiofibular ligament inserts into the upper part of the lateral malleolar fossa in the posteroinferior portion of the fibula. This ligament extends below the pos-

terior surface of the tibia, contacting the posterior aspect of the talus. It contains a proportion of yellow elastic fibers, accounting for its yellowish color, and its internal surface is covered by a synovial membrane.

Medial Complex. The medial or tibial collateral ligament of the ankle is the strong, triangular or fan-shaped deltoid ligament. The deltoid ligament often is divided into superficial and deep portions (Fig. 70–421). The superficial portion of the ligament originates mainly from the anterior colliculus of the tibial malleolus. This portion of the deltoid ligament is divided further into three sets of fibers which, in an anterior to posterior direction, are the tibionavicular, tibiocalcaneal, and posterior tibiotalar fibers. The anterior or tibionavicular part of the superficial portion of the deltoid ligament consists of fibers that pass from their tibial attachment site to the tuberosity of the navicular bone and the medial margin of the plantar calcaneonavicular ligament. The middle or tibiocalcaneal part consists of fibers that descend almost in a perpendicular direction from the medial malleolus to the whole length of the sustentaculum tali of the calcaneus. The posterior tibiotalar part of the superficial portion of the deltoid ligament has fibers that pass laterally and backward to attach to the medial side of the talus and to its medial tubercle. This part is deeper in location than the anterior and middle parts and sometimes is considered together with the deep portion of the deltoid ligament. The deep portion of the deltoid ligament extends from the tip of the medial malleolus to the entire nonarticular medial surface of the body of the talus. The tendons of the tibialis posterior and flexor digitorum longus muscles are located superficial to the deltoid ligament.

The fibers of the deep portion of the deltoid ligament prevent the talus from being displaced laterally. If the deep portion remains intact, displacement of a fractured distal portion of the fibula or tibiofibular diastasis does not occur.[1208] The tibionavicular component of the superficial portion of the deltoid ligament suspends the inferior calcaneonavicular or spring ligament which, in turn, supports the head of the talus; the tibiocalcaneal portion of the superfi-

FIGURE 70–421. Tibial collateral ligament: Normal anatomy. See text for details. (From Kelikian H, and Kelikian AS: Disorders of the Ankle. Philadelphia, WB Saunders Co, 1985, p 20.)

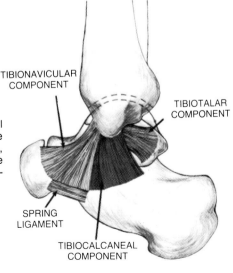

TIBIONAVICULAR
COMPONENT

TIBIOTALAR
COMPONENT

SPRING
LIGAMENT

TIBIOCALCANEAL
COMPONENT

A

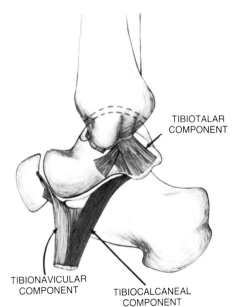

TIBIOTALAR
COMPONENT

TIBIONAVICULAR
COMPONENT

TIBIOCALCANEAL
COMPONENT

B

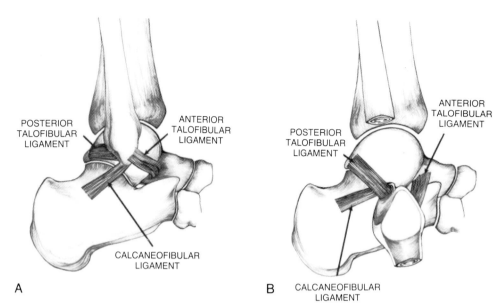

A

B

FIGURE 70–422. Lateral ligamentous complex of the ankle: Normal anatomy. See text for details. (From Kelikian H, and Kelikian AS: Disorders of the Ankle. Philadelphia, WB Saunders Co, 1985, p 20.)

cial portion of the deltoid ligament prevents the calcaneus from assuming a valgus alignment.[1208]

Lateral Complex. The lateral ligamentous complex of the ankle is referred to as the fibular collateral ligament, consisting of three components, or fasciculi, all of which

attach to the lateral (fibular) malleolus (Figs. 70–422 and 70–423). One component connects the lateral malleolus to the calcaneus and is designated the calcaneofibular ligament. Two components connect the lateral malleolus to the anterolateral and posterolateral surfaces of the talus and are

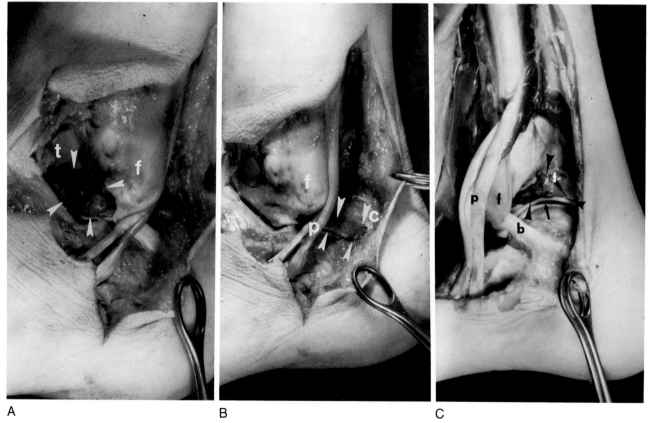

A   B   C

FIGURE 70–423. Lateral ligamentous complex of the ankle. Normal anatomy. Dissection identifying the major lateral ligaments of the ankle (ligaments are painted with tantalum). The anterior talofibular ligament **(A)** (arrowheads) extends from the distal end of the fibula (f) to the talus (t). The calcaneofibular ligament **(B)** (arrowheads) originates from the posterior aspect of the distal fibula (f) and inserts on the superior aspect of the calcaneus (c). It is intimate with the tendons of the peroneal muscles (p). The posterior talofibular ligament **(C)** (arrowheads) extends from the fibula (f) to the talus (t). Note its relationship to the calcaneofibular ligament (b), peroneal tendons (p), and posterior subtalar joint (arrow). (Courtesy of J. Kaye, M.D., New York, New York.)

designated the anterior talofibular and posterior talofibular ligaments, respectively. These two ligaments fuse with the capsule of the ankle joint, whereas the calcaneofibular ligament does not.[1208] Owing to their location in an anteroposterior plane, these three components of the lateral ligamentous complex of the ankle sometimes are referred to as the anterior (anterior talofibular), middle (calcaneofibular), and posterior (posterior talofibular) segments, or bands.

The anterior talofibular ligament passes from the anterior margin of the fibular malleolus in a forward and medial direction to attach to the lateral articular facet and lateral aspect of the neck of the talus. This component of the lateral ligamentous complex is the weakest and is injured most often. When intact, the anterior talofibular ligament prevents forward displacement of the talus. This ligament passes over a ridge related to the anterior border of the lateral articular facet of the talar body, a part of the ligament that is vulnerable to injury. The intimacy of the anterior talofibular ligament with the joint capsule explains the inevitable occurrence of capsular disruption in cases of anterior talofibular ligament disruption, and the location of the perforating branch of the peroneal artery close to the superficial margin of the anterior talofibular ligament explains the occasional occurrence of traumatic aneurysms of this vessel in cases of anterior talofibular ligament disruption.[1208]

The calcaneofibular ligament is long and rounded, and it extends across two joints (the talocrural and posterior subtalar joints) from a depression in front of the apex of the lateral malleolus, in an inferior and posterior direction, to attach to a tubercle on the lateral surface of the calcaneus. The tendons of the peroneus longus and peroneus brevis muscles and their sheath cross over this ligament. The calcaneofibular ligament is lax in the standing position and is taut during inversion of the calcaneus. This ligament serves to stabilize the posterior subtalar joint.

The posterior talofibular ligament is a strong, horizontally oriented structure that passes from the lower part of the fossa of the lateral malleolus to the lateral tubercle of the posterior process of the talus. One slip of this ligament, designated the tibial slip, passes obliquely upward, to attach to the medial malleolus. The posterior talofibular ligament has some features in common with the transverse tibiofibular ligament of the inferior tibiofibular syndesmosis[1208]: both structures are located in the coronal plane, both arise from the fossa of the lateral malleolus, and both are deeply seated and partially invested by a synovial membrane. These structures are intimately related when the foot is in a position of plantar flexion, and they are separated by a space (through which the talus is visible) when the foot is in a position of dorsiflexion.

Pathologic Considerations. Injuries to the ligaments about the ankle are one of the most frequently encountered consequences of trauma. They typically are seen in young adults, particularly those involved in sports such as basketball and soccer.[1245] The lateral ligamentous complex is injured more commonly than the medial or tibiofibular complex. Of the lateral ligaments, the anterior talofibular ligament is affected most frequently, either alone or in combination with an injury of the calcaneofibular ligament.[1246] Indeed, a predictable sequence of injury may be observed, beginning with involvement of the anterior talofibular ligament and followed by involvement of the calca-

neofibular and finally the posterior talofibular ligaments. As acute injuries to the ligaments of the ankle may be complicated by chronic dysfunction of the joint, accurate and early diagnosis is important. Clinical assessment employs local palpation of the ligaments, often combined with stress testing, in order to determine which individual ligaments are injured. Diffuse swelling leads to diagnostic problems in some cases, and severe pain in the acute stage may limit the usefulness of stress maneuvers designed to identify patterns of talar displacement unless the patient is examined under general anesthesia.

The classification of ligamentous injuries is based upon the specific site or sites of involvement and their severity. The severity of the injury may be categorized as grade I, II, or III. Grade I injuries are the least severe, apparently, representing failure of some of the tendinous fibers; grade III injuries are the most severe, associated with complete ligamentous disruption and instability of the ankle joint; and grade II injuries are intermediate in severity. Instability of the ankle implies abnormal joint motion during the application of varus or valgus stress or positive results during an anterior drawer test (in which the talus moves in a forward direction when anterior stress is placed on the calcaneus).[1247] These stress tests, discussed in Chapter 68, require meticulous technique such that each of the ligaments about the ankle is tested individually. Furthermore, the results of stress testing may be unreliable in the acute stage of injury.[1248]

With regard to the lateral ligamentous complex of the ankle, isolated tears of the anterior talofibular ligament are encountered most commonly. In approximately 40 per cent of cases in which this ligament is disrupted, an associated tear of the calcaneofibular ligament is evident.[1208] Isolated tears of the calcaneofibular ligament (i.e., without an associated tear of the anterior talofibular ligament) are very rare, as such tears represent the second stage of disruption of the lateral ligamentous complex. When the calcaneofibular ligament is disrupted, associated abnormalities may include avulsion of the base of the fifth metatarsal bone and tears of the medial layer of the common peroneal tendon sheath.[1208] Furthermore, as the pattern of injury to the lateral side of the ankle continues, the capsule of the posterior subtalar joint and the lateral talocalcaneal ligament also are torn. The usual mechanism of injury to the lateral ligamentous complex of the ankle is plantar flexion of the foot and inversion at the ankle. Such injuries predominate in young men and in women who wear high-heeled shoes. The posterior talofibular ligament rarely is torn; one mechanism of injury relates to a dislocation of the talus that is not accompanied by a fracture of the distal portion of the fibula.[1208]

Stress radiography (Fig. 70–424) applied to assessment of the lateral ligaments of the ankle employs inversion forces with the foot in a neutral position, in a position of plantar flexion, or in both positions. As indicated in Chapter 68, the angle of talar tilt is increased relative to the uninjured side. An anterior drawer sign also can be used, in which a positive response is characterized by forward movement of the talus (7 or 8 mm) with respect to the tibia.

Injuries to the medial side of the ankle include avulsion fractures of the medial malleolus or disruption of the deltoid ligament. Widening of the ankle mortise is encountered more commonly when the deltoid ligament is torn, as fractures of the malleoli are characterized by normal ligamen-

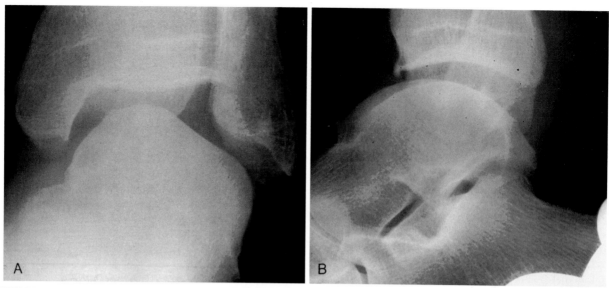

FIGURE 70–424. Lateral ligamentous complex of the ankle: Stress radiography.
 A Talar tilt. An inversion force applied to the ankle with the foot in plantar flexion is associated with abnormal displacement and angulation of the talus with widening of the lateral aspect of the joint.
 B Anterior drawer sign. Forward stress applied to the heel is associated with abnormal anterior movement of the talus with respect to the tibia. Tibial and talar osteophytes also are seen.

tous connections between the malleoli and the talus.[1208] Thus, rupture of the deltoid ligament implies more severe injury, and it may be accompanied not only by widening of the mortise of the talocrural joint, but also by significant injuries to the lateral ligaments of the ankle and entrapment of the tendon of the tibialis posterior muscle. Partial tears of the deltoid ligament, with involvement only of its superficial portion, are seen occasionally, although complete tears involving both the superficial and deep portions of the ligament are encountered more frequently. These complete tears commonly are accompanied by fractures of the lateral malleolus and by lateral or posterolateral displacement of the talus. With routine radiography, the altered position of the talus may be evident, or the bone may appear to be tilted medially. Occasionally, however, at the time of routine radiography, the displaced talus may have assumed a more normal relationship with the tibia. This has led to such designations as "invisible injury to the deltoid ligament" or "silent displacement of the talus."[1208, 1249, 1250] When displacement of the talus is evident, a widened clear space (the distance between the talar body and the medial malleolus) of the ankle is seen radiographically. Disruption of the deltoid ligament is suggested when this clear space measures 3 mm or more.[1208]

Unusual patterns of posttraumatic deficiency of the deltoid ligament are described. A rupture of the deep portion of the ligament may be accompanied by an avulsion fracture of the medial malleolus at the site of attachment of its superficial portion.[1251, 1252] Partial tears of the anterior part of the superficial portion of the deltoid ligament (i.e., tibionavicular part) also may occur.

Diastasis of the distal portions of the tibia and fibula relates to injury of the ligaments of the inferior tibiofibular syndesmosis and the adjacent fibers of the crural interosseous membrane. Diastasis may occur in an anterior-to-posterior direction (open book injury) or in a posterior-to-anterior direction. Kelikian[1208] has defined three types of tibiofibular diastasis: intercalary diastasis, the least common

type, involves disruption of the lowermost fibers of the crural interosseous membrane with intact ligaments of the tibiofibular syndesmosis; anterior tibiofibular diastasis, the most common type, represents the open book injury, in which the anterior ligaments of the tibiofibular syndesmosis are disrupted; and total tibiofibular diastasis, intermediate in frequency, leads to complete disruption of all four syndesmotic ligaments and tearing of the crural interosseous membrane to the level of the associated fracture of the fibula. Intercalary diastasis is an injury of children, occurring prior to closure of the physis in the distal portion of the tibia. Associated physeal injuries of the tibia are seen. Anterior tibiofibular diastasis, leading to disruption of the anterior portion of the syndesmotic ligaments, is associated with external rotation of the talus, disruption of some of the fibers of the interosseous ligament, capsular injury, and in some cases, spiral fractures of the fibula at any level (e.g., Maisoneuve fracture of the proximal portion of the fibula). The diagnosis is facilitated by the presence of associated fractures, not only of the fibula, but also of the anterior tubercle of the tibia, of the posterior margin of the distal portion of the tibia, and of the medial malleolus.[1208] Total tibiofibular diastasis, which is caused by excessive abduction or external rotation at the ankle, is accompanied almost universally by suprasyndesmotic fractures of the fibula and, in some cases, by an avulsion fracture of the medial malleolus or disruption of the deltoid ligament.

With regard to therapy, the great majority of injuries to the lateral ligamentous complex of the ankle are treated conservatively with aggressive and early rehabilitation. Surgical treatment usually is reserved for athletes who wish to resume a preinjury level of activity. With regard to medial ligamentous injuries, conservative therapy also is employed if, following reduction, the ankle mortise is intact. When this mortise remains widened, surgical exploration and repair often are required. Syndesmotic injuries commonly necessitate surgical intervention.

Imaging Considerations. Initial assessment of injuries

to the medial, lateral, and syndesmotic ligaments about the ankle requires routine radiography, which allows detection of any accompanying fractures (see Chapter 68), and radiography obtained during the application of stress (see Fig. 70–424). Complementary imaging methods involve predominantly arthrography and MR imaging.

Arthrography. Under normal circumstances, ankle arthrography results in opacification of the articular cavity without evidence of extra-articular leak except for filling of the tendon sheath of the flexor hallucis longus or the flexor digitorum longus, or both, in approximately 20 per cent of patients[1253–1257] (Fig. 70–425). The posterior subtalar joint will be opacified in approximately 10 per cent of patients. All other patterns of contrast extravasation are regarded as abnormal.

The normal ankle arthrogram reveals three recesses (Fig. 70–425). In the region of the syndesmosis between distal portions of the tibia and fibula, a small vertical recess, best delineated on oblique radiographs, extends 1 to 2.5 cm in height and is approximately 4 mm in width.[1256] Additional

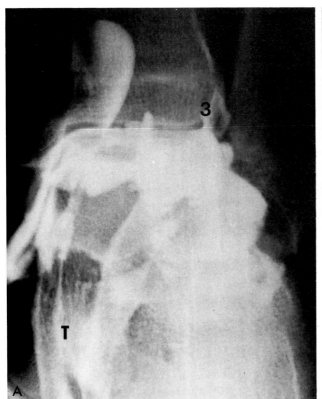

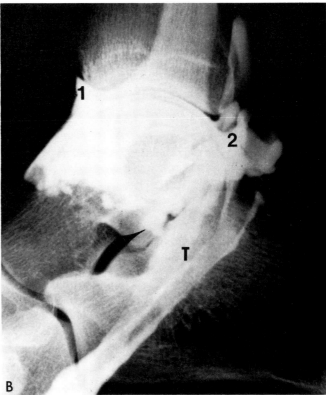

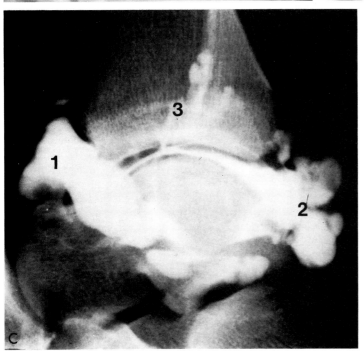

FIGURE 70–425. Normal ligaments of the ankle: Arthrography.

A, B Anteroposterior **(A)** and lateral **(B)** views of a normal arthrogram. The tibiotalar joint has been opacified. Note the normal recesses: anterior recess (1), posterior recess (2), and syndesmotic recess (3). Filling of the medial tendon sheaths (T) and posterior subtalar joint (arrowhead) is a normal finding.

C Lateral view of a normal arthrogram from another patient showing prominent (but normal) anterior (1), posterior (2), and syndesmotic (3) recesses.

anterior and posterior recesses are best observed on lateral radiographs. All three recesses should be smooth and well delineated.

Arthrographic abnormalities associated with ligamentous injuries have been well described[1253–1267] (Fig. 70–426). With tears of the anterior talofibular ligament, contrast material will be seen both inferior and lateral to the distal fibula on frontal radiographs and anterior to the distal fibula on lateral radiographs. Occasionally, on anteroposterior views, the contrast material will overlie the syndesmosis. With tears of the calcaneofibular ligament, contrast material fills the peroneal tendon sheaths as the inner aspect of the sheaths also is torn.[1268–1272] Tears of the calcaneofibular ligament are associated with tears of the anterior talofibular ligament, so that the arthrographic findings of both ligament injuries are apparent. The posterior talofibular ligament also may be injured in these instances.

Contrast opacification of the peroneal tendon sheaths, although always an abnormal finding on ankle arthrograms,[1269] is not specific for calcaneofibular ligament disruption.[1268] Isolated filling of these sheaths is most compatible with a new or old injury to this ligament, whereas such filling combined with leakage of contrast material distal and lateral to the lateral malleolus suggests combined ruptures of the anterior talofibular and calcaneofibular ligaments or an anterior talofibular ligament rupture associated with disruption of the peroneal tendon sheaths. Opacification of the sheaths may be prevented by blood or fibrin clot so that false-negative arthrograms are encountered.[1268, 1272] With injury to the anterior tibiofibular ligament, extravasation of contrast material occurs between distal tibia and fibula, beyond the syndesmotic recess. Its arthrographic appearance may simulate that of capsular rupture.[1273] The arthrographic appearance of injuries to the deltoid ligament is characterized by extravasation of contrast material beyond the medial confines of the joint. Syndesmotic tears are associated with such extravasation between the tibia and the fibula.[1267]

The amount of extravasation of contrast material following any of these ligament tears depends on many factors, including the volume of contrast material injected, the degree of surrounding soft tissue injury, the presence of scar tissue from previous injuries, and the length of time from injury to arthrography.[1253] Arthrography performed after considerable delay may not reveal the presence of ligamentous injury; arthrography performed after appropriate conservative or operative therapy may not demonstrate previously evident abnormalities.[1254]

Ankle arthrography is a reliable method of delineating these ligamentous injuries. Its reported accuracy is 75 to 90 per cent.[1257, 1258] Some observers report less success, particularly in diagnosing double injuries of the lateral ligaments.[1255] In these cases, massive extravasation related to one injury may obscure extravasation related to a second injury. The combination of ankle arthrography and peroneal tenography may improve diagnostic accuracy in patients with combined lesions of both the anterior talofibular and calcaneofibular ligaments.[1266]

MR Imaging. MR imaging has been used to evaluate ligamentous injuries about the ankle.[1274–1279, 1421] Although standard spin echo MR sequences[1275] have been employed, three-dimensional Fourier transform gradient recalled MR sequences may provide superior information, owing to the ability to obtain thin contiguous sections.[1274, 1421] Furthermore, earlier investigations employing MR imaging usually studied the ankle in a neutral position, with no regard to placing the ligaments paraxial to the imaging plane. The value of plantar flexion of the foot as a means to allow better delineation of some of these ligaments with MR imaging was emphasized in one report.[1275] In 1992, Schneck and coworkers[1276, 1277] provided the most detailed description of MR imaging techniques that allowed optimal visualization of the ankle ligaments. Based on a cadaveric study,[1276] these investigators analyzed the appearance of the normal ligaments, employing spin echo MR images and various positions of the foot. They concluded that: (1) transaxial images with the foot taped into dorsiflexion of 10 to 20 degrees provided optimized visualization of the anterior, posterior, and inferior tibiofibular ligaments and of the anterior and posterior talofibular ligaments and provided an overview of the deltoid ligaments; (2) coronal MR images provided full length views of various parts of the deltoid ligament; (3) transaxial images with the foot taped into plantar flexion of 40 to 50 degrees provided optimized visualization of the calcaneofibular ligament and of some parts of the deltoid ligament; and (4) sagittal images provided the best full length views of the calaneonavicular (spring) ligament.

Whether the ankle ligaments are evaluated with the foot in a neutral position, plantar flexed, or dorsiflexed, or combinations of these positions, three MR imaging planes are required to fully evaluate all the ligaments of the ankle. The normal ligaments are thin and of low signal intensity. The anterior talofibular ligament is the easiest to identify, particularly in transaxial MR images (Fig. 70–427). Similarly, the posterior talofibular ligament is identified most readily in the transaxial plane (although it also is seen in coronal images), and its posterior aspect is intimately related to the peroneal longus tendon and its sheath (Fig. 70–427). A parallel arrangement of individual fibers separated by fibrofatty tissue may be evident. In the sagittal plane, the posterior talofibular ligament produces one or more foci of low signal intensity adjacent to the posterior surface of the talus, an appearance that simulates that of an intraarticular body. The calcaneofibular ligament is best evaluated in transaxial and coronal MR images (Fig. 70–427), although it is not seen in approximately 20 per cent of normal ankles. The peroneus longus and peroneus brevis tendons are located just superficial to the calcaneofibular ligament, and the synovial sheath of the peroneal tendons is attached to this ligament.

The deltoid ligament is seen regularly and often in its entirety in coronal MR images (Fig. 70–428), particularly those obtained with 20 to 40 degrees of plantar flexion of the foot. In the coronal plane, however, inhomogeneity of signal intensity within some portions of the deltoid ligament may be encountered normally, perhaps related to partial volume artifact created by periligamentous collections of fatty or fibrocartilaginous tissue.[1195] Transaxial MR images also are useful in studying both the superficial and deep portions of the deltoid ligament at any single level. Furthermore, the transaxial MR images show the relationship of the deltoid ligament to nearby tendons and neurovascular structures.

The tibiofibular ligaments are best evaluated in the transaxial plane, particularly in images located within 1 cm of

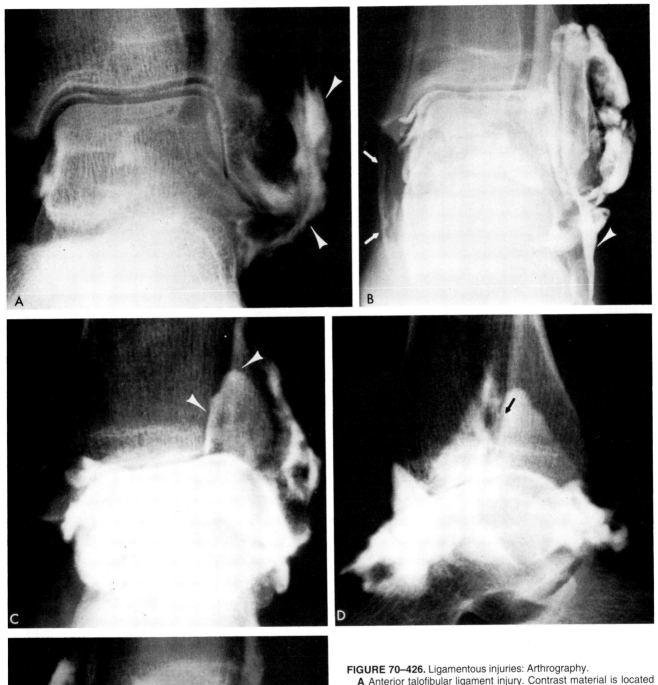

FIGURE 70–426. Ligamentous injuries: Arthrography.

A Anterior talofibular ligament injury. Contrast material is located inferior and lateral to the tip of the fibula (arrowheads). On a lateral view (not shown), the contrast material was anterior to the distal fibula.

B Anterior talofibular and calcaneofibular ligament injuries. In addition to extravasation of contrast material lateral to the distal fibula, there is visualization of the peroneal tendon sheaths (arrowhead). Normal filling of the medial tendon sheaths is noted (arrows).

C, D Distal anterior tibiofibular ligament injury. Oblique **(C)** and lateral **(D)** views reveal extravasation between the distal tibia and fibula (arrowheads). The normal clear zone anterior to the distal fibula has been obliterated (arrow).

E Deltoid ligament injury. There is contrast material that is extravasated beneath and medial to the medial malleolus (arrowhead).

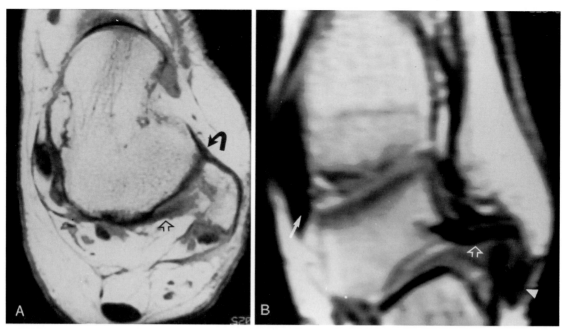

FIGURE 70–427. Normal ligaments of the ankle: MR imaging. Anterior and posterior talofibular ligaments and calcaneofibular ligament. A transaxial T1-weighted (TR/TE, 600/20) spin echo MR image **(A)** and a coronal T1-weighted (TR/TE, 600/20) spin echo MR image **(B)** show the anterior talofibular ligament (curved arrow), posterior talofibular ligament (open arrows), calcaneofibular ligament (arrowhead), and tibiotalar ligament (straight solid arrow).

the tibial plafond.[1276] Both the anterior and posterior tibiofibular ligaments are identifiable (Fig. 70–429), although analysis of several consecutive transaxial images often is required. Mink[1280] has emphasized the difficulty that may be encountered in proper identification of the tibiofibular and talofibular ligaments in the transaxial MR images, owing in part to the oblique course of the anterior tibiofibular ligament, and the tibial attachment site of the posterior tibiofibular ligament that may be seen in transaxial images in which the remaining portion of the tibia no longer is visible. This investigator noted the importance of two os-

seous landmarks, the talus and the fibula, that can be used to allow correct identification of each of the talofibular and tibiofibular ligaments in the transaxial plane[1280]:

1. *Talus*. At the level of its dome, the talus is nearly rectangular in configuration; this is the level at which the tibiofibular ligaments are observed. More distally, the talus is more elongated in shape, and a portion of the sinus tarsi usually is visible; this is the level at which the talofibular ligaments are observed.

2. *Fibula*. At the level of the distal portion of the fibular

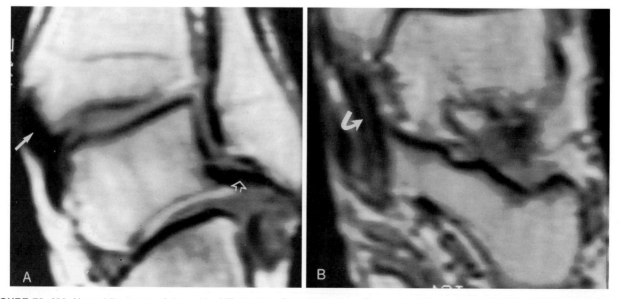

FIGURE 70–428. Normal ligaments of the ankle: MR imaging. Deltoid ligament. Two coronal T1-weighted (TR/TE, 600/20) spin echo MR images show portions of the tibiotalar (solid straight arrow) and tibiocalcaneal (solid curved arrow) ligaments. In **A**, note visualization of the posterior talofibular (open arrow) ligament.

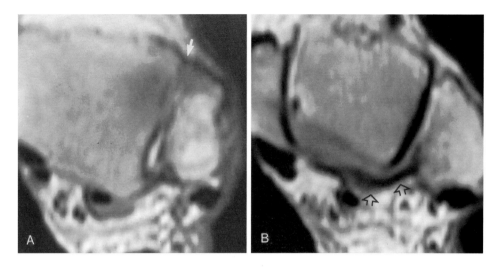

FIGURE 70–429. Normal ligaments of the ankle: MR imaging. Tibiofibular ligaments. Two transaxial T1-weighted (TR/TE, 600/20) spin echo MR images, with **A** located at a level slightly above **B**, show the anterior tibiofibular (solid arrow) and posterior tibiofibular (open arrows) ligaments.

shaft, the fibula has a flattened medial border; the tibiofibular ligaments are observed at this level. At the level of the malleolar fossa (appearing as a deep indentation along the medial border of the lateral malleolus), the talofibular ligaments are seen.

The MR imaging findings associated with disruption of the ligaments about the ankle include interruption of a portion or an entire ligament, ligament laxity or waviness, thickening and irregularity of the ligament, surrounding hemorrhage and edema (in acute injuries), and accumulation of abnormal amounts of fluid in adjacent joints and tendon sheaths[1277, 1279, 1280] (Figs. 70–430 to 70–433). The abnormalities of the ligament itself are the most important diagnostic findings; the presence of a joint effusion or fluid in a tendon sheath is not specific for the diagnosis of ligamentous disruption. Inability to visualize a ligament may indicate a tear, but the reliability of this finding depends upon the ligament being considered and the technical aspects of the MR imaging examination. For example, the anterior tibiofibular and calcaneofibular ligaments are not identified universally in MR imaging examinations of the ankle, so that their nonvisualization cannot be used as a reliable sign of injury.[1280] Inability to visualize the deltoid ligament, however, indicates a strong likelihood of its disruption.

Additional diagnostic problems related to assessment of ligamentous integrity with MR imaging include heterogeneous signal intensity, creating a striated appearance in normal ligaments (particularly the posterior talofibular and posterior tibiofibular ligaments and the deep portion of the deltoid ligament), the appearance of the normal posterior talofibular and posterior tibiofibular ligaments in the sagittal MR images that may simulate that of intra-articular bodies, and an irregular and frayed superior edge of the normal posterior talofibular ligament that may simulate a tear.[1195, 1199, 1280]

A potential role exists for MR arthrography employing intra-articular (talocrural joint) injection of a gadolinium compound or saline as a means to assess ligamentous injuries about the ankle, although this role has yet to be proved (Fig. 70–431).

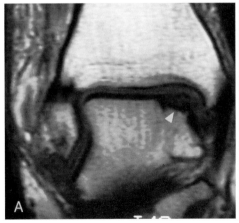
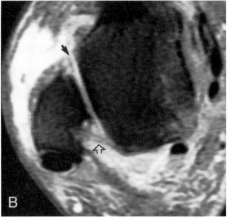

FIGURE 70–430. Injuries of the talofibular ligaments: MR imaging. Acute complete tear of the anterior talofibular ligament and acute partial tear of the posterior talofibular ligament.
  A A coronal T1-weighted (TR/TE, 600/20) spin echo MR image reveals subcutaneous edema laterally and an osteochondral fracture of the talus (arrowhead).
  B A transaxial proton density–weighted (TR/TE, 2000/20) spin echo MR image obtained with chemical presaturation of fat (ChemSat) at a level just below the ankle shows soft tissue edema and hemorrhage (of high signal intensity), complete disruption of the anterior talofibular ligament (solid arrow), and attenuation of the posterior talofibular ligament (open arrow).
  (Courtesy of C. Sebrechts, M.D., San Diego, California.)

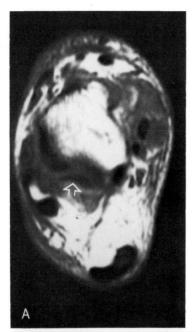

FIGURE 70–431. Injuries of the talofibular and calcaneofibular ligaments: MR imaging and MR arthrography.

A Acute complete tear of the anterior talofibular ligament. In a transaxial T1-weighted (TR/TE, 650/20) spin echo MR image, the anterior talofibular ligament is not seen, although some of the fibers of the posterior talofibular ligament are identified (open arrow). (Courtesy of J. Beltran, M.D., New York, New York.)

B Acute complete tear of the anterior talofibular ligament. A transaxial T1-weighted (TR/TE, 600/16) spin echo MR image, obtained after the injection of a gadolinium compound into the ankle, reveals failure to visualize the anterior talofibular ligament and anterolateral extravasation of fluid.

C Acute complete tears of the anterior talofibular and calcaneofibular ligaments. In a transaxial MR arthrographic image with parameters identical to those in **B**, findings include a torn anterior talofibular ligament (arrow) and fluid in the peroneal tendon sheath (arrowhead), evidence of a tear of the calcaneofibular ligament.

(**B, C**, Courtesy of V. Chandnani, M.D., Honolulu, Hawaii.)

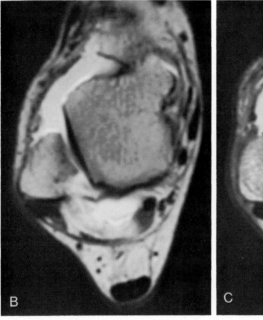

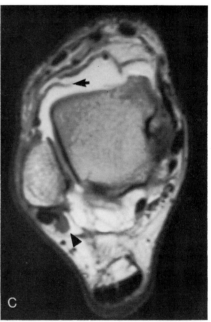

Sinus Tarsi Syndrome. Between the two subtalar joints, the posterior subtalar and talocalcaneonavicular joints, a cone-shaped region is found, designated the tarsal sinus and tarsal canal (Fig. 70–434). The apex of the cone is located posteromedially, representing the tarsal canal, and the expanded anterolateral portion of the cone represents the tarsal sinus. The contents of the tarsal canal and sinus include fat, an arterial anastomosis with branches from the posterior tibial and peroneal arteries, joint capsules, nerve endings, and five ligaments. These ligaments are the medial, intermediate, and lateral roots of the inferior extensor retinaculum; the cervical ligament; and the ligament of the tarsal canal (talocalcaneal interosseous ligament).[1281] Injury to these structures leads to a syndrome, termed the sinus tarsi

syndrome, that is associated with lateral foot pain, tenderness, and hindfoot instability.

The ligaments of the tarsal sinus and canal, particularly the cervical and the talocalcaneal interosseous ligaments, serve to limit inversion and to maintain alignment between the talus and the calcaneus.[1282] The cervical ligament is located at the lateral margin of the sinus tarsi. It originates from the superior surface of the calcaneus, medial to the origin of the extensor digitorum brevis muscle. From here, it extends in a superior and medial direction to attach to the tubercle on the inferior and lateral aspects of the talar neck. The cervical ligament is taut when the foot is inverted. The talocalcaneal interosseous ligament (ligament of the tarsal canal) extends from the sulcus tali to the sulcus calcanei. It

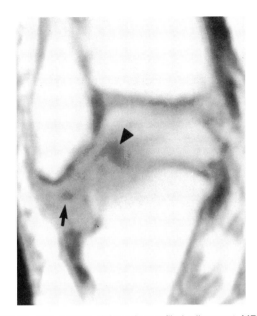

FIGURE 70–432. Injuries of the calcaneofibular ligament: MR imaging. Acute complete tear of the calcaneofibular ligament. A coronal T1-weighted (TR/TE, 550/20) spin echo MR image reveals a few residual fibers of the calcaneofibular ligament (arrow). Note the soft tissue mass of intermediate signal intensity about the torn ligament. Some of the fibers of the posterior talofibular ligament (arrowhead) are seen. (Courtesy of J. Beltran, M.D., New York, New York.)

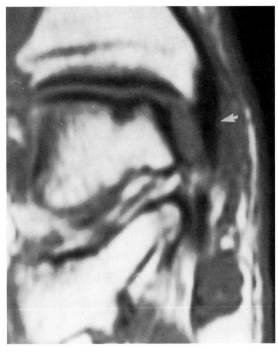

FIGURE 70–433. Injuries of the deltoid ligament: MR imaging. Acute complete tear of the tibiotalar and tibiocalcaneal parts of the deltoid ligament. A coronal T1-weighted (TR/TE, 550/20) spin echo MR image shows the proximal portion of the deltoid ligament (arrow). Neither its tibiotalar or tibiocalcaneal segment can be identified, however. A talar lesion also is evident. (Courtesy of J. Beltran, M.D., New York, New York.)

FIGURE 70–434. Ligaments of the tarsal sinus and canal: Normal anatomy. A superior view of the calcaneus is provided by removal of the talus. See text for details. (From Williams PL, Warwick R [Eds]: Gray's Anatomy. 36th British edition. Edinburgh, Churchill Livingstone, 1980, p 465.)

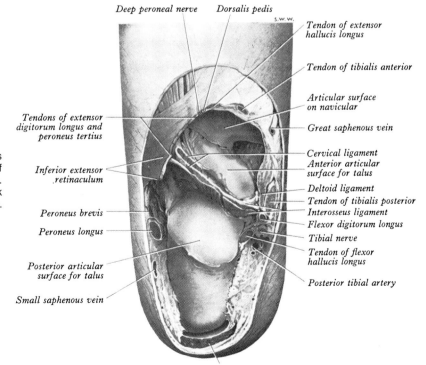

is located just anterior to the posterior subtalar joint and is smaller than the cervical ligament. This ligament is taut when the foot is everted. The lateral root of the inferior extensor retinaculum attaches to the calcaneus at the external aspect of the tarsal sinus; the medial root of this retinaculum extends deep within the tarsal sinus, attaching to the calcaneus just anterior to the calcaneal attachment site of the ligament of the tarsal canal and to the talus in common with the ligament of the tarsal canal; and the intermediate root of the inferior extensor retinaculum attaches to the calcaneus within the tarsal sinus, just posterior to the attachment site of the cervical ligament.[1281, 1282] Experimentally induced tears of the cervical ligament and ligament of the tarsal canal produce minor degrees of instability of the hindfoot.[1283]

The sinus tarsi syndrome leads to pain and tenderness, particularly in the lateral side of the foot, and a sensation of hindfoot weakness and instability.[1283] In approximately 70 per cent of affected persons, an inversion injury to the ankle occurs which, in some cases, results in tears of various components of the lateral ligamentous complex of the ankle.[1284, 1285] The high association of tarsal sinus and canal injury and that of the lateral ligaments of the ankle requires careful analysis of the sinus tarsi in all patients in whom inversion injuries of the ankle have occurred. Such analysis may be difficult, owing to the lack of clinical and routine radiographic findings that are sensitive to subtalar injury. In patients with a clinically serious ankle injury, negative results from stress tests (such as the anterior drawer and inversion stress tests) should arouse suspicion of an underlying subtalar sprain. Arthrography and MR imaging allow more direct assessment of the subtalar joints and the tarsal sinus and canal.

Arthrographic analysis of the tarsal sinus and canal requires contrast opacification of the posterior subtalar joint.[1285–1288] The basis of a positive arthrographic examination is the obliteration of the normal synovial recesses present about the talocalcaneal interosseous ligament. The changes apparently relate to synovial hyperplasia and may not be present immediately after trauma. Another arthrographic finding is leakage of contrast material into the sinus tarsi.[1285] This abnormality apparently reflects disruption of

fibers of the talocalcaneal interosseous ligament and possibly the cervical ligament as well. Further arthrographic findings include retraction of normal joint recesses, limited articular distention, lateral capsular leakage of contrast material, ganglion cysts, and abnormalities indicative of tears of the anterior talofibular and calcaneofibular ligaments.[1285, 1288] In one study, approximately 70 per cent of cases of chronic sinus tarsi syndrome had abnormal arthrograms.[1289]

MR imaging has been employed to study the normal contents of the tarsal sinus and canal and to investigate patients with the sinus tarsi syndrome[1274, 1280, 1281, 1422] (Fig. 70–435). The sagittal, coronal, and transaxial MR images all are important in analyzing the sinus tarsi. The cervical ligament and portions of the inferior extensor retinaculum are seen in all normal ankles, and the interosseous ligament is evident in most normal ankles. Fluid collections with increased signal intensity in T2-weighted spin echo MR images normally are evident in the recesses about the talocalcaneal interosseous ligament, although the absence of these recesses with MR imaging (as opposed to arthrography) does not allow a diagnosis of the sinus tarsi syndrome.[1281] MR imaging findings of this syndrome include poor definition of soft tissue structures (including the cervical and talocalcaneal interosseous ligaments), edema or fibrosis, and abnormal fluid collections[1280, 1281] (Figs. 70–436 and 70–437). Abnormalities of adjacent structures, such as the anterior talofibular ligament, calcaneofibular ligament, and tibialis posterior tendon, also may be evident.[1281] The MR imaging appearance of the abnormal tarsal sinus and canal are consistent with the known pathologic findings.[1281] Chronic synovitis, inflammation, fibrosis, and synovial cysts are recognized pathologic abnormalities in the sinus tarsi syndrome.[1284]

Impingement Syndromes

Several impingement syndromes may lead to restricted motion of the ankle joint. These can be divided into three types: anterior, posterior, and anterolateral impingement syndromes.

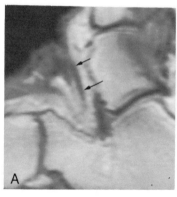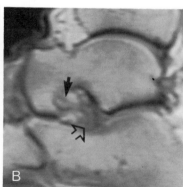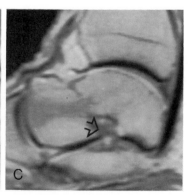

FIGURE 70–435. Normal tarsal sinus and canal: MR imaging. Three sagittal T1-weighted (TR/TE, 600/20) spin echo MR images are shown, with **A** being the most lateral, **B** being intermediate in position, and **C** being the most medial.
    A The medial root of the extensor retinaculum (solid arrows) extends from the extensor tendons to its insertion in the tarsal sinus.
    B Just medial to **A**, the cervical ligament (solid arrow) extends from the talus to the calcaneus. A portion of the talocalcaneal interosseous ligament (open arrow) also is seen.
    C Just medial to **B**, a portion of the talocalcaneal interosseous ligament (open arrow) is noted.
    (Courtesy of D. Goodwin, M.D., and D. Salonen, M.D., San Diego, California.)

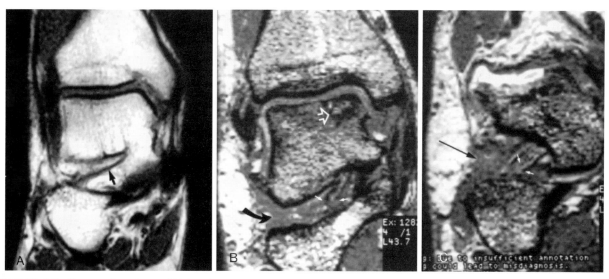

FIGURE 70–436. Sinus tarsi syndrome: MR imaging.

A Normal appearance. A coronal T1-weighted (TR/TE, 500/18) spin echo MR image reveals the normal talocalcaneal interosseous ligament (arrow), which is surrounded by fat.

B, C Sinus tarsi syndrome. Coronal reconstructions from a three-dimensional GRASS MR image (TR/TE, 30/10; flip angle, 70 degrees), with **B** being slightly more posterior than **C**, show diffuse infiltration of the tarsal sinus (black arrows). In **B**, partial disruption of the talocalcaneal interosseous ligament has led to a wavy, discontinuous appearance (solid white arrows). A small osteochondral fracture of the medial talar dome (open white arrow) is seen. In **C** partial disruption of the cervical ligament (white arrows) is evident.

(From Klein MA, Spreitzer AM: Radiology *186:*233, 1993.)

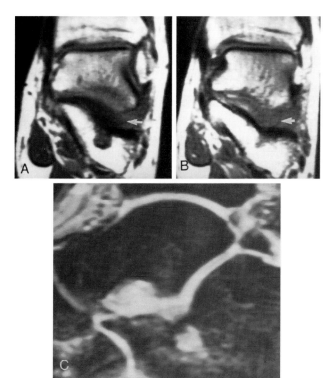

FIGURE 70–437. Sinus tarsi syndrome: MR imaging.

A, B Two coronal T1-weighted (TR/TE, 500/20) spin echo MR images show diffuse infiltration of the tarsal sinus with tissue of intermediate signal intensity (arrows) and loss of definition of the talocalcaneal interosseous ligament. A cystic lesion of the calcaneus is evident in **A**.

C In the same patient, a sagittal MPGR MR image (TR/TE, 1000/20; flip angle, 40 degrees) shows high signal intensity in the tarsal sinus and calcaneal cyst and absence of visualization of the ligaments of the tarsal canal and sinus.

(Courtesy of J. Beltran, M.D., New York, New York.)

Anterior Impingement Syndrome. The anterior impingement syndrome results from impingement of the anterior aspect of the tibia against the superior portion of the neck of the talus.[1290] The condition first was described in 1943 by Morris,[1291] who used the term athlete's ankle. It commonly is observed in young athletic persons, particularly baseball, soccer and (American) football players, and professional dancers.[1292–1296] Any athlete who uses repetitive and forceful dorsiflexion in movements of the ankle may be susceptible to this syndrome. Clinical findings include pain and tenderness in the anterior region of the ankle, findings accentuated with dorsiflexion of the joint. Restricted motion may be an accompanying clinical manifestation. Routine radiography reveals osteophytes in the anterior surface of the tibia or the neck of the talus, or in both sites[1290] (Fig. 70–438). Arthroscopic resection of the osteophytes may lead to symptomatic relief and increased ankle motion.[1290, 1297]

Posterior Impingement Syndrome. The posterior impingement syndrome relates to the presence of an os trigonum (Fig. 70–439) or a prominent process, Stieda's process, in the posterior surface of the talus (see previous discussion). Symptoms are common, owing to limitation of plantar flexion at the ankle, and for athletes such as professional ballet dancers, the condition may be disabling, requiring excision of the os trigonum or the prominent posterior process of the talus (which may be intact or fractured). Accompanying inflammation in the sheath about the flexor hallucis longus tendon may be evident. Findings may be unilateral or bilateral in distribution.

Anterolateral Impingement Syndrome. The anterolateral impingement syndrome generally occurs in young persons who have sustained an injury to the lateral ligaments of the ankle.[1298–1302] A complete or partial tear of the anterior talofibular ligament (or other lateral ligaments) is associated

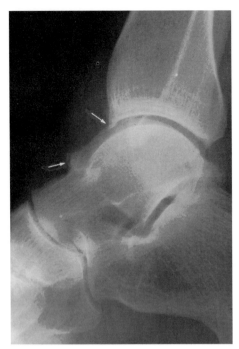

FIGURE 70–438. Anterior impingement syndrome: Routine radiography. Observe osteophytes (arrows) involving the anterior surface of the tibia and the talus.

with intra-articular hemorrhage and hyperplasia of the synovial membrane that extends into the articular gutter in the lateral aspect of the ankle. Entrapment of the synovial membrane or reactive hyalinized connective or scar tissue between the talus and fibula or tibia may lead to cartilage erosion in the anterolateral portion of the talar dome.[1280]

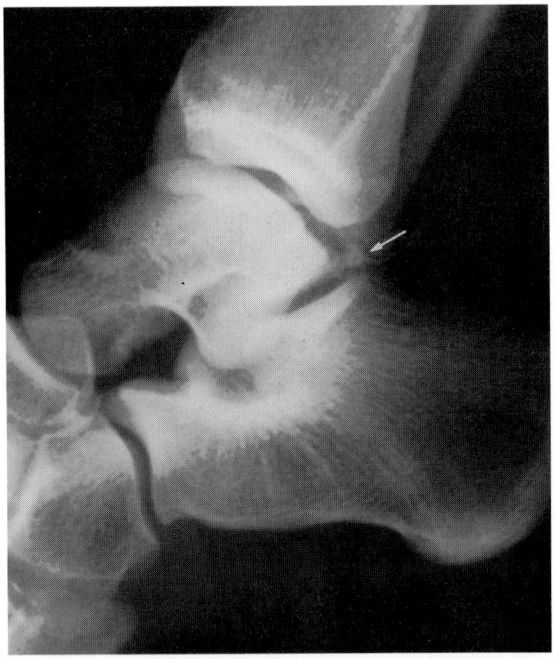

MR imaging reveals the mass, which commonly is of intermediate signal intensity in both T1-weighted and T2-weighted spin echo MR images. At arthroscopy, the hyalinized mass usually is associated with lesions of either the anterior talofibular ligament or the anterior tibiofibular syndesmotic ligament. Resection of the meniscus-like tissue may be curative.[1297, 1301] Additional causes of soft tissue lesions in this or other portions of the ankle include localized nodular synovitis, diffuse pigmented villonodular synovitis, idiopathic synovial (osteo)chondromatosis, ganglion cysts, and idiopathic arthrofibrosis.[1297]

Synovial and Capsular Abnormalities

Adhesive Capsulitis. Although far better known in the glenohumeral joint, posttraumatic adhesive capsulitis is encountered in the ankle. Restriction of ankle motion is detected on clinical examination. Arthrography delineates a decrease in the articular capacity, with resistance to injection of contrast material, obliteration of the normal anterior and posterior recesses or the tibiofibular syndesmosis, opacification of lymphatic vessels, and extravasation of contrast material along the needle tract (Fig. 70–440). The relationship of this condition to posttraumatic arthrofibrosis of the ankle and to causes of the anterolateral impingement syndrome is not clear.

Synovitis. In common with other joints, the ankle may be affected in a variety of systemic rheumatic diseases and local processes. Rheumatoid arthritis, the seronegative spondyloarthropathies, hemophilia, gout, and calcium pyrophosphate dihydrate crystal deposition disease are among the systemic disorders that may involve the ankle. Pigmented villonodular synovitis, idiopathic synovial (osteo)-chondromatosis (Fig. 70–441), and infection are among the monoarticular processes that may localize to the ankle.

FIGURE 70–439. Posterior impingement syndrome: Routine radiography. In a 14 year old ballet student with pain during plantar flexion of the foot, a lateral radiograph of the foot in plantar flexion shows approximation of the surfaces of the tibia and calcaneus with an adjacent os trigonum (arrow). The os trigonum was excised with relief of pain. (Courtesy of G. Greenway, M.D., Dallas, Texas.)

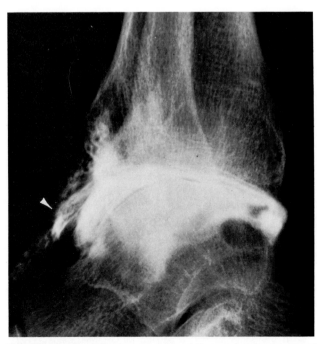

FIGURE 70–440. Adhesive capsulitis: Arthrography. On the lateral view, there is no filling of normal anterior and posterior recesses, and extravasation of contrast material is seen along the needle track (arrowhead).

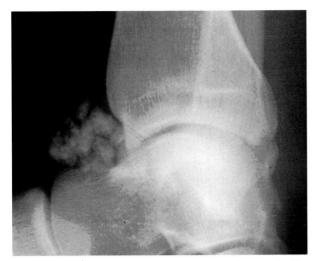

FIGURE 70–441. Idiopathic synovial (osteo)chondromatosis: Routine radiography. Note multiple ossified bodies involving the anterior aspect of the ankle.

Involvement of surrounding structures such as tendons, tendon sheaths, and bursae, and the formation of para-articular synovial cysts may be evident. Giant cell tumors of the tendon sheath are observed about the ankle or in the foot[1364] (Fig. 70–442). These disorders are discussed and illustrated elsewhere in this work.

Muscle Abnormalities

Muscle abnormalities occurring about the ankle and foot are similar to those observed in other anatomic regions.

Inflammatory, infectious, and traumatic disorders may involve the muscles of the foot and ankle, either in isolation or in combination with changes elsewhere (see Chapters 35, 64, and 67).

Accessory and Anomalous Muscles. Although accessory and anomalous muscles occur elsewhere in the body, those in the foot and ankle have received the greatest attention.

An accessory soleus muscle appears to represent a frequent finding, especially on MR imaging examinations. Affected persons commonly are asymptomatic, although soft tissue fullness or a mass and occasionally pain and swelling following exercise may be seen, especially in teenagers and young adults.[1303–1308] Accentuation of foot deformity has been noted in patients with equinovarus conditions who also have an accessory soleus muscle.[1307]

The origin and insertion sites of an accessory soleus muscle vary.[1308] The muscle may arise from the proximal third of the fibula, the oblique soleal line of the tibia, the aponeurosis of the flexor digitorum longus muscle, the anterior portion of the normal soleus muscle, or combinations of these structures.[1305, 1309, 1310] The insertion sites of the accessory soleus muscle include the Achilles tendon and the superior and medial surfaces of the calcaneus.[1311] The diagnosis of this accessory muscle can be provided by routine radiography (Fig. 70–443), CT (Fig. 70–443), and MR imaging (Figs. 70–443 to 70–445). Of these techniques, MR imaging appears to be best.[1308] MR imaging confirms that the abnormal tissue has signal intensity charactertistics identical to those of normal muscle, unless intramuscular hemorrhage or a hematoma is present. Treatment of symp-

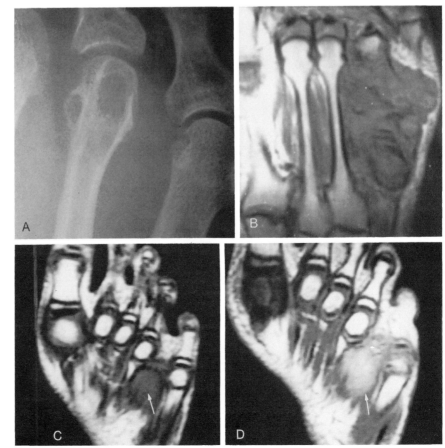

FIGURE 70–442. Giant cell tumor of tendon sheath: Routine radiography and MR imaging.

A, B In a 63 year old man, a routine radiograph **(A)** reveals erosion of the fourth metatarsal head. A transverse T1-weighted (TR/TE, 588/34) spin echo MR image **(B)** shows the extent of the mass, which is of low signal intensity.

C, D In a 7 year old girl, a transverse T1-weighted (TR/TE, 600/11) spin echo MR image **(C)** reveals a mass (arrow) of low signal intensity between the fourth and fifth metatarsal bones. A transverse T1-weighted (TR/TE, 600/12) spin echo MR image obtained after the intravenous administration of a gadolinium compound **(D)** shows an increase in signal intensity in the mass (arrow).

(Courtesy of G. Greenway, M.D., Dallas, Texas.)

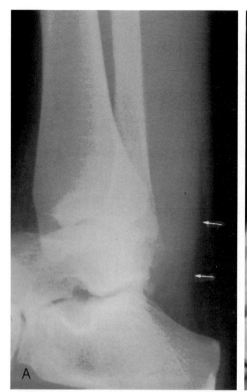
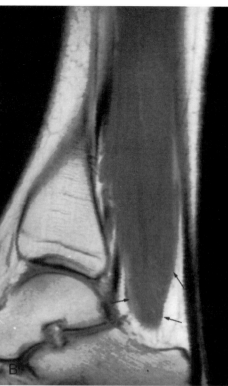
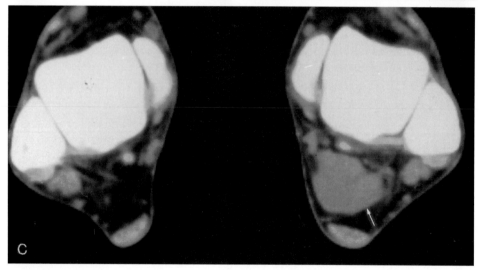

FIGURE 70–443. Accessory soleus muscle: Routine radiography, CT scanning, and MR imaging.

A, B A lateral radiograph **(A)** and a sagittal T1-weighted (TR/TE, 600/16) spin echo MR image **(B)** show the accessory muscle (arrows). (Courtesy of G. Greenway, M.D., Dallas, Texas.)

C In a second patient, a transaxial CT scan reveals the accessory soleus muscle (arrow). Compare with the opposite side. (Courtesy of A. Newberg, M.D., Boston, Massachusetts.)

tomatic patients with an accessory soleus muscle includes fasciotomy of the muscle sheath or excision of the muscle, owing to the belief that the condition may predispose to a localized compartment syndrome.[1309]

The peroneus quartus muscle, also designated the peroneus accessorius, peroneus externus, and peroneus calcaneus externus muscle, has been associated with chronic pain and swelling about the ankle.[1308, 1312–1314] Its reported frequency, based on results of cadaveric dissections, has varied from approximately 12 to 22 per cent.[1315] Its site of origin may include the distal lateral portion of the fibula and the peroneus brevis or longus muscle, and its site of insertion may include the phalanges or metatarsal bone of the fifth toe, the calcaneus, the cuboid bone, and the lateral retinaculum of the ankle.[1308] Accurate diagnosis again is provided by MR imaging.[1308]

The flexor digitorum longus accessorius is a third anomalous muscle with variable sites of origin and insertion.[1308] It may arise from the tibia, fibula, or interosseous membrane, or combinations of these structures, and it may insert into the flexor digitorum longus tendon at various levels. Clinical manifestations usually are absent. An anomalous flexor hallucis longus muscle also has been described.[1316]

Abnormalities of the Plantar Soft Tissues

Plantar Fasciitis. The plantar aponeurosis is a thick, strong band of tissue extending from the calcaneus posteriorly to the region of the metatarsal heads and beyond. It is composed of a prominent central part and lateral and medial parts (Fig. 70–446). The central part of the plantar aponeurosis originates as a narrow tissue attaching to the

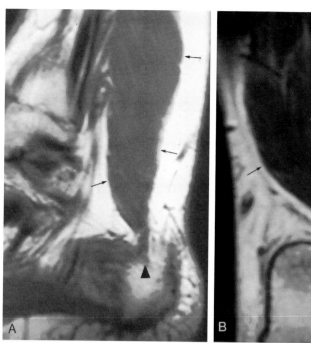

FIGURE 70–444. Accessory soleus muscle: MR imaging. A sagittal T1-weighted (TR/TE, 600/20) spin echo MR image **(A)** and a coronal T1-weighted (TR/TE, 800/25) spin echo MR image **(B)** show the accessory soleus muscle (arrows), which is attaching to the medial aspect of the calcaneus (arrowheads). (Courtesy of V. Chandnani, M.D., Honolulu, Hawaii.)

medial process of the tuberosity of the calcaneus. As it extends distally, it broadens and, near the metatarsal heads, divides into five processes, each with superficial and deep components, and each extending into one toe. The lateral part of the plantar aponeurosis, which is inferior to the abductor digiti minimi muscle, has a thick proximal portion that extends between the lateral process of the calcaneal tuberosity and the base of the fifth metatarsal bone. It is thinner distally, with bands that extend to the plantar plate of the fourth and fifth toes. The medial part of the plantar

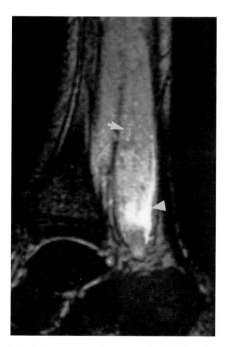

FIGURE 70–445. Accessory soleus muscle: MR imaging. A sagittal MPGR MR image (TR/TE, 517/11; flip angle, 15 degrees) reveals an accessory soleus muscle (arrow) with distal high signal intensity (arrowhead) related to hemorrhage following an injury. (Courtesy of S. Moreland, M.D., San Diego, California.)

aponeurosis is located inferior to the abductor hallucis muscle. It is thin and continuous proximally with the flexor retinaculum, laterally with the central part of the plantar aponeurosis, and medially with the fascia dorsalis pedis.

Plantar fasciitis represents inflammation of the plantar fascia and the perifascial structures.[1365] Its causes may be divided into three categories[1318-1320]: mechanical, degenerative, and systemic. Mechanical factors associated with plantar fasciitis include pes cavus, a pronated foot, and an externally rotated lower extremity.[1317] Such factors, particularly when present in active persons, may predispose to inflammation of the plantar fascia. Degenerative causes of plantar fasciitis include atrophy of the heel pad and age-related increases in foot pronation. Systemic causes include a wide variety of rheumatic disorders, especially rheumatoid arthritis and the seronegative spondyloarthropathies. As the factors responsible for plantar fasciitis vary, the pathologic findings also are variable. In the setting of predisposing mechanical factors and overuse syndromes (cases associated with participation in competitive sports), tearing of some of the fibers of the plantar fascia may occur.[1321-1323] These abnormalities initially predominate at the site of origin of the plantar fascia and are accompanied by a local inflammatory reaction. Histologic findings include angiofibroblastic hyperplasia, collagen degeneration and necrosis, and matrix calcification.[1324, 1325] With chronicity, the entire course of the plantar aponeurosis may be affected, with thickening and nodularity. Clinical findings include pain and tenderness localized to the regions of inflammation. Dorsiflexion of the toes may lead to an excerbation of the findings, owing to stretching of the fibers of the plantar fascia. Conservative therapy is the preferred treatment in the early stages of plantar fasciitis; in chronic cases or in those that do not respond to conservative measures, surgical therapy, consisting of release of the origin of the plantar fascia with decompression of the lateral plantar nerve, may be required.[1322]

Although bone scintigraphy may reveal regions of increased accumulation of the radiopharmaceutical agent at

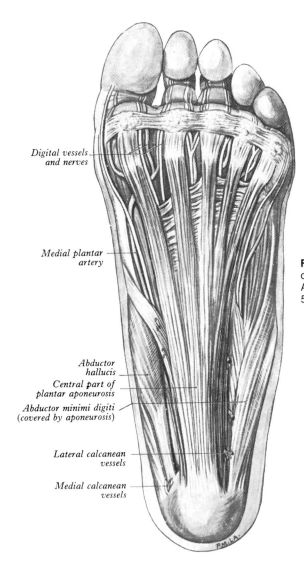

Digital vessels and nerves

Medial plantar artery

Abductor hallucis

Central part of plantar aponeurosis

Abductor minimi digiti (covered by aponeurosis)

Lateral calcanean vessels

Medial calcanean vessels

FIGURE 70–446. Plantar aponeurosis and related structures: Normal anatomy. See text for details. (From Williams PL, Warwick R [Eds]: Gray's Anatomy. 36th British edition. Edinburgh, Churchill Livingstone, 1980, p 579.)

the site of inflammation, the increased scintigraphic activity may be more widespread, producing a nonspecific pattern. MR imaging, however, appears to be both sensitive and specific in the diagnosis of plantar fasciitis (Figs. 70–447 and 70–448), and it may be useful in cases in which the clinical diagnosis is in doubt. MR imaging abnormalities of plantar fasciitis include thickening of the plantar fascia (which may grow to a thickness of 7 or 8 mm, when compared with the 3 or 4 mm thickness that characterizes normal plantar fascia) and intrafascial alterations in signal intensity.[1326] In T1-weighted spin echo MR images, foci of intermediate signal intensity may be seen within the plantar fascia, which normally is of uniform low signal intensity. In T2-weighted spin echo and STIR MR images, areas of high signal intensity may be evident in the plantar fascia and subcutaneous tissue. Alterations in the signal intensity in the marrow of the calcaneus, reflecting edema, also may be apparent.

Plantar fasciitis is but one of the many causes of plantar heel pain. Other causes of heel pain include rupture of the plantar fascia, nerve entrapment syndromes, atrophy or inflammation of the fat pad, tendinitis and tenosynovitis, calcaneal stress fractures, infections, and tumors (Fig. 70–449).

Plantar Fibromatosis. Plantar fibromatosis is a common condition associated with fibrous proliferation and replacement of portions of the plantar aponeurosis. The disorder is seen in persons of all ages and is more common in men. Lesions may be solitary or multiple and unilateral or bilateral in distribution.[1327, 1328] Affected persons usually are asymptomatic, the nodules being discovered by palpation. Mild pain and discomfort in the plantar aspect of the foot after walking or prolonged standing may be evident, however. An association of plantar fibromatosis with other conditions associated with proliferation of fibrous tissue, such as Dupuytren's contractures of the hand, Peyronie's disease of the penis, and keloids, has been suggested but is not proved.[1329] Plantar fibromatosis may become more extensive over a number of years, with gradual enlargement of the nodules and an increased number of nodules, although contractures of the toes generally do not occur.[1330] On physical examination, the masses are firm and fixed to the plantar fascia. They may be treated conservatively or removed surgically.

Histologically, the lesions are composed of fibroblasts separated by variable amounts of collagen tissue. They may infiltrate surrounding structures, leading to difficulty in defining the full extent of the lesions, but plantar fibromatosis

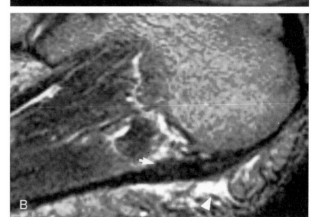

FIGURE 70–447. Plantar fasciitis: MR imaging.

A Normal plantar fascia. A sagittal proton density–weighted (TR/TE, 2000/20) spin echo MR image shows the normal thin plantar fascia (arrows) and overlying subcutaneous fibrous septa.

B Plantar fasciitis. A sagittal T2-weighted (TR/TE, 2000/80) spin echo MR image reveals subcutaneous edema (arrowhead) and focally thickened plantar fascia (arrow). A plantar calcaneal enthesophyte also is present.

(From Berkowitz JF, et al: Radiology *179:*665, 1991.)

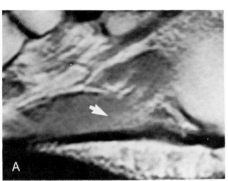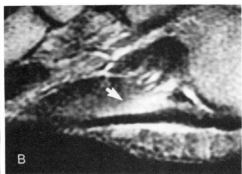

FIGURE 70–448. Plantar fasciitis: MR imaging. Sagittal proton density–weighted (TR/TE, 2500/20) **(A)** and T2-weighted (TR/TE, 2500/80) **(B)** spin echo MR images show altered signal intensity (arrows) deep to the plantar fascia with high signal intensity both deep and superficial to the plantar fascia in **B**. (Courtesy of M. Schweitzer, M.D., Philadelphia, Pennsylvania.)

FIGURE 70–449. Cavernous hemangioma: MR imaging. Sagittal T1-weighted (TR/TE, 700/20) **(A)** and T2-weighted (TR/TE, 2000/80) **(B)** spin echo MR images reveal the tumor (arrows), which is of high signal intensity in **B**. It involved the flexor digitorum brevis and abductor digiti minimi muscles and displaced the plantar fascia. (Courtesy of C. Chen, M.D., Kaohsiung, Taiwan.)

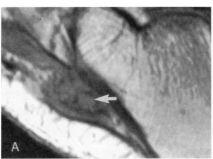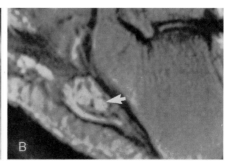

does not undergo malignant transformation. Three phases of the disorder have been defined[1329]: an initial proliferative phase is associated with increased fibroblastic activity and cellular proliferation; an involutional (active) phase is associated with the formation of nodules; and a residual phase is accompanied by reduced fibroblastic activity, maturation of collagen, and tissue contracture.

With MR imaging, single or multiple nodules in the plantar fascia and subcutaneous tissue are observed. The lesions are of low signal intensity in T1-weighted spin echo images and of low to intermediate signal intensity on T2-weighted spin echo MR images. In some cases, regions of high signal intensity are seen in T2-weighted spin echo or STIR MR images.[1329]

Abnormalities of Nerves

Entrapment Neuropathies. Entrapment neuropathies occurring in the foot and ankle are described in Chapter 77. The most important of these relate to compression of the posterior tibial nerve in the medial aspect of the ankle (i.e., the tarsal tunnel syndrome) and entrapment of the deep peroneal nerve.

The tarsal tunnel is located behind and below the medial malleolus; its floor is bony and its roof is formed by the flexor retinaculum. The resulting fibro-osseous channel allows passage of the tendons of the tibialis posterior, flexor digitorum longus, and flexor hallucis longus muscles, the posterior tibial artery and vein, and the posterior tibial nerve. Causes of compression of the posterior tibial nerve within the tarsal tunnel include tumors of nerves and other structures, tenosynovitis, ganglion cysts (Fig. 70–450), post-traumatic fibrosis, and dilated or tortuous veins. Many of the causes can be defined with CT or MR imaging.[1331–1334]

Entrapment of the deep peroneal nerve in the ankle and foot may occur in several different locations. The most common site of compression is beneath the inferior extensor retinaculum, a condition referred to as the anterior tarsal tunnel syndrome.[1335, 1336] The typical site of involvement is subjacent to the superior edge of this retinaculum, close to the extensor hallucis longus tendon. Entrapment of the nerve in a more distal location may relate to osteophytes that form at the talonavicular, naviculocuneiform, or tarso-metatarsal joints or to an os intermetatarseum.[1337] Deep peroneal nerve entrapment may occur in skiers, owing to tight-fitting ski boots, or in soccer players who kick the ball

with the dorsum of the foot.[1336, 1337] Clinical findings vary according to the site of entrapment but may include pain, numbness, muscle weakness, and paresthesia.

Sural nerve entrapment may occur in the ankle, generally related to fibrosis occurring as a response to an ankle sprain, fracture (e.g., calcaneal or fifth metatarsal fracture), Achilles tendon rupture, or a ganglion cyst.[1337–1339] Entrapment of the superficial peroneal nerve, particularly in the distal portion of the leg and ankle, also occurs, especially as a result of fibrosis secondary to ankle injuries.[1337]

Interdigital Neuromas. Interdigital neuromas, or Morton's neuromas, are not true tumors but rather represent a fibrotic response that occurs in and about the plantar digital nerves.[1340–1342] Interdigital neuromas are encountered most frequently in young and middle-aged persons, especially women. A unilateral distribution predominates but is not universal. The interspace between the third and fourth toes is affected most commonly. The third plantar digital nerve may be most vulnerable, owing to its large size and relatively fixed position.[1337] Clinical findings include pain at the level of the metatarsophalangeal joint that may radiate into the adjacent toes. Trauma with resulting fibrosis appears to be important in the pathogenesis of this condition. Because of its persistently low signal intensity in both T1-weighted and T2-weighted spin echo MR images (see Chapter 77), interdigital neuromas generally can be differentiated from true neuromas, which show high signal intensity in T2-weighted spin echo MR images (Fig. 70–451).

Abnormalities of Subchondral Bone

The major abnormalities affecting the subchondral bone about the ankle are discussed elsewhere in this work. These include osteochondral fractures and osteochondritis dissecans of the talus (see Chapter 67), fracture-dislocations (see Chapter 68), stress fractures (see Chapter 67), transient or migratory bone marrow edema or osteoporosis (see Chapter 51), osteonecrosis (see Chapters 79 and 80), osteomyelitis (see Chapters 64 and 66), and tumors and tumor-like conditions (see Chapter 83). Imaging evaluation of these conditions usually begins with routine radiography. Bone scintigraphy provides a sensitive but nonspecific means of further evaluation of these processes, particularly if they are radiographically occult. CT allows more specific assessment of most lesions, and MR imaging provides both sensitivity and specificity in their analysis (Fig. 70–452).

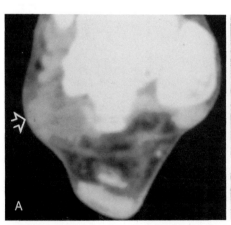
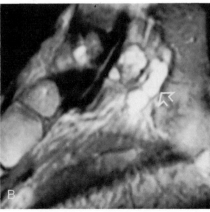

FIGURE 70–450. Ganglion cysts: CT scanning and MR imaging. Both of these ganglion cysts, which developed in the medial aspect of the ankle, led to compression of the posterior tibial nerve. A transaxial CT scan **(A)** in one patient and a sagittal T2-weighted (TR/TE, 2000/75) spin echo MR image **(B)** in a second patient show the location of the ganglion cysts (open arrows). (**A** Courtesy of C. Chen, M.D., Kaohsiung, Taiwan; **B** Courtesy of S. Eilenberg, M.D., San Diego, California.)

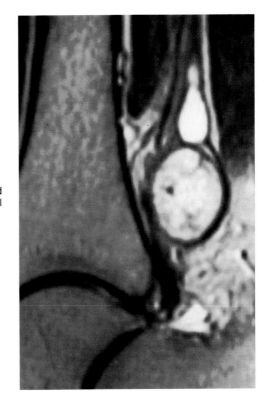

FIGURE 70–451. Neurilemoma of tibial nerve: MR imaging. A sagittal T2-weighted (TR/TE, 3000/100) fast spin echo MR image shows the large tumor of high signal intensity. (Courtesy of P. Kindynis, M.D., Geneva, Switzerland.)

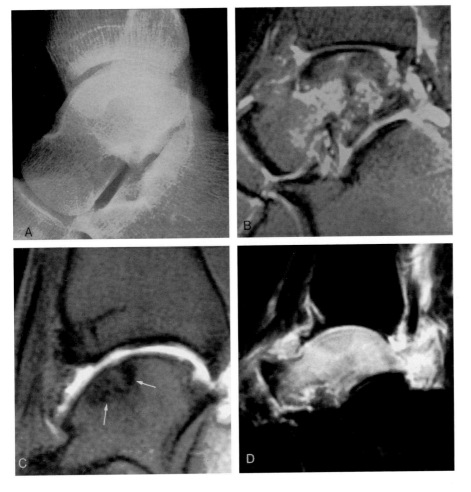

FIGURE 70–452. Abnormalities of subchondral bone: MR imaging.

A, B Occult talar fracture. Although the routine radiograph **(A)** fails to document a fracture, a sagittal T2-weighted (TR/TE, 2000/80) spin echo MR image **(B)** confirms the presence of a comminuted fracture of the talus. (Courtesy of G. Greenway, M.D., Dallas, Texas.)

C Osteochondritis dissecans of the talus. A sagittal T1-weighted (TR/TE, 500/20) spin echo MR image obtained with chemical presaturation of fat (ChemSat) and following the intra-articular administration of a gadolinium compound reveals the location of the lesion (arrows) in the lateral aspect of the talar dome and thinning of the adjacent articular cartilage.

D Transient bone marrow edema. A sagittal T1-weighted (TR/TE, 650/19) spin echo MR image obtained with chemical presaturation of fat (ChemSat) following the intravenous administration of a gadolinium compound shows high signal intensity in the talus and adjacent soft tissues. (Courtesy of S. Eilenberg, M.D., San Diego, California.)

SUMMARY

In this chapter, a summary of some of the more important internal derangements and related conditions occurring in six anatomic regions is provided. Abnormalities of articular cartilage, subchondral bone, synovial membrane, joint capsule, ligaments, tendons, muscles, and nerves are emphasized, with particular attention to anatomy and concepts of pathology and pathophysiology. These abnormalities are delineated with a variety of imaging methods, which include routine radiography, arthrography, tenography, bursography, bone scintigraphy, conventional tomography, CT scanning, conventional arthrotomography, computed arthrotomography, and MR imaging. Although clinical assessment forms the foundation of correct diagnosis of many of these conditions, the contributions of these imaging methods are significant.

References

1. Stein J (Ed): The Random House Dictionary of the English Language. The Unabridged Edition. New York, Random House, 1970, p 389.
2. Mikic ZD: Detailed anatomy of the articular disc of the distal radioulnar joint. Clin Orthop 245:123, 1989.
3. Bogumill GP: Anatomy of the wrist. In DM Lichtman (Ed): The Wrist and Its Disorders. Philadelphia, WB Saunders Co, 1988, p 14.
4. Palmer AK: The distal radioulnar joint. In DM Lichtman (Ed): The Wrist and Its Disorders. Philadelphia, WB Saunders Co, 1988, p 220.
5. Palmer AK, Werner FW: The triangular fibrocartilage complex of the wrist—anatomy and function. J Hand Surg 6:153, 1981.
6. Palmer AK, Werner FW: Biomechanics of the distal radioulnar joint. Clin Orthop 187:26, 1984.
7. Mayfield JK: Pathogenesis of wrist ligament instability. In DM Lichtman (Ed): The Wrist and Its Disorders. Philadelphia, WB Saunders Co, 1988, p 53.
8. Taleisnik J: The ligaments of the wrist. J Hand Surg 1:110, 1976.
9. Mayfield JK, Johnson RP, Kilcoyne RF: The ligaments of the human wrist and their functional significance. Anat Rec 186:417, 1976.
10. Kauer JMG: Functional anatomy of the wrist. Clin Orthop 149:9, 1980.
11. Berger RA, Landsmeer JMF: The palmar radiocarpal ligaments: A study of adult and fetal human wrist joints. J Hand Surg [Am] 15:847, 1990.
12. Smith DK: Volar carpal ligaments of the wrist: Normal appearance on multiplanar reconstructions of three-dimensional Fourier transform MR imaging. AJR 161:353, 1993.
13. Mizuseki T, Ikuta Y: The dorsal carpal ligaments: their anatomy and function. J Hand Surg [Br] 14:91, 1989.
14. Smith DK: Dorsal carpal ligaments of the wrist: Normal appearance on multiplanar reconstructions of three-dimensional Fourier transform MR imaging. AJR 161:119, 1993.
15. Mesgarzadeh M, Schneck CD, Bonakdarpour A: Carpal tunnel: MR imaging. Part I. Normal anatomy. Radiology 171:743, 1989.
16. Zeiss J, Skie M, Ebraheim N, et al: Anatomic relations between the median nerve and flexor tendons in the carpal tunnel: MR evaluation in normal volunteers. AJR 153:533, 1989.
17. Zeiss J, Jakab E, Khimji T, et al: The ulnar tunnel at the wrist (Guyon's canal): Normal MR anatomy and variants. AJR 158:1081, 1992.
18. Gross MS, Gelberman RH: The anatomy of the distal ulnar tunnel. Clin Orthop 196:238, 1985.
19. Kaplan E: Functional and Surgical Anatomy of the Hand. 2nd Ed. Philadelphia, JB Lippincott, 1965.
20. Lampe E: Surgical anatomy of the hand with special reference to infections and trauma. Clin Symp 21:66, 1969.
21. Scheldrup E: Tendon sheath patterns in hand. Surg Gynecol Obstet 93:161, 1951.
22. Ekenstam FA: Anatomy of the distal radioulnar joint. Clin Orthop 275:14, 1992.
23. Kauer JMG: The distal radioulnar joint. Anatomic and functional considerations. Clin Orthop 275:37, 1992.
24. Linscheid RL: Biomechanics of the distal radioulnar joint. Clin Orthop 275:46, 1992.
25. Nathan R, Schneider LH: Classification of distal radioulnar disorders. Hand Clin 7:239, 1991.
26. Palmer AK: Triangular fibrocartilage complex lesions: A classification. J Hand Surg [Am] 14:594, 1989.
27. Ekenstam F, Hagert CG: Anatomical studies of the geometry and stability of the distal radioulnar joint. Scand J Plast Reconstr Surg 19:17, 1985.
28. Vesely DG: The distal radio-ulnar joint. Clin Orthop 51:75, 1967.
29. Bowers WH: Problems of the distal radioulnar joint. Adv Orthop Surg 7:289, 1984.
30. Milch H: So-called dislocation of the lower end of the ulna. Ann Surg 116:282, 1942.
31. Weigl K, Spira E: The triangular fibrocartilage of the wrist joint. Reconstr Surg Traumatol 11:139, 1969.
32. Gilula LA, Palmer AK: Is it possible to diagnose a tear at arthrography or MR imaging? Radiology 187:581, 1993.
33. Zlatkin MB, Chao PC, Osterman AL, et al: Chronic wrist pain: Evaluation with high-resolution MR imaging. Radiology 173:723, 1989.
34. Golimbu CN, Firooznia H, Melone CP Jr, et al: Tears of the triangular fibrocartilage of the wrist: MR imaging. Radiology 173:731, 1989.
35. Skahen JR III, Palmer AK, Levinsohn EM, et al: Magnetic resonance imaging of the triangular fibrocartilage complex. J Hand Surg [Am] 15:552, 1990.
36. Greenan T, Zlatkin MB: Magnetic resonance imaging of the wrist. Semin Ultrasound CT MR 11:267, 1990.
37. Cerofolini E, Luchetti R, Pederzini L, et al: MR evaluation of triangular fibrocartilage complex tears in the wrist: Comparison with arthrography and arthroscopy. J Comput Assist Tomogr 14:963, 1990.
38. Dalinka MK, Meyer S, Kricun ME, et al: Magnetic resonance imaging of the wrist. Hand Clin 7:87, 1991.
39. Kang HS, Kindynis P, Brahme SK, et al: Triangular fibrocartilage and intercarpal ligaments of the wrist: MR imaging. Cadaveric study with gross pathologic and histologic correlation. Radiology 181:401, 1991.
40. Brahme SK, Resnick D: Magnetic resonance imaging of the wrist. Rheum Dis Clin North Am 17:721, 1991.
41. Schweitzer ME, Brahme SK, Hodler J, et al: Chronic wrist pain: Spin-echo and short tau inversion recovery MR imaging and conventional and MR arthrography. Radiology 182:205, 1992.
42. Metz VM, Schratter M, Dock WI, et al: Age-associated changes of the triangular fibrocartilage of the wrist: Evaluation of the diagnostic performance of MR imaging. Radiology 184:217, 1992.
43. Mikic ZD: Age changes in the triangular fibrocartilage of the wrist joint. J Anat 126:367, 1978.
44. Mikic Z, Somer L, Somer T: Histologic structure of the articular disk of the human distal radioulnar joint. Clin Orthop 275:29, 1992.
45. Metz VM, Mann FA, Gilula LA: Three-compartment wrist arthrography: correlation of pain site with location of uni- or bidirectional communications. AJR 160:819, 1993.
46. Metz VM, Mann FA, Gilula LA: Lack of correlation between site of wrist pain and location of noncommunicating defects shown by three-compartment wrist arthrography. AJR 160:1239, 1993.
47. Friedman SL, Palmer AK: The ulnar impaction syndrome. Hand Clin 7:295, 1991.
48. Mann FA, Wilson AJ, Gilula LA: Radiographic evaluation of the wrist: What does the hand surgeon want to know? Radiology 184:15, 1992.
49. Bell MJ, Hill RJ, McMurtry RY: Ulnar impingement syndrome. J Bone Joint Surg [Br] 67:126, 1985.
50. King GJ, McMurtry RY, Rubenstein JD, et al: Kinematics of the distal radioulnar joint. J Hand Surg [Am] 11:798, 1986.
51. Adams BD: Partial excision of the triangular fibrocartilage complex articular disk: A biomechanical study. J Hand Surg [Am] 18:334, 1993.
52. Törnvall AH, Ekenstam FA, Hagert CG, et al: Radiologic examination and measurement of the wrist and distal radio-ulnar joint. New aspects. Acta Radiol Diagn 27:581, 1986.
53. Mino DE, Palmer AK, Levinsohn EM: The role of radiography and computerized tomography in the diagnosis of subluxation and dislocation of the distal radioulnar joint. J Hand Surg 8:23, 1983.
54. Mino DE, Palmer AK, Levinsohn EM: Radiography and computerized tomography in the diagnosis of incongruity of the distal radio-ulnar joint. J Bone Joint Surg [Am] 67:247, 1985.
55. Olerud C, Kongsholm J, Thuomas K-A: The congruence of the distal radioulnar joint. A magnetic resonance imaging study. Acta Orthop Scand 59:183, 1988.
56. Pirela-Cruz MA, Goll SR, Klug M, et al: Stress computed tomography analysis of the distal radioulnar joint: A diagnostic tool for determining translational motion. J Hand Surg [Am] 16:75, 1991.
57. Linscheid RL, Dobyns JH, Beabout JW, et al: Traumatic instability of the wrist. Diagnosis, classification, and pathomechanics. J Bone Joint Surg [Am] 54:1612, 1972.
58. Dobyns JH, Linscheid RL, Chao EYS, et al: Traumatic instability of the wrist. In Instructional Course Lectures. American Academy of Orthopaedic Surgeons. Vol. 24, p 182. St Louis, CV Mosby, 1975.
59. Logan SE, Nowak MD, Gould PL, et al: Biomechanical behavior of the scapholunate ligament. Biomed Sci Instrum 22:81, 1986.
60. Taleisnik J: Carpal instability. J Bone Joint Surg [Am] 70:1262, 1988.
61. Herbert TJ, Faithfull RG, McCann DJ, et al: Bilateral arthrography of the wrist. J Hand Surg [Br] 15:233, 1990.
62. Wilson AJ, Gilula LA, Mann FA: Unidirectional joint communications in wrist arthrography: An evaluation of 250 cases. AJR 157:105, 1991.
63. Gilula LA, Hardy DC, Totty WG, et al: Fluoroscopic identification of torn intercarpal ligaments after injection of contrast material. AJR 149:761, 1987.
64. Manaster BJ: Digital wrist arthrography: Precision in determining the site of radiocarpal-midcarpal communication. AJR 147:563, 1986.
65. Belsole RJ, Quinn SF, Greene TL, et al: Digital subtraction arthrography of the wrist. J Bone Joint Surg [Am] 72:846, 1990.
66. Mitchell DG, Kressel HY: MR imaging of early avascular necrosis. Radiology 169:281, 1988.
67. Mitchell DG: Using MR imaging to probe the pathophysiology of osteonecrosis. Radiology 171:25, 1989.

68. Mitchell DG, Rao VM, Dalinka MK, et al: Femoral head avascular necrosis: Correlation of MR imaging, radiographic staging, radionuclide imaging and clinical findings. Radiology *162*:709, 1987.

69. Koenig H, Lucas D, Meissner R: The wrist: A preliminary report on high-resolution MR imaging. Radiology *160*:463, 1986.

70. Reinus WR, Conway WF, Totty WG, et al: Carpal avascular necrosis: MR imaging. Radiology *160*:689, 1986.

71. Sowa DT, Holder LE, Patt PG, et al: Application of magnetic resonance imaging to ischemic necrosis of the lunate. J Hand Surg [Am] *14*:1008, 1989.

72. Gelberman RH, Wolock BS, Siegel DB: Fractures and non-unions of the carpal scaphoid. J Bone Joint Surg [Am] *71*:1560, 1989.

73. Wilton TJ: Soft-tissue interposition as a possible cause of scaphoid non-union. J Hand Surg [Br] *12*:50, 1987.

74. Kerluke L, McCabe SJ: Nonunion of the scaphoid: A critical analysis of recent natural history studies. J Hand Surg [Am] *18*:1, 1993.

75. Szabo RM, Manske D: Displaced fractures of the scaphoid. Clin Orthop *230*:30, 1988.

76. Dias JJ, Taylor M, Thompson J, et al: Radiographic signs of union of scaphoid fractures. An analysis of inter-observer agreement and reproducibility. J Bone Joint Surg [Br] *70*:299, 1988.

77. Gooding GAW: Tenosynovitis of the wrist: a sonographic demonstration. J Ultrasound Med *7*:225, 1988.

78. John V, Nau HE, Nahsen HC, et al: CT of carpal tunnel syndrome. ÁJNR *4*:770, 1983.

79. Merhar GL, Clark RA, Schneider HJ, et al: High-resolution computed tomography of the wrist in patients with carpal tunnel syndrome. Skel Radiol *15*:549, 1986.

80. Zucker-Pinchoff B, Hermann G, Srinivasan R: Computed tomography of the carpal tunnel: a radioanatomical study. J Comput Assist Tomogr *5*:525, 1981.

81. Mesgarzadeh M, Schneck CD, Bonakdarpour A, et al: Carpal tunnel: MR imaging. Part II. Carpal tunnel syndrome. Radiology *171*:749, 1989.

82. Middleton WD, Kneeland JB, Kellman GM, et al: MR imaging of the carpal tunnel: Normal anatomy and preliminary findings in the carpal tunnel syndrome. AJR *148*:307, 1987.

83. Fullerton GD, Cameron IL, Ord VA: Orientation of tendons in the magnetic field and its effect on T2 relaxation times. Radiology *155*:433, 1985.

84. Erickson SJ, Cox IH, Hyde JS, et al: Effect of tendon orientation on MR imaging signal intensity: A manifestation of the ''magic angle'' phenomenon. Radiology *181*:389, 1991.

85. Campbell JD, Feagin JA, King P, et al: Ulnar collateral ligament injury of the thumb: treatment with glove spica cast. Am J Sports Med *20*:29, 1992.

86. Stener B: Displacement of the ruptured ulnar collateral ligament of the metacarpophalangeal joint of the thumb. J Bone Joint Surg [Am] *68*:1320, 1986.

87. Resnick D, Danzig LA: Arthrographic evaluation of injuries of the first metacarpophalangeal joint: Gamekeeper's thumb. AJR *126*:1046, 1976.

88. Linscheid RL: Arthrography of the metacarpophalangeal joint. Clin Orthop *103*:91, 1974.

89. Bowers WH, Hurst LC: Gamekeeper's thumb. Evaluation by arthrography and stress roentgenography. J Bone Joint Surg [Am] *59*:519, 1977.

90. Spaeth HJ, Abrams RA, Bock GW, et al: Gamekeeper thumb: Differentiation of nondisplaced and displaced tears of the ulnar collateral ligament with MR imaging. Work in progress. Radiology *188*:553, 1993.

91. Morrey BF, An K-N: Functional anatomy of the ligaments of the elbow. Clin Orthop *201*:84, 1985.

92. Middleton WD, Macrander S, Kneeland JB, et al: MR imaging of the normal elbow: Anatomic considerations. AJR *149*:543, 1987.

93a. Bunnell DH, Fisher DA, Bassett LW, et al: Elbow joint: Normal anatomy on MR images. Radiology *165*:527, 1987.

93b. Cirincione RJ, Baker BE: Tendon ruptures with secondary hyperparathyroidism. A case report. J Bone Joint Surg [Am] *57*:852, 1975.

94. Match RM, Corrylos EV: Bilateral avulsion fracture of the triceps tendon insertion from skiing with osteogenesis imperfecta tarda. Am J Sports Med *11*:99, 1983.

95. Jorgensen U, Hinge K, Rye B: Rupture of the distal biceps brachii tendon. J Trauma *26*:1061, 1986.

96. Levy M, Fischel RE, Stern GM: Triceps tendon avulsion with or without fracture of the radial head—a rare injury? J Trauma *18*:677, 1978.

97. Davis WM, Jassine Z: An etiologic factor in the tear of the distal tendon of the biceps brachii. J Bone Joint Surg [Am] *38*:1365, 1956.

98. Farrar EL III, Lippert FG: Avulsion of the triceps tendon. Clin Orthop *161*:242, 1981.

99. Barr LL, Babcock DS: Sonography of the normal elbow. AJR *157*:793, 1991.

100. Murphy BJ: MR imaging of the elbow. Radiology *184*:525, 1992.

101. Schwab GH, Bennett JB, Woods GW, et al: Biomechanics of elbow instability: The role of the medial collateral ligament. Clin Orthop *146*:42, 1980.

102. Sojbjerg JO, Ovesen J, Nielsen S: Experimental elbow instability after transection of the medial collateral ligament. Clin Orthop *218*:186, 1987.

103. Hotchkiss RN, Weiland AJ: Valgus stability of the elbow. J Orthop Res *5*:372, 1987.

104. Mirowitz SA, London SL: Ulnar collateral ligament injury in baseball pitchers: MR imaging evaluation. Radiology *185*:573, 1992.

105. Morrey BF, Tanaka S, An KNA: Valgus stability of the elbow: a definition of primary and secondary constraints. Clin Orthop *201*:84, 1991.

106. Kuroda S, Sakamaki K: Ulnar collateral ligament tears of the elbow joint. Clin Orthop *208*:266, 1986.

107. Bora FW, Osterman AL: Compression neuropathy. Clin Orthop *163*:20, 1982

108. Vanderpool DW, Chalmers J, Lamb DW, et al: Peripheral compression lesions of the ulnar nerve. J Bone Joint Surg [Br] *50*:792, 1968.

109. Feindel W, Stratford J: Cubital tunnel compression. Can Med Assoc J *78*:351, 1958.

110. Osborne GV: Surgical treatment of tardy ulnar neuritis. J Bone Joint Surg [Br] *39*:782, 1957.

111. St John JN, Palmaz JC: The cubital tunnel in ulnar entrapment neuropathy. Radiology *158*:119, 1986.

112. Rosenberg ZS, Beltran J, Cheung YY, et al: The elbow: MR features of nerve disorders. Radiology *188*:235, 1993.

113. Lichter R, Jacobson T: Tardy palsy of the posterior interosseous nerve with Monteggia fracture. J Bone Joint Surg [Am] *57*:124, 1975.

114. Millender LH, Nalebuff EA, Holdsworth DE: Posterior interosseous nerve syndrome secondary to rheumatoid synovitis. J Bone Joint Surg [Am] *55*:753, 1973.

115. Yates C, Sullivan JA: Arthrographic diagnosis of elbow injuries in children. J Pediatr Orthop *7*:54, 1987.

116. Jaramillo D, Laor T, Zaleske DJ: Indirect trauma to the growth plate: Results of MR imaging after epiphyseal and metaphyseal injury in rabbits. Radiology *187*:171, 1993.

117. Jaramillo D, Hoffer FA: Cartilaginous epiphysis and growth plate: Normal and abnormal MR imaging findings. AJR *158*:1105, 1992.

118. Leffert RD, Dorfman HD: Antecubital cyst in rheumatoid arthritis—surgical findings. J Bone Joint Surg [Am] *54*:1555, 1972.

119. Ehrlich GE, Guttmann GG: Valvular mechanisms in antecubital cysts of rheumatoid arthritis. Arthritis Rheum *16*:259, 1973.

120. Ehrlich GE: Antecubital cysts in rheumatoid arthritis—a corollary to popliteal (Baker's) cysts. J Bone Joint Surg [Am] *54*:165, 1972.

121. Pirani M, Lange-Mechlen I, Cockshott WP: Rupture of a posterior synovial cyst of the elbow. J Rheumatol *9*:94, 1982.

122. Ogilvie-Harris DJ, Schemitsch E: Arthroscopy of the elbow for removal of loose bodies. Arthros: J Arthros Rel Surg *9*:5, 1993.

123. O'Driscoll SW, Morrey BF: Arthroscopy of the elbow. Diagnostic and therapeutic benefits and hazards. J Bone Joint Surg [Am] *74*:84, 1992.

124. O'Brien SJ, Arnoczky SP, Warren RF, et al: Developmental anatomy of the shoulder and anatomy of the glenohumeral joint. *In* CA Rockwood, Jr and FA Matsen III (Eds): The Shoulder. Philadelphia, WB Saunders Co, 1990, p. 1.

125. Cone RO, Danzig L, Resnick D, et al: The bicipital groove: a radiographic, anatomic, and pathologic study. AJR *141*:781, 1983.

126. Saha AK: Dynamic stability of the glenohumeral joint. Acta Orthop Scand *42*:491, 1971.

127. Sarrafian SK: Gross and functional anatomy of the shoulder. Clin Orthop *173*:11, 1983.

128. Saha AK: Mechanism of shoulder movements and a plea for the recognition of the ''zero position'' of the glenohumeral joint. Clin Orthop *173*:3, 1983.

129. Friedman RJ, Hawthorne KB, Genez BM: The use of computerized tomography in the measurement of glenoid version. J Bone Joint Surg [Am] *74*:1032, 1992.

130. Petersson CJ, Redlund-Johnell I: Joint space in normal glenohumeral radiographs. Acta Orthop Scand *54*:274, 1983.

131. Petersson CJ, Redlund-Johnell I: The subacromial space in normal shoulder radiographs. Acta Orthop Scand *55*:57, 1984.

132. Gradoyevitch B: Coracoclavicular joint. J Bone Joint Surg *21*:918, 1939.

133. Nutter PD: Coracoclavicular articulations. J Bone Joint Surg *23*:177, 1941.

134. Wertheimer LG: Coracoclavicular joint. J Bone Joint Surg [Am] *30*:570, 1948.

135. Redlund-Johnell I: The costoclavicular joint. Skel Radiol *15*:25, 1986.

136. Cockshott WP: The coracoclavicular joint. Radiology *131*:313, 1979.

137. Uhthoff HK, Piscopo M: Anterior capsular redundancy of the shoulder: Congenital or traumatic? An embryological study. J Bone Joint Surg [Br] *67*:363, 1985.

138. Killoran PJ, Marcove RC, Freiberger RH: Shoulder arthrography. AJR *103*:658, 1968.

139. Weston WJ: Subdeltoid bursa. Australas Radiol *17*:214, 1973.

140. Weston WJ: The enlarged subdeltoid bursa in rheumatoid arthritis. Br J Radiol *42*:481, 1969.

141. Mitchell MJ, Causey G, Berthoty DP, et al: Peribursal fat plane of the shoulder: Anatomic study and clinical experience. Radiology *168*:699, 1988.

142. DePalma AF: Surgical anatomy of the acromioclavicular and sternoclavicular joints. Surg Clin North Am *43*:1541, 1963.

143. Weston WJ: Arthrography of the acromioclavicular joint. Australas Radiol *18*:213, 1974.

144. DePalma AF, Callery G, Bennett GA: Shoulder joint: variational anatomy and degenerative lesions of the shoulder joint. AAOS Instructional Course Lectures *6*:255, 1949.

145. O'Brien SJ, Neves MC, Rozbuck RS, et al: The anatomy and histology of the inferior glenohumeral complex of the shoulder. Paper presented at the Annual Meeting of the Shoulder and Elbow Society, February 1989, Las Vegas, Nevada.

146. Moseley HF, Overgaard B: The anterior capsular mechanism in recurrent anterior dislocation of the shoulder. Morphological and clinical studies with special reference to the glenoid labrum and gleno-humeral ligaments. J Bone Joint Surg [Br] *44*:913, 1962.

147. Turkel SJ, Panio MW, Marshall JL, et al: Stabilizing mechanisms preventing anterior dislocation of the glenohumeral joint. J Bone Joint Surg [Am] *63*:1208, 1981.

148. Schwartz RE, O'Brien SJ, Warren RF, et al: Capsular restraints to anterior-posterior motion of the abducted shoulder: a biomechanical study. Orthop Trans 12:727, 1988.

149. Edelson JG, Taitz C, Grishkan A: The coracohumeral ligament. Anatomy of a substantial but neglected structure. J Bone Joint Surg [Br] 73:150, 1991.

150. Neer CS II, Satterlee CC, Dalsey RM, et al: The anatomy and potential effects of contracture of the coracohumeral ligament. Clin Orthop 280:182, 1992.

151. Basmajian JV, Bazant FJ: Factors preventing downward dislocation of the adducted shoulder joint. J Bone Joint Surg [Am] 41:1182, 1959.

152. Ovesen J, Nielsen S: Experimental distal subluxation in the glenohumeral joint. Arch Orthop Trauma Surg 104:78, 1985.

153. Cooper DE, Arnoczky SP, O'Brien SJ, et al: Anatomy, histology, and vascularity of the glenoid labrum. An anatomical study. J Bone Joint Surg [Am] 74:46, 1992.

154. Prodromos CC, Ferry JA, Schiller AL: Histological studies of the glenoid labrum from fetal life to old age. J Bone Joint Surg [Am] 72:1344, 1990.

155. Rafii M, Minkoff J, Bonamo J, et al: CT arthrography of shoulder instabilities in athletes. Am J Sports Med 16:352, 1988.

156. McNeish LM, Callaghan JJ: CT arthrography of the shoulder: variations of the glenoid labrum. AJR 149:963, 1987.

157. Neumann CH, Petersen SA, Jahnke AH: MR imaging of the labral-capsular complex: Normal variations. AJR 157:1015, 1991.

158. Bankart ASB: Recurrent or habitual dislocation of the shoulder joint. Br Med J 2:132, 1923.

159. Bankart ASB: The pathology and treatment of recurrent dislocation of the shoulder joint. Br J Surg 26:23, 1938.

160. McLaughlin HL, Cavallaro WU: Primary anterior dislocation of the shoulder. Am J Surg 80:615, 1950.

161. Jobe CM: Gross anatomy of the shoulder. In CA Rockwood Jr and FA Matsen III (Eds): The Shoulder. Philadelphia, WB Saunders Co, 1990, p 34.

162. Kronberg M, Németh G, Broström L-A: Muscle activity and coordination in the normal shoulder. Clin Orthop 257:76, 1990.

163. Keating JF, Waterworth P, Shaw-Dunn J, et al: The relative strengths of the rotator cuff muscles. A cadaver study. J Bone Joint Surg [Br] 75:137, 1993.

164. Bassett RW, Browne AO, Morrey BF, et al: Glenohumeral muscle force and moment mechanics in a position of shoulder instability. J Biomech 23:405, 1990.

165. Kannus P, Jozsa L: Histopathological changes preceding spontaneous rupture of a tendon. A controlled study of 891 patients. J Bone Joint Surg [Am] 73:1507, 1991.

166. Brewer BJ: Aging of the rotator cuff. Am J Sports Med 7:102, 1979.

167. Clark J, Sidles JA, Matsen FA: The relationship of the glenohumeral joint capsule to the rotator cuff. Clin Orthop 254:29, 1990.

168. Harryman DT, Sidles JA, Harris SL, et al: The role of the rotator interval capsule in passive motion and stability of the shoulder. J Bone Joint Surg [Am] 74:53, 1992.

169. Rothman RH, Parke WW: The vascular anatomy of the rotator cuff. Clin Orthop 41:176, 1965.

170. Brooks CH, Revell WJ, Heatley FW: A quantitative histological study of the vascularity of the rotator cuff tendon. J Bone Joint Surg [Br] 74:151, 1992.

171. Sarkar K, Taine W, Uhthoff HK: The ultrastructure of the coracoacromial ligament in patients with chronic impingement syndrome. Clin Orthop 254:49, 1990.

172. Dines DM, Warren RF, Inglis AE, et al: The coracoid impingement syndrome. J Bone Joint Surg [Br] 72:314, 1990.

173. Edelson JG, Zuckerman J, Hershkovitz I: Os acromiale: Anatomy and surgical implications. J Bone Joint Surg [Br] 74:551, 1993.

174. Gagey N, Ravaud E, Lassau JP: Anatomy of the acromial arch: correlation of anatomy and magnetic resonance imaging. Surg Radiol Anat 15:63, 1993.

175. Edelson JG, Taitz C: Anatomy of the coraco-acromial arch. Relation to degeneration of the acromion. J Bone Joint Surg [Br] 74:589, 1992.

176. Bigliani LH, Morrison DS, April EW: The morphology of the acromion and its relationship to rotator cuff tears. Orthop Trans 10:228, 1986.

177. Neer CS, Poppen NK: Supraspinatus outlet. Orthop Trans 11:234, 1987.

178. Kitchel SH, Butters KA, Rockwood CA: The shoulder impingement syndrome. Orthop Trans 8:510, 1984.

179. Rockwood CA Jr, Lyons FR: Shoulder impingement syndrome: Diagnosis, radiographic evaluation and treatment with a modified Neer acromioplasty. J Bone Joint Surg [Am] 75:409, 1993.

180. Beaton LE, Anson BJ: Variation of the origin of the m. trapezius. Anat Rec 83:41, 1942.

181. Neer CS II: Anterior acromioplasty for the chronic impingement syndrome in the shoulder. A preliminary report. J Bone Joint Surg [Am] 54:41, 1972.

182. Neer CS II: Impingement lesions. Clin Orthop 173:70, 1983.

183. Neer CS II, Bigliani LU, Hawkins RJ: Rupture of the long head of the biceps related to subacromial impingement. Orthop Trans 1:111, 1977.

184. Neer CS II, Welsh RP: The shoulder in sports. Orthop Clin North Am 8:583, 1977.

185. Matsen FA III, Arntz CT: Subacromial impingement. In CA Rockwood Jr and FA Matsen III (Eds): The Shoulder. Philadelphia, WB Saunders Co, 1990, p 623.

186. Rathbun JB, Macnab I: The microvascular pattern of the rotator cuff. J Bone Joint Surg [Br] 52:540, 1970.

187. Sigholm G, Styf J, Körner L, et al: Pressure recording in the subacromial bursa. J Orthop Res 6:123, 1988.

188. Fu FH, Harner CD, Klein AH: Shoulder impingement syndrome. A critical review. Clin Orthop 269:162, 1991.

189. Jobe FW, Kvitne RS: Shoulder pain in the overhand or throwing athlete: The relationship of anterior instability and rotator cuff impingement. Orthop Rev 18:963, 1989.

190. Miniaci A, Fowler PJ: Impingement in the athlete. Clin Sports Med 12:91, 1993.

191. Fowler PJ, Webster MS: Shoulder pain in highly competitive swimmers. Orthop Trans 7:170, 1983.

192. Hawkins RJ, Abrams JS: Impingement syndrome in the absence of rotator cuff tear (Stages 1 and 2). Orthop Clin North Am 18:373, 1987.

193. Berens DL, Lockie LM: Ossification of the coraco-acromial ligament. Radiology 74:802, 1959.

194. Cone RO III, Resnick D, Danzig L: Shoulder impingement syndrome: Radiographic evaluation. Radiology 150:29, 1984.

195. Kieft GJ, Bloem JL, Rozing PM, et al: Rotator cuff impingement syndrome: MR imaging. Radiology 166:211, 1988.

196. Seeger LL, Gold RH, Bassett LW, et al: Shoulder impingement syndrome: MR findings in 53 shoulders. AJR 150:343, 1988.

197. Seeger L: Magnetic resonance imaging of the shoulder. Clin Orthop 244:48, 1989.

198. Chandnani V, Ho C, Gerharter J, et al: MR findings in asymptomatic shoulders: A blind analysis using symptomatic shoulders as controls. Clin Imag 16:25, 1992.

199. Epstein RE, Schweitzer ME, Frieman BG, et al: Hooked acromion: Prevalence on MR images of painful shoulders. Radiology 187:479, 1993.

200. Kaplan PA, Bryans KC, Davick JP, et al: MR imaging of the normal shoulder: Variants and pitfalls. Radiology 184:519, 1992.

201. Gartsman GM: Arthroscopic acromioplasty for lesions of the rotator cuff. J Bone Joint Surg [Am] 72:169, 1990.

202. Hurley J, Bronstein R: Shoulder arthroscopy in the athlete. Practical applications. Sports Med 15:133, 1993.

203. Owen RS, Iannotti JP, Kneeland JB, et al: Shoulder after surgery: MR imaging with surgical validation. Radiology 186:443, 1993.

204. Matsen FA III, Arntz CT: Rotator cuff tendon failure. In CA Rockwood Jr and FA Matsen III (Eds): The Shoulder. Philadelphia, WB Saunders Co, 1990, p 647.

205. Cofield RH: Rotator cuff disease of the shoulder. J Bone Joint Surg [Am] 67:974, 1985.

206. Patte D: Classification of rotator cuff lesions. Clin Orthop 254:81, 1990.

207. Keyes EL: Observations on rupture of the supraspinatus tendon. Based upon a study of 73 cadavers. Ann Surg 97:849, 1933.

208. Wilson CL, Duff GL: Pathologic study of degeneration and rupture of the supraspinatus tendon. Arch Surg 47:121, 1943.

209. Cotton RE, Rideout DF: Tears of the humeral rotator cuff. A radiological and pathological necropsy study. J Bone Joint Surg [Br] 46:314, 1964.

210. Fukuda H, Mikasa M, Ogawa K, et al: The partial thickness tear of the rotator cuff. Orthop Trans 7:137, 1983.

211. Pettersson G: Rupture of the tendon aponeurosis of the shoulder joint in anterior inferior dislocation. Acta Chir Scand (Suppl) 77:1, 1942.

212. Gerber C, Krushell RJ: Isolated rupture of the tendon of the subscapularis muscle. Clinical features in 16 cases. J Bone Joint Surg [Br] 73:389, 1991.

213. Neviaser RJ, Neviaser TJ, Neviaser JS: Concurrent rupture of the rotator cuff and anterior dislocation of the shoulder in the older patient. J Bone Joint Surg [Am] 70:1308, 1988.

214. McAuliffe TB, Dowd GS: Avulsion of the subscapularis tendon. A case report. J Bone Joint Surg [Am] 69:1454, 1987.

215. Lohr JF, Uhthoff HK: The microvascular pattern of the supraspinatus tendon. Clin Orthop 254:35, 1990.

216. Meyer AW: The minute anatomy of attrition lesions. J Bone Joint Surg [Am] 13:341, 1931.

217. Brewer BJ: Aging of the rotator cuff. Am J Sports Med 7:102, 1979.

218. Ozaki J, Fujimoto S, Nakagawa Y, et al: Tears of the rotator cuff of the shoulder associated with pathological changes in the acromion. A study in cadavera. J Bone Joint Surg [Am] 70:1224, 1988.

219. Hijioka A, Suzuki K, Nakamura T, et al: Degenerative change and rotator cuff tears. An anatomical study in 160 shoulders of 80 cadavers. Arch Orthop Trauma Surg 112:61, 1993.

220. Ogata S, Uhthoff HK: Acromial enthesopathy and rotator cuff tear. A radiologic and histologic postmortem investigation of the coracoacromial arch. Clin Orthop 254:39, 1990.

221. Kjellin I, Ho CP, Cervilla V, et al: Alterations in the supraspinatus tendon at MR imaging: correlation with histopathologic findings in cadavers. Radiology 181:837, 1991.

222. Jim YF, Hsu HC, Chang CY, et al: Coexistence of calcific tendinitis and rotator cuff tear: an arthrographic study. Skel Radiol 22:183, 1993.

223. Bloom RA: The active abduction view: a new maneuvre in the diagnosis of rotator cuff tears. Skel Radiol 20:255, 1991.

224. Kotzen LM: Roentgen diagnosis of rotator cuff tear. Report of 48 surgically proven cases. AJR 112:507, 1971.

225. DeSmet AA, Ting YM: Diagnosis of rotator cuff tear on routine radiographs. J Can Assoc Radiol 28:54, 1977.

226. Golding C: Radiology and orthopedic surgery. J Bone Joint Surg [Br] 48:320, 1966.

227. Garcia JF: Arthrographic visualization of rotator cuff tears. Optimal application of stress to the shoulder. Radiology 150:595, 1984.

228. Kilcoyne RF, Matsen FA III: Rotator cuff tear measured by arthropneumotomography. AJR *140*:315, 1983.

229. Beltran J, Gray L, Bools JC, et al: Rotator cuff lesions of the shoulder: Evaluation by direct sagittal CT arthrography. Radiology *160*:161, 1986.

230. Blum A, Boyer B, Regent D, et al: Direct coronal view of the shoulder with arthrographic CT. Radiology *188*:677, 1993.

231. Stiles RG, Resnick D, Sartoris DJ, et al: Rotator cuff disruption: Diagnosis with digital arthrography. Radiology *168*:705, 1988.

232. Resnik CS, Fronek J, Frey C, et al: Intra-articular pressure determination during glenohumeral joint arthrography. Preliminary investigation. Invest Radiol *19*:45, 1984.

233. Bjorkenheim J-M, Paavolainen P, Ahovuo J, et al: The intraarticular pressure during shoulder arthrography. A diagnostic aid in rotator cuff tear. Acta Orthop Scand *58*:128, 1987.

234. Craig EV: The geyser sign and torn rotator cuff: Clinical significance and pathomechanics. Clin Orthop *191*:213, 1984.

235. Craig EV: The acromioclavicular joint cyst. An unusual presentation of a rotator cuff tear. Clin Orthop *202*:189, 1986.

236. Goldman AB, Ghelman B: The double-contrast shoulder arthrogram. A review of 158 studies. Radiology *127*:655, 1978.

237. Mink JH, Harris E, Rappaport M: Rotator cuff tears: Evaluation using double-contrast shoulder arthrography. Radiology *157*:621, 1985.

238. Killoran PJ, Marcove RC, Freiberger RH: Shoulder arthrography. AJR *103*:658, 1957.

239. Fukuda H, Mikasa M, Yamanaka K: Incomplete thickness rotator cuff tears diagnosed by subacromial bursography. Clin Orthop *223*:51, 1987.

240. Preston BJ, Jackson JP: Investigation of shoulder disability by arthrography. Clin Radiol *28*:259, 1977.

241. Burk DL, Karasick D, Kurtz AB, et al: Rotator cuff tears: prospective comparison of MR imaging with arthrography, sonography, and surgery. AJR *153*:87, 1989.

242. Davis SJ, Teresi LM, Bradley WG, et al: Effect of arm rotation on MR imaging of the rotator cuff. Radiology *181*:265, 1991.

243. Huber DJ, Sauter R, Mueller E, et al: MR imaging of the normal shoulder. Radiology *158*:405, 1986.

244. Kneeland JB, Middleton WD, Carrera WD, et al: MR imaging of the shoulder: Diagnosis of rotator cuff tears. AJR *149*:333, 1987.

245. Reeder JD, Andelman S: The rotator cuff tear: MR evaluation. Magn Res Imag *5*:331, 1987.

246. Evancho AM, Stiles RG, Fajman WA, et al: MR imaging diagnosis of rotator cuff tears. AJR *151*:751, 1988.

247. Zlatkin MB, Reicher MA, Kellerhouse LE, et al: The painful shoulder: MR imaging of the glenohumeral joint. J Comput Assist Tomogr *12*:995, 1988.

248. Buirski G: Magnetic resonance imaging in acute and chronic rotator cuff tears. Skel Radiol *19*:109, 1990.

249. Seeger LL, Ruszkowski JT, Bassett LW, et al: MR imaging of the normal shoulder: Anatomic correlation. AJR *148*:83, 1987.

250. Middleton WD, Kneeland JB, Carrera GF, et al: High-resolution MR imaging of the normal rotator cuff. AJR *148*:559, 1987.

251. Neumann CH, Holt RG, Steinbach LS, et al: MR imaging of the shoulder: Appearance of the supraspinatus tendon in asymptomatic volunteers. AJR *158*:1281, 1992.

252. Mirowitz SA: Normal rotator cuff: MR imaging with conventional and fat-suppression techniques. Radiology *180*:735, 1991.

253. Vahlensieck M, Pollack M, Lang P, et al: Two segments of the supraspinous muscle: Cause of high signal intensity at MR imaging? Radiology *186*:449, 1993.

254. Liou JTS, Wilson AJ, Totty WG, et al: The normal shoulder: Common variations that simulate pathologic conditions at MR imaging. Radiology *186*:435, 1993.

255. Zlatkin MB, Iannotti JP, Roberts MC, et al: Rotator cuff tears: Diagnostic performance of MR imaging. Radiology *172*:223, 1989.

256. Holt RG, Helms CA, Steinbach L, et al: Magnetic resonance imaging of the shoulder: rationale and current applications. Skel Radiol *19*:5, 1990.

257. Rafii M, Firooznia H, Sherman O, et al: Rotator cuff lesions: Signal patterns at MR imaging. Radiology *177*:817, 1990.

258. Meyer SJF, Dalinka MK: Magnetic resonance imaging of the shoulder. Semin Ultrasound CT MR *11*:253, 1990.

259. Iannotti JP, Zlatkin MB, Esterhai JL, et al: Magnetic resonance imaging of the shoulder. Sensitivity, specificity, and predictive value. J Bone Joint Surg [Am] *73*:17, 1991.

260. Nelson MC, Leather GP, Nirschl RP: Evaluation of the painful shoulder. A prospective comparison of magnetic resonance imaging, computerized tomographic arthrography, ultrasonography, and operative findings. J Bone Joint Surg [Am] *73*:707, 1991.

261. Hodler J, Terrier B, von Schulthess GK, et al: MRI and sonography of the shoulder. Clin Radiol *43*:323, 1991.

262. Farley TE, Neumann CH, Steinbach LS, et al: Full-thickness tears of the rotator cuff of the shoulder: Diagnosis with MR imaging. AJR *158*:347, 1992.

263. Hodler J, Kursunoglu-Brahme S, Snyder SJ, et al: Rotator cuff disease: Assessment with MR arthrography versus standard MR imaging in 36 patients with arthroscopic confirmation. Radiology *182*:431, 1992.

264. Karzel RP, Snyder SJ: Magnetic resonance arthrography of the shoulder. A new technique of shoulder imaging. Clin Sports Med *12*:123, 1993.

265. Fritz RC, Stoller DW: Fat-suppression MR arthrography of the shoulder. Radiology *185*:614, 1992.

266. Palmer WE, Brown JH, Rosenthal DI: Rotator cuff: Evaluation with fat-suppressed MR arthrography. Radiology *188*:683, 1993.

267. Andrews JR, Broussard TS, Carson WG: Arthroscopy of the shoulder in the management of partial tears of the rotator cuff: A preliminary report. Arthroscopy *1*:117, 1985.

268. Itoi E, Tabata S: Incomplete rotator cuff tears. Results of operative treatment. Clin Orthop *284*:128, 1992.

269. Traughber PD, Goodwin TE: Shoulder MRI: Arthroscopic correlation with emphasis on partial tears. J Comput Assist Tomogr *16*:129, 1992.

270. Flannigan B, Kursunoglu-Brahme S, Snyder S, et al: MR arthrography of the shoulder: Comparison with conventional MR imaging. AJR *155*:829, 1990.

271. Samilson RL, Binder WF: Symptomatic full thickness tears of the rotator cuff: An analysis of 292 shoulders in 276 patients. Orthop Clin North Am *6*:449, 1975.

272. Neer CS, Marberry TA: On the disadvantages of radical acromionectomy. J Bone Joint Surg [Am] *63*:416, 1981.

273. Ellman H, Hanker G, Bayer M: Repair of the rotator cuff. End-result study of factors influencing reconstruction. J Bone Joint Surg [Am] *68*:1136, 1986.

274. Ellman H: Diagnosis and treatment of incomplete rotator cuff tears. Clin Orthop *254*:64, 1990.

275. Calvert PT, Packer NP, Stoker DJ, et al: Arthrography of the shoulder after operative repair of the torn rotator cuff. J Bone Joint Surg [Br] *68*:147, 1986.

276. Mack LA, Nyberg DA, Matsen FA III, et al: Sonography of the postoperative shoulder. AJR *150*:1089, 1988.

277. Luck JV Jr, Andersson GBJ: Occupational shoulder disorders. *In* CA Rockwood Jr and FA Matsen III (Eds): The Shoulder. Philadelphia, WB Saunders Co, 1990, p 1088.

278. Nirschl RP, Pettrone F: Tennis elbow: The surgical treatment of lateral epicondylitis. J Bone Joint Surg [Am] *61*:832, 1979.

279. Burk DL Jr, Karasick D, Mitchell DG, et al: MR imaging of the shoulder: Correlation with plain radiography. AJR *154*:549, 1990.

280. Murnaghan JP: Frozen shoulder. *In* CA Rockwood Jr and FA Matsen III (Eds): The Shoulder. Philadelphia, WB Saunders Co, 1990, p 837.

281. Lundberg BJ: The frozen shoulder. Acta Orthop Scand (Suppl) *119*:1, 1969.

282. Kay N: The clinical diagnosis and management of frozen shoulders. Practitioner *225*:164, 1981.

283. Withers RJW: The painful shoulder: review of one hundred personal cases with remarks on the pathology. J Bone Joint Surg *31*:414, 1949.

284. Reeves B: Arthrographic changes in frozen and post-traumatic stiff shoulders. Proc R Soc Med *59*:827, 1966.

285. Neviaser JS: Adhesive capsulitis of the shoulder. A study of the pathological findings in periarthritis of the shoulder. J Bone Joint Surg *27*:211, 1945.

286. McLaughlin HL: On the frozen shoulder. Bull Hosp Jt Dis *12*:383, 1951.

287. Simmonds FA: Shoulder pain with particular reference to the frozen shoulder. J Bone Joint Surg *31*:834, 1949.

288. Macnab I: Rotator cuff tendinitis. Ann R Coll Surg Engl *53*:271, 1973.

289. Lippman RK: Frozen shoulder; periarthritis; bicipital tenosynovitis. Arch Surg *47*:283, 1943.

290. Lidström A: Den "frusna" skuldran. Nord Med *69*:125, 1963.

291. Weber J, Kecskés S: Arthrografie bei Periarthritis humeroscapularis. ROFO *124*:573, 1976.

292. Andrén L, Lundberg BJ: Treatment of rigid shoulders by joint distention during arthrography. Acta Orthop Scand *36*:45, 1965.

293. Binder AI, Balgen DY, Hazleman BL, et al: Frozen shoulder: An arthrographic and radionuclear scan assessment. Ann Rheum Dis *43*:365, 1984.

294. Resnick D: Frozen shoulder. Ann Rheum Dis *44*:805, 1985.

295. Resnik CS, Fronek J, Frey C, et al: Intra-articular pressure determination during glenohumeral joint arthrography. Preliminary investigation. Invest Radiol *19*:45, 1984.

296. Gilula LA, Schoenecker PL, Murphy WA: Shoulder arthrography as a treatment modality. AJR *131*:1047, 1978.

297. Wright MG, Richards AJ, Clarke MB: 99-m pertechnetate scanning in capsulitis. Lancet *2*:1265, 1975.

298. Ogilvie-Harris DJ, Wiley AM: Arthroscopic surgery of the shoulder. J Bone Joint Surg [Am] *68*:201, 1986.

299. Neviaser TJ: Arthroscopy of the shoulder. Orthop Clin North Am *18*:361, 1987.

300. Howell SM, Galinat BJ, Renzi AJ, et al: Normal and abnormal mechanics of the glenohumeral joint in the horizontal plane. J Bone Joint Surg [Am] *70*:227, 1988.

301. Matsen FA III, Thomas SC, Rockwood CA Jr: Glenohumeral instability. *In* CA Rockwood Jr and FA Matsen III (Eds): The Shoulder. Philadelphia, WB Saunders Co, 1990, p 526.

302. Rowe CR, Zarins B: Recurrent transient subluxation of the shoulder. J Bone Joint Surg [Am] *63*:863, 1981.

303. Kazar B, Relovszky E: Prognosis of primary dislocation of the shoulder. Acta Orthop Scand *40*:216, 1969.

304. Galinat BJ, Warren RF, Buss DD: Pathophysiology of shoulder instability. *In* JB McGinty (Ed): Operative Arthroscopy. New York, Raven Press, 1991.

305. Stiles RG, Otte MT: Imaging of the shoulder. Radiology *188*:603, 1993.

306. Cyprien JM, Vasey HM, Burdet A, et al: Humeral retrotorsion and glenohumeral relationship in the normal shoulder and in recurrent anterior dislocation. Clin Orthop *175*:8, 1983.

307. Brewer BJ, Wubben RC, Carrera GF: Excessive retroversion of the glenoid cavity. A cause of non-traumatic posterior instability of the shoulder. J Bone Joint Surg [Am] *68*:724, 1986.

308. Pavlov H, Warren RF, Weiss CB Jr, et al: The roentgenographic evaluation of anterior shoulder instability. Clin Orthop 194:153, 1985.

309. El-Khoury GY, Albright JP, Abu Yousef MM, et al: Arthrotomography of the glenoid labrum. Radiology 131:333, 1979.

310. Braunstein EM, O'Connor G: Double-contrast arthrotomography of the shoulder. J Bone Joint Surg [Am] 64:192, 1982.

311. Kleinman PK, Kanzaria PK, Goss TP, et al: Axillary arthrotomography of the glenoid labrum. AJR 141:993, 1984.

312. McGlynn FJ, El-Khoury GY, Albright JP: Arthrography of the glenoid labrum in shoulder instability. J Bone Joint Surg [Am] 64:506, 1982.

313. El-Khoury GY, Kathol MH, Chandler JB, et al: Shoulder instability: Impact of glenohumeral arthrotomography on treatment. Radiology 160:669, 1986.

314. Kneisl JS, Sweeney HJ, Paige ML: Correlation of pathology observed in double contrast arthrotomography and arthroscopy of the shoulder. Arthroscopy 4:21, 1988.

315. Kinnard P, Tricoire J-L, Levesque R-Y, et al: Assessment of the unstable shoulder by computed arthrography. A preliminary report. Am J Sports Med 11:157, 1983.

316. Shuman WP, Kilcoyne RF, Matsen FA, et al: Double-contrast computed tomography of the glenoid labrum. AJR 141:581, 1983.

317. Deutsch AL, Resnick D, Mink JH, et al: Computed and conventional arthrotomography of the glenohumeral joint: Normal anatomy and clinical experience. Radiology 143:603, 1984.

318. Resnik CS, Deutsch AL, Resnick D, et al: Arthrotomography of the shoulder. RadioGraphics 4:963, 1984.

319. Rafii M, Firooznia H, Golimbu C, et al: CT arthrography of the capsular structures of the shoulder. AJR 146:361, 1986.

320. Wilson AJ, Totty WG, Murphy WA, et al: Shoulder joint: Arthrographic CT and long-term follow-up, with surgical correlation. Radiology 173:329, 1989.

321. Pennes DR, Jonsson K, Buckwalter K, et al: Computed arthrotomography of the shoulder: Comparison of examinations made with internal and external rotation of the humerus. AJR 153:1017, 1989.

322. Ribbans WJ, Mitchell R, Taylor GJ: Computerised arthrotomography of primary anterior dislocation of the shoulder. J Bone Joint Surg [Br] 72:181, 1990.

323. Pappas AM, Goss TP, Kleinman PK: Symptomatic shoulder instability due to lesions of the glenoid labrum. Am J Sports Med 11:279, 1983.

324. McNiesh LM, Callaghan JJ: Pictorial essay. CT arthrography of the shoulder: variations of the glenoid labrum. AJR 149:963, 1987.

325. Rafii M, Firooznia H: Variations of normal glenoid labrum. AJR 152:201, 1989.

326. Seeger LL, Gold RH, Bassett LW: Shoulder instability: Evaluation with MR imaging. Radiology 168:695, 1988.

327. Habibian A, Stauffer A, Resnick D, et al: Comparison of conventional and computed arthrotomography with MR imaging in the evaluation of the shoulder. J Comput Assist Tomogr 13:968, 1989.

328. Munk PL, Holt RG, Helms CA, et al: Glenoid labrum: Preliminary work with use of radial-sequence MR imaging. Radiology 173:751, 1989.

329. Gross ML, Seeger LL, Smith JB, et al: Magnetic resonance imaging of the glenoid labrum. Am J Sports Med 18:229, 1990.

330. Legan JM, Burkhard TK, Goff WB II, et al: Tears of the glenoid labrum: MR imaging of 88 arthroscopically confirmed cases. Radiology 179:241, 1991.

331. Garneau RA, Renfrew DL, Moore TE, et al: Glenoid labrum: Evaluation with MR imaging. Radiology 179:519, 1991.

332. Imhoff A, Perrenoud A, Neidl K: MRI bei Schulterinstabilitat-Korrelation zum Arthro-CT und zur Arthroskopie der Schulter. Arthroskopie 5:122, 1992.

333. Gudinchet F, Naggar L, Ginalski JM, et al: Magnetic resonance imaging of nontraumatic shoulder instability in children. Skel Radiol 21:19, 1992.

334. McCauley TR, Pope CF, Jokl P: Normal and abnormal glenoid labrum: Assessment with multiplanar gradient-echo MR imaging. Radiology 183:35, 1992.

335. Hajec PC, Baker LL, Sartoris D, et al: MR arthrography: Pathologic investigation. Radiology 163:141, 1987.

336. Danzig LA, Greenway G, Resnick D: The Hill-Sachs lesion. An experimental study. Am J Sports Med 8:328, 1980.

337. Workman TL, Burkhard TK, Resnick D, et al: Hill-Sachs lesion: Comparison of detection with MR imaging, radiography, and arthroscopy. Radiology 185:847, 1992.

338. Snyder SJ: Superior labrum anterior and posterior lesions of the shoulder. Proceed Ann Meeting Arthrosc Surg Shoulder, San Diego, 1989.

339. Andrews JR, Carson WG Jr, McLeod WD: Glenoid labrum tears related to the long head of the biceps. Am J Sports Med 13:337, 1985.

340. Yoneda M, Hirooka A, Saito S, et al: Arthroscopic stapling for detached superior glenoid labrum. J Bone Joint Surg [Br] 73:746, 1991.

341. Snyder S, Karzel RP, Del Pizzo W, et al: SLAP lesions of the shoulder. Arthroscopy 6:274, 1990.

342. Hunter JC, Blatz DJ, Escobedo EM: SLAP lesions of the glenoid labrum: CT arthrographic and arthroscopic correlation. Radiology 184:513, 1992.

343. Hodler J, Kursunoglu-Brahme S, Flannigan B, et al: Injuries of the superior portion of the glenoid labrum involving the insertion of the biceps tendon: MR imaging findings in nine cases. AJR 159:565, 1992.

344. Cartland JP, Crues JV III, Stauffer A, et al: MR imaging in the evaluation of SLAP injuries of the shoulder: Findings in 10 patients. AJR 159:787, 1992.

345. Detrisac DA, Johnson LL: Arthroscopic Shoulder Anatomy. Thorofare, NJ, Slack Inc, 1986, p 71.

346. DePalma AF: Surgery of the Shoulder. 3rd ed. Philadelphia, JB Lippincott, 1983, p 211.

347. Matthews LS, Terry G, Vetter WL: Shoulder anatomy for the arthroscopist. Arthroscopy 1:83, 1985.

348. Neviaser TJ: The GLAD lesion: Another cause of anterior shoulder pain. J Arthrosc Rel Surg 9:22, 1993.

349. Neviaser TJ: The anterior labroligamentous periosteal sleeve avulsion lesion: a cause of anterior instability of the shoulder. J Arthrosc Rel Surg 9:17, 1993.

350. Rowe CR, Zarins B, Ciullo JV: Recurrent anterior dislocation of the shoulder after surgical repair: apparent causes of failure and treatment. J Bone Joint Surg [Am] 66:159, 1984.

351. Hovelius L, Thorling J, Fredin H: Recurrent anterior dislocation of the shoulder: results after the Bankart and Putti-Platt operations. J Bone Joint Surg [Am] 61:566, 1979.

352. Singson RD, Feldman F, Bighani LU, et al: Recurrent shoulder dislocation after surgical repair: Double-contrast CT arthrography. Work in progress. Radiology 164:425, 1987.

353. Burkhead WZ Jr: The biceps tendon. In CA Rockwood Jr and FA Matsen III (Eds): The Shoulder. Philadelphia, WB Saunders Co, 1990, p 791.

354. Meyer AW: Spontaneous dislocation of the tendon of the long head of the biceps brachii. Arch Surg 13:109, 1926.

355. Meyer AW: Spontaneous dislocation and destruction of the tendon of the long head of the biceps brachii. Arch Surg 17:493, 1928.

356. Abbott LC, Saunders LB: Acute traumatic dislocation of the tendon of the long head of the biceps brachii: report of 6 cases with operative findings. Surgery 6:817, 1939.

357. Cone RO, Danzig L, Resnick D, et al: The bicipital groove: radiographic, anatomic, and pathologic study. AJR 41:781, 1983.

358. Hitchcock HH, Bechtol CO: Painful shoulder. Observations on the role of the tendon of the long head of the biceps brachii in its causation. J Bone Joint Surg [Am] 30:263, 1948.

359. Habermeyer P, Kaiser E, Knappe M, et al: Functional anatomy and biomechanics of the long biceps tendon. Unfallchirurg 90:319, 1987.

360. O'Donohue D: Subluxating biceps tendon in the athlete. Clin Orthop 164:26, 1982.

361. Middleton WD, Remus WR, Totty WG, et al: Ultrasonographic evaluation of the rotator cuff and biceps tendon. J Bone Joint Surg [Am] 68:440, 1986.

362. Collier SG, Wynn-Jones CH: Displacement of the biceps with subscapularis avulsion. J Bone Joint Surg [Br] 72:145, 1990.

363. Levinsohn EM, Santelli ED IV: Bicipital groove dysplasia and medial dislocation of the biceps brachii tendon. Skel Radiol 20:419, 1991.

364. Slätis P, Aalto K: Medial dislocation of the tendon of the long head of the biceps brachii. Acta Orthop Scand 50:73, 1979.

365. Chan TW, Dalinka MK, Kneeland JB, et al: Biceps tendon dislocation: Evaluation with MR imaging. Radiology 179:649, 1991.

366. Cervilla V, Schweitzer ME, Ho C, et al: Medial dislocation of the biceps brachii tendon: Appearance at MR imaging. Radiology 180:523, 1991.

367. Kernwein GA, Roseberg B, Sneed WR Jr: Arthrographic studies of shoulder joint. J Bone Joint Surg [Am] 39:1267, 1957.

368. Samilson R, Raphael RL, Post L, et al: Arthrography of the shoulder joint. Clin Orthop 20:21, 1961.

369. Lindbloom K: Arthrography and roentgenography in ruptures of the tendons of the shoulder joint. Acta Radiol 20:548, 1939.

370. Fritz RC, Helms CA, Steinbach LS, et al: Suprascapular nerve entrapment: Evaluation with MR imaging. Radiology 182:437, 1992.

371. Jobe FW, Tibone JE, Jobe CM, et al: The shoulder in sports. In CA Rockwood Jr and FA Matsen III (Eds): The Shoulder. Philadelphia, WB Saunders Co, 1990, p 961.

372. Callahan JD, Scully TB, Shapiro SA, et al: Suprascapular nerve entrapment. A series of 27 cases. J Neurosurg 74:893, 1991.

373. Ganzhorn RW, Hocker JT, Horowitz M, et al: Suprascapular-nerve entrapment. J Bone Joint Surg [Am] 63:492, 1981.

374. Garcia G, McQueen D: Bilateral suprascapular-nerve entrapment syndrome. J Bone Joint Surg [Am] 63:491, 1981.

375. Thompson RC, Schneider W, Kennedy T: Entrapment neuropathy of the inferior branch of the suprascapular nerve by ganglia. Clin Orthop 166:185, 1982.

376. Demaio M, Drez D Jr, Mullins RC, et al: The inferior transverse scapular ligament as a possible cause of entrapment neuropathy of the nerve to the infraspinatus. A brief note. J Bone Joint Surg [Am] 73:1061, 1991.

377. Takagishi K, Maeda K, Ikeda T, et al: Ganglion causing paralysis of the suprascapular nerve. Diagnosis by MRI and ultrasonography. Acta Orthop Scand 62:391, 1991.

378. Cahill BR, Palmer RE: Quadrilateral space syndrome. J Hand Surg 8:65, 1983.

379. Francel TJ, Dellon AL, Compbell JN: Quadrilateral space syndrome: diagnosis and operative decompression technique. Plast Reconstr Surg 87:911, 1991.

380. Redler MR, Ruland LJ III, McCue FC III: Quadrilateral space syndrome in a throwing athlete. Am J Sports Med 14:511, 1986.

381. Cormier PJ, Matalon TAS, Wolin PM: Quadrilateral space syndrome: A rare cause of shoulder pain. Radiology 167:797, 1988.

382. Linker CS, Helms CA, Fritz RC: Quadrilateral space syndrome: Findings at MR imaging. Radiology 188:675, 1993.

383. Johnstone WH, Keats TE, Lee ME: The anatomic basis for the superior acetabular roof notch. "Superior acetabular notch." Skel Radiol 8:25, 1982.

384. Wiberg G: Studies on dysplastic acetabula and congenital subluxation of the

hip joint—with special reference to the complication of osteoarthritis. Acta Chir Scand (Suppl) 58:1, 1939.

385. Hooper JC, Jones EW: Primary protrusion of the acetabulum. J Bone Joint Surg [Br] 53:23, 1971.

386. Armstrong P, Saxton H: Iliopsoas bursa. Br J Radiol 45:493, 1972.

387. Chandler SB: The iliopsoas bursa in man. Anat Rec 58:235, 1934.

388. Staple TW: Arthrographic demonstration of the iliopsoas bursa extension of the hip joint. Radiology 102:515, 1972.

389. Guerra J Jr, Armbuster TG, Resnick D, et al: The adult hip: An anatomic study. Part II. The soft-tissue landmarks. Radiology 128:11, 1978.

390. Weston WJ: The bursae deep to gluteus medius and minimus. Australas Radiol 14:325, 1970.

391. Paterson I: The torn acetabular labrum: a block to reduction of a dislocated hip. J Bone Joint Surg [Br] 39:306, 1957.

392. Dameron TB: Bucket-handle tear of the acetabular labrum accompanying posterior dislocation of the hip. J Bone Joint Surg [Am] 41:131, 1959.

393. Altenberg AR: Acetabular labrum tears: a cause of hip pain and degenerative osteoarthritis. South Med J 70:174, 1977.

394. Dorrell JH, Catterall A: The torn acetabular labrum. J Bone Joint Surg [Br] 68:400, 1986.

395. Suzuki S, Awaya G, Okada Y, et al: Arthroscopic diagnosis of ruptured acetabular labrum. Acta Orthop Scand 57:513, 1986.

396. Ikeda T, Awaya G, Suzuki S, et al: Torn acetabular labrum in young patients. Arthroscopic diagnosis and management. J Bone Joint Surg [Br] 70:13, 1988.

397. Klaue K, Durnin CW, Ganz R: The acetabular rim syndrome. A clinical presentation of dysplasia of the hip. J Bone Joint Surg [Br] 73:423, 1991.

398. Ueo T, Hamabuchi M: Hip pain caused by cystic deformation of the labrum acetabulare. Arthritis Rheum 27:947, 1984.

399. Matsui M, Ohzono K, Saito S: Painful cystic degeneration of the limbus in the hip. A case report. J Bone Joint Surg [Am] 70:448, 1988.

400. McBeath AA, Neidhart DA: Acetabular cyst with communicating ganglion: a case report. J Bone Joint Surg [Am] 58:267, 1976.

401. Lagier R, Seigne JM, Mbakop A: Juxta-acetabular mucoid cyst in a patient with osteoarthritis of the hip secondary to dysplasia. Intern Orthop (SICOT) 8:19, 1984.

402. Haller J, Resnick D, Greenway G, et al: Juxtaacetabular ganglionic (or synovial) cysts: CT and MR features. J Comput Assist Tomogr 13:976, 1989.

403. Silver DAT, Cassar-Pullicino VN, Morrissey BM, et al: Gas-containing ganglia of the hip. Clin Radiol 46:257, 1992.

404. Murphy WA, Siegel MJ, Gilula LA: Arthrography in the diagnosis of unexplained chronic hip pain with regional osteopenia. AJR 129:283, 1977.

405. Brower AC, Kransdorf MJ: Imaging of hip disorders. Radiol Clin North Am 28:955, 1990.

406. Beltran J, Caudill JL, Herman LA, et al: Rheumatoid arthritis: MR imaging manifestations. Radiology 165:153, 1987.

407. Yulish BS, Lieberman JM, Newman AJ, et al: Juvenile rheumatoid arthritis: Assessment with MR imaging. Radiology 165:149, 1987.

408. Warren R, Kaye JJ, Salvati EA: Arthrographic demonstration of an enlarged iliopsoas bursa complicating osteoarthritis of the hip—a case report. J Bone Joint Surg [Am] 57:413, 1975.

409. O'Connor DS: Early recognition of iliopectineal bursitis. Surg Gynecol Obstet 57:674, 1933.

410. Steinbach LS, Schneider R, Goldman AB, et al: Bursae and abscess cavities communicating with the hip. Diagnosis using arthrography and CT. Radiology 156:303, 1985.

411. Chaiamnuay P, Davis P: An unusual case of inguinal swelling. Arthritis Rheum 27:239, 1984.

412. Weinreb JC, Cohen JM, Maravilla KR: Iliopsoas muscles: MR study of normal anatomy and disease. Radiology 156:435, 1985.

413. Penkava RR: Iliopsoas bursitis demonstrated by computed tomography. AJR 135:175, 1980.

414. Peters JC, Coleman BG, Turner ML, et al: CT evaluation of enlarged iliopsoas bursa. AJR 135:392, 1980.

415. Janus CL, Hermann G: Enlargement of the iliopsoas bursa: Unusual cause of cystic mass on pelvic sonogram. J Clin Ultrasound 10:133, 1982.

416. Helfgott SA: Unusual features of iliopsoas bursitis. Arthritis Rheum 31:1331, 1988.

417. Li KC, Higgs J, Aisen AM, et al: MRI in osteoarthritis of the hip: Gradations of severity. Magn Res Imag 6:229, 1988.

418. Hodler J, Trudell D, Pathria MN, et al: Width of the articular cartilage of the hip: Quantification by using fat-suppression spin-echo MR imaging in cadavers. AJR 159:351, 1992.

419. Mitchell DG, Rao VM, Dalinka MK, et al: Femoral head avascular necrosis: correlation of MR imaging, radiographic staging, radionuclide imaging, and clinical findings. Radiology 162:709, 1987.

420. Mitchell DG, Joseph PM, Fallon M, et al: Chemical-shift MR imaging of the femoral head: an in vitro study of normal hips and hips with avascular necrosis. AJR 148:1159, 1987.

421. Lang P, Jergesen HE, Moseley ME, et al: Avascular necrosis of the femoral head: high field strength MR imaging with histologic correlation. Radiology 169:517, 1988.

422. Vande Berg BE, Malghem JJ, Labaisse MA, et al: MR imaging of avascular necrosis and transient marrow edema of the femoral head. RadioGraphics 13:501, 1993.

423. Curtiss PH Jr, Kincaid WE: Transient demineralization of the hip in pregnancy: a report of three cases. J Bone Joint Surg [Am] 41:1327, 1959.

424. Wilson AJ, Murphy WA, Hardy DC, et al: Transient osteoporosis: transient bone marrow edema? Radiology 167:757, 1988.

425. Hofman S, Engel A, Neuhold A, et al: Bone marrow oedema syndrome and transient osteoporosis of the hip. An MRI-controlled study of treatment by core decompression. J Bone Joint Surg [Br] 75:210, 1993.

426. Solomon L: Bone-marrow oedema syndrome. J Bone Joint Surg [Br] 75:175, 1993.

427. Turner DA, Templeton AC, Selzer PM, et al: Femoral capital osteonecrosis: MR finding of diffuse marrow abnormalities without focal lesions. Radiology 171:135, 1989.

428. Fairclough J, Colhoun E, Johnston D, et al: Bone scanning for suspected hip fractures. A prospective study in elderly patients. J Bone Joint Surg [Br] 69:251, 1987.

429. Matin P: The appearance of bone scans following fractures, including immediate and long-term studies. J Nucl Med 20:1227, 1979.

430. Matin P: Bone scintigraphy in the diagnosis and management of traumatic injury. Semin Nucl Med 13:104, 1983.

431. Slavin JD, Mathews J, Spencer RP: Bone imaging in the diagnosis of fractures of the femur and pelvis in the sixth to tenth decades. Clin Nucl Med 11:328, 1986.

432. Holder LE, Schwarz C, Wernicke PG, et al: Radionuclide bone imaging in the early detection of fractures of the proximal femur (hip): Multifactorial analysis. Radiology 174:509, 1990.

433. Rizzo PF, Gould ES, Lyden JP, et al: Diagnosis of occult fractures about the hip. Magnetic resonance imaging compared with bone-scanning. J Bone Joint Surg [Am] 75:395, 1993.

434. Speer KP, Spritzer CE, Harrelson JM, et al: Magnetic resonance imaging of the femoral head after acute intracapsular fracture of the femoral neck. J Bone Joint Surg [Am] 72:98, 1990.

435. Quinn SF, McCarthy JL: Prospective evaluation of patients with suspected hip fracture and indeterminate radiographs: Use of T1-weighted MR images. Radiology 187:469, 1993.

436. Deutsch AL, Mink JH, Waxman AD: Occult fractures of the proximal femur: MR imaging. Radiology 170:113, 1989.

437. Lyons JC, Peterson LFA: The snapping iliopsoas tendon. Mayo Clin Proc 59:327, 1984.

438. Nunziata A, Blumenfeld I: Cadeva a resorte. A proposito de una variedad. Prensa Med Argent 38:1997, 1951.

439. House AJG: Orthopaedists and ballet. Clin Orthop 89:52, 1972.

440. Schaberg JE, Harper MC, Allen WC: The snapping hip syndrome. Am J Sports Med 12:361, 1984.

441. Silver SF, Connell DG, Duncan CP: Case report 550. Skel Radiol 18:327, 1989.

442. Staple TW, Jung D, Mork A: Snapping tendon syndrome: Hip tenography with fluoroscopic monitoring. Radiology 166:873, 1988.

443. Harper MC, Schaberg JE, Allen WC: Primary iliopsoas bursography in the diagnosis of disorders of the hip. Clin Orthop 221:238, 1987.

444. Brantigan OC, Voshell AF: The tibial collateral ligament: Its function, its bursae, and its relation to the medial meniscus. J Bone Joint Surg 25:121, 1943.

445. Walmsley R: Joints. In GJ Romanes (Ed): Cunningham's Textbook of Anatomy. 11th Ed. London, Oxford University Press, 1972.

446. Doppman JL: Baker's cyst and the normal gastrocnemiosemimembranosus bursa. AJR 94:646, 1965.

447. Wilson PD, Eyre-Brook AL, Francis JD: A clinical and anatomical study of the semimembranosus bursa in relation to popliteal cyst. J Bone Joint Surg 20:963, 1938.

448. Wolfe RD, Colloff B: Popliteal cysts. An arthrographic study and review of the literature. J Bone Joint Surg [Am] 54:1057, 1972.

449. Guerra J Jr, Newell JD, Resnick D, et al: Gastrocnemio-semimembranosus bursal region of the knee. AJR 136:593, 1981.

450. Dalinka MK, Garofola J: The infrapatellar synovial fold: A cause for confusion in the evaluation of the anterior cruciate ligament. AJR 127:589, 1976.

451. Resnick D, Newell JD, Guerra J Jr, et al: Proximal tibiofibular joint: Anatomic-pathologic-radiographic correlation. AJR 131:133, 1978.

452. Weston WJ: The deep infrapatellar bursa. Australas Radiol 17:212, 1973.

453. Weston WJ: The extrasynovial and capsular fat pads on the posterior aspect of the knee joint. Skel Radiol 2:87, 1977.

454. Lindgren PG, Willén R: Gastrocnemio-semimembranosus bursa and its relation to the knee joint. Acta Radiol 18:497, 1977.

455. Harrison RB, Wood MB, Keats TE: The grooves of the distal articular surface of the femur—a normal variant. AJR 126:751, 1976.

456. Jacobsen K: Landmarks of the knee joint on the lateral radiograph during rotation. ROFO 125:399, 1976.

457. Ravelli A: Zum Roetgenbild des menschlichen Kniegelenkes. ROFO 71:614, 1949.

458. Danzig LA, Newell JD, Guerra J Jr, et al: Osseous landmarks of the normal knee. Clin Orthop 156:201, 1981.

459. Blumensaat C: Die Lageabweichugen und Verrenkungen der Kniescheibe. Ergebn Chir Orthop 31:149, 1938.

460. Jacobsen K, Bertheussen K, Gjerloff CC: Characteristics of the line of Blumensaat. Acta Orthop Scand 45:764, 1974.

461. Hall FM: Radiographic diagnosis and accuracy in knee joint effusions. Radiology 115:49, 1975.

462. Butt WP, Lederman H, Chuang S: Radiology of the suprapatellar region. Clin Radiol 34:511, 1983.

463. Engelstad BL, Friedman EM, Murphy WA: Diagnosis of joint effusion on lateral and axial projections of the knee. Invest Radiol *3*:188, 1981.

464. Lewis RW: Roentgenographic study of soft tissue pathology in and about the knee joint. AJR *65*:200, 1951.

465. Bachman AL: Roentgen diagnosis of knee-joint effusion. Radiology *46*:462, 1946.

466. Harris RD, Hecht HL: Suprapatellar effusions. A new diagnostic sign. Radiology *97*:1, 1970.

467. Friedman AC, Naidich TP: The fabella sign: Fabella displacement in synovial effusion and popliteal fossa masses. Radiology *127*:113, 1978.

468. Harris ED Jr: Biology of the joint. *In* WN Kelley, ED Harris Jr, S Ruddy, and CB Sledge (Eds): Textbook of Rheumatology. 2nd Ed. Philadelphia, WB Saunders Co, 1985, p 254.

469. Pedowitz RA, Gershuni DH, Crenshaw AG, et al: Intraarticular pressure during continuous passive motion of the human knee. J Orthop Res *7*:530, 1989.

470. Knight AD, Levick JR: Physiological compartmentation of fluid within the synovial cavity of the rabbit knee. J Physiol *331*:1, 1982.

471. Schweitzer ME, Falk A, Berthoty D, et al: Knee effusion: Normal distribution of fluid. AJR *159*:361, 1992.

472. Kaneko K, De Mony EH, Robinson AE: Distribution of joint effusion in patients with traumatic knee joint disorders: MRI assessment. Clin Imag *17*:176, 1993.

473. Schweitzer ME, Falk A, Pathria M, et al: MR imaging of the knee: Can changes in the intracapsular fat pads be used as a sign of synovial proliferation in the presence of an effusion? AJR *160*:823, 1993.

474. Gillquist J, Hagberg G, Oretorp N: Arthroscopy in acute injuries of the knee joint. Acta Orthop Scand *48*:190, 1977.

475. Noyes FR, Basset RW, Grood ES, et al: Arthroscopy in acute traumatic hemarthrosis of the knee. J Bone Joint Surg [Am] *62*:687, 1980.

476. Davie B: The significance and treatment of haemarthrosis of the knee following trauma. Med J Aust *1*:1355, 1969.

477. Wilkinson A: Traumatic haemarthrosis of the knee. Lancet *2*:13, 1965.

478. Weinberger A, Schumacher HR: Experimental joint trauma: Synovial response to blunt trauma and inflammatory reaction to intraarticular injections of fat. J Rheumatol *8*:380, 1981.

479. Baer AN, Wright EP: Lipid laden macrophages in synovial fluid: A late finding in traumatic arthritis. J Rheumatol *14*:848, 1987.

480. Lawrence C, Seife B: Bone marrow in joint fluid: A clue to fracture. Ann Intern Med *74*:740, 1971.

481. Berk RN: Liquid fat in the knee joint after trauma. N Engl J Med *277*:1411, 1967.

482. Kling DH: Fat in traumatic effusions of the knee joint. Am J Surg *6*:71, 1929.

483. Gregg JR, Nixon JE, DiStefano V: Neutral fat globules in traumatized knees. Clin Orthop *132*:219, 1978.

484. Graham J, Goldman JA: Fat droplets and synovial fluid leukocytes in traumatic arthritis. Arthritis Rheum *21*:76, 1978.

485. Rabinowitz JL, Gregg JR, Nixon JE: Lipid composition of the tissues of human knee joints. II. Synovial fluid in trauma. Clin Orthop *190*:292, 1984.

486. Pierce CB, Eaglesham DC: Traumatic lipohemarthrosis of the knee. Radiology *39*:655, 1942.

487. Saxton HM: Lipohaemarthrosis. Br J Radiol *35*:122, 1962.

488. Arger PH, Oberkircher PE, Miller WT: Lipohemarthrosis. AJR *121*:97, 1974.

489. Train JS, Hermann G: Lipohemarthrosis: Its occurrence with occult cortical fracture of the knee. Orthopedics *3*:416, 1980.

490. Sacks BA, Rosenthal DI, Hall FM: Capsular visualization in lipohemarthrosis of the knee. Radiology *122*:31, 1977.

491. Egund N, Nilsson LT, Wingstrand H, et al: CT scans and lipohaemarthrosis in hip fractures. J Bone Joint Surg [Br] *72*:379, 1990.

492. Kier R, McCarthy SM: Lipohemarthrosis of the knee: MR imaging. J Comput Assist Tomogr *14*:395, 1990.

493. Kursunoglu-Brahme S, Riccio T, Weisman MH, et al: Rheumatoid knee: Role of gadopentetate-enhanced MR imaging. Radiology *176*:831, 1990.

494. Singson RD, Zalduondo FM: Value of unenhanced spin-echo MR imaging in distinguishing between synovitis and effusion. AJR *159*:569, 1992.

495. Drapé J-L, Thelen P, Gay-Depassier P: Intra-articular diffusion of Gd-DOTA after intravenous injection in the knee: MR imaging evaluation. Radiology *188*:227, 1993.

496. Winalski CS, Aliabadi P, Wright RJ, et al: Enhancement of joint fluid with intravenously administered gadopentetate dimeglumine: Technique, rationale, and implications. Radiology *187*:179, 1993.

497. Patel D: Arthroscopy of the plicae-synovial folds and their significance. Am J Sports Med *6*:217, 1978.

498. Pipkin G: Knee injuries: The role of the suprapatellar plica and suprapatellar bursa in simulating internal derangements. Clin Orthop *74*:161, 1971.

499. Harty M, Joyce JJ III: Synovial folds in the knee joint. Orthop Rev *7*:91, 1977.

500. Deutsch AL, Resnick D, Dalinka MK, et al: Synovial plicae of the knee. Radiology *141*:627, 1981.

501. Apple JS, Martinez S, Hardaker WT, et al: Synovial plicae of the knee. Skel Radiol *7*:251, 1982.

502. Jackson RW: The sneaky plicae. J Rheumatol *7*:251, 1982.

503. Jouanin T, Dupont JY, Halimi P, et al: The synovial folds of the knee joint: Anatomical study based on the dissection of 200 knee joints. Anat Clin *4*:47, 1982.

504. Kinnard P, Levesque RY: The plica syndrome. A syndrome of controversy. Clin Orthop *183*:141, 1984.

505. Dorfmann H, Orengo Ph, Amarenco G: Pathology of the synovial folds in the knee. The value of arthroscopy. Rev Rhum Mal Osteoartic *50*:324, 1983.

506. Harrewyn JM, Algnan M, Renoux M, et al: Pathological synovial folds in the knee joint (synovial plica). Arthroscopic treatment. Rev Rhum Mal Osteoartic *49*:3, 1982.

507. Gray DJ, Gardner E: Prenatal development of the human knee and superior tibiofibular joints. Am J Anat *86*:235, 1950.

508. Pipkin G: Lesions of the suprapatellar plica. J Bone Joint Surg [Am] *32*:363, 1950.

509. Patel D: Plica as a cause of anterior knee pain. Orthop Clin North Am *17*:273, 1986.

510. Aprin H, Shapiro J, Gershwind M: Arthrography (plica views). A noninvasive method for diagnosis and prognosis of plica syndrome. Clin Orthop *183*:90, 1984.

511. Frija G, Halimi Ph, Dupont JY, et al: Expression radiologique des plicae du genou. Ann Radiol *25*:375, 1982.

512. Schäfer H: Synovialfalten des kniegelenkes. Die Plica parapatellaris medialis. Fortschr Röntgenstr *147*:640, 1987.

513. Boven F, De Boeck M, Potvliege R: Synovial plicae of the knee on computed tomography. Radiology *147*:805, 1983.

514. Hodge JC, Ghelman B, O'Brien SJ, et al: Synovial plicae and chondromalacia patellae: Correlation of results of CT arthrography with results of arthroscopy. Radiology *186*:827, 1993.

515. Richmond JC, McGinty JB: Segmental arthroscopic resection of the hypertrophic mediopatellar plica. Clin Orthop *178*:185, 1983.

516. Nottage WM, Sprague NF III, Auerbach BJ, et al: The medial patellar plica syndrome. Am J Sports Med *11*:211, 1983.

517. Vaughan-Lane T, Dandy DJ: The synovial shelf syndrome. J Bone Joint Surg [Br] *64*:475, 1982.

518. Jackson RW, Marshall DJ, Fujisawa Y: The pathologic medial shelf. Orthop Clin North Am *13*:307, 1982.

519. Dory MA: Arthrographic recognition of the mediopatellar plica of the knee. Radiology *150*:608, 1984.

520. Thijn CJP, Hillen B: Arthrography and the medial compartment of the patellofemoral joint. Skel Radiol *11*:183, 1984.

521. Hardaker WT Jr, Whipple TL, Bassett FM III: Diagnosis and treatment of the plica syndrome of the knee. J Bone Joint Surg [Am] *62*:221, 1980.

522. Dalinka MK, Garofola J: The infrapatellar synovial fold: A cause for confusion in the evaluation of the anterior cruciate ligament. AJR *127*:589, 1976.

523. Klein W: The medial shelf of the knee. A follow-up study. Arch Orthop Traum Surg *102*:67, 1983.

524. Schulitz KP, Hille E, Kochs W: The importance of the mediopatellar synovial plica for chondromalacia patellae. Arch Orthop Traum Surg *102*:37, 1983.

525. Moller H: Incarcerating mediopatellar synovial plica syndrome. Acta Orthop Scand *52*:357, 1981.

526. Reid GD, Glasgow M, Gordon DA, et al: Pathological plicae of the knee mistaken for arthritis. J Rheumatol *7*:573, 1980.

527. Cooke TD, Wyllie J: Anatomic separation of the suprapatellar pouch spares its involvement by rheumatoid synovitis in the knee. Rheumatol Int *1*:99, 1981.

528. Amatuzzi MM, Fazzi A, Varella MH: Pathologic synovial plica of the knee. Results of conservative management. Am J Sports Med *18*:466, 1990.

529. San Dretto MA, Wartinbee DR, Carrerra GF, et al: Suprapatellar plica synovialis: A common arthrographic finding. J Can Assoc Radiol *33*:163, 1982.

530. Zeiss J, Booth RL Jr, Woldenberg LS, et al: Post-traumatic synovitis presenting as a mass in the suprapatellar bursa of the knee. MRI appearance. Clin Imag *17*:81, 1993.

531. Reider B, Marshall JL, Warren RF: Persistent vertical septum in the human knee joint. J Bone Joint Surg [Am] *63*:1185, 1981.

532. Darlington D, Hawkins CF: Nail-patella syndrome with iliac horns and hereditary nephropathy. Necropsy report and anatomical dissection. J Bone Joint Surg [Br] *49*:164, 1967.

533. Burleson RJ, Bickel WH, Dahlin DC: Popliteal cyst: Clinico-pathologic survey. J Bone Joint Surg [Am] *38*:1265, 1956.

534. Rauschning W: Anatomy and function of the communication between knee joint and popliteal bursae. Ann Rheum Dis *39*:354, 1980.

535. Rauschning W, Fredriksson BA, Wilander E: Histomorphology of idiopathic and symptomatic popliteal cysts. Clin Orthop *164*:306, 1982.

536. Lindgren PG, Willen R: Gastrocnemio-semimembranosus bursa and its relation to the knee joint. I. Anatomy and histology. Acta Radiol Diagn *18*:497, 1977.

537. Baker WM: Formation of synovial cysts in leg in connection with disease of knee joint. St. Bartholomew's Hosp Rep *13*:245, 1877.

538. Wigley RD: Popliteal cysts: Variations on a theme of Baker. Semin Arthritis Rheum *12*:1, 1982.

539. Gristina AG, Wilson PD: Popliteal cysts in adults and children: Review of 90 cases. Arch Surg *88*:357, 1964.

540. Hoffman BK: Cystic lesions of popliteal space. Surg Gynecol Obstet *116*:551, 1963.

541. Jayson MIV, Dixon AS: Intra-articular pressure in rheumatoid arthritis of the knee. III. Pressure changes during joint use. Ann Rheum Dis *29*:401, 1970.

542. Taylor AR, Rana NA: A valve. An explanation of the formation of popliteal cysts. Ann Rheum Dis *32*:419, 1973.

543. Lindgren PG, Rauschning W: Clinical and arthrographic studies on the valve mechanism in communicating popliteal cysts. Arch Orthop Traum Surg *95*:245, 1979.

544. Palmer DG: Anteromedial synovial cysts at the knee joint in rheumatoid disease. Australas Radiol *16*:79, 1972.

545. Seidl G, Scherak O, Hofner W: Antefemoral dissecting cysts in rheumatoid arthritis. Radiology *133*:343, 1979.

546. Shepherd JR, Helms CA: Atypical popliteal cyst due to lateral synovial herniation. Radiology *140*:66, 1981.

547. O'Dell JR, Andersen PA, Hollister JR, et al: Anterior tibial mass: An unusual complication of popliteal cysts. Arthritis Rheum *27*:113, 1984.

548. Corbetti F, Schiavon F, Fiocco U, et al: Unusual antefemoral dissecting cyst. Br J Radiol *58*:675, 1985.

549. Thevenon A, Hardouin P, Duquesnoy B: Popliteal cyst presenting as an anterior tibial mass. Arthritis Rheum *28*:477, 1985.

550. Podgorski M, Edmonds J: Bidirectional knee joint rupture. J Rheumatol *12*:1180, 1985.

551. Eyanson S, Macfarlane JD, Brandt KD: Popliteal cyst mimicking thrombophlebitis as the first indication of knee disease. Clin Orthop *144*:215, 1979.

552. Schmidt MC, Workman JB, Barth WF: Dissection or rupture of a popliteal cyst. A syndrome mimicking thrombophlebitis in rheumatic diseases. Arch Intern Med *134*:694, 1974.

553. Swett HA, Jaffe RB, McIff EB: Popliteal cysts: Presentation as thrombophlebitis. Radiology *115*:613, 1975.

554. Solomon L, Berman L: Synovial rupture of knee joint. J Bone Joint Surg [Br] *54*:460, 1972.

555. Gordon GV, Edell S, Brogadir SP, et al: Baker's cysts and true thrombophlebitis. Report of two cases and review of the literature. Arch Intern Med *139*:40, 1979.

556. Patrone NA, Ramsdell GM: Baker's cyst and venous thrombosis. South Med J *74*:768, 1981.

557. Iacano V, Gauvin G, Zimbler S: Giant synovial cyst of the calf and thigh in a patient with granulomatous synovitis. Clin Orthop *115*:220, 1976.

558. Pallardy G, Fabre P, Ledoux-Lebard G, et al: L'arthrographie du genou dans l'étude des bursites et des kystes synoviaux. J Radiol Electrol Med Nucl *50*:481, 1969.

559. Shapiro RF, Resnick D, Castles JJ, et al: Fistulization of rheumatoid joints. Spectrum of identifiable syndromes. Ann Rheum Dis *34*:489, 1975.

560. Perri JA, Rodnan GP, Mankin HJ: Giant synovial cysts of the calf in patients with rheumatoid arthritis. J Bone Joint Surg [Am] *50*:709, 1968.

561. Fedullo LM, Bonakdarpour A, Moyer RA, et al: Giant synovial cysts. Skel Radiol *12*:90, 1984.

562. Hertzanu Y, Mendelsohn DB, Firer P: Calcified bodies in a giant Baker's cyst. S Afr Med J *65*:973, 1984.

563. Rosenthal DI, Schwartz AN, Schiller AL: Case report 179. Skel Radiol *7*:142, 1981.

564. Kattapuram SV: Case report 181. Skel Radiol *7*:279, 1982.

565. McLeod BC, Charters JR, Straus AK, et al: Gas-like radiolucencies in a popliteal cyst. Rheumatol Int *3*:143, 1983.

566. Wilson AJ, Ford LT, Gilula LA: Migrating mouse: A sign of dissecting popliteal cyst. AJR *150*:867, 1988.

567. Molpus WM, Shah HR, Nicholas RW, et al: Case report 731. Skel Radiol *21*:266, 1992.

568. Lapayowker MS, Cliff MM, Tourtelotte CD: Arthrography in the diagnosis of calf pain. Radiology *95*:319, 1970.

569. Pastershank SP, Mitchell DM: Knee joint bursal abnormalities in rheumatoid arthritis. J Can Assoc Radiol *28*:199, 1977.

570. Wolfe RD, Colloff B: Popliteal cysts. An arthrographic study and review of the literature. J Bone Joint Surg [Am] *54*:1057, 1972.

571. Bryan RS, DiMichele JD, Ford GL Jr: Popliteal cysts. Arthrography as an aid to diagnosis and treatment. Clin Orthop *50*:203, 1967.

572. Grepl J: Beitrag zur positiven Arthrographie bei pathologischen Veränderungen der Bursae popliteae. ROFO *119*:84, 1973.

573. Clark JM: Arthrography diagnosis of synovial cysts of the knee. Radiology *115*:480, 1975.

574. Cooperberg PL, Tsang I, Truelove L, et al: Grey scale ultrasound in the evaluation of rheumatoid arthritis of the knee. Radiology *126*:759, 1978.

575. Ambanelli U, Manganelli P, Nervetti A, et al: Demonstration of articular effusions and popliteal cysts with ultrasound. J Rheumatol *3*:134, 1976.

576. Carpenter JR, Hattery RR, Hunder GG, et al: Ultrasound evaluation of the popliteal space. Comparison with arthrography and physical examination. Mayo Clin Proc *51*:498, 1976.

577. Rudikoff JC, Lynch JJ, Philipps E, et al: Ultrasound diagnosis of Baker cyst. JAMA *235*:1054, 1976.

578. Moore CP, Sarti DA, Lovie JS: Ultrasonographic demonstration of popliteal cysts in rheumatoid arthritis. A noninvasive technique. Arthritis Rheum *18*:577, 1975.

579. Meire HB, Lindsay DJ, Swinson DR, et al: Comparison of ultrasound and positive contrast arthrography in the diagnosis of popliteal and calf swellings. Ann Rheum Dis *33*:221, 1974.

580. Szer IS, Klein-Gitelman M, DeNardo BA, et al: Ultrasonography in the study of prevalence and clinical evolution of popliteal cysts in children with knee effusions. J Rheumatol *19*:458, 1992.

581. Pathria MN, Zlatkin M, Sartoris DJ, et al: Ultrasonography of the popliteal fossa and lower extremities. Radiol Clin North Am *26*:77, 1988.

582. Fam AG, Wilson SR, Holmberg S: Ultrasound evaluation of popliteal cysts in osteoarthritis of the knee. J Rheumatol *9*:428, 1982.

583. Lukes PJ, Herberts P, Zachrisson BE: Ultrasound in the diagnosis of popliteal cysts. Acta Radiol Diagn *21*:663, 1980.

584. Gompels BM, Darlington LG: Evaluation of popliteal cysts and painful calves with ultrasonography: Comparison with arthrography. Ann Rheum Dis *41*:355, 1982.

585. Harper J, Schubert F, Benson MD, Hayes P: Ultrasound and arthrography in the detection of ruptured Baker's cysts. Australas Radiol *26*:281, 1982.

586. Hermann G, Yeh H-C, Lehr-Janus C, Berson BL: Diagnosis of popliteal cyst: Double-contrast arthrography and sonography. Am J Roentgenol *137*:369, 1981.

587. Levin MH, Nordyke RA, Ball JJ: Demonstration of dissecting popliteal cysts by joint scans after intra-articular isotope injections. Arthritis Rheum *14*:591, 1971.

588. Abdel-Dayem HM, Barodawala YK, Papademetriou T: Scintigraphic arthrography. Comparison with contrast arthrography and future applications. Clin Nucl Med *7*:516, 1982.

589. Lamki L: Baker's cyst. Radionuclide arthrographic findings. Clin Nucl Med *10*:147, 1985.

590. Wallner RJ, Dadparvar S, Croll MN, Brady LW: Demonstration of an infected popliteal (Baker's) cyst with three-phase skeletal scintigraphy. Clin Nucl Med *10*:153, 1985.

591. Cooper RA: Computerized tomography (body scan) of Baker's cyst. J Rheumatol *5*:184, 1978.

592. Schwimmer M, Edelstein G, Heiken JP, Gilula LA: Synovial cysts of the knee: CT evaluation. Radiology *154*:175, 1985.

593. Lee KR, Tines SC, Price HI, De Smet AA, Neff JR: The computed tomographic findings of popliteal cysts. Skel Radiol *10*:26, 1983.

594. Lee KR, Tines SC, Yoon JW: CT findings of suprapatellar synovial cysts. J Comput Assist Tomogr *8*:296, 1984.

595. Grepl J: Wert der positiven Arthrographie zur Diagnostik und Pathogenese retrofemoraler Bakerzvsten. Z Orthop *120*:1, 1982.

596. Dixon AS, Grast C: Acute synovial rupture in rheumatoid arthritis: Clinical and experimental observations. Lancet *1*:742, 1964.

597. Tait GBW, Bach F, Dixon AS: Acute synovial rupture: Further observations. Ann Rheum Dis *24*:273, 1965.

598. Hull RG, Rennie JAN, Eastmond CJ, et al: Nuclear magnetic resonance (NMR) tomographic imaging for popliteal cysts in rheumatoid arthritis. Ann Rheum Dis *43*:56, 1984.

599. Lieberman JM, Yulish BS, Bryan PJ, et al: Magnetic resonance imaging of ruptured Baker's cyst. J Can Assoc Radiol *39*:295, 1988.

600. Fielding JR, Franklin PD, Kustan J: Popliteal cysts: a reassessment using magnetic resonance imaging. Skel Radiol *20*:433, 1991.

601. Dungan DH, Seeger LL, Grant EG: Case report 707. Skel Radiol *21*:52, 1992.

602. Barbaric ZL, Young LW: Synovial cyst in juvenile rheumatoid arthritis. AJR *116*:655, 1972.

603. Toyama WM: Familial popliteal cysts in children. Am J Dis Child *124*:586, 1972.

604. Rauschning W, Lindgren PG: Popliteal cysts (Baker's cysts) in adults. I. Clinical and roentgenological results of operative excision. Acta Orthop Scand *50*:583, 1979.

605. DeSmet AA, Neff JR: Knee arthrography for the preoperative evaluation of juxta-articular masses. Radiology *143*:633, 1982.

606. Griffiths HT, Elston CW, Colton CL, et al: Popliteal masses masquerading as popliteal cysts. Ann Rheum Dis *43*:60, 1984.

607. Bogumill GP, Bruno PD, Barrick EF: Malignant lesions masquerading as popliteal cysts. A report of three cases. J Bone Joint Surg [Am] *63*:474, 1981.

608. Littlejohn GO, Brand CA, Ada A, et al: Popliteal cysts and deep venous thrombosis: Tc-99m red blood cell venography. Radiology *155*:237, 1985.

609. Giyanani VL, Grozinger KT, Gerlock AJ Jr, et al: Calf hematoma mimicking thrombophlebitis: Sonographic and computed tomographic appearance. Radiology *154*:779, 1985.

610. Robb D: Obstruction of the popliteal artery by synovial cyst. Br J Surg *48*:221, 1960.

611. Haid SP, Conn J, Bergan JJ: Cystic adventitial disease of the popliteal artery. Arch Surg *101*:765, 1970.

612. Shute K, Rothnie NG: The aetiology of cystic arterial disease. Br J Surg *60*:397, 1973.

613. Firooznia H, Golimbu C, Rafii M, et al: Computerized tomography in diagnosis of compression of the common peroneal nerve by ganglion cysts. Comput Radiol *7*:343, 1983.

614. Gambari PI, Giuliani G, Poppi M, et al: Ganglionic cysts of the peroneal nerve at the knee: CT and surgical correlation. J Comput Assist Tomogr *14*:801, 1990.

615. Muckart RD: Compression of the common peroneal nerve by intramuscular ganglion from the superior tibio-fibular joint. J Bone Joint Surg [Br] *58*:241, 1976.

616. Barrie HJ, Barrington TW, Colwill JC, et al: Ganglion migrans of the proximal tibiofibular joint causing lesions in the subcutaneous tissue, muscle, bone, or peroneal nerve. Report of three cases and review of the literature. Clin Orthop *149*:211, 1980.

617. Burk DL Jr, Dalinka MK, Kanal E, et al: Meniscal and ganglion cysts of the knee: MR evaluation. AJR *150*:331, 1988.

618. Present DA, Hudson TM, Enneking WF: Computed tomography of extraosseous ganglia. Clin Orthop *202*:249, 1986.

619. Matsumoto K, Hukuda S, Ogata M: Juxta-articular bone cysts at the insertion of the pes anserinus. Report of two cases. J Bone Joint Surg [Am] *72*:286, 1990.

620. Zeiss J, Coombs RJ, Booth RL Jr, et al: Chronic bursitis presenting as a mass

in the pes anserinus bursa: MR diagnosis. J Comput Assist Tomogr *17*:137, 1993.

621. Muckle DS, Monahan P: Intra-articular ganglion of the knee. Report of two cases. J Bone Joint Surg [Br] *54*:520, 1972.

622. Caan P: Zystenbildung (Ganglion) im Ligamentum cruciatum anti genus. Deutsche Zeitschrift Chir *186*:403, 1924.

623. Sjovall H: Ein Fall von Ganglion in einem rupturierten Ligamentum cruciatum genus post. Acta Chir Scand *87*:331, 1942.

624. Levine J: A ganglion of the anterior cruciate ligament. Surgery *24*:836, 1948.

625. Chang W, Rose DJ: Ganglion cysts of the anterior cruciate ligament. A case report. Bull Hosp Joint Dis *48*:182, 1988.

626. Yasuda K, Majima T: Intra-articular ganglion blocking extension of the knee: Brief report. J Bone Joint Surg [Br] *70*:837, 1988.

627. Kaempffe F, D'Amato C: An unusual intra-articular ganglion of the knee with intraosseous extension. A case report. J Bone Joint Surg [Am] *71*:773, 1989.

628. Brown MF, Dandy DJ: Intra-articular ganglia in the knee. J Arthrosc Rel Res *6*:322, 1990.

629. Garcia A, Hodler J, Vaughn L, et al: Case report 677. Skel Radiol *20*:373, 1991.

630. McLaren DB, Buckwalter KA, Vahey TN: The prevalence and significance of cyst-like changes at the cruciate ligament attachments in the knee. Skel Radiol *21*:365, 1992.

631. Wolfe RD, Giuliano VJ: Double-contrast arthrography in the diagnosis of pigmented villonodular synovitis of the knee. AJR *110*:793, 1970.

632. Greenfield MM, Wallace KM: Pigmented villonodular synovitis. Radiology *54*:350, 1950.

633. Sanderud A: Pigmented villonodular synovitis. Acta Orthop Scand *24*:155, 1955.

634. Crittenden JJ, Jones DM, Santarelli AG: Knee arthrogram in synovial chondromatosis. Radiology *94*:133, 1970.

635. Prager RJ, Mall JC: Arthrographic diagnosis of synovial chondromatosis. AJR *127*:344, 1976.

636. Resnick D, Oliphant M: Hemophilia-like arthropathy of the knee associated with cutaneous and synovial hemangiomas. Report of 3 cases and review of the literature. Radiology *114*:323, 1975.

637. Forrest J, Staple TW: Synovial hemangioma of the knee. Demonstration by arthrography and arteriography. AJR *112*:512, 1971.

638. Weitzman G: Lipoma arborescens of the knee. Report of a case. J Bone Joint Surg [Am] *47*:1030, 1965.

639. Burgan DW: Lipoma arborescens of the knee. Another cause of filling defects on a knee arthrogram. Radiology *101*:583, 1971.

640. Hermann G, Hochberg F: Lipoma arborescens: Arthrographic findings. Orthopedics *3*:19, 1980.

641. Armstrong SJ, Watt I: Lipoma arborescens of the knee. Br J Radiol *62*:178, 1989.

642. Martinez D, Millner PA, Coral A, et al: Case report 745. Skeletal Radiol *21*:393, 1992.

643. Pudlowski RM, Gilula LA, Kyriakos M: Intra-articular lipoma with osseous metaplasia. Radiographic-pathologic correlation. AJR *132*:471, 1979.

644. Renström P, Johnson RJ: Anatomy and biomechanics of the menisci. Clin Sports Med *9*:523, 1990.

645. Arnoczky SP: Gross and vascular anatomy of the meniscus and its role in meniscal healing, regeneration, and remodeling. *In* VC Mow, SP Arnoczky, and DW Jackson (Eds): Knee Meniscus: Basic and Clinical Foundations. New York, Raven Press, 1992, p 1.

646. Sintzoff SA Jr, Gevenois PA, Andrianne Y, et al: Transverse geniculate ligament of the knee: Appearance at plain radiography. Radiology *180*:259, 1991.

647. Heller L, Langman J: The meniscofemoral ligaments of the human knee. J Bone Joint Surg [Br] *46*:307, 1964.

648. Kaplan EB: The lateral meniscofemoral ligaments of the knee joint. Bull Hosp Joint Dis *17*:176, 1956.

649. Hassine D, Feron JM, Henry-Feugeas MC, et al: The meniscofemoral ligaments: magnetic resonance imaging and anatomic correlations. Surg Radiol Anat *14*:59, 1992.

650. Ingman AM, Ghosh P, Taylor TKF: Variation of collagenous and non-collagenous proteins of human knee joint menisci with age and degeneration. Gerontologia *20*:212, 1974.

651. Adams ME, Hukins DWL: The extracellular matrix of the meniscus. *In* VC Mow, SP Arnoczky, and DW Jackson (Eds): Knee Meniscus. Basic and Clinical Foundations. New York, Raven Press, 1992, p 15.

652. Bullough PG, Munuera L, Murphy J, et al: The strength of the menisci of the knee as it relates to their fine structure. J Bone Joint Surg [Am] *52*:564, 1970.

653. Peters TJ, Smillie IS: Studies on the chemical composition of the menisci of the knee joint with special reference to the horizontal cleavage lesion. Clin Orthop *86*:245, 1972.

654. Radin EL, Paul IL: Does cartilage compliance reduce skeletal impact loads? Arthritis Rheum *13*:139, 1970.

655. Voloshin AS, Wosk J: Shock absorption of meniscectomized and painful knees: A comparative in-vivo study. J Biomed Eng *5*:157, 1983.

656. Kurosawa H, Fukuboyashi T, Nakajima H: Load-bearing mode of the knee: Physical behavior of the knee joint with or without menisci. Clin Orthop *149*:283, 1980.

657. Krause WE, Pope MD, Johnson RJ, et al: Mechanical changes in the knee after meniscectomy. J Bone Joint Surg [Am] *58*:599, 1976.

658. Di Carlo EF: Pathology of the meniscus. *In* SP Arnoczky and DW Jackson

(Eds): Knee Meniscus: Basic and Clinical Foundations. New York, Raven Press, 1992, p 117.

659. Hough AJ, Webber RJ: Pathology of the meniscus. Clin Orthop *252*:32, 1990.

660. Fahmy NRM, William EA, Noble J: Meniscal pathology and osteoarthritis of the knee. J Bone Joint Surg [Br] *65*:24, 1983.

661. Sokoloff L, Varma AA: Chondrocalcinosis in surgically resected joints. Arthritis Rheum *31*:750, 1988.

662. Noble J, Hamblen DL: The pathology of the degenerative meniscus lesion. J Bone Joint Surg [Br] *57*:180, 1975.

663. Adams ME, Billingham MEJ, Muir H: The glycosaminoglycans in menisci in experimental and natural osteoarthritis. Arthritis Rheum *26*:69, 1983.

664. Ricklin P, Ruttimann A, Del Buono MS: Meniscus Lesions: Diagnosis, Differential Diagnosis, and Therapy. 2nd Ed. New York, Grune and Stratton, 1983.

665. Shogry MEC, Pope TL Jr: Vacuum phenomenon simulating meniscal or cartilaginous injury of the knee at MR imaging. Radiology *180*:513, 1991.

666. Hodler J, Haghighi P, Pathria MN, et al: Meniscal changes in the elderly: Correlation of MR imaging and histologic findings. Radiology *184*:221, 1992.

667. Day B, Mackenzie WG, Shim SS, et al: The vascular and nerve supply of the human meniscus. Arthroscopy *1*:58, 1985.

668. Ferrer-Roca O, Vilalta C: Lesions of the meniscus. Part I. Macroscopic and histologic findings. Clin Orthop *146*:289, 1980.

669. Crues JV III, Stoller DW: The menisci. *In* JH Mink, MA Reicher, and JV Crues III (Eds): Magnetic Resonance Imaging of the Knee. New York, Raven Press, 1987, p 55.

670. Levinsohn EM, Baker BE: Prearthrotomy diagnostic evaluation of the knee: review of 100 cases diagnosed by arthrography and arthroscopy. AJR *134*:107, 1980.

671. Grenier R, du Tremblay P: Clinical judgement versus arthrography for diagnosing knee lesions. Can J Surg *23*:186, 1980.

672. Selby B, Richardson ML, Nelson BD, et al: Sonography in the detection of meniscal injuries of the knee: Evaluation in cadavers. AJR *149*:549, 1987.

673. McDonnell CH III, Jeffrey RB Jr, Bjorkengren AG, et al: Intraarticular sonography for imaging the knee menisci: Evaluation in cadaveric specimens. AJR *159*:573, 1992.

674. Selby B, Richardson ML, Montana MA, et al: High resolution sonography of the menisci of the knee. Invest Radiol *21*:332, 1986.

675. Marymont JV, Lynch MA, Henning CE: Evaluation of meniscus tears of the knee by radionuclide imaging. Am J Sports Med *11*:432, 1983.

676. Collier BD, Johnson RP, Carrera GF, et al: Chronic knee pain assessed by SPECT: Comparison with other modalities. Radiology *157*:795, 1985.

677. Passariello R, Trecco F, de Paulis F, et al: Meniscal lesions of the knee joint: CT diagnosis. Radiology *157*:29, 1985.

678. Steinbach LS, Helms CA, Sims RE, et al: High resolution computed tomography of knee menisci. Skel Radiol *16*:11, 1987.

679. Manco LG, Lozman J, Coleman ND, et al: Noninvasive evaluation of knee meniscal tears: Preliminary comparison of MR imaging and CT. Radiology *163*:727, 1987.

680. Manco LG, Kavanaugh JH, Lozman J, et al: Diagnosis of meniscal tears using high-resolution computed tomography. Correlation with arthroscopy. J Bone Joint Surg [Am] *69*:498, 1987.

681. Manco LG, Berlow ME, Czajka J, et al: Bucket-handle tears of the meniscus: Appearance at CT. Radiology *168*:709, 1988.

682. Manco LG, Berlow ME: Meniscal tears—comparison of arthrography, CT, and MRI. CRC Crit Rev Diagn Imag *29*:151, 1989.

683. Lindblom K: Arthrography of the knee, a roentgenographic and anatomical study. Acta Radiol Suppl *74*:7, 1948.

684. Montgomery CE: Synovial recesses in knee arthrography. AJR *121*:86, 1974.

685. Russell E, Hamm R, LePage JR, et al: Some normal variations of knee arthrograms and their anatomical significance. J Bone Joint Surg [Am] *60*:66, 1978.

686. Nicholas JA, Freiberger RH, Killoran PJ: Double contrast arthrography of the knee. Its value in the management of 225 knee derangements. J Bone Joint Surg [Am] *52*:203, 1970.

687. Heiser S, LaBriola JH, Meyers MH: Arthrography of the knee. Radiology *79*:822, 1962.

688. McIntyre JL: Arthrography of the lateral meniscus. Radiology *105*:531, 1972.

689. Jelaso DV: The fascicles of the lateral meniscus: An anatomic-arthrographic correlation. Radiology *114*:335, 1975.

690. Wickstrom KT, Spitzer RM, Olsson HE: Roentgen anatomy of the posterior horn of the lateral meniscus. Radiology *116*:617, 1975.

691. Fetto JF, Marshall JL, Ghelman B: An anomalous attachment of the popliteus tendon to the lateral meniscus. Case report. J Bone Joint Surg [Am] *59*:548, 1977.

692. Pavlov H, Goldman AB: The popliteus bursa: An indicator of subtle pathology. AJR *134*:313, 1980.

693. Freiberger RH, Killoran PJ, Cardona G: Arthrography of the knee by double contrast method. AJR *97*:736, 1966.

694. Butt WP, McIntyre JL: Double contrast arthrography of the knee. Radiology *92*:487, 1969.

695. Ringertz HG: Arthrography of the knee. I. Localization of lesions. Acta Radiol Diagn *14*:138, 1973.

696. Ringertz HG: Arthrography of the knee. II. Isolated and combined lesions. Acta Radiol Diagn *17*:235, 1976.

697. Hall FM: Buckled meniscus. Radiology *126*:89, 1978.

698. Bramson RT, Staple TW: Double contrast knee arthrography in children. AJR *123*:838, 1975.

699. Stenström R: Diagnostic arthrography of traumatic lesions of the knee joint in children. Ann Radiol *18*:391, 1975.

700. Saddawi ND, Hoffman BK: Tear of the attachment of a normal medial meniscus of the knee in a four year old child. J Bone Joint Surg [Am] *52*:809, 1970.

701. Shakespeare DT, Rigby HS: The bucket-handle tear of the meniscus. A clinical and arthrographic study. J Bone Joint Surg [Br] *65*:383, 1983.

702. Kean DM, Worthington BS, Preston BJ, et al: Nuclear magnetic resonance imaging of the knee: examples of normal anatomy and pathology. Br J Radiol *56*:355, 1983.

703. Moon KL Jr, Genant HK, Helms CA, et al: Musculoskeletal applications of nuclear magnetic resonance. Radiology *147*:161, 1983.

704. Li KC, Henkelman RM, Poon PY, et al: MR imaging of the normal knee. J Comput Assist Tomogr *8*:1147, 1984.

705. Reicher MA, Rauschning W, Gold RH, et al: High-resolution magnetic resonance imaging of the knee joint: Normal anatomy. AJR *145*:895, 1985.

706. Reicher MA, Bassett LW, Gold RH: High-resolution magnetic resonance imaging of the knee joint: Pathologic correlations. AJR *145*:903, 1985.

707. Burk DL Jr, Kanal E, Brunberg JA, et al: 1.5-T surface-coil MRI of the knee. AJR *147*:293, 1986.

708. Soudry M, Lanir A, Angel D, et al: Anatomy of the normal knee as seen by magnetic resonance imaging. J Bone Joint Surg [Br] *68*:117, 1986.

709. Turner DA, Prodromos CC: Magnetic resonance imaging of knee injuries. Semin Ultrasound CT MR *7*:339, 1986.

710. Gallimore GW Jr, Harms SE: Knee injuries: High-resolution MR images. Radiology *160*:457, 1986.

711. Harms SE, Muschler G: Three-dimensional MR imaging of the knee using surface coils. J Comput Assist Tomogr *10*:773, 1986.

712. Beltran J, Noto AM, Mosure JC, et al: The knee: Surface-coil MR imaging at 1.5 T. Radiology *159*:747, 1986.

713. Mandelbaum BR, Finerman GAM, Reicher MA, et al: Magnetic resonance imaging as a tool for evaluation of traumatic knee injuries. Anatomical and pathoanatomical correlations. Am J Sports Med *14*:361, 1986.

714. Reicher MA, Hartzman S, Duckwiler GR, et al: Meniscal injuries: Detection using MR imaging. Radiology *159*:753, 1986.

715. Reicher MA, Hartzman S, Bassett LW, et al: MR imaging of the knee. Part I. Traumatic disorders. Radiology *162*:547, 1987.

716. Cruess JV III, Mink J, Levy TL, et al: Meniscal tears of the knee: Accuracy of MR imaging. Radiology *164*:445, 1987.

717. Stoller DW, Martin C, Crues JV III, et al: Meniscal tears: Pathologic correlation with MR imaging. Radiology *163*:731, 1987.

718. Bellon EM, Keith MW, Coleman PE, et al: Magnetic resonance imaging of internal derangements of the knee. RadioGraphics *8*:95, 1988.

719. Mesgarzadeh M, Schneck CD, Bonakdarpour A: Magnetic resonance imaging of the knee and correlation with normal anatomy. RadioGraphics *8*:707, 1988.

720. Tyrrell RL, Gluckert K, Pathria M, et al: Fast three-dimensional MR imaging of the knee: Comparison with arthroscopy. Radiology *166*:865, 1988.

721. Herman LJ, Beltran J: Pitfalls in MR imaging of the knee. Radiology *167*:775, 1988.

722. Haggar AM, Froelich JW, Hearshen DO, et al: Meniscal abnormalities of the knee: 3DFT fast-scan GRASS MR imaging. AJR *150*:1341, 1988.

723. Spritzer CE, Vogler JB, Martinez S, et al: MR imaging of the knee: Preliminary results with a 3DFT GRASS pulse sequence. AJR *150*:597, 1988.

724. Silva I Jr, Silver DM: Tears of the meniscus as revealed by magnetic resonance imaging. J Bone Joint Surg [Am] *70*:199, 1988.

725. Van Heuzen EP, Golding RP, Van Zanten TEG, et al: Magnetic resonance imaging of meniscal lesions of the knee: Clin Radiol *39*:658, 1988.

726. Watanabe AT, Carter BC, Teitelbaum GP, et al: Normal variations in MR imaging of the knee: Appearance and frequency. AJR *153*:341, 1989.

727. Mink JH, Deutsch AL: Magnetic resonance imaging of the knee. Clin Orthop *244*:29, 1989.

728. Bassett LW, Grover JS, Seeger LL: Magnetic resonance imaging of knee trauma. Skel Radiol *19*:401, 1990.

729. Rothschild PA, Domesek JM, Kaufman L, et al: MR imaging of the knee with a 0.064-T permanent magnet. Radiology *175*:775, 1990.

730. Manaster BJ: Magnetic resonance imaging of the knee. Semin Ultrasound CT MR *11*:307, 1990.

731. Kursunoglu-Brahme S, Resnick D: Magnetic resonance imaging of the knee. Orthop Clin North Am *21*:561, 1990.

732. Reeder JD, Matz SO, Becker L, et al: MR imaging of the knee in the sagittal projection: Comparison of three-dimensional gradient-echo and spin-echo sequences. AJR *153*:537, 1989.

733. Solomon SL, Totty WG, Lee JKT: MR imaging of the knee: Comparison of three-dimensional FISP and two-dimensional spin-echo pulse sequences. Radiology *173*:739, 1989.

734. Gay SB, Chen NC, Burch JJ, et al: Multiplanar reconstruction in magnetic resonance evaluation of the knee. Comparison with film magnetic resonance interpretation. Invest Radiol *28*:142, 1993.

735. Harms SE, Flamig DP, Fisher CF, et al: New method for fast MR imaging of the knee. Radiology *173*:743, 1989.

736. Hajek PC, Baker LL, Sartoris DJ, et al: MR arthrography: Anatomic-pathologic investigation. Radiology *163*:141, 1987.

737. Hajek PC, Sartoris DJ, Neumann C, et al: Potential contrast agents for MR arthrography: in vitro evaluation and practical observations. AJR *149*:97, 1987.

738. Engel A: Magnetic resonance knee arthrography. Enhanced contrast by gado-linium complex in the rabbit and in humans. Acta Orthop Scand (Supplement 240) *61*:3, 1990.

739. Boden SD, Labropoulos PA, Vailas JC: MR scanning of the acutely injured knee: Sensitive, but is it cost effective? Arthroscopy *6*:306, 1990.

740. Ruwe PA, Wright J, Randall RL, et al: Can MR imaging effectively replace diagnostic arthroscopy? Radiology *183*:335, 1992.

741. Spiers ASD, Meagher T, Ostlere SJ, et al: Can MRI of the knee affect arthroscopic practice? A prospective study of 58 patients. J Bone Joint Surg [Br] *75*:49, 1993.

742. Noble J: Unnecessary arthroscopy. Editorial. J Bone Joint Surg [Br] *74*:797, 1992.

743. Senghas RE: Indications for magnetic resonance imaging. Editorial. J Bone Joint Surg [Am] *73*:1, 1991.

744. Boden SD, Davis DO, Dina TS, et al: A prospective and blinded investigation of magnetic resonance imaging of the knee. Abnormal findings in asymptomatic subjects. Clin Orthop *282*:177, 1992.

745. Munk PL, Helms CA, Genant HK, et al: Magnetic resonance imaging of the knee: Current status, new directions. Skel Radiol *18*:569, 1989.

746. Buckwalter KA, Braunstein EM, Janizek DB, et al: MR imaging of meniscal windows: Narrow versus conventional window width photography. Radiology *187*:827, 1993.

747. Quinn SF, Brown TR, Szumowski JKT: Menisci of the knee: Radial MR imaging correlated with arthroscopy in 259 patients. Radiology *185*:577, 1992.

748. Heron CW, Calvert PT: Three-dimensional gradient-echo MR imaging of the knee: Comparison with arthroscopy in 100 patients. Radiology *183*:839, 1992.

749. Araki Y, Ootani F, Tsukaguchi I, et al: MR diagnosis of meniscal tears of the knee: Value of axial three-dimensional Fourier transformation GRASS images. AJR *158*:587, 1992.

750. Aubel S, Heyd RL, Thaete FL, et al: MR knee imaging: Axial 3DFT GRASS pulse sequence versus spin-echo imaging for detecting meniscal tears. Magn Reson Imag *10*:531, 1992.

751. Vahey TN, Bennett HT, Arrington LE, et al: MR imaging of the knee: Pseudotear of the lateral meniscus caused by the meniscofemoral ligament. AJR *154*:1237, 1990.

752. Mesgarzadeh M, Moyer R, Leder DS, et al: MR imaging of the knee: Expanded classification and pitfalls to interpretation of meniscal tears. Radio-Graphics *13*:489, 1993.

753. Carpenter WA: Meniscofemoral ligament simulating tear of the lateral meniscus: MR features. J Comput Assist Tomogr *14*:1033, 1990.

754. Lee JK, Yao L: Tibial collateral ligament bursa: MR imaging. Radiology *178*:855, 1991.

755. Chew FS: Medial meniscal flounce: Demonstration on MR imaging of the knee. AJR *155*:199, 1990.

756. Davis SJ, Teresi LM, Bradley WG, et al: The ''notch'' sign: Meniscal contour deformities as indicators of tear in MR imaging of the knee. J Comput Assist Tomogr *14*:975, 1990.

757. Turner DA, Rapoport ML, Erwin WD, et al: Truncation artifact: A potential pitfall in MR imaging of the menisci of the knee. Radiology *179*:629, 1991.

758. Negendank WG, Fernandez-Madrid FR, Heilbrun LK, et al: Magnetic resonance imaging of meniscal degeneration in asymptomatic knees. J Orthop Res *8*:311, 1990.

759. Kaplan PA, Nelson NL, Garvin KL, et al: MR of the knee: The significance of high signal in the meniscus that does not clearly extend to the surface. AJR *156*:333, 1991.

760. De Smet AA, Norris MA, Yandow DR, et al: MR diagnosis of meniscal tears of the knee: Importance of high signal in the meniscus that extends to the surface. AJR *161*:101, 1993.

761. Dillon EH, Pope CF, Jokl P, et al: Follow-up of grade 2 meniscal abnormalities in the stable knee. Radiology *181*:849, 1991.

762. Kursunoglu-Brahme S, Schwaighofer B, Gundry C, et al: Jogging causes acute changes in the knee joint: An MR study in normal volunteers. AJR *154*:1233, 1990.

763. Shellock FG, Deutsch AL, Mink JH, et al: Do asymptomatic marathon runners have an increased prevalence of meniscal abnormalities? An MR study of the knee in 23 volunteers. AJR *157*:1239, 1991.

764. Shellock F, Mink JH: Knees of trained long-distance runners: MR imaging before and after competition. Radiology *179*:635, 1991.

765. Brunner MC, Flower SP, Evancho AM, et al: MRI of the athletic knee. Findings in asymptomatic professional basketball and collegiate football players. Invest Radiol *24*:72, 1989.

766. Reinig JW, McDevitt ER, Ove PN: Progression of meniscal degenerative changes in college football players: Evaluation with MR imaging. Radiology *181*:255, 1991.

767. Glashow JL, Katz R, Schneider M, et al: Double-blind assessment of the value of magnetic resonance imaging in the diagnosis of anterior cruciate and meniscal lesions. J Bone Joint Surg [Am] *71*:113, 1989.

768. Boeree NR, Watkinson AF, Ackroyd CE, et al: Magnetic resonance imaging of meniscal and cruciate injuries of the knee. J Bone Joint Surg [Br] *73*:452, 1991.

769. De Smet AA, Norris MA, Yandow DR, et al: Diagnosis of meniscal tears of the knee with MR imaging: Effect of observer variation and sample size on sensitivity and specificity. AJR *160*:555, 1993.

770. Quinn SF, Brown TF: Meniscal tears diagnosed with MR imaging versus arthroscopy: How reliable a standard is arthroscopy? Radiology *181*:843, 1991.

771. Singson RD, Feldman F, Staron R, et al: MR imaging of displaced bucket-handle tear of the medial meniscus. AJR *156*:121, 1991.

772. Weiss KL, Morehouse HT, Levy IM: Sagittal MR images of the knee: A low-signal band parallel to the posterior cruciate ligament caused by a displaced bucket-handle tear. AJR *156*:117, 1991.

773. Haramati N, Staron RB, Rubin S, et al: The flipped meniscus sign. Skel Radiol *22*:273, 1993.

774. Woods GW, Chapman DR: Reparable posterior meniscocapsular disruption in anterior cruciate ligament injuries. Am J Sports Med *12*:381, 1984.

775. El-Khoury GY, Usta HY, Berger RA: Meniscotibial (coronary) ligament tears. Skel Radiol *11*:191, 1984.

776. Becton JL, Young HH: Cysts of the semilunar cartilage of the knee. Arch Surg *90*:708, 1985.

777. Lantz B, Singer KM: Meniscal cysts. Clin Sports Med *9*:707, 1990.

778. Parisien JS: Arthroscopic treatment of cysts of the menisci. A preliminary report. Clin Orthop *257*:154, 1990.

779. Passler JM, Hofer HP, Peicha G, et al: Arthroscopic treatment of meniscal cysts. J Bone Joint Surg [Br] *75*:303, 1993.

780. Glasgow MMS, Allen PW, Blakeway C: Arthroscopic treatment of cysts of the lateral meniscus. J Bone Joint Surg [Br] *75*:299, 1993.

781. Hernandez FJ: Cysts of the semilunar cartilage of the knee. A light and electron microscopic study. Acta Orthop Scand *47*:436, 1976.

782. Burgan DW: Arthrographic findings in meniscal cysts. Radiology *101*:579, 1971.

783. Wroblewski M: Trauma and the cystic meniscus: Review of 500 cases. Injury *4*:319, 1971.

784. Raine GET, Gonet LCL: Cysts of the menisci of the knee. Postgrad Med J *48*:49, 1972.

785. Spence KF Jr, Robertson RJ: Medial meniscal cysts. Orthopedics *9*:1093, 1986.

786. Mills CA, Henderson IJP: Cysts of the medial meniscus. Arthroscopic diagnosis and management. J Bone Joint Surg [Br] *75*:293, 1993.

787. Ferrer-Roca O, Vilalta C: Lesions of the menisci. Part II. Horizontal cleavages and lateral cysts. Clin Orthop *146*:301, 1980.

788. Barrie HJ: The pathogenesis and significance of meniscal cysts. J Bone Joint Surg [Br] *61*:184, 1979.

789. Coral A, van Holsbeeck M, Adler RS: Imaging of meniscal cyst of the knee in three cases. Skel Radiol *18*:451, 1989.

790. Enis JE, Ghandur-Mnaymneh L: Cyst of the lateral meniscus causing erosion of the tibial plateau. A case report. J Bone Joint Surg [Am] *61*:441, 1979.

791. Kay SP, Gold RH, Bassett LW: Meniscal pneumatocele. A case report of spontaneous, persistent intra-articular and juxta-articular gas. J Bone Joint Surg [Am] *67*:1117, 1985.

792. Chen W-C, Wu J-J, Chang C-Y, et al: Computed tomography of a meniscal cyst. Orthopedics *10*:1569, 1987.

793. De Flaviis L, Scaglione P, Nessi P, et al: Ultrasound in degenerative cystic meniscal disease of the knee. Skel Radiol *19*:441, 1990.

794. Buckwalter JA, Dryer RF, Mickelson MR: Arthrography in juxtaarticular cysts of the knee. Two cases diagnosed by delayed roentgenograms. J Bone Joint Surg [Am] *61*:465, 1979.

795. Schafer H: Das Meniskusganglion. Früherkennung durch Ausmessung standardisierter Arthrogramme. ROFO *136*:505, 1982.

796. Hall FM: Arthrography of the discoid lateral meniscus. AJR *128*:993, 1977.

797. Haveson SB, Rein BI: Lateral discoid meniscus of the knee: Arthrographic diagnosis. AJR *109*:581, 1970.

798. Smillie IS: The congenital discoid meniscus. J Bone Joint Surg [Br] *30*:671, 1948.

799. Kaplan EB: Discoid lateral meniscus of the knee joint. Nature, mechanism and operative treatment. J Bone Joint Surg [Am] *39*:77, 1957.

800. Fisher AGT: The disk-shaped external semilunar cartilage. Br Med J *1*:688, 1936.

801. Cave EF, Staples OS: Congenital discoid meniscus. A cause of internal derangement of the knee. Am J Surg *54*:371, 1941.

802. Jeannopoulos CL: Observations on discoid menisci. J Bone Joint Surg [Am] *32*:649, 1950.

803. Dickhaut SC, DeLee JC: The discoid lateral-meniscus syndrome. J Bone Joint Surg [Am] *64*:1068, 1982.

804. Murdoch G: Congenital discoid medial semilunar cartilage. J Bone Joint Surg [Br] *38*:564, 1956.

805. Riachi E, Phares A: An unusual deformity of the medial semilunar cartilage. J Bone Joint Surg [Br] *45*:146, 1963.

806. Richmond DA: Two cases of discoid medial cartilage. J Bone Joint Surg [Br] *40*:268, 1958.

807. Ross JA, Tough ICK, English TA: Congenital discoid cartilage. Report of a case of discoid medial cartilage with an embryological note. J Bone Joint Surg [Br] *40*:262, 1958.

808. Weiner B, Rosenberg N: Discoid medial meniscus: Association with bone changes in the tibia. A case report. J Bone Joint Surg [Am] *56*:171, 1974.

809. Resnick D, Goergen TG, Kaye JJ, et al: Discoid medial meniscus. Radiology *121*:575, 1976.

810. Dickason JM, Del Pizzo W, Blazina ME, et al: A series of ten discoid medial menisci. Clin Orthop *168*:75, 1982.

811. Johnson RG, Simmons EH: Discoid medial meniscus. Clin Orthop *167*:176, 1982.

812. Hermann G, Berson BL: Discoid medial meniscus: Two cases of tears presenting as locked knee due to athletic trauma. Am J Sports Med *12*:74, 1984.

813. Comba D, Quaglia F, Magliano GE: Massive discoid medial meniscus. A case report. Acta Orthop Scand *56*:340, 1985.

814. Philippon J: Étude des malformations congénitales méniscales par arthropneumographie. J Radiol Electrol Med Nucl *40*:1, 1959.

815. Moes CAF, Munn JD: The value of knee arthrography in children. J Can Assoc Radiol *16*:226, 1965.

816. Nathan PA, Cole SC: Discoid meniscus—a clinical and pathological study. Clin Orthop *64*:107, 1969.

817. Schonholtz GJ, Koenig TM, Prince A: Bilateral discoid medial menisci: A case report and literature review. J Arthrosc *9*:315, 1993.

818. Dashefsky JH: Discoid lateral meniscus in three members of a family. J Bone Joint Surg [Am] *53*:1208, 1971.

819. Busch MT: Meniscal injuries in children and adolescents. Clin Sports Med *9*:661, 1990.

820. Woods GW, Whelan JM: Discoid meniscus. Clin Sports Med *9*:695, 1990.

821. Kulowski J, Rickett HW: The relation of discoid meniscus to cyst formation and joint mechanics. J Bone Joint Surg *29*:900, 1947.

822. Engber WD, Mickelson MR: Cupping of the lateral tibial plateau associated with a discoid meniscus. Orthopedics *4*:904, 1981.

823. Weiner B, Rosenberg N: Discoid medial meniscus: Association with bone changes in the tibia. A case report. J Bone Joint Surg [Am] *56*:171, 1974.

824. Aichroth PM, Patel DV, Marx CL: Congenital discoid lateral meniscus in children. A follow-up study and evolution of management. J Bone Joint Surg [Br] *73*:932, 1991.

825. Berson BL, Hermann G: Torn discoid menisci of the knee in adults. Four case reports. J Bone Joint Surg [Am] *61*:303, 1979.

826. Howe MA, Buckwalter KA, Braunstein EM, et al: Case report 483. Skel Radiol *17*:293, 1988.

827. Silverman JM, Mink JH, Deutsch AL: Discoid menisci of the knee: MR imaging appearance. Radiology *173*:351, 1989.

828. Blacksin MF, Greene B, Botelho G: Bilateral diskoid medial menisci diagnosed by magnetic resonance imaging: A case report. Clin Orthop *285*:214, 1992.

829. Neuschwander DC, Drez D Jr, Finney TP: Lateral meniscal variant with absence of the posterior coronary ligament. J Bone Joint Surg [Am] *74*:1186, 1992.

830. Symeonides PP, Ioannides G: Ossicles in the knee menisci. Report of three cases. J Bone Joint Surg [Am] *54*:1288, 1972.

831. Weaver JB: Calcification and ossification of the menisci. J Bone Joint Surg *24*:873, 1942.

832. Rosen IE: Unusual intrameniscal lunulae. Three case reports. J Bone Joint Surg [Am] *40*:925, 1958.

833. Glass RS, Barnes WM, Kells DU, et al: Ossicles of knee menisci. Report of seven cases. Clin Orthop *111*:163, 1975.

834. Bernstein RM, Olsson HE, Spitzer RM, et al: Ossicle of the meniscus. AJR *127*:785, 1976.

835. Mariani PP, Puddo G: Meniscal ossicle. A case report. Am J Sports Med *9*:392, 1981.

836. Pederson HE: The ossicles of the semilunar cartilages of rodents. Anat Rec *105*:1, 1949.

837. Mitrovic DR: Ossification of human menisci. Arthritis Rheum *34*:638, 1991.

838. Richmond JC, Sarno RC: Arthroscopic treatment of medial meniscal avulsion fractures. Arthroscopy *4*:117, 1988.

839. Richmond JC, Sarno RC: Posttraumatic intracapsular bone fragments: Association with meniscal tears. AJR *150*:159, 1988.

840. Radin EL, de Lamotte F, Maquet P: Role of the menisci in the distribution of stress in the knee. Clin Orthop *185*:290, 1984.

841. Kurosawa H, Fukubayashi T, Nakajima H: Load-bearing mode of the knee joint: Physical behavior of the knee joint with or without menisci. Clin Orthop *149*:283, 1980.

842. Korkala O, Karaharju E, Gronblad M, et al: Articular cartilage after meniscectomy. Rabbit knees studied with the scanning electron microscope. Acta Orthop Scand *55*:273, 1984.

843. Jackson JP: Degenerative changes in the knee after meniscectomy. Br Med J *2*:525, 1968.

844. Appel H: Late results after meniscectomy in the knee joint. A clinical and roentgenologic follow-up investigation. Acta Orthop Scand (Suppl *133*):6, 1970.

845. Tapper EM, Hoover NW: Late results after meniscectomy. J Bone Joint Surg [Am] *51*:517, 1969.

846. Noble J, Erat K: In defense of the meniscus. A prospective study of 200 meniscectomy patients. J Bone Joint Surg [Br] *62*:7, 1980.

847. Shapiro F, Glimcher MJ: Induction of osteoarthrosis in the rabbit knee joint: Histologic changes following meniscectomy and meniscal lesions. Clin Orthop *147*:287, 1980.

848. Arnoczky SP, Warren RF: The microvasculature of the meniscus and its response to injury—an experimental study in the dog. Am J Sports Med *11*:131, 1983.

849. De Haven KE: Peripheral meniscal repair: an alternative to meniscectomy. J Bone Joint Surg [Br] *63*:463, 1981.

850. Hamberg P, Gillquist J, Lysholm J: Suture of new and old peripheral meniscal tears. J Bone Joint Surg [Am] *65*:193, 1983.

851. Gershuni DH, Skyhar MJ, Danzig LA, et al: Experimental models to promote healing of tears in the avascular segment of canine knee menisci. J Bone Joint Surg [Am] *71*:1363, 1989.

852. De Young DJ, Flo GL, Tvedten H: Experimental medial meniscectomy in

dogs undergoing cruciate ligament repair. J Am Anim Hosp Assoc 16:639, 1980.

853. Kim JM, Moon MS: Effects of synovectomy upon regeneration of meniscus in rabbits. Clin Orthop 141:287, 1979.

854. Burr DB, Radin EL: Meniscal function and the importance of meniscal regeneration in preventing late medial compartment osteoarthrosis. Clin Orthop 171:121, 1982.

855. Arnoczky SP, Warren RN, Kaplan N: Meniscal remodeling following partial meniscectomy: an experimental study in the dog. Arthroscopy 1:248, 1985.

856. Northmore-Ball MD, Dandy DJ, Jackson RW: Arthroscopic, open partial, and total meniscectomy. J Bone Joint Surg [Br] 65:400, 1983.

857. Tregonning RJA: Closed partial meniscectomy. Early results for single tears with meniscal symptoms. J Bone Joint Surg [Br] 65:378, 1983.

858. Goodfellow JW: Closed meniscectomy. J Bone Joint Surg [Br] 65:373, 1983.

859. Heatley FW: The meniscus—can it be repaired? J Bone Joint Surg [Br] 62:397, 1980.

860. Cabaud HE, Rodkey WG, Fitzwater JE: Medial meniscus repairs. An experimental and morphologic study. Am J Sports Med 9:129, 1981.

861. Danzig L, Resnick D, Gonsalves M, et al: Blood supply to the normal and abnormal menisci of the human knee. Clin Orthop 172:271, 1983.

862. Doyle JR, Eisenberg JH, Orth MW: Regeneration of knee menisci: A preliminary report. J Trauma 6:50, 1966.

863. Smillie IS: Observations on the regeneration of the semilunar cartilages in man. Br J Surg 31:398, 1944.

864. Goldenberg RR: Refracture of a regenerated internal semilunar cartilage. J Bone Joint Surg 17:1054, 1935.

865. Massare C, Bard M, Tristant H: Intérét de l'arthrographie du genou dans les gonalgies après meniscectomie. Revue de 200 dossiers personnels. J Radiol Electrol Med Nucl 55:401, 1974.

866. Debnam JW, Staple TW: Arthrography of the knee after meniscectomy. Radiology 113:67, 1974.

867. Laasonen EM, Wilppula E: Why a meniscectomy fails. Acta Orthop Scand 47:672, 1976.

868. Dandy DJ, Jackson RW: The diagnosis of problems after meniscectomy. J Bone Joint Surg [Br] 57:349, 1975.

869. Yu JS, Resnick D: Imaging of the knee. Curr Opin Orthop 4:56, 1993.

870. Smith DK, Totty WG: The knee after partial meniscectomy: MR imaging features. Radiology 176:141, 1990.

871. Kent RH, Pope CF, Lynch JK, et al: Magnetic resonance imaging of the surgically repaired meniscus: six month follow-up. Magn Res Imag 9:335, 1991.

872. Deutsch AL, Mink JH, Fox JM, et al: Peripheral meniscal tears: MR findings after conservative treatment or arthroscopic repair. Radiology 176:485, 1990.

873. Farley TE, Howell SM, Love KF, et al: Meniscal tears: MR and arthographic findings after arthroscopic repair. Radiology 180:517, 1991.

874. Odgaard A, Pedersen CM, Bentzen SM, et al: Density changes at the proximal tibia after medial meniscectomy. J Orthop Res 7:744, 1989.

875. Burks RT: Gross anatomy. In D Daniel, W Akeson, and J O'Connor (Eds): Knee Ligaments: Structure, Function, Injury, and Repair. New York, Raven Press, 1990, p 59.

876. Warren LF, Marshall JL, Girgis F: The prime static stabilizers of the medial side of the joint. J Bone Joint Surg [Am] 56:665, 1974.

877. Hughston JC, Eilers AF: The role of the posterior oblique ligament in repairs of acute medial (collateral) ligament tears of the knee. J Bone Joint Surg [Am] 55:923, 1973.

878. Brantigan OC, Voshell AF: The mechanics of the ligaments and menisci of the knee joint. J Bone Joint Surg 23:44, 1941.

879. Grood ES, Noyes FR, Butler DL, et al: Ligamentous and capsular restraints preventing medial and lateral laxity in intact human cadaver knees. J Bone Joint Surg [Am] 63:1257, 1981.

880. Markolf KL, Mensch JS, Amstutz HC: Stiffness and laxity of the knee—the contributions of the supporting structures. A quantitative in vitro study. J Bone Joint Surg [Am] 58:583, 1976.

881. Seering WP, Piziali RL, Nagel DA, et al: The function of the primary ligaments of the knee in varus-valgus and axial rotation. J Biomech 13:785, 1980.

882. Shoemaker SC, Markolf KL: Effects of joint load on the stiffness and laxity of ligament-deficient knees. An in vitro study of the anterior cruciate and medial collateral ligaments. J Bone Joint Surg [Am] 67:136, 1985.

883. Hughston JC, Andrews JR, Cross MJ, et al: Classification of knee ligament instabilities: Part I: The medial compartment and cruciate ligaments. J Bone Joint Surg [Am] 58:159, 1976.

884. Hughston JC, Andrews JR, Cross MJ, et al: Classification of knee ligament instabilities. Part II: The lateral compartment. J Bone Joint Surg [Am] 58:173, 1976.

885. Andrews JR, Axe MJ: The classification of knee ligament instability. Orthop Clin North Am 16:69, 1985.

886. Indelicato PA: Injury to the medial capsuloligamentous complex. In JA Feagin (Ed): The Crucial Ligaments. Diagnosis and Treatment of Ligamentous Injuries About the Knee. New York, Churchill Livingstone, 1988, p 197.

887. O'Donoghue DH: Surgical treatment of fresh injuries to major ligaments of the knee. J Bone Joint Surg [Am] 32:721, 1950.

888. Turner DA, Prodromos CC, Petasnick JP, et al: Acute injury of the ligaments of the knee: Magnetic resonance evaluation. Radiology 154:717, 1985.

889. Tehranzadeh J, Kerr R, Amster J: Magnetic resonance imaging of tendon and ligament abnormalities: Part II. Pelvis and lower extremities. Skel Radiol 21:79, 1992.

890. Garvin GJ, Munk PL, Vellet AD: Tears of the medial collateral ligament: magnetic resonance imaging findings and associated injuries. J Can Assoc Radiol 44:199, 1993.

891. Yao L, Lee JK: Avulsion of the posteromedial tibial plateau by the semimembranosus tendon: Diagnosis with MR imaging. Radiology 172:513, 1989.

892. Seebacher JR, Inglis AE, Marshall JL, et al: The structure of the posterolateral aspect of the knee. J Bone Joint Surg [Am] 64:536, 1982.

893. Reider B, Marshall JL, Koslin RT, et al: The anterior aspect of the knee joint. J Bone Joint Surg [Am] 63:351, 1981.

894. Terry GC, Hughston JD, Norwood LA: The anatomy of the iliopatellar band and iliotibial tract. Am J Sports Med 14:39, 1986.

895. Last RJ: The popliteus muscle and the lateral meniscus. J Bone Joint Surg [Br] 32:93, 1950.

896. Cohn AK, Mains DB: Popliteal hiatus of the lateral meniscus. Am J Sports Med 7:221, 1979.

897. De Lee JC, Riley MB, Rockwood CA Jr: Acute posterolateral rotary instability of the knee. Am J Sports Med 11:199, 1983.

898. Shoemaker SC, Daniel DM: The limits of knee motion. In vitro studies. In D Daniel, W Akeson, and J O'Connor (Eds): Knee Ligaments. Structure, Function, Injury, and Repair. New York, Raven Press, 1990, p 153.

899. Sebastianelli WJ, Hanks GA, Kalenak A: Isolated avulsion of the biceps femoris insertion. A case report. Clin Orthop 259:200, 1990.

900. Rose DJ, Parisien JS: Popliteus tendon rupture. Case report and review of the literature. Clin Orthop 226:113, 1988.

901. Tria AJ, Johnson CD, Zawadsky JP: The popliteus tendon. J Bone Joint Surg [Am] 71:714, 1989.

902. Geissler WB, Corso SR, Caspari RB: Isolated rupture of the popliteus with posterior tibial nerve palsy. J Bone Joint Surg [Br] 74:811, 1992.

903. Naver L, Aalberg JR: Avulsion of the popliteus tendon: a rare cause of chondral fracture and hemarthrosis. Am J Sports Med 13:423, 1985.

904. Orava S: Iliotibial tract friction syndrome in athletes: an uncommon exertion syndrome on the lateral side of the knee. Br J Sports Med 12:69, 1978.

905. Martens M, Libbrecht P, Burssens A: Surgical treatment of the iliotibial band friction syndrome. Am J Sports Med 17:651, 1989.

906. Noble CA: Iliotibial band friction syndrome in runners. Am J Sports Med 8:232, 1980.

907. Murphy BJ, Hechtman KS, Uribe JW, et al: Iliotibial band friction syndrome: MR imaging findings. Radiology 185:569, 1992.

908. Segond P: Recherches cliniques et experimentales sur les epanchements sanguirs du genou par entorse. Prog Med 7:297, 1879.

909. Johnson LL: Lateral capsular ligament complex: anatomical and surgical considerations. Am J Sports Med 7:156, 1979.

910. Weber WN, Neumann CH, Barakos JA, et al: Lateral tibial rim (Segond) fractures: MR imaging characteristics. Radiology 180:731, 1991.

911. Ficat RP, Hungerford DS: Disorders of the Patello-femoral Joint. Baltimore, Williams & Wilkins, 1977.

912. Reider B, Marshall JL, Koslin B, et al: The anterior aspect of the knee joint: an anatomic study. J Bone Joint Surg [Am] 63:351, 1981.

913. Wiberg G: Roentgenographic and anatomic studies of the femoropatellar joint, with special reference to chondromalacia patellae. Acta Orthop Scand 12:319, 1941.

914. Goodfellow JW, Hungerford DS, Zindel M: Patellofemoral mechanics and pathology. I. Functional anatomy of the patellofemoral joint. J Bone Joint Surg [Br] 58:287, 1976.

915. Goodfellow JW, Hungerford DS, Woods C: Patellofemoral joint mechanics and pathology. II. Chondromalacia patellae. J Bone Joint Surg [Br] 58:291, 1976.

916. Outerbridge RE: Further studies on the etiology of chondromalacia patellae. J Bone Joint Surg [Br] 46:179, 1964.

917. Delgado-Martins H: A study of the position of the patella using computerized tomography. J Bone Joint Surg [Br] 61:443, 1976.

918. Hungerford DS, Barry M: Biomechanics of the patellofemoral joint. Clin Orthop 144:9, 1979.

919. Martens M, Wouters P, Burssens A, et al: Patellar tendinitis: Pathology and results of treatment. Acta Orthop Scand 53:445, 1982.

920. Blazina ME, Kerlan RK, Jobe FW, et al: Jumper's knee. Orthop Clin North Am 4:665, 1973.

921. Roels J, Martens M, Mulier JC, et al: Patellar tendinitis (jumper's knee). Am J Sports Med 6:362, 1978.

922. Bodne D, Quinn SF, Murray WT, et al: Magnetic resonance images of chronic patellar tendinitis. Skel Radiol 17:24, 1988.

923. El-Khoury GY, Wira RL, Berbaum KS, et al: MR imaging of patellar tendinitis. Radiology 184:849, 1992.

924. Kahn D, Wilson MA: Bone scintigraphic findings in patellar tendinitis. J Nucl Med 28:1768, 1987.

925. Mourad K, King J, Guggiana P: Computed tomography and ultrasound imaging of jumper's knee—patellar tendinitis. Clin Radiol 39:162, 1988.

926. Davies SG, Baudouin CJ, King JB, et al: Ultrasound, computed tomography and magnetic resonance imaging in patellar tendinitis. Clin Radiol 43:52, 1991.

927. O'Keefe D: Ultrasound in clinical orthopaedics. J Bone Joint Surg [Br] 74:488, 1992.

928. Scranton PE Jr, Farrar EL: Mucoid degeneration of the patellar ligament in athletes. J Bone Joint Surg [Am] 74:435, 1992.

929. Siwek CW, Rao JP: Ruptures of the extensor mechanism of the knee joint. J Bone Joint Surg [Am] 63:932, 1981.

930. Scuderi C: Quadriceps tendon rupture. Am J Surg 95:626, 1958.
931. Levy M, Seelefreund M, Maor P, et al: Bilateral spontaneous and simultaneous rupture of the quadriceps tendon in gout. J Bone Joint Surg [Br] 53:510, 1971.
932. Potasman I, Bassan HN: Multiple tendon ruptures in systemic lupus erythematosus. Case report and review of the literature. Ann Rheum Dis 43:347, 1984.
933. Lotem N, Robson MD, Rosenfield JB: Spontaneous rupture of the quadriceps tendon in patients on chronic hemodialysis. Ann Rheum Dis 33:428, 1974.
934. Newburg A, Wales L: Radiographic diagnosis of quadriceps tendon rupture. Radiology 125:367, 1977.
935. Walker LG, Glick H: Bilateral spontaneous quadriceps tendon ruptures. A case report and review of the literature. Orthop Rev 8:867, 1989.
936. Ramsey RH, Mueller GE: Quadriceps tendon rupture: a diagnostic trap. Clin Orthop 70:161, 1970.
937. Berlin RC, Levinsohn EM, Chrisman H: The wrinkled patellar tendon: an indication of abnormality in the extensor mechanism of the knee. Skel Radiol 20:181, 1991.
938. Kuivila TE, Brems JJ: Diagnosis of acute rupture of the quadriceps tendon by magnetic resonance imaging. A case report. Clin Orthop 262:236, 1991.
939. Smason JB: Post-traumatic fistula connecting prepatellar bursa with knee joint. Report of a case. J Bone Joint Surg [Am] 54:1553, 1972.
940. Jelaso DV, Morris GA: Rupture of the quadriceps tendon: Diagnosis by arthrography. Radiology 116:621, 1975.
941. Aprin H, Broukhim B: Early diagnosis of acute rupture of the quadriceps tendon by arthrography. Clin Orthop 195:185, 1985.
942. Laine H, Harjula A, Peltokaillio P: Ultrasound in the evaluation of the knee and patellar regions. J Ultras Med 6:33, 1987.
943. Zeiss J, Saddemi SR, Ebraheim NA: MR imaging of the quadriceps tendon: Normal layered configuration and its importance in cases of tendon rupture. AJR 159:1031, 1992.
944. Schutzer SF, Ramsby GR, Fulkerson JP: The evaluation of patellofemoral pain using computerised tomography: A preliminary report. Clin Orthop 204:286, 1986.
945. Insall JN, Falvo KA, Wise DN: Chondromalacia patellae. J Bone Joint Surg [Am] 58:1, 1976.
946. Insall JN, Salvati E: Patella position in the normal knee joint. Radiology 101:101, 1971.
947. Insall J, Goldberg V, Salvati E: Recurrent dislocation and the high-riding patella. Clin Orthop 88:67, 1972.
948. Blumensaat C: Die lageabweichungen und verrenkugen der kniescheibe. Ergeb Chir Orthop 31:149, 1938.
949. Brattstrom H: Patella alta in non-dislocated knee joints. Acta Orthop Scand 41:578, 1970.
950. Labelle H, Laurin CA: Radiological investigation of normal and abnormal patellae. J Bone Joint Surg [Br] 57:530, 1975.
951. Blackburne JS, Peel TE: A new method of measuring patellar height. J Bone Joint Surg [Br] 59:241, 1977.
952. de Carvalho A, Andersen AH, Toop S, et al: A method for assessing the height of the patella. Int Orthop 9:195, 1985.
953. Gresalmer RP, Meadows S: The modified Insall-Salvati ratio for assessment of patellar height. Clin Orthop 282:170, 1992.
954. Merchant AC, Mercer RL, Jacobsen RM, et al: Roentgenographic analysis of patellofemoral congruence. J Bone Joint Surg [Am] 56:1391, 1974.
955. Laurin CA, Dussault R, Levesque HP: The tangential x-ray investigation of the patellofemoral joint: x-ray technique, diagnostic criteria, and interpretation. Clin Orthop 144:16, 1979.
956. Conway WF, Hayes CW, Loughran T, et al: Cross-sectional imaging of the patellofemoral joint and surrounding structures. RadioGraphics 11:195, 1991.
957. Inoue M, Shino K, Hirose H, et al: Subluxation of the patella: Computed tomography of patellofemoral congruence. J Bone Joint Surg [Am] 70:1331, 1988.
958. Martinez S, Korokken M, Fondren FB, et al: Diagnosis of patellofemoral malalignment by computed tomography. J Comput Assist Tomogr 7:1050, 1983.
959. Stanford W, Phelan J, Kathol MH, et al: Patellofemoral joint motion: Evaluation by ultrafast computed tomography. Skel Radiol 17:487, 1988.
960. Shellock FG, Mink JH, Fox JM: Patellofemoral joint: Kinematic MR imaging to assess tracking abnormalities. Radiology 168:551, 1988.
961. Shellock FG, Mink JH, Deutsch AL, et al: Patellar tracking abnormalities: Clinical experience with kinematic MR imaging in 130 patients. Radiology 172:799, 1989.
962. Shellock FG, Foo TKF, Deutsch AL, et al: Patellofemoral joint: Evaluation during active flexion and ultrafast spoiled GRASS MR imaging. Radiology 180:581, 1991.
963. Shellock FG, Mink JH, Deutsch AL, et al: Kinematic MR imaging of the patellofemoral joint: Comparison of passive positioning and active movement techniques. Radiology 184:574, 1992.
964. Shellock FG, Mink JH, Deutsch AL, et al: Patellofemoral joint: Identification of abnormalities with active-movement, "unloaded" versus "loaded" kinematic MR imaging techniques. Radiology 188:575, 1993.
965. Brossman J, Muhle C, Schröder C, et al: Patellar tracking patterns during active and passive knee extension: Evaluation with motion-triggered cine MR imaging. Radiology 187:205, 1993.
966. Niitsu M, Akisada M, Anno I, et al: Moving knee joint: Technique for kinematic MR imaging. Radiology 174:569, 1990.
967. Hughston JC, Deese M: Medial subluxation of the patella as a complication of lateral release. Am J Sports Med 16:383, 1988.
968. Hughston JC: Patellar subluxation: a recent history. Clin Sports Med 8:153, 1989.
969. Kirsch MD, Fitzgerald SW, Friedman H, et al: Transient lateral patellar dislocation: Diagnosis with MR imaging. AJR 161:109, 1993.
970. Gilbert TJ, Johnson E, Detlie T, et al: Patellar dislocation: Medial retinacular tears, avulsion fractures, and osteochondral fragments. Orthopedics 16:732, 1993.
971. Aleman O: Chondromalacia post-traumatica patellae. Acta Chir Scand 63:149, 1928.
972. Ficat RP, Phillippe J, Hungerford DS: Chondromalacia patellae. A system of classification. Clin Orthop 144:55, 1979.
973. Jackson RW: Etiology of chondromalacia patellae. Instr Course Lect 25:36, 1976.
974. Outerbridge RE: The etiology of chondromalacia patellae. J Bone Joint Surg [Br] 43:752, 1961.
975. Arnoczky SP, Warren RF: Anatomy of the cruciate ligaments. In JA Feagin Jr (Ed): The Crucial Ligaments. New York, Churchill Livingstone, 1988, p 179.
976. Dye SF, Cannon WD Jr: Anatomy and biomechanics of the anterior cruciate ligament. Clin Sports Med 7:715, 1988.
977. Girgis FG, Marshall JL, Monajem ARS: The cruciate ligaments of the knee joint. Anatomical, functional, and experimental analysis. Clin Orthop 106:216, 1975.
978. Kennedy JC, Hawkins RJ, Willis RB, et al: Tension studies of human knee ligaments. Yield point, ultimate failure, and disruption of the cruciate and tibial collateral ligaments. J Bone Joint Surg [Am] 58:350, 1976.
979. Arnoczky SP: Anatomy of the anterior cruciate ligament. Clin Orthop 172:19, 1983.
980. Odensten M, Gillquist J: Functional anatomy of the anterior cruciate ligament and a rationale for reconstruction. J Bone Joint Surg [Am] 67:257, 1985.
981. Cabaud HE: Biomechanics of the anterior cruciate ligaments. Clin Orthop 172:26, 1983.
982. Hodler J, Haghighi P, Trudell D, et al: The cruciate ligaments of the knee: Correlation between MR appearance and gross and histologic findings in cadaveric specimens. AJR 159:357, 1992.
983. Danylchuk KD, Finlay JB, Kreck JP: Microstructural organization of human and bovine cruciate ligaments. Clin Orthop 131:294, 1978.
984. Cooper RR, Misol S: Tendon and ligament insertion: a light and electron microscopic study. J Bone Joint Surg [Am] 52:1, 1970.
985. Kennedy JC, Weinberg HW, Wilson AS: The anatomy and function of the anterior cruciate ligament. J Bone Joint Surg [Am] 56:223, 1974.
986. Markolf KL, Mensch JS, Amstutz HC: Stiffness and laxity of the knee—contributions of the supporting structures. A quantitative in vitro study. J Bone Joint Surg [Am] 58:583, 1976.
987. Grood ES, Stowers SF, Noyes FR: Limits of motion in the human knee: Effect of sectioning the posterior cruciate ligament and posterolateral structures. J Bone Joint Surg [Am] 70:88, 1988.
988. Daniel DM, Stone ML: Diagnosis of knee ligament injury: Tests and measurements of joint laxity. In JA Feagin Jr (Ed): The Crucial Ligaments. New York, Churchill Livingstone, 1988, p 287.
989. Balkfors B: The course of knee-ligament injuries. Acta Orthop Scand 198:1, 1982.
990. Fetto JF, Marshall JL: The natural history and diagnosis of anterior cruciate ligament insufficiency. Clin Orthop 147:29, 1980.
991. Feagin JA, Curl WW: Isolated tear of the anterior cruciate ligament: 5-year follow-up study. Am J Sports Med 4:95, 1976.
992. Feagin JA: The syndrome of the torn anterior cruciate ligament. Orthop Clin North Am 10:81, 1979.
993. Arnold JA, Coker TP, Heaton LM, et al: Natural history of anterior cruciate tears. Am J Sports Med 7:305, 1979.
994. Noyes FR, Mooar PA, Matthews DS, et al: The symptomatic anterior cruciate deficient knee. Part I: The long-term functional disability in athletically active individuals. J Bone Joint Surg [Am] 65:154, 1983.
995. Noyes FR, Grood ES: Diagnosis of knee ligament injuries: Clinical concepts. In JA Feagin Jr (Ed): The Crucial Ligaments. New York, Churchill Livingstone, 1988, p 261.
996. Malcolm LL, Daniel DM, Stone ML, et al: The measurement of anterior knee laxity after ACL reconstructive surgery. Clin Orthop 196:35, 1985.
997. Daniel DM, Malcolm LL, Losse G, et al: Instrumented measurement of anterior laxity of the joint. J Bone Joint Surg [Am] 67:720, 1985.
998. Noyes FR, Bassett RW, Grood ES, et al: Arthroscopy in acute traumatic hemarthrosis of the knee. J Bone Joint Surg [Am] 62:687, 1980.
999. Gillquist J, Hagberg G, Oretorp N: Arthroscopy in acute injuries of the knee joint. Acta Orthop Scand 48:190, 1977.
1000. De Haven KE: Diagnosis of acute knee injuries with hemarthrosis. Am J Sports Med 8:9, 1980.
1001. Meyers MH, McKeever FM: Fracture of the intercondylar eminence. J Bone Joint Surg [Am] 41:209, 1959.
1002. Eady JL, Cardenas CD, Sopa D: Avulsion of the femoral attachment of the anterior cruciate ligament in a seven-year-old child. J Bone Joint Surg [Am] 64:1376, 1982.
1003. Stallenberg B, Gevenois PA, Sintzoff SA Jr, et al: Fracture of the posterior aspect of the lateral tibial plateau: Radiographic sign of anterior cruciate ligament tear. Radiology 187:821, 1993.

1004. Losee RE, Johnson TR, Southwick WO: Anterior subluxation of the lateral tibial plateau. J Bone Joint Surg [Am] 60:1015, 1978.

1005. Galway HR, MacIntosh DL: The lateral pivot shift: a symptom and sign of anterior cruciate ligament insufficiency. Clin Orthop 147:45, 1980.

1006. Cobby MJ, Schweitzer ME, Resnick D: The deep lateral femoral notch: An indirect sign of a torn anterior cruciate ligament. Radiology 184:855, 1992.

1007. Warren RF, Kaplan N, Bach BR: The lateral notch sign of anterior cruciate ligament insufficiency. Am J Knee Surg 1:119, 1988.

1008. Mittler S, Freiberger RH, Harrison-Stubbs M: A method of improving cruciate ligament visualization in double contrast arthrography. Radiology 102:441, 1972.

1009. Arcomano JP, Anetrella LJ: Visualizing the anterior cruciate ligament. AJR 138:1189, 1982.

1010. Reider B, Clancy W, Langer LO: Diagnosis of cruciate ligament injury using single contrast arthrography. Am J Sports Med 12:451, 1984.

1011. Dalinka MK, Gohel VK, Rancier L: Tomography in the evaluation of the anterior cruciate ligament. Radiology 108:31, 1973.

1012. Pavlov H, Torg JS: Double contrast arthrographic evaluation of the anterior cruciate ligament. Radiology 126:661, 1978.

1013. Pavlov H, Freiberger RH: An easy method to demonstrate the cruciate ligaments by double contrast arthrography. Radiology 126:817, 1978.

1014. Pavlov H, Warren RF, Sherman MF, et al: The accuracy of double-contrast arthrographic evaluation of the anterior cruciate ligament. A retrospective review of one hundred and sixty-three knees with surgical confirmation. J Bone Joint Surg [Am] 65:175, 1983.

1015. Pavlov H: The radiographic diagnosis of the anterior cruciate ligament deficient knee. Clin Orthop 172:57, 1983.

1016. Brody GA, Pavlov H, Warren RF, et al: Plica synovialis infra-patellaris: Arthrographic sign of anterior cruciate ligament disruption. AJR 140:767, 1983.

1017. Braunstein EM: Anterior cruciate ligament injuries: A comparison of arthrographic and physical diagnosis. AJR 138:423, 1982.

1018. Fitzgerald SW, Remer EM, Friedman H, et al: MR evaluation of the anterior cruciate ligament: Value of supplementing sagittal images with coronal and axial images. AJR 160:1233, 1993.

1019. Remer EM, Fitzgerald SW, Friedman H, et al: Anterior cruciate ligament injury: MR imaging diagnosis and patterns of injury. RadioGraphics 12:901, 1992.

1020. Buckwalter KA, Pennes DR: Anterior cruciate ligament: Oblique sagittal MR imaging. Radiology 175:276, 1990.

1021. Vellet AD, Fowler P, Marks P, et al: Accuracy of non-orthogonal MR imaging in acute disruption of the anterior cruciate ligament. Radiology 173(P):233, 1989.

1022. Mink JH, Levy T, Crues JV III: Tears of the anterior cruciate ligament and menisci of the knee: MR imaging evaluation. Radiology 167:769, 1988.

1023. Niitsu M, Anno I, Fukubayashi T, et al: Tears of the cruciate ligaments and menisci: Evaluation with cine MR imaging. Radiology 178:859, 1991.

1024. Lee JK, Yao L, Phelps CT, et al: Anterior cruciate ligament tears: MR imaging compared with arthroscopy and clinical tests. Radiology 166:861, 1988.

1025. Vahey TN, Broome DR, Kaye KJ, et al: Acute and chronic tears of the anterior cruciate ligament: Differential features at MR imaging. Radiology 181:251, 1991.

1026. Kaye JJ: Ligament and tendon tears: Secondary signs. Radiology 188:616, 1993.

1027. Tung GA, Davis LM, Wiggens ME, et al: Tears of the anterior cruciate ligament: Primary and secondary signs at MR imaging. Radiology 188:661, 1993.

1028. Boeree NR, Ackroyd CE: Magnetic resonance imaging of anterior cruciate ligament rupture. A new diagnostic sign. J Bone Joint Surg [Br] 74:614, 1992.

1029. Schweitzer ME, Cervilla V, Kursunoglu-Brahme S, et al: The PCL line: An indirect sign of anterior cruciate ligament injury. Clin Imag 16:43, 1992.

1030. Vahey TN, Hunt JE, Shelbourne KD: Anterior translocation of the tibia at MR imaging: A secondary sign of anterior cruciate ligament tear. Radiology 187:817, 1993.

1031. Murphy BJ, Smith RL, Uribe JW, et al: Bone signal abnormalities in the posterolateral tibia and lateral femoral condyle in complete tears of the anterior cruciate ligament: A specific sign? Radiology 182:221, 1992.

1032. Kaplan PA, Walker CW, Kilcoyne RF, et al: Occult fracture patterns of the knee associated with anterior cruciate ligament tears: Assessment with MR imaging. Radiology 183:835, 1992.

1033. McDaniel WJ, Dameron TB: Untreated ruptures of the anterior cruciate ligament: a follow-up. J Bone Joint Surg [Am] 62:696, 1980.

1034. McDaniel WJ, Dameron TB: The untreated anterior cruciate ligament rupture. Clin Orthop 172:158, 1983.

1035. Beynnon BD, Johnson RJ, Fleming BC: The mechanics of anterior cruciate ligament reconstruction. In DW Jackson (Ed): The Anterior Cruciate Ligament: Current and Future Concepts. New York, Raven Press, 1993, p 259.

1036. Johnson RJ, Beynnon BD, Nichols CE, et al: Current concepts review: the treatment of injuries to the anterior cruciate ligament. J Bone Joint Surg [Am] 74:140, 1992.

1037. Noyes FR, Butler D, Grood E, et al: Biomechanical analysis of human ligament grafts used in knee ligament repairs and reconstruction. J Bone Joint Surg [Am] 66:344, 1984.

1038. Noyes FR, Butler D, Paulos LE, et al: Intra-articular cruciate reconstruction: 1. Perspectives on graft strength, vascularization, and immediate motion after replacement. Clin Orthop 172:71, 1983.

1039. McFarland EG, Morrey BF, An KN, et al: The relationship of vascularity and water content to tensile strength in a patellar tendon replacement of the anterior cruciate in dogs. Am J Sports Med 14:436, 1986.

1040. Yasuda K, Tomiyama Y, Ohkoshi Y, et al: Arthroscopic observations of autogenetic quadriceps and patellar tendon grafts after anterior cruciate ligament reconstruction of the knee. Clin Orthop 246:217, 1989.

1041. Clancy WG, Ray M, Zoltan J: Nonoperative or operative treatment of acute anterior cruciate ligament tears. J Bone Joint Surg [Am] 70:1483, 1988.

1042. Grood ES, Hefzy MS, Butler DL, et al: On the placement and the initial tension of anterior cruciate ligament substitutes. Trans Orthop Res Soc 8:92, 1983.

1043. Burns GS, Howell SM: The effect of tibial hole placement and roofplasty on impingement of anterior cruciate ligament reconstructions. Trans Orthop Res 17:656, 1992.

1044. Hefzy MS, Grood ES: Sensitivity of insertion locations on length patterns of anterior cruciate ligament fibers. J Biomech Eng 108:73, 1986.

1045. Paulos LE, Rosenberg TD, Drawbert J, et al: Infrapatellar contracture syndrome: an unrecognized cause of knee stiffness with patella entrapment and patella infera. Am J Sports Med 15:331, 1987.

1046. Jackson DW, Schaefer RK: Cyclops syndrome: loss of extension following intra-articular ACL reconstruction. Arthroscopy 6:171, 1990.

1047. Manaster BJ, Remley K, Newman AP, et al: Knee ligament reconstruction: Plain film analysis. AJR 150:337, 1988.

1048. Howell SM, Clark JA: Tibial tunnel placement in anterior cruciate ligament reconstructions and graft impingement. Clin Orthop 283:187, 1992.

1049. Christen B, Jakob RP: Fractures associated with patellar ligament grafts in cruciate ligament surgery. J Bone Joint Surg [Br] 74:617, 1992.

1050. Bonamo JJ, Krinick RM, Sporn AA: Rupture of the patellar ligament after use of its central third for anterior cruciate ligament reconstruction: a report of two cases. J Bone Joint Surg [Am] 66:1294, 1984.

1051. McCarroll JR: Fracture of the patella during a golf swing following reconstruction of the anterior cruciate ligament: a case report. Am J Sports Med 11:26, 1983.

1052. Moeser P, Bechtold RE, Clark T, et al: MR imaging of anterior cruciate ligament repair. J Comput Assist Tomogr 13:105, 1989.

1053. Rak KM, Gillogly SD, Schaefer RA, et al: Anterior cruciate ligament reconstruction: Evaluation with MR imaging. Radiology 178:553, 1991.

1054. Allgayer B, Gradinger R, Lehner K, et al: Die Kernspintomgraphic zur Beurteilung des vorderen Kreuzbandersatzes mit Sehnentransplantaten. Fortschr Röntgenstr 155:294, 1991.

1055. Autz G, Goodwin C, Singson RD: Magnetic resonance evaluation of anterior cruciate ligament repair using the patellar tendon double bone block technique. Skel Radiol 20:585, 1991.

1056. Howell SM, Berns GS, Farley TE: Unimpinged and impinged anterior cruciate ligament grafts: MR signal intensity measurements. Radiology 179:639, 1991.

1057. Yamato M, Yamagishi T: MRI of patellar tendon anterior cruciate ligament autografts. J Comput Assist Tomogr 16:604, 1992.

1058. Sanchis-Alfonso V, Martinez-Sanjuan V, Gastaldi-Orquin E: The value of MRI in the evaluation of the ACL deficient knee and in the post-operative evaluation after ACL reconstruction. Europ J Radiol 16:126, 1993.

1059. Coupens SD, Yates CK, Sheldon C, et al: Magnetic resonance imaging evaluation of the patellar tendon after use of its central one-third for anterior cruciate ligament reconstruction. Am J Sports Med 20:332, 1992.

1060. Fowler PJ, Messieh SS: Isolated PCL injuries in athletes. Am J Sports Med 15:553, 1987.

1061. Bianchi M: Acute tears of the PCL: Clinical study and results of operative treatment in 27 cases. Am J Sports Med 11:308, 1983.

1062. Cross MJ, Powell JF: Long-term followup of PCL rupture: a study of 116 cases. Am J Sports Med 12:292, 1984.

1063. Fanelli GC: Posterior cruciate ligament injuries in trauma patients. J Arthrosc Rel Surg 9:291, 1993.

1064. Barton TM, Torg JS, Das M: PCL insufficiency: a review of the literature. Sports Med 1:419, 1984.

1065. Grover JS, Bassett LW, Gross ML, et al: Posterior cruciate ligament: MR imaging. Radiology 174:527, 1990.

1066. Campbell CJ: The healing of cartilage defects. Clin Orthop 64:45, 1969.

1067. Landells JW: The reactions of injured human articular cartilage. J Bone Joint Surg [Br] 39:548, 1957.

1068. Harris ED Jr: Biology of the joint. In WN Kelley, ED Harris Jr, S Ruddy, and CB Sledge (Eds): Textbook of Rheumatology. Philadelphia, WB Saunders Co, 1985, p 254.

1069. Meachim G: Light microscopy of Indian ink preparations of fibrillated cartilage. Ann Rheum Dis 31:457, 1972.

1070. Byers PD, Contepomi CA, Farker TA: A postmortem study of the hip joint. Ann Rheum Dis 29:15, 1970.

1071. Anderson PW, Maslin P: Tomography applied to knee arthrography. Radiology 110:271, 1974.

1072. Thomas RH, Resnick D, Alazraki NP, et al: Compartmental evaluation of osteoarthritis of the knee. A comparative study of available diagnostic modalities. Radiology 116:585, 1975.

1073. Kaufmann J, Langlotz M: Ist die idiopathische Chondropathia patellae mit radiologischen methoden Diagnostizierbar? ROFO 141:422, 1984.

1074. Horns JW: The diagnosis of chondromalacia by double contrast arthrography of the knee. J Bone Joint Surg [Am] 59:119, 1977.

1075. Thijn CJP: Double contrast arthrography in meniscal lesions and patellar chondropathy. Radiol Clin Biol 45:345, 1976.

1076. Rau WS, Kauffmann G: Röntgendiagnostik des Knorpelschadens am Kniegelenk. Radiologe 18:451, 1978.

1077. Reichelt A, Hehne HJ, Rau WS, et al: Die doppel Kontrast-arthrographie bei der Chondropathia patellae—klinische und experimentelle Studie zur Pathogenese und Diagnostik. Z Orthop 117:746, 1979.

1078. Reiser M, Karpf P-M, Bernett P: Diagnosis of chondromalacia patellae using CT arthrography. Eur J Radiol 2:181, 1982.

1079. Boven F, Bellemans M-A, Geurts J, et al: A comparative study of the patellofemoral joint on axial roentgenogram, axial arthrogram, and computed tomography following arthrography. Skel Radiol 8:179, 1982.

1080. Boven F, Bellemans M-A, Geurts J, et al: The value of computed tomography scanning in chondromalacia patellae. Skel Radiol 8:183, 1982.

1081. Hayes CW, Sawyer RW, Conway WF: Patellar cartilage lesions: in vitro detection and staging with MR imaging and pathologic correlation. Radiology 176:479, 1990.

1082. Yulish BS, Montanez J, Goodfellow DB, et al: Chondromalacia patellae: assessment with MR imaging. Radiology 164:763, 1987.

1083. Hodler J, Resnick D: Chrondromalacia patellae. AJR 158:101, 1992.

1084. McCauley TR, Kier R, Lynch KJ, et al: Chondromalacia patellae: diagnosis with MR imaging. AJR 158:101, 1992.

1085. Handelberg F, Shahabpour M, Casteleyn P: Chondral lesions of the patella evaluated with computed tomography, magnetic resonance imaging, and arthroscopy. Arthroscopy 6:24, 1990.

1086. Wojtys E, Wilson M, Buckwalter K, et al: Magnetic resonance imaging of knee hyaline cartilage and intraarticular pathology. Am J Sports Med 15:455, 1987.

1087. Lehner KB, Rechl HP, Gmeinwieser JK, et al: Structure, function and degeneration of bovine hyaline cartilage: assessment with MR imaging in vitro. Radiology 170:495, 1989.

1088. Wolff SD, Chesnick S, Frank JA, et al: Magnetization transfer contrast imaging of the knee. Radiology 179:623, 1991.

1089. Chandnani VP, Ho C, Chu P, et al: Knee hyaline cartilage evaluated with MR imaging: a cadaveric study involving multiple imaging sequences and intraarticular injection of gadolinium and saline solution. Radiology 178:557, 1991.

1090. Totterman S, Weiss SL, Szumowski J, et al: MR fat suppression technique in the evaluation of normal structure of the knee. J Comput Assist Tomogr 13:473, 1989.

1091. König H, Sauter R, Deimling M, et al: Cartilage disorders: comparison of spin-echo, CHESS, and FLASH sequence MR images. Radiology 164:753, 1987.

1092. Speer KP, Spritzer CE, Goldner JL, et al: Magnetic resonance imaging of traumatic knee articular cartilage injuries. Am J Sports Med 19:396, 1991.

1093. Tyrrell RL, Gluckert K, Pathria M, et al: Fast three-dimensional MR imaging of the knee: comparison with arthroscopy. Radiology 166:865, 1988.

1094. Heron CW, Calvert PT: Three-dimensional gradient-echo MR imaging of the knee: comparison with arthroscopy in 100 patients. Radiology 183:839, 1992.

1095. Reiser MF, Bongartz G, Erlemann R, et al: Magnetic resonance in cartilaginous lesions of the knee joint with three-dimensional gradient-echo imaging. Skel Radiol 17:465, 1988.

1096. Gylys-Morin VM, Hajek PC, Sartoris DJ, et al: Articular cartilage defects: detectability in cadaver knees with MR. AJR 148:1153, 1987.

1097. Kramer J, Stiglbauer R, Engel A, et al: MR contrast arthrography (MRA) in osteochondrosis dissecans. J Comput Assist Tomogr 16:254, 1992.

1098. Modl JM, Sether LA, Haughton VM, et al: Articular cartilage: correlation of histologic zones with signal intensity at MR imaging. Radiology 181:853, 1991.

1099. Recht MP, Kramer J, Marcelis S, et al: Abnormalities of articular cartilage in the knee: Analysis of available MR techniques. Radiology 187:473, 1993.

1100. Rubenstein JD, Kim JK, Morava-Protzner I, et al: Effects of collagen orientation on MR imaging characteristics of bovine articular cartilage. Radiology 188:219, 1993.

1101. Maroudas A: Physicochemical properties of articular cartilage. In MAR Freeman (Ed): Adult Articular Cartilage. London, Pitman Medical, 1979, pp 215–290.

1102. Maroudas A, Weinberg PD, Parker KH: The distributions and diffusivities of small ions in chondroitin sulphate, hyaluronate and some proteoglycan solutions. Biophys Chem 32:257, 1988.

1103. Maroudas A, Schneiderman R, Popper O: The role of water, proteoglycan, and collagen in solute transport in cartilage. In KE Kuettner, R Schleyerbach, JG Peyron, and VC Hascall (Eds): Articular Cartilage and Osteoarthritis. New York, Raven Press, 1992, pp 355–372.

1104. Maroudas A: Distribution and diffusion of solutes in articular cartilage. Biophys J 10:365, 1970.

1105. Torzilli PA, Adams TC, Mis RJ: Transient solute diffusion in articular cartilage. J Biomech 2:203, 1987.

1106. Burstein D, Gray ML, Hartman AL, et al: Diffusion of small solutes in cartilage as measured by nuclear magnetic resonance (NMR) spectroscopy and imaging. J Orthop Res 11:465, 1993.

1107. Brandt KD, Adams ME: Exuberant repair of articular cartilage damage. Effect of anterior cruciate ligament transection in the dog. Trans Orthop Res Society 14:584, 1989.

1108. Vignon E, Arlot M, Hartman D, et al: Hypertrophic repair of articular cartilage in experimental osteoarthrosis. Ann Rheum Dis 42:82, 1983.

1109. Braunstein EM, Brandt KD, Albrecht M: MRI demonstration of hypertrophic articular cartilage repair in osteoarthritis. Skel Radiol 19:335, 1990.

1110. Adams ME, Brandt KD: Hypertrophic repair of canine articular cartilage in osteoarthritis after anterior cruciate ligament transection. J Rheumatol 18:428, 1991.

1111. Pritzker KPH: Posttraumatic cartilage hypertrophy: Edema or repair? J Rheumatol 18:314, 1991.

1112. Brandt KD, Braunstein EM, Visco DM, et al: Anterior (cranial) cruciate ligament transection in the dog: A bona fide model of osteoarthritis, not merely of cartilage injury and repair. J Rheumatol 18:436, 1991.

1113. Yao L, Sinha S, Seeger LL: MR imaging of joints: Analytic optimization of GRE techniques at 1.5 T. AJR 158:339, 1992.

1114. Hayes CW, Conway WF: Evaluation of articular cartilage: Radiographic and cross-sectional imaging techniques. RadioGraphics 12:409, 1992.

1115. De Smet AA, Monu JUV, Fisher DR, et al: Signs of patellar chondromalacia on sagittal T2-weighted magnetic resonance imaging. Skel Radiol 21:103, 1992.

1116. Hodler J, Berthiaume M-J, Schweitzer ME, et al: Knee joint hyaline cartilage defects: A comparitive study of MR and anatomic sections. J Comput Assist Tomogr 16:597, 1992.

1117. Brown TR, Quinn SF: Evaluation of chondromalacia of the patellofemoral compartment with axial magnetic resonance imaging. Skel Radiol 22:325, 1993.

1118. Tien RD: Fat-suppression MR imaging in neuroradiology: Techniques and clinical application. AJR 158:369, 1992.

1119. Koskinen SK, Komu M, Aho HJ, et al: MR imaging of patellar cartilage degeneration at 0.02T. Study of 23 cadaveric patellae. Acta Radiol 32:514, 1991.

1120. Nakanishi K, Inoue M, Harada K, et al: Subluxation of the patella: evaluation of patellar articular cartilage with MR imaging. Br J Radiol 65:662, 1992.

1121. Chan WP, Lang P, Stevens MP, et al: Osteoarthritis of the knee: Comparison of radiography, CT, and MR imaging to assess extent and severity. AJR 157:799, 1991.

1122. McAlindon TEM, Watt I, McCrae F, et al: Magnetic resonance imaging in osteoarthritis of the knee: correlation with radiographic and scintigraphic findings. Ann Rheum Dis 50:14, 1991.

1123. Bongartz G, Bock E, Horbach T, et al: Degenerative cartilage lesions of the hip: magnetic resonance evaluation. Magn Res Imag 7:179, 1989.

1124. Wolff SD, Balaban RS: Magnetization transfer contrast (MTC) and tissue water proton relaxation in vivo. Magn Reson Med 10:135, 1989.

1125. Wolff SD, Eng J, Balaban RS: Magnetization transfer contrast: Method for improving contrast in gradient-recalled-echo images. Radiology 179:133, 1991.

1126. Wolff SD, Chesnick S, Frank JA, et al: Magnetization transfer contrast: MR imaging of the knee. Radiology 179:623, 1991.

1127. Milgram JW: Radiologic and Histologic Pathology of Nontumorous Diseases of Bones and Joints. Northbrook, IL, Northbrook Publishing Company, Inc. 1990, pp 265, 281.

1128. Milgram JW: The classification of loose bodies in human joints. Clin Orthop 124:282, 1977.

1129. Milgram JW: The development of loose bodies in human joints. Clin Orthop 124:292, 1977.

1130. Milgram JW: Radiological and pathological manifestations of osteochondritis dissecans of the distal femur. Radiology 126:305, 1978.

1131. Nelson DW, DiPaola J, Colville M, et al: Osteochondritis dissecans of the talus and knee: Prospective comparison of MR and arthroscopic classifications. J Comput Assist Tomogr 14:804, 1990.

1132. Adam G, Bühune M, Prescher A, et al: Stability of osteochondral fragments of the femoral condyle: magnetic resonance imaging with histopathologic correlation in an animal model. Skel Radiol 20:601, 1991.

1133. Lehner K, Heuck A, Rodammer G, et al: MRI bei der Osteochondrosis dissecans. ROFO 147:191, 1987.

1134. De Smet AA, Fisher DR, Graf BK, et al: Osteochondritis dissecans of the knee: Value of MR imaging in determining lesion stability and the presence of articular cartilage defects. AJR 155:549, 1990.

1135. Mesgarzadeh M, Sapega AA, Bonakdarpour A, et al: Osteochondritis dissecans: Analysis of mechanical stability with radiography, scintigraphy, and MR imaging. Radiology 165:775, 1987.

1136. Vellet AD, Marks PH, Fowler PJ, et al: Occult posttraumatic osteochondral lesions of the knee: Prevalence, classification, and short-term sequelae evaluated with MR imaging. Radiology 178:271, 1991.

1137. Yao L, Lee JK: Occult intraosseous fracture: Detection with MR imaging. Radiology 167:749, 1988.

1138. Lynch TCP, Crues JV III, Morgan FW, et al: Bone abnormalities of the knee: Prevalence and significance at MR imaging. Radiology 171:761, 1989.

1139. Mink JH, Deutsch AL: Occult cartilage and bone injuries of the knee: Detection, classification, and assessment with MR imaging. Radiology 170:823, 1989.

1140. Thompson RC Jr, Vener MJ, Griffiths HJ, et al: Scanning electron-microscopic and magnetic resonance-imaging studies of injuries to the patellofemoral joint after acute transarticular loading. J Bone Joint Surg [Am] 75:704, 1993.

1141. Deutsch AL, Mink JH, Rosenfelt FP, et al: Incidental detection of hematopoietic hyperplasia on routine knee MR imaging. AJR 152:333, 1989.

1142. Schuck JE, Czarnecki DJ: MR detection of probable hematopoietic hyperplasia involving the knees, proximal femurs, and pelvis. AJR 153:655, 1989.

1143. Shellock FG, Morris E, Deutsch AL, et al: Hematopoietic bone marrow hyperplasia: High prevalence on MR images of the knee in asymptomatic marathon runners. AJR 158:335, 1992.

1144. Lang PL, Fritz R, Vahlensieck M, et al: Residuales und rekonvertiertes hämatopoetisches Knochenmark im distalen Femur. ROFO *156*:89, 1992.

1145. Lang PL, Fritz R, Majumdar S, et al: Hematopoietic bone marrow in the adult knee: spin-echo and opposed-phase gradient-echo MR imaging. Skel Radiol *22*:95, 1993.

1146. Freund E: Chondromatosis of the joints. Arch Surg *34*:670, 1937.

1147. Dandy DJ, O'Carroll PF: The removal of loose bodies from the knee under arthroscopic control. J Bone Joint Surg [Br] *64*:473, 1982.

1148. Ramsey PL, Hamilton W: Changes in tibiotalar area of contact caused by lateral talar shift. J Bone Joint Surg [Am] *58*:356, 1976.

1149. Skinner EH: The mathematical calculation of progress in fractures at the ankle and wrist. Surg Gynecol Obstet *18*:238, 1914.

1150. Joy G, Patzakis MJ, Harvey JP Jr: Precise evaluation of the reduction of severe ankle fractures. Technique and correlation with end results. J Bone Joint Surg [Am] *56*:979, 1974.

1151. Hutter CG Jr, Scott W: Tibial torsion. J Bone Joint Surg [Am] *31*:511, 1949.

1152. Goergen TG, Danzig LA, Resnick D, et al: Roentgenographic evaluation of the tibiotalar joint. J Bone Joint Surg [Am] *59*:874, 1977.

1153. Jonsson K, Fredin HO, Cederlund CG, Bauer M: Width of the normal ankle joint. Acta Radiol Diagn *25*:147, 1984.

1154. Kaye JJ, Bohne WHO: A radiographic study of the ligamentous anatomy of the ankle. Radiology *125*:659, 1977.

1155. Towbin R, Dunbar JS, Towbin J, et al: Teardrop sign: Plain film recognition of ankle effusion. AJR *134*:985, 1980.

1156. Hall FM: Pitfalls in the diagnosis of ankle joint effusion. AJR *136*:637, 1981.

1157. Resnick D: Radiology of the talocalcaneal articulations. Anatomic considerations and arthrography. Radiology *111*:581, 1974.

1158. Rhea JT, De Luca SA, Sheehan J: Radiographic anatomy of the tarsal bones. Med Radiogr Photogr *59*:2, 1983.

1159. Mehrez M, el-Geneidy S: Arthrography of the ankle. J Bone Joint Surg [Br] *52*:308, 1970.

1160. Olson RW: Arthrography of the ankle: Its use in the evaluation of ankle sprains. Radiology *92*:1439, 1969.

1161. Faure C: The skeleton of the anterior foot. Anatomia Clin *3*:49, 1981.

1162. Palmer DG: Tendon sheaths and bursae involved by rheumatoid disease at the foot and ankle. Australas Radiol *14*:419, 1970.

1163. Teng MMH, Destouet JM, Gilula LA, et al: Ankle tenography: A key to unexplained symptomatology. Part I. Normal tenographic anatomy. Radiology *151*:575, 1984.

1164. Gilula LA, Oloff L, Caputi R, et al: Ankle tenography: A key to unexplained symptomatology. Part II. Diagnosis of chronic tendon disabilities. Radiology *151*:581, 1984.

1165. Meurman KOA: Bursa tendinis musculi flexoris hallucis longi. ROFO *136*:27, 1982.

1166. Resnick D, Goergen TG: Peroneal tenography in previous calcaneal fractures. Radiology *115*:211, 1975.

1167. Sutro CJ: The os calcis, the tendo-achillis and the local bursae. Bull Hosp Joint Dis *27*:76, 1966.

1168. Weston WJ: The bursa deep to the tendo achillis. Australas Radiol *14*:327, 1970.

1169. Lieber GA, Lemont H: The posterior triangle of the ankle. Determination of its true anatomical boundary. J Am Podiatr Assoc *72*:363, 1982.

1170. Goodman LR, Shanser JD: The pre-Achilles fat pad: An aid to early diagnosis of local systemic disease. Skel Radiol *2*:81, 1977.

1171. Minns RJ, Hunter JAA: The mechanical and structural characteristics of the tibiofibular interosseous membrane. Acta Orthop Scand *47*:236, 1976.

1172. Schweitzer ME, Resnick D: Normal anatomy of the foot and ankle. *In* AL Deutsch, JH Mink, and R Kerr (Eds): MRI of the Foot and Ankle. New York, Raven Press, 1992, p 33.

1173. Jaffe WL, Gannon PJ, Laitman JT: Paleontology, embryology, and anatomy of the foot. *In* MH Jahss (Ed): Disorders of the Foot and Ankle. 2nd Ed. Philadelphia, WB Saunders Co, 1991, p 3.

1174. Mink JH: Tendons. *In* AL Deutsch, JH Mink, and R Kerr (Eds): MRI of the Foot and Ankle. New York, Raven Press, 1992, p 135.

1175. Jahss MH: Tendon disorders of the foot and ankle. *In* MH Jahss (Ed): Disorders of the Foot and Ankle. 2nd Ed. Philadelphia, WB Saunders Co, 1991, p 1461.

1176. Cheung Y, Rosenberg ZS, Magee T, et al: Normal anatomy and pathologic conditions of ankle tendons: Current imaging techniques. RadioGraphics *12*:429, 1992.

1177. Morti R: Dislocation of the peroneal nerve. Am J Sports Med *5*:19, 1977.

1178. Murr S: Dislocation of the peroneal tendon with marginal fracture of the lateral malleolus. J Bone Joint Surg [Br] *43*:563, 1965.

1179. Thompson FM, Patterson AH: Rupture of the peroneus longus tendon. Report of three cases. J Bone Joint Surg [Am] *71*:293, 1989.

1180. Martinoli C, Derchi LE, Pastorino C, et al: Analysis of echotexture of tendons with US. Radiology *186*:839, 1993.

1181. Solomon MA, Gilula LA, Oloff LM, et al: CT scanning of the foot and ankle. 2. Clinical applications and review of the literature. AJR *146*:1204, 1986.

1182. Rosenberg ZS, Feldman F, Singson RD: Peroneal tendon injuries: CT analysis. Radiology *161*:743, 1986.

1183. Szczukowski M, St Pierre RK, Fleming LL, et al: Computerized tomography in the evaluation of peroneal tendon dislocation. A report of two cases. Am J Sports Med *11*:444, 1983.

1184. Keyser CK, Gilula LA, Hardy DC, et al: Soft-tissue abnormalities of the foot and ankle: CT diagnosis. AJR *150*:845, 1988.

1185. Baker KS, Gilula LA: The current role of tenography and bursography. AJR *154*:129, 1990.

1186. Deyerle WM: Long term follow-up of fractures of the os calcis. Diagnostic peroneal synoviagram. Orthop Clin North Am *4*:213, 1973.

1187. Abraham E, Stirnaman JE: Neglected rupture of the peroneal tendons causing recurrent sprains of the ankle. Case report. J Bone Joint Surg [Am] *61*:1247, 1979.

1188. Evans GA, Frenyo SK: The stress-tenogram in the diagnosis of ruptures of the lateral ligament of the ankle. J Bone Joint Surg [Br] *61*:347, 1979.

1189. Teng MMH, Destouet JM, Gilula LA, et al: Ankle tenography: A key to unexplained symptomatology. Part I. Normal tenographic anatomy. Radiology *151*:575, 1984.

1190. Reinus WR, Gilula LA, Lesiak LF, et al: Tenography in unresolved ankle tenosynovitis. Orthopedics *10*:497, 1987.

1191. Beltran J, Noto AM, Mosure JC, et al: Ankle: Surface coil MR imaging at 1.5T. Radiology *161*:203, 1986.

1192. Hajek PC, Baker LL, Bjorkengren A, et al: High-resolution magnetic resonance imaging of the ankle: normal anatomy. Skel Radiol *15*:536, 1986.

1193. Kneeland JB, Macrandar S, Middleton WD, et al: MR imaging of the normal ankle: Correlation with anatomic sections. AJR *151*:117, 1988.

1194. Rosenberg ZS, Cheung Y, Jahss M: Computed tomography and magnetic resonance imaging of ankle tendons: An overview. Foot Ankle *8*:297, 1988.

1195. Noto AM, Cheung Y, Rosenberg ZS, et al: MR imaging of the ankle: Normal variants. Radiology *170*:121, 1989.

1196. Berquist TH: Magnetic resonance imaging of the foot and ankle. Semin Ultrasound CT MR *11*:327, 1990.

1197. Kier R, McCarthy S, Dietz MJ, et al: MR appearance of painful conditions of the ankle. RadioGraphics *11*:401, 1991.

1198. Klein MA: Reformatted three-dimensional Fourier transform gradient-recalled echo MR imaging of the ankle: Spectrum of normal and abnormal findings. AJR *161*:831, 1993.

1199. Link SC, Erickson SJ, Timins ME: MR imaging of the ankle and foot: Normal structures and anatomic variants that may simulate disease. AJR *161*:607, 1993.

1200. Rosenberg ZS, Cheung Y, Jahss MH, et al: Rupture of posterior tibial tendon: CT and MR imaging with surgical correlation. Radiology *169*:229, 1988.

1201. Schweitzer ME, Caccese R, Karasick D, et al: Posterior tibial tendon tears: Utility of secondary signs for MR imaging diagnosis. Radiology *188*:655, 1993.

1202. Weinstabl R, Stiskal M, Neuhold A, et al: Classifying calcaneal tendon injury according to MRI findings. J Bone Joint Surg [Br] *73*:683, 1991.

1203. Neuhold A, Stiskal M, Kainberger F, et al: Degenerative Achilles tendon disease: assessment by magnetic resonance and ultrasonography. Eur J Radiol *14*:213, 1992.

1204. Liem MD, Zegel HG, Balduini FC, et al: Repair of Achilles tendon ruptures with a polylactic acid implant: Assessment with MR imaging. AJR *156*:769, 1991.

1205. Kettlekamp DB, Alexander HH: Spontaneous rupture of the posterior tibial tendon. J Bone Joint Surg [Am] *51*:759, 1969.

1206. Jahss MH: Spontaneous rupture of the tibialis posterior tendon: clinical findings, tenographic studies, and a new technique of repair. Foot Ankle *3*:158, 1982.

1207. Johnson KA: Tibialis posterior tendon rupture. Clin Orthop *177*:140, 1983.

1208. Kelikian H, Kelikian AS: Disorders of the Ankle. Philadelphia, WB Saunders Co, 1985.

1209. Lagergren C, Lindholm A: Vascular disruption in the achilles tendon and angiographic and microangiographic study. Acta Chir Scand *116*:481, 1985.

1210. Schmidt-Rohlfing B, Graf J, Schneider U, et al: The blood supply of the Achilles tendon. Int Orthop (SICOT) *16*:29, 1992.

1211. Quinn SF, Murray WT, Clark RA, et al: Achilles tendon: MR imaging at 1.5T. Radiology *164*:767, 1987.

1212. Christensen IB: Rupture of the Achilles tendon: Analysis of 57 cases. Acta Chir Scand *106*:50, 1953.

1213. Marcus DS, Reicher MA, Kellerhouse LE: Achilles tendon injuries: The role of MR imaging. J Comput Assist Tomogr *13*:480, 1989.

1214. Keene JS, Lash EG, Fisher DR, et al: Magnetic resonance imaging of achilles tendon ruptures. Am J Sports Med *17*:333, 1989.

1215. Reinig JW, Dorwart RH, Roden WC: MR imaging of a ruptured Achilles tendon. J Comput Assist Tomogr *9*:1131, 1985.

1216. Kellam JF, Hunter GA, McElwain JP: Review of the operative treatment of Achilles tendon rupture. Clin Orthop *201*:80, 1985.

1217. Beskin JL, Sanders RA, Hunter SC, et al: Surgical repair of Achilles tendon ruptures. Am J Sports Med *15*:1, 1987.

1218. Inglis AE, Sculco TP: Surgical repair of ruptures of the tendo Achilles. Clin Orthop *156*:160, 1981.

1219. Rooks MD: Tendon, vascular, nerve, and skin injuries. *In* JS Gould (Ed): Operative Foot Surgery. Philadelphia, WB Saunders Co, 1994, p 515.

1220. Funk DA, Cass JR, Johnson KA: Acquired adult flat foot secondary to posterior tibial tendon pathology. J Bone Joint Surg [Am] *68*:95, 1986.

1221. Goldner JL, Keats PK, Bassett FH III, et al: Progressive talipes equinovalgus due to trauma or degeneration of the posterior tibial tendon and medial plantar ligaments. Orthop Clin North Am *15*:39, 1974.

1222. Scheller AD, Kasser JR, Quigley TB: Tendon injuries about the ankle. Orthop Clin North Am *11*:801, 1980.

1223. Frey C, Shereff M, Greenridge N: Vascularity of the posterior tibial tendon. J Bone Joint Surg [Am] *72*:884, 1990.

1224. Stein R: Rupture of the posterior tibial tendon in closed ankle fractures: Possible prognostic value of a medial bone flake. Report of two cases. J Bone Joint Surg [Am] 67:493, 1985.

1225. Hamilton WG: Conditions seen in classical ballet and modern dance. In JS Gould (Ed): Operative Foot Surgery. Philadelphia, WB Saunders Co, 1994, p 954.

1226. Gould N: Stenosing tenosynovitis of the flexor hallucis longus tendon at the great toe. Foot Ankle 2:46, 1981.

1227. Sammarco GJ, Miller ED: Partial rupture of the flexor hallucis longus tendon in classical ballet dancers. J Bone Joint Surg [Am] 61:149, 1979.

1228. Howse AJG: Posterior block of the ankle joint in dancers. Foot Ankle 3:81, 1982.

1229. Hamilton WG: Stenosing tenosynovitis of the flexor hallucis longus tendon and posterior impingement upon the os trigonum in ballet dancers. Foot Ankle 3:74, 1982.

1230. Hamilton WG: Foot and ankle injuries in dancers. Clin Sports Med 7:143, 1988.

1231. Lapidus PW: Indirect subcutaneous rupture of the anterior tibial tendon. Report of two cases. Bull Hosp Joint Dis 2:119, 1941.

1232. Moberg E: Subcutaneous rupture of the tendon of the tibialis anterior muscle. Acta Chir Scand 95:455, 1947.

1233. Mensor MC, Ordway GI. Traumatic subcutaneous rupture of the tibialis anterior tendon. J Bone Joint Surg [Am] 35:675, 1953.

1234. Kojima Y, Kataoka Y, Suzuki S: Dislocations of the peroneal tendons in neonates and infants. Clin Orthop 266:180, 1991.

1235. Eckert WR, Davis EA: Acute rupture of the peroneal retinaculum. J Bone Joint Surg [Am] 58:670, 1976.

1236. Oden R: Tendon injuries about the ankle resulting from skiing. Clin Orthop 216:63, 1987.

1237. Rosenberg Z, Feldman F, Singson R: Peroneal tendon injuries: CT analysis. Radiology 161:743, 1986.

1238. Trevino S, Gould N, Korson R: Surgical treatment of stenosing tenosynovitis at the ankle. Foot Ankle 2:37, 1981.

1239. Zeiss J, Saddemi SR, Ebraheim NA: MR imaging of the peroneal tunnel. J Comput Assist Tomogr 13:840, 1989.

1240. Deyerle WM: Long term follow-up of fractures of the os calcis. Orthop Clin North Am 4:213, 1973.

1241. Thompson F, Patterson A: Rupture of the peroneus longus tendon: Report of three cases. J Bone Joint Surg [Am] 71:293, 1989.

1242. Munk RL, Davis PH: Longitudinal rupture of the peroneus brevis tendon. J Trauma 16:803, 1976.

1243. Peacock KC, Resnick EJ, Thoder JJ: Fracture of the os peroneum with rupture of the peroneus longus tendon. Clin Orthop 202:223, 1984.

1244. Schon LC, Ouzounian TJ: The ankle. In MH Jahss (Ed): Disorders of the Foot and Ankle. 2nd Ed. Philadelphia, WB Saunders Co, 1991, p 1417.

1245. Kannus P, Renstrom P: Treatment for acute tears of the lateral ligaments of the ankle. J Bone Joint Surg [Am] 73:305, 1991.

1246. Siegler S, Block J, Schneck CD: The mechanical characteristics of the collateral ligaments of the human ankle joint. Foot Ankle 8:234, 1988.

1247. Frost HM, Hanson CA: Technique for testing the drawer sign at the ankle. Clin Orthop 123:49, 1977.

1248. Raatikainen T, Putkonen M, Puranen J: Arthrography, clinical examination, and stress radiograph in the diagnosis of acute injury to the lateral ligaments of the ankle. Am J Sports Med 20:2, 1992.

1249. Gaston SR, McLaughlin HL: Complex fractures of the lateral malleolus. J Trauma 1:69, 1961.

1250. Staples OS: Injuries to the medial ligaments of the ankle. J Bone Joint Surg [Am] 42:1287, 1960.

1251. Pankovich AM, Shivaram MS: Anatomical basis of variability in injuries of the medial malleolus and the deltoid ligament. I. Anatomical studies. Acta Orthop Scand 50:217, 1979.

1252. Pankovich AM, Shivaram MS: Anatomical basis of variability in injuries of the medial malleolus and the deltoid ligament. II. Clinical studies. Acta Orthop Scand 50:225, 1979.

1253. Olson RW: Arthrography of the ankle: Its use in the evaluation of ankle sprains. Radiology 92:1439, 1969.

1254. Broström L, Liljedahl SO, Lindvall N: Sprained ankles. II. Arthrographic diagnosis of recent ligament ruptures. Acta Chir Scand 129:485, 1965.

1255. Spiegel PK, Staples OS: Arthrography of the ankle joint: Problems in diagnosis of acute lateral ligament injuries. Radiology 114:587, 1975.

1256. Arner O, Ekengren K, Hulting B, et al: Arthrography of the talocrural joint: Anatomic, roentgenographic and clinical aspects. Acta Chir Scand 113:253, 1957.

1257. Fordyce AJW, Horn CV: Arthrography in recent injuries of the ligament of the ankle. J Bone Joint Surg [Br] 54:116, 1972.

1258. Ala-Ketola L, Puranen J, Koivisto E, et al: Arthrography in the diagnosis of ligament injuries and classification of ankle injuries. Radiology 125:63, 1977.

1259. Mehrez M, El Geneidy S: Arthrography of the ankle. J Bone Joint Surg [Br] 52:308, 1970.

1260. Fussell ME, Godley DR: Ankle arthrography in acute sprains. Clin Orthop 93:278, 1973.

1261. Sanders HWA: Ankle arthrography and ankle distortion. Radiol Clin Biol 46:1, 1977.

1262. Gordon RB: Arthrography of the ankle joint. Experience in 107 studies. J Bone Joint Surg [Am] 52:1623, 1970.

1263. Percy EC, Hill RO, Callaghan JE: The "sprained" ankle. J Trauma 9:972, 1969.

1264. Sauser DD, Nelson RC, Lavine MH, et al: Acute injuries of the lateral ligaments of the ankle: Comparison of stress radiography and arthrography. Radiology 148:653, 1983.

1265. Haller J, Resnick D, Sartoris D, et al: Arthrography, tenography, and bursography of the ankle and foot. Clin Podiatr Med Surg 5:893, 1988.

1266. Bleichrodt RP, Kingma LM, Binnendijk B, et al: Injuries of the lateral ankle ligaments: Classification with tenography and arthrography. Radiology 173:347, 1989.

1267. Wrazidlo W, Karl E-L, Koch K: Die arthrographische Diagnostik der vorderen Syndesmosenruptur am oberen Sprunggelenk. ROFO 148:492, 1988.

1268. van Moppes FI, van den Hoogenband CR, van Engelshoven JMA, et al: Arthrography, talar tilt and surgical findings after inversion trauma of the ankle. ROFO 134:413, 1981.

1269. van Moppes FI, van den Hoogenband CR: The significance of the peroneus tendon sheath in ankle arthrography. ROFO 132:573, 1980.

1270. Vuust M: Arthrographic diagnosis of ruptured calcaneofibular ligament. I. A new projection tested on experimental injury post mortem. Acta Radiol Diagn 21:123, 1980.

1271. Vuust M, Niedermann B: Arthrographic diagnosis of ruptured calcaneofibular ligament. II. Clinical evaluation of a new method. Acta Radiol Diagn 21:231, 1980.

1272. Lindholmer E, Andersen A, Andersen SB, et al: Arthrography of the ankle. Value in diagnosis of rupture of the calcaneofibular ligament. Acta Radiol Diagn 24:217, 1983.

1273. van Moppes FI, Meijer F, van den Hoogenband CR: Arthrographic differential diagnosis between ruptures of the anterior talofibular ligament, the joint capsule and the anterior tibiofibular ligament. ROFO 133:534, 1980.

1274. Beltran J, Munchow AM, Khabiri H, et al: Ligaments of the lateral aspect of the ankle and sinus tarsi: An MR imaging study. Radiology 177:455, 1990.

1275. Erickson SJ, Smith JW, Ruiz ME, et al: MR imaging of the lateral collateral ligament of the ankle. AJR 156:131, 1991.

1276. Schneck CD, Mesgarzadeh M, Bonakdarpour A, et al: MR imaging of the most commonly injured ankle ligaments. Part I. Normal anatomy. Radiology 184:499, 1992.

1277. Schneck CD, Mesgarzadeh M, Bonakdarpour A: MR imaging of the most commonly injured ankle ligaments. Part II. Ligament injuries. Radiology 184:507, 1992.

1278. Oloff LM, Sullivan BT, Heard GS, et al: Magnetic resonance imaging of traumatized ligaments of the ankle. J Am Podiatr Med Assoc 82:25, 1992.

1279. Cardone BW, Erickson SJ, Den Hartoy BD, et al: MRI of injury to the lateral collateral ligamentous complex of the ankle. J Comput Assist Tomogr 17:102, 1993.

1280. Mink JH: Ligaments of the ankle. In AL Deutsch, JH Mink, and R Kerr (Eds): MRI of the Foot and Ankle. New York, Raven Press, 1992, p 173.

1281. Klein MA, Spreitzer AM: MR imaging of the tarsal sinus and canal: Normal anatomy, pathologic findings, and features of the sinus tarsi syndrome. Radiology 186:233, 1993.

1282. Cahill DR: The anatomy and function of the contents of the human tarsal sinus and canal. Anat Rec 153:1, 1965.

1283. Kjaersgaard-Anderson P, Wethelund JO, Helmig P, et al: The stabilizing effect of the ligamentous structures in the sinus and canalus tarsi on movements in the hind foot: an experimental study. Am J Sports Med 16:512, 1988.

1284. Lowe A, Schilero J, Kanat IO: Sinus tarsi syndrome: a postoperative analysis. J Foot Surg 24:108, 1985.

1285. Meyer J-M, Garcia J, Hoffmeyer P, et al: The subtalar sprain. A roentgenographic study. Clin Orthop 226:169, 1988.

1286. Meyer JM: L'arthrographie de l'articulation sous-astragalienne postérieure et de l'articulation de Chopart. Thèse Méd Genève, No 3318, 1973.

1287. Meyer JM, Lagier R: Post-traumatic sinus tarsi syndrome. An anatomical and radiological study. Acta Orthop Scand 48:121, 1977.

1288. Goosens M, De Stoop N, Claessens H, et al: Posterior subtalar joint arthrography. A useful tool in the diagnosis of hindfoot disorders. Clin Orthop 249:248, 1989.

1289. Taillard W, Meyer JM, Garcia J, et al: The sinus tarsi syndrome. Int Orthop 5:117, 1981.

1290. Ogilvie-Harris DJ, Mahomed N, Demazière A: Anterior impingement of the ankle treated by arthroscopic removal of bony spurs. J Bone Joint Surg [Br] 75:437, 1993.

1291. Morris LH: Athlete's ankle. J Bone Joint Surg 25:220, 1943.

1292. McMurray TP: Footballer's ankle. J Bone Joint Surg [Br] 32:68, 1950.

1293. King JW, Tullos H, Stanley R, et al: Lesions of the feet in athletes. South Med J 64:45, 1971.

1294. Brodelius A: Osteoarthritis of the talar joints in footballers and ballet dancers. Acta Orthop Scand 30:309, 1960.

1295. O'Donoghue DH: Impingement exostoses of the talus and tibia. J Bone Joint Surg [Am] 39:835, 1957.

1296. Hardaker WT Jr, Margello S, Goldner JL: Foot and ankle injuries in theatrical dancers. Foot Ankle 6:59, 1985.

1297. Ferkel RD, Scranton PE Jr: Arthroscopy of the ankle and foot. J Bone Joint Surg 75:1233, 1993.

1298. Bassett FH, Gates H, Billys J, et al: Talar impingement by the anteroinferior tibiofibular ligament. J Bone Joint Surg [Am] 72:55, 1990.

1299. Ferkel R, Fischer S: Progress in ankle arthroscopy. Clin Orthop 240:210, 1988.

1300. McCarroll J, Schrader J, Shelbourne K, et al: Meniscoid lesions of the ankle in soccer players. Am J Sports Med *15*:255, 1987.

1301. Martin D, Curl W, Baker C: Arthroscopic treatment of chronic synovitis of the ankle. Arthroscopy *5*:110, 1989.

1302. Wolin I, Glassman F, Sideman S, et al: Internal derangement of the talofibular component of the ankle. Surg Gynecol Obstet *91*:193, 1950.

1303. Dunn AW: Anomalous muscles simulating soft tissue tumors in the lower extremities. Report of three cases. J Bone Joint Surg [Am] *47*:1397, 1965.

1304. Ger E, Sedlin E: The accessory soleus muscle. Clin Orthop *116*:200, 1976.

1305. Gordon SL, Matheson DW: The accessory soleus. Clin Orthop *97*:129, 1973.

1306. Paul MA, Imanse J, Golding RP, et al: Accessory soleus muscle mimicking a soft tissue tumor. A report of 2 patients. Acta Orthop Scand *62*:609, 1991.

1307. Danielsson LG, El-Haddad I, Sabri T: Clubfoot with supernumerary soleus muscle. Report of 2 cases. Acta Orthop Scand *61*:371, 1990.

1308. Buschmann WR, Cheung Y, Jahss MH: Magnetic resonance imaging of anomalous leg muscles: Accessory soleus, peroneus quartus and the flexor digitorum longus accessorius. Foot Ankle *12*:109, 1991.

1309. Percy EC, Telep GN: Anomalous muscles in the leg: soleus accessorium. Am J Sports Med *12*:447, 1984.

1310. Beasley AW: The accessory soleus. Aust N Zeal J Surg *49*:86, 1979.

1311. Lorentzon R, Wirell S: Anatomic variations of the accessory soleus muscle. Acta Radiol *28*:627, 1987.

1312. White AA, Johnson DJ, Griswold DM: Chronic ankle pain associated with the peroneus accessorius. Clin Orthop *103*:53, 1974.

1313. Wachter S, Beekman S: Peroneus quartus: A case report. J Am Podiatr Assoc *73*:523, 1983.

1314. Regan TP, Hughston JC: Chronic ankle ''sprain'' secondary to anomalous peroneal tendon. Clin Orthop *123*:55, 1977.

1315. Sobel M, Levy ME, Bohne WHO: Congenital variations of the peroneus quartus muscle: an anatomic study. Foot Ankle *11*:81, 1990.

1316. Moorman CT III, Monto RR, Bassett FH III: So-called trigger ankle due to an aberrant flexor hallucis longus muscle in a tennis player. A case report. J Bone Joint Surg [Am] *74*:294, 1992.

1317. Kwong PK, Kay D, Voner RT, et al: Plantar fasciitis. Mechanics and pathomechanics of treatment. Clin Sports Med *7*:119, 1988.

1318. McBryde AM: Plantar fasciitis. Instr Course Lect *33*:278, 1984.

1319. Bordelon RL: Subcalcaneal pain. Clin Orthop *177*:49, 1983.

1320. Leach RE, Dilorio E, Harney RA: Pathologic hindfoot conditions in the athlete. Clin Orthop *177*:116, 1983.

1321. Graham CE: Painful heel syndrome: Rationale of diagnosis and treatment. Foot Ankle *3*:261, 1983.

1322. Baxter DE, Thigpen CM: Heel pain—operative results. Foot Ankle *5*:16, 1984.

1323. Furey JG: Plantar fasciitis: The painful heel syndrome. J Bone Joint Surg [Am] *57*:672, 1975.

1324. Clancy WG Jr: Tendinitis and plantar fasciitis in runners. Orthopedics *6*:217, 1983.

1325. Snider MP, Clancy WG Jr, McBeath AA: Plantar fascia release for chronic plantar fasciitis in runners. Am J Sports Med *11*:215, 1983.

1326. Berkowitz JF, Kier R, Rudicel S: Plantar fasciitis: MR imaging. Radiology *179*:665, 1991.

1327. Aviles E, Arlen M, Miller T: Plantar fibromatosis. Surgery *69*:117, 1971.

1328. Allen RA, Woolner LB, Ghormley RK: Soft-tissue tumors of the sole. With special reference to plantar fibromatosis. J Bone Joint Surg [Am] *37*:14, 1955.

1329. Lee TH, Hecht PJ: Plantar fibromatosis. J Bone Joint Surg [Am] *75*:1080, 1993.

1330. Pickren JW, Smith AG, Stevenson TW Jr, et al: Fibromatosis of the plantar fascia. Cancer *4*:846, 1951.

1331. Erickson SJ, Quinn SF, Kneeland JB, et al: MR imaging of the tarsal tunnel and related spaces: Normal and abnormal findings with anatomic correlation. AJR *155*:323, 1990.

1332. Kerr R, Frey C: MR imaging in tarsal tunnel syndrome. J Comput Assist Tomogr *15*:280, 1991.

1333. Zeiss J, Ebraheim N, Rusin J: Magnetic resonance imaging in the diagnosis of tarsal tunnel syndrome. Case report. Clin Imag *14*:123, 1990.

1334. Zeiss J, Fenton P, Ebraheim N, et al: Normal magnetic resonance anatomy of the tarsal tunnel. Foot Ankle *10*:214, 1990.

1335. Dellon AL: Deep peroneal nerve entrapment on the dorsum of the foot. Foot Ankle *11*:73, 1990.

1336. Schon LC, Baxter DE: Neuropathies of the foot and ankles in athletes. Clin Sports Med *9*:489, 1990.

1337. Kerr R: Spectrum of disorders. *In* AL Deutsch, JH Mink, and R Kerr (Eds): MRI of the Foot and Ankle. New York, Raven Press, 1992, p 345.

1338. Raynor KJ, Raczka EK, Stone PA, et al: Entrapment of the sural nerve. J Am Podiatr Med Assoc *76*:401, 1986.

1339. Pringle RM, Protheroe K, Mukherjee SK: Entrapment neuropathy of the sural nerve. J Bone Joint Surg [Br] *56*:465, 1974.

1340. Addante JB, Peicott PS, Wong KY, et al: Interdigital neuromas. Results of surgical excision of 152 neuromas. J Am Podiatr Med Assoc *76*:493, 1986.

1341. Reed RJ, Bliss BO: Morton's neuroma. Arch Pathol *95*:123, 1973.

1342. Mann RA, Reynolds JC: Interdigital neuroma—a critical clinical analysis. Foot Ankle *3*:238, 1983.

1343. Whipple TL, Geissler WB: Arthroscopic management of wrist triangular fibrocartilage complex injuries in the athlete. Orthopedics *16*:1061, 1993.

1344. Whipple TL, Marotta JJ, Powell JH III: Techniques of wrist arthroscopy. Arthroscopy *2*:244, 1986.

1345. Rominger MB, Bernreuter WK, Kenney PJ, et al: MR imaging of anatomy and tears of wrist ligaments. RadioGraphics *13*:1233, 1993.

1346. Gold RH, Seeger LL, Yao L: Imaging shoulder impingement. Skel Radiol *22*:555, 1993.

1347. Prietto C: Arthroscopic shoulder treatment—what can and cannot be done. West J Med *159*:484, 1993.

1348. Chandnani VP, Yeager TD, DeBerardino T, et al: Glenoid labral tears: Prospective evaluation with MR imaging, MR arthrography, and CT arthrography. AJR *161*:1229, 1993.

1349. Maffulli N, Binfield PM, King JB, et al: Acute haemarthrosis of the knee in athletes. A prospective study of 106 cases. J Bone Joint Surg [Br] *75*:945, 1993.

1350. Johnson DP, Eastwood DM, Witherow PJ: Symptomatic synovial plicae of the knee. J Bone Joint Surg [Am] *75*:1485, 1993.

1351. Kaplan PA, Dussault RG: Magnetic resonance imaging of the knee: Menisci, ligaments, tendons. Top Magn Reson Imaging *5*:228, 1993.

1352. Vande Berg B, Malghem J: Arthrographic pseudotear of the anterior horn of the lateral meniscus caused by a displaced meniscal fragment. Skel Radiol *22*:600, 1993.

1353. Applegate GR, Flannigan BD, Tolin BS, et al: MR diagnosis of recurrent tears in the knee: Value of intraarticular contrast material. AJR *161*:821, 1993.

1354. Schweitzer ME, Mitchell DG, Ehrlich SM: The patellar tendon: thickening, internal signal, buckling, and other MR variants. Skel Radiol *22*:411, 1993.

1355. Koskinen SK, Taimela S, Nelimarkka O, et al: Magnetic resonance imaging of patellofemoral relationships. Skel Radiol *22*:403, 1993.

1356. Virolainen H, Visuri T, Kuusela T: Acute dislocation of the patella: MR findings. Radiology *189*:243, 1993.

1357. Lance E, Deutsch AL, Mink JH: Prior lateral patellar dislocation: MR imaging findings. Radiology *189*:905, 1993.

1358. Kapelov SR, Teresi LM, Bradley WG, et al: Bone contusions of the knee: Increased lesion detection with fast spin-echo MR imaging with spectroscopic fat saturation. Radiology *189*:901, 1993.

1359. Covey DC, Sapega AA: Injuries of the posterior cruciate ligament. J Bone Joint Surg [Am] *75*:1376, 1993.

1360. Fu FH, Harner CD, Johnson DL, et al: Biomechanics of knee ligaments. Basic concepts and clinical application. J Bone Joint Surg [Am] *75*:1716, 1993.

1361. Poulton TB, Murphy WD, Duerk JL, et al: Bone marrow reconversion in adults who are smokers: MR imaging findings. AJR *161*:1217, 1993.

1362. Myllymäki T, Tikkakoski T, Typpö T, et al: Carpet-layer's knee. An ultrasonagraphic study. Acta Radiol Diagn *34*:496, 1993.

1363. Karasick D, Schweitzer ME: Tear of the posterior tibial tendon causing asymptomatic flatfoot: Radiologic findings. AJR *161*:1237, 1993.

1364. Demouy EH, Kaneko K, Bear HM, et al: Giant cell tumor of the plantar tendon sheath: Role of MR imaging in diagnosis. Case report. Clin Imag *17*:153, 1993.

1365. DeMaio M, Paine R, Mangine RE, et al: Plantar fasciitis. Orthopedics *16*:1153, 1993.

1366. Coel M, Yamada CY, Ko J: MR imaging of patients with lateral epicondylitis of the elbow (tennis elbow): Importance of increased signal of the anconeus muscle. AJR *161*:1019, 1993.

1367. Goupille P, Anger C, Cotty P, et al: Diagnostic value of plain radiographs in rotator cuff tear. Rev Rhum [Engl Ed.] *60*:359, 1993.

1368. Recht MP, Resnick D: Magnetic resonance-imaging studies of the shoulder. Diagnosis of lesions of the rotator cuff. J Bone Joint Surg [Am] *75*:1244, 1993.

1369. Ryu KN, Lee SW, Rhee YG, et al: Adhesive capsulitis of the shoulder joint: Usefulness of dynamic sonography. J Ultrasound Med *12*:445, 1993.

1370. Smith AM, McCauley TR, Jokl P: SLAP lesions of the glenoid labrum diagnosed with MR imaging. Skel Radiol *22*:507, 1993.

1371. Sennwald GR, Zdravkovic V, Oberlin C: The anatomy of the palmar scaphotriquetral ligament. J Bone Joint Surg [Br] *76*:147, 1994.

1372. Sugimoto H, Shinozaki T, Ohsawa T: Triangular fibrocartilage in asymptomatic subjects: Investigations of abnormal MR signal intensity. Radiology *191*:193, 1994.

1373. Haramati N, Deutsch A: Proximal wrist imaging. Clin Imag *18*:79, 1994.

1374. Smith DK, Snearly WN: Lunotriquetral interosseous ligament of the wrist: MR appearances in asymptomatic volunteers and arthrographically normal wrists. Radiology *191*:199, 1994.

1375. Sugimoto M, Miyaji N, Ohsawa T: Carpal tunnel syndrome: Evaluation of median nerve circulation with dynamic contrast-enhanced MR imaging. Radiology *190*:459, 1994.

1376. Jelinek JS, Kransdorf MJ, Shmookler BM, et al: Giant cell tumor of the tendon sheath: MR findings in nine cases. AJR *162*:919, 1994.

1377. Bianchi S, Abdelwahab IF, Zwass A, et al: Ultrasonographic evaluation of wrist ganglia. Skeletal Radiol *23*:201, 1994.

1378. Fitzgerald SW, Curry DR, Erickson SJ, et al: Distal biceps tendon injury: MR imaging diagnosis. Radiology *191*:203, 1994.

1379. Falchook FS, Zlatkin MB, Erbacher GE, et al: Rupture of the distal biceps tendon: Evaluation with MR imaging. Radiology *190*:659, 1994.

1380. Rijke AM, Goitz HT, McCue FC, et al: Stress radiography of the medial elbow ligaments. Radiology *191*:213, 1994.

1381. Paavolainen P, Ahovuo J: Ultrasonography and arthrography in the diagnosis of tears of the rotator cuff. J Bone Joint Surg [Am] *76*:335, 1994.

1382. Patten RM, Spear RP, Richardson ML: Diagnostic performance of magnetic resonance imaging for the diagnosis of rotator cuff tears using supplementary images in the oblique sagittal plane. Invest Radiol *29*:87, 1994.

1383. Patten RM: Tears of the anterior portion of the rotator cuff (the subscapularis tendon): MR imaging findings. AJR *162*:351, 1994.

1384. Minkoff J, Cavaliere G: Glenohumeral instabilities and the role of magnetic resonance imaging techniques. The orthopedic surgeon's perspective. MRI Clin North Am *1*:105, 1993.

1385. Richards RD, Sartoris DJ, Pathria MN, et al: Hill-Sachs lesion and normal humeral groove: MR imaging features allowing their differentiation. Radiology *190*:665, 1994.

1386. Tirman PFJ, Stauffer AE, Crues JU III, et al: Saline magnetic resonance arthrography in the evaluation of glenohumeral instability. J Arthrosc Rel Surg *9*:550, 1993.

1387. Palmer WE, Brown JH, Rosenthal DI: Labral-ligamentous complex of the shoulder: Evaluation with MR arthrography. Radiology *190*:645, 1994.

1388. Schweitzer ME: MR arthrography of the labral-ligamentous complex of the shoulder. Radiology *190*:641, 1994.

1389. van Leersum M, Schweitzer ME: Magnetic resonance imaging of the biceps complex. MRI Clin North Am *1*:77, 1993.

1390. Tirman PFJ, Feller JF, Janzen DL, et al: Association of glenoid labral cysts with labral tears and glenohumeral instability: Radiologic findings and clinical significance. Radiology *190*:653, 1994.

1391. Jiang C-C, Shih TTF: Epiphyseal scar of the femoral head: Risk factor of osteonecrosis. Radiology *191*:409, 1994.

1392. Richardson ML: Answer. AJR *162*:1244, 1994

1393. Haramati N, Staron RB, Barax C, et al: Magnetic resonance imaging of occult fractures of the proximal femur. Skeletal Radiol *23*:19, 1994.

1394. Peterfy CG, Majumdar S, Lang P, et al: MR imaging of the arthritic knee: Improved discrimination of cartilage, synovium, and effusion with pulsed saturation transfer and fat-suppressed T1-weighted sequences. Radiology *191*:413, 1994.

1395. Kramer J, Recht M, Deely DM, et al: MR appearance of idiopathic synovial osteochondromatosis. J Comput Assist Tomogr *17*:772, 1993.

1396. Bylski-Austrow DJ, Malumed J, Meade T, et al: Knee joint contact pressure decreases after chronic meniscectomy relative to the acutely meniscectomized joint: A mechanical study in the goat. J Orthop Res *11*:796, 1993.

1397. Haramati N, Staron RB, Cushin S, et al: Value of the coronal plane in MRI of internal derangement of the knee. Skeletal Radiol *23*:211, 1994.

1398. Rubin DA, Kneeland JB, Listerud J, et al: MR diagnosis of meniscal tears of the knee: Value of fast spin echo vs conventional spin-echo pulse sequences. AJR *162*:1131, 1994.

1399. Zobel MS, Borrello JA, Siegel MJ, et al: Pediatric knee MR imaging: Pattern of injuries in the immature skeleton. Radiology *190*:397, 1994.

1400. DeSmet AA, Graf BK: Meniscal tears missed on MR imaging: Relationship to meniscal tear patterns and anterior cruciate ligament tears. AJR *162*:905, 1994.

1401. Ganey TM, Ogden JA, Abou-Madi N, et al: Meniscal ossification. II. The normal pattern in the tiger knee. Skeletal Radiol *23*:173, 1994.

1402. Ogden JA, Ganey TM, Arrington JA, et al: Meniscal ossification. I. Human. Skeletal Radiol *23*:167, 1994.

1403. DeHaven KE, Arnoczky SP: Meniscal repair. Part I: Basic science indications for repair, and open repair. J Bone Joint Surg [Am] *76*:140, 1994.

1404. Frank CB, Bray R, Chimich D, et al: Abnormality of the contralateral ligament after injuries of the medial collateral ligament. An experimental study in rabbits. J Bone Joint Surg [Am] *76*:403, 1994.

1405. Vanek J: Posteromedial fracture of the tibial plateau is not an avulsion injury. A case report and experimental study. J Bone Joint Surg [Br] *76*:290, 1994.

1406. Veltri DM, Warren RF: Posterolateral instability of the knee. J Bone Joint Surg [Am] *76*:460, 1994.

1407. Bianchi S, Zwass A, Abdelwahab IF, et al: Diagnosis of tears of the quadriceps tendon of the knee: Value of sonography. AJR *162*:1137, 1994.

1408. Brossman J, Muhle C, Büll CC, et al: Evaluation of patellar tracking in patients with suspected patellar malalignment: Cine MR imaging vs arthroscopy. AJR *162*:361, 1994.

1409. Owens TC: Posteromedial pivot shift of the knee: a new test for rupture of the posterior cruciate ligament. A demonstration in six patients and a study of anatomical specimens. J Bone Joint Surg [Am] *76*:532, 1994.

1410. Leach WJ, King JB: Posterior reattachment of the torn anterior cruciate ligament. J Bone Joint Surg [Br] *76*:159, 1994.

1411. Chan WP, Peterfy C, Fritz RC, et al: MR diagnosis of complete tears of the anterior cruciate ligament of the knee: Importance of anterior subluxation of the tibia. AJR *162*:355, 1994.

1412. McCauley TR, Moses M, Kier R, et al: MR diagnosis of tears of anterior cruciate ligament of the knee: Importance of ancillary findings. AJR *162*:115, 1994.

1413. Kaneko K, Demouy EH, Brunet ME: Correlation between occult bone lesions and meniscoligamentous injuries in patients with traumatic knee joint disease. Clin Imag *17*:253, 1993.

1414. Moyen B, Lerat J-L: Artificial ligaments for anterior cruciate replacement. A new generation of problems. J Bone Joint Surg [Br] *76*:173, 1994.

1415. Sonia AH, Fitzgerald SW, Friedman H, et al: Posterior cruciate ligament injury: MR imaging diagnosis and patterns of injury. Radiology *190*:455, 1994.

1416. Broderick LS, Turner DA, Renfrew DL, et al: Severity of articular cartilage abnormality in patients with osteoarthritis: Evaluation with fast spin-echo MR vs arthroscopy. AJR *162*:99, 1994.

1417. Munk PL, Vellet AD: Lesions of cartilage and bone around the knee. Top Magn Res Imaging *5*:249, 1993.

1418. Schweitzer ME, van Leersum M, Ehrlich SS, et al: Fluid in normal and abnormal ankle joints: Amount and distribution as seen on MR images. AJR *162*:111, 1994.

1419. Bude RO, Adler RS, Bassett DR, et al: Heterozygous familial hypercholesterolemia: Detection of xanthomas in the Achilles tendon with US. Radiology *188*:567, 1993.

1420. Bude RO, Adler RS, Bassett DR: Diagnosis of Achilles tendon xanthoma in patients with heterozygous familial hypercholesterolemia: MR vs sonography. AJR *162*:913, 1994.

1421. Klein MA: MR imaging of the ankle: Normal and abnormal findings in the medial collateral ligament. AJR *162*:377, 1994.

1422. Rule J, Yao L, Seeger LL: Spring ligament of the ankle: Normal MR anatomy. AJR *161*:1241, 1993.

1423. Beltran J, Rosenberg ZS, Kawelblum M, et al: Pediatric elbow fractures: MRI evaluation. Skeletal Radiol *23*:277, 1994.

1424. Otis JC, Jiang C-C, Wickiewicz TL, et al: Changes in the moment arms of the rotator cuff and deltoid muscles with abduction and rotation. J Bone Joint Surg [Am] *76*:667, 1994.

1425. Haygood TM, Langlotz CP, Kneeland JB, et al: Categorization of acromial shape: Interobserver variability with MR imaging and conventional radiography. AJR *162*:1377, 1994.

1426. Kanecko K, DeMouy EH, Brunet ME: MR evaluation of rotator cuff impingement: Correlation with confirmed full-thickness rotator cuff tears. J Comput Assist Tomogr *18*:225, 1994.

1427. Liu SH, Osti L, Mirzayan R: Ganglion cysts of the anterior cruciate ligament: A case report and review of the literature. J Arthrosc Rel Surg *10*:110, 1994.

1428. Nokes SR, Koonce TW, Montanez J: Ganglion cysts of the cruciate ligaments of the knee: Recognition on MR images and CT-guided aspiration. AJR *162*:1503, 1994.

1429. Vangsness CT Jr, Ghaderi B, Hohl M, et al: Arthroscopy of meniscal injuries with tibial plateau fractures. J Bone Joint Surg [Br] *76*:488, 1994.

1430. Hall FM: MR diagnosis of recurrent meniscal tears: How soon we forget. AJR *162*:1502, 1994.

1431. Engle CP, Noguchi M, Ohland KJ, et al: Healing of the rabbit medial collateral ligament following an O'Donoghue triad injury. Effects of anterior cruciate ligament reconstruction. J Orthop Res *12*:357, 1994.

1432. Astrom M, Westlin N: Blood flow in the human Achilles tendon assessed by laser Doppler flowmetry. J Orthop Surg *12*:246, 1994.

1433. Masterson E, Jagannathan S, Borton D, et al: Pes planus in childhood due to tibialis posterior tendon injuries. J Bone Joint Surg [Br] *76*:444, 1994.

71

Physical Injury: Sports Related Abnormalities

Helene Pavlov, M.D.

SPORTS INJURY: DEFINITION AND GENERAL CONSIDERATIONS

Sports related physical abuse and athletic injuries "represent a potential health problem of a magnitude far outweighing many reportable infectious diseases in the U.S. today."[1] However, in an epidemiologic study of sports injury in school age children (8 to 17 years of age), only 31 per cent of documented sports injuries required professional treatment; hence, a high prevalence of sports injuries is not necessarily indicative of injury severity.[2] The Research Committee of the American Orthopaedic Society for Sports Medicine reviewed the definition of an athletic injury and found that because no common definition was being used, reported injury rates of various studies were not comparable.[3] Noyes and coworkers[3] developed the following definition for tracking sports injuries and assessing the rate of injuries other than inconsequential bumps and bruises: "Injury/illness would be entered if it is sports related and: (1) injury/illness keeps a player out of practice or competition on the day following the injury, (2) injury/illness requires medical attention [by a physician or trainer] or dental care of any kind beyond icing or wrapping . . . all concussions, nerve injuries, no matter how transient, and eye injuries are included."

SITES AND PATTERNS OF SPORTS RELATED INJURIES

The way in which an athletic injury is defined, the specific sport popular in the region, and the sex and age of the participants all are factors to be considered in attempting to interpret the results of studies on the epidemiology and incidence of sports injuries. In adults, a 2 to 1 male-female ratio of injuries has been reported.[4] In high school, athletic injuries predominate in male students, with the overwhelm-

TABLE 71–1. Ten Most Common Overuse Injuries

Adult Males		Adult Females		Male Children		Female Children	
Injury	Per Cent	Injury	Per Cent	Injury	Per Cent	Injury	Per Cent
Achilles tendinitis or bursitis	18	Achilles tendinitis or bursitis	16	Osgood-Schlatter disease	18	Nonspecific knee synovitis	16
Jumper's knee	15	Nonspecific knee synovitis	16	Sever's disease	8	Shin splint syndrome	15
Iliotibial tract friction syndrome	14	Patellar chondromalacia	9	Ankle overpronation, flatfoot, or both	8	Osgood-Schlatter disease	13
Meniscus lesion	12	Knee instability	9	Achilles tendinitis or bursitis	7	Ankle overpronation, flatfoot, or both	11
Shin splint syndrome	10	Shin splint syndrome	9	Nonspecific knee synovitis	7	Lower back insufficiency	11
Flexor tendinitis of the foot	8	Plantar fasciitis	9	Ankle instability with synovitis	5	Ankle instability with synovitis	9
Supraspinatus tendinitis	7	Tightened neck musculature, spasm	9	Hamstring syndrome	5	Achilles tendinitis or bursitis	7
Nonspecific knee synovitis	6	Jumper's knee	7	Trochanteric bursitis	5	Extensor tendinitis of the foot	7
Knee instability	5	Osgood-Schlatter disease	7	Shin splint syndrome	4	Sever's disease	5
Extensor tendinitis of the foot	5	Flexor tendinitis of the foot	7	Osteochondritis dissecans of the knee	3	Patellar chondromalacia	5

Adapted from Kannus P, et al: Clin Pediatr *27*:333, 1988.

ing number of injuries occurring in football and wrestling. In those sports in which both sexes participate, the injury rate is more uniform between the sexes, although the number of days lost to injury is greater for women.[5] Kannus and associates reported the 10 most common overuse injuries in male and female adults and children (Table 71–1)[6] and the 10 most common sites of athletic injuries in adults (Table 71–2).[4]

By any definition, physical injuries resulting from sports related activities have escalated over the past two decades, as evidenced by the exponential increase in the number of sports medicine specialists and facilities around the nation. Sports injuries have been reported in association with almost every sport imaginable—for example, ice skating,[7–9] ice hockey,[10–12] skiing,[13–15] racquet sports,[16–19] handball,[20, 21] lacrosse,[22] rugby, soccer, and (American) football,[23–29] row-

ing,[30] bicycling,[31, 32] mountain climbing,[33] running,[34] track and field,[35] parachuting,[36] aerobics,[37] basketball,[38] horseback riding,[39] gymnastics,[40, 41] ballet,[42, 43] golf,[44] snowboarding,[45] sailboarding,[46] and swimming.[47] The increase in sports related injuries is multifactorial, with two major factors being responsible: (1) the increase in the number of persons participating in recreational and competitive sports related activities, and (2) the increase in the use of newer diagnostic methods, especially MR imaging, permitting earlier detection and documentation of "occult" osseous injuries and muscle, tendon, ligament, and other soft tissue injuries. As a consequence, sprains and strains that previously were diagnosed clinically from subjective information now are being confirmed objectively.

CAUSES OF SPORTS RELATED INJURIES

Injury to the musculoskeletal system results when load exceeds tissue tolerance. Athletic injuries that occur during contact sports (hockey and football) result from a single load; injuries include fractures, dislocations, bone bruises, and muscle, tendon, and ligament ruptures. More commonly, sports related injuries result from noncontact activities. Factors contributing to injury include body malalignment (leg length discrepancy, broad pelvis, femoral anteversion, knock knees, external tibial torsion, foot pronation); inappropriate style (running on an embankment, running in one direction on a circular track); poor footwear or shoe repair; a change in a routine exercise activity (increased distance, speed, intensity, and so forth), and intense competition and training programs (hill training) without sufficient warmup or rest periods (Table 71–3).[48–50] These factors and the athlete's desire to "push through the pain" result in loads that exceed the body's limitations or in

TABLE 71–2. Ten Most Common Sites of Injury in Adults

Men		Women	
Injury Site	Per Cent	Injury Site	Per Cent
Knee	27	Knee	29
Ankle	10	Ankle	10
Lower back	9	Lower back	9
Shoulder	7	Lower leg	6
Achilles tendon	7	Metatarsal region	3
Lower leg	4	Toes	3
Hip	3	Calf	3
Elbow	3	Achilles tendon	3
Heel	3	Sole	2
Calf	3	Hip	2

Adapted from Kannus P, et al: Br J Sports Med *21*:37, 1987.

TABLE 71–3. Factors Contributing to Stress Injuries

Training Errors
Running on embankment
Running in one direction in circular track
Hard or soft surfaces
Sudden change in routine (intensity, speed, endurance)
Hill training
Improper or insufficient rest period (warm up, cool down)

Body Habitus
Broad pelvis
Leg-length discrepancy
Femoral anteversion
Knock knees
External tibial torsion
Foot pronation
Muscle imbalances
Normal variants (juxta-articular ossicles, transitional vertebrae)

Equipment
Inappropriate for sport
Poor fitting equipment
Poor shoe repair

overuse; typical injuries include stress reactions or fractures, musculotendinous strains, and ligament sprains.[48–52]

Thirty to 50 per cent of all sports injuries are due to overuse.[48, 51, 52] An overuse injury is not associated with a sudden event but is insidious and results when a physiologic load exceeds the body's tolerance because of repetition (i.e., repetitive cyclic loading).[53] Repetitive cyclic loading can be compared analogously to bending a paper clip back and forth repeatedly until it snaps. One bend does not produce discontinuity, but the repetitive bending, without increasing the strength of the load, eventually weakens the site and results in failure. Repetitive action on the musculoskeletal system has the same effect as that on the metal paper clip except that the musculoskeletal system is dynamic living tissue that responds to the stress in an attempt to prevent failure.[49, 54–62] The ability to adapt to these repetitive demands depends on the magnitude of each load, the frequency of the repetitions, the duration of the cycles, the frequency of the rest periods, and the tolerance level and condition of the tissue being stressed. The smaller the individual load, the greater the number of load cycles that may be tolerated. Repeated loads that are within the physiologic range of repair create improved tolerance of the musculoskeletal system and the anticipated rewards of an exercise regimen; repeated overloading results in an inflammatory tissue response that produces weakening and fatigue of the involved body tissue, increased susceptibility to injury, and, with continued stress, injury.[48, 49] In addition, whereas the repeated loads of athletic activity increase the strength of both the muscles and the bone, the muscles tone and strengthen faster than the skeleton; therefore, continued ''overloading'' activities produce additional stress on the bones.[49, 55–61]

Five major types of load exist: traction, compression, bending, twisting, and shearing.[62] *Traction* loads result in muscle, tendon, or ligament rupture when the intrinsic tensile strength is exceeded. *Compression* loads typically are responsible for cartilaginous and osseous injuries. *Bending* loads usually are responsible for osseous fracture originating at the maximum point of tensile stress. In older persons, a fracture typically propagates across the shaft to the site of compressive stresses on the concave side, in comparison to the situation in younger persons, in whom a fracture may not propagate unless the stresses are continued or intensified. *Twisting* (torsion) loads are responsible for osseous fracture or ligamentous rupture (i.e., a spiral fracture of the proximal portion of the humerus in a professional pitcher or an anterior cruciate ligament rupture in a skier or a football player). *Shear* stress loads typically are responsible for joint surface injuries (e.g., a tear of the knee menisci or osteochondral fracture).

Clinically, athletic injuries have poorly localized symptoms with poorly defined pain, although with various imaging methods these injuries typically have a specific presentation and occur in predictable sites (Table 71–2). The site of musculoskeletal injury is determined by the athletic activity (e.g., skier's knee, basketball foot, runner's foot, gymnastic back, tennis elbow). The resultant injury varies according to the athlete's age and the corresponding musculoskeletal development (i.e., elasticity and strength of the various components). Muscular strength and the elasticity of tendons and ligaments decrease after the age of approximately 30 years, and the strength of bone decreases after approximately 50 years of age; hence, the same athletic pursuit results in different injuries in the skeletally immature person, the young adolescent, the adult, and the elderly athlete. In the skeletally immature patient, the physeal cartilage is weaker than the joint capsule; therefore, injuries through the growth plate (physis) or apophysis are more common. Similarly, the physeal cartilage is weaker than the tendon and ligaments, and a violent rapid loading of a muscle, sufficient to produce a tendon rupture in an adult, typically will result in an apophyseal bony avulsion in the adolescent athlete. The adolescent athlete also is prone to chondral and osteochondral fractures (in comparison to the adult, who suffers stress fractures), and the elderly patient is prone to tendon and ligament ruptures and osteoarthritis.

In this chapter a discussion of musculoskeletal sports related injury patterns will be limited to the appendicular skeleton and divided into (1) osseous injuries, including stress reactions or fractures, epiphyseal or apophyseal injuries, avulsion fractures, bone bruises, chondral or osteochondral injuries, fractures and dislocations, symptomatic normal variants, and osteoarthritis; and (2) soft tissue injuries including muscle, musculotendinous, tendon and ligament ruptures, cartilage tears, bursitis, nerve injuries, and other miscellaneous soft tissue conditions.

OSSEOUS INJURIES

Stress Reaction and Stress Fractures

Stress reactions and stress fractures occur in well-trained and professional as well as in recreational athletes.[63, 64] Stress reactions and stress fractures represent the bony response to repetitive cyclic overloading and can involve both cortical and cancellous bone. These injuries occur in predictable sites according to the specific athletic involvement (Table 71–4).[7, 30, 42–44, 49, 56–61, 64–132] Prior to the appearance of radiographic signs, a ^{99m}Tc radionuclide bone scan is useful to confirm or exclude a site of suspected stress reaction,[133–138] and three-phase skeletal imaging is helpful in assessing blood flow and soft tissue hyperemia and bone turnover.[139–142] MR imaging may confirm or exclude the pres-

TABLE 71–4. Common Sites of Stress Injuries and Associated Activities

	Location	Activity	References
Sesamoids	Medial—middle to distal	Standing, running, football	65–70
Metatarsal	Second, third—shaft	Running, marching, ballet, skating	7, 42, 56, 57, 71–75
	Fifth—distal to tuberosity	Running, basketball	76–79
Navicular	Central third—dorsal and proximal	Basketball, running	56, 80–83
Calcaneus	Posterior—dorsal	Running, jumping, marching	56, 57, 60, 84, 85
Fibula	Proximal	Jumping, parachuting	86, 87
	Supramalleolar	Running, marching	56, 57, 88
Tibia	Posterior—junction of proximal and middle or junction of distal and middle thirds	Running, marching, aerobics, ballet, basketball	42, 56–61, 74, 89–94
	Anterior—midshaft	Ballet, basketball, running	42, 43, 49, 56, 57, 60, 93, 94
	Proximal	Standing, running	95, 96
Patella	Midpole	Jumping, basketball, hurdling	97–99
Femur	Femoral neck	Running, long-distance running, ballet	42, 100–105
	Shaft—junction of proximal and middle thirds	Long-distance running, ballet	42, 56, 105–109
Pelvis	Junction of pubis and ischium	Long-distance running	56, 110–112
Sacrum	Proximal	Running, aerobics	49, 113–115
Spine	Pars (lumbar)	Ballet, gymnastics, running, weight-lifting	116, 117
Ribs	First rib	Backpacking, weight-lifting, pitching	118, 119
	Lower ribs	Golf, rowing	30, 44, 120
Clavicle	Medial	Carrying heavy weights	121
Scapula	Coracoid	Golf, trapshooting	122
Humerus	Shaft	Pitching, tennis, wrestling, shotputting	123–125
Radius	Shaft	Pitching	126, 127
Ulna	Shaft	Shoveling, rowing, pitching, body building, wheelchair athletics	56, 128–130
Hamate	Hook	Golf, tennis, batting	56, 92, 131
Scaphoid	Waist	Shotputting, gymnastics	132

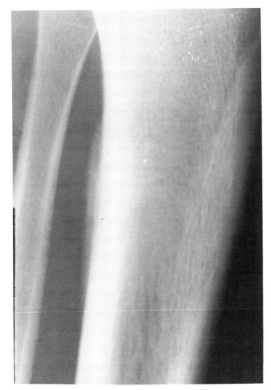

FIGURE 71–1. Stress reaction. An oblique fluoroscopic spot film of the proximal portion of the tibia demonstrates periosteal and endosteal reaction of the posterior cortex of the tibia at the junction of the proximal and middle thirds. This is a classic site for a stress reaction or stress fracture. (From Pavlov H, et al: RadioGraphics *1*:17, 1981.)

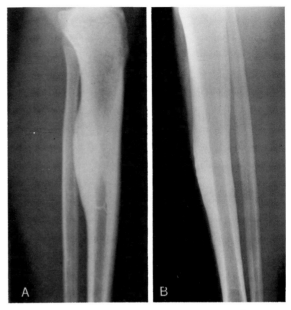

FIGURE 71–2. Mature cortical hypertrophy. Hypertrophy occurs as a result of the increased stress demands of athletics. Typical sites include the posterior cortex of the proximal portion of the tibia, at the junction of the proximal and middle thirds **(A)**, and the anterior midshaft of the tibia **(B)**. The smooth endosteal surface (as demonstrated in **B**) suggests that this response is mature. (**B**, From Pavlov H, Torg JS: The Running Athlete. Chicago, Year Book, 1987.)

ence of bone marrow edema, periosteal reaction, and, in most instances, fracture.[143–151]

A stress reaction is not evident in cancellous bone on plain radiographs but appears "hot" on the radionuclide bone scan. In cortical bone, a stress reaction is identified radiographically as a localized area of periosteal and endosteal response (Fig. 71–1). This local response can heal without sequelae or progress, either to a localized area of mature cortical hyperostosis or to an identifiable stress fracture, depending on the magnitude of the response and the stress demand.[152] If the bone response is greater than the demand on the bone, the localized area of periosteal and endosteal reaction matures, resulting in cortical hypertrophy that strengthens the bone at the site required (Fig. 71–2). Bone responds according to Wolff's law in an effort to improve the tolerance level for the new and increased load (Fig. 71–3).[49, 153–154] Stress on bone produces a progressive deformity. If the deformity is within the elastic range of the bone, the bone returns to its original configuration when the deforming force relaxes. When the bone becomes stressed beyond the elastic range, permanent deformity occurs as a result of microfractures.[49, 153, 154] With continued or intensified stress, the number of microfractures increases and progresses, and, as the fatigue point is exceeded, structural failure and complete (and, sometimes, catastrophic) fracture occurs.[49, 155, 156]

In cancellous bone, a stress fracture is identified radiographically as a linear radiodense area oriented perpendicular to the trabeculae (Fig. 71–4).[152] The radiodense region represents collapsed trabeculae, osteoblastic activity, and

endosteal callus. The calcaneus and the ends of the long tubular bones are examples of cancellous bone. A cortical stress fracture is identified as a radiolucent line within an area of cortical hyperostosis (Fig. 71–5). The radiolucent fracture line can be oriented perpendicular or parallel to the long axis of the bone.[56–60, 91–93] Cortical stress fractures occur during the period of active periosteal and endosteal re-

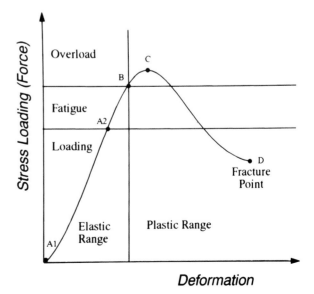

FIGURE 71–3. Wolff's law. The deformation of a structure increases proportionately to the stress loading force to point B. Within the elastic range, the structure returns to its original conformation without damage. Beyond the elastic range, additional stress produces permanent deformity. Microfractures begin at point C, and failure occurs at point D. (From Daffner RH, Pavlov H: AJR *159*:245, 1992. Copyright 1992, American Roentgen Ray Society.)

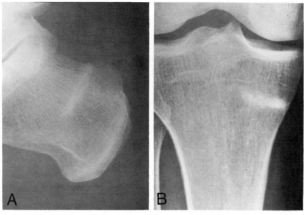

FIGURE 71–4. Cancellous stress fracture. The linear area of radiodensity is oriented perpendicular to the direction of the trabeculae. Typical sites for these stress fractures include the calcaneus **(A)** and proximal portion of the tibia **(B)**. (From Pavlov H, Torg JS: The Running Athlete. Chicago, Year Book, 1987.)

sponse (stress reaction) when the bone is weakened temporarily and the demand exceeds the bone tolerance. The stress on the bone results in localized cortical changes representing gradual and progressive resorption of circumferential lamellar bone and its replacement by dense osteonal bone.[133, 157–159] When the resultant localized cortical response and hypertrophy are massive, the radiolucent stress fracture line may be obscured on plain radiographs. In those patients in whom it is necessary to confirm or exclude a stress fracture within the localized area of cortical response, coned views to the area of concern, overpenetrated radiographs, conventional tomography or CT scanning, or MR imaging may be helpful.[91, 144–151, 160–166] In MR images, acute cortical and cancellous stress fractures are of low signal intensity on T1-weighted spin echo images and of high signal intensity on the T2-weighted spin echo or T2*-weighted gradient echo sequences. Fast spin echo sequences using fat suppression and short tau inversion recovery (STIR) sequences are especially sensitive to subacute hemorrhage and surrounding bone marrow edema.[147, 150] Bone marrow edema can be extensive, extend-

ing far from the fracture site. The linear fracture appears as a signal void on all pulse sequences. Because MR imaging is multiplanar, the orientation of the fracture should not limit its demonstration; however, the fracture line is not always evident in MR images, and, if necessary, a CT examination may help document cortical or trabecular disruption.[49, 161, 162] A chronic stress reaction with solid thick cortical hypertrophy appears as a localized area of low signal intensity in T2-weighted spin echo MR images.[144]

Stress Fracture Complications

Stress reactions and stress fractures are responsible for downtime and interruption of training regimens and professional careers as well as for insinuations and claims of malingering from coaches and managers. When undetected, untreated, or denied by the patient, stress fractures can have serious complications, including propagation to a complete fracture, delayed union or nonunion, and contralateral injuries.

Propagation to Complete Fractures

All stress reactions can progress to stress fractures and all stress fractures can propagate to complete fractures if the pain is ignored or if the activity is intensified. Two sites at which stress fracture propagation to a complete fracture is especially common are the femoral neck and the tarsal navicular bone. A stress fracture of the proximal portion of the femur is first manifested as vague hip or groin pain aggravated by weight-bearing. The fracture usually occurs in the medial aspect of the femoral neck, just proximal to the lesser trochanter, and has a cancellous stress fracture pattern (i.e., a linear radiodense region oriented perpendicular to the long axis of the bone) (Fig. 71–6A). Prior to the appearance of any radiographic manifestations, the hip is extremely vulnerable and, when there is a high index of clinical suspicion, a bone scan or MR imaging examination is recommended before the patient is permitted to continue or to increase his or her athletic endeavors (Fig. 17–6B). If undetected, the fracture may propagate to a complete intraarticular fracture requiring surgical intervention.[100–109]

Tarsal navicular stress fractures are characterized by

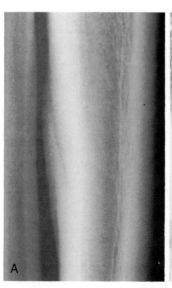

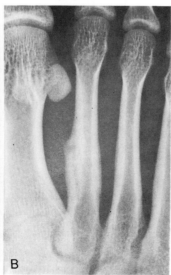

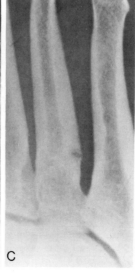

FIGURE 71–5. Cortical stress fracture. The linear radiolucent fracture line occurs within an area of periosteal and endosteal new bone formation. Fractures can be oriented parallel or perpendicular to the long axis of the bone, as seen in these examples: at the posterior cortex of the proximal end of the tibia at the junction of the proximal and middle thirds **(A)**, at the base of the second metatarsal bone **(B)**, and at the base of the fourth metatarsal bone **(C)**. (From Pavlov H, Torg JS: The Running Athlete. Chicago, Year Book, 1987.)

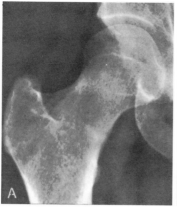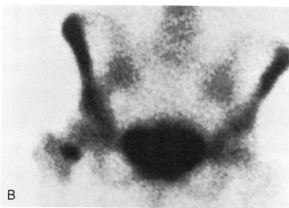

FIGURE 71–6. Stress fracture of the proximal portion of the femur. The typical radiographic pattern is a faint radiodense line in the medial cortex, just proximal to the lesser trochanter **(A)**. On radionuclide bone scan **(B)**, the classic stress fracture pattern of the proximal end of the femur is a focal area of augmented uptake at its medial aspect, just proximal to the lesser trochanter. **(B,** From Pavlov H, Torg HS: The Running Athlete. Chicago, Year Book, 1987.)

poorly localized pain in the medial arch of the foot, primarily in runners and basketball players.[80–83] The fracture occurs in the sagittal plane at the junction of the middle and lateral thirds (Fig. 71–7). Typically, the fracture starts in the proximal dorsal articular surface and, if untreated, propagates distally and plantarly. The partial fracture usually is not evident on routine radiographs, even when films are coned to the navicular bone. When there is a strong clinical suspicion of a navicular stress fracture, a radionuclide bone scan with plantar views is indicated. In plantar views, a navicular stress fracture reveals augmented radionuclide uptake that conforms to the configuration of the navicular bone.[80] To confirm that the uptake is due to a fracture or to evaluate the extent of the fracture, anatomic anteroposterior conventional tomography through the dorsal aspect of the navicular bone, or a CT scan or MR imaging examination performed tangential (true transaxial sections and coronal sections) to the dorsal surface of the navicular bone is recommended.[80, 164–166] Unlike the partial fracture, a complete tarsal navicular stress fracture usually is evident in routine frontal views of the foot; however, the midfoot must be penetrated adequately, and the separate lateral navicular fragment must not be misinterpreted as a separate tarsal bone. Nonunion and ischemic necrosis of the lateral fragment further complicate this injury (Fig. 71–7*B*).[80, 81]

Delayed Healing

Delayed healing or nonunion, defined radiographically as sclerosis bordering the fracture margins partially or completely, is a not uncommon complication of stress fractures.[167] Several stress fracture sites have predictable healing complications, including those in flat bones, the tarsal navicular bone, the anterior cortex of the midportion of the tibia, and the base of the fifth metatarsal bone, distal to the tuberosity.

The radiographic detection of a fracture nonunion is common in the flat or irregular bones. Examples include the first rib in backpackers or pitchers (Fig. 71–8)[118] and the junction of the ischium and pubis in female long-distance or marathon runners.[110–112] Despite the radiographic appearance of fracture nonunion, however, these injuries usually heal without surgical intervention, provided that the patient discontinues the offending activity for 2 to 3 months (Fig. 71–9).[110] Stress fractures in flat bones can be very subtle radiographically in the early stages, and a radionuclide bone scan is indicated early after symptoms first appear to allow identification of the injury and prevent further healing complications.

The partial tarsal navicular stress fracture propagates to a complete fracture, and the complete fracture can result in

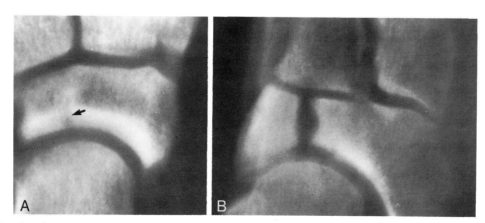

FIGURE 71–7. Tarsal navicular stress fracture.
  A Partial tarsal navicular stress fracture. Anatomic anteroposterior conventional tomogram demonstrates a classic partial stress fracture (arrow) in the dorsal aspect of the proximal articular border of the navicular bone. The fracture is linear and at the junction of the middle and lateral thirds of the bone.
  B Ischemic necrosis and nonunion of a complete tarsal navicular stress fracture. The lateral fragment is dense and sclerosis completely borders the fracture margin, consistent with nonunion. (From Pavlov H, et al: Radiology *148*:641, 1983.)

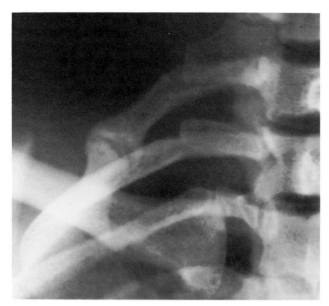

FIGURE 71–8. Stress fracture of the right first rib with delayed healing. A radiolucent fracture line with sclerosis bordering the fracture margin is observed. (From Pavlov H: South Orthop J *1*:241, 1992. Reprinted by permission from the Journal of the Southern Orthopaedic Association.)

nonunion or ischemic necrosis of the lateral fragment, or both (Fig. 71–7).

Stress fractures in the anterior cortex of the midshaft of the tibia occur commonly in ballet dancers and basketball players, theoretically as a consequence of the repeated impacts with the floor during repetitive leaping.[42, 49, 94] Multiple partial stress fractures in various stages of healing in the anterior tibial cortex are a less debilitating condition clinically than the single cortical stress fracture (Fig. 71–

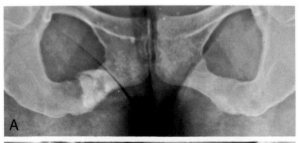

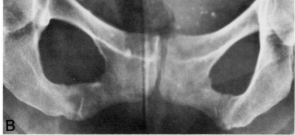

FIGURE 71–9. Pubic stress fracture with delayed healing.
A Sclerosis is present along the margins of the stress fracture of the right ischium, at the junction with the inferior pubic ramus.
B Forty-one months after a 2 to 3 month cessation of marathon participation, the stress fracture on the right has healed without surgical intervention. Note, however, there is now a contralateral injury on the left secondary to the patient's resumption of marathon participation.
(From Pavlov H, et al: J Bone Joint Surgery [Am] *64*:1020, 1982.)

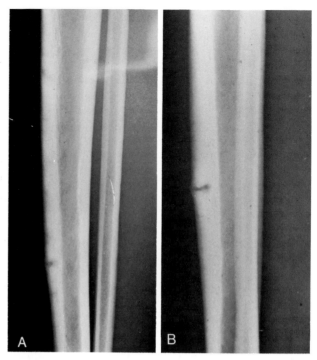

FIGURE 71–10. Anterior tibial stress fracture.
A Multiple horizontal radiolucent stress fractures at various stages of healing.
B The "dreaded black line" (i.e., a single linear radiolucent fracture line within a localized area of cortical hyperostosis).
(From Pavlov H, Torg JS: The Running Athlete. Chicago, Year Book, 1987.)

10). The single horizontal fracture line, which is completely surrounded by bone sclerosis, is known as the "dreaded black line" (Fig. 71–10*B*). Occasionally, the linear aspect of the fracture may become ovoid secondary to bone resorption around the fracture margins. A radiolucent area in the mid–anterior tibial cortex should be interpreted with respect to the patient's clinical manifestations and should not be confused with a bone abscess or osteoid osteoma. Biopsy should be avoided as it can result in further weakening of the bone and an increase in the risk of a complete fracture.[49] The appearance of a horizontal partial cortical fracture completely surrounded by sclerosis is most common. This appearance is not limited to the anterior cortex of the tibia and, indeed, can occur in the cortex of any bone. Treatment of a "dreaded black line" may require surgical intervention.

A stress fracture in the base of the fifth metatarsal bone, distal to the tuberosity, is common in runners and basketball players.[76–79] This fracture is prone to delayed healing and propagation to a complete fracture owing to the poor vascularity at this site.[76–79] A non–weight-bearing cast applied for 6 to 8 weeks is recommended as effective treatment. This fracture is not difficult to detect radiographically and should be distinguished from the more common avulsion injury of the tuberosity in the base of the fifth metatarsal bone, which usually heals without difficulty.[168, 169]

Contralateral Injuries

Abnormalities in the contralateral bone result when the athlete is injured and, in response, changes his or her gait to shift the forces away from the painful injured side. This altered activity increases the intensity of the forces onto the nonpainful side, which, if there is an insufficient period of adaptation, will result in injury to the side opposite the original injury (Fig. 71–9).[49, 56, 110]

Epiphyseal or Apophyseal Injuries

Athletic activities are the second most common cause of fractures in school children and the most common in youngsters between 15 and 24 years of age.[170] The epiphyseal complex is involved in 6 to 15 per cent of fractures of long bones in children under 16 years of age.[171–175] Eighty per cent of epiphyseal injuries result from a shearing force to the epiphyseal center or force applied through the ligament or capsule, or both[176, 177]; only 20 per cent of epiphyseal injuries result from compression. An epiphyseal separation in the skeletally immature athlete is analogous to a dislocation or ligamentous injury in the adult.[178–181] The joint capsule and ligaments are two to five times stronger than the physis; and forces that would produce a ligamentous injury in an adult typically result in an epiphyseal separation or fracture in the skeletally immature patient.[178, 182]

Epicondylitis-Apophysitis

In the skeletally immature athlete, hyperemia and forces that would produce cortical hypertrophy and traction enthesophytes in the adult result in accelerated maturity of the growth center, early or delayed closure of the physis, or epicondylitis-apophysitis.[18, 183–186] Epicondylitis-apophysitis is a focal fragmentation at the bony origin or insertion sites of a tendon or ligament secondary to repetitive microtrauma (Fig. 71–11A). A bone scan may help confirm the injury pattern with increased focal isotope uptake; however, because the open physis normally has accentuated uptake, careful comparison with the other side is essential (Fig. 71–11B). An MR imaging study may help identify associated soft tissue injuries.

Epiphyseal and apophyseal injuries are common in the elbow and the knee. In the elbow, the superior aspect of the olecranon apophysis, the medial epicondyle, and the lateral epicondyle frequently are affected.[18, 183, 184, 186] In the knee, two common sites for apophysitis are the origin and insertion of the patellar tendon (e.g., jumper's knee and Osgood-Schlatter disease, respectively). Jumper's knee represents a chronic form of stress applied to the origin of the patellar

tendon. It is diagnosed by irregularities of the inferior pole of the patella and thickening and irregularity of the proximal portion of the patellar tendon.[187–192] Osgood-Schlatter disease represents a chronic form of stress at the insertion of the patellar tendon and is diagnosed on plain radiographs by fragmentation of the tibial tubercle, swelling of the soft tissues over the anterior aspect of the tibial tubercle, and thickening and loss of the posterior definition of the patellar tendon (Fig. 71–12).[193–197] With MR imaging, a distended deep infrapatellar bursa may be identified in addition to other findings.[198] After skeletal maturity, an intratendinous ossicle may be present just proximal to the tibial tubercle, which, if symptomatic, may require removal.[199]

Physeal Injuries

Acute and stress induced sports related epiphyseal fractures are not uncommon. An active youngster with clinical symptoms of an acute ligamentous injury, with soft tissue swelling around the joint or a joint effusion, must be evaluated for an epiphyseal fracture.

In the knee of a young adolescent, painful medial instability occurring after an acute "clipping" injury during football may be misdiagnosed clinically as a medial collateral ligament injury if subtle widening of the medial aspect of the physis of the distal portion of the femur is not recognized radiographically.[200, 201] The clinically detected medial joint compartment widening and "instability" actually occur in the medial aspect of the femoral physis, not at the level of the joint. A crosstable lateral view of the knee is indicated in a young patient with an acute injury and a joint effusion but without an obvious fracture on the radiograph. A lipohemarthrosis (fat-fluid level) evident in the crosstable radiographic projection helps to confirm an intra-articular fracture. The vertical fracture component of a Salter-Harris type III injury is identified best on an oblique view or on an overpenetrated anteroposterior view.[200–201] Stress views should be avoided as the entire medial femoral condylar fragment may be dislodged (Fig. 71–13A). The extent of physeal involvement (Salter-Harris classification) and the associated soft tissue and cartilage injuries may be determined on MR imaging examination (Fig. 71–13B).

A not uncommon physeal stress lesion occurs in the proximal end of the humerus in young baseball pitchers (e.g., "Little League shoulder"). This condition is identi-

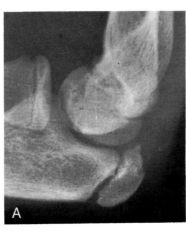
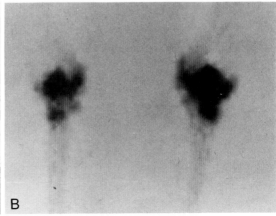

FIGURE 71–11. Olecranon apophysitis.

A The superior aspect of the olecranon apophysis is pointed, irregular, and fragmented in this symptomatic young athlete.

B Radionuclide bone scan confirms the asymmetry with increased isotope uptake on the symptomatic side.

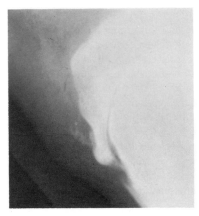

FIGURE 71–12. Osgood-Schlatter disease. The classic radiographic appearance consists of thickening of the patellar tendon with loss of definition posteriorly, fragmentation of the tubercle, and superficial soft tissue swelling over the tibial tubercle. Radiographic findings must be correlated with the patient's symptoms. (From Pavlov H, Torg JS: The Running Athlete. Chicago, Year Book, 1987.)

fied in the lateral aspect of the proximal humeral physis by widening associated with sclerotic margins and metaphyseal irregularity (Fig. 71–14).[202–209] These osseous changes usually resolve without a growth disturbance if the child stops pitching.[18, 184, 206]

Other sites of stress related physeal injuries occur in the distal ends of the radius and ulna in gymnasts,[210–214] the distal portion of the femur,[215] and the proximal end of the tibia.[216]

Apophyseal (Avulsion) Fractures

Avulsion injuries occur in young adult or adolescent athletes just prior or subsequent to apophyseal fusion. Apophyses form the bony projections in which tendons and ligaments originate and insert. Almost all apophyseal injuries are secondary to force transmitted through the tendon, ligament, or capsule.[176–179] The musculotendinous unit is stronger than the open or recently fused physis, and a strong muscular pull results in a bone avulsion, as opposed to the muscle injury expected from the same activity in the skeletally mature patient.[179–182]

Avulsion fractures in the young athlete are common. Patients usually have poorly defined symptoms. An acute avulsion fracture is diagnosed radiographically as a cres-

centic osseous fragment displaced from the bone of origin; MR imaging may allow identification of associated muscle injury. The majority of avulsion injuries occur in the pelvis.[217–219] Avulsion of the ischial tuberosity as a result of a violent hamstring tendon pull is the most common type of pelvic avulsion injury and occurs in those sports that require violent hip flexion while the knee is extended (e.g., cheerleading, hurdling, and high jumping) (Fig. 71–15).[217–220] Avulsion of the anterior inferior iliac spine, at the site of the reflected head of the rectus femoris muscle (Fig. 71–16),[217–220] is another frequent injury. A radiograph obtained in a young athletic patient with pelvic or groin pain should include the entire pelvis or, at a minimum, the entire symptomatic hemipelvis to allow identification of all major musculotendinous attachment sites. This is especially important for identifying an avulsion fracture of the iliac crest related to abdominal muscle insertion[221–223] or a fracture of the anterior superior iliac spine; either of these injuries may be manifested as hip or groin pain and can be missed if only hip films are obtained (Fig. 71–17). The anterior superior iliac spine is avulsed by the sartorius muscle as a result of knee flexion while the hip is extended (e.g., in kicking sports, such as soccer).[217–219, 224] The adductor muscle group, which arises from the pubic bone and inserts in the posterior aspect and midshaft of the femur, is subject to both acute avulsion injuries (gracilis syndrome) and overloading injuries (osteitis pubis) as a consequence of sideways kicks (soccer) and adduction (ice skating) (Fig. 71–18).[225–228] In some instances, this injury can result in instability at the symphysis pubis, which may be detected radiographically in flamingo views, which are anteroposterior views of the symphysis obtained while the patient stands alternately on one foot and then on the other.[229]

In the knee, avulsion at the site of attachment of the cruciate ligaments may occur instead of a ligament rupture in the skeletally immature patient. Avulsion at the site of insertion of either of these ligaments usually can be identified in the lateral view of the knee, whereas avulsion at the site of origin of these ligaments is evident in the tunnel view. A Segond fracture (capsular sign) is an avulsion of the inferior attachment of the meniscocapsular portion of the lateral capsular ligament and, although this fracture fragment is not significant clinically, it indicates that a twisting injury has occurred that almost always is associated with a rupture of the anterior cruciate ligament (Fig. 71–19).[230–233]

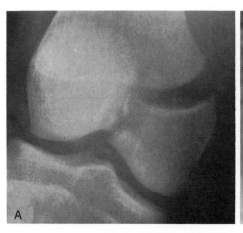

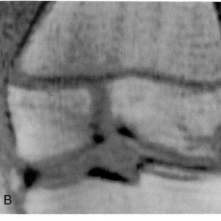

FIGURE 71–13. Salter-Harris type III fracture of the distal portion of the femur.

A Stress views should be avoided as the entire medial condyle can become displaced.

B A coronal T1-weighted (TR/TE, 516/16) spin echo MR image of a Salter-Harris type III fracture of the distal portion of the femur demonstrates the horizontal component through the medial aspect of the physis and the vertical component.

(*A,* from Pavlov H, Torg JS: The Running Athlete. Chicago, Year Book, 1987.)

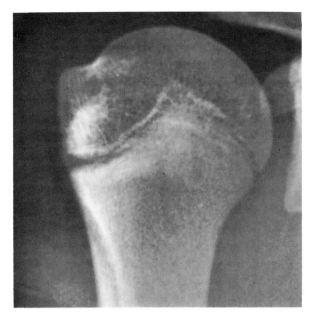

FIGURE 71–14. Little League shoulder (Salter-Harris type I fracture). A routine radiograph demonstrates mild widening of the lateral aspect of the physis with sclerosis along the metaphyseal aspect.

Avulsion injuries about the ankle and foot usually result from twisting injuries. Clinically, these injuries usually appear as nonlocalized foot or ankle pain. To identify these injuries, care must be used in obtaining the radiographs of patients with diffuse foot or ankle pain to ensure that the calcaneus is included in the frontal view of the ankle and that the soft tissues adjacent to the hindfoot are visualized in the frontal view of the foot. This is especially necessary

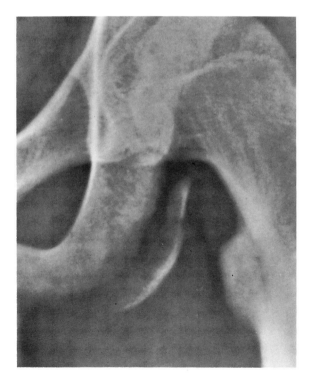

FIGURE 71–15. Avulsion of the ischial tuberosity. Note the classic crescent-shaped osseous avulsion fragment from the lateral aspect of the physis secondary to the pull of the origin of the hamstring muscles. (From Pavlov H, Torg JS: The Running Athlete. Chicago, Year Book, 1987.)

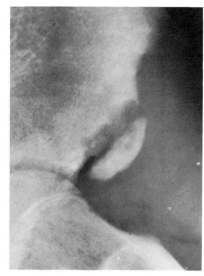

FIGURE 71–16. Avulsion fracture of the reflected head of the rectus femoris muscle. (From Pavlov H, Torg JS: The Running Athlete. Chicago, Year Book, 1987.)

to allow identification of an avulsion injury in the lateral distal aspect of the calcaneus.[234, 235]

Complications. In certain situations, a small avulsion fracture may be indistinguishable radiographically from a normal secondary center of ossification (juxta-articular ossicle). Acutely, such a fracture may be diagnosed accurately because bone margins are sharp and the fragments fit together; however, if a small fracture fragment heals as a separate fragment, its borders become rounded and smooth (Fig. 71–20). A radionuclide bone scan is helpful to determine if a juxta-articular ossicle is an old or an acute fracture fragment and if it is the source of symptoms. An MR imaging examination may allow identification of associated ligamentous or tendinous injury.

Young athletes with avulsion injuries typically do not come to medical attention immediately but wait several

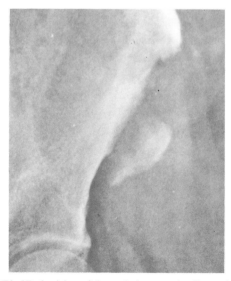

FIGURE 71–17. Avulsion of the anterior superior iliac spine. This avulsion injury may not be included on a routine radiographic view of the hip if the fragment is not significantly displaced inferiorly. (From Pavlov H: Radiol Clin North Am 28:435, 1990.)

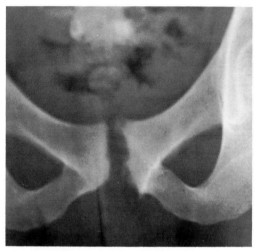

FIGURE 71–18. Gracilis syndrome or osteitis pubis. Unilateral irregularity of the symphyseal margin with hypertrophy, osteophytes, and widening of the physis is diagnostic. Occasionally, a separate osseous fragment may be present inferiorly, owing to an avulsion of the origin of the gracilis muscle. (From Pavlov H, Torg JS: The Running Athlete. Chicago, Year Book, 1987.)

weeks until competition or tryouts are over, at which time the specific insult may not be remembered. Two to 3 weeks after an avulsion injury, healing callus already may be present radiographically (Fig. 71–21). The callus can be extensive and poorly organized and, if clinical history is unavailable, the healing process noted in both the radiographs and the biopsy specimen can be misinterpreted as evidence of tumor; hence, biopsy is discouraged.[236] A detailed history and repeat radiographs in 2 weeks usually are sufficient to establish the traumatic cause.

Occasionally, extensive heterotopic ossification, or a traction excrescence, which projects toward the joint, can form and may cause mechanical limitation of joint motion (Fig. 71–22).[217, 218]

Persistent stress and traction on an apophysis, with or without a single violent avulsion, can result in an apophyseal separation or nonunion, or both. Apophyseal nonunion is diagnosed radiographically by widening of the growth plate, with smooth sclerotic margins and loss of normal interdigitation of apposing bone surfaces. The olecranon apophysis, for example, may fail to unite with the remaining portions of the ulna in Little League pitchers, a situation that may require surgical intervention (Fig. 71–23).[237–239]

Chondral and Osteochondral Injuries

Cartilage is composed of collagen and 60 to 80 per cent water. Joint cartilage is lubricated and protected from injury by two mechanisms: (1) a "weeping" mechanism in high loads, by which interstitial fluid weeps out and accepts the bulk of the load, and (2) a boundary phenomenon in low loads, by which a proteoglycan lubricating fraction forms on apposing surfaces of the joint to keep them apart.[48, 240] The underlying cancellous bone protects the cartilage by its ability to deform as a response to the stress.[240] Shearing, rotatory, or tangentially aligned impaction forces produce chondral or osteochondral fractures in one or both apposing joint surfaces, and injuries usually are oriented parallel to the joint surface (Fig. 71–24).[241–243]

Early chondral changes include softening of the cartilage, or chondromalacia. Although the term is used most frequently in relation to the posterior aspect of the patella, it is applicable to cartilage changes in all articular surfaces. Cartilage injuries range from chondromalacia, which typically occurs in the adolescent or young athlete, to thinning and denudation of the cartilage secondary to osteoarthritis, which typically occurs in older athletes. A pure chondral injury is not evident in routine plain films, and arthrography with or without arthrotomography, CT scanning after arthrography, and MR imaging are helpful to document the extent of injury (Fig. 71–25).[244–250] Multiple MR imaging techniques have been suggested to demonstrate cartilage lesions.[251–255] When the subchondral bone is involved, plain radiographs may be diagnostic, although the findings usually are subtle. A radionuclide bone scan is recommended to confirm the presence of a suspected lesion on plain film, whereas the extent of injury usually is demonstrated better in MR images.

Patellofemoral pain syndrome is a frequent complaint in active persons, especially teenagers and young adults, and accounts for 10 per cent of visits to a sports medicine clinic.[256] This is a common complaint in runners, although not long-distance runners.[257–259] The onset of symptoms typically is insidious and complaints may be bilateral.[257] A slight female predominance has been reported.[260] Patellofemoral pain syndrome[249, 258–260] is an enigma, and the dif-

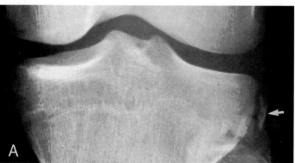
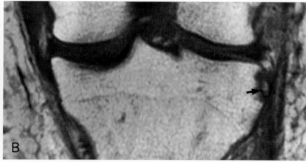

FIGURE 71–19. Segond fracture. This fracture almost always is associated with a tear of the anterior cruciate ligament secondary to the twisting mechanism responsible for both injuries.

A On routine views, the fracture (arrow) is identified as a longitudinal sliver of bone adjacent to the lateral tibial plateau.

B In a coronal T1-weighted spin echo MR image (TR/TE, 500/12), a bone fragment (arrow) is identified at the margin of the lateral tibial plateau. The soft tissues in this region are poorly defined as a result of edema and hemorrhage.

(From Pavlov H, Torg JS: The Running Athlete. Chicago, Year Book, 1987.)

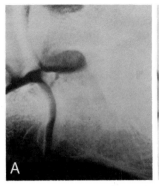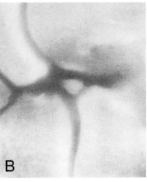

FIGURE 71–20. Avulsion injury of calcaneus.

A Acute avulsion injury from the origin of the bifurcate ligament. The margins between the separate fracture fragments at the anterior spine of the calcaneus are sharp and the bones fit together.

B An os calcaneus secondarius or an old fracture fragment that has healed. The margins of the fragments are rounded and smooth.

(From Pavlov H, Torg JS: The Running Athlete. Chicago, Year Book, 1987.)

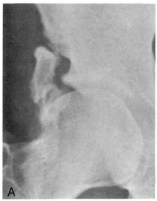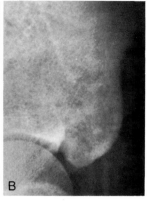

FIGURE 71–22. Avulsion injury with bone formation.

A Posttraumatic ossification. Heterotopic ossification secondary to an avulsion of the reflected head of the rectus femoris muscle is seen.

B Posttraumatic exostosis. An exostosis that points toward the joint in the superolateral aspect of the acetabulum is a result of an old avulsion of the reflected head of the rectus femoris muscle.

(From Pavlov H, Torg JS: The Running Athlete. Chicago, Year Book, 1987.)

ferential diagnosis includes chondromalacia patellae (Fig. 71–25),[257–263] abnormal patellar tracking,[255, 264–273] plica syndrome,[274–278] patellalgia (patellofemoral arthralgia),[279] and chondromalacia or osteochondral lesions in the femoral side of the patellofemoral joint.[280]

Osteochondral injuries include osteochondritis dissecans and osteochondral fractures, which are overlapping phenomena with similar radiographic appearances and clinical presentations.[244–248, 250, 281–283] Osteochondritis dissecans occurs in adolescents and may or may not be related to acute or chronic repetitive trauma.[284–287] Although trauma is the most likely cause of osteochondritis dissecans, a family history has been identified.[288–290] An osteochondral injury

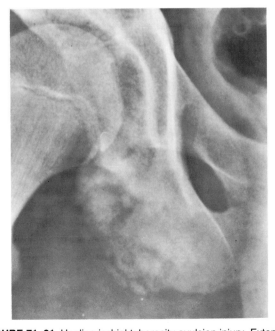

FIGURE 71–21. Healing ischial tuberosity avulsion injury. Extensive callus formation and a mottled appearance at the site of ischial tuberosity avulsion are present. Interpretation of the radiograph and the pathologic specimen (if a biopsy was performed) can be difficult without clinical history. (From Pavlov H, Torg JS: The Running Athlete. Chicago, Year Book, 1987.)

usually is the result of a single traumatic episode, but the exact time of injury is not always determinable or remembered by the patient, as subchondral bone is insensitive to pain. The radiographic pattern of either osteochondritis dissecans or osteochondral fracture is that of a crescent-shaped radiolucent defect within which cartilage (radiolucent), degenerative fragmented calcification, or a well-corticated osteochondral body may be evident.[241–248] Evaluation of the extent of the cartilaginous component can be accomplished by arthrotomography or MR imaging.[248–250, 291–293] Loosening of the fragment is best identified by the demonstration of contrast material or synovial fluid between the fragment and the defect in the bone.[248, 250] Most loose chondral or osteochondral fragments attach to the synovium and are reabsorbed[283]; however, if they remain as intra-articular bodies, they may cause locking and subsequent osteoarthritis.[241–243, 294–297] Whenever an intra-articular body is identified, the site of origin should be sought (Fig. 71–26).

In athletes, the elbow, the knee, and the talus are common sites for chondral and osteochondral fractures.[297–299] Osteochondritis dissecans in the capitulum of the distal end of the humerus is one of the conditions referred to as ''Little Leaguer's elbow'' and occurs primarily in male pitchers between 5 and 10 years of age. This injury is a result of valgus stress and extensor thrust and is manifested as tenderness along the medial joint line, with swelling and decreased joint motion.[18, 183, 205, 208, 300] Osteochondritis of the radial head, including condensation, fragmentation, and articular incongruity, can result in osteoarthritic changes and, with marked deformity, excision of the radial head may be indicated. Intra-articular bodies are a not infrequent complication of osteochondritis dissecans, and removal of these bodies may be required.[205, 206, 208]

Osteochondral injuries in the knee usually result from sudden pivoting on the knee while weight-bearing. In the femur, the typical site for osteochondritis dissecans or osteochondral fracture is the medial femoral condyle (85 per cent), with the intercondylar aspect of the medial femoral condyle being affected most commonly (69 per cent).[285] The frequency of lateral femoral condylar involvement is

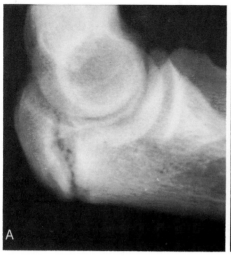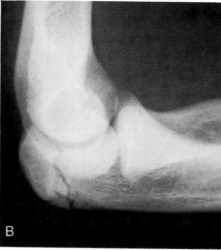

FIGURE 71–23. Nonunion of the olecranon apophysis.

A Sclerosis bordering the physeal margin and loss of sharp interdigitation suggest delayed union or nonunion.

B Normal appearance.

(From Pavlov H, et al: AJR *136*: 819, 1981. Copyright 1981, American Roentgen Ray Society.)

reported as 15 to 30 per cent.[285, 295, 301] Involvement of the anterior aspect of the lateral femoral condyle may be manifested by symptoms consistent with chondromalacia patellae or patellar pain syndrome.[256–264, 267–280] This lesion occurs just distal to the physeal plate and corresponds to the level of the patella. Although it is evident in the lateral view, it is overlooked easily. The lesion is better identified in Merchant views.[265, 266] In a radionuclide bone scan, the augmented uptake is confined to the femoral side of the patellofemoral joint and, as with all osteochondral injuries, can be identified in conventional tomograms or CT scans after arthrography or with MR imaging (Fig. 71–27).[280]

Osteochondral lesions of the talus occur secondary to an inversion injury (71 per cent) and usually while playing sports (52 per cent).[299] Patients complain of pain, locking, and either limitation or inability to participate in sports.

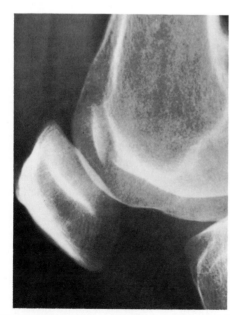

FIGURE 71–24. Shearing type osteochondral fracture of the anterior aspect of the medial femoral condyle. The fracture fragment is aligned tangentially to the joint surface.

Bone Bruises

A bone bruise is an occult intraosseous fracture that is manifested as severe focal pain after an acute impact (compression) or twisting injury.[151, 302–304] Compression forces deform the elastic cartilage, producing hemorrhage and disruption of the weaker underlying trabecular bone. A bone bruise is not evident on plain radiographs, is "hot" on a radionuclide bone scan, and, on MR images, has a geographic stellate pattern of low signal intensity on T1-weighted spin echo sequences and correspondingly high signal intensity on T2-weighted spin echo or T2*-weighted gradient echo sequences (Fig. 71–28). These injuries have increased conspicuity on fast spin echo proton density sequences performed with fat suppression. The high signal intensity corresponds to regions of hemorrhage and edema associated with the microfracture. Typically, the T2-weighted changes regress more rapidly than those on the T1-weighted spin echo MR sequences. The articular cartilage is normal.[151, 302]

Bone bruises predominate at sites of ligamentous attachment in the ends of the bones. Those occurring in the anterior to midportion of the lateral femoral condyle, the posterior aspect of the lateral tibial plateau, and the proximal portion of the lateral aspect of the tibia, distal to the plateau, are associated with an acute anterior cruciate ligament tear (Fig. 71–29).[305–311]

Fractures and Dislocations

True fractures and fracture-dislocations from sports activities usually result from collisions and falls occurring in contact sports. Athletics is the most common cause of fractures in young people between 15 and 24 years of age.[170] Classic injuries are fractures of the ribs and clavicle in hockey and football; olecranon fractures from skateboard and rollerblade falls; supracondylar fractures from bicycling and gymnastic accidents; metacarpal fractures in volleyball and basketball players; and fractures of the hook of the hamate bone in golfers. Fibular head dislocations, which may occur in parachute jumpers,[312] are extremely difficult

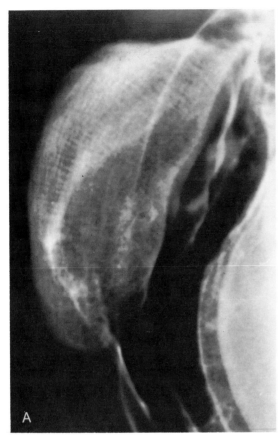

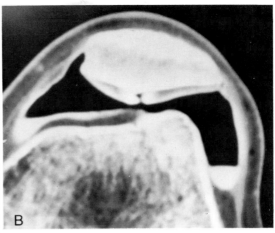

FIGURE 71–25. Chondromalacia patellae.

A In an arthrographic image, the posterior articular cartilage of the patella is wavy and irregular, with a focal linear appearance of contrast material on the cartilaginous surface, indicating a fissure.

B With CT arthrography, a fissure is identified in the posterior articular cartilage at the apex of the patella. Increased absorption of contrast medium is seen along its margins.

(From Pavlov H: South Orthop J *1*:241, 1992. Reprinted by permission from the Journal of the Southern Orthopaedic Association.)

FIGURE 71–26. Intra-articular bodies and osteochondral injury. Whenever an osteochondral defect is identified, intra-articular bodies should be sought, and the converse.

A On a lateral radiograph, large intra-articular bodies are identified in the suprapatellar bursa, and an osteochondral defect is evident in the weight-bearing aspect of the medial femoral condyle.

B In a sagittal T2-weighted spin echo MR image (TR/TE, 2000/80) an osteochondral defect (arrow) is present in the weight-bearing aspect of the medial femoral condyle and is defined by the presence of a large joint effusion.

C In a more lateral T2-weighted (TR/TE, 2000/80) image, an intra-articular body (arrow) is outlined by the joint fluid anterior to the femoral condyle.

(**A**, From Pavlov H, Torg JS: The Running Athlete. Chicago, Year Book, 1987.)

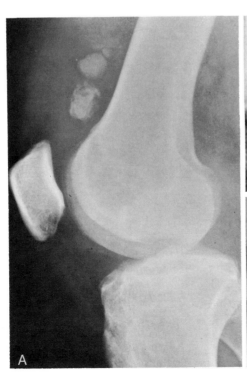

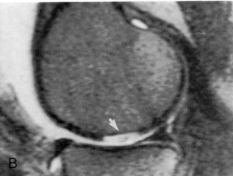

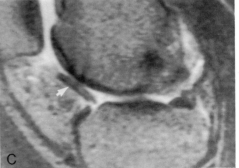

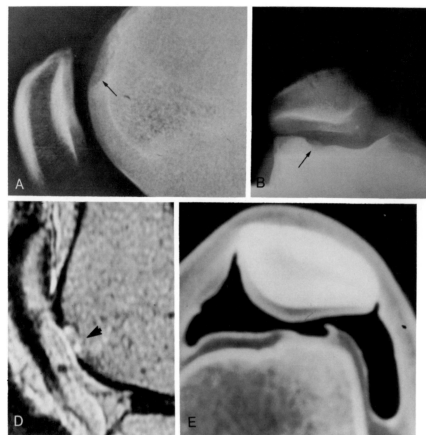

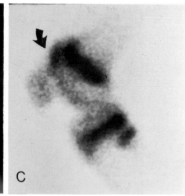

FIGURE 71–27. Osteochondral lesion at the anterior aspect of the lateral femoral condyle.

A In the routine lateral view, the lesion (arrow) is easily overlooked.

B In the Merchant view, the osteochondral defect on the anterior aspect of the lateral femoral condyle is identified (arrow).

C In a radionuclide bone scan, localized isotope uptake (arrow) is confined to the femoral side of the patellofemoral joint, distinct from the physeal uptake.

D With MR imaging, the lesion (arrow) is evident on the T2-weighted spin echo sequence (TR/TE, 2000/80).

E With CT arthrography, a purely cartilaginous lesion is evident at the anterior aspect of the lateral femoral condyle.

(**C,** From Cayea PD, et al: AJR *137*:1145, 1981. Copyright 1981, American Roentgen Ray Society.)

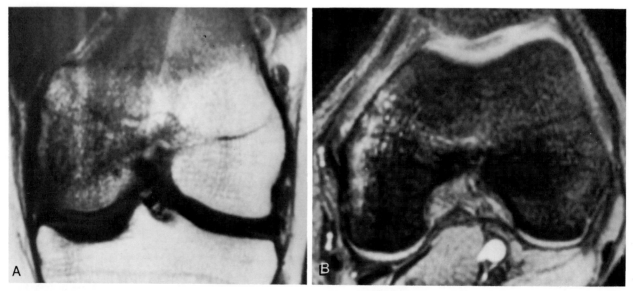

FIGURE 71–28. Bone bruise.

A In a T1-weighted spin echo MR image (TR/TE, 500/12), a geographic area of decreased signal intensity within the medial femoral condyle is identified in the coronal plane.

B In the transaxial multiplanar gradient recalled (MPGR) sequence (TR/TE, 350/18; flip angle, 30 degrees), high signal intensity is seen along the medial femoral condylar margin, indicative of hemorrhage, edema, and associated microfracture.

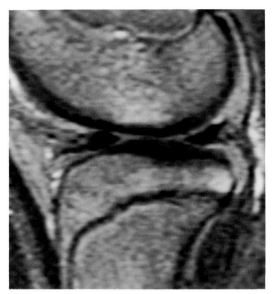

FIGURE 71–29. Classic bone bruise pattern associated with anterior cruciate ligament injury. High signal intensity is identified on the T2-weighted spin echo MR image (TR/TE, 2000/80) in the posterior and middle aspect of the proximal part of the lateral tibia and the middle to anterior aspects of the lateral femoral condyle.

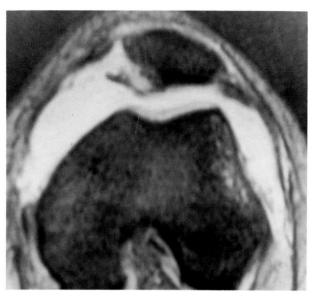

FIGURE 71–31. Acutely relocated patellar dislocation. In a transaxial multiplanar gradient recalled (MPGR) sequence (TR/TE, 350/18; flip angle, 30 degrees), a fracture of the medial facet of the patella is identified and the fragment is seen to be surrounded by joint fluid. Irregularity and disruption of the medial patellar retinaculum also are present, in addition to a contusion and flattening of the lateral femoral condyle.

to diagnose radiographically and usually require clinical suspicion and comparison with the contralateral knee.

Patella

In the knee, spontaneous fractures of the patella, including bilateral involvement, have been reported after violent quadriceps muscle contraction while the knee is flexed, as in basketball and tennis players.[97–99, 313]

Patellar subluxations or dislocations relate to abnormal patellar tracking or a twisting injury. The position of the patella has been defined by multiple radiographic criteria.[265–271, 273] Abnormal patellar tracking may be demonstrated on a Merchant view[265, 266] or transaxial imaging using CT scans or MR images (Fig. 71–30).[255, 271, 273] Evidence of a prior patellar dislocation that has relocated can be obtained radiographically by observing flattening of the medial facet of the patella or a separate osseous dense area adjacent to the medial facet of the patella and, in some instances, a congruent flattening of the lateral aspect of the lateral femoral condyle.[314] Similar findings have been de-

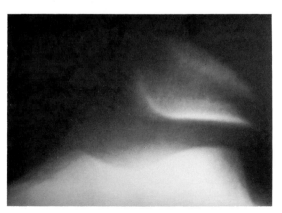

FIGURE 71–30. Abnormal patellar tracking. On a Merchant view, abnormal patellar tracking is seen.

scribed on MR images and include disruption of the medial retinaculum, contusion or osteochondral injury of the lateral femoral condyle, medial patellar contusion, and joint effusion (Fig. 71–31).[271]

Shoulder

Fractures of the humerus from athletic activities occur with violent muscular contractions.[315, 316] Spiral fractures have been reported during the preparatory phase of pitching from the rotational force on the humeral shaft[186] in young amateur pitchers[186] and also in adolescent tennis players,[125, 185] wrist wrestlers, and shotputters[123, 124]; professional pitchers typically have compensatory cortical hypertrophy that results from these stresses.[183, 184, 186]

Shoulder (glenohumeral joint) instability without a history of dislocation is a frequent complaint of athletes, especially those involved in sports requiring throwing movements, weight-lifters, swimmers, football players, wrestlers, and boxers.[317–324] Anterior instability is the most common complaint, although the sensations of posterior and multidirectional instability are not infrequent. The stability of the glenohumeral joint depends on the integrity of the rotator cuff, the muscles of the shoulder girdle, and the glenohumeral ligament–labral complex. Typically, the capsular and anterior ligaments are redundant in patients who have had a dislocation or have clinical signs of instability, and the labrum often is hypoplastic.[324]

A fracture-dislocation of the shoulder usually is a result of contact activities with the most common traumatic dislocation of the glenohumeral joint being anterior. Once the shoulder is relocated, the radiographs in these patients may be normal or demonstrate Hill-Sachs and Bankart lesions.[325–327] The Hill-Sachs lesion is a compression fracture of the posterolateral aspect of the humeral head, best observed in the frontal view of the shoulder with the humerus

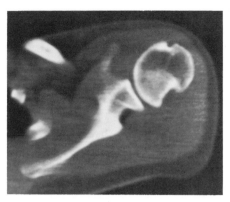

FIGURE 71–32. Hill-Sachs deformity. In a transaxial CT image, the Hill-Sachs deformity is readily apparent in the posterolateral aspect of the left humerus.

in internal rotation, in a Stryker notch view,[317] or with transaxial imaging (Fig. 71–32). The presence or absence of marrow edema on the MR imaging examination identifies the injury as acute or chronic, respectively. The Bankart lesion is a compression injury of the anterior margin of the glenoid rim, which, if osseous, is best identified in a West Point view (a modified prone axillary view).[317, 327, 328] In most instances, however, the Bankart lesion requires double contrast arthrotomography, CT arthrography,[329–331] or MR imaging for detection. In MR images, the surrounding ligaments and joint capsule also can be examined.[332–335]

Sesamoid Bones

Sesamoid fractures result from repetitive stress in ballet dancers[65] and long-distance runners[68, 70] and may occur after acute hyperextension of the metatarsophalangeal joints in football players when tackled from behind on a plantar-flexed foot.[66–68, 336] A stress fracture usually can be distinguished from a bipartite sesamoid bone because multipartite sesamoid bones are larger than unipartite ones, the fragments are smooth and rounded (unlike fracture margins, which are jagged), and fracture fragments fit together (Fig. 71–33). Diastasis of a bipartite sesamoid bone is a not infrequent injury in football players.[336] Osteonecrosis of a sesamoid bone occasionally complicates these injuries.[66–69]

Symptomatic Normal Variants

Normal variants refer to developmental conditions (e.g., juxta-articular ossicles, bipartite sesamoid bones, bipartite patella, transitional vertebra) that, although present from birth, become symptomatic as a consequence of repetitive cyclic loading activity, which changes the dynamic relationship between the skeletal elements. When symptoms are present, sclerosis may be identified radiographically at the margins of the bone fragments or ossicles (Fig. 71–34). Increased accumulation of the radiopharmaceutical agent during bone scintigraphy confirms abnormal motion of the fragmented bone and reactive changes. Common symptomatic normal variants include the os supranaviculare, os supratalare, os intermetatarseum, and os tibialis externa (accessory navicular bone). The os trigonum or a long Stieda's process in the posterior aspect of the talus may be compromised between the calcaneus and the posterior tibial lip in

forced plantar flexion of the foot (e.g., deep knee pliés in dancers or duckwalking in football players). This injury typically is recurrent unless the accessory bone is removed.[337]

Degenerative Conditions

Osteoarthritis occurring after sports related activities is moot. Some reports state that preponderance of premature osteoarthritis of the lower extremities is no greater in runners than in nonrunners.[338–341] Other reports have shown acute articular changes with jogging, such as transient joint effusions.[342] Still other studies report that excessive repetitive cyclic loading activities result in osteoarthritic changes earlier than expected owing to hypertrophy and pathologic stresses on the synovium, which may produce metaplasia of the synovium, joint incongruity, and intra-articular bodies.[183] Early degenerative changes are expected if a compensatory process has occurred, such as a leg length discrepancy or scoliosis, that places unequal stress on one side of the body. The site of degenerative arthritis is dependent on the sport (i.e., football players have osteoarthritis in the knee, pitchers have degenerative changes in the glenohumeral joint and elbow). Osteoarthritis consisting of joint space narrowing, sclerosis on both sides of the joint, subchondral cysts, osteophytes, and intra-articular bodies usually is evident radiographically in the older athlete while earlier findings may be evident in MR images. Enthesophytes at sites of musculotendinous and ligamentous attachment result from chronic repetitive irritation, bleeding and inflammation, periostitis, or microavulsions. These enthesophytes are especially common in the elbow on the medial aspect of the coronoid tubercle as a consequence of the pull of the ulnar collateral ligament and joint capsule about the elbows of professional pitchers and tennis players. Decreased range of motion and, in rare instances, irritation of the ulnar nerve may be evident. An enthesophyte in the medial aspect of the coracoid tubercle is present in 75 per cent of professional baseball pitchers (Fig. 71–35).[183]

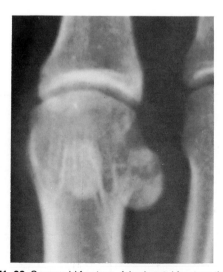

FIGURE 71–33. Sesamoid fracture. A horizontal fracture through the lateral sesamoid is seen. The overall size of the sesamoid approximates that of the medial sesamoid, the fracture fragments fit together, and the margins are irregular and jagged.

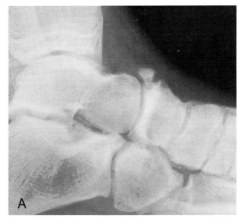

FIGURE 71–34. Symptomatic normal variants.

A Sclerosis and osteophytes are seen between the os supranaviculare and the proximal articular border of the navicular bone, indicating motion.

B, C On plain film **(B)** and bone scan **(C),)** a large os tibialis externa with mild soft tissue swelling is associated with a corresponding area of localized isotope uptake.

(From Pavlov H, Torg JS: The Running Athlete. Chicago, Year Book, 1987.)

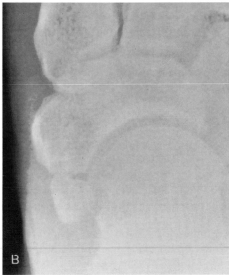

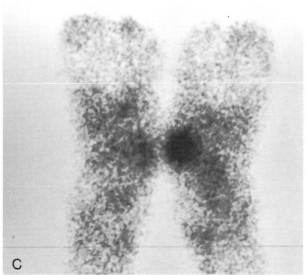

SOFT TISSUE INJURIES

Sports related soft tissue injuries include muscle injuries, musculotendinous strains, ligament sprains, cartilage (meniscal) tears, bursitis, nerve injuries, and miscellaneous conditions including fascial injuries and superficial soft tissue bruises. The causes of soft tissue injuries may be direct or indirect. Indirect injuries can be acute (due to sudden extreme overloading), chronic (due to overuse), or acute on chronic.[343] Definitions applicable to soft tissue injury are indicated in Table 71–5.

Muscle Injuries

Muscle injuries account for approximately 10 to 30 per cent of all athletic injuries. The mildest injury is a muscle cramp from dehydration and minute muscle rupture, bleeding, or impaired circulation. Muscle soreness, pain, tenderness, and swelling can occur after strenuous training. Eccentric (stretching or lengthening) and concentric (isometric or shortening) muscle action has been shown by MR imaging to respond differently to exercise; increased signal in-

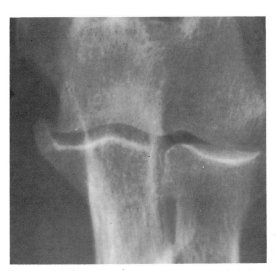

FIGURE 71–35. Traction osteophyte in a professional pitcher in the medial aspect of the coronoid tubercle.

TABLE 71–5. Definitions of Soft Tissue Injuries

Contusion	Bruised skin and underlying soft tissues secondary to edema and bleeding
Hemorrhage	Poorly defined soft tissue bleeding
Hematoma	Well-defined and restricted blood collection
Strain	Inflammation or rupture at the musculotendinous junction or muscle
Sprain	Inflammation or rupture of a ligament

tensity on T2-weighted spin echo sequences has been identified after intense exercise in muscles performing concentric actions, whereas no change has been observed in muscles performing eccentric action.[344, 345] This increased signal intensity reflects muscle edema.[345] An increase in the total muscle water, predominantly in the extracellular space, has been shown to occur in the groin adductor muscle groups and also at the origin of the hamstring muscles in long-distance runners. This is a benign condition that resolves quickly.[346, 347]

Delayed onset muscle soreness, often designated DOMS, is a condition of skeletal muscle occurring after muscular exertion in which soreness progresses in the first 24 to 48 hours after exercise and resolves within 7 days.[346, 348, 349] The muscle has decreased capacity to produce force during this period.[349] Abnormal MR imaging findings, with prolongation of T1 and T2 times and increase in signal intensity in T1- and T2-weighted sequences, may last up to 3 weeks longer than the clinical symptoms.[346] No gross fiber disruption[350] occurs, and there is an absence of focal hematoma, fascial herniation, and subsequent fibrous or fatty infiltration.[346]

Muscles are injured by both impact (direct) (e.g., football) and overloading (indirect) (e.g., running).[351, 352] A muscle rupture occurs from either distraction or compression. Distraction injuries result primarily from overstretching and affect the superficial parts of the muscles at their insertions and origins; these are discussed in the section on muscle strains.[351, 352] Compression injuries (muscle contusion) result from direct impact and affect primarily the deep parts of the muscles.[353]

A classic example of a compression muscle injury is a quadriceps muscle rupture occurring after direct impact of the contracted muscle by a fellow football player's helmet. Compression injuries from direct trauma result in intramuscular or intermuscular hematoma. *Intramuscular* hematoma occurs from bleeding within the fascia or muscle sheath. The increased intramuscular pressure compresses the blood vessels and limits the extent of bleeding. Usually marked pain and impaired mobility occur, and muscle function may be absent. Muscle swelling secondary to edema or hemor-

rhage can produce an acute compartment syndrome when it exceeds the capacity of the surrounding inelastic fascia. This is a not uncommon complication in the calf, in which four compartments are present: an *anterior* compartment; the *deep* (flexor digitorum longus, flexor hallucis longus, and tibialis posterior muscles) and *superficial* (soleus and superficial gastrocnemius muscles) compartments, posterior to the interosseous membrane; and the *lateral* compartment (peroneus longus and peroneus brevis muscles), each of which contain nerves and blood vessels. *Intermuscular hematoma* develops between the muscles after a muscle sheath or fascial injury. Swelling occurs distant to the damaged area and, depending on where the blood collects, usually is evident clinically 24 to 48 hours after the injury. Muscle function typically returns.

An acute muscle injury is evident clinically and on transaxial imaging by its asymmetry with the contralateral side.[354] The specific site of injury is best identified on MR imaging[346] using STIR[346, 355, 356] or a hybrid fat suppression sequence,[357] which increases conspicuity (Fig. 71–36). Contused muscle has primarily interstitial edema and a feathery appearance, with only slight distortion of muscle architecture. A subacute hemorrhage within the muscle is demonstrated as a region of high signal intensity on T1-weighted and T2-weighted spin echo sequences, whereas an older injury, with hemosiderin deposition, will be of low signal intensity on the T2-weighted spin echo sequence. Associated muscle retraction and atrophy are best identified in the T1-weighted spin echo images as regions of high signal intensity secondary to fatty infiltration.

Chronic muscle hematoma may result in myositis ossificans, which represents self-limiting soft tissue ossification within the skeletal muscle. On plain radiographs, myositis ossificans may be evident 2 to 6 weeks after the onset of symptoms by the presence of faint calcific shadows.[358] A well-defined ossific area, with a circumscribed edge and oriented parallel to the long axis of the adjacent tubular bone, usually is apparent within 6 to 8 weeks (Fig. 71–37).[358] The dense rim, characteristic of myositis ossificans, is present after 4 to 6 weeks and is identified more readily on plain films or CT scans than on MR images.[359–363] On

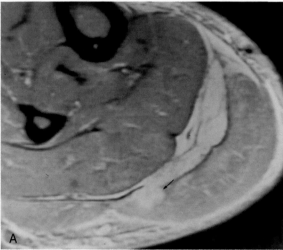
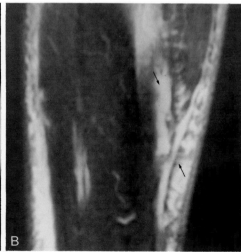

FIGURE 71–36. Muscle injury. In a transaxial proton density fast spin echo MR image (TR/TE, 3500/18) **(A)** and a sagittal T2-weighted fast spin echo MR image (TR/TE, 4500/102) **(B)** obtained with fat suppression, a focal area of high signal intensity (arrows) is evident in the distal aspect of the medial head of the gastrocnemius muscle with diffuse increased signal intensity of the surrounding muscle.

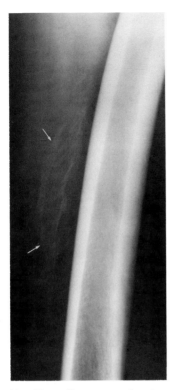

FIGURE 71–37. Myositis ossificans secondary to a chronic quadriceps muscle injury. The heterotopic ossification (arrows) is oriented parallel to the long axis of the adjacent bone and has a peripheral rim of calcification. (From Pavlov H, et al: RadioGraphics *1*:17, 1981.)

MR imaging, myositis ossificans varies in appearance depending on the histologic findings that change with the passage of time. Edema surrounds the lesion in the early stages, fluid-fluid levels are evident in an intermediate-aged lesion, and a well-defined lesion with an inhomogeneous signal intensity is typical of a mature lesion.[363, 364]

Musculotendinous Strains

Distraction or overstretching produces muscle injuries in the superficial aspect of the muscle (i.e., muscle strains). Muscle strains are very common in the lower extremities of athletes.[16, 22, 26, 38, 40, 351, 352, 365] The site of musculotendinous injury depends on the athlete's age; musculotendinous junction injuries occur more commonly in the young adult and adult athlete, whereas tendon injuries are more common in the adult and elderly athlete.[365, 366] The myotendinous junction is vulnerable when tension is applied quickly, when it is applied obliquely, when the muscle is maximally innervated and under tension before loading, or when the tendon is weak with respect to the muscle.[48, 351, 352, 366–370] The musculotendinous junction is especially vulnerable in those muscles that cross two joints (e.g., hamstrings, quadriceps, gastrocnemius).[367] Muscle strains typically localize to a single muscle within a group of synergists (e.g., the adductor longus, rectus femoris, and the medial head of the gastrocnemius).[365]

A myotendinous junction injury is characterized by inflammation and edema and, to a lesser extent, hemorrhage.[352, 365, 366, 370] On CT scans, hypodensity at the muscu-

lotendinous unit has been identified 1 to 2 days after the injury, suggesting inflammation and edema, not bleeding.[371] On MR images, muscle strains are confirmed by the presence of areas of high signal intensity on T2-weighted spin echo sequences.[356, 372, 373] When disruption occurs at the myotendinous junction, fluid may collect at the site of disruption and dissect along the epimysium and subcutis remote from the musculotendinous junction.[365] Highly trained marathon runners, however, have mild MR imaging changes at the myotendinous junction.[346]

Muscle strains are graded[368] as follows: grade one (mild)—less than 5 per cent fiber disruption and no loss of strength or restriction of movement; grade two (moderate)—50 per cent disruption and partial loss of strength; and grade three (severe)—complete musculotendinous rupture, with or without muscle retraction and with loss of strength and function.

Muscle strains result from the same activities that cause an avulsion injury in the slightly younger athlete and, similarly, are especially common in the pelvis and lower extremity; as examples, the adductor muscle group is overloaded in soccer players, ice skaters, skiers, hockey players, hurdlers, and high jumpers; the hamstring muscles are ruptured from forceful knee flexion while the hip is extended, as in sprinters; and the iliopsoas muscle is injured with sit-ups, rowing, uphill running, and hurdling, with the rupture occurring distally near the lesser trochanter. In the shoulder, overuse of the deltoid muscle occurs near its attachment to the humerus in swimmers using vigorous backward arm movements (e.g., butterfly strokes) and also in rowers and throwers. The pectoralis major muscle, which inserts into the anterior surface of the upper humerus, can rupture near its insertion during bench pressing and wrestling.

Shoulder

Throwing Mechanism. Pitching causes hypertrophy of both the bones (humerus) and the muscles (pectoralis major, latissimus dorsi, and forearm flexors). Racquet sports, especially the serve in tennis, reproduce the throwing mechanism and lead to the same types of injuries.[183, 185] The tendons of the shoulder and the ligaments of the elbow are at risk from the throwing mechanism. The throwing mechanism has three phases: the wind-up (cocking), the acceleration stage, and the follow-through.[208, 209] During wind-up, the humerus is brought into external rotation, placing the triceps and the anterior capsular structures and tendon of the long head of the biceps brachii muscle under tension, while the flexor and extensor muscles of the elbow are contracted. The acceleration stage (from the end of wind-up to ball release) is divided into two phases: the first phase produces valgus stress on the elbow (distraction of the medial side and compression of the lateral side) as the shoulder and elbow are brought forward with the forearm and hand left behind; the second phase, in which the shoulder rotates internally and the forearm and hand are snapped forward, can injure the internal shoulder rotators (latissimus dorsi and pectoralis major muscles) and, less commonly, cause spiral fractures of the shaft of the humerus. The flexors stabilize the elbow. The final stage of throwing starts with ball release and is characterized by rotation of the forearm into pronation, causing rotational and shearing forces on the lateral side of the elbow and compression on the posterior aspect of the elbow.[208, 209]

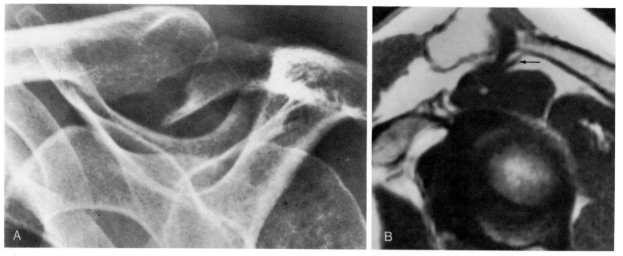

FIGURE 71–38. Shoulder impingement syndrome.

A A supraspinatus outlet view of the shoulder demonstrates an extremely prominent enthesophyte on the undersurface of the acromion process anteriorly.

B In a T1-weighted spin echo MR image (TR/TE, 600/15), the enthesophyte (arrow) is seen to compress the superior aspect of the supraspinatus muscle.

Impingement Syndrome. The impingement syndrome is pain produced by repetitive movements of the arm at or above the horizontal plane and when the arm is abducted at 40 to 120 degrees.[274] Pitchers and swimmers using the crawl or butterfly stroke may complain of pain during forward and inward motions of the arm. The impingement syndrome currently is theorized to result from the compression of the rotator cuff tendons between the humeral head and the coracoacromial arch.[374, 375] The disorder is associated with subacromial bursitis or rotator cuff inflammation with or without degenerative changes at the insertion site of the supraspinatus tendon,[374–379] proliferative changes (an enthesophyte) on the undersurface of the acromion process anteriorly, osteoarthritis of the acromioclavicular joint, calcification in the rotator cuff, degenerative changes of the lesser tuberosity, and narrowing of the acromiohumeral space (Fig. 71–38).[375–379] Three stages of changes in the supraspinatus tendon have been described: stage 1, reversible edema and hemorrhage; stage 2, chronic fibrosis; and stage 3, disruption.[379–381]

A coracoid impingement syndrome also has been reported and is associated with use of the overhead position of the arm while in medial rotation, as in tennis players and weight-lifters. These patients have severe pain over the coracoid process associated with a painful audible click.[382]

Rotator Cuff Tear. A rotator cuff tear results from a single traumatic episode in both middle-aged and older athletes, in comparison to athletes younger than 40 years, in whom a rotator cuff tear usually is associated with an acute glenohumeral joint dislocation.[383] The integrity of the rotator cuff can be evaluated by arthrography or sonography, although the specific tendons (the supraspinatus, infraspinatus, teres minor, and subscapularis) can be assessed individually in MR images.[384–388] The supraspinatus tendon is ruptured most frequently.

The subscapularis tendon is an important component in internal humeral rotation, and throwers, weight-lifters, racquet ball players, and wrestlers are subject to complete tendon tears, partial tendon tears, and tendinitis. The sub-

scapularis tendon is best evaluated with transaxial MR imaging.

Calcific tendinitis in the rotator cuff is identified on plain films as an amorphous collection of calcific density. Most frequently, calcification occurs in the supraspinatus tendon, located superior to the greater tuberosity of the humerus in all views. In MR images, calcification within the tendon is identified as an area of signal void on all sequences and may be associated with tendinitis or tenosynovitis.

Biceps Tendon and SLAP Injuries. Subluxation or dislocation of the tendon of the long head of the biceps brachii muscle from the bicipital groove is a common cause of shoulder disability in throwers.[389] The tendon normally moves within the groove, being maintained within the groove by the transverse humeral ligament. If the groove is tight, the tendon can become irritated and a tenovaginitis can result.[389–392] Bicipital tendinitis or dislocation of the tendon of the long head of the biceps brachii muscle occurs in gymnasts, tennis and badminton players, wrestlers, and rowers, especially in persons who are 40 to 50 years old.[390, 391]

SLAP lesions (superior labrum anterior, posterior) refer to injuries of the superior portion of the glenoid labrum at the insertion of the biceps tendon to the superior labral complex. The biceps tendon reportedly decelerates the arm during throwing, resulting in strenuous forces being placed upon it.[393] SLAP injuries result from excessive stress on the biceps tendon as it inserts into the glenoid labrum.[393–395] SLAP injuries usually are manifested by pain and clicking and, occasionally, instability after acute pitching or racquet sport activity, catching a heavy falling object, or falling on an outstretched hand. The degree of involvement of the biceps tendon varies,[395] and SLAP lesions can occur in the absence of capsular injuries.[393, 396–399] Four grades of SLAP lesions have been established: 1, superior glenoid labrum fraying with an intact biceps tendon; 2, avulsion of the labral-biceps anchor; 3, bucket-handle tear of the superior glenoid fossa with intact labral-biceps anchor; and 4, bucket-handle tear of the superior glenoid fossa and exten-

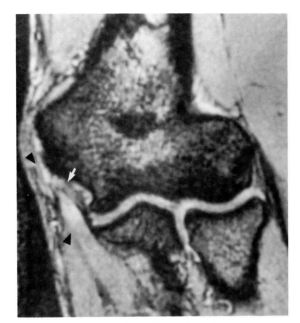

FIGURE 71–39. Golfer's elbow. Coronal gradient echo sequence (TR/TE, 50/15; flip angle, 10 degrees) demonstrates increased signal intensity within the proximal aspect of the common flexor tendon (arrowheads) and in the tissues surrounding the medial epicondyle. Mild increased signal intensity also is present in the proximal attachment of the ulnar collateral ligament (arrow), indicating partial injury. The extensor tendon and radial collateral ligament are normal.

sion of the tear into the proximal portion of the biceps tendon.[400] SLAP lesions can be evaluated with CT scanning[393] or MR imaging.[395, 396]

Elbow

Flexion contractures of the elbow are present in 50 per cent of professional athletes.[208, 209] Injuries to the lateral side of the elbow, collectively known as "tennis elbow," are manifested as pain overlying the radiohumeral joint owing to repetitive rotatory forearm motion, compression, and shearing forces. In athletes over 40 years old, edematous changes or thickening of the common extensor tendon results, and traction enthesophytes are common. Injuries to the medial side of the elbow occur most commonly secondary to forceful flexion and distraction. Although this is known as "Little League elbow," it also occurs in golfers and tennis players who use exaggerated top spin requiring excessive pronation of the forearm. The common flexor-pronator group is the first line of defense to the valgus strain of throwing while the ligaments are still lax and can become inflamed (myositis) or ruptured (Fig. 71–39).[400, 401]

Triceps tendon injury usually results from a fall or forceful throwing in the adult. Rupture of the distal portion of the biceps tendon, which inserts along the ulnar aspect of the radius, represents 3 per cent of all biceps tendon ruptures and occurs as a result of forced flexion against strong resistance.[400] Avulsion of the distal portion of the tendon from the radial tuberosity[403–405] and partial tendon rupture[406] have been identified. Clinically, this injury results in proximal retraction of the biceps tendon and a mass in the upper aspect of the arm.

Knee

The extensor mechanism of the knee consists of the quadriceps femoris muscles and tendons, the patella, and the patellar tendon. The quadriceps is made up of four muscles: rectus femoris, vastus medialis, vastus intermedius, and vastus lateralis, with tendon fibers from each joining to form a single tendon that inserts in the superior border of the patella. Quadriceps tendon ruptures are most common in the fourth and fifth decades of life.[407] Injury results from forceful contraction against forced knee flexion or against excessive resistance, as with landing from a jump.[407, 408] Injury also may occur on executing a quick change in stride while running or attempting to kick a ball forcibly and then catching the foot.[407] The normal tendon does not rupture under stress.[409] Loss of extensor function is unusual with direct injuries but does occur with indirect trauma and takes place when the medial and lateral expansions of the tendon rupture.[407, 410] Because the tendon is formed from four tendons, it has a laminated appearance in MR images, and diagnosing partial tears of this tendon can be difficult.[411]

The patellar tendon is the least common cause of extensor mechanism disruption and most typically is injured in the young athlete.[407, 410, 412] The tendon usually ruptures at its origin in the inferior pole of the patella.[408, 413] Patellar tendon ruptures and tendinitis are associated with sudden knee extension, such as in running, jumping, and kicking, and injuries typically are associated with an increase in speed or strength training.[187–192] Evaluation of the tendon can be done on plain films, ultrasonograms, CT scans, and MR images (Fig. 71–40).[414–416]

Ankle and Foot

Achilles tendon injury is common in middle-aged (third to fifth decade) male athletes.[417–421] Tendinitis affects primarily joggers, with ruptures occurring in both "weekend jocks" and well-trained athletes.[417] The most vulnerable site of injury, because of its poor vascularity, is the musculotendinous junction, which is 2 to 5 cm proximal to the tendi-

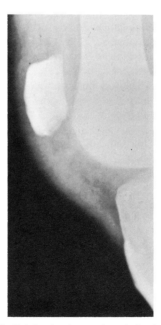

FIGURE 71–40. Patellar tendon rupture. Lateral radiograph, using soft tissue technique, demonstrates elongation of the patellar tendon. The tendon is thickened with poor definition posteriorly, and the patella is high-riding. (From Pavlov H, Torg JS: The Running Athlete. Chicago, Year Book, 1987.)

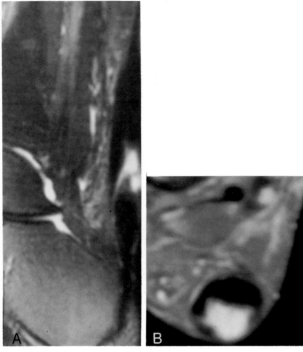

FIGURE 71–41. Acute Achilles tendon rupture. In a sagittal T2-weighted fast spin echo MR image with fat suppression (TR/TE, 3750/102) **(A)** and in a transaxial proton density fast spin echo sequence with fat suppression (TR/TE, 5000/19) **(B)**, the abnormal morphology and high signal intensity within the tendon indicate an acute disruption at the typical site, 2 to 5 cm proximal to its insertion in the calcaneus. The injury involves approximately 75 per cent of the tendon girth.

nous insertion in the calcaneus.[422] An Achilles tendon rupture is a clinical diagnosis and, although the tendon can be identified on plain films, it is imaged more completely with ultrasonography[423, 424] or MR imaging.[356, 425, 426] With MR imaging, the tendon injury can be graded, and an acute injury can be distinguished from a chronic one (Fig. 71–41).[417, 427] Typically, the injury pattern in MR images is consistent with fluid, not hemorrhage.[356]

In the foot, the tibialis posterior tendon is subject to mechanical pressure where it lies behind the medial malleolus and is injured in runners, skaters, skiers, and those who have or require excessive pronation of the foot. These injuries frequently are found in middle-aged women in their fifth and sixth decades. When this tendon is injured, progressive disabling flatfoot deformity results.[428–432] Injuries to the flexor hallucis longus tendon and tendinitis are seen primarily in ballet dancers at the site where the tendon passes through the tarsal tunnel. An aberrant extension of the muscle belly of the flexor hallucis longus muscle into the region of the flexor retinaculum has been reported as a cause of locking (''trigger ankle'') in a tennis player.[433]

Ligament Sprains

Ligaments attach bone to bone and are a frequent source of pain and instability in the young adult and adult athlete. Inflammation of the ligamentous attachment to bone from repeated stresses may produce bleeding, periosteal irritation, bone fragmentation, and traction enthesophytes. If guarding can be eliminated, stress films, with comparison to the opposite side, may confirm the existence of ligamentous laxity or joint instability. Although intra-articular ligaments can be evaluated arthrographically, MR imaging is a noninvasive method of visualizing both intra- and extra-articular ligaments directly and distinguishing acute from chronic injury.[434–439] Ligament injuries occur in all joints but are most prevalent in the knees, ankles, elbows, and metacarpophalangeal joint of the thumb of athletes.

Knee

The knee has four main ligaments. The most critical ligament responsible for knee stability is the anterior cruciate ligament, which extends from the intercondylar aspect of the lateral femoral condyle to insert in the anterior aspect of the tibial plateau just anterior to the tibial spines. This ligament can be evaluated by double contrast arthrography[440–443] or MR imaging.[435, 444–447] In MR images, the normal anterior cruciate ligament is of slightly higher signal intensity than the posterior cruciate ligament. In the sagittal view, the anterior edge of the ligament normally is straight. The anterior cruciate ligament is injured primarily from external rotation and abduction with hyperextension of the knee or from forced internal rotation with the knee in full extension. In younger persons, avulsion fractures occur at either its site of insertion or its site of origin and are identified on the routine lateral or notch view, respectively. An acute anterior cruciate ligament injury has been noted to be associated with specific sites of bone bruises and fractures of the tibia and femur (Fig. 71–29).[306–311]

Posterior cruciate ligament tears are less common than those of the anterior cruciate ligament. Athletic injuries to the posterior cruciate ligament result from forced hyperextension of the knee,[448] valgus angulation of the knee after anterior cruciate ligament and medial collateral ligament ruptures,[448, 449] or hyperflexion of the knee.[450] Injuries to the posterior cruciate ligament usually are associated with a tear of the anterior cruciate ligament or the collateral ligaments or with posterolateral abnormalities involving the meniscus, popliteus tendon, or capsule.[451]

The medial collateral ligament ruptures as a consequence of valgus force on a flexed knee and is a common injury in football players and skiers (Fig. 71–42). The ligament has a superficial and deep component, and complete medial collateral ligament tears are associated with tears of the medial and posterior portions of the joint capsule, the anterior cruciate ligament, and the medial meniscus. A chronic medial collateral ligament injury is referred to as Pellegrini-Stieda disease[452, 453] and is manifested on plain radiographs as calcification within the soft tissues adjacent to the medial femoral condyle, at the joint line, or less often at the distal tibial attachment of the ligament. In MR images, this calcification appears as a signal void on all sequences.

The lateral ligamentous complex of the knee is primarily an extra-articular structure. Posteriorly, an extracapsular fibular collateral ligament extends from the lateral femoral condyle to join with the biceps femoris tendon and forms the conjoint tendon, which inserts in the fibular head. Anteriorly, the iliotibial band inserts in Gerdy's tubercle of the tibia. The only intra-articular portion of the lateral ligamentous complex is the meniscocapsular attachment of the lateral meniscus. It is this latter component that is responsible for the Segond avulsion fracture (Fig. 71–19).[231–234]

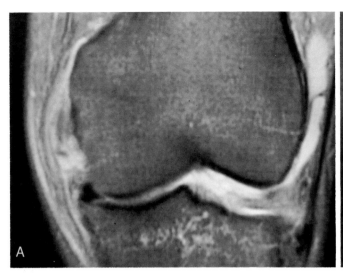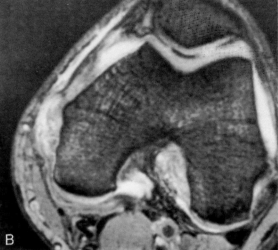

FIGURE 71–42. Torn medial collateral ligament. Coronal, fast spin echo MR image with fat suppression (TR/TE, 4000/18) **(A)** and a transaxial multiplanar gradient recalled (MPGR) MR image (TR/TE, 400/16; flip angle, 30 degrees) **(B)** show a poorly demarcated elongated area of high signal intensity adjacent to the medial femoral condyle, consistent with a tear of the medial collateral ligament. The medial patellar retinaculum appears intact.

Ankle and Foot

Ankle injuries account for approximately 10 per cent of emergency room visits and radiographic requests.[454-456] Injuries of the ligaments of the ankle, especially the lateral ligaments, are extremely common in athletes.[457-460] Three distinct lateral ligaments exist: the anterior talofibular, the calcaneofibular, and the posterior talofibular ligaments.[461] Anterior talofibular ligament injury is the most common ankle injury resulting from supination and inward rotation of the foot and occurs as an isolated finding in 70 per cent of ankle ligament injuries. A tear of the calcaneofibular ligament is a frequently associated injury, however. Fewer than 10 per cent of ankle injuries involve the large medial deltoid ligament, which extends from the medial malleolus to insert in the navicular, the calcaneus, and the talus. A deltoid ligament injury usually results from pronation of the foot (sole of the foot turned outward).

Elbow

Injuries to the ulnar collateral ligament occur in throwing athletes, including baseball pitchers, javelin throwers, and tennis players.[183, 462-464] The ulnar collateral ligament complex is the primary contributor in resisting valgus stress applied to the elbow.[464] The repetitive nature of throwing results in ulnar collateral ligament trauma, including microtears, hemorrhage, and edema, both within and around the ligament (Fig. 71–39).[465, 466] When this ligament is injured, athletes have medial joint pain and tenderness that are accentuated by throwing.[465] Symptoms of ulnar nerve compression may accompany an injury of the ulnar collateral ligament.[466] The radial collateral ligament, which originates in the lateral epicondyle and inserts in the annular ligament, does not contribute to stability of the elbow to the same degree as the ulnar collateral ligament.[464]

Thumb

The ulnar collateral ligament of the metacarpophalangeal joint of the thumb frequently is injured, which may be associated with an avulsion injury of the base of the proximal phalanx (gamekeeper's thumb) (Fig. 71–43). This injury accounts for approximately 6 per cent of all skiing injuries and occurs when the ski pole is planted.[467] It also is seen in football, hockey, wrestling, and baseball participants. The damage results from violent abduction of the thumb and can be diagnosed on the basis of findings seen in stress radiographs or MR images.[467-472]

Meniscal Injuries

Meniscal injuries may occur in association with all athletic endeavors and in patients of all ages; however, meniscal tears are seen predominantly in football players and skiers. In recreational runners, MR images have shown increased signal intensity in the menisci and knee joint

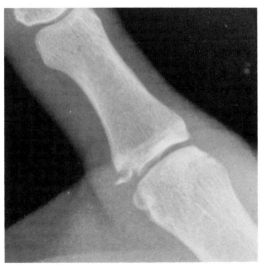

FIGURE 71–43. Gamekeeper's thumb. Avulsion fracture related to the phalangeal attachment of the ulnar collateral ligament of the metacarpophalangeal joint is seen.

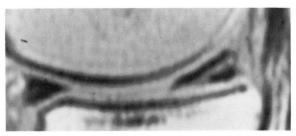

FIGURE 71–44. Meniscal tear. In a sagittal proton density spin echo MR image using meniscal windows (TR/TE, 2000/12), a linear region of high signal intensity extends to the inferior articular surface of the posterior horn of the medial meniscus, and the inner rim of the posterior horn is slightly blunted and oriented inferiorly.

effusions,[342] whereas meniscal degeneration actually has been shown to be delayed in long-distance runners.[340, 473] In an MR imaging study of marathon runners, the prevalence of meniscal tears was found to be no higher than that reported for sedentary persons and was equal to that for nonrunning athletes.[474] These findings suggest an adaptive response of the meniscal cartilage to prolonged training.[474, 475]

The diagnosis of meniscal injuries may be made clinically, arthroscopically, arthrographically, with arthrography combined with CT, and with MR imaging. An advantage of the MR imaging examination when compared to arthrography is that it does not require an intra-articular injection or application of stress to a painful knee. The normal meniscus is a triangular structure with a smooth surface that is of low signal intensity in all MR imaging sequences as it consists of uniform fibrocartilaginous tissue. Not infrequently, however, increased signal intensity is present within the meniscus, which has led to the establishment of a grading system. Menisci demonstrating low signal intensity (grade 0) are normal. An amorphous, globular, nonlinear area of increased signal intensity that does not extend to an articular surface is categorized as grade 1, and a linear increase in signal intensity that does not extend to an articular surface is categorized as grade 2; both are normal findings and do not indicate a meniscal tear. A linear increase in signal intensity that extends to an articular surface is categorized as grade 3 and indicates a meniscal tear (Fig. 71–44).[435–437, 476] Loss of the normal meniscal contour without a sharp inner rim also is representative of a torn meniscus. A full description of the MR imaging findings of meniscal tears is provided in Chapter 70.

Bursitis

A bursa is a sac formed by two layers of synovial tissue located at sites of friction between a bone and a tendon or superficial to a bone or tendon. Bursitis indicates inflammation and edema, usually as a result of repetitive trauma from friction or external pressure. Clinically suspected bursitis is confirmed on MR imaging by a focal area of high signal intensity on the T2-weighted spin echo sequences. Calcific bursitis is identified on plain films as an amorphous radiodense collection and in MR images as an area of signal void.

Several bursal injuries are associated with sports activities. In the knee, bursae occur superficial to the patellar

tendon (prepatellar) and tibial tubercle (infrapatellar) and also deep or posterior to the patellar tendon, inferior to Hoffa's fat pad. The pes anserina bursa is located deep to the semitendinosus, gracilis, and sartorius tendon insertions in the proximal medial portion of the tibia. The iliotibial bursa is located deep to the iliotibial band.

At the posterior aspect of the heel, a bursa is present on either side of the insertion of the Achilles tendon. The superficial tendo Achillis bursa is an acquired bursa, posterior to the insertion site of the Achilles tendon, which is irritated by the wearing of athletic footwear, such as golf, hockey, or tennis shoes. A deep, retrocalcaneal bursa lies between the Achilles tendon and the posterior process of the calcaneus. Retrocalcaneal bursitis is diagnosed in plain radiographs by loss of the normal lucent shadow at the inferiormost aspect of the preachilles fat pad or in MR images by high signal intensity on T2-weighted spin echo sequences. The constellation of superficial tendo Achillis bursitis, retrocalcaneal bursitis, and thickening of the Achilles tendon at its site of insertion is termed Haglund's syndrome (Fig. 71–45).[477, 478] Haglund's syndrome originally was described in golfers and hockey players and is associated with the type of footwear used in these sports.[478]

In the shoulder, calcific bursitis is frequent in the subacromial-subdeltoid bursa. This can be distinguished from calcific tendinitis as the calcific bursal mass does not move with the humerus during internal and external rotation of the arm.

Nerve Injuries

The peripheral nerves can be affected by direct trauma, repetitive motion and loading, muscular hypertrophy, ganglia, or irritation by posttraumatic bone excrescences. Decreased flexibility has been implicated in nerve entrapment syndromes in athletes.[48] Acute denervation of muscle is not demonstrated reliably by MR imaging; subacute denervation has prolonged T1 and T2 values; and chronically denervated muscles show atrophy and fatty infiltration in T1-weighted images.[479] Any and all peripheral nerves are at risk. Suprascapular nerve injuries occur in the groove on the upper edge of the scapula from a direct blow to the scapula or external pressure, as with backpacking. Ganglia also have been reported in this area, both with and without symptoms (Fig. 71–46).[480–484] Injuries to the axillary nerve typically occur as a result of shoulder dislocation. The long thoracic nerve is injured in combination with an injury of the pectoralis major muscle in wrestling, weight-lifting, tennis,[485–487] and ballet, owing to warm-up or stretching exercises.[488]

Compression of the ulnar nerve in the cubital tunnel at the elbow results from direct trauma, repetitive blunt trauma, a lateral ulnar shift with chronic valgus stress, arthritis, recurring subluxation or dislocation, or muscle compression.[489] In throwing sports and in the tennis serve, the nerve can be stretched or can slide out of its groove, resulting in mechanical irritation and ulnar nerve palsy or paresis.[489] Direct pressure on the ulnar nerve at Guyon's canal produces "handlebar palsy" in cyclists.[490, 491]

Tarsal tunnel syndrome is an entrapment of the tibialis posterior nerve or any of its branches[492] and is characterized by paresthesias and burning pain along the plantar surface of the foot that intensifies with weight-bearing. Pain also

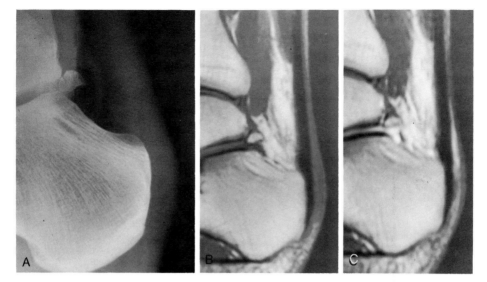

FIGURE 71–45. Haglund's disease.

A On the routine lateral view of the foot, a superficial soft tissue swelling is seen at the insertion of the Achilles tendon (superficial tendo Achillis bursitis), the Achilles tendon is poorly defined and thickened (tendinitis), and loss of the normal lucent retrocalcaneal recess between the Achilles tendon and the extreme superior aspect of the bone (retrocalcaneal bursitis) is observed.

B Sagittal T1-weighted spin echo MR image (TR/TE, 500/16) demonstrates soft tissue thickening posterior to the Achilles tendon. Fat does not extend between the calcaneus and the tendon. The Achilles tendon has normal low signal intensity.

C Sagittal T2-weighted spin echo MR image (TR/TE, 2000/70) demonstrates high signal intensity posterior to the Achilles tendon, consistent with superficial tendo Achillis bursitis.

may be noted in the medial plantar aspect of the heel or proximally along the medial part of the calf. The syndrome is a result of compression or constriction of the nerve either from a valgus or varus deformity or from scar formation within the tarsal tunnel. The tarsal tunnel extends from the level of the medial malleolus to the navicular bone along the medial wall of the calcaneus.

The sinus tarsi syndrome is characterized by chronic pain over the lateral aspect of the foot and a feeling of hindfoot instability.[493, 494] In 70 per cent of patients it is caused by supination or inversion injury and, hence, is associated with injury to the lateral ligaments of the ankle. MR imaging allows direct visualization of the ligaments of the sinus tarsi and surrounding structures.[495–497]

Miscellaneous Injuries

Snapping Hip Syndrome

In the hip, the iliopsoas bursa lies between the lesser tuberosity and the iliopsoas insertion, anterior to the hip joint, and iliopsoas bursitis occasionally is referred to or associated with the "snapping hip" syndrome. In the snapping hip syndrome an audible snapping sound occurs with hip motion. Specifically, a snap is heard when the hip is flexed while in adduction and with the knee in extension. It is produced by altered motion of the fascia lata or gluteus maximus muscle over the greater trochanter[498–504] or the iliopsoas tendon as it passes over the iliopectineal eminence of the pubis. The snapping also has been attributed to a fibrous band in the gluteus maximus muscle; the fibrosis was caused by a prior injection.[505]

Iliotibial Band Friction Syndrome

The iliotibial band friction syndrome appears as poorly defined pain in the lateral and distal aspects of the thigh or knee pain just proximal to the joint line.[506–512] This syndrome is seen in long-distance runners, cyclists, football players, or weightlifters. It is believed that the pain is caused by friction of the iliotibial tract over the lateral

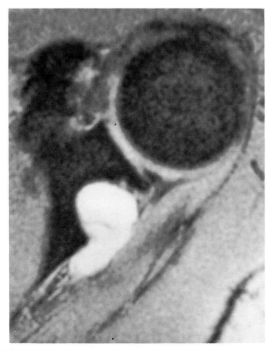

FIGURE 71–46. Suprascapular ganglion cyst. A large cystic collection in the posterior aspect of the scapular spinoglenoid fossa is identified clearly in a transaxial multiplanar gradient recalled (MPGR) MR image (TR/TE, 350/20; flip angle, 30 degrees). No associated atrophy of the infraspinatus muscle is present.

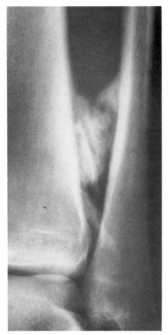

FIGURE 71–47. Old injury of the tibiofibular syndesmosis. Almost complete osseous bridging has occurred between the tibia and the fibula at the distal aspect of the interosseous membrane. (From Pavlov H, Torg JS: The Running Athlete. Chicago, Year Book, 1987.)

femoral epicondyle and a resultant inflammatory response.[506–508] In South Africa, 52 per cent of 200 consecutive knee injuries in long-distance runners were diagnosed as being this syndrome.[509] On MR imaging, increased signal intensity on T2-weighted images, representing fluid, is identified deep to the iliotibial band, adjacent to the lateral femoral epicondyle. This fluid must be distinguished from fluid in the joint.[506, 507, 510–512]

Plantar Fasciitis

The plantar fascia is a multilayered fibrous aponeurosis that runs from the plantar and medial part of the calcaneus to the ligaments attaching to the toes. As the toes are extended, the aponeurosis is stretched and the longitudinal arch is stabilized. Plantar fasciitis is a low grade inflammation of the plantar fascia and perifascial structures.[513] Symptoms are insidious pain located medial or plantar to the calcaneus that typically is associated with running and the presence of a calcaneal enthesophyte.[514] The enthesophyte seldom is the causative factor of plantar fasciitis, although it may cause symptoms if the heel pad is atrophied from aging or repeated steroid injections.[513] A bone scan or MR image is helpful in localizing abnormality within the soft tissues prior to the appearance of radiographic changes.

Injury of the Tibiofibular Syndesmosis

The tibiofibular syndesmosis is injured in combination with a deltoid ligament rupture or a fracture of the fibula or medial malleolus. Hypertrophic ossification and osseous bridging of the tibia and fibula may result (Fig. 71–47). Injury also is associated with stress fractures of the tibia and fibula and tibialis posterior tendinitis.[515–517]

Turf Toe

Plantar capsular ligament sprain of the metatarsophalangeal joint of the great toe (''turf toe'') is a sports related

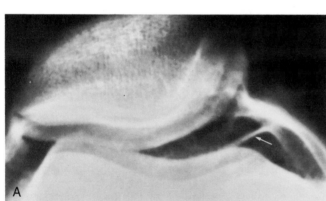

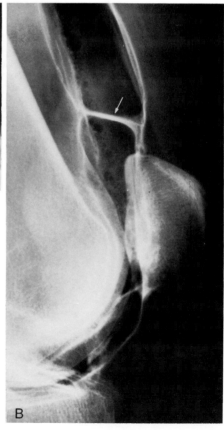

FIGURE 71–48. Plica syndrome.
  A Medial plica (arrow) of normal thickness is identified in a Merchant view after double contrast arthrography.
  B The suprapatellar (arrow) and infrapatellar plicae are documented in the lateral view of the knee after double contrast arthrography.

hyperextension injury usually associated with play on artificial turf.[336, 518, 519] Swelling and pain at this joint occur. Diastasis of a bipartite or fractured sesamoid bone is a frequent associated finding.[336]

Plica Syndrome

Plicae are intra-articular bands of fibrous tissue within the knee representing normal embryologic remnants, which, when thickened, may contribute to anterior knee pain.[274–278] The medial patellar and infrapatellar plicae are identified in the transaxial MR images. Thickening of the medial plica is said to be associated with pain along the medial aspect of the patellofemoral joint and produces symptoms of chondromalacia (referred to as "pseudochondromalacia").[272] The suprapatellar plica is best demonstrated in the sagittal MR images or with arthrography (Fig. 71–48).

SUMMARY

The beneficial effects of athletic pursuits and exercise on the musculoskeletal system result in the physical rewards of increased endurance and increased bone and muscular strength. Athletic abuse and overuse result in the breakdown of components of the musculoskeletal system. Overuse injuries result from repetitive microtrauma. The specific location and severity of an athletic injury depend on the type and level of activity, the age of the patient, and the training regimen. Athletic activities should be monitored continuously to ensure steady improvement and success without permanent physical injury and failure. Sports injuries can be prevented provided that coaches, managers, trainers, parents, and athletes understand and emphasize skill development and fitness in proper proportions. Early confirmation of injury and determination of the extent of damage are critical as injuries typically are more responsive to conservative treatment in the earlier phases, and prolonged immobilization or surgical repair can be prevented. Unrecognized injuries and "running through the pain" result in further complications and injuries to the contralateral side. Late diagnosis and treatment are responsible for chronic disabling pain, prolonged immobilization, extensive surgical downtime, and eventual osteoarthritis, all of which can destroy a professional athletic career or seriously interfere with the endeavors of an amateur sports enthusiast.

References

1. Kraus JF, Conroy C: Mortality and morbidity from runners in sports and recreation. Annu Rev Publ Health 5:163, 1984.
2. Back FJC, Wietze BME, Kemper ABA: Sports injuries in school-age children. An epidemiologic study. Am J Sports Med 17:234, 1989.
3. Noyes FR, Lindenfeld TN, Marshall MT: What determines an athletic injury (definition)? Who determines an injury (occurrence)? Am J Sports Med 16(Suppl 1):S65, 1988.
4. Kannus P, Nittymäki S, Järvinen M: Sports injuries in women: A one year prospective follow-up study in an outpatient sports clinic. Br J Sports Med 21:37, 1987.
5. McLain LG, Reynolds S: Sports injuries in a high school. Pediatrics 84:446, 1989.
6. Kannus P, Nittymäki S, Järvinen M: Athletic overuse injuries in children. Clin Pediatr 27:333, 1988.
7. Pecina M, Bojanic I, Dubravcic S: Stress factors in figure skaters. Am J Sports Med 18:277, 1990.
8. Williamson DM, Lowdon IMR: Ice-skating injuries. Injury 17:205, 1986.
9. Bernard AA, Corlett S, Thomsen E, et al: Ice skating accidents and injuries. Injury 19:191, 1988.
10. Lorentzon R, Wedren H, Pietilä T: Incidence, nature, and causes of ice hockey injuries. A three-year prospective study of a Swedish elite ice hockey team. Am J Sports Med 16:392, 1988.
11. Lorentzon R, Wedren H, Pietilä T, et al: Injuries in international ice hockey. A prospective, comparative study of injury incidence and injury types in international and Swedish elite ice hockey. Am J Sports Med 16:389, 1988.
12. Sim FH, Simonet WT, Melton LJ, et al: Ice hockey injuries. Am J Sports Med 15:S86, 1988.
13. Matter P, Ziegler WJ, Holzach P: Skiing accidents in the past 15 years. J Sports Sci 5:319, 1987.
14. Morrow PL, McQuillen EN, Eaton LA: Downhill ski fatalities: The Vermont experience. J Trauma 28:95, 1988.
15. Steinbrück K: Frequency and aetiology of injury in cross-country skiing. J Sports Sci 5:187, 1987.
16. Berson BL, Rolnick AM, Ramos CL, et al: An epidemiologic study of squash injuries. Am J Sports Med 9:103, 1981.
17. Maylack FH: Epidemiology of tennis, squash, and racquetball injuries. Clin Sports Med 7:233, 1988.
18. Gregg JR, Torg E: Upper extremity injuries in adolescent tennis players. Clin Sports Med 7:371, 1988.
19. Chard MD, Lachmann SM: Racquet sports-patterns of injury presenting to a sports injury clinic. Br J Sports Med 21:150, 1987.
20. Hoeberigs HJ, van Galen WCC, Philipsen H: Pattern of injury in handball and comparison of injured versus noninjured handball players. Int J Sports Med 7:333, 1986.
21. Nielsen AB, Yde J: An epidemiologic and traumatologic study of injuries in handball. Int J Sports Med 9:341, 1988.
22. Mueller FO, Blyth CS: A survey of 1981 college lacrosse injuries. Physician Sportsmed 10:87, 1982.
23. Ekstrand J, Nigg BM: Surface-related injuries in soccer. Sports Med 8:56, 1989.
24. Keller CS, Noyes FR, Buncher CR: The medical aspects of soccer injury epidemiology. Am J Sports Med 15:S105, 1987.
25. Thompson RR: A study of the type and cost of football injuries. Minn Med 69:656, 1986.
26. Pritchett JW: High cost of high school football injuries. Am J Sports Med 8:197, 1980.
27. Nicholas JA, Rosenthal PP, Gleim GW: A historical perspective of injuries in professional football. JAMA 260:939, 1988.
28. Halpern B, Thompson N, Curl WW, et al: High school football injuries: Identifying the risk factors. Am J Sports Med 15:S113, 1987.
29. Gibbs N: Injuries in professional rugby league. A three-year professional rugby league football club. Am J Sports Med 21:696, 1993.
30. McKenzie DC: Stress fracture of the rib in an elite oarsman. Int J Sports Med 10:220, 1989.
31. Kiburz D, Jacobs R, Reckling F, et al: Bicycle accidents and injuries among adult cyclists. Am J Sports Med 14:416, 1986.
32. Tucci JJ, Barone JE: A study of urban bicycling accidents. Am J Sports Med 16:181, 1988.
33. Addiss DG, Baker SP: Mountaineering and rock-climbing injuries in US national parks. Ann Emerg Med 18:975, 1989.
34. Marti B, Vader JP, Minder CE, et al: On the epidemiology of running injuries. The 1984 Bern Grand-Prix study. Am J Sports Med 16:285, 1988.
35. Watson MD, DiMartino PP: Incidence of injuries in high school track and field athletes and its relation to performance ability. Am J Sports Med 15:251, 1987.
36. Ellitsgaard N: Parachuting injuries: A study of 110,000 sports jumps. Br J Sports Med 21:13, 1987.
37. Rothenberger LA, Chang JI, Cable TA: Prevalence and types of injuries in aerobic dancers. Am J Sports Med 16:403, 1988.
38. Apple DV, O'Toole J, Annis C: Professional basketball injuries. Physician Sportsmed 10:81, 1982.
39. Whitlock MR, Whitlock J, Johnston B: Equestrian injuries: A comparison of professional and amateur injuries in Berkshire. Br J Sports Med 21:25, 1987.
40. Garrick JG, Requa RK: Epidemiology of women's gymnastic injuries. Am J Sports Med 8:261, 1980.
41. McAuley E, Hudash G, Shields K, et al: Injuries in women's gymnastics. The state of the art. Am J Sports Med 5:558, 1987.
42. Schneider HJ, King AY, Brownson JL, et al: Stress injuries and development changes of lower extremities in ballet dancers. Radiology 113:627, 1974.
43. Mussbaum AR, Treves ST, Micheli L: Bone stress lesions in ballet dancers. Scientific assessment. AJR 150:851, 1988.
44. Rasad S: Golfer's fracture of the ribs. Report of three cases. AJR 120:901, 1974.
45. Bladin C, Giddings P, Robinson M: Australian snowboard injury data base study. A four year prospective study. Am J Sports Med 21:701, 1993.
46. McCormick DP, Davis AL: Injuries in sailboard enthusiasts. Br J Sports Med 22:95, 1988.
47. Richardson AB, Jobe PW, Collins HR: The shoulder in competitive swimming. Am J Sports Med 8:159, 1980.
48. Herring SA, Nilson KL: Introduction to overuse injuries. Clinics Sports Med 6:225, 1992.
49. Daffner R, Pavlov H: Stress fractures: Current concepts. AJR 159:245, 1992.
50. Brody DM: Running injuries. Clin Symp 39:22, 1987.
51. Orava S: Exertion injuries due to sports and physical exercise. A clinical and statistical study of nontraumatic overuse injuries of the musculoskeletal system of athletes and keep-fit athletes. Thesis, University of Ouler, Finland, 1980.
52. Renstrom P, Johnson RJ: Overuse injuries in sports: A review. Sports Med 2:316, 1985.
53. McKeag DB: The concept of overuse: The primary care aspects of overuse syndromes in sports medicine. Primary Care 1:43, 1984.

54. Jones HH, Priest JD, Hayes WC, et al: Humeral hypertrophy in response to exercise. J Bone Joint Surg Am 59:204, 1977.

55. Kuusela T, Kurri J, Virtama P: Stress response of the tibial cortex: A longitudinal radiographic study. Ann Clin Res 16(Suppl 40):14, 1984.

56. Devas MB: Stress Fractures. London, Churchill Livingstone, 1975.

57. Daffner RH: Stress fractures: Current concepts. Skel Radiol 2:221, 1978.

58. Matheson GO, Clement DB, McKenzie DC, et al: Stress fractures in athletes: A study of 320 cases. Am J Sports Med 15:46, 1987.

59. Daffner RH, Martinez S, Gehweiler JA Jr, et al: Stress fractures of the proximal tibia in runners. Radiology 142:63, 1982.

60. Wilson ES, Katz FN: Stress fractures: An analysis of 250 consecutive cases. Radiology 92:481, 1969.

61. Devas MB: Stress fractures of the tibia in athletes or "shin soreness." J Bone Joint Surg [Br] 40:227, 1958.

62. Rogers LF: Skeletal Biomechanics. In LF Rogers (Ed): Radiology of Skeletal Trauma. 2nd Ed. Vol 1. New York, Churchill Livingstone, 1992, p 20.

63. Aspergren D, Cox JM, Benak DR: Detection of stress fractures in athletes and nonathletes. J Manipulative Physiol Ther 12:298, 1989.

64. Daffner RH, Martinez S, Gehweiler JA: Stress fractures in runners. JAMA 247:1039, 1982.

65. Sammarco GG, Miller EH: Forefoot conditions in dancers. Part II. Foot Ankle 3:93, 1982.

66. Coker JP, Arnold JA, Weber DL: Traumatic lesions of the metatarsophalangeal joints of the great toe in athletes. Am J Sports Med 6:326, 1978.

67. Potter HG, Pavlov H, Abrahams TG: The hallux sesamoid revisited. Skel Radiol 21:437, 1992.

68. Taylor JAM, Sartoris DJ, Huang GS, et al: Painful conditions affecting the first metatarsal sesamoid bones. RadioGraphics 13:817, 1993.

69. Guebert GM, Thompson JR: Sesamoid stress fractures of the foot. Chiro Sports Med 1:24, 1987.

70. Parra G: Stress fractures of the sesamoids of the foot. Clin Orthop 18:281, 1960.

71. Micheli LJ, Sohn RS, Solomon R: Stress fractures of the second metatarsal involving Lisfranc's joint in ballet dancers. J Bone Joint Surg [Am] 67:1372, 1985.

72. Protzman RR, Griffis CG: Stress fractures in men and women undergoing military training. J Bone Joint Surg [Am] 59:825, 1977.

73. Harrington T, Crichton KJ, Anderson IF: Overuse ballet injury of the base of the 2nd metatarsal. A diagnostic problem. Am J Sports Med 21:591, 1993.

74. Greaney RB, Gerber FH, Laughlan RL: Distribution and natural history of stress fractures in US Marine recruits. Radiology 146:339, 1983.

75. Grusd R: Pseudofractures and stress fractures. Semin Roentgenol 13:81, 1978.

76. Lehman RC, Torg JS, Pavlov H, et al: Fractures of the base of the 5th metatarsal distal to the tuberosity: A review. Foot Ankle 7:245, 1987.

77. Torg JS, Balduini FC, Zelko RR, et al: Fractures of the base of the 5th metatarsal distal to the tuberosity. J Bone Joint Surg [Am] 66:209, 1984.

78. Jones R: Fracture of the base of the 5th metatarsal bone by indirect violence. Am Surg 35:697, 1902.

79. Zelko RR, Torg JS, Rachun A: Proximal diaphyseal fractures of the 5th metatarsal—treatment of the fractures and their complications in athletes. Am J Sports Med 7:95, 1979.

80. Pavlov H, Torg JS, Freiberger RH: Tarsal navicular stress fractures. Radiology 148:641, 1983.

81. Torg JS, Pavlov H, Cooley LH, et al: Stress fractures of the tarsal navicular. J Bone Joint Surg [Am] 64:700, 1982.

82. Goergen TG, Venn-Watson EA, Rossman DJ, et al: Tarsal navicular stress fractures in runners. AJR 136:201, 1981.

83. Towne LC, Blazina ME, Cozen LN: Fatigue fracture of the tarsal navicular. J Bone Joint Surg [Am] 51:376, 1970.

84. Hopson CN, Perry DR: Stress fractures of the calcaneus in women Marine recruits. Clin Orthop 128:159, 1977.

85. Kroening PM, Shelton ML: Stress fractures. AJR 89:1281, 1963.

86. Symeonides PP: High stress fractures of the fibula. J Bone Joint Surg [Br] 62B:192, 1980.

87. Burrows HJ: Fatigue fractures of the fibula. J Bone Joint Surg [Br] 30:266, 1948.

88. Devas MB, Sweetnan R: Stress fractures of the fibula. J Bone Joint Surg [Br] 38:818, 1956.

89. Hallel T, Amit S, Segal D: Fatigue fractures of tibial and femoral shaft in soldiers. Clin Orthop 118:35, 1976.

90. Orava S, Puranen J, Ala-Ketola L: Stress fractures caused by physical exercise. Acta Orthop Scand 49:19, 1978.

91. Allen JG: Longitudinal stress fractures of the tibia: Diagnosis with CT. Radiology 167:799, 1988.

92. Bowerman JW: Radiology and Injury in Sport. New York, Appleton-Century-Crofts, 1977.

93. Devas MB: Longitudinal stress fractures: Another variety seen in long bones. J Bone Joint Surg [Br] 42:508, 1960.

94. Daffner RH: Anterior tibial striations. AJR 143:651, 1984.

95. Satku K, Kumar VP, Chacha PB: Stress fracture around the knee in elderly patients: A cause of acute pain in the knee. J Bone Joint Surg [Am] 72:918, 1990.

96. Manco LG, Schneider R, Pavlov H: Insufficiency fractures of the tibial plateau. AJR 140:1211, 1983.

97. Devas MB: Stress fractures of the patella. J Bone Joint Surg [Br] 42:71, 1960.

98. Hensal F, Nelson T, Pavlov H, et al: Bilateral patellar fractures from indirect trauma. A case report. Clin Orthop 178:207, 1983.

99. Higgens TT: Fractures of both patella by muscular action. Br Med J 1:1006, 1925.

100. Wolfgang GL: Stress fracture of the femoral neck in a patient with open capital femoral epiphyses. J Bone Joint Surg [Am] 59:680, 1987.

101. Erne P, Burchardt A: Femoral neck fatigue fracture. Arch Orthop Trauma Surg 97:312, 1980.

102. Blickenstaff LD, Morris JM: Fatigue fracture of the femoral neck. J Bone Joint Surg [Am] 48:1031, 1966.

103. Devas MB: Stress fractures of the femoral neck. J Bone Joint Surg [Br] 47:728, 1965.

104. Skinner HB, Cook SD: Fatigue failure stress of the femoral neck. A case report. Am J Sports Med 10:245, 1982.

105. Lombardo SJ, Benson DW: Stress fractures of the femur in runners. Am J Sports Med 10:219, 1982.

106. Provost RA, Morris JM: Fatigue fracture of the femoral shaft. J Bone Joint Surg [Am] 51:487, 1969.

107. Luchini MA, Sarokhan AJ, Micheli LJ: Acute displaced femoral-shaft fractures in long distance runners. J Bone Joint Surg [Am] 65:689, 1983.

108. Butler JE, Brown SL, McConnel BG: Subtrochanteric stress fractures in runners. Am J Sports Med 10:228, 1982.

109. Hershman EB, Lombardo J, Bergfeld JA: Femoral shaft stress fractures in athletes. Clin Sports Med 1:111, 1990.

110. Pavlov H, Nelson TL, Warren RF, et al: Stress fractures of the pubic ramus. A review of 12 cases. J Bone Joint Surg [Am] 64:1020, 1982.

111. Tehranzadeh J, Kurth LA, Elyaderani MK, et al: Combined pelvic stress fracture and avulsion of the adductor longus in a middle distance runner. Am J Sports Med 10:108, 1982.

112. Kim SM, Park CH, Gartland JJ: Stress fracture of the pubic ramus in a swimmer. Clin Nucl Med 12:118, 1987.

113. Czarnecki DJ, Till EW, Minikel JL: Unique sacral stress fracture in a runner (letter). AJR 151:1255, 1988.

114. Hoang T-A, Nguyen TH, Daffnere RH, et al: Case report 491: Stress fracture of the right sacrum. Skel Radiol 17:364, 1988.

115. Schneider R, Yacovone J, Ghelman B: Unsuspected sacral fractures: Detection by radionuclide bone scanning. AJR 144:337, 1985.

116. Abel MS: Jogger's fracture and other stress fractures of the lumbo-sacral spine. Skel Radiol 13:221, 1985.

117. Laferty JF, Winter WG, Ganilaro SA: Fatigue characteristics of posterior elements of vertebra. J Bone Joint Surg [Am] 59:154, 1977.

118. Gurtler R, Pavlov H, Torg JS: Stress fracture of the ipsilateral first rib in a pitcher. Am J Sports Med 13:277, 1985.

119. Lankenner PA Jr, Micheli LJ: Stress fracture of the first rib. J Bone Joint Surg [Am] 67:159, 1985.

120. Holden DL, Jackson DW: Stress fractures of the ribs in female rowers. Am J Sports Med 12:342, 1985.

121. Kaye JJ, Nance EP, Green NE: Fatigue fracture of the medial aspect of the clavicle. Radiology 144:89, 1982.

122. Sandrock AR: Another sports fatigue fracture. Stress fracture of the coracoid process of the scapula. Radiology 117:274, 1975.

123. Whitaker JH: Arm wrestling fracture—a humerus twist. Am Sports Med 5:67, 1977.

124. Santavirta S, Kiviluoto O: Transverse fracture of the humerus in a shotputter. A case report. Am J Sports Med 5:122, 1977.

125. Rettig AC, Betty HF: Stress fracture in the humerus in an adolescent tennis tournament player. Am J Sports Med 13:55, 1985.

126. Farquharson-Roberts MA, Fulford PC: Stress fractures of the radius. J Bone Joint Surg [Br] 62:194, 1980.

127. Perry CR, Perry HM, Burdge RE: Stress fracture of the radius following a fracture of the ulna diaphysis. Clin Orthop 187:193, 1984.

128. Kendall HK: Stress fractures of the diaphysis of the ulna in a body builder. Am J Sports Med 12:405, 1984.

129. Kitchin ID: Fatigue fracture of the ulna. J Bone Joint Surg [Br] 30:622, 1948.

130. Tanabe S, Nakahira J, Bando E, et al: Fatigue fracture of the ulna occurring in pitchers of fast-pitch softball. Am J Sports Med 19:317, 1991.

131. Stark HH, Jobe FW, Boyes JH, et al: Fracture of the hook of the hamate in athletes. J Bone Joint Surg [Am] 59:575, 1977.

132. Hanks GA, Kalenak A, Bowman LS, et al: Stress fractures of the carpal scaphoid. J Bone Joint Surg [Am] 71:938, 1989.

133. Roub LW, Gumerman LW, Hanley EN, et al: Bone stress: A radionuclide imaging prospective. Radiology 132:431, 1979.

134. Geslien GE, Thrall JH, Espinosa JL, et al: Early detection of stress fractures using ^{99m}Tc-polyphosphate. Radiology 121:683, 1976.

135. Prather JI, Nusynowitz ML, Snowdy HA, et al: Scintigraphic findings in stress fractures. J Bone Joint Surg [Am] 59:869, 1977.

136. Norfray JF, Schlachter L, Kernahan WT Jr, et al: Early confirmation of stress fractures in joggers. JAMA 243:1647, 1980.

137. Wilcox JR, Moniot AL, Green JP: Bone scanning in the evaluation of exercise-related stress injuries. Radiology 123:699, 1977.

138. Papanicolaou N, Wilkinson RH, Emans JB, et al: Bone scintigraphy and radiography in young athletes with low back pain. AJR 145:1039, 1985.

139. Martire JR, Levinsohn EM: Imaging of Athletic Injuries: A Multimodality Approach. New York, McGraw-Hill, 1992.

140. Rupani HD, Holder LE, Espinola DA, et al: Three-phase radionuclide bone imaging in sports medicine. Radiology 156:187, 1985.

141. Rockett J, Bridges J: Anterior tibial stress fracture: Case report. J Nucl Med Tech *18*:186, 1990.
142. Rockett JF, Freeman BL III: Stress fracture of the patella: Confirmation by triple-phase bone imaging. Clin Nucl Med *15*:873, 1990.
143. Stafford SA, Rosenthal DI, Gebhardt MC, et al: MRI in stress fracture. AJR *147*:553, 1986.
144. Lee JK, Yao L: Stress fractures: MR imaging. Radiology *169*:217, 1988.
145. Deutsch AL, Mink JH, Waxman AD: MR imaging of occult fractures of the proximal femur. Radiology *170*:113, 1989.
146. Deutsch AL, Mink JH: Magnetic resonance imaging of musculoskeletal injuries. Radiol Clin North Am *27*:983, 1989.
147. Mink JH, Deutsch AL: Occult osseous and cartilaginous injuries about the knee: MR assessment, detection, and classification. Radiology *170*:823, 1989.
148. Brahme SK, Cervilla V, Vint V, et al: Magnetic resonance appearance of sacral insufficiency fractures. Skel Radiol *19*:489, 1990.
149. Laroche M, Rousseau H, Jacquemier J-M, et al: Unusual stress fracture on the roof of the acetabulum: Magnetic resonance imaging. J Rheumatol *18*:115, 1991.
150. Meyers SP, Wiener SN: Magnetic resonance imaging features of fractures using the short tau inversion recovery (STIR) sequence: Correlation with radiographic findings. Skel Radiol *20*:499, 1991.
151. Lynch TC, Crues JV III, Morgan FW, et al: Bone abnormalities in the knee: Prevalence and significance of MR imaging. Radiology *171*:761, 1989.
152. Savoca CL: Stress fractures: A classification of the earliest radiographic signs. Radiology *100*:519, 1971.
153. Chamay A, Tschantz P: Mechanical influence in bone remodeling: Experimental research on Wolff's law. J Biomech *5*:173, 1972.
154. Wright TM, Hayes WC: The fracture mechanics of fatigue crack propagation in compact bone. J Biomed Res *7*:637, 1976.
155. Carter DR, Caler WE: Cycle-dependent and time-dependent bone fracture with repeated loading. J Biomech Eng *105*:166, 1983.
156. Chamay A: Mechanical and morphological aspects of experimental overload and fatigue in bone. J Biomech *3*:263, 1970.
157. Resnick D, Niwayama G (eds): Physical Injury. Diagnosis of Bone and Joint Disorders. 2nd Ed. Vol 5. Philadelphia, W B Saunders, 1988, p 2776.
158. Sweet DE, Allman RM: RPC of the month from the AFIP. Radiology *99*:687, 1971.
159. Johnson LC: Morphologic analysis in pathology: The kinetics of disease and general biology of bone. *In* H Frost (Ed): Bone Biodynamics. Boston, Little, Brown and Company, 1964, p 607.
160. Murcia M, Brennan RE, Edeiken J: Computed tomography of stress fracture. Skel Radiol *8*:193, 1982.
161. Somer K, Meurman KOA: Computed tomography of stress fractures. J Comput Assist Tomogr *6*:109, 1982.
162. Pavlov H: Athletic injuries. Radiologic Clin North Am *28*:435, 1990.
163. Pavlov H, Torg JS, Hersh A, et al: The roentgen examination of runners' injuries. RadioGraphics *1*:17, 1981.
164. Ting A, King W, Yocum L, et al: Stress fractures of the tarsal navicular in long-distance runners. Clin Sports Med *7*:89, 1988.
165. Khan K, Fuller PJ, Brukner PD, et al: Outcome of conservative and surgical management of navicular stress fracture in athletes. Eighty-six cases proven with computerized tomography. Am J Sports Med *20*:657, 1992.
166. Kiss ZS, Khan KM, Fuller PJ: Stress fractures of the tarsal navicular bone. CT findings in 55 cases. AJR *160*:111, 1993.
167. Orava S, Hulkko A: Delayed unions and nonunions of stress fractures in athletes. Am J Sports Med *16*:378, 1988.
168. Keene JS, Lange RH: Diagnostic dilemmas in foot and ankle injuries. JAMA *256*:247, 1986.
169. Richli WR, Rosenthal DI: Avulsion fracture of the 5th metatarsal: Experimental study of pathomechanics. AJR *143*:889, 1984.
170. Rogers LF: Special considerations in children. *In* LF Rogers (Ed): Radiology of Skeletal Trauma. 2nd Ed. Vol 1. New York, Churchill Livingstone, 1992, p 110.
171. Compere EL: Growth arrest in long bones as result of fractures that include the epiphysis. JAMA *105*:2140, 1953.
172. Larson RL, McMahan RO: The epiphyses and the childhood athlete. JAMA *196*:607, 1966.
173. Ogden JA: Injury to the growth mechanisms of the immature skeleton. Skel Radiol *6*:237, 1981.
174. Sakakida K: Clinical observations on the epiphyseal separation of long bones. Clin Orthop *34*:119, 1964.
175. Salter RB, Harris WR: Injuries involving the epiphyseal plate. J Bone Joint Surg [Am] *45*:587, 1968.
176. Bright RW, Elmore SM: Physical properties of epiphyseal plate cartilage. Surg Forum *19*:463, 1968.
177. Rogers LF: Special considerations in children. *In* LF Rogers (Ed): Radiology of Skeletal Trauma. 2nd Ed. Vol 1. New York, Churchill Livingstone, 1992, p 119.
178. Rogers LF: The radiography of epiphyseal injuries. Radiology *96*:289, 1970.
179. O'Donoghue DH: Treatment of Injuries to Athletes. Philadelphia, WB Saunders Co, 1962.
180. Ozonoff MB: Pediatric Orthopedic Radiology. Philadelphia, WB Saunders Co, 1979.
181. Smith L: A concealed injury to the knee. J Bone Joint Surg [Am] *44*:1659, 1962.
182. Rogers LF: Special considerations in children. *In* LF Rogers (Ed): Radiology of Skeletal Trauma. 2nd Ed. Vol 1. New York, Churchill Livingstone, 1992, p 117.
183. Gore RM, Rogers LF, Bowerman J, et al: Osseous manifestations of elbow stress associated with sports activities. AJR *134*:971, 1980.
184. Torg JS: Little League: The theft of a care free youth. Phys Sports Med *1*:72, 1973.
185. Priest SD, Nagel PA: Tennis shoulder. Am J Sports Med *4*:28, 1976.
186. Tullos HS, Erwin WD, Woods GW, et al: Unusual lesions of the pitching arm. Clin Orthop *88*:169, 1972.
187. Tarsney FJ: Catastrophic jumpers knee. Am J Sports Med *9*:60, 1981.
188. Tibone JE, Lombardo SJ: Bilateral fractures of the inferior poles of the patellae in a basketball player. Am J Sports Med *9*:215, 1981.
189. Blazina ME, Kerlan RK, Jobe FW, et al: Jumper's knee. Orthop Clin North Am *4*:665, 1973.
190. Grossman RB, Nicholas JA: Common disorders of the knee. Orthop Clin North Am *8*:619, 1977.
191. Martens M, Wouters P, Burssens A, et al: Patellar tendonitis: Pathology and results of treatment. Acta Orthop Scand *53*:445, 1982.
192. Roels J, Martens M, Mulier JC, et al: Patellar tendinitis (jumper's knee). Am J Sports Med *6*:362, 1978.
193. Ogden JA, Southwick WO: Osgood-Schlatter's disease and tibial tuberosity development. Clin Orthop *116*:180, 1976.
194. Osgood RB: Lesions of the tibial tubercle occurring during adolescence. Boston Med Surg J *148*:114, 1903.
195. Scotti DM, Sadhu UK, Heimberg F, et al: Osgood-Schlatter's disease, an emphasis on soft tissue changes in roentgen diagnosis. Skel Radiol *4*:21, 1979.
196. Nimityoungskul P, Montague WL, Anderson EP: Avulsion fracture of the tibial tuberosity in late adolescence. J Trauma *28*:505, 1988.
197. Jaramillo D, Wilkinson RH: Avulsing injuries of the tibial tubercle. Contemp Diagn Radiol *13*:1, 1990.
198. Rosenberg ZS, Kawelblum M, Cheung YY, et al: Osgood-Schlatter's lesion: Fracture or tendinitis? Scintigraphic, CT, and MR imaging features. Radiology *185*:853, 1992.
199. Pavlov H, Torg JS: The Running Athlete: Roentgenograms and Remedies. Chicago, Year Book Medical Publishers, 1987, p 223.
200. Torg JS, Pavlov H, Morris YB: Salter-Harris type III fracture of the medial femoral condyle occurring in the adolescent athlete. J Bone Joint Surg [Am] *63*:586, 1981.
201. Rogers LF, Jones S, Davis AR, et al: "Clipping injury." Fracture of the epiphysis in the adolescent football player: An occult lesion of the knee. AJR *121*:69, 1979.
202. Adams JE: Little League shoulder: Osteochondrosis of proximal humeral epiphyses in boy baseball pitchers. California Med *105*:22, 1966.
203. Barnett LS: Little League shoulder syndrome: Proximal humeral epiphyseolysis in adolescent baseball pitchers: a case report. J Bone Joint Surg [Am] *67*:495, 1985.
204. Dotter WE: Little Leaguer's shoulder: A fracture of proximal epiphyseal cartilage of the humerus due to baseball pitching. Guthrie Clin Bull *23*:68, 1953.
205. Torg JS, Pollack H, Sweterlitsch P: The effect of competitive pitching in the shoulders and elbows of preadolescent baseball players. Pediatrics *49*:267, 1972.
206. Torg JS: The Little League pitcher. Am Fam Physician *6*:71, 1972.
207. Hansen NM: Epiphyseal changes in the proximal humerus of an adolescent baseball pitcher: A case report. Am J Sports Med *10*:180, 1982.
208. Tullos HS, King JW: Lesions of the pitching arm in adolescents. JAMA *220*:264, 1972.
209. Tullos HS, King JW: Throwing mechanism in sports. Orthop Clin North Am *4*:709, 1973.
210. Carter SR, Aldridge MJ: Stress injury of the distal radial growth plate. J Bone Joint Surg [Br] *70*:834, 1988.
211. Fliegel CP: Stress related widening of the growth plate in adolescents. Ann Radiol *29*:37, 1985.
212. Rogers LF, Braunstein E, DeSmet AA, et al: All-Star sports medicine film panel. RadioGraphics *8*:235, 1988.
213. Roy S, Caine D, Singer KM: Stress changes of the distal radial epiphysis in young gymnasts. Am J Sports Med *13*:301, 1985.
214. Ruggles DL, Peterson HA, Scott SG: Radial growth plate injury in a female gymnast. Med Sci Sports Exercise *23*:393, 1991.
215. Godshall KW, Hansen CA, Rising DC: Stress fractures through the distal femoral epiphysis in athletes. Am J Sports Med *9*:114, 1981.
216. Cahill BR: Stress fracture of the proximal tibial epiphysis: A case report. Am J Sports Med *5*:186, 1977.
217. Pavlov H, Torg JS: The Running Athlete: Roentgenograms and Remedies. Chicago, Year Book Medical Publishers, 1986, p 294.
218. Fernbach SK, Wilkinson RH: Avulsion injuries of the pelvis and proximal femur. AJR *137*:581, 1981.
219. Metzmaker JN, Pappas AM: Avulsion fractures of the pelvis. Am J Sports Med *13*:349, 1985.
220. Muckle DS: Associated factors in recurrent groin and hamstring injuries. Br J Sports Med *16*:37, 1982.
221. Godshall RW, Hansen CA: Incomplete avulsion of a portion of the iliac epiphysis. J Bone Joint Surg [Am] *55*:1301, 1973.
222. Lombardo SJ, Retting AC, Kerlan RK: Radiographic abnormalities of the iliac apophysis in adolescent athletes. J Bone Joint Surg [Am] *65*:444, 1983.
223. Clancy WG Jr, Folz AS: Iliac apophysitis and stress fractures in adolescent runners. Am J Sports Med *4*:214, 1976.

224. Khoury MB, Kirks DR, Martinze S, et al: Bilateral avulsion fractures of the anterior superior iliac spines in sprinters. Skel Radiol *13*:65, 1985.

225. Cochraine GM: Osteitis pubis in athletes. Br J Sports Med *5*:233, 1971.

226. Wiley JJ: Traumatic osteitis pubis: The gracilis syndrome. Am J Sports Med *11*:360, 1983.

227. Schneider R, Kaye JJ, Ghelman B: Adductor avulsive injuries near the symphysis pubis. Radiology *120*:567, 1976.

228. Harris NH, Murray RG: Lesions of the symphysis pubis in athletes. J Bone Joint Surg [Br] *56*:563, 1974.

229. Rogers LF: The Pelvis. *In* LF Rogers (Ed): Radiology of Skeletal Trauma. 2nd Ed. Vol 2. New York, Churchill Livingstone, 1992, p 1087.

230. Segond P: Recherches cliniques et experimentales, sur les epanchements sanguins du genou par entorse. Prog Med *7*:297, 319, 340, 379, 400, 419, 879, 1836.

231. Woods GW, Stanley RF, Tullos HS: Lateral capsular sign: X-ray clue to a significant knee instability. Am J Sports Med *7*:27, 1979.

232. Goldman AB, Pavlov H, Rubenstein D: The Segond fracture of the proximal tibia: A small avulsion that reflects major ligamentous damage. AJR *151*:1163, 1988.

233. Weber WN, Neumann CH, Barakos JA, et al: Lateral rim (Segond) fractures: MR imaging characteristics. Radiology *180*:731, 1991.

234. Norfray LF, Rogers LF, Adams GP, et al: Common calcaneal avulsion fracture. AJR *134*:119, 1980.

235. Pavlov H: Imaging of the foot and ankle. Radiol Clin North Am *28*:991, 1990.

236. Goergen TG, Resnick D, Riley RR: Post-traumatic abnormalities of the pubic bone simulating malignancy. Radiology *126*:85, 1978.

237. Torg JS, Mayer RA: Non-union of a stress fracture through olecranon epiphyseal plate observed in an adolescent baseball pitcher. A case report. J Bone Joint Surg [Am] *59*:264, 1977.

238. Pavlov H, Torg JS, Jacobs B, et al: Non-union of the olecranon epiphysis. Report of two cases in adolescent baseball pitchers. AJR *136*:819, 1981.

239. Wilkerson RD, Johns JC: Non-union of an olecranon stress fracture in an adolescent gymnast. Am J Sports Med *18*:432, 1990.

240. Rodman GP, Schumacher HR (Eds): Primer on the Rheumatic Diseases. Atlanta, Arthritis Foundation, 1983.

241. Milgram JW: Radiological and pathological manifestations of osteochondritis dissecans of the distal femur. Radiology *126*:305, 1978.

242. Milgram JW: Injury to articular cartilage joint surfaces: Displaced fractures of underlying bone. Clin Orthop *206*:236, 1986.

243. Milgram JW, Rodgers LS, Miller JW: Osteochondral fractures: Mechanism of injury and fate of fragments. AJR *130*:651, 1978.

244. O'Donoghue D: Chondral and osteochondral fractures. J Trauma *6*:469, 1966.

245. Conventry MB: Osteochondral fractures of the femoral condyles. Surg Gynecol Obstet *100*:591, 1955.

246. Kennedy JC, Grainger RW, McGraw RW: Osteochondral fractures of the femoral condyles. J Bone Joint Surg [Br] *48*:436, 1966.

247. Pavlov H, Schneider R: Extrameniscal abnormalities as diagnosed by knee arthrography. Radiol Clin North Am *19*:287, 1981.

248. Schneider R: Extra-meniscal lesions. *In* RH Freiberger, JJ Kaye (Eds): Arthrography. New York, Appleton-Century-Crofts, 1979.

249. Minkoff J, Fein L: The role of radiography in the evaluation and treatment of common anarthrotic disorders of the patellofemoral joint. Clin Sports Med *8*:203, 1989.

250. Gilley JS, Gelman MI, Edson DM, et al: Chondral fractures of the knee, arthrographic, arthroscopic, and clinical manifestations. Radiology *138*:51, 1981.

251. Konig H, Sauter R, Deimling M, et al: Cartilage disorders: Comparison of spin echo, CHESS and FLASH sequence MR images. Radiology *164*:753, 1987.

252. McCauley TR, Kier R, Lynch KJ, et al: Chondromalacia patellae: Diagnosis with MR imaging. AJR *158*:101, 1992.

253. Yulish BS, Montanez J, Goodfellow DB, et al: Chondromalacia patellae: Assessment with MR imaging. Radiology *164*:763, 1987.

254. Recht MP, Kramer J, Marcelis S, et al: Abnormalities of articular cartilage in the knee: Analysis of available MR techniques. Radiology *87*:473, 1993.

255. Nakanishi K, Inoue M, Harada K: Subluxation of the patella: Evaluation of patellar articular cartilage with MR imaging. Br J Radiol *65*:662, 1992.

256. Kannus P, Ahu H, Järvinen M, et al: Computerized recording of visits to an outpatient sports clinic. Am J Sports Med *151*:79, 1987.

257. Cox JS: Patellofemoral problems in runners. Clinics Sports Med *4*:699, 1985.

258. Outerbridge RD: The etiology of chondromalacia patellae. J Bone Joint Surg [Br] *43*:752, 1961.

259. Ficat RP, Philippe J, Hungerford DS: Chondromalacia patellae: A system of classification. Clin Orthop *144*:55, 1979.

260. Goodfellow J, Hunderford DS, Woods C: Patellofemoral joint mechanics and pathology. 2. Chondromalacia patellae. J Bone Joint Surg [Br] *58*:291, 1976.

261. Insall J, Falvo KA, Wise DW: Chondromalacia patella. J Bone Joint Surg [Am] *58*:1, 1976.

262. Dehaven KE, Dolan WA, Mayer PJ: Chondromalacia patellae in athletes. Am J Sports Med *7*:5, 1979.

263. Wiles P, Andrews PS, Devas MB: Chondromalacia of the patella. J Bone Joint Surg [Br] *38*:95, 1956.

264. Insall J: Chondromalacia patella: Patellar malalignment syndrome. Orthop Clin North Am *10*:117, 1979.

265. Merchant AC, Mercer RL, Jacobsen RM, et al: Roentgenographic analysis of patellofemoral congruence. J Bone Joint Surg [Am] *56*:1391, 1974.

266. Bradley WG, Ominsky SH: Mountain view of the patella. AJR *136*:53, 1981.

267. Insall J, Salvati E: Patella position in the normal knee joint. Radiology *101*:101, 1971.

268. Blackburne JS, Peel TE: A new method of measuring patellar height. J Bone Joint Surg [Br] *59*:241, 1977.

269. Brattström H: Shape of the intercondylar groove normally and in recurrent dislocation of patella. Acta Orthop Scand 68(Suppl)*5*:148, 1964.

270. Kannus PA: Long patellar tendon: Radiographic sign of patellofemoral pain syndrome—a prospective study. Radiology *185*:859, 1992.

271. Kirsch MD, Fitzgerald SW, Friedman H: Transient lateral patella dislocation: Diagnosis with MR imaging. AJR *161*:109, 1993.

272. Rydholm A: Pseudochondromalacia of the patellae. Acta Orthop Scand *49*:205, 1978.

273. Brossmann J, Muhle C, Schroder C, et al: Patellar tracking patterns during active and passive knee extension: Evaluation with motion-triggered ciné MR imaging. Radiology *187*:205, 1993.

274. Dandy DJ: Anatomy of the medial suprapatellar plica and medial synovial shelf. Arthroscopy *6*:79, 1990.

275. Patel D: Arthroscopy of the plicae—synovial folds and their significance. Am J Sports Med *6*:217, 1978.

276. Hardaker WT, Whipple TL, Bassett EH: Diagnosis and treatment of the plica syndrome of the knee. J Bone Joint Surg [Am] *62*:221, 1980.

277. Patel D: Plica as a cause of anterior knee pain. Orthop Clin North Am *17*:273, 1986.

278. Boven F, DeBoeck M, Potviege R: Synovial plicae of the knee on computed tomography. Radiology *147*:805, 1983.

279. Percy EC, Strother RT: Patellalgia. Phys Sports Med *13*:43, 1985.

280. Cayea P, Pavlov H, Sherman MJ, et al: A lucent articular lesion in the lateral femoral condyle: A source of patellar femoral pain in the athletic adolescent. AJR *137*:1145, 1981.

281. Aichroth P: Osteochondral fractures and their relations to osteochondritis dissecans of the knee. J Bone Joint Surg [Br] *53*:448, 1971.

282. Linden B: Osteochondritis dissecans of the femoral condyles. J Bone Joint Surg [Am] *59*:769, 1977.

283. Makin M: Osteochondral fracture of the lateral femoral condyle. J Bone Joint Surg [Am] *33*:262, 1951.

284. Green JP: Osteochondritis dissecans of the knee. J Bone Joint Surg [Br] *48*:82, 1966.

285. Aichroth P: Osteochondritis dissecans of the knee. J Bone Joint Surg [Br] *53*:440, 1971.

286. Mollan RAB: Osteochondritis dissecans of the knee. Acta Orthop Scand *48*:517, 1977.

287. Pappas AM: Osteochondritis dissecans. Clin Orthop *158*:59, 1981.

288. Pick M: Familial osteochondritis dissecans. J Bone Joint Surg [Br] *37*:142, 1955.

289. Stougaard J: Familial occurrence of osteochondritis dissecans. J Bone Joint Surg [Br] *46*:542, 1964.

290. Stougaard J: The hereditary factor in osteochondritis dissecans. J Bone Joint Surg [Br] *43*:256, 1961.

291. Kramer J, Stiglbauer R, Engel A: MR contrast arthrography (MRA) in osteochondrosis dissecans. J Comput Assist Tomogr *16*:254, 1992.

292. Deutsch A: Osteochondral injuries of the talar dome. *In* AL Deutsch, JM Menk, R Kerr (Eds): MRI of the Foot and Ankle. New York, Raven Press, 1992, p 115.

293. Gylys-Morin VM, Hajek PC, Sartoris DJ, et al: Articular cartilage defects: Detectability in cadaver knees with MR. AJR *148*:1153, 1987.

294. Matthewson MH, Dandy DJ: Osteochondral fractures of the lateral femoral condyle. J Bone Joint Surg [Br] *60*:199, 1978.

295. Rosenberg NJ: Osteochondral fracture of the lateral femoral condyle. J Bone Joint Surg [Am] *46*:1013, 1964.

296. Lipscomb PR Jr, Lipscomb PR Sr, Bryan RS: Osteochondritis dissecans of the knee with loose fragments. J Bone Joint Surg [Am] *60*:235, 1978.

297. Newberg AH: Osteochondral fractures of the dome of the talus. Br J Radiol *52*:105, 1979.

298. Thompson JP, Looner R: Osteochondral lesions of the talus in a sports medicine clinic. A new radiographic technique and surgical approach. Am J Sports Med *12*:460, 1984.

299. Loomer R, Fisher E, Lloyd-Smith R, et al: Osteochondral lesions of the talus. Am J Sports Med *21*:13, 1993.

300. Sampson S, Akelman E, Garroway RJ, et al: Traumatic injury to the upper extremity. *In* D Deer: Principles of Orthopaedic Practice. New York, McGraw-Hill, 1989, p 536.

301. Linden B: The incidence of osteochondritis dissecans in the condyles of the femur. Acta Orthop Scand *47*:664, 1976.

302. Mink JH, Deutsch AL: Occult cartilage and bone injuries of the knee: Detection, classification, and assessment with MR imaging. Radiology *170*:823, 1989.

303. Lee JK, Yao L: Occult intraosseous fracture: Magnetic resonance appearance versus age of injury. Am J Sports Med *17*:620, 1989.

304. Yao L, Lee JK: Occult intraosseous fracture: Detection with MR imaging. Radiology *167*:749, 1988.

305. Losee RE, Johnson TR, Southwick WO: Anterior subluxation of the lateral tibial plateau. J Bone Joint Surg [Am] *60*:1015, 1978.

306. Stallenberg B, Genenois PA, Sintzoff SA, et al: Fracture of the posterior aspect of the lateral tibial plateau: Radiographic sign of anterior cruciate ligament tear. Radiology *187*:821, 1993.

307. Vellet AD, Marks PH, Fowlere PJ, et al: Occult post traumatic osteochondral

lesions of the knee: Prevalence, classification, and a short term sequelae evaluated with MR imaging. Radiology *178*:271, 1991.

308. Weber WN, Neumann CH, Barakas JA, et al: Lateral tibial rim (Segond) fractures: MR imaging characteristics. Radiology *180*:731, 1991.

309. Rosen MA, Jackson DW, Berger PE: Occult osseous lesions documented by magnetic resonance imaging associated with anterior cruciate ligament ruptures. Arthroscopy *7*:45, 1991.

310. Murphy BJ, Smith RL, Uribe JW, et al: Bone signal abnormalities in the posterolateral tibia and lateral femoral condyle in complete tears of the anterior cruciate ligament: A specific sign? Radiology *182*:221, 1992.

311. Kaplan PA, Walker CW, Kilcoyne RF, et al: Occult fracture patterns of the knee associated with anterior cruciate ligament tears: Assessment with MR imaging. Radiology *183*:835, 1992.

312. Conforty B, Tal E, Margulies Y: Anterior dislocation of the head of the fibula. J Trauma *20*:902, 1980.

313. Steinke CR: Simultaneous fractures of both patella. Am Surg *58*:510, 1913.

314. Freiberger RH, Kotzen LM: Fracture of the medial margin of the patella: A finding diagnostic of lateral dislocation. Radiology *88*:902, 1967.

315. Peltokallio P, Peltokallio V, Vaalasti T: Fractures of the humerus from muscular violence in sport. J Sports Med *8*:21, 1968.

316. Gregersen HN: Fractures of the humerus from muscular violence. Acta Orthop Scand *42*:506, 1971.

317. Pavlov H, Warren RF, Weiss CB Jr: The roentgen evaluation of anterior shoulder instability. Clin Orthop *184*:153, 1985.

318. Protzman RR: Anterior instability of the shoulder. J Bone Joint Surg [Am] *62*:909, 1980.

319. Lombardo SJ, Jobe FW, Keilan RK, et al: Posterior shoulder lesions in throwing athletes. Am J Sports Med *5*:106, 1977.

320. Pappas AM, Goss TP, Kleinman PK: Symptomatic shoulder instability due to lesions of the glenoid labrum. Am J Sports Med *11*:279, 1983.

321. Rome CR, Zarins B: Recurrent transient subluxation of the shoulder. J Bone Joint Surg [Am] *63*:863, 1981.

322. Nevaisir TJ: Weight lifting risks and injuries to the shoulder. Clin Sports Med *10*:615, 1991.

323. Gross ML, Brenner SL, Esformes I, et al: Anterior shoulder instability in weight lifters. Am J Sports Med *21*:599, 1993.

324. McMaster WC: Anterior glenoid labrum damage: A painful lesion in swimmers. Am J Sports Med *14*:383, 1986.

325. Hill HA, Sachs MD: The grooved defect of the humeral head. A frequently unrecognized complication of dislocation of the shoulder joint. Radiology *35*:690, 1940.

326. Bankart ASB: Recurrent or habitual dislocation of the shoulder. Br Med J *2*:1132, 1906.

327. Bankart ASB: The pathology and treatment of recurrent dislocation of the shoulder joint. Br J Surg *26*:23, 1938–39.

328. Rokous JR, Feagin JA, Abbott HG: Modified axillary roentgenogram, a useful adjunct in the diagnosis of recurrent instability of the shoulder. Clin Orthop *82*:84, 1972.

329. Goldman AB, Dines DM, Warren RF (Eds): Shoulder Arthrography—Technique, Diagnosis and Clinical Correlation. Boston, Little, Brown, and Company, 1982.

330. Shuman WP, Kilcoyne RF, Matsen FA, et al: Double contrast computed tomography of the glenoid labrum. AJR *141*:581, 1983.

331. Zlatkin MB, Bjorkengren AG, Gylys-Morin V, et al: Cross-sectional imaging of the capsular mechanism of the glenohumeral joint. AJR *150*:15, 1988.

332. Seeger LL, Gold RH, Bassett LW: Shoulder instability: Evaluation with MR imaging. Radiology *168*:695, 1988.

333. Kieft GS, Bloem JL, Rosen PM, et al: MR imaging of recurrent anterior dislocation of the shoulder: Comparison with CT arthrography. AJR *150*:1083, 1988.

334. Munk PL, Halt RG, Helms CA, et al: Glenoid labrum: Preliminary work with use of radial-sequence MR imaging. Radiology *173*:751, 1989.

335. McCauley TR, Pope CF, Jokl P: Normal and abnormal glenoid labrum: Assessment with multi planar gradient echo MR imaging. Radiology *183*:35, 1992.

336. Rodeo SA, Warren RF, O'Brien SJ, et al: Diastasis of bipartite sesamoids of the first metatarsal phalangeal joint simulating turf toe in professional football players. Foot Ankle *14*:425, 1993.

337. Pavlov H, Torg JS: The Running Athlete: Roentgenograms and Remedies. Chicago, Year Book Medical Publishers, 1987, pp 38, 40–43, 67–71.

338. Panush RS, Schmidt C, Caldwell JR, et al: Is running associated with degenerative joint disease? JAMA *255*:1152, 1986.

339. Lane NE, Bloch DA, Jones HH, et al: Long distance running, bone density, and osteoarthritis. JAMA *255*:1147, 1986.

340. Shellock FG, Mink JH: Knees of trained long distance runners: MR imaging before and after competition. Radiology *179*:635, 1991.

341. Sohn RS, Micheli LJ: The effect of running on the pathogenesis of osteoarthritis of the hips and knees. Clin Orthop *198*:106, 1985.

342. Kursunoglu-Brahme S, Schwaighofer B, Gundry C, et al: Jogging causes acute changes in the knee joint: An MR study in normal volunteers. AJR *154*:1233, 1990.

343. Kellett J: Acute soft tissue injuries—a review of the literature. Med Sci Sports Exerc *18*:489, 1986.

344. Shellock FG, Fukunaga T, Mink JH, et al: Acute effects of exercise on MR imaging of skeletal muscle. Concentric vs. eccentric actions. AJR *156*:765, 1991.

345. McCully K, Shellock FG, Bank WJ, et al: The use of nuclear magnetic resonance to evaluate muscle injury. Med Sci Sports Exerc *24*:537, 1992.

346. Fleckenstein JL, Weatherall PT, Parkey RW, et al: Sports-related muscle injuries: Evaluation with MR imaging. Radiology *172*:793, 1989.

347. Fleckenstein JL, Canby RC, Parkey RW, et al: Acute effects of exercise on MR imaging of skeletal muscle in normal volunteers. AJR *151*:231, 1988.

348. Hough T: Ergographic studies in muscular soreness. Am J Physiol *7*:76, 1902.

349. Armstrong RB: Mechanisms of exercise-induced delayed onset muscular soreness: A brief review. Med Sci Sports Exerc *16*:529, 1984.

350. Newham DJ, McPhail G, Mills KR, et al: Ultrastructural changes after concentric and eccentric contractions of human muscle. J Neurol Sci *61*:109, 1983.

351. Garrett WE, Lohnes J: Cellular and matrix response to mechanical injury at the myotendinous junction. In WB Leadbetter, JA Buckwalter, SL Gordon (Eds): Sports-induced Inflammation. Park Ridge, Ill, American Academy of Orthopaedic Surgeons, 1990, p 215.

352. Garrett WE, Tidball J: Myotendinous junction: Structure, function and failure. In SI-Y Woo, JA Buckwalter (Eds): Injury and Repair of Musculoskeletal Soft Tissues. Park Ridge, Ill, American Academy of Orthopaedic Surgeons, 1988, p 171.

353. Garrett WE Jr: Muscle strain injuries: Clinical and basic aspects. Med Sci Sports Exerc *22*:436, 1990.

354. Shirkheda A, Mauro MA, Stabb EV, et al: Soft tissue hemorrhage in hemophilic patients: Computed tomography and ultrasound study. Radiology *147*:811, 1983.

355. Greco A, McNamara MT, Escher MB, et al: Spin-echo and STIR MR imaging of sports related muscle injuries at 1.5T. J Comput Assist Tomogr *15*:994, 1991.

356. Ehman RL, Berquist TH: Magnetic resonance imaging of musculoskeletal trauma. Radiol Clin North Am *24*:291, 1986.

357. Hernandez RJ, Keim DR, Chenevert TL, et al: Fat-suppressed MR imaging of myositis. Radiology *182*:217, 1992.

358. Ackerman LV: Extra-osseous localized non-neoplastic bone and cartilage formation (so-called myositis ossificans). J Bone Joint Surg [Am] *40*:279, 1958.

359. Amendola MA, Glazer GM, Agha FP, et al: Myositis ossificans circumscripta: Computed tomographic diagnosis. Radiology *149*:775, 1983.

360. Heiken JP, Lee JKT, Smathers RL, et al: CT of benign soft-tissue masses of the extremities. AJR *142*:575, 1984.

361. Zeanah WR, Hudson TM: Myositis ossificans: Radiologic evaluation of two cases with diagnostic computed tomograms. Clin Orthop *168*:187, 1982.

362. Hudson TM: Radiologic-Pathologic Correlation of Musculoskeletal Lesions. Baltimore, Williams & Wilkins, 1987, p 589.

363. Kransdorf MJ, Meis JM, Jelinek JS: Myositis ossificans: MR appearance with radiologic-pathologic correlation. AJR *157*:1243, 1991.

364. Tsai JC, Dalinka MK, Fallon MD, et al: Fluid-fluid level—a nonspecific finding in tumors of bone and soft tissue. Radiology *175*:779, 1990.

365. Speer KP, Lahnes J, Garret WE: Radiographic imaging of muscle strain injuries. Am J Sports Med *21*:89, 1993.

366. Garrett WE, Safran MR, Seaber AV: Biomechanical comparison of stimulated and nonstimulated skeletal muscle pulled to failure. Am J Sports Med *15*:448, 1987.

367. Dooms GC, Fisher MG, Hricak H, et al: MR imaging of intramuscular hemorrhage. J Comput Assist Tomogr *9*:908, 1985.

368. O'Donoghue DO: Treatment of Injuries to Athletes. Philadelphia, WB Saunders Co, 1984, p 51.

369. Barfred T: Experimental rupture of the Achilles tendon: Comparison of various experimental ruptures in rats. Acta Orthop Scand *41*:528, 1971.

370. Nikolaou PK, Macdonald BL, Glisson RR: Biomechanical and histological evaluation of muscle after controlled strain injury. Am J Sports Med *15*:9, 1987.

371. Genett WE Jr, Rich FR, Nikolaou PK, et al: Computed tomography of hamstring muscle strains. Med Sci Sports Exerc *21*:506, 1991.

372. Alexandeer IJ, Johnson KA, Berquist TH: Magnetic resonance imaging in the diagnosis of disruption of the posterior tibial tendon. Foot Ankle *8*:144, 1987.

373. Daffner RH, Reimer BL, Lupetin AR, et al: Magnetic resonance imaging in acute tendon ruptures. Skel Radiol *15*:619, 1986.

374. Kessel L, Watson M: The painful arc syndrome. J Bone Joint Surg [Br] *59*:166, 1977.

375. Bland JH, Merritt JA, Bouskey DR: The painful shoulder. Semin Arthritis Rheum *71*:21, 1977.

376. Resnick D: Shoulder pain. Orthop Clin North Am *14*:81, 1983.

377. Cone RO, Resnick D, Danzig L: Shoulder impingement syndrome: Radiographic evaluation. Radiology *150*:29, 1984.

378. Neer CS III: Anterior acromioplasty for the chronic impingement syndrome of the shoulder: A preliminary report. J Bone Joint Surg [Am] *54*:41, 1972.

379. Neer CS III: Impingement lesions. Clin Orthop *173*:70, 1983.

380. Seeger LL, Gold RH, Bassett LW, et al: Shoulder impingement syndrome: MR findings in 53 shoulders. AJR *150*:343, 1988.

381. Kieft JJ, Bloem AL, Razing PM, et al: Rotator cuff impingement syndrome: MR imaging. Radiology *166*:211, 1988.

382. Dines DM, Warren RF, Inglis AE: The coracoid impingement syndrome. J Bone Joint Surg [Br] *72*:314, 1990.

383. Neer CS: Shoulder Reconstruction. Philadelphia, WB Saunders Co, 1990, p 41.

384. Killoran PJ, Marcove RC, Freiberger RH: Shoulder arthrography. AJR *103*:658, 1968.

385. Ghelman B, Goldman AB: The double contrast shoulder arthrogram: Evaluation of rotator cuff tears. Radiology *124*:251, 1977.

386. Goldman AB, Ghelman B: The double contrast shoulder arthrogram. A review of 158 studies. Radiology 127:655, 1978.

387. Burk JDL, Karasick D, Kurtz AB, et al: Rotator cuff tears: Prospective comparison of MR imaging with arthrography, sonography and surgery. AJR 153:87, 1989.

388. Zlatkin MB, Jannotti JP, Roberts MC, et al: Rotator cuff tears: Diagnostic performance of MR imaging. Radiology 172:225, 1989.

389. O'Donoghue DH: Subluxing biceps tendon in the athlete. J Sports Med 20:29, 1973.

390. Nevaiser RJ: Lesions of the biceps and tendinitis of the shoulder. Orthop Clin North Am 11:318, 1989.

391. Nevaiser RJ: Painful conditions affecting the shoulder. Clin Orthop 173:63, 1983.

392. Goldman AB: Calcific tendinitis of the long head of the biceps brachii distal to the glenohumeral joint: Plain film radiographic findings. AJR 153:1011, 1989.

393. Hunter JC, Blatz DJ, Escobedo EM: SLAP lesions of the glenoid labrum: CT arthrographic and arthroscopic correlation. Radiology 184:513, 1992.

394. Andrews JA, Carson WG, McLeod WD: Glenoid labrum tears related to the long head of the biceps. Am J Sports Med 13:337, 1985.

395. Cartland JP, Crues JV III, Stauffer A, et al: MR imaging in the evaluation of SLAP injuries of the shoulder: Findings in 10 patients. AJR 159:787, 1992.

396. Gross ML, Seager LL, Smith JB, et al: Magnetic resonance imaging of the glenoid labrum. Am J Sports Med 18:229, 1990.

397. Snyder SJ, Karzel RP, Del Pizzo W, et al: SLAP lesions of the shoulder. Arthroscopy 6:274, 1990.

398. Pappas AM, Goss TP, Kleinman PK: Symptomatic shoulder instability due to lesions of the glenoid labrum. Am J Sports Med 11:279, 1983.

399. McMaster WG: Anterior glenoid labrum damage: A painful lesion in swimmers. Am J Sports Med 14:383, 1986.

400. Gilcreest EL: Rupture of muscle and tendons, particularly subcutaneous rupture of the biceps flexor cubiti. JAMA 84:1819, 1933.

401. Mirowitz SA, London SL: Ulnar collateral ligament injury in baseball pitchers: MR imaging evaluation. Radiology 185:573, 1992.

402. Bennett JB, Tullos HS: Ligamentous and articular injuries in the athlete. In BF Morrey (Ed): The Elbow and Its Disorders. Philadelphia, WB Saunders Co, 1985, p 505.

403. Dobbie RP: Avulsion of the lower biceps brachii tendon. Analysis of fifty-one previously unreported cases. Am J Surg 51:662, 1941.

404. Hovelius L, Josefsson G: Rupture of the distal biceps tendon. Report of five cases. Acta Orthop Scand 48:280, 1977.

405. Postacchini F, Puddu G: Subcutaneous rupture of the distal biceps brachii tendon. A report of seven cases. J Sports Med 15:81, 1975.

406. Nielson K: Partial rupture of the distal biceps brachii tendon. A case report. Acta Orthop Scand 58:287, 1987.

407. Nance EP, Kaye JJ: Injuries of the quadriceps mechanism. Radiology 142:301, 1982.

408. Larson RL: Dislocations and ligamentous injuries of the knee. In CA Rockwood Jr, DP Green (Eds): Fractures. Vol 2. Philadelphia, JB Lippincott, 1975, p 1182.

409. Hohl M: Fractures about the knee. In CA Rockwood Jr, DP Green (Eds): Fractures. Vol 2. Philadelphia, JB Lippincott, 1975, p 1131.

410. Watson-Jones R: Injuries of the knee. In JN Wilson, R Watson-Jones (Eds): Fractures and Joint Injuries. 5th Ed. Vol 2. New York, Churchill Livingstone, 1976, p 1012.

411. Zeiss J, Sadaemi SR, Ebraheim NA: MR imaging of the quadriceps tendon: Normal layered configuration and its importance in cases of tendon rupture. AJR 159:1031, 1992.

412. Turek SL: Orthopaedics. Principles and Their Application. 3rd Ed. Philadelphia, JB Lippincott, 1977, p 1182.

413. Kamali M: Bilateral traumatic rupture of the infrapatella tendon. Clin Orthop 142:131, 1979.

414. Davis SG, Baudouin CJ, King JB, et al: Ultrasound, computed tomography, and magnetic resonance imaging in patellar tendinitis. Clin Radiol 43:52, 1991.

415. Bodne D, Quinn SF, Murray WT, et al: Magnetic resonance images of chronic patellar tendinitis. Skel Radiol 17:24, 1988.

416. El-Khoury G, Wira RL, Berbaum KS, et al: MR imaging of patellar tendinitis. Radiology 84:849, 1992.

417. Quinn SF, Murray WT, Clark RA, et al: Achilles tendon: MR imaging at 1.5T. Radiology 164:767, 1987.

418. Clement PB, Taunton JE, Smart GW: Achilles tendinitis and peritendinitis: Etiology and treatment. Am J Sports Med 12:179, 1984.

419. Cetti R, Christensen SE: Surgical treatment under local anaesthesia of Achilles tendon upture. Clin Orthop 173:204, 1973.

420. Stein SR, Leuken CA: Closed treatment of Achilles tendon ruptures. Orthop Clin North Am 7:241, 1976.

421. Inglis AE, Scott WN, Sculco TP, et al: Ruptures of the tendo Achillis. J Bone Joint Surg [Am] 58:990, 1976.

422. Lagengren C, Lindholm A: Vascular distribution in the Achilles tendon: An angiographic and micro-angiographic study. Acta Chir Scand 116:491, 1958.

423. Blei LC, Nirschl RP, Grant EG: Achilles tendon: US diagnosis of pathologic conditions. Radiology 159:765, 1986.

424. Fornage B: Achilles tendon: US examination. Radiology 159:759, 1986.

425. Belthax J, Noto AM, Mosure JC, et al: Ankle: Surface coil MR imaging at 1.5T. Radiology 161:203, 1986.

426. Rosenberg ZS, Cheung Y, Jahss MH: Computed tomography scan and magnetic resonance imaging of ankle tendons: An overview. Foot Ankle 8:297, 1988.

427. Daffner RH, Riemer BL, Lupetin AR, et al: Magnetic resonance imaging in acute tendon ruptures. Skel Radiol 15:619, 1986.

428. Jahss MH: Spontaneous rupture of the tibiales posterior tendon: Clinical findings, tenographic studies, and a new technique of repair. Foot Ankle 3:158, 1982.

429. Johnson KA: Tibialis posterior tendon rupture. Clin Orthop 177:140, 1983.

430. Mann RA: Rupture of the posterior tibial tendon causing flat foot: Surgical treatment. J Bone Joint Surg [Am] 67:556, 1985.

431. Funk DA, Cass RJ, Johnson KA: Acquired adult flat foot secondary to posterior tibial-tendon pathology. J Bone Joint Surg [Am] 68:95, 1986.

432. Rosenberg ZS, Cheung Y, Jahss MH: Rupture of posterior tibial tendon: CT and MR imaging and surgical correlation. Radiology 169:229, 1988.

433. Moorman CT III, Monto R, Bassett FH, et al: So-called trigger ankle due to aberrant flexor hallucis longus muscle in a tennis player—a case report. J Bone Joint Surg [Am] 74:294, 1992.

434. Turner PA, Prodromos CC, Petasnick JP, et al: Acute injury of the ligaments of the knee: Magnetic resonance evaluation. Radiology 154:717, 1985.

435. Mink JH, Levy T, Crues JV III: Tears of the anterior cruciate ligament and menisci of the knee: MR imaging evaluation. Radiology 167:769, 1988.

436. Jackson DW, Jennings LD, Maywood RM, et al: Magnetic resonance imaging of the knee. Am J Sports Med 16:2938, 1988.

437. Crues JV, Mink J, Levy TL, et al: Meniscal tears of the knee: Accuracy of MR imaging. Radiology 64:445, 1987.

438. Schneck CD, Mesgarzadeh M, Bonakdarpour A: MR imaging of the most commonly injured ankle ligaments. Part II. Ligament injuries. Radiology 184:507, 1992.

439. Polly DW, Callaghan JJ, Sikes RA, et al: The accuracy of selective magnetic resonance imaging compared with findings of arthroscopy of the knee. J Bone Joint Surg [Am] 70:192, 1988.

440. Liljedahl S-O, Lindvall N, Wetterfos J: Early diagnosis and treatment of the anterior cruciate ligament. A clinical and arthroraphic study of forty-eight cases. J Bone Joint Surg [Am] 47:1503, 1956.

441. Pavlov H, Freiberger, RH: An easy method to demonstrate the cruciate ligaments by double contrast arthrography. Radiology 126:817, 1978.

442. Pavlov H, Torg JS: Double contrast arthrographic evaluation of the anterior cruciate ligament. Radiology 132:389, 1979.

443. Pavlov H, Warren R, Sherman MF, et al: The accuracy of double contrast arthrographic evaluation of the anterior cruciate ligament. A retrospective review of 163 knees with surgical correlation. J Bone Joint Surg [Am] 65:175, 1983.

444. Berquist TH (Ed): Magnetic Resonance of the Musculoskeletal System. 2nd Ed. New York, Raven Press, 1990, p 227.

445. Lee JK, Yao L, Phelps CT, et al: Anterior cruciate ligament tears: MR imaging compared with arthroscopy and clinical tests. Radiology 166:861, 1988.

446. Moeser P, Bechtold RE, Clark T, et al: MR imaging of anterior cruciate ligament repair. J Comput Assist Tomogr 13:105, 1989.

447. Reicher MA, Hartzman S, Bassett LW, et al: MR imaging of the knee. Part I. Traumatic disorders. Radiology 162:547, 1987.

448. Cross MJ, Powell JF: Long term follow-up of PCL ruptures: A study of 116 cases. Am J Sports Med 121:292, 1984.

449. Bianchi M: Acute tears of the PCL: Clinical study and results of operative treatment in 27 cases. Am J Sports Med 11:308, 1983.

450. Fowlere PJ, Messieh SS: Isolated PCL injuries in athletes. Am J Sports Med 15:553, 1987.

451. Grover JS, Bassett LW, Gross ML, et al: Posterior cruciate ligament: MR imaging. Radiology 174:507, 1990.

452. Nachlas IW, Olpp JL: Para-articular calcification (Pellegrini-Stieda) in afflictions of the knee. Surg Gynecol Obstet 81:206, 1945.

453. Norman A, Dorfman HD: Juxtacortical circumscribed myositis ossificans: Evolution and radiographic features. AJR 96:301, 1970.

454. Cox JS: Surgical and nonsurgical treatment of acute ankle sprains. Clin Orthop 198:118, 1985.

455. Crim JR, Bassett LW: The ankle and foot. In LW Bassett, RH Gold, LL Seeger (Eds): MRI Atlas of the Musculoskeletal System. London, Martin Dunitz, 1989, p 266.

456. deLacey G, Bradbooke S: Rationalizing requests for X-ray examination of acute ankle injuries. Br Med J 1:1597, 1979.

457. Brand RL, Blank HM, Cox JS: The natural history of inadequately treated ankle sprains. Am J Sports Med 6:248, 1977.

458. Dumeron TB: Management of acute ankle sprains. South Med J 70:1166, 1977.

459. Fiore RD, Leard JS: A functional approach in the rehabilitation of the ankle and rear foot. Athletic Training 15:231, 1980.

460. Balduini FC, Begso JJ, Torg JS, et al: Management and rehabilitation of ligamentous injuries to the ankle. Sports Med 4:364, 1987.

461. Kjaersgaard-Andersen P, Wethelund JO, Nielsen S: Lateral talocalcaneal instability following section of the calcaneofibular ligament: A kinesiologic study. Foot Ankle 7:355, 1987.

462. Mirowitz SA, London SL: Ulnar collateral ligament injury in baseball pitchers: MR imaging evaluation. Radiology 185:573, 1992.

463. Murphy BJ: MR imaging of the elbow. Radiology 184:525, 1992.

464. Priest JD, Jones HA, Nagel DA: Elbow injuries in highly skilled tennis players. J Sports Med Phys Fitness 2:137, 1974.

465. Jabe FW, Nuber G: Throwing injuries of the elbow. Clin Sports Med 5:621, 1986.

466. Bennett JB, Tuelos HSS: Ligamentous and articular injuries in the athlete. In BF Morrey (Ed): The Elbow and Its Disorders. Philadelphia, WB Saunders Co, 1985, p 502.

467. Campbell JD, Feagin JA, King P, et al: Ulnar collateral ligament injury of the thumb: Treatment in the glove spica cast. Am J Sports Med 20:29, 1992.
468. Linscheid RL: Arthrography of the metacarpophalangeal joint. Clin Arthrop 103:91, 1974.
469. Bowers WH, Hurst LC: Gamekeeper's thumb: Evaluation by arthrography and stress roentgenography. J Bone Joint Surg [Am] 59:519, 1977.
470. Resnick D, Danzig LA: Arthrographic evaluation of injuries of the first metacarpophalangeal joint: Gamekeeper's thumb. AJR 126:1046, 1976.
471. Spaeth HJ, Abrams RA, Bock GW, et al: Gamekeeper thumb: Differentiation of nondisplaced and displaced tears of the ulnar collateral ligament with MR imaging work in progress. Radiology 188:553, 1993.
472. Louis DS, Buckwalter KA: Magnetic resonance imaging of the collateral ligaments of the thumb. J Hand Surg [Am] 14:739, 1989.
473. Brunner MC, Flower SP, Evancho AM, et al: MRI of the athletic knee: Findings in asymptomatic professional basketball and collegiate football players. Invest Radiol 24:72, 1989.
474. Shellock FG, Deutsch AL, Mink JH, et al: Do asymptomatic marathon runners have an increased prevalence of meniscal abnormalities? An MR study of the knee in 23 volunteers. AJR 157:1239, 1991.
475. Vailas AC, Zernicke RF, Matsuda J, et al: Adaptation of rat knee meniscus to prolonged exercise. J Appl Physiol 60:1031, 1986.
476. DeSmet AA, Nairis MA, Yandaw DR, et al: MR diagnosis of meniscal tears of the knee: Importance of high signal in the meniscus that extends to the surface. AJR 161:101, 1993.
477. Pavlov H, Heneghan MA, Hersh A, et al: Haglund's deformity: Diagnosis and differential diagnosis of posterior heel pain. Radiology 144:83, 1982.
478. Haglund P: Beitrag zur Klinik der Achillessehne. Z Orthop Chir 49:49, 1927.
479. Fleckenstein JL, Watumull L, Conner KE, et al: Denervated human skeletal muscle: MR imaging evaluation. Radiology 187:213, 1993.
480. Ganzhorn RW, Hockere JT, Horowitz M, et al: Suprascapular nerve entrapment. J Bone Joint Surg [Am] 63:492, 1981.
481. Neviaser TJ, Ain BR, Neviaser RJ: Suprascapular nerve denervation secondary to attenuation by a ganglion cyst. J Bone Joint Surg [Am] 68:627, 1986.
482. Takagishi K, Maeda K, Ikeda T, et al: Ganglion causing paralysis of the suprascapular nerve. Acta Orthop Scand 62:391, 1991.
483. Hussamy OD, Bynum DF Jr: Ganglion cyst of the shoulder joint presenting as a painful axillary mass: Case report. Cont Orth 27:123, 1993.
484. Fritz RC, Helms CA, Steinbach LS, et al: Suprascapular nerve entrapment: Evaluation with MR imaging. Radiology 182:437, 1992.
485. Foo CL, Swann M: Isolation paralysis of the serratus anterior. J Bone Joint Surg [Br] 65:552, 1983.
486. Goodman CE, Kenrick MM, Blum MV: Long thoracic nerve palsy. A follow-up study. Arch Phys Med Rehabil 56:352, 1975.
487. Gregg JR, Labosky D, Hartz M, et al: Serratus anterior paralysis in the young athlete. J Bone Joint Surg [Am] 61:805, 1979.
488. White SM, Witten CM: Long thoracic nerve palsy in a professional ballet dancer. Am J Sports Med 21:626, 1993.
489. Rosenberg ZS, Beltran J, Theung YY, et al: The elbow: MR features of nerve disorders. Radiology 188:235, 1993.
490. Burke ER: Ulnar neuropathy in bicyclists. Phys Sports Med 9:53, 1981.
491. Eckman PB, Perlstein G, Attrocchi PH: Ulnar neuropathy in bicycle riders. Arch Neurol 32:130, 1975.
492. Henricson AS, Westlin NE: Chronic calcaneal pain in athletes: Entrapment of the calcaneal nerve? Am J Sports Med 12:152, 1984.
493. O'Connor D: Sinus tarsi syndrome: A clinical entity (Abstr). J Bone Joint Surg [Am] 40:720, 1958.
494. Taillard W, Meyer JM, Garcia J, et al: The sinus tarsi syndrome. Int Orthop 5:117, 1981.
495. Klein MA, Spreitzer AM: MR imaging of the tarsal sinus and canal: Normal anatomy, pathologic findings and features of the sinus tarsi syndrome. Radiology 186:233, 1993.
496. Meyer JM, Garcia J, Hoffmeyer P, et al: The subtalar sprain: A roentgenographic study. Clin Orthop 226:169, 1988.
497. Beltran J, Munchow AM, Khabiri H: Ligaments of the lateral aspect of the ankle and sinus tarsi: An MR imaging study. Radiology 177:455, 1990.
498. Binnie JF: Snapping hip. Am Surg 58:59, 1913.
499. Dickson AM: Bilateral snapping hip. Am J Surg 6:97, 1929.
500. Jones FW: The anatomy of snapping hip. J Orthop Surg 2:1, 1920.
501. Mayer L: Snapping hip. Surg Gynecol Obstet 29:425, 1919.
502. Lyon JC, Peterson LF: The snapping iliopsoas tendon. Mayo Clin Proc 59:327, 1984.
503. Schaberg JE, Harper MC, Allen WC: The snapping hip syndrome. Am J Sports Med 12:361, 1984.
504. Staple TW, Jung D, Mork A: Snapping tendon syndrome: Hip tomography with fluoroscopic monitoring. Radiology 166:873, 1988.
505. Brignall CG, Brown RM, Stainsby GD: Fibrosis of the gluteus maximus as a cause of snapping hip. J Bone Joint Surg [Am] 75:909, 1993.
506. Murphy B, Hechtman KS, Uribe JW, et al: Iliotibial band friction syndrome: MR imaging findings. Radiology 185:569, 1992.
507. Orava S: Iliotibial tract fraction syndrome in athletes: An uncommon exertion syndrome on the lateral side of the knee. Br J Sports Med 12:69, 1978.
508. Noble CA: The treatment of iliotibial band friction syndrome. Br J Sports Med 13:51, 1979.
509. Noble CA: Proceedings of the International Sports Medicine Federation, Brazil, 1978.
510. Noble CA: Iliotibial band friction syndrome in runners. Am J Sports Med 8:232, 1980.
511. Martens M, Libbrecht P, Burssens A: Surgical treatment of the iliotibial band friction syndrome. Am J Sports Med 17:651, 1989.
512. McNichol K, Taunton JE, Clement DB: Iliotibial tract friction syndrome in athletes. Can J Appl Sport Sci 6:76, 1981.
513. Kwong PK, Kay D, Voner RT: Plantar fasciitis: Mechanics and pathomechanics of treatment. Foot and ankle injuries. Clin Sports Medicine 7:119, 1988.
514. Bassiouni M: Incidence of calcaneal spurs in osteoarthrosis and rheumatoid arthritis, and in control patients. Ann Rheum Dis 24:490, 1965.
515. Henry JH, Anderson J, Cothren CC: Tibiofibular synostosis in professional basketball players. Am J Sports Med 21:619, 1993.
516. Flandry F, Sanders RA: Tibiofibular synostosis: An unusual case of skin splint like pain. Am J Sports Med 15:280, 1987.
517. Whiteside LA, Reynolds RC, Ellsasser JC: Tibiofibular synostosis and recurrent ankle sprains in high performance athletes. Am J Sports Med 6:204, 1978.
518. Bowers KD Jr, Martin RB: Turf-toe—a shoe-surface–related football injury. Med Sci Sports 8:81, 1976.
519. Bowers KD, Martin RB: Impact absorption, new and old Astroturf at West Virginia University. Med Sci Sports 6:217, 1974.

72

Thermal and Electrical Injuries

Donald Resnick, M.D.

Exposure of the human body to extremes in temperature or to electricity can lead to significant abnormalities. Osseous and articular structures may participate in the body's response to such insult, and the changes that are induced may be irreparable. This chapter summarizes musculoskeletal manifestations of thermal and electrical injury.

FROSTBITE

Terminology and General Abnormalities

Local damage can follow nonfreezing (immersion foot) and freezing (frostbite) injuries.[1] *Immersion foot* is related to prolonged exposure to low but not freezing temperatures in combination with persistent dampness.[2] Typical examples of immersion foot occur in soldiers (trench foot) and in survivors of shipwrecks. Contributory to the tissue injury in this entity are prolonged exposure to cold and dampness, immobility and dependency of the extremities, semistarvation, dehydration, and exhaustion. Singly or in combination, these factors lead to hypoxic injury in response to decreased blood flow to the affected body part. Plasma escapes through the injured capillary wall, producing edema, which further compromises the integrity of the vascular supply to nerve and muscle tissue. The resulting clinical manifestations pass through three distinct stages: an ischemic stage of hours to days in which cold, pulseless, and anesthetic extremities are seen; a hyperemic stage lasting 1 to 12 weeks in which a bounding, pulsatile circulation is associated with tissue swelling, blistering, and weeping; and a post-hyperemic recovery phase, with restoration of normal vascular tones, skin color, and temperature. Although gangrene and necrosis of skin are frequent in the hyperemic stage, and induration and fibrosis of subcutaneous tissue with limitation of joint motion may be seen for several years after the injury, complete recovery from immersion foot is common.

Frostbite differs from immersion foot in that blood vessels are injured severely or irreparably, the circulation of blood ceases, and the vascular beds within the frozen tissue are occluded by thrombi and cellular aggregation.[3] Frostbite results from exposure to cold air that usually is at a temperature below $-13°C$ (8°F). Once the freezing process has been initiated, it progresses rapidly, and tissue located superficially, such as that in the ears, nose, and digits, is damaged increasingly by the formation of tiny crystals of ice. The involved cutaneous areas are firm or hard, white, and numb. In part, the cutaneous injury consists of a separation of the epidermal-dermal interface.[3]

Musculoskeletal Abnormalities

Pathogenesis. The development and progression of frostbite injuries are directly related to abnormality in circulation.[4-8] During the period of exposure, vascular spasm in the involved extremities is evident. With warming or thawing of the injured parts, vasodilation leads to increased permeability of the vascular wall, transudation of fluid, perivascular edema, and intravascular stasis, with agglutination of erythrocytes and deposition of fibrin. In this latter stage, vasoconstriction may persist in less damaged areas.

Angiography can be used to assess these vascular changes.[9-12] Varying degrees of vasospasm as well as vascular stenosis and occlusion can be identified. Proliferation of collateral vessels involving both arterial and venous components occurs in the recovery phase.[5, 13] Transcatheter

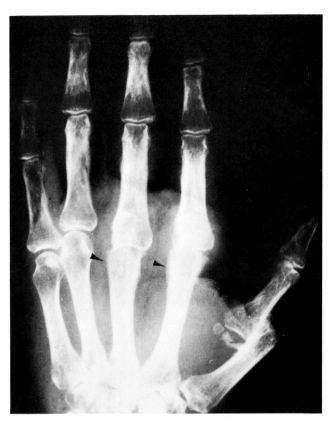

FIGURE 72–1. Frostbite: Early changes. Note soft tissue swelling, osteoporosis, periostitis (arrowheads), osteolysis, and subluxation of metacarpophalangeal joints. (Courtesy of M. Dalinka, M.D., Philadelphia, Pennsylvania.)

administration of sympathetic blocking agents may have a role in the treatment of vasospasm complicating frostbite.[9]

Radiographic Abnormalities. Bony and articular manifestations of frostbite apparently are related to cellular injury and necrosis from the freezing process itself or from the vascular insufficiency it produces.[14] Findings are most marked in the hands and the feet, and their severity depends on the length of exposure and the prevailing temperature.

Initially, no abnormality may be apparent. Early radiographic manifestations include soft tissue swelling and loss of tissue, especially at the tips of the digits; osteoporosis and periostitis may occur at a slightly later stage (Fig. 72–1). In the hand, the findings predominate in the four medial digits; sparing of the thumb is characteristic although not invariable and can be attributed to clenching of the fist with the thumb clasped in the palm during the exposure to cold.

Late skeletal manifestations are variable (Fig. 72–2). In children, epiphyseal abnormalities are frequent.[14–20] The epiphyseal injuries involve primarily the distal phalanges,[86] although other phalangeal epiphyses and, rarely, metacarpal (or metatarsal) epiphyses can be affected. Fragmentation, destruction, and disappearance of epiphyseal centers are seen. Premature physeal fusion also is noted, resulting in brachydactyly.[65, 66, 93] Metaphyseal irregularities consist of expansion and coarse trabeculation. Secondary infection of bone or joint can develop. Injury to articular cartilage can lead to an arthritis that is symptomatic and disabling.[63] Chondrocyte injury may relate to vascular changes or direct effect of the depressed temperature.

Interphalangeal joint abnormalities eventually may simulate those of osteoarthritis[16, 21–23, 88] (Fig. 72–3). Unilateral or bilateral changes with joint space narrowing, sclerosis, osteophytosis, and soft tissue hypertrophy are seen. Juxta-articular punched-out cystic defects also may be observed.[22] Deformity and deviation can result from uneven digital involvement.[20, 66, 67] Tuftal resorption of terminal phalanges can be traced to loss of overlying soft tissue structures. Unilateral changes and the presence of subchondral cysts may aid in differentiating frostbite arthritis from osteoarthritis.[63, 64] Acute bouts of interphalangeal arthritis occurring years after the exposure to cold temperatures have been described.[64]

Frostbite injury of the ears can become manifest as calcification and ossification of the pinna.[24, 25] Cartilage calcification at this site after cold injury must be differentiated from that due to mechanical trauma, hyperparathyroidism, calcium pyrophosphate dihydrate crystal deposition disease, gout, Addison's disease, alkaptonuria, and acromegaly.[25]

Other Diagnostic Techniques

The role of arteriography in the diagnosis and treatment of frostbite has been noted earlier. In addition, scintiscanning with bone-seeking pharmaceutical agents can be used to assess the viability of involved osseous tissue.[26, 87] The uptake of radionuclide in the region of frostbite depends on the integrity of the vascular tree; absence of such uptake indicates bone that lacks vascular perfusion, providing useful information to the surgeon.[68] Persistent perfusion defects indicate nonviable tissue, whereas reperfusion, which may be evident on studies performed weeks after the injury, indicates tissue viability.[69] The use of ^{99m}Tc-pertechnetate, rather than technetium diphosphonates, appears to have advantages, allowing the recognition of soft tissue damage (Fig. 72–4); it is recommended that an initial scan be performed within 24 to 48 hours after the injury and a repeat examination be performed 7 to 10 days later.[69] Triple phase bone scanning appears to offer advantages over standard techniques, and it may provide a useful indicator of tissue viability as early as 2 days after cold injury.[89] The perfusion and blood pool images demonstrate the ischemic tissue at risk, whereas the delayed bone scan images demonstrate the extent of deep tissue and bone infarction. The poorest prognosis is associated with abnormalities on all three phases of the examination and the absence of uptake of the radionuclide by bone in the delayed images.[89] Radionuclide examinations also have been used to identify rhabdomyolysis after frostbite.[70]

Thermography is an additional technique that has been applied to the evaluation of tissue damage after frostbite.[71]

Phalangeal Microgeodic Syndrome

A distinctive self-limiting syndrome has been described in infants and children, presumably related to cold injury.[72–77] Observed principally in Japan but also seen elsewhere (e.g., Scotland, Israel), the disorder, which also is termed "winter fingers," occurs sporadically and exclusively in the colder months of the year, resolves spontaneously, and has a good prognosis. Swelling, redness, heat, and mild pain occur in the fingers of one or both hands. Small cystic lesions, accompanied by soft tissue swelling and minimal

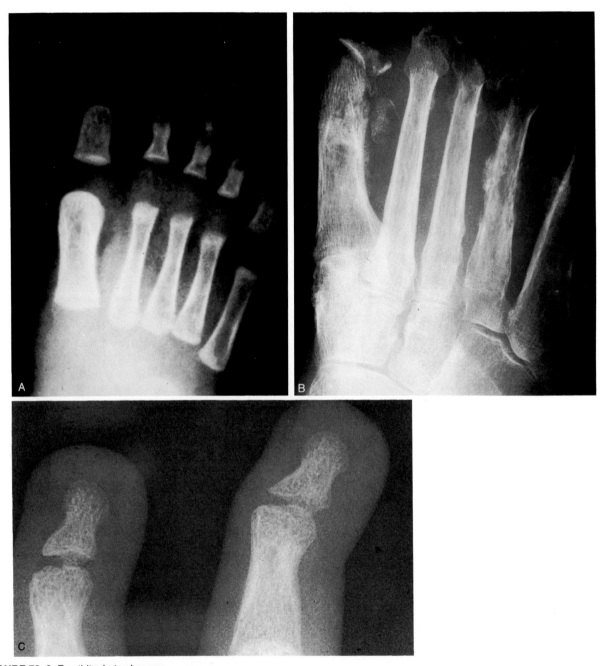

FIGURE 72–2. Frostbite: Late changes.

  A This baby was left as a newborn on a doorstep in subzero weather. At the time this radiograph was taken, the child's chronologic age was 11 months, although the skeletal bone age is markedly retarded. Also note amputation of multiple phalanges in the toes. (Courtesy of R. Fellow, M.D., Fairbanks, Alaska.)

  B This 75 year old man had a previous history of severe frostbite involving the hands and the feet. Recently, he had developed soft tissue swelling and infection in the lower extremity. The changes on this radiograph, which include soft tissue swelling, acro-osteolysis, and poorly defined destruction of the metatarsals with periostitis, can be attributed to frostbite or infection, or both.

  C Epiphyseal destruction and disappearance can occur after frostbite in children. (Courtesy of M. Dalinka, M.D., Philadelphia, Pennsylvania.)

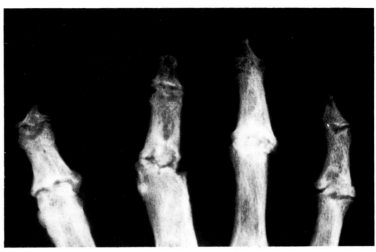

FIGURE 72–3. Frostbite: Interphalangeal joint abnormalities. In addition to acro-osteolysis, osseous and cartilaginous destruction is evident in the proximal interphalangeal and distal interphalangeal joints. Subchondral erosion and collapse, sclerosis, osteophytosis, and joint space narrowing with or without intra-articular bony ankylosis simulate the findings of inflammatory (erosive) osteoarthritis. (Courtesy of M. Dalinka, M.D., Philadelphia, Pennsylvania.)

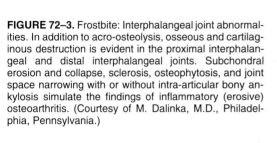

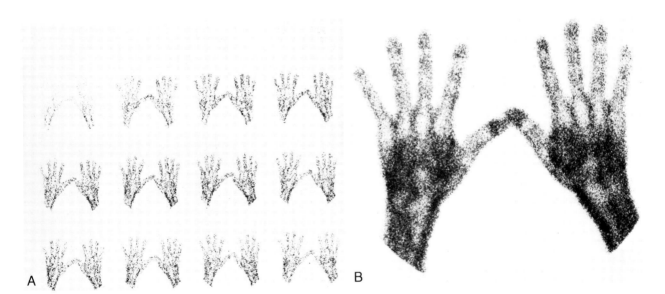

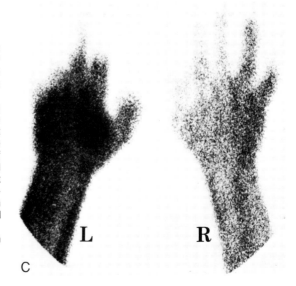

FIGURE 72–4. Frostbite: Scintigraphic abnormalities—^{99m}Tc pertechnetate.

A, B Normal study. Both the flow images **(A)** and the immediate static image **(B)** are shown. In **A,** observe the filling of the radial and ulnar arteries, palmar arch, and digital arteries. In **B,** note the normal soft tissue perfusion. The vascular structures are distinct, with diminished activity in the midpalmar and web spaces.

C In a 62 year old alcoholic man who had been exposed to freezing temperatures with his hands unprotected for 3 hours, a static image shows the following features: in the left hand, marked hyperemia, absent perfusion of the fourth and fifth digits, and diminished perfusion in the middle and distal phalanges of the second digit and the distal phalanx of the first digit; in the right hand, hyperemia in the midpalmar region and the fourth and fifth digits, and diminished perfusion in the distal phalanx of the fifth digit. Eventually, the left fourth and fifth fingers required amputation at the level of the metacarpophalangeal joints, and the right fifth finger and the distal parts of the left thumb and index fingers required debridement.

(From Salami Z, et al: AJR *142*:415, 1984. Copyright 1984, American Roentgen Ray Society.)

periostitis, particularly in the middle phalanges, are seen on the radiographs. These subsequently disappear, although residual bone sclerosis may be evident. Histologically, fibrous tissue in the marrow and periosteal bone formation are noted. Acute inflammation is lacking.

Although the precise cause of this syndrome is unclear, it has been postulated to relate to an injury analogous to frostbite but with a less severe degree of tissue cooling. Its occurrence in winter months and the selection of fingers (and rarely toes) support this concept, although sparing of the thumb, as seen in frostbite, is not evident and it has been described in locations in which mild winters are characteristic.[77] Of further interest, similar osseous abnormalities have been related to exposure to caterpillars of the *Macrothylasia rubi* variety.[84]

The radiographic manifestations of the phalangeal microgeodic syndrome resemble those seen in the hands of patients with sickle cell anemia, sarcoidosis, fat necrosis, and infection. In one case of this syndrome, *Brucella melitensis* was grown from one of the phalangeal lesions.[95]

Differential Diagnosis

The normal occurrence of sclerosis of one or more epiphyses (ivory epiphyses) should not be misinterpreted as evidence of epiphyseal necrosis after frostbite. Thiemann's disease (epiphyseal acrodysplasia) is a poorly defined condition occurring predominantly in men in their late teens, in which swelling of the fingers is associated with epiphyseal irregularity, sclerosis, and fragmentation, particularly of the proximal and middle phalanges.[27–29] Although a dominant inheritance has been noted in some patients with Thiemann's disease, its exact cause is unknown. The distribution of epiphyseal abnormalities (changes predominate in proximal and middle phalanges, especially in the third finger, with sparing of the distal phalanges) differs from that in frostbite. Rarely, Volkmann's ischemia apparently can be associated with physeal growth arrest.[15]

Ungual tuftal resorption can occur in a variety of conditions other than frostbite, including collagen vascular disease, epidermolysis bullosa, neuropathic osteoarthropathy, hyperparathyroidism, sarcoidosis, and psoriatic arthritis. In these conditions, the thumb frequently is affected, and other, more diagnostic findings generally are present.

THERMAL BURNS

General Abnormalities

Thermal injury results in coagulative tissue necrosis.[30] An inflammatory response is evoked, with subsequent changes in cellular structure and configuration.[31] The thickness of burn injury is related to the magnitude of the heat exposure. A second degree burn implies that coagulative necrosis involves only the epidermis and part of the dermis, and that elements are available for epithelial regeneration; a third degree burn implies death of tissue to such an extent that epithelial regeneration cannot occur.[32] In both second and third degree burns, massive outpouring of protein-rich fluid is due to both endothelial capillary damage and interference with normal lymphatic absorption. Secondary bacterial invasion is frequent and may contribute to ischemic

necrosis of tissue by the presence of perivascular infiltration and arterial thrombosis.

Musculoskeletal Abnormalities

Thermal burns can produce significant skeletal and soft tissue abnormalities. Such abnormalities generally are more frequent and severe in children than in adults, perhaps related to a more exuberant response of the immature skeleton to injury.[33] The changes may involve the bone, the joint, or the periarticular tissue; the pathogenesis of many of the findings is not clear.[33–38]

The frequency of radiographic changes after burns depends on the severity of the thermal injury and the method of radiographic examination. Schiele and associates[39] observed osteoporosis in 34 per cent and heterotopic calcification and ossification in 23 per cent of 70 patients with upper extremity burns.

Radiographic Abnormalities. Early radiographic alterations include soft tissue loss, osteoporosis, and periostitis; late alterations include articular and periarticular changes and growth disturbances.

Soft Tissue Loss. Necrosis of soft tissue after a burn produces a decrease in its outline on radiographic examination. This finding can occur during the acute stage or in chronic stages subsequent to further loss of skin and subcutaneous structures.

Osteoporosis. Osteoporosis is the most frequent bony response to thermal burns[33–35] (Fig. 72–5). It may be local-

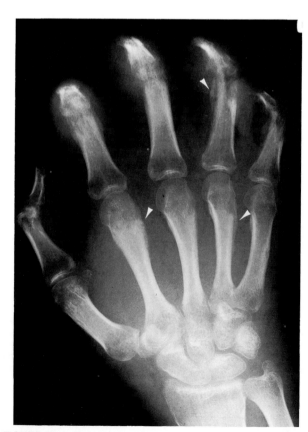

FIGURE 72–5. Thermal burn: Early changes. The early radiographic findings in this patient who had burned his hand include diffuse soft tissue swelling, soft tissue and bony loss in the digits, severe periarticular osteoporosis, and periostitis, especially of the phalanges and metacarpal bones (arrowheads).

ized to the burned area or more generalized. The pathogenesis of such osteoporosis probably includes immobilization and disuse, a reflex vasomotor response, or a metabolic reaction to tissue destruction. Osteoporosis is more extensive in cases of severe burn or long immobilization.

In the burned region, localized hyperemia can produce osteoporosis, which, depending on the distribution of the burn, can be unilateral or bilateral, although symmetric changes are somewhat unusual. Osteoporosis can appear within a period of weeks to months after injury, and with increased mobilization of the patients during the recovery phase, the finding may diminish or disappear completely.

Periostitis. Generally, periosteal bone formation appears within a period of months after the injury in those bones that underlie severely burned areas[33] (Fig. 72–5). It represents a local response to periosteal irritation and in tubular bones produces diaphyseal and metaphyseal changes that are similar to those in hypertrophic osteoarthropathy.

Osteophytosis. Periarticular osseous excrescences that attach to the underlying bone are more frequent in adults than in children. Although they cannot always be differentiated clearly from soft tissue calcification and ossification, these outgrowths may contain recognizable trabeculae and appear to arise from the subjacent bone. They are most prevalent about the elbow, where they appear at the articular margins of the olecranon or coronoid process (Fig. 72–6). They lie in the planes of ligaments and correspond histologically to new bone formation in a fibrous connective tissue stroma.[33] Osteophytes invariably are associated with adjacent burns of the soft tissue and are a response to the thermal injury itself or to the stress of nearby atrophic ligaments. Their course is variable; they may gradually decrease in size or progress, leading to complete osseous bridging of the articulation.[62]

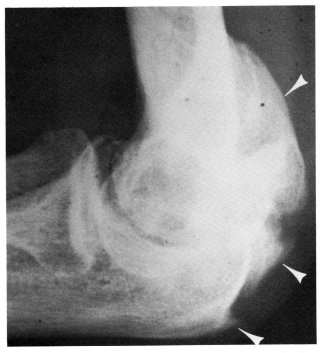

FIGURE 72–6. Thermal burn: Osteophytes, soft tissue calcification, and ossification. Several months after a thermal burn, local ossification (arrowheads) appears along the posterior surface of the humerus and ulna.

Periarticular Calcification and Ossification. The appearance of irregular periarticular calcification is not infrequent within 1 month or more after thermal injury. The deposits create poorly defined and flocculent radiodense areas that are separate from the underlying bone. They are found most commonly about the elbow, near the radial head, or along the anterior and posterior surfaces of the distal end of the humerus.[39] Calcification can remain unchanged in extent or become incorporated into enlarging areas of soft tissue ossification.

Periarticular ossification is a recognized complication of thermal burns, occurring with a reported frequency of 0.6 to 23 per cent of patients.[90] Such variation may relate to differences in the patient population being studied, to the methods of detection, or to the specific site and type of tissue involved.[90] Periarticular ossification most commonly is encountered about the elbow and, with lesser frequency, about the hip and shoulder (Fig. 72–6).[92] Such ossification usually becomes evident in the second or third month after injury,[33, 91] although it occasionally may occur as early as the fourth or fifth week.[39] The relationships among heterotopic bone formation, periarticular calcification, and osteophytosis are not clear, although all three abnormalities may represent various stages of the same process and frequently occur at the same location. Heterotopic ossification is intimately associated with the surrounding musculature, although it does not appear to replace the muscle tissue. The bony ridges commonly attach to the adjacent osseous structure. One common pattern of ossification is from the olecranon process to the medial epicondylar ridge of the humerus, along the medial border of the triceps muscle.[91] Other patterns about the elbow include anterior ossification in the plane of the brachialis muscle extending from the anterior surface of the humerus to the coronoid process; ossification in the plane of the biceps brachii muscle and its attachment to the radius; and ossification between the radius and ulna.[91] About the shoulder, sheets of bone in the plane of the rotator cuff, subscapularis muscle, pectoralis major muscle, or glenohumeral joint capsule may be observed.[91] When extensive, ossification is accompanied by a decrease in joint mobility.[85] Heterotopic ossification tends to regress once the burn has healed.[91]

The pathogenesis of heterotopic calcification and ossification occurring after burns is unknown. Although the deposits may be prominent in proximity to the area of burn, calcification and bone formation also can be observed in the contralateral unburned extremity.[33, 40] Thus, superimposed mechanical trauma, immobility, and vascular alterations may be important in the development of periarticular calcific and ossific deposits after burns (as well as after neurologic injury). In this regard, Schiele and colleagues[39] were unable to detect a correlation between the occurrence of heterotopic ossification and either the percentage of total body surface burned or the average extent of third degree burns, suggesting that factors other than the burn itself were important in the appearance of periarticular radiodense shadows.

Acromutilation. Acromutilation with partial or complete loss of phalanges can be a prominent finding when the hand or the foot is burned[36, 39] (Fig. 72–7). Adjacent soft tissue loss is typical.

Abnormalities in Bone Growth. Increased bone growth can be seen in children who are burned, presumably as a

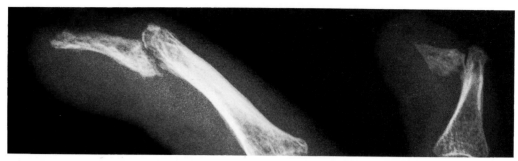

FIGURE 72–7. Thermal burn: Acromutilation. Observe the terminal phalangeal destruction of two burned digits. Joint destruction and subluxation also are evident.

result of hyperemia. Even in adults, a similar phenomenon has been observed.[33]

Articular Abnormalities. Progressive destruction of one or more joints with eventual fibrous or bony ankylosis can be evident after thermal burns.[33, 39, 41, 42] Destruction may appear within a period of a few weeks, and ankylosis may develop within a few months. These changes can occur either close to the initial site of injury or at a remote site. The elbow, the hip, the ankle, and the joints of the hand are affected most typically (Fig. 72–8).

Initially, fusiform soft tissue swelling and osteoporosis can be observed about the involved joint. Progressive loss of interosseous space and subchondral irregularity are seen. Eventually, intra-articular osseous fusion may result.

Thermal injury, mechanical trauma, infection, neuropathic osteoarthropathy, and immobilization have all been considered possible factors in the pathogenesis of these articular changes. The fact that joint alterations can occur in areas that are not burned indicates that agents other than the thermal injury itself must be implicated in their pathogenesis. Although minor or significant mechanical trauma may occur during positioning or movement of the burn patient, and even can lead to fracture, subluxation, and dislocation,[78] this factor does not appear to be responsible for many of the articular manifestations of burns. Bacteremia with hematogenous dissemination of infection to bones and joints may account for some of the destructive articular changes,[33, 39, 43] although the lack of substantial pathologic evidence of joint sepsis and the poor correlation between the degree of sepsis and the amount of articular destruction are noteworthy. Nerve injury leading to neuropathic osteoarthropathy does not appear to be a significant factor in these joint manifestations, although such injuries do occur.[79]

Chondral lysis and atrophy after immobilization due to interference with normal pathways of cartilaginous nutrients may be a prominent cause of the joint space loss and ankylosis that accompany thermal burns.[42] Indeed, immobilization and compression of joint surfaces have been found experimentally to cause acute necrosis of cartilage.[44–46] Closely applied cartilaginous surfaces can be associated with chondrocyte death and chondral degeneration, whereas unapposed cartilage may remain relatively viable. During immobilization of burn patients, the intimacy of the articular surfaces and the stasis of the synovial fluid may produce chondrolysis.[42] A similar phenomenon may accompany paralysis or immobilization for treatment of slipped capital femoral epiphyses[47, 48] or scoliosis.[49]

Contractures. Contractures due to soft tissue and muscular changes in the burn patient are frequent, especially about the elbow and the hand.[32, 50] Joint malalignment, subluxation, and dislocation as well as disuse osteoporosis may be evident (Fig. 72–9).

Differential Diagnosis

The radiographic features of osteoporosis, periarticular calcification and ossification, joint space loss, intra-articular bony ankylosis, and contracture that are encountered in burn patients also may be seen after paralysis (or immobilization). Heterotopic ossification in these situations is identical; it may occur in the area of the thermal injury or neurologic defect, although it also may be noted in remote locations, suggesting that common factors may be operational. Accurate differential diagnosis often depends on appropriate clinical history.

In some patients with thermal burns, articular abnormalities resemble those in pyogenic arthritis and may reflect an accompanying bacteremia with septic embolization.

Phalangeal tuftal resorption or destruction occurring after burns must be differentiated from similar changes occurring in association with frostbite, collagen vascular disorders, and articular diseases.

ELECTRICAL BURNS

General Abnormalities

Electricity can produce severe injury or death. The extent of bodily harm depends on the type of electricity, the voltage, the water content of tissues, and the points of entry and exit of the charge.[51, 52, 94] Alternating currents produce tetanization of muscles and sweating; direct currents produce electrolytic changes in the tissues.[53] Alternating currents are estimated to be approximately four to five times more dangerous than direct currents; fatal electrocution can be produced by exposure to household circuits of 115 volts at 60 cycles.[53]

The pathway of the current influences the body's response to injury. Electrical injury associated with a relatively short route from a point of entry in an arm to a point of exit in a finger is associated with less tissue damage than an injury in which the electricity enters the head and exits at the foot. The duration of contact also is crucial. With alternating currents, muscular contraction occurring after injury may prevent the person's releasing the source of

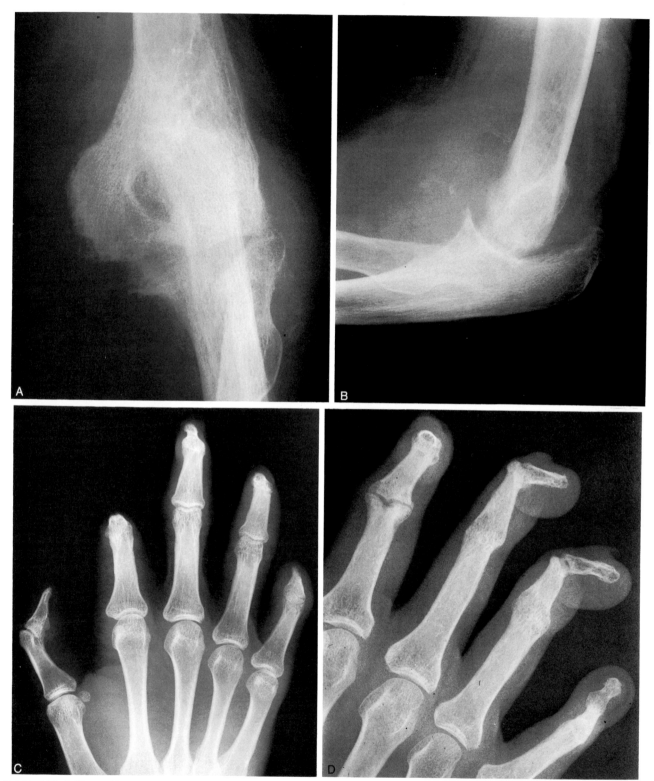

FIGURE 72–8. Thermal burn: Articular abnormalities.

A, B This 54 year old man developed destructive changes of the elbow after severe burns. Findings, which include osteoporosis, soft tissue swelling, an effusion, and osteolysis and fragmentation of the humerus, radius, and ulna, simulate those of infection or neuropathic osteoarthropathy.

C, D Two examples of articular and osseous changes following burns of the hand. Note osteolysis with deformity of phalanges and intraarticular osseous fusion.

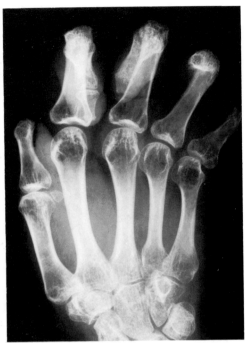

FIGURE 72–9. Thermal burn: Contractures. Flexion contractures of the digits, osteolysis, and osteoporosis represent the sequelae of a burn that had occurred many years previously.

electricity, leading to more prolonged and severe tissue damage. Furthermore, the electrical conductivity of tissues influences their susceptibility to injury from electricity. Structures with a high water content, such as the vascular tree, the muscles, and the perspiring skin, are good conductors, whereas the bones are tissues of high resistance.

Electrical energy is converted to heat in traversing the skin.[53] Resulting burns are accentuated by vascular spasm, leading to electrical necrosis. Death from low voltage elec-

trical injury (below 200 volts) usually is due to ventricular fibrillation; death related to high voltage electricity (greater than 1000 volts) is due to inhibition of the respiratory center in the brain.[54]

Musculoskeletal Abnormalities

Severe injury induced by electricity is much more common in adults than in children because of the increased occupational risk in the former age group. In young children, injuries commonly relate to low voltage current sources, such as extension cords and small appliances; in older children, high tension electrical injuries are a major hazard.[81] The hand, because of its grasping function, is the most commonly affected area in the body. Severe skin burns are encountered at the point of entry and exit of the electrical charge. Osseous and articular changes relate to the effects of heat, mechanical trauma from accompanying uncoordinated muscle spasm, neural and vascular tissue damage, infection, disuse or immobilization, and, perhaps, a specific effect of the electricity itself.[55]

Initial radiographic features include loss of cutaneous, subcutaneous, and osseous tissues owing to tissue charring. Other findings are soft tissue hematomas; compression fractures of the spine, dislocation of joints, and avulsions at tendinous insertions related to muscle spasm; and various fractures due to accompanying falls[56, 82, 83] (Fig. 72–10). Small, rounded osseous dense lesions resembling wax drippings may be attributable to melting of the bone from the intense heat.[56] Focal tiny disruptions in bony continuity (microfractures) also may be a direct effect of the heat.[57, 58] They can possess a zigzag contour with discrete margins and may occur anywhere along the route of electricity. Osteolysis and periostitis also are encountered[55] (Fig. 72–11). Epiphyseal fragmentation and osteochondral fractures may be noted.[56]

Delayed musculoskeletal alterations, which may appear

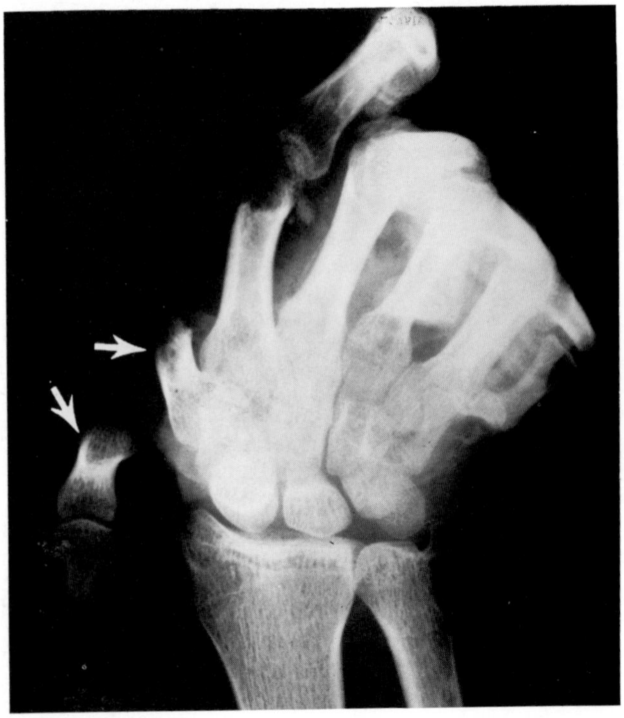

FIGURE 72–10. Electrical burn. This man developed changes in the hands after touching a high tension wire. The severe alterations in the left hand resulted from sustained grasping of the wire. They include contracture, soft tissue injury, subluxation, dislocation, and fracture (arrows). The right hand was affected similarly.

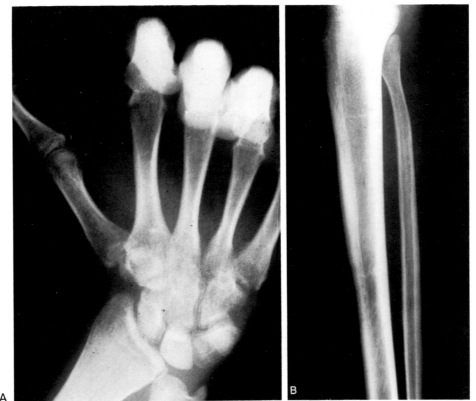

FIGURE 72–11. Electrical burn. A 21 year old man came into contact with a high tension wire, resulting in a severe injury to both hands (entrance wounds) and to the pretibial regions (exit wounds).

A A radiograph of a hand reveals contractures of multiple digits and periarticular osteoporosis.

B Osteolysis of the mid-diaphysis of the tibia reflects bony changes at the point of exit of the electric current.

(Courtesy of J. Barry, M.D., Seattle, Washington, and J. Ogden, M.D., Tampa, Florida.)

months or years later, are related predominantly to ischemia.[59] Osteonecrosis, which develops at sites distal to the entry and exit wounds, may be attributed to periosteal stripping or damage to the vascular wall with thrombosis. Medullary lucent areas in the diaphyses and metaphyses of tubular bones, endosteal resorption with medullary expansion, cystic rarefactions, cortical sequestration, and epiphyseal collapse and fragmentation can be evident (Fig. 72–12). Accelerated bone growth and premature fusion of damaged physes may follow electrical injury in children.[61] De-

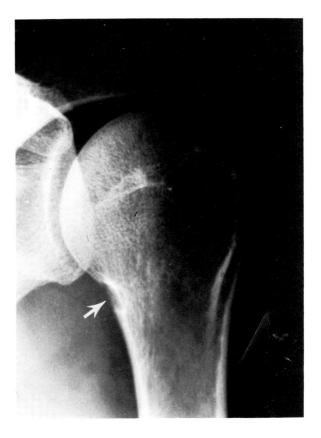

FIGURE 72–12. Electrical burn. A 48 year old woman developed an electrical injury with a point of entrance in the hand and a point of exit in the shoulder. The small, eccentric, cortical lucent lesion (arrow) evident in the proximal end of the humerus months later is consistent with bone lysis at the exit point after an electrical burn.

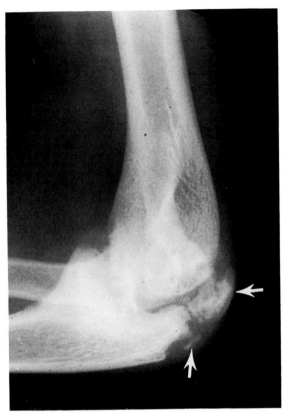

FIGURE 72–13. Electrical burn. Bony fragmentation, periarticular calcification and ossification (arrows), and joint contracture occur at sites remote from an electrical burn. (Courtesy of J. Barry, M.D., Seattle, Washington, and J. Ogden, M.D., Tampa, Florida.)

formities such as clinodactyly are described.[80] Secondary infection with osteomyelitis and septic arthritis, nonunion of pathologic fractures, neuropathic osteoarthropathy, and contracture with joint subluxation or dislocation also have been described. Periarticular calcification and ossification (Fig. 72–13), and intra-articular bony ankylosis may eliminate joint motion.[55] Some of these osseous and soft tissue changes have been reproduced experimentally.[60]

Differential Diagnosis

The radiographic findings occurring after this type of injury represent a combination of thermal, mechanical, and electrical effects on bones and joints. They are complicated by vascular and neurologic damage and secondary infection. The resulting radiographic picture is nonspecific; some of the imaging abnormalities are identical to those occurring after trauma from any cause, whereas others resemble those of septic arthritis, neuropathic osteoarthropathy, osteoporosis, thermal burns, frostbite, and neurologic deficit.

SUMMARY

The radiographic features of the skeleton after thermal and electrical injuries can be varied (Table 72–1). In many cases, they are not specific and must be interpreted with knowledge of the mechanism of injury. Of particular interest are the appearance of epiphyseal abnormalities in frostbite, periarticular calcification and ossification after thermal burns, and pathologic fractures in the electrocuted person.

TABLE 72–1. Radiographic Findings Associated with Thermal and Electrical Injuries

Soft tissue swelling, loss, or contracture
Osteoporosis
Acro-osteolysis
Periostitis
Epiphyseal injury and growth disturbance
Articular abnormalities
Periarticular calcification and ossification
Osteolysis, osteosclerosis, and fracture

References

1. Meryman HT: Tissue freezing and local cold injury. Physiol Rev *37*:233, 1957.
2. Ungley CC: The immersion foot syndrome. Adv Surg *1*:209, 1949.
3. Brauer RW, Behnke AR: Hypothermia and cold injury. *In* TR Harrison, et al (Eds): Principles of Internal Medicine. 4th Ed. New York, McGraw-Hill Book Co, 1962, p 835.
4. Bellman S, Adams-Ray J: Vascular reactions after experimental cold injury. A microangiographic study on rabbit ears. Angiology *7*:339, 1956.
5. Hurley LA: Angioarchitectural changes associated with rapid rewarming subsequent to freezing injury. Angiology *8*:19, 1957.
6. Martinez A, Golding M, Sawyer PN, et al: The specific arterial lesions in mild and severe frostbite: Effect of sympathectomy. J Cardiovasc Surg *7*:495, 1966.
7. Edwards EA, Leeper RW: Frostbite: An analysis of seventy-one cases. JAMA *149*:1199, 1952.
8. Quintanilla R, Krusen FH, Essex HE: Studies on frostbite with special reference to treatment and the effect on minute blood vessels. Am J Physiol *149*:149, 1947.
9. Gralino BJ, Porter JM, Rosch J: Angiography in the diagnosis and therapy of frostbite. Radiology *119*:301, 1976.
10. Tishler J: The soft tissue and bone changes in frostbite injuries. Radiology *102*:511, 1972.
11. Smith SP, Walker WF: Arteriography in cold injury. Br J Radiol *37*:471, 1964.
12. Erikson U, Ponten B: The possible value of arteriography supplemented by a vasodilator agent in the early assessment of tissue viability in frostbite. Injury *6*:150, 1974.
13. Likhoded VI: Angiografiia v diagnostike otmorozhenii. Vestn Khir *110*:90, 1973.
14. Bigelow DR, Ritchie GW: The effects of frostbite in childhood. J Bone Joint Surg [Br] *45*:122, 1963.
15. Bennett RB, Blount WP: Destruction of epiphyses by freezing. JAMA *105*:661, 1935.
16. Dreyfuss JR, Glimcher MJ: Epiphyseal injury following frostbite. N Engl J Med *253*:1065, 1955.
17. Florkiewicz L, Kozlowski K: Symmetrical epiphyseal destruction by frostbite. Arch Dis Child *37*:51, 1962.
18. Thelander HE: Epiphyseal destruction by frostbite. J Pediatr *36*:105, 1950.
19. Wenzl JE, Burke EC, Bianco AJ: Epiphyseal destruction from frostbite of the hands. Am J Dis Child *114*:668, 1967.
20. Selke AC Jr: Destruction of phalangeal epiphyses by frostbite. Radiology *93*:859, 1969.
21. Ellis R, Short JG, Simonds BD: Unilateral osteoarthritis of the distal interphalangeal joints following frostbite. A case report. Radiology *93*:857, 1969.
22. Blair JR, Schatzki P, Orr KD: Sequelae to cold injury in one hundred patients. A follow-up study four years after occurrence of cold injury. JAMA *163*:1203, 1957.
23. Schumacher HR Jr: Unilateral osteoarthritis of the hand. JAMA *191*:246, 1965.
24. Sessions DG, Stallings JO, Mills WJ Jr, et al: Frostbite of the ear. Laryngoscope *81*:1223, 1971.
25. Yeh CW, Chan KF: Case report 87. Skel Radiol *4*:49, 1979.
26. Lisbona R, Rosenthall L: Assessment of bone viability by scintiscanning in frostbite injuries. J Trauma *16*:989, 1976.
27. Thiemann H: Juvenile Epiphysenstorungen. ROFO *14*:79, 1909.
28. Giedion A: Acrodysplasias: Cone-shaped epiphyses, peripheral dysostosis, Thiemann's disease, and acrodysostosis. Progr Pediatr Radiol *4*:325, 1973.
29. Shaw EW: Avascular necrosis of the phalanges of the hand (Thiemann's disease). JAMA *156*:711, 1954.
30. Order SE, Moncrief JA: The Burn Wound. Springfield, Ill, Charles C Thomas, 1965.
31. Foley FD: Pathology of cutaneous burns. Surg Clin North Am *50*:1201, 1970.
32. Brown HC: Current concepts of burn pathology and mechanisms of deformity in the burned hand. Orthop Clin North Am *4*:987, 1973.
33. Evans EB, Smith JR: Bone and joint changes following burns. A roentgenographic study—preliminary report. J Bone Joint Surg [Am] *41*:785, 1959.
34. Owens N: Osteoporosis following burns. Br J Plast Surg *1*:245, 1949.
35. Colson P, Stagnara P, Houot H: L'ostéoporose chez les brûlés membres. Lyon Chir *48*:950, 1953.
36. Rabinov D: Acromutilation of the fingers following severe burns. Radiology *77*:968, 1961.
37. Boyd BM Jr, Roberts WM, Miller GR: Peri-articular ossification following burns. South Med J *52*:1048, 1959.

38. Evans EB: Orthopaedic measures in the treatment of severe burns. J Bone Joint Surg [Am] 48:643, 1966.
39. Schiele HP, Hubbard RB, Bruck HM: Radiographic changes in burns of the upper extremity. Radiology 104:13, 1972.
40. Johnson JTH: Atypical myositis ossificans. J Bone Joint Surg [Am] 39:189, 1957.
41. Schwartz EE, Weiss W, Plotkin R: Ankylosis of the temporomandibular joint following burn. JAMA 235:1477, 1976.
42. Pellicci PM, Wilson PD Jr: Chondrolysis of the hips associated with severe burns. A case report. J Bone Joint Surg [Am] 61:592, 1979.
43. Artz CP, Reiss E: The Treatment of Burns. Philadelphia, WB Saunders Co, 1957, p 169.
44. Thaxter TH, Mann RA: Factors contributing to the degeneration of immobilized normal synovial joints in rats. J Bone Joint Surg [Am] 46:921, 1964.
45. Trias A: Effects of persistent pressure on the articular cartilage. An experimental study. J Bone Joint Surg [Br] 43:376, 1961.
46. Salter RB, Field P: The effects of continuous compression on living articular cartilage. J Bone Joint Surg [Am] 42:31, 1960.
47. Cruess RL: The pathology of acute necrosis of cartilage in slipping of the capital femoral epiphysis. A report of two cases with pathological sections. J Bone Joint Surg [Am] 45:1013, 1963.
48. Maurer RC, Larsen IJ: Acute necrosis of cartilage in slipped capital femoral epiphysis. J Bone Joint Surg [Am] 52:39, 1970.
49. Heppenstall RB, Marvel JP Jr, Chung SMK, et al: Chondrolysis of the hip joint—usual and unusual presentations. J Bone Joint Surg [Am] 55:1308, 1973.
50. Jackson D: Acquired vertical talus due to burn contractures. A report of two cases. J Bone Joint Surg [Br] 60:215, 1978.
51. Maclachlan W: Electrical injuries. J Ind Hyg 16:52, 1934.
52. Langworthy OR, Kouwenhoven WB: An experimental study of abnormalities produced in the organism by electricity. J Ind Hyg 12:31, 1930.
53. Bennett IL Jr: Electrical injury. In TR Harrison, et al (Eds): Principles of Internal Medicine. 4th Ed. New York, McGraw-Hill Book Co, 1962, p 855.
54. Pearl FL: Electric shock: Presentation of cases and review of the literature. Arch Surg 27:227, 1933.
55. Brinn LB, Moseley JE: Bone changes following electrical injury. Case report and review of literature. AJR 97:682, 1966.
56. Kolar J, Vrabec R: Roentgenological bone findings after high voltage injury. ROFO 92:385, 1960.
57. Jellinek S: Roentgen bone changes found in the treatment of electrical accidents. Wien Med Wochenschr 79:543, 1929.
58. Jellinek S: Changes in electrically injured bones: Examined microscopically and by x-rays. Br J Radiol 31:23, 1926.
59. Barber JW: Delayed bone and joint changes following electrical injury. Radiology 99:49, 1971.
60. Granberry WM, Janes JM: The effect of electrical current on the epiphyseal cartilage: A preliminary experimental study. Proc Mayo Clin 38:87, 1963.
61. Ogden JA, Southwick WO: Electrical injury involving the immature skeleton. Skel Radiol 6:187, 1981.
62. Clark GS, Naso F, Ditunno JF Jr: Marked bone spur formation in a burn amputee patient. Arch Phys Med Rehabil 61:189, 1976.
63. Carrera GF, Kozin F, McCarty DJ: Arthritis after frostbite injury in children. Arthritis Rheum 22:1082, 1979.
64. Glick R, Parhami N: Frostbite arthritis. J Rheumatol 6:456, 1979.
65. Carrera GF, Kozin F, Flaherty L, et al: Radiographic changes in the hands following childhood frostbite injury. Skel Radiol 6:33, 1981.
66. Brown FE, Spiegel PK, Boyle WE Jr: Digital deformity: An effect of frostbite in children. Pediatrics 71:955, 1983.
67. McKendry RJR: Frostbite arthritis. Can Med Assoc J 125:1128, 1981.
68. Purdue GF, Lewis SA, Hunt JL: Pyrophosphate scanning in early frostbite injury. Am Surg 49:619, 1983.
69. Salimi Z, Vas W, Tang-Barton P, et al: Assessment of tissue viability in frostbite by 99mTc pertechnetate scintigraphy. AJR 142:415, 1984.
70. Rosenthall L, Kloiber R, Gagnon R, et al: Frostbite with rhabdomyolysis and renal failure: Radionuclide study. AJR 137:387, 1981.
71. Foray J, Schmitt M, Renaud S: Thermographie et gelures de montagne. Chirurgie 106:301, 1980.
72. Maroteaux P: Cinq observations d'une affection microgeodique des phalanges du nourrisson d'etiologie inconnue. Ann Radiol 13:229, 1970.
73. Sweet EM, Smith MGH: "Winter fingers." Bone infarction in Scottish children as a manifestation of cold injury. Ann Radiol 22:71, 1979.
74. MacCarthy J, O'Brien N: Phalangeal microgeodic syndrome of infancy. Arch Dis Child 51:472, 1976.
75. Sugiura Y, Kaneko M, Kataoka O, et al: Bone changes of unknown etiology affecting phalanges of fingers in children. Pediatr Radiol 4:243, 1976.
76. Kaibara N, Masuda S, Katsuk I, et al: Phalangeal microgeodic syndrome in childhood: Report of seven cases and review of the literature. Eur J Pediatr 136:41, 1981.
77. Meller Y, Bar-Ziv J, Goldstein J, et al: Phalangeal microgeodic syndrome in childhood. A case report. Acta Orthop Scand 53:553, 1982.
78. Jay MS, Saphyakhajon P, Scott R, et al: Bone and joint changes following burn injury. Clin Pediatr 20:734, 1981.
79. Salisbury RE, Dingeldein GP: Peripheral nerve complications following burn injury. Clin Orthop 163:92, 1982.
80. Fingerhut A, Brocard M, Ronat R: Clinodactylie par brulure electrique. Quelques reflexions à propos de deux cas. Ann Chir Main 1:347, 1982.
81. Thompson JC, Ashwal S: Electrical injuries in children. Am J Dis Child 137:231, 1983.
82. Salem MI: Bilateral anterior fracture-dislocation of the shoulder joints due to severe electric shock. Injury 14:361, 1983.
83. Beswick DR, Morse SD, Barnes AU: Bilateral scapular fractures from low-voltage electrical injury. Ann Emerg Med 11:676, 1982.
84. Schmidt H, Barfred T: Caterpillar dermatitis of the palm associated with osteitis of finger bones. Acta Derm Venereol 59(Suppl 89):157, 1979.
85. Seth MK, Khurana JK: Bony ankylosis of the elbow after burns. J Bone Joint Surg [Br] 67:747, 1985.
86. Nakazato T, Ogino T: Epiphyseal destruction of children's hands after frostbite: A report of two cases. J Hand Surg [Am] 11:289, 1986.
87. Salimi Z, Wolverson MK, Herbold DR, et al: Frostbite: Experimental assessment of tissue damage using Tc-99m pyrophosphate. Work in progress. Radiology 161:227, 1986.
88. Kolář J: Locomotor consequences of electrical and radiation injuries, burns, and freezings. Clin Rheumatol 3:99, 1989.
89. Mehta RC, Wilson MA: Frostbite injury: Prediction of tissue viability with triple-phase bone scanning. Radiology 170:511, 1989.
90. Puzas JE, Miller MD, Rosier RN: Pathologic bone formation. Clin Orthop 245:269, 1989.
91. Evans EB: Heterotopic bone formation in thermal burns. Clin Orthop 263:94, 1991.
92. Elledge ES, Smith AA, McManus WF, et al: Heterotopic bone formation in burned patients. J Trauma 28:684, 1988.
93. Reed MH: Growth disturbances in the hands following thermal injuries in children. 2. Frostbite. J Can Assoc Radiol 39:95, 1988.
94. Nafs FJE, Aromir FC, Carreira IS, et al: High tension electrical burns. A review of 85 patients. Eur J Plast Surg 16:84, 1993.
95. Howard CB, Alkrinawi S, Gadalia A, et al: Bone infection resembling phalangeal microgeodic syndrome in children. A case report. J Hand Surg [Br] 18:491, 1993.

73

Radiation Changes

Murray K. Dalinka, M.D.,
and Tamara Miner Haygood, Ph.D., M.D.

The use of x-rays in diagnosis and therapy became well established shortly after Roentgen discovered these rays in 1895. Equipment for producing x-rays and forming photographic images was widely available, and within a year of Roentgen's publication of his discovery, the new technique was in clinical use, chiefly for diagnosis of fractures and localization of metallic foreign bodies.[1] Not everyone was pleased, however. An editorial in the London *Pall Mall Gazette* expressed indignation over the possibility of looking at others not merely without their clothing, but without their very flesh:

> We are sick of the röntgen ray; . . . you can see other people's bones with the naked eye, and also see through eight inches of solid wood. On the revolting indecency of this there is no need to dwell. But what we seriously put before the attention of the Government . . . that it will call for legislative restriction of the severest kind. Perhaps the best thing would be for all civilised nations to combine to burn all works on the röntgen rays, to execute all the discov-

erers, and to corner all the tungstate in the world and whelm it in the middle of the ocean.[2]

It soon became apparent to scientists that x-rays posed a threat to health as well as to privacy. Some of the deleterious effects of radiation were noted as early as 6 months following Roentgen's initial description, with the development of pigmentation, telangiectasia, fibrosis, alopecia, scarring, ulceration, and dermatitis.[2] Radiation-induced neoplasia was described in 1902 in a 33 year old demonstrator of x-ray tubes.[3]

Nonetheless, radiation, both x-rays and the natural emission of radium, found more uses in diagnosis, in therapy, and outside of medicine. Radium was even used recreationally to make objects, including food and drink, glow in the dark.[4] As people were exposed to radiation in large numbers and in varying ways, more of radiation's harmful effects became known. The widely publicized plight of radium watch dial painters in the 1930s was the beginning of the end of the American public's love of radiation. Now, though dial painters no longer lick radioactive paintbrushes and children no longer wiggle their toes in shoe-store fluoroscopes, the public has an exaggerated idea of risk[5] of radiation exposure.

This chapter describes the effects of radiation on the musculoskeletal system and attempts to relate them both in a historical context and in the context of the amount and type of exposure needed to produce them. It also discusses radiographic diagnosis and evaluation of radiation effects.

RADIUM

During the early twentieth century, the public had many opportunities for exposure to radium and related isotopes. Often exposure was occupational. Workers who painted luminous dials on watches pointed the paintbrushes with their lips and teeth, causing them to ingest luminous paint containing radium (^{226}Ra) and mesothorium (^{228}Ra). The average mixture of the isotopes was approximately 6 to 1 (mesothorium to radium), and the radiation dosage for the mixture was 10 times that of radium.[6] The fluorescence of the watch dials came from the bombardment of the zinc sulfide in the paint by the alpha particles of radium and mesothorium.

Radium has a half-life of 1622 years and emits continuous radiation, mostly alpha particles with a range of 40 μm in tissue. Mesothorium has a half-life of 6.7 years, and thorium, its major daughter product, has a half-life of 52 seconds.

Radium was used therapeutically, both orally and intravenously, in the treatment of many ailments between 1910 and 1930. Most parenteral and oral radium preparations were not contaminated with mesothorium.[7, 8] Radithor, a patent medicine, however, included mesothorium in approximately a 1:1 ratio with radium.[9] Radium became so popular that it was mixed into beverages and used in toothpaste and cleansers.[4]

Orally ingested radium is deposited mainly in the outer cortex of bone, with an irregular and generalized distribution.[10] With parenteral administration, the early peak blood level leads to "flush labeling" with an unequal distribution.[7] Both radium and mesothorium are deposited like calcium in the skeleton and can be leached back into the blood stream, becoming bound elsewhere in the skeletal system and causing deleterious effect wherever they go.

In 1924 Blum described radium jaw, a type of osteomyelitis, in radium dial painters.[11] In 1929 Martland and Humphries described osseous neoplasms in radium dial workers.[10] Similar neoplasms were later found as a consequence of oral and parenteral radium administration.[8] Squamous cell carcinomas of the mastoids and paranasal sinuses have been reported in dial workers.[7] This is not surprising in view of the proximity of the epithelium to underlying bone. These and other health problems in occupationally exposed persons eventually ended the popularity of radium use among the general public.[4]

Many of the deaths in radium dial workers were secondary to severe aplastic anemia. Loutit postulated that this anemia may have been aleukemic leukemia.[12] He thought that radium might have a direct effect on the bone marrow.[12]

A general correlation is seen between the bony lesions produced and the body burden of radium acquired. With a body burden of less than 0.1 μg of ^{226}Ra, no radiographic changes occur.[13] Bone neoplasms have been reported with doses greater than 0.4 μg of uncontaminated radium.[8] With time, the number and severity of osseous lesions increase.[7]

When large quantities of radium are deposited in bone for more than 20 years, mostly dead osteoid tissue remains. Normal bone physiology becomes erratic and large resorption cavities are formed.[8, 13] These cavities contain gelatinous material with osteoid-like matrix and appear as sharply defined bone lesions resembling those of multiple myeloma. They occur in the long bones (Fig. 73–1) and skull (Fig. 73–2) and increase in size with time. These areas of cortical resorption are due to constant alpha particle irradiation.[7]

Metaphyseal sclerosis is frequent, particularly in patients who ingest radium prior to physeal closure.[7] Areas of increased density probably represent the deposition of new bone on unresorbed trabeculae, a manifestation of bone ischemia due to vascular changes in the central arteries of

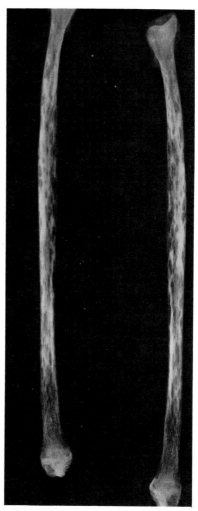

FIGURE 73–1. Radiograph of specimen from radium dial worker showing both fibulae with multiple resorption cavities within the shafts. Note the well-defined lucent lesions somewhat resembling those of multiple myeloma.

the haversian canals. These density changes may simulate those of Paget's disease, but the bone is of normal size.[7] Large areas of osteonecrosis indistinguishable from ischemic necrosis from other causes may be seen. Pathologic fractures can occur, and frequently they heal normally. Osteosarcomas (Fig. 73–3) and fibrosarcomas, sometimes multicentric, are seen. The average latent period of these sarcomas is 23 years. Carcinomas of the paranasal sinuses and mastoids also have been reported.[7]

THORIUM

Thorium dioxide in dextran (Thorotrast) was introduced as a contrast agent in 1928 and was widely used in the United States between 1930 and the early 1950s.[14, 15] Its clinically inert properties and high atomic number made it the agent of choice for hepatolienography, peripheral and cerebral angiography, and the opacification of body cavities.[15]

Extravasation of Thorotrast at the site of injection leads to continuous alpha particle irradiation, resulting in an expanding cicatricial mass, which invades contiguous struc-

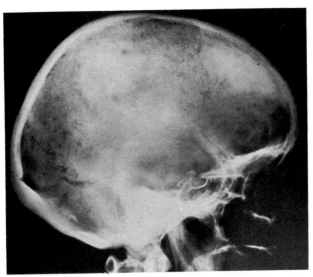

FIGURE 73–2. Skull of radium dial worker demonstrating multiple small lucent areas within the calvarium, mainly in the parietal region, simulating the lesions in multiple myeloma. (From Dalinka MK, et al: *Semin Roentgenol* 9:29, 1974.)

tures, leading to tissue destruction and vascular compromise.[16, 17] In addition to these "Thorotrastomas" (i.e., Thorotrast granulomas), sarcomas, including extraskeletal chondrosarcomas and osteosarcomas, have been described at the extravasation sites.[16, 18, 19]

Thorotrast is a colloidal suspension that is phagocytized by the reticuloendothelial system, with 70 per cent deposited in the liver, 20 per cent in the spleen, and 1.5 to 3 per cent in the subendosteal cancellous bone.[20] It has a physical half-life of 1.4×10^{10} years and a biologic half-life of 400 years; hence, the liver, spleen, and bone marrow are subjected to continuous low-dose alpha radiation. The reticuloendothelial system and adjacent tissues are therefore at risk for radiation-induced neoplasia, particularly hemangioendothelial sarcoma of the liver.[20]

Jee and coworkers have studied the distribution of thorium and its daughter products in bone.[21] Histologic and autoradiographic studies demonstrated that most of the Thorotrast was deposited along the endosteum. The weekly bone marrow exposure of a 25 ml injection of Thorotrast was calculated at 0.3 centigray (cGy) (rad).[22] Irradiation leads to thickened trabeculae and sclerosis adjacent to the endosteum, probably owing to vascular ischemia. Diffuse osteosclerosis, bone marrow aplasia, and osteomalacia have been described by Murphy and colleagues.[23]

The injection of Thorotrast into growing children may give rise to a "bone-within-bone" or "ghost vertebra" appearance[24] (Fig. 73–4). The Thorotrast deposition causes constant alpha radiation and temporary growth arrest. The size of the ghost vertebra corresponds to the vertebral size at the time of injection.[24]

Sindelar and associates reviewed five patients with skeletal sarcomas after Thorotrast injection. Four patients had osteosarcomas and one had a vertebral fibrosarcoma.[25] These tumors occurred at least 16 years after administration of the contrast agent. Three of these patients demonstrated thorium within the vicinity of the tumor on autoradiography.

EFFECTS OF RADIATION THERAPY

Bone Growth

The effects of radiation on bone growth were first demonstrated in 1903, when Perthes showed that the growth of chick wings was retarded by radiation.[26, 27] In 1906, Fösterling demonstrated gross impairment of the growth of rabbits after radiation to the upper half of the body.[28] The effects of radiation on bone growth in humans were reported in the German literature in 1929 by Hueck and Spiess[29, 30]; Desjardins[31] and Bisgard and Hunt[32] reported similar changes in the United States.

The epiphysis is the area of the bone most sensitive to radiation.[26, 33, 34] Microscopic changes may occur with a dose as low as 300 cGy, and decreased growth can occur with as little as 400 cGy.[26] The histologic changes can be demonstrated as early as 2 to 4 days after therapy.[34] The early radiation effects are in the zone of provisional calcification, which shows a decrease in the number of chondrocytes and an abnormal columnar arrangement of the cartilage cells. Swelling, pyknosis, and fragmentation of the chondrocytes occur, as well as chondrocyte degeneration with irregular, faintly stained cells.[34] With a low dose of 600 to 1200 cGy, rapid histologic recovery occurs. Secondary changes are limited, but some residua may remain.[35]

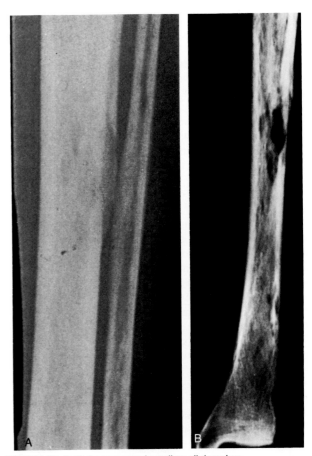

FIGURE 73–3. Osteosarcoma in radium dial worker.

A Radiograph demonstrating a lytic lesion in tibia with poorly defined resorption cavities in the shaft.

B Radiograph of amputated specimen showing lytic osteosarcoma. The resorption cavities now are well visualized.

(From Dalinka MK, et al: *Semin Roentgenol* 9:29, 1974.)

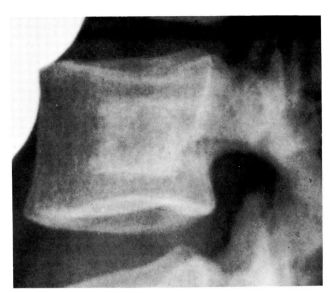

FIGURE 73–4. Coned-down view of lumbar vertebra showing bone-within-bone appearance in patient injected with Thorotrast at the age of 3 years. (From Teplick JG, et al: Radiology *129*:657, 1978.)

With 1200 cGy or more, the damage is increased and is maximal to the chondroblasts. Delayed changes take 6 months or longer to appear and are dose related.[34, 36] Late changes may occur secondary to vascular damage and include premature cartilage degeneration and bone marrow atrophy.[34] Although these changes had been attributed to vascular damage,[34] other studies have shown that the underlying vasculature is normal and the changes are related to cellular injury.[37] The dose-related changes are decreased with protraction. Growth impairment is related to the age of the animal or patient, with the effect of the given dose being greater at a younger age. The greater the growth potential of a particular bone, the more drastic is the effect. Any skeletal part capable of growth that is exposed to 2000 cGy or more will show growth disturbances.[38]

Rubin and Casarett have shown that when the entire bone is irradiated, a decrease in overall size and diameter is seen, simulating osteogenesis imperfecta.[34] If only the epiphysis is irradiated, growth deformity with a decrease in width resembling achondroplasia occurs. Irradiation of the metaphysis leads to a bowing deformity, whereas diaphyseal irradiation causes a narrow shaft with normal cortical diameter.

The effects of radiation generally are independent of their method of production and can be produced by internal or external sources.[39, 40] Actually, with radium or radioactive isotopes, the effects tend to be greater than with external radiation.[41] In growing bone the quality of radiation is of little significance, as cartilage is almost of water density and there is no differential absorption.[29, 42] The larger the field irradiated, the greater the effects.

Reidy and coworkers showed that a decrease occurring in overall length and growth rate slowed after epiphyseal irradiation in dogs.[33] In pediatric patients, irradiation of the growing epiphysis or apophysis may cause shortening of long bones or hypoplasia of the ilium. In the 1930s and early 1940s this property was used deliberately to decrease growth in the longer limbs of patients with unequal limb

length.[43–45] In the 1930s, case reports also began to appear of limb shortening complicating therapeutic irradiation.[29, 46] In 1950 Frantz reported a patient with marked shortening of an extremity after treatment of a soft tissue hemangioma.[43] The treated bone had a decrease in shaft diameter, cortical thickness, and overall bone length. Despite decreased use of radiation in childhood malignancies owing to development of chemotherapeutic regimens that have partially replaced radiation, leg-length discrepancy remains a problem in long-term survivors of lower extremity and pelvic tumors. Robertson and colleagues found leg-length inequality in 12 of 67 patients who underwent pelvic or lower extremity irradiation and survived to skeletal maturity. Seven of the 12 had a discrepancy in leg length sufficient to cause symptoms.[47]

Growth arrest may occur in flat bones as in long bones. When the skull or face is included in the radiation field, facial deformities may result, which can be difficult to correct and are damaging psychologically.[48, 49]

Widening of the growth plate has been described as early as 1 to 2 months after treatment (Fig. 73–5). If mild, this returns to normal after approximately 6 months.[50] Joint space widening also has been reported 8 to 10 months after therapy. Metaphyseal changes, including irregularity (Fig. 73–6), fraying, and sclerosis (Fig. 73–7), may resemble superficially those of rickets (Fig. 73–8). Patients with metaphyseal changes may develop a broad band of increased density, which may be a manifestation of repair. Its absence may predict substantial limb shortening. These metaphyseal alterations can resolve, leading to normal trabeculae.

In humans, the diaphysis is relatively resistant to radiation, and periosteal new bone formation is affected less than enchondral bone formation.[26] Dawson thought that growth impairment did not occur after radiation of the shaft of long bones if the epiphysis was spared.[26] The degree of sensitivity depended on the bone involved.[26] Osteoporosis was a frequent and nonspecific finding.[26]

Slipped Capital Femoral Epiphysis

Wolf and associates[51] and Rubin and Casarett[34] have reported slipped capital femoral epiphysis as a sequel to radiation therapy (Fig. 73–9). In these patients, the femoral head was included in the field of therapy. The damaged growth plate was not able to withstand the shearing stresses of growth, leading to epiphyseal slippage.[29, 51, 52] Radiation-induced slipped epiphyses usually occur at an earlier age than the idiopathic variety[51] and may be seen in patients who do not conform to the typical age and body habitus of most children with idiopathic slipped capital femoral epiphysis.[53] Ryan and Walters[55] and Dickerman and colleagues[54] believe that the chemotherapy administered along with the radiation may contribute to the toxicity to the growth cartilage, leading to the slipped capital femoral epiphysis. In one study,[56] significant radiation-induced abnormalities of the pediatric hip were found in eight of 44 patients, aged 16 years or younger at the time of therapy; these changes consisted of aseptic necrosis (six patients), slipped capital femoral epiphysis (three patients), and osteosarcoma (one patient). Six of these eight patients also received chemotherapy, however, which may have had a synergistic ef-

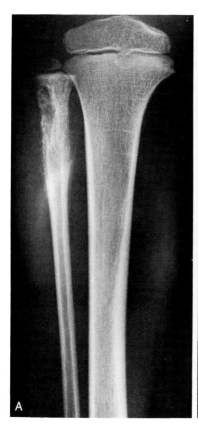
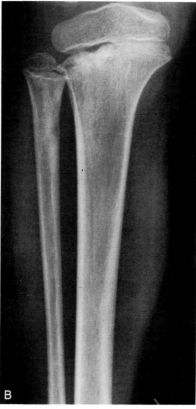

FIGURE 73–5. Ewing's tumor prior to and after radiation therapy.
 A Ewing's tumor of proximal portion of the fibula with destructive metaphyseal and diaphyseal lesion and layered periosteal new bone formation.
 B Same patient 6 months after radiation therapy. There is widening of the cartilaginous growth plate in the lateral aspect of the tibia and adjacent fibula. Note the dense metaphyseal band in the tibia.

fect.[56] Walker and collaborators advocated prophylactic percutaneous pinning in patients with a widened physeal plate and metaphyseal sclerosis as a means of preventing epiphyseal slippage.[53]

Rarely, changes secondary to radiation therapy in children may not be manifest clinically until adulthood. Bilateral ischemic necrosis of the femoral head has been reported in a 25 year old patient who was treated with 2200 cGy to the pelvis at the age of 13 months.[57] Other changes occurring when the acetabulum or femoral head, or both, are included in the radiation port include iliac hypoplasia, acetabular dysplasia, coxa vara and coxa valga, and leg shortening.[36, 57]

Scoliosis

Engel produced scoliosis in rabbits, dogs, and goats by implanting radium needles unilaterally in the spine.[58] They found loss of vertebral height and destruction of the adjacent bone marrow in the irradiated area. The disc cartilage was two to three times thicker on the irradiated side as it hypertrophied to compensate for the bone loss.

Arkin and Simon used radon seeds and asymmetric external beam irradiation to produce scoliosis in rabbits.[59] A single dose of 1000 cGy was sufficient. Histologically, the vertebra demonstrated an absence of cartilaginous columns and an irregular zone of provisional calcification. No gross or microscopic evidence of necrosis, inflammation, or marrow fibrosis was found.

Arkin and colleagues reported the first case of radiation-induced scoliosis in humans.[60] The patient developed an isolated lumbar scoliosis with uniform wedging of the vertebral bodies after therapy to the back for melanotic nevi.

In 1952, Neuhauser and coworkers described the effects of radiation on the growing spine in 45 patients treated for abdominal malignancies, with autopsy data for 11 patients and radiographic data for 34 patients.[38] The radiographic findings were dose related. No radiologic abnormalities were seen in patients treated with less than 1000 cGy. Those children receiving 1000 to 2000 cGy developed changes secondary to growth arrest. These changes, which occurred 9 to 12 months after therapy, consisted of horizontal lines of increased density, which were parallel to the vertebral endplates; on occasion, a "bone-within-bone" appearance was noted. These abnormalities were not confined to the treatment field and hence were related to the general effect on bone growth. Alternatively, irreversible changes of irregularity and scalloping of the vertebral endplates were confined to the irradiated area and became evident at a dose between 2000 and 3000 cGy. They were associated with decreased vertebral height and abnormality of bone contour (Fig. 73–10). The changes were more severe in patients treated prior to the age of 2 years; hence, the effects of radiation were believed to be both dose- and age-related.

The earliest histologic changes occur in the zone of provisional calcification. The gross aberrations are not detected until the osseous changes take place, usually at least a year after therapy.[35] Bony abnormalities may occur earlier if the patient is treated with over 3000 cGy or prior to 18 months of age.[34, 61]

Neuhauser and associates found a mild, nonprogressive scoliosis to be common in their patients, and they suggested that radiation of the entire vertebral body would eliminate the scoliosis (Fig. 73–11).[38] These authors and later Whitehouse and Lampe[62] suggested that spinal complications could be minimized by protracting the course of radiation

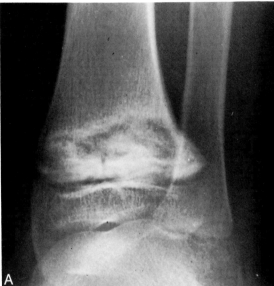

FIGURE 73–6. Radiation-induced lesion of distal tibial metaphysis in patient after therapy for Ewing's tumor of proximal end of the tibia.

A Six months after completion of therapy, a lucent lesion is observed in the distal metaphysis, which is well defined, having sclerotic margins. A small fracture also is present.

B Six months after **A,** the lesion has filled in with normal-appearing bone. A lucent band is present at the proximal extent of the lesion.

C Five months after **B,** little change has occurred in the appearance of the lesion.

(Reprinted with permission from Dalinka MK, Mazzeo VP Jr: CRC Crit Rev Diagn Imaging *23*:235, 1985. Copyright CRC Press, Inc, Boca Raton, FL.)

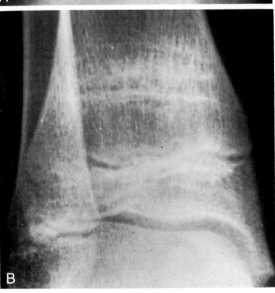

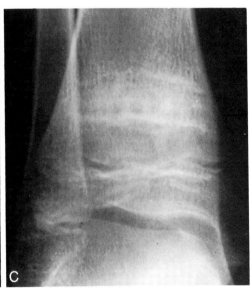

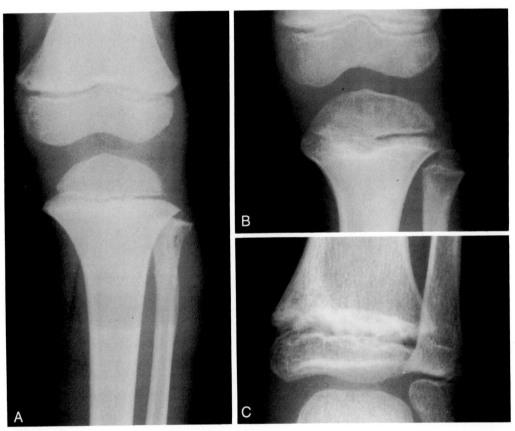

FIGURE 73–7. Radiation therapy for Ewing's tumor.

A Frontal view of the knee shows destructive lesion in the proximal portion of the fibula, which represented a Ewing's tumor.

B Fifteen months after whole bone radiation for Ewing's sarcoma, the lesion in the fibula has healed. Slight widening of the growth plate is seen, mainly in the tibia.

C In this same patient, metaphyseal sclerosis extending to the diaphysis with slight widening of the growth plate is evident in the distal portion of the tibia.

(Courtesy of P. Borns, M.D., Philadelphia, Pennsylvania.)

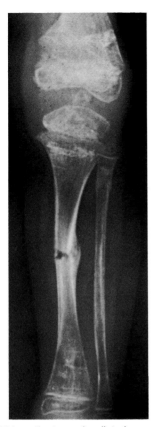

FIGURE 73–8. This patient was irradiated approximately 2 years prior to this film for leukemia and knee pain. The treated field included most of the tibia as well as the knee. A fracture through the midshaft of the tibia is seen with periosteal reaction about it. Periosteal reaction also is noted about the midshaft of the fibula. Metaphyseal irregularity of the distal end of the femur is present, with deformity secondary to radiation therapy. Diffuse osteopenia also is present. (Courtesy of P. Borns, M.D., Wilmington, Delaware.)

It also has become apparent that radiation-induced scoliosis can be progressive, particularly when high doses are given to young patients.[68] Progression occurs during the adolescent growth spurt.[68] In Riseborough and colleagues' study, adolescent progression of scoliosis occurred despite treatment with Milwaukee bracing. Surgical therapy with Harrington rods was necessary in eight of 57 scoliotic patients. The degree of scoliosis was not proportional to the changes in the vertebral body. Kyphosis occurred in 21 of 81 patients and usually was associated with scoliosis. An increased prevalence of pseudarthrosis occurred after surgical therapy for kyphoscoliosis. Other authors also have noted the development of postradiation kyphosis.[69]

Scoliosis is most likely to be the consequence of a combination of factors, including "fall off" at the edge of the x-ray beam, changes in the small blood vessels, and fibrosis of the overlying soft tissues.[48, 61, 70]

Radiation-induced decrease in axial growth of the vertebral bodies may occur independently of development of scoliosis.[42, 71] This usually takes place after irradiation of patients less than 6 years old or at puberty. The decreased growth might be overlooked if sitting heights are not measured. Children receiving more than 3500 cGy show a decrease in sitting height, whereas those receiving less than 2500 cGy do not.

The effects of radiation on growing bone have important radiotherapeutic implications. Growth disturbances largely are independent of the quality of radiation.[29, 42] The major radiation changes occur in the fine physeal blood vessels and chondroblasts, which both are of unit density material and therefore affected equally by all types of radiation.

In radiotherapy, the radiation field size should be as small as possible. When treating the spine, the entire vertebral body is included. The iliac crest apophysis should be shielded if possible, as it is responsible for 40 per cent of the growth of the ilium.

Radiation Necrosis

The pathologic effects of radiation are independent of their method of production. The effects of radiation in mature bone are mainly on the osteoblasts, with the primary event being decreased matrix production.[72, 73] Immediate or delayed cell death, injury with recovery, arrest of cellular division, abnormal repair, or neoplasia may occur.[39, 40] These changes may be seen after exposure to either internal or external sources of radiation.

Ewing used the term "radiation osteitis" to define the effects of radiation on bone.[74] He classified radiation changes into different stages, which were dose related. Abnormalities included temporary cessation of growth with recovery, periostitis, bone sclerosis with increased fragility, ischemic necrosis, and infection with osteoradionecrosis. Ewing also described a loss of vascularity associated with obliterative periarteritis and endarteritis. Some later studies have contradicted these findings and have found that blood vessels are not altered significantly after high doses of radiation.[34, 75]

Rubin and Casarett thought that osteonecrosis of mature bone and cartilage was due to a combination of irradiation, infection, and trauma, with irradiation causing a susceptibility to damage by other noxious stimuli.[75]

Howland and coworkers believed that radiation causes

with small daily doses. Vaeth and coworkers, studying patients who had been irradiated for Wilms' tumor, believed that the scoliosis was mild and nonprogressive.[63] Incidentally, they also found that four of six women in their series conceived after therapy, and all six had normal menses.

In many later series, however, scoliosis occurred despite therapy to the entire vertebral body (Figs. 73–12 and 73–13) and even megavoltage therapy.[64–66] Nonetheless, scrupulous inclusion of the entire vertebral body may mitigate the resulting scoliosis. Mayfield and collaborators, studying a group of long-term survivors of neuroblastoma, found that asymmetric irradiation was associated with more frequent deformities and more severe curves.[67] Other factors also may affect the severity of scoliosis. Rubin and coworkers[34, 61] and Katzman and associates[76] stated that the scoliosis was more severe if osseous involvement was present prior to therapy. In Mayfield and coworkers' series, severity of scoliosis varied not only with symmetric or asymmetric inclusion of the vertebral body but also with dose. Fifty-seven per cent of children treated at an average age of 17 months with orthovoltage radiation had radiation-induced spinal deformity. In general, a dose less than 2000 cGy produced no deformity. A dose between 2000 and 3000 cGy was associated with a scoliosis of not more than 20 degrees. A dose of over 3000 cGy produced a curvature greater than 20 degrees.[67]

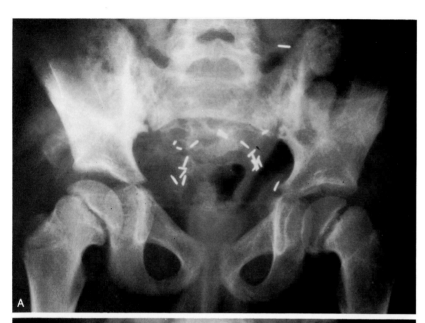

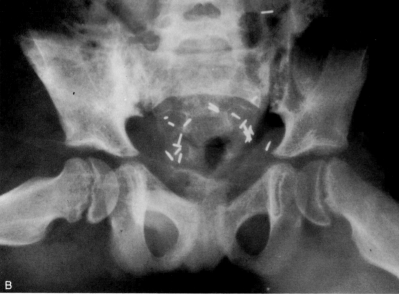

FIGURE 73–9. Slipped capital femoral epiphysis after radiation therapy. **A,** Anteroposterior (AP) view. **B,** Frog-leg lateral view of the pelvis in an 8 year old child after radiation therapy for an embryonal rhabdomyosarcoma. The pelvis was treated with 5940 centigrays (cGy) with a femoral shield added at 4500 cGy. Note the slipped epiphysis on the left side. The right sacroiliac joint has sclerotic margins also secondary to the radiation therapy. (Courtesy of A. Newburg, M.D., Boston, Massachusetts.)

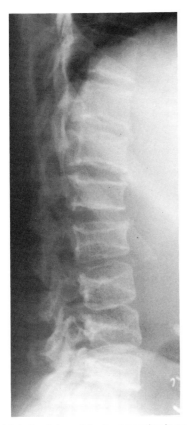

FIGURE 73–10. Lateral view of the lumbar spine in patient irradiated for Ewing's tumor at an early age. The five lumbar vertebrae are decreased considerably in height. The height of the twelfth dorsal vertebra also is decreased slightly. The other thoracic vertebrae appear normal as they were not included within the irradiated field.

bone atrophy, not necrosis; secondary infection must be present for true necrosis to occur.[72, 73] The atrophy is followed by repair. Attempts at regeneration result in the deposition of new bone on the unresorbed ischemic trabeculae.[96] A mottled appearance results with a mixture of osteoporosis, increased density, and coarse trabeculation.[96] Fractures through the osteopenic bone may heal normally, as true necrosis is absent.[77]

The osseous changes are secondary to destruction of the osteoblasts, which disappear after therapy.[37, 72] Vascular damage may contribute to the late radiation changes.[75] The bony abnormalities are dependent on the dosage, quality of the x-ray beam, method of fractionation, length of time after therapy, specific bone or bones involved, and the superimposition of trauma or infection.[75]

The quality of the x-ray beam determines the energy absorption and hence the radiation effect. With orthovoltage therapy, bone absorbs more energy per unit volume than other tissues. This increase in absorption may be as high as 30 to 40 per cent.[78] The high calcium content of bone may lead to secondary effects from the scattered radiation.[78] This causes more damage to the periosteum, blood vessels, and endosteal cells than if they were surrounded by soft tissues. With orthovoltage, the changes are caused mainly by the photoelectric effect, which mostly is scattered radiation dependent on the third power of the atomic number. With supervoltage therapy, the Compton effect predominates, and it is independent of the atomic number of the tissue

irradiated. The absorbed dose in bone is similar to the exposure dose. Supervoltage therapy also may allow effective tumor doses to be reached with smaller fields, causing less damage to the surrounding structures.

Radiation effects in mature bone, like those in growing bone, are dose related—the larger the dose, the greater the effect. In the 1940s Woodard and Coley[79] found that permanent damage to mature bone was very unusual at doses below 3000 cGy. Doses between 3000 and 5000 cGy caused permanent damage, and at doses over 5000 cGy cell death and permanent devitalization of bone occurred. The issue was complicated, however, by inconsistent reporting of doses by various authors.[79] In 1969, Ellis derived a formula relating the total dose, number of fractions, and treatment time to a nominal single dose (NSD).[80] The empirically derived formula is as follows:

$$TD = NSD \times N^{0.24} \times T^{0.11}$$
(Total dose)   (Number of fractions)   (Treatment time in days)

This formula was based on extensive clinical data and radiobiologic principles.[80] The NSD is of value in comparing different treatment regimens.[80, 81] Montague believed that the margin of tolerance was narrow and clinical trials were necessary before changes in fractionation were established.[82] Individual and geometric field variations were such that complete reliance should not be placed on empirical formulas.

Rubin[83] attempted to define radiation tolerance doses using minimal and maximal values. A minimal tolerance dose (TD5/5) is that which produces not more than 5 per cent of serious complications in the first 5 years after treatment. The maximal tolerance dose (TD50/5) is that dose which produces 50 per cent of serious complications during the first 5 years after treatment. Using these definitions, the value of TD5/5 for cartilage and bone during growth is 1000 and 2000 cGy, respectively, whereas the TD50/5 is 3000 cGy for each tissue. For adult cartilage and bone, however, TD5/5 (necrosis, fracture) is 6000 cGy in each case, and the TD50/5 is 10,000 and 15,000 cGy, respectively. This points to the greater sensitivity of bone and cartilage in children than in adults.

The temporal relationships vary with different bones. Mandibular osteonecrosis frequently become manifest within a year after therapy, whereas in most other sites the latent period is longer. Minimal changes usually occur at least a year after treatment and are slowly progressive. When fractures occur in irradiated bone, other radiation changes usually are present.

In a series of 100 patients, Bragg and coworkers found that the vast majority of cases of radiation osteitis occurred in the mandible (32 per cent), with the clavicle (18 per cent), humeral head (14 per cent), ribs (9 per cent), and femur (9 per cent) also well represented.[78]

Regional Effects

Mandible. Osteonecrosis is considerably more common in the mandible than in the maxilla because of its compact bone and poor blood supply.[84–86] The mandible, owing to its superficial location, receives a large dose of radiation in the treatment of intraoral cancer.[87] A high complication rate

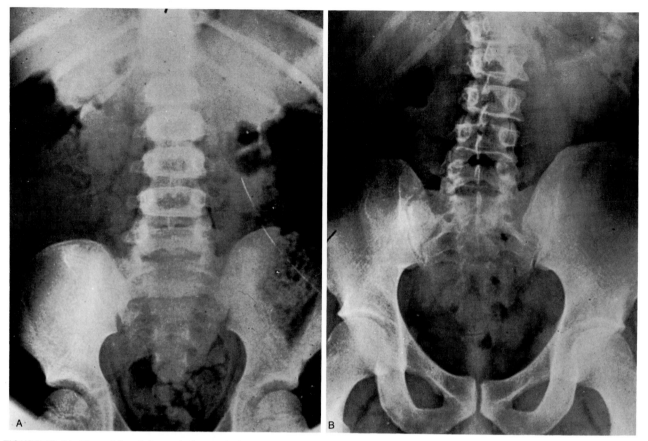

FIGURE 73–11. Films of the abdomen before and after therapy for a right-sided Wilms' tumor.
   A Normal film taken in July 1938, prior to therapy.
   B Film taken 26 years later, demonstrating a levoscoliosis. The right sides of the vertebral bodies are decreased in height, and the pedicles are decreased in size. The right iliac crest is hypoplastic. Note that the intervertebral discs are thickened, probably representing hypertrophy because of the decrease in bone size.

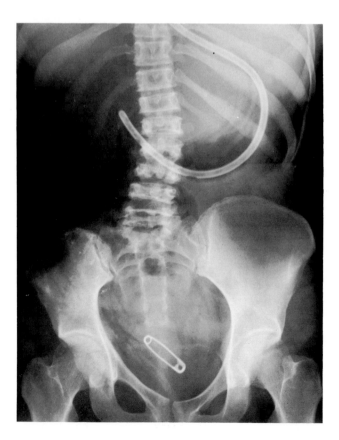

FIGURE 73–12. Another patient irradiated for a right-sided Wilms' tumor in childhood. Note the severe decrease in the height of the vertebral bodies and a slight scoliosis convex to the left. The ribs and iliac crest on the right side also are hypoplastic. The long tube was present because of intestinal obstruction, which later was shown to be secondary to radiation enteritis.

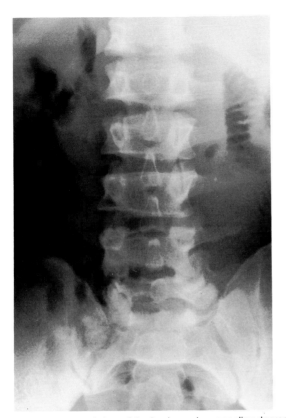

FIGURE 73–13. Frontal view of the lumbar spine revealing decrease in the height of the right side of T12, L1, L2, and L3 vertebrae with compensatory increase in the right side of the intervertebral discs in a patient whose entire lumbar spine was included in the radiation field during therapy for a Wilms' tumor.

is considered an acceptable risk when treating a potentially curable but also potentially fatal lesion.[88]

The prevalence of osteonecrosis increases with an increasing mandibular dose. It varies with the treatment method and is least common with parallel opposing fields.[88] Osteonecrosis is more common when the tumor involves or is adjacent to bone.[89] In one series of 176 patients treated with supervoltage therapy for tonsillar lesions, 66 developed mandibular necrosis.[88] The necrosis usually was of a mild and temporary nature. Mandibular necrosis may be aseptic or septic (Fig. 73–14); the aseptic or simple type usually is of no consequence.[84]

Patients with carcinoma of the oral cavity have a high prevalence of poor oral hygiene, smoking, and alcoholism.[90] Considerable controversy exists regarding the role of dental extraction in radiation therapy. Grossly carious teeth should be removed prior to treatment. Teeth with periodontal disease without opposing teeth should be extracted if they are within the treatment field.[84] The extraction should take place prior to therapy so that the tooth bed can heal before irradiation begins. Salvageable teeth should be preserved.[89] After treatment, good oral care is imperative, as radiation decreases salivary function and mandibular vascularity.[88] If teeth are removed after therapy, the trauma and bare sockets predispose to infection. In a study of 183 patients receiving radiation for oral (lip or mucous membrane) carcinoma, 5.5 per cent developed osteomyelitis of the mandible.[91]

Mandibular osteonecrosis may be difficult to differentiate from tumor recurrence.[78] Recurrence and osteoradionecrosis usually both occur within a year after therapy. Pain, ulceration, bleeding, and weight loss are common to both.[75] Mandibular necrosis frequently becomes manifest as a poorly defined destructive lesion without sequestration (Fig. 73–15). The absence of a soft tissue mass helps in the differentiation of necrosis from tumor recurrence, but an inflammatory mass may be present with osteonecrosis. Cortical destruction is frequent. The necrosis is confined to the treated area. Radiation necrosis may progress slowly or heal with vigorous conservative therapy. Hyperbaric oxygenation and intraoral mandibular surgery sometimes are necessary.[92]

Skull. Camp and Moreton[93] believed that a relatively low prevalence of radiation change occurred in the calvarium after therapy. In a more recent study of 92 patients irradiated for pituitary lesions, however, 17 (18.5 per cent) had radiation injury of the calvarium.[91] The minimum absorbed dose in these patients was 3600 cGy. A linear relationship was seen between absorbed dose and radiation injury. The longer the follow-up, the greater the rate of radiation changes.

The typical finding in the calvarium is a mixed region of lysis and sclerosis (Fig. 73–16), which starts in the epicenter of the radiation portal and extends outward to the margins of the portal.[91] Even when the overlying skin remains intact, conductive or sensorineural hearing loss or facial palsy may occur if the temporal bone is involved. If soft tissue necrosis is associated with the calvarial changes, osteomyelitis, mastoiditis, or meningitis may occur.[94, 95]

Shoulder. Radiation changes in the shoulder girdle after therapy for breast carcinoma have been reported in 1 to 3 per cent of patients.[96] With the advent of supervoltage therapy, the prevalence and severity of these changes have decreased.[72]

Osteopenia is common after irradiation but occurs in a substantial number of patients treated by radical mastectomy alone.[97] Osteopenia frequently is associated with a coarse, disorganized trabecular pattern, which may resemble Paget's disease superficially.[98]

Rib fractures are common and may be subtle. The early finding frequently is a sharp change in alignment with or without a fracture line. The lesions frequently occur in the anterior or anterolateral aspects of the ribs and usually are multiple[99] (Figs. 73–17 and 73–18). This may happen because this region is a watershed area between the territory supplied by the internal mammary artery and that supplied by the intercostal artery. Involvement of the posterior rib surfaces also is common (Fig. 73–18). The edges of the fracture fragments frequently are resorbed, and they may show sclerotic or pointed ends (Fig. 73–17). Fractures frequently are painless, and the resorption may be progressive.[87] The fractures may heal spontaneously with increased bony density.[99] Involved osseous structures frequently show other changes at the time of fracture (Figs. 73–18 and 73–19).

Clavicular fractures commonly are associated with rib fractures and also may be associated with adjacent bone resorption.[78] Symptoms usually are minimal unless associated ulceration or infection of the skin is present. Slaughter stated that osseous infection may lead to rapid clavicular destruction simulating malignancy[100]; however, this may occur in the absence of infection.[78] Scapular fractures can

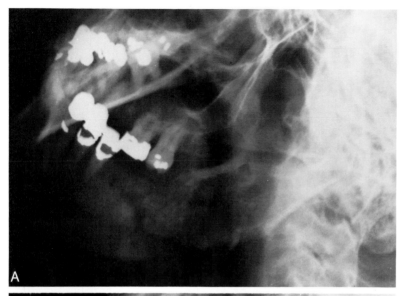

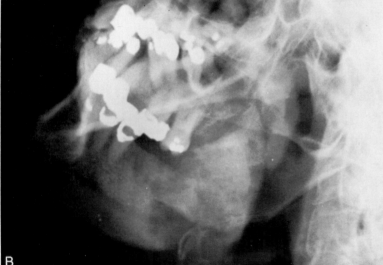

FIGURE 73–14. Septic radiation necrosis of the mandible.

A Extensive destruction of the mandible with a pathologic fracture is observed.

B Six months after conservative therapy, a decrease in mandibular abnormality has occurred.

FIGURE 73–15. Oblique view of mandible in patient previously treated for carcinoma of the floor of the mouth. There is a poorly defined destructive lesion in the body of the mandible, with a pathologic fracture. No discernible soft tissue mass is present. This represents mandibular necrosis.

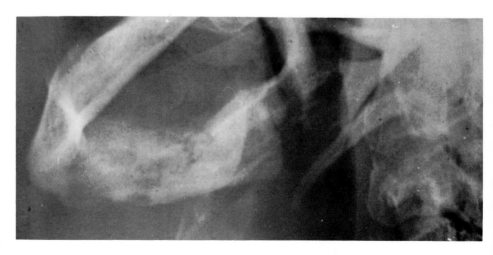

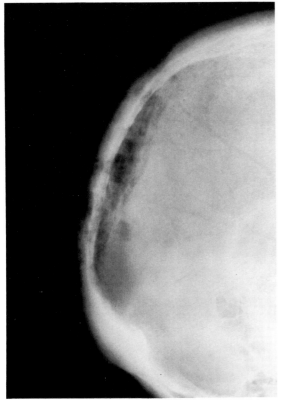

FIGURE 73–16. Radiation necrosis of the skull after treatment of basal cell carcinoma. Note that the edges of the lesion are sharp and that the area of necrosis is well defined and relatively superficial. (Reprinted with permission from Dalinka MK, Mazzeo VP Jr: CRC Crit Rev Diagn Imaging 23:235, 1985. Copyright CRC Press, Inc, Boca Raton, FL.)

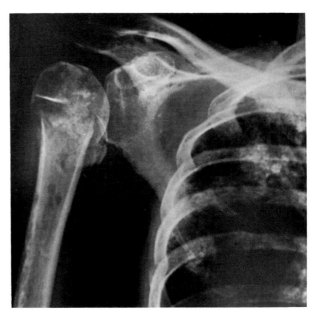

FIGURE 73–18. Radiation necrosis. Examination of the shoulder 10 years after radiation for carcinoma of the breast reveals pathologic fractures of the right humerus and multiple ribs. The lucent lesions in the proximal humeral shaft also are secondary to radiation necrosis. (From Dalinka MK, et al: Semin Roentgenol 9:29, 1974.)

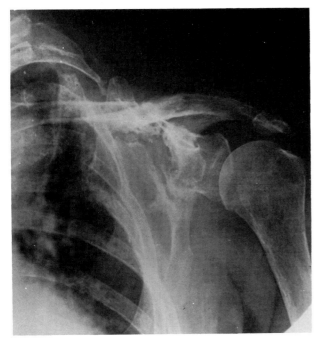

FIGURE 73–17. Changes of radiation necrosis after orthovoltage therapy and radical mastectomy for carcinoma of the breast. A pathologic fracture is present in the scapula. Multiple rib fractures are present, with resorption of the edges of the second rib and a large gap in the first rib. Pathologic fractures are observed in the posterior fourth and fifth ribs. Diffuse osteopenia is seen in the proximal humeral shaft. (From Dalinka MK, et al: Semin Roentgenol 9:29, 1974.)

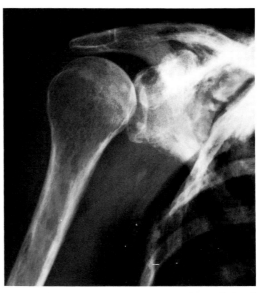

FIGURE 73–19. Right shoulder many years after radiation therapy for carcinoma of the breast. Pathologic fractures are present in the ribs. Multiple radiolucent areas are present in the proximal humeral shaft, as is patchy sclerosis of the scapula, ribs, and clavicle. The well-defined radiolucent channel projected over the scapula and lateral to the ribs represents a long-standing cutaneous sinus tract. (Reprinted with permission from Dalinka MK, Mazzeo VP Jr: CRC Crit Rev Diagn Imaging 23:235, 1985. Copyright CRC Press, Inc, Boca Raton, FL.)

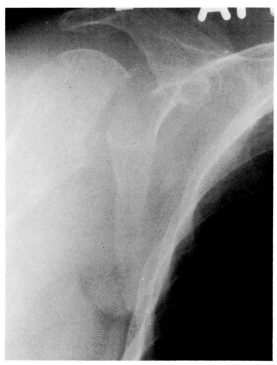

FIGURE 73–20. Ischemic necrosis of the head of the humerus with destruction of its medial margin secondary to radiation therapy for carcinoma of the breast.

be associated with rib and clavicular fractures, but the fragments usually are not resorbed (Fig. 73–17). Fractures about the shoulder girdle frequently progress to nonunion, as affected patients are relatively asymptomatic and the fragments are not immobilized.[78]

In a study involving 158 patients treated for carcinoma of the breast,[91] radiation injury to the ribs or clavicle, or both, was seen in 11 patients (7 per cent) with a minimum dose of 4500 cGy. Similar changes occurred in 4.6 per cent of 238 patients treated for carcinoma of the lung with a minimum dose of 5000 cGy after linear accelerator therapy.

Radiation necrosis of the humerus (Fig. 73–18) can be seen 7 to 10 years after therapy.[37] Associated findings in the ribs, clavicle, and scapula are frequent. DeSantos and

Libshitz state that humeral necrosis almost always is symptomatic.[96] Changes may include resorption cavities, fractures, and ischemic necrosis of the humeral head (Fig. 73–20). Histologically no osteoblasts are present. New bone formation is absent and blood vessels, including capillaries are normal.[37]

In one report,[101] two cases of slipped proximal humeral epiphysis were described as a complication of therapy for Ewing's sarcoma. The relative infrequency of this lesion in comparison to its femoral counterpart is attributable to the lack of weight-bearing and decreased stress in the upper extremities compared with the lower extremities.

Pelvis. Fractures of the femoral neck occuring after radiation therapy to the pelvis (Figs. 73–21 and 73–22) were first reported in the late 1920s in the German literature.[102] Dalby and coworkers[103] and others[77, 78, 100, 102] later reported similar findings in the United States. Patients in these series all were treated with orthovoltage therapy, and lateral fields were used in most cases except for the series by Dalby and associates.[103] Fractures occurred in approximately 2 per cent of patients treated with pelvic radiation.[77] The fractures usually were subcapital and occurred in osteopenic bone. They were unilateral or bilateral (Figs. 73–21 and 73–22). Bonfiglio believed that they were stress or insufficiency fractures.[77] Baerwolff and Buchhorn stated that even with supervoltage therapy the femoral neck receives approximately 65 per cent of the parametrial dose.[91, 104] Fractures of the femoral neck have been reported to occur after as little as 1540 cGy and as early as 5 months after therapy.[102] Diparc and associates[105] determined that a bimodal pattern existed for radiation-induced fractures of the femoral neck; the peaks in this pattern occur between 0 and 6 months and between 24 and 30 months after the end of treatment. Sclerotic changes in the femoral neck with increased trabecular density frequently were present prior to fracture.[102]

Pain, frequently in the knee or groin, commonly precedes the onset of the fractures, which, as indicated previously, usually are subcapital.[75] The average radiation dose is estimated to be 3000 cGy. Vascular damage is not sufficient to prevent repair, and fractures heal with routine treatment, with adequate callus formation.[77] Ischemic necrosis may occur (Fig. 73–23) but is rare after fractures in irradiated bone.

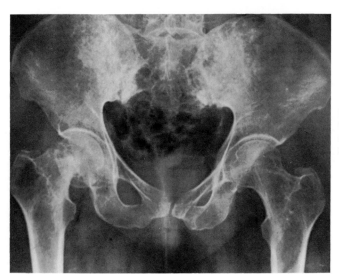

FIGURE 73–21. Fracture of right femoral neck 4 years after therapy for carcinoma of the cervix. The patient was treated with 2500 cGy external radiation plus two applications of radium. Sclerotic changes are present about both sacroiliac joints with adjacent calcification.

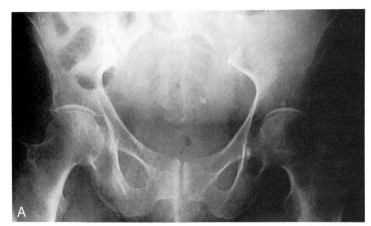

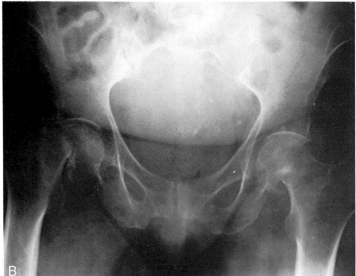

FIGURE 73–22. Bilateral femoral neck fractures after radiation therapy to the pelvis.

   A Anteroposterior view of the pelvis prior to radiation therapy.

   B Similar view of the pelvis 4 months after therapy illustrating a displaced fracture of the right femoral neck and a nondisplaced fracture on the left.

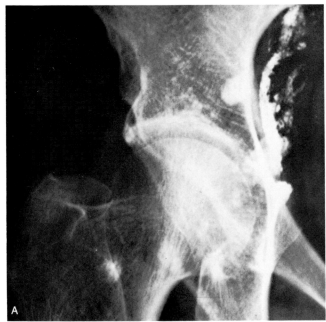

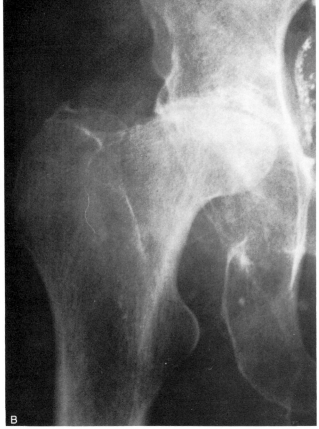

FIGURE 73–23. Radiation necrosis after treatment for carcinoma of the cervix.

   A Anteroposterior view of right hip prior to therapy shows no evidence of abnormality. Note contrast medium within lymphatic vessels from lymphangiogram.

   B Same patient 9 months after therapy. The femoral head has collapsed and marked narrowing of the hip joint is seen.

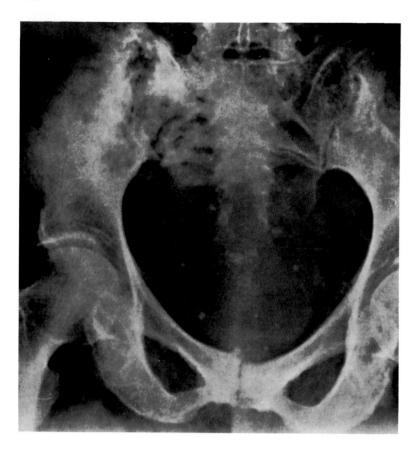

FIGURE 73–24. Radiation necrosis 10 years after radiation therapy for carcinoma of the cervix. The right sacroiliac joint is widened and markedly irregular. Radiation changes in the symphysis pubis simulate osteitis pubis. This patient was treated with 7000 cGy externally using the betatron and 3290 mg-hours of radium for carcinoma of the cervix. The patient died of a ruptured necrotic bladder and also had radiation necrosis of the bowel. (From Dalinka MK, et al: Semin Roentgenol 9:29, 1974.)

The sacroiliac joints may be wide and irregular, with sclerosis about the joint margins (Fig. 73–24). This sclerosis, which often is bilateral and symmetric, may extend from the region of the joint to the ilium, simulating osteitis condensans ilii[75, 106] (Fig. 73–25). Fractures may extend from the middle of the posterior superior iliac crest through the iliac wing[75] (Figs. 73–26 and 73–27). Sacral fractures also are encountered.

Cooper and collaborators[107] studied 12 patients with stress fractures of the sacrum; all were postmenopausal and 50 per cent had had prior radiation therapy. None of these patients reported any significant trauma to account for their sacral fractures. Five of the six patients who had received radiation had additional pelvic fractures with the pubic or iliac bones typically being involved. The primary finding was linear sclerosis running vertically in the sacral alae, parallel and adjacent to the sacroiliac joints. Transverse fractures also may develop as a secondary complication from continued stress on the weakened sacrum. Bone scintigraphy in these patients may demonstrate vertically oriented lines of increased activity running through the sacrum on one or both sides. The lines may be joined by a trans-

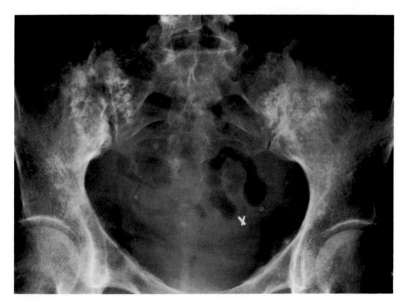

FIGURE 73–25. Radiation changes about the sacroiliac joint after therapy for carcinoma of the cervix. Note the irregular sclerotic areas near the sacroiliac joint and the wavy periosteal new bone along the arcuate (iliopubic) line of the pelvis. Radiation changes in the bladder also were evident. (Reprinted with permission from Dalinka MK, Mazzeo VP Jr: CRC Crit Rev Diagn Imaging 23:235, 1985. Copyright CRC Press, Inc, Boca Raton, FL.)

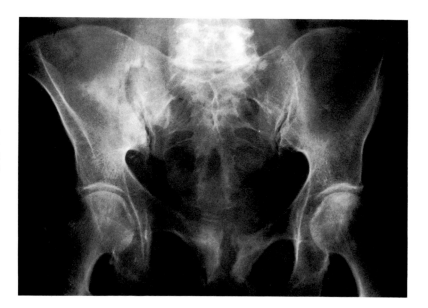

FIGURE 73–26. Radiation changes of the bony pelvis. Note widening and irregularity about the symphysis pubis and the right sacroiliac joint. A fracture extends from the right sacroiliac joint to the iliac bone.

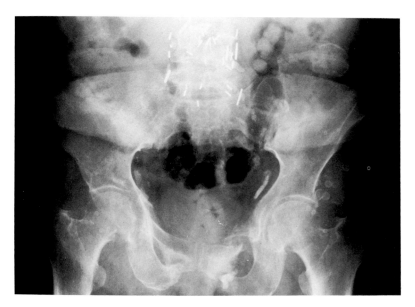

FIGURE 73–27. Multiple pelvic fractures after radiation therapy and surgery for carcinoma of the cervix. Note the bilateral fractures about the symphysis pubis and the symmetric fractures of the iliac wings.

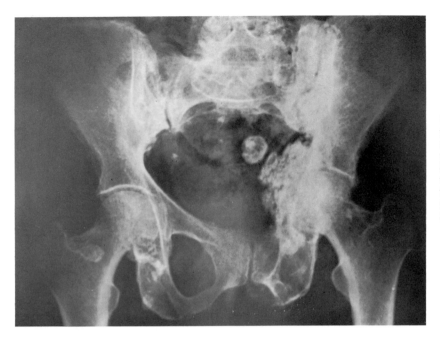

FIGURE 73–28. Pelvic changes after radiation therapy. A radiograph of the pelvis prior to therapy was normal. A radiograph obtained 23 years after therapy reveals extensive soft tissue calcification about the pelvis. The left hemipelvis is deformed secondary to a previous ischial fracture. Sclerosis is present about both sacroiliac joints, particularly on the left side. Protrusio acetabuli also is seen on the left.

verse line to create an H-shaped area of increased activity.[108] CT scanning may show these fractures to advantage.[109] Similar changes may be demonstrated by MR imaging.[110]

Occasionally soft tissue calcifications occur, and they are not associated with masses or underlying bony destruction (Fig. 73–28), which differentiates them from radiation-induced sarcoma.[96]

Changes in the symphysis pubis simulating osteitis pubis (Fig. 73–24) can occur, as may fractures about the pubic rami or ischium. These may be secondary to the high dosage of internal radiation to the anterior pelvis. Fractures can occur anywhere in the pelvis, particularly if the patient is re-treated (Fig. 73–29).

Protrusio acetabuli has been reported after irradiation. This can occur after orthovoltage or supervoltage therapy.

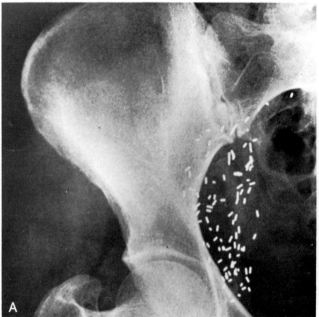

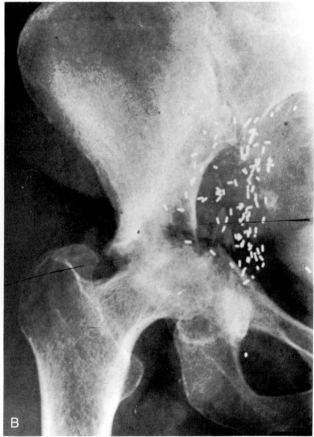

FIGURE 73–29. Radiation necrosis after retreatment.

A Radon seeds implanted in the right parametrial area for recurrent cervical carcinoma.

B Same patient 10 years later, revealing fracture through the medial wall of the acetabulum with loss of the joint space and large cyst formation.

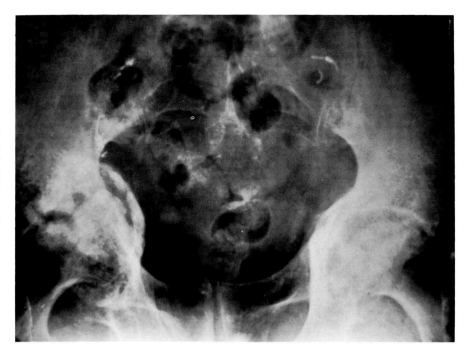

FIGURE 73–30. Protrusio acetabuli after treatment of prostatic carcinoma with 7000 cGy. A considerable degree of protrusio acetabuli is present on the right side with an acetabular fracture and loss of the joint space. Mild protrusio acetabuli is present on the left. (From Hasselbacher P, Schumacher HR: J Rheumatol *41*:189, 1977.)

In one case, it was seen after irradiation for transitional cell carcinoma of the prostatic urethra[111] (Fig. 73–30). The mechanism of acetabular protrusion in these patients is unclear but may be related to remodeling and revascularization of weakened, previously irradiated bone.[112] Associated calcification in the peritoneum is easily seen with CT scanning (Fig. 73–31). Osteonecrosis of the acetabulum leading to destruction of the hip joint and requiring hip prostheses has been reported after radiation therapy of cervical and anal carcinoma.[113]

The changes secondary to pelvic irradiation have decreased markedly with increased awareness in using supervoltage therapy. Use of lateral fields in pelvic cancer has long since been abandoned.[75] The femoral neck usually is shielded during treatment; the fields for the pelvis are smaller, and re-treatment is rare.

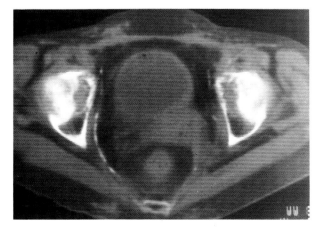

FIGURE 73–31. A transaxial CT scan in a patient who had received radiation for carcinoma of the cervix shows calcification in the region of the pelvic peritoneum. The region of soft tissue density between the bladder and the rectum suggests recurrent tumor, but the exact cause is unproved.

Radiation changes usually are easy to differentiate from recurrence or spread of disease. Metastases may involve the lateral pelvic walls from direct extension or the vertebral bodies via spread to the retroperitoneal lymph nodes.[75, 106] Hematologic dissemination frequently occurs to sites outside the treatment field and is associated with multiple lesions.[75, 106] Radiation-induced tumors occur after long latent periods and frequently are associated with soft tissue masses or characteristic osseous lesions.

Sternum. Morris and coworkers reported sternal changes after therapy for Hodgkin's disease and compared the changes subsequent to megavoltage to those occurring after orthovoltage therapy.[114] The prevalence and severity of the changes were related directly to the dose and length of follow-up examination and were best explained by damage to the microvascular structures, similar to that seen in sickle cell disease with infarction.[114]

Mild changes consisted of osteoporosis, abnormal bony trabeculae, and localized bone necrosis with sclerosis. Moderate changes included the development of localized pectus excavatum and necrosis involving more than one sternal segment. Severe changes were defined as complete osseous necrosis of one or more sternal segments with deformity.[114] The changes were more common and more severe in those patients treated with orthovoltage therapy.[114] Similar changes have been reported in adults as a consequence of mediastinal[115] and chest radiation (Fig. 73–32).

Miscellaneous Sites. Radiation changes in other areas usually follow a similar pattern. Well-defined lucent shadows are sometimes identified within the field of therapy.[116] These can occur in normal bone after therapy for a soft tissue lesion (Figs. 73–33 to 73–35) or in bone previously treated for an osseous lesion (Figs. 73–36 and 73–37). Small areas of trabecular sclerosis may occur, as can larger areas of ischemic necrosis, and these may be complicated by superimposed infection (Fig. 73–38). Bragg and coworkers have described faint sclerosis in radiation-induced phalangeal lesions.[78]

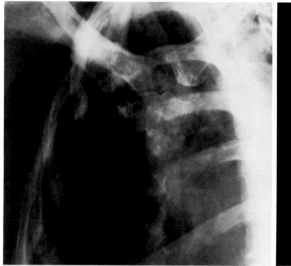
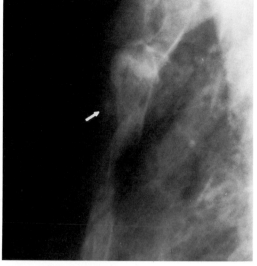

FIGURE 73–32. Radiation changes in the sternum after treatment of carcinoma of the breast.

A An oblique film of the sternum demonstrates mixed osteolytic and osteosclerotic lesions involving the entire sternum. Note that the anterior ribs also are affected extensively.

B Lateral view in the same patient demonstrates a small sequestrum-like radiodense area anterior to the upper portion of the sternum (arrow).

Articular cartilage is relatively radioresistant. Although Dawson has stated that osteoarthritis does not occur after radiotherapy,[26] severe cartilaginous destruction occasionally can be seen with joint space narrowing and osteophyte formation. This may represent secondary degenerative arthritis caused by destructive changes with collapse of the subchondral bone. However, it may be a direct effect of radiation therapy[117] (Figs. 73–23 and 73–39).

Radiation-Induced Neoplasms

Benign Neoplasms. Benign radiation-induced neoplasms occur almost exclusively in patients who are treated during childhood,[26, 28] especially those who were younger than 2

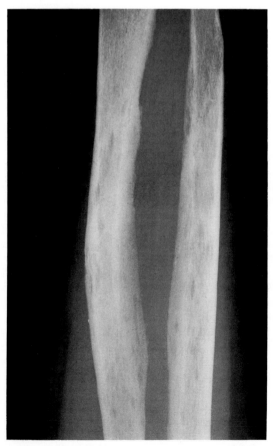

FIGURE 73–33. Anteroposterior view of forearm revealing multiple lucent lesions within the shaft of the radius and ulna, representing radiation necrosis occurring after therapy for a soft tissue tumor.

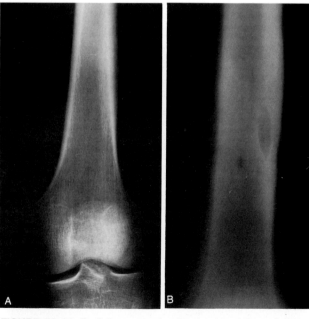

FIGURE 73–34. Radiation necrosis after treatment for soft tissue liposarcoma.

A Normal femur.

B Same patient 2 years after therapy, revealing resorption cavities within the femur secondary to radiation.

(Courtesy of F. Hall, M.D., Boston, Massachusetts.)

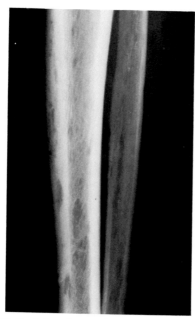

FIGURE 73–35. Radiation changes in the tibia and fibula after treatment for varicose veins. Approximately 50 years after this therapy, radiolucent lesions are observed in these long bones. (Courtesy of G. Beauregard, M.D., Montreal, Quebec, Canada.)

years old[57] at treatment, because in infancy and early childhood the rapidly growing mesenchymal tissue is more vulnerable to radiation.[118] Osteochondromas (exostoses) are the most common benign radiation-induced tumors reported in humans.[119] They occur exclusively in children[29] and can be seen in any bone in the irradiated field (Figs. 73–40 to 73–42), usually within 5 years after the radiation therapy. They were first reported in 1950 after radiation therapy for a soft tissue hemangioma.[43]

Radiation-induced exostoses are identical histologically and radiologically to spontaneously occurring osteochondromas.[36] To date there has been no well-documented, published case of malignant degeneration; however, we have seen such a case, which was shared with us by colleagues at another hospital in Philadelphia. In this case a radiation-induced pelvic osteochondroma was transformed into a chondrosarcoma. Radiation-induced exostoses generally have been reported with doses ranging from 1600 to 6425 cGy,[120] although Murphy and Blount reported an exostosis in a patient who received 125 cGy during the first week of life,[120] and Sanger and associates[118] reported three patients treated prior to the age of 2 years who developed osteochondromas with doses of less than 1000 cGy. All five of Murphy and Blount's exostoses arose at the periphery of the irradiated field.[120]

In rabbits, enchondromas histologically indistinguishable from those in Ollier's disease have been produced by internal or external radiation.[70, 121] Their production represents an aberration of epiphyseal development similar to that seen in spontaneously developing enchondromas. A failure of cellular differentiation occurs with a persistence of undifferentiated cartilage in the metaphysis.[70, 121] Although radiation-induced enchondromas have not been reported in humans, other benign tumors may occur rarely. Cohen and D'Angio reported a benign osteoblastoma in one patient and an unusual benign cartilaginous tumor in another.[122]

Malignant Neoplasms. Radiation-induced neoplasia was first reported in 1902 by Frieben, who reported a case of squamous cell carcinoma of the skin with lymph node metastases.[2, 3] Other early workers described cases of squamous cell carcinoma of the skin occurring after radiation dermatitis and continuous x-ray exposures.[2] In 1922 Beck reported three patients who developed osteosarcoma after radiation therapy for tuberculous arthritis.[123, 124] Martland and Humphries in 1929 reported on the development of osteosarcomas in radium dial workers.[10]

In the laboratory, osteosarcomas have been produced by external radiation[125, 126] as well as by bone-seeking radionuclides.[127] Fabrikant and Smith have shown that in mice osteosclerotic changes frequently precede the development of osteosarcomas.[127] These investigators produced sarcomas using both alpha and beta emitters and showed that the osseous changes were independent of the method of production. The location of the tumors was mainly in the long bones after irradiation with phosphorus-32, a beta emitter.[127] Tumors induced by the alpha emitters plutonium-239 and americium-211 had a more widespread distribution.[127] King and coworkers[126] believed that combined radiographic and scintigraphic techniques should be used for the early detection of radiation-induced osteosarcomas.

Arlen and coworkers[128] and others[129–131] have shown that radiation osteitis frequently is present adjacent to radiation-induced tumors. This was present in 50 per cent of Arlen

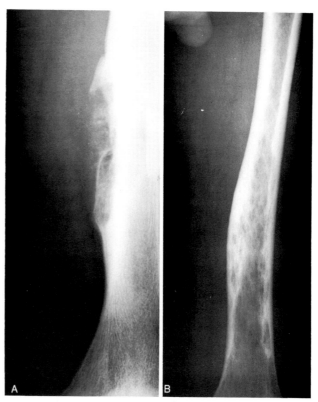

FIGURE 73–36. Ewing's tumor followed by late radiation necrosis.
  A Oblique view of femur demonstrates destructive diaphyseal lesion with saucerization, perpendicular periosteal new bone formation, and a large soft tissue mass. Codman's triangles are present at both edges of the lesion.
  B Same patient 31 years later, revealing multiple well-defined lucent areas in the shaft of the femur secondary to radiation necrosis.

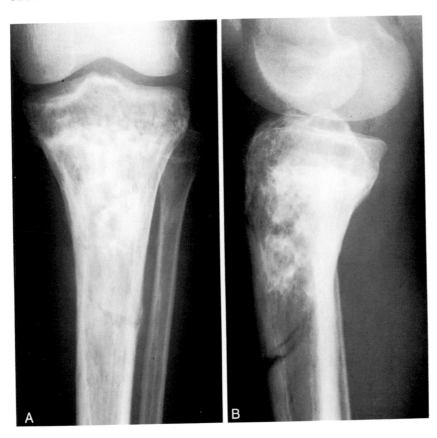

FIGURE 73–37. Ewing's tumor followed by radiation-induced necrosis. Frontal **(A)** and lateral **(B)** radiographs of a patient who was radiated for Ewing's tumor 9 years previously show areas of osteosclerosis, which represent radiation necrosis with ischemic bone. The fracture occurred secondary to trauma.

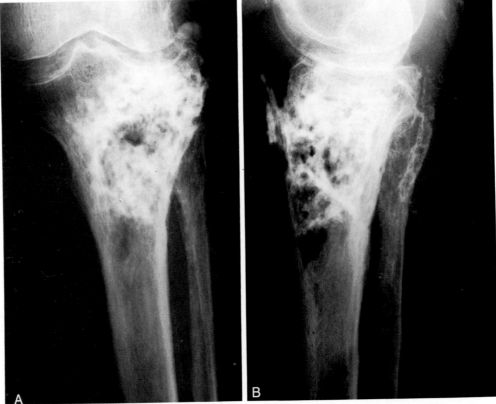

FIGURE 73–38. Osteomyelitis in irradiated bone. Radiographs in a patient who received radiation therapy for a giant cell tumor over 30 years previously show a radiolucent area in the tibia, which is secondary to infection related to *Staphylococcus aureus*.

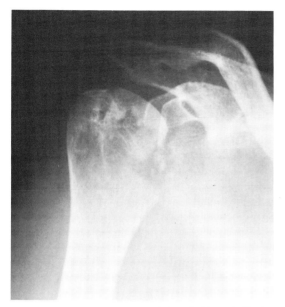

FIGURE 73–39. Destruction of the subchondral bone in the humeral head, loss of joint space, and soft tissue calcification are seen after radiation therapy. (Courtesy of M. Pitt, M.D., Birmingham, Alabama.)

and colleagues' cases[128] and in 10 of 11 patients in Steiner's series.[128] In humans as well as animals, bony changes usually precede the development of radiation-induced tumors (Fig. 73–43). Cruz and associates stated that these changes usually occur in the areas of intermediate radiation damage, as heavily damaged areas lack the capability to regenerate.[132] Young and Liebscher[133] furthered this idea by stating that if radiation is given in excess of that needed to sterilize bone, the neoplasm could not develop. Radiation-induced neoplasms form in the areas that receive radiation sufficient to induce mutation, but not enough to destroy the regenerating capacity of the bone.

Cahan and collaborators established the following criteria for the diagnosis of radiation-induced sarcoma[124]:

1. Microscopic or radiologic evidence of a nonmalignant condition.
2. Sarcoma must arise within the irradiated field.

3. A long latent period must be present—at least 4 years.
4. Histologic proof of sarcoma must be available.

Arlen and coworkers modified these criteria slightly by stating that a malignant tumor with different histologic pattern from the primary lesion should also be considered radiation induced[128] (Fig. 73–44). In a series of 50 radiation-induced sarcomas, two were osteosarcomas that arose in areas of treated round cell tumors: one Ewing's tumor and one reticulum cell sarcoma.[128]

Radiation-induced sarcomas can arise in either soft tissue or bone as well as in areas that either were previously normal or were involved by the condition being treated. Histologically a radiation-induced sarcoma is identical to a spontaneously occurring sarcoma[134] (Fig. 73–45). Prior to the mid-1980s, osteosarcoma was the most common radiation-induced sarcoma in most series.[124, 125, 135] Generally a single tumor appears, but one case has been reported of four separate osteosarcomas occurring synchronously in the tibia and fibula of a 10 year old girl who had been irradiated at the age of 2 years for an embryonal rhabdomyosarcoma of the calf.[136]

Since the mid-1980s malignant fibrous histiocytoma has become established as a histologic entity. It now is the most frequent diagnosis in many series of radiation-induced malignancies, and even in studies in which osteosarcoma retains its place as the most common tumor, malignant fibrous histiocytoma often is not far behind. Many soft tissue tumors that would once have been considered fibrosarcomas are now being called malignant fibrous histiocytoma.[137–144]

Chondrosarcomas occasionally have been reported[145, 146] and account for approximately 9 per cent of radiation-induced tumors.[32] Feintuch reported a patient with fibrous dysplasia, which degenerated into chondrosarcoma after radiation.[147] Unusual bone tumors with confusing histologic features also may occur after irradiation.[148]

Although this chapter mainly is concerned with musculoskeletal radiation-induced disease, it must be remembered that other tissues also may undergo malignant change. Bilateral breast cancer has been reported in two young women who as adolescents had received whole-lung irradiation as part of an experimental protocol for treatment of osteosarcoma.[150]

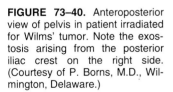

FIGURE 73–40. Anteroposterior view of pelvis in patient irradiated for Wilms' tumor. Note the exostosis arising from the posterior iliac crest on the right side. (Courtesy of P. Borns, M.D., Wilmington, Delaware.)

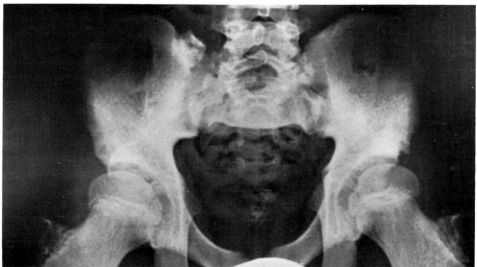

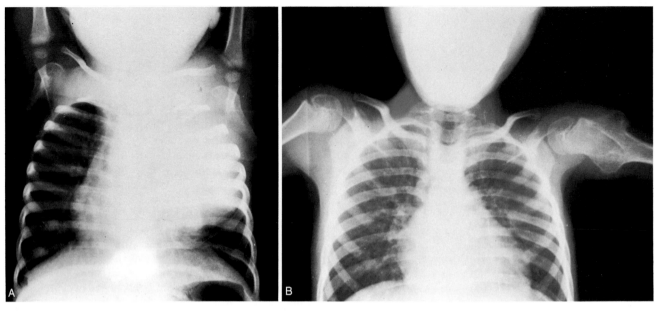

FIGURE 73–41. Exostoses secondary to radiation therapy.
A Left posterior mediastinal neuroblastoma, which was biopsied, partially excised, and treated with 2500 cGy tumor dose.
B Same patient 8 years later, revealing two benign exostoses in the left humerus.
(From Berdon WE, et al: AJR *93*:565, 1964. Copyright 1964, American Roentgen Ray Society.)

The evidence that radiation can induce sarcomas is overwhelming. Sarcomas have been reported with doses as low as 800 cGy for the treatment of bursitis.[38] Radiation-induced sarcomas usually require a dose of at least 3000 cGy

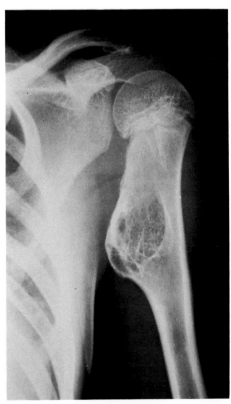

FIGURE 73–42. Radiation-induced exostosis in the proximal portion of the humerus after radiation therapy. This appearance is identical to that of a spontaneously occurring osteochondroma. (Courtesy of W. E. Berdon, M.D., New York, New York.)

in 3 weeks, with a threshold appearing at about 1000 cGy.[134] In children, a higher prevalence of radiation-induced tumors would be expected because of the longer potential period at risk.[131] The latent period does not seem to differ between children and adults, however.[151] It varies between 4 and 42 years, with an average of 11 years[129] (Fig. 73–46). These tumors have been produced by supervoltage as well as orthovoltage therapy.

Sarcomas have been produced in the skull after pituitary radiation[152, 153] and therapy for retinoblastoma.[154, 155] Sagerman and coworkers believed that the minimal risk for developing osteosarcoma after irradiation for retinoblastoma was 1.5 per cent of survivors.[154] However, two of their 23 patients developed osteosarcoma outside the irradiated field, which may indicate an increased prevalence of osteosarcoma in patients with retinoblastoma.[154] Other studies of children with retinoblastoma have strongly suggested the association of this disease with osteosarcoma as well as other tumors, particularly Ewing's sarcoma, perhaps indicating a genetic abnormality, as the tumor may arise outside the treatment field.[156–158]

In the 1960s and 1970s the prevalence of radiation-induced sarcoma was thought to range from 0.1 per cent of 5 year survivors[159] to 0.2 per cent of 10 year survivors from breast carcinoma.[134, 160] More recent reports, however, indicate increasing risk, possibly due to longer survival times for many patients with these tumors.[144] The reported risk of this complication in 5 year survivors of Hodgkin's disease has been 0.9 per cent.[161] A multicenter study of 9170 survivors of childhood cancer found a cumulative risk of bone cancer of 2.8 per cent over 20 years in irradiated patients.[162]

Radiation-induced bone sarcoma may arise in previously normal or abnormal bone. In one series of 50 radiation-induced sarcomas, 35 patients had preexisting bone disease.[128] A large decrease has taken place in the use of radiation for benign disease, and most patients with radia-

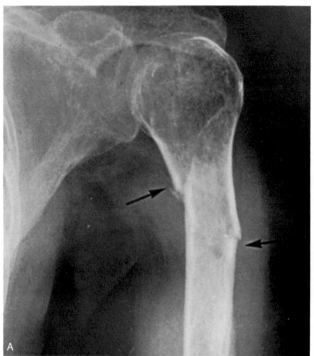

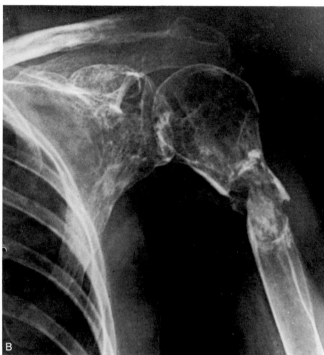

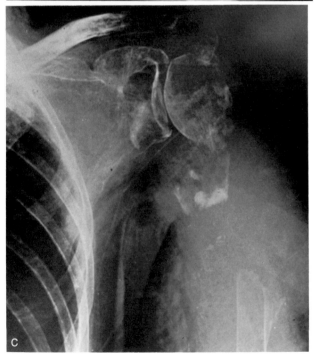

FIGURE 73–43. Sarcoma arising in irradiated bone.

A Pathologic fracture (arrows) of proximal portion of the humerus 6 years after radiation therapy for carcinoma of the breast.

B Same patient 2 years later, revealing pseudarthrosis of the humerus with radiation changes in the scapula and humerus.

C Same patient 6 years after **B,** showing an undifferentiated radiation-induced sarcoma of the humerus.

(**A, C,** From Dalinka MK, et al: Semin Roentgenol *9*:29, 1974.)

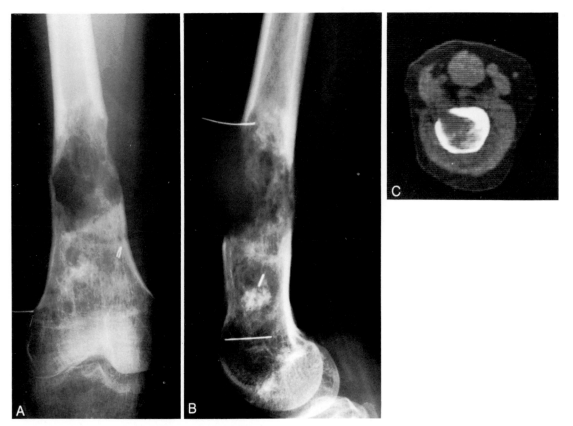

FIGURE 73–44. Osteosarcoma arising in bone previously irradiated for Ewing's sarcoma.

A, B Frontal and lateral radiographs of the femur reveal a poorly defined destructive lesion with a large soft tissue mass. A calcific area distal to the main destructive lesion represents infarcted bone, which probably is related to the radiation therapy.

C Transaxial CT scan shows extensive destruction of the femur and a large soft tissue mass.

(Reprinted with permission from Dalinka MK, Mazzeo VP Jr: CRC Crit Rev Diagn Imaging 23:235, 1985. Copyright CRC Press, Inc, Boca Raton, FL.)

tion-induced malignancies have had normal bones prior to therapy.

Radiation necrosis usually can be differentiated from sarcoma arising in irradiated bone, although occasional cases may cause difficulty. It may not be possible to distinguish a new radiation-induced sarcoma from recurrence of the original tumor. Sarcoma, necrosis, and recurrences all occur within the field of radiation and may be seen years after treatment. The presence of pain, a soft tissue mass, or a new focal lucent area favors the diagnosis of recurrent or new neoplasia, whereas their absence favors radiation necrosis. The relative lack of change on serial radiographs favors the diagosis of radiation necrosis, though healing, remodeling, and development of osteoradionecrosis are dynamic processes that will themselves produce radiographic changes (Fig. 73–47). Ehara and coworkers found that progressive bone healing continued for 2 years in patients irradiated successfully for Ewing's sarcoma (Figs. 73–5 and 73–36).[163, 164]

Radiation is used extensively in the management of painful myelomatous and metastatic lesions (Fig. 73–48). Patients are treated symptomatically with relatively low doses, frequently with large fractions. A favorable clinical response often is followed by sclerosis in the treated area, with partial or complete healing of the metastatic focus.

Radiation in Benign Disease

Recognition of the inherent dangers and complications of radiation therapy has led to more conservative use of radiotherapy than was practiced early in this century. Occasion-

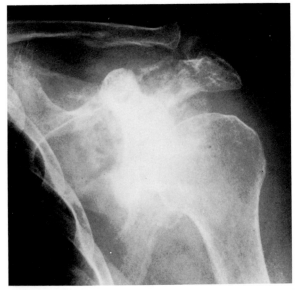

FIGURE 73–45. Radiation-induced osteosarcoma of the scapula. Radiologic and histologic findings were identical to those of a spontaneously occurring osteosarcoma.

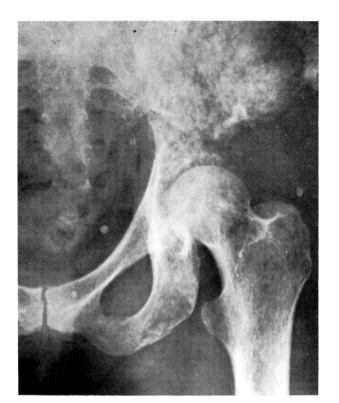

FIGURE 73–46. Anteroposterior view of pelvis with osteosarcoma of left iliac wing 17 years after therapy for cervical carcinoma. (From Dalinka MK, et al: Semin Roentgenol 9:29, 1974.)

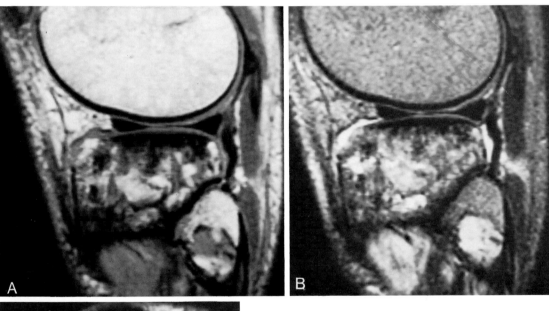

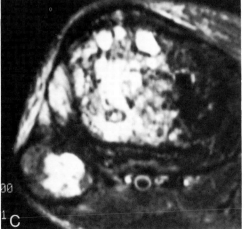

FIGURE 73–47. Radiation change with MR imaging. This patient had undergone radiation therapy for a tibial lymphoma 2 years previously. The radiographic appearance (not shown) of mixed lytic and sclerotic patches in both tibia and fibula is mirrored in the mottled signal pattern seen on MR imaging. Areas of signal void probably represent extremely dense sclerotic bone without mobile protons. This appearance was unchanged for more than a year, which, together with involvement of both the tibia and the fibula, suggests radiation change rather than new or recurrent tumor. **A,** Proton density sagittal (TR/TE, 1600/16) image. **B,** T2-weighted sagittal (TR/TE, 1600/60) image. **C,** T2-weighted transaxial fast spin echo (TR/TE, 4000/80) image.

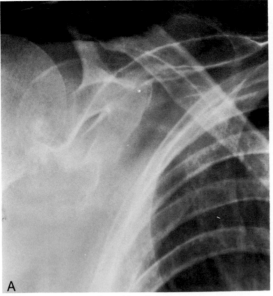

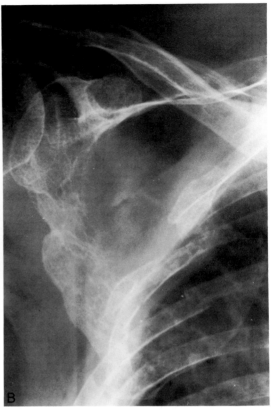

FIGURE 73–48. Healing of irradiated lesion in plasma cell myeloma.

A Destructive lesions of the lower border of the scapula and adjacent ribs are seen.

B After radiation therapy, healing of the destructive scapular lesions is seen. Multiple rib lesions with pathologic fractures now are identified.

(Reprinted with permission from Dalinka MK, Mazzeo VP Jr: CRC Crit Rev Diagn Imaging *23*:235, 1985. Copyright CRC Press, Inc., Boca Raton, FL.)

ally aggressive benign lesions in inaccessible areas, particularly the spine, still are treated by irradiation. Patients with histiocytosis frequently are given low dose radiation, usually 550 to 600 cGy.[165] After therapy, the lytic lesions frequently heal and appear normal (Fig. 73–49).

Total doses of 700 to 2000 cGy have been used to decrease ectopic bone formation in high-risk patients undergoing total hip arthroplasty.[166–170] This therapy, sometimes used in conjunction with nonsteroidal anti-inflammatory drugs, prevents heterotopic ossification in approximately 90 per cent of such patients. As yet, there are no definite reported complications of this therapy. Animal models, however, suggest a potential for impaired biologic fixation of porous prostheses.[171, 172] In addition, Pellegrini

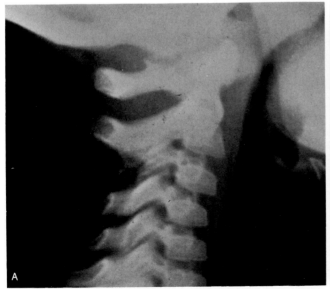

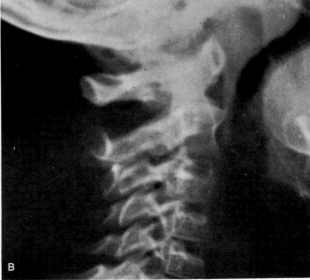

FIGURE 73–49. Healing of eosinophilic granuloma of spine after radiation therapy.
A A destructive lesion is seen involving the spinous process and the lamina of C3.
B Same patient after 600 cGy of radiation therapy, showing complete healing of the destructive osseous lesion.

74. Ewing J: Radiation osteitis. Acta Radiol 6:399, 1926.
75. Rubin P, Casarett GW: Mature cartilage and adult bone. *In* Clinical Radiation Pathology. Vol 2. Philadelphia, WB Saunders Co, 1968, p 557.
76. Katzman H, Waugh T, Berdon W: Skeletal changes following irradiation of childhood tumors. J Bone Joint Surg [Am] 51:825, 1969.
77. Bonfiglio M: The pathology of fractures of the femoral neck following irradiation. AJR 70:449, 1953.
78. Bragg DG, Shidnia H, Chu FCH, et al: The clinical and radiographic aspects of radiation osteitis. Radiology 97:103, 1970.
79. Woodard HQ, Coley BL: The correlation of tissue dose and clinical response in irradiation of bone tumors and of normal bone. AJR 57:464, 1947.
80. Ellis F: Dose, time and fractionation, a clinical hypothesis. Clin Radiol 20:1, 1969.
81. Kim JH, Chu FCH, Pope RA, et al: Time dose factors in radiation induced osteitis. AJR 120:684, 1974.
82. Montague ED: Experience with altered fractionation in radiation therapy of breast cancer. Radiology 90:962, 1968.
83. Rubin P: The radiographic expression of radiotherapeutic injury: An overview. Semin Roentgenol 9:5, 1974.
84. Guttenberg SA: Osteoradionecrosis of the jaw. Am J Surg 127:326, 1974.
85. Marciani RD, Bowden CM Jr: Osteoradionecrosis of the maxilla: Report of a case. J Oral Surg 31:56, 1973.
86. Parker RG: Tolerance of mature bone and cartilage in clinical radiation therapy. Front Radiat Ther Oncol 6:312, 1972.
87. Dalinka MK, Edeiken J, Finkelstein JB: Complications of radiation therapy: Adult bone. Semin Roentgenol 9:29, 1974.
88. Grant BP, Fletcher GH: Analysis of complications following megavoltage therapy for squamous cell carcinomas of the tonsillar area. AJR 96:28, 1966.
89. Bedwinek JM, Shukovsky LJ, Fletcher GH, et al: Osteonecrosis in patients treated with definitive radiotherapy for squamous cell carcinomas of the oral cavity and naso- and oropharynx. Radiology 119:665, 1976.
90. Cheng VST, Wang CC: Osteonecrosis of the mandible resulting from external megavoltage radiation therapy. Radiology 112:685, 1974.
91. Shimanovskaya K, Shiman A: Radiation Injury of Bone. New York, Pergamon Press, 1983.
92. Mainous EG, Hart GB: Osteoradionecrosis of the mandible treated with hyperbaric oxygen. Arch Otolaryngol 101:173, 1975.
93. Camp JD, Moreton RD: Radiation necrosis of the calvarium. Report of 5 cases. Radiology 45:213, 1945.
94. Guida RA, Finn DG, Buchalter IH, et al: Radiation injury to the temporal bone. Am J Otol 11:6, 1990.
95. Sikand A, Longridge N: CSF otorrhea complicating osteoradionecrosis of the temporal bone. J Otolaryngol 20:209, 1991.
96. DeSantos LA, Libshitz HI: Adult bone. *In* HI Libshitz (Ed): Diagnostic Roentgenology of Radiotherapy Change. Baltimore, Williams & Wilkins, 1979.
97. Langlands AO, Souter WA, Samuel E, et al: Radiation osteitis following irradiation for breast cancer. Clin Radiol 28:93, 1977.
98. Meyer JE: Thoracic effects of therapeutic irradiation for breast carcinoma. AJR 130:877, 1978.
99. Paul LW, Pohle EA: Radiation osteitis of the ribs. Radiology 38:543, 1942.
100. Slaughter DP: Radiation osteitis and fractures following irradiation with report of five cases of fractured clavicle. AJR 48:201, 1942.
101. Edeiken BS, Libshitz HI, Cohen MA: Slipped proximal humeral epiphysis: A complication of radiotherapy to the shoulder in children. Skel Radiol 9:123, 1982.
102. Gratzek FR, Holmstrom EG, Rigler LG: Post-irradiation bone changes. AJR 53:62, 1945.
103. Dalby RG, Jacox HW, Miller NF: Fracture of the femoral neck following irradiation. Am J Obstet Gynecol 32:50, 1936.
104. Baerwolff G, Buchhorn P: Beitrag zur Frage der Schenkelhalsfracturen bei gynäkologischen Röntgen-Tielenbestrahlungen. Strahlentherapie 99:72, 1956.
105. Diparc J, Frot B, Casdambide D: Radiation induced lesions of the hip. Chirurgie 100:183, 1974.
106. Rubin P, Probhasawat D: Characteristic bone lesions in post irradiated carcinoma of the cervix—metastases versus osteonecrosis. Radiology 76:703, 1961.
107. Cooper KL, Beabout JW, Swee RG: Insufficiency fractures of the sacrum. Radiology 156:15, 1985.
108. Lundin B, Björkholm E, Lundell M, et al: Insufficiency fractures of the sacrum after radiotherapy for gynaecological malignancy. Acta Oncol 29:211, 1990.
109. Rafii M, Firoozina H, Golimbu C, et al: Radiation induced fractures of sacrum: CT diagnosis. J Comput Assist Tomogr 12:231, 1988.
110. Bromlie V, Lien HH, Iverson T, et al: Radiation-induced insufficiency fractures of the sacrum: Evaluation with MR imaging. Radiology 188:241, 1993.
111. Hasselbacher P, Schumacher HR: Bilateral protrusio acetabuli following pelvic irradiation. J Rheumatol 4:189, 1977.
112. Hall FM, Mauch PM, Levene MB, et al: Protrusio acetabuli following pelvic irradiation. AJR 132:291, 1979.
113. Deleeuw HW, Pottenger LA: Osteonecrosis of the acetabulum following radiation therapy. J Bone Joint Surg [Am] 70:293, 1988.
114. Morris LL, Cassady JR, Jaffe N: Sternal changes following mediastinal irradiation for childhood Hodgkin's disease. Radiology 115:701, 1975.
115. Mullan F: Occasional notes: Seasons of survival: Reflections of a physician with cancer. N Engl J Med 313:270, 1985.
116. Paling MR, Herdt JR: Radiation osteitis: A problem of recognition. Radiology 137:339, 1980.
117. Murphy W: Personal communication. 1979.
118. Saenger EL, Silverman F, Sterling TD, et al: Neoplasia following therapeutic irradiation for benign conditions in childhood. Radiology 74:889, 1960.
119. Libshitz HI, Cohen MA: Radiation induced osteochondromas. Radiology 142:643, 1982.
120. Murphy FD Jr, Blount WP: Cartilaginous exostoses following irradiation. J Bone Joint Surg [Am] 44:662, 1962.
121. Spiess H: Exostotische Dysplasie durch Strahlenwirkung? Dtsch Med Wochenschr 35:1483, 1957.
122. Cohen J, D'Angio GJ: Unusual bone tumors after roentgen therapy of children. AJR 86:502, 1961.
123. Beck A: Zur Frage des Röntgensarkoms, zugleich ein Beitrag zur Pathogenese des Sarkoms. Münch Med Wochenschr 69:623, 1922.
124. Cahan WG, Woodard HQ, Higinbotham NL, et al: Sarcoma arising in irradiated bone: Report of eleven cases. Cancer 1:3, 1948.
125. Brady LW: Radiation induced sarcomas of bone. Skel Radiol 41:72, 1979.
126. King MA, Casarett GW, Weber DA, et al: A study of irradiated bone. III. Scintigraphic and radiographic detection of radiation-induced osteosarcomas. J Nucl Med 21:426, 1980.
127. Fabrikant JI, Smith CLD: Radiographic changes following the administration of bone seeking radionuclides. Br J Radiol 37:53, 1964.
128. Arlen M, Higinbotham NL, Huvos AG, et al: Radiation induced sarcoma of bone. Cancer 28:1087, 1971.
129. Mindell ER, Shah NK, Webster JH: Post radiation sarcoma of bone and soft tissues. Orthop Clin North Am 8:821, 1977.
130. Steiner GC: Postradiation sarcoma of bone. Cancer 18:603, 1965.
131. Tountas AA, Fornasier VL, Harwood AR, et al: Post irradiation sarcoma of bone—a perspective. Cancer 43:182, 1979.
132. Cruz MN, Coley BL, Stewart FW: Post-radiation bone sarcoma: Report of eleven cases. Cancer 10:72, 1957.
133. Young JW, Liebscher LA: Postirradiation osteogenic sarcoma with unilateral metastatic spread within the field of irradiation. Skel Radiol 8:279, 1982.
134. Kim JH, Chu FCH, Woodard HQ, et al: Radiation induced soft tissue and bone sarcoma. Radiology 129:501, 1978.
135. Tefft M, Vawter GF, Mitus A: Second primary neoplasms in children. AJR 103:800, 1968.
136. Tillotson C, Rosenberg A, Gebhardt M, et al: Postradiation multicentric osteosarcoma. Cancer 62:67, 1988.
137. Vanel D, Hagay C, Rebibo G, et al: Study of three radio-induced malignant fibrohistiocytomas of bone. Skel Radiol 9:174, 1983.
138. Weatherby RP, Dahlin DC, Ivins JC: Postradiation sarcoma of bone. Review of 78 Mayo Clinic cases. Mayo Clin Proc 56:294, 1981.
139. Huvos AG, Woodard HQ, Cahan WG, et al: Postradiation osteogenic sarcoma of bone and soft tissues. Cancer 55:1244, 1985.
140. Ros PR, Viamonte M, Rynlin A: Malignant fibrous histiocytoma: Mesenchymal tumor of ubiquitous origin. AJR 142:753, 1984.
141. Brady MS, Gaynor JJ, Brennan MF: Radiation-associated sarcoma of bone and soft tissue. Arch Surg 127:1379, 1992.
142. Davidson T, Westbury G, Harmer CL: Radiation-induced soft-tissue sarcoma. Br J Surg 73:308, 1986.
143. Laskin WB, Silverman TA, Enzinger FM: Postradiation soft tissue sarcomas: An analysis of 53 cases. Cancer 62:2330, 1988.
144. Smith J: Postradiation sarcoma of bone in Hodgkin disease. Skel Radiol 16:524, 1987.
145. Fitzwater JE, Cabaud HE, Fan GH: Irradiation induced chondrosarcoma. A case report. J Bone Joint Surg [Am] 58:1037, 1976.
146. Peimer CA, Yuan HA, Sagerman RH: Post radiation chondrosarcoma, a case report. J Bone Joint Surg [Am] 58:1033, 1976.
147. Feintuch TA: Chondrosarcoma arising in a cartilagenous area of previously irradiated fibrous dysplasia. Cancer 31:877, 1973.
148. Cohen J, D'Angio GJ: Unusual bone tumors after roentgen therapy of children. AJR 86:502, 1961.
149. Glicksman AS, Toker C: Osteogenic sarcoma following radiotherapy for bursitis. Mt Sinai J Med 43:163, 1976.
150. Ivins JC, Taylor WF, Wold LE: Elective whole-lung irradiation in osteosarcoma treatment: appearance of bilateral breast cancer in two long-term survivors. Skel Radiol 16:133, 1987.
151. Sim FH, Cupps RE, Dahlin DC, et al: Post radiation sarcoma of bone. J Bone Joint Surg [Am] 54:1479, 1972.
152. Amine ARC, Sugar O: Suprasellar osteogenic sarcoma following radiation for pituitary adenoma: Case report. J Neurosurg 44:88, 1976.
153. Sparagana M, Eells RW, Stefani S, et al: Osteogenic sarcoma of the skull: A rare sequela of pituitary irradiation. Cancer 29:1376, 1972.
154. Sagerman RH, Cassady JR, Tretter P, et al: Radiation induced neoplasia following external beam therapy for children with retinoblastoma. AJR 105:529, 1969.
155. Pagani JJ, Bassett LW, Winter J, et al: Osteogenic sarcoma after retinoblastoma radiotherapy. AJR 133:399, 1979.
156. Varela-Duran J, Dehner LP: Postirradiation osteosarcoma in childhood. Am J Pediatr Hematol-Oncol 2:263, 1980.
157. Draper GJ, Sanders BM, Kingston JE: Second primary neoplasms in patients with retinoblastoma. Br J Cancer 53:661, 1986.
158. Helton KJ, Fletcher BD, Kun LE, et al: Bone tumors other than osteosarcoma after retinoblastoma. Cancer 71:2847, 1993.
159. Phillips TL, Sheline GE: Bone sarcomas following radiation therapy. Radiology 81:992, 1963.
160. Hatfield PM, Schulz MD: Post irradiation sarcoma: Including five cases after x-ray therapy of breast carcinoma. Radiology 96:593, 1970.

161. Halperin EC, Greenberg MS, Suite HD: Sarcoma of bone and soft tissue following treatment of Hodgkin's disease. Cancer 53:232, 1984.

162. Tucker MA, D'Angio GJ, Boice JD Jr, et al: Bone sarcomas linked to radiotherapy and chemotherapy in children. N Engl J Med 317:588, 1987.

163. Ehara S, Kattapuram SV, Egglin TK: Ewing's sarcoma: Radiographic pattern of healing and bony complications in patients with long-term survival. Cancer 68:1531, 1991.

164. Lorigan JG, Libshitz HI, Peuchot M: Radiation-induced sarcoma of bone: CT findings in 19 cases. AJR 153:791, 1989.

165. Smith DG, Nesbit ME Jr, D'Angio GJ, et al: Histiocytosis X: Role of radiation therapy in management with special reference to dose levels employed. Radiology 106:419, 1973.

166. Coventry MB, Scanlon PW: The use of radiation to discourage ectopic bone. J Bone Joint Surg [Am] 63:201, 1984.

167. DeFlitch CJ, Stryker JA: Postoperative hip irradiation in preventions of heterotopic ossification: Causes of treatment failure. Radiology 188:265, 1993.

168. Lo TCM, Healy WL, Covall DJ, et al: Heterotopic bone formation after hip surgery: Prevention with single-dose postoperative hip irradiation. Radiology 168:851, 1988.

169. Seegenschmiedt MH, Goldmann AR, Martus P, et al: Prophylactic radiation therapy for prevention of heterotopic ossification after hip arthroplasty: Results in 141 high-risk hips. Radiology 188:257, 1993.

170. Warren SB, Brooker AF Jr: Excision of heterotopic bone followed by irradiation after total hip arthroplasty. J Bone Joint Surg [Am] 74:201, 1992.

171. Konski A, Weiss C, Rosier R, et al: The use of postoperative irradiation for the prevention of heterotopic bone after total hip replacement with biological fixation (porous coated) prosthesis: an animal model. Int J Radiat Oncol Biol Phys 18:861, 1990.

172. Summer DR, Turner TM, Pierson RH, et al: Effects of radiation on fixation of non-cemented porous-coated implants in a canine model. J Bone Joint Surg [Am] 72:1527, 1990.

173. Pellegrini VD Jr, Konski AA, Gastel JA, et al: Prevention of heterotopic ossification with irradiation after total hip arthroplasty: Radiation therapy with a single dose of eight hundred centigray administered to a limited field. J Bone Joint Surg [Am] 74:186, 1992.

174. Anderson MJ, Keyak JH, Skinner HB: Compressive mechanical properties of human cancellous bone after gamma irradiation. J Bone Joint Surg [Am] 74:747, 1992.

175. Loty B, Courpied JP, Tomeno B, et al: Bone allografts sterilised by irradiation: Biological properties, procurement and results of 150 massive allografts. Int Orthop 14:237, 1990.

176. Deeths TM, Stanley RJ: Parametrial calcification in cervical carcinoma patients treated with radioactive gold. AJR 127:511, 1976.

177. Ramsey RG, Zacharias CE: MR Imaging of the spine after radiation therapy: Easily recognizable effects. AJR 144:1131, 1985.

178. Glazer HS, Lee JKT, Levitt RG, et al: Radiation fibrosis: Differentiation from recurrent tumor by MR imaging—work in progress. Radiology 156:721, 1985.

74

Disorders Due to Medications and Other Chemical Agents

Donald Resnick, M.D.

Significant musculoskeletal changes can result from medications and other chemical agents. The effects of some of these agents, such as heavy metals (Chapter 76), aluminum (Chapter 57), vitamins A, C, and D (Chapter 75), tryptophan (Chapter 34), deferoxamine (Chapter 59), phenytoin (Chapter 53), polyvinyl chloride (Chapter 94), and alcohol (Chapter 78), are discussed elsewhere. In this chapter, consideration is given to the musculoskeletal alterations that may accompany administration of certain teratogenic drugs, corticosteroids and other anti-inflammatory agents, fluorine, dopamine, calcium gluconate, milk-alkali, prostaglandins, retinoic acid, and some anticoagulants. The nonspecific al-

terations that may result from the trauma associated with the administration process itself will not be considered, although, for example, subcutaneous injection of drugs can lead to infection, calcification, pseudomalignant soft tissue reaction, and even introduction of foreign material.[1-4] Intramuscular injections, especially in the thigh and gluteal area, can produce neurologic damage, particularly in infants,[174-178] and intravenous, intra-articular, and intradiscal injections may be complicated by local or distant infections.

TERATOGENIC DRUGS

It is a well-recognized fact that medications administered to the pregnant woman can affect the fetus. This problem is becoming increasingly important, as it has been estimated that more than 80 per cent of expectant mothers take at least one drug during pregnancy.[5-7] Certain of the drugs act on the somatic cells of the developing organism during vulnerable periods of embryogenesis and organogenesis and are termed teratogens. The teratogenicity of a drug depends on several factors, including its chemical and pharmacologic properties, the duration of its use, the modification of the drug by the mother, the access of the drug to the fetus, the developmental stage of the fetus at the time of exposure, a possible genetic susceptibility to the agent, and the effect of the drug on fetal metabolism.[8] Some substances are known to be teratogenic, whereas others are suspected of possessing this property.[9] Of particular importance are four chemicals that appear to be teratogenic to the musculoskeletal system.[10]

Thalidomide

The thalidomide disaster became evident in the reports of McBride in 1961[11] and Lenz and Knapp in 1962.[12] This drug was used to induce sleep in the pregnant woman, and when its ingestion occurred in the first trimester, particularly between days 34 and 50 after the start of the last menstrual period,[12] thalidomide exposure produced reduction deformities of the limbs. The anomalies included dysplasia of the thumb and radial hemimelia, phocomelia, or complete four limb amelia and were associated with hypoplasia or aplasia of the external ear and canal, congenital heart defects, gastrointestinal tract atresia or stenosis, and capillary hemangioma of the face.[10] The teratogenic effect of thalidomide may be related to inhibition of the early mesodermal precursors of the anlagen of the developing parts[10] or a chemical injury to the neural crest, which inhibits migration of its cells to the sensory nerve of the appropriate segment so that the tissues normally supplied by that nerve are deficient in growth.[13, 14, 162]

Although abnormalities in the appendicular skeleton predominate in thalidomide embryopathy, peculiar spinal alterations also may be observed.[303] Irregularity of the contour of the vertebral bodies and anterior fusion between adjacent vertebrae are encountered.[304] The resulting radiographic findings simulate those of Scheuermann's disease (see Chapter 81) and idiopathic progressive noninfectious anterior vertebral fusion.[304] This last condition occurs in the first decade of life and may be asymptomatic or accompanied by spinal cord compression occurring secondary to acute kyphosis.

Anticonvulsants

When administered to expectant mothers, anticonvulsant medications, especially phenytoin,[15–17, 183] may lead to congenital anomalies in infants, including hypoplasia of the distal phalanges, a digitate thumb, cleft palate, a decrease in head circumference, and peculiar facies.[10] The teratogenic potential of the anticonvulsants is not accepted uniformly by all investigators.[18]

Alcohol

Infants born to severely and chronically alcoholic women may reveal the fetal alcohol syndrome, consisting of prenatal and postnatal growth deficiency and delayed development.[10, 19–21] Findings may include clinodactyly, camptodactyly, congenital dislocation of the hip, pectus excavatum or carinatum, radioulnar synostosis, scoliosis and vertebral fusion.[19–21, 179, 180] A possible relationship of this syndrome to chondrodysplasia punctata (Conradi-Hünermann disease) has been reported.[181] An association of the fetal alcohol syndrome (as well as the fetal phenytoin syndrome) with adrenal neoplasms has been suggested.[161]

The precise cause of the fetal alcohol syndrome is unclear. Although ethanol appears to be the principal agent responsible for the findings, a potential role for acetaldehyde, the primary metabolite of ethanol, also is possible. Acetaldehyde is intensely cytoxic, mutagenic, and teratogenic, and it inhibits DNA synthesis and amino acid transport across the placenta.[182]

Folic Acid Antagonists

Fetal malformations have been associated with maternal exposure to folic acid antagonists, especially aminopterin, and include cranial dysplasia and foot and hand anomalies.[22]

Other Drugs

A number of reports implicate other drugs as teratogens. Examples include the potential role of warfarin (Coumadin) in the development of chondrodysplasia punctata (Conradi-Hünermann disease, chondrodystrophica calcificans congenita)[23, 24] and of estrogen and progestogen in certain congenital abnormalities.[25] Large doses of some vitamins, including vitamin A (which is being used to control severe acne in teenagers), have been accompanied by teratogenic effects.[284] It is certain that additional examples of teratogenic agents will be identified in the future; in this regard, the warning of Wilson[8] should be noted: "All chemicals are capable of producing some embryotoxic effect under the right conditions of dosage, developmental stage and species selection."

CORTICOSTEROIDS AND OTHER ANTI-INFLAMMATORY AGENTS

In 1949, Hench and colleagues[26] isolated a hormone of the adrenal cortex, compound E, and reported on its beneficial properties in the treatment of rheumatoid arthritis. In the subsequent decades, the anti-inflammatory characteristics of this agent (cortisone) became well known, as did certain of its side effects.

The complications of cortisone therapy can become manifest in almost all systems of the body, including the skeleton (Table 74–1). Detrimental effects include osteoporosis, osteonecrosis, neuropathic-like articular destruction, osteomyelitis, septic arthritis, tendinous and soft tissue injury, periarticular and capsular calcification, and abnormalities in the distribution of fat.

Osteoporosis

The occurrence of generalized osteoporosis in patients receiving systemic corticosteroids has been noted by many observers (Chapters 20 and 51). Stress (insufficiency) fractures occur that heal with extensive callus formation.[27, 28] Collapse of single or multiple vertebral bodies with condensation of bone at the superior and inferior surfaces (Figs. 74–1 and 74–2) and infractions of ribs particularly are characteristic and are relatively asymptomatic in these steroid-medicated patients, who lack normal protective pain responses. The contribution of osteoporosis in periarticular locations to subchondral bony collapse and disintegration has been emphasized by some investigators[29] but is not accepted universally.[30] The radiologic diagnosis of insufficiency fractures related to corticosteroid therapy frequently

TABLE 74–1. Musculoskeletal Abnormalities Associated with Corticosteroid Medication

Osteoporosis
Osteonecrosis
Neuropathic-like arthropathy
Osteomyelitis (septic arthritis)
Tendinous injury or rupture
Soft tissue atrophy
Intra-articular calcification
Periarticular calcification
Accumulation of fat

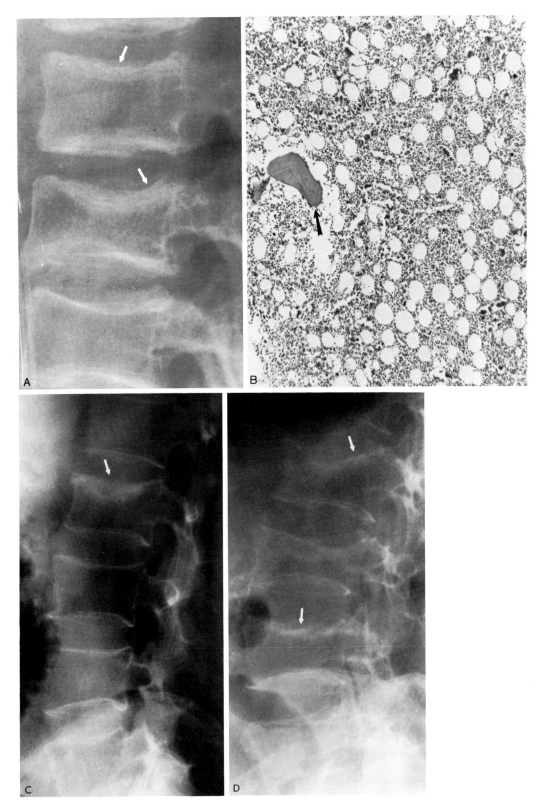

FIGURE 74–1. Steroid-induced osteoporosis.

A A lateral radiograph of the lumbar spine reveals biconcave deformities of multiple vertebral bodies with bony condensation at the superior and inferior aspects of each vertebra (arrows). This appearance can be seen with exogenous or endogenous hypercortisolism.

B A photomicrograph (90 ×) indicates sparse bony trabeculae (arrow) surrounded by marrow.

C, D In another patient being treated with corticosteroids, radiographs of the lumbar spine obtained several months apart reveal osteoporosis, progressive collapse of vertebral bodies, and bony condensation (arrows) on the superior aspect of multiple collapsed vertebrae.

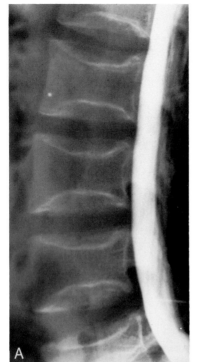

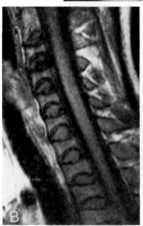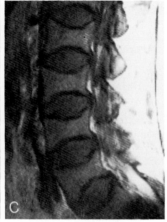

FIGURE 74-2. Steroid-induced osteoporosis. This 22 year old woman had received systemic corticosteroid therapy for many months as a child, and she developed cushingoid features, with deposition of fat in the shoulders and back and muscle weakness.

A A lateral radiograph obtained during a lumbar myelogram (accomplished for investigation of low back pain) reveals osteopenia, biconcave deformities of multiple vertebral bodies, and well-defined subchondral bone plates.

B, C Sagittal T1-weighted (TR/TE, 200/26) spin echo MR images of the cervical spine **(B)** and lumbar spine **(C)** show the biconcave deformities to good advantage. The signal intensity of the bone marrow reflects the presence of hematopoietic tissue and is within normal limits.

(Courtesy of G. Greenway, M.D., Dallas, Texas.)

is difficult, owing to the associated generalized osteopenia, the presence of skeletal alterations of the underlying process (such as rheumatoid arthritis) for which the medication was administered, a lack of clinical manifestations, and, in some cases, the involvement of skeletal sites (such as the sacrum) that are visualized suboptimally on radiographs. Although bone scintigraphy can be used to enhance the diagnostic accuracy, falsely negative results may be encountered.[184] CT and MR imaging are very useful in detect-

ing such fractures in anatomically complex regions, such as the sacrum (Chapters 51 and 67).

Assessment of the exact role of corticosteroid medication in the production of osteoporosis is difficult because many of the conditions for which the drug is used are themselves associated with bone loss.[285] This particularly is true in the inflammatory arthritides, in which immobilization and disuse are additional factors leading to osteoporosis.[31] It seems probable that accelerated bone loss is associated with the use of corticosteroids in noninflammatory conditions and that it also is evident in inflammatory disorders, particularly when the patients are more than 50 years old. In the latter situation, however, the anti-inflammatory action of the drug could decrease the bone loss associated with the inflammation, and, in some cases, the net result may be a reduction in local bone turnover.[32] Although reports have been conflicting, steroid-induced osteoporosis may be more significant in patients who are elderly, in women, and in those receiving larger cumulative doses[167, 286, 305] and may be uninfluenced by the exact schedule of the therapeutic regimen.[168, 185]

The precise mechanism by which corticosteroids lead to bone loss is not known, although the drug can influence calcium metabolism by affecting renal tubular reabsorption of calcium, bone cell kinetics, intestinal absorption of calcium, and endocrine function.[186] Currently, it is believed that two primary mechanisms are involved in glucocorticoid-induced osteopenia: direct inhibition of bone formation and indirect stimulation of bone resorption resulting from increased parathyroid hormone secretion secondary to diminished intestinal absorption of calcium.[185, 187, 189] Both cortical and trabecular bone is lost, depending on the skeletal site,[188] and the process is partially reversible once the corticosteroids are no longer administered.[190, 191]

Osteonecrosis

Although osteonecrosis is a recognized complication of steroid therapy, it should not be equated with the term steroid arthropathy.[33] Steroid arthropathy indicates structural joint damage occurring in association with local or systemic administration of steroids; it may relate to osteoporosis and bony collapse, perhaps accelerated by the absence of pain sensation (after oral, parenteral, topical, or, most strikingly, intra-articular administration of steroids), or it may relate to osteonecrosis (after oral, parenteral, subcutaneous,[192] intra-articular,[306, 307] or topical administration of steroids). It is not always possible to distinguish which of the two processes is operational even on radiographic and pathologic examination, and in many cases, both may be occurring simultaneously.

Since the report of Pietrogrande and Mastromarino in 1957,[34] descriptions of steroid-induced osteonecrosis have been numerous.[27–30, 35–46, 192–196] In some cases, the reports are complicated by the fact that the underlying disease for which the corticosteroids had been used, such as systemic lupus erythematosus,[165, 308–310] may itself be capable of producing osteonecrosis, although the occurrence of bone necrosis in steroid-treated patients with conditions not associated with necrosis (asthma, tuberculosis, pemphigus, and thrombocytopenia purpura) also is well recognized. Furthermore, in some patients, such as those with lymphoma, chemotherapeutic agents given in conjunction with the corticosteroids may contribute to bone necrosis (Chapter 62).

The true frequency of steroid-induced osteonecrosis is difficult to determine because of the many variables that are included in the various studies. In patients receiving corticosteroids after renal transplantation, the frequency appears to be approximately 5 to 10 per cent[47, 311]; this complication probably is less frequent in other conditions. In many reviews of patients with osteonecrosis, steroid medications have been implicated in 20 to 35 per cent of cases. The occurrence of steroid-induced bone necrosis appears to be related directly to the dosage level and the duration of the medication and may become prominent in many persons after prolonged high intake.[39, 44] It is less frequent after short-term (7 to 18 days) high dose steroid therapy.[193–195, 312] Other factors that may be important include the mode and the schedule of steroid administration. In general, the frequency of ischemic necrosis in association with corticosteroid therapy is greater when (1) divided, rather than single, daily doses are used; (2) long-term (greater than 6 months), rather than short-term, treatment is employed; (3) high dose, rather than low dose, therapy is used; and (4) an associated disorder is present that itself causes avascular necrosis.[196] Such factors, although important, are not accepted universally as events predisposing to ischemic necrosis of bone, and exceptions to these general rules are reported commonly. In fact, the occurrence of osteonecrosis has been observed during replacement steroid therapy in patients in whom cortisol levels are depressed as a result of endocrine dysfunction.[197]

The onset of symptoms and signs related to osteonecrosis usually is delayed for a period of 2 to 3 years after administration of the drug. Although it is uncommon to recognize clinical and radiographic manifestations of this complication within 6 months of the onset of the therapy, occasional examples of more acute bony necrosis are seen, and the rapidity of the radiographic and pathologic changes may be striking.[44] Single or multiple osseous sites can be affected; the femoral head, the humeral head, the distal end of the femur, and the proximal part of the tibia, in decreasing order of frequency, are altered most commonly (Figs. 74–3 and 74–4). About the knee, involvement of the lateral femoral condyle has been reported to be more frequent than that of the medial femoral condyle,[316, 317] a pattern of distribution that differs from that seen in spontaneous osteonecrosis, and steroid-induced necrosis of the upper pole of the patella has been described.[318, 362] Unusual sites of involvement have included the acetabulum,[319] the lunate bone,[320] the talus (Fig. 74–5), and the metatarsal heads (Fig. 74–6). In general, although one site may be involved at the time of initial clinical presentation, there is a tendency for more widespread abnormalities to appear over a period of time. In fact, it is expected that approximately 30 to 50 per cent of patients who reveal steroid-induced osteonecrosis of one femoral head later will demonstrate changes on the contralateral side.

Radiographic and pathologic characteristics of osteonecrosis due to corticosteroids are not unique, being evident in cases of bony necrosis due to other causes (Chapter 79). Osteoporosis, patchy osteonecrosis, subchondral radiolucent lines (crescent sign), osseous collapse, and fragmentation are recognized. Preservation of joint space also is typical during the early stages of the process.

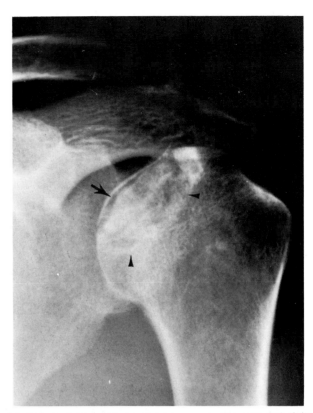

FIGURE 74–3. Steroid-induced osteonecrosis: Proximal end of the humerus. Abnormalities consist of flattening of the humeral head with a subchondral radiolucent line (crescent sign) (arrow), surrounding osteolysis and osteosclerosis (arrowheads), and relative preservation of joint space.

As observed in ischemic necrosis in general, bone scanning is more sensitive than plain film radiography in detecting sites of osseous necrosis in patients receiving corticosteroids.[198] Radionuclide examinations allow an earlier diagnosis of the complication and identify its complete distribution more accurately. Findings include an initial ''cold'' stage with decreased accumulation of the bone-seeking radiopharmaceutical agent,[199] followed by a stage with increased uptake of the radionuclide.[200] The value of CT as a sensitive indicator of ischemic necrosis of bone is questionable, but that of MR imaging in this condition has been established (Chapter 80) (Figs. 74–7 and 74–8).[311, 313]

The pathogenesis of steroid-associated osteonecrosis is not clear (Table 74–2). Osteoporosis leading to microfractures and eventual bony collapse (mechanical factors) and vascular compromise due to compression from marrow ac-

TABLE 74–2. Pathogenesis of Steroid-Induced Osteonecrosis

Theory	Possible Mechanisms
Mechanical	Osteoporosis leading to microfractures and osseous collapse
Vascular	Vascular compression from marrow accumulation of fat
	Fat embolization following steroid-induced fatty liver
	Vasculitis
	Hyperviscosity

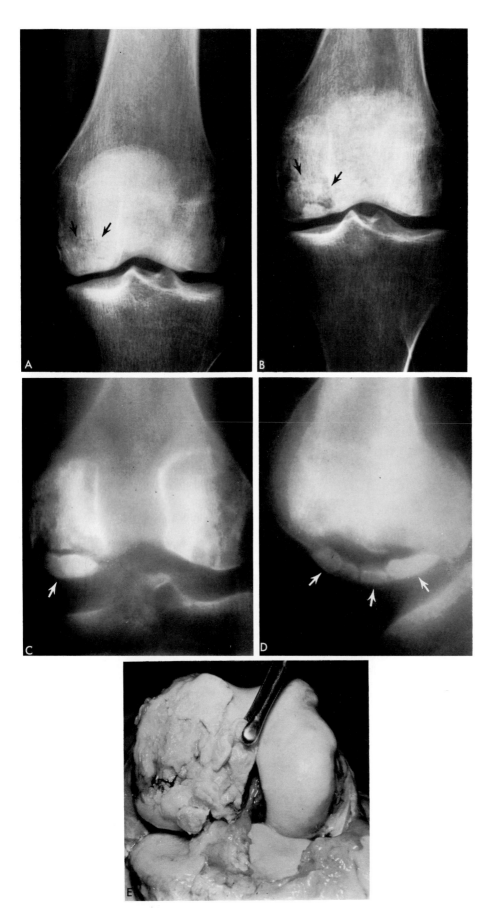

FIGURE 74–4. Steroid-induced osteonecrosis: Distal end of the femur. Progressive changes in a 1 year period are illustrated in a young patient who was treated with corticosteroids after renal transplantation. Both knees were affected similarly.

A An initial film indicates a subtle radiolucent line (arrows) in the medial femoral condyle, indicating definite osteonecrosis.

B One year later, considerable fragmentation (arrows) of the articular surface is seen.

C, D Frontal and lateral conventional tomograms demonstrate the fragmentation of the osseous surface with the creation of multiple intra-articular bony pieces (arrows).

E An operative photograph of the distal femoral condylar surface reveals the severity of the osteocartilaginous abnormalities on the medial side.

(**E,** Courtesy of R. Convery, M.D., San Diego, California.)

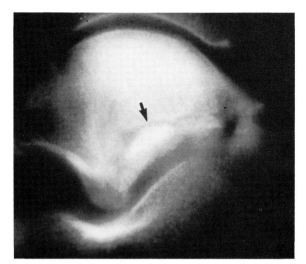

FIGURE 74–5. Steroid-induced osteonecrosis: Talus. A conventional tomogram in the lateral projection shows sclerosis, mainly in the proximal portion of the bone, and a subchondral radiolucent line (arrow). (Courtesy of A. Nemcek, M.D., Chicago, Illinois.)

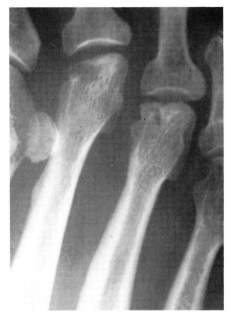

FIGURE 74–6. Steroid-induced osteonecrosis: Metatarsal heads. Observe sclerosis, radiolucent zones, and collapse of the second and third metatarsal heads. (Courtesy of M. Murphey, M.D., Washington, D.C.)

cumulation of adjacent relatively inelastic fat cells, fat embolization, vasculitis, or hyperviscosity (vascular factors) are frequently proposed mechanisms for this complication.[314] The mechanical theory gained support from Frost's observation that trabecular cracks can be observed in subchondral bone prior to collapse,[48] whereas the vascular theory is supported by demonstrated alterations in coagulation mechanisms and viscosity,[49, 50] by changes similar to those of giant cell arteritis in the soft tissues about the necrotic bone,[51] by documented increases in marrow fat cell size and intrafemoral pressure,[201] by elevation of cholesterol content

in necrotic regions,[202] and by identification of fat globules in subchondral vessels in areas of osteonecrosis.[38, 52] The importance of intravascular fatty deposits in the production of osteonecrosis has been further popularized by Jones and his collaborators,[53–56] who emphasized the following sequence of events: corticosteroid-induced fatty liver, systemic fatty embolization, infarction of bone, and osteone-

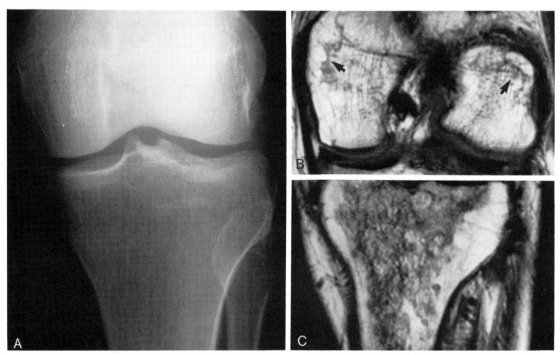

FIGURE 74–7. Steroid-induced osteonecrosis: Distal end of the femur and proximal portion of the tibia. MR imaging.
   A The routine radiograph is normal.
   B, C Two coronal T1-weighted (TR/TE, 750/20) MR images show characteristic findings of osteonecrosis involving both femoral condyles (arrows) and tibia.

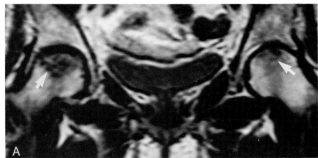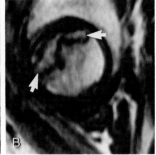

FIGURE 74–8. Steroid-induced osteonecrosis: Femoral heads. MR imaging. This 62 year old woman had received intraocular corticosteroids for glaucoma. Coronal **(A)** proton density (TR/TE, 2000/30) and sagittal **(B)** T1-weighted (TR/TE, 600/12) spin echo MR images reveal bilateral osteonecrosis of the femoral heads (arrows). The sagittal image in **B** is of the right femoral head. Note the serpentine regions of low signal intensity.

crosis. This hypothesis was partially confirmed by Jaffe and coworkers,[57] who detected significant intraosseous fat embolization in rabbits that were given systemic corticosteroids, an observation that also was supported in other investigations.[43] Some studies have documented swelling and death of osteocytes in areas of necrosis, changes that may relate to intracellular accumulation of lipid.[314] Currently, the theory of fat embolization or of fatty infiltration in the bone marrow is accepted most widely, although an ancillary role of altered mechanical forces acting on weakened osteoporotic bone or vulnerability of vascular circulation at certain sites, such as the proximal part of the femur, or both factors, may be important.

Additional analgesics may be associated with drug-induced arthropathy and osteonecrosis.[14, 29, 58, 287, 315] These medications include phenylbutazone and indomethacin. The pathogenesis of the articular abnormalities that are evident after treatment with nonsteroidal anti-inflammatory agents is presumed to be similar to that after corticosteroid administration. Such manifestations in the hip, which have been designated analgesic hip, also may relate to other factors such as calcium phosphate crystal deposition (see Chapter 45).

Changes in the diaphyses and metaphyses of tubular bones are encountered less frequently than epiphyseal alterations in patients being treated with steroids or other anti-inflammatory agents.[298] Wilkenfeld and Sliwinski[59] noted osteolytic lesions of both humeri in a rheumatoid arthritis patient who was receiving corticosteroids and cyclophosphamide that on biopsy were characterized by fatty cellular infiltration and cortical thinning. This finding is consistent with the corticosteroid-induced fatty overgrowth of the bone marrow that has been observed experimentally.[60, 201]

Osteonecrosis of vertebral bodies in association with steroid medications has been recognized. Radiolucent linear shadows in the subchondral bone reflect fractures of necrotic bone and are reminiscent of the radiolucent areas that appear at other sites of osteonecrosis, such as the femoral and humeral heads (Fig. 74–9).[163, 164] The phenomenon is termed the vacuum vertebral body. Although it is not associated universally with ischemic necrosis of bone, it is most suggestive of that diagnosis, and the finding eliminates the

alternative diagnoses of infection and neoplasm almost completely.

Neuropathic-like Articular Destruction

A neuropathic-like, rapidly progressive joint disease characterized by severe osseous and cartilaginous destruction represents one variety of steroid arthropathy that appears most typically after intra-articular injection of the drug[33, 61–64] (Table 74–3). It may be associated with osteoporosis, osteonecrosis, and an underlying articular disorder, such as rheumatoid arthritis or degenerative joint disease (Figs. 74–10 and 74–11). Although any joint can be affected,[363] it is the hip and the knee that are involved most frequently. The rapidity of the process may be remarkable, with the transition in a short period of time from a joint with minor alterations (perhaps due to underlying osteoarthritis or rheumatoid arthritis) to one with significant osseous collapse and fragmentation. Gouged-out areas of bony destruction have been compared to animal bites, the "bite" sign.[61]

The pathogenesis of the process is not certain. Although osteonecrosis may be an accompanying feature, it does not appear to be the initial event in this articular manifestation; joint space narrowing, contour defects, and eburnation may appear before osseous collapse and fragmentation become evident. The process resembles an infection, but organisms

TABLE 74–3. Steroid-Induced Neuropathic-like Alterations

Possible Pathogenesis	Characteristics
Neuropathic osteoarthropathy due to sensory loss induced by medication	Usually evident after intra-articular administration of drug
	Predilection for the hip and the knee
Osteonecrosis	Rapid onset and progression
	Osseous defects ("bites"), collapse, and fragmentation
	Cartilaginous destruction

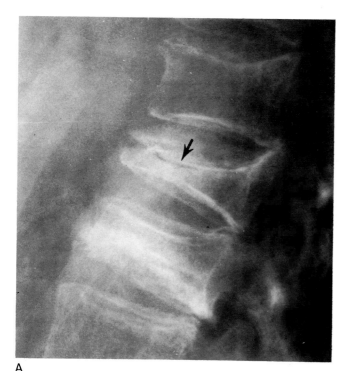

A

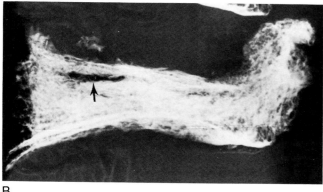

B

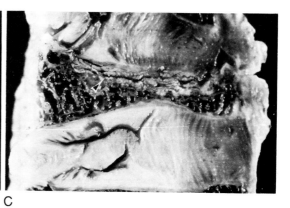

C

FIGURE 74–9. Steroid-induced osteonecrosis: Vertebral bodies.

A Observe collapse of multiple osteoporotic lumbar vertebral bodies, reactive sclerosis of endplates, and a radiolucent line or crescent within the bone (arrow). The last-mentioned finding differs from a vacuum intervertebral disc, in which the radiolucent collection is located in the disc itself.

B, C A radiograph and photograph of a spinal section show a radiolucent collection (arrow) that corresponds in position to a fracture (arrowhead) in a collapsed vertebral body.

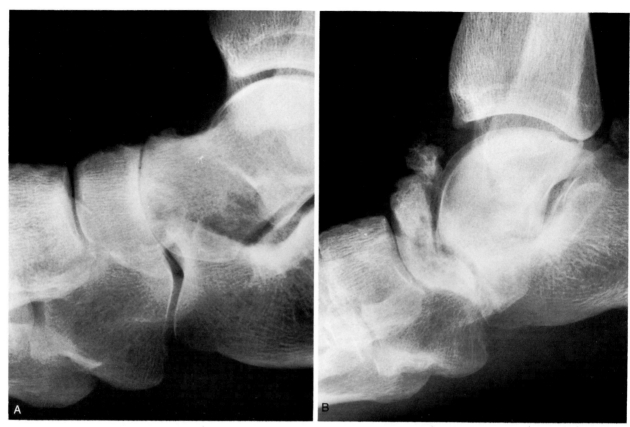

FIGURE 74–10. Steroid-induced neuropathic-like arthropathy. This patient with rheumatoid arthritis had had repeated injections of corticosteroids into the talonavicular space. Radiographs obtained 2 years apart indicate progressive abnormalities. The initial film **(A)** demonstrates joint space narrowing, sclerosis, and subchondral cyst formation, whereas the later film **(B)** reveals fragmentation of the talus and navicular bone. The findings are unlike uncomplicated rheumatoid arthritis and resemble neuropathic changes.

are not recovered from the joint in most instances. Crystal accumulation (see later discussion) is another potential causative factor. The fact that there is a relative absence of pain in the presence of severe osseous and cartilaginous destruction may indicate that the analgesic effect of the

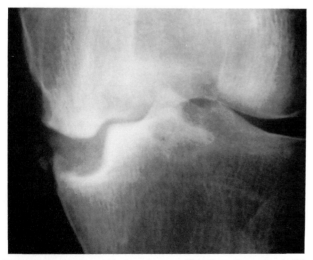

FIGURE 74–11. Steroid-induced neuropathic-like arthropathy. In this 70 year old woman with rheumatoid arthritis, multiple steroid injections into the knee were associated with significant bone abnormalities. Note the gouged-out area of destruction in the medial tibial plateau.

steroid medication may be fundamental to the pathogenesis of the articular changes. The joint destruction, therefore, may relate to neuropathic osteoarthropathy created by the steroid-induced obscuration of pain and may be aggravated by the steroid-related osteoporosis of the neighboring bone. Recurrent trauma in this painless situation can lead to disintegration of weakened subchondral bone and acceleration of any underlying articular disorder. Cartilaginous destruction can appear as a secondary event in a joint that reveals increasing incongruity of apposing articular surfaces, although a direct effect of the corticosteroids on the articular cartilage also may be important.[204, 299] Experimentally, cartilaginous fibrillation and cystic degeneration in hyaline cartilage or fibrocartilage[206] (including the intervertebral disc)[288, 289] can accompany intra-articular, systemic, or intramuscular steroid injection[65, 66] (Fig. 74–12). Inhibition of protein and polysaccharide synthesis by the chondrocyte can be evident.[67–69, 203, 205] The detrimental effect of the corticosteroid is influenced by the choice of a soluble versus an insoluble form of hydrocortisone (the latter appears to be more harmful) and, in the case of intra-articular administration, whether the drug is injected into a cartilage-containing cavity or into a nearby inflamed lining tissue (the latter is less harmful).[207]

The ability of steroids to provoke neuropathic-like changes is not accepted universally. Gibson and colleagues[70] were unable to document significant joint changes in monkeys that were subjected to intra-articular steroid

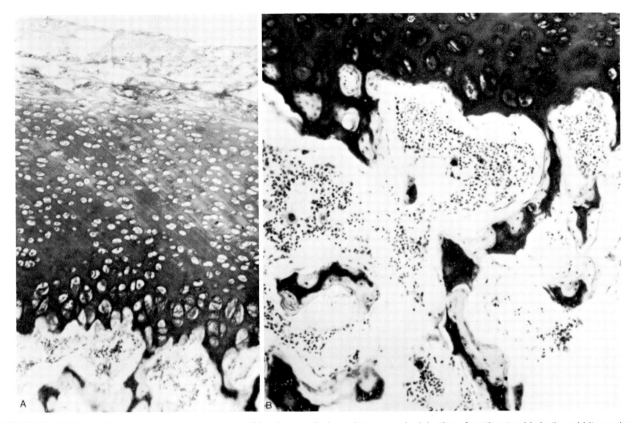

FIGURE 74–12. Steroid-induced cartilaginous abnormalities. Intra-articular or intramuscular injection of corticosteroids in the rabbit may lead to significant abnormalities.
 A After 13 daily intramuscular injections of cortisone, superficial cartilage fibrillation, a decrease in hypertrophic cells, and poor organization of subchondral trabeculae can be seen (160×).
 B Twelve days after intra-articular methylprednisolone administration, the zone of hypertrophic cells is shallow, the calcified matrix is not remodeled in the normal dentate pattern, and osteoblasts are few and spindle-shaped (160×).
 (From Shaw NE, Lacey E: J Bone Joint Surg [Br] *55*:197, 1973.)

injections. They emphasized the anecdotal nature of many of the previous reports of pseudoneuropathic steroid-induced joint changes in humans[62, 64, 71, 72] and the inconsistency of the reported changes in other series,[73, 74] although these investigators did concede that the medication might have a harmful effect on cartilage already compromised by inflammatory disease,[75] especially if administered at frequent intervals. It appears that the risk from the judicious use of intra-articular corticosteroids is small.[204]

Osteomyelitis and Septic Arthritis

Bone and joint infections can complicate steroid therapy, although such complications are rare. Septic arthritis can appear after oral, intravenous, or intra-articular administration[76–79] and can affect any joint, particularly the knee. Single or multiple joints may be involved, and bacterial organisms, especially *Staphylococcus aureus,* predominate. Similarly, osteomyelitis can appear alone or in conjunction with septic arthritis. The initiation and spread of infection are promoted by the medication's interference with normal host defense mechanisms; in addition, direct inoculation of joint, bone, or soft tissue can result from the usage of contaminated needles or syringes during the injection process. Rarely, nonseptic joint effusions may be identified in patients receiving steroid medications, especially those who have had renal transplantations.[169] In these cases, the synovial fluid may be colorless and have an unusually low protein content.

Tendinous and Soft Tissue Injury

Tendinous rupture has been described in association with systemically or locally administered corticosteroids,[80–85, 208, 209, 300] but it is not certain if the complication relates to the effect of steroids or the disease process for which the steroids are being used (Fig. 74–13). Experimental evidence suggests that steroids may induce changes in healthy tendons and that they may inhibit the healing process of unhealthy tendons.[86, 88, 210] Langhoff and colleagues[86] reported the dissolution of fibrocytes and fibroblasts after injection of methylprednisolone into tendons, although Phelps and coworkers[87] were unable to confirm a change in the biochemical properties of rabbit patellar tendons after corticosteroid injection. Wrenn and associates[88] found that corticosteroid therapy inhibited partially the healing process of tendons, decreasing the amount of fibrous tissue, reducing the tendon strength, and delaying regeneration of the tendon sheath. Similar results were reported by Kapetanos.[210] Hydrocortisone injection into a tendon also has been associated with fatty degeneration and collagen necrosis.[89, 90] At this time, it appears likely that steroids, particularly when administered locally, accelerate degeneration and rupture of a tendon that is already the site of a pathologic process;

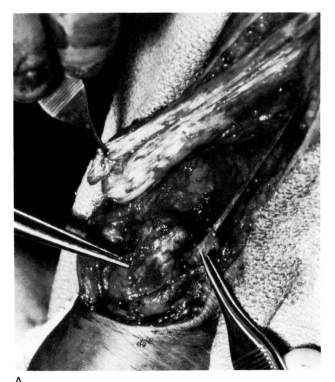

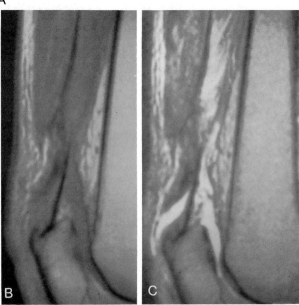

FIGURE 74–13. Steroid-induced tendon injury.

A Achilles tendon. The upper forceps holds the proximal torn end of the Achilles tendon in a patient who had received steroid injections adjacent to this tendon. (Courtesy of R. Convery, M.D., San Diego, California.)

B, C Quadriceps tendon. In this patient on a long-term systemic steroid regimen, sagittal proton density (TR/TE, 2500/20) **(B)** and T2-weighted (TR/TE, 2500/80) **(C)** MR images show rupture of the quadriceps tendon with peritendinous extravasation of fluid and a joint effusion.

whether or not similar complications can occur in healthy tendons after steroid administration is not certain, although reports of tendon rupture in patients receiving corticosteroids for nonrheumatic disorders support this possibility.[208] Locally administered steroids also may have a detrimental effect on ligaments, decreasing the strength of ligamentous attachments to bone.[166]

Atrophy of subcutaneous tissues may appear after local application of various steroid preparations, especially triamcinolone; this can occur when the medication is applied topically or when it is injected in or beneath the skin.[91–95, 321] Rarely, intra-articular injection can lead to periarticular (perilymphatic) skin atrophy.[96] Although some recovery of the cutaneous tissue may occur after a number of years, complete restoration of the local fat is not common.

Intra-articular and Periarticular Calcification

The occurrence of calcification in and around joints that have been injected with corticosteroid preparations was observed by McCarty in 1972[211] and has been further documented in other reports.[212–214, 293, 322] Gilsanz and Bernstein[212] demonstrated this pattern of calcification in 20 patients with juvenile chronic arthritis and, in all instances, the affected joint had been the site of one or more injections of corticosteroids, suggesting that it was the therapy, rather than the underlying disease, that was the important etiologic event. The knee was involved most commonly, and the calcified deposits occurred in the infrapatellar fat pad and, less frequently, the synovial membrane, joint capsule, and adjacent ligaments. In a report by Dalinka and associates,[213] triamcinolone hexacetonide was the specific corticosteroid preparation that, when injected on multiple occasions into the joint, led to subsequent calcification. Interphalangeal joints of the hands, which otherwise appeared normal or were the sites of osteoarthritis, were affected. Capsular or intra-articular linear or cloud-like radiodense shadows were seen, and pathologic examination indicated that hydroxyapatite was the likely chemical nature of the crystalline material. Such crystals also were demonstrated by McCarty[211] in the calcifications that were evident in the rheumatoid arthritis patients who were receiving triamcinolone hexacetonide. This investigator observed soft tissue calcific collections within 1 or 2 years after corticosteroid injections in approximately 50 per cent of joints and suggested that leakage of the drug was the most plausible explanation of such calcifications, which occurred along the needle tract. Stelling and Keats[214] reported intra-articular calcifications in the knee in two patients who had received long-term steroid therapy (an oral prednisone preparation in one patient and intra-articular medication in the other). Chondrocalcinosis and speckled calcific foci were evident in the recesses of the joint.

These reports appear to document a definite association of calcification in the synovial membrane, joint capsule, periarticular tissue, and, perhaps, cartilage in patients receiving intra-articular corticosteroid injections, especially if multiple injections are given for a period of years. Large joints or small joints, such as those in the hand, may be involved (Fig. 74–14). The responsible crystal is hydroxyapatite,[293] which itself can cause joint inflammation, and the typical radiographic findings are cloudlike radiodense collections within the joint and curvilinear and punctate calcifications in the articular capsule and surrounding soft tissues. Periarticular and intra-articular calcification also may be observed after systemic administration of corticosteroids,[214, 323] and epidural calcification may be encountered after intradiscal injections of corticosteroids.[324]

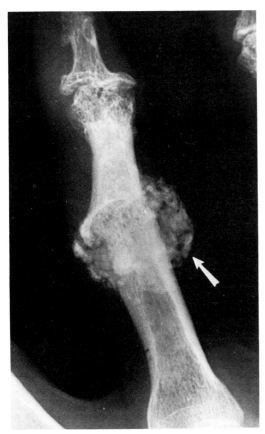

FIGURE 74–14. Steroid-induced intra-articular and periarticular calcification. In a 57 year old woman with osteoarthritis of the interphalangeal joints of both hands, multiple intra-articular injections of triamcinolone hexacetonide were followed by the development of intra-articular and periarticular calcifications (arrow), presumably related to hydroxyapatite crystal deposition. (Courtesy of M. Dalinka, M.D., Philadelphia, Pennsylvania.)

Accumulation of Fat

Endogenous or exogenous excess of corticosteroids leads to abnormal accumulations of fat. Mediastinal lipomatosis represents one manifestation of this phenomenon,[215–217] which may resolve if the steroid dosage is lowered or terminated. Similarly, paraspinal localization of fat produces characteristic radiographic findings consisting of widening of the paraspinal lines and a lobulated or masslike contour, generally in a bilateral distribution, simulating the abnormalities of lymphoma, metastatic disease, or neurogenic tumor.[218] CT or MR imaging documents the extent of involvement and the fatty nature of the abnormal accumulations of tissue.[218, 219]

Although the masses of fat in the thorax and paraspinal regions as well as elsewhere (face, neck, trunk, presacral and episternal areas)[220] rarely lead to clinical manifestations, epidural lipomatosis in patients receiving corticosteroid therapy (as well as those with Cushing's disease) may produce neurologic complications,[221–223, 294, 325–331] including paraplegia.[222, 325] Cord compression is a far more common complication of epidural lipomatosis in exogenous as opposed to endogenous (Cushing's disease) steroid excess.[330] Very rarely, similar epidural deposits are encountered in the absence of a history of corticosteroid use or of clinical

evidence of endocrinopathy.[332, 333] Myelography, CT, or MR imaging is an appropriate diagnostic technique.[331, 333] Remarkable improvement can be expected after laminectomy, removal of the adipose tissue, and cessation of the drug.

FLUORINE

Chronic fluorine intoxication (fluorosis) arises when the drinking water contains fluoride in concentrations higher than 4 parts per million (ppm)[97–100]; fluorosis occurs as an endemic problem in certain regions of the world, especially India, where it was first described in the 1930s,[101] and sporadically in almost a worldwide distribution. The entity also may appear in industrial workers who are exposed to fluorine compounds over a period of years,[171, 334] in laboratory personnel who have inhaled fluorine vapors, in patients receiving medications containing high doses of fluorine, such as niflumic acid (a nonsteroidal anti-inflammatory agent),[173] and in persons who habitually drink fluorine-containing wine (wine fluorosis).[114, 116] Bone changes also are recognized in patients with osteoporosis who are treated with sodium fluoride, although these changes are less striking, are modified by the underlying metabolic disease, and are considered separately in the discussion that follows. It is the well-documented intoxication by fluorine that has generated interest and criticism in public health programs for the prevention of dental caries.[98] Paradoxically, the cumulative effects of fluorine may be detrimental not only to the skeleton but also to the dental tissues. The investigation of Smith and Hodge[102] has revealed that although fluoride concentration in 1 ppm can reduce dental caries, a level of 2 ppm or more can lead to mottled enamel and of 8 ppm can produce osteosclerosis in 10 per cent of persons, and a concentration greater than 100 ppm may induce growth disturbances, kidney damage, or death.

As summarized by Grandjean,[224] the fate of fluoride particles depends on their size and solubility and the pattern of exposure. For example, in workers employed in the aluminum industry, in which cryolite is used, inhalation of insoluble or sparingly soluble fluoride particles is accompanied by pulmonary accumulation, whereas soluble forms reach the blood stream within hours; fluoride dust entering the gastrointestinal tract is dissolved by the action of gastric acid and passive intestinal absorption takes place. Approximately 50 per cent of the absorbed fluoride is excreted, mainly in the urine, and approximately 99 per cent of the fluoride retained in the body is deposited in the calcified tissue. The biologic half-life for bone fluoride is about 8 years, owing to the slow rate of turnover of skeletal tissues. With cessation of the exposure to fluoride and with continued, although slow, metabolism of bone tissue, excretion of fluoride can lead to an improvement in the pulmonary and skeletal manifestations of the disease. Radiographic improvement of the osseous abnormalities has been documented (see later discussion).[225]

Clinical manifestations of acute fluoride exposure include nausea, vomiting, constipation, loss of appetite, and toxic nephritis; manifestations in more prolonged cases of exposure include joint pain and restriction of motion, back stiffness, restriction of respiratory movements, functional dyspnea, dental alterations, paraplegia, and palpable thickening of the bones, including the clavicle, tibia, and ulna.[224]

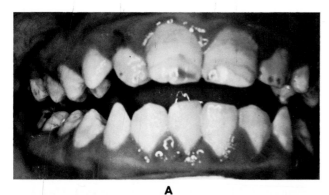

A

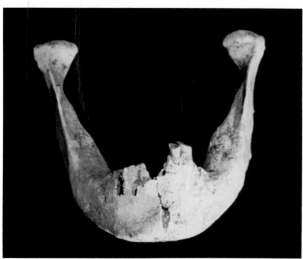

B

FIGURE 74–15. Fluorosis: Dental and mandibular abnormalities.

A Depressions, discoloration, and opaque flecks are evident in this person with fluorosis. (Courtesy of R. Smith, D.D.S., San Francisco, California.)

B Observe osseous expansion and irregularity of the bone surface. The mandible has a "chalky" appearance. (Courtesy of D. Ortner, Ph.D., Washington, D.C.)

Dental Fluorosis

Mottled enamel is an early dental sign of fluoride intoxication.[98, 103–105] The teeth appear polished and hard and contain minute opaque flecks, which may be scattered about the tooth surface (Fig. 74–15). Progression of the dental changes leads to depressions or pits of variable size and discoloration.[106] Radiographs outline hypoplasia, irregular dental roots, and periapical sclerosis and root resorption.

Skeletal Fluorosis

Radiographic Abnormalities. Involvement of the axial skeleton is characteristic[98, 99, 107–113, 335, 364, 367] (Table 74–4) (Figs. 74–16 to 74–18). Changes are most marked in the spine, the pelvis, and the ribs. Although osteopenia can appear initially, particularly in children, osteosclerosis usually appears first. Increasing trabecular condensation eventually creates a radiodense or chalky appearance throughout the thorax, vertebral column, and pelvis with obscuration of bony architecture. The skull and tubular bones of the appendicular skeleton are relatively spared in this sclerotic process.

Vertebral osteophytosis can lead to encroachment on the

TABLE 74–4. Radiographic Abnormalities in Fluorosis

Hypoplasia and irregularity of dental structures
Osteosclerosis
Vertebral osteophytosis
Ligamentous calcification
Periostitis

spinal canal and intervertebral foramina. In the axial skeleton, hyperostosis and bony excrescences develop at sites of ligamentous attachment, especially in the iliac crests, ischial tuberosities, and inferior margins of the ribs. Calcification of paraspinal and intraspinal ligaments, including the posterior longitudinal ligament,[335, 336] and the sacrotuberous and iliolumbar ligaments can be noted.

In the appendicular skeleton, osteopenia with or without growth recovery lines may be an early finding.[367] Periosteal thickening, calcification of ligaments, and excrescences at ligamentous and muscular attachments to bone also can be seen at one or more sites, particularly near the interosseous membranes of the forearm and leg, the calcaneus, the posterior surface of the femur, the tibial tuberosity, and the proximal portion of the humerus (Figs. 74–19 and 74–20).[337] In some cases, the degree of periosteal bone formation can become profound and is termed periostitis deformans.[114, 115] This variety of fluorosis can lead to unilateral or bilateral cloaks of undulating periosteal bone, which may surround the humeri, femora, ulnae, radii, tibiae, fibuli, metatarsals, metacarpals, and phalanges and is associated with cortical thickening, medullary diminution with endos-

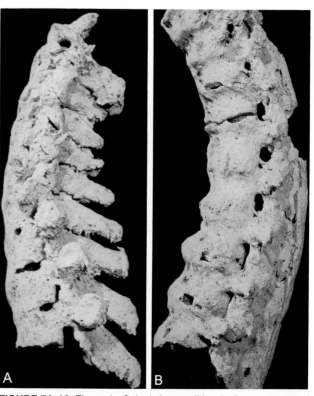

A   **B**

FIGURE 74–16. Fluorosis: Spinal abnormalities. In these macerated specimens, note extensive vertebral osteophytosis and ligamentous ossification. The neural foramina are narrowed. (Courtesy of D. Ortner, Ph.D., Washington, D.C.)

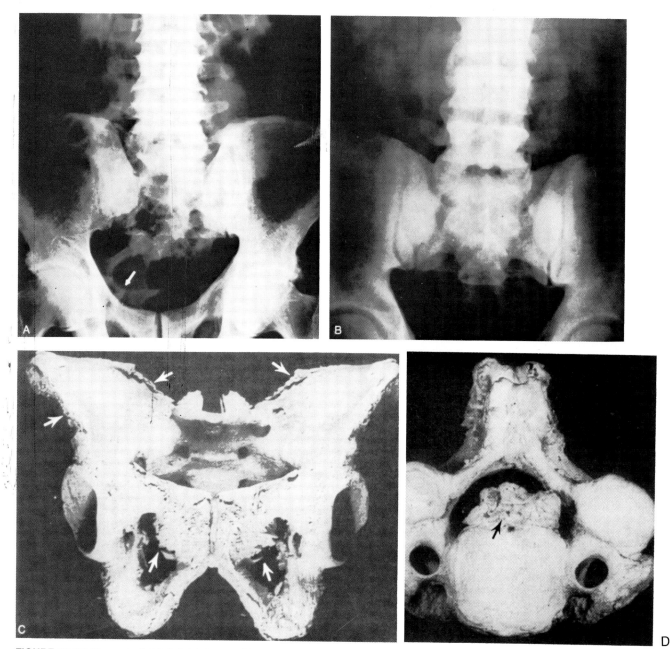

FIGURE 74–17. Fluorosis: Axial skeletal abnormalities.

A Osteosclerosis with a coarsened trabecular pattern, vertebral osteophytosis, and sacrotuberous ligament ossification (arrow) are the observed radiographic changes.

B Osteosclerosis and vertebral osteophytosis are evident in a different patient with fluorosis. Note the bony eburnation about the sacroiliac joints.

C A macerated pelvis of a 45 year old farmer from India with fluorosis reveals proliferation at ligamentous attachments, especially about the iliac crests and the ischial and pubic rami (arrows).

D In the same patient as in **C,** a photograph of the inferior surface of the third cervical vertebra reveals calcification and ossification of the posterior longitudinal ligament (arrow) and osseous overgrowth about the spinous processes and articular pillars.

(**C, D** From Singh A, et al: J Bone Joint Surg [Br] *44*:806, 1982.)

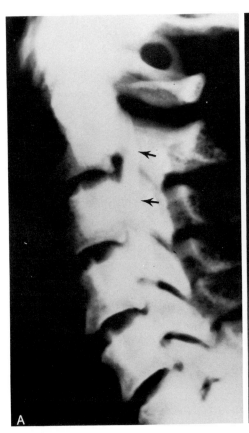
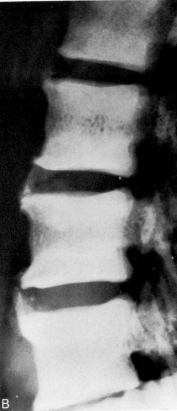

FIGURE 74–18. Fluorosis: Axial skeletal abnormalities. In this 47 year old woman, an extreme increase in radiodensity of the cervical and lumbar spine is observed. Note spinal osteophytes and ossification of the posterior longitudinal ligament (arrows). (Courtesy of G. Beauregard, M.D., Montreal, Quebec, Canada.)

teal bone formation, "invading" osteophytes that extend into tendons, fasciae, or muscles, and periarticular excrescences, especially about the hip, the knee, or the elbow. Soft tissue ossification resembling myositis ossificans and cartilaginous atrophy and ulceration have been noted.[115]

Pathologic Abnormalities. Histopathologic assessments of skeletal fluorosis have been inconsistent. Although cortical thickening with narrowing of the marrow cavity, decreased bone resorption, and virtual absence of osteoclasts have been noted in some reports,[107] other authors have cited an increase in bone surfaces lined by osteoid and striking evidence of osseous resorption (Fig. 74–21).[117] Accelerated bone formation and resorption may occur simultaneously; irregular laying down of periosteal bone on the surface may be associated with an increased rate of resorption, as indicated by cancellization of the cortex, the presence of enlarged haversian canals (resorption tunnels), and an increased number of lacunae.[118] Tetracycline studies have indicated that subperiosteal bony deposition may create disordered or irregular lamellae,[98, 119] whereas histologic investigations have indicated an increase in resorption surfaces that correlates with plasma levels of alkaline phosphatase, bone fluoride, and the radiologic findings of coarse osseous striations.[117] It has been suggested that the concomitant increase in bone formation and osteoclastic resorption in skeletal fluorosis is caused by overactivity of parathyroid hormone,[117] a suggestion that is supported by clinical, laboratory, and radiologic data.[120] Fluorine can influence the response of bone to parathyroid hormone and calcitonin markedly, an action that appears to be mediated, in large part, by an effect on bone mineral.[121, 122] The fluoroapatite crystals, which are of large size, may be more stable and

less reactive in surface exchange reactions,[117] increasing the resistance of bone to the actions of parathyroid hormone.[120] Whether this structural change is a major factor in inciting parathyroid stimulation is not known, although animal experiments indicating that an increase in circulating hormone can appear within days of fluoride administration[123] suggest that other mechanisms also are important in the production of elevated parathyroid hormone levels in association with skeletal fluorosis.

The mechanical properties of bone in fluorosis also have been studied, although not without disagreement.[172] Fluoride affects bone strength in at least two ways: Fluoride ions replace the hydroxyl ions in bone crystals to form fluoroapatite; and high serum levels of fluoride cause an increase in osteoblast activity.[338] Evans and Wood[124] discovered that certain characteristics, such as tensile strength, tensile strain, energy required for fracture, and modulus of elasticity, were less in fluorotic human bone specimens than in normal bone specimens, whereas other characteristics, such as compressive strength and compressive strain, were increased in the fluorotic bone. Franke and colleagues[125] observed an increase in bone strength in fluorosis, an effect that was related to an increase in the amount of osseous tissue, although methodology in this latter experiment later was challenged by Lindahl and Lindwall.[126] Turner and colleagues[338] reported a positive effect on bone strength for lower fluoride intakes and a negative influence on bone strength for higher fluoride intakes. Chemical analysis of fluorotic bone has indicated elevated fluoride and carbonate content and reduced citrate and magnesium content.[127] The fluoride content may decrease slowly after exposure has ceased.[128]

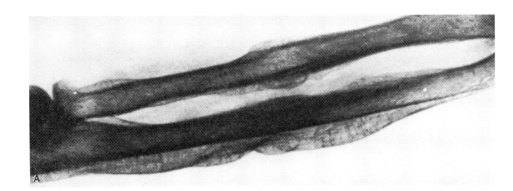

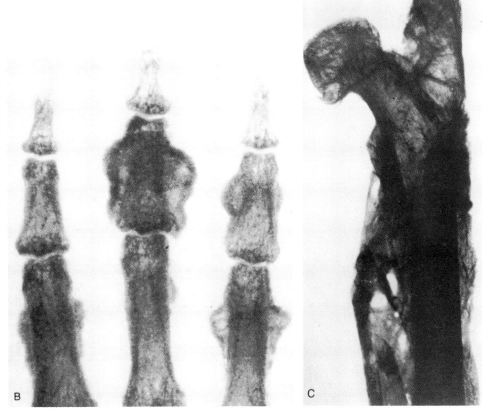

FIGURE 74–19. Fluorosis: Appendicular skeletal abnormalities. Extensive periosteal proliferation of the radius, ulna, proximal end of the femur, and phalanges can be noted in fluorosis. A striking appearance consisting of enlarged and undulating osseous contours is seen. (From Soriano M, Manchon F: Radiology *87*:1089, 1966.)

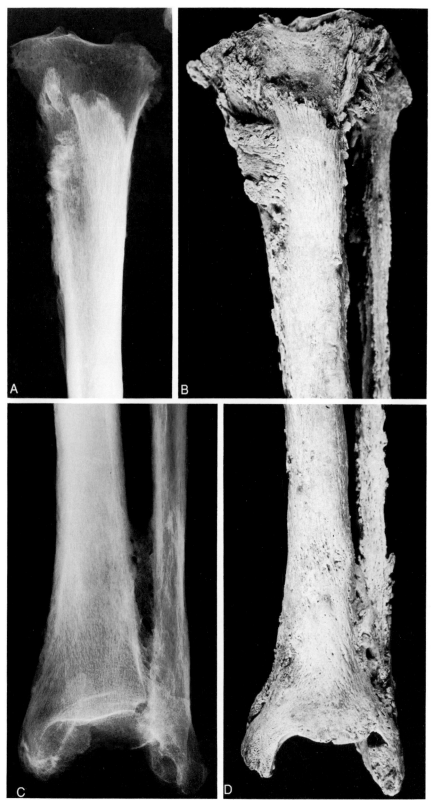

FIGURE 74–20. Fluorosis: Appendicular skeletal abnormalities.

A, B Changes in the proximal portions of the tibia and fibula include exuberant periosteal proliferation, especially in the area of the tibial tuberosity.

C, D In the same cadaver, similar alterations affect the distal portions of the bones, particularly in the region of the interosseous membrane.

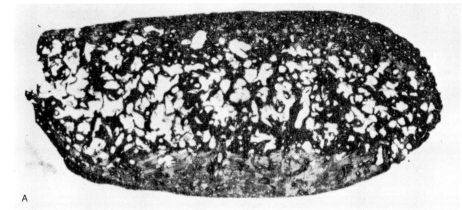

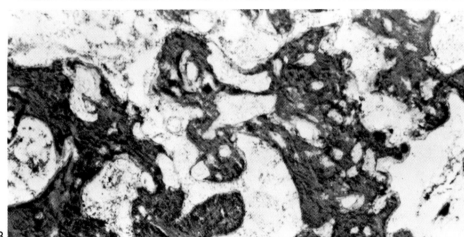

FIGURE 74–21. Skeletal fluorosis: Pathologic abnormalities.

A A photograph of a cross section of a fluorotic rib reveals cortical thickening and prominent trabeculae in the medullary cavity.

(**A,** From Singer L, et al: Clin Orthop *99*:303, 1974.)

B An iliac crest biopsy from a patient with fluorosis indicates a filigree pattern of trabecular bone, with loops and bridges of osteoid and internal resorption (50×).

(**B,** From Faccini JM, Teotia SPS: Calcif Tissue Res *16*:45, 1974.)

Complications. Advanced stages of fluorosis can lead to significant and crippling abnormalities, including kyphosis, restricted spinal and chest motion, and contractures and deformities of extraspinal joints such as the hips and the knees.[98] A high frequency of genu valgum deformity has been cited in some reports.[129] Neurologic complications include paresthesias, muscular weakening and wasting, sensory disturbances, and paralysis.[98] Although neurologic and musculoskeletal complications are reported more frequently in adults with fluorosis, they also are evident in some children with the disease.[170]

Reversibility of Skeletal Abnormalities. The identification of less striking radiographic abnormalities of the skeleton in retired workers who had been exposed to fluoride while employed is consistent with the concept that such abnormalities are reversible. This concept has been supported in an investigation by Grandjean and Thomsen[225] in which four patients who had been employed as cryolite workers were reexamined 8 to 15 years after the fluoride exposure had ended. Extensive fading of the sclerotic changes in the pelvis, ribs, and vertebrae was seen (Fig. 74–22). The resulting radiographic appearance, consisting of a coarsened trabecular pattern without increased radiodensity, resembled that of Paget's disease. The degree of cortical bone thickening and calcification of muscle insertions and ligaments remained unchanged. It appears likely that the improvement in the skeletal alterations relates to continued excretion of the fluoride, especially in the urine.

Fluoride Treatment of Osteoporosis. Sodium fluoride has been used in the treatment of osteoporosis for approximately 25 years.[226–229] The rationale for its use is the ability of fluoride to stimulate new bone formation through increased osteoblastic activity[230] and to depress bone resorption through the deposition of relatively stable fluoroapatite, which is less active in surface exchange reactions.[117] Histologic evaluation of osseous tissue in osteoporotic patients receiving sodium fluoride reveals cortical and trabecular new bone formation juxtaposed on underlying normal lamellar bone; the new bone shows increased osteocytic cellularity, irregular arrangement of the osteocytes, and enlarged osteocyte lacunae.[231] Additional findings are increases in trabecular bone volume, trabecular osteoid surface, and trabecular osteoid volume and prominent osteoclastic resorptive activity.[231] The morphologic changes indicate the deposition of new bone that possesses abnormal matrix characteristics.

Radiographic changes accompany these histologic alterations and appear to occur in direct proportion to the duration of the treatment.[232] The first detectable changes are noted at least 1 year after the start of the fluoride therapy (Fig. 74–23). Findings include pronounced bone radiodensity, cortical thickening, coarsening of the trabecular pattern, and partial obliteration of the medullary space, and they are observed principally in the axial skeleton, especially the spine and the pelvis[339]; ligamentous calcification, a frequent finding in industrial and endemic fluorosis, is not a feature of iatrogenic fluorosis.[232] The abnormalities simulate those of Paget's disease, myelofibrosis, and renal osteo-

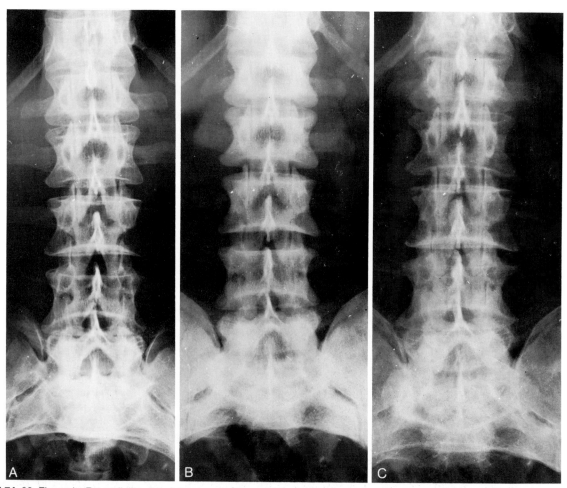

FIGURE 74–22. Fluorosis: Reversibility of skeletal abnormalities. Radiographs of the lumbar spine from 1957 **(A),** 1967 **(B),** and 1982 **(C),** of a man who had been employed as a cryolite worker in Copenhagen. No skeletal abnormalities are seen in **(A),** after 12 years of employment. Ten years later, in **B,** generalized increased radiodensity of the spine and pelvis is observed. Fifteen years later and 9 years after the cessation of exposure, in **C,** the radiodensity of the bone is decreased, although a coarsened trabecular pattern is evident. (From Grandjean P, Thomsen G: Br J Industr Med 40:456, 1983.)

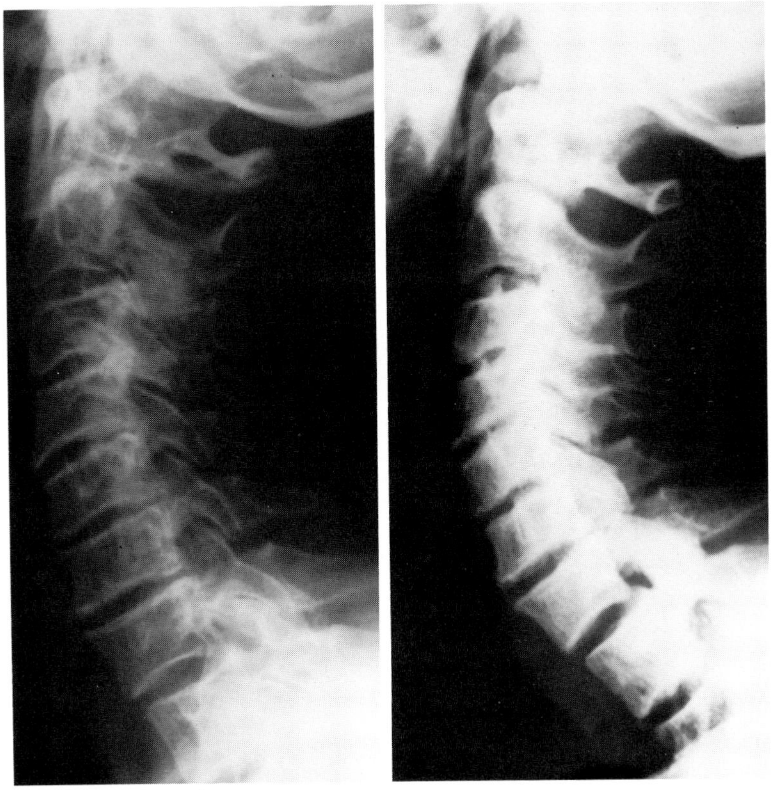

FIGURE 74–23. Fluoride treatment of osteoporosis. Radiographs obtained 5 years apart of a 70 year old woman with osteoporosis who began receiving sodium fluoride at the time the initial study **(A)** was obtained. At this time, osteoporosis is evident. Five years later **(B)**, note the increase in skeletal radiodensity and the coarsened trabecular pattern. (Courtesy of V. Vint, M.D., San Diego, California.)

A   B

dystrophy. In the appendicular skeleton, periosteal and endosteal bone formation are particularly prominent in areas of high mechanical stress.[295]

The osseous changes occurring during fluoride therapy for osteoporosis, particularly those in the appendicular skeleton, can be well evaluated with scintigraphy.[233, 340] An increased uptake of the bone-seeking radionuclide in total skeletal scintigrams has been seen within 4 to 20 months after the initiation of the therapy; new areas of increased accumulation of the radiopharmaceutical agent correspond in location to metaphyseal regions of tubular bones and the small bones of the appendicular skeleton. It is suggested that such changes indicate increased bone formation (rather than augmented blood flow) and predominate in areas under greater mechanical stress.[233] Concurrently, an increase of activity of serum alkaline phosphatase is seen. Furthermore, bone pain and rheumatic complaints have been associated with sodium fluoride therapy, and they correspond in location to sites of increased radionuclide activity.[233] In some instances, the cause of the pain as well as of the scintigraphic abnormality appears to be a stress fracture.[290]

Although the radiographic appearance of osteoporotic bone in patients receiving sodium fluoride is one of progressive osteosclerosis, it is not clear if a commensurate increase in osseous strength occurs. In fact, fractures of the vertebral bodies and tubular bones are reported during fluoride treatment.[234–236, 341] The femoral neck is a common site of fracture in this situation, and the fractures may be bilateral. Other sites of fracture include the pubic rami, greater trochanter of the femur, tibia, and fibula. Vertebral fractures may appear earlier than those in the tubular bones.[341] The precise cause of this complication is unclear; the relative

importance of the underlying osteoporosis and that of fluoride-induced osteomalacia are not known, although Riggs and collaborators[236] found fewer compression fractures of the spine in osteoporotic patients receiving sodium fluoride compared with those who received a placebo. These results and others[226, 227, 235] suggest that the sclerotic bone is not so strong as it looks but probably is stronger than it was before treatment began.[232]

Differential Diagnosis. The combination of findings noted on radiographs of patients with skeletal fluorosis is virtually diagnostic. Osteosclerosis, osteophytosis, and ligamentous calcification represent a useful triad of abnormalities that are evident on pelvis and spine radiographs. The other alterations that occur in both axial and extra-axial locations, such as periostitis and osseous excrescences at sites of tendinous and ligamentous attachment, provide additional clues to the correct diagnosis.

Osteosclerosis alone is not diagnostic of fluorosis, being evident in skeletal metastasis, myelofibrosis, mastocytosis, certain hemoglobinopathies, renal osteodystrophy, Paget's disease, congenital disorders, and other conditions. Likewise, vertebral osteophytosis or similar outgrowths can accompany many diseases, including fluorosis, spondylosis deformans, diffuse idiopathic skeletal hyperostosis, ankylosing spondylitis, the spondylitis of psoriasis, Reiter's syndrome, and inflammatory bowel disorders, acromegaly, neuropathic osteoarthropathy, and alkaptonuria. Proliferative changes at ligamentous and tendinous insertions in bones are apparent not only in fluorosis but also in diffuse idiopathic skeletal hyperostosis, hypoparathyroidism, X-linked hypophosphatemic osteomalacia, and certain plasma cell dyscrasias. Periostitis similar to that seen in fluorosis

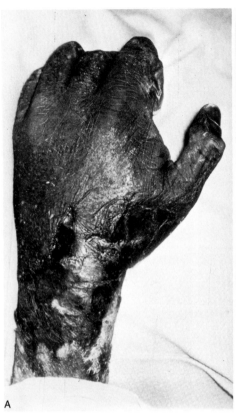

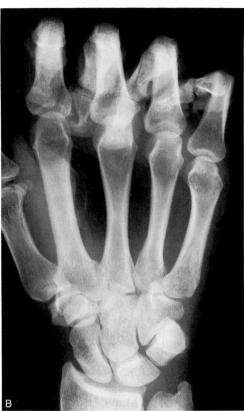

FIGURE 74–24. Dopamine-induced gangrene. A 46 year old man, admitted to the hospital with severe hypotension, was given a dopamine infusion of 8 to 16 μg/kg/min. He developed progressive cyanosis of both hands and both feet. He required bilateral below-the-knee amputations and a unilateral below-the-elbow amputation.

A A photograph of the left hand indicates the severity of the necrosis.

B A radiograph reveals the extent of soft tissue contracture. The bones are intact.

can be detected in hypertrophic osteoarthropathy, pachydermoperiostosis, and thyroid acropathy. Thus, each individual radiographic finding of skeletal fluorosis can be apparent in other disorders as well; it is the combination of findings in fluorosis that is diagnostic.

DOPAMINE AND RELATED SUBSTANCES

Dopamine is a direct-acting catecholamine that at lower doses dilates the mesenteric, renal, cerebral, and coronary vessels and at high doses has a vasoconstrictor action due to stimulation of alpha receptors.[130–132] Use of this drug in large amounts can be associated with ischemic necrosis and gangrene.[133–137] These complications, which may be more severe in patients with underlying vascular diseases, such as diabetes mellitus and atherosclerosis, in unusual circumstances can require amputation of one or more extremities[138, 139] (Fig. 74–24).

Gangrene also may occur during the course of treatment with other vasoconstrictive drugs. Ergotamine and its derivatives, such as methysergide, which have been used in the treatment of migraine headaches to reduce the vasodilation and excessive pulsation of the branches of the external carotid artery, can lead to vasoconstriction of peripheral vessels and gangrene.[140–144] Administration of vasopressin (Pitressin) can induce gangrene, soft tissue calcification, and perhaps osteonecrosis (Fig. 74–25).[145, 237] Repeated self-administered injections of epinephrine into the thighs of asthmatic persons have eventuated in gangrene and massive soft tissue calcification, perhaps attributable to capillary spasm, decreased vascularity, and pH alterations.[4, 14, 238]

CALCIUM GLUCONATE

Intravenous administration of calcium gluconate has been used in the treatment of neonatal tetany and neonatal asphyxia. Subcutaneous masses of calcification can appear at

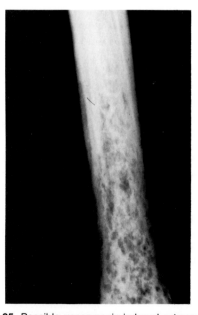

FIGURE 74–25. Possible vasopressin-induced osteonecrosis. This elderly woman with carcinoma of the breast had required extensive surgery and irradiation, pituitary ablation, and vasopressin medication for over 10 years. The changes in the femoral shaft consisting of patchy sclerosis apparently are related to osteonecrosis. (Courtesy of W. Murphy, M.D., Houston, Texas.)

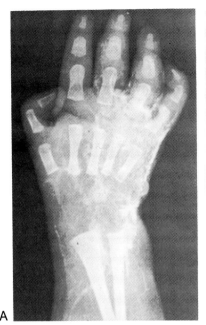
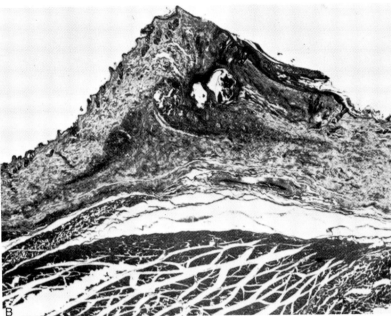

FIGURE 74–26. Calcium gluconate extravasation.

 A This 3 lb 6 oz black infant received an infusion of calcium gluconate into a vein in the dorsum of the hand that subsequently infiltrated into the soft tissues. A radiograph taken approximately 1 week later reveals extensive linear and platelike subcutaneous deposits with vascular calcification.

 B A cross section of the skin, subcutaneous tissue, and muscle of a rabbit 37 days after subcutaneous injection of 4 ml calcium gluconate reveals a calcium-filled inclusion cyst in the upper dermis with adjacent calcification in fibrous tissue (9×).

 (From Berger PE, et al: AJR *121*:109, 1974, American Roentgen Ray Society.)

sites of recent or previous injections.[146, 147, 239, 240] Clinical findings include erythema and bulla formation, becoming evident in a period of days, which may be followed by skin sloughing and secondary infection.[242] Calcification, which is related to tissue necrosis,[241] can be noted within 4 or 5 days or as late as 3 weeks after injection (Fig. 74–26). It is amorphous and can be localized or distributed along fascial planes. Vascular calcification also may be apparent. With healing, clinical and radiologic manifestations may disappear. The radiographic changes simulate those in subcutaneous fat necrosis and hematomas following trauma.[146]

MILK-ALKALI

In 1949, Burnett and coworkers[148] observed six patients with chronic peptic ulcer disease and renal insufficiency in whom excessive intake of milk and alkali (for a few to many years) led to metastatic calcification. These patients revealed hypercalcemia without hypercalciuria or hypophosphatemia, normal serum alkaline phosphatase levels, azotemia, and mild alkalosis. Although all six persons revealed clinical improvement after the withdrawal of milk and alkali from the diet, the calcification persisted and none of the patients survived. These investigators postulated that the following sequence of events was important: excessive intake of milk and alkali, kidney damage, fixation in urinary calcium excretion, hypercalcemia, supersaturation of calcium phosphate, and calcinosis.

Other reports of this complication soon appeared,[149–151] and the reversibility of both clinical and radiologic findings and the importance of renal insufficiency with the simultaneous ingestion of milk and alkali were emphasized.[152] Poppel and Zeitel[153] outlined the radiographic manifestations of

milk-drinker's syndrome; unilateral or bilateral periarticular deposits predominate, which are amorphous and vary in size from small nodules to bulky tumors (Fig. 74–27). Widespread calcification in blood vessels, kidneys, ligaments, and falx cerebri also are observed, and the osseous tissues are normal.[154–159]

Wenger and associates[160] summarized their experiences at the University of Chicago; 35 patients with the milk-alkali syndrome were detected among 33,000 patients who were hospitalized for the management of peptic ulcer disease. They noted that the syndrome might appear within several days to weeks after the start of therapy with calcium carbonate, milk, and cream, the interval averaging 1 week. The typical clinical manifestations were nausea, vomiting, anorexia, weakness, headache, and dizziness. No definite relationship with primary hyperparathyroidism was detected, although the exact mechanism could not be determined.

Orwoll[243] recently has summarized the major features of this syndrome. It occurs principally in middle-aged men (the male to female ratio is about 4 to 1) who are ingesting milk and calcium carbonate, or calcium carbonate alone, for abdominal pain or heartburn. Although hypercalcemia, alkalosis, and renal impairment represent the classic triad of the syndrome, the clinical characteristics are variable and may include acute (toxemia), intermediate (Cope's syndrome), and chronic (Burnett's syndrome) forms. It is the chronic pattern that is associated with (1) major metabolic consequences consisting of renal failure with hyperphosphatemia, alkalosis, and hypercalcemia and (2) diffuse calcification in the soft tissues, kidneys, eyes, and other regions. After a period in which some of these consequences are reversible, irreversible renal disease and soft tissue calcification appear.[291]

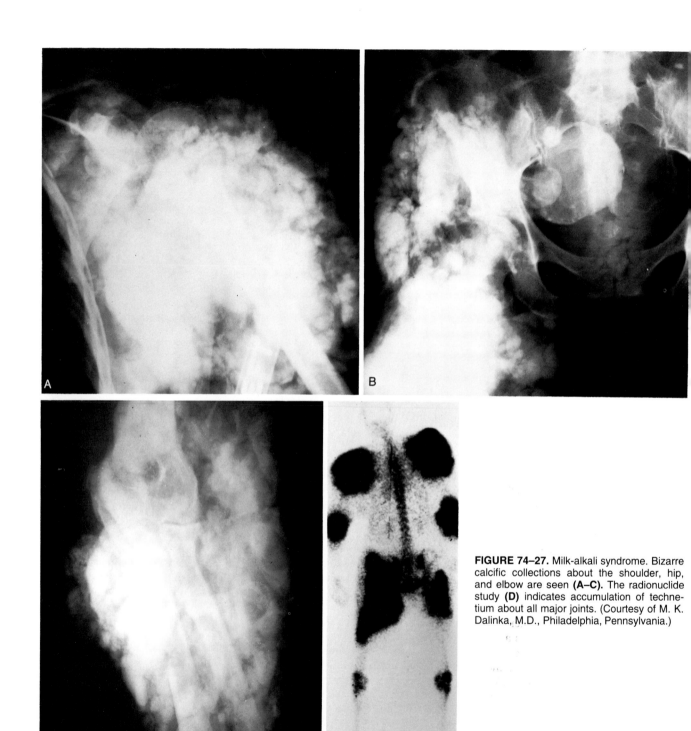

FIGURE 74–27. Milk-alkali syndrome. Bizarre calcific collections about the shoulder, hip, and elbow are seen **(A–C)**. The radionuclide study **(D)** indicates accumulation of technetium about all major joints. (Courtesy of M. K. Dalinka, M.D., Philadelphia, Pennsylvania.)

Although the ingestion of calcium and absorbable alkali is fundamental to the occurrence of the milk-alkali syndrome, questions remain as to its precise pathogenesis and, specifically, to its relationship to primary hyperparathyroidism. The two conditions may coexist, and overt hyperparathyroidism may lead to an exacerbation of the milk-alkali syndrome. Surgical exploration of the neck in some patients with the latter syndrome has documented the absence of gross pathologic and histologic evidence of parathyroid gland hyperplasia or adenoma, suggesting that the milk-alkali syndrome, although accompanied by laboratory features of hyperparathyroidism, is a distinct entity.[244]

The differential diagnosis of periarticular calcific deposits accompanying the milk-alkali syndrome includes collagen vascular disorders, hyperparathyroidism, renal osteodystrophy, hypervitaminosis D, and idiopathic tumoral calcinosis.

PROSTAGLANDINS

Prostaglandin E_1 commonly is used to maintain the patency of the ductus arteriosus in neonates with ductus-dependent congenital heart disease, including interruption or coarctation of the aortic arch, pulmonary atresia complex, and tetralogy of Fallot.[245] Although the duration of prostaglandin E_1 administration usually is confined to the period of time that is required to allow stabilization of the infant's condition prior to surgical intervention, longer periods of infusion occasionally are required. A variety of complications have been encountered during and after prostaglandin E_1 therapy; these include damage of the ductus, hypotension, hyperthermia, diarrhea, apnea, bradycardia, and flushing and edema of the skin.[248] One further complication, related to the musculoskeletal system, was described in reports from Japan in 1980[246, 247]: new bone formation appearing as periostitis and cortical thickening. The existence of this abnormality subsequently has been confirmed in other investigations.[249–252, 292, 301, 342–344, 368]

Periosteal bone formation is characteristic of long-term (40 days or more) prostaglandin E_1 infusion, although it also may be seen with short-term (9 to 14 days) therapy[249, 292] as well as with prostaglandin E_2 therapy.[251, 345] Affected sites include the ribs, tubular bones, and, to a lesser extent, mandible, clavicle, scapula, and pelvis. Although multiple areas may be involved, a symmetric distribution is not present uniformly. Periostitis varies in intensity from subtle and localized osseous deposits to widespread and severe alterations leading to enlargement of the bone (Figs. 74–28 and 74–29). Additional findings include soft tissue swelling and the presence of an unossified zone at the margins of the cranial sutures that simulates the appearance of sutural diastasis.[344] Generally the process is self-limited, with no apparent effect on subsequent bone growth and development; complete resolution commonly is seen over a 6 month to 1 year period.[249, 346]

As summarized by Ringel and associates,[249] bone resorption represents a well-documented effect of prostaglandin administration and, experimentally, periosteal bone formation occurs in response to long-term prostaglandin E_1 infusions.[253] As prostaglandins are cleared rapidly during the first passage through the lungs, bone changes would not be anticipated when they are administered intravenously to a healthy infant.[344]

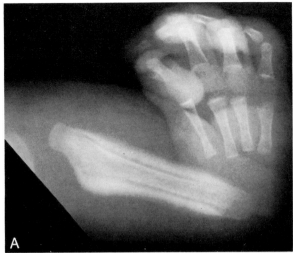

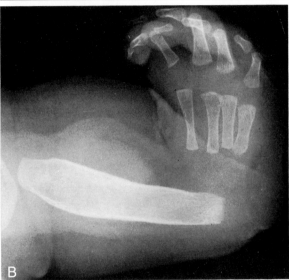

FIGURE 74–28. Prostaglandin periostitis. This male infant was noted to have multiple congenital abnormalities at birth. A cardiac catheterization confirmed the presence of a severe tetralogy of Fallot. An infusion of prostaglandin E_1 was begun when the patient was 3 weeks old and maintained for 7 weeks, after which it was discontinued. Bone changes were observed initially in the ribs and clavicle after 20 days of therapy.

A A radiograph of the forearm, obtained when the infant was 43 days old, reveals extensive periosteal elevation in the ulna. Note the absence of the radius, a finding of the VATER syndrome.

B At 6 months of age, the periosteal bone has been incorporated into the diaphysis of the ulna.

(From Poznanski AK, et al: Skel Radiol *14*:20, 1985.)

The differential diagnosis of the osseous alterations includes physiologic periostitis, trauma,[347, 348] Caffey's disease, congenital syphilis, hypervitaminosis A, scurvy, hypertrophic osteoarthropathy, leukemia, and skeletal metastasis.

RETINOIDS

Natural and synthetic forms of vitamin A, known collectively as retinoids, have been employed in the treatment of various dermatologic disorders, including severe refractory cystic and conglobate acne and keratinizing dermatoses, such as lamellar ichthyosis.[254, 255, 349, 350] Although the administration of one of these synthetic forms, isotretinoin (13-

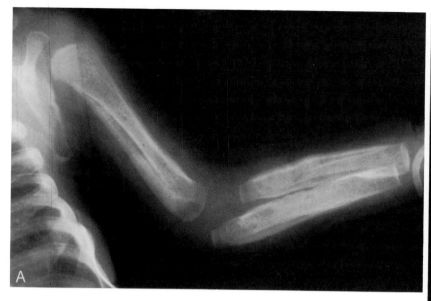

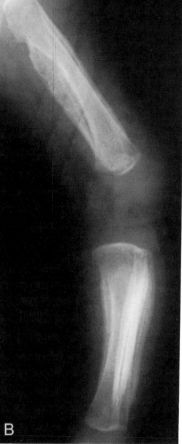

FIGURE 74–29. Prostaglandin periostitis. In a 3 month old infant receiving prostaglandin E$_1$ infusions, exuberant periosteal new bone is observed in the ribs, humerus, radius, ulna, femur, tibia, and fibula. (Courtesy of T. Broderick, M.D., Orange, California.)

cis-retinoic acid, Accutane), in short-term low doses results in the remission of many cases of cystic acne, long-term administration of this agent (or other agents such as tretinoin, etretinate, and acitretin) in higher doses may be required in some of these dermatologic disorders, especially ichthyosis. Reports indicate that the long-term use of isotretinoin is associated with skeletal hyperostosis resembling that seen in chronic vitamin A intoxication.[256, 257, 302] Pennes and collaborators[257] observed such hyperostosis in six of eight patients, aged 5 to 26 years, within 1 year after the initiation of high dosage retinoid therapy. Both axial and appendicular skeletal sites were affected. Vertebral alterations predominated in the cervical region, although thoracic and lumbar spinal changes also were evident. The findings, which usually were subtle and required comparison with previous radiographic studies for identification, consisted of pointed osseous excrescences arising from the anterior and posterior margins of the vertebral bodies, which, with time, progressed to larger osteophytic outgrowths (Figs. 74–30 and 74–31). In the appendicular skeleton, pointlike hyperostosis was seen at the corners and promontories of bones, such as the tarsal navicular and calcaneus. Bilateral and symmetric changes occurred more frequently than unilateral abnormalities. Clinical manifestations were absent or mild, confined to joint stiffness, and serologic testing for the histocompatibility antigen HLA-B27 was negative in all patients. Although Pennes and coworkers did not identify instances of premature physeal fusion, this complication has been recognized by others in patients receiving isotre-

tinoin[258, 351] and is a known complication of hypervitaminosis A (see Chapter 75).

Adverse musculoskeletal manifestations related to isotretinoin therapy have been recognized in other reports as well.[351, 352] Initial clinical trials documented that 15 per cent of approximately 500 patients receiving 13-cis-retinoic acid orally developed diffuse arthralgias and myalgias.[259] Vertebral hyperostosis similar to that described earlier, ossification of the anterior and posterior longitudinal ligaments and atlanto-occipital ligaments (Fig. 74–32), and nasal bone osteophytosis have been related to such therapy in additional patients.[260, 261, 296, 351] Acute arthritis leading to joint effusions[262, 365] and isotretinoin embryopathy occurring in the infants born to women who had taken the drug[263, 264] are additional evidence supporting the occurrence of significant musculoskeletal alterations in response to 13-cis-retinoic acid therapy.

The evolution of skeletal hyperostosis caused by this chemical agent has been studied by Pennes and coworkers.[352] In general, the earliest appearing hyperostoses became the largest with time, although in some instances, the outgrowths ceased growing at some sites and progressed at others. The severity of skeletal involvement appeared independent of dose and may have been related to the patient's age at the initiation of therapy (the older the patient at the start of therapy, the more severe the abnormalities). Spinal involvement occurred earlier and was more pronounced than extraspinal involvement, and the most prominent appendicular hyperostoses were evident at the tendinous and

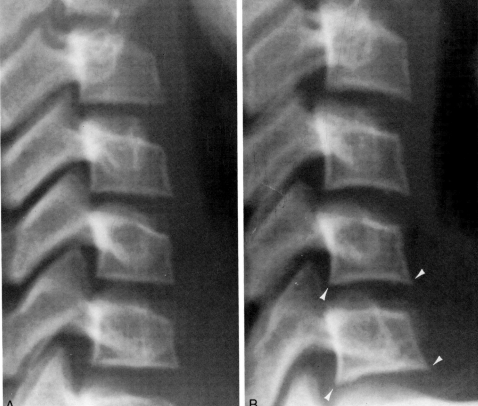

FIGURE 74–30. Isotretinoin hyperostosis. In this patient, a lateral radiograph of the cervical spine obtained prior to therapy **(A)** and another after 1 year of therapy **(B)** are shown. A definite interval change can be noted. In **B,** observe the "pointing" of the bone at the anteroinferior and posteroinferior portions of the vertebral bodies (arrowheads). (From Pennes DR, et al: Radiology *141*:979, 1984.)

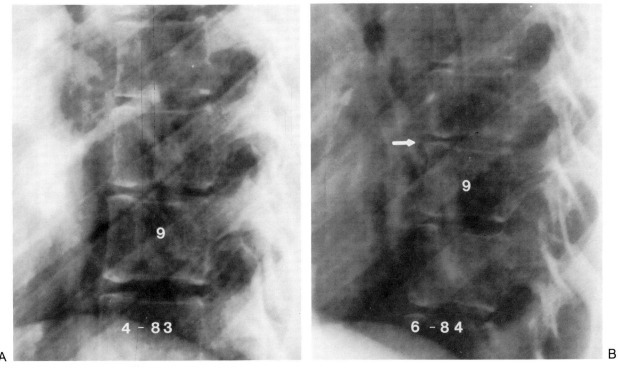

FIGURE 74–31. Isotretinoin hyperostosis. In this patient, note the interval change that occurred during isotretinoin (Accutane) therapy. It is the ninth thoracic vertebral body (arrow) that is principally affected. Changes are subtle. (Courtesy of R. F. Kilcoyne, M.D., Denver, Colorado.)

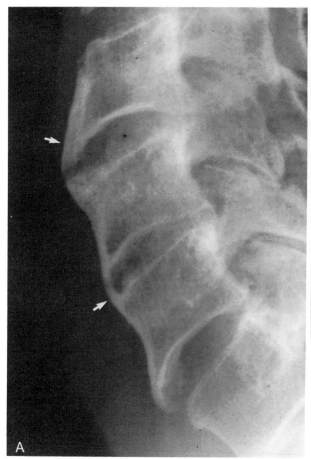
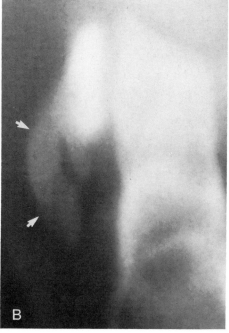

FIGURE 74–32. Isotretinoin hyperostosis. In two different patients, prominent ligamentous ossification is apparent (arrows) in the midcervical spine (**A**) and about the anterior arch of the atlas (**B**). (**A**, Courtesy of J. Mink, M.D., Los Angeles, California; **B**, courtesy of J. Lawson, M.D., New Haven, Connecticut.)

aponeurotic insertions in the calcaneus. In the calcaneus, bilateral changes eventually predominated, whereas at other extraspinal locations, asymmetric or unilateral enthesophytes generally were encountered.

Although its application to the treatment of dermatologic disorders is more recent, etretinate also may lead to skeletal hyperostosis.[350, 353, 354] In one study, more than 80 per cent of patients revealed radiographic evidence of hyperostosis after 5 years of etretinate therapy, and such hyperostosis predominated in extraspinal sites.[302] The therapeutic toxicity of one additional agent, acitretin, appears to be similar to that of etretinate.[350]

The relationship of the skeletal alterations occurring after administration of isotretinoin (or similar agents) to those of diffuse idiopathic skeletal hyperostosis has received attention.[257, 265] Spinal and extraspinal changes in both disorders are similar in terms of distribution and morphology, although those of diffuse idiopathic skeletal hyperostosis generally are more extensive. In cats, high doses of retinol induce skeletal changes similar to those of diffuse idiopathic skeletal hyperostosis, and it has been suggested that a higher free retinol fraction exists in the plasma of patients with the latter disease and that retinol is responsible for the bone lesions.[265]

ADDITIONAL CHEMICALS

Phenytoin (*Dilantin*) has been associated with calvarial thickening[266] and enlargement of the heel pad,[267] findings resembling those of acromegaly. Dilantin,[268] along with *heparin*,[269–273, 297] *alcohol*,[274] and *methotrexate*,[275] can lead to skeletal osteopenia (Fig. 74–33) (see Chapters 51 and 53). With long-term methotrexate therapy for childhood neoplasms, especially acute lymphocytic leukemia, severe osteopenia and multiple fractures in the tubular bones of the lower extremities (and to a lesser extent, the upper extremities) are seen; additional findings include growth recovery lines and radiodense areas in the metaphyses and epiphyses, simulating the changes of scurvy (Fig. 74–34).[275] The abnormalities occur within a period of months (2 to 24 months) after the initiation of the therapy. The cause of the osteopenia is not known, although the antifolic acid action of the drug probably is important; increased bone resorption, rather than decreased bone formation, apparently is involved.[275] Another chemotherapeutic agent used in the treatment of tumors, *ifosfamide,* has been associated with hypophosphatemic rickets,[356–358, 366] and nitrogen-containing *biphosphates,* used in the treatment of a variety of skeletal disorders, may lead to bandlike metaphyseal sclerosis and concentric epiphyseal and apophyseal sclerosis when administered to children.[359]

Disulfiram (Antabuse), used in the treatment of alcoholism, has been accompanied by myalgia,[276] arthritis,[277, 278] the carpal tunnel syndrome,[278] and arteritis.[279] *Propranolol and oxprenolol,* as well as other beta-blocking medications, have been linked to arthritis.[280, 281] *Anticoagulants,* particularly heparin, can be associated with sudden, unexpected bleeding leading to large hematomas in a variety of sites.[282, 283, 355]

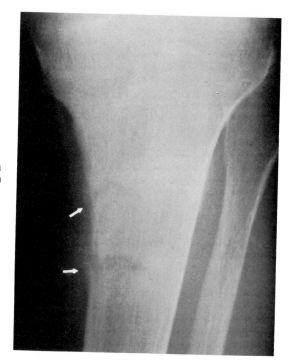

FIGURE 74–33. Phenytoin (Dilantin)-induced osteomalacia. In this adult with a seizure disorder, long-term Dilantin therapy has resulted in osteomalacia with Looser's zones, or insufficiency fractures (arrows).

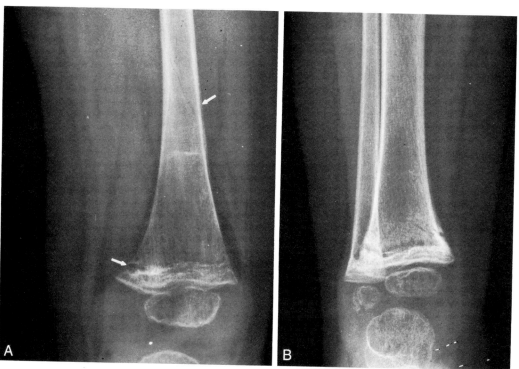

FIGURE 74–34. Methotrexate osteopathy. An 18 month old boy with acute lymphocytic leukemia was treated with a variety of drugs, including methotrexate. Approximately 2 years later, these radiographs were obtained because the patient had pain and weakness in the legs. Findings in **A** include osteopenia, periostitis, and fractures both in the diaphysis and in the metaphysis of the left femur (arrows). A growth recovery line is seen. In **B,** observe osteopenia, growth recovery lines, and a fracture of the metaphysis of the right tibia. Although these fractures healed well, additional ones occurred subsequently. (From Schwartz AM, Leonidas JC: Skel Radiol *11*:13, 1984.)

Additional chemical agents associated with musculoskeletal complications include *pentazocine,* an analgesic drug that may lead to cutaneous abnormalities (abnormal pigmentation, ulceration, and loss of sensation) and local (at sites of intramuscular injections) or diffuse myopathy[360]; and *quinolones,* which have been associated with arthralgias, arthritis, myalgias, tendinitis, and spontaneous tendon ruptures.[361]

SUMMARY

A survey of some of the musculoskeletal manifestations associated with certain medications and chemical substances indicates that at times the therapeutic regimen indeed may be more detrimental than the disease. A variety of teratogenic drugs can lead to significant fetal anomalies. Corticosteroids and other anti-inflammatory agents can produce osteoporosis, osteonecrosis, and neuropathic-like alterations. Osteosclerosis, periostitis, osseous excrescences, ligamentous calcification, and dental abnormalities can accompany fluorosis. Injection of dopamine and related substances may lead to gangrene, requiring amputation, whereas soft tissue calcification may appear after calcium gluconate injection or milk and alkali ingestion. New bone formation is seen in some patients receiving prostaglandins or isotretinoin.

References

1. Keats TE: Post-injection calcification of the deltoid muscle. J Can Assoc Radiol 29:165, 1978.
2. Goldman AB: Myositis ossificans circumscripta: A benign lesion with a malignant differential diagnosis. AJR 126:32, 1976.
3. Imray TJ, Hiramatsu Y: Radiographic manifestations of Japanese acupuncture. Radiology 115:625, 1975.
4. Murray RO: Radiological importance of soft tissue lesions related to skeletons. Ann R Coll Surg 54:109, 1974.
5. Forfar JO, Nelson MM: Epidemiology of drugs taken by pregnant women: Drugs that may affect the fetus adversely. Clin Pharmacol Ther 14:632, 1973.
6. Bleyer WA, Au WYW, Lange WA, et al: Studies on the detection of adverse drug reaction in the newborn. 1. Fetal exposure to maternal medications. JAMA 213:2046, 1970.
7. Hill RM: Drugs ingested by pregnant women. Clin Pharmacol Ther 14:654, 1973.
8. Wilson JG: Factors determining the teratogencity of drugs. Ann Rev Pharmacol 14:205, 1974.
9. Wilson JG: Present status of drugs as teratogens in man. Teratology 7:3, 1973.
10. Harris JM III, Pashayan HM: Teratogenesis. Orthop Clin North Am 7:281, 1976.
11. McBride WG: Thalidomide and congenital anomalies. Lancet 2:1358, 1961.
12. Lenz W, Knapp K: Thalidomide embryopathy. Arch Environ Health 5:100, 1962.
13. McCredie J, McBride WG: Some congenital abnormalities: Possibly due to embryonic peripheral neuropathy. Clin Radiol 24:204, 1973.
14. Murray RO: Iatrogenic lesions of the skeleton. AJR 126:5, 1976.
15. Loughnan PM, Gold H, Vance JC: Phenytoin teratogenicity in man. Lancet 1:70, 1973.
16. Hill RM, Verniaud WM, Horning MG, et al: Infants exposed in utero to antiepileptic drugs. A prospective study. Am J Dis Child 127:645, 1974.
17. Monson RR, Rosenberg L, Hartz SC, et al: Diphenylhydantion and selected congenital malformations. N Engl J Med 289:1049, 1973.
18. Lowe CR: Congenital malformations among infants born to epileptic women. Lancet 1:9, 1973.
19. Palmer RH, Quellette EM, Warner L, et al: Congenital malformations in offspring of a chronic alcoholic mother. Pediatrics 53:490, 1974.
20. Ferrier PE, Nicod I, Ferrier S: Fetal alcohol syndrome. Lancet 2:1496, 1973.
21. Jones KL, Smith DW: Recognition of the fetal alcohol syndrome in early infancy. Lancet 2:999, 1973.
22. Milunsky A, Graef JW, Gaynor MF: Methotrexate-induced congenital malformations. J Pediatr 72:790, 1968.
23. Becker MH, Genieser NB, Finegold M, et al: Chondrodysplasia punctata. Is maternal warfarin therapy a factor? Am J Dis Child 129:356, 1975.
24. Shaul WL, Emery H, Hall JG: Chondrodysplasia punctata and maternal warfarin use during pregnancy. Am J Dis Child 129:360, 1975.
25. Greenberg G, Inman WHW: Hormonal pregnancy tests and congenital malformations. Br Med J 2:191, 1975.
26. Hench PS, Kendall EC, Slocumb CH, et al: Effect of hormone of adrenal cortex (17-hydroxy-11-dehydro cortisone, compound E) and of pituitary adrenocorticotropic hormone on rheumatoid arthritis: Preliminary report. Ann Rheum Dis 8:97, 1949.
27. Murray RO: Radiological bone changes in Cushing's syndrome and steroid therapy. Br J Radiol 33:1, 1960.
28. Murray RO: Steroids and skeleton. Radiology 77:729, 1961.
29. Solomon L: Drug-induced arthropathy and necrosis of the femoral head. J Bone Joint Surg [Br] 55:246, 1973.
30. Fisher DE, Bickel WH: Corticosteroid-induced avascular necrosis. A clinical study of seventy-seven patients. J Bone Joint Surg [Am] 53:859, 1971.
31. Saville PD, Kharmosh O: Osteoporosis of rheumatoid arthritis. Influence of age, sex and corticosteroids. Arthritis Rheum 10:423, 1967.
32. Heaney RP, Walch JJ, Steffes P, et al: Periarticular bone remodeling in rheumatoid arthritis. Calcif Tissue Res 2(Suppl):33, 1968.
33. Sweetman R: Corticosteroid arthropathy and tendon rupture. J Bone Joint Surg [Br] 51:397, 1969.
34. Pietrogrande V, Mastromarino R: Osteopatia da prolungata trattamento cortisonico. Ortop Traum Appar Mot 25:791, 1957.
35. Gold EW, Fox OD, Weissfeld S, et al: Corticosteroid-induced avascular necrosis: An experimental study in rabbits. Clin Orthop 135:272, 1978.
36. Cruess RL: Cortisone-induced avascular necrosis of the femoral head. J Bone Joint Surg [Br] 59:308, 1977.
37. Cruess RL: Steroid-induced avascular necrosis of the head of the humerus. Natural history and management. J Bone Joint Surg [Br] 58:313, 1976.
38. Fisher DE, Bickel WH, Holley KE: Histologic demonstration of fat emboli in aseptic necrosis associated with hypercortisonism. Mayo Clin Proc 44:252, 1969.
39. Velayos EE, Leidholt JD, Smyth CJ, et al: Arthropathy associated with steroid therapy. Ann Intern Med 64:759, 1966.
40. Smyth CJ, Leidholt JD: Steroid arthropathy of the hip. Clin Orthop 90:50, 1973.
41. Fisher DE: The role of fat embolism in the etiology of corticosteroid-induced avascular necrosis. Clinical and experimental results. Clin Orthop 130:68, 1978.
42. Cruess RL: Experience with steroid-induced avascular necrosis of the shoulder and etiologic considerations regarding osteonecrosis of the hip. Clin Orthop 130:86, 1978.
43. Cruess RL, Ross D, Crawshaw E: The etiology of steroid-induced avascular necrosis of bone. A laboratory and clinical study. Clin Orthop 113:178, 1975.
44. Heimann WG, Freiberger RH: Avascular necrosis of the femoral and humeral heads after high-dosage corticosteroid therapy. N Engl J Med 263:672, 1960.
45. Boksenbaum M, Mendelson CG: Aseptic necrosis of the femoral head associated with steroid therapy. JAMA 184:262, 1963.
46. Serre H, Simon L: Le role de la corticothérapie dans l'osteo-necrose primitive de la téte femoral chez l'adulte. Presse Med 69:1995, 1961.
47. Harrington KD, Murray WR, Kountz SL, et al: Avascular necrosis of bone after renal transplantation. J Bone Joint Surg [Am] 53:203, 1971.
48. Frost HM: The etiodynamics of aseptic necrosis of the femoral head. In Proceedings of the Conference on Aseptic Necrosis of the Femoral Head. St Louis, National Institute of Health, 1964, p 393.
49. Boettcher WG, Bonfiglio M, Hamilton HH, et al: Nontraumatic necrosis of the femoral head. Part I. Relation of altered hemostasis to etiology. J Bone Joint Surg [Am] 52:312, 1970.
50. Cosgriff SW: Thromboembolic complications associated with ACTH and cortisone therapy. JAMA 147:924, 1951.
51. Merle d'Aubigne R, Postel M, Mazabraud A, et al: Idiopathic necrosis of the femoral head in adults. J Bone Joint Surg [Br] 47:612, 1965.
52. Fisher DE, Bickel WH, Holley KE, et al: Corticosteroid-induced aseptic necrosis. II. Experimental study. Clin Orthop 84:200, 1972.
53. Jones JP, Engleman EP, Steinbach HL, et al: Fat embolization as a possible mechanism producing avascular necrosis. Arthritis Rheum 8:449, 1965.
54. Jones JP, Sakovich L: Fat embolism of bone: A roentgenographic and histological investigation with use of intra-arterial lipiodol in rabbits. J Bone Joint Surg [Am] 48:149, 1966.
55. Jones JP, Engleman EP: Fat embolization complicating hypercortisonism. Arthritis Rheum 8:448, 1965.
56. Jones JP, Engleman EP, Najarian JS: Systemic fat embolism after renal homotransplantation and treatment with corticosteroids. N Engl J Med 273:1453, 1965.
57. Jaffe WL, Epstein M, Heyman N, et al: The effect of cortisone on femoral and humeral head in rabbits. Clin Orthop 82:221, 1972.
58. Arora JS: Indomethacin arthropathy of hips. Proc R Soc Med 61:669, 1968.
59. Wilkenfeld MJ, Sliwinski AJ: Fatty lesions of both humeri in a patient on corticosteroids and cyclophosphamide. Arthritis Rheum 22:199, 1979.
60. Sakai T, Cruess RL: Effect of cortisone on the lipids of bone matrix in the rat. Proc R Soc Exp Bio Med 124:490, 1967.
61. Miller WT, Restifo RA: Steroid arthropathy. Radiology 86:652, 1966.
62. Chandler GN, Jones DT, Wright V, et al: Charcot's arthropathy following intraarticular hydrocortisone. Br Med J 1:952, 1959.
63. Steinberg CL, Duthe RB, Piva AE: Charcot-like arthropathy following intraarticular hydrocortisone. JAMA 181:851, 1962.
64. Bently G, Goodfellow JW: Disorganization of the knees following intra-articular hydrocortisone injections. J Bone Joint Surg [Br] 51:498, 1969.
65. Salter RB, Gross A, Hall JH: Hydrocortisone arthropathy—an experimental investigation. Can Med Assoc J 97:374, 1967.

66. Shaw NE, Lacey E: The influence of corticosteroids on normal and papain-treated articular cartilage in the rabbit. J Bone Joint Surg [Br] 55:197, 1973.

67. Mankin HJ, Conger KA: The acute effects of intra-articular hydrocortisone on articular cartilage in rabbits. J Bone Joint Surg [AM] 48:1383, 1966.

68. Moskowitz RW, Davis W, Sammarco J, et al: Experimentally induced cortico-steroid arthropathy. Arthritis Rheum 13:236, 1970.

69. Mankin HJ, Zarins A, Jaffe WL: The effect of systemic corticosteroids on rabbit articular cartilage. Arthritis Rheum 15:593, 1972.

70. Gibson T, Burry HC, Poswillo D, et al: Effect of intra-articular corticosteroid injections on primate cartilage. Ann Rheum Dis 36:74, 1977.

71. Zachariae L: Deleterious effects of corticosteroids administered topically, in particular intra-articularly. Acta Orthop Scand 36:127, 1965.

72. Alarcon-Segovia D, Ward LE: Marked destructive changes occurring in os-teoarthritic finger joints after intra-articular injection of corticosteroids. Arthritis Rheum 9:443, 1966.

73. Wright V, Chandler GN, Morison RAH, et al: Intra-articular therapy in osteo-arthritis. Comparison of hydrocortisone acetate and hydrocortisone tertiary butyl-acetate. Ann Rheum Dis 19:257, 1960.

74. Keagy RD, Keim HA: Intra-articular steroid therapy: Repeated use in patients with chronic arthritis. Am J Med Sci 253:45, 1967.

75. Chandler GN, Wright V: Deleterious effect of intra-articular hydrocortisone. Lancet 2:661, 1958.

76. Rabinowitz MS: Pyarthrosis of knee joint following intra-articular hydrocorti-sone. Bull Hosp Joint Dis 16:158, 1955.

77. Thomet M: Le danger des injections intra-articulaires d'hydrocortisone. Praxis 46:152, 1957.

78. Mills LC, Boylston BF, Greene JA, et al: Septic arthritis as a complication of orally given steroid therapy. JAMA 164:1310, 1957.

79. Tondreau RL, Hodes PJ, Schmidt ER Jr: Joint infections following steroid therapy: Roentgen manifestations. AJR 82:258, 1959.

80. Ismail AM, Balakrishnan R, Rajakumar MK: Rupture of patellar ligament after steroid infiltration. J Bone Joint Surg [Br] 51:503, 1969.

81. Melmed EP: Spontaneous bilateral rupture of the calcaneal tendon during ste-roid therapy. J Bone Joint Surg [Br] 47:104, 1965.

82. Bedi SS, Ellis W: Spontaneous rupture of the calcaneal tendon in rheumatoid arthritis after local steroid injection. Ann Rheum Dis 29:494, 1970.

83. Morgan J, McCarty DJ: Tendon ruptures in patients with systemic lupus erythe-matosus treated with corticosteroids. Arthritis Rheum 17:1033, 1974.

84. Halpern AA, Horowitz BG, Nagel DA: Tendon ruptures associated with corti-costeroid therapy. West J Med 127:378, 1977.

85. Smaill GB: Bilateral rupture of achilles tendons. Br Med J 1:1657, 1961.

86. Langhoff J, Krahl H, Langhoff I: Mikroskopische unde submikroskopische Veranderungen an Kaninchensehen nach lokaler Injektion von 6-Methylpred-nisolon. Bruns Beitr Klin Chir 218:736, 1971.

87. Phelps D, Sonstegard DA, Matthews LS: Corticosteroid injection effects on the biomechanical properties of rabbit patellar tendons. Clin Orthop 100:345, 1974.

88. Wrenn RN, Goldner JL, Markee JL: An experimental study of the effect of cortisone on the healing process and tensile strength of tendons. J Bone Joint Surg [Am] 36:588, 1954.

89. Salter RB, Murray D: Effect of hydrocortisone on musculoskeletal tissue. J Bone Joint Surg [Br] 51:195, 1969.

90. Balasubramaniam P, Prathrap K: The effect of injection of hydrocortisone into rabbit calcaneal tendons. J Bone Joint Surg [Br] 54:729, 1972.

91. Goldman L: Reactions following intralesional and sublesional injections of corticosteroids. JAMA 182:613, 1962.

92. Fisherman EW, Feinberg AR, Feinberg SM: Local subcutaneous atrophy. JAMA 179:971, 1962.

93. Beardwell A: Subcutaneous atrophy after local corticosteroid injection. Br Med J 3:600, 1967.

94. Schetman D, Hambrick GW Jr, Wilson CE: Cutaneous changes following local injection of triamcinolone. Arch Dermatol 88:820, 1963.

95. Rostron PKM, Calver RF: Subcutaneous atrophy following methylprednisolone injection in Osgood-Schlatter epiphysitis. J Bone Joint Surg [Am] 61:627, 1979.

96. Gottlieb NL, Penneys NS, Brown HE Jr: Periarticular perilymphatic skin atro-phy after intra-articular corticosteroid injections. JAMA 240:559, 1978.

97. Singh A, Jolly SS: Endemic fluorosis. Q J Med 30:357, 1961.

98. Singh A, Jolly SS, Bansal BC, et al: Endemic fluorosis. Epidemiological, clinical and biochemical study of chronic fluorine intoxication in Panjab (India). Medicine 42:229, 1963.

99. Singh A, Dass R, Hayreh SS, et al: Skeletal changes in endemic fluorosis. J Bone Joint Surg [Br] 44:806, 1962.

100. Singh A, Vazirani SJ, Jolly SS, et al: Endemic fluorosis. Postgrad Med J 38:150, 1962.

101. Shortt HE, McRobert GR, Barnard TW, et al: Endemic fluorosis in the Madras presidency. Ind J Med Res 25:553, 1937.

102. Smith FA, Hodge HC: Fluoride toxicity. In JC Muhler, MK Hine (Eds): Fluo-rine and Dental Health. Bloomington, Indiana University Press, 1959.

103. Dean HT: Distribution of mottled enamel in the United States. Pub Health Rep 48:703, 1933.

104. McClure FJ, Likins RC: Fluorine in human teeth studied in relation to fluorine in the drinking water. J Dent Res 30:172, 1951.

105. Smith MC, Lantz EM, Smith HV: The cause of mottled enamel. Science 74:244, 1931.

106. Siddiqui AH: Fluorosis in Nalgonda district Hyderabad-Deccan. Br Med J 2:1408, 1955.

107. Roholm K: Fluorine Intoxication. A Clinical Hygienic Study with a Review of the Literature and Some Experimental Investigations. London, HK Lewis & Company, Ltd, 1937.

108. Stevenson CA, Watson AR: Fluoride osteosclerosis. AJR 78:13, 1957.

109. Stevenson CA, Watson AR: Roentgenologic findings in fluoride osteosclerosis. Arch Indust Health 21:340, 1960.

110. Linsman JF, McMurray CA: Fluoride osteosclerosis from drinking water. Ra-diology 40:474, 1943.

111. Moller PF, Gudjonsson SV: Massive fluorosis of bones and ligaments. Acta Radiol 13:269, 1932.

112. Largent EJ, Bovard PG, Heyroth FF: Roentgenographic changes and urinary fluoride excretion among workmen engaged in the manufacture of inorganic fluorides. AJR 65:42, 1951.

113. Leone NC, Stevenson CA, Hilbish TF, et al: A roentgenologic study of a human population exposed to high fluoride domestic water. AJR 74:874, 1955.

114. Soriano M: Periostitis deformans (un nuevo tipo de fluorosis osea en el hombre) la fluorosis vinica. Rev Clin Esp 97:375, 1965.

115. Soriano M, Manchon F: Radiological aspects of a new type of bone fluorosis, periostitis deformans. Radiology 87:1089, 1966.

116. Johnson FF, Fischer LL: Report on fluorine in wine. Am J Pharm 107:512, 1939.

117. Faccini JM, Teotia SPS: Histopathological assessment of endemic skeletal fluo-rosis. Calcif Tissue Res 16:45, 1974.

118. Aggarwal ND: Structure of human fluorotic bone. J Bone Joint Surg [Am] 55:331, 1973.

119. Singh A, Jolly SS, Bansal BC: Skeletal fluorosis and its neurological compli-cations. Lancet 1:197, 1961.

120. Teotia SPS, Teotia M: Secondary hyperparathyroidism in patients with endemic skeletal fluorosis. Br Med J 1:637, 1973.

121. Messer HH, Armstrong WD, Singer L: Fluoride, parathyroid hormone and calcitonin: Inter-relationships in bone calcium metabolism. Calcif Tissue Res 13:217, 1973.

122. Messer HH, Armstrong WD, Singer L: Fluoride, parathyroid hormone, and calcitonin: Effects on metabolic processes involved in bone resorption. Calcif Tissue Res 13:227, 1973.

123. Faccini JM: Fluoride and bone. Calcif Tissue Res 3:1, 1969.

124. Evans FG, Wood JL: Mechanical properties and density of bone in a case of severe endemic fluorosis. Acta Orthop Scand 47:489, 1976.

125. Franke J, Runge H, Grau P, et al: Physical properties of fluorosis bone. Acta Orthop Scand 47:20, 1976.

126. Lindahl O, Lindwall L: Physical properties of fluorosis bone. Critical com-ments. Acta Orthop Scand 49:382, 1978.

127. Singer L, Armstrong WD, Zipkin I, et al: Chemical composition and structure of fluorotic bone. Clin Orthop 99:303, 1974.

128. Baud CA, Lagier R, Boivin G, et al: Value of the bone biopsy in the diagnosis of industrial fluorosis. Virchows Arch (Pathol Anat Histol) 380:283, 1978.

129. Krishnamachari KAVR, Krishnaswamy K: Genu valgum and osteoporosis in an area of endemic fluorosis. Lancet 2:877, 1973.

130. Reid PR, Thompson WL: The clinical use of dopamine in the treatment of shock. Johns Hopkins Med J 137:265, 1975.

131. Goldberg LI: Dopamine—clinical uses of an endogenous catecholamine. N Engl J Med 291:707, 1974.

132. Stetson JB, Reading GP: Avoidance of vascular complications associated with the use of dopamine. Can Anaesth Soc J 24:727, 1977.

133. Holzer J, Karliner JS, O'Rourke RA, et al: Effectiveness of dopamine in patients with cardiogenic shock. Am J Cardiol 32:79, 1973.

134. Boltax RS, Dineen JP, Scarpa FJ: Gangrene resulting from infiltrated dopamine solution. N Engl J Med 296:823, 1977.

135. Buchanan N, Cane RD, Miller N: Symmetrical gangrene of the extremities associated with the use of dopamine subsequent to ergometrine administration. Intensive Care Med J 3:55, 1977.

136. Green SI, Smith JW: Dopamine gangrene. N Engl J Med 294:114, 1976.

137. Alexander CS, Sako Y, Mikulic E: Pedal gangrene associated with the use of dopamine. N Engl J Med 293:591, 1975.

138. Golbranson F, Vance R, Vandell R, et al: Multiple extremity amputations in hypotensive patients treated with dopamine. JAMA 243:1145, 1980.

139. Ebels T, Homan van der Heide JN: Dopamine-induced ischaemia. Lancet 2:762, 1977.

140. Graham JR: Methysergide for prevention of headache. N Engl J Med 270:67, 1964.

141. Johnson TD: Severe peripheral arterial constriction, acute ischemia of a lower extremity with use of methysergide and ergotamine. Arch Intern Med 117:237, 1966.

142. Imrie CW: Arterial spasm associated with oral ergotamine therapy. Br J Clin Pract 27:457, 1973.

143. Ureles A, Rob C: Acute ischemia of a limb complicating methysergide maleate therapy. JAMA 183:1041, 1963.

144. Vaughan-Lane T: Gangrene induced by methysergide and ergotamine. A case report. J Bone Joint Surg [Br] 61:213, 1979.

145. Twiford TW Jr, Granmayeh M, Tucker MJ: Gangrene of the feet associated with mesenteric intra-arterial vasopressin. AJR 130:558, 1978.

146. Berger PE, Heidelberger KP, Poznanski AK: Extravasation of calcium gluco-nate as a cause of soft tissue calcification in infancy. AJR 121:109, 1974.

147. Harris V, Ramamurthy RS, Pildes RS: Late onset of subcutaneous calcifications after intravenous injections of calcium gluconate. AJR 123:845, 1975.

148. Burnett CH, Commons RR, Albright F, Howard JE: Hypercalcemia without hypercalcuria or hypophosphatemia, calcinosis, and renal insufficiency. N Engl J Med *240*:787, 1949.

149. Miller JM, Freeman I, Heath WH: Calcinosis due to treatment of duodenal ulcer. JAMA *148*:198, 1952.

150. McQueen EG: "Milk poisoning" and "calcium gout." Lancet *2*:67, 1952.

151. Wermer P, Kuschner M, Riley EA: Reversible metastatic calcification associated with excessive milk and alkali intake. Am J Med *14*:108, 1953.

152. Dworetzky M: Reversible metastatic calcification (milk-drinker's syndrome). JAMA *155*:830, 1954.

153. Poppel MH, Zeitel BE: Roentgen manifestations of milk drinker's syndrome. Radiology *67*:195, 1956.

154. Snapper I, Bradley WG, Wilson VE: Metastatic calcification and nephrocalcinosis from medical treatment of peptic ulcer. Arch Intern Med *93*:807, 1954.

155. Foltz EE: Calcinosis complicating peptic ulcer therapy. Gastroenterology *27*:50, 1954.

156. Ogle JC, Harvey CM Jr: Hypercalcemia and renal impairment following milk and alkali therapy for peptic ulcer. South Med J *48*:126, 1955.

157. Scholz DA, Keating FR Jr: Milk-alkali syndrome. Review of eight cases. Arch Intern Med *95*:460, 1955.

158. Kessler E: Hypercalcemia and renal insufficiency secondary to excessive milk and alkali intake. Ann Intern Med *42*:324, 1955.

159. Rodnan G, Johnson H: Chronic renal failure in association with the excessive intake of calcium and alkali. Gastroenterology *27*:584, 1954.

160. Wenger J, Kirsner JB, Palmer WL: The milk-alkali syndrome. Hypercalcemia, alkalosis and temporary renal insufficiency during milk-antacid therapy for peptic ulcer. Am J Med *24*:161, 1958.

161. Seeler RA, Israel JN, Royal JE, et al: Ganglioneuroblastoma and fetal hydantoin-alcohol syndromes. Pediatrics *63*:524, 1979.

162. Hamanishi C: Congenital short femur. Clinical, genetic, and epidemiological comparison of the naturally occurring condition with that caused by thalidomide. J Bone Joint Surg [Br] *62*:307, 1980.

163. Maldague B, Noel H, Malghem J: The intravertebral vacuum cleft: A sign of ischemic vertebral collapse. Radiology *129*:23, 1978.

164. Maldague B, Malghem J, Huaux JP, et al: Ischemic collapse of the vertebral body: Myth or reality. J Belge Radiol *62*:61, 1979.

165. Zizic TM, Hungerford DS, Stevens MB: Ischemic bone necrosis in systemic lupus erythematosus. I. The early diagnosis of ischemic necrosis of bone. Medicine *59*:134, 1980.

166. Oxlund H: The influence of a local injection of cortisol on the mechanical properties of tendons and ligaments and the indirect effect on skin. Acta Orthop Scand *51*:231, 1980.

167. Gluck O, Murphy W, Hahn T, et al: Risk factors for steroid-induced bone loss (Abstr). Arthritis Rheum *23*:681, 1980.

168. Gluck O, Hahn T, Hahn B: Comparison of bone loss in patients receiving alternate or daily glucocorticoid therapy (Abstr). Arthritis Rheum *23*:681, 1980.

169. Weinstein J: Benign joint effusion associated with glucocorticosteroid therapy. J Rheumatol *7*:245, 1980.

170. Christie DP: The spectrum of radiographic bone changes in children with fluorosis. Radiology *136*:85, 1980.

171. Boillat MA, Garcia J, Velebit L: Radiological criteria of industrial fluorosis. Skel Radiol *5*:161, 1950.

172. Alhava EM, Olkkonen H, Kauranen P, et al: The effect of drinking water fluoridation on the fluoride content, strength and mineral density of human bone. Acta Orthop Scand *51*:413, 1980.

173. Meunier PJ, Courpron P, Smoller JS, et al: Niflumic acid-induced skeletal fluorosis: Iatrogenic disease or therapeutic perspective for osteoporosis? Clin Orthop *148*:304, 1980.

174. Coumbes MA, Clark WK, Gregory CF, et al: Sciatic nerve injuries in infants. Recognition and prevention of impairment resulting from intragluteal injections. JAMA *173*:1336, 1960.

175. Fahrni WH: Neonatal sciatic injury. J Bone Joint Surg [Br] *32*:42, 1950.

176. Giles FH, French JH: Post-injection sciatic nerve palsies in infants and children. J Pediatr *58*:195, 1961.

177. Curtiss PH Jr, Tucker JH: Sciatic palsy in premature infants. A report and followup study of 10 cases. JAMA *174*:1586, 1960.

178. Bigos SJ, Coleman SS: Foot deformities secondary to gluteal injection in infancy. J Pediatr Orthop *4*:560, 1984.

179. Aragona J, Lee CY: Scoliosis in fetal alcohol syndrome: A case report. Orthopedics *4*:1141, 1981.

180. Tredwell SJ, Smith DF, Macleod PJ, et al: Cervical spine anomalies in fetal alcohol syndrome. Spine *7*:331, 1982.

181. Maroteaux P, Lavollay B, Bomsell F, et al: Chondrodysplasie ponctuée et intoxication alcoolique maternelle. Arch Fr Pediatr *41*:547, 1984.

182. Kumar SP: Fetal alcohol syndrome. Mechanisms of teratogenesis. Ann Clin Lab Sci *12*:254, 1982.

183. Hiilesmaa VK, Teramo K, Granstrom ML, et al: Fetal head growth retardation associated with maternal antiepileptic drugs. Lancet *2*:165, 1981.

184. Scott S, Alazraki N, Manaster B: Failure of bone scanning to detect fractures in a woman on chronic steroid therapy. Skel Radiol *12*:204, 1984.

185. Gluck OS, Murphy WA, Hahn TJ, et al: Bone loss in adults receiving alternate day glucocorticoid therapy. A comparison with daily therapy. Arthritis Rheum *24*:892, 1981.

186. Crilly RG: Pathogenesis and management of glucocorticoid osteoporosis. Geriatr Med Today *3*:111, 1984.

187. Hahn TJ, Halstead LR, Teitelbaum SL, et al: Altered mineral metabolism in glucocorticoid-induced osteopenia: Effect of 25-hydroxy vitamin D administration. J Clin Invest *64*:655, 1979.

188. Jee WSS, Black HE, Gotcher JE: Effect of dichloromethane diphosphonate on cortisol-induced bone loss in young adult rabbits. Clin Orthop *156*:39, 1981.

189. Hahn TJ: Drug-induced disorders of vitamin D and mineral metabolism. Clin Endocrinol Metab *9*:107, 1980.

190. Riggs BL, Jowsey J, Kelly P: Quantitative microradiographic study of bone remodeling in Cushing's syndrome. Metabolism *15*:773, 1966.

191. Litvin Y, Hage S, Catane R, et al: Reversibility of glucocorticoid-induced osteopenia. A case report. Clin Nucl Med *7*:269, 1982.

192. Roseff R, Canoso JJ: Femoral osteonecrosis following soft tissue corticosteroid infiltration. Am J Med *77*:1119, 1984.

193. Taylor LJ: Multifocal avascular necrosis after short-term high-dose steroid therapy. A report of three cases. J Bone Joint Surg [Br] *66*:431, 1984.

194. Anderton JM, Helm R: Multiple joint osteonecrosis following short-term steroid therapy. Case report. J Bone Joint Surg [Am] *64*:139, 1982.

195. McCluskey J, Gutteridge DH: Avascular necrosis of bone after high doses of dexamethasone during neurosurgery. Br Med J *284*:333, 1982.

196. Richards JM, Santiago SM, Klaustermeyer WB: Aseptic necrosis of the femoral head in corticosteroid-treated pulmonary disease. Arch Intern Med *140*:1473, 1980.

197. Williams PL, Corbett M: Avascular necrosis of bone complicating replacement therapy. Ann Rheum Dis *42*:276, 1983.

198. Conklin JJ, Alderson PO, Zizic TM, et al: Comparison of bone scan and radiograph sensitivity in the detection of steroid-induced ischemic necrosis of bone. Radiology *147*:221, 1983.

199. Burt RW, Matthews TJ: Aseptic necrosis of the knee: Bone scintigraphy. AJR *138*:571, 1982.

200. D'Ambrosia RD, Shoji H, Riggins RS, et al: Scintigraphy in the diagnosis of osteonecrosis. Clin Orthop *128*:139, 1978.

201. Wang G-J, Rawles JG, Hubbard SL, et al: Steroid-induced femoral head pressure changes and their response to lipid-clearing agents. Clin Orthop *174*:298, 1983.

202. Boskey AL, Raggio CL, Bullough PG, et al: Changes in the bone tissue lipids in persons with steroid- and alcohol-induced osteonecrosis. Clin Orthop *172*:289, 1983.

203. Higuchi M, Masuda T, Susuda K, et al: Ultrastructure of the articular cartilage after systemic administration of hydrocortisone in the rabbit: An electron microscopic study. Clin Orthop *152*:296, 1980.

204. Gray RG, Gottlieb NL: Intra-articular corticosteroids. An updated assessment. Clin Orthop *177*:235, 1983.

205. Silbermann M, Lewinson D, Toister Z: Early cartilage response to systemic glucocorticoid administration: An ultrastructural study. Metab Bone Dis Rel Res *2*:267, 1980.

206. Ishikawa K: Effect of intra-articular corticosteroid on the meniscus. A histological and histochemical study in rabbit knees. J Bone Joint Surg [Am] *63*:120, 1981.

207. Sedgwick AD, Sin YM, Moore AR, et al: Effects of local administration of hydrocortisone on cartilage degradation in vivo. Ann Rheum Dis *43*:418, 1984.

208. Haines JF: Bilateral rupture of the Achilles tendon in patients on steroid therapy. Ann Rheum Dis *42*:652, 1983.

209. Kleinman M, Gross AE: Achilles tendon rupture following steroid injection. Report of three cases. J Bone Joint Surg [Am] *65*:1345, 1983.

210. Kapetanos G: The effect of the local corticosteroids on the healing and biomechanical properties of the partially injured tendon. Clin Orthop *163*:170, 1982.

211. McCarty DJ: Treatment of rheumatoid joint inflammation with triamcinolone hexacetonide. Arthritis Rheum *15*:157, 1972.

212. Gilsanz V, Bernstein BH: Joint calcification following intra-articular corticosteroid therapy. Radiology *151*:647, 1984.

213. Dalinka MK, Stewart V, Bomalaski JS, et al: Periarticular calcifications in association with intra-articular corticosteroid injections. Radiology *153*:615, 1984.

214. Stelling CB, Keats TE: Synovial calcifications associated with long-term steroid therapy for chronic arthritis. South Med J *77*:1455, 1984.

215. Koerner JH, Sun DC: Mediastinal lipomatosis secondary to steroid therapy. AJR *98*:461, 1966.

216. Price JE, Rigler LG: Widening of the mediastinum resulting from fat accumulation. Radiology *96*:497, 1970.

217. Van de Putte LBA, Wagenaar JPM, San KH: Pericardiac lipomatosis in exogenous Cushing syndrome. Thorax *28*:653, 1973.

218. Streiter ML, Schneider HJ, Proto AV, et al: Steroid-induced thoracic lipomatosis: paraspinal involvement. AJR *139*:679, 1982.

219. Bein ME, Mancuso AA, Mink JH, et al: Computed tomography in the evaluation of mediastinal lipomatosis. J Comput Assist Tomogr *2*:379, 1978.

220. Sowerbutts JG: Some uses of presacral oxygen insufflation. J Fac Radiologists *10*:201, 1959.

221. Lee M, Lekias J, Gubbay SS, et al: Spinal cord compression by extradural fat after renal transplantation. Med J Austr *1*:201, 1975.

222. Kaneda K, Yamaura I, Kamikozuru M, et al: Paraplegia as a complication of corticosteroid therapy. A case report. J Bone Joint Surg [Am] *66*:783, 1984.

223. Guegan Y, Fardoun R, Launois B, et al: Spinal cord compression by extradural fat after prolonged corticosteroid therapy. Case report. J Neurosurg *56*:267, 1982.

224. Grandjean P: Occupational fluorosis through 50 years: Clinical and epidemiological experiences. Am J Industr Med *3*:227, 1982.

225. Grandjean P, Thomsen G: Reversibility of skeletal fluorosis. Br J Indust Med *40*:456, 1983.

226. Rich C, Ensinck J: Effects of sodium fluoride on calcium metabolism. Nature *191*:184, 1961.

227. Jowsey J, Riggs BL, Kelly PJ, et al: Effect of combined therapy with sodium fluoride, vitamin D and calcium in osteoporosis. Am J Med *53*:43, 1972.

228. Franke J, Rempel H, Franke M: Three years' experience with sodium-fluoride therapy of osteoporosis. Acta Orthop Scand *45*:1, 1974.

229. Riggs BL, Jowsey J: Treatment of osteoporosis with fluoride. Semin Drug Treat *2*:27, 1972.

230. Jowsey J, Schenk RK, Reutter FW: Some results of the effect of fluoride on bone tissue in osteoporosis. J Clin Endocrinol Metab *28*:869, 1968.

231. Vigorita VJ, Suda MK: The microscopic morphology of fluoride-induced bone. Clin Orthop *177*:274, 1983.

232. El-Khoury GY, Moore TE, Albright JP, et al: Sodium fluoride treatment of osteoporosis: Radiologic findings. AJR *139*:39, 1982.

233. Schulz EE, Libanati CR, Farley SM, et al: Skeletal scintigraphic changes in osteoporosis treated with sodium fluoride: Concise communication. J Nucl Med *25*:651, 1984.

234. Inkovaara J, Heikinheimo R, Jarvinen K, et al: Prophylactic fluoride treatment and aged bones. Br Med J *3*:73, 1975.

235. Riggs BL, Hodgson SF, Hoffman DL, et al: Treatment of primary osteoporosis with fluoride and calcium. Clinical tolerance and fracture occurrence. JAMA *243*:446, 1980.

236. Riggs BL, Seeman E, Hodgson SF, et al: The effect of the fluoride/calcium regimen on vertebral fracture occurrence in postmenopausal osteoporosis: Comparison with conventional therapy. N Engl J Med *306*:446, 1982.

237. Adam A, Rakhit G, Beeton S, et al: Extensive subcutaneous calcification following injections of pitressin tannate. Br J Radiol *57*:921, 1984.

238. Teo WS, Balasubramaniam P: Gas gangrene after intramuscular injection of adrenaline. Clin Orthop *174*:206, 1983.

239. Propst-Proctor SL, Jones RB, Nagel DA: Iatrogenic soft-tissue calcification in an extremity. A case report. J Bone Joint Surg [Am] *64*:449, 1982.

240. Wolfe MS, North ER: Extravasation of injected calcium solution leading to calcifications in the upper extremity of the neonate. Report of a case. J Bone Joint Surg [Am] *65*:558, 1983.

241. Dalinka MK: Letter to the editor. J Bone Joint Surg [Am] *66*:152, 1984.

242. Ravenel SDB: Cellulitis from extravasation of calcium gluconate simulating osteomyelitis. Am J Dis Child *137*:402, 1983.

243. Orwoll ES: The milk-alkali syndrome: Current concepts. Ann Intern Med *97*:242, 1982.

244. Carroll PR, Clark OH: Milk alkali syndrome. Does it exist and can it be differentiated from primary hyperparathyroidism? Ann Surg *197*:427, 1983.

245. Freed MD, Heymann MA, Lewis AB, et al: Prostaglandin E$_1$ in infants with ductus arteriosus–dependent congenital heart disease. Circulation *64*:899, 1981.

246. Ueda K, Saito A, Nakano H, et al: Cortical hyperostosis following long-term administration of prostaglandin E$_1$ in infants with congenital heart disease. J Pediatr *97*:834, 1980.

247. Sone K, Tashiro M, Fujinaga T, et al: Long-term low-dose prostaglandin E$_1$ administration. J Pediatr *97*:866, 1980.

248. Moulaert AJ, Gittenberger AC, Harinck E: Prostaglandin and damage to ductus arteriosus. Lancet *1*:703, 1977.

249. Ringel RE, Haney PJ, Brenner JI, et al: Periosteal changes secondary to prostaglandin administration. J Pediatr *103*:251, 1983.

250. Ringel RE, Brenner JI, Haney PJ, et al: Prostaglandin-induced periostitis: A complication of long-term PGE$_1$ infusion in an infant with congenital heart disease. Radiology *142*:657, 1982.

251. Benz-Bohm G, Emons D, Schickendantz S, et al: Kortikale Hyperostosen unter langerfristiger Prostaglandin E$_2$-thrapie. Radiologe *24*:72, 1984.

252. Dekel S, Francis MJO: Cortical hyperostosis after administration of prostaglandin E$_1$. J Pediatr *99*:500, 1981.

253. Dietrich JW, Raisz LG: Prostaglandin in calcium and bone metabolism. Clin Orthop *11*:228, 1975.

254. Peck GL, Yoder FW: Treatment of lamellar ichthyosis and other keratinising dermatoses with an oral synthetic retinoid. Lancet *2*:1172, 1976.

255. Voorhees JJ, Orfanos CE: Oral retinoids: Broad spectrum dermatologic therapy in the 1980's. Arch Dermatol *117*:418, 1981.

256. Pittsley RA, Yoder FW: Retinoid hyperostosis: Skeletal toxicity associated with long-term administration of 13-cis-retinoic acid for refractory ichthyosis. N Engl J Med *308*:1012, 1983.

257. Pennes DR, Ellis CN, Madison KC, et al: Early skeletal hyperostoses secondary to 13-cis-retinoic acid. AJR *141*:979, 1984.

258. Milstone LM, McGuire J, Ablow RC: Premature epiphyseal closure in a child receiving oral 13-cis-retinoic acid. J Am Acad Dermatol *7*:663, 1982.

259. Windhorst DB, Nigra T: General clinical toxicology of oral retinoids. J Am Acad Dermatol *6*:675, 1982.

260. Accutane (isotretinoin) in the treatment of severe, recalcitrant cystic acne. Roche Scientific Summary *32*, 1982.

261. Novick NL, Lawson W, Schwartz IS: Bilateral nasal bone osteophytosis associated with short-term oral isotretinoin therapy for cystic acne vulgaris. Am J Med *77*:736, 1984.

262. Matsuoka LY, Wortsman J, Pepper JJ: Acute arthritis during isotretinoin treatment for acne. Arch Intern Med *144*:1870, 1984.

263. Rosa FW: Teratogenicity of isotretinoin. Lancet *2*:513, 1983.

264. Fernhoff PM, Lammer EJ: Craniofacial features of isotretinoin embryopathy. J Pediatr *105*:595, 1984.

265. Abiteboul M, Arlet J: Retinol-related hyperostosis. AJR *144*:435, 1985.

266. Kattan KR: Calvarial thickening after Dilantin medication. AJR *110*:102, 1970.

267. Kattan KR: Thickening of the heel-pad associated with long-term Dilantin therapy. AJR *124*:52, 1975.

268. Dent CE, Richens A, Rowe DJF, et al: Osteomalacia with long-term anticonvulsant therapy in epilepsy. Br Med J *4*:69, 1970.

269. Sackler JP, Liu L: Heparin-induced osteoporosis. Br J Radiol *46*:548, 1973.

270. Megard M, Cuche M, Grapeloux A, et al: Ostéoporose de l'héparinothérapie. Nouv Presse Med *11*:261, 1982.

271. Rafii M, Firoozina H, Golimbu C, et al: Pathologic fracture in systemic mastocytosis. Clin Orthop *180*:260, 1983.

272. Squires JW, Pinch LW: Heparin-induced spinal fractures. JAMA *241*:2417, 1979.

273. Thompson RC: Heparin osteoporosis. An experimental model using rats. J Bone Joint Surg [Am] *55*:606, 1973.

274. Dalen N, Feldreich AL: Osteopenia in alcoholism. Clin Orthop *99*:201, 1974.

275. Schwartz AM, Leonidas JC: Methotrexate osteopathy. Skel Radiol *11*:13, 1984.

276. Ekvarn S, Jonsson M, Lindquist NG, et al: Disulfiram-induced myocardial and skeletal-muscle degeneration in rats. Lancet *2*:770, 1977.

277. Black D: An allergic reaction to disulfiram implant. Br J Addict *74*:88, 1979.

278. Howard JF: Arthritis and carpal tunnel syndrome associated with disulfiram (Antabuse) therapy. Arthritis Rheum *25*:1494, 1982.

279. Telerman-Toppet N, Vanaise A, Six R, et al: A propos d'un cas de périarterite nouleuse après implantation de disulfiram. Acta Clin Belg *30*:101, 1975.

280. Savola J: Arthropathy induced by beta blockade. Br Med J *287*:1256, 1983.

281. Machtey I: Polyarthritis following propranolol. Arthritis Rheum *24*:568, 1981.

282. Tysvaer AT: Computerized tomography and surgical treatment of femoral compression neuropathy. Report of two cases. J Neurosurg *57*:137, 1982.

283. Pastakia B, Horvath K, Kurtz D, et al: Giant rectus sheath hematomas of the pelvis complicating anticoagulant therapy: CT findings. J Comput Assist Tomogr *8*:1120, 1984.

284. Hall JG: Vitamin A: A newly recognized human teratogen. Harbinger of things to come? J Pediatr *105*:583, 1984.

285. Als OS, Gotfredsen A, Christiansen C: The effect of glucocorticoids on bone mass in rheumatoid arthritis patients. Influence of menopausal state. Arthritis Rheum *28*:369, 1985.

286. Dykman TR, Gluck OS, Murphy WA, et al: Evaluation of factors associated with glucocorticoid-induced osteopenia in patients with rheumatic diseases. Arthritis Rheum *28*:361, 1985.

287. Newman NM, Ling RSM: Acetabular bone destruction related to nonsteroidal anti-inflammatory drugs. Lancet *1*:11, 1985.

288. Higuchi M, Abe K: Effects of hydrocortisone on the vertebral cartilage plate in mice. A light and electron microscope study. Spine *10*:297, 1985.

289. Higuchi M, Abe K: Ultrastructure of the nucleus pulposus in the intervertebral disc after systemic administration of hydrocortisone in mice. Spine *10*:638, 1985.

290. Schnitzler CM, Solomon L: Trabecular stress fractures during fluoride therapy for osteoporosis. Skel Radiol *14*:276, 1985.

291. Schuman CA, Jones HW III: The "milk-alkali" syndrome: Two case reports with discussion of pathogenesis. Q J Med *55*:119, 1985.

292. Poznanski AK, Fernbach SK, Berry TE: Bone changes from prostaglandin therapy. Skel Radiol *14*:20, 1985.

293. Ohira T, Ishikawa K: Hydroxyapatite deposition in articular cartilage by intra-articular injections of methylprednisolone. A histological, ultrastructural, and x-ray–microprobe analysis in rabbits. J Bone Joint Surg [Am] *68*:509, 1986.

294. Ferrandez D, Martin-Dupont P, Pompougnac E, et al: Lipomatose extra-durale compressive induite par al corticothérapie. Sem Hôp Paris *61*:3327, 1985.

295. Schulz EE, Engstrom H, Sauser DD, et al: Osteopososis: Radiographic detection of fluorine-induced extra-axial bone formation. Radiology *159*:457, 1986.

296. Kilcoyne RF, Cope R, Cunningham W, et al: Minimal spinal hyperostosis with low-dose isotretinoin therapy. Invest Radiol *21*:41, 1986.

297. Crisp AJ, Wright JK, Hazleman BL: Effects of heparin, histamine, and salmon calcitonin on mouse calvarial bone resorption. Ann Rheum Dis *45*:422, 1986.

298. Shpall EJ, Efremidis AP, Kasambalides E, et al: Case report 352. Skel Radiol *15*:170, 1986.

299. Rusanen M, Grönblad M, Korkala O: Scanning electron microscopical study of the effects of crystalloid and water-soluble glucocorticoids on articular cartilage. Scand J Rheumatol *15*:47, 1986.

300. Price AE, Evanski PM, Waugh TR: Bilateral simultaneous Achilles tendon ruptures. A case report and review of the literature. Clin Orthop *213*:249, 1986.

301. Williams JL: Periosteal hyperostosis resulting from prostaglandin therapy. Eur J Radiol *6*:231, 1986.

302. DiGiovanna JJ, Helfgott RK, Gerber LH, et al: Extraspinal tendon and ligament calcification associated with long-term therapy with etretinate. N Engl J Med *315*:1177, 1986.

303. Nicholas PJR, Boldero JC, Goodfellow JW, et al: Abnormalities of the vertebral column associated with thalidomide-induced limb deformities. Orthopaedics *1*:71, 1968.

304. Smith JRG, Martin IR, Shaw DG, et al: Progressive non-infectious anterior vertebral fusion. Skel Radiol *15*:599, 1986.

305. Sambrook PN, Cohen ML, Eisman JA, et al: Effects of low dose corticosteroids on bone mass in rheumatoid arthritis: A longitudinal study. Ann Rheum Dis *48*:535, 1989.

306. Laroche M, Arlet J, Mazieres B: Osteonecrosis of the femoral and humeral heads after intraarticular corticosteroid injections. J Rheumatol *17*:549, 1990.

307. McCarty DJ, McCarthy G, Carrera G: Intraarticular corticosteroids possibly

leading to osteonecrosis and marrow fat induced synovitis. J Rheumatol *18*:1091, 1991.

308. Ono K, Tohjima T, Komazawa T: Risk factors of avascular necrosis of the femoral head in patients with systemic lupus erythematosus using high-dose corticosteroid therapy. Clin Orthop *277*:89, 1992.

309. Weiner ES, Abeles M: Aseptic necrosis and glucocorticoids in systemic lupus erythematosus: A reevaluation. J Rheumatol *16*:604, 1989.

310. Weiner ES, Abeles M: More on aseptic necrosis and glucocorticoids in systemic lupus erythematosus. J Rheumatol *17*:119, 1990.

311. Tervonen O, Mueller DM, Matteson EL, et al: Clinically occult avascular necrosis of the hip: Prevalence in an asymptomatic population at risk. Radiology *182*:845, 1992.

312. O'Brien TJ, Mack GR: Multifocal osteonecrosis after short-term high-dose corticosteroid therapy. A case report. Clin Orthop *279*:176, 1992.

313. Kalunian KC, Hahn BH, Bassett L: Magnetic resonance imaging identifies early femoral head ischemic necrosis in patients receiving systemic glucocorticoid therapy. J Rheumatol *16*:959, 1989.

314. Humphreys S, Spencer JD, Tighe JR, et al: The femoral head in osteonecrosis. A quantitative study of osteocyte population. J Bone Joint Surg [Br] *71*:205, 1989.

315. Pope TL Jr, Keats TE, de Lange EE, et al: Case report 426. Skel Radiol *16*:342, 1987.

316. Kelman GJ, Williams GW, Colwell CW Jr, et al: Steroid-related osteonecrosis of the knee. Two case reports and a literature review. Clin Orthop *257*:171, 1990.

317. Havel PE, Ebraheim NA, Jackson WT: Steroid-induced bilateral avascular necrosis of the lateral femoral condyles. A case report. Clin Orthop *243*:166, 1989.

318. Yamaguchi H, Masuda T, Sasaki T, et al: Steroid-induced osteonecrosis of the patella. Clin Orthop *229*:201, 1988.

319. Kida Y, Katoh Y, Yamada H, et al: Extensive osteonecrosis of the acetabulum in a patient who had rheumatoid arthritis. A case report. J Bone Joint Surg [Am] *73*:930, 1991.

320. Culp RW, Schaffer JL, Osterman L, et al: Kienböck's disease in a patient with Crohn's enteritis treated with corticosteroids. J Hand Surg [Am] *14*:294, 1989.

321. Reis ND, Karkabi S, Zinman C: Metatarsophalangeal joint dislocation after local steroid injection. J Bone Joint Surg [Br] *71*:864, 1989.

322. Gerster J-C, Fallet GH: Periarticular hydroxyapatite deposition after corticosteroid injections. J Rheumatol *14*:1156, 1987.

323. Kubota RT, Resnik CS: Periarticular calcification in immunosuppressed cardiac transplant patients. Invest Radiol *23*:113, 1988.

324. Menei P, Fournier D, Alhayek G, et al: Granulome nécrotico-inflammatoire calcifé après nucléorthèse à l'hexacétonide de triamcinolone. Rev Rhum *58*:605, 1991.

325. Jungreis CA, Cohen WA: Spinal cord compression induced by steroid therapy: CT findings. J Comput Assist Tomogr *11*:245, 1987.

326. Kaplan JG, Barasch E, Hirschfeld A, et al: Spinal epidural lipomatosis: A serious complication of iatrogenic Cushing's syndrome. Neurology *39*:1031, 1989.

327. Arroyo IL, Barron KS, Brewer EJ Jr: Spinal cord compression by epidural lipomatosis in juvenile rheumatoid arthritis. Arthritis Rheum *31*:447, 1988.

328. Taborn J: Epidural lipomatosis as a cause of spinal cord compression in polymyalgia rheumatica. J Rheumatol *18*:286, 1991.

329. Haid RW Jr, Kaufman HH, Schochet SS Jr, et al: Epidural lipomatosis simulating an epidural abscess: Case report and literature review. Neurosurgery *21*:744, 1987.

330. Doppman JL: Epidural lipomatosis. Radiology *171*:581, 1989.

331. Quint DJ, Boulos RS, Sanders WP, et al: Epidural lipomatosis. Radiology *169*:485, 1988.

332. Rawlins BA, DiGiacinto GV: Epidural compression in the spinal canal caused by excessive adipose tissue. A case report. Clin Orthop *275*:140, 1992.

333. Gero BT, Chynn KY: Symptomatic spinal epidural lipomatosis without exogenous steroid intake. Report of a case with magnetic resonance imaging. Neuroradiology *31*:190, 1989.

334. Németh L, Zsögön E: Occupational skeletal fluorosis. Clin Rheumatol *3*:81, 1989.

335. Bruns BR, Tytle T: Skeletal fluorosis. A report of two cases. Orthopedics *11*:1083, 1988.

336. Subbarao B, Taraknath VR, Sista VN: Ossification of the posterior longitudinal ligament and fluorosis. J Bone Joint Surg [Br] *74*:469, 1992.

337. Prost A, Caumon JP, Maugars Y, et al: Périostite déformante par fluorose subaiguë. Une observation de cause originale. Rev Rhum Mal Osoteoartic *55*:709, 1988.

338. Turner CH, Akhter MP, Heaney RP: The effects of fluoridated water on bone strength. J Orthop Res *10*:581, 1992.

339. Schnitzler CM, Sweet MBE, Blumenfeld TS, et al: Radiographic features of the spine in fluoride therapy for osteoporosis. J Bone Joint Surg [Br] *69*:190, 1987.

340. Weingrad TR, Eymontt MJ, Martin JH, et al: Periostitis due to low-dose fluoride intoxication demonstrated by bone scanning. Clin Nucl Med *16*:59, 1991.

341. Schnitzler CM, Wing JR, Gear KA, et al: Bone fragility of the peripheral skeleton during fluoride therapy for osteoporosis. Clin Orthop *261*:268, 1990.

342. Rowley RF, Lawson JP: Case report 701. Skel Radiol *20*:617, 1991.

343. Drvaric DM, Parks WJ, Wyly JB, et al: Prostaglandin-induced hyperostosis. A case report. Clin Orthop *246*:300, 1989.

344. Kassner EG: Drug-related complications in infants and children: Imaging features. AJR *157*:1039, 1991.

345. Jørgensen HRI, Svanholm H, Høst A: Bone formation induced in an infant by systemic prostaglandin-E_2 administration. Acta Orthop Scand *59*:464, 1988.

346. Høst A, Halken S, Andersen PE Jr: Reversibility of cortical hyperostosis following long-term prostaglandin E_1 therapy in infants with ductus-dependent congenital heart disease. Pediatr Radiol *18*:149, 1988.

347. Wood BP: Infant ribs: Generalized periosteal reaction resulting from vibrator chest physiotherapy. Radiology *162*:811, 1987.

348. Hussain M, Wood BP: Periosteal new bone of ribs with associated extremity fractures after high-frequency jet ventilation. Radiology *183*:875, 1992.

349. Boyd AS: An overview of the retinoids. Am J Med *86*:568, 1989.

350. Goldfarb MT, Ellis CN, Voorhees JJ: Retinoids in dermatology. Mayo Clin Proc *62*:1161, 1987.

351. Lawson JP, McGuire J: The spectrum of skeletal changes associated with long-term administration of 13-cis-retinoic acid. Skel Radiol *16*:91, 1987.

352. Pennes DR, Martel W, Ellis CN, et al: Evolution of skeletal hyperostosis caused by 13-cis-retinoic acid therapy. AJR *151*:967, 1988.

353. Bologna C, Poirier JL, Herisson C, et al: Enthésopathies ossifiantes des hanches et du rachis induites par l'etrétinate au cours d'un rhumatisme psoriasique périphérique. Rev Rhum Mal Osteoartic *58*:595, 1991.

354. Guit GL, Obermann WR, van der Schroeff JG, et al: Cortical hyperostosis and enthesopathy due to long-term etretinate administration. Diagn Imaging Clin Med *55*:214, 1986.

355. Jackson S: Femoral neuropathy secondary to heparin induced intrapelvic hematoma. A case report and review of the literature. Orthopedics *10*:1049, 1987.

356. Skinner R, Pearson AD, Price L, et al: Nephrotoxicity after ifosfamide. Arch Dis Child *65*:732, 1990.

357. Burk CD, Restaino I, Kaplan BS, et al: Ifosfamide-induced renal tubular dysfunction and rickets in children with Wilms' tumor. J Pediatr *117*:331, 1990.

358. Silberzweig JE, Haller JO, Miller S: Ifosfamide: A new cause of rickets. AJR *158*:823, 1992.

359. van Meerten ELP, Kroon HM, Papapoulous SE: Epi- and metaphyseal changes in children caused by administration of biphosphonates. Radiology *184*:249, 1992.

360. De Schepper AMA, Degryse HRM: Imaging findings in a patient with pentazocine-induced myopathy. AJR *154*:343, 1990.

361. Ribard P, Audisio F, Kahn M-F, et al: Seven Achilles tendinitis including 3 complicated by rupture during fluoroquinolone therapy. J Rheumatol *19*:1479, 1992.

362. Mitzuta H, Kubota K, Shiraishi M, et al: Steroid-related bilateral osteonecrosis of the patella. Arthroscopy *9*:114, 1993.

363. Parikh JR, Houpt JB, Jacobs S, et al: Charcot's arthropathy of the shoulder following intraarticular corticosteroid injections. J Rheumatol *20*:885, 1993.

364. Mithal A, Trived N, Gupta SK, et al: Radiological spectrum of endemic fluorosis: Relationship with calcium intake. Skel Radiol *22*:257, 1993.

365. Hughes RA: Arthritis precipitated by isotretinoin treatment for acne vulgaris. J Rheumatol *20*:1241, 1993.

366. Sweeney LE: Hypophosphataemic rickets after ifosfamide treatment in children. Clin Radiol *47*:345, 1993.

367. Wang Y, Yin Y, Gilula LA, et al: Endemic fluorosis of the skeleton: Radiographic features in 127 cases. AJR *162*:93, 1994.

368. Woo K, Emery J, Peabody J: Cortical hyperostosis: A complication of prolonged prostaglandin infusion in infants awaiting cardiac transplantation. Pediatrics *93*:417, 1994.

75

Hypervitaminosis and Hypovitaminosis

Donald Resnick, M.D.

Vitamins are biologically active organic compounds that are not synthesized by the body and are obtained from exogenous sources, mainly the diet. Vitamins, which are essential for normal growth and development, can be classified according to whether they are fat soluble (vitamins A, D, E, and K) or water soluble (vitamins B_1, B_2, niacin, B_6 or pyridoxine, folic acid, cyanocobalamin, C or ascorbic acid, biotin, and pantothenic acid). Musculoskeletal manifestations accompany deficiencies and excesses of certain vitamins. A classic example of a disorder that illustrates the fundamental dependence of normal osseous development and maturation on vitamin intake is rickets, which is due to a deficiency in vitamin D or its active metabolites (Chapter 53). In addition, excessive levels of the vitamins D and A and depressed levels of the vitamins A and C can produce characteristic changes in the skeleton, which will be illustrated on the following pages.

HYPERVITAMINOSIS A

Vitamin A poisoning appears in both children and adults. Its clinical and radiologic manifestations are influenced by the acute or chronic nature of the vitamin abuse. In infants and children, short-term or long-term ingestion of excessive amounts of vitamin A are due, in many cases, to the actions of an overly concerned or enthusiastic parent and may be accompanied by significant skeletal alterations. In adults, extraskeletal changes predominate, and the affected person can reveal prominent dermatologic aberrations in addition to anorexia and weight loss.[1–3] The detrimental effects of certain natural and synthetic forms of vitamin A that are used in both children and adults in the treatment of dermatologic disorders are discussed in Chapter 74.

Acute Poisoning

After a massive dose of vitamin A (several hundred thousand units), acute clinical findings can develop. These were first alluded to by Kane,[4] an Arctic explorer, who in 1856 recorded transient symptoms of vertigo and headache that followed the ingestion of polar bear liver, a substance that contains a high concentration of vitamin A.[5, 6] Approximately one century later, nausea, vomiting, headache, drowsiness, and irritability were noted in adults with acute hypervitaminosis A resulting from ingestion of shark liver, also rich in this vitamin.[7] The findings of acute intoxication due to vitamin A were further delineated in 1954 by Marie and See[8] in children who developed drowsiness, vomiting, and bulging of the fontanelles from accidental overdose of vitamin drops. The symptoms and signs cleared within a few days after the cessation of vitamin A intake.

Bulging of the fontanelles can appear within 12 hours after vitamin ingestion, usually disappearing after 36 to 48 hours[9, 10]; the acute hydrocephalus may be attributable to an increase in production or a decrease in absorption of cerebrospinal fluid.[30] Although skull films can reveal widening of the sutures, the finding is transient, and the ocular fundi and cerebral electroencephalogram generally are normal.

Subacute and Chronic Poisoning

Chronic vitamin A poisoning was first recorded in a child in 1944 by Josephs,[11] and several years later, its association with soft tissue swellings of the extremities and radiographic osseous abnormalities was recognized.[12] The skeletal changes were described in detail later,[13] and a similar condition occurring in adults was noted.[14] In both age groups, anorexia and itching represent nonspecific early findings of the disorder. After a period of weeks or months, hard and tender soft tissue nodules appear in the extremities, particularly in the forearms. Additional manifestations include dry scaly skin, coarse and sparse hair, hepatosplenomegaly, and digital clubbing. An elevated serum vitamin A level is diagnostic in this clinical setting, and rapid diminution and disappearance of the symptoms and signs follow withdrawal of vitamin A intake.[9]

Radiographic signs are characteristic. With a few exceptions,[89, 90] they are virtually confined to children, usually appearing near the end of the first year of life, although infants and teenagers occasionally can reveal similar abnormalities. Cortical thickening of the tubular bones is a constant finding and usually is related to the areas in which soft tissue nodules are present.[9, 12, 15–18] Typically, hyperostosis is observed in the ulnae and metatarsal bones, producing a wavy or undulating diaphyseal contour; metaphyseal and epiphyseal segments do not participate in the cortical thickening (Fig. 75–1). The clavicles, tibiae, and fibulae not uncommonly are affected[100]; involvement of the femora, humeri, metacarpal bones, and ribs is less constant, and changes in the mandible rarely are observed. Scintigraphy, using bone seeking radiopharmaceutical agents, further documents this characteristic distribution of abnormalities (Fig. 75–2).[91, 92] Microscopic examination indicates that subperiosteal deposition of bone accounts for the increased thickening of the cortices.[9]

Additional findings may appear in the epiphyseal and metaphyseal segments of tubular bones that may lead to crippling deformities.[19–21] The distal ends of the femora are altered most commonly. Cupping, shortening, and splaying of the metaphyses, irregularity and narrowing of the cartilaginous growth plates, and hypertrophy and premature fusion of the epiphyseal ossification centers can be noted (Fig. 75–3). Although the areas of cortical hyperostosis may gradually disappear after removal of the excess vitamin A, the damage to the epiphyseal cartilage may be irreversible if the poisoning has been protracted. Flexion contractures, short stature, and leg length discrepancies may ensue. Furthermore, scoliosis and fractures have been recorded,[20] although the relationship of these findings to hypervitaminosis A is not clear.

As in cases of acute poisoning, increased intracranial pressure has been noted in association with chronic hypervitaminosis A.[6, 22, 88] In those cases in which chronic hypervitaminosis A appears in the first 6 months of life, the skull may be poorly mineralized and have relatively dense sutural margins.[23] After this age, cranial findings include widening of the sutures with elongation of the head, hyperostosis in the occipital and the temporal bones, and ventricular dilation.[24]

Certain effects of vitamin A on the skeleton have been observed in the laboratory.[93] In weaning rats and guinea pigs, premature maturation and vascularization of the cartilaginous growth plates can be produced with excessive intake of vitamin A. Premature closure of the plates can produce early cessation of growth in these animals.[25] Furthermore, an accelerated remodeling of the transverse diameter of the tubular bones, particularly in the juxtaepiphyseal areas, can lead to osseous fracture.[26] Transplacental effects of high doses of vitamin A on fetal bones in mice have included shortening of the diaphyses of the tubular bones and an increase in calcification of the epiphyseal cartilage.[104] On the basis of organ cultures, Dingle and associates[27–29] have postulated that vitamin A produces ac-

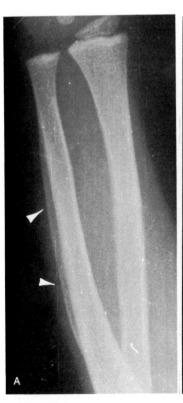
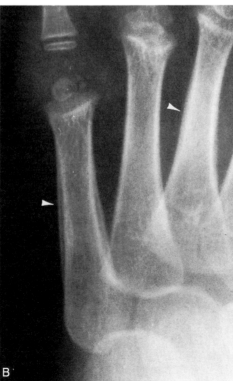

FIGURE 75–1. Hypervitaminosis A: Periostitis and cortical hyperostosis.
  A Note periosteal bone formation in the diaphysis of the ulna (arrowheads).
  B In a different child, periosteal proliferation is evident in the diaphyses of multiple metatarsals (arrowheads).
  (**A,** Courtesy of F. Silverman, M.D., Stanford, California.)

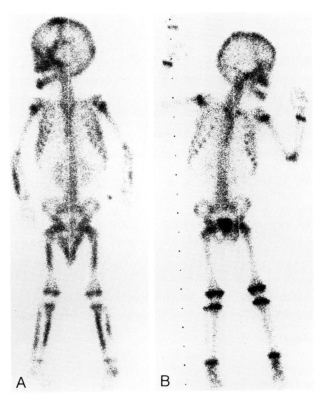

FIGURE 75–2. Hypervitaminosis A: Scintigraphic abnormalities. A 3 year old boy, who had been eating a high protein, low carbohydrate diet supplemented with vitamins A, D, E, and K, developed discomfort on standing, muscle spasm, and abdominal pain. Physical examination documented desquamation of the skin and loss of hair. Radiographs (not shown) revealed diastasis of the cranial sutures without evidence of periostitis in the tubular bones. There was evidence of marked elevation of serum vitamin A levels.

A An initial bone scan, using ^{99m}Tc-methylene diphosphonate, shows an abnormally increased accumulation of the radionuclide in the diaphyseal regions of the ulnae, femora, tibiae, and fibulae and along the sutures of the calvaria. The megavitamin therapy was discontinued. Five weeks later, periostitis became visible in the shafts of the tibiae and fibulae.

B A repeat bone scan using the same radiopharmaceutical agent accomplished 4 months after **A** is normal.

(From Miller JH, Hayon II: AJR *144*:767, 1985. Copyright 1985, American Roentgen Ray Society.)

tivation or release of cell proteases, which destroy extracellular cartilage matrix.[20] The simultaneous administration of cortisone to animals receiving high doses of vitamin A may prevent the cartilaginous destruction.[30]

In cats, excessive intake of vitamin A has been associated with postural changes, hyperostosis in the cervical spine, exostoses in the thoracic and lumbar regions, pelvic girdle, hips, and ribs, and ankylosis of peripheral joints, such as the elbows and shoulders.[93] A similar condition, caused by feeding large amounts of raw liver, has been described as a naturally occurring disorder of cats.[94, 95] It is these observations that have led to speculation regarding a potential role of hypervitaminosis A in the pathogenesis of diffuse idiopathic skeletal hyperostosis (see Chapter 41), speculation that has been promoted further by reports that link osseous outgrowths of the vertebrae with the administration of medications containing vitamin A derivatives (see Chapter 74).

The condition that produces skeletal changes that most resemble those of chronic hypervitaminosis A is infantile cortical hyperostosis (Caffey's disease) (Table 75–1). In

vitamin A intoxication, cortical hyperostosis usually becomes manifest no earlier than the end of the first year of life (whereas infantile cortical hyperostosis may produce changes in the first 6 months of life), mandibular and facial involvement is unusual (whereas these areas typically are affected in infantile cortical hyperostosis), metatarsal alterations are frequent (whereas these bones generally are spared in infantile cortical hyperostosis), and biochemical analysis of the blood reveals marked elevation of vitamin A concentration.[31]

HYPOVITAMINOSIS A

Vitamin A dietary deficiency in a pregnant woman can lead to an abortion or stillbirth of the fetus, or, in less severe cases, birth of a child who may reveal ophthalmic defects. Chronic vitamin A deficiency in infancy, childhood, or adulthood produces a variety of epithelial alterations, including dry and scaly skin, photophobia, night blindness, and dry conjunctivae; in infancy, additional manifestations include a susceptibility to infection, anemia, cranial nerve injury, and growth retardation.[33, 34] Increased intracranial pressure of unknown pathogenesis is observed in this condition,[24, 32, 34, 35] which in infants below the age of 6 months may lead to widening of the cranial sutures with bulging fontanelles.[36, 37]

Additional skeletal changes in vitamin A deficiency are recognized in experimental situations.[31] In animals deprived of vitamin A, stimulation of periosteal and endosteal bone formation[38] and retardation of endochondral bone formation[39] can lead to the appearance of short and thick tubular bones and may contribute to neural damage due to the effect of osseous pressure on neurologic tissue in the bones that are encasing the nervous system.[31] Furthermore, in experimental and nonexperimental situations, vitamin A de-

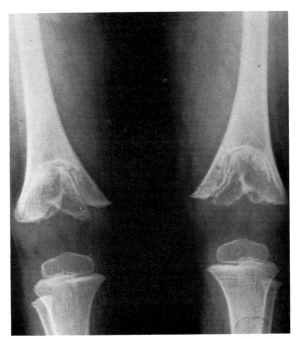

FIGURE 75–3. Hypervitaminosis A: Metaphyseal and epiphyseal changes. Observe the striking splaying and cupping of the distal femoral metaphyses, with narrowing of the cartilaginous growth plates and hypertrophy and invagination of the epiphyses.

TABLE 75–1. Hypervitaminosis A Versus Infantile Cortical Hyperostosis (Caffey's Disease)

	Hypervitaminosis A	Infantile Cortical Hyperostosis
Age of onset	End of first year of life	First 6 months of life
Findings	Soft tissue nodules Periostitis and hyperostosis Metaphyseal changes Growth disturbances Increased intracranial pressure	Soft tissue nodules Periostitis and hyperostosis Growth disturbances
Sites of hyperostosis (descending order of frequency)	Ulnae Metatarsals Clavicles Tibiae Fibulae Metacarpals Other tubular bones Ribs	Mandible Clavicles Scapulae Ribs Tubular bones
Etiology	Vitamin A poisoning	Unknown; possibly a viral disease

ficiency may have a dramatic effect on dental development.[40–42]

HYPOVITAMINOSIS C (SCURVY)

A long-term deficiency of dietary vitamin C (ascorbic acid) results in scurvy. This disease can be divided into those cases that develop in infancy or childhood (infantile scurvy) and those that occur in adults (adult scurvy).

Infantile Scurvy

Infantile scurvy occurs in babies who are fed pasteurized or boiled milk[9]; the process of heating the milk leads to disruption of vitamin C and the appearance of the disorder. Clinically apparent disease develops after deficiency of the vitamin has existed for 4 to 10 months; thus, it is exceedingly unusual to detect this disorder in infants below the age of 4 months, the manifestations generally becoming apparent at 8 to 14 months of age. There are reports of scurvy appearing in the first and second months of life,[43–45] however, although the authenticity of some of these cases is open to question.[9] Prior to the appearance of hemorrhagic tendencies, infants with scurvy can develop nonspecific findings, including a failure to thrive and digestive alterations. The onset of pale skin with petechial hemorrhages, swollen, red, and ulcerated gums, palatal petechiae, hematuria, melena, hematemesis, and secondary infections, when combined with characteristic radiographic changes and depressed levels of serum ascorbic acid, ensures accurate diagnosis; this hemorrhagic tendency, which is a hallmark of the disease, may be related to a lack of intercellular cement substance in the endothelial layer of the capillaries. Additional clinical findings of infantile scurvy include inactivity, soft tissue swelling due to edema and hemorrhage, and costochondral tenderness and prominence.

Metaphyseal Changes. Skeletal alterations result from a depression of normal cellular activity, which is manifested in the collagen of the bony tissues.[31, 46] The activity of the osteoblast is reduced, thereby leading to a decrease in the formation of bony matrix, which is most marked in areas of active endochondral bone growth (ends of tubular bones and costochondral junctions). In the region of the cartilaginous growth plate, proliferating cartilage cells are reduced in number, modified osteoblasts are identified, and a disorganization of the growth zone is evident. An irregular arrangement of cartilage cells appears in the proliferating zone of the plate, and a small area of the adjacent metaphysis contains a trabecular latticework of calcified cartilage matrix that is strikingly free of borders of osseous tissue[31] (Fig. 75–4). A sparsity of newly formed trabeculae is evident in this junctional region, and a brittleness of trabecular structure is demonstrated. Extensive resorption of cortical and spongy bone contributes to a tendency to fracture through this zone, leading to evidence of fresh and remote hemorrhage. The abnormal marrow in the junctional area is termed "Gerüstmark," and the entire zone consists of detritus ("Trümmerfeldzone").[31] Lateral extension of the heavy provisional zones of calcification in conjunction with elevation and stimulation of the adjacent periosteal membrane produces small spicules or excrescences of the metaphysis.

A radiograph of the end of an involved tubular bone will reveal several zones (Table 75–2) (Fig. 75–5). A radiodense line borders on the growth plate, representing the sclerotic provisional zone. On its metaphyseal side between the provisional zone of calcification and the heavy spongiosa deeper in the shaft is a transverse band of diminished density, the "scurvy" line. Small beaklike outgrowths of the metaphysis, incomplete or complete separation of the plate from the shaft due to subepiphyseal marginal clefts and

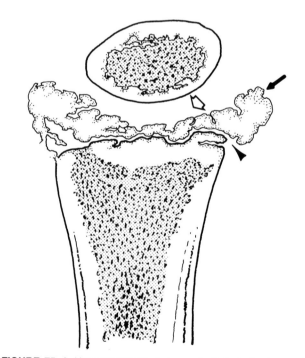

FIGURE 75–4. Hypovitaminosis C (scurvy): Pathologic abnormalities. The changes in the ends of tubular bones consist of an irregular arrangement of cartilage cells in the proliferating zone of the growth plate (open arrow), a metaphyseal area containing a latticework of calcified cartilage that is free of osseous tissue (solid arrow), and a decrease in trabeculae, fracture, and detritus in the junctional area (arrowhead). Metaphyseal excrescences can develop.

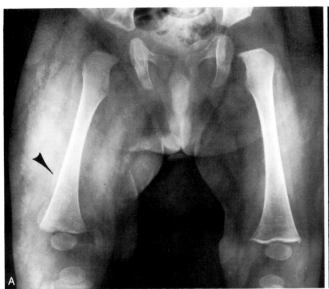
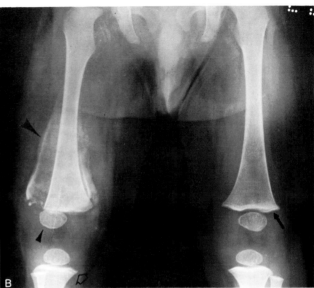
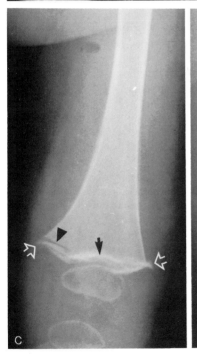
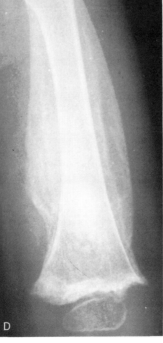

FIGURE 75–5. Hypovitaminosis C (scurvy): Radiographic abnormalities.

A, B At the ends of tubular bones, osteoporosis, a thick sclerotic metaphyseal line beneath which is a radiolucent line ("scurvy line") (solid arrow), small beaklike excrescences (open arrow), epiphyseal displacement (small arrowhead), and subperiosteal hemorrhage with periostitis (large arrowheads) can be noted.

C, D Radiographs obtained 1 month apart show, initially **(C),** a sclerotic metaphyseal line (arrow), beaklike excrescences (open arrows) and a metaphyseal radiolucent line (arrowhead). Subsequently **(D),** a thicker band of metaphyseal sclerosis and periostitis is seen. A sclerotic line about the epiphysis also is seen both in **C** and in **D.**

(A, B, Courtesy of F. Silverman, M.D., Stanford, California.)

TABLE 75–2. Hypovitaminosis C (Scurvy): Radiographic-Pathologic Correlation

Radiographic Finding	Pathologic Finding
Transverse metaphyseal line of increased density	Prominent thickened provisional zone of calcification
Transverse metaphyseal line of decreased density ("scurvy" line)	Decrease in trabeculae and detritus in junctional area of metaphysis ("Trümmerfeldzone")
Metaphyseal excrescences or beaks	Lateral extension of the heavy provisional zone of calcification with periosteal elevation and stimulation
Subepiphyseal infractions ("corner" or "angle" sign)	Decrease and brittleness of trabeculae in junctional area with fracture and hemorrhage
Periostitis	Subperiosteal hemorrhage with elevation and stimulation of periosteum
Epiphyseal shell of increased density with central lucency (Wimberger's sign of scurvy)	Prominent thickened provisional zone of calcification with atrophy of central spongiosa

infractions ("corner" or "angle" sign), extensive physiolysis with osseous malalignment,[97] and periosteal elevation with new bone formation due to subperiosteal hemorrhage complete the distinctive radiographic picture of the meta-epiphyseal regions of tubular bones (and costochondral junctions).[9] These changes are most marked in areas of active endochondral bone formation, such as the distal end of the femur, the proximal and distal ends of the tibia and fibula, the distal end of the radius and ulna, the proximal end of the humerus, and the sternal ends of the ribs.

Epiphyseal Changes. In the ossification centers of the epiphyses of tubular bones and in the carpus and tarsus, similar but less marked alterations are seen.[102] Persistence and thickening of the provisional zone of calcification produce a radiodense shell around the ossification center that is accentuated by central rarefaction owing to atrophy of the adjacent spongiosa (Wimberger's sign of scurvy).[9] These epiphyseal abnormalities, which do not include infraction or fracture, invariably are combined with the metaphyseal changes that were outlined previously.

Diaphyseal Changes. Atrophy of spongiosa in the shafts of tubular bones accounts for a nonspecific decreased radiodensity and a "ground glass" appearance of the diaphyses. Cortical diminution is common and often severe, yet fracture of the shafts is unusual. Subperiosteal hemorrhage is most frequent in the larger tubular bones, such as the femur, the tibia, and the humerus, although similar but less extensive bleeding may appear in other sites, including the flat bones of the calvarium and shoulder girdle.[9] The degree of hemorrhage is variable and can produce focal or diffuse elevation of the periosteal membrane. The entire length of the diaphysis may be affected; epiphyseal hemorrhage is exceedingly rare. Radiographically, soft tissue masses of increased density, displacement of adjacent bones, and small or large shells of periosteal bone, particularly during the healing phase of the disease, are observed.

Articular Changes. Hemarthrosis is a rare manifestation of scurvy,[47, 48] demonstrating a predilection for the large weight-bearing joints of the lower extremities. A bloody

effusion and thickened synovial membrane with hemosiderin deposition in the macrophages of the deep connective tissue can be observed. Hemarthrosis and intrasynovial hemorrhage can be attributed to loss of the structural integrity of the collagen tissue in the synovial membrane coupled with the trauma of normal activity.[48]

Dental Changes. Cyst formation and hemorrhage in the enamel and interruptions of the lamina dura may be dental manifestations of scurvy in humans.[49, 50] In animals, dental changes in experimental vitamin C deficiency can be prominent, with arrested growth and hemorrhage.[31]

Growth Disturbances. Permanent growth disturbances after scurvy are unusual despite the frequency and severity of epiphyseal separations. Central segmental metaphyseal cupping in a bilateral or unilateral distribution can lead to intrusion of the epiphysis into the exaggerated concavity of the metaphysis and apparent early fusion of the growth plate.[51, 52, 96] This complication is not frequent, however, and the degree of limb shortening may be minimal. The pathogenesis of metaphyseal cupping is not clear, although impaired ossification in the central portion of the growth plate due to interruption of vascular supply, perhaps related to periosteal stripping, has been suggested as one possible mechanism for this alteration.[51] The change may be accentuated by osseous weakening of the neighboring metaphyseal bone.[53] Similar cupping may be observed after trauma, infection, irradiation, immobilization, and vitamin A poisoning, as well as in sickle cell anemia and hereditary bone disorders.[54]

Effects of Therapy. With treatment of the disease, radiographic signs may accompany healing scurvy.[55] Thickening of the cortex, increased density of the radiolucent zone of the metaphysis, transverse densities within the shaft due to burying of the thickened provisional zone of calcification, massive subperiosteal bone formation, which later merges with the underlying cortex, spontaneous shifting of the diaphysis to realign with the displaced epiphysis, and increased density of the epiphysis all can be observed.[9] Circular central radiolucent foci in the epiphyseal ossification centers corresponding to the original outline of the osteoporotic epiphyses have been noted.

Differential Diagnosis. The appearance of a radiolucent metaphyseal band in scurvy does not represent a pathognomonic finding. Other chronic illnesses, such as leukemia and neuroblastoma, can produce bony atrophy in this region. The identification of radiodense lines at the metaphysis and about the epiphysis, metaphyseal fractures, osseous beaks, epiphyseal displacements, and diaphyseal periostitis allows an accurate diagnosis of scurvy. Leukemia can lead to periostitis and diaphyseal destruction in combination with bandlike metaphyseal radiolucency, but fracture and epiphyseal separation are not identified. Syphilis produces symmetric destructive foci in the metaphyses, particularly in the proximal tibia, but the distinctive findings are not confused with those of scurvy. Metaphyseal changes also can accompany rubella, cytomegalic inclusion disease, toxoplasmosis, and a variety of traumatic and dysplastic disorders.

Adult Scurvy

Currently, scurvy rarely is encountered in adults, although it may be observed in severely malnourished per-

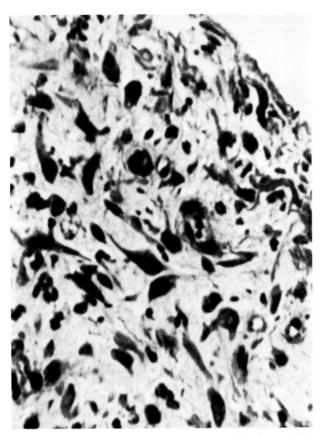

FIGURE 75–6. Hypovitaminosis C (scurvy): Articular abnormalities. In a 56 year old man with scurvy, knee hemarthrosis appeared. The synovial membrane shows many elongated fibroblasts and smaller erythrocytes scattered throughout the interstitium (360×). (From Bevelaqua P, et al: JAMA 235:1874, 1976. Copyright 1976, American Medical Association.)

sons, especially the elderly. The findings require a protracted period of vitamin deficiency for clinical expression.[49] Nonspecific weakness, anorexia, weight loss, and fatigue generally antedate the more diagnostic hemorrhagic manifestations, such as petechiae and ecchymoses of the skin, subcutaneous tissues, and gums.[56]

Hemarthrosis and bleeding at synchondroses can be observed in adult scurvy[48, 57, 105] (Fig. 75–6). Such hemarthrosis has been associated with collapse of subchondral bone, especially in the femoral head.[106, 107] This collapse may relate to ischemic necrosis of bone produced by vascular compromise effected by the hemarthrosis or to osteopenia and subsequent fractures of subarticular bone. Osteoporosis is prominent in the axial skeleton, especially the spine, and in the tubular bones of the appendicular skeleton. In the vertebral column, biconcave deformities of vertebral bodies, condensation of bone at the superior and inferior vertebral margins, and central rarefaction are identical to changes of osteoporosis accompanying a wide spectrum of disorders; in the extremities, cortical thinning can be associated with mild periosteal proliferation. The cranium also may be osteoporotic in adult-onset scurvy.

HYPERVITAMINOSIS D

Excessive intake of vitamin D can be associated with clinical and radiologic manifestations in both children and

adults. Initial reports noted findings of intoxication in infants and young children who had been given excessive levels of vitamin D for the treatment of rickets and other skeletal disorders[58]; similar intoxication in adults later was identified in patients who were receiving inordinate amounts of vitamin D for the therapy of Paget's disease or rheumatoid arthritis.[31, 59, 60]

Musculoskeletal Abnormalities

Vitamin D poisoning can be acute or chronic. The level of the vitamin that is required to produce toxic symptoms and signs is extremely variable; patients with preexisting renal or gastrointestinal dysfunction are especially susceptible.[31] Acute clinical manifestations may appear within 3 to 9 days after massive doses (4 to 18 million units per day) of the vitamin and include vomiting, fever, dehydration, abdominal cramps, bone pain and tenderness, convulsions, and coma.[61] With chronic poisoning, lassitude, thirst, anorexia, and polyuria are followed by vomiting, abdominal pain, and diarrhea.[9] Laboratory analysis indicates albuminuria, hematuria, hypercalciuria, and hypercalcemia. With the onset of renal insufficiency, the levels of serum phosphorus and nonprotein nitrogen become elevated.

In infants and in children, metaphyseal bands of increased density, reflecting heavy calcifications of the matrix of the proliferating cartilage, alternating with areas of increased lucency are evident in the tubular bones.[62] Cortical thickening due to periosteal apposition[63] may be observed at certain sites, and osteoporosis and thinning of the cortices may be evident at other locations. Widespread osteosclerosis also has been noted.[64] Metastatic calcification of viscera, blood vessels, periarticular structures, muscles, laryngeal and tracheal cartilage, the falx cerebri, and the tentorium cerebelli can be noted.[63, 65, 66]

In adults, hypervitaminosis D can lead to focal or generalized osteoporosis. The bones of the appendicular skeleton, the spine, the pelvis, and even the skull reveal varying degrees of bone loss. Massive soft tissue calcification can become apparent, especially in patients with rheumatoid arthritis or gout being treated with excessive amounts of the vitamin, and this frequently is combined with severe osteoporosis. Lobulated, smooth, amorphous masses of calcium are evident in periarticular regions, bursae, tendon sheaths, joint capsules, and intra-articular cavities[31, 67, 101] (Fig. 75–7). On pathologic evaluation, thick white granular calcareous material, usually representing calcium hydroxyapatite, is identified, and an inflammatory reaction in the bursal wall or adjacent soft tissues can be seen. In patients with rheumatoid arthritis or gout, calcification of soft tissue nodules or tophi is observed.

Experimentally, toxic doses of vitamin D administered to animals lead to osteoporosis, subperiosteal bone resorption, metaphyseal sclerosis, hypercalcemia, hyperphosphatemia, and metastatic calcification,[68, 69, 108] although smaller doses cause little effect on calcium and phosphorus balance.[70] It is not known precisely why metastatic calcification occurs at specific sites; previous tissue degeneration does not appear to be an essential factor,[71] although local alkalinity may favor deposition of calcium phosphate.[31] Experimentally, withdrawal of the vitamin can be followed by reversion to normal serum levels and metabolic balance of cal-

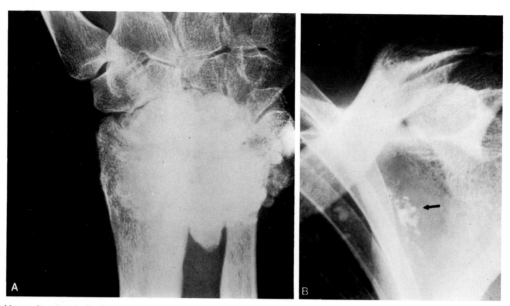

FIGURE 75–7. Hypervitaminosis D: Soft tissue abnormalities.
  A In a patient with rheumatoid arthritis who was treated with vitamin D, note massive soft tissue calcification about the wrist.
  B In a different patient without articular disease, small calcific deposits in the soft tissue are evident (arrow).

cium and phosphorus with recalcification of bone and resorption of metastatic calcific deposits.[72]

Metastatic soft tissue calcification accompanies a variety of disorders, including hypervitaminosis D, milk-alkali syndrome, hyperparathyroidism, plasma cell myeloma, and skeletal metastasis.[73, 74, 98] Furthermore, soft tissue calcinosis can be evident in various collagen vascular disorders, and dystrophic calcification can occur after tissue injury or devitalization from any cause. Periarticular deposits are most characteristic of hypervitaminosis D, milk-alkali syndrome, hyperparathyroidism, renal osteodystrophy, collagen vascular disorders, and idiopathic tumoral calcinosis.

Chronic Idiopathic Hypercalcemia

Idiopathic infantile hypercalcemia first was described in 1952.[75, 76] The major clinical manifestations of this disorder include a peculiar facies, anorexia, hypotonia, mental and physical retardation, and vomiting. Radiographically, a generalized increase in skeletal density is observed.[77, 78] Although the exact pathogenesis of chronic idiopathic hypercalcemia is not known, the disease may relate to the excessive ingestion of vitamin D over prolonged periods by infants who are slightly sensitive to this vitamin.[79, 80]

In 1963, Black and Bonham-Carter[81] noted that infants with a facies similar to that of patients with idiopathic hypercalcemia could reveal supravalvular aortic stenosis and mental retardation (Williams' syndrome), an observation that subsequently was verified by numerous investigators. Furthermore, the vascular manifestations that were encountered in these patients were varied and included, in addition to supravalvular aortic stenosis, stenosis of the branches of the aorta, the peripheral pulmonary vessels, or the carotid arteries and aortic hypoplasia.[24]

The detection of hypercalcemia and these variable vascular anomalies suggests that vitamin D excess or hypersensitivity in the expectant mother may represent a fundamental cause of congenital malformations of the cardiovascular system of the fetus. Clinical evidence supporting this con-

cept includes the detection of elevated levels of vitamin D in the blood of some infants with idiopathic hypercalcemia, osteosclerosis, and aortic stenosis[82–86]; supporting experimental findings include the observations of Friedman and Roberts[87] in the offspring of pregnant rabbits given high doses of vitamin D. These investigators noted an elevated level of serum calcium and aortic lesions similar to supravalvular aortic stenosis in some of the newborn rabbits. In addition, disturbances in the development of the bones of the face and cranium were evident.

OTHER VITAMINOSES

Vitamin K deficiency can lead to hemorrhagic manifestations in the infant, consisting of bleeding from the nose, gastrointestinal tract, umbilical stump, and sites of skin puncture, as well as within the brain. Rarely, hemarthrosis is observed.[99] This vitamin deficiency is more frequent in breast-fed infants than in those fed cow's milk or formula owing to the low concentration of vitamin K in breast milk.[99] Soft tissue calcification may follow intramuscular *vitamin E* injection.[103]

SUMMARY

Deficiencies and excesses of certain vitamins may have a pronounced effect on the musculoskeletal system. In addition to vitamin D deficiency leading to rickets, hypervitaminosis A and D and hypovitaminosis C (scurvy) are examples of vitamin-related disorders that affect the osseous, articular, or soft tissue structures.

References

1. Jeghers H, Marraro H: Hypervitaminosis A: Its broadening spectrum. Am J Clin Nutr 6:335, 1958.
2. Sulzberger MG, Lazar MP: Hypervitaminosis A. JAMA 146:788, 1951.
3. DiBenedetto RJ: Chronic hypervitaminosis A in an adult. JAMA 201:700, 1967.
4. Kane EK: Arctic Explorations in the Years 1853, 1854, 1855. Philadelphia, Childs & Peterson Publishers, 1856, p 392.

5. Rodahl K, Moore T: The vitamin A content and toxicity of bear and seal liver. Biochem J 37:166, 1943.

6. Feldman MH, Schlezinger NS: Benign intracranial hypertension associated with hypervitaminosis A. Arch Neurol 22:1, 1970.

7. Lonie TC: Excess vitamin A as a cause of food poisoning. NZ Med J 49:680, 1950.

8. Marie J, See G: Acute hypervitaminosis A of the infant: Its clinical manifestations with benign acute hydrocephalus and pronounced bulge of the fontanel; a clinical and biologic study. Am J Dis Child 87:731, 1954.

9. Caffey J: Pediatric X-Ray Diagnosis. 7th Ed. Chicago, Year Book Medical Publishers, 1978, p 1466.

10. Moore LA, Sykes JF: Cerebrospinal fluid pressure and vitamin A deficiency. Am J Physiol 130:684, 1940.

11. Josephs HW: Hypervitaminosis A and carotenemia. Am J Dis Child 67:33, 1944.

12. Toomey JA, Morisette RA: Hypervitaminosis A. Am J Dis Child 73:473, 1947.

13. Caffey J: Chronic poisoning due to excess of vitamin A. Description of the clinical and roentgen manifestations in seven infants and young children. Pediatrics 5:672, 1950.

14. Sulzberger MB, Lazar MP: Hypervitaminosis A: Report of a case in an adult. JAMA 146:788, 1951.

15. Dickey LB, Bradley EJ: Hypervitaminosis A. Stanford Med Bull 6:345, 1948.

16. Woodard WK, Miller LJ, Legant O: Acute and chronic hypervitaminosis A in a 4 month old infant. J Pediatr 59:260, 1961.

17. Tunell R, Pierson B: Chronic vitamin A intoxication in infants. Acta Paediatr Scand 50:319, 1961.

18. Pickup JD: Hypervitaminosis A. Arch Dis Child 31:229, 1956.

19. Pease CN: Focal retardation and arrestment of growth due to vitamin A intoxication. JAMA 182:980, 1962.

20. Ruby LK, Mital MA: Skeletal deformities following chronic hypervitaminosis A. A case report. J Bone Joint Surg [Am] 56:1283, 1974.

21. Perrson B, Tunell R, Ekengren K: Chronic vitamin A intoxication during the first half year of life; description of five cases. Acta Paediatr Scand 54:49, 1965.

22. Grossman LA: Increased intracranial pressure: Consequence of hypervitaminosis A. South Med J 65:916, 1972.

23. Arena JM, Sarazen P Jr, Baylin GJ: Hypervitaminosis A: Report of an unusual case with marked craniotabes. Pediatrics 8:788, 1951.

24. Taybi H: Vitamin deficiency and intoxication. In TH Newton, DG Potts (Eds): Radiology of the Skull and Brain. Vol 1. The Skull. St Louis, CV Mosby Co, 1971, p 678.

25. Wolbach SB: Vitamin-A deficiency and excess in relation to skeletal growth. J Bone Joint Surg 29:171, 1947.

26. Wolke RE, Nielsen SW: Pathogenesis of hypervitaminosis A in growing porcine bone. Lab Invest 16:639, 1967.

27. Dingle JT, Lucy JA, Fell HB: Studies on the mode of action of excess vitamin A. 1. Effect of excess of vitamin A on the metabolism and composition of embryonic chick-limb cartilage grown in organ culture. Biochem J 79:497, 1961.

28. Lucy JA, Dingle JT, Fell HB: Studies on the mode of action of excess vitamin A. 2. A possible role of intracellular proteases in the degradation of cartilage matrix. Biochem J 79:500, 1961.

29. Dingle JT: Studies on the mode of action of excess vitamin A. 3. Release of a bound protease by the action of vitamin A. Biochem J 79:509, 1961.

30. Thomas L, McCluskey RT, Li J, et al: Prevention by cortisone of the changes in cartilage induced by an excess of vitamin A in rabbits. Am J Pathol 42:271, 1963.

31. Jaffe HL: Metabolic, Degenerative and Inflammatory Diseases of Bones and Joints. Philadelphia, Lea & Febiger, 1972, p 448.

32. Bass MH: The relation of vitamin A intake to cerebrospinal fluid pressure; a review. J Mt Sinai Hosp 24:713, 1957.

33. Bass MH, Caplan J: Vitamin A deficiency in infancy. J Pediatr 47:690, 1955.

34. Keating JP, Feigin RD: Increased intracranial pressure associated with probable vitamin A deficiency in cystic fibrosis. Pediatrics 46:41, 1970.

35. Eaton HD: Chronic bovine hypo- and hypervitaminosis A and cerebrospinal fluid pressure. Am J Clin Nutr 22:1070, 1969.

36. Cornfeld D, Cooke RE: Vitamin A deficiency: Case report; unusual manifestations in a 5½ month old baby. Pediatrics 10:33, 1952.

37. Bass MH, Fisch GR: Increased intracranial pressure with bulging fontanel; a symptom of vitamin A deficiency in infants. Neurology 11:1091, 1961.

38. Mellanby E: Skeletal changes affecting the nervous system produced in young dogs by diets deficient in vitamin A. J Physiol 99:467, 1941.

39. Wolbach SB, Bessey OA: Vitamin A deficiency and the nervous system. Arch Pathol 32:689, 1941.

40. Boyle PE: Manifestations of vitamin A deficiency in a human toothgerm. J Dent Res 13:39, 1933.

41. Orten AU, Burn CG, Smith AH: Effects of prolonged chronic vitamin A deficiency in the rat with special reference to odontomas. Proc Soc Exp Biol Med 36:82, 1937.

42. Burn CG, Orten AU, Smith AH: Changes in the structure of the developing tooth in rats maintained on a diet deficient in vitamin A. Yale J Biol Med 13:817, 1941.

43. Jackson D, Park EA: Congenital scurvy. J Pediatr 7:741, 1935.

44. Burns RR: The unusual occurrence of scurvy in an eight week old infant. AJR 89:923, 1963.

45. Dennis JM, Mercado R: Scurvy following folic acid antagonist therapy. Radiology 67:412, 1956.

46. Wolbach SB, Howe PR: Intercellular substances in experimental scorbutus. Arch Pathol 1:1, 1926.

47. Pirani CL, Bly CG, Sutherland K: Scorbutic arthropathy in the guinea pig. Arch Pathol 49:710, 1950.

48. Bevelaqua FA, Hasselbacher P, Schumacher HR: Scurvy and hemarthrosis. JAMA 235:1874, 1976.

49. Crandon JH, Lund CC, Dill DB: Experimental human scurvy. N Engl J Med 223:353, 1940.

50. Boyle PE: The tooth germ in acute scurvy. J Dent Res 14:172, 1934.

51. Silverman FN: Recovery from epiphyseal invagination: Sequel to an unusual complication of scurvy. J Bone Joint Surg [Am] 52:384, 1970.

52. Sprague PL: Epiphyseo-metaphyseal cupping following infantile scurvy. Pediatr Radiol 4:122, 1976.

53. Siffert RS: The growth plate and its affections. J Bone Joint Surg [Am] 48:546, 1966.

54. Caffey J: Traumatic cupping of the metaphyses of growing bones. AJR 108:451, 1970.

55. McLean S, McIntosh R: Healing in infantile scurvy as shown by x-ray. Am J Dis Child 36:875, 1928.

56. Mitra ML: Vitamin-C deficiency in the elderly and its manifestations. J Am Geriatr Soc 18:67, 1970.

57. Joffe N: Some radiological aspects of scurvy in the adult. Br J Radiol 34:429, 1961.

58. Thatcher L: Hypervitaminosis-D with report of a fatal case in a child. Edinburgh Med J 38:457, 1931.

59. Wells HG, Holley SW: Metastatic calcification in osteitis deformans. (Paget's disease of bone). Arch Pathol 34:435, 1942.

60. Danowski TS, Winkler AW, Peters JP: Tissue calcification and renal failure produced by massive dose vitamin D therapy of arthritis. Ann Intern Med 23:22, 1945.

61. Ruziczka O: Injuries due to overdosage of vitamin D. Wien Klin Wochenschr 64:964, 1952.

62. Ross SG: Vitamin D intoxication in infancy. A report of four cases. J Pediatr 41:815, 1952.

63. Swoboda W: Die rontgensymptomatik der vitamin-D-intoxikation im kindesalter. ROFO 77:534, 1952.

64. DeWind LT: Hypervitaminosis D with osteosclerosis. Arch Dis Child 36:373, 1961.

65. Debre R: Toxic effects of overdosage of vitamin D_2 in children. Am J Dis Child 75:787, 1948.

66. Holman CB: Roentgenologic manifestations of vitamin D intoxication. Radiology 59:805, 1952.

67. Christensen WR, Liebman C, Sosman MC: Skeletal and peri-articular manifestations of hypervitaminosis D. AJR 65:27, 1951.

68. Kreitmair H, Moll T: Hypervitaminose nach grossen dosen vitamin D. Much Med Wochenschr 75:1113, 1928.

69. Shohl AT, Goldblatt H, Brown HB: The pathological effects upon rats of excess irradiated ergosterol. J Clin Invest 8:505, 1930.

70. Bauer W, Marble A, Claflin D: Studies on mode of action of irradiated ergosterol; its effect on calcium, phosphorus and nitrogen metabolism of normal individuals. J Clin Invest 11:1, 1932.

71. Ham AW: Mechanism of calcification in the heart and aorta in hypervitaminosis D. Arch Pathol 14:613, 1932.

72. Steck IE, Deutsch H, Reed CI, et al: Further studies on intoxication with vitamin D. Ann Intern Med 10:951, 1937.

73. Barr DP: Pathological calcification. Physiol Rev 12:593, 1932.

74. Bauer JM, Freyberg RH: Vitamin D intoxication with metastatic calcification. JAMA 130:1208, 1946.

75. Fanconi G, Girardet P: Chronische Hypercalcämie kombiniert mit Osteodklerose, Hyperazotämie, Minderwuchs, und kongenitalen missbildungen. Helv Paediatr Acta 7:314, 1952.

76. Schlesinger B, Butler N, Black J: Chronische Hypercalcämie kombiniert mit Osteosklerose, hyperazotämie, Minderwuchs, und kongenitalen missbildungen. Helv Paediatr Acta 7:335, 1952.

77. Shiers JA, Neuhauser EBD, Bowman JR: Idiopathic hypercalcemia. AJR 78:19, 1957.

78. Singleton EB: The radiographic features of severe idiopathic hypercalcemia of infancy. Radiology 68:721, 1957.

79. Forbes GB, Cafarelli C, Manning J: Vitamin D and infantile hypercalcemia. Pediatrics 42:203, 1968.

80. Fraser D, Kidd BSL, Kooh SW, et al: A new look at infantile hypercalcemia. Pediatr Clin North Am 13:503, 1966.

81. Black JA, Bonham-Carter RE: Association between aortic stenosis and facies of severe infantile hypercalcemia. Lancet 2:745, 1963.

82. Garcia RE, Friedman WF, Kaback MM, et al: Idiopathic hypercalcemia and supravalvular aortic stenosis. N Engl J Med 271:117, 1964.

83. Kurlander GJ, Petry EL, Taybi H, et al: Supravalvular aortic stenosis; roentgen analysis of twenty-seven cases. AJR 98:782, 1966.

84. Seelig MS: Vitamin D and cardiovascular, renal, and brain damage in infancy and childhood. Ann NY Acad Sci 147:537, 1969.

85. Friedman WF: Vitamin D as a cause of the supravalvular aortic stenosis syndrome. Am Heart J 73:718, 1967.

86. Manios SG, Antener I: A study of vitamin D metabolism in idiopathic hypercalcemia of infancy. Acta Paediatr Scand 55:600, 1966.

87. Friedman WF, Roberts WC: Vitamin D and the supravalvular aortic stenosis syndrome; the transplacental effects of vitamin D on the aorta of the rabbit. Circulation 34:77, 1966.

88. Mahoney CP, Margolis T, Knauss TA, et al: Chronic vitamin A intoxication in infants fed chicken liver. Pediatrics 65:893, 1980.

89. Fumich RM, Essig GW: Hypervitaminosis A. Case report in an adolescent soccer player. Am J Sports Med 11:34, 1983.

90. Gerber A, Raab A, Sobel A: Vitamin A poisoning in adults. Am J Med 30:729, 1954.

91. James MB, Leonard JC, Fraser JJ Jr, et al: Hypervitaminosis A: A case report. Pediatrics 69:112, 1982.

92. Miller JH, Hayon II: Bone scintigraphy in hypervitaminosis A. AJR 144:767, 1985.

93. Mazierces B: Vitamin A, bone and joint. Clin Rheumatol 1:239, 1982.

94. Seawright AH, English PB, Gartner RJW: Hypervitaminosis A of the cat. Adv Vet Sci Comp Med 14:1, 1970.

95. English PB, Seawright AH: Deforming cervical spondylosis of the cat. Aust Vet J 40:376, 1964.

96. Hallel T, Malkin C, Garti R: Epiphyseometaphyseal cupping of the distal femoral epiphysis following scurvy in infancy. Clin Orthop 153:166, 1980.

97. Nerubay J, Pilderwasser D: Spontaneous bilateral distal femoral physiology due to scurvy. Acta Orthop Scand 55:18, 1984.

98. Stewart VL, Herling P, Dalinka MK: Calcification in soft tissues. JAMA 250:78, 1983.

99. Naveh Y, Berant M, Bialik V: Vitamin K deficiency presenting with hemarthrosis. Case report. J Pediatr Orthop 4:630, 1984.

100. Gamble JG, Ip SC: Hypervitaminosis A in a child from megadosing. J Pediatr Orthop 5:219, 1985.

101. Butler RC, Dieppe PA, Keat ASC: Calcinosis of joints and periarticular tissues associated with vitamin D intoxication. Ann Rheum Dis 44:494, 1985.

102. Boeve WJ, Martijn A: Case report 406. Skel Radiol 16:67, 1987.

103. Barak M, Herschkowitz S, Montag J: Soft tissue calcification: A complication of vitamin E injection. Pediatrics 77:382, 1986.

104. Atkins I, Cohen I, Schwartz Z, et al: Transplacental effects of vitamin A on fetal bones in mice—follow-up studies on postnatal recovery. J Orthop Res 6:704, 1988.

105. Haslock I: Spontaneous hemarthrosis of the shoulder associated with destructive arthropathy. J Orthop Rheumatol 5:121, 1992.

106. Shetty A, Buckingham RB, Killian PJ, et al: Hemarthrosis and femoral head destruction in an adult diet faddist with scurvy. J Rheumatol 15:12, 1988.

107. Sudbury S, Ford P: Femoral head destruction in scurvy. J Rheumatol 17:1108, 1990.

108. Jiang Y, Wang Y, Zhao J, et al: Bone remodeling in hypervitaminosis D3. Radiologic-microangiographic-pathologic correlations. Invest Radiol 26:213, 1991.

76

Heavy Metal Poisoning and Deficiency

Donald Resnick, M.D.

Poisoning with certain heavy metals can produce characteristic musculoskeletal alterations. One of the most well recognized changes associated with ingestion, inhalation, or injection of lead or other heavy metals is the appearance of radiodense lines at the ends of tubular bones or along the contours of flat and irregular bones. These lines must be differentiated from the transverse radiodense areas that commonly are observed at some of these locations in persons who have not been poisoned with metals. This chapter first reviews the nature and appearance of growth recovery lines and subsequently describes the radiographic changes of the skeleton associated with heavy metal poisoning. Included also is a discussion of the skeletal manifestations associated with deficiencies of some of the trace elements. The role of copper in Wilson's disease, of iron in hemochromatosis and anemia, and of calcium in osteoporosis is discussed elsewhere in the textbook.

TRANSVERSE OR STRESS LINES (OF PARK OR HARRIS)

The appearance of opaque transverse lines that extend across the metaphyses of tubular bones is a common radiographic phenomenon[1, 2] that may be observed in children and adults (Fig. 76–1). They often are referred to as Park or Harris lines (as a tribute to the contributions of these two investigators)[3–6] and as transverse or growth arrest lines.[4, 7] A historical summary[8–40] of the numerous early investigations of these lines, which is tabulated by Garn and colleagues[2] (Table 76–1), emphasizes that they have been recognized in both healthy and sick persons, that similar lines have been encountered in patients who have been poisoned with a variety of heavy metals, that the lines may be used as a determinant of growth potential and magnitude, that they may be produced experimentally in animals restricted to specific dietary intakes, and that their exact pathogenesis is not uniformly agreed on by all investigators. It now generally is recognized that these transverse radiodense lines can be evident at birth or during infancy and that they do not appear after growth has ceased but that, once formed, they persist into adult life. They are without local symptoms and signs. Similar lines can appear about the margins of the round and the flat bones and in both the appendicular and the axial portions of the skeleton (Fig. 76–2). The radiodense lines are more frequent and prominent as sites of rapid bone growth, such as the femora and tibiae about the knee. Although they usually are symmetric and widespread in distribution, atypical patterns are encountered.

In the tubular bones, single or multiple lines of increased density parallel the contours of the nearby provisional zones of calcification. Although the pathogenesis of the dense lines is not certain, it is the close proximity and similarity between the lines and the growth plate that have suggested that the bands are related to a disturbance of normal growth patterns. Indeed, the term ''arrest'' lines, which still is applied to these dense shadows, underscores the early belief that their appearance signified an arrest in normal growth. As shown by Park and his associates,[3, 4] however, they are more properly termed ''recovery'' lines, indicating periods of renewed or increased growth, presumably after a period of inhibited growth of the bone. The discovery of the radiodense bands suggests a previous occurrence of an episode

TABLE 76–1. Historical Summary of Early Published Studies on Lines and Bands

Date	Author	Summary of Findings	Date	Author	Summary of Findings
1874	Wegener[8]	Produced transverse bands of trabeculae by administration of phosphorus to rabbits and chickens.	1953	Park and Richter[4]	Indicated that although initiation of a transverse line is caused by cessation of cartilage growth, thickening is caused by lag of cartilage cell maturation behind resumed osteoblastic activity in recovery phase.
1877	Gies[9]	Produced transverse bands by administration of arsenic to rabbits.			
1903	Ludloff[10]	Reported transverse striations in radiographs of legs of normal individuals.	1955	Hewitt, Westropp, and Acheson[25]	Demonstrated statistically significant association between transverse lines in radiographs of knees and periods of illness in 650 normal children.
1904	Lehndorff[11]	Described transverse striations in scurvy.	1956	Jones and Dean[26]	Reported that more children with kwashiorkor had transverse lines on distal end of radius than normal children and followed development of these lines in serial radiographs.
1918	Phemister[12]	Described radiopaque transverse bands in long bones after administration of phosphorus.			
1921	Stettner[13]	Interpreted transverse lines as lines of arrested growth.	1956	Dreizen, Currie, Gilley, and Spies[27]	Found transverse lines and nutritive status not to be significantly associated, although relation between resorption of lines and nutritive status was reported.
1924	Asada[14]	Reported experimental production of lines by encasing extremities in plaster.			
1926	Harris[5]	Reviewed earlier literature on lines, used lines to demonstrate nonexistence of interstitial growth, explained their presence as manifestations of arrested growth, and discussed their formation with reference to vitamins.	1959	Acheson[28]	Suggested that in starvation and illness, withdrawal of growth hormone is primary cause of slowing of cartilage growth.
			1960	Goff[29]	Reviewed previous uses of transverse lines to elucidate relative growth, and gave additional examples of their utility.
1927	Eliot, Souther, and Park[15]	Concluded from histologic studies that transverse lattice formation might be regarded as temporary halting of cartilage growth but with continuation of osteoblastic activity.	1962	Platt and Steward[30]	Produced transverse lines in growing pigs subjected to low-protein diets.
1931	Harris[6]	Presented historical review, case histories and illustrations of various clinical conditions and experimental evidence indicating that transverse stratum first appears as calcification in proliferative zone of cartilage.	1964	Dreizen, Spirakis, and Stone[31]	Indicated in longitudinal study of 679 children that frequency of transverse lines on distal end of radius reached a maximum by 5 years of age and decreased thereafter.
1931	Park, Jackson, and Kajdi[16]	Reported radiopaque bands following lead poisoning and suggested that lead produced more densely packed trabeculae.	1964	Park[3]	Presented summary and review of work by him and his colleagues on formation and distribution of transverse lines and their distinction from bands produced by phosphorus and heavy metals.
1933	Park, Jackson, Goodwin, and Kajdi[17]	Discussed transverse formations in lead poisoning and distinguished these "bands" from transverse lines.	1964	Wells[32]	Showed prevalence of transverse tibial lines in skeletal remains of children and adults.
1933	Harris[18]	Presented essentially a repetition of his earlier article.[6]	1965	Roche[33]	Used transverse lines to demonstrate articular apposition at nonepiphyseal ends of metacarpals.
1938	Sontag[19]	Reported striae in tarsal bones of 1 month old infants, and attributed their presence to shift from prenatal to postnatal environment.	1966	Marshall[34]	Found presence of new transverse lines on radius to be associated with illness and inoculation and discussed their use in paleopathology.
1941	Stammel[20]	Reported two persons with multiple lines and bands on vertebrae, round bones, epiphyses, and phalanges, as well as major long bones and pelvis.	1967	Gahn and Schwager[35]	Showed persistent transverse lines on distal end of tibiae of adults into ninth decade, with decreasing frequency after sixth decade in both sexes.
1941	Siegling[21]	Used radiopaque lines to determine growth loci in epiphyses of long bones.	1967	Gray[36]	Observed radiopaque lines in 30 per cent of 133 Egyptian mummies, and suggested ". . . a general poor state of health during adolescence in ancient Egypt."
1942	Gill and Abbott[22]	Described shifting proportions of relative growth at both ends of tibia and femur between prenatal and postnatal life in child whose mother had been given bismuth during pregnancy.	1968	Gahn, Hempy, and Schwager[37]	Used transverse lines on distal end of tibia in longitudinal series to partition relative contribution of proximal and distal ends of diaphyseal and epiphyseal growth increments.
1945	Caffey[23]	Reported lines in sites of accelerated growth, and doubted that growth retardation is essential to development of these lines.	1968	Cornwell and Littleton[38]	Identified radiopaque lines on tibia as subcortical, reaching from endosteal surface to endosteal surface, as confirmed by transaxial conventional tomograms and bone sections.
1952	Follis and Park[24]	Distinguished between lattice formation, or zones of increased density, and transverse strata, or lines of increased density—the former being primarily a defect in resorptional activity by osteoblasts, whereas in the latter, a cessation of cartilaginous growth is primary.	1968	Schwager[39]	Reported statistically significant, low order associations between episodes of disease and trauma in childhood and appearance of new transverse lines in succeeding period.
			1968	McHenry[40]	Showed high frequency of transverse lines on distal end of femur in prehistoric populations and demonstrated such lines to be manifestations of bony lattice within marrow cavity.

(From Garn SM, Silverman FN, Hertzog KP, Rohmann CG: Med Radiogr Photogr *44*:60, 1968.)

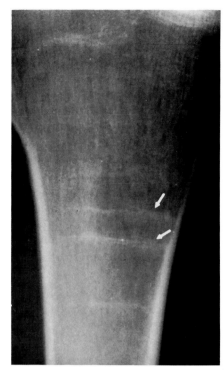

FIGURE 76–1. Transverse or stress lines: Appendicular skeleton. In the proximal tibia, multiple transverse radiodense lines extend almost completely across the medullary cavity (arrows).

or episodes of trauma or infection. The lines also may be related to significant prenatal injury or stress.[151] Although this association between disease or stress and linear radiodense shadows is useful, certain limitations must be recognized[2]: The association is significant but of low order; the disease-line association is highest in the earliest age group (3 to 18 months); and, despite the fact that a new line may be encountered after episodes of trauma or disease, it also may be observed without such an episode.

Anatomically, the transverse bands consist of horizontally oriented trabeculae that cross the medullary cavity partially or completely at right angles to the normal longitudinally directed trabecular structures (Fig. 76–3). Histologically, the bands are composed of thickened, transversely oriented, interconnected trabecular networks, with more typical, longitudinally arranged trabeculae on either side.[122] According to Park,[3, 4] during the initial stage of growth arrest, the osteoblasts form a very thin transverse bony template beneath the zone of proliferative cartilage. With resurgence of growth during the recovery phase, cartilaginous proliferation and increased osteoblastic activity contribute to the thickening and metaphyseal migration of the transverse line, which, at this stage, can be recognized radiographically. Thus, these radiodense areas are not growth arrest lines but are postarrest, poststress, or growth recovery lines.

In most of the investigations related to growth arrest lines, little attention has been given to the mature skeleton and, in fact, the presence of similar radiodense shadows in the adult has been regarded as rare. This is incorrect, as transversely or obliquely oriented radiodense lines regularly are encountered in the tubular bones of adults with osteopenia. These lines, which are termed bone bars or reinforcement lines, are discussed more fully in Chapter 51. They

are especially frequent in the distal portion of the femur and the tibia in persons with long-term osteoporosis, as is seen after neurologic injury, amputation, or prolonged disuse. Although in some cases, bone bars may reflect the unmasking of normal trabeculae or growth recovery lines owing to ongoing, adjacent loss of bone, the fact that they may localize to focal pathologic areas, such as an osteoma or osteochondroma, suggests that bone bars or reinforcement lines relate to trabecular buttressing in response to stress. Furthermore, they are more typical of chronic osteoporosis than of acute bone loss, as in reflex sympathetic dystrophy. Bone bars should be regarded as an adaptive response of chronically weakened bone to normal or abnormal stress, not as a manifestation of growth disturbance.

LEAD POISONING

General Abnormalities

Lead poisoning results from prolonged ingestion of lead-containing materials, such as paint; inhalation of fumes from burning storage batteries or similar substances[41, 123]; or, rarely, absorption of the material from bullets or buckshot that is contained within a serous cavity after a wound.[58–60, 67–73, 138, 139, 153] Lead poisoning also may occur in the fetus of a mother exposed to lead as lead may cross the placenta as early as the twelfth to fourteenth week of gestation.[63] Delayed dental and skeletal development, lead lines, and osteosclerosis may be evident in infants with congenital lead poisoning.

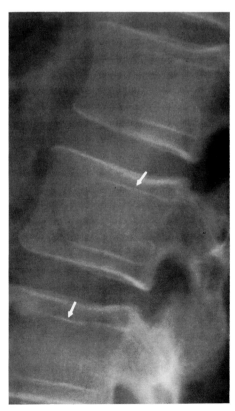

FIGURE 76–2. Transverse or stress lines: Axial skeleton. In multiple vertebral bodies, observe radiodense lines paralleling the superior and inferior osseous margins (arrows), creating a bone-within-bone appearance.

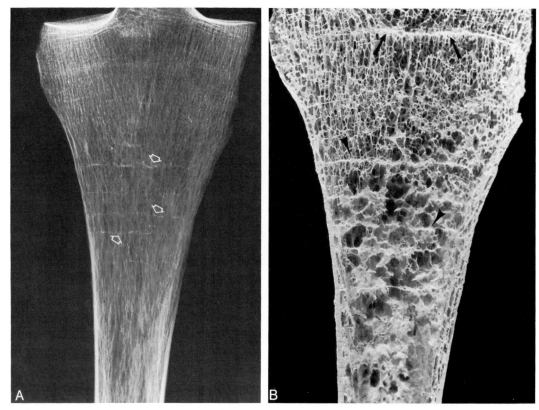

FIGURE 76–3. Transverse growth recovery lines: Anatomic correlation. A radiograph **(A)** and photograph **(B)** of a coronal section of a macerated tibia show multiple wavy radiodense lines (open arrows) representing trabecular bands (arrowheads). They are parallel to the physeal scar (solid arrows).

The onset of symptoms and signs after chronic lead poisoning may be abrupt. Poorly localized, cramping abdominal pain, encephalopathy with convulsions, delirium, coma or death, peripheral neuritis with muscular paralysis, and mild anemia are recognized clinical manifestations of the disorder.[42, 43] Examining the urine for porphyrin is a useful screening test for establishing the diagnosis. Other chemical tests of blood and urine also can be used for diagnostic purposes. It has been suggested that children with reduced serum levels of 1,25-dihydroxyvitamin D may demonstrate increased intestinal absorption of lead.[64]

Musculoskeletal Abnormalities in Infants and Children

Lead poisoning is associated with the appearance of thick transverse radiodense lines in the metaphyses of growing tubular bones.[14, 17, 44] It is suggested that the metaphyseal radiodense lines do not appear until the level of lead in the blood attains a concentration of 70 to 80 μg/dl.[74] Some investigators, however, have found lower concentrations of lead (approximately 50 μg/dl) in the blood of patients with such lines.[132] The pathogenesis and morphology of these lead lines differ from those of the transverse or stress lines of Park or Harris. Although some authors have suggested that the increased radiodensity of the metaphysis in cases of lead poisoning is due to laying down of lead within the cartilaginous matrix (''leadification''),[17] it seems more probable that deposition of calcium is the basis of the transverse lines; even though lead is deposited in the metaphysis,

it is in very minute amounts relative to the content of calcium.[44] Caffey[1] terms the process chondrosclerosis and notes the presence of trabeculae composed of calcified thick cartilaginous cores covered by thin sleeves of endosteal bone almost devoid of osteoblasts. The process may be initiated by oligemia of the metaphyseal segment of the cartilage plate owing to a prolonged decrease in blood flow in the metaphyseal arteries.

The lead lines that almost are invariable in chronic infantile and juvenile plumbism are not an early manifestation of the process and, therefore, are of little diagnostic aid. The radiodense zones are especially prominent in the bones about the knees (Fig. 76–4); identification of density in the proximal fibular metaphysis may be particularly helpful in establishing a radiographic diagnosis of lead poisoning,[132] as similar changes in the distal end of the femur and proximal portion of the tibia can be seen in apparently healthy children. Radiodense lines also can be evident at other sites, particularly in the wrist (Fig. 76–5). Single transverse bands predominate; however, multiple lines may result from several episodes of lead poisoning. Even the axial skeleton may be affected (Fig. 76–6). In both axial and extra-axial sites, the radiodense line, originally appearing in the metaphysis or adjacent to the physis, migrates into the substance of the bone at a rate that varies directly with the velocity of bone growth: in the distal portion of the radius and in the proximal portion of the femur, the rate of migration is 10 mm each year; in the distal portion of the femur, the rate is 22 mm each year; and in the iliac crest, migration of the lines occurs at the rate of 5 mm each year.[74] In the

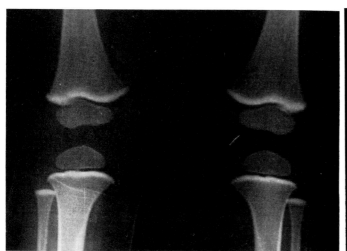

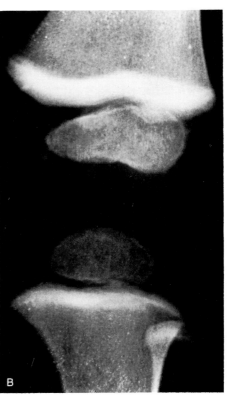

A

FIGURE 76–4. Lead poisoning: Knee.

A In this child, observe the transverse radiodense bands of the metaphyses of femur, tibia, and fibula. (Courtesy of F. Silverman, M.D., Stanford, California.)

B An enlargement of this region in another patient indicates radiodense bands in the metaphyses of the same bones.

B

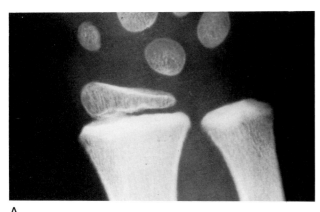

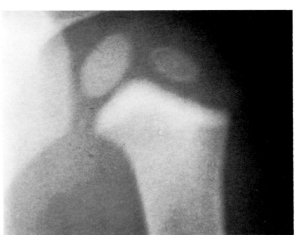

A

FIGURE 76–5. Lead poisoning: Wrist and shoulder. In two different children, radiodense metaphyseal bands are identified in the distal end of the radius and ulna and the proximal portion of the humerus.

B

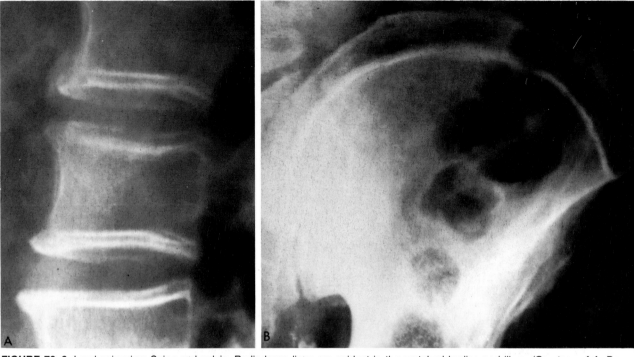

FIGURE 76–6. Lead poisoning: Spine and pelvis. Radiodense lines are evident in the vertebral bodies and ilium. (Courtesy of A. Brower, M.D., Norfolk, Virginia.)

absence of continued lead poisoning, the migrating lead lines decrease in radiodensity and disappear in approximately 4 years.[74]

An additional manifestation of plumbism is failure of normal modeling of the tubular bones, which is most prominent in the femora.[45] Widening of the metaphyses can resemble the changes in Pyle's disease and may persist for months or years before resolving spontaneously.

Lead poisoning can be associated with clinical and radiologic signs of increased intracranial pressure.[46] Mild pleocytosis and an increase in the protein content of the cerebrospinal fluid are frequent, and decompression craniotomy may be required to sustain life.[47] Widening of the cranial sutures, especially the coronal and sagittal sutures, may be evident in as many as 10 per cent of cases of chronic lead poisoning.[48]

Musculoskeletal Abnormalities in Adults

Lead intoxication related to retained lead missiles within the body commonly is overlooked as a diagnostic possibility in patients with protean clinical manifestations, such as anemia, encephalopathy, nephropathy, neuropathy, and abdominal pain. Bullets, shrapnel, and buckshot are potential sources of the lead, and the resulting clinical findings may be intermittent, delayed for as long as 50 years after the injury,[71] and exacerbated in the presence of acidosis, infection, alcoholism, thyrotoxicosis, arthritis, and hyperparathyroidism.[67] As metallic lead is insoluble, lead intoxication is a rare complication of retained lead missiles. The absorption of lead from the missile generally requires that it be located in a cystic cavity, typically a synovium-lined joint. In this regard, previous reports have documented lead poisoning in patients in whom missiles were retained in the hip, knee, ankle, elbow, glenohumeral joint, and small

joints of the hands and feet[67, 68, 73, 153]; in these cases, localized synovial reaction leading to symptoms and signs of arthritis may occur.[72, 76, 124, 136] It is assumed that some factor in the synovial fluid leads to accelerated solution of the lead.[67] Dissolution of lead by synovial fluid has been demonstrated in vivo and in vitro.[58] Such synovial fluid in cases of lead arthropathy is gray and without characteristics of inflammation. Synovial hypertrophy, chronic inflammation and fibrosis, and discrete particles of lead in the synovial membrane and the articular cartilage are the pathologic findings[124] (Fig. 76–7). A radical synovectomy may lead to a decrease in serum levels of lead.[73] In other patients, localized or systemic manifestations are associated with lead missiles that are retained in extra-articular locations, including soft tissues, bursal sacs, pseudarthroses,[140] bones,[67, 71] and spinal tissues.[69, 70, 152] In some of these instances, multiple pellet gunshot wounds had been sustained, suggesting that the large surface area of the numerous pellets may have been an important factor in the subsequent lead absorption.[73, 133] Pathologically, encapsulation with fibrous or hypovascular tissue is observed about lead fragments in soft tissue or osseous sites.

Radiographic evidence of dissolution of lead missiles is provided by progressive fragmentation, enlargement, and migration of the radiodense foci (Fig. 76–8), which, in a joint, can lead to initial findings resembling a lead arthrogram (plumbogram)[73, 77, 78] that subsequently disappear.[76] In the vertebral column, enlarging radiodense areas in the spinal canal,[70] intervertebral disc,[69] and adjacent connective tissues[69] may be accompanied by osseous and cartilaginous destruction (Fig. 76–9).

Saturnine gout also is termed the "moonshine malady"[49] because of the appearance of the condition in moonshiners whose home-brewed liquor contained an appreciable quantity of lead.[50, 51] Saturnine gout appears to be an expression

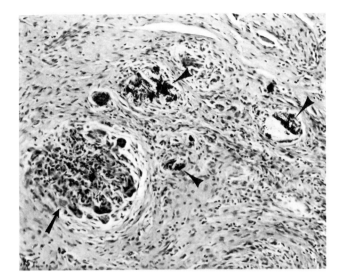

FIGURE 76–7. Lead poisoning: Retained lead missile. Histologic abnormalities that may accompany retained intra-articular bullets include hyperplasia of the synovial membrane, an inflammatory response that is focally granulomatous (arrow), and deposition of lead in the synovium (arrowheads). (Hematoxylin and eosin stain, 200×.) (From Sclafani SJA, et al: Radiology *156*:299, 1985.)

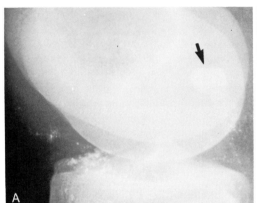
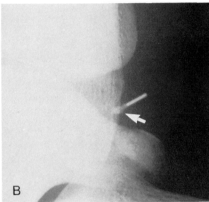

FIGURE 76–8. Lead poisoning: Radiographic abnormalities.

A In this 23 year old man, observe fragmentation of a missile (arrow), with opaque fragments present in the knee joint.

B In a 37 year old man with ankle pain, dissolution (arrow) of the tip of a needle that had been present for several years is seen. An arthrogram (not shown) confirmed that only the needle tip was present in the joint.

FIGURE 76–9. Lead poisoning: Retained lead missile. Systemic symptoms were associated with resorption of a lead bullet in the paraspinal region. Note the central radiodense bullet and the surrounding fragments. Paraspinal soft tissue swelling is seen.

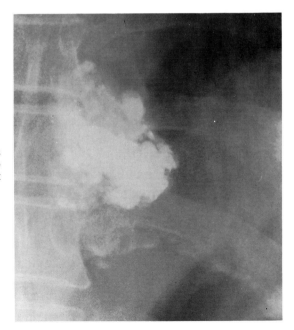

of renal injury from lead in which a tubular defect leading to uric acid retention becomes evident.

Differential Diagnosis

Radiodense lines in the metaphyses of tubular bones can be seen as a normal variant,[1] as an indication of previous stress, in heavy metal poisoning, including lead poisoning, and in the healing stages of leukemia, rickets, and scurvy (Table 76–2).[75] Similar findings may accompany hypothyroidism, hypervitaminosis D, and transplacental infections (rubella, cytomegalic inclusion disease, herpes simplex, toxoplasmosis, and syphilis). Metaphyseal flaring or widening is seen not only in lead poisoning but also in various anemias (sickle cell anemia, thalassemia), storage disorders (Gaucher's disease, Niemann-Pick disease), and congenital syndromes (Pyle's disease, multiple familial exostoses, osteopetrosis, Ollier's disease), and as a normal variant.

PHOSPHORUS POISONING

Phosphorus poisoning had previously been seen in rachitic and tuberculous children who were being treated with phosphorized cod liver oil,[52, 53] although it rarely is encountered today. It may be reproduced experimentally by feeding metallic (yellow) phosphorus to growing rats. Single or multiple deep bands of increased radiodensity are produced in the ends of growing tubular bones and within flat or irregular bones and persist for many years. The phosphorus shadow is caused by numerous and closely packed trabeculae that are composed of solid bone or small central cartilaginous cores surrounded by heavy sleeves of endosteal bone containing many osteoblasts.[1] Caffey indicates that the process is an osteosclerosis that differs from the chondrosclerosis that is evident in lead (or bismuth) poisoning and concludes that the lines result from chronic hyperemia in the metaphyseal side of the cartilaginous growth plate caused by excessive blood flow in terminal metaphyseal vessels.

BISMUTH POISONING

In the pregnant woman with syphilis, injected bismuth may cross the placenta and enter the fetal circulation to be deposited in the skeleton.[54–56] Single or multiple radiodense bands or lines in the metaphyses of the tubular bones in cases of bismuth poisoning share radiographic and morphologic characteristics with those that appear in cases of lead poisoning.[57] The radiographic findings may resemble syphilitic osteochondritis, and differentiation of this condition from bismuth poisoning in the fetus of a syphilitic mother

TABLE 76–2. Some Causes of Radiodense Metaphyseal Lines

Stress lines of Park or Harris
Heavy metal poisoning
Leukemia
Rickets
Scurvy
Hypothyroidism
Hypoparathyroidism
Hypervitaminoses
Transplacental infections

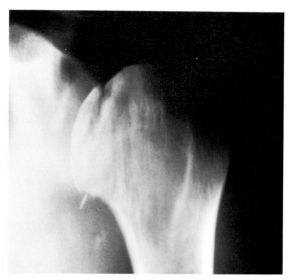

FIGURE 76–10. Bismuth poisoning: Ischemic necrosis of bone. This 68 year old woman, who had been taking bismuth nitrate for constipation, developed encephalopathy with myoclonic movements. Elevated levels of bismuth were found in the blood. Observe ischemic necrosis involving the humeral head with osseous fragmentation. (Courtesy of J. P. Mabille, M.D., Dijon, France.)

who has received bismuth during pregnancy can be difficult.[1] In adults, radiographic abnormalities simulating those of osteonecrosis have been described in cases of bismuth poisoning (Fig. 76–10).[65, 79] It is not clear if ischemic necrosis of bone represents a direct effect of bismuth on bone, a complication of myoclonic movements owing to encephalopathy, or an incidental finding.

ALUMINUM TOXICITY

The oral or parenteral administration of aluminum compounds may lead to its deposition in the body's tissues and, in some sites—such as the brain and bones—to toxic effects.[84] This situation can arise in nonuremic adults, some of whom have peptic ulcer disease, who are ingesting large amounts of aluminum carbonate[80, 141]; in uremic patients who ingest aluminum salts as phosphate binders and whose renal clearance of aluminum is reduced or who are undergoing hemodialysis in which the tap water is contaminated or in which aluminum hydroxide is present in the Redy sorbent cartridge[81, 82, 142, 143]; and in patients who have lost small bowel function and are maintained on chronic total parenteral nutrition.[83]

The toxic effects of aluminum on the brain and bone have been well studied in patients with chronic renal failure who are maintained on regular hemodialysis or, rarely, peritoneal dialysis (Chapter 57). Accumulation of aluminum in the lysosomes of cerebral tissue appears to play a major role in dialysis encephalopathy, a syndrome consisting of dementia, speech disorder, seizures, and dyspraxia.[85–91] Furthermore, bone toxicity, manifested clinically as pain, tenderness, and deformity, is accompanied by the accumulation of aluminum in osseous tissue[92, 93, 125, 144]; similar accumulation within joints, indicating that aluminum is able to cross the synovial barrier, suggests a potential role for this element in the articular manifestations of hemodialyzed patients, a concept supported by the known articular toxicity of aluminum compounds in animals.[94]

Osteopenia (related to osteomalacia), Looser's zones (insufficiency fractures), and complete fractures affecting the ribs, spine, and tubular bones are the principal radiographic manifestations of aluminum-induced osteopathy.[90, 93, 95–98, 134, 137] Periosteal new bone in the shafts of the tibiae and fibulae and in the pelvis also has been observed.[126] In children, rickets-like metaphyseal abnormalities appear.[127, 144] Although subperiosteal resorption of bone has been described in some patients,[98] this finding may be subtle or entirely absent. Histologic analysis documents the presence of excessive amounts of lamellar osteoid and the deposition of aluminum mainly at the interface between mineralized bone and excessive osteoid.[96–98] This observation strongly supports a primary role of aluminum in causing the osseous abnormalities; indirect evidence for this role includes a high frequency of osteopathy when the dialysate or ambient water contains elevated concentrations of aluminum,[129] an association of this osteopathy with aluminum-induced encephalopathy and myopathy, a response of the bone changes to chelating agents,[95, 98, 99] and the reversal of the abnormalities after the removal of sources of aluminum contamination.[90, 127]

The mechanism by which aluminum alters mineralization of bone is not known. In experimental situations, aluminum accumulation has been observed in the tissues of both normal and uremic rats receiving intraperitoneal aluminum chloride; however, aluminum-induced osteomalacia was documented only in the uremic group of animals, suggesting that aluminum is deposited differently in uremic bones as a result of either quantitative or qualitative changes in the osteoid tissue or a hyperparathyroid state.[84] The relationship of aluminum osteopathy and parathyroid function is not clear; some investigators have found a positive correlation between serum levels of parathyroid hormone and aluminum,[100] whereas others believe that aluminum toxicity occurs independently of hyperparathyroidism.[101] In fact, parathyroid hormone levels in the serum in some of the patients with aluminum-induced bone changes have been reported as low or even undetectable,[83, 103] and a functional hypoparathyroidism may exist that is related to the toxic effects of aluminum in the parathyroid glands.[83] Some authors believe that elevated parathyroid hormone levels offer protection against the toxic effects of aluminum.[104] Aluminum also may interfere with the orderly deposition of bone by forming insoluble complexes with phosphates and by inhibiting the precipitation of calcium apatite.[93] Furthermore, in vitro investigations have documented that aluminum inhibits the production of inorganic pyrophosphatase, and it may displace calcium from protein-binding sites.[102]

Although overwhelming evidence exists supporting a toxic role of aluminum in the osteomalacia associated with hemodialysis (as well as peritoneal dialysis and chronic parenteral nutrition), elevated levels of bone aluminum have been observed in dialysis patients who do not have osteomalacia.[104] Such inconsistencies may be explained by the variability of osseous sites of aluminum deposition, which have included the mineralization front, the cement lines of mineralized bone, and areas about the osteocytes; in some locations, this deposition may be unaccompanied by an interference with bone mineralization.[104] Furthermore, in some investigations, intraosseous deposition of aluminum produces an osteopathy that is characterized by decreased osteoid production and not by the classic histologic picture of osteomalacia.[128]

POISONING FROM OTHER METALS

In experimental and in clinical situations, other heavy metals, such as radium, gold, mercury, magnesium, and silver, may lead to metaphyseal changes.[1, 149, 150] In addition, metallic mercury emboli in arterial and venous circulation can appear after blood sampling using mercury-sealed syringes and after accidents or suicide attempts and can lead to mercurialism, mercury abscesses, and local ischemia.[61–62, 66, 130, 145] Synovial inflammation with an effusion can follow mercury contamination of a joint.[105]

COPPER DEFICIENCY

In 1953, Baxter and collaborators[106, 107] described a skeletal disorder observed in puppies that were fed a diet low in copper. The bone changes, which resembled scurvy, consisted of osteopenia, fractures, and epiphyseal displacements and healed completely when supplements of copper were included in the animals' food. A human disorder associated with hypocupremia subsequently was reported in infants who are malnourished,[108–110] those receiving long-term parenteral nutrition,[111–114, 116] or those who were born prematurely and are maintained on diets low in copper.[113, 115] Radiographic findings include osteopenia, metaphyseal radiodense lines and spurs, fractures, and physeal disruptions with malalignment of the epiphysis and metaphysis. Periostitis, which may become profound, also is observed. Reversal of the osseous abnormalities occurs when copper supplementation is employed.

Menkes' syndrome (kinky hair syndrome) is an inherited disorder, with an X-linked pattern of transmission, that relates to a defect in copper absorption from the gut.[117–119, 146] Obliteration or tortuosity of arteries occurs in the brain and in other tissues.[131] Radiographic findings are similar to those in nutritional copper deficiency, consisting of osteopenia, flaring of the ends of the tubular bones, metaphyseal cupping and irregularity, and osseous spurs. The changes resemble those of rickets and the abused child syndrome. The early introduction of copper supplementation may improve the prognosis of this syndrome.

ZINC DEFICIENCY

As zinc, along with other heavy metals, appears to be essential for normal bone metabolism, its deficiency probably leads to osteoporosis and growth disturbances as well as anemia and hepatosplenomegaly.[120, 121] Analysis of the precise effects of zinc deficiency is difficult, owing to the presence of other deficiencies as well.[116]

DEFICIENCIES OF OTHER TRACE ELEMENTS

Direct evidence supporting the nutritional consequences of deficiencies of such trace elements as chromium, cobalt, molybdenum, and manganese is difficult to obtain, although symptoms, signs, and serologic abnormalities related to such deficiencies may be observed experimentally in animals.[135, 147] Magnesium deficiency leads to tetany, similar to that associated with hypocalcemia. It also is accompanied by abnormal patterns of formation of bone mineral[148] and calcium pyrophosphate dihydrate crystal deposition (see Chapter 44).

SUMMARY

In some cases of heavy metal poisoning, radiodense lines or bands may appear in the metaphyses of tubular bones and within flat or irregular bones. The resulting radiographic findings, which are observed most characteristically in lead, phosphorus, and bismuth poisoning, must be differentiated from normal variants, stress lines of Park or Harris, and changes in various metabolic, endocrine, and infectious disorders. Significant radiographic abnormalities also are observed in the aluminum accumulation that accompanies dialysis, in nutritional or inherited deficiencies of copper, and, possibly, in deficiencies of other trace elements as well.

References

1. Caffey J: Pediatric X-Ray Diagnosis. 7th Ed. Chicago, Year Book Medical Publishers, 1978, p 1125.
2. Garn SM, Silverman FN, Hertzog KP, et al: Lines and bands of increased density. Their implication to growth and development. Med Radiogr Photogr 44:58, 1968.
3. Park EA: The imprinting of nutritional disturbances on the growing bone. Pediatrics 33:815, 1964.
4. Park EA, Richter CP: Transverse lines in bone: The mechanism of their development. Bull Johns Hopkins Hosp 93:234, 1953.
5. Harris HA: The growth of the long bones in childhood with special reference to certain bony striations of the metaphysis and to the role of the vitamins. Arch Intern Med 38:785, 1926.
6. Harris HA: Lines of arrested growth in the long bones in childhood. Correlation of histological and radiographic appearances in clinical and experimental conditions. Br J Radiol 4:561, 622, 1931.
7. Schwager PM: The frequency of appearance of transverse lines in the tibia in relation to chronic illnesses. Am J Phys Anthropol 29:130, 1968.
8. Wegener G: Ueber das normale and pathologische Wachstum der Rohrenknochen. Eine dritische Untersuchung auf experimenteller und casiustischer Grundlage. Arch Pathol Anat 61:44, 1874.
9. Gies T: Experimentelle Untersuchungen über den Einfluss des Arsens auf den Organismus. Arch Exp Pathol Pharmakol 8:175, 1877.
10. Ludloff K: Ueber Wachstum und Architektur der unteren Femurepiphyse und oberen tibiaepiphyse. Ein beitrag zur Röntgendiagnostik. Bruns Beitr Klin Chir 38:64, 1903.
11. Lehndorff H: Zur kenntniss des Morbus Barlow. Röntgenbefund Arch Kinderheilk 38:161, 1904.
12. Phemister DB: The effect of phosphorus on growing, normal and diseased bones. JAMA 70:1737, 1918.
13. Stettner E: Uber die Beziehungen der Ossifikation des Handskeletts zu Alter und Langenwachstum bei gesunden und kranken Kindern von der Geburt bis zur Pubertat. Arch Kinderheilk 68:342, 439, 1920; 69:27, 1921.
14. Asada T: Uber die Entstehung und pathologische Bedeutung der im Röntgenbild des Rohrenknochens am diaphysaende zum vorschein kommenden parallelen Querlinienbildung. Mitt Med Fak Univ Kyushu Fukuoka 9:43, 1924.
15. Eliot MM, Souther SP, Park EA: Transverse lines in x-ray plates of the long bones of children. Bull Johns Hopkins Hosp 41:364, 1927.
16. Park EA, Jackson D, Kajdi L: Shadows produced by lead in x-ray pictures of growing skeleton. Am J Dis Child 41:485, 1931.
17. Park EA, Jackson D, Goodwin TC, et al: X-ray shadows in growing bones produced by lead; their characteristics, cause, anatomical counterpart in bone and differentiation. J Pediatr 3:265, 1933.
18. Harris HA: Bone Growth in Health and Disease: The Biological Principles Underlying the Clinical, Radiological and Histological Diagnosis of Perversions of Growth and Disease in the Skeleton. London, Oxford University Press, 1933, p 3.
19. Sontag LW: Evidences of disturbed prenatal and neonatal growth in bones of infants aged one month. Am J Dis Child 55:1248, 1938.
20. Stammel CA: Multiple striae parallel to epiphyses and ring shadows around bone growth centers. AJR 46:497, 1941.
21. Siegling JA: Growth of epiphyses. J Bone Joint Surg 23:23, 1941.
22. Gill GG, Abbott LRC: A practical method of predicting the growth of the femur and tibia in the child. Arch Surg 45:286, 1942.
23. Caffey J: Pediatric X-ray Diagnosis. A Textbook for Students and Practitioners of Pediatrics, Surgery & Radiology. Chicago, Year Book Medical Publishers, 1945, p 597.
24. Follis RH Jr, Park EA: Some observations on bone growth with particular respect to zones and transverse lines of increased density in the metaphysis. AJR 68:709, 1952.
25. Hewitt D, Westropp CK, Acheson RM: Oxford child health survey: Effect of childish ailments on skeletal development. Br J Prev Soc Med 9:179, 1955.
26. Jones PRM, Dean RFA: The effects of kwashiorkor on the development of the bones of the hand. J Trop Pediatr 2:51, 1956.
27. Dreizen S, Currie C, Gilley EJ, et al: Observations on the association between nutritive failure, skeletal maturation rate and radiopaque transverse lines in the distal end of the radius in children. AJR 76:482, 1956.
28. Acheson RM: Effects of starvation, septicaemia, and chronic illness on the growth cartilage plate and metaphysis of the immature rat. J Anat 93:123, 1959.
29. Goff CW: Surgical Treatment of Unequal Extremities. Publication 418, American Lecture Series, Monograph in the Bannerstone Division of American Lectures in Orthopaedic Surgery. Springfield, Ill, Charles C Thomas, 1960, p 3.
30. Platt BS, Steward RJC: Transverse trabeculae and osteoporosis in bones in experimental protein-calorie deficiency. Br J Nutr 16:483, 1962.
31. Dreizen S, Spirakis CN, Stone RE: The influence of age and nutritional status on "bone scar" formation in the distal end of the growing radius. Am J Phys Anthropol 22:295, 1964.
32. Wells C: Les lignes de Harris et les maladies anciennes. Scalpel 117:665, 1964.
33. Roche AF: The sites of elongation of human metacarpals and metatarsals. Acta Anat 61:193, 1965.
34. Marshall WA: Problems in relating radiopaque transverse lines in the radius to the occurrence of disease. Symp Soc Hum Biol 8:245, 1966.
35. Garn SM, Schwager PM: Age dynamics of persistent transverse lines in the tibia. Am J Phys Anthropol 27:375, 1967.
36. Gray PHK: Radiography of ancient Egyptian mummies. Med Radiogr Photogr 43:34, 1967.
37. Garn SM, Hempy HO III, Schwager PM: Measurement of localized bone growth employing natural markers. Am J Phys Anthropol 28:105, 1968.
38. Cornwell WS, Littleton JT: An investigation of transverse lines by axial tomography (Abstr). Am J Phys Anthropol 29:130, 1968.
39. Schwager PM: The frequency of appearance of transverse lines in the tibia in relation to childhood illnesses (Abstr). Am J Phys Anthropol 29:130, 1968.
40. McHenry H: Transverse lines in long bones of prehistoric California Indians. Am J Phys Anthropol 29:1, 1968.
41. Browder AA, Joselow MM, Louria DB: The problem of lead poisoning. Medicine 52:121, 1973.
42. Jones RR: Symptoms in early stages of industrial plumbism. JAMA 104:195, 1935.
43. Aub JC, Fairhall LT, Minot AS, et al: Lead poisoning. Medicine 4:1, 1925.
44. Leone AJ Jr: On lead lines. AJR 103:165, 1968.
45. Pease CN, Newton GG: Metaphyseal dysplasia due to lead poisoning in children. Radiology 79:233, 1962.
46. Greengard J: Lead poisoning in childhood: Signs, symptoms, current therapy, clinical expression. Clin Pediatr 5:269, 1966.
47. McLaurin RL, Nichols JB Jr: Extensive cranial decompression in the treatment of severe lead encephalopathy. Pediatrics 20:653, 1957.
48. Freeman R: Chronic lead poisoning in children; a review of 90 children diagnosed in Sydney 1948–1967. Med J Aust 1:640, 1970.
49. Klinenberg JR: Saturnine gout—a moonshine malady. N Engl J Med 280:1238, 1969.
50. Emmerson BT: The clinical differentiation of lead gout from primary gout. Arthritis Rheum 11:623, 1968.
51. Ball GV, Sorensen LB: Pathogenesis of hyperuricemia in saturnine gout. N Engl J Med 280:1199, 1969.
52. Hess AE, Weinstock M: The value of elementary phosphorus in rickets. Am J Dis Child 32:483, 1926.
53. Phemister BD: The effect of phosphorus in growing normal and diseased bone. JAMA 70:1737, 1918.
54. Heyman A: Systemic manifestations of bismuth toxicity; observations on 4 patients with pre-existent kidney disease. Am J Syph Gonorr Vener Dis 28:721, 1944.
55. Caffey J: Changes in the growing skeleton after the administration of bismuth. Am J Dis Child 53:56, 1937.
56. Whitridge J Jr: Changes in the long bones of newborn infants following the administration of bismuth during pregnancy. Am J Syph Gonorr Vener Dis 24:223, 1940.
57. Russin LA, Stadler HE, Jeans PC: The bismuth lines in the long bones in relation to linear growth. J Pediatr 21:211, 1942.
58. Leonard MH: The solution of lead of synovial fluid. Clin Orthop 64:255, 1969.
59. Switz DM, Elmorshidy ME, Deyerle WM: Bullets, joints, and lead intoxication. A remarkable and instructive case. Arch Intern Med 136:939, 1976.
60. Windler EC, Smith RB, Bryan WJ, et al: Lead intoxication and traumatic arthritis of the hip secondary to retained bullet fragments. A case report. J Bone Joint Surg [Am] 60:254, 1978.
61. Buxton JT Jr, Hewett JC, Gadsden RH, et al: Metallic mercury embolism. JAMA 193:573, 1965.
62. Naidich TP, Bartelt D, Wheeler PS, et al: Metallic mercury emboli. AJR 117:886, 1973.
63. Pearl M, Boxt LM: Radiographic findings in congenital lead poisoning. Radiology 136:83, 1980.

64. Rosen JF, Chesney RW, Hamstra A, et al: Reduction in 1,25-dihydroxyvitamin D in children with increased lead absorption. N Engl J Med *302*:1128, 1980.

65. Gaucher A, Netter P, Faure G, et al: Les ostéoarthropathies "bismuthiques." Intérêt du dosage du bismuth osseux. Rev Rhum Mal Osteoartic *47*:31, 1980.

66. Krohn IT, Solof A, Mobini J, et al: Subcutaneous injection of metallic mercury. JAMA *243*:548, 1980.

67. Linden MA, Manton WI, Stewart RM, et al: Lead poisoning from retained bullets. Pathogenesis, diagnosis, and management. Ann Surg *195*:305, 1982.

68. Beazley WC, Rosenthal RE: Lead intoxication 18 months after a gunshot wound. Clin Orthop *190*:199, 1984.

69. Grogan DP, Bucholz RW: Acute lead intoxication from a bullet in an intervertebral disc space. A case report. J Bone Joint Surg [Am] *63*:1180, 1981.

70. Saniforth P, Watt I: Extradural "plumboma." A rare cause of acquired spinal stenosis. Br J Radiol *55*:772, 1982.

71. DiMaio VJM, Garriott JC, DiMaio SM, et al: A fatal case of lead poisoning due to a retained bullet. Am J Forensic Med Pathol *4*:165, 1983.

72. Primm DD Jr: Lead arthropathy—progressive destruction of a joint by a retained bullet. Case report. J Bone Joint Surg [Am] *66*:292, 1984.

73. Roberts RD, Wong SW, Theil GB: An unusual case of lead arthropathy. Arthritis Rheum *26*:1048, 1983.

74. Sachs HK: The evolution of the radiologic lead line. Radiology *139*:81, 1981.

75. Frager DH, Subbarao K: The "bone within a bone." JAMA *249*:77, 1983.

76. Weston WJ: The vanishing lead arthrogram—plumbography. Aust Radiol *24*:80, 1980.

77. Weston WJ: The lead arthrogram—plumbography. Skel Radiol *2*:169, 1978.

78. Sentura HR: The roentgen findings in increased lead absorption due to retained projectiles. AJR *47*:381, 1942.

79. Mabille JP, Gaudet M, Charpin JF: Ostéonécrose de la tête humérale au cours de l'encéphalopathie bismuthique. Ann Radiol *23*:515, 1980.

80. Recker RR, Blotcky AJ, Leffler JA, et al: Evidence for aluminum absorption from the gastrointestinal tract and bone deposition by aluminum carbonate ingestion with normal renal function. J Lab Clin Med *90*:810, 1977.

81. Parkinson IS, Ward MK, Feest TG, et al: Fracturing dialysis osteodystrophy and dialysis encephalopathy. Lancet *1*:406, 1979.

82. Pierides AM, Frohnert PP: Aluminum related dialysis osteomalacia and dementia after prolonged use of Redy cartridge. Trans Am Soc Artif Intern Organs *27*:629, 1981.

83. Ott SM, Maloney NA, Klein GL, et al: Aluminum is associated with low bone formation in patients receiving chronic parenteral nutrition. Ann Intern Med *98*:910, 1983.

84. Chan Y-L, Alfrey AC, Posen S, et al: Effect of aluminum on normal and uremic rats: Tissue distribution, vitamin D metabolites, and quantitative bone histology. Calif Tissue Int *35*:344, 1983.

85. Alfrey AC: Dialysis encephalopathy syndrome. Ann Rev Med *29*:93, 1978.

86. Lederman RJ, Henry CE: Progressive dialysis encephalopathy. Ann Neurol *4*:199, 1978.

87. Alfrey AC, LeGendre GR, Kaehny WD: The dialysis encephalopathy syndrome: Possible aluminum intoxication. N Engl J Med *294*:184, 1976.

88. McDermott JR, Smith AI, Ward MK, et al: Brain-aluminum concentration in dialysis encephalopathy. Lancet *1*:901, 1978.

89. Rozas VV, Port FK, Rutt WM: Progressive dialysis encephalopathy from dialysate aluminum. Arch Intern Med *138*:1375, 1978.

90. Prior JC, Cameron EC, Knickerbocker WJ, et al: Dialysis encephalopathy and osteomalacic bone disease. A case-controlled study. Am J Med *72*:33, 1982.

91. Bertholf RL, Roman JM, Brown S, et al: Aluminum hydroxide-induced osteomalacia, encephalopathy and hyperaluminemia in CAPD. Treatment with desferrioxamine. Perit Dialys Bull, Jan-Mar 1984, p 30.

92. Ellis HA, McCarty JH, Herrington J: Bone aluminum in haemodialysed patients and in rats injected with aluminum chloride: Relationship to impaired bone mineralization. J Clin Pathol *32*:832, 1979.

93. Walker GS, Aaron JE, Peacock M, et al: Dialysate aluminum concentration and renal bone disease. Kidney Int *21*:411, 1983.

94. Netter P, Kessler M, Burnel D, et al: Aluminum in the joint tissues of chronic renal failure patients treated with regular hemodialysis and aluminum compounds. J Rheumatol *11*:66, 1984.

95. Sebes JI, Pinstein ML, Massie JD, et al: Radiographic manifestations of aluminum-induced bone disease. AJR *142*:424, 1984.

96. Llewellyn CH, Resnik CS, Brower AC: Case report 288. Skel Radiol *12*:223, 1984.

97. Skinner HB, Harris JR, Cook SD, et al: Bilateral sequential tibial and fibular fatigue fractures associated with aluminum intoxication osteomalacia. A case report. J Bone Joint Surg [Am] *65*:843, 1983.

98. Xipell JM, Ham KN, Brown DJ, et al: Case report 294. Skel Radiol *12*:298, 1984.

99. Brown DJ, Dawborn JK, Ham KN, et al: Treatment of dialysis osteomalacia with desferrioxamine. Lancet *2*:343, 1982.

100. Mayor GH, Keiser JA, Makdani D, et al: Aluminum absorption and distribution: Effect of parathyroid hormone. Science *197*:1187, 1977.

101. Hodsman AB, Sherrard DJ, Wong EGC, et al: Vitamin-D–resistant osteomalacia in hemodialysis patients lacking secondary hyperparathyroidism. Ann Intern Med *94*:629, 1981.

102. Ihle B, Buchanan M, Stevens B, et al: Aluminum-associated bone disease: Clinico-pathologic correlation. Am J Kidney Dis *2*:255, 1982.

103. Cannata JB, Briggs JD, Junior BJR, et al: Effect of acute aluminum overload on calcium and parathyroid-hormone metabolism. Lancet *1*:501, 1983.

104. McCarthy JT, Kurtz SB, McCall JT: Elevated bone aluminum content in dialysis patients without osteomalacia. Mayo Clin Proc *60*:315, 1985.

105. Theodorou SD, Vlachos P, Vamvasakis E: Knee joint injury by mercury from a broken thermometer. Case report and review of the literature. Clin Orthop *160*:159, 1981.

106. Baxter JH, Van Wyk JJ: A bone disorder associated with copper deficiency. I. Gross morphological, roentgenological and chemical observations. Bull Johns Hopkins Hosp *93*:1, 1953.

107. Baxter JH, Van Wyk JJ, Follis RH Jr: A bone disorder associated with copper deficiency. II. Histological and chemical studies on the bones. Bull Johns Hopkins Hosp *93*:25, 1953.

108. Sturgeon P, Brubacker C: Copper deficiency in infants. A syndrome characterized by hypocupremia, iron deficiency anemia and hypoproteinemia. Am J Dis Child *92*:254, 1956.

109. Ashkenazai A, Levin S, Djaldetti M, et al: The syndrome of neonatal copper deficiency. Pediatrics *52*:525, 1971.

110. Cordano A, Baertl JM, Graham GG: Copper deficiency in infancy. Pediatrics *34*:324, 1964.

111. Karpel JT, Peden VH: Copper deficiency in long term parenteral nutrition. J Pediatr *80*:32, 1972.

112. Heller RM, Kirchner SG, O'Neil JA, et al: Skeletal changes of copper deficiency in infants receiving prolonged total parenteral nutrition. J Pediatr *92*:947, 1978.

113. Levy J, Berdon WE, Abramson SJ: Epiphyseal separation simulating pyarthrosis, secondary to copper deficiency in an infant receiving total parenteral nutrition. Br J Radiol *57*:636, 1984.

114. Allen TM, Manoli A II, LaMont RL: Skeletal changes associated with copper deficiency. Clin Orthop *168*:206, 1982.

115. Griscom NT, Craig NJ, Neuhauser EBD: Systemic bone disease developing in small premature infants. Pediatrics *48*:883, 1971.

116. McGill LC, Boas RN, Zerella JT: Extremity swelling in an infant with copper and zinc deficiency. J Pediatr Surg *15*:746, 1980.

117. Danks DM, Campbell PE, Stevens BJ, et al: Menkes' kinky hair syndrome. An inherited defect in copper absorption with widespread effects. Pediatrics *50*:188, 1972.

118. Wesenberg RL, Gwinn JL, Barnes GR Jr: Radiological findings in the kinky hair syndrome. Radiology *92*:500, 1969.

119. Adams PC, Strand RD, Bresnan MJ, et al: Kinky hair syndrome: Serial study of radiological findings with emphasis on the similarity to the battered child syndrome. Radiology *112*:401, 1974.

120. Castro-Magana M, Collipp PJ, Chen S-Y, et al: Zinc nutritional status, androgens, and growth retardation. Am J Dis Child *135*:322, 1981.

121. Gordon EF, Gordon RC, Passal DB: Zinc metabolism: Basic, clinical, and behavioral aspects. J Pediatr *99*:341, 1981.

122. Ogden JA: Growth slowdown and arrest lines. J Pediatr Orthop *4*:409, 1984.

123. Christoffersson JO, Schutz A, Ahlgren L, et al: Lead in finger-bone analysed in vivo in active and retired lead workers. Am J Ind Med *6*:447, 1984.

124. Sclafani SJA, Vuletin JC, Twersky J: Lead arthropathy: Arthritis caused by retained intra-articular bullets. Radiology *156*:299, 1985.

125. Charhon SA, Chavassieux PM, Meunier PJ, et al: Serum aluminum concentration and aluminum deposits in bone in patients receiving haemodialysis. Br Med J *290*:1613, 1985.

126. Chambers SE, Winney RJ: Periosteal new bone in patients on intermittent haemodialysis: An early indicator of aluminum-induced osteomalacia? Clin Radiol *36*:163, 1985.

127. Andreoli SP, Smith JA, Bergstein JM: Aluminum bone disease in children: Radiographic features from diagnosis to resolution. Radiology *156*:663, 1985.

128. de Vernejoul MC, Belenguer R, Halkidou H, et al: Histomorphometric evidence of deleterious effect of aluminum on osteoblasts. Bone *6*:15, 1985.

129. Chan Y-L, Furlong J, Cornish CJ, et al: Dialysis osteodystrophy. A study involving 94 patients. Medicine *64*:296, 1985.

130. Cassar-Pullicino VN, Taylor DN, Fitz-Patrick JD: Multiple metallic mercury emboli. Br J Radiol *58*:470, 1985.

131. Farrelly C, Stringer DA, Daneman A, et al: CT manifestations of Menkes' kinky hair syndrome (trichopoliodystrophy). J Can Assoc Radiol *35*:406, 1984.

132. Blickman JG, Wilkinson RH, Graef JW: The radiologic "lead band" revisited. AJR *146*:245, 1986.

133. Selbst SM, Henretig F, Fee MA, et al: Lead poisoning in a child with gunshot wound. Pediatrics *77*:413, 1986.

134. Garrett P, McWade M, O'Callaghan J: Radiological assessment of aluminum-related bone disease. Clin Radiol *37*:63, 1986.

135. Strause LG, Hegenauer J, Saltman P, et al: Effects of long-term dietary manganese and copper deficiency on rat skeleton. J Nutr *116*:135, 1986.

136. Viegas SF, Calhoun JH: Lead poisoning from a gunshot wound to the hand. J Hand Surg [Am] *11*:729, 1986.

137. Williams JW, Vera SR, Peters, TG, et al: Biliary excretion of aluminum in aluminum osteodystrophy with liver disease. Ann Intern Med *104*:782, 1986.

138. Hollerman JJ, Fackler ML, Coldwell DM, et al: Gunshot wounds: 1. Bullets, ballistics, and mechanisms of injury. AJR *155*:685, 1990.

139. Hollerman JJ, Fackler ML, Coldwell DM, et al: Gunshot wounds: 2. Radiology. AJR *155*:691, 1990.

140. Jensen SP, Richardson ML, Conrad EU, et al: Case report 608. Skel Radiol *19*:233, 1990.

141. Neumann L, Jensen BG: Osteomalacia from Al and Mg antacids. Report of a case of bilateral hip fracture. Acta Orthop Scand *60*:361, 1989.

142. Kassner EG: Dry-related complications in infants and children: Imaging features. AJR *157*:1039, 1991.

143. Kriegshauser JS, Swee RG, McCarthy JT, et al: Aluminum toxicity in patients undergoing dialysis: Radiographic findings and prediction of bone biopsy results. Radiology *164*:399, 1987.

144. Hernandez RJ, Sedman AB, Smid DM, et al: Radiographic manifestations of experimental aluminum toxicity in growing bone. Skel Radiol *16*:209, 1987.

145. Spizarny DL, Renzi P: Metallic mercury pulmonary emboli. J Can Assoc Radiol *38*:60, 1987.

146. Gerdes A-M, Tonnesen T, Pergament E, et al: Variability in clinical expression of Menkes syndrome. Eur J Pediatr *148*:132, 1988.

147. Svensson O, Engfeldt B, Reinholt FP, et al: Manganese rickets. A biochemical and stereologic study with special reference to the effect of phosphate. Clin Orthop *218*:302, 1987.

148. Boskey AL, Rimnac CM, Bansal M, et al: Effect of short-term hypomagnesemia on the chemical and mechanical properties of rat bone. J Orthop Res *10*:774, 1992.

149. Lamm C, Norton KI, Murphy RJC, et al: Congenital rickets associated with magnesium sulfate infusion for tocolysis. J Pediatr *113*:1078, 1988.

150. Cumming WA, Thomas VJ: Hypermagnesemia: A cause of abnormal metaphyses in the neonate. AJR *152*:1071, 1989.

151. Edwards DK III: Skeletal growth lines on radiographs of newborn infants: Prevalence and possible association with obstetric abnormalities. AJR *161*:141, 1993.

152. Conway JE, Crofford TE, Terry AF, et al: Cauda equina syndrome occurring nine years after a gunshot injury to the spine. J Bone Joint Surg [Am] *75*:760, 1993.

153. Farber JM, Rafii M, Schwartz D: Lead arthropathy and elevated serum levels of lead after a gunshot wound of the shoulder. AJR *162*:385, 1994.

77

Neuromuscular Disorders

Donald Resnick, M.D.

Osseous, articular, and soft tissue changes accompany many neuromuscular disorders. Although the specific response of the musculoskeletal system depends to some degree on the nature of the disorder, certain general abnormalities are evident in many of the diseases. These alterations, which include osteoporosis, fractures, soft tissue atrophy or hypertrophy, growth disturbances and deformities due to altered muscular forces, growth plate and epiphyseal changes, soft tissue, bone, and joint infections, heterotopic ossification, cartilage and muscle atrophy, spondylopathy, synovitis, and capsular abnormalities, are discussed in this chapter. Neuropathic osteoarthropathy, which also may accompany neurologic disorders, is described in Chapter 78.

Imaging of the brain and spinal cord (Chapter 12) allows direct visualization of some of the primary disease processes that account for these generalized abnormalities of the musculoskeletal system. In other instances, such as entrapment peripheral neuropathies, imaging of the extremities is capable of identifying the causative disease process.

GENERAL ABNORMALITIES

Osteoporosis and Fractures

Profound osteoporosis accompanies immobilization, disuse, or paralysis. It can affect the entire skeleton or a portion of it, according to the cause or the circumstances[1, 2] (Fig. 77–1). The pathogenesis of the osteoporosis is not clear (Chapters 51 and 52), although the bone atrophy accompanying muscle paralysis due to conditions of the central nervous system, spinal cord, or peripheral nerves may be similar in its cause to that which follows muscular inactivity due to long-standing debilitating diseases, immobilization of a fracture, or weightlessness. It appears that immobilization causes stasis of blood flow, changes in arterial and venous blood gases with accumulation of carbon dioxide within bone, and an increase in intraosseous venous pressure.[3–5, 123] The alterations in bone circulation can modify cellular differentiation and function[6, 7]; initially, osteoclastic activity may be stimulated and osteoblastic activity may be reduced.[126, 127] Bone resorption predominates over bone formation, although subsequent osteoblastic activation allows repair of the bone resorption.[8, 9] In tubular bones, all three cortical envelopes (periosteal, intracortical or haversian, and endosteal envelopes) appear to participate in bone loss.[10] The contribution of each cortical envelope as well as trabecular bone[11] to osseous resorption and formation is influenced by the nature of the underlying disorder, the length of the observation period after immobilization or paralysis, the method of evaluation, and the integrity of certain endocrine glands.[12, 13, 117]

The radiographic counterpart of the altered cellular dynamics is osteopenia (Chapter 51). The axial and appendicular skeleton participates in this process. A generalized or localized, uniform or patchy, diffuse or periarticular decrease in spongy bone density is associated with diminution of the cortex and accentuation of stress trabeculae in the peripheral or central skeleton or in both. Several types of fractures are seen. Muscle weakness leads to frequent episodes of falling or stumbling, resulting in fractures of the tubular bones in the lower extremity[128] or, if the patient tries to stop the fall, in the upper extremity. Seizures are

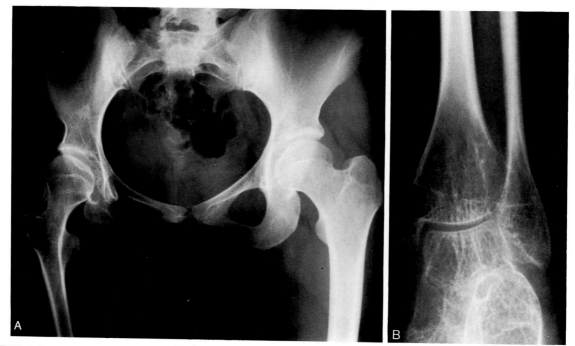

FIGURE 77–1. Osteoporosis, bony underdevelopment, and soft tissue atrophy: Patients with poliomyelitis.
A Note osteoporosis and underdevelopment of the hemipelvis and femur on the right, paralyzed side. Coxa valga and external rotation of the femur and stress changes at the contralateral sacroiliac joint also are noted.
B In the ankle, thin or slender diaphyses, soft tissue atrophy, and periarticular osteoporosis are prominent.

associated with direct forces on bone as a result of a fall or with indirect forces on bone due to uncontrolled and violent muscle contraction[129, 130]; typical sites of fractures accompanying seizures are the spine, proximal portion of the femur, acetabulum, and shoulder region,[308, 309, 331] although unusual sites of fracture or dislocation also are encountered.[332] "Spontaneous" fractures may be encountered as a result of bony atrophy and weakening aggravated by altered patterns of ambulation, spasticity, contractures, deformities, and, in some instances, vigorous physical therapy[14–17, 131, 132]; excessive callus formation can appear in the healing phase,[111, 112, 133, 333, 334] probably the result of continued active or passive motion at the fracture site[16, 17] (Figs. 77–2 and 77–3). Soft tissue ossification[134] and synostosis[135] about sites of fracture are seen. Insufficiency fractures also may be evident (Fig. 77–4). Furthermore, focal areas of cortical resorption can develop, such as in the ribs (Fig. 77–5), owing to pressure erosion from apposing bone or muscle atrophy with loss of normal mechanical stress.[18, 19, 116]

The occurrence of the reflex sympathetic syndrome in patients with neuromuscular disease is discussed later in this chapter.

Soft Tissue and Muscle Atrophy and Hypertrophy

Soft tissue atrophy with muscle wasting and fatty infiltration accompanies most neuromuscular disorders, particularly denervation, and such fatty infiltration and loss of muscle volume can be detected on radiographs of the extremities.[108] In certain primary muscle disorders such as muscular dystrophy and congenital myotonia, however, the actual bulk of the musculature is increased.[20, 21] In the former condition, fatty infiltration of muscle is evident, and

additional radiographic signs include congestive heart failure, osteoporosis, and a peculiar increased anteroposterior thickness of the diaphysis of the fibula.[22]

CT has been used to document the extent of muscle abnormality that occurs in neuromuscular disorders.[136–139, 310] Fatty replacement of muscle in paraspinal regions is a normal age-progressive phenomenon, most prominent in women, that is exaggerated in neuromuscular diseases[136] as well as in spinal ankylosis (Fig. 77–6). It is more severe in the lower portions of the spine and is symmetric in muscular dystrophy and asymmetric or unilateral in paralytic disorders such as poliomyelitis.[136] With regard to the musculature of the appendicular skeleton, neural diseases generally are manifested as initial atrophy of muscle and a subsequent decrease in radiodensity; primary muscle disorders are characterized by decreased radiodensity followed by atrophy.[137] A decrease in attenuation values on the CT display indicates the presence of intramuscular fat cells, which, in some cases, are smaller than the normal fat cells of the body.[139] In some specific situations, muscle hypertrophy occurs alone or in combination with atrophy. In all instances, CT abnormalities parallel in distribution the pathologic aberrations of the individual neuromuscular disorder.

The response of muscle to denervation deserves special emphasis. Injury to peripheral nerves related to trauma or other causes leads to a spectrum of muscle abnormalities that appear to be time dependent. Such abnormalities can be studied with well-established nonimaging techniques such as electromyography or newer imaging methods such as ultrasonography,[335] CT, and MR imaging.[336, 337, 471] With regard to MR imaging, Fleckenstein and coworkers[337] described findings in the subacute and chronic stages of denervation that were dissimilar, suggesting that this method

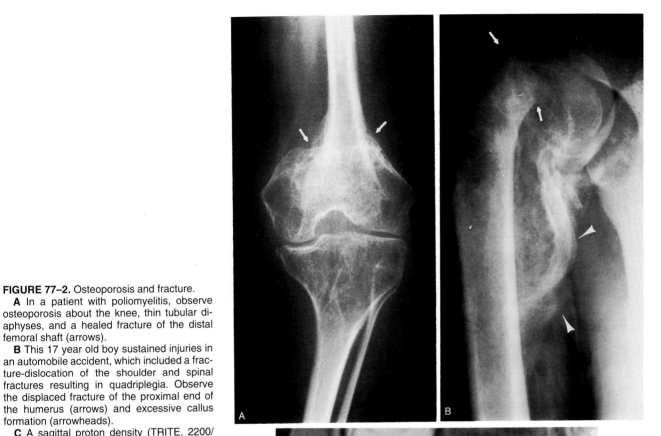

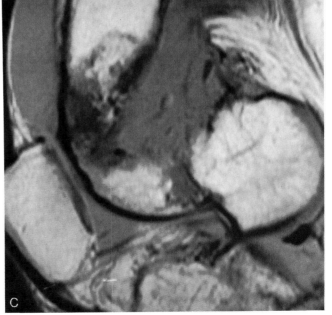

FIGURE 77–2. Osteoporosis and fracture.

A In a patient with poliomyelitis, observe osteoporosis about the knee, thin tubular diaphyses, and a healed fracture of the distal femoral shaft (arrows).

B This 17 year old boy sustained injuries in an automobile accident, which included a fracture-dislocation of the shoulder and spinal fractures resulting in quadriplegia. Observe the displaced fracture of the proximal end of the humerus (arrows) and excessive callus formation (arrowheads).

C A sagittal proton density (TRITE, 2200/20) MR image in a 49 year old man with paraplegia shows a supracondylar and intercondylar fracture of the femur and knee effusion that resulted from vigorous physical therapy.

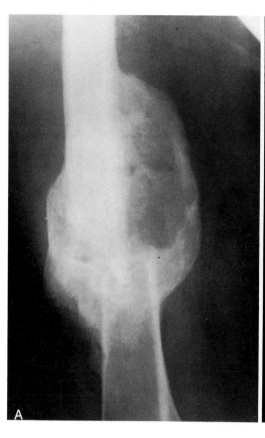
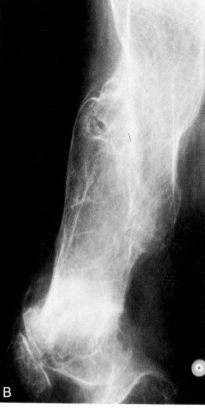

FIGURE 77–3. Osteoporosis and fracture.

A In a 24 year old man who became comatose at the time of an automobile accident, subsequent healing of a femoral fracture is associated with exuberant callus and solid bone union.

B A quadriplegic 56 year old man with a femoral fracture reveals an extraordinary amount of new bone, which has resulted in a bone-within-bone appearance.

could be used to monitor the muscle changes occurring in these two stages of the process, although MR imaging was not sensitive to alterations in muscle occurring in the acute phase of the process (i.e., the first few weeks after injury). In this investigation, muscles of patients with subacute denervation revealed prolonged T1 and T2 values, which con-

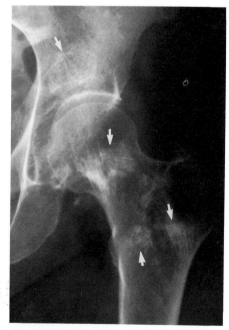

FIGURE 77–4. Osteoporosis and fracture. In this 86 year old woman with hemiplegia, insufficiency fractures have resulted in bone sclerosis in the acetabulum and proximal portion of the femur (arrows).

tributed to conspicuous hyperintensity on short tau inversion recovery (STIR) images.[337] The resulting appearance was similar to that occurring in a variety of other conditions such as myonecrosis, intramuscular hemorrhage, polymyositis, muscle edema secondary to tumors, effects of ionizing radiation, and exertional muscle injuries. Uetani and associates[471] also noted high signal intensity in affected muscles in T2-weighted spin echo images during the subacute stages of denervation. On the basis of results from studies in animals,[338] the progressively increased signal intensity of subacutely denervated skeletal muscle at a longer echo time is consistent with an increase in the extracellular water space.[337] Chronically denervated muscles showed marked atrophy, variable changes on STIR images, and conspicuous fatty infiltration (Fig. 77–6) on T1-weighted spin echo MR images.[337] Serial MR imaging studies revealed that subacutely denervated muscles may progress to fatty replacement but also may return to normal.[337]

Paradoxically, in rare instances, a muscle's response to denervation is enlargement, not atrophy (Fig. 77–7). Such enlargement can relate to two processes: true hypertrophy, which is enlargement due to an increase in size of the remaining innervated muscle fibers; and pseudohypertrophy, which is enlargement related to accumulation of fat within the muscle.[339–341] The inciting neurologic insult in such cases may be disease of the anterior horn cells, radiculopathy secondary to herniation of an intervertebral disc, disease of peripheral nerves, or other causes. Although any site may be involved, most reported cases of hypertrophy or pseudohypertrophy have described involvement of the calf musculature. A slowly enlarging painful or painless extremity may be mistaken for evidence of a tumor. CT and MR imaging can be used to differentiate between true

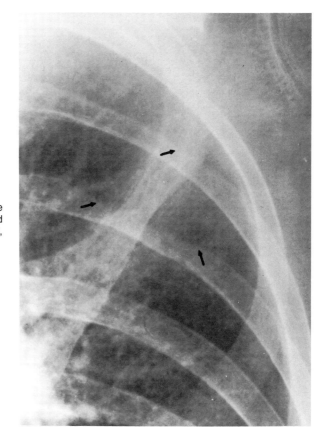

FIGURE 77–5. Rib resorption. Observe long, superficial erosions in the superior portion of two upper ribs (arrows). An incidental finding is a bifid anomaly of the anterior aspect of an additional rib. (Courtesy of C. Resnik, M.D., Baltimore, Maryland.)

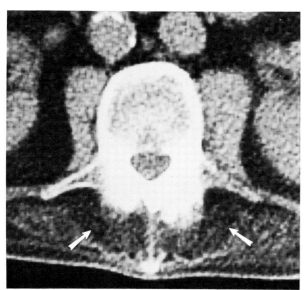

FIGURE 77–6. Muscle atrophy.

A In this patient with ankylosing spondylitis, note fatty replacement of paraspinal muscles (arrows). Compare their appearance to the relatively normal appearance of the psoas muscles. (Courtesy of M. Sage, M.D., Bedford Park, South Australia.)

B, C In this patient, chronic denervation about the shoulder has resulted from cervical spine disease. Coronal oblique T2-weighted (TR/TE, 2000/80) (**B**) and sagittal oblique proton density-weighted (TR/TE, 2000/17) (**C**) spin echo MR images show atrophy and fatty infiltration of the supraspinatus and infraspinatus muscles. (Courtesy of H. M. Fritts, M.D., Minneapolis, Minnesota.)

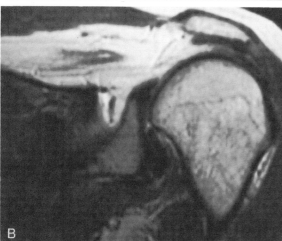

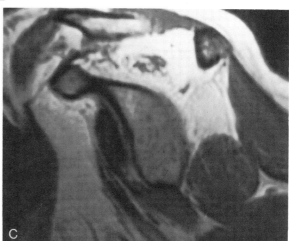

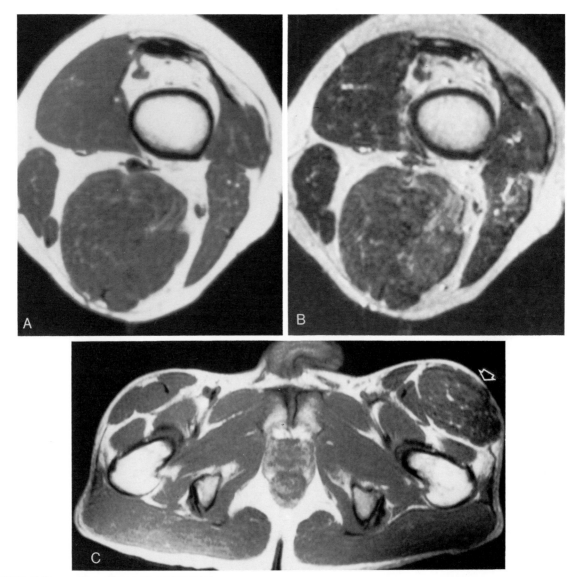

FIGURE 77–7. Denervation with muscle enlargement.

A, B True hypertrophy. Transaxial T1-weighted (TRITE, 600/17) (**A**) and T2-weighted (TRITE, 2500/90) (**B**) spin echo MR images show an enlarged semimembranosus muscle with signal intensity similar to that of the other muscles. The cause of denervation was a herniated intervertebral disc. (Courtesy of J. T. Makley, M.D., and C. A. Petersilge, M.D., Cleveland, Ohio.)

C True hypertrophy and pseudohypertrophy. Subsequent to a stab wound of the left thigh, this 32 year old man developed a painful mass in the injured area. A transaxial T1-weighted (TRITE, 770/15) spin echo MR image shows an enlarged left tensor fasciae latae muscle (arrow) with signal intensity similar to that of other muscles, although foci of intramuscular fat are seen. (Courtesy of C. A. Petersilge, M.D., Cleveland, Ohio.)

hypertrophy and pseudohypertrophy, revealing findings of normal but enlarged muscle tissue in the former situation and of excessive amounts of intramuscular fat in the latter situation.

Myonecrosis (rhabdomyolysis), which is associated with compression of musculature as a result of coma (or prolonged sleep), can be unifocal or multifocal and unilateral or bilateral; areas of hypodensity are observed in the involved musculature on CT scans.[140, 342, 343] Hypoacoustic echogenicity is evident with ultrasonography in cases of myonecrosis,[140, 141] and increased accumulation of bone-seeking radionuclides, perhaps related to calcification,[142] is the corresponding scintigraphic abnormality.[141, 296, 344, 345] A similar radionuclide pattern accompanies the muscle damage associated with extreme exercise.[143]

Growth Disturbances and Deformities Due to Altered Muscular Forces

Activity is essential to the normal growth and development of bones. With inactivity from any cause, muscle contraction diminishes or is lost, and, in the immature skeleton, the growth cartilage, which loses the healthy intermittent compression that everyday activity brings, is damaged. Although the specific alterations of growth may vary from one disorder to another, certain changes are common and well recognized. Neonates with muscle hypotonia or flaccidity and inactive children who spend most of their time in a horizontal position can reveal vertebral bodies with increased vertical dimensions and narrowed intervertebral discs.[23–25, 297] The increase in the height index (ratio of superoinferior diameter to anteroposterior diameter) is approximately proportional to the degree of inactivity; the presence of an inhibitory effect of the compressive force of weight-bearing on the potential longitudinal growth of vertebral bodies may be lost in prolonged recumbency. The similarity of the resulting radiographic appearance of the vertebral bodies in the immobilized child to that of certain animals, such as dogs, with horizontally oriented vertebral columns is of interest in this regard. The reported occurrence of increased height of vertebral bodies in young children with Down's syndrome suggests that genetic mechanisms also may affect bone development.[26]

Similarly, an increase in the neck-shaft angle of the femur, producing coxa valga (Figs. 77–8 and 77–9), can result from muscular imbalance or a decrease in weight-bearing, particularly in very young children.[23, 24, 27–29] In severe cases, subluxation or dislocation of the hip may occur[30, 31, 144, 298, 319] (Fig. 77–10). The opposite situation, coxa vara, develops when the normal amount of upward muscle pull exceeds the force that can be resisted by weakened bone, such as in osteomalacia and Paget's disease.[24]

The pathogenesis of the many abnormalities that appear in the hip and proximal portion of the femur in association with neuromuscular disease in the skeletally immature patient is complex, depending not only on muscle power imbalance but also on anatomic characteristics of the regional growth zones, the latter being well summarized by Siffert,[145] whose observations are repeated here (Fig. 77–9). Skeletal development proceeds by proliferation of growth cartilage in both the acetabulum and the femoral head and neck. Two sites of such cartilage are present in the acetab-

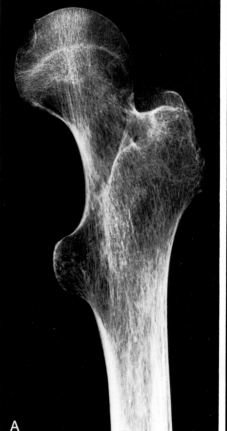
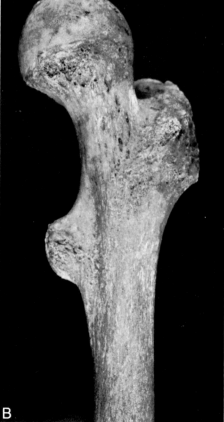

FIGURE 77–8. Coxa valga. Observe the increase in the neck-shaft angle of the femur, a typical finding of neuromuscular disease.

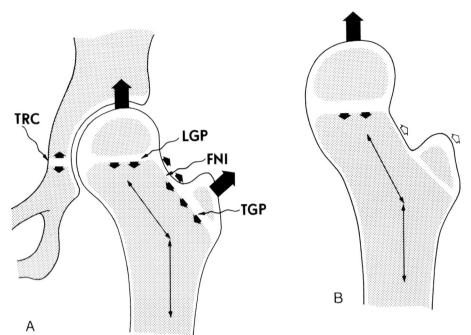

A

B

FIGURE 77–9. Pathogenesis of coxa valga.

A Normal. The growth zones in this region are the articular cartilage, the longitudinal growth plate (LGP), the femoral neck isthmus (FNI), and the trochanteric growth plate (TGP). The triradiate cartilage (TRC) is present on the acetabular side of the joint. The direction of growth is indicated by small and large bold arrows. The double-headed arrows indicate the normal neck-shaft angle.

B Coxa valga. A weakness in the abductor musculature reduces the growth stimulus to the trochanteric growth plate and the femoral neck isthmus (open arrows). The horizontally oriented longitudinal growth plate continues to lengthen the femoral neck in line with the femoral shaft (small and large bold arrows). A valgus angulation results (double-headed arrows).

(Modified from Siffert RS: Clin Orthop *160*:14, 1981.)

ulum, the articular surface of the acetabulum and the triradiate cartilage. Normal growth at the former site depends on proper placement of the femoral head within the acetabulum; hence, growth is modified in the presence of subluxated or dislocated femoral heads (Chapter 86) and internal abnormalities of the femoral head, including Legg-Calvé-Perthes disease (Chapter 81). Normal growth at the triradiate cartilage, which extends among the ilium, ischium, and pubis, allows the acetabulum to keep pace with the enlarging femoral head.

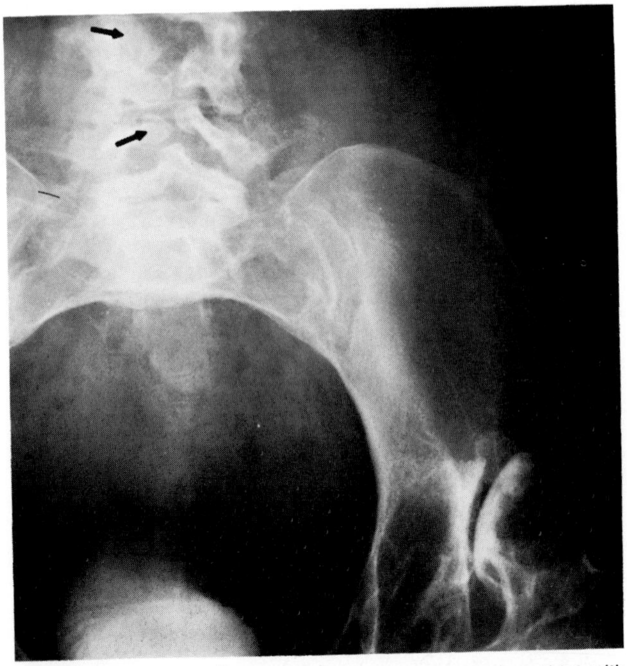

FIGURE 77–10. Dislocation of the hip. In a paraplegic patient with spina bifida (arrows) and meningomyelocele, note the dislocated left femoral head, which is flattened and sclerotic. A neurogenic bladder also is apparent.

The growth zones of the proximal portion of the femur include the articular cartilage; the longitudinal growth plate, horizontally oriented between the epiphysis and the metaphysis; the femoral neck isthmus, in the lateral portion of the neck, which connects the longitudinal growth plate with the trochanteric growth plate and contributes to lateral widening of the neck; and the trochanteric growth plate, located between the greater trochanter and the femoral neck (Fig. 77–9A). One additional cartilaginous zone, in the lesser trochanter, is less influential in its effect on the growth of the proximal femur.

In neuromuscular disease, abductor muscle weakness reduces the growth stimulus to the trochanteric growth plate and femoral neck isthmus.[145] The horizontally oriented longitudinal growth plate contributes to elongation of the femoral neck and to a gradual shift to a coxa valga position (Fig. 77–9B). A thin, vertically oriented femoral neck is the radiographic hallmark of such neuromuscular disease. Abnormalities of the iliopsoas muscle, which attaches to the lesser trochanter, appear to contribute little to the development of femoral neck deformity, although spasticity in this muscle may increase the likelihood of subluxation or dislocation of the hip in the presence of coxa valga.[145, 146]

The severe muscle imbalance, consisting of the absence of hip extensors and abductors and the presence of functioning hip flexors and adductors, that characterizes many of the neuromuscular diseases leads to displacement of the femoral head in a superolateral direction with respect to the acetabulum. Additional etiologic factors in this femoral migration include "bow-stringing" of the iliopsoas tendon and valgus deformity of the femoral neck.[144] The degree of displacement is variable, although complete dislocations are frequent. In cases of subluxation of the femoral head, an osseous notch may be observed in the superolateral aspect of the femoral head, presumably related to bone molding produced by the superior portion of the joint capsule.[147] In the presence of spastic paralysis, a triangular appearance of the femoral head has been described, consisting of flattening in the medial portion of the femoral head (related to an indentation produced by a hypertrophied, taut ligamentum teres) and flattening in the superolateral portion of the femoral head (related to pressure exerted by the abductor muscle mass).[311]

Coxa vara deformity also is reported in children with sensory-deficient neuromuscular disorders, such as spina bifida.[148, 149] It is accompanied by spontaneous separation of the femoral metaphysis and epiphysis owing to disruption of the longitudinal growth plate and fragmentation of the femoral neck. With healing, a coxa vara deformity is seen. The pathogenesis of the changes appears to be microtrauma attributable to the sensory deficit, and the physeal abnormalities are reminiscent of those seen in neuropathic osteoarthropathy (Chapter 78).

Additional examples of the effects of altered muscular activity on neighboring bone can be identified easily (Fig. 77–11). In the child with cerebral palsy, scoliosis, lordosis, and pelvic obliquity (Chapter 89) may result from unbalanced spine and hip muscle contraction and spasticity[32, 150,] [151, 312]; external rotation of the upper femur with a prominent lesser trochanter results from the exaggerated pull of the iliopsoas muscle; flexion contractures of the hips and the knees with abnormal stress in the quadriceps mechanism may lead to patella alta, an elongated patellar shape, and fragmentation of the lower pole of the patella[33–36, 152] and the tibial tuberosity.[36] An exaggerated pull of the flexor muscles of the leg relative to the extensors can produce equinus at the ankle.[37, 38] In the child with poliomyelitis or peroneal muscle atrophy, a pes cavus deformity is attributable to altered muscular function and stress.[153–155]

Obstetric trauma, particularly that related to a breech presentation, may result in an injury to the brachial plexus. Most commonly, an Erb-Duchenne type of paralysis of the upper arm, due to damage of the fifth and sixth cervical roots, is seen; less commonly, a Klumpke's type of paralysis, related to injury of the seventh and eighth cervical and first thoracic roots, is apparent.[346] The affected newborn will fail to move his or her arm, a finding also evident in cases of birth-related clavicular fractures. Although the ultimate

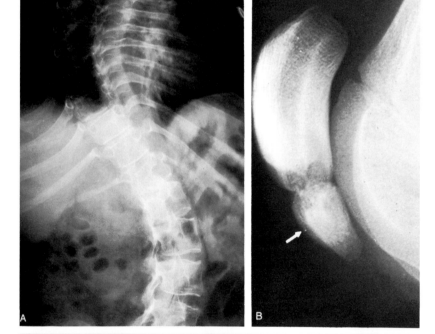

FIGURE 77–11. Additional osseous effects related to altered muscular activity.

A Scoliosis in cerebral palsy. Note the prominent scoliotic curvatures, which were associated with considerable pelvic obliquity.

B Patellar fragmentation in cerebral palsy. Observe the large fragment of the inferior pole of the patella (arrow) caused by altered stress in the quadriceps mechanism.

C Pes cavus deformity in poliomyelitis. Observe the exaggerated arch of the foot, soft tissue atrophy, and osteoporosis.

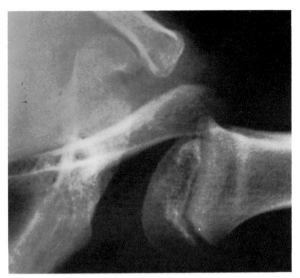

FIGURE 77–12. Erb-Duchenne paralysis. Observe scapular deformity, a shallow glenoid fossa, an elongated acromion, and an inferiorly directed coracoid process. The arm is abducted.

prognosis of such paralysis is good, with full recovery reported in more than 90 per cent of patients,[347] persistent paralysis is accompanied by a variety of shoulder deformities. These include hypoplasia and elevation of the scapula, a shallow glenoid fossa, an inferiorly directed coracoid process, and an abnormally tapered acromion[348, 349] (Fig. 77–12). The findings resemble those associated with congenital hypoplasia of the glenoid neck (see Chapter 90).

Growth Plate and Epiphyseal Changes

Premature closure of the growth plate, particularly in the metatarsals and knees, is noted in patients with poliomyelitis[39, 40] (Fig. 77–13). Currarino[41] noted evidence of prema-

ture fusion of one or more epiphyses in 9 per cent of 250 patients with poliomyelitis, in all cases limited to the feet or the knees. Unilateral or bilateral changes occur, always corresponding to sites that are involved in the neurologic disease; the fourth metatarsal is affected most frequently. The altered epiphyses in the foot or the knee can be buried in the adjacent metaphyses (ball-and-socket epiphyses), and, after epiphyseal fusion, the involved bone is shortened. Although the pathogenesis of the change is not known, chronic growth plate trauma from angular deformity and muscular and osseous weakening may be responsible for the premature epiphyseal fusion.

Premature physeal closure can become evident in other neuromuscular diseases, and it may be associated with epiphyseal overgrowth (ballooning), findings resembling those of hemophilia or juvenile chronic arthritis.[156] Factors such as altered patterns of stress and hyperemia probably are important in the development of these changes.

Epiphyseal and metaphyseal trauma is a recognized manifestation in patients with certain neurologic disorders (meningomyelocele and congenital insensitivity to pain) owing to their sensory deficiency, osteoporosis, and musculoligamentous laxity [42–49, 113, 114, 350–354] (Chapter 78). After injury, the absence of significant pain allows continued activity, and neuropathic alterations appear, characterized by metaphyseal and growth plate hemorrhage, epiphyseal displacement, widening and irregularity of the cartilaginous plate, metaphyseal and epiphyseal fragmentation, and periosteal bone formation. The appearance may simulate that of rickets or infection.

Osseous, Articular, and Soft Tissue Infection

The immobilized and debilitated patient with neuromuscular disease frequently develops generalized or localized infections. Skin breakdown over pressure points is a common and frustrating problem in these patients[50–52] (Fig. 77–

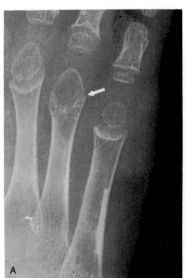
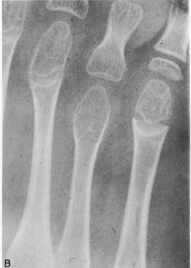
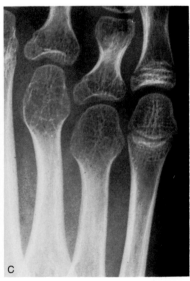

FIGURE 77–13. Premature closure of the growth plate in a patient with poliomyelitis.
   A In the initial film, the growth plate of the fourth metatarsal bone is partially closed (arrow), whereas those of the third and fifth metatarsal bones still are open. Furthermore, the fourth metatarsal bone is shortened, and considerable osteoporosis is evident.
   B Five years later, note the solid fusion of the fourth metatarsal epiphysis and the shortening of the digit. Observe fusion of the growth plate of the proximal phalanx of the fourth toe.
   C At this stage, closure of the growth plate of the third metatarsal bone has produced shortening of this digit as well.

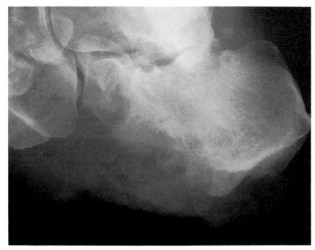

FIGURE 77–14. Soft tissue and bone infection. A large decubitus ulcer in the soft tissues of the posterior and plantar aspects of the foot has led to osteomyelitis of the calcaneus.

14), and with penetration of the subcutaneous and fascial tissue, infection may reach the underlying bones and joints. The ischial tuberosities, the femoral trochanters, the hip joints, and other bony protuberances are affected most typically, and the characteristic radiographic findings of osteomyelitis or septic arthritis (or both) ensue (Chapters 64 and 65). The degree of osteolysis in these cases may become extreme,[53] the bone loss being aggravated by factors other than infection, such as disuse, the trauma of continual pressure, and neuropathy. CT and MR imaging are useful in the delineation of the extent of bone and soft tissue involvement.[157, 158]

The frequency of sacroiliac joint abnormality in paralyzed persons has been attributed, at least in part, to chronic pelvic sepsis resulting in osseous contamination. This articular manifestation is discussed later in this chapter.

Heterotopic Ossification

Heterotopic new bone formation is a well-documented complication of central nervous system and spinal cord disorders.[54–59, 358] It is reported most commonly in association with paraplegia secondary to spinal cord trauma, in which it may be observed in 16 to 53 per cent of cases.[60–65, 159, 355] Less frequently, heterotopic ossification is evident after acute anoxia, head injury,[124] cerebrovascular accident, encephalomyelitis, poliomyelitis, multiple sclerosis, neoplastic disease, and tetanus.[58, 59, 63, 66–71, 356, 472] It occurs in both flaccid and spastic forms of paralysis and is more common and severe in young men.

In general, ossification appears 2 to 6 months after injury. It has been evident as early as 19 days after trauma, however.[61, 65, 299] Furthermore, in children, the onset of heterotopic ossification commonly occurs more than 1 year after the injury.[359] Single or multiple, unilateral or bilateral sites may be affected. The areas involved most typically are the hip (Fig. 77–15), the knee (Fig. 77–16), and the shoulder (Fig. 77–17)[320]; less commonly, the elbow (Fig. 77–18)[109] and the small joints of the hand and the foot are altered.[59, 160, 464] Although ossification almost always is seen in a paralyzed limb or limbs, this association is not constant.

The clinical manifestations are variable. Many patients have no symptoms or signs other than those of the primary neurologic disorder itself. Other patients develop pain, swelling, and restricted joint motion, simulating the findings of an acute arthritis.[321, 357] In some persons, synovitis occurs prior to radiographically apparent ossification.[161, 162, 300] Aspiration of articular contents may reveal clear yellow or serosanguineous synovial fluid with a meager number of erythrocytes or leukocytes.[59, 60] Additional laboratory findings may be unrewarding, although elevation of the serum alkaline phosphatase level has been observed.[72] The frequency of certain histocompatibility antigens in patients with heterotopic ossification appears to be identical to that

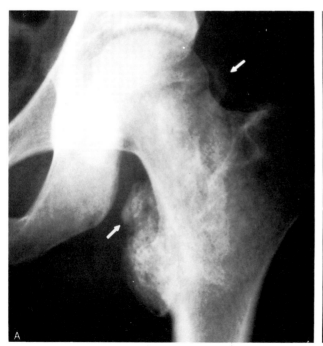
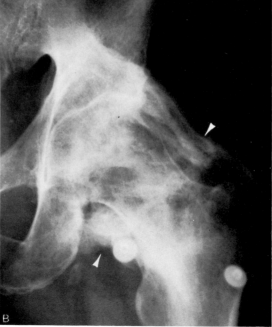

FIGURE 77–15. Heterotopic ossification: The hip. Two examples of ossification of varying severity about the hip. The deposits begin as poorly defined opaque areas (solid arrows) and progress to radiodense lesions of considerable size possessing trabecular pattern (arrowheads).

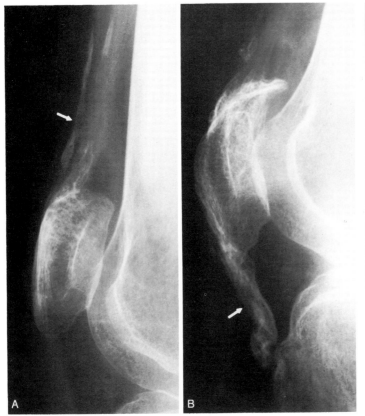

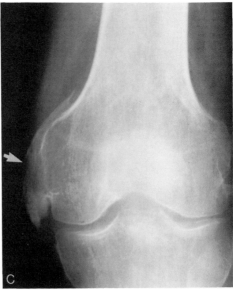

FIGURE 77–16. Heterotopic ossification: The knee. Three examples of soft tissue and tendinous ossification (arrows) about the knee.

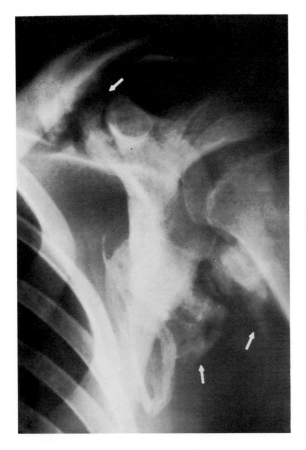

FIGURE 77–17. Heterotopic ossification: The shoulder. Deposits of varying size also can be noted about the shoulder (arrows).

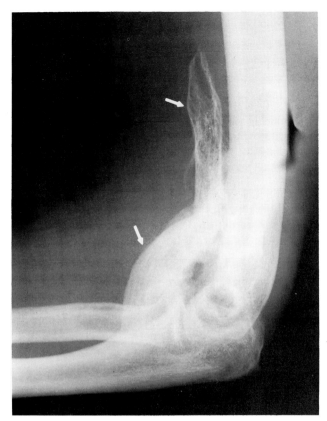

FIGURE 77–18. Heterotopic ossification: The elbow. Striking mature ossification (arrows) has produced "ankylosis" along the anterior aspect of the elbow.

in healthy persons,[73, 163, 165] although some reports have suggested otherwise.[164, 166]

Radiographic examination delineates initially poorly defined periarticular radiodense areas that do not contain recognizable trabeculae. The collections enlarge, merge with the underlying bone in the form of an irregular excrescence, and demonstrate trabecular architecture. Eventually, complete periarticular osseous bridging may result,[167] associated with significant loss or absence of joint motion. In some instances, ossification develops at a distance from a joint and eventually it merges with the subjacent bone, forming a peculiar excrescence. Exceptionally, spontaneous regression of heterotopic ossification is observed,[168] a phenomenon that is more frequent in children.[359]

Scintigraphic examination also may be used to determine the evolution of this process and the maturity of the heterotopic ossification.[57, 74, 75, 299, 361] This determination is important, as surgical removal of immature new bone frequently is followed by recurrence of the abnormal deposits, whereas excision of mature ossification is not associated with such recurrence.[301] Images obtained with bone-seeking pharmaceutical agents reveal an acute phase with increased radionuclide activity occurring as early as 2 weeks after the neurologic insult, prior to the appearance of clinical or radiographic abnormalities; a subacute phase with a rapid increase in activity; a chronic active immature phase with a steady state of increased activity; a chronic active maturing phase with decreased activity; and a chronic mature phase with a return of the normal scan.[57] The time necessary for the bone scan to pass from one stage to the next appears to

be variable, but operative intervention should not be contemplated before the activity of the radionuclide begins to diminish. Supplementing the study with a scintigraphic examination with a bone marrow-seeking agent may further document the maturity of the deposited bone; the accumulation of radionuclide in this study indicates mature marrow-containing ectopic bone.

CT has been employed to study areas of neurogenic heterotopic ossification.[362] Ossification progresses from an early appearance of soft tissue density of lower attenuation than muscle to a calcific density paralleling radiographic and scintigraphic evidence of bone formation. Persistent soft tissue regions of low density adjacent to areas of ossification may be present for years. These regions may represent immature connective tissue that maintains its potential for ossification.[362] Descriptions of the MR imaging appearance of heterotopic ossification have related mainly to cases of trauma (posttraumatic myositis ossificans) and have indicated some variability in the findings, which appear to be time dependent.[363, 364] Patterns of signal intensity are consistent with the presence of ossific shells, marrow fat, hemorrhage and edema of soft tissues, or fibrosis, or combinations of these constituents.

Histologically, the maturing heterotopic ossification consists of essentially normal bone with haversian canals, osteoblasts, blood vessels, and marrow.[60, 61, 76, 77]

The cause of the ectopic bone formation is unknown.[59] Local factors, such as continuous pressure, decubitus ulceration, and trauma from vigorous therapy, have been emphasized by some investigators[122, 169, 170]; however, the occurrence of heterotopic ossification in areas remote from the pressure points or the decubitus ulcers and in the absence of physical manipulation has been documented. Systemic factors, such as hypoproteinemia, elevated serum levels of growth hormone,[171] and urinary tract infections, also have been implicated,[77] but studies have failed to confirm this.[61] The appearance of excessive callus formation around fractures as well as at sites of insertion of intramedullary nails[360] in some paralyzed patients has suggested that an exaggerated healing response or bone-forming tendency may be operational,[112] but this, too, appears unlikely.[54] A genetic predisposition to bone formation also has been postulated as a cause of ossification in these patients (as well as in those with diffuse idiopathic skeletal hyperostosis),[78] but results of histocompatibility antigen determinations have not been rewarding.[73, 121] It also has been theorized that denervation stimulates the connective tissue to recover its embryonic osteogenic function,[79] but the exact basis for this stimulation and the variability of this response in different persons remain unexplained.

The common factor in heterotopic ossification in neurologic disorders is immobilization. The deposition of calcium and bone may relate to vascular stasis,[125] perhaps in Batson's paravertebral plexus (which has tributaries in the appendicular skeleton as well),[80] but the exact pathogenesis of such ossification and why it is present in some persons and absent in others remain mysteries.

Heterotopic ossification of soft tissues is not confined to patients with neuromuscular disease. Burns, mechanical trauma, and venous stasis (varicosities) can lead to similar changes. In addition, a progressive form of ossification of unknown cause, myositis (fibrodysplasia) ossificans progressiva, also is recognized.

Cartilage Atrophy

Articular cartilage is nourished predominantly by diffusion of synovial fluid[81–84] (Fig. 77–19). A subchondral route for nutrition of the innermost portion of the cartilaginous surface appears probable on the basis of data from experimental studies in animals.[85, 86] This latter process may be more prominent in the immature skeleton than in the mature skeleton owing to differences in the anatomic configuration of the junctional region between articular cartilage and subchondral bone; nutrition in the young animal may be enhanced by the presence of prominent vascular buds extending from the subchondral circulation into the cartilage mass, whereas in the older animal, mature cortical bone may separate the cartilage from the subchondral vascular spaces.[87, 118] These experimental observations indeed may have relevance to chondral nutrition in the human.[88] The diffusion into cartilage of nutrients from the synovial fluid and subchondral bone is aided by the pliability and hydrophilic characteristics of the chondral surface[89, 90] and depends on a pumping action that develops during normal activity.[91] Cartilage acts somewhat like a sponge that gives off fluid when squeezed and takes up fluid when relaxed.[174] Alternating periods of squeezing and relaxing of cartilage accompany joint movement.

Immobilization leads to significant changes in cartilaginous nutrition. The production of synovial fluid is greatly curtailed.[92] In animals, progressive contracture of capsular and pericapsular structures and encroachment on the joint by intra-articular fibrofatty connective tissue are observed.[93–96] At sites at which the articular surfaces are in contact, chondral fibrillation, erosion, and necrosis with liquefaction are identified.[94–98, 110] The subchondral bone may be thickened and invaded by proliferating primitive mesenchymal tissue from the marrow spaces, which replaces the deep layer of articular cartilage.[95, 99] Repair of

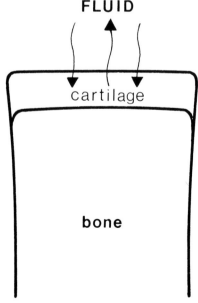

FIGURE 77–19. Normal cartilage nutrition. The predominant mechanism of cartilage nutrition is derived from a pumping action in which synovial fluid diffuses into and out of the chondral substance. A subchondral route of nutrition is present but of less magnitude.

chondral elements may follow short periods of immobilization.[100]

Similar events may accompany immobilization of human joints.[101, 102] In the knee, prolonged immobilization is associated with proliferation of fibrofatty tissue, which subsequently envelops intra-articular ligaments and obliterates the articular lumen and is associated with gradual resorption of peripheral cartilage[102] (Fig. 77–20). In areas of apposed articular surfaces, fibrillation and cystic defects appear within the cartilage, and a reparative effort associated with proliferation and transchondral extension of primitive mesenchymal tissue within the marrow and with endochondral ossification may result in total replacement of articular cartilage and intra-articular fibrous or bony ankylosis.[102] Both intra-articular and periarticular changes are important in the limitation of joint motion that follows long-term immobilization.[95–102]

These observations in animals and humans suggest that the chondral alterations occurring after immobilization result from a decrease in cartilage nutrition due to the presence of an atrophic synovial membrane and the absence of normal movement with a concomitant decrease in fluid diffusion. A decrease in loading of the cartilage attributable to absence of contraction of the muscles that span the joint may contribute to these alterations[119]; muscle stimulation may lessen or prevent cartilage deterioration if it is accomplished electrically during the period of immobilization,[172] and moderate exercise after such a period can lead to reversal of some of the cartilaginous alterations.[173] The radiographic counterpart of these chondral changes is a loss of interosseous (joint) space in the patient with neurologic disease (Fig. 77–21). Although this may be observed in any paralyzed body part, changes are especially characteristic in the hip, the knee, and the sacroiliac joint. Pool[91] noted significant joint space narrowing (by at least 50 per cent) of the hip articulation in 12.5 per cent of 200 patients with flaccid paralysis, in some cases within 2 years of injury; the frequency of this abnormality in spastic paralysis probably is less because of the muscular tension across the joint.[175] Characteristically, diffuse loss of interosseous space is evident with axial migration of the femoral head, although narrowing of the superolateral aspect of the articulation may be prominent in some persons because of associated lateral subluxation of the femoral head. Accompanying osteoporosis may be evident.

Changes also may be observed in one or both sacroiliac joints, although the interpretation of the alterations in this location has been a matter of debate (Fig. 77–22). In 1950, Abel[103] reported radiographic changes of the sacroiliac joint in 98 of 160 patients (61 per cent) with traumatic paraplegia. The abnormalities consisted of periarticular osteoporosis and joint space narrowing, which, in some cases, progressed to intra-articular bony ankylosis. On biopsy of the sacroiliac joint in one patient, atrophic bone with vascular marrow, cartilaginous denudation, and osseous fusion were noted. Abel cited the radiographic and histologic similarity of sacroiliac joint involvement in paraplegia to that in ankylosing spondylitis, perhaps indicating a common pathogenesis in both disorders. Mason and colleagues subsequently suggested that chronic genitourinary tract infection might produce the osteoarticular lesions of ankylosing spondylitis as a result of dissemination of infection via the

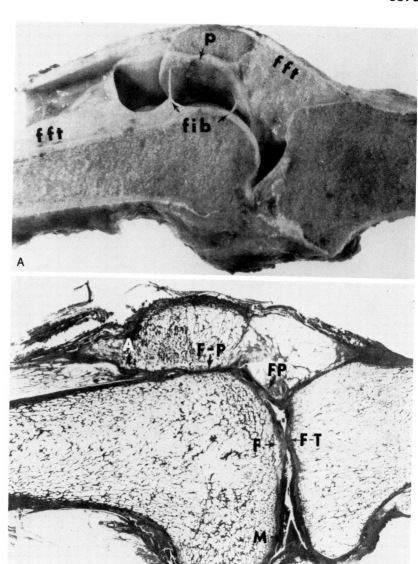

FIGURE 77–20. Cartilage atrophy: Pathologic abnormalities.

A On a photograph of a sagittal section of an immobilized knee (period of immobilization, over 12 months), note fibrofatty tissue (fft) filling the inferior portion of the joint cavity as well as a portion of the suprapatellar pouch. Fibrous septa (fib) extend from the femoral condyle to the patella. The patellar articular cartilage (p) is irregular.

B On a photomicrograph (1×) of a similar sagittal section in a different patient (period of immobilization, 16 months), note osteoporosis. Replacement of the articular cartilages of the femoral condyle, patella, and tibia by fibrous connective tissue is apparent. Small islands of cartilage remain in the patella (A), the femoral condyle (F), and the tibia. Mature fibrous connective tissue, in which ossification is occurring, joins the femoral condyle and the patella (F-P), and the femoral condyle and the tibia (F-T). Obliteration of portions of the joint cavity as well as the suprapatellar pouch by fibrofatty tissue (FP) is evident.

(From Enneking WF, Horowitz M: J Bone Joint Surg [Am] *54*:973, 1972.)

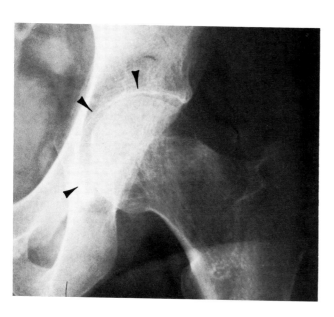

FIGURE 77–21. Cartilage atrophy: Radiologic abnormalities. A typical example of symmetric loss of the joint space (arrowheads) in the hip due to cartilage atrophy resulting from paralysis is presented.

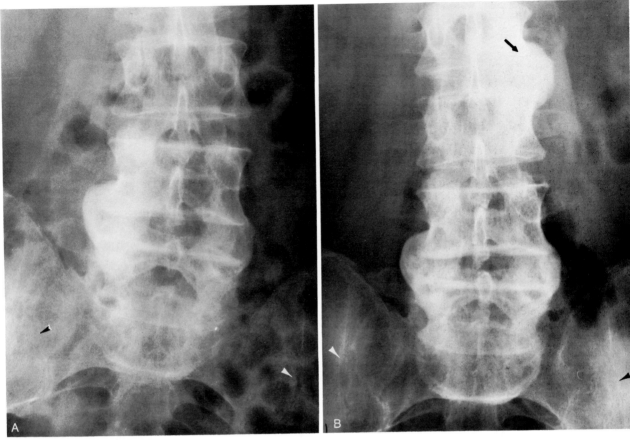

FIGURE 77–22. Sacroiliac joint and spinal abnormalities.

A, B In this patient, who had been quadriplegic for over 5 years, radiographs obtained 2 years apart indicate loss of interosseous space in both sacroiliac joints (arrowheads) and spinal ossification. One of the vertebral outgrowths appeared during the period of paralysis (arrow). Whether these excrescences represent typical osteophytes or heterotopic bone formation is not clear.

paravertebral venous plexus,[104] a mechanism that also would be operational in paralyzed persons. In 1965, Wright and colleagues[105] studied 38 paraplegic men, noting sacroiliac joint abnormalities on radiographs of 12 (32 per cent) of these patients. Major osseous erosion, complete bony ankylosis of the joint, or spondylitis was not evident, thus creating a radiographic picture that differed from that in ankylosing spondylitis. Furthermore, these investigators found that the sacroiliac joint changes were not related to the presence or severity of genital infection, leading them to postulate that sacroiliac articular alterations in paraplegia are attributable not to sacroiliitis or chronic infection but to damage by the severe mechanical stresses to which the pelvis is subjected acting on osteoporotic bone. The differing pathogeneses of sacroiliac joint changes in paralysis and ankylosing spondylitis were further underscored by histocompatibility antigen typing of 54 paraplegic or quadriplegic patients, 24 of whom had abnormal radiographs of the sacroiliac articulations.[106] Although the sacroiliac joint alterations were more severe in quadriplegic than in paraplegic patients,[106] no association was found between these alterations and any of the HLA antigens of the A and B loci in either group.

Thus, the pathogenesis of sacroiliac joint changes in paralyzed persons remains a mystery. The findings may relate to a combination of cartilage atrophy due to immobilization and subchondral osseous collapse due to weakening and fracture of osteoporotic bone. Sacroiliac joint abnormalities may be more common in patients with high spinal levels of paraplegia than in those with paraplegia involving lower levels, perhaps related to more severe limitation of trunk mobility in the former persons.[115] The abnormalities appear to be more frequent and severe in patients with paralysis of longer duration.[120] Rarely, they are combined with changes in the spine, including syndesmophytes, interspinous ossification, osteophytes, and intervertebral discal calcification.[120]

Spondylopathy

A variety of spinal abnormalities occur in paralyzed persons. Some of these represent neuropathic osteoarthropathy, consisting of disc space loss, bone sclerosis, fragmentation, osteophytosis, and subluxation, and are similar to those appearing in diabetes mellitus, syringomyelia, and syphilis[365–367] (see Chapter 78). In other instances, bone outgrowths of the spine develop whose characteristics resemble those of the paravertebral ossification that accompanies psoriasis or Reiter's syndrome, the flowing ossification of diffuse idiopathic skeletal hyperostosis, or the thin excrescences of ankylosing spondylitis[120] (Figs. 77–23 and 77–24). Diffuse increased radiodensity of the spine may accompany these changes, and the sacroiliac joints may appear normal. The cause of these findings is not clear, although they appear to be unrelated to the level of paralysis, appearing both in quadriplegic and in paraplegic pa-

fibers and fascial planes. Pain is not a prominent feature, although foot deformities related to the nerve injury are apparent. The cause of the calcification is not known.

SPECIFIC TYPES OF NEUROMUSCULAR DISEASE

Peripheral Neuropathies

Although a complete discussion of peripheral neuropathy is beyond the scope of this textbook and is available readily elsewhere,[190–192] an overview of the subject is presented here. Peripheral neuropathies represent primary disorders of peripheral motor, sensory, and autonomic neurons and are accompanied by muscle weakness, muscle atrophy, sensory change, or autonomic dysfunction, or any combination of these. They can be classified further on the basis of a precise cause or relationship to an underlying disease, pathologic characteristics of the neural alterations, site of involvement, or clinical course, but classification commonly is accomplished using designations of mononeuropathy, multiple mononeuropathies, and polyneuropathies (Table 77–1). Such designations are useful as they imply specific pathogenetic mechanisms and, in turn, specific causes.[193] Accurate diagnosis requires meticulous neurologic examination to elucidate the exact distribution of the motor and sensory nerve abnormalities, which, ultimately, allows localization of the pathologic process to one or more regions of the body.

Mononeuropathy can be produced by physical injury, whether related to laceration, contusion, traction, or compression, or by electricity and radiation.[194] Examples of these mechanisms include axillary nerve involvement resulting from a dislocation of the glenohumeral joint, long thoracic nerve involvement producing the winged scapula, ulnar nerve involvement from nerve entrapment at the elbow, median nerve involvement related to the carpal tunnel syndrome, radial nerve involvement attributable to ''Saturday night palsy,'' sciatic nerve involvement occurring in association with trauma or gluteal injections, and posterior tibial nerve involvement from entrapment in the tarsal tunnel.[193] *Multiple mononeuropathies* imply dysfunction of several individual nerve trunks at different times and may be observed in leprosy, uremia, diabetes mellitus, inflammatory-immunologic disorders, necrotizing angiopathies, and other conditions.[194] *Polyneuropathies* are associated with a large number of disorders, including nutritional deficiencies, anemias, conditions related to toxins and drugs, infection, diabetes mellitus, uremia, amyloidosis, rheumatoid arthritis, systemic lupus erythematosus, polyarteritis nodosa, acromegaly, hypothyroidism, syphilis, sarcoidosis, alcoholism, dysproteinemias, Refsum's disease, Fabry's disease, Charcot-Marie-Tooth disease, and the Guillain-Barré syndrome.[193]

Entrapment Neuropathies. Peripheral nerve entrapment syndromes involve the compression of a short segment of a single nerve at a specific site frequently as a result of the vulnerability of that nerve as it passes through a fibro-osseous tunnel or an opening in fibrous or muscular tissue. Any or all portions of the nerve, including the nerve fibers, Schwann cells, endoneurium, perineurium, epineurium, and intraneural microvessels, may be injured, accounting for the variability of the pathologic features, which range from a transient conduction block through total demyelination to neural fibrosis and wallerian degeneration.[195] A classification system of the severity of injury was introduced by Seddon[373] in 1943 and still is used today. Three levels of injury were described: neurapraxia, which results from mild compression and is related to local injury of the myelin sheath without axonal involvement; axonotmesis, which occurs with more severe compression and leads to axonal injury as well as focal demyelination; and neurotmesis, which relates to severe compression and is accompanied by disruption of all elements of the nerve. Recovery generally is complete in cases of neurapraxia, delayed and less satisfactory in cases of axonotmesis, and incomplete in cases of neurotmesis.[374] Clinical manifestations, consisting of motor and sensory abnormalities, vary not only according to the severity of the injury but also according to the specific nerve that is affected, and accurate diagnosis depends on knowledge of the anatomic course of the peripheral nerve and the results of electromyography, motor and sensory nerve conduction and velocity studies, and imaging examinations.[196, 197]

Complicating the accurate diagnosis of entrapment neuropathy is the existence of numerous syndromes that relate

---

TABLE 77—1. Classification of Peripheral Neuropathies

Type	Characteristics	Pathophysiology	Common Cause
Mononeuropathy	Involves one cranial or peripheral nerve or nerve root	Trauma Compression Entrapment Infarction	Common peroneal palsy Carpal tunnel syndrome Diabetes mellitus
Multiple mononeuropathy	Involves several nerves Contiguous nerves	 Neoplastic invasion Infarction	 Invasion of the brachial plexus by cancer Diabetes mellitus
	Noncontiguous nerves	Infarction	Diabetes mellitus Vasculitis
Polyneuropathy	Involves the longest nerves first; distal, symmetric	Toxic-metabolic	Alcohol-nutritional Diabetes mellitus Uremia Systemic cancer
		Inflammatory or immune (or both)	Guillain-Barré syndrome

(From Sherman DG: Peripheral neuropathies. *In* JG Stein [Ed]: Internal Medicine. Boston, Little, Brown, 1983, p 872.)

to varying degrees of compression of nerves at multiple sites and levels.[375] Indeed, more than two decades ago, Upton and McComas[376] introduced the concept of a double crush phenomenon, in which a single nerve was involved at two different levels. These authors, noting an association between cervical disc disease and the carpal tunnel syndrome and between the thoracic outlet and cubital tunnel syndromes, suggested that a proximal source of nerve compression renders the distal aspect of the nerve more vulnerable to compression at a second anatomic site.[375, 377] They further implied that a given nerve could be entrapped at more than two sites (i.e., multiple crush syndrome) and that two nerves (e.g., median and ulnar nerves) could be compressed in a single extremity (i.e., multiple entrapment neuropathies). Finally, these investigators suggested that certain situations (such as stretching of a proximal portion of a nerve) or diseases (such as diabetes mellitus) would render a nerve more susceptible to compression or damage.[375] Subsequent to this landmark publication, additional investigations both in humans and in animals have confirmed the clinical importance of double and multiple crush syndromes and, further, have sustained the view that the symptoms and signs of such syndromes may be far more devastating than those encountered in cases of single sites of nerve compression.[378] The mechanism behind the double crush phenomenon may relate to changes in axoplasmic flow with associated decreased transport of neurotrophic substances.[375, 379]

The clinical manifestations of entrapment neuropathies, as indicated previously, vary with the specific site or sites of involvement. In addition, in some cases the manifestations are persistent and in others they occur only with certain maneuvers of the extremity. The latter situation often is referred to as dynamic compression neuropathy.[375] One example of this is the occurrence of the carpal tunnel syndrome when the wrist is placed in an extended or flexed position and the absence of nerve compression when the wrist is in a neutral position. Changes in the shape of the carpal tunnel occur during such modifications of wrist position.[473] Basic to the concept of dynamic nerve compression is the normal excursion and free gliding of a nerve in its soft tissue bed during positional changes of an extremity. Displacement or fixation of a nerve in this bed leads to decreased mobility; movement of the extremity in this situation results in a secondary traction injury to the nerve just proximal and distal to the point of displacement or tethering.[375] Any clinical tests used in the diagnosis of dynamic nerve compression are applied more appropriately in extremity positions known to provoke the nerve compression. A variety of provocative clinical tests have been described during which gentle pressure on the nerve at the site of entrapment is accompanied by paresthesias in the distribution of that nerve. These provocative tests can be used to diagnose (1) entrapment of the median nerve in the carpal tunnel (pressure proximal to carpal tunnel, Phalen's test) or proximal portion of the forearm (pressure over proximal forearm, resisted elbow flexion, and pronation and finger flexion); (2) entrapment of the ulnar nerve in Guyon's canal (pressure proximal to Guyon's canal) or in the cubital tunnel (pressure proximal to the cubital tunnel, elbow flexion); (3) entrapment of the radial nerve in the arcade of Frohse (i.e., posterior interosseous nerve syndrome) (pressure applied during supination) or forearm (pressure over the junction of the brachioradialis and exten-

sor carpi radialis tendons, forearm pronation); (4) entrapment of components of the brachial plexus in the supraclavicular region (elevation of the arms above the head, pressure over the brachial plexus in the interscalene area); (5) or other conditions.[375] These provocative tests, when applied carefully and combined with data derived from the clinical history and routine physical examination, aid in the assessment of entrapment neuropathies. The initial diagnostic step is the identification of the specific nerve or nerves that are affected. Entrapment neuropathies typically involve the median, ulnar, radial, musculocutaneous, suprascapular, dorsoscapular, or brachial plexus nerves in the upper extremities (Fig. 77–26) and the sciatic, common peroneal, posterior tibial, femoral, saphenous, lateral femoral cutaneous, obturator, ilioinguinal, or genitofemoral nerve in the lower extremity (Table 77–2) (Fig. 77–27). Imaging studies, particularly MR imaging, provide supplementary information in some cases that delineate a specific and sometimes treatable cause of the compression neuropathy.

Median Nerve. Entrapment of the *median nerve* occurs most frequently in the wrist as the carpal tunnel syndrome, but it also may develop in the region of the distal portion of the humerus or proximal portion of the forearm.[198, 199]

Ligament of Struthers. In approximately 1 per cent of limbs, the ligament of Struthers connects an anomalous bony excrescence (the supracondylar process), arising from the anterior surface of the distal portion of the humerus, to the medial epicondyle of the humerus (Fig. 77–28). Although a supracondylar process usually is an incidental finding on radiographs and is unassociated with symptoms and signs, compromise of the median nerve is a possible complication, especially in patients who have had trauma to the area.[198, 200, 201]

Pronator Syndrome. An entrapment neuropathy of the median nerve can occur in the antecubital area where the nerve passes between the two heads of the pronator teres muscle and then under the edge of the flexor digitorum sublimis muscle (Fig. 77–29). Clinical manifestations include an aching pain in the forearm, often initiated by repetitive movements of the elbow, as occurs in weightlifting, tennis, needlework, and writing.[380] Clumsiness or weakness of the hand, numbness and paresthesias in the distribution of the median nerve, painful pronation, tenderness, firmness or enlargement of the pronator teres muscle, weakness of the flexor pollicis longus and abductor pollicis brevis muscles, and thenar atrophy also may be observed.[381] The anatomic basis of this syndrome includes hypertrophy of the pronator muscle, trapping by the lacertus fibrosus (bicipital aponeurosis) from the biceps tendon, or an aberrant median artery or a fibrous component of the flexor carpi radialis muscle originating from the ulna.[195, 198, 199, 202, 203, 382]

Anterior Interosseous Nerve Syndrome (Kiloh-Nevin Syndrome). The anterior interosseous nerve is the largest branch of the median nerve and is purely motor, supplying the flexor pollicis longus, the pronator quadratus, and the radial part of the flexor digitorum profundus muscles.[198] Its compression leads to weakness of the thumb and index finger and occurs on an idiopathic basis, after radial or supracondylar humeral fractures, in association with thrombosed vessels or enlarged bursae or, most commonly, as a result of aberrant fibrous bands.[198, 204–209, 380]

Carpal Tunnel Syndrome. The most frequent entrapment syndrome of the median nerve occurs as the nerve passes

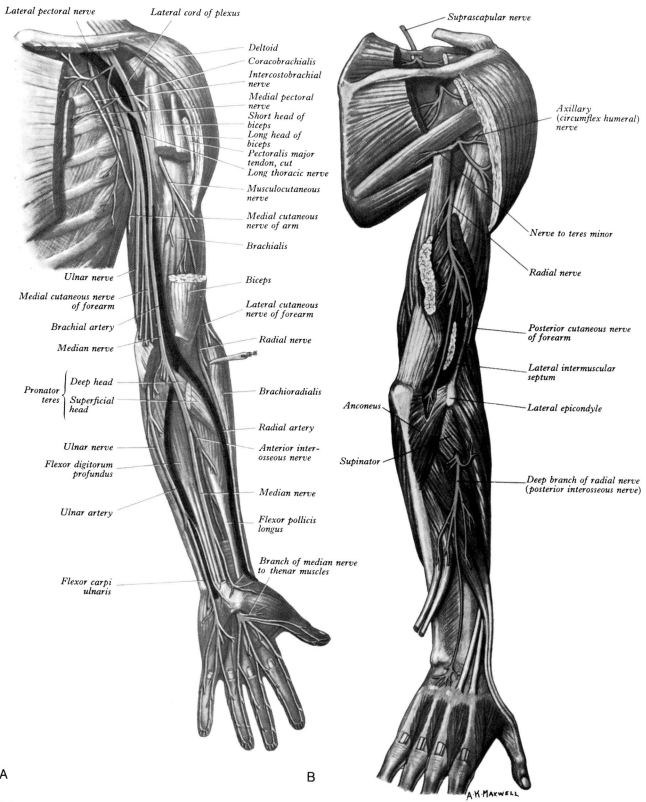

FIGURE 77–26. The nerves of the upper limb.
 A Dissection, anterior aspect.
 B Dissection, posterior aspect.
(From Williams PL, Warwick R: Gray's Anatomy. 36th Ed. Philadelphia, WB Saunders Co, 1980, pp 1099, 1100.)

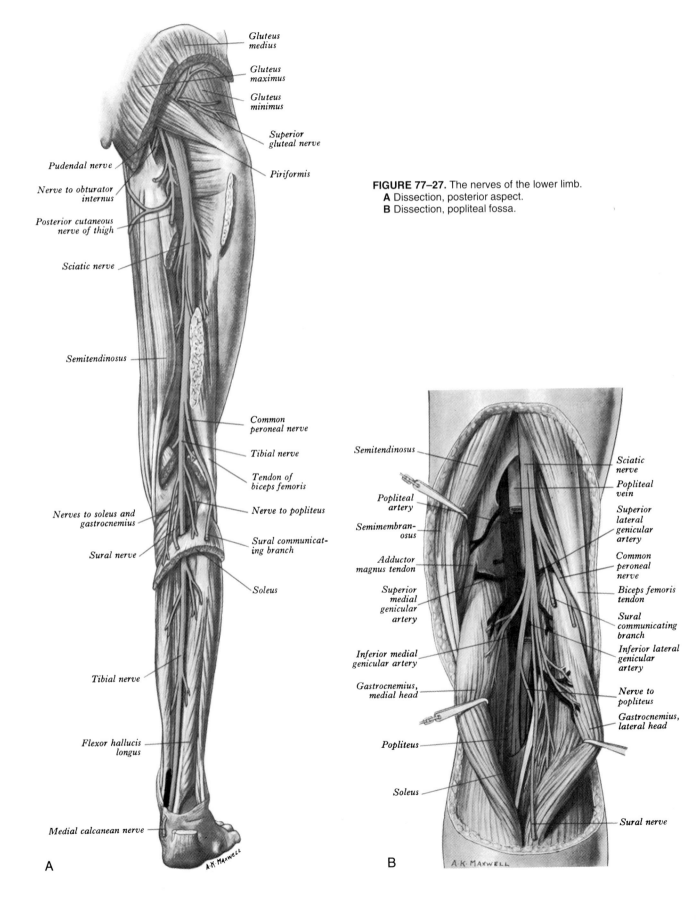

FIGURE 77–27. The nerves of the lower limb.
A Dissection, posterior aspect.
B Dissection, popliteal fossa.

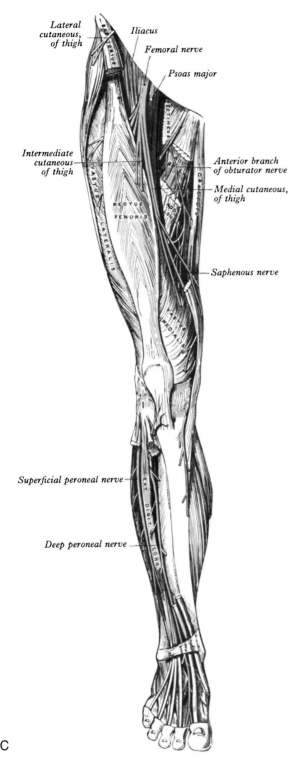

C

FIGURE 77–27 *Continued*
C Dissection, anterior aspect.
(From Williams PL, Warwick R: Gray's Anatomy. 36th Ed. Philadelphia, WB Saunders Co, 1980, pp 1109, 1113.)

through the narrow fibro-osseous tunnel that exists between the carpal bones and a roof consisting of the inelastic transverse carpal ligament.[198, 199, 210] Although specific radiologic projections, such as the carpal tunnel view, allow analysis of the osseous components of this passageway, delineation

of the fibrous roof and the structures within the canal requires ultrasonography,[389] CT,[211, 212, 323] or MR imaging[313, 314, 324, 383–389, 473, 474] (Fig. 77–30).

Causes of the carpal tunnel syndrome are many (Fig. 77–31), including gout, calcium pyrophosphate dihydrate crystal deposition disease, hydroxyapatite crystal deposition disease, acromegaly, hypothyroidism, amyloidosis, rheumatoid arthritis, paraplegia, ganglion cysts, neuromas and other tumors (Fig. 77–32), infection, thrombosis of the median artery, fibrosis of the tendon sheaths, muscle and bone anomalies, hemorrhage, and trauma (Table 77–3). Many of the cases occur on an idiopathic basis, however.[195, 197–199, 213–221, 390, 391, 394, 395, 397] Most patients are between the ages of 35 and 65 years, although children may be affected.[392, 393] More than 80 per cent of affected patients are older than 40 years.[475] Women are affected more frequently than men and, although bilateral involvement is common, the dominant hand usually is involved first and more severely.[198] Aggravating factors include occupations that require a great deal of repetitive hand and wrist motion,[222, 396] pregnancy,[223] and use of oral contraceptive agents.[224] Clinical findings include sensory and motor deficits with numbness and paresthesias of the thumb, index, middle, and one half of the ring finger and atrophy and weakness of the thenar muscles.[399] Pain in the forearm, shoulder, and neck also may be evident. Soft tissue loss of the digits and acro-osteolysis have been observed.[398] Physical examination documents a positive Tinel's sign (paresthesias after percussion of the nerve in the volar aspect of the wrist) and reproduction of pain and paresthesias with the Phalen maneuver, accomplished by flexing the patient's hand at the wrist for longer than 1 min.[196, 325] Nerve conduction tests reveal typical motor or sensory impairment, or both.

The analysis of carpal tunnel syndrome using MR imaging deserves emphasis. Proper interpretation of MR images requires knowledge of the osseous and soft tissue components of the carpal tunnel. This tunnel represents a narrow channel approximately 6 cm long extending from the wrist to the midportion of the palm, through which pass the nine extrinsic finger flexor tendons and the median nerve.[374] The dorsal portion of the carpal tunnel is formed by a concave arch of carpal bones covered by the intrinsic and extrinsic wrist ligaments; the volar portion of the canal is formed by the transverse carpal ligament.[399] This ligament, which is 2.5 to 3.5 mm thick and 3 to 4 cm wide, is attached to the tuberosity of the scaphoid and the crest of the trapezium on the radial side and to the pisiform and the hook of the hamate on the ulnar side.[399] The median nerve normally becomes superficial to the flexor digitorum superficialis muscle bellies approximately 5 cm proximal to the transverse carpal ligament and ordinarily lies superficial in the carpal tunnel and volar to the flexor digitorum superficialis tendons of the index and long fingers.[399] In the palm, the median nerve divides into five branches. The first, and most radial, is the motor branch that supplies the thenar muscles; the remaining four branches supply sensation to the thumb, index, and middle fingers and the radial half of the ring finger.[374]

The narrowest part of the carpal canal is located 2 to 4 cm distal to the wrist crease.[374] At this site, which corresponds to the palmar oriented prominence of the capitate bone, the width of the carpal canal is approximately 10

Text continued on page 3392

TABLE 77–2. Some Nerve Entrapment Syndromes

Nerve	Site (Syndrome)	Causes or Findings
Median	Distal end of humerus	Supracondylar spur, ligament of Struthers
	Elbow (pronator syndrome)	Abnormality of pronator teres, flexor digitorum sublimis, or biceps
	Elbow (anterior interosseous nerve syndrome, Kiloh-Nevin syndrome)	Fracture of humerus or radius, fibrous band, or idiopathic
	Wrist (carpal tunnel syndrome)	Systemic and local factors or idiopathic
	Wrist (sublimis syndrome, pseudo–carpal tunnel syndrome)	Sublimis muscle belly
Ulnar	Elbow (cubital tunnel syndrome, tardy ulnar palsy)	Fracture, arthritis, cubitus valgus, trochlear hypoplasia
	Wrist (ulnar tunnel syndrome, Guyon's canal syndrome)	Fracture, ganglion, arthritis, ulnar artery abnormalities
Radial	Axilla (Saturday night palsy, sleep palsy)	Alcoholism, drug addiction, prolonged sleep with abnormal position of arm
	Distal end of humerus	Fracture involving spiral groove
	Elbow (posterior interosseous nerve syndrome)	Fracture, dislocation, rheumatoid arthritis, tumor, fibrous band
Suprascapular	Shoulder	Scapular fracture, glenohumeral joint dislocation, ganglion, tumor
Plantar and interdigital	Foot (Morton's metatarsalgia)	Digital nerve compression and ischemia, digital neuroma
Posterior tibial	Ankle (tarsal tunnel syndrome)	Sprain, fracture, arthritis, tumor, ganglion, venous tortuosity
Common peroneal	Knee	Sprain, fracture, use of casts, surgery, ganglion, fabella, popliteal cyst
Lateral femoral cutaneous	Anterior superior iliac spine (meralgia paresthetica)	Trauma, pelvic fracture, pelvic tilt
Femoral	Inguinal region	Trauma, tumor, abscess, aneurysm, bleeding
Obturator	Obturator canal	Hernia, inflammation
Sciatic	Sciatic foramen (including piriformis syndrome)	Hip surgery, gluteal injection, tumor
	Knee	Popliteal cyst
Brachial plexus	Neck and shoulder (thoracic outlet syndrome, scalenus anticus syndrome)	Fracture, dislocation, tumor, infection, surgery, injection, cervical rib

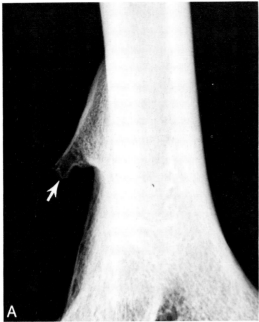

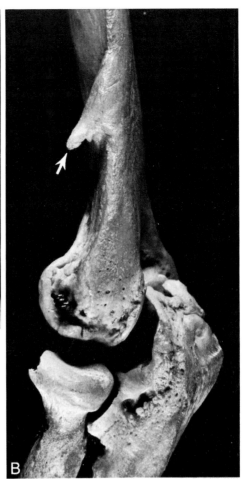

FIGURE 77–28. Entrapment of the median nerve: Supracondylar process. This bony outgrowth (arrows) arises from the anterior surface of the distal portion of the humerus. The ligament of Struthers may extend from its tip to the medial epicondyle of the humerus, leading to compromise of the median nerve.

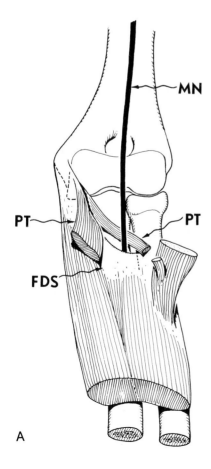

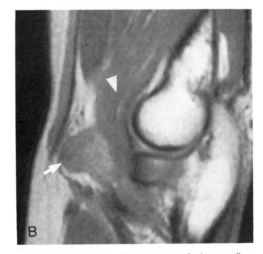

FIGURE 77–29. Entrapment of the median nerve: Pronator syndrome.

A The median nerve (MN) normally passes between the two heads of the pronator teres muscle (PT) and then under the edge of the flexor digitorum sublimis muscle (FDS). It may be compromised in this region. (Reprinted by permission from Thompson WAL, Kopell HP: N Engl J Med 260:1261, 1959.)

B In this 42 year old woman with signs of compression of the median nerve, a sagittal proton density (TR/TE, 1800/20) spin echo MR image reveals a ganglion (arrow) arising from the proximal radioulnar joint located, in part, in front of the brachialis muscle (arrowhead) (Courtesy of S. K. Brahme, M.D., La Jolla, California.)

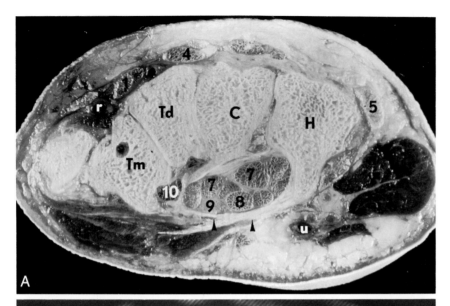

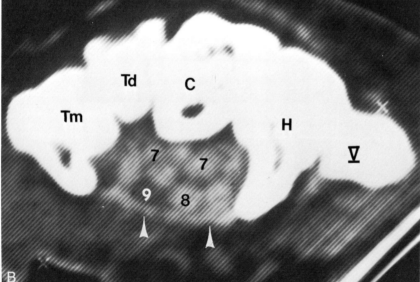

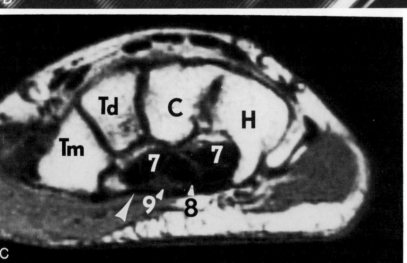

FIGURE 77–30. Entrapment of the median nerve: Carpal tunnel syndrome—normal sectional anatomy. Photograph **(A),** CT scan **(B),** and T1-weighted (TR/TE, 600/20) spin echo MR image **(C)** at the level of the hook of the hamate. Observe the position of the median nerve (9) and the transverse carpal ligament (arrowheads). H, Hamate; C, capitate; Td, trapezoid; Tm, trapezium; 4, digital extensors; 5, extensor carpi ulnaris; 7, flexor digitorum profundus; 8, flexor digitorum superficialis; 10, flexor carpi radialis; u, ulnar artery; r, radial artery; V, base of fifth metacarpal. **(A, B,** From Cone RO, et al: Invest Radiol *18*:546, 1983.)

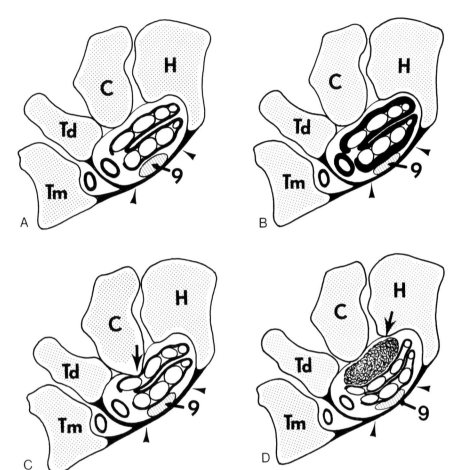

FIGURE 77–31. Entrapment of the median nerve: Carpal tunnel syndrome—potential causes.

A Normal. The median nerve (9) and transverse carpal ligament (arrowheads) are indicated. H, Hamate; C, capitate; Td, trapezoid; Tm, trapezium.

B Tenosynovitis.

C Osseous spur (arrow).

D Mass (arrow).

(From Lipscomb TR: J Musculoskel Med 1(8):35, 1984.)

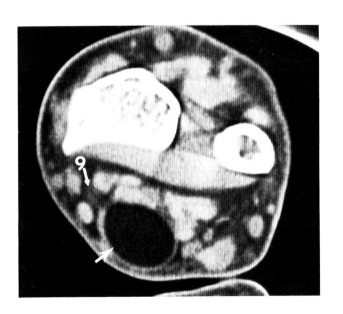

FIGURE 77–32. Entrapment of the median nerve: Carpal tunnel syndrome—Lipoma. This 61 year old man developed an enlarging mass in the palmar aspect of the forearm and wrist and a carpal tunnel syndrome. A transaxial CT scan at the level of the distal portions of the radius and ulna shows the mass (arrow) whose attenuation value was—100 Hounsfield units. The position of the median nerve (9) is indicated. At surgery, an 18 × 14 × 35 mm lipoma, located adjacent to the median nerve, was excised.

TABLE 77–3. Some Causes of the Carpal Tunnel Syndrome

Synovitis
  Rheumatoid arthritis
  Scleroderma
  Systemic lupus erythematosus
  Dermatomyositis
  Seronegative spondyloarthropathies
  Granulomatous and nongranulomatous infections
  Hemophilia
  Crystal deposition diseases

Infiltrative Diseases
  Amyloidosis
  Myxedema
  Acromegaly
  Mucopolysaccharidoses

Trauma
  Fractures and dislocations
  Repetitive and prolonged stress

Tumors and Tumor-like Lesions
  Neuromas
  Lipomas
  Synovial cysts
  Ganglia
  Multiple myeloma

Anatomic Factors
  Small carpal canal
  Thick transverse carpal ligament
  Anomalous nerves, muscles, bursae

Medical and Surgical Procedures
  Arteriovenous fistulae
  Artery punctures, catheterizations

Miscellaneous
  Diabetes mellitus
  Polymyalgia rheumatica
  Hemorrhage
  Hypoparathyroidism
  Pregnancy
  Use of oral contraceptives
  Gynecologic surgery
  Osteoarthritis
  Pyridoxine deficiency
  Paget's disease
  Idiopathic

mm.[475] Variations occur in the carpal canal width and area in asymptomatic men and women, however, although the cross sectioned area and width tend to be decreased in patients with the carpal tunnel syndrome, findings that may be more prominent in the proximal portion of the canal.[394] Compression of the median nerve in the carpal tunnel occurs when there is too little space or too much tissue, or both, within the tunnel.[399] Patients with the carpal tunnel syndrome have elevated intracarpal tunnel pressure, which increases further with flexion or extension of the wrist. These wrist positions generally produce a decrease in the transverse dimension, the anteroposterior dimension, or the cross-sectional area of the carpal tunnel, or combinations of these parameters.[473] Such elevations in pressure are responsible for nerve ischemia, which in turn leads to epineurial edema.[399] Local edema fluid may be dispersed within the epineurium, or it may cause enlargement of the median nerve. Persistent ischemia contributes to epineural fibrosis that may be responsible for irreversibility of the process.

In 1989, Mesgarzadeh and coworkers[384, 385] provided a detailed description of MR imaging findings of the carpal tunnel in normal persons and in those with the carpal tunnel syndrome. The MR imaging appearance of the structures in the normal carpal tunnel in the neutral position and with flexion and extension of the wrist was further delineated by Zeiss and associates[386] in the same year. Both studies emphasized the value of the transaxial plane in the assessment of the median nerve, although supplementary data were provided by coronal and sagittal imaging. In the neutral position, the normal median nerve typically is situated in one of two standard positions: either anterior to the superficial flexor tendon of the index finger or interposed more posterolaterally between this tendon and the flexor pollicus longus tendon.[386] During wrist extension, the nerve always maintains or assumes an anterior position between the superficial index finger flexor and the flexor retinaculum, while the flexor tendons move posteriorly; during wrist flexion, the tendons shift anteriorly toward the retinaculum, and the median nerve either remains in its anterior position between the superficial index finger flexor and retinaculum or becomes interposed between the superficial flexor tendons of the index finger and thumb or middle and ring fingers.[386, 387] When positioned anteriorly, the median nerve may appear flattened in an anteroposterior plane between the tendon and the flexor retinaculum, a finding that is most evident in wrist flexion and least evident in wrist extension; interposed median nerves may be either round or flattened in a mediolateral plane.[386] In general, however, the size of the normal median nerve is fairly constant within the carpal tunnel, although it may appear slightly smaller at the level of the pisiform bone.[384]

As defined by Mesgarzadeh and colleagues,[385] four general findings characterize the MR imaging appearance of the carpal tunnel syndrome: swelling of the medial nerve, best evaluated at the level of the pisiform bone; flattening of the median nerve, judged most reliably at the level of the hamate bone; palmar bowing of the flexor retinaculum, best visualized at the level of the hamate bone; and increase signal intensity of the median nerve on T2-weighted spin echo MR images (Fig. 77–33). Additional MR imaging findings of the carpal tunnel syndrome that were noted in this investigation were cause specific and included evidence of tenosynovitis, synovial hypertrophy in rheumatoid arthritis, ganglion cysts (Fig. 77–34), a persistent median artery, an increased amount of fatty tissue, and a large adductor pollicis muscle. Other investigators have confirmed the general and cause specific MR imaging abnormalities of the carpal tunnel syndrome,[388, 389] although the alterations may be subtle and changes in size and configuration of the median nerve may require quantitative assessment. Furthermore, the clinical impact of MR imaging in cases of carpal tunnel syndrome needs additional study.[466]

Supplementary techniques may aid in the diagnosis of the carpal tunnel syndrome with MR imaging. These techniques include assessment of the carpal tunnel during flexion and extension of the wrist,[473] with or without the intravenous injection of a gadolinium compound,[474] and MR imaging after provocative movement of the wrist.

Incision of the flexor retinaculum, the carpal tunnel release, commonly is used in the treatment of carpal tunnel syndrome. This can be accomplished with open surgery or endoscopic control.[476] It is an operation not without complications, including residual or recurrent compression of the median nerve. Such complications may reflect the presence of fibrous fixation of the nerve leading to traction neuropa-

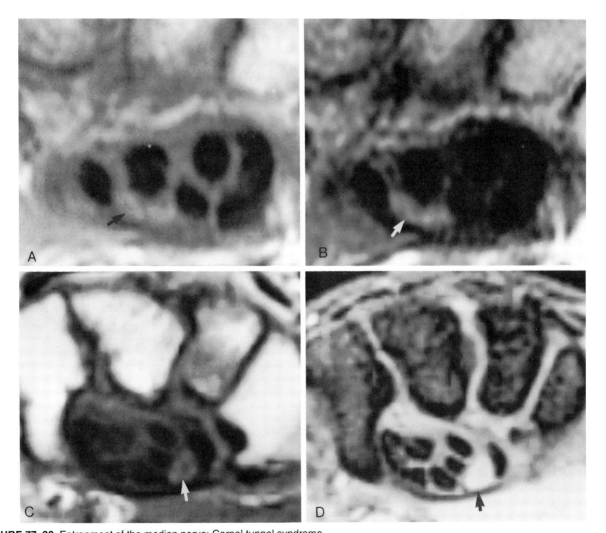

FIGURE 77–33. Entrapment of the median nerve: Carpal tunnel syndrome.

A, B Transverse proton density (TR/TE, 1800/20) **(A)** and T2-weighted (TR/TE, 1800/70) **(B)** spin echo MR images at the level of the metacarpal bases reveal enlargement and flattening of the median nerve (arrows) with subtle increased signal intensity in **B.** (Courtesy of C. Sebrechts, M.D., San Diego, California.)

C, D Transverse T1-weighted (TR/TE, 417/20) spin echo **(C)** and multiplanar gradient recalled (MPGR) (TR/TE, 550/20; flip angle, 20 degrees) **(D)** MR images at the level of the hook of the hamate show a prominent median nerve (arrows), which shows increased signal intensity in **D,** and volar bowing of the flexor retinaculum. Tenosynovitis also is present. (Courtesy of S. Moreland, M.D., La Jolla, California.)

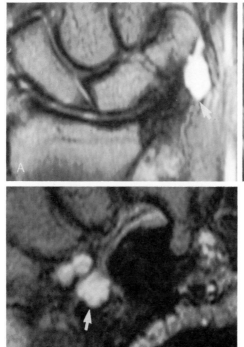
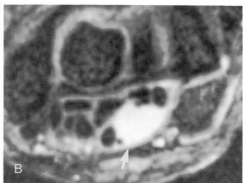

FIGURE 77–34. Entrapment of the median nerve: Carpal tunnel syndrome—ganglia.

A, B A coronal T2-weighted (TR/TE, 2000/80) spin echo MR image (A) and a transverse multiplanar gradient recalled (MPGR) image (TR/TE, 550/17; flip angle, 20 degrees) (B) show high signal intensity in a synovial cyst (arrows) that arose from the pisiform-triquetral joint and extended into the carpal tunnel.

C In this patient, a transverse T2-weighted (TR/TE, 2200/80) spin echo MR image shows a recurrent ganglion (arrow) adjacent to the median nerve.

thy or of congenital variation or anomalies of the median nerve, tendons, and adjacent muscles.[400] The role of MR imaging in the assessment of postoperative residual or recurrent carpal tunnel syndrome is not clear, although reports indicate that the technique may outline incomplete incision of the flexor retinaculum, persistent neuritis of the median nerve, excessive fat within the carpal tunnel, and the development of neuromas[385, 467] (Fig. 77–35). After carpal tunnel release, a change in shape and an increase in volume of the carpal tunnel occur, which must be taken into account when assessing postoperative MR images.

Sublimis Syndrome (Pseudo-carpal Tunnel Syndrome). Compromise of a more proximal portion of the median nerve may relate to its compression by the lateral border of the sublimis muscle belly.[225] Clinical findings resemble those of a true carpal tunnel syndrome.

Ulnar Nerve. Entrapment of the *ulnar nerve* occurs most commonly near the elbow or wrist[196, 199, 401] and rarely in the forearm.[226]

Cubital Tunnel Syndrome. Ulnar nerve entrapment is seen most frequently at the level of the cubital tunnel. In this location, the ulnar nerve extends through a fibro-osseous canal formed by the medial epicondyle and an aponeurotic band bridging the dual origin of the flexor carpi ulnaris muscle.[227, 405] This condition probably is the second most common compressive neuropathy of the upper extremity (after the carpal tunnel syndrome).[404] Typical causes of compression of the ulnar nerve in the cubital tunnel are trauma[195, 197] and progressive cubitus valgus deformity (tardy ulnar nerve palsy), although additional causes include nerve subluxation, osteoarthritis, rheumatoid arthritis, synovial cysts, prolonged bedrest, flexion deformity of the elbow, anomalous muscles, trochlear hypoplasia, aneurysms, and masses as well as idiopathic entrapment.[197, 227–231, 402, 403] (Fig. 77–36). Persons at risk include athletes involved in sports that involve a throwing motion and musicians who must maintain prolonged flexion of the elbow.[475]

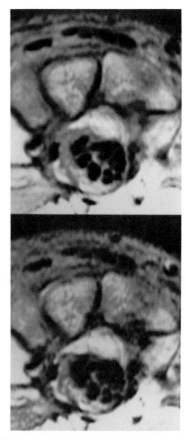

FIGURE 77–35. Entrapment of the median nerve: Recurrent carpal tunnel syndrome. Transverse proton density (TR/TE, 1800/20) (top) and T2-weighted (TR/TE, 1800/70) (bottom) spin echo MR images show evidence of prior incision of the flexor retinaculum with volar migration of the contents of the carpal tunnel, a vertically oriented median nerve, and subtle evidence of proliferative synovitis. This 43 year old woman had persistent symptoms of median nerve compression after the operative procedure. (Courtesy of S. K. Brahme, M.D., La Jolla, California.)

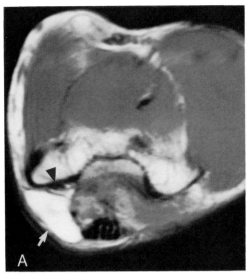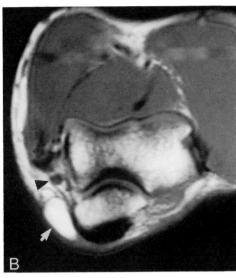

FIGURE 77–36. Entrapment of the ulnar nerve: Cubital tunnel syndrome. A lipoma (arrows) adjacent to the ulnar nerve (arrowheads) is well shown in these transverse proton density (TR/TE, 2000/20) spin echo MR images. It led to clinical findings of ulnar nerve entrapment in this 36 year old man. (Courtesy of Z. Rosenberg, M.D., New York, New York.)

Clinical findings are sensory deficits and weakness of the flexor carpi ulnaris muscle, flexor digitorum profundus muscle of the fourth and fifth fingers, and intrinsic hand muscles.[196] A positive Tinel's sign follows percussion of the ulnar nerve at the level of the elbow, and the nerve itself may be palpable, enlarged, and tender. Axial radiographs may reveal medial trochlear osteophytes or medial incongruity of the elbow joint, or both.[304] Conservative measures may be used to treat this condition, although operative intervention with either local decompression or anterior transposition of the nerve may be required.[475]

Guyon's Canal Syndrome (Ulnar Tunnel Syndrome). An entrapment neuropathy of the ulnar nerve may occur in the wrist where the nerve enters the palm through the canal of Guyon, the ulnar tunnel (Figs. 77–37 and 77–38). The walls of the canal consist of the pisiform bone medially and the hook of the hamate laterally.[199] The floor of the canal is composed of the flexor retinaculum and the origin of the hypothenar muscles, and the roof is composed of the volar carpal ligament, palmaris brevis muscle, and fibers from the palmar fascia.[232] The contents of the canal are the ulnar nerve, ulnar artery, and fatty tissue; no flexor tendons pass through the canal.[410] The ulnar nerve, after giving rise to the dorsal cutaneous branch, enters the canal medial to the artery. Within the canal, the ulnar nerve divides into superficial sensory and deep motor branches.[410]

The most frequent causes of ulnar nerve entrapment in Guyon's canal are ganglia and accidental, occupational, or recreational (bicycling) trauma.[233, 234] Fractures of the hook of the hamate also may lead to such entrapment. Although there are no tendons in this canal, tenosynovitis (as in rheumatoid arthritis) within the carpal tunnel can compress the ulnar nerve just proximal to Guyon's canal.[196] Additional causes are anomalous muscles, pisiform-hamate coalition, calcinosis, Dupuytren's contracture, and ulnar artery abnormalities.[195, 406–409] Predominant clinical manifestations may be motor or sensory, or both, influenced by the site of nerve compromise and the type of nerve fibers that are involved.[197, 199, 305]

MR imaging can be used to study the normal Guyon's canal and its abnormalities.[384, 411] In one study, the normal ulnar nerve had a mean diameter of 3 mm and bifurcated an average distance of 12 mm from the proximal margin of the pisiform bone.[411] The precise role of this imaging technique in the evaluation of the ulnar tunnel syndrome is not established, however.

Double Crush Syndrome. A type of double crush syndrome relates to entrapment of the ulnar nerve occurring concomitantly with disease of the lower cervical spine or the thoracic outlet syndrome.[196, 375]

Radial Nerve. Entrapment of the *radial nerve* may occur in the axilla, elbow, or proximal portion of the forearm. Five distinct syndromes of radial nerve compression occur at these three different sites: Near the wrist, either the superficial radial nerve or the posterior interosseous nerve may be compressed; near the elbow, the posterior interosseous syndrome or radial tunnel syndrome may appear; and high radial nerve compression occurs proximally in the arm.[412] Four of these situations deserve emphasis.

Saturday Night Palsy. Persons who sleep with the arm held in an improper position such that pressure is exerted on the proximal medial aspect of the extremity may develop radial nerve dysfunction owing to its compression in the axilla or spiral groove of the humerus.[195–197] This type of sleep palsy is particularly common in alcoholics and drug abusers and in patients using crutches. Weakness of the triceps, brachioradialis, and extensors and supinators of the hand and wrist is seen.[196] Similar findings may occur with tourniquet injuries and after humeral fractures.

Entrapment in the Spiral Groove of the Humerus. Compression of the radial nerve may occur between the origins of the lateral and medial heads of the triceps muscle where it winds around the humerus in close proximity to the bone.[197] Humeral fractures are one of the potential causes of this type of nerve entrapment.[326, 468]

Posterior Interosseous Nerve Syndrome. Compression of the posterior interosseous nerve, a purely motor branch of the radial nerve, occurs just distal to the elbow as the nerve passes into the supinator muscle (Fig. 77–39).[415] Causes of this compression neuropathy include dislocations of the elbow,[235] fractures,[236] rheumatoid arthritis,[237] soft tissue tumors,[238, 413] ganglia,[414] and traumatic or developmental fibrous bands.[195] Partial or complete inability to extend the digits at the metacarpophalangeal joints, similar to that noted with extensor tendon rupture, is the major finding.[196]

Radial Tunnel Syndrome. At the elbow, radial nerve

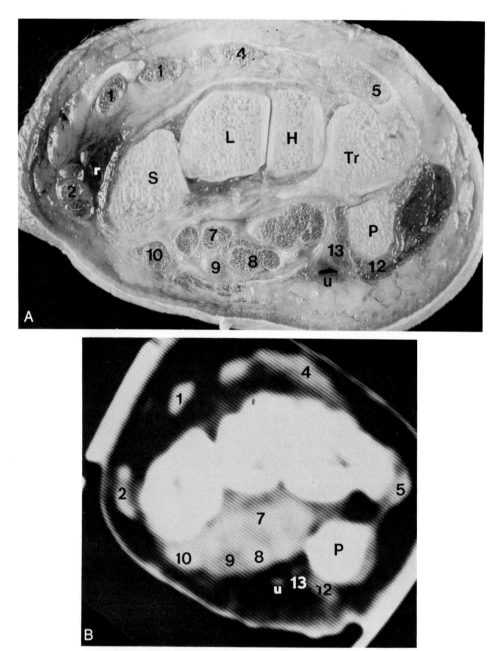

FIGURE 77–37. Entrapment of the ulnar nerve: Guyon's canal syndrome (ulnar tunnel syndrome)—normal sectional anatomy. Photograph **(A)** and CT scan **(B)** at the level of the pisiform-triquetral joint. The plane of section is slightly more proximal than that shown in Figure 77–30. The position of the ulnar nerve (13) and ulnar artery (u) within Guyon's canal is shown. S, Scaphoid; L, lunate; H, hamate; Tr, triquetrum; P, pisiform; 1, extensor carpi radialis and brevis; 2, abductor pollicis longus and brevis; 4, digital extensors; 5, extensor carpi ulnaris; 7, flexor digitorum profundus; 8, flexor digitorum superficialis; 9, median nerve; 10, flexor carpi radialis; 12, flexor carpi ulnaris; r, radial artery. (From Cone RO, et al: Invest Radiol *18:*546, 1983.)

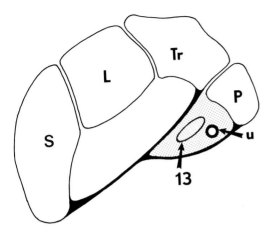

FIGURE 77–38. Entrapment of the ulnar nerve: Guyon's canal syndrome (ulnar tunnel syndrome)—normal sectional anatomy. Observe the ulnar nerve (13) and ulnar artery (u). S, scaphoid; L, lunate; Tr, triquetrum; P, pisiform. (From Grundberg AB: J Hand Surg [Br] *9:*72, 1984.)

compression may result in pain referred to the lateral aspect of the humerus, elbow, and dorsal region of the wrist without muscle weakness.[412] Causes leading to this syndrome are similar to those producing the posterior interosseous nerve syndrome (the syndromes sometimes are considered together as variations of a single entity), although tumors rarely are implicated.[412, 416] This syndrome may occur after radial head excision.[416]

Suprascapular Nerve. Entrapment of the *suprascapular nerve* occurs most commonly as it passes through the suprascapular notch. This nerve, which contains motor and sensory fibers, arises from the upper trunk of the brachial plexus, runs deep to the trapezius and omohyoid muscles, and enters the supraspinous fossa through the suprascapular notch, passing below the superior transverse scapular ligament.[239, 417] After the suprascapular nerve passes through the notch, it supplies the supraspinatus and infraspinatus muscles and the articular branches to both the glenohumeral and acromioclavicular joints.[417] Sensory and sympathetic nerve fibers innervate two thirds of the shoulder capsule. The most frequent site of nerve encroachment is at the point where the suprascapular nerve traverses the suprascapular notch adjacent to the suprascapular ligament; variability of the size and shape of the notch and ligament, together with the angulation of the nerve as it crosses the superior portion of the notch, predisposes the nerve to injury at this point.[418] As the nerve continues over the lateral part of the scapular spine and spinoglenoid notch and under the inferior transverse ligament and the spinoglenoid ligament to the infraspinatus fossa, other sites of entrapment are possible but rare.[418, 419] Potential causes of suprascapular nerve entrapment include a scapular fracture or glenohumeral joint dislocation, occupational or recreational stress (as in weightlifting), ganglia, tumors, developmental anomalies of the notch, or any condition that leads to traction on the nerve, allowing its compression by the osseous or ligamentous edges of the foramen.[199, 239–242, 327, 418, 422] The major clinical findings, which may be unilateral or bilateral, are shoulder pain and weakness and atrophy of the supraspinatus and infraspinatus muscles, with limited external rotation and abduction of the humerus.

Entrapment neuropathy of the suprascapular nerve by a ganglion deserves special emphasis.[420, 421] Most affected pa-

tients are young men involved in jobs requiring manual labor or are weightlifters. Such ganglia arising at the scapular notch compress both motor branches of the suprascapular nerve, resulting in weakness or atrophy of both the supraspinatus and the infraspinatus muscles; ganglia arising near the spinoglenoid notch affect a more distal segment of the nerve, resulting in selective involvement of the infraspinatus muscle. Ultrasonography, CT, and MR imaging can be used to diagnose such ganglia.[420, 423] On MR images a fluid-filled mass communicating with the joint, muscle atrophy, and in some cases a rotator cuff tear are evident[423] (Fig. 77–40). Associated tears of the glenoid labrum also are observed, suggesting that the pathogenesis of some of these ganglion cysts is similar to that of meniscal cysts about the knee (see Chapter 70).

Axillary Nerve. The axillary nerve arises from the posterior cord of the brachial plexus, its fibers being derived from the fifth and sixth cervical nerves. It is located behind the axillary artery and anterior to the subscapularis muscle. At the lower margin of this muscle, the axillary nerve extends backward and, in company with the posterior circumflex humeral vessels, enters the quadrilateral space, which is bounded above by the teres minor muscle, below by the teres major muscle, medially by the long head of the triceps muscle, and laterally by the surgical neck of the humerus. Although rare, a quadrilateral space syndrome produced by compression of the posterior circumflex hu-

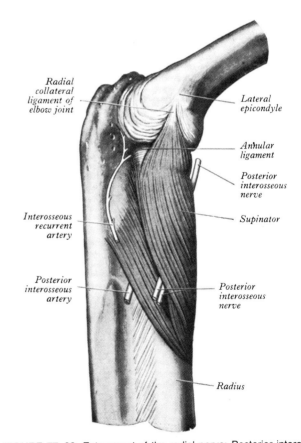

FIGURE 77–39. Entrapment of the radial nerve: Posterior interosseous nerve syndrome—normal anatomy. Compression of this purely motor branch of the radial nerve occurs distal to the elbow as the nerve passes into the supinator muscle. (From Williams PL, Warwick R: Gray's Anatomy. 36th Ed. Philadelphia, WB Saunders Co, 1980, p 582.)

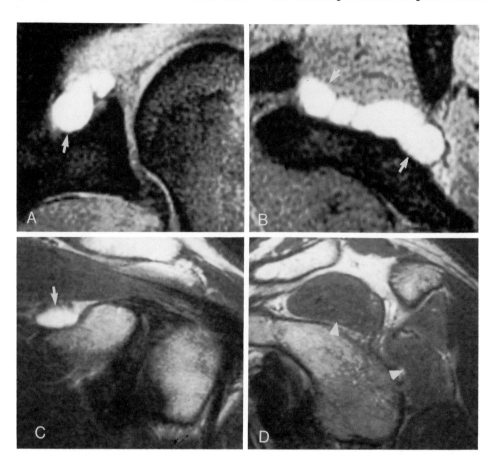

FIGURE 77–40. Entrapment of the suprascapular nerve: Ganglia.

A, B Coronal oblique multiplanar gradient recalled (MPGR) (TR/TE, 540/15; flip angle, 25 degrees) **(A)** and sagittal oblique multiplanar gradient recalled (MPGR) (TR/TE, 580/18; flip angle, 20 degrees) **(B)** MR images show the ganglion (arrows) located deep to the supraspinatus and infraspinatus muscles. (Courtesy of P. Kindynis, M.D., Geneva, Switzerland.)

C, D Coronal oblique T2-weighted (TR/TE, 2500/96) **(C)** and sagittal oblique T2-weighted (TR/TE, 2500/96) **(D)** spin echo MR images reveal the ganglion (arrow) and subtle changes in signal intensity in the supraspinatus and infraspinatus muscles (arrowheads). (Courtesy of S. Eilenberg, M.D., San Diego, California.)

meral artery and the axillary nerve or one or more of its major branches has been described.[417, 424] The syndrome predominates in young men and women, usually being seen in the third or fourth decade of life, and is more common in the dominant upper extremity. Symptoms include paresthesias in the upper extremity and anterior shoulder pain that may interfere with daily physical activity. Asymmetry in peripheral pulses in the arm may be encountered. Subclavian arteriography usually is diagnostic.[424] MR imaging also allows accurate diagnosis (see Chapter 70).

Medial or Lateral Plantar Nerves. Entrapment of the *medial or lateral plantar nerves* of the foot (Fig. 77–41) as a result of injury to these nerves near the transverse intertarsal ligament leads to local weakness and burning sensation. In this location, a neuroma may develop. This is especially common between the third and fourth toes, where it is termed a Morton's neuroma[243]; the second most common location is between the second and third toes. Resulting symptoms and signs are known as Morton's metatarsalgia.[244] The precise cause of Morton's neuralgia is not clear; nerve ischemia[245] or entrapment[244, 246] has been implicated. The taut transverse metatarsal ligament appears to play a critical role in the compression of the interdigital nerve, and the compressive effect may be augmented by an enlarged forefoot bursa that may occur in such diseases as rheumatoid arthritis.[425] Histologic and electron microscopic analysis reveals edema of the endoneurium, perineural fibrosis, and axonal degeneration and necrosis.[426] These findings are consistent with nerve damage secondary to mechanical impingement. An inflammatory response within the affected nerve may result from such impingement.

Ultrasonography[427] and MR imaging[428] may be used in the diagnosis of a Morton's neuroma. The typical sonographic appearance is that of an ovoid, hypoechoic mass oriented parallel to the long axis of the metatarsal bones.[427] The MR imaging characteristics include a mass with decreased signal intensity, well demarcated from adjacent fat tissue, on T1-weighted spin echo MR images, a mass that is isointense or slightly hypointense to fat tissue on T2-weighted spin echo images, and evidence of intermetatarsal bursitis[428] (Fig. 77–42). The relatively low signal intensity of the lesions on T2-weighted images, which differs from the high signal intensity of true neuromas on such images, is consistent with their fibrous composition.[429] MR imaging accomplished with fat suppression techniques after the intravenous administration of gadolinium-based contrast agents may lead to improved detection of Morton's neuromas.[469]

Posterior Tibial Nerve. Compression of the *posterior tibial nerve* at the medial aspect of the ankle results in the tarsal tunnel syndrome.[195–197, 243, 247–249, 430–433] The tarsal tunnel is located behind and below the medial malleolus; its floor is bony and its roof is formed by the flexor retinaculum.[248] The resulting fibro-osseous channel allows passage of the tibialis posterior, flexor digitorum longus and flexor hallucis longus muscles and the posterior tibial artery and vein, in addition to the posterior tibial nerve (Fig. 77–43). Trauma is the leading cause of this compression neuropathy; tissue scarring after an ankle sprain or osseous deformity after a calcaneal fracture is a common cause. Additional causes are synovial inflammation (especially in rheumatoid arthritis), foot deformities including pes planus

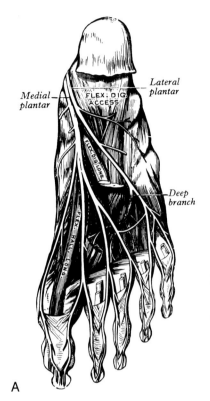

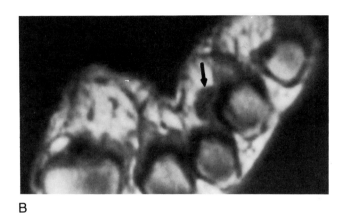

FIGURE 77–41. Entrapment of the medial and lateral plantar nerves.

A Normal anatomy. A dissection of the plantar aspect of the foot has been accomplished. (From Williams PL, Warwick R: Gray's Anatomy, 36th Ed. Philadelphia, WB Saunders Co, 1980, p 1114.)

B Morton's neuroma. Observe the neuroma (arrow) between the third and fourth toes on a coronal T1-weighted (TR/TE, 600/25) spin echo MR image obtained with the patient prone.

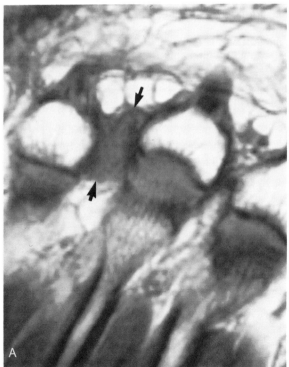

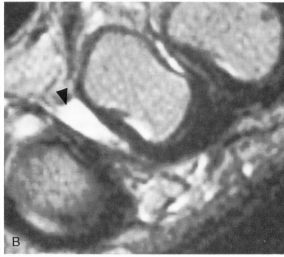

FIGURE 77–42. Morton's neuroma.

A An oblique transverse T1-weighted (TR/TE, 500/27) spin echo MR image shows the neuroma (arrows), of low signal intensity, in the web space between the third and fourth toes.

B An oblique coronal T2-weighted (TR/TE, 2500/80) spin echo MR image reveals a fluid-filled intermetatarsal bursa (arrowhead) at a level just proximal to the neuroma.

(From Erickson SJ, et al: Radiology *181*:833, 1991.)

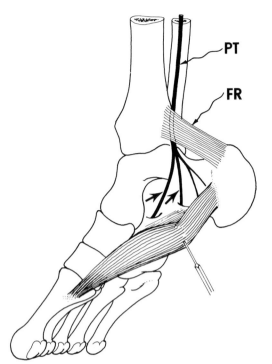

FIGURE 77–43. Entrapment of the posterior tibial nerve: Tarsal tunnel syndrome—normal anatomy. The posterior tibial nerve (PT) passes beneath the flexor retinaculum (FR), and then divides into various nerves including the medial and lateral plantar nerves (arrows). (Reprinted by permission from Kopell HP, Thompson WAL: N Engl J Med 262:56, 1960.)

and talocalcaneal coalition, benign tumors (neurilemoma, lipoma, ganglion), an os trigonum, and dilated or tortuous veins, although spontaneously developing neuropathy also is described.[248] An insidious onset of pain and burning sensation aggravated by activity in the plantar aspect of the foot is typical. The clinical manifestations may be modified in instances in which additional nerve lesions involve the same limb[434] and compression involves the deep peroneal nerve under the inferior extensor retinaculum on the dorsum of the foot and ankle (anterior tarsal tunnel syndrome).[435]

MR imaging represents an effective technique in the assessment of the tarsal tunnel syndrome. The complex normal anatomy of the tarsal tunnel as delineated with MR imaging has been the subject of several investigations, to which the interested reader should refer.[436, 437] Coronal, transaxial, and oblique transaxial imaging planes are most useful, allowing identification of the flexor retinaculum, the fine septa deep to the retinaculum, the contents of the tunnel, the separating septum between the medial and lateral plantar nerves distal to the retinaculum, and the three terminal branches of the posterior tibial nerve[437] (Fig. 77–44). In instances of the tarsal tunnel syndrome, MR imaging can provide information regarding its cause, including the documentation of the presence and nature of an extrinsic mass[437–439] (Figs. 77–45 and 77–46). In this fashion, neurogenic tumors, ganglia, tenosynovitis, posttraumatic fibrosis, varicosities, muscle hypertrophy, fractures, and other types of pathologic conditions can be outlined. CT and ultrasonography also can be used for this purpose. MR imaging, however, appears to be the best of these techniques and can be used to document causes of ineffectual operative treatment of the tarsal tunnel syndrome.[440]

Common Peroneal Nerve. Compression of the *common peroneal nerve or its branches* (deep, superficial, recurrent) occurs near the knee (Fig. 77–47). This nerve is derived from the sciatic nerve, passes from the popliteal region to the lateral aspect of the fibular neck, and divides into its three branches.[243] Entrapment of the common peroneal nerve, although relatively infrequent, typically occurs as it winds around the neck of the fibula[197]; causes of such entrapment are injury with stretching or traction of the nerve, popliteal cysts, total knee arthroplasty, high tibial osteotomy, arthroscopic surgery of the knee, tight casts, masses, and ganglia[250, 251] (Fig. 77–48), as well as a normal, enlarged, or malpositioned fabella.[252, 253, 441, 442, 470] Transient lesions are caused by habitual sitting with the legs crossed or sleeping on a firm mattress.[195] Clinical findings include impaired dorsiflexion and eversion of the foot and impaired extension of the toes, resulting in a footdrop.[197] Inversion of the foot produces pain.[243] Rarely, entrapment of one or more of the branches of the common peroneal nerve, rather than the entire nerve, occurs.[254, 255]

Lateral Femoral Cutaneous Nerve. Compression of the *lateral femoral cutaneous nerve* leads to a syndrome termed meralgia paresthetica, consisting of burning pain and hypesthesia in the anterolateral aspect of the thigh.[195–197, 243] This sensory nerve is derived from the second and third lumbar nerve roots and enters the thigh through an opening formed by the attachment of the inguinal ligament to the superior anterior iliac spine.[195] It is in the latter region that entrapment may occur, owing to direct trauma (such as a fracture of the anterior surface of the ilium), harvesting of a bone graft from the iliac crest, or a pelvic tilt (related to a shift of the trunk or a shortened lower extremity).[196] A similar syndrome can relate to midlumbar spinal stenosis, however.[443]

Femoral Nerve. Entrapment of the *femoral nerve,* arising from the second, third, and fourth lumbar nerve roots, is rare but occurs in the inguinal region of the pelvis (Fig. 77–27C). Causes include an inguinal hernia, surgical scar, psoas abscess, pelvic tumor, lymphoma, iliopsoas bursitis, bleeding (hemophilia and anticoagulant therapy),[256] aneurysms of the external iliac and femoral arteries, and trauma.[196, 197, 444, 445] Clinical manifestations are pain and tenderness in the groin, atrophy and weakness of the quadriceps muscle, diminution or absence of the knee jerk reflex, and sensory loss in the anteromedial aspect of the thigh.

Obturator Nerve. Compression of the *obturator nerve* occurs in the obturator canal, an osseofibrous tunnel whose roof is the obturator groove of the pubic bone and whose floor is composed of the obturator muscles separated by the obturator membrane.[243] This nerve supplies the adductor musculature, its bone margin, a portion of the hip joint, and a cutaneous region in the medial aspect of the thigh and knee. Causes of compression of the obturator nerve include an obturator hernia and inflammation (as in osteitis pubis).[243]

Sciatic Nerve. The *sciatic nerve,* the largest in diameter in the body, is derived from the sacral plexus, which is formed from the fourth and fifth lumbar and first and second sacral roots. As a single trunk, it exits the pelvis by traversing the greater sciatic foramen, below the piriformis muscle, and then descends between the greater trochanter of the femur and the ischial tuberosity, deep to the gluteus

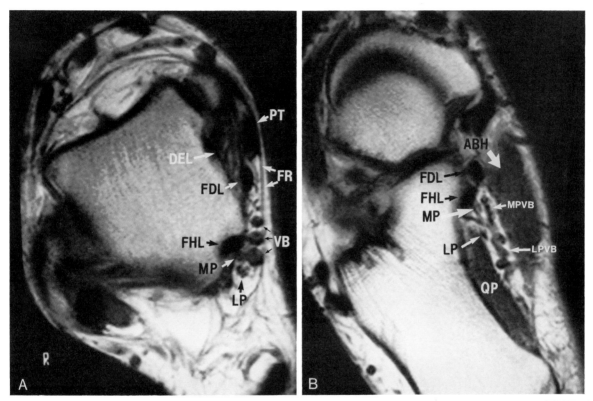

FIGURE 77–44. Entrapment of the posterior tibial nerve: Tarsal tunnel syndrome—normal anatomy. Transverse T1-weighted (TR/TE, 600/20) spin echo MR images through the tibiotalar **(A)** and talocalcaneal **(B)** portions of the tarsal tunnel are shown. In **A,** note the position of the posterior tibial tendon (*PT*) and flexor retinaculum (*FR*). The medial plantar (*MP*) and lateral plantar (*LP*) nerves lie deep to the vascular bundles (*VB*). The medial plantar nerve is in close proximity to the flexor hallucis longus tendon (*FHL*). The deltoid ligament (*DEL*) and flexor digitorum longus muscle (*FDL*) are seen. In **B,** the lateral plantar neurovascular bundle (*LPVB*) and medial plantar neurovascular bundle (*MPVB*) lie deep to the abductor hallucis muscle (*ABH*), and beneath these bundles lie the medial plantar (*MP*) and lateral plantar (*LP*) nerves. Other identified structures are the quadratus plantae muscle (*QP*), the flexor hallucis longus tendon (*FHL*), and the flexor digitorum longus muscle (*FDL*). The roof of the tarsal tunnel is formed in **A** by the flexor retinaculum and in **B** by the abductor hallucis muscle. (From Kerr R, et al: J Comput Assist Tomogr *15*:280, 1991.)

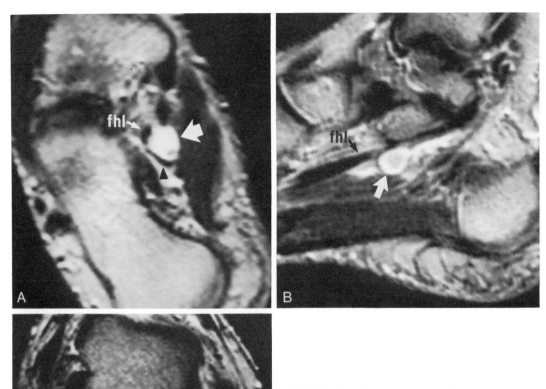

FIGURE 77–45. Entrapment of the posterior tibial nerve: Tarsal tunnel syndrome.

A, B Neurilemoma. Transverse **(A)** and sagittal **(B)** T2-weighted (TR/TE, 1800/80) spin echo MR images demonstrate a mass (arrows) of high signal intensity adjacent to the flexor hallucis longus (*fhl*) tendon, compressing the medial plantar neurovascular bundle (arrowhead, **A**).

C Blunt trauma. A transverse T2-weighted (TR/TE, 1800/80) spin echo MR image reveals a calcaneal contusion and fluid (arrows) within the tarsal tunnel, overlying the neurovascular bundle (*NVB*).

From Kerr R, et al: J Comput Assist Tomogr *15*:280, 1991.)

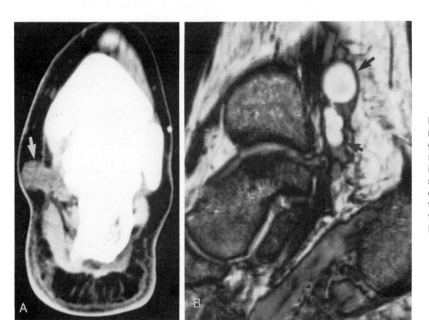

FIGURE 77–46. Entrapment of the posterior tibial nerve: Tarsal tunnel syndrome—ganglion. A ganglion (arrows) occurring on the medial and posterior portions of the ankle in this 48 year old man is shown on a soft tissue image of a coronal CT scan **(A)** and on a sagittal gradient recalled acquisition in the steady state (GRASS) image obtained with volumetric acquisition (TR/TE, 30/12; flip angle, 40 degrees) **(B).** (Courtesy of G. Bock, M.D., Winnipeg, Manitoba, Canada.)

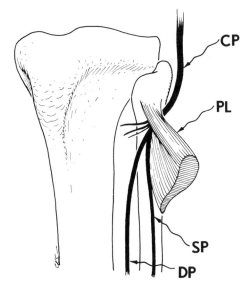

FIGURE 77–47. Entrapment of the common peroneal nerve and its branches: Normal anatomy. On this posterior view, observe that the common peroneal nerve (CP) winds around the back of the fibula in intimate association with the peroneus longus muscle (PL) and then divides into the deep peroneal nerve (DP) and the superficial peroneal nerve (SP). (Reprinted by permission from Kopell HP, Thompson WAL: N Engl J Med *262*:56, 1960.)

maximus muscle (Fig. 77–27A). In the back of the thigh, above the popliteal fossa, it divides into two large branches, the tibial nerve and the common peroneal nerve. The course of the sciatic nerve and its major branches is well shown with CT, ultrasonography, and MR imaging.[257–260, 315, 446] Although a prolapsed intervertebral disc is the most common cause of sciatica, entrapment neuropathies of the sciatic nerve also are encountered.

The proximal portion of the sciatic nerve infrequently is compressed. Slightly more distally, compression neuropathy of the sciatic nerve may be produced by immobility, prolonged squatting, Paget's disease of the ischium, avulsion of the ischial tuberosity, fractures about and dislocations of the hip, posttraumatic ossification in the biceps femoris muscle, intramuscular injections, and hip surgery.[196, 261–263, 447] Below the sciatic foramen, a piriformis syndrome represents a distinct pattern of nerve compression in which symptoms and signs resemble those of discal herniation.[196, 448–451] It appears to be caused by enlargement, inflammation, or anatomic variations of the piriformis muscle. As the sciatic nerve usually passes between the piriformis muscle above and the gemellus muscles below, nerve entrapment is not unexpected in these situations.

The lower portion of the sciatic nerve in the region of the knee may be compressed by synovial cysts in the popliteal fossa, a recognized complication of rheumatoid arthritis.[264]

Plexus Neuropathies. Plexus neuropathies can occur in regions other than the sacral area. Tumors, infections, trauma, surgical and diagnostic procedures, and injections can involve all or some of the branches of the brachial plexus, leading to thoracic outlet, scalenus anticus, costoclavicular, and other syndromes.[328] Anatomic variations, such as a cervical rib, may contribute to these neuropathies.[329] Symptoms and signs vary according to the precise

site of involvement, and CT and MR imaging are helpful in delineating the nature of the lesion.[259, 260, 452–455]

Hereditary Neuropathies. Slowly progressive peripheral neuropathies that are hereditary can be differentiated according to the specific type of neurons that are affected predominantly: sensory neurons, motor neurons, and autonomic neurons. Although classification of these disorders on the basis of specific neuron involvement is logical, it is complicated, as many of the diseases affect more than one type of neuron. A more useful system may be to divide the disorders into three categories: those that involve sensory and autonomic neurons; those that involve sensory and motor neurons; and those that affect only motor neurons.[265] These disorders differ also in their mode of inheritance, age of onset, natural history and prognosis, distribution of abnormalities, and pathologic alterations. Some, such as those with prominent sensory loss, produce neuropathic osteoarthropathy, the features of which are discussed in Chapter 78. Contained here is the author's attempt to summarize the major features of the important hereditary peripheral neuropathies, a task that is made difficult because of changing terminology, inconsistencies and inadequacies in the literature, and the previous use of such vague terms as indifference or insensitivity to pain.[266]

Hereditary Sensory and Autonomic Neuropathies. The *hereditary sensory and autonomic neuropathies* are a number of disorders that have in common dysfunction of sensory neurons and, in some cases, autonomic neurons as well. Indifference or insensitivity to pain accounts for the appearance of neuropathic osteoarthropathy (Chapter 78). Four different types have been recognized (Table 77–4).

Type I. Type I neuropathy also is termed hereditary sensory radicular neuropathy, acrodystrophic neuropathy, mutilating acropathy, and hereditary perforating ulcers of the feet.[267–269] It is inherited as a dominant trait, varies in severity, has predilection for the lower extremities, and leads to

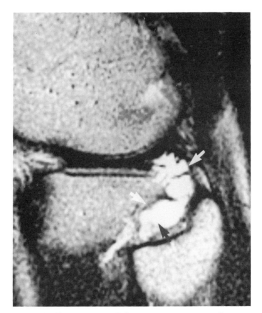

FIGURE 77–48. Entrapment of the common peroneal nerve and its branches: Ganglion. A sagittal T2-weighted (TR/TE, 2200/80) spin echo MR image shows the ganglion (arrows), of high signal intensity, in close proximity to the proximal tibiofibular joint.

TABLE 77–4. Hereditary Sensory Neuropathies

Type	Mode of Inheritance	Age of Onset	Distinctive Features
I	Dominant	Late childhood or adulthood	Lower extremity involvement, foot ulcerations, neuropathic osteoarthropathy
II	Recessive	Infancy or childhood	Upper and lower extremities, ulcerations, fractures, neuropathic osteoarthropathy
III	Recessive	Infancy or childhood	Jewish children, dysautonomia, neuropathic osteoarthropathy, ischemic necrosis, osteomyelitis, self-mutilation
IV	Recessive	Infancy or childhood	Anhidrosis, mental retardation, self-mutilation, neuropathic osteoarthropathy, ischemic necrosis, fractures, osteoporosis

sensory loss complicated by perforating lesions of the soft tissues and foot deformities. Burning feet may be a prominent symptom.[270] Sporadic cases also have been reported.

Type II. Type II disorder, which also is termed congenital sensory neuropathy, is inherited as a recessive trait, appears in infancy and childhood, predominates in the distal portions of the upper and lower extremities, and leads to soft tissue ulcerations and fractures in the extremities.[194] Absence of myelinated fibers in the cutaneous nerves is a prominent pathologic feature.

Type III. Type III disorder also is termed familial dysautonomia of Riley-Day. This inherited disease is seen principally in Jewish infants and children,[271, 272] although non-Jewish persons also may be affected.[273] Peripheral sensory, motor, and autonomic neurons are involved. Clinical manifestations include poor feeding, repeated episodes of vomiting and pulmonary infections, autonomic disturbances (defective lacrimation and temperature control, excessive perspiration, and hypertension), areflexia, insensitivity to pain, and early death.[194] Neuropathic osteoarthropathy,[272] abnormalities of spinal curvature,[275] osteomyelitis,[273] and ischemic necrosis of bone[275] are seen. Disintegration of large portions of the articular surfaces of the femoral head, femoral condyles, and tarsus, leading to subluxations, may be evident. Associated skeletal dysplasia has been reported.[276]

Type IV. Type IV, a recessively inherited disorder, is associated with sensory neuropathy, insensitivity to pain, mental retardation, and anhidrosis[277–280] and has been attributed to an abnormality of the neural crest.[278] Clinical manifestations generally appear in the first years of life. Neuropathic osteoarthropathy, periostitis, fractures, epiphyseal displacement, disintegration and necrosis, and osteoporosis may be observed.[281]

Hereditary Motor and Sensory Neuropathies. *Hereditary motor and sensory neuropathies* represent several distinct progressive inherited disorders.[265]

Type I. Type I is a dominantly inherited, hypertrophic form of peroneal muscular atrophy (Charcot-Marie-Tooth disease).[282] It varies in severity but frequently is mild, and some patients have no obvious symptoms or signs.[283] When present, clinical manifestations generally occur in the first or second decade of life. Affected patients reveal a high

plantar arch, hammer toes, and a high-stepping, awkward gait caused by paresis of the dorsiflexor muscles of the ankle and instability of the ankle joint.[194, 456] Markedly reduced or absent tendon reflexes, pes cavus,[284] scoliosis,[316] tremors, foot ulcerations, and distal muscle atrophy may be identified. Sensory loss is mild. Nerve biopsy shows extensive segmental demyelination and, sometimes, hypertrophic changes,[265] and palpably enlarged peripheral nerves are detected in approximately 25 per cent of cases.[194] Spinal nerve roots also may be enlarged.[306, 330, 457]

Type II. Type II disorder, which usually is inherited as a dominant trait,[285] represents the neuronal pattern of peroneal muscular atrophy (Charcot-Marie-Tooth disease).[283] Its onset typically is in the second decade of life, although a wide variation in the age of onset is reported. Clinical manifestations are symmetric muscle weakness and atrophy in the feet and ankles, difficulty in standing and walking, and, inconstantly, pes cavus and hammer toes; the upper extremity is affected subsequently.[194] Tendon reflexes are diminished in intensity, although generally they are present.[283] Compared with patients with type I disease, persons with type II disease may be older at the time of the disease onset, reveal lesser degrees of tremor, ataxia, upper limb involvement, and sensory loss, and do not have nerve thickening.[265]

Other Types. Additional motor and sensory neuropathies have been described, including recessively inherited hypertrophic neuropathy or Dejerine-Sottas neuropathy (onset in infancy, short stature, enlarged nerves, distal extremity involvement), Refsum's disease (autosomal recessive inheritance, onset in childhood or adulthood, ataxia, night blindness, ichthyosis, skeletal deformities, elevated levels of phytanic acid in the serum, muscles, and organs, and early demise), and neuropathies combined with optic atrophy or retinitis pigmentosa.[194, 265, 458]

Hereditary Motor Neuropathies. *Hereditary motor neuropathies* represent a group of chronic neurologic disorders with selective involvement of the anterior horn cells of the spinal cord and lower brain stem and, in some cases, the motor neurons of the corticospinal tract.[286] Sensory deficits and cerebellar dysfunction are absent. These neuropathies are further divided into those diseases in which prominent changes in upper neurons are combined with muscle atrophy and weakness (amyotrophic lateral sclerosis) and those in which upper neuron disease is lacking and slowly progressive muscle weakness and wasting occur (progressive muscular atrophy).[286] Two specific types of progressive muscular atrophy deserve emphasis.

Werdnig-Hoffman Disease. Werdnig-Hoffman disease manifests autosomal recessive inheritance or occurs sporadically. It begins in infancy and early childhood and appears clinically as hypotonia, severe weakness, areflexia, tremors and fasciculations, and normal sensation; proximal muscles are affected more severely than distal ones, and the lower extremities are weaker than the upper extremities.[287] Muscle biopsy indicates neurogenic atrophy. Orthopedic complications include scoliosis, pelvic tilt, coxa valga, plastic bowing of the ribs, and subluxation or dislocation of the hips.[287–289, 463]

Wohlfart-Kugelberg-Welander Disease. Wohlfart-Kugelberg-Welander disease, an autosomal recessive disorder, differs from Werdnig-Hoffman disease in its older age of onset (late childhood, adolescence, or adulthood) and slower course, affecting mainly proximal muscles, especially in the lower extremities. Scoliosis, joint contractures, mild acetabular dysplasia, and coxa valga are apparent.[287]

Friedreich's Ataxia

Friedreich's ataxia is one form of spinocerebellar degeneration. It usually is a recessive disorder that begins in childhood or adolescence, becoming manifest as progressive ataxia, dysarthria, and nystagmus with impairment of vibratory and position sensation and diminished or absent reflexes.[283] Cardiomyopathy may lead to the patient's death in the third or fourth decade of life.[283] Many specific causes of this disease (Friedreich's syndrome) exist, including inborn errors of metabolism, disorders of lipid or oxidative metabolism, aminocidurias, and the partial deficiency of hypoxanthine phosphoribosyltransferase.[286]

Orthopedic complications include severe scoliosis (50 to 75 per cent of cases), coxa valga deformity, subluxation of the hips, instability of the knees and ankles, and pes cavus.[283, 290, 307, 317] Painful muscle spasms occur in some patients, usually in the second decade of life.[477]

Muscle Diseases

Diseases of muscle can be classified as congenital or genetic, metabolic, inflammatory or infectious, traumatic, neoplastic, and of miscellaneous type.[291] Many of these are considered elsewhere in this textbook, so that the discussion here will be restricted to a summary of the muscular dystrophies. Diseases of muscle are better evaluated with CT or MR imaging[318, 459–461] than with routine radiography. Ultrasonography also has been used for such evaluation.[462]

Muscular Dystrophies. The universal clinical finding in the inherited myopathies is weakness, and the pathologic abnormalities are limited to the skeletal musculature (and, rarely, the cardiac musculature), in which necrosis and regeneration of muscle fibers and their replacement with fibrous connective tissue and fat are observed.[292] Additional histologic aberrations are characteristic (although not diagnostic) of individual dystrophies, such as pseudohypertrophy (due to both true enlargement of the muscle fibers and fatty and fibrous replacement of muscle) in Duchenne muscular dystrophy and ring fibers and sarcoplasmic masses in myotonic dystrophy.

The muscular dystrophies can be separated into several forms on the basis of their genetic patterns and such clinical manifestations as age of onset of the disease, distribution of muscle involvement, and the presence or absence of muscle hypertrophy (Table 77–5). Recognized types are the Duchenne (pseudohypertrophic), Becker's (benign pseudohypertrophic), facioscapulohumeral, limb-girdle, ocular or oculopharyngeal, myotonic, and distal dystrophies.[291] Of these patterns, Duchenne muscular dystrophy is most common and has the greatest relevance to the musculoskeletal system.[293–295]

Duchenne muscular dystrophy is characterized by an X-linked recessive inheritance (affecting boys only), disease onset in the first decade of life, weakness in the proximal muscles (especially those in the hips and shoulders), and mild mental retardation.[291] The muscles of the calf are large and firm and have a rubbery consistency. The disease is progressive, leading to incapacitation by adolescence. Serum levels of creatine kinase are markedly elevated.

Foot deformities, including pes planus and equinovarus, occur relatively early in the course of the disease owing to tightening of the Achilles tendon, and progressive contractures appear in the hips and knees. Subsequently, spinal deformities consisting of scoliosis and kyphosis are seen. Respiratory failure, pneumonia, and cardiac decompensation are causes of the patient's demise, commonly by the third decade of life.

Becker's muscular dystrophy resembles Duchenne dystrophy, but the onset of symptoms occurs later and the condition is less severe. Men are affected exclusively.

TABLE 77–5. Classification of Human Muscular Dystrophies

	Duchenne Dystrophy	Facioscapulohumeral Dystrophy	Limb-Girdle Dystrophy	Myotonic Dystrophy
Genetic pattern	X-linked recessive	Autosomal dominant	Autosomal recessive	Autosomal dominant
Age at onset	Before age 5 years	Adolescence	Adolescence	Early or late
First symptoms	Pelvic	Shoulders	Pelvic	Distal; hands or feet
Pseudohypertrophy	+	−	−	−
Predominant early weakness	Proximal	Proximal	Proximal	Distal
Progression	Relatively rapid; incapacitated in adolescence	Slow	Variable	Slow
Facial weakness	−	+	−	Occasional
Ocular, oropharyngeal weakness	−	−	−	Occasional
Myotonia	−	−	−	+
Cardiomyopathy	− or late	−	−	Arrhythmia, conduction block
Associated disorders	None (? mental retardation)	None	None	Cataracts; testicular atrophy and baldness in men
Serum enzyme levels	Very high	Slight or no increase	Slight or no increase	Slight or no increase

(From Rowland LP: Diseases of muscle and neuromuscular junction. *In* PB Beeson, W McDermott, JB Wyngaarden [Eds]: Cecil Textbook of Medicine. 15th Ed. Philadelphia, WB Saunders Co, 1979, p 916.)

TABLE 77–6. Musculoskeletal Abnormalities in Paralysis

Osteoporosis
Soft tissue and muscle atrophy or hypertrophy
Osseous deformities
Growth disturbances
"Stress" fragmentation of bone
Epiphyseal and metaphyseal fracture or fragmentation
Infection
Heterotopic ossification
Cartilage atrophy
Spondylopathy
Synovitis
Abnormalities of joint capsule
Reflex sympathetic dystrophy

Facioscapulohumeral muscular dystrophy has an autosomal dominant pattern of inheritance and affects both men and women. It appears in adolescence, with characteristic weakness of the shoulder girdle musculature. The scapulae are positioned abnormally, with a "winged" appearance. Additional manifestations relate to muscle involvement in the trunk, pelvis, legs, and face.

Limb-girdle muscular dystrophy is an autosomal recessive disorder of boys and girls. Initial manifestations, including a waddling gait and difficulty in walking, relate to weakness of the pelvic girdle. Disease progression is variable, but other areas, such as the shoulders and extremities, may become involved. Scoliosis, coxa valga, and equinovarus deformities are seen.[293]

Myotonic dystrophy is a syndrome of variable severity with an autosomal dominant genetic pattern. Its onset may occur in children or be delayed until adolescence or beyond. Weakness predominates in the distal portions of the extremities, especially the hands, sternocleidomastoid muscles, and face. Myotonia, a delay in muscle relaxation, is best exemplified by the patient's inability to unclasp the hand.

SUMMARY

The musculoskeletal abnormalities accompanying neuromuscular disorders include osteoporosis, soft tissue atrophy, growth disturbances, deformities, growth plate injuries, infection, heterotopic ossification, cartilage atrophy, synovitis, clubbing, joint capsule alterations, and neuropathic osteoarthropathy (Table 77–6). Typical radiographic changes are encountered that are easy to interpret when an adequate clinical history is provided. Although the pathogenesis of some of the findings is clear, that of heterotopic ossification and sacroiliac joint and spinal alterations is unknown.

Some specific types of neuromuscular disease lead to characteristic clinical and imaging findings. Of particular importance, entrapment neuropathies occur at vulnerable sites along the course of the peripheral nerves as well as in plexuses. Hereditary neuropathies of sensory neurons produce neuropathic osteoarthropathy, which is discussed further in the following chapter.

References

1. Albright F, Burnett CH, Cope O, et al: Acute atrophy of bone (osteoporosis) simulating hyperparathyroidism. J Clin Endocrinol *1*:711, 1941.
2. Eichler J: Inaktivitätsosteoporose. Z Rheumaforsch *31*:367, 1972.
3. Little K: Bone Behavior. London, Academic Press, 1973.
4. Benassy J, Mazabraud J, Diverres JC: L'osteogenese neurogene. Rev Chir Orthop *49*:95, 1963.
5. Trueta J: The dynamics of bone circulation. *In* HM Frost (Ed): Bone Dynamics. Boston, Little, Brown, 1964, p 245.
6. Dhem A: Les mécanismes des destruction du tissue osseux. Acta Orthop Belg *39*:423, 1973.
7. Andrew C, Basset L: Biophysical principles affecting bone structure. *In* GH Bourne (Ed): Biochemistry and Physiology of Bone. Vol 3. New York, Academic Press, 1971, p 584.
8. Chantraine A: Actual concept of osteoporosis in paraplegia. Paraplegia *16*:51, 1978.
9. Rasmussen H, Bordier P: The cellular basis of metabolic bone disease. N Engl J Med *289*:25, 1973.
10. Uhthoff HK, Jaworski ZFG: Bone loss in response to long-term immobilization. J Bone Joint Surg [Br] *60*:420, 1978.
11. Griffiths HJ, Bushueff B, Zimmerman RE: Investigation of the loss of bone mineral in patients with spinal cord injury. Paraplegia *14*:207, 1976.
12. Burkhart JM, Jowsey J: Parathyroid and thyroid hormones in the development of immobilization osteoporosis. Endocrinology *81*:1053, 1967.
13. Minaire P, Meunier P, Edouard C, et al: Quantitative histological data on disuse osteoporosis. Comparison with biological data. Calcif Tissue Res *17*:57, 1974.
14. Eichenholtz N: Management of long-bone fractures in paraplegic patients. J Bone Joint Surg [Am] *45*:299, 1963.
15. McIvor WC, Samilson RL: Fractures in patients with cerebral palsy. J Bone Joint Surg [Am] *44*:858, 1966.
16. Handelsman JE: Spontaneous fractures in spina bifida. J Bone Joint Surg [Br] *54*:381, 1972.
17. Miller PR, Glazer DA: Spontaneous fractures in the brain-crippled, bedridden patient. Clin Orthop *120*:138, 1976.
18. Bernstein C, Loeser WD, Manning LE: Erosive rib lesions in paralytic poliomyelitis. Radiology *70*:368, 1958.
19. Woodlief RM: Superior marginal rib defects in traumatic quadriplegia. Radiology *126*:673, 1978.
20. Litt RE, Altman DH: Significance of the muscle cylinder ratio in infancy. AJR *100*:80, 1967.
21. Furukawa T, Peter JB: The muscular dystrophies and related disorders. I. The muscular dystrophies. JAMA *239*:1537, 1978.
22. Harris VJ, Harris WS: Increased thickness of the fibula in Duchenne muscular dystrophy. AJR *98*:744, 1966.
23. Houston CS, Zaleski WA: The shape of vertebral bodies and femoral necks in relation to activity. Radiology *89*:59, 1967.
24. Houston CS: The radiologist's opportunity to teach bone dynamics. J Can Assoc Radiol *29*:232, 1978.
25. Gooding CA, Neuhauser EBD: Growth and development of the vertebral body in the presence and absence of normal stress. AJR *93*:388, 1965.
26. Rabinowitz JG, Moseley JE: The lateral lumbar spine in Down's syndrome: A new roentgen feature. Radiology *83*:74, 1964.
27. Stevenson FH: The osteoporosis of immobilization in recumbency. J Bone Joint Surg [Br] *34*:256, 1952.
28. Lamb DW, Pollock GA: Hip deformities in cerebral palsy and their treatment. Dev Med Child Neurol *4*:488, 1962.
29. Baker LD, Dodelin R, Bassett FH: Pathological changes in the hip in cerebral palsy; incidence, pathogenesis, and treatment. A preliminary report. J Bone Joint Surg [Am] *44*:1331, 1962.
30. Tachdjian MO, Minear WL: Hip dislocation in cerebral palsy. J Bone Joint Surg [Am] *38*:1358, 1956.
31. Sharrard WJW, Allen JMH, Heaney SH, et al: Surgical prophylaxis of subluxation and dislocation of the hip in cerebral palsy. J Bone Joint Surg [Br] *57*:160, 1975.
32. Samilson R, Bechard R: Scoliosis in cerebral palsy: Incidence, distribution of curve patterns, and thoughts on etiology. Curr Pract Orthop Surg *5*:183, 1973.
33. Saupe E: Beitrag zur Patella bipartita. ROFO *28*:37, 1921.
34. Roberts WM, Adams JP: The patellar-advancement operation in cerebral palsy. J Bone Joint Surg [Am] *35*:958, 1953.
35. Kaye JJ, Freiberger RH: Fragmentation of the lower pole of the patella in spastic lower extremities. Radiology *101*:97, 1971.
36. Rosenthal RK, Levine DB: Fragmentation of the distal pole of the patella in spastic cerebral palsy. J Bone Joint Surg [Am] *59*:934, 1977.
37. Baker LD, Hill LM: Foot alignment in the cerebral palsy patient. J Bone Joint Surg [Am] *46*:1, 1964.
38. Sharrard WJW, Bernstein S: Equinus deformity in cerebral palsy. A comparison between elongation of the tendocalcaneus and gastrocnemius recession. J Bone Joint Surg [Br] *54*:272, 1972.
39. Ross D: Disturbance of longitudinal growth associated with prolonged disability of the lower extremity. J Bone Joint Surg [Am] *30*:103, 1948.
40. Ratliff AH: The short leg in poliomyelitis. J Bone Joint Surg [Br] *41*:56, 1959.
41. Currarino G: Premature closure of epiphyses in the metatarsals and knees: A sequel of poliomyelitis. Radiology *87*:424, 1966.
42. Edvardsen P: Physeo-epiphyseal injuries of lower extremities in myelomeningocele. Acta Orthop Scand *43*:550, 1972.
43. Gyepes MT, Newbern DH, Neuhauser EBD: Metaphyseal and physeal injuries in children with spina bifida and meningomyeloceles. AJR *95*:168, 1965.
44. Poznanski AK: Diagnostic clues in the growing ends of bone. J Can Assoc Radiol *29*:7, 1978.
45. Nellhaus G: Neurogenic arthropathies (Charcot's joints) in children. Clin Pediatr *14*:647, 1975.

46. Drummond RP, Rose GK: A twenty-one-year review of a case of congenital indifference to pain. J Bone Joint Surg [Br] 57:241, 1975.
47. Franklyn PP: Congenital indifference to pain. Ann Radiol 15:343, 1972.
48. Gold RH, Mirra JM: Case report 45. Skel Radiol 2:127, 1977.
49. Schneider R, Goldman AB, Bohne WHO: Neuropathic injuries to the lower extremities in children. Radiology 128:713, 1978.
50. Shea JD: Pressure sores. Classification and management. Clin Orthop 112:89, 1975.
51. Enis JE, Sarmiento A: The pathophysiology and management of pressure sores. Orthop Rev 2:25, 1973.
52. Griffith BH: Pressure sores. Mod Trends Plast Surg 2:150, 1966.
53. Abel MS, Smith GR: The case of the disappearing pelvis. Radiology 111:105, 1974.
54. Rosin AJ: Ectopic calcification around joints of paralysed limbs in hemiplegia, diffuse brain damage, and other neurological diseases. Ann Rheum Dis 34:499, 1975.
55. Hsu JD, Sakimura I, Stauffer ES: Heterotopic ossification around the hip joint in spinal cord injured patients. Clin Orthop 112:165, 1975.
56. Wharton GW, Morgan TH: Ankylosis in the paralyzed patient. J Bone Joint Surg [Am] 52:105, 1970.
57. Tibone J, Sakimura I, Nickel VL, et al: Heterotopic ossification around the hip in spinal cord-injured patients. J Bone Joint Surg [Am] 60:769, 1978.
58. Roberts PH: Heterotopic ossification complicating paralysis of intracranial origin. J Bone Joint Surg [Br] 50:70, 1968.
59. Goldberg MA, Schumacher HR: Heterotopic ossification mimicking acute arthritis after neurologic catastrophies. Arch Intern Med 137:619, 1977.
60. Nicholas JJ: Ectopic bone formation in patients with spinal cord injury. Arch Phys Med Rehabil 54:354, 1973.
61. Hardy AG, Dickson JW: Pathological ossification in traumatic paraplegia. J Bone Joint Surg [Br] 45:76, 1963.
62. Furman R, Nicholas JJ, Jivoff L: Elevation of the serum alkaline phosphatase coincident with ectopic-bone formation in paraplegic patients. J Bone Joint Surg [Am] 52:1131, 1970.
63. Liberson M: Soft tissue calcification in cord lesions. JAMA 152:1010, 1953.
64. Dejerine Mme, Ceillier A: Para-osteoarthropathies des paraplegiques par lesions medullaires: Etude clinique et radiographique. Ann Med 5:497, 1918.
65. Abramson AS: Bone disturbances in injuries to the spinal cord and cauda equina (paraplegia): Their prevention by ambulation. J Bone Joint Surg [Am] 30:982, 1948.
66. Money RA: Ectopic para-articular ossification after head injury. Med J Aust 1:125, 1972.
67. Hossack DW, King A: Neurogenic heterotopic ossification. Med J Aust 1:326, 1967.
68. Freiberg JA: Para-articular calcification and ossification following acute anterior poliomyelitis in an adult. J Bone Joint Surg [Am] 34:339, 1952.
69. Storey G, Tegner WS: Paraplegic para-articular calcification. Ann Rheum Dis 14:176, 1955.
70. Gunn DR, Young WB: Myositis ossificans as a complication of tetanus. J Bone Joint Surg [Br] 41:535, 1959.
71. Rosin AJ: Peri-articular calcification in a hemiplegic limb: A rare complication of a stroke. J Am Geriatr Soc 18:916, 1970.
72. Nechwatal E: Early recognition of heterotopic calcifications by means of alkaline phosphatase. Paraplegia 11:79, 1973.
73. Weiss S, Grosswasser Z, Ohri A, et al: Histocompatibility (HLA) antigens in heterotopic ossification associated with neurological injury. J Rheumatol 6:88, 1979.
74. Donath A, Muheim G, Rossier A: Valeurs des scintigraphies iteratives dans l'évaluation des calcifications ectopiques des paraplegiques. Radiol Clin Biol 43:387, 1974.
75. Muheim G, Donath A, Rossier AB: Serial scintigrams in the course of ectopic bone formation in paraplegic patients. AJR 118:865, 1973.
76. Miller LF, O'Neill CJ: Myositis ossificans in paraplegics. J Bone Joint Surg [Am] 31:283, 1949.
77. Damanski M: Heterotopic ossification in paraplegia: A clinical study. J Bone Joint Surg [Br] 43:286, 1961.
78. Shapiro RF, Utsinger PD, Wiesner KB, et al: HLA-B27 and modified bone formation. Lancet 1:230, 1976.
79. Radt P: Peri-articular ectopic ossification in hemiplegics. Geriatrics 25:142, 1970.
80. Major P, Resnick D, Greenway G: Heterotopic ossification in paraplegia: A possible disturbance of the paravertebral venous plexus. Radiology 136:797, 1980.
81. Brower TD, Akahoshi Y, Orlic P: The diffusion of dyes through articular cartilage in vivo. J Bone Joint Surg [Am] 44:456, 1962.
82. Maroudas A, Bullough P, Swanson SAV, et al: The permeability of articular cartilage. J Bone Joint Surg [Br] 50:166, 1968.
83. Mankin HJ: Localization of tritiated cytidine in articular cartilage of immature and adult rabbits after intra-articular injection. Lab Invest 12:543, 1963.
84. Bollet AJ: An essay on the biology of osteoarthritis. Arthritis Rheum 12:152, 1969.
85. McKibbin B, Holdsworth FW: The nutrition of immature joint cartilage in the lamb. J Bone Joint Surg [Br] 48:793, 1966.
86. Hodge JA, McKibbin B: The nutrition of mature and immature cartilage in rabbits. An autoradiographic study. J Bone Joint Surg [Br] 51:140, 1969.
87. Ogata K, Whiteside LA, Lesker PA: Subchondral route for nutrition to articular

cartilage in the rabbit. Measurement of diffusion with hydrogen gas in vivo. J Bone Joint Surg [Am] 60:905, 1978.
88. Greenwald AS, Haynes DW: A pathway for nutrients from the medullary cavity to the articular cartilage of the human femoral head. J Bone Joint Surg [Br] 51:747, 1979.
89. Reynolds JJ: Degradation processes in bone and cartilage. Calcif Tissue Res 4(Suppl):52, 1970.
90. Thaxter TH, Mann RA, Anderson CE: Degeneration of immobilized knee joints in rats: Histological and autoradiographic study. J Bone Joint Surg [Am] 47:567, 1965.
91. Pool WH Jr: Cartilage atrophy. Radiology 112:47, 1974.
92. Thompson RC Jr, Bassett CA: Histological observations on experimentally induced degeneration of articular cartilage. J Bone Joint Surg [Am] 52:435, 1970.
93. Ginsberg JM, Eyring EJ, Curtiss PH Jr: Continuous compression of rabbit articular cartilage producing loss of hydroxyproline before loss of hexosamine. J Bone Joint Surg [Am] 51:467, 1969.
94. Hall MC: Cartilage changes after experimental relief of contact in the knee joint of the mature rat. Clin Orthop 64:64, 1969.
95. Evans EB, Eggers GWN, Butler JK, et al: Experimental immobilization and remobilization of rat knee joints. J Bone Joint Surg [Am] 42:737, 1960.
96. Akeson WH, Woo SLY, Amiel D, et al: The connective tissue response to immobility: Biochemical changes in peri-articular connective tissue of the immobilized rabbit knee. Clin Orthop 93:356, 1973.
97. Trias A: Effect of persistent pressure on the articular cartilage. An experimental study. J Bone Joint Surg [Br] 43:376, 1961.
98. Salter RB, Field P: The effects of continuous compression on living articular cartilage: An experimental investigation. J Bone Joint Surg [Am] 42:31, 1960.
99. Finsterbush A, Friedman B: Early changes in immobilized rabbits knee joints: A light and electron microscopic study. Clin Orthop 92:305, 1973.
100. Finsterbush A, Friedman B: Reversibility of joint changes produced by immobilization in rabbits. Clin Orthop 111:290, 1975.
101. Baker WD, Thomas TG, Kirkaldy-Willis WH: Changes in the cartilage of the posterior intervertebral joints after anterior fusion. J Bone Joint Surg [Br] 51:736, 1969.
102. Enneking WF, Horowitz M: The intra-articular effects of immobilization on the human knee. J Bone Joint Surg [Am] 54:973, 1972.
103. Abel MS: Sacroiliac joint changes in traumatic paraplegics. Radiology 55:235, 1950.
104. Mason RM, Murray RS, Oates JK, et al: Prostatitis and ankylosing spondylitis. Br Med J 1:748, 1958.
105. Wright V, Catterall RD, Cook JB: Bone and joint changes in paraplegic men. Ann Rheum Dis 24:419, 1965.
106. Hunter T, Hildahl CR, Smith NJ, et al: Histocompatibility antigens in paraplegic or quadriplegic patients with sacroiliac joint changes. J Rheumatol 6:92, 1979.
107. Hermann E: Acute arthritis in hemiplegics. Scand J Rheumatol 1:87, 1972.
108. Pálvölgyi R: Roentgenmorphological muscle changes in anterior horn cell lesions. ROFO 130:338, 1979.
109. Roberts JB, Pankratz DG: The surgical treatment of heterotopic ossification at the elbow following long coma. J Bone Joint Surg [Am] 61:760, 1979.
110. Lagenskiold A, Michelsson JE, Videman T: Osteoarthritis of the knee in the rabbit produced by immobilization. Acta Orthop Scand 50:1, 1979.
111. Heuwinkel R: Zur Ätiologie und Pathogenese der Knochenneubildungen bei Hirnverletzen und Paraplegiken. I. Das lokale Milieu—untersuchungen im Frakturhamatom. Unfallheikunde 82:252, 1979.
112. Heuwinkel R, Schneider H-M: Zur Ätiologie und Pathogenese der Knochenneubildungen bei Hirnverletzen und Paraplegikern. II. Histochemie der frakturnahen Weichgewebe (Enzymmuster im Bereich der heilenden Fraktur). Unfallheilkunde 82:349, 1979.
113. Townsend PF, Cowell HR, Steg NL: Lower extremity fractures simulating infection in myelomeningocele. Clin Orthop 144:255, 1979.
114. Wenger DR, Jeffcoat BT, Herring JA: The guarded prognosis of physeal injury in paraplegic children. J Bone Joint Surg [Am] 62:241, 1980.
115. Khan MA, Kushner I, Freehafer AA: Sacroiliac joint abnormalities in paraplegics. Ann Rheum Dis 38:317, 1979.
116. Wignall KB, Williamson BRJ: The chest x-ray in quadriplegia: A review of 119 patients. Clin Radiol 31:81, 1980.
117. Hancock DA, Reed GW, Atkinson PJ: Bone and soft tissue changes in paraplegic patients. Paraplegia 17:267, 1979–1980.
118. Ogata K, Whiteside LA: Barrier to material transfer at the bone-cartilage interface. Measurement with hydrogen gas in vivo. Clin Orthop 145:273, 1979.
119. Palmoski MJ, Colyer RA, Brandt KD: Joint motion in the absence of normal loading does not maintain normal articular cartilage. Arthritis Rheum 23:325, 1980.
120. Bhate DV, Pizarro AJ, Seitam A, et al: Axial skeletal changes in paraplegics. Radiology 133:55, 1979.
121. Hunter T, Dubo HI, Hildahl CR, et al: Histocompatibility antigens in patients with spinal cord injury or cerebral damage complicated by heterotopic ossification. Rheumatol Rehabil 19:97, 1980.
122. Michelsson JE, Granroth G, Andersson LC: Myositis ossificans following forcible manipulation of the leg. J Bone Joint Surg [Am] 62:811, 1980.
123. Chantraine A, Van Ouwenaller C, Hachen HJ, et al: Intra-medullary pressure and intra-osseous phlebography in paraplegia. Paraplegia 17:391, 1979.
124. Garland DE, Blum CE, Waters RL: Periarticular heterotopic ossification in

head-injured adults. Incidence and location. J Bone Joint Surg [Am] 62:1143, 1980.

125. Seigel RS: Heterotopic ossification in paraplegia. Radiology 137:259, 1980.

126. Minaire P, Meunier P, Edouard C, et al: Histomorphometric study of acute osteoporosis in paraplegic patients. Paraplegia 20:281, 1982.

127. Wronski TJ, Morey ER: Inhibition of cortical and trabecular bone formation in the long bones of immobilized monkeys. Clin Orthop 181:269, 1983.

128. Christodoulou NA, Dretaski EK: Significance of muscular disturbances in the location of fractures of the proximal femur. Clin Orthop 187:215, 1984.

129. Lovelock JE, Monaco LP: Central acetabular fracture dislocations: An unusual complication of seizures. Skel Radiol 10:91, 1983.

130. Remec PT, Evarts CM: Bilateral central dislocation of the hip. A case report. Clin Orthop 181:118, 1983.

131. Rafii M, Firooznia H, Golimbu C, et al: Bilateral acetabular stress fractures in a paraplegic patient. Arch Phys Med Rehabil 63:240, 1982.

132. Nottage WM: A review of long-bone fractures in patients with spinal cord injuries. Clin Orthop 155:65, 1981.

133. Aro H, Eerola E, Aho AJ, et al: Healing of experimental fractures in the denervated limbs of the rat. Clin Orthop 155:211, 1981.

134. Garland DE, Miller G: Fractures and dislocations about the hip in head-injured adults. Clin Orthop 186:154, 1984.

135. Garland DE, Dowling V: Forearm fractures in the head-injured adult. Clin Orthop 176:190, 1983.

136. Hadar H, Gadoth N, Heifetz M: Fatty replacement of lower paraspinal muscles: Normal and neuromuscular disorders. AJR 141:895, 1983.

137. Hawley RJ, Schellinger D, O'Doherty DS: Computed tomographic patterns of muscles in neuromuscular disease. Arch Neurol 41:383, 1984.

138. Bulcke JAL, Herpels V: Diagnostic scanning in neuromuscular diseases. Radiologe 23:523, 1983.

139. Termote J-L, Baert A, Crolla D, et al: Computed tomography of the normal and pathologic muscle system. Radiology 137:439, 1980.

140. Vukanovic S, Hauser H, Curati WL: Myonecrosis induced by drug overdose: Pathogenesis, clinical aspects and radiological manifestations. Eur J Radiol 3:314, 1983.

141. Kaplan GN: Ultrasound appearance of rhabdomyolysis. AJR 134:375, 1980.

142. Akmal M, Goldstein D, Telfer M, et al: Resolution of muscle calcification in rhabdomyolysis and renal failure. Ann Intern Med 89:928, 1978.

143. Matin P, Lang G, Carretta R, et al: Scintigraphic evaluation of muscle damage following extreme exercise: Concise communication. J Nucl Med 24:308, 1983.

144. Breed AL, Healy PM: The midlumbar myelomeningocele hip: Mechanism of dislocation and treatment. J Pediatr Orthop 2:15, 1982.

145. Siffert RS: Patterns of deformity of the developing hip. Clin Orthop 16:14, 1981.

146. McKibbin B: The action of the iliopsoas muscle in the newborn. J Bone Joint Surg [Br] 50:161, 1968.

147. Howard CB, Williams LA: A new radiological sign in the hips of cerebral palsy patients. Clin Radiol 35:317, 1984.

148. Weisl H: Coxa vara in spina bifida. J Bone Joint Surg [Br] 65:128, 1983.

149. Dias LS, Locher FG, Mazur JM, et al: Femoral neck abnormalities in spina bifida. Clin Orthop 184:164, 1984.

150. Mayfield JK, Erkkila JC, Winter RB: Spine deformity subsequent to acquired childhood spinal cord injury. J Bone Joint Surg [Am] 63:1401, 1981.

151. Letts M, Shapiro L, Mulder K, et al: The windblown hip syndrome in total body cerebral palsy. J Pediatr Orthop 4:55, 1984.

152. Lloyd-Roberts GC, Jackson AM, Albert JS: Avulsion of the distal pole of the patella in cerebral palsy. A cause of deteriorating gait. J Bone Joint Surg [Br] 67:252, 1985.

153. Eilert RE: Cavus foot in cerebral palsy. Foot Ankle 4:185, 1984.

154. Jahss MH: Evaluation of the cavus foot for orthopedic treatment. Clin Orthop 181:52, 1983.

155. Rothschild H, Shoji H, McCormick D: Heel deformity in hereditary spastic paraplegia. Clin Orthop 160:48, 1981.

156. Richardson ML, Helms CA, Vogler JB III, et al: Skeletal changes in neuromuscular disorders mimicking juvenile rheumatoid arthritis and hemophilia. AJR 143:893, 1984.

157. Firoosnia H, Rafii M, Golimbu C, et al: Computerized tomography of pelvic osteomyelitis in patients with spinal cord injuries. Clin Orthop 181:126, 1983.

158. Firooznia H, Rafii M, Golimbu C, et al: Computerized tomography in diagnosis of pelvic abscess in spinal-cord-injured patients. Comput Radiol 7:335, 1983.

159. Blane CE, Perkash I: True heterotopic bone in the paralyzed patient. Skel Radiol 7:21, 1981.

160. Henderson HP, Reid DAC: Para-articular ossification in the hand. Hand 13:239, 1981.

161. Good AE, Solsky MA, Gulati SM: Heterotopic ossification simulating acute arthritis: a patient with stable, chronic neurologic disease. J Rheumatol 10:124, 1983.

162. Barron M, Stern J, Lander P: Heterotopic ossification heralded by a knee effusion. J Rheumatol 10:961, 1983.

163. Garland DE, Alday B, Venos KG: Heterotopic ossification and HLA antigens. Arch Phys Med Rehabil 65:531, 1984.

164. Larson JM, Michalski JP, Collacott EA, et al: Increased prevalence of HLA-B27 in patients with ectopic ossification following traumatic spinal cord injury. Rheumatol Rehabil 20:193, 1981.

165. Ohry A: Paraosteoarthropathies and HLA. Arch Phys Med Rehabil 61:427, 1980.

166. Minaire P, Betuel H, Girard R, et al: Neurologic injuries, paraosteoarthropathies and human leukocyte antigens. Arch Phys Med Rehabil 61:214, 1980.

167. Nielsen BF: Myositis ossificans articulating with the pelvis. A case report. Acta Orthop Scand 56:86, 1985.

168. Van der Linden AJ: Spontaneous regression of neurogenic heterotopic ossification. Int Orthop (SICOT) 8:25, 1984.

169. Chantraine A, Minaire P: Para-osteo-arthropathies. Scand J Rehabil Med 13:31, 1981.

170. Izumi K: Study of ectopic bone formation in experimental spinal cord injured rabbits. Paraplegia 21:351, 1983.

171. Sazbon L, Sack J, Najenson T, et al: Growth hormone and periarticular new bone formation—a causal relationship? Scand J Rehabil Med 15:43, 1982.

172. Burr DB, Frederickson RG, Pavlinch C, et al: Intracast muscle stimulation prevents bone and cartilage deterioration in cast-immobilized rabbits. Clin Orthop 189:264, 1984.

173. Palmoski MJ, Brandt KD: Running inhibits the reversal of atrophic changes in canine knee cartilage after removal of a leg cast. Arthritis Rheum 24:1329, 1981.

174. Troyer H: Experimental models of osteoarthritis: A review. Semin Arthritis Rheum 11:362, 1982.

175. Andersen J, Breidahl P: Cartilage atrophy following spinal cord damage. Aust Radiol 25:98, 1981.

176. Rizk TE, Christopher RP, Pinals RS, et al: Arthrographic studies in painful hemiplegic shoulders. Arch Phys Med Rehabil 65:254, 1984.

177. Hakuno A, Sashika H, Ohkawa T, et al: Arthrographic findings in hemiplegic shoulders. Arch Phys Med Rehabil 65:706, 1984.

178. Bruckner FE, Nye CJS: Prospective study of adhesive capsulitis of the shoulder ("frozen shoulder") in a high risk population. Q J Med 198:191, 1981.

179. Nepomuceno CS, Miller JM III: Shoulder arthrography in hemiplegic patients. Arch Phys Med Rehabil 55:49, 1974.

180. Lev-Toaff AS, Karasick D, Rao VM: "Drooping shoulder"—nontraumatic causes of glenohumeral subluxation. Skel Radiol 12:34, 1984.

181. Shai G, Ring H, Costeff H, et al: Glenohumeral malalignment in the hemiplegic shoulder. An early radiologic sign. Scand J Rehabil Med 16:133, 1984.

182. Miglietta O, Lewitan A, Ragoff JB: Subluxation of the shoulder in hemiplegic patients. NY State J Med 59:457, 1959.

183. Najenson T, Pikielny SS: Malalignment of the glenohumeral joint following hemiplegia. A review of 500 cases. Ann Phys Med 8:96, 1966.

184. Basmajian JV, Bazant FJ: Factors preventing downward dislocation of the adducted shoulder joint. An electromyographic and morphological study. J Bone Joint Surg [Am] 41:1182, 1959.

185. Davis SW, Petrillo CR, Eichberg RD, et al: Shoulder-hand syndrome in a hemiplegic population: 5-year retrospective study. Arch Phys Med Rehabil 58:353, 1977.

186. Tepperman PS, Greyson D, Hilbert L, et al: Reflex sympathetic dystrophy in hemiplegia. Arch Phys Med Rehabil 65:442, 1984.

187. Wainapel SF, Freed MM: Reflex sympathetic dystrophy in quadraplegia: A case report. Arch Phys Med Rehabil 65:35, 1984.

188. Greyson ND, Tepperman PS: Three-phase bone studies in hemiplegia with reflex sympathetic dystrophy and the effect of disuse. J Nucl Med 25:423, 1984.

189. Osterman K, Lindholm TS: Massive ectopic calcification of the leg following nerve injury. Arch Orthop Trauma Surg 102:82, 1983.

190. Dyck PJ, Thomas PK, Lambert EH: Peripheral Neuropathy. Philadelphia, WB Saunders Co, 1975.

191. Kopell HP, Thompson WAL: Peripheral Entrapment Neuropathies. 2nd Ed. Huntington, New York, RE Krieger, 1976.

192. Sunderland S: Nerves and Nerve Injuries. Edinburgh, E & S Livingstone, 1968.

193. Sherman DG: Peripheral neuropathies. In JH Stein (Ed): Internal Medicine. Boston, Little, Brown, 1983, p 871.

194. Dyck PJ: Diseases of the peripheral nervous system. In PB Beeson, W McDermott, JB Wyngaarden (Eds): Cecil Textbook of Medicine. 15th Ed. Philadelphia, WB Saunders Co, 1979, p 899.

195. Bora FW Jr, Osterman AL: Compression neuropathy. Clin Orthop 163:20, 1982.

196. Nakano KK: Entrapment neuropathies. In WN Kelley, ED Harris Jr, S Ruddy, CB Sledge (Eds): Textbook of Rheumatology. 2nd Ed. Philadelphia, WB Saunders Co, 1985, p 1754.

197. Reddy MP: Peripheral nerve entrapment syndromes. Am Fam Physician 28:133, 1983.

198. Wertsch JJ, Melvin J: Median nerve anatomy and entrapment syndromes: A review. Arch Phys Med Rehabil 63:623, 1982.

199. Thompson WAL, Kopell HP: Peripheral entrapment neuropathies of the upper extremities. N Engl J Med 260:1261, 1959.

200. Spinner M, Spencer PS: Nerve compression lesions of upper extremity. Clin Orthop 104:46, 1974.

201. Smith RV, Fisher RG: Struthers ligament: Source of median nerve compression above elbow: Case report. J Neurosurg 38:778, 1973.

202. Johnson RK, Spinner M, Shrewsbury MM: Median nerve entrapment syndrome in the proximal forearm. J Hand Surg 4:48, 1979.

203. Bell GE Jr, Goldner JL: Compression neuropathy of the median nerve. South Med J 49:966, 1956.

204. Farber JS, Bryan RS: The anterior interosseous nerve syndrome. J Bone Joint Surg [Am] 50:521, 1968.

205. Kaplan EB, Spinner M: The anterior interosseous nerve syndrome. J Bone Joint Surg [Am] *51*:1677, 1969.
206. Rask MR: Anterior interosseous nerve entrapment. Clin Orthop *142*:176, 1979.
207. Stern MB: The anterior interosseous nerve syndrome (the Kiloh-Nevin syndrome). Clin Orthop *187*:223, 1984.
208. Fearn CB, Goodfellow JW: Anterior interosseous nerve palsy. J Bone Joint Surg [Br] *47*:91, 1965.
209. Spinner M: Anterior interosseous nerve syndrome: With special attention to its variations. J Bone Joint Surg [Am] *52*:84, 1970.
210. Takechi H, Kono M: The osseous structure of the carpal groove. Anat Clin *5*:153, 1983.
211. Zucker-Pinchoff B, Hermann G, Srinivasan R: Computed tomography of the carpal tunnel: A radioanatomical study. J Comput Assist Tomogr *5*:525, 1981.
212. Cone RO, Szabo R, Resnick D, et al: Computed tomography of the normal soft tissues of the wrist. Invest Radiol *18*:546, 1983.
213. Mayers LB: Carpal tunnel syndrome secondary to tuberculosis. Arch Neurol *10*:426, 1964.
214. Robbins H: Anatomical study of the median nerve in the carpal tunnel and etiologies of the carpal-tunnel syndrome. J Bone Joint Surg [Am] *45*:953, 1963.
215. Schiller F, Kolb FO: Carpal tunnel syndrome in acromegaly. Neurology *4*:271, 1954.
216. Thompkins DG: Median neuropathy in the carpal tunnel caused by tumor-like conditions. Report of two cases. J Bone Joint Surg [Am] *49*:737, 1967.
217. Haque I-U: Carpal tunnel syndrome due to an anomalous distal end of the radius. A case report. J Bone Joint Surg [Am] *64*:943, 1982.
218. Dorwart BB: Carpal tunnel syndrome: A review. Semin Arthritis Rheum *14*:134, 1984.
219. Graham RA: Carpal tunnel syndrome. A statistical analysis of 214 cases. Orthopedics *6*:1283, 1983.
220. Lipscomb PR: Carpal tunnel syndrome: Guide to office diagnosis. J Musculoskel Med *1*:35, 1984.
221. Phalen GS: Reflection on 21 years' experience with carpal-tunnel syndrome. JAMA *212*:1365, 1970.
222. Cannon LJ, Bernacki EJ, Walter SD: Personal and occupational factors associated with carpal tunnel syndrome. J Occup Med *23*:255, 1981.
223. Gould JS, Wissinger HA: Carpal tunnel syndrome in pregnancy. South Med J *71*:144, 1978.
224. Lin R, Lin E, Engel J, et al: Histo-mechanical aspects of carpal tunnel syndrome. Hand *15*:305, 1983.
225. Gardner RC: Confirmed case and diagnosis of pseudocarpal-tunnel (sublimis) syndrome. N Engl J Med *282*:858, 1970.
226. Holtzman RNN, Mark MH, Patel MR, et al: Ulnar entrapment neuropathy in the forearm. J Hand Surg [Am] *9*:576, 1984.
227. Vanderpool DW, Chalmers J, Lamb DW, et al: Peripheral compression lesions of the ulnar nerve. J Bone Joint Surg [Br] *50*:792, 1968.
228. Feindel W, Stratford J: Cubital tunnel compression. Can Med Assoc J *78*:351, 1958.
229. Osborne GV: Surgical treatment of tardy ulnar neuritis. J Bone Joint Surg [Br] *39*:782, 1957.
230. Balagtas-Balmaseda OM, Grabois M, Balmaseda PF, et al: Cubital tunnel syndrome in rheumatoid arthritis. Arch Phys Med Rehabil *64*:163, 1983.
231. Tanabu S, Yamauchi Y, Fukushima M: Hypoplasia of the trochlea of the humerus as a cause of ulnar-nerve palsy. Report of two cases. J Bone Joint Surg [Am] *67*:151, 1985.
232. Grundberg AB: Ulnar tunnel syndrome. Hand [Br] *9*:72, 1984.
233. Kleinert HE, Hayes JE: The ulnar tunnel syndrome. Plast Reconstr Surg *47*:21, 1971.
234. Dupont C, Cloutier GE, Prevost Y, et al: Ulnar tunnel syndrome at the wrist. J Bone Joint Surg [Am] *47*:757, 1965.
235. Morris AH: Irreducible Monteggia lesion with radial nerve entrapment. J Bone Joint Surg [Am] *56*:1744, 1974.
236. Lichter R, Jacobson T: Tardy palsy of the posterior interosseous nerve with Monteggia fracture. J Bone Joint Surg [Am] *57*:124, 1975.
237. Millender LH, Nalebuff EA, Holdsworth DE: Posterior interosseous nerve syndrome secondary to rheumatoid synovitis. J Bone Joint Surg [Am] *55*:753, 1973.
238. Wu KT, Jordon FR, Eckert C: Lipoma, a cause of paralysis of the deep radial (posterior interosseous) nerve: Report of a case and review of the literature. Surgery *75*:790, 1974.
239. Garcia G, McQueen D: Bilateral suprascapular-nerve entrapment syndrome. Case report and review of the literature. J Bone Joint Surg [Am] *63*:491, 1981.
240. Ganzhorn RW, Hocker JT, Horowitz M, et al: Suprascapular-nerve entrapment. J Bone Joint Surg [Am] *63*:492, 1981.
241. Yoon TN, Grabois M, Guillen M: Suprascapular nerve injury following trauma to the shoulder. J Trauma *21*:652, 1981.
242. Sarno JB: Suprascapular nerve entrapment. Surg Neurol *20*:493, 1983.
243. Koppell HP, Thompson WAL: Peripheral entrapment neuropathies of the lower extremity. N Engl J Med *262*:56, 1960.
244. Guiloff RJ, Scadding JW, Klenerman L: Morton's metatarsalgia. Clinical, electrophysiological and histological observations. J Bone Joint Surg [Br] *66*:586, 1984.
245. Nissen KI: Plantar digital neuritis: Morton's metatarsalgia. J Bone Joint Surg [Br] *30*:84, 1948.
246. Gauthier G: Thomas Morton's disease: A nerve entrapment syndrome. Clin Orthop *142*:90, 1979.
247. Lam SJS: Tarsal tunnel syndrome. J Bone Joint Surg [Br] *49*:87, 1967.

248. Radin EL: Tarsal tunnel syndrome. Clin Orthop *181*:167, 1983.
249. McGuigan L, Burke D, Fleming A: Tarsal tunnel syndrome and peripheral neuropathy in rheumatoid disease. Ann Rheum Dis *42*:128, 1983.
250. Firooznia H, Golimbu C, Rafii M, et al: Computerized tomography in diagnosis of compression of the common peroneal nerve by ganglionic cysts. Comput Radiol *7*:343, 1983.
251. Stack RE, Younku AJ Jr, McCarty CS: Compression of the common peroneal nerve by ganglion cysts: Report of nine cases. J Bone Joint Surg [Am] *47*:773, 1965.
252. Mangieri JV: Peroneal-nerve injury from an enlarged fabella. J Bone Joint Surg [Am] *55*:395, 1973.
253. Takebe K, Hirohata K: Peroneal nerve palsy due to fabella. Arch Orthop Trauma Surg *99*:91, 1981.
254. Tibrewal SB, Goodfellow JW: Peroneal nerve palsy at the level of the lower third of leg. J R Soc Med *77*:72, 1984.
255. Gessini L, Jandola B, Pietrangeli A: The anterior tarsal syndrome. Report of four cases. J Bone Joint Surg [Am] *66*:786, 1984.
256. Tysvaer AT: Computerized tomography and surgical treatment of femoral compression neuropathy. J Neurosurg *57*:137, 1982.
257. Lanzieri CF, Hilal SK: Computed tomography of the sacral plexus and sciatic nerve in the greater sciatic foramen. AJR *143*:165, 1984.
258. Pech P, Haughton V: A correlative CT and anatomic study of the sciatic nerve. AJR *144*:1037, 1985.
259. Powers SK, Norman D, Edwards MSB: Computerized tomography of peripheral nerve lesions. J Neurosurg *59*:131, 1983.
260. Stewart JD, Schmidt B, Wee R: Computed tomography in the evaluation of plexopathies and proximal neuropathies. Can J Neurol Sci *10*:244, 1983.
261. Scheinberg L, Allensworth M: Sciatic neuropathy in infants related to antibiotic injections. Pediatrics *19*:261, 1957.
262. Giles FH, French JH: Post-injection sciatic nerve palsies in infants and in children. J Pediatr *58*:195, 1961.
263. Bigos SJ, Coleman SS: Foot deformities secondary to gluteal injection in infancy. J Pediatr Orthop *4*:560, 1984.
264. Nakano KK: Entrapment neuropathy from Baker's cyst. JAMA *239*:135, 1978.
265. Thomas PK: Inherited neuropathies. Mayo Clin Proc *58*:476, 1983.
266. Dyck PJ, Mellinger JF, Reagan TJ, et al: Not ''indifference to pain'' but varieties of hereditary sensory and autonomic neuropathy. Brain *106*:373, 1983.
267. Shahriaree H, Kotcamp WW, Sheikh S, et al: Hereditary perforating ulcers of the foot. ''Hereditary sensory radicular neuropathy.'' Clin Orthop *140*:189, 1979.
268. Banna M, Foster JB: Roentgenologic features of acrodystrophic neuropathy. AJR *115*:186, 1972.
269. Dyck PJ, Stevens JC, O'Brien P, et al: Neurogenic arthropathy and recurring fractures with subclinical inherited neuropathy. Neurology *33*:357, 1983.
270. Dyck PJ, Low PA, Stevens JC: ''Burning feet'' as the only manifestation of dominantly inherited sensory neuropathy. Mayo Clin Proc *58*:426, 1983.
271. Riley CM: Familial dysautonomia. Adv Pediatr *9*:157, 1957.
272. Brunt PW: Unusual cause of Charcot joint in early adolescence (Riley-Day syndrome). Br Med J *4*:277, 1967.
273. Klebanoff MA, Neff JM: Familial dysautonomia associated with recurrent osteomyelitis in a non-Jewish girl. J Pediatr *96*:75, 1980.
274. Orbeck H, Oftedal G: Familial dysautonomia in a non-Jewish child. Acta Paediatr Scand *66*:777, 1977.
275. Mitnick JS, Axelrod FB, Genieser NB, et al: Aseptic necrosis in familial dysautonomia. Radiology *142*:89, 1982.
276. Axelrod FB, Pearson J, Tepperberg J, et al: Congenital sensory neuropathy with skeletal dysplasia. J Pediatr *102*:727, 1983.
277. Swanson A: Congenital insensitivity to pain with anhydrosis. Arch Neurol *8*:299, 1966.
278. Brown J, Podosin R: A syndrome of the neural crest. Arch Neurol *15*:294, 1966.
279. Mazar A, Herold HZ, Vardy PA: Congenital sensory neuropathy and anhydrosis: Orthopaedic complications and management. Clin Orthop *118*:184, 1976.
280. Vardy PA, Greenberg LW, Kachel C, et al: Congenital insensitivity to pain with anhydrosis. Am J Dis Child *133*:1153, 1979.
281. Gold RH, Mirra JM: Case report 45. Skel Radiol *2*:127, 1977.
282. Dyck PJ, Lambert EH: Lower motor and primary sensory neuron diseases with peroneal muscle atrophy. I. Neurologic, genetic, and electrophysiologic findings in hereditary polyneuropathies. Arch Neurol *18*:603, 1968.
283. Shapiro F, Bresnan MJ: Orthopaedic management of childhood neuromuscular disease. Part II. Peripheral neuropathies, Friedreich's ataxia, and arthrogryposis multiplex congenita. J Bone Joint Surg [Am] *64*:949, 1982.
284. Sabir M, Lyttle D: Pathogenesis of Charcot-Marie-Tooth disease. Clin Orthop *184*:223, 1984.
285. Harding AE, Thomas PK: Genetic aspects of hereditary motor and sensory neuropathy (types I and II). J Med Genet *17*:329, 1980.
286. Rosenberg RN: Inherited degenerative diseases of the nervous system. *In* PB Beeson, W McDermott, JB Wyngaarden (Eds): Cecil Textbook of Medicine. 15th Ed. Philadelphia, WB Saunders Co, 1979, p 764.
287. Shapiro F, Bresnan MJ: Orthopaedic management of childhood neuromuscular disease. Part I: Spinal muscular atrophy. J Bone Joint Surg [Am] *64*:785, 1982.
288. Evans GA, Drennan JC, Russman BS: Functional classification and orthopaedic management of spinal muscular atrophy. J Bone Joint Surg [Br] *63*:516, 1981.
289. Schwentker EP, Gibson DA: The orthopaedic aspects of spinal muscular atrophy. J Bone Joint Surg [Am] *58*:32, 1976.

290. Makin M: The surgical management of Friedreich's ataxia. J Bone Joint Surg [Am] 35:425, 1953.
291. Seybold ME, Sherman DC: Muscle diseases. In JH Stein (Ed): Internal Medicine. Boston, Little, Brown, 1983, p 874.
292. Rowland LP: Diseases of muscle and neuromuscular junction. In PB Beeson, W McDermott, JB Wyngaarden (Eds): Cecil Textbook of Medicine. 15th Ed. Philadelphia, WB Saunders Co, 1979, p 914.
293. Shapiro F, Bresnan MJ: Orthopaedic management of childhood neuromuscular disease. Part III. Diseases of muscle. J Bone Joint Surg [Am] 64:1102, 1982.
294. Gibson DA, Koreska J, Robertson D, et al: The management of spinal deformity in Duchenne's muscular dystrophy. Orthop Clin North Am 9:437, 1978.
295. Robin GC, Brief LP: Scoliosis in childhood muscular dystrophy. J Bone Joint Surg [Am] 53:466, 1971.
296. Haseman MK, Kriss JP: Selective, symmetric, skeletal muscle uptake of Tc-99m pyrophosphate in rhabdomyolysis. Clin Nucl Med 10:180, 1985.
297. Donaldson JS, Gilsanz V, Gonzalez G, et al: Tall vertebrae at birth: A radiographic finding in flaccid infants. AJR 145:1293, 1985.
298. Howard CB, McKibbin B, Williams LA, et al: Factors affecting the incidence of hip dislocation in cerebral palsy. J Bone Joint Surg [Br] 67:530, 1985.
299. Orzel JA, Rudd TG: Heterotopic bone formation: Clinical, laboratory, and imaging correlation. J Nucl Med 26:125, 1985.
300. Yue CC, Regier A, Kushner I: Heterotopic ossification presenting as arthritis. J Rheumatol 12:769, 1985.
301. Garland DE, Hanscom DA, Keenan MA, et al: Resection of heterotopic ossification in the adult with head trauma. J Bone Joint Surg [Am] 67:1261, 1985.
302. Needs CJ, Webb J, Tyndall A: Paralysis and unilateral arthritis: Is the association established? Clin Rheumatol 4:176, 1985.
303. Weiner SR, Bassett LW, Reichman RP: Protective effect of poliomyelitis on psoriatic arthritis. Arthritis Rheum 28:703, 1985.
304. St John JN, Palmaz JC: The cubital tunnel in ulnar entrapment neuropathy. Radiology 158:119, 1986.
305. Gross MS, Gelberman RH: The anatomy of the distal ulnar tunnel. Clin Orthop 196:238, 1985.
306. Miura T, Hirabuki N, Imakita S, et al: Radiological findings in a case of Charcot-Marie-Tooth disease. Br J Radiol 58:1017, 1985.
307. Daher YH, Lonstein JE, Winter RB, et al: Spinal deformities in patients with Friedreich ataxia: A review of 19 patients. J Pediatr Orthop 5:553, 1985.
308. Aubart F, Fares J, Chaise F: Fracture du cotyle avec luxation intrapelvienne au décours d'une crise comitiale. A propos de 2 cas dont 1 bilatéral. Rev Chir Orthoped 72:143, 1986.
309. Duus BR: Fractures caused by epileptic seizures and epileptic osteomalacia. Injury 17:31, 1986.
310. Calò M, Crisi G, Martinelli C, et al: CT and the diagnosis of myopathies. Preliminary findings in 42 cases. Neuroradiology 28:53, 1986.
311. Sauser DD, Hewes RC, Root L: Hip changes in spastic cerebral palsy. AJR 146:1219, 1986.
312. Winter RB, Pinto WC: Pelvic obliquity. Its causes and its treatment. Spine 11:225, 1986.
313. Weiss KL, Betran J, Shamam OM, et al: High-field MR surface-coil imaging of the hand and wrist. Part I. Normal anatomy. Radiology 160:160, 1986.
314. Weiss KL, Betran J, Lubbers LM: High-field MR surface-coil imaging of the hand and wrist. Part II. Pathologic correlations and clinical relevance. Radiology 160:147, 1986.
315. Gebarski KS, Gebarski SS, Glazer GM, et al: The lumbosacral plexus: Anatomic-radiologic-pathologic correlation using CT. RadioGraphics 6:401, 1986.
316. Daher YH, Lonstein JE, Winter RB, et al: Spinal deformities in patients with Charcot-Marie-Tooth disease. A review of 12 patients. Clin Orthop 202:219, 1986.
317. Labelle H, Tohmé S, Duhaime M, et al: Natural history of scoliosis in Friedreich's ataxia. J Bone Joint Surg [Am] 68:564, 1986.
318. Murphy WA, Totty WG, Carroll JE: MRI of normal and pathologic skeletal muscle. AJR 146:565, 1986.
319. Lau JHK, Parker JC, Hsu LCS, et al: Paralytic hip instability in poliomyelitis. J Bone Joint Surg [Br] 68:528, 1986.
320. Wenner SM: Heterotopic ossification of the shoulder following head injury. A case report. Clin Orthop 212:231, 1986.
321. Ragone DJ Jr, Kellerman WC, Bonner FJ Jr: Heterotopic ossification masquerading as deep venous thrombosis in head-injured adult: complications of anticoagulation. Archiv Phys Med Rehab 67:339, 1986.
322. Bohannon RW, Larkin PA, Smith MB, et al: Shoulder pain in hemiplegia: Statistical relationship with five variables. Archiv Phys Med Rehab 67:514, 1986.
323. Merhar GL, Clark RA, Schneider HJ, et al: High-resolution computed tomography of the wrist in patients with carpal tunnel syndrome. Skel Radiol 15:549, 1986.
324. Middleton WD, Kneeland JB, Kellman GM, et al: MR imaging of the carpal tunnel: Normal anatomy and preliminary findings in the carpal tunnel syndrome. AJR 148:307, 1987.
325. Gellman H, Gelberman RH, Tan AM, et al: Carpal tunnel syndrome. An evaluation of the provocative diagnostic tests. J Bone Joint Surg [Am] 68:735, 1986.
326. Bostman O, Bakalim G, Vainionpaa S, et al: Radial palsy in shaft fracture of the humerus. Acta Orthop Scand 57:316, 1986.
327. Hadley MN, Sonntag VKH, Pittman HW: Suprascapular nerve entrapment. A summary of seven cases. J Neurosurg 64:843, 1986.

328. Nichols HM: Anatomic structures of the thoracic outlet. Clin Orthop 207:13, 1986.
329. Adson AW: Surgical treatment for symptoms produced by cervical ribs and the scalenus anticus muscle. Clin Orthop 207:3, 1986.
330. Morano JU, Russell WF: Nerve root enlargement in Charcot-Marie-Tooth disease: CT appearance. Radiology 161:784, 1986.
331. Phen HT, Kumar NVG, Ireland J: Bilateral central dislocation of the hip following a cerebrovascular accident. J Bone Joint Surg [Br] 71:703, 1989.
332. Dastgeer GM, Mikolich DJ: Fracture-dislocation of manubriosternal joint: An unusual complication of seizures. J Trauma 27:91, 1987.
333. Perkins R, Skirving AP: Callus formation and the rate of healing of femoral fractures in patients with head injuries. J Bone Joint Surg [Br] 69:521, 1987.
334. Spencer RF: The effect of head injury on fracture healing. A quantitative assessment. J Bone Joint Surg [Br] 69:525, 1987.
335. Gunreben G, Bogdahn U: Real-time sonography of acute and chronic muscle denervation. Muscle Nerve 14:654, 1991.
336. Shabas D, Gerard G, Rossi D: Magnetic resonance imaging examination of denervated muscle. Comput Radiol 11:9, 1987.
337. Fleckenstein JL, Watumull D, Conner KE, et al: Denervated human skeletal muscle: MR imaging evaluation. Radiology 187:213, 1993.
338. Polak JF, Jolesz FA, Adams DF: Magnetic resonance imaging of skeletal muscle prolongation of T1 and T2 subsequent to denervation. Invest Radiol 23:365, 1988.
339. Montagna P, Martinelli P, Rasi F, et al: Muscular hypertrophy after chronic radiculopathy. Arch Neurol 41:397, 1984.
340. Pareyson D, Morandi L, Scaioli R, et al: Neurogenic muscle hypertrophy: Report of two cases. J Neurol 236:292, 1989.
341. Bernat JL, Ochoa JL: Muscle hypertrophy after partial denervation: A human case. J Neurol Neurosurg Psychiatry 41:719, 1978.
342. Barloon TJ, Zachar CK, Harkens KL, et al: Rhabdomyolysis: Computed tomography findings. J Comput Tomogr 12:193, 1988.
343. Farmlett EJ, Fishman EK, Magid D, et al: Computed tomography in the assessment of myonecrosis. J Can Assoc Radiol 38:278, 1987.
344. Timmons JH, Hartshorne MF, Peters VJ, et al: Muscle necrosis in the extremities: Evaluation with Tc-99m pyrophosphate scanning—a retrospective review. Radiology 167:173, 1988.
345. Ludmer LM, Chandeysson P, Barth WF: Diphosphonate bone scan in an unusual case of rhabdomyolysis: A report and literature review. J Rheumatol 20:382, 1993.
346. Sever JW: Obstetric paralysis, its etiology, pathology, clinical aspects and treatment, with a report of four hundred and seventy cases. Am J Dis Child 12:553, 1916.
347. Greenwald AG, Schute PC, Shiveley JL: Brachial plexus birth palsy: A 10-year report on the incidence and prognosis. J Pediatr Orthop 4:689, 1984.
348. Pollock AN, Reed MH: Shoulder deformities from obstetrical brachial plexus paralysis. Skel Radiol 18:295, 1989.
349. Kattan KR, Spitz HB: Roentgen findings in obstetrical injuries to the brachial plexus. Radiology 91:462, 1968.
350. Westcott MA, Dynes MC, Remer EM, et al: Congenital and acquired orthopedic abnormalities in patients with myelomeningocele. RadioGraphics 12:1155, 1992.
351. Dirschl DR, Greene WB: Pseudotumor of the distal part of the femur in a patient who had myelomeningocele. A case report. J Bone Joint Surg [Am] 74:935, 1992.
352. Roberts JA, Bennet GC, MacKenzie JR: Physeal widening in children with myelomeningocele. J Bone Joint Surg [Br] 71:30, 1989.
353. Lock TR, Aronson DD: Fractures in patients who have myelomeningocele. J Bone Joint Surg [Am] 71:1153, 1989.
354. Pfeil J, Fromm B, Carstens C, et al: Frakturen und Epiphysenver letzungen bei kindern mit Myelomeningocele. Z Orthop 128:551, 1990.
355. Garland DE: Clinical observations on fractures and heterotopic ossification in the spinal cord and traumatic brain injured populations. Clin Orthop 233:86, 1988.
356. An HS, Ebraheim N, Kim K, et al: Heterotopic ossification and pseudoarthrosis in the shoulder following encephalitis. A case report and review of the literature. Clin Orthop 219:291, 1987.
357. Kun EW, Barr WG: Heterotopic ossification presenting as acute arthritis. J Rheumatol 19:994, 1992.
358. Puzas JE, Miller MD, Rosier RN: Pathologic bone formation. Clin Orthop 245:269, 1989.
359. Garland DE, Shimoyama ST, Lugo C, et al: Spinal cord insults and heterotopic ossification in the pediatric population. Clin Orthop 245:303, 1989.
360. Keret D, Harcke T, Mendez AA, et al: Heterotopic ossification in central nervous system-injured patients following closed nailing of femoral fractures. Clin Orthop 256:254, 1990.
361. Garland DE: A clinical perspective on common forms of acquired heterotopic ossification. Clin Orthop 263:13, 1991.
362. Bressler EL, Marn CS, Gore RM, et al: Evaluation of ectopic bone by CT. AJR 148:931, 1987.
363. DeSmet AA, Norris MA, Fisher DR: Magnetic resonance imaging of myositis ossificans: analysis of seven cases. Skel Radiol 21:503, 1992.
364. Kransdorf MJ, Meis JM, Jelinek JS: Myositis ossificans: MR appearance with radiographic-pathologic correlation. AJR 157:1243, 1991.
365. Schwartz HS: Traumatic Charcot spine. J Spinal Dis 3:269, 1990.

366. Kapila A, Lines M: Neuropathic spinal arthropathy: CT and MR findings. J Comput Assist Tomogr *11*:736, 1987.

367. Harrison MJ, Sacher M, Rosenblum BR, et al: Spinal Charcot arthropathy. Neurosurgery *29*:273, 1991.

368. Sethi S, Sequeira W: Sparing effect of hemiplegia on scleroderma. Ann Rheum Dis *49*:999, 1990.

369. Pariser KM, Canoso JJ: Remitting, seronegative (A) symmetrical synovitis with pitting edema—two cases of RS₃PE syndrome. J Rheumatol *18*:1260, 1991.

370. Van Langenberghe HVK, Hogan BM: Degree of pain and grade of subluxation in the painful hemiplegic shoulder. Scand J Rehabil Med *20*:161, 1988.

371. Gellman H, Eckert RR, Botte MJ, et al: Reflex sympathetic dystrophy in cervical spinal cord injury patients. Clin Orthop *233*:126, 1988.

372. Bayley JC, Cochran TP, Sledge CB: The weight-bearing shoulder. The impingement syndrome in paraplegics. J Bone Joint Surg [Am] *69*:676, 1987.

373. Seddon H: Three types of nerve injury. Brain *66*:237, 1943.

374. Shuman S, Osterman L, Bora FW: Compression neuropathies. Semin Neurol *7*:76, 1987.

375. Mackinnon SE: Double and multiple "crush" syndromes. Double and multiple entrapment neuropathies. Hand Clin *8*:369, 1992.

376. Upton ARM, McComas AJ: The double crush in nerve entrapment syndromes. Lancet *2*:259, 1973.

377. Mariano KA, McDougle MA, Tanksley GW: Double crush syndrome: Chiropractic care of an entrapment neuropathy. J Manip Physiol Ther *14*:262, 1991.

378. Dellon AL, MacKinnon SE: Chronic nerve compression model for the double crush hypothesis. Ann Plast Surg *26*:259, 1991.

379. Nemoto K, Matsumoto N, Kenichi T, et al: An experimental study on the "double crush" hypothesis. J Hand Surg [Am] *12*:552, 1987.

380. Gerstner DL, Omer GE Jr: Peripheral entrapment neuropathies in the upper extremity. Part I: Key differential findings, median nerve syndromes. J Musculoskel Med *5*:14, 1988.

381. Fuss FK, Wurzl GH: Median nerve entrapment. Pronator teres syndrome. Surgical anatomy and correlation with symptom patterns. Surg Radiol Anat *12*:267, 1990.

382. Jones NF, Ming NL: Persistent median artery as a cause of pronator syndrome. J Hand Surg [Am] *13*:728, 1988.

383. Richman JA, Gelberman RH, Rydevik BL, et al: Carpal tunnel volume determination by magnetic resonance imaging three-dimensional reconstruction. J Hand Surg [Am] *12*:712, 1987.

384. Mesgarzadeh M, Schneck CD, Bonakdarpour A: Carpal tunnel: MR imaging. Part I. Normal anatomy. Radiology *171*:743, 1989.

385. Mesgarzadeh M, Schneck CD, Bonakdarpour A, et al: Carpal tunnel: MR imaging. Part II. Carpal tunnel syndrome. Radiology *171*:749, 1989.

386. Zeiss J, Skie M, Ebraheim N, et al: Anatomic relations between the median nerve and flexor tendons in the carpal tunnel: MR evaluation in normal volunteers. AJR *153*:533, 1989.

387. Skie M, Zeiss J, Ebraheim NA, et al: Carpal tunnel changes and median nerve compression during wrist flexion and extension seen by magnetic resonance imaging. J Hand Surg [Am] *15*:934, 1990.

388. Healy C, Watson JD, Longstaff A, et al: Magnetic resonance imaging of the carpal tunnel. J Hand Surg [Br] *15*:243, 1990.

389. Buchberger W, Judmaier W, Birbamer G, et al: Carpal tunnel syndrome: Diagnosis with high-resolution sonography. AJR *159*:793, 1992.

390. Dickinson JC, Kleinert JM: Acute carpal-tunnel syndrome caused by a calcified median artery. A case report. J Bone Joint Surg [Am] *73*:610, 1991.

391. Kato H, Ogino T, Nanbu T, et al: Compression neuropathy of the motor branch of the median nerve caused by palmar ganglion. J Hand Surg [Am] *16*:751, 1991.

392. McDonnell JM, Makley JT, Horwitz SJ: Familial carpal-tunnel syndrome presenting in childhood. Report of two cases. J Bone Joint Surg [Am] *69*:928, 1987.

393. Poilvache P, Carlier A, Rombouts JJ, et al: Carpal tunnel syndrome in childhood: Report of five new cases. J Pediatr Orthop *9*:687, 1989.

394. Papaioannou T, Rushworth G, Atar D, et al: Carpal canal stenosis in men with idiopathic carpal tunnel syndrome. Clin Orthop *285*:210, 1992.

395. Gellman H, Chandler DR, Petrasek J, et al: Carpal tunnel syndrome in paraplegic patients. J Bone Joint Surg [Am] *70*:517, 1988.

396. Barnhart S, Rosenstock L: Carpal tunnel syndrome in grocery workers. A cluster of a work-related illness. West J Med *147*:37, 1987.

397. Spinner RJ, Bachman JW, Amadio PC: The many faces of carpal tunnel syndrome. Mayo Clin Proc *64*:829, 1989.

398. Huaux JP, Rombouts JJ, Knoops P, et al: Pertes de substances digitales et syndrome du canal carpien. A propos de trois observations. Ann Chir Main *5*:249, 1986.

399. Omer GE Jr: Median nerve compression at the wrist. Hand Clin *8*:317, 1992.

400. Hunter JM: Recurrent carpal tunnel syndrome, epineural fibrous fixation, and traction neuropathy. Hand Clin *7*:491, 1991.

401. Gerstner DL, Omer GE Jr: Peripheral entrapment neuropathies in the upper extremity. Part 2. Recognizing and treating ulnar and radial nerve syndromes. J Musculoskel Med *5*:37, 1988.

402. Bruijn JD, Koning J: Compression of the ulnar nerve by an aneurysm. A case of late complication after a supracondylar fracture. Acta Orthop Scand *63*:223, 1992.

403. Mainard D, Saury Ph, Delagoutte JP: Compression du nerf cubital au coude par un kyste synovial d'origine rhumatoide. Rev Rhum Mal Osteoartic *58*:611, 1991.

404. Rayan GM: Proximal ulnar nerve compression. Cubital tunnel syndrome. Hand Clin *8*:325, 1992.

405. O'Driscoll SW, Horii E, Carmichael SW, et al: The cubital tunnel and ulnar neuropathy. J Bone Joint Surg [Br] *73*:613, 1991.

406. Berkowitz AR, Melone CP Jr, Belsky MR: Pisiform-hamate coalition with ulnar neuropathy. J Hand Surg [Am] *17*:657, 1992.

407. Robinson D, Aghasi MK, Halperin N: Ulnar tunnel syndrome caused by an accessory palmaris muscle. Orthop Rev *18*:345, 1989.

408. Thurman RT, Jindal P, Wolff TW: Ulnar nerve compression in Guyon's canal caused by calcinosis in scleroderma. J Hand Surg [Am] *16*:739, 1991.

409. Salzberg CA, Weinberg H: Dupuytren's disease as a cause of ulnar tunnel syndrome. J Hand Surg [Am] *12*:91, 1987.

410. Moneim MS: Ulnar nerve compression at the wrist. Ulnar tunnel syndrome. Hand Clin *8*:337, 1992.

411. Zeiss J, Jakab E, Khimji T, et al: The ulnar tunnel at the wrist (Guyon's canal): Normal MR anatomy and variants. AJR *158*:1081, 1992.

412. Eaton CJ, Lister GD: Radial nerve compression. Hand Clin *8*:345, 1992.

413. Werner C-O: Paralysis of the posterior interosseous nerve caused by tumour: Brief report. J Bone Joint Surg [Br] *69*:670, 1987.

414. McCollam SM, Corley FG, Green DP: Posterior interosseous nerve palsy caused by ganglions of the proximal radioulnar joint. J Hand Surg [Am] *13*:725, 1988.

415. Fuss FK, Wurzl GH: Radial nerve entrapment at the elbow: Surgical anatomy. J Hand Surg [Am] *16*:742, 1991.

416. Crawford GP: Late radial tunnel syndrome after excision of the radial head. A report of two cases. J Bone Joint Surg [Am] *70*:1416, 1988.

417. Post M, Grinblat E: Nerve entrapment about the shoulder girdle. Hand Clin *8*:299, 1992.

418. Kaspi A, Yanai J, Pick CG, et al: Entrapment of the distal suprascapular nerve. An anatomical study. Int Orthop (SICOT) *12*:273, 1988.

419. Demaio M, Drez D Jr, Mullins RC: The inferior transverse scapular ligament as a possible cause of entrapment neuropathy of the nerve to the infraspinatus. A brief note. J Bone Joint Surg [Am] *73*:1061, 1991.

420. Ogino T, Minami A, Kato H, et al: Entrapment neuropathy of the suprascapular nerve by a ganglion. A report of three cases. J Bone Joint Surg [Am] *73*:141, 1991.

421. Takagishi K, Maeda K, Ikeda T, et al: Ganglion causing paralysis of the suprascapular nerve. Diagnosis by MRI and ultrasonography. Acta Orthop Scand *62*:391, 1991.

422. Callahan JD, Scully TB, Shapiro SA, et al: Suprascapular nerve entrapment. A series of 27 cases. J Neurosurg *74*:893, 1991.

423. Fritz RC, Helms CA, Steinbach LS, et al: Suprascapular nerve entrapment: Evaluation with MR imaging. Radiology *182*:437, 1992.

424. Cormier PJ, Matalon TAS, Wolin PM: Quadrilateral space syndrome: A rare cause of shoulder pain. Radiology *167*:797, 1988.

425. Alexander IJ, Johnson KA, Parr JW: Morton's neuroma: A review of recent concepts. Orthopedics *10*:103, 1987.

426. Shereff MJ, Grande DA: Electron microscopic analysis of the interdigital neuroma. Clin Orthop *271*:296, 1991.

427. Redd RA, Peters VJ, Emery SF, et al: Morton neuroma: Sonographic evaluation. Radiology *171*:415, 1989.

428. Erickson SJ, Canale PB, Carrera GF, et al: Interdigital (Morton) neuroma: High-resolution MR imaging with a solenoid coil. Radiology *181*:833, 1991.

429. Sartoris DJ, Brozinsky S, Resnick D: Magnetic resonance images: interdigital or Morton's neuroma. J Foot Surg *28*:78, 1989.

430. Taguchi Y, Nosaka K, Yasuda K, et al: The tarsal tunnel syndrome. Report of two cases of unusual cause. Clin Orthop *217*:247, 1987.

431. Havens RT, Kaloogian H, Thul JR, et al: A correlation between os trigonum syndrome and tarsal tunnel syndrome. J Am Podiatr Assoc *76*:450, 1986.

432. Takakura Y, Kitada C, Sugimoto K, et al: Tarsal tunnel syndrome. Causes and results of operative intervention. J Bone Joint Surg [Br] *73*:125, 1991.

433. Francis H, March L, Terenty T, et al: Benign joint hypermobility with neuropathy: Documentation and mechanism of tarsal tunnel syndrome. J Rheumatol *14*:577, 1987.

434. Sammarco GJ, Chalk DE, Feibel JH: Tarsal tunnel syndrome and additional nerve lesions in the same limb. Foot Ankle *14*:71, 1993.

435. Zongzhao L, Jiansheng Z, Li Z: Anterior tarsal tunnel syndrome. J Bone Joint Surg [Br] *73*:470, 1991.

436. Zeiss J, Fenton P, Ebraheim N, et al: Normal magnetic resonance anatomy of the tarsal tunnel. Foot Ankle *10*:214, 1990.

437. Erickson SJ, Quinn SF, Kneeland JB, et al: MR imaging of the tarsal tunnel and related spaces: Normal and abnormal findings with anatomic correlation. AJR *155*:323, 1990.

438. Zeiss J, Ebraheim N, Rusin J: Magnetic resonance imaging in the diagnosis of tarsal tunnel syndrome. Case report. Clin Imaging *14*:123, 1990.

439. Kerr R, Frey C: MR imaging in tarsal tunnel syndrome. J Comput Assist Tomogr *15*:280, 1991.

440. Zeiss J, Fenton P, Ebraheim N, et al: Magnetic resonance imaging for ineffectual tarsal tunnel surgical treatment. Clin Orthop *264*:264, 1991.

441. Curley P, Eyres K, Brezinova V, et al: Common peroneal nerve dysfunction after high tibial osteotomy. J Bone Joint Surg [Br] *72*:405, 1990.

442. Gambari PI, Giuliani G, Poppi M, et al: Ganglionic cysts of the peroneal nerve at the knee: CT and surgical correlation. J Comput Assist Tomogr *14*:801, 1990.

443. Guo-Xiang J, Wei-Dong X, Ai-Hao W: Spinal stenosis with meralgia paraesthetica. J Bone Joint Surg [Br] 70:272, 1988.

444. Létourneau L, Dessureault M, Carette S: Rheumatoid iliopsoas bursitis presenting as unilateral femoral nerve palsy. J Rheumatol 18:462, 1991.

445. Apter S, Hertz M, Rubinstein ZJ, et al: Femoral neuropathy: The role of computed tomography in diagnosis and management in 27 patients. Clin Radiol 40:30, 1989.

446. Graif M, Seton A, Nerubai J, et al: Sciatic nerve: Sonographic evaluation and anatomic-pathologic considerations. Radiology 181:405, 1991.

447. Gadelrab RR: Sciatic nerve entrapment in an osseous tunnel as a late complication of fracture dislocation of the hip. Orthopedics 13:1262, 1990.

448. Hughes SS, Goldstein MN, Hicks DG, et al: Extrapelvic compression of the sciatic nerve. J Bone Joint Surg [Am] 74:1553, 1992.

449. Jankiewicz JJ, Hennrikus WL, Houkom JA: The appearance of the piriformis muscle syndrome in computed tomography and magnetic resonance imaging. Clin Orthop 262:205, 1991.

450. Vandertop WP, Bosma NJ: The piriformis syndrome. A case report. J Bone Joint Surg [Am] 73:1095, 1991.

451. Chen W-S: Sciatica due to piriformis pyomyositis. Report of a case. J Bone Joint Surg [Am] 74:1546, 1992.

452. de Verdier HJ, Colletti PM, Terk MR: MRI of the brachial plexus: A review of 51 cases. Comput Med Imaging Graph 17:45, 1993.

453. Blair DN, Rapoport S, Sostman HD, et al: Normal brachial plexus: MR imaging. Radiology 165:763, 1987.

454. Rapoport S, Blair DN, McCarthy SM, et al: Brachial plexus: Correlation of MR imaging with CT and pathologic findings. Radiology 167:161, 1988.

455. Castagno AA, Shuman WP: MR imaging in clinically suspected brachial plexus tumor. AJR 149:1219, 1987.

456. Mann RA, Missirian J: Pathophysiology of Charcot-Marie-Tooth disease. Clin Orthop 234:221, 1988.

457. Choi SK, Bowers RP, Buckthal PE: MR imaging in hypertrophic neuropathy: A case of hereditary motor and sensory neuropathy, type I (Charcot-Marie-Tooth). Clin Imaging 14:204, 1990.

458. Bird TD: Hereditary motor-sensory neuropathies. Charcot-Marie-Tooth syndrome. Neurol Clin 7:9, 1989.

459. Schreiber A, Smith WL, Ionasescu V, et al: Magnetic resonance imaging of children with Duchenne muscular dystrophy. Pediatr Radiol 17:495, 1987.

460. Liu G-C, Jong Y-J, Chiang C-H, et al: Duchenne muscular dystrophy: MR grading system with functional correlation. Radiology 186:475, 1993.

461. Bárány M, Siegel IM, Venkatasubramanian PN, et al: Human leg neuromuscular diseases: P-31 MR spectroscopy. Radiology 172:503, 1989.

462. Lamminen A, Jääskeläinen J, Rapola J, et al: High-frequency ultrasonography of skeletal muscle in children with neuromuscular disease. J Ultrasound Med 7:505, 1988.

463. Caro PA, Borden S IV: Plastic bowing of the ribs in children. Skel Radiol 17:255, 1988.

464. Flipo RM, Castelain V, Sutter B, et al: Heterotopic ossification of the hands in patients with neurologic disorders. A report of two cases. Rev Rhum Mal Osteoartic [Engl Ed] 60:378, 1993.

465. Park Y-H, Huang G-S, Taylor JA, et al: Patterns of vertebral ossification and pelvic abnormalities in paralysis: A study of 200 patients. Radiology 188:561, 1993.

466. Rosenbaum RB: The role of imaging in the diagnosis of carpal tunnel syndrome. Invest Radiol 28:1059, 1993.

467. Murphy RX Jr, Chernofsky MA, Osborne MA, et al: Magnetic resonance imaging in the evaluation of persistent carpal tunnel syndrome. J Hand Surg [Am] 18:113, 1993.

468. Foster RJ, Swiontkowski MF, Bach AW, et al: Radial nerve palsy caused by open humeral shaft fractures. J Hand Surg [Am] 18:121, 1993.

469. Terk MR, Kwong PK, Suthar M, et al: Morton neuroma: Evaluation with MR imaging performed with contrast enhancement and fat suppression. Radiology 189:239, 1993.

470. Rodeo SA, Sobel M, Weiland AJ: Deep peroneal-nerve injury as a result of arthroscopic meniscectomy. A case report and review of the literature. J Bone Joint Surg [Am] 75:1221, 1993.

471. Uetani M, Hayashi K, Matsunaga N, et al: Denervated skeletal muscle: MR imaging. Work in progress. Radiology 189:511, 1993.

472. Luisto M, Zitting A, Tallroth K: Hyperostosis and osteoarthritis in patients surviving after tetanus. Skeletal Radiol 23:31, 1994.

473. Yoshioka S, Okuda Y, Tamai K, et al: Changes in carpal tunnel shape during wrist joint motion. MRI evaluation of normal volunteers. J Hand Surg [Br] 18:620, 1993.

474. Sugimoto H, Miyaji N, Ohsawa T: Carpal tunnel syndrome: Evaluation of median nerve circulation with dynamic contrast-enhanced MR imaging. Radiology 190:459, 1994.

475. Gelberman RH, Eaton R, Urbaniak JR: Peripheral nerve compression. J Bone Joint Surg [Am] 75:1854, 1993.

476. Rowland EB, Kleinert JM: Endoscopic carpal-tunnel release in cadavers. J Bone Joint Surg [Am] 76:266, 1994.

477. Shapiro F, Specht L: The diagnosis and orthopaedic treatment of childhood spinal muscle atrophy, peripheral neuropathy, Friedreich ataxia, and arthrogryposis. J Bone Joint Surg [Am] 75:1699, 1993.

78

Neuropathic Osteoarthropathy

Donald Resnick, M.D.

The report that first acknowledged the relationship of arthropathy and neural disease was that of Mitchell[1] in 1831, in which a patient with a spinal disorder ("caries of the lumbar spine") developed a peripheral joint affliction that did not respond to the "usual treatment by leeches, purgatives, and cooling diaphoretics."[2] Thirty-seven years later, in 1868, Charcot[3] described an apparent cause-and-effect relationship between primary lesions of the central nervous system and certain arthropathies, naming the condition "l'arthropathie des ataxiques." Charcot continued to study and to characterize the disorder during the next 15 years,[4–6] and although his description virtually was confined to patients with tabes dorsalis, the name "Charcot joint" has become synonymous with all articular abnormalities related to neurologic deficits, regardless of the nature of the primary disease.[7] Other terms applied to this disorder are neuroarthropathy and neurotrophic or neuropathic joint disease.[126] None of these terms is ideal, however, as the initial event in some types of this disorder occurs not in the joint itself but in the adjacent bone or even at some distance from the articulation. It would appear that the designations *neuropathic osteoarthropathy* and *neuropathic bone and joint disease* are applied more suitably to a problem that may arise first either in an osseous or in an articular site.

ETIOLOGY AND PATHOGENESIS

Central (upper motor neuron) and peripheral (lower motor neuron) lesions can lead to neuropathic osteoarthropa-

thy. Included in a list of central lesions that may produce neuropathic osteoarthropathy are syphilis, syringomyelia, meningomyelocele, trauma, multiple sclerosis, Charcot-Marie-Tooth disease, congenital vascular anomalies, and other causes of cord compression, injury, or degeneration; peripheral causes include diabetes mellitus, alcoholism, amyloidosis, infection (tuberculosis, yaws, leprosy), pernicious anemia, trauma, and intra-articular or systemic administration of steroids.[7] Additionally, specific syndromes leading to congenital insensitivity to pain and dysautonomia produce similar alterations.

Despite the prominent role that neurologic disorders play in the development of neuropathic osteoarthropathy, no uniform agreement exists on the pathogenesis of the articular changes. In fact, after early reports of this disorder, two fundamental theories of pathogenesis arose. The "French theory,"[8] as supported by Mitchell[1] and Charcot,[3] held that joint changes were the result of damage to the central nervous system trophic centers, which controlled nutrition of the bones and the joints, leading to atrophy of osseous and articular structures. This theory was challenged immediately by Volkmann, who maintained that unusual mechanical stresses about a weight-bearing joint in an ataxic person led to recurrent subclinical trauma.[8] This latter concept was later championed by Virchow and became known as the "German theory."

Eloesser[9] in 1917, on the basis of the results of a series of small (and not always successful) experiments, supported the role of trauma in the development of neuropathic joints. He noted that cats' joints rendered anesthetic by posterior sensory nerve section remained intact, whereas those joints that were subjected to additional damage developed neuropathic-like alterations. Furthermore, chemical analysis and in vitro stress studies of both denervated and normal bones failed to reveal any atrophy or inherent osseous weakening, "making untenable Charcot's theory that atrophic disturbance causing a wasting of the bone [was] at the root of these arthropathies," and suggesting that Charcot joints were caused by "the sudden response of an anesthetic joint to . . . acute trauma."[2] The results of other investigations supported this concept[10] and demonstrated the obvious pattern of repetitive trauma resulting in intra-articular osseous fragments that arises in an anesthetic joint.[11]

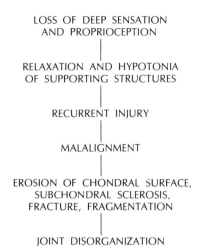

LOSS OF DEEP SENSATION
AND PROPRIOCEPTION

|

RELAXATION AND HYPOTONIA
OF SUPPORTING STRUCTURES

|

RECURRENT INJURY

|

MALALIGNMENT

|

EROSION OF CHONDRAL SURFACE,
SUBCHONDRAL SCLEROSIS,
FRACTURE, FRAGMENTATION

|

JOINT DISORGANIZATION

FIGURE 78–1. Pathogenesis of neuropathic osteoarthropathy. The probable sequential steps in the development of the disease are indicated.

Although additional theories emphasized the contributory role of lesions of the autonomic nervous system,[12] vascular insufficiency,[13] or infection[14] in the production of neuropathic osteoarthropathy, the current consensus supports the prominent role of misuse or abuse of insensitive joints in this condition (Fig. 78–1). Loss of the protective sensations of pain and proprioception leads to relaxation of the supporting structures and chronic instability of the joint. In this setting, the daily stresses of normal movement produce injury, malalignment, and abnormal joint loading. Cumulative injury leads to progressive degeneration and disorganization of the articulation.[15]

The radiographic and pathologic features reflect the joint disorganization with excessive cartilaginous and osseous destruction. The appearances may vary with the specific cause of the neurologic deficit, however. Productive (or hypertrophic) changes commonly are associated with central spinal cord lesions, such as trauma, tumor, or congenital malformations, and with diseases that commonly spare the sympathetic nervous system, such as tabes dorsalis and syringomyelia. Destructive (or atrophic) manifestations typically are linked to peripheral nerve injuries and related to trauma, alcoholism, and diabetes, which presumably affect postganglionic nerve segments carrying sympathetic vasoconstrictive as well as sensory and motor fibers.[16] Hypertrophic abnormalities are encountered most frequently in, but are not limited to, the spine and proximal sites in the lower extremities; atrophic abnormalities typically are encountered in, but are not confined to, non–weight-bearing locations and the forefoot.[161] The existence in neuropathic osteoarthropathy of a neurally mediated vascular reflex leading to increased osteoclastic bone resorption in hyperemic areas that are devoid of vasoconstrictive impulses has been postulated by Johnson.[17] Angiography may confirm the existence of hypervascularity,[18] although the increased blood flow may promote both lysis and sclerosis about the neuropathic joint. Associated osteonecrosis could be caused by mechanical compromise of the vascular supply produced by osseous fragmentation.[16]

Proponents of a neurovascular cause for neuropathic osteoarthropathy cite the inconclusive results of Eloesser's classic experiment in cats.[125] They emphasize that osteoclastic resorption of bone due to hyperemia could explain all of the radiographic changes of this disease, which could be considered neurotrophic rather than neurotraumatic in nature. This mechanism is supported by histologic evidence of hypervascularity of bone, osteoclastic activity, and dilation of haversian canals, as well as radiologic evidence of osteolysis and fracture at sites not subject to unusual trauma.[125]

What, then, is the true pathogenesis of neuropathic osteoarthropathy? Although the initial, or triggering, event is not clear, considerable evidence has been accumulated that both mechanical and vascular factors contribute to the subsequent disintegration of the joint. It certainly is possible that both the temporal relationship and the relative contribution of one factor as compared with the other are disease-dependent. In certain disorders, a neurotraumatic event may be followed by vascular alterations and together they lead to productive and resorptive bone abnormalities; in other disorders, initial hypervascularity and its effect on bone may make a specific area more vulnerable to normal and abnormal mechanical forces. What is clear is that loss of normal neurologic function renders a joint (and adjacent bone) susceptible to a sequence of pathologic and radiologic alterations that ultimately may produce its disintegration. Instability of the joint prior to the neurologic dysfunction may make this sequence more likely.[128]

GENERAL RADIOGRAPHIC AND PATHOLOGIC ABNORMALITIES

Although the pathologic and radiologic features of advanced neuropathic osteoarthropathy indeed are characteristic,[10, 15, 19] early features may simulate those of osteoarthritis (Fig. 78–2). Thus, cartilaginous fibrillation and erosion, subchondral trabecular thickening, and osteophytosis on pathologic examination, and joint space narrowing, sclerosis, and osseous excrescences on radiographic examination are similar to findings in degenerative joint disease. The presence of an enlarging and persistent effusion, minimal subluxation, fracture, and fragmentation should alert the radiologist to the possibility of neuropathic osteoarthropathy[20]; similarly, the finding of considerable amounts of cartilaginous and osseous debris attached to and incorporated into the synovial membrane (detritic synovitis) in a patient who is presumed to have degenerative joint disease should suggest to a pathologist that the changes may indeed represent joint manifestations of neuropathic disease (Table 78–1). These early changes may show rapid progression, suggesting that microfractures exist that evolve quickly into gross fragmentation,[16, 21] and the joint may appear to fall apart in a matter of days or weeks[22] (Fig. 78–3). The rapid nature of the evolving neuropathic process also has been verified experimentally,[9] and in clinical situations, acute subluxations or dislocations may be encountered.[23] It is the

TABLE 78–1. Some Causes of Detritic Synovitis

Neuropathic osteoarthropathy
Osteonecrosis
Calcium pyrophosphate dihydrate crystal deposition disease
Psoriatic arthritis
Osteoarthritis
Osteolysis with detritic synovitis

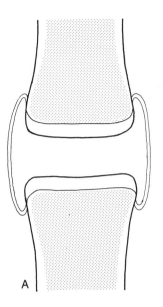

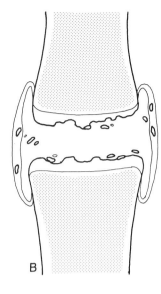

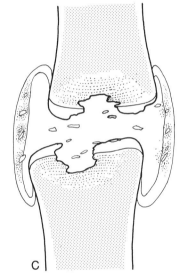

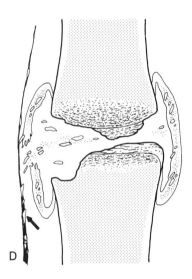

FIGURE 78–2. General radiographic and pathologic abnormalities: Stages of neuropathic osteoarthropathy.

A A normal synovial joint is illustrated.

B Initially, cartilaginous fibrillation and fragmentation can be observed; some of the cartilaginous debris remains attached to the chondral surface, some is displaced into the articular cavity, and some becomes embedded in the synovial membrane.

C Subsequently, osseous and cartilaginous destruction becomes more extensive, the embedded pieces of cartilage and bone producing local synovial irritation. Bony eburnation and subluxation also are evident.

D Eventually, large portions of the chondral coat are lost, sclerosis is extreme, capsular rupture can occur, and shards of bone can dissect along the soft tissue planes (arrow).

focal disruption of chondral and osseous surfaces in the early stages of neuropathic osteoarthropathy that leads to collections of bone and cartilage debris, which are ground into the synovial and subsynovial tissues (Fig. 78–4), and that produces radiographic and pathologic clues to the nature of the articular abnormality sometimes months to years before gross fragmentation becomes evident.[24]

When a joint is the site of more advanced abnormalities, diagnostic radiographic features appear, consisting of depression, absorption, and shattering of subchondral bone, osseous proliferation in the form of significant sclerosis and osteophytosis, intra-articular osseous fragments, subluxation, massive soft tissue enlargement and effusion, and fracture of neighboring bones (Figs. 78–5 and 78–6). On pathologic examination, the capsule is found to be thickened irregularly by fibrous tissue and ossified, the synovial membrane is indurated, with villous transformation, and considerable fluid and connective tissue adhesions are evident within the joints.[15] In the synovial membrane, fragments of cartilage and bone may reveal growth activity. In addition, diffuse metaplasia of the synovium with formation of car-

tilage and calcification of cartilage within the deeper layers of the membrane can be noted.[25] The embedded and metaplastic osteocartilaginous bodies in the synovium of neuropathic joints produce radiographically detectable calcific and ossific dense lesions, which eventually may become far removed from the joint itself[26, 27] (Fig. 78–7). This latter phenomenon represents migration of bone shards into the distant recesses of an enlarging joint cavity, into a neighboring synovial cyst,[162] or along muscle tissue planes. In some instances, the radiodense shadows later disappear.[26]

The articular ends of the bones that are contained within a neuropathic joint become devoid of cartilage, the surface being replaced by fibrous tissue or fibrocartilage.[15] The exposed subchondral bone appears eburnated and shiny, and it may be deformed, distorted, or worn away by the apposing articular surface. Marginal osteophytes can reach considerable size, although others fragment and disintegrate. Malalignment with angular deformity, subluxation, or dislocation leads to increased stress on the articular bone, contributing to sclerosis and gross fractures (Fig. 78–8). Fracture lines can originate in the subchondral region and

Text continued on page 3420

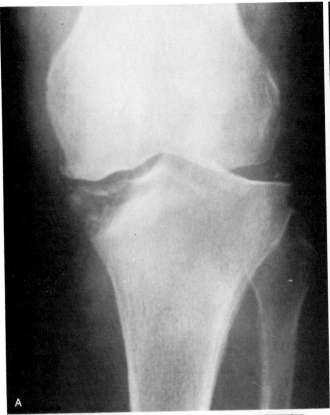
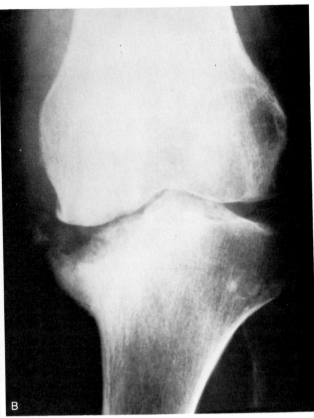

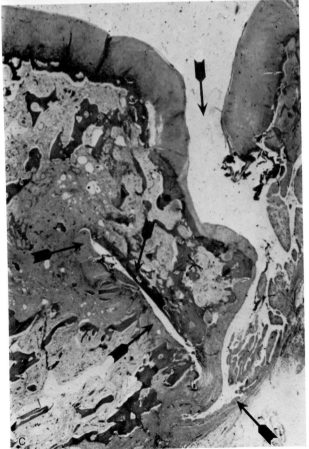

FIGURE 78–3. General radiographic and pathologic abnormalities of neuropathic osteoarthropathy: Rapid progression of disease.

A, B The appearance and progression of articular destruction can occur rapidly. Initial foci of chondral and osseous destruction can lead to fragmentation and collapse in a period of weeks. This is a patient with tabes dorsalis.

C This photomicrograph (3×) of the articular margin of the talus of a diabetic patient demonstrates unhealed linear microfractures, which are not visible to the naked eye or on radiographs of specimen slices (arrows). The extension of the microfracture through the subarticular bone and the cavitation at the fracture site suggest motion between adjacent surfaces.

(**C,** From Feldman F, et al: Radiology *111*:1, 1974.)

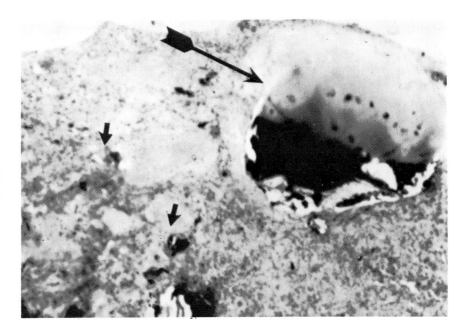

FIGURE 78–4. General radiographic and pathologic abnormalities of neuropathic osteoarthropathy: Detritic synovitis. Note the large fragment of recognizable articular cartilage and subchondral bone embedded within the synovium (large arrow). Other fragments of bone and cartilage are visible (small arrows) (52×). (From Feldman F, et al: Radiology *111*:1, 1974.)

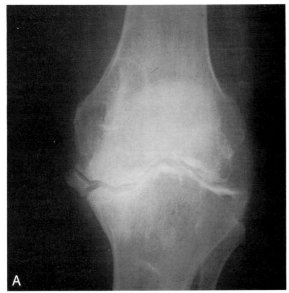

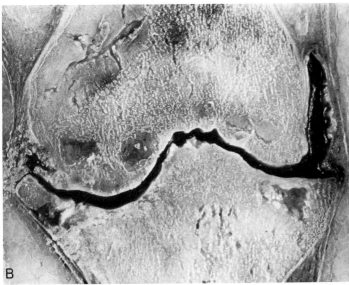

FIGURE 78–5. General radiographic and pathologic abnormalities of neuropathic osteoarthropathy: Intermediate lesions. A frontal radiograph **(A)** and a photograph **(B)** of a coronal section of the knee show joint space narrowing due to cartilage destruction, depression and fragmentation of the articular surface, especially in the tibia, and intraosseous cysts. Note the blood in the joint cavity. (Presumptive diagnosis.)

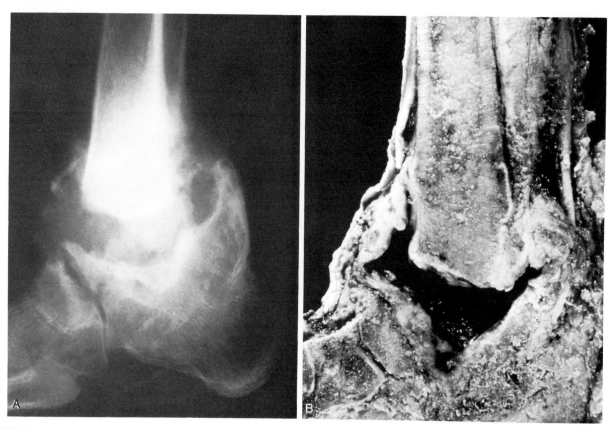

FIGURE 78–6. General radiographic and pathologic abnormalities of neuropathic osteoarthropathy: Advancing lesions.

　A Note soft tissue swelling and considerable fragmentation and resorption of the talus, tibia, and fibula, with extreme sclerosis, osteophytosis, and intra-articular osseous bodies.

　B On a sagittal section of the amputated extremity, the degree of osseous resorption and fragmentation is apparent, as are synovial and capsular hypertrophy and distention.

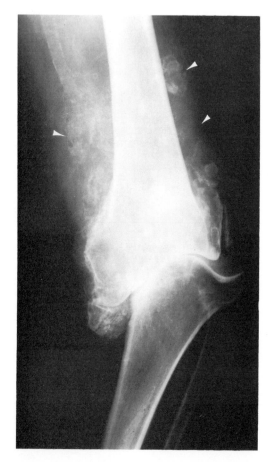

FIGURE 78–7. General radiographic and pathologic abnormalities of neuropathic osteoarthropathy: Migration of bony shards. In this patient with syphilis, numerous fragments of bone originating from the destroyed articular surfaces have moved into the far recesses of the joint or migrated along adjacent tissue planes (arrowheads).

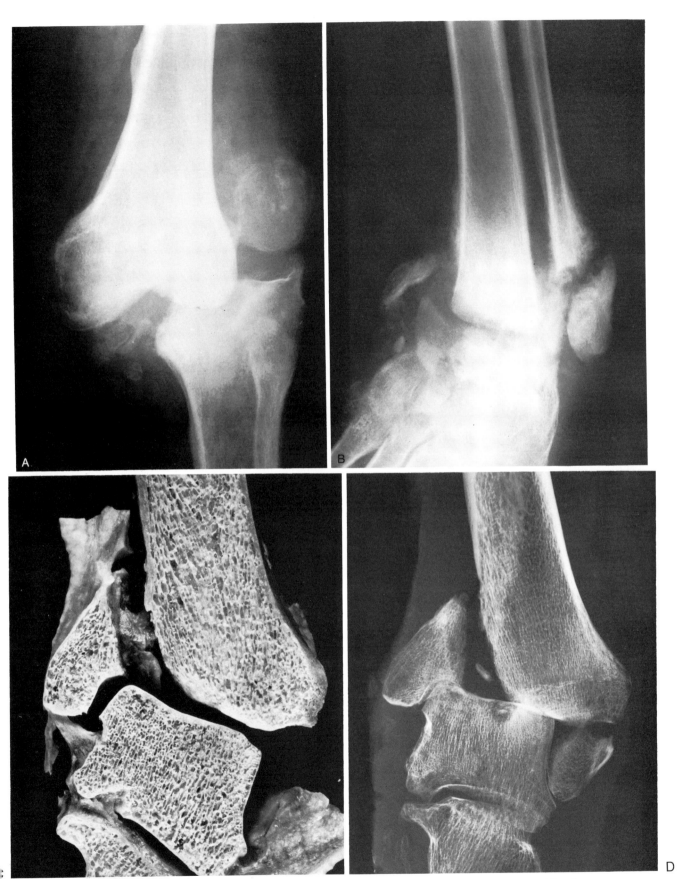

FIGURE 78–8. General radiographic and pathologic abnormalities of neuropathic osteoarthropathy: Fractures and subluxations.

  A Gross disorganization of the joint in a tabetic patient is characterized by lateral subluxation of the tibia on the femur, lateral patellar dislocation, soft tissue swelling, osseous fragmentation and sclerosis, and periostitis.

  B In a different patient with the same disease, note the angular deformity of the ankle with fragmentation, sclerosis, and fractures. Periostitis and soft tissue swelling are evident.

  C, D This patient with diabetes mellitus developed spontaneous fractures of the distal ends of the tibia and fibula, which became displaced in the following few weeks. After amputation, a photograph **(C)** and radiograph **(D)** of a coronal section of the specimen indicate severe displacement and angulation. The patient had been relatively asymptomatic during this period.

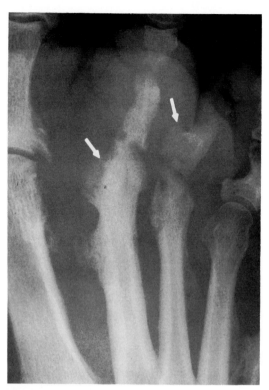

FIGURE 78–9. General radiographic and pathologic abnormalities of neuropathic osteoarthropathy: Superimposed infection. In diabetic patients, neuropathic changes in superficial joints such as the metatarsophalangeal joints frequently are complicated by osteomyelitis and septic arthritis. In such instances, the poorly defined contour of the involved bones (arrows) usually allows diagnosis of both conditions.

extend extra-articularly, or they may occur at a site distant from the joint (e.g., the diaphysis of a tubular bone). Fracture repair with periostitis is encountered, and the exuberant callus may merge with the endosteal sclerosis and marginal osteophytic lips; in some patients, delayed healing or even pseudarthroses develop at sites of fracture or, after healing, refracture occurs.

In long-standing neuropathic osteoarthropathy, the resulting radiographic picture is that of a disorganized joint, characterized by simultaneously occurring bone resorption and formation. The degree of sclerosis, osteophytosis, and fragmentation in this disorder is greater than that in any other process. Yet, the bone shards and irregular articular surfaces that are produced by the considerable osseous fragmentation and collapse accompanying this disease generally are well defined and sharp.[161] Poorly marginated, "fuzzy" bone contours, as occur in osteomyelitis and septic arthritis, are not evident unless infection has become superimposed on the neuropathic process.[129] This last-mentioned complication, however, is not infrequent, especially in diabetic patients and in those joints that are located superficially in the body (e.g., metatarsophalangeal joints) (Fig. 78–9).[127] Intra-articular bony fusion is an uncommon manifestation of neuropathic osteoarthropathy at any site, with the exception of the spine. In fact, attempts at arthrodesis or arthroplasty in this disease frequently, but not invariably, are unsuccessful (Fig. 78–10).[130, 163, 164]

SPECIFIC DISORDERS

Although Charcot's original description of neuropathic osteoarthropathy emphasized its occurrence in tabes dorsalis,[3–6] Charcot anticipated that similar abnormalities might accompany other neurologic processes, and, in fact, he described neuropathic changes in two non-tabetic patients with spinal injuries and hemiplegia.[2] Subsequent reports of neuropathic osteoarthropathy in poliomyelitis,[28] syringomyelia,[2] peripheral nerve injuries,[29] and diabetes mellitus[30] confirmed the accuracy of this anticipation. It now is known that neuropathic osteoarthropathy can accompany many disorders that lead to sensory disturbances, including the use of intra-articular or oral corticosteroids.[31] Although some motor function is fundamental in the pathogenesis of the lesions, patients with both sensory and motor loss can develop neuropathic osteoarthropathy, presumably related to vigorous physical therapy.

Although the radiographic and pathologic features of this condition generally are similar in these various disorders, certain subtle differences can be evident. Furthermore, the distribution of the abnormalities varies among these disorders, providing an important clue to a proper specific diagnosis (Table 78–2).

Tabes Dorsalis

It is estimated that 5 to 10 per cent of patients with tabes dorsalis will reveal neuropathic osteoarthropathy.[15] The joints of the lower extremity are affected in 60 to 75 per cent of cases; those of the upper extremity or elsewhere are involved in the remaining instances. The knee (Figs. 78–3A, B, 78–7, and 78–8A), hip (Fig. 78–11A), ankle (Fig. 78–8B), shoulder, and elbow (Fig. 78–11B) are altered, in

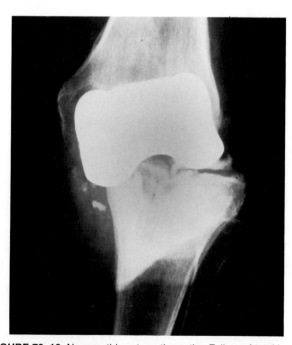

FIGURE 78–10. Neuropathic osteoarthropathy: Failure of total knee arthroplasty. Replacement of the knee in a 73 year old man with tabes dorsalis failed owing to fragmentation of the polyethylene tibial component. Subluxation is evident.

TABLE 78–2. Common Sites of Involvement in Neuropathic Osteoarthropathy

Disease	Site of Involvement
Tabes dorsalis	Knee, hip, ankle, spine
Syringomyelia	Glenohumeral joint, elbow, wrist, spine
Diabetes mellitus	Metatarsophalangeal, tarsometatarsal, intertarsal joints
Alcoholism	Metatarsophalangeal, interphalangeal joints
Amyloidosis	Knee, ankle
Meningomyelocele	Ankle, intertarsal joints
Congenital sensory neuropathy, hereditary sensory radicular neuropathy	Knee, ankle, intertarsal, metatarsophalangeal, interphalangeal joints
Idiopathic	Elbow, shoulder

descending order of frequency. Other involved sites include the joints of the forefoot, midfoot, vertebral column, and fingers, and the temporomandibular and sternoclavicular joints.[15, 16, 32–34] Monoarticular involvement predominates but polyarticular alterations are not unusual, and bilateral symmetric changes affecting as many as eight joints may be encountered.[15]

Most typically, painless swelling, deformity, weakness, and instability represent the clinical manifestations of tabetic neuropathic osteoarthropathy. Affected joints indeed may be painful, however, although the mild nature of the discomfort appears relatively insignificant in the face of extensive soft tissue swelling. The soft tissue prominence results from sizeable joint effusions, dissection of fluid into periarticular structures, and capsular and soft tissue hypertrophy. In some instances, patients show evidence of a spontaneous fracture of the neighboring bone, which, when combined with significant capsular and ligamentous laxity, leads to considerable deformity or angulation. The radiographs will reveal typical features of neuropathic osteoarthropathy, including exuberant eburnation and fragmentation. Scintigraphy accomplished with bone-seeking radiopharmaceutical agents shows areas of increased accumulation of the radionuclide (Fig. 78–12). Abnormalities in certain laboratory parameters, such as the *Treponema pallidum* Immobilization (TPI) test, the fluorescent treponemal antibody absorption (FTA-ABS) test, the Venereal Disease Research Laboratory (VDRL) test, and the Automated Reagin Test (ART), although not entirely without false-positive and false-negative results, provide important clues to the specific diagnosis. Additional laboratory abnormalities are less specific—for example, findings of anemia may indicate accompanying vascular injury.[157]

Axial neuropathic osteoarthropathy is not uncommon in tabes[7, 16, 35–40, 165] and may represent 20 per cent of all cases of neuropathic disease encountered in tabetic patients. It most frequently is seen in men and in the sixth and seventh decades of life, predominantly in the lumbar spine, less commonly in the thoracic spine, and rarely in the cervical spine.[7, 16, 41, 131] One or more vertebrae can be affected. As opposed to the situation in peripheral neuropathic osteoarthropathy, axial involvement often is symptomatic, leading

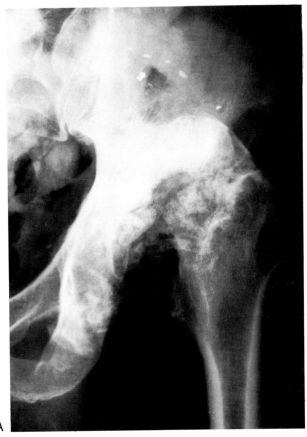

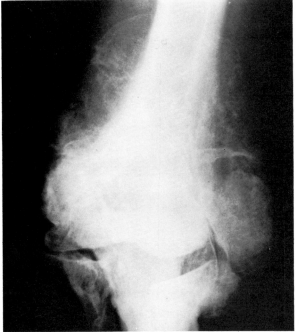

FIGURE 78–11. Tabes dorsalis: Neuropathic osteoarthropathy of the appendicular skeleton. Examples of neuropathic joint disease of the hip **(A)** and the elbow **(B)** are shown. Sclerosis and fragmentation are prominent, and deformities, subluxation, and dislocation may be evident.

A

B

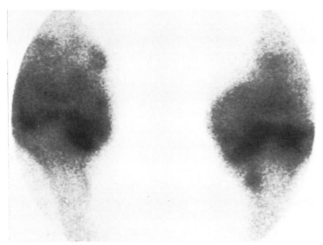

FIGURE 78–12. Tabes dorsalis: Neuropathic osteoarthropathy of the appendicular skeleton—scintigraphy. In this 78 year old man with extensive radiographic abnormalities of both knees, abnormal accumulation of the bone-seeking radionuclide is evident bilaterally, especially in the medial portion of the tibiae.

Fracture with osseous fragmentation in spinal and paraspinal locations as well as malalignment also can be evident. The resulting radiographic findings, when severe, are unique to this disorder, differing from the spinal manifestations of degenerative joint disease, infection, skeletal metastasis, and Paget's disease (Table 78–3).

Less commonly, osteolytic or destructive changes predominate in axial neuropathic osteoarthropathy. These can appear acutely and progress rapidly, leading to significant bony dissolution in a period of weeks or months. Anterior (intervertebral discs and vertebral bodies) or posterior (apophyseal joints) structures can be affected more extensively, and the irregular destructive changes that ensue can produce osseous surfaces resembling the pieces of a jigsaw puzzle.[16] The appearance of this lytic variety of neuropathic disease can resemble that in infection or skeletal metastasis.

Pathologic features in axial and appendicular skeletal sites of tabetic neuropathic osteoarthropathy resemble those of other neuropathic disorders (Fig. 78–14). Initial stress fractures or microfractures precede the more extensive destructive and productive changes. Degeneration of adjacent nerves and superimposed infection can be encountered.

Syringomyelia

It has been estimated that 20 to 25 per cent of patients with syringomyelia develop neuropathic osteoarthropathy.[15, 36, 44–49] Although the radiographic and pathologic characteristics of neuropathic bone and joint disease in syringomyelia resemble those of tabes, striking differences in the distribution of the abnormalities can be noted. Neuropathic changes in syringomyelia are common in the joints of the upper extremity,[132, 133, 158] especially the glenohumeral articulation (Figs. 78–15 and 78–16), the elbow (Fig. 78–17A), and the joints of the wrist and fingers (Fig. 78–17B). Approximately 75 to 80 per cent of syringomyelia patients with neuropathic osteoarthropathy demonstrate abnormalities in one or more of these sites; the remainder have changes in the articulations of the lower extremity, the spine, or, rarely, elsewhere, such as the sternoclavicular joint.[132] In the lower extremity, the knee, the ankle, and the

to significant pain; this symptom is related to the preservation of some nerve fibers and the compression of nerve roots by intervertebral disc herniation, osteophytes, or debris.[7, 16, 42, 43] Clinical signs include abnormal spinal curvature (kyphosis or scoliosis) and motor and sensory disturbances. Rarely, paraplegia is evident.[42, 43]

Radiographic features of tabetic axial neuropathic disease may be productive or destructive.[16] In the former group, changes such as intervertebral disc space and apophyseal joint narrowing, sclerosis, and osteophytosis can simulate findings in degenerative joint disease. The productive alterations of neuropathic osteoarthropathy generally are more exaggerated than those of degenerative joint disease, however, representing "osteoarthritis with a vengeance."[16] Thus, eburnation may be florid, intervertebral disc space narrowing may be complete, osteophytes can reach mammoth proportions, and apophyseal joint subluxation with neighboring bony sclerosis can be profound (Fig. 78–13).

TABLE 78–3. Axial Neuropathic Osteoarthropathy and Its Differential Diagnosis

	Neuropathic Osteoarthropathy	Intervertebral (Osteo)Chondrosis	Infection	CPPD Crystal Deposition Disease[1]
Sites of involvement	One or more levels Predominates in thoracolumbar spine[2]	Frequently widespread Cervical, thoracic, or lumbar spine	Frequently one level Predominates in thoracolumbar spine	Widespread Cervical, thoracic, or lumbar spine
Intervertebral disc spaces	Narrowed or obliterated	Narrowed	Narrowed or obliterated	Calcification; narrowed
Bony sclerosis	May be extreme	Usually mild to moderate	Variable[3]	Variable[5]
Osteophytosis	May be massive	Absent or moderate in size	Usually absent	Variable
Bony fragmentation	May be extreme	Absent or minimal	Usually absent	Variable[6]
Subluxation, angulation	Common	Rare	Variable[4]	Variable
Paravertebral mass	Usually absent	Absent	Common	Absent

[1]CPPD, Calcium pyrophosphate dihydrate.
[2]Influenced by the specific underlying disorder.
[3]Sclerosis more typical in pyogenic spondylitis and in black patients with tuberculous spondylitis.
[4]In tuberculosis, kyphosis may become prominent.
[5]Discal calcification may appear without sclerosis, or disc space loss may be combined with moderate or severe sclerosis.
[6]In some patients, fragmentation and deformity may be severe, especially in the cervical spine.

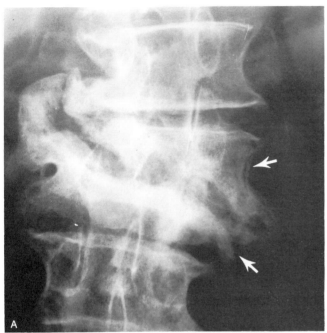

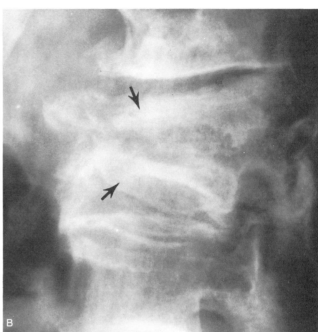

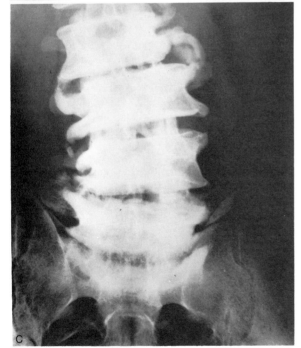

FIGURE 78–13. Tabes dorsalis: Neuropathic osteoarthropathy of the axial skeleton.

A, B Localized disease. Frontal and lateral radiographs of the lumbar spine reveal extensive disorganization involving two vertebral bodies (arrows) and the intervening intervertebral disc. Note the loss of intervertebral disc space, sclerosis, and osteophytosis. The resulting osseous contours are relatively well defined.

C Generalized disease. An example of widespread abnormalities in the lumbar spine consisting of loss of height of multiple intervertebral discs, extreme sclerosis, osteophytes, subluxation, and vertebral angulation is shown.

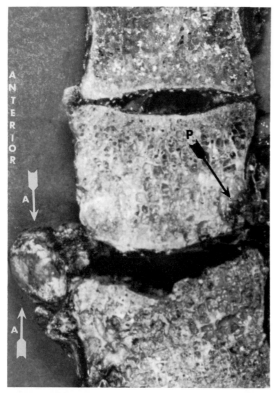

FIGURE 78–14. Tabes dorsalis: Neuropathic osteoarthropathy of the axial skeleton. A photograph of a sagittal section of the lumbar spine in a syphilitic patient reveals subarticular fractures, particularly evident in the lower vertebral body, with crumbling bone margins and displacement of detritus into adjacent paravertebral tissue (arrows marked A). Note the loss of bone along the posterior margin of the upper vertebra (arrow marked P). (From Feldman F, et al: Radiology *111*:1, 1974.)

hip are affected with approximately equal frequency; in both the upper and lower limbs, bilateral symmetric changes are not so common as in tabes.[15] Changes in the spine are most characteristic in the cervical region, although localized alterations in the thoracic and lumbar segments, including scoliosis,[134] are encountered.

Generally, neuropathic osteoarthropathy occurs during the later phases of syringomyelia, although occasionally joint findings may be the initial or predominant manifestation of the disease. Accompanying or preceding neurologic changes due to spinal cord damage are variable and include decreased reflexes, ataxia, bladder disturbances, muscle atrophy, and spastic weakness or paralysis.[118] Myelography, CT,[133, 166] and MR imaging[135, 136] can demonstrate spinal cord enlargement, especially in the cervical region (Figs. 78–16*B, C* and 78–18), and laboratory analysis can indicate increases in cerebrospinal fluid pressure and protein content.

The clinical, radiographic, and pathologic alterations of neuropathic osteoarthropathy in syringomyelia are similar to those in tabes,[160] although the frequency of spontaneous fractures of the diaphyses and metaphyses of tubular bones may be somewhat less in the former disease. Rapid and painless swelling of the affected region appears.[50] The degree of fragmentation and sclerosis of the humeral head can be striking, and these changes may be associated with fractures of neighboring bones, including the scapula, clavicle,

and ribs. In the spine, productive or destructive changes can predominate, and the appearance in the initial stages of the disease can simulate degenerative joint disease.

Diabetes Mellitus

The complexity of diabetic neuropathic osteoarthropathy is well known.[30, 51–65] The first description of a typical painless "Charcot joint" in a patient with diabetes mellitus belongs to Jordan in 1936,[66] an association that subsequently was emphasized by Bailey and Root in 1947.[67] Since the latter report, countless descriptions of "neuropathic," "neuroarthropathic," "osteoarthropathic," "osteopathic," "neurogenic," and "atrophic" articular changes in this disease have appeared, and the wide variation of terms applied to the alterations reflects a continuing debate as to their pathogenesis.[30] Loss of pain and loss of proprioceptive sensation appear to be of major importance in diabetic neuropathic osteoarthropathy,[68] and, in the presence of repetitive micro- or macrotrauma, promote the changes. Ischemia has been reported to be important[69] despite the preservation of peripheral pulses[30, 70]; small blood vessel disease may act synergistically with other factors, such as neuropathy, trauma, or infection, to further promote the osteoarticular alterations. Adequate blood supply is a prerequisite for the occurrence of osteolysis,[63] however, and the prominent role of vascular insufficiency in the initiation of diabetic neuropathic osteoarthropathy remains controversial.[30] That infectious processes commonly are superimposed on neuropathic changes in diabetic patients is well recognized,[53, 71] especially in superficially located joints. The addition of suppuration to neuropathic osteoarthropathy can accentuate and accelerate the joint destruction, although recovery from the infection may be followed by remarkable reconstitution of the bony architecture.[30]

As was indicated earlier in this chapter, considerable evidence exists that the findings of neuropathic osteoarthropathy in diabetes mellitus relate, at least in part, to a neurally initiated vascular reflex that leads to increased blood flow.[167] Numerous studies of arterial circulation in the foot in cases of diabetic neuropathy have documented a significant increase in vascularity,[168–171] and the skin temperatures in the insensitive limb in diabetes have been documented to be higher than those in controls.[169, 172] Arteriovenous shunting is associated with the increased blood flow, and prominent turgid veins and bounding arterial pulses over the dorsum of the foot in diabetic neuropathy are observed commonly.[167] These shunts, in combination with sympathetic nerve dysfunction that decreases vascular tone owing to an effect on arterial smooth muscle, contribute to marked hypervascularity. Such hypervascularity may be accompanied by an increase in bone resorption, osteopenia, and bone fragility.[167] Fractures and subchondral bone collapse, known findings in diabetic neuropathic osteoarthropathy, may reflect the terminal event occurring when repetitive mechanical trauma is applied to a foot (or other site) containing bones made weak and vulnerable by hypervascularity.

Although the exact frequency of neuropathic bone and joint changes in diabetic persons is not clear, this disease has overtaken both syphilis and syringomyelia as the leading cause of neuropathic osteoarthropathy. Sinha and coworkers[30] noted neuropathic alterations in 0.15 per cent of

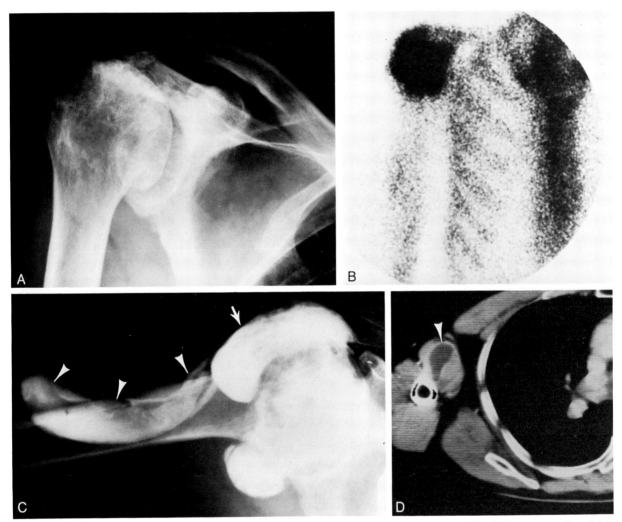

FIGURE 78–15. Syringomyelia. A 66 year old man with a 30 year history of syringomyelia developed swelling in the upper portion of the right arm. A venogram was normal.

A The plain film shows bone sclerosis and cyst formation in the humeral head and deformity of the glenoid region of the scapula.

B A bone scan reveals intense uptake of the radionuclide about the right shoulder.

C Arthrography confirms a full-thickness tear of the rotator cuff, allowing visualization of the subacromial (subdeltoid) bursa (arrow), and a synovial cyst (arrowheads) arising from the bicipital tendon sheath.

D A transaxial CT scan at the level of the upper portion of the humerus shows a cystic area of decreased attenuation (arrowhead) anterior to the humeral diaphysis, representing the synovial cyst.

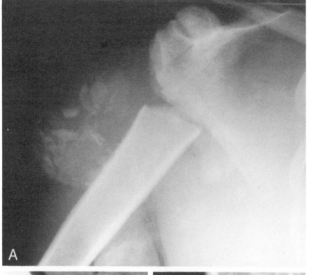

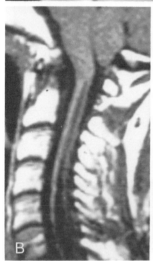
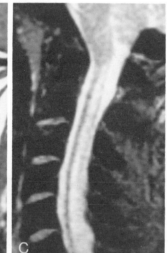

FIGURE 78–16. Syringomyelia. A 52 year old woman developed enlargement of the right arm over a 1 year period. On physical examination, the right upper extremity was insensitive.

A A radiograph of the right shoulder reveals dissolution of the humeral head with bone fragmentation. The shaft of the humerus is displaced inferiorly.

B A sagittal T1-weighted (TR/TE, 300/20) spin echo MR image shows cavitation in the cervical spinal cord, manifested as a region of low signal intensity, and downward displacement of the brain stem.

C A sagittal gradient echo image (MPGR; TR/TE, 450/14; flip angle, 15 degrees) also demonstrates the region of cord cavitation. (Courtesy of G. Greenway, M.D., Dallas, Texas.)

68,000 consecutive hospital admissions of diabetic patients, although these investigators speculated that the true prevalence was greater because of the asymptomatic nature of the lesions. Typically, diabetic neuropathic osteoarthropathy appears in a man or woman with long-standing diabetes mellitus, generally in the fifth to seventh decades of life. Changes in younger and older patients, however, can occur.[72, 137] The joints of the forefoot and midfoot are altered most commonly, although the ankle, knee, spine, and joints of the upper extremity, in descending order of frequency, can be affected.[52] Painless soft tissue swelling,[138] skin ulceration, and joint deformity are encountered. Mono- or polyarticular involvement can occur; spontaneous arrest of clinical and radiographic changes at one site may be followed by the onset and progressive growth of alterations at a previously unaffected joint.[30]

Destructive or resorptive bony abnormalities can predominate, depending on the location of the neuropathic changes.[54] In the intertarsal or tarsometatarsal joints, osseous fragmentation, sclerosis, and subluxation or dislocation can be prominent, and the complete disintegration of one or more tarsal bones can occur rapidly.[54, 119, 120, 173, 174] Rapidly progressive alterations may be initiated by a minor

traumatic event[175, 176] (Figs. 78–19 and 78–20). Calcaneal fragmentation is typical (Fig. 78–21), and fracture lines may extend from the plantar aspect of the bone into the subtalar joints. Fractures of the calcaneus related to avulsion by the Achilles tendon are seen.[207] Talar disruption and dorsolateral displacement of the metatarsal bones in relation to the cuneiform and cuboid bones also are characteristic, and the resulting radiographic picture may resemble that which is observed in an acute Lisfranc's fracture-dislocation[65] (Fig. 78–22). At the metatarsophalangeal joints, osseous resorption is frequent, leading to partial or complete disappearance of the metatarsal heads and proximal phalanges with tapering or "pencil-pointing" of phalangeal and metatarsal shafts[54, 62, 63] (Fig. 78–23). Flattening and fragmentation of the metatarsal heads are particularly characteristic and may resemble the changes of Freiberg's infraction (Fig. 78–24).[139, 177] Occasionally, the bases of the proximal phalanges may broaden (Fig. 78–25), forming a cup,[54] an appearance which has been termed "intrusion," "mortar and pestle," "bulbous," "pencil and cup," or "balancing pagoda."[64] With continued forefoot involvement, progressive resorption of phalanges and dorsiflexion and shortening of the toes appear. Concomitant ulceration of soft tis-

Text continued on page 3431

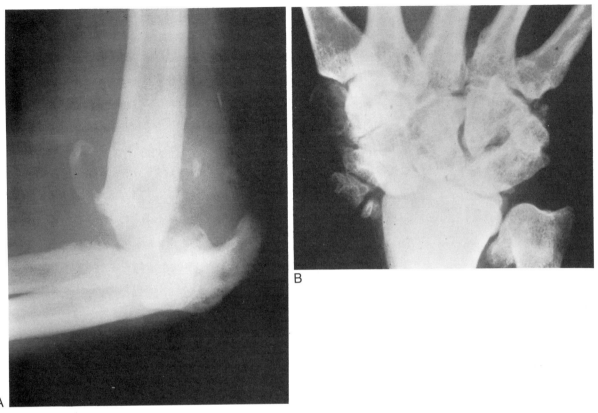

FIGURE 78–17. Syringomyelia.
   A A lateral radiograph indicates the classic features of neuropathic osteoarthropathy, consisting of soft tissue swelling, subluxation of the radius and ulna with relation to the humerus, extensive osseous resorption and fragmentation, sclerosis, and adjacent bony debris.
   B In another patient, note the resorption, flattening, and sclerosis of the distal ends of the radius and ulna, fragmentation, and carpal malalignment.

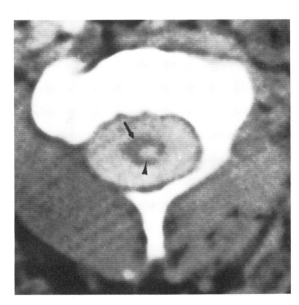

FIGURE 78–18. Syringomyelia: Spinal cord involvement. A transaxial CT scan of the cervical region after the introduction of metrizamide shows an atrophic spinal cord (arrow) and a contrast medium–filled cystic cavity (arrowhead).

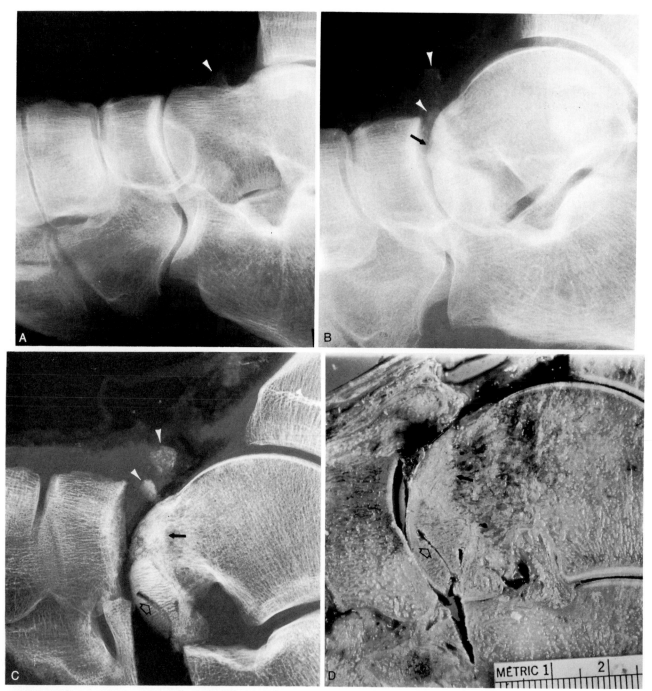

FIGURE 78–19. Diabetes mellitus: Intertarsal joints. A 32 year old patient with diabetes mellitus developed neuropathic osteoarthropathy without signs of infection.

  A An initial radiograph reveals a talar outgrowth (arrowhead) but otherwise is unremarkable.

  B Four months later, resorption and sclerosis of the articular surface of the distal portion of the talus (arrow) are associated with fragmentation (arrowheads) of the dorsal surface of the bone, including the previously noted outgrowth.

  C, D A radiograph and photograph of a sagittal section of the amputated foot show the sclerosis (solid arrows) and fragmentation (arrowheads). An artifact produced by the band-saw (open arrows) also is evident.

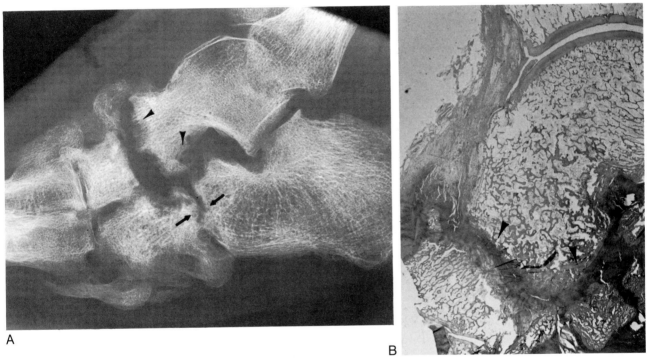

FIGURE 78–20. Diabetes mellitus: Intertarsal and tarsometatarsal joints. This 55 year old patient with diabetes mellitus had signs of neuropathic osteoarthropathy and infection, with soft tissue ulcerations.

A A lateral sagittal section of the amputated foot reveals extensive involvement of the anterior talocalcaneonavicular joint (arrowheads) and calcaneocuboid joint (arrows). The poorly marginated osseous destruction and fragmentation are evident. Most of the navicular bone has been resorbed.

B A photomicrograph (2×) of the section in **A** indicates fibrous ankylosis of the talocalcaneonavicular joint (arrowheads) and subchondral sclerosis. Observe the intact articular cartilage of the ankle joint.

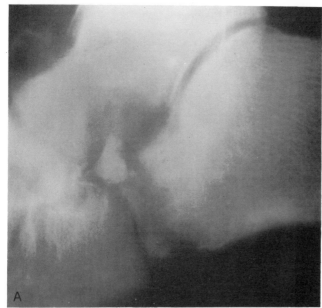

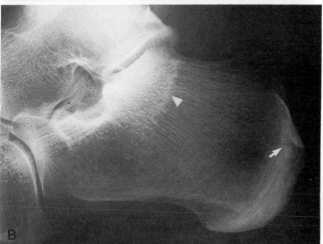

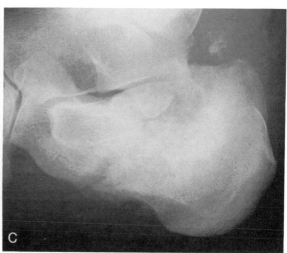

FIGURE 78–21. Diabetes mellitus. Calcaneus.

A A conventional tomogram reveals multiple fractures of the anterior portion of the calcaneus and superior surface of the talus. Bone sclerosis is evident.

B, C In a different patient, radiographs obtained 4 months apart show initial fractures of the posterior aspect of the calcaneus (arrow) and subtalar region (arrowhead) and subsequent collapse of the bone.

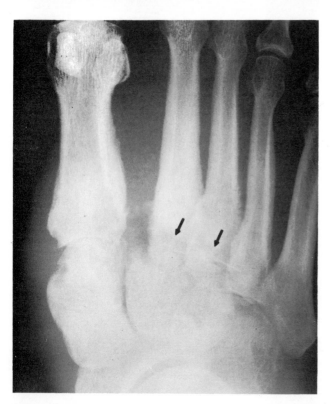

FIGURE 78–22. Diabetes mellitus: Tarsometatarsal joints. Note the lateral displacement of the bases of the metatarsals (arrows) with respect to the tarsals. This finding, combined with soft tissue swelling and fragmentation, represents a neuropathic Lisfranc's fracture-dislocation.

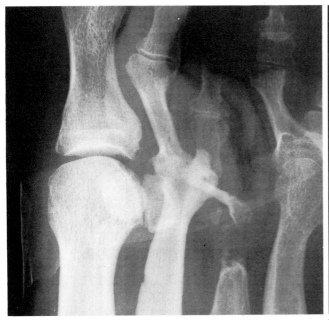
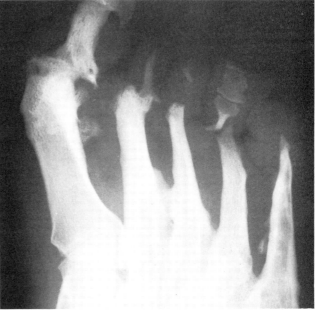

A   B

FIGURE 78–23. Diabetes mellitus: Metatarsophalangeal and interphalangeal joints.
A, B Neuropathic osteoarthropathy and infection in the forefoot of a diabetic patient can combine to produce bizarre abnormalities consisting of osteolysis of distal metatarsals and proximal phalanges, with tapering of the osseous contours.

sues over a bony prominence due to downward subluxation of the proximal phalangeal head leads to osteomyelitis or septic arthritis, or both.

Although less frequent than changes in the forefoot or midfoot, ankle involvement can be detected.[56, 60] A history of severe trauma is common in diabetic persons with ankle changes,[30] and significant fragmentation, eburnation, and dislocation can be seen. Knee abnormalities are rare indeed (Fig. 78–26).

Reports of changes in the bones and joints of the upper extremities are limited.[59, 64] Sensory neuropathy is not infre-

quent in the upper limbs[73, 74] and apparently can lead to neuropathic abnormalities in the glenohumeral joint, elbow, wrist, and hand. The changes in the shoulder consist of joint space loss, humeral head deformity, subchondral lysis and sclerosis, cystic changes, and subluxation[59] (Fig. 78–27). Although fragmentation may be less frequent and prominent about the joints of the upper limbs, patients with severe bone fracture, eburnation, and dissolution are seen (Fig. 78–28). Flexion contracture of the hand can accompany diabetic neuropathy. Subchondral and periarticular cystic bony changes about the shoulder and the hands are

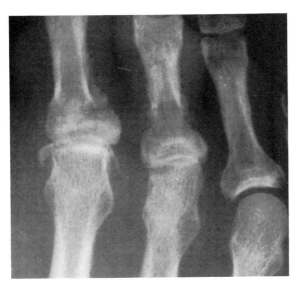
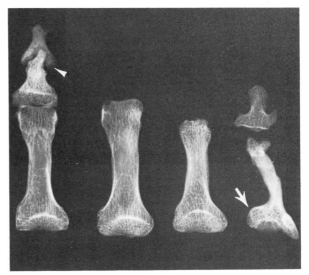

FIGURE 78–24. Diabetes mellitus: Metatarsophalangeal joints. Observe collapse of the second and third metatarsal heads, resembling the findings of Freiberg's infraction. Fractures in the bases of the proximal phalanges also are evident. (Courtesy of A. D'Abreu, M.D., Porte Alegre, Brazil.)

FIGURE 78–25. Diabetes mellitus: Phalangeal abnormalities in the foot. A radiograph of the macerated phalanges reveals expansion of the base of the proximal phalanx of the fifth toe (arrow) and a "pencil and cup" appearance about the distal interphalangeal joint of the second toe (arrowhead). The terminal phalanx in this digit is pointed.

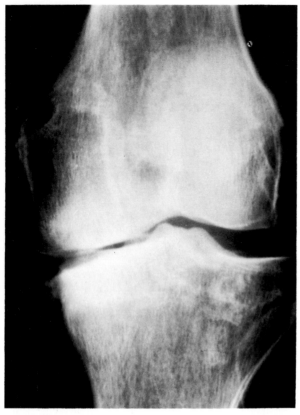

FIGURE 78–26. Diabetes mellitus: Knee. Neuropathic abnormalities in this diabetic patient consist of sclerosis and flattening of the medial femoral condyle and tibial plateau. The changes easily could be interpreted as degenerative joint disease, although they are slightly more severe.

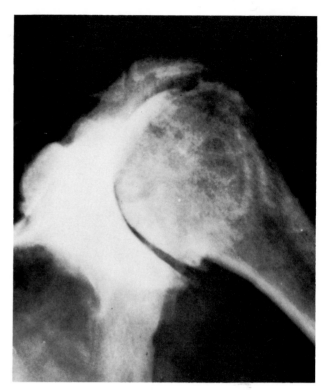

FIGURE 78–27. Diabetes mellitus: Glenohumeral joint. The findings include joint space narrowing, sclerosis, cyst formation, and osteophytosis. Although these changes might be misinterpreted as osteoarthritis, the history of diabetes mellitus, the presence of neurologic abnormality on clinical examination, and the degree of sclerosis on radiographic examination should suggest the correct diagnosis. Furthermore, severe osteoarthritis of the glenohumeral joint is unusual.

more frequent in diabetic than in nondiabetic persons, although their relationship to neuropathic or "degenerative" disease remains speculative.[59]

Diabetic axial neuropathic osteoarthropathy may be generalized or localized.[16, 75] The resulting radiographic changes, which include destruction of vertebral bodies, sclerosis, osteophytosis, fragmentation, bony ankylosis, and spinal angulation, resemble those in tabes or syringomyelia (Figs. 78–29 and 78–30).

The pathologic aberrations accompanying neuropathic osteoarthropathy in the diabetic patient do not differ significantly from those in other neurologic disorders.[30, 72, 76, 77] Articular cartilage and osseous destruction with the appearance of debris in intra-articular and intrasynovial locations is typical. Alterations in the blood vessels and nerves of diabetic patients also have been recorded.[78, 79]

Alcoholism

Although peripheral neuropathy may be evident in as many as 30 per cent of alcoholic patients who are examined at a hospital,[80] reports of neuropathic osteoarthropathy in these persons are infrequent. Only a few descriptions of this complication in alcoholic patients had appeared[81, 82] prior to the report by Thornhill and colleagues[80] of 10 such patients with neuropathic changes in the feet. These patients had prolonged histories of heavy alcoholic intake and revealed soft tissue ulceration, edema, increased skin pigmentation,

and peripheral neuropathy, in addition to radiographic changes consistent with neuropathic osteoarthropathy. The radiographic findings included soft tissue swelling, atrophy of phalangeal and metatarsal bones, osteolysis of terminal phalanges, subluxation, sclerosis, and pathologic fractures, and they were reminiscent of those accompanying diabetic neuropathic disease. Infection was frequent (e.g., *Staphylococcus albus*), although its role in the neuropathic disorder

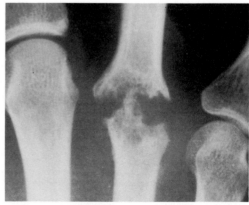

FIGURE 78–28. Diabetes mellitus: Metacarpophalangeal joint. In this unusual example, osteolysis of portions of the metacarpal head and base of the proximal phalanx is seen. (Courtesy of A. Brower, M.D., Washington, D.C.)

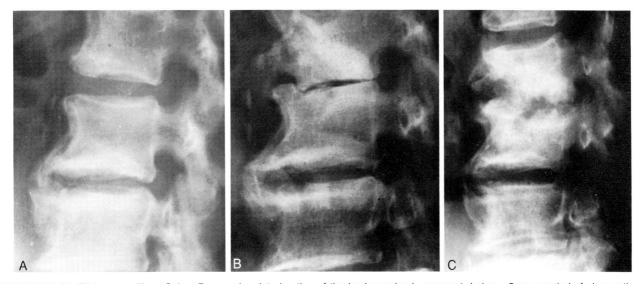

FIGURE 78–29. Diabetes mellitus: Spine. Progressive deterioration of the lumbar spine is apparent during a 3 year period of observation. Initially **(A)**, the changes at the lower lumbar level resemble degenerative disc disease. Subsequently **(B, C)**, this level deteriorates very slowly but, one level above, rapid destruction of the intervertebral disc and bone is evident. The vacuum phenomenon in the upper disc as well as the well-defined and sclerotic bone in **B** makes infection unlikely. In **C**, the pattern of discal destruction is identical to that of infection, although the latter was not apparent clinically. (Courtesy of U.S. Naval Hospital, San Diego, California.)

could not be ascertained. Furthermore, the frequency and contribution of diabetes mellitus to the clinical and radiographic features in this study were not clear.

In a report by Bjorkengren and colleagues,[178] five chronic alcoholic patients in whom the coexistence of diabetes mellitus was excluded by laboratory methods developed neuropathic osteoarthropathy of the feet. Radiographic alterations included hypertrophic changes at the tarsal joints in four, bone fragmentation at the tarsal and metatarsal regions in three, fracture-dislocation at the tarsometatarsal joint in two, and multiple pathologic fractures in one patient (Fig. 78–31).

Amyloidosis

Neuropathy, which is encountered in certain variants of amyloidosis,[83, 84] not commonly is associated with neuropathic osteoarthropathy despite an impairment of sensory more than of motor function. Occasionally, patients with amyloidosis with or without additional plasma cell dyscrasias will develop neuropathic bone and joint disease.[85, 86] The knee and the ankle appear to be the predominant sites of involvement. Vascular amyloid infiltration in nerve tissue can be demonstrated on histologic examination[86] (see Chapter 60).

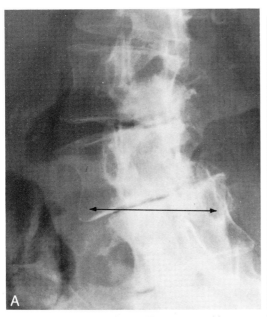

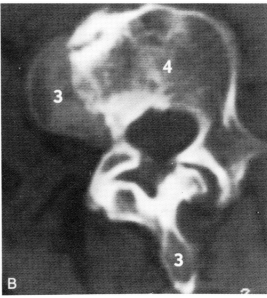

FIGURE 78–30. Diabetes mellitus: Spine. This 60 year old woman with adult-onset diabetes mellitus, treated with insulin, developed rapidly progressive lumbar scoliosis with mild low back pain and a feeling of "uneasiness." A frontal radiograph of the lumbar spine **(A)** and a transaxial CT scan **(B)** at the approximate level indicated in **A** show severe rotary scoliosis with considerable loss of discal height, bone sclerosis, and vertebral subluxation. In **B**, labeled structures include the third (3) and fourth (4) lumbar vertebral bodies and posterior elements. Observe the subluxation at the apophyseal joints between these two vertebrae.

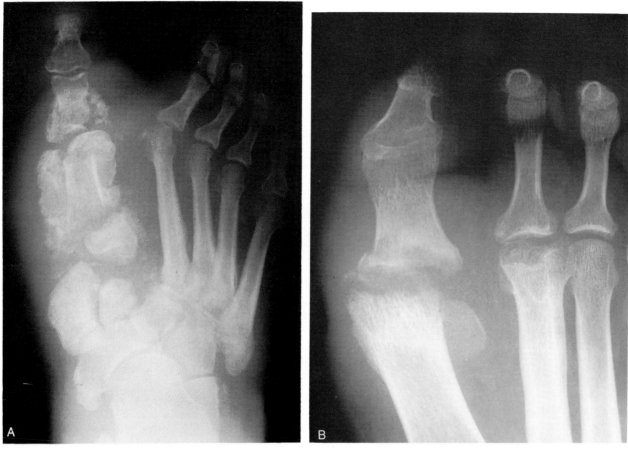

FIGURE 78–31. Alcoholism.

A This man with chronic alcoholism who had severe peripheral neuropathy developed painless swelling and subsequent infection (staphylococcal) of the foot. He was not diabetic. The radiographic findings are consistent with neuropathic osteoarthropathy with or without osteomyelitis, although the extent of such changes in association with alcoholic neuropathy indeed is unusual. Observe soft tissue swelling, fracture, fragmentation, and new bone formation about the metatarsal bone and phalanx of the great toe, fragmentation of the cuneiforms, and lateral displacement of the metatarsal bases. The bony detritus appears remarkably well defined.

B In a different patient with alcoholic neuropathic osteoarthropathy, changes in the forefoot, including soft tissue swelling, collapse and fragmentation of metatarsal heads, and thickening of the shaft of the second metatarsal bone, resemble those occurring in diabetes mellitus.

Congenital Indifference to Pain

Congenital indifference to pain first was described in 1932 by Dearborn.[87] It now is recognized that indifference or insensitivity to pain is a feature common to several distinct hereditary sensory neuropathies that differ in their patterns of inheritance, precise clinical manifestations, and prognosis (see Chapter 77). Although pain sensation is decreased in all of these disorders, normal perception of touch and temperature and normal tendon reflexes may be present. It has been postulated that in some types of congenital indifference to pain, the abnormalities lie somewhere in the cerebral cortex; the nerve endings in the skin and periosteum may be normal.[88]

In most of these syndromes, the neurologic deficit can be recognized in infancy or childhood. A decreased or absent reaction to pain, scars on the tongue or finger related to burns or infections, corneal opacities resulting from unnoticed foreign bodies, and aggressive behavior may be found.[89] Self-mutilation with amputation of fingers and toes is encountered.[155] These clinical manifestations, coupled with progressive deformities, may lead to radiographic evaluation with demonstration of typical skeletal abnormalities[89–96] (Fig. 78–32).

Schneider and coworkers[95] and other investigators[140, 141] have characterized the skeletal lesions in the syndromes of congenital indifference to pain (and related disorders) into fractures of the metaphysis and diaphysis of long bones, epiphyseal separations, neuropathic osteoarthropathy, and soft tissue ulcerations. These injuries, which often are unrecognized and untreated, can lead to severe disability and generally are more frequent in the lower extremity than in the upper extremity. Diaphyseal and metaphyseal fractures relate to both osteoporosis and neurologic deficit; the bony fragments can heal, with abundant callus formation, although displacement with deformity or osteomyelitis can appear. Epiphyseal separations are the result of chronic trauma or stress, as the growth plate represents the weak link in the child's skeleton; widening and irregularity of the growth plate, lysis and sclerosis of the metaphysis, periostitis and callus, and variable degrees of epiphyseal displacement are recognized. Neuropathic osteoarthropathy is especially common in the knee, ankle, and tarsal areas, although multiple sites, including those in the spine,[183] can be affected; fragmentation and sclerosis can be prominent. Fracture and collapse of the lateral femoral condyle may have diagnostic significance. Soft tissue ulcerations appear at the pressure areas on weight-bearing joints or over bony prom-

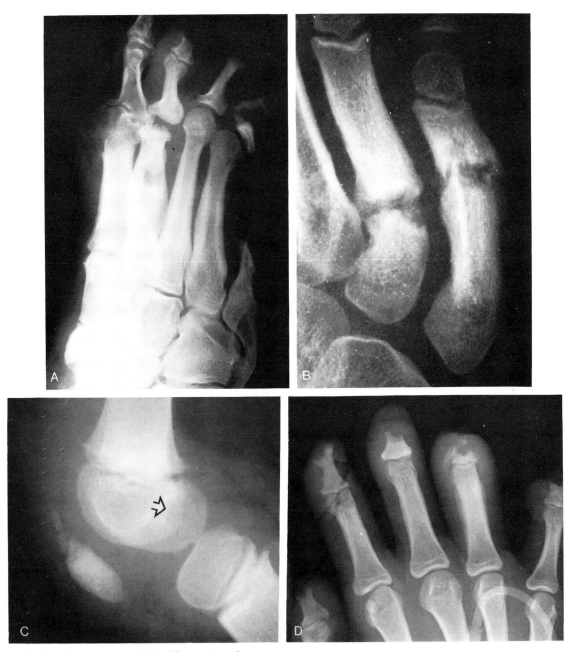

FIGURE 78–32. Syndromes of congenital indifference to pain.

A In this woman, observe the resorption and tapering of metatarsals and phalanges of the foot, with periostitis, sclerosis, and fragmentation. The changes are consistent with neuropathic osteoarthropathy, although infection also is probable. (Courtesy of M. Pallayew, M.D., Montreal, Quebec, Canada.)

B This 10 year old boy developed fractures of multiple metatarsals in both feet, which failed to heal and which later were associated with deformity.

C In this 7 year old boy, fragmentation of the lateral femoral condyle (arrow) and patella is associated with a joint effusion and intra-articular osseous bodies. The opposite side (not shown) was affected similarly.

D In a 17 year old patient, osteolysis and autoamputation of multiple phalanges are evident. The opposite hand was involved similarly. (Courtesy of M. Mitchell, M.D., Halifax, Nova Scotia, Canada.)

inences; the ulcers may deepen and lead to contamination of underlying bones and joints.

Many of the lesions may heal with proper supervision and treatment. Recurrent osteomyelitis, fractures, dislocations, and progressive joint or skeletal deformity can be seen, however.[89, 94, 122]

It should be emphasized that overt neurologic symptoms and signs may be absent in children and adolescents with some types of congenital insensitivity to pain, although careful and detailed clinical examination often will detect subclinical sensory neuropathy.[142] Therefore, the presence of unusual fractures and physeal abnormalities on radiographs should stimulate a search for subtle neurologic deficit, especially if clinical findings appear mild compared with the severity of the radiologic alterations. Virtually identical skeletal abnormalities are seen in all of the syndromes of congenital insensitivity to pain, such as in familial dysautonomia or the Riley-Day syndrome, which is characterized by autonomic dysfunction, sensory and motor disturbance, and spinal deformities[97–99, 107, 143]; in congenital sensory neuropathy with anhidrosis, which is characterized by a probable autosomal recessive mode of inheritance, inability to detect noxious stimuli, defective intelligence, and reduced temperature and touch sensation[100, 101, 121, 179–181]; in congenital sensory neuropathy without anhidrosis, which is inherited as a recessive trait, appearing in early life with predominant involvement of the lower extremities; and in hereditary sensory radicular neuropathy (acrodystrophic neuropathy), which is characterized by sensory neuropathy, trophic ulceration, and severe neuropathic skeletal alterations.[102–104, 117, 182]

Meningomyelocele (Spinal Dysraphism)

Skeletal abnormalities are detected in patients with various types of spinal dysraphism.[95, 105–109] Sensory impairment resulting from spina bifida and meningomyelocele is the most frequent underlying cause of neuropathic osteoarthropathy in childhood, principally affecting the ankle and the tarsal joints.[146] In active children, changes may appear in the first 3 years of life. These changes are identical to those in the syndromes of congenital indifference to pain and include osteoporosis, diaphyseal and metaphyseal fractures, injuries of the growth plate, epiphyseal separations, persistent effusions, articular destruction, and soft tissue ulcerations[123, 124, 144, 145, 159, 184–190] (Fig. 78–33).

As indicated in Chapter 77, coxa valga deformity is a common finding in neuromuscular disease, owing to muscular imbalance. In spinal dysraphism, however, coxa vara deformity develops as a sequel to disruption of the physis in the femoral neck.[147, 148] The femoral metaphysis becomes situated lateral and superior to the capital epiphysis and, with healing, typical coxa vara is seen. Ischemic necrosis of the proximal femoral capital epiphysis itself also is described, apparently as an iatrogenic complication of prolonged abduction splintage of unstable hips.[147]

Other Diseases

Numerous other causes of neuropathic skeletal alterations exist. These include spinal cord or peripheral nerve injury,[95, 110, 156] myelopathy of pernicious anemia,[111] Charcot-Marie-Tooth disease,[112] Arnold-Chiari malformation,[191] neurofibromatosis,[192] arachnoiditis,[113, 114] intraspinal tumors,[149] degenerative spinal disease,[150] paraplegia, quadriplegia, familial interstitial hypertrophic polyneuropathy of Dejerine and Sottas, chronic inflammatory demyelinating polyradiculoneuropathy,[193] limb replantation,[194] leprosy (Fig. 78–34),[195] and yaws. An idiopathic variety of neuropathic osteoarthropathy of the elbow and shoulder also has been identified[115, 116, 196, 197] (Fig. 78–35). Neuropathic-like changes that follow intra-articular injection of steroids are discussed in Chapter 74.

Although the imaging manifestations associated with paralysis are addressed fully in Chapter 77, a few observations regarding neuropathic-like changes occurring in patients with chronic paraplegia and quadriplegia are appropriate here. As classic descriptions of the pathogenesis of neuropathic osteoarthropathy emphasize the occurrence of movement with repeated trauma of insensitive bones and joints, the observation of such osteoarthropathy in paralyzed patients who lack both sensation and motor function initially may seem contradictory. Movement in the setting of paralysis, however, is initiated by physical therapy as well as by daily activities such as the transfer of the paralyzed patient from his or her bed to a wheelchair. This movement, when combined with decreased muscle tone, ligament laxity, and absence of normal proprioceptive reflexes, may lead to fractures of articular cartilage or subchondral bone or even extra-articular osseous sites. Most reports of neuropathic osteoarthropathy occurring in paralyzed patients have indicated predilection for the spine,[198–200] although other regions may be affected.[201] Areas of the vertebral column distal to the level of paralysis typically are involved, and improper fracture healing, which in some cases is accompanied by pseudarthrosis, may lead to bone and disc fragmentation and to collapse and development of a large paraspinal mass. Previous laminectomies may further render the spine unstable and accentuate the neuropathic abnormalities.[202] Differentiation of true neuropathic spinal alterations in paralysis from a variety of patterns of vertebral ossification that occur in this clinical setting, and which may be unrelated to neuropathic osteoarthropathy, sometimes is difficult.

MAGNETIC RESONANCE IMAGING ABNORMALITIES

Little meaningful data have been accumulated with regard to the role of MR imaging in the assessment of neuropathic osteoarthropathy. Some attention, however, has been given to the MR imaging findings in diabetic patients with soft tissue and bone infections of the foot and the differentiation of such infection from neuropathic abnormalities (also see Chapter 64). In an investigation evaluating osteomyelitis of the foot in diabetic patients using MR imaging (as well as routine radiography and bone scintigraphy), Yuh and coworkers[203] emphasized some differences in the MR appearance of infection and that of neuropathic osteoarthropathy. MR changes in osteomyelitis were characterized by signal intensity in bone that was similar to that of muscle but higher than that of tendon sheaths on T1-weighted spin echo MR images (Fig. 78–36) and that was similar to soft tissue edema on T2-weighted spin echo and short tau inversion recovery (STIR) images. The patterns of signal intensity in acute trauma in these patients were identical to those of osteomyelitis, presumably related to the

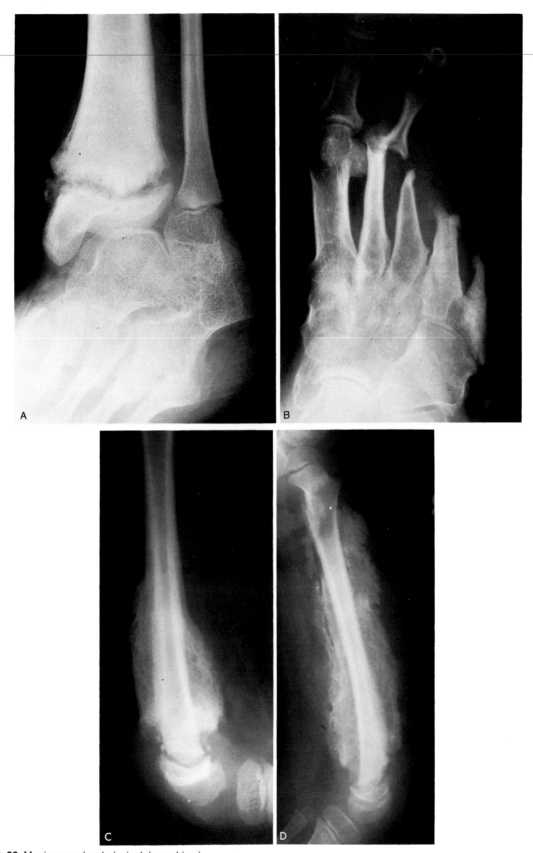

FIGURE 78–33. Meningomyelocele (spinal dysraphism).
  A In this child with a meningomyelocele, note an epiphyseal separation of the distal end of the tibia, with a widened and irregular growth plate, sclerosis, and periostitis.
  B In a 20 year old man with a meningomyelocele, progressive osteolysis of metatarsals and phalanges occurred over a period of years. Some of the findings may be related to secondary infection or surgical intervention. (Courtesy of F. Feldman, M.D., New York, New York.)
  C, D Lateral radiographs of the femora in this child with a meningomyelocele reveal irregular and widened distal femoral growth plates, fracture and fragmentation, and exuberant periostitis. (Courtesy of J. E. L. Desautels, M.D., Calgary, Alberta, Canada.)

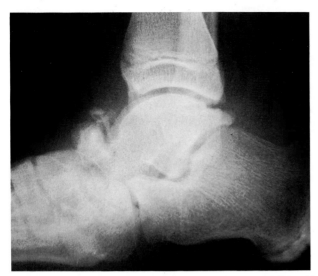

FIGURE 78–34. Leprosy. Tarsal disintegration, as in this 13 year old boy with involvement of the talus and navicular, is characteristic of leprosy.

presence of edema associated with acute fractures and dislocations. Chronic fractures, however, were not accompanied by a significant increase in signal intensity within the bone marrow. Beltran and coworkers[204] confirmed the presence of low signal intensity on T1- and T2-weighted spin echo MR images about areas of neuropathic osteoarthropathy in the feet of diabetic patients. Deficiencies in this latter study included a small study population (14 diabetic patients) and the lack of absolute confirmation of the presence or absence of infection in some of the patients.

Despite the encouraging results of these preliminary investigations, diagnostic problems are expected to be encountered in the differentiation of osteomyelitis and neuropathic osteoarthropathy in patients with diabetes mellitus (and other conditions using MR and other imaging techniques). Several reasons explain this. First, in the ambulatory diabetic patient, recurrent and ongoing neuropathic changes are encountered, and edema may be observed in both the adjacent bones and the soft tissues. Such edema in neuropathic osteoarthropathy has similar, if not identical, signal intensity patterns as those encountered in infection. Second, sympathetic joint effusions are observed consistently in the foot in diabetic patients and must be differentiated from findings of septic arthritis. Third, neuropathic bone and joint changes and infection frequently coexist in the involved foot in diabetes, and sorting out the MR characteristics of one condition from the other may prove difficult. Although the application of additional MR imaging methods such as the intravenous administration of gadolinium contrast agent may be useful in some patients with neuropathic osteoarthropathy, evidence of this is not available currently. Indeed, enhancement of signal intensity after such administration is encountered in cases of neuropathic bone and joint disease (Fig. 78–37).

DIFFERENTIAL DIAGNOSIS

When severe, neuropathic osteoarthropathy is associated with radiographic changes that are almost pathognomonic. Bony eburnation, fracture, subluxation, and joint disorganization can be more profound in this disorder than in any

other condition. It is the mild and moderate stages of neuropathic bone and joint disease that can be confused with other diseases.

In the joints of the appendicular skeleton, joint space loss, sclerosis, and fragmentation in early stages of neuropathic osteoarthropathy can resemble changes in osteoarthritis. With the progressive flattening and deformity of the articular surfaces, the production of numerous intra-articular osseous dense areas, and the appearance of increasing sclerosis and osteophytosis, the diagnosis of neuropathic osteoarthropathy becomes more obvious. In calcium pyrophosphate dihydrate crystal deposition disease, a neuropathic-like arthropathy characterized by joint space narrowing, eburnation, and fragmentation can appear, especially in the knee, the wrist, and the metacarpophalangeal joints. The identification of articular and periarticular calcification; the involvement of specific areas of the joint, such as the radiocarpal compartment of the wrist, the patellofemoral compartment of the knee, and the talonavicular space of the midfoot; and the variability of osteophyte formation are helpful clues to the accurate diagnosis of pyrophosphate arthropathy. Neuropathic osteoarthropathy and calcium pyrophosphate dihydrate crystal deposition disease can appear in the same person, however (see Chapter 44). Intra-articular deposition of calcium hydroxyapatite crystals may lead to progressive destruction of a joint, especially in the shoulder, with fracture and dissolution of bone (see Chapter 45). A similar appearance in the shoulder has been reported

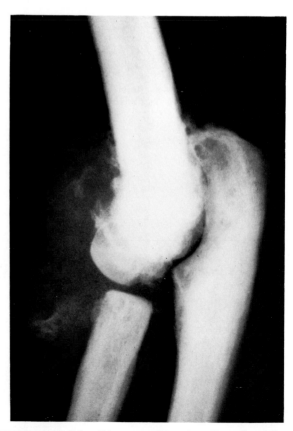

FIGURE 78–35. Idiopathic neuropathic osteoarthropathy of the elbow. This middle-aged man developed a neurologic deficit and progressive painless elbow deformity. No underlying disease could be detected. The changes of severe sclerosis and fragmentation are consistent with neuropathic osteoarthropathy.

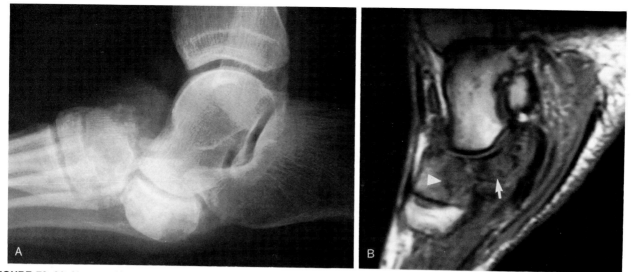

FIGURE 78–36. Neuropathic osteoarthropathy: MR imaging. Diabetes mellitus. A 68 year old man developed progressive collapse of the midfoot with rupture of the tibialis posterior tendon.

A A lateral radiograph demonstrates plantar dislocation of the talus and navicular bone. Fragmentation of the cuneiform bones is apparent.

B A sagittal T1-weighted (TR/TE, 750/20) spin echo MR image reveals low signal intensity in the navicular (arrow) and cuneiform (arrowhead) bones. With T2 weighting (not shown), inhomogeneous signal intensity with areas of low and high signal intensity was evident in the marrow of these bones.

FIGURE 78–37. Neuropathic osteoarthropathy: MR imaging. Syringomyelia.

A A disorganized elbow joint with bone resorption, fragmentation and sclerosis, and multiple intra-articular osseous bodies is evident.

B, C Coronal oblique T1-weighted (TR/TE, 500/30) spin echo MR images are shown. In **B,** prior to the intravenous injection of gadolinium contrast agent, a distorted elbow joint contains material of low signal intensity, presumably representing a combination of fluid and pannus. In **C,** after administration of gadolinium agent, the fluid remains of low signal intensity (arrow), and the pannus exhibits high signal intensity (arrowhead).

(Courtesy of H. S. Kang, M.D., Seoul, Korea.)

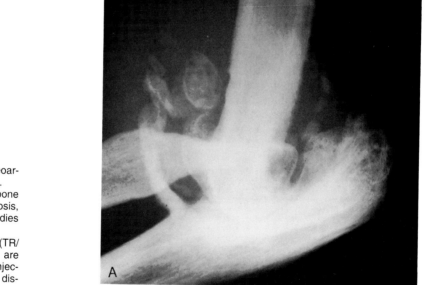

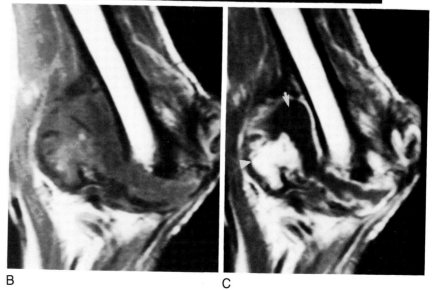

as a manifestation of an idiopathic "rapid destructive arthropathy,"[151, 152] of idiopathic "chondrolysis,"[153] and of the "senescent hemorrhagic shoulder."[154] The precise cause of these syndromes, which probably are identical to each other, is not known, although the fact that they are seen in elderly women and affect the glenohumeral joint suggests that hydroxyapatite crystal deposition may be a common factor. Furthermore, a condition of rapidly destructive osteoarthritis of the hip,[205, 206] as well as of other joints, also may relate to deposition of calcium hydroxyapatite crystals (see Chapters 39 and 45).

Bony fragmentation and collapse also are manifestations of osteonecrosis, posttraumatic osteoarthritis, intra-articular steroid arthropathy, neglected infection, and alkaptonuria. Additional clinical and radiographic manifestations in these latter disorders usually ensure proper differential diagnosis.

In the joints of the axial skeleton, early findings of neuropathic osteoarthropathy, such as intervertebral disc space narrowing and vertebral sclerosis, resemble those of intervertebral osteochondrosis, infection, or alkaptonuria. With the appearance of significant fragmentation, sclerosis, and osteophytosis, the diagnosis of axial neuropathic disease is not difficult (Table 78–3).

Once the radiographic findings are interpreted as those of neuropathic osteoarthropathy, identification of the underlying disorder usually depends on the location of the changes. Although considerable overlap occurs in the distribution patterns of the various diseases, tabes typically produces changes in the hip, the knee, the ankle, and the spine; diabetes mellitus leads to alterations in the midfoot and forefoot; syringomyelia affects the articulations of the upper extremity and cervical spine; and the syndromes of congenital indifference to pain and meningomyelocele commonly localize in the joints of the lower extremity. The presence of metaphyseal and growth plate destruction in the immature skeleton especially is characteristic of congenital indifference to pain and meningomyelocele.

SUMMARY

The effect of the deprivation of sensory feedback on the musculoskeletal system can be profound. The anesthetized joint or bone that is subject to continuing stress deteriorates progressively, leading to specific radiographic abnormalities. These changes, which include articular space narrowing, bony eburnation, osteophytosis, fragmentation, fracture, and subluxation, can accompany a variety of disorders but are most common in tabes dorsalis, diabetes mellitus, and syringomyelia. When severe, the resulting radiographic picture is diagnostic, although in earlier stages the findings may resemble those of osteoarthritis, calcium pyrophosphate dihydrate crystal deposition disease, calcium hydroxyapatite crystal deposition disease, osteonecrosis, or, in the spine, intervertebral (osteo)chondrosis.

References

1. Mitchell JK: On a new practice in acute and chronic rheumatism. Am J Med Sci 8:55, 1831.
2. Kidd JG Jr: The Charcot joint: Some pathologic and pathogenetic considerations. South Med J 67:597, 1974.
3. Charcot JM: Sur quelques arthropathies qui paraissent d'épendre d'une lésion du cerveau ou de la moelle épinière. Arch Physiol Norm Pathol 1:161, 1868.
4. Charcot JM: Lectures on the Diseases of the Nervous System. Vol 2. Edited and translated by S Sigerson. London, The New Sydenham Society, 1881, p 47.
5. Charcot JM: Ataxie locomotrice progressive: Arthropathie de l'épaule gauche. Resultats necropsiques. Arch Physiol Norm Pathol 2:121, 1869.
6. Charcot JM, Joffrov A: Note sur une lésion de la substance grise de la moelle épinière observée dans un cas d'arthropathie née a l'ataxie locomotrice progressive. Arch Physiol Norm Pathol 3:306, 1870.
7. Goldman AB, Freiberger RH: Localized infectious and neuropathic diseases. Semin Roentgenol 14:19, 1979.
8. Delano PJ: The pathogenesis of Charcot's joint. AJR 56:189, 1946.
9. Eloesser L: On the nature of neuropathic affections of the joints. Ann Surg 66:201, 1917.
10. Potts WJ: Pathology of Charcot joints. Ann Surg 86:596, 1927.
11. Leriche R, Brenckmann E: Recherches experimentales sur le mécanisme de formation de la chondromatose articulaire et de l'arthrite deformante. Presse Med 2:1441, 1928.
12. Foster D, Bassett R: Neurogenic arthropathy (Charcot joint) associated with diabetic neuropathy. Arch Neurol Psychiatry 57:173, 1947.
13. Parsons H, Norton W: The management of diabetic neuropathic joints. N Engl J Med 244:935, 1951.
14. Hodgson J, Pugh D, Young H: Roentgenologic aspects of certain lesions of bone: Neurotropic or infectious? Radiology 50:65, 1948.
15. Jaffe HL: Metabolic, Degenerative and Inflammatory Diseases of Bones and Joints. Philadelphia, Lea & Febiger, 1972, p 847.
16. Feldman F, Johnson AM, Walter JF: Acute axial neuroarthropathy. Radiology 111:1, 1974.
17. Johnson LC: Discussion. Arthritis Rheum 9:358, 1966.
18. Rabaiotti A, Rossi L, Schittone N, et al: Le alterazioni vascolari nell'arthropatia tabetica. Ann Radiol (Diagn) 33:115, 1960.
19. Soto-Hall R, Halderman KO: The diagnosis of neuropathic joint disease (Charcot joint). An analysis of forty cases. JAMA 114:2076, 1940.
20. Katz I, Rabinowitz JG, Dziadiw R: Early changes in Charcot's joints. AJR 86:965, 1961.
21. Johnson JTH: Neuropathic fractures and joint injuries. Pathogenesis and rationale of prevention and treatment. J Bone Joint Surg [Am] 49:1, 1967.
22. Norman A, Robbins H, Milgram JE: The acute neuropathic arthropathy—a rapid severely disorganizing form of arthritis. Radiology 90:1159, 1968.
23. Stewart A, Kettelkamp DB, Brandt KD: Acute joint dislocation—an early feature of neuropathic arthropathy. Arthritis Rheum 19:1367, 1976.
24. Horwitz T: Bone and cartilage debris in the synovial membrane. Its significance in the early diagnosis of neuroarthropathy. J Bone Joint Surg [Am] 30:579, 1948.
25. Lloyd-Roberts GC: The role of capsular changes in osteoarthritis of the hip joint. J Bone Joint Surg [Br] 35:627, 1953.
26. Harrison RB: Charcot's joints: Two new observations. AJR 128:807, 1977.
27. Forrester DM, Magre G: Migrating bone shards in dissecting Charcot joints. AJR 130:1133, 1978.
28. Steindler A: The tabetic arthropathies. JAMA 96:250, 1931.
29. Philips H, Rosenheck C: Neuro-arthropathies of peripheral nerve injury origin. JAMA 86:169, 1926.
30. Sinha S, Munichoodappa C, Kozak GP: Neuro-arthropathy (Charcot joints) in diabetes mellitus. Medicine 51:191, 1972.
31. Alarcon-Segovia D, Ward LE: Charcot-like arthropathy in rheumatoid arthritis. Consequence of overuse of a joint repeatedly injected with hydrocortisone. JAMA 193:1052, 1965.
32. Beetham WP Jr, Kaye RL, Polley HF: Charcot joints. A case of extensive polyarticular involvement, and discussion of certain clinical and pathologic features. Ann Intern Med 58:1002, 1963.
33. Key JA: Clinical observations on tabetic arthropathies (Charcot joints). Am J Syph 16:429, 1932.
34. Pomeranz MM, Rothberg AS: A review of 58 cases of tabetic arthropathy. Am J Syph 25:103, 1941.
35. Frewin DB, Downey JA, Feldman F, et al: Neuropathic arthropathy: A report of two cases. Aust NZ J Med 3:587, 1973.
36. Brain R, Wilkinson M: Cervical arthropathy in syringomyelia, tabes dorsalis, and diabetes. Brain 81:275, 1958.
37. Campbell DJ, Doyle JO: Tabetic Charcot's spine: Report of 8 cases. Br Med J 1:1018, 1954.
38. Herndon RF: Three cases of tabetic Charcot's spine. J Bone Joint Surg 9:605, 1927.
39. Holland HW: Tabetic spinal arthropathy. Proc R Soc Med 46:747, 1953.
40. Thomas DF: Vertebral osteoarthropathy or Charcot's disease of the spine. Review of the literature and a report of two cases. J Bone Joint Surg [Br] 34:248, 1952.
41. Cutting PEJ: A case of Charcot's disease of the cervical spine. Br Med J 1:311, 1949.
42. McNeel DP, Ehni G: Charcot joint of the lumbar spine. J Neurosurg 30:55, 1969.
43. Ramani PS, Sengupta RP: Cauda equina compression due to tabetic arthropathy of the spine. J Neurol Neurosurg Psychiatry 36:260, 1973.
44. Meyer GA, Stein J, Poppel MH: Rapid osseous changes in syringomyelia. Radiology 69:415, 1957.
45. Skall-Jansen J: Osteoarthropathy in syringomyelia. Analysis of seven cases. Acta Radiol 38:382, 1952.
46. Tully JC Jr, Latteri A: Paraplegia, syringomyelia tarda and neuropathic arthrosis of the shoulder: A triad. Clin Orthop 134:244, 1978.

47. Villiaumey J, Caron JP, Larget-Piet B, et al: Arthropathie destructive de l'épaule révélatrice d'un syndrome syringomyélique chez un malade atteint d'une paraplégie post-traumatique. Rev Rhum Mal Osteoartic 40:279, 1973.

48. Von Cube N, Lincke HO: Akuter Verlauf bei Arthropathia Syringomyelica. Ein kasuistischer Beitrag zur Differentialdiagnose der akuten Schultergelenksaffektion. Z Orthop 116:745, 1978.

49. Heyser K, Günther E, Rumpf P: Progrediente Nekrose am Humeruskopf bei Syringomyelie. ROFO 123:280, 1975.

50. Sackellares JC, Swift TR: Shoulder enlargement as the presenting sign in syringomyelia. JAMA 236:2878, 1976.

51. Sheppe WM: Neuropathic (Charcot) joints occurring in diabetes mellitus. Ann Intern Med 39:625, 1953.

52. Clouse ME, Gramm HF, Legg M, et al: Diabetic osteoarthropathy: Clinical and roentgenographic observations in 90 cases. AJR 121:22, 1974.

53. Pogonowska MJ, Collins LC, Dobson HL: Diabetic osteopathy. Radiology 89:265, 1971.

54. Kraft E, Spyropoulos E, Finby N: Neurogenic disorders of the foot in diabetes mellitus. AJR 124:17, 1975.

55. Shagan BP, Friedman SA, Allesandri R: Diabetic osteopathy: Report of a relentlessly progressive case with clinico-pathologic correlations. J Am Geriatr Soc 21:561, 1973.

56. Forgacs S: Stages and roentgenological picture of diabetic osteoarthropathy. ROFO 126:36, 1977.

57. Gray RG, Gottlieb NL: Rheumatic disorders associated with diabetes mellitus: Literature review. Semin Arthritis Rheum 6:19, 1976.

58. Meltzer AD, Skversky N, Ostrum BJ: Radiographic evaluation of soft-tissue necrosis in diabetics. Radiology 90:300, 1968.

59. Campbell WL, Feldman F: Bone and soft tissue abnormalities of the upper extremity in diabetes mellitus. AJR 124:7, 1975.

60. Lippmann HI, Perotto A, Farrar R: The neuropathic foot of the diabetic. Bull NY Acad Med 52:1159, 1976.

61. Clouse ME, Gramm HF, Legg M, et al: Diabetic osteoarthropathy. Clinical and roentgenographic observations in 90 cases. AJR 121:22, 1974.

62. Gondos B: Roentgen observations in diabetic osteopathy. Radiology 91:6, 1968.

63. Gondos B: The pointed tubular bone. Its significance and pathogenesis. Radiology 105:541, 1972.

64. Schwarz GS, Berenyi MR, Siegel MW: Atrophic arthropathy and diabetic neuritis. AJR 106:523, 1969.

65. Giesecke SB, Dalinka MK, Kyle GC: Lisfranc's fracture-dislocation: A manifestation of peripheral neuropathy. AJR 131:139, 1978.

66. Jordan WR: Neuritic manifestations in diabetes mellitus. Arch Intern Med 57:307, 1936.

67. Bailey CC, Root HF: Neuropathic foot lesions in diabetes mellitus. N Engl J Med 236:397, 1947.

68. Eichenholtz SN: Charcot Joints. Springfield, Ill, Charles C Thomas, 1966.

69. Parsons H, Norton WS: Management of diabetic neuropathic joints. N Engl J Med 244:935, 1951.

70. Boehm HJ Jr: Diabetic Charcot joints. N Engl J Med 267:185, 1962.

71. Lippman EM, Grow JL: Neurogenic arthropathy associated with diabetes mellitus. J Bone Joint Surg [Am] 37:971, 1955.

72. Robillard R, Gagnon PA, Alarie P: Diabetic neuroarthropathy. Report of 4 cases. Can Med Assoc J 91:795, 1974.

73. Ellenberg M: Diabetic neuropathy of upper extremities. J Mt Sinai Hosp 35:134, 1968.

74. Chochinov RH, Ullyot GLE, Moorhouse JA: Sensory perception thresholds in patients with juvenile diabetes and their close relatives. N Engl J Med 286:1233, 1972.

75. Zucker G, Marder MJ: Charcot spine due to diabetic neuropathy. Am J Med 12:118, 1952.

76. King ESJ: On some aspects of the pathology of hypertrophic Charcot's joints. Br J Surg 18:113, 1930.

77. Lister J, Maudsley RH: Charcot joints in diabetic neuropathy. Lancet 2:1110, 1951.

78. Fagerberg SE: Diabetic neuropathy: Clinical and histological study on the significance of vascular affections. Acta Med Scand Suppl 345:1, 1959.

79. Woltman HW, Wilder RM: Diabetes mellitus: Pathologic changes in spinal cord and peripheral nerves. Arch Intern Med 44:576, 1929.

80. Thornhill HL, Richter RW, Shelton ML, et al: Neuropathic arthropathy (Charcot forefeet) in alcoholics. Orthop Clin North Am 4:7, 1973.

81. Chappet V, Mouriquand G: Arthropathies nerveuses et maux perforants de causes diverses (tabes, diabete, alcoolisme). Bull Soc Med Hôp Lyon 2:523, 1903.

82. Classon JN: Neuropathic arthropathy with ulceration. Ann Surg 159:891, 1964.

83. Schlesinger AS, Duggins VA, Masucci EF: Peripheral neuropathy in familial primary amyloidosis. Brain 85:357, 1962.

84. Andrade C: A peculiar form of peripheral neuropathy. Brain 75:408, 1952.

85. Scott RB, Elmore SM, Brackett NC, et al: Neuropathic joint disease (Charcot joints) in Waldenström's macroglobulinemia with amyloidosis. Am J Med 54:535, 1973.

86. Peitzman SJ, Miller JL, Ortega L, et al: Charcot arthropathy secondary to amyloid neuropathy. JAMA 235:1345, 1976.

87. Dearborn GV: A case of congenital general pure analgesia. J Nerv Ment Dis 75:612, 1932.

88. Feindel W: Note on the nerve endings in a subject with arthropathy and congenital absence of pain. J Bone Joint Surg [Br] 35:402, 1953.

89. Murray RO: Congenital indifference to pain with special reference to skeletal changes. Br J Radiol 30:2, 1957.

90. Silverman FN, Gilden JJ: Congenital insensitivity to pain; a neurologic syndrome with bizarre skeletal lesions. Radiology 72:176, 1959.

91. Sandell LJ: Congenital indifference to pain. J Fac Radiol 9:50, 1958.

92. Franklyn PP: Congenital indifference to pain. Ann Radiol 15:343, 1972.

93. Siegelman S, Heimann WG, Manin MC: Congenital indifference to pain. AJR 97:242, 1966.

94. Drummond RP, Rose GK: A twenty-one year review of a case of congenital indifference to pain. J Bone Joint Surg [Br] 57:241, 1975.

95. Schneider R, Goldman AB, Bohne WH: Neuropathic injuries to the lower extremities in children. Radiology 128:713, 1978.

96. Van der Houwen H: A case of neuropathic arthritis caused by indifference to pain. J Bone Joint Surg [Br] 43:314, 1961.

97. Riley CR: Familial autonomic dysfunction. JAMA 149:1532, 1952.

98. Kirkpatrick RH, Riley CR: Roentgenographic findings in familial dysautonomia. Radiology 68:654, 1957.

99. Levine DB, Axelrod F: The occurrence of spinal deformities in familial dysautonomia (Abstr). Clin Orthop 105:298, 1974.

100. Pinsky L, DiGeorge AM: Congenital familial sensory neuropathy with anhidrosis. J Pediatr 68:1, 1966.

101. Gold RH, Mirra JM: Case report 45. Skel Radiol 2:127, 1977.

102. Heller IH, Robb P: Hereditary sensory neuropathy. Neurology 5:15, 1955.

103. Pallis C, Schneeweiss J: Hereditary sensory radicular neuropathy. Am J Med 32:110, 1962.

104. Banna M, Foster JB: Roentgenologic features of acrodystrophic neuropathy. AJR 115:186, 1972.

105. Gyepes MT, Newbern DH, Neuhauser EBD: Metaphyseal and physeal injuries in children with spina bifida and meningomyeloceles. AJR 95:168, 1965.

106. Korhonen BJ: Fractures in myelodysplasia. Clin Orthop 79:145, 1971.

107. Brunt PW: Unusual cause of Charcot's joints in early adolescence (Riley-Day syndrome). Br Med J 4:277, 1967.

108. Nellhaus G: Neurogenic arthropathies (Charcot's joints) in children. Description of a case traced to occult spinal dysraphism. Clin Pediatr 14:647, 1975.

109. Edvardsen P: Physeo-epiphyseal injuries of lower extremities in myelomeningocele. Acta Orthop Scand 43:550, 1972.

110. Slabaugh PB, Smith TK: Neuropathic spine after spinal cord injury. J Bone Joint Surg [Am] 60:1005, 1978.

111. Halonen PI, Jarvinen KAJ: On the occurrence of neuropathic arthropathies in pernicious anaemia. Ann Rheum Dis 7:152, 1948.

112. Bruckner FE, Kendall BE: Neuroarthropathy in Charcot-Marie-Tooth disease. Ann Rheum Dis 28:577, 1969.

113. Wolfgang GL: Neurotrophic arthropathy of the shoulder—a complication of progressive adhesive arachnoiditis. A case report. Clin Orthop 87:217, 1972.

114. Nissenbaum M: Neurotrophic arthropathy of the shoulder secondary to tuberculous arachnoiditis. A case report. Clin Orthop 118:169, 1976.

115. Meyn M Jr, Yablon IG: Idiopathic arthropathy of the elbow. Clin Orthop 97:90, 1973.

116. Blanford AT, Keane SP, McCarty DJ, et al: Idiopathic Charcot joint of the elbow. Arthritis Rheum 21:723, 1978.

117. Shahriaree H, Kotcamp WW, Sheikh S, et al: Hereditary perforating ulcers of the foot. "Hereditary sensory radicular neuropathy." Clin Orthop 140:189, 1979.

118. William B: Orthopaedic features in the presentation of syringomyelia. J Bone Joint Surg [Br] 61:314, 1979.

119. El-Khoury GY, Kathol MH: Neuropathic fractures in patients with diabetes mellitus. Radiology 134:313, 1980.

120. Newman JH: Spontaneous dislocation in diabetic neuropathy. A report of six cases. J Bone Joint Surg [Br] 61:484, 1979.

121. Vardy PA, Greenberg LW, Kachel C, et al: Congenital insensitivity to pain with anhidrosis. Am J Dis Child 133:1153, 1979.

122. Roberts JM, Taylor J, Burke S: Recurrent dislocation of the hip in congenital indifference to pain. J Bone Joint Surg [Am] 62:829, 1980.

123. Townsend PF, Cowell HR, Steg NL: Lower extremity fractures simulating infection in myelomeningocele. Clin Orthop 144:255, 1979.

124. Wenger DR, Jeffcoat BT, Herring JA: The guarded prognosis of physeal injury in paraplegic children. J Bone Joint Surg [Am] 62:241, 1980.

125. Brower AC, Allman RM: Pathogenesis of the neurotrophic joint. Neurotraumatic versus neurovascular. Radiology 139:349, 1981.

126. Klawans HL: Neurological manifestations of systemic diseases. In PJ Vinken, GW Bruyn (Eds): Handbook of Clinical Neurology. New York, North Holland Publishing Co, 1979, p 431.

127. Rubinow A, Spark EC, Canoso JJ: Septic arthritis in a Charcot joint. Clin Orthop 147:203, 1980.

128. O'Connor BL, Palmoski MJ, Brandt KD: Neurogenic acceleration of degenerative joint lesions. J Bone Joint Surg [Am] 67:562, 1985.

129. Goodman MA, Swartz W: Infection in a Charcot joint. A case report. J Bone Joint Surg [Am] 67:642, 1985.

130. Sprenger TR, Foley CJ: Hip replacement in a Charcot joint. A case report and historical review. Clin Orthop 165:191, 1982.

131. Wirth CR, Jacobs RL, Rolander SD: Neuropathic spinal arthropathy. A review of the Charcot spine. Spine 5:558, 1980.

132. Daffner RH, Gehweiler JA Jr: Case report 236. Skel Radiol 10:113, 1983.

133. Batnitzky S, Price HI, Gaughan MJ, et al: The radiology of syringohydromyelia. RadioGraphics 3:585, 1983.

134. Baker AS, Dove J: Progressive scoliosis as the first presenting sign of syringomyelia. Report of a case. J Bone Joint Surg [Br] 65:472, 1983.

135. Pojunas K, Williams AL, Daniels DL, et al: Syringomyelia and hydromyelia: Magnetic resonance evaluation. Radiology 153:679, 1984.

136. Yeates A, Brant-Zawadski M, Norman D, et al: Nuclear magnetic resonance imaging of syringomyelia. Am J Neuroradiol 4:234, 1983.

137. Esses S, Langer F, Gross A: Charcot's joints: A case report in a young patient with diabetes. Clin Orthop 156:183, 1981.

138. Goldman F: Identification, treatment, and prognosis of Charcot joint in diabetes mellitus. J Am Podiatry Assoc 72:485, 1982.

139. Reinhardt K: The radiological residua of healed diabetic arthropathies. Skel Radiol 7:167, 1981.

140. Greider TD: Orthopedic aspects of congenital insensitivity to pain. Clin Orthop 172:177, 1983.

141. Fath MA, Hassanein MR, James JIP: Congenital absence of pain. A family study. J Bone Joint Surg [Br] 65:186, 1983.

142. Dyck PJ, Stevens JC, O'Brien PC, et al: Neurogenic arthropathy and recurring fractures with subclinical inherited neuropathy. Neurology 33:357, 1983.

143. Mitnick JS, Axelrod FB, Genieser NB, et al: Aseptic necrosis in familial dysautonomia. Radiology 142:89, 1982.

144. Kumar SJ, Cowell HR, Townsend P: Physeal, metaphyseal, and diaphyseal injuries of the lower extremities in children with myelomeningocele. J Pediatr Orthop 4:25, 1984.

145. Wolverson MK, Sundaram M, Graviss ER: Spina bifida and unilateral focal destruction of the distal femoral epiphysis. Skel Radiol 6:119, 1981.

146. Malhotra D, Puri R, Owen R: Valgus deformity of the ankle in children with spina bifida aperta. J Bone Joint Surg [Br] 66:381, 1984.

147. Weisl H: Coxa vara in spina bifida. J Bone Joint Surg [Br] 65:128, 1983.

148. Dias LS, Locher FG, Mazur JM, et al: Femoral neck abnormalities in spina bifida. Clin Orthop 184:164, 1984.

149. Robinson SC, Sweeney JP: Cauda equina lipoma presenting as acute neuropathic arthropathy of the knee. A case report. Clin Orthop 178:210, 1983.

150. Chalmers IM, Lochead JA: Neuropathic arthropathy secondary to severe degenerative spinal disease. J Rheumatol 9:465, 1982.

151. Lequesne M, Fallut M, Coulomb R, et al: Rapid destructive arthropathy of the shoulder. Rev Rhum Mal Osteoartic 50:359, 1983.

152. Camus JP, Prier A, Merlet CL, et al: Les ostéoarthropathies destructices non tumorales de l'épaule. Sem Hop Paris 59:1225, 1983.

153. Kahan A, Amor B, Benhamou C-L: Rapidly progressive idiopathic chondrolysis simulating tuberculosis of the shoulder. J Rheumatol 10:291, 1983.

154. de Seze S, Hubault A, Rampon S: L'épaule senile hemorragique. L'actualité. Rhumatologique Presenteé au Practicen, Paris, 1967, p 107.

155. Gwathmey FW, House JH: Clinical manifestations of congenital insensitivity of the hand and classification of syndromes. J Hand Surg [Am] 9:863, 1984.

156. Sobel JW, Bohlman HH, Freehafer AA: Charcot's arthropathy of the spine following spinal cord injury. A report of five cases. J Bone Joint Surg [Am] 67:771, 1985.

157. Boynton EL, Paley D, Gross AE, et al: False aneurysm in a Charcot hip. J Bone Joint Surg [Am] 68:462, 1986.

158. Resnik CS, Reed WW: Hand, wrist, and elbow arthropathy in syringomyelia. J Can Assoc Radiol 36:325, 1985.

159. Citron ND, Paterson FWN, Jackson AM: Neuropathic osteonecrosis of the lateral femoral condyle in childhood. A report on four cases. J Bone Joint Surg [Br] 68:96, 1986.

160. Mau H, Nebinger G: Die Schultergelenks-arthropathie bei der Syringomyelie. Z Orthop 124:157, 1986.

161. Brower AC: The acute neuropathic joint. Arthritis Rheum 31:1571, 1988.

162. Thompson JS, Kaufman RL, Beardmore TD: Pseudothrombophlebitis in neuropathic arthropathy. J Rheumatol 16:1606, 1989.

163. Katthagen B-D, Boos N: Zur endoprothetischen Versorgung bei tabischer Arthropathie. Z Orthop 126:48, 1988.

164. Robb JE, Rymaszewski LA, Reeves BF, et al: Total hip replacement in a Charcot joint: Brief report. J Bone Joint Surg [Br] 70:489, 1988.

165. Harrison MJ, Sacher M, Rosenblum BR, et al: Spinal Charcot arthropathy. Neurosurgery 29:273, 1991.

166. Kolawole T, Banna M, Hawass N, et al: Neuropathic arthropathy as a complication of post-traumatic syringomyelia. Br J Radiol 60:702, 1987.

167. Edelman SV, Kosofsky EM, Paul RA, et al: Neuro-osteoarthropathy (Charcot's joint) in diabetes mellitus following revascularization surgery. Three case reports and a review of the literature. Arch Intern Med 147:1504, 1987.

168. Edmonds ME: The neuropathic foot in diabetes. I. Blood flow. Diabetic Med 3:111, 1986.

169. Archer AG, Roberts VL, Watkins PJ: Blood-flow patterns in diabetic neuropathy. Diabetologia 27:563, 1984.

170. Gunderson HLG: Peripheral blood flow and metabolic control in juvenile diabetes. Diabetologia 10:225, 1974.

171. Edmonds ME, Roberts VL, Watkins PJ: Blood flow in the diabetic neuropathic foot. Diabetologia 22:9, 1982.

172. Ward JD: The diabetic leg. Diabetologia 22:141, 1982.

173. Jensen BN, Christensen KS: Diabetic osteoarthropathy: Rapid osteoarthropathic progression in the tarsal and tarso-metatarsal joints. J Orthop Rheumatol 5:179, 1992.

174. Lesko P, Maurer RC: Talonavicular dislocations and midfoot arthropathy in neuropathic diabetic feet. Clin Orthop 240:226, 1989.

175. Slowman-Kovacs SD, Braunstein EM, Brandt KD: Rapidly progressive Charcot arthropathy following minor joint trauma in patients with diabetic neuropathy. Arthritis Rheum 33:412, 1990.

176. Clohisy DR, Thompson RC Jr: Fractures associated with neuropathic arthropathy in adults who have juvenile-onset diabetes. J Bone Joint Surg [Am] 70:1192, 1988.

177. Nguyen VD, Keh RA, Daehler RW: Freiberg's disease in diabetes mellitus. Skel Radiol 20:425, 1991.

178. Bjorkengren AG, Weisman M, Pathria MN, et al: Neuroarthropathy associated with chronic alcoholism. AJR 151:743, 1988.

179. Hasegawa Y, Ninomiya M, Yamada Y, et al: Osteoarthropathy in congenital sensory neuropathy with anhidrosis. Clin Orthop 258:232, 1990.

180. Guille JT, Forlin E, Bowen JR: Charcot joint disease of the shoulder in a patient who had familial sensory neuropathy with anhidrosis. A case report. J Bone Joint Surg [Am] 74:1415, 1992.

181. Okono T, Inque A, Izumo S: Congenital insensitivity to pain with anhidrosis. A case report. J Bone Joint Surg [Am] 72:279, 1990.

182. Ahmed SS, Kaji S, Samesimi K, et al: Osteoarthropathy in hereditary sensory radicular neuropathy. A case report. Acta Orthop Scand 61:92, 1990.

183. Piazza MR, Bassett GS, Bunnell WP: Neuropathic spinal arthropathy in congenital insensitivity to pain. Clin Orthop 236:175, 1988.

184. Roberts JA, Bennet GC, Mackenzie JR: Physeal widening in children with myelomeningocele. J Bone Joint Surg [Br] 71:30, 1989.

185. Lock TR, Aronson DD: Fractures in patients who have myelomeningocele. J Bone Joint Surg [Am] 71:1153, 1989.

186. Pfeil J, Fromm B, Carstens C, et al: Frakturen und Epiphysenverletzungen bei Kindren mit Myelomeningocele. Z Orthop 128:551, 1990.

187. Dirschi DR, Greene WB: Pseudotumor of the distal part of the femur in a patient who had myelomeningocele. A case report. J Bone Joint Surg [Am] 74:935, 1992.

188. Kjaerulff H, Hejgaard N: Neuropathic osteonecrosis of the knee in childhood. Two cases of myelomeningocele. Acta Orthop Scand 58:436, 1987.

189. Hyre HM, Stelling CB: Radiographic appearance of healed extremity fractures in children with spinal cord lesions. Skel Radiol 18:189, 1989.

190. Westcott MA, Dynes MC, Remer EM, et al: Congenital and acquired orthopedic abnormalities in patients with myelomeningocele. RadioGraphics 12:1155, 1992.

191. Davis RP, Ko KR, Sachdev VP: Charcot shoulder as the initial symptom in Arnold-Chiari malformation with hydromyelia: Case report. Mt Sinai J Med 55:406, 1988.

192. McCann PD, Herbert J, Feldman F, et al: Neuropathic arthropathy associated with neurofibromatosis. A case report. J Bone Joint Surg [Am] 74:1411, 1992.

193. Gardner D, Toth J, Aube M: Neuropathic arthropathy associated with chronic inflammatory demyelinating polyradiculoneuropathy. J Can Assoc Radiol 40:117, 1989.

194. Jackson A, Reilly M, Watson S: Radiological appearances following limb replantation: A report of 5 cases. Skel Radiol 21:155, 1992.

195. Horibe S, Tada K, Nagano J: Neuroarthropathy of the foot in leprosy. J Bone Joint Surg [Br] 70:481, 1988.

196. Mitchell ML, Lally JF, Ackerman LV, et al: Case report 697. Skel Radiol 20:550, 1991.

197. Kuur E: Two cases of Charcot's shoulder arthropathy. Acta Orthop Scand 58:581, 1987.

198. Kalen V, Isono SS, Cho CS, et al: Charcot arthropathy of the spine in long-standing paraplegia. Spine 12:42, 1987.

199. Kapila A, Lines M: Neuropathic spinal arthropathy: CT and MR findings. J Comput Assist Tomogr 11:736, 1987.

200. Schwartz HS: Traumatic Charcot spine. J Spinal Dis 3:269, 1990.

201. Pattrick M, Doherty M: Rapidly destructive hip disease following ipsilateral hemiparesis: Report of two cases. Ann Rheum Dis 46:477, 1987.

202. Luke DL, Bridwell KH: "Silent" spinal dislocation in a Charcot spine occurring postlaminectomy: Case report and review of literature. J Spinal Dis 3:87, 1990.

203. Yuh WTC, Corson JD, Baraniewski HM, et al: Osteomyelitis of the foot in diabetic patients: Evaluation with plain film, 99mTc-MDP bone scintigraphy, and MR imaging. AJR 152:795, 1989.

204. Beltran J, Campanini S, Knight C, et al: The diabetic foot: Magnetic resonance imaging evaluation. Skel Radiol 19:37, 1990.

205. Rosenberg ZS, Shankman S, Steiner GC, et al: Rapidly destructive osteoarthritis: Clinical, radiographic, and pathologic features. Radiology 182:213, 1992.

206. Komiya S, Inque A, Sasaguri Y, et al: Rapidly destructive arthropathy of the hip. Studies on bone resorptive factors in joint fluid with a theory of pathogenesis. Clin Orthop 284:273, 1992.

207. Kathol MH, El-Khoury GY, Moore TE, et al: Calcaneal insufficiency avulsion fractures in patients with diabetes mellitus. Radiology 180:725, 1991.

SECTION

XV

Osteonecrosis and Osteochondrosis

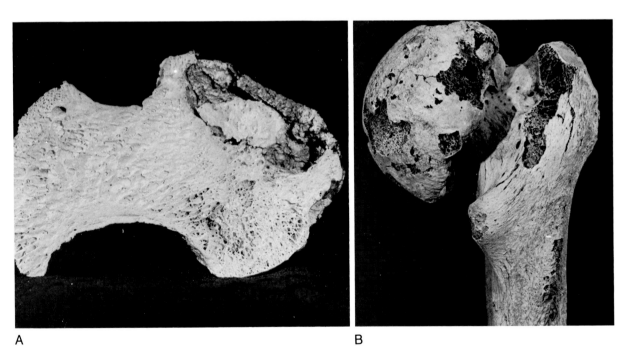

A

B

A Ischemic necrosis of bone: Typical features in the femoral head include collapse of the articular surface, subchondral fractures, and sequestration.
B Legg-Calvé-Perthes disease: An enlarged, mushroom-like appearance of the femoral head is evident. (From Ortner DJ, Putschar WGJ: Identification of Pathological Conditions in Human Skeletal Remains. Washington, DC, Smithsonian Institution Press, 1981.)

79

Osteonecrosis: Pathogenesis

Donald E. Sweet, M.D., and John E. Madewell, M.D.

The concepts and terminology of bone necrosis (osteonecrosis) have undergone considerable evolution over the past two centuries.[3, 46, 54, 67, 87, 88, 102, 165, 180, 183, 202, 203] Russell's classic essay on "disease of the bones termed necrosis," published in 1794, describes in great detail the sequestration of bone in osteomyelitis.[102] As currently used, osteonecrosis indicates the occurrence of ischemic death of the cellular constituents of bone and marrow. The purpose of this chapter is to focus attention on the sequential morpho-

logic reparative response to the infarcted foci, primarily in the adult femoral head, its consequences, and the radiographic correlation. To accomplish this, terminology, principles of infarction, the marrow cavity, associations and mechanisms of osteonecrosis, and the histologic-radiographic correlation of the host response are discussed.

TERMINOLOGY

For most of the nineteenth century, "osteonecrosis" was regarded as septic in origin.[3, 102] Failure to appreciate the radiographic appearance of bone sequestra as of relative, rather than absolute, increased density resulted in the equating of almost any unexplained increased bone density on a radiograph with osteonecrosis. A large group of these radiographic entities known under a variety of eponyms (Fig. 79–1) were eventually brought together under the term osteochondrosis[16, 136] despite histologic absence of dead bone in many of them.[67]

Continued negative bacteriologic studies from well-documented cases of bone necrosis led to the use of the term aseptic necrosis.[88, 89] Subsequent observations indicated the necrotic bone foci were not only aseptic but also avascular; hence the terms ischemic necrosis, avascular necrosis, and bone infarction were suggested. By convention, the term ischemic necrosis generally is applied to areas of epiphyseal or subarticular involvement, whereas "bone infarct" usually is reserved for metaphyseal and diaphyseal involvement. The literature on ischemic bone necrosis indicates, however, considerable overlap and lack of uniformity in applied terminology.

PRINCIPLES OF INFARCTION

Ischemic necrosis of bone, like infarction in other organ systems, results from a significant reduction in or obliteration of the affected area's blood supply.[98] Cessation of blood flow may be initiated in any part of the vascular network: arterial, capillary, sinusoidal, or venous. Eventually the flow of blood from the arterial side of the system will be compromised. One of the following phenomena

The opinions or assertions contained herein are the private views of the authors and are not to be construed as official, or as reflecting the views of the United States Departments of the Army, of the Air Force, of the Navy, or of Defense.

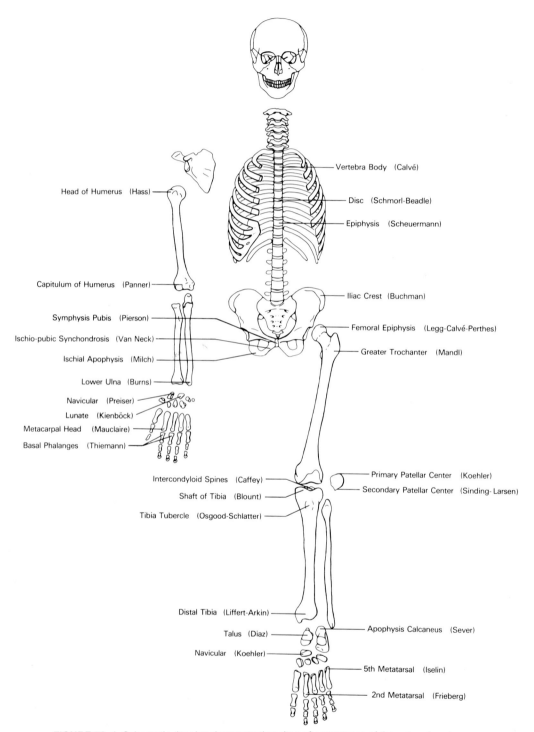

FIGURE 79–1. Schematic drawing demonstrating sites of occurrence of the osteochondroses.

usually can be demonstrated or inferred as impeding blood flow: (1) intraluminal obstruction (e.g., thromboembolic disorders, sludging of blood cells, or stasis); (2) vascular compression (e.g., external mechanical pressure or vasospasm); or (3) physical disruption of the vessel (e.g., trauma). These factors can act alone or in combination.

The type of compromised vessel and the architectural arrangement of the involved organ's vascular network both are key factors determining the effect of blood flow interruption.[98] For example, in the absence of collateral circulation, arterial occlusion produces a bloodless infarct, as is encountered frequently in the heart, kidney, and brain. Organs with collateral circulation, such as the liver and lungs, are less susceptible to infarction by arterial occlusion; when infarction occurs, the necrotic area frequently is relatively small and usually is hemorrhagic. Infarction resulting from venous obstruction generally is hemorrhagic, as in the small bowel after mesenteric vein thrombosis. Small arteriole or capillary blockade with microinfarction in a number of organ systems has been associated with subacute bacterial endocarditis and disseminated intravascular coagulation.[80] Organs with extensive sinusoidal vascular beds, such as the spleen and medullary cavity of bone, are at particular risk for infarction without evidence of arterial or venous occlusion in disorders such as sickle cell disease.

Cell death from anoxia is not immediate, but rather occurs through progressive stages of ischemic injury. For the purposes of this discussion, the term ''anoxia'' shall be extended to include an absence or decrease in all metabolites essential for cell viability and function. Subdivision of the cellular changes of progressive ischemic injury and death into three stages is arbitrary and is done to facilitate understanding of the possible disposition of these cells. These stages are defined as follows[96]: stage 1, cessation of intracellular metabolic activity at a chemical level; stage 2, alteration or interruption of intracellular enzyme systems; stage 3, disruption or dissolution of intracellular nuclear and cytoplasmic ultrastructure. Dissolution of intracellular structural integrity is irreversible and results in cell death.[96]

With reversal of anoxia, the lag period between the earliest ischemic cell changes and irreversible cell death makes possible the revival and return to normal for cells in stage 1. The more severely injured cells of stage 2 may survive, but their rehabilitation rarely permits approximation of normal function. Once cells reach stage 3, they cannot survive.[67] The fate of dead cells usually is progressive autolysis, with eventual removal and either restoration or reconstruction by the combined effort of the host's inflammatory and reparative responses.[97]

The production of ischemic injury or necrosis and the rapidity with which cell death occurs depend on the sensitivity of the individual cell type as well as the degree and duration of anoxia. Neurons in the central nervous system, under normal homeostatic conditions, survive only 3 to 5 min of complete anoxia before damage becomes irreversible. The sensitivity of the cellular elements of bone and marrow to anoxia varies. The use of ^{3}H-cytidine and ^{3}H-thymidine studies as a measure of continued bone and marrow cell activity after anoxia under controlled circumstances seems to have produced a fairly reliable baseline.[46, 73] Some questions remain unanswered, however, regarding marrow fat cells. The hematopoietic elements generally are acknowledged to be the first to undergo anoxic death (in

from 6 to 12 hours), followed by bone cells (osteocytes, osteoclasts, and osteoblasts) (in 12 to 48 hours) and, subsequently, marrow fat cells (48 hours to 5 days).[53, 67, 72, 99, 125, 126] Although some variations occur in the sensitivity of osteocytes, osteoclasts, and osteoblasts to anoxia, as a group they appear to undergo cell death after 12 to 48 hours of anoxia.

The variation in cell sensitivity of the different cellular constituents of bone and the marrow cavity makes it possible for temporary anoxia to result in the death of hematopoietic elements without necessarily being sufficient to cause osteocytic or marrow fat cell death. By extension, foci of hematopoietic and osteocytic death could be present without ischemic necrosis of marrow fat. Once ischemic marrow fat cell death occurs, the involved segment of bone and marrow can clearly be labeled infarcted.

Infarcts, including those in bone, are three-dimensional and can be subdivided into four zones: a central zone of cell death surrounded by successive zones of ischemic injury, active hyperemia, and finally normal tissue.[98] The ischemic zone reflects a gradation of hypoxic injury ranging from severe cell damage immediately adjacent to the central zone of cell death to marginal cellular alterations adjacent to the hyperemic zone. Once ischemic necrosis is established, the breakdown products of dying and severely damaged cells provoke the initial inflammatory response, characterized by vasodilation, transudation of fluid, fibrin precipitation, and local infiltration of inflammatory cells. This response forms the basis for development of the hyperemic zone and also represents the initial step of repair, removal, and reconstruction of the infarcted area.[97]

Bone infarcts occurring in the metadiaphyseal intramedullary cavity (Fig. 79–2) have a central core of dead marrow and bone surrounded by zones of ischemically injured marrow and bone, active hyperemia, and viable marrow and bone. Those infarcts occurring within an epiphysis or small, round bone demonstrate a similar three-dimensional pattern, except that one surface is covered almost always by compact subchondral bone and articular cartilage. Articular cartilage receives the bulk of its nourishment from the synovial fluid, and its viability therefore initially usually is not affected significantly by the underlying osteonecrosis, except for the cartilage cells below the tidemark, which may die. Because the osteonecrotic segment is by definition avascular, repair begins along its outer perimeter at the junction between the ischemic zone surrounding the dead area and the viable area with an intact circulation (the hyperemic zone). This reparative response results in the progressive development of a reactive margin (interface) between the dead zone and adjacent viable tissues. The reactive interface generally encompasses the bulk of the ischemically injured zone and adjacent hyperemic zone.[67]

Because tissue death essentially is a cellular phenomenon, mineralized bone matrix does not appear to be altered materially by ischemic necrosis directly. What changes, if any, occur within the matrix or affect the stress-bearing capability of bone as a direct result of anoxia (in the absence of cell activity) are controversial and have yet to be fully clarified.[40, 41] From a practical point of view, bone structure initially is unaltered as a direct result of osteocyte death or osteonecrosis. The x-ray absorbing quality of bone (density) is based on attenuation of the x-ray beam by the total amount of bone matrix and mineral content (especially

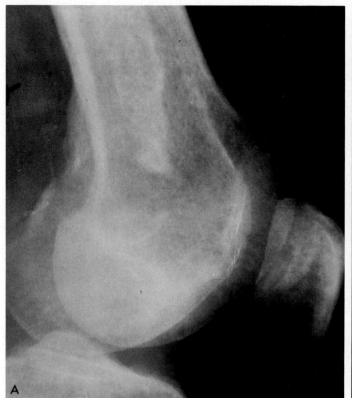

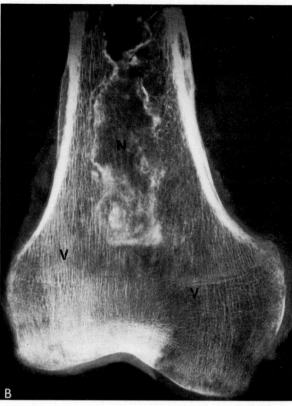

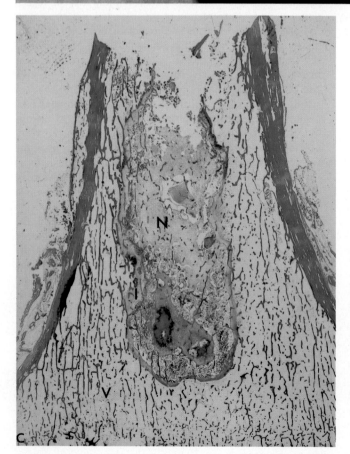

FIGURE 79–2. Intramedullary bone infarct.

A Lateral radiographic view of the distal portion of the femur demonstrates an irregular but discrete area of increased endosteal density, which is most pronounced at the periphery of the lesion.

B Specimen radiograph of the coronally sectioned distal end of the femur reveals unaltered density within the central necrotic zone (N), which is separated from the adjacent viable bone and marrow (V) by an irregular linear margin of increased density. Note the localized area of increased density that appears to be within the inferior portion of the infarct.

C Macroscopic section (2×, hematoxylin and eosin stain) shows the essentially unchanged but slightly opacified central necrotic zone (N) separated from the adjacent viable endosteal cavity (V) by a narrow, more darkly stained reactive ischemic zone (I). The dark-stained areas correspond to the dense areas in the specimen radiograph. The distal radiodense areas in the specimen radiograph reflect poor quality ischemic bone formation within the outer reactive fibrous zone, which appears to lie within the infarct. This is because the plane of section has cut into a portion of the posterior reactive margin. The immediately necrotic area around this region shows large numbers of cholesterol crystals due to fat breakdown.

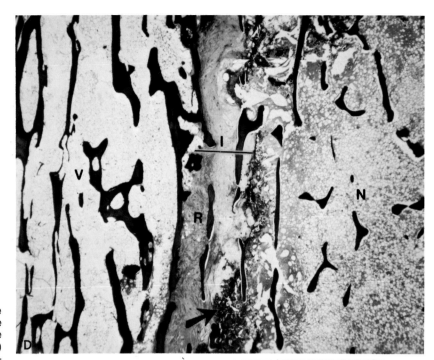

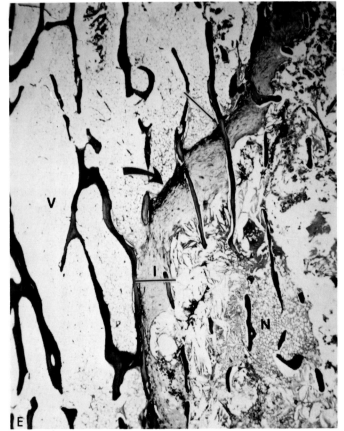

FIGURE 79–2. *Continued*

D Photomicrograph (18×) demonstrates the ischemic zone (I, horizontal line), of which the reactive interface (R) is part, separating the slightly opacified infarcted marrow and bone (N) from the surrounding viable endosteal components (V). Dystrophic mineralization (arrow) lies just inside the reactive ischemic zone.

E Photomicrograph (18×) of the reactive ischemic margin (I, horizontal line) separating necrotic (N) from viable (V) bone and marrow. Atypical ischemic fiber bone formation is also seen (curved arrow). Essentially unaltered cancellous bone traverses all three zones (straight arrow).

(Armed Forces Institute of Pathology Neg. Nos. 65-5966-3, 79-5408, 79-15021-3, 79-15021-1,2.)

calcium), not on cellular viability. Therefore, any alteration in bone density—either a real increase or decrease in radiographic density—is an indication of viability requiring osteoblastic or osteoclastic cell activity, respectively, and initially will be perceived in the viable bone and marrow surrounding the osteonecrotic segment.

MARROW CAVITY

The medullary cavity is an admixture of cancellous bone, hematopoietic marrow, fatty marrow, and sinusoidal vascular bed confined by a nonexpandable shell of cortical bone. Radiographically, ischemic necrosis of bone is encountered most commonly within the epiphyseal (especially the femoral and humeral heads) and metadiaphyseal marrow cavities of adult long tubular bones.[33] Occasional involvement of the distal femoral condyles,[127, 164] small round bones of the wrist and ankle, and other sites is seen.[60]

The primary function of cancellous bone is to support the subarticular bony plate and transmit biomechanical force from the articular surface to the cortical shaft. For this reason, cancellous bone tends to be more concentrated in the epiphyseal and, to a lesser degree, the metaphyseal ends of long bones. Little cancellous bone remains in the diaphysis of long bones. The amount and architectural orientation of cancellous bone will, in large part, be determined by the changing biomechanical requirements of each bone.

Because the femoral head is a major area of clinical concern, the architectural arrangement of its cancellous bone is of particular interest. For example, the stress-diffusing characteristics of the growth plate interposed between the articular surface and cortical shaft in a growing bone result in a tightly packed, crossing pattern of cancellous bone throughout the epiphysis (Fig. 79–3A). Under these circumstances, the metaphyseal cancellous bone supports the growth plate, and the growth plate in turn provides the base of support for the epiphyseal cancellous bone supporting the articular surface. Closure of the growth plate is followed by extensive architectural reorganization (remodeling) of the epiphyseal and, to a lesser extent, the metaphyseal cancellous bone such that they become a continuum (Fig. 79–3B). This normally results in a somewhat wedge-shaped orientation of tightly packed and thicker cancellous bone trabeculae supporting the articular surface directly beneath the anterolateral weight-bearing segment of the femoral head. Similar but less dramatic findings are encountered in the humeral head and femoral condyles.[127]

The arterial, sinusoidal, and venous vascular network of bone has been well demonstrated by previous anatomic studies[116–118] and need not be detailed here. The extensive arterial supply to adult long tubular bones, including the nutrient artery with its ascending and descending diaphyseal branches and the penetrating metaphyseal and epiphyseal (retinacular) arteries, as well as the superficial periosteal vessels and the diffuse intramedullary sinusoidal vascular bed, provides excellent collateral circulation. This fact is underscored by experimental data indicating the inability to produce bone infarcts by isolated occlusion of either the

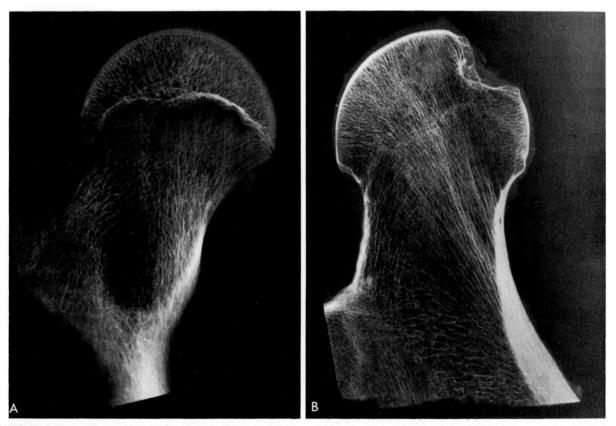

FIGURE 79–3. Normal femoral heads. Specimen radiograph of the femoral head and neck from a patient with closing capital femoral physis **(A)** and a patient with a closed **(B)** capital femoral physeal growth plate. Note the differing amounts and orientations of cancellous bone, especially in the epiphysis of each patient. This reflects the changing mechanical requirements as the growth plate closes. (Armed Forces Institute of Pathology Neg. Nos. 79-6007, 79-6008.)

nutrient, metaphyseal, epiphyseal, or periosteal arterial supply.[118]

The sinusoidal vascular bed of the intramedullary canal, which supplies the bulk of the marrow and cancellous bone, originates from the terminal branches of the arterial network penetrating the bony cortex. Venous outflow also is extensive, as evidenced by numerous perforating channels exiting from the cortex.[27, 50]

Despite the extensive circulation available to the metadiaphyseal cortex and intramedullary cavity, the epiphyseal ends of long bones have limited arterial access and venous outflow because much of their surface is covered by articular cartilage. This fact is reflected by reductions in both blood flow through the epiphyseal sinusoidal vascular bed and intraosseous marrow pressure (blood perfusion pressure) compared with those in the metadiaphyseal intramedullary cavity.[112] Arterial access to the epiphysis is further compromised in the growing skeleton, as the epiphysis is separated from the metaphysis by the growth plate. Although occasional small arterioles penetrate the physeal growth plate (physis), little or no significant collateral circulation exists between a developing epiphysis and its adjacent metaphysis.[116, 118] In the absence of collateral circulation, the likelihood of a single or dominant artery supplying an entire epiphysis or a significant segment of an epiphysis is increased. The small carpal and tarsal bones also are covered to a large extent by articular cartilage. In many respects, their ossification centers are analogous to the developing epiphyses of a long bone with regard to blood supply. Compromise of a dominant artery[140] supplying a developing epiphysis or small round bone ossification center is a possible mechanism for Legg-Calvé-Perthes disease (femoral head),[159, 172] Köhler's disease (tarsal navicular bone), and Kienböck's disease (lunate bone).

Development of a sinusoidal vascular bed appears to be an important prerequisite for the emergence of normal hematopoietic activity—witness the confinement of the bulk of extramedullary hematopoiesis in the fetus (except in extreme circumstances) to the liver and spleen, both of which have well-developed sinusoidal vascular beds.

Each bone develops its own sinusoidal vascular bed and marrow cavity as it grows. The sinusoids are seen readily via the microscope in areas of active enchondral bone formation. In regions of active hematopoiesis, the sinusoids appear packed with erythroid and myeloid elements. The expansive sinusoidal space available during active hematopoiesis, however, becomes predominantly a potential space in areas of fatty marrow. Rapid discharge of hematopoietic elements provides the ability to increase blood flow more quickly through areas of active hematopoietic marrow than through fatty marrow.[67, 74] Experimental studies indicate that the rate of blood flow through fatty marrow and fatty tissue is considerably reduced per unit area over that of other tissues, such as skeletal muscle and skin.[44]

The relative amounts and localization of hematopoietic or fatty marrow depend primarily on hematopoietic demand. This demand largely is a function of age. The marrow cavities of all bones in the newborn and young child are actively engaged in hematopoiesis. As the total marrow volume increases with skeletal growth, normal hematopoietic demand eventually can be satisfied by the marrow capacity of the axial skeleton. Therefore, the marrow cavities of the adolescent and adult appendicular skeleton nor-

mally contain predominantly fatty marrow, unless some special circumstance requires increased hematopoiesis.

Thus, both radiographic and anatomic observations indicate that ischemic necrosis of bone, either avascular necrosis or bone infarction, occurs almost invariably within areas of predominantly fatty marrow (Figs. 79–2 and 79–4). The converse is equally true; ischemic necrosis in areas of normal active hematopoiesis is distinctly unusual except in sickle cell disease and related hemoglobinopathies, or following complete traumatic disruption of the arterial blood supply. Ischemic necrosis of cortical bone is relatively rare and occurs only when there is extensive interruption of the arterial blood supply, as in osteomyelitis (Fig. 79–5).

ISCHEMIC BONE NECROSIS: ASSOCIATIONS AND MECHANISMS

A variable group of clinical situations are associated with the development of avascular necrosis and bone infarction.[211] These include traumatic disruption of the blood supply (femoral head dislocation and subcapital femoral neck fracture), the hemoglobinopathies (sickle cell disease), exogenous corticosteroid therapy and Cushing's disease, alcoholism, Gaucher's disease, dysbaric disorders, pregnancy, and irradiation. Patients with collagen vascular disorders, such as systemic lupus erythematosus and rheumatoid arthritis, and patients who have had renal transplants or have lymphoproliferative disorders also are at risk for osteonecrosis. The vast majority of patients within the last three groups usually have received significant corticosteroid or immunosuppressive therapy, or both. Patients with pancreatitis and gout also have been reported to be at risk for osteonecrosis. The prevalence of chronic alcoholism in both of these patient populations may be a significant factor.

The sequestrum of osteomyelitis, although no longer generally regarded in the context of osteonecrosis, is a manifestation of ischemic bone death occurring as a consequence of compressive and destructive suppuration that isolates a segment of bone from its blood supply (Fig. 79–5). The sequestration of cortical bone is accomplished by obliteration of the sinusoidal bed, disruption of the metaphyseal and nutrient arterial supply, and stripping of the periosteum with its penetrating periosteal arteries from the cortical surface by pus.

Finally, a sizeable group of patients with osteonecrosis exists in whom none of the foregoing conditions are implicated; for this group, the term idiopathic osteonecrosis is reserved. The label "idiopathic" may reflect unknown history (e.g., "closet alcoholism") as much as unknown cause. Interestingly, rare instances of multiple "idiopathic" bone infarcts in several members of a family over one or more generations have been encountered, suggesting a hereditary predisposition in some cases.[114, 211]

Femoral Head Dislocation

Subluxation of the adult femoral head invariably ruptures the ligamentum teres, disrupting the arterial supply to the femoral head. In addition, the superior retinacular arteries may be compromised partially or totally.[106] Patients with dislocations[131] and delayed reductions[30] appear to be at greater risk for the development of ischemic necrosis. Re-

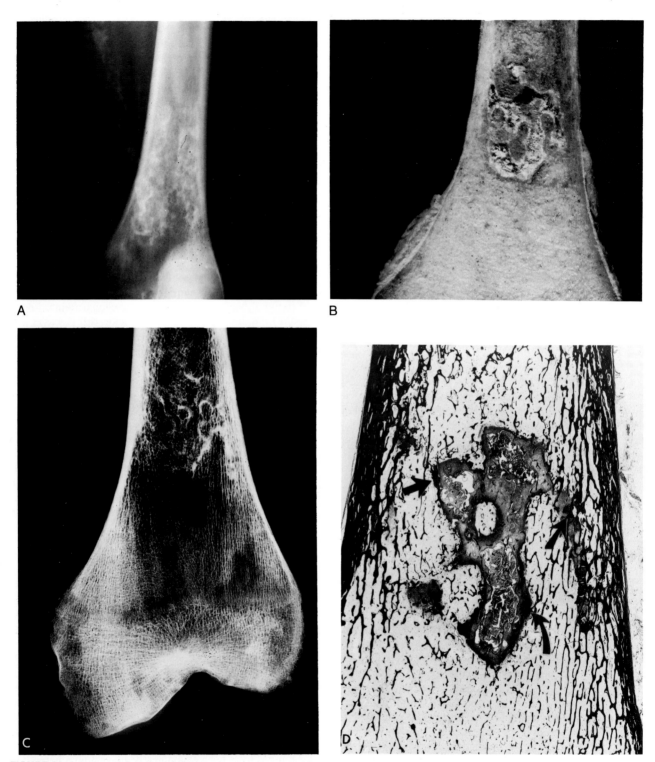

FIGURE 79–4. Intramedullary bone infarct.

A Clinical radiograph of the distal portion of the femur demonstrates an intramedullary infarct, characterized by curly, smokelike wisps of increased density primarily at the margins.

B Slightly reduced gross photograph of the coronally sectioned femur shows an irregular, yellow, necrotic area of infarction within fatty marrow.

C Specimen radiograph of the gross section correlates the curly wisps of increased density with the margins of the infarct. The scattered radiolucent foci distal to the infarct are probably secondary to active hyperemia (reflex vascular osteoporosis).

D Macrosection (4×) reveals the dense margin of the infarct to be the result of ischemic bone formation (curved arrow), dystrophic mineralization (tapered arrow), and focal trabecular reinforcement (straight arrow). Note: The relatively small size of the infarct in **B, C,** and **D** as compared with the clinical radiograph **(A)** reflects the plane of section.

(Armed Forces Institute of Pathology Neg. Nos. 76-2218-2, 79-15023, 79-5413, 79-15024.)

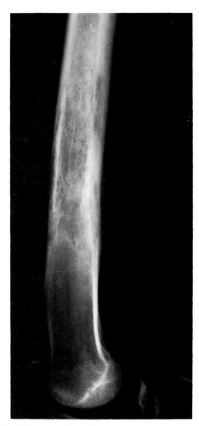

FIGURE 79–5. Osteomyelitis with cortical sequestrum. Lateral view of the distal end of the femur shows a motheaten area of bone lysis with apparent radiodensity of the inner anterior cortex. Intracortical destruction of bone just anterior to this sequestrum is also seen. (Armed Forces Institute of Pathology Neg. No. 73-11186-8.)

duction of the femoral head returns the bone to its normal stress-bearing orientation. This will not restore blood flow through the ligamentum teres but may relieve any vascular embarrassment that had occurred as a result of twisting or stretching of the retinacular vessels.[106, 108] Whether or not ischemic necrosis develops under these circumstances depends on the availability of sufficient collateral circulation to augment the blood supply reduced by the damaged extraosseous arterial vessels. Ischemic necrosis of the femoral head following subluxation usually is confined to the anterolateral weight-bearing segment, although occasionally more extensive areas or the entire head will be involved.[114]

Femoral Neck Fracture

Intracapsular femoral neck fractures result in extensive interruption of blood flow to the femoral head. The sinusoidal vascular bed is interrupted[106] and the subsynovial retinacular vessels, including the lateral epiphyseal, superior metaphyseal, and inferior metaphyseal arterial extensions,[117] also may be disrupted or damaged severely.[19, 83, 105] The only remaining blood supply available to the femoral head may be within the ligamentum teres, provided that it was functional prior to fracture.[19, 91, 105]

The prevalence of ischemic necrosis after intracapsular femoral neck fractures depends on the reestablishment of adequate blood flow from the remaining intact vasculature, revascularization (ingrowth) by new vessels in the femoral head,[19, 105] or both. Available data indicate between 60 and

75 per cent of femoral heads removed under the circumstances described previously will demonstrate evidence of ischemic necrosis.[12, 18, 125] This is particularly true if there has been significant displacement or excessive rotation of the fractured fragments.[48] Both displacement and rotation are likely to increase the severity of damage to the retinacular vessels.

Reestablishment of blood flow to a portion of the femoral head through the ligamentum teres occurs in 50 to 60 per cent of patients, but only rarely will it supply the entire femoral head.[19, 89, 91, 103, 105, 106] Unfortunately, a small percentage of normal patients have no functional blood flow through the ligamentum teres, and in some patients the fracture disrupts the ligament.[21] Under these circumstances revascularization must occur from the femoral neck.

Close approximation of the fracture edges provides the opportunity to reestablish blood flow by local revascularization across the fracture site with ingrowth of new vessels from the retinacular group.[4, 19, 21, 105] The higher prevalence of ischemic necrosis that follows displaced femoral neck fractures suggests persistent motion (instability) across the fracture site continually ruptures the anastomosing vascular channels bridging the fracture.[19, 105] Should the fractured segment fail to unite, the reestablishment of blood flow to the femoral head will be impaired significantly.[23, 107] The extent and distribution of necrosis within the femoral head tend to vary considerably after fracture. The majority of infarcts are localized to the anterolateral weight-bearing segment, but more extensive involvement is fairly common.[20] Not infrequently, the entire femoral head dies. The latter is most likely to occur with nonunion of the fractured neck[7, 17, 23, 48, 107, 114] (Fig. 79–6).

In the absence of a reestablished blood supply, no reparative response can occur, and the femoral head, though dead, will remain unchanged both anatomically and radiographically for a time.[46, 88–90, 107] This radiographic pattern was encountered more frequently prior to hip nailing, when patients with femoral neck fractures were treated by immobilization. The progressive disuse osteoporosis of the adjacent viable pelvis and femur resulted in a necrotic femoral head that appeared relatively dense.[103] With hip nailing and rapid weight-bearing, early radiographic identification of avascular necrosis became more difficult.[11, 17, 48] This identification is further complicated by the cancellous bone remodeling that normally follows in response to the altered mechanics created by fracture.[46]

Sickle Cell Disease

Sickle cell disease, sickle cell trait, and the other related hemoglobinopathies are associated with localized areas of epiphyseal and metadiaphyseal bone infarction.[5, 28, 29, 82, 84, 94] Sludging of sickled erythrocytes within the sinusoidal vascular bed results in functional occlusion. The localized anoxia further aggravates the sickling process, increasing the likelihood of additional vessel occlusion and extension of the involved area. If the process becomes sufficiently extensive, infarction will occur. Because this process frequently takes place within areas of active hematopoiesis, localized areas of intramedullary bone infarction may be found throughout the skeleton.[22, 28, 156, 170, 173, 185] In most cases, however, the foci of osteonecrosis are encountered in the epiphyseal and metadiaphyseal marrow cavities of long tub-

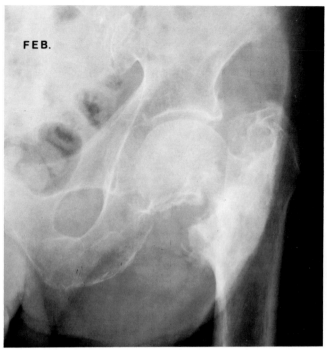
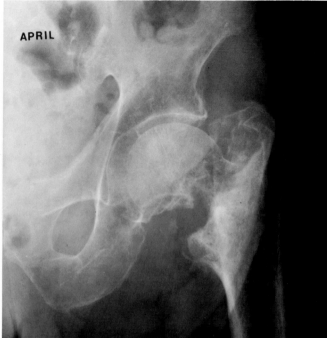

A   B

FIGURE 79–6. Fracture of femoral neck with fibrous nonunion.

A, B Radiographs of an ununited femoral neck fracture taken 2 months apart with slight difference in technique. No significant change has occurred over the 2 months, suggesting an impaired repair process.

C Macroscopic section (2×) of the femoral head demonstrates extensive ischemic necrosis and only a partial fibrous union. Note the subchondral area of ischemic necrosis (N) surrounded by a fairly well defined reactive fibrous interface (R). The remaining portion of the femoral head is an admixture of ischemic necrosis (n) and injury and revascularization (r). This suggests extension of the original infarct and is likely to have been the result of the fracture's failure to unite properly and reestablish adequate blood flow. The increased bone density at the peripheral margin adjacent to the fibrous nonunion indicates viability and mechanical reinforcement (straight arrows).

D Photomicrographic view (2×) of the subchondral area of ischemic necrosis shows unaltered dead cancellous bone, lipid cysts (C), and partially opacified necrotic fat (O).

E Photomicrograph (28×) of a reactive interface demonstrates dead fat superiorly (N), the fibrous interface (R), and surrounding revitalized cancellous bone and fat (V). Some reactive fiber bone reinforcement is seen within the reactive interface (curved arrow).

F Photomicrograph (40×) of the outer margin of a reactive interface, showing fibrous modulation of marrow fat (R), lipid cyst formation (C), increased vascularity and new vessel formation, and revascularization surrounded by an inflammatory cell infiltrate (arrow).

(Armed Forces Institute of Pathology Neg. Nos. 64-2229-2,5; 79-15317; 79-15318-1,2; 79-15316.)

ular bones,[28] especially the distal segments of the humerus, tibia, and femur.[170]

Reestablishment of the vascular supply depends on stabilization of the infarcted area and reversal of the sickling phenomenon, allowing resumption of blood flow. The precise nature of the "bone within bone" radiographic appearance (Fig. 79–7A) occasionally encountered in sickle cell disease during childhood remains incompletely resolved, but it probably represents infarction of the internal third of the cortex; the latter's vascular supply is an extension of the sinusoidal vascular bed.[8, 28] Sickle cell disease frequently is complicated by superimposed osteomyelitis (Fig. 79–7B), especially due to Salmonella organisms.[56, 185] Exclusion of cortical sequestration by infection is essential prior to ascribing the "bone within bone" appearance to ischemic bone necrosis.[8, 47]

Corticosteroid Therapy

The increased prevalence of ischemic necrosis in patients receiving corticosteroid therapy and in persons with Cushing's disease is well established.[9, 14, 38, 45, 51, 52] Even patients receiving short-term high dose corticosteroid treatment for cerebral edema or long-term soft tissue corticosteroid infil-

tration appear at risk for ischemic necrosis.[150, 196, 197, 205] Considerable experimental work has been undertaken in an attempt to explain the mechanism of osteonecrosis associated with corticosteroid therapy.[39, 70, 121, 220] Much attention has been focused on the presence of microscopic fat emboli in the end-arteries of bone and other organ systems.[30, 39, 70, 71, 188] It has been proposed that the fat emboli and hyperlipidemia observed in this clinical setting are derived from a fatty liver.[37, 55] Interestingly, isolated occurrences of osteonecrosis associated with various types of nonsteroid-induced hyperlipidemia have been reported.[129, 187] Other investigators have proposed steroid-induced osteoporosis or osteomalacia with subsequent microfracture as a cause of osteonecrosis.[40, 41, 68, 75, 95] Until recently little attention has been paid to alterations in marrow fat cells.[67] Experimental evidence indicates a significant increase in individual marrow fat cell size associated with high dose corticosteroid therapy.[12, 142, 184, 193, 203] Similar morphologic findings, including elevated lipid content, have been described in the osteonecrotic femoral heads of both steroid-treated and alcoholic patients.[135] The increasing fat cell mass is not accommodated completely by an equivalent loss of trabecular and cortical bone. Because the marrow cavity is encased by a nonexpansile shell of bone (compartmental effect), any in-

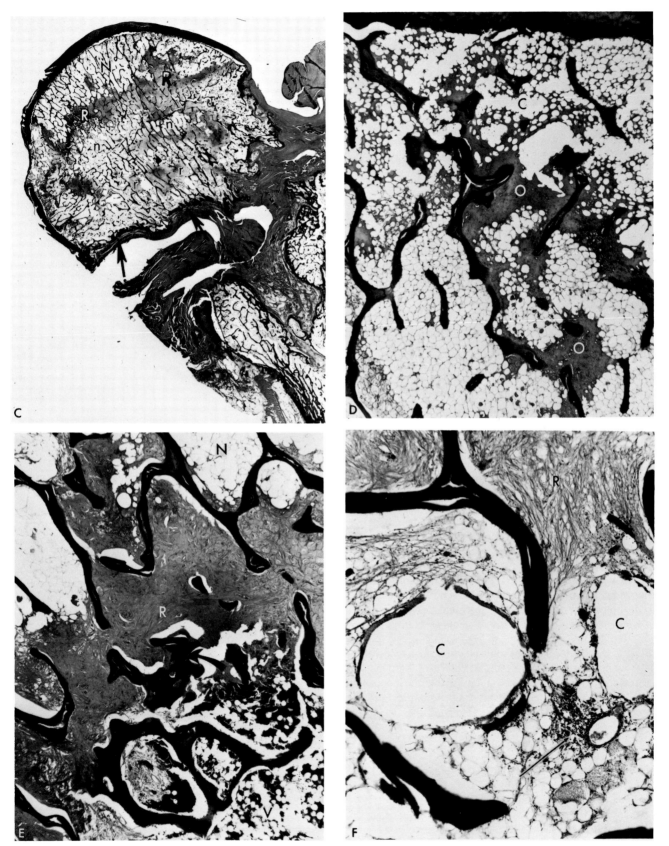

FIGURE 79–6. *Continued*

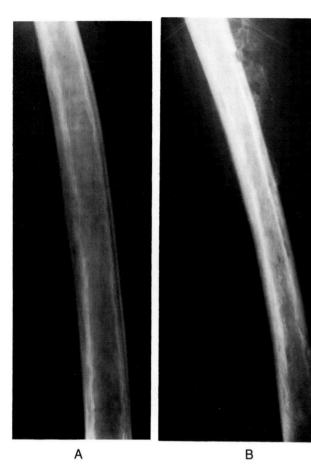

A   B

FIGURE 79–7. Sickle cell disease.
A Sickle cell disease without osteomyelitis. Lateral view of midfemur demonstrates a bone-within-bone appearance. This is noted by the radiolucent area splitting the anterior cortex with a radiodense line on both surfaces.
B Sickle cell disease with osteomyelitis. Lateral view of femur showing a bone-within-bone appearance as well as patchy bone destruction in the cortex and extensive periosteal new bone formation.
(Armed Forces Institute of Pathology Neg. Nos. 68-4951-1, 70-69023.)

crease in marrow fat cell mass not accommodated by bone loss must occur at the expense of the remaining marrow constituents, especially the sinusoidal vascular bed, because hematopoietic activity normally is scant in areas of fatty marrow.[121] The resulting mechanical infringement on the sinusoidal vascular bed will impede blood flow (venous stasis) and increase intraosseous marrow pressure.[122]

Recent clinical and experimental studies have demonstrated significantly increased intraosseous marrow pressures within the femoral heads of patients and rabbits treated with corticosteroids.[57, 122] Perfusion of the marrow sinusoidal vascular bed depends on hydrostatic pressure from the pumping action of the heart and the elastic recoil of arteries.[49] Any increase in intraosseous pressure not compensated for by an increase in hydrostatic pressure will result in the compromise of marrow sinusoidal blood flow and venous stasis, increasing the risk of infarction. This is further supported by success in modifying the course or actually preventing the emergence of ischemic necrosis through use of core decompression biopsies.[151–153, 165, 203]

Alcoholism

Ischemic necrosis, especially of the femoral head, in association with chronic alcoholism is fairly common.[6, 68, 85] The prevalence among alcoholics may not be as high as expected.[160] Metadiaphyseal infarcts are rare. It has been suggested that the alcoholic fatty liver is associated with systemic fat emboli, which may lodge in bone.[69] Similar mechanisms to those outlined for corticosteroid necrosis also have been proposed for osteonecrosis in chronic alcoholism.[67]

Studies on alcohol abuse–associated ischemic necrosis indicate a higher lipid content, especially cholesterol, in the osteonecrotic segment of bone than in uninvolved bony segments and, perhaps more importantly, a higher lipid content than in the bones of normal and osteoarthritic controls. The highest lipid content values were encountered in patients with combined steroid and alcohol use.[135] Increased fat cell size and intramedullary pressure also have been described in osteonecrotic femoral heads in patients with a history of alcohol abuse in comparison to those of normal controls.[58] Elevated intraosseous marrow pressures likewise have been recorded in normal-appearing femoral heads of alcoholic patients who have ischemic necrosis in the contralateral femoral head.[58]

Gaucher's Disease

Histologic examination of the bone marrow in Gaucher's disease reveals sinusoids packed with lipid (glucocerebroside)-containing histiocytes termed Gaucher's cells. An increasing number of Gaucher's cells results in progressive obstruction of the flow of blood through the sinusoids, leading to osteonecrosis.[62, 67] Both ischemic necrosis and metadiaphyseal infarcts are encountered in this disorder.[1, 2, 64, 101, 115]

Dysbaric Disorders

On the basis of accumulating evidence, the risk of osteonecrosis under dysbaric conditions appears to be related directly to the depth of dive, number of dives, uncontrolled decompression, and low oxygen concentrations.[167, 179, 186] Even current decompression standards have been challenged as not being uniformly protective.[171] Osteonecrosis of both the epiphyseal and metadiaphyseal medullary cavities is seen in association with dysbaric disorders.[100, 123] Radionuclide scintigraphy currently is used to detect evidence of early osteonecrosis under dysbaric conditions.[178, 189] Many, but not all, observers still regard dysbaric osteonecrosis to be the result of gas (nitrogen) embolization after rapid decompression.[26, 34, 92, 120] Partial pressures of dissolved gases demand eventual equilibrium among the atmosphere, blood, and interstitial and intracellular compartments. Invariably, a relative time lag occurs in the equalization of partial pressures across vessel walls and cell membranes during both compression and decompression.[26] Experimental studies reveal fat cells to have a fivefold increased ability to absorb dissolved nitrogen,[44] and individual marrow fat cell volume increases under these circumstances.[191, 206] Because both blood flow and the capillary–fat cell surface area are relatively reduced, the ability to transport nitrogen away from fatty tissue is only about half that of other tissues.[44] This will result in nitrogen bubbles appearing within fat cells if the rate of decompression exceeds the transporting ability of the circulation.[43] Although fat cells in soft tissue have room to expand under these circumstances, as already noted the marrow fat cells are confined by a nonexpansile shell of bone.[67] As a result, the potential for a dramatic increase in intraosseous marrow pressure and venous stasis during decompression is significant. The accumulation of undissolved nitrogen gas bubbles in interstitial and vascular spaces undoubtedly plays a role, as evidenced by the endothelial injury and platelet and fibrinogen consumption associated with decompression sickness.[201] However, failure of equalization of pressure across the marrow fat cell membrane with subsequent expansion and rupture of the fat cell may be a more significant causative factor of osteonecrosis in this condition (see Chapter 80).

Pregnancy

Women appear to be at risk for developing ischemic necrosis of the femoral head during the last trimester of pregnancy.[190, 210] As might be expected, in most cases the typical radiographic signs do not become apparent until after delivery.[130] Hip pain during the third trimester may be the only clinical finding. Venous stasis with increased intramedullary pressure secondary to impaired venous drainage caused by the gravid uterus and engorged pelvic venous plexus has been suggested as the likely etiologic factor.

Radiation-induced Osteonecrosis

Depending on the dosage of radiation therapy, a direct cytotoxic effect may occur especially on the more sensitive hematopoietic marrow constituents.[21, 25, 65, 81, 124] Although the actual mechanism remains controversial, the long-term radiation effects resulting in osteonecrosis are mediated through damage to the bones' vascularity.[61, 66, 148]

Collagen Vascular Disorders

The relatively high prevalence of ischemic bone necrosis in systemic lupus erythematosus[161, 166, 199, 209] and rheumatoid arthritis is likely related to corticosteroid therapy.[21, 32, 110] Vasculitis with interruption of the arterial blood supply has

been suggested as a possible additional mechanism[119] for at least some of the patients with collagen vascular disorders not treated with steroids who develop osteonecrosis.[109, 110, 113]

Renal Transplantation and Chemotherapy

Osteonecrosis, especially in the femoral heads and condyles, humeral heads, and occasionally other sites, is a significant complication of renal transplantation.[24, 128, 195] There seems little doubt that corticosteroids and other immunosuppressive agents used to control rejection are the major etiologic factors in the genesis of osteonecrosis under these circumstances.[162, 163, 204] Underlying metabolic bone changes associated with chronic renal disease, however, also may be a contributing factor, as evidenced by the apparent increased frequency of this abnormality in hypophosphatemia and the protective effect of active vitamin D metabolites.[146, 175, 176, 198] Histomorphometric analysis of iliac bone biopsy specimens indicates the presence of metabolic bone changes and impaired repair capabilities, factors that also may be significant in the genesis of osteonecrosis, even in the absence of renal dysfunction.[131]

Patients with lymphoproliferative disorders also appear to be at risk for developing osteonecrosis, presumably as a result of corticosteroid and combined chemotherapy.[147, 192] The marrow packing effect of these disorders and associated tumor necrosis may contribute to osseous abnormality.

Chronic Pancreatitis and Gout

Necrosis of the peritoneal and mesenteric fat is a well-recognized complication of acute pancreatitis.[77] Similar findings have been demonstrated in the brain, kidney, subcutaneous tissue, and bone marrow at autopsy.[77, 132] Disseminated small areas of fat necrosis in bone, presumably the result of circulating lipases,[86] have been described as a complication of acute pancreatitis.[59] Typical patterns of femoral head and intramedullary bone infarcts are observed only rarely, however.[42, 78] The recognized association of pancreatitis and alcoholism requires close scrutiny to exclude the latter as a possible contributing mechanism in this patient population.

What relationship, if any, exists to explain the apparent association between gout and ischemic necrosis, other than alcoholism, remains obscure.[6, 76, 79]

Circulation, Intraosseous Marrow Pressure, and Weight-Bearing

Several of the clinical situations outlined previously seem to be associated with an alteration of marrow constituents and an increase in intraosseous marrow pressure. Because the marrow cavity is encased by a rigid bony shell, any increase in one marrow component, in terms of either cell number or volume, must take place at the expense of the remaining marrow elements. It is increasingly apparent against this background, that the cellular composition of marrow and its relationship to the sinusoidal vascular bed are fundamental to understanding the mechanisms of nontraumatic ischemic necrosis and bone infarction. The predominance of metadiaphyseal bone infarcts in the intertrochanteric area and distal end of the femur, the proximal portion of the tibia, and the proximal part of the humerus (all areas of fatty marrow in adults) and the relatively high prevalence of ischemic necrosis in the femoral head and, to a lesser extent, the humeral head and femoral condyles of adults (also areas of predominantly fatty marrow and densely packed cancellous bone) underscore an important relationship between the fatty marrow and the sinusoidal vascular bed.

The foregoing observations leave unexplained the predominant localization of ischemic necrosis of the femoral head to the anterolateral weight-bearing subchondral bony segment. This indicates something unique about the weight-bearing area of the femoral head or its vascular supply, or of both, that places it at higher risk for ischemic necrosis. If increased intraosseous pressure with venous stasis is as significant a factor in the development of osteonecrosis as accumulating data would suggest,[57, 58, 175, 209] the ability to decompress the marrow space would be an equally important factor in the prevention of osteonecrosis.[151–153, 165, 203] This ability to decompress the marrow space depends largely on regional anatomic structure, especially bony architecture and vascular outflow.[50] The humeral head, the femoral condyles, and especially the femoral head are at an anatomic disadvantage for decompression. They represent large spheres covered by articular surface, perched on narrow metaphyseal necks. Therefore, relatively few venous channels penetrating the bony cortex are directly available for decompression. For this reason, any increase in pressure within these large spheres must be funneled through the narrow metaphyseal neck for decompression, a situation analogous to rush-hour traffic on a one lane bridge.

The subchondral weight-bearing area of the femoral head and, to a lesser extent, of the femoral condyles is at a special disadvantage for decompression. In response to the mechanical requirements of weight-bearing, greater amounts of more tightly packed cancellous bone are present within these areas. This creates a baffle effect, which further restricts the ability to decompress the marrow space in comparison with the more open adjacent subchondral areas. Trabecular deformation that normally occurs during weight-bearing also will compress the marrow space to some degree and should result in a localized, temporary increase in intraosseous pressure. This situation may be aggravated further by the morphologic profile of reduced trabecular bone, thickened osteoid seams, and indolent calcification dynamics noted in specimens from iliac bone biopsies of patients with normal renal function and osteonecrosis.[131] In some instances of idiopathic osteonecrosis, the aforementioned changes have been accompanied by decreased concentrations of 1,25-dihydroxyvitamin D_3. Such findings suggest a possible quantitative or qualitative deficiency in the bone architecture, which undoubtedly would potentiate the altered pressure effects of deformation.[144, 158, 168] In either event, the increased intraosseous pressure would tend to remain concentrated in this area because of the tightly structured bone architecture. This, coupled with a clinical situation in which the intraosseous pressure already is elevated, could transform an area of bone that is ischemic and marginally profused into an area of functional anoxia with resultant infarction.

Finally, angiographic studies in high risk patients with symptoms suggesting impending or emerging ischemic necrosis of the femoral head, irrespective of cause, have demonstrated "transient" obstruction (thrombosis or oblitera-

tion) of the lateral branches of the left medial femoral circumflex artery where they penetrate the cortex (Fig. 79–8A,B). Follow-up angiograms in these patients demonstrate "revascularization" and vascular blushes along the fibroreactive or reparative interface (Fig. 79–8C,D).[212] The explanation for this apparent obstructive thrombosis remains incompletely resolved, but it could be the result of increased intraosseous marrow pressure, predisposing to thrombosis through reduced arterial blood flow. The reduced arterial flow already has been demonstrated experimentally in areas of increased intramedullary pressure. Involvement of the vascular branches that represent the primary blood supply to the weight-bearing zone of the femoral head may explain the localization of ischemic necrosis to this site.[222, 224]

HISTOLOGIC-RADIOGRAPHIC CORRELATION OF THE HOST RESPONSE

Once osteonecrosis or ischemic injury is an established anatomic fact, the body sets into motion the initial inflammatory host response as the first step toward revival, rehabilitation, or removal and reconstruction (repair).

Anything modifying the ability of the host to generate an adequate circulatory response (e.g., increased intraosseous pressure), inflammatory response (e.g., corticosteroids) or metabolic response will be a major factor affecting the morphologic, radiographic, and clinical manifestations of osteonecrosis repair. Structural disruption either prior to the development of osteonecrosis (e.g., femoral neck fracture) or during its repair will alter the stress-transmitting capabilities of the involved bone significantly.[137, 138] This disruption consequently will result in superimposed bone remodeling to meet the changing mechanical requirements in addition to the inflammatory reparative process. It is the interaction of these various factors that is responsible for the relatively wide-ranging anatomic and radiographic changes observed in patients with osteonecrosis.

Within the limits of this chapter, it will not be possible to illustrate all the routine radiographic variations that can emerge as part of the host response to ischemic necrosis of the adult femoral head. Attention will be focused on the progressive histologic changes of the host reparative response to the osteonecrotic segment and their reflection in the radiograph. The discussion will consider each of five anatomic phases, from cell death to articular collapse, stages not dissimilar from previously outlined radiographic and clinical stages of ischemic necrosis.[35, 111]

Phase I: Cellular Death and the Initial Host Response

The recognition of cell death in osteonecrosis by light microscopy has long been a subject of considerable discussion. Proper histologic analysis can be complicated by improper fixation and decalcification of the tissue specimen, both of which can result in marked artifactual distortion of cells. Although functional cell death may have occurred, documentation of cell death is not possible histologically until sufficient cytoplasmic (coagulation) or nuclear (pyknosis, karyorrhexis, and karyolysis) changes occur to cause the cellular constituents to lose their morphologic and staining characteristics.[96] This feature is exemplified in a femoral

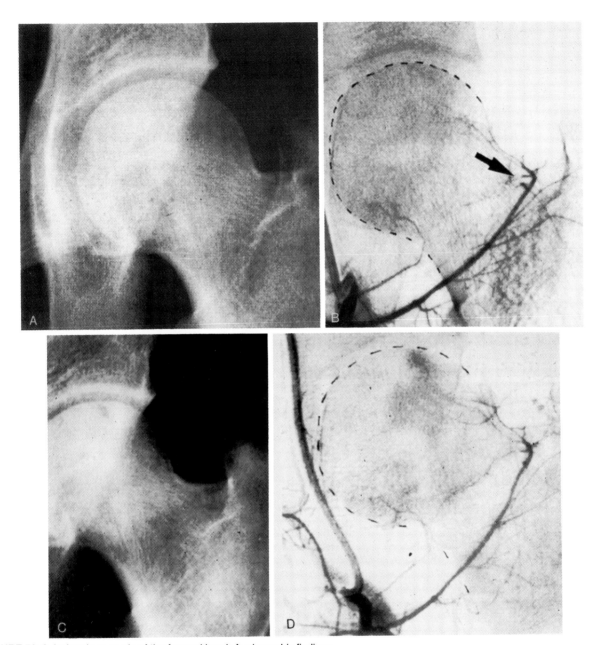

FIGURE 79–8. Ischemic necrosis of the femoral head: Angiographic findings.

A Anteroposterior radiograph of the left hip, demonstrating an essentially normal appearing femoral head and hip joint in a patient with impending ischemic necrosis. Note that the plain film radiographic features of ischemic necrosis are not yet recognizable.

B Anteroposterior angiogram of the left hip, obtained at the same time as the plain film in **A.** Note what appears to represent complete blockage of two branches of the lateral extent of the left medial femoral circumflex artery as they penetrate the femoral neck (arrow). The vascular blush seen within the femoral head, including the weight-bearing zone, owes its presence to the remaining penetrating branches of the left circumflex vasculature.

C Anteroposterior radiograph of the same left hip as in **A** several months later. The plain film appearance clearly demonstrates the presence of ischemic necrosis, as evidenced by the central area of relatively increased density in the weight-bearing zone, encompassed by a thin lucent reactive fibrous margin (reparative interface). The latter also appears partially surrounded by a thin zone of actual increased density (sclerosis).

D Anteroposterior angiogram of the left hip undertaken at the same time as the plain film in **C.** Note that the previously occluded medial circumflex artery branches seen in **B** now are revascularized, and that the predominant vascular blush is confined to the reactive interface at the perimeter of the osteonecrotic segment. In fact, the osteonecrotic segment appears avascular.

(From Atsumi T, et al: Clin Orthop *246:*186–194, 1989.)

head from a 73 year old woman that was resected 24 hours after femoral neck fracture (Fig. 79–9). Aside from the fracture (Fig. 79–9A) and acute hemorrhage adjacent to the fracture site (Fig. 79–9C), no abnormal radiographic, gross pathologic, or histologic findings were observed (Fig. 79–9B–D). The hematopoietic marrow, osteocytes, and marrow fat appear unremarkable. Although the clinical setting indicates anoxia of the femoral head has been present for 24 hours, necrosis cannot be confirmed by light microscopy in this specimen. Six hours of anoxia generally is regarded as sufficient to result in death of the hematopoietic marrow.[125] Forty-eight to 72 hours may elapse before the degree of cell autolysis is sufficient to be recognized histologically, however (see Fig. 79–10D). Thus, in this case the time interval between the onset of anoxia and resection is not sufficient even for the most sensitive marrow elements to demonstrate morphologic evidence of anoxic damage.

Clinical and experimental studies suggest osteocytes, osteoblasts, and osteoclasts may survive approximately 6 to 48 hours of anoxia before irreversible visible cell damage and death occur.[72] Because viable osteocytes within bony lacunae frequently appear pyknotic, pyknosis alone is not a reliable sign of cell death under this circumstance.[21] Generally empty osteocytic lacunae have been presumed to reflect cell death. Because there is a normal attrition of osteocytes with age,[63] the presence of empty osteocytic lacunae does not necessarily indicate osteonecrosis. Even with functional death of osteocytes, complete autolysis, as evidenced by empty osteocytic lacunae, may take from 48 hours to 4 weeks or longer to occur.[21, 67, 72] Thus, the presence or absence of osteocytes in lacunae cannot be considered a reliable indication of either cell viability or cell death in the early stages of osteonecrosis. However, complete absence of osteocytes within localized areas of trabecular bone is a reasonably reliable indicator of previous or existing ischemic necrosis, if artifactual loss can be excluded.

These considerations are exemplified in the femoral head of a 69 year old man resected 72 hours after a femoral neck fracture (Fig. 79–10). Aside from the fracture, neither the clinical nor the specimen radiographs (Fig. 79–10A,B) show any alteration in the subchondral or trabecular bone architecture. The macroscopic section shows evidence of hemorrhage along the fracture site and both hyperemic and avascular areas within the substance of the femoral head (Fig. 79–10C). The high power view of the microscopic section reveals an autolytic ghostlike appearance (necrosis) in the hematopoietic elements (Fig. 79–10D). Many of the osteocytic lacunae within the bone trabeculae also appear empty, suggesting bone death (Fig. 79–10D). No alteration of marrow fat cells is evident.

Little attention has been focused on the marrow fat cells' ability to survive anoxia. Estimates of marrow fat cell survivability after complete anoxia range from 2 to 5 days or more.[67] Histologically, marrow fat cell death may be reflected by no appreciable structural change other than loss of its nucleus, a feature that frequently is difficult to identify under normal conditions because of nuclear eccentricity and section thickness relative to cell size. Loss of nuclei, disruption of a cluster of fat cells (forming lipid cysts), and partial opacification of fat cells generally are considered to reflect cell death. Such findings are exemplified in the femoral head resected from a 71 year old man 5 days after subcapital femoral neck fracture (Fig. 79–11). The gross photograph shows characteristic pale areas of avascularity partly surrounded by a hyperemic zone (Fig. 79–11A). No alteration is observed in the specimen radiograph (Fig. 79–11B). The macroscopic section shows the expected hemorrhage along the fracture site, with focal areas of hyperemia but no alteration in bony architecture (Fig. 79–11C). The high power view of the microscopic section reveals the presence of large lipid cysts and necrotic hematopoietic elements (Fig. 79–11D). The lipid cysts are surrounded partially by lightly opacified but otherwise unaltered fat cells. No viable osteoblasts or osteoclasts are seen. A few osteocytic lacunae are empty, whereas others appear to contain nuclei. The findings in this case reflect unequivocal ischemic necrosis, despite the incomplete osteocyte loss.

In the early stages, histologically recognizable death of the hematopoietic elements, and especially marrow fat, is the most reliable light microscopic sign of osteonecrosis. The presence or absence of osteocytic nuclei (empty lacunae) is of lesser importance because of the wide variations in their rates of autolysis after functional death. However, uniformly empty osteocytic lacunae are important findings in the evaluation of the late stages of osteonecrosis, when they may be the only reliable histologic marker left, indicating the extent of the original infarcted area.

Hence, the first phase of osteonecrosis, cell death and initial host response, is characterized by microscopic changes in the hematopoietic elements, the osteocytic cellular constituents, and the marrow fat cells. Although the "central" zone of cell death usually is distinguishable from the surrounding viable zone by the fifth day of complete anoxia, the ischemic zone between the zone of cell death and viable tissue is not well defined histologically. During this phase, the gross appearance of the unsectioned femoral head is unaltered. Sectioning of the femoral head may reveal gross areas of apparent avascularity and hyperemia. However, no recognizable gross architectural or radiographic changes are observed in the cancellous and subchondral bone or overlying articular surface. Therefore, no radiographically recognizable evidence of osteonecrosis would be anticipated during phase I on plain films.

Phase II: Cell Modulation in the Ischemic Zone and Hyperemia

Although the initial phase, cell death, is entirely a reflection of anoxia, phase II, marked by cell modulation and hyperemia, is dependent primarily on the availability of an adequate blood supply within the viable tissue surrounding the osteonecrotic and ischemic zones. In the case of a femoral neck fracture, this requires either reestablishing blood flow through existing vascular spaces or revascularization by new vessels. In the presence of adequate circulation, the breakdown products of dying and severely damaged cells initiate the host's inflammatory response, characterized by vascular dilation, transudation of fluid, fibrin precipitation, and local infiltration of inflammatory cells. During this phase, two morphologically identifiable alterations become manifest. One is perceived radiographically (Fig. 79–12A), the other microscopically (Fig. 79–12B,C).

Histologically, the ischemic marrow between the central core of osteonecrosis and the surrounding viable tissue initially is characterized by modulation of ischemically injured marrow fat cells that have not undergone anoxic death (Fig.

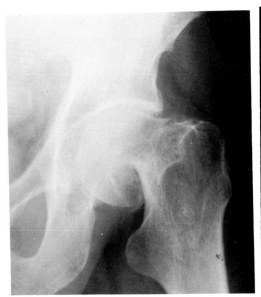

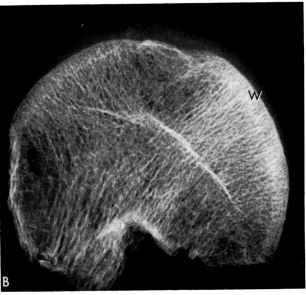

A

B

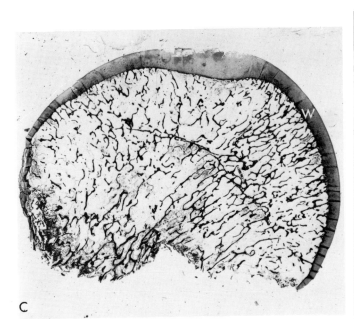

C

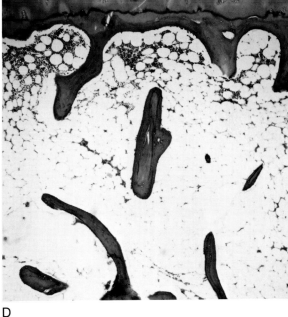

D

FIGURE 79–9. Fracture of the femoral neck (24 hours).

   A Clinical radiograph demonstrates a femoral neck fracture without dislocation.

   B Specimen radiograph (2.5×) of the coronally sectioned femoral head resected 24 hours after fracture reveals a normal appearing subchondral plate and underlying cancellous bone. The concentration and orientation of the supporting trabecular bone in the weight-bearing area (W) are normal.

   C Macroscopic section (2.5×) reveals an intact articular surface and subchondral plate. Note the orientation (W) of the cancellous bony architecture underlying the weight-bearing area. The marrow is predominantly fatty, with scattered areas of hematopoietic activity. Acute hemorrhage is present along the fracture line inferiorly.

   D Photomicrograph (40×) shows the "tidemark" separating the articular cartilage from the subchondral bony plate as well as the underlying cancellous bone marrow. Although portions of the marrow and cancellous bone presumably have been anoxic for 24 hours, no histologic changes suggestive of cell death or ischemic injury are present. The focal areas of appositional bone formation on the preexisting cancellous trabeculae are part of normal remodeling and are not related to the fracture or ischemia.

   (Armed Forces Institute of Pathology Neg. Nos. 66-3884, 79-5414, 79-15019, 79-15020.)

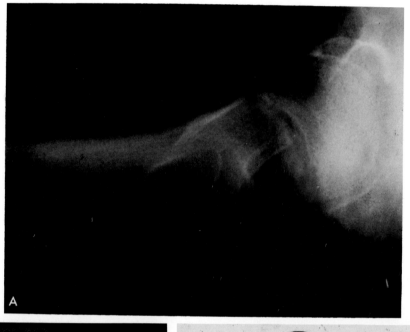

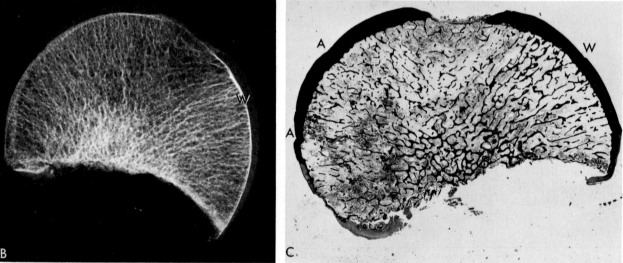

FIGURE 79–10. Fracture of the femoral neck (72 hours).

  A Clinical radiograph demonstrates a subcapital femoral neck fracture with minimal displacement of the femoral head.

  B Specimen radiograph (2.5×) of the coronally sectioned femoral head resected 72 hours after fracture reveals an intact subchondral plate and normal appearing cancellous bone. Some normal trabecular coarsening has occurred in the weight-bearing area (W) and a lucent area is present adjacent to the fovea.

  C Macroscopic section (2.5×) from the femoral head reveals an intact and normal appearing articular surface. A slight artifactual buckling (A) of the articular surface is seen inferiorly, which has resulted from processing. Although the cancellous bone appears unremarkable, extensive areas of altered marrow (slightly darker staining) are observed throughout the specimen.

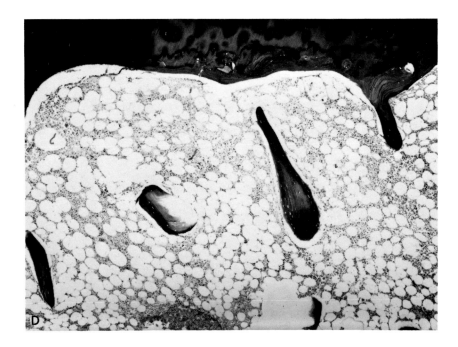

FIGURE 79–10. *Continued*

D Photomicrograph (40×) shows essentially normal appearing articular cartilage, tidemark, and subchondral plate. The ghostlike appearance of the hematopoietic and myelopoietic marrow indicates anoxic death and accounts for the altered staining characteristics in **C.** Many of the osteocytic lacunae appear empty. The marrow fat cells are essentially unchanged. The recently formed appositional bone on the surface of the cancellous bone reflects remodeling that antedates the fracture.

(Armed Forces Institute of Pathology Neg. Nos. 79-5407-1,2; 79-15017; 79-15018.)

79–12*D*). Within the immediately adjacent viable bone and marrow, evidence of increased vascularity and perivascular inflammatory cell infiltration can be identified (Fig. 79–12*C*). Radiographically, the generalized active hyperemia* in response to the injured and dying cells results in osteoporosis (mediated through osteoclastic activity) of the adjacent viable bone.

These changes are exemplified in the femoral head segment removed from a patient 2 months after a subcapital femoral neck fracture (Fig. 79–12). Considerable hemorrhage and some bone loss are seen along the fracture site (Fig. 79–12*B*). The specimen radiograph shows a small, wedge-shaped area of apparently increased bone density characterized by tightly packed but uniform-appearing cancellous bone trabeculae (Fig. 79–12*A*). The area of apparent increased radiodensity represents the zone of osteonecrosis and ischemic injury (Fig. 79–12*B–D*). The surrounding cancellous bone appears less radiodense and is characterized by considerable bone loss with focally coarsened trabeculae (Fig. 79–12*A*). The altered bone density is not appreciated easily in the histologic sections (Fig. 79–12*B,C*). The slightly opacified and spindled appearance of the marrow fat cells is characteristic of ischemically dead and injured fat tissue (Fig. 79–12*D*). The cancellous bone in the area of ischemic and dead fat is devoid of osteocytes (Fig. 79–12*D*), indicating cellular bone death. Of interest are the small tongues of cartilage below the tidemark, which are devoid of chondrocytes, indicating focal cartilage death as well (Fig. 79–12*D*). The osteonecrotic area also fails to demonstrate either osteoblastic or osteoclastic activity, which would be necessary for any radiographically

perceptible changes in bone architecture (Fig. 79–12*D*). Therefore, the radiodense-appearing wedge in the specimen radiograph is relative and does not represent a true increase in bony density (Fig. 79–12*A*). The adjacent areas of less dense bone reflect a vascular-induced bone loss analogous to the reflex vascular osteoporosis (Fig. 79–12*A*) seen in other clinical situations. Hence, it is the active hyperemia within the viable tissue surrounding the ischemic and osteonecrotic segment that results in osteoporosis and represents the first recognizable plain film radiographic alteration in osteonecrosis, the dead area remaining unchanged.

Phase III: Emergence of the Reactive Interface

Phase III is characterized morphologically by the development of a reactive interface (margin) about the osteonecrotic zone. The reactive interface begins to emerge during phase II as marrow fat cells in the ischemic zone undergo cellular alteration. Because the infarcted zone is completely avascular and the ischemic zone sufficiently anoxic, neither area is able to support osteoblasts or osteoclasts. Accordingly, initial repair must begin at the junction between the outer margin of the ischemic zone and the adjacent viable zone. The reactive interface demonstrates an increase in vascularity associated with infiltration of inflammatory cells along the outer viable margin (Fig. 79–12*C*) and with further modulation of ischemic marrow fat toward fibroblastic cells (Fig. 79–13*D–F*). During this phase, atypical-appearing ischemic fiber bone may be elaborated in the modulating fibrous tissue, or even as an appliqué on the surface of preexisting dead bone trabeculae within the ischemic zone (Figs. 79–13*E,G* and 79–14*D*). The progressive loss of mechanical support due to resorption and disruption of cancellous bone within the reactive interface stimulates compensatory reinforcement of adjacent viable cancellous bone (Fig. 79–13*D*) by osteoblastic activity. While the above

---

*Hyperemia means an excess of blood in a part. Active hyperemia refers to a rapidly flowing increased blood supply to an area. Active hyperemia in bone favors osteoclastic resorption of bone, whereas passive hyperemia (engorgement and slow flow) tends to favor osteoblastic activity.[67, 114]

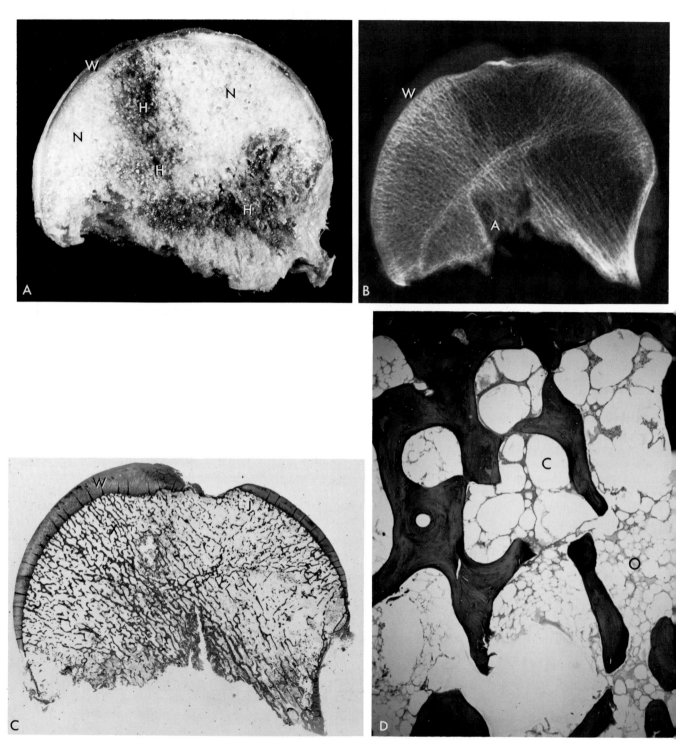

FIGURE 79–11. Fracture of the femoral neck (5 days).

A Gross photograph (2.5×) of the coronally sectioned femoral head reveals two pale, wedge-shaped avascular areas (N) surrounded in part by a darkened hyperemic zone (H). The articular surface and subchondral plate appear unremarkable.

B Specimen radiograph (2.5×) of the sectioned femoral head reveals a normal subchondral plate and underlying cancellous bony architecture. Note the weight-bearing aspect (W). The disorganized trabeculae inferiorly represent an artifact (A) of surgical removal.

C Macroscopic section (2.5×) reveals an intact articular surface, subchondral plate, and normal underlying cancellous bone with coarsening beneath the weight-bearing area (W). There is evidence of hemorrhage along the fracture line, but the remaining marrow appears unremarkable at low power.

D Photomicrograph (40×) of the subchondral area shows the tidemark, subchondral plate, and normal appearing cancellous bone. Striking lipid cyst formation (C), opacification of marrow fat cells (O), and dissolution of hematopoietic cells are seen, indicating ischemic death of all marrow elements. Occasional osteocytic lacunae appear empty.

(Armed Forces Institute of Pathology Neg. Nos. 79-15016-1, 79-5217, 79-15016-2, 79-15015.)

change slowly evolves in the reactive interface, sustained active hyperemia results in progressive osteoporosis in the remaining viable portion of the femoral head.

This sequence of change is exemplified in the femoral head of a 79 year old woman removed 3 days after "femoral neck fracture" (Fig. 79–13A). The well-developed reactive interface indicates the osteonecrotic focus dates well beyond 3 days and probably developed somewhere between 3 and 6 months ago (Fig. 79–13B–D). In this case, it is possible the active hyperemic response to the infarcted area has sufficiently weakened the viable cancellous bone in the femoral neck to the point of fracture (Fig. 79–13B). The area of slightly altered density in the clinical radiograph (Fig. 79–13A) is demonstrated more clearly in the specimen radiograph (Fig. 79–13C) and in the macroscopic section (Fig. 79–13D). The infarcted zone reveals a slightly more dense appearance than the remainder of the femoral head. This appearance is due to the vascular-induced osteoporosis (active hyperemia) within the viable areas (Fig. 79–13C). The infarcted zone is essentially unchanged histologically (Fig. 79–13D); therefore, the relatively dense appearance of this area (Fig. 79–13C) is apparent rather than real. However, the reactive interface (margin) about the infarcted zone also demonstrates a pattern of altered density on the specimen radiograph (Fig. 79–13C). The increase in density within the reactive interface is primarily a reflection of ischemic coarse-textured fiber bone formation between, and adjacent to, dead cancellous bone (Fig. 79–13E–G). The areas of decreased density within the reactive interface are due to osteoclastic activity removing injured or previously dead cancellous bone (Fig. 79–13D). This case also demonstrates evidence of extension of a previous area of ischemic necrosis (Fig. 79–13D,E). In Figure 79–13D,E, a small zone of subchondral ischemic necrosis surrounded by a fibrous reactive interface is identified (arrow). This area has been surrounded subsequently by a second zone of ischemic necrosis and a second reactive interface. The emergence of a second reactive interface outside the old infarct indicates the initial reactive area is now dead and will remain unchanged until repair progresses to that level.

Because the osteonecrotic (infarcted) segment during this phase is characterized by an apparent increase in radiographic density, the vascular-induced osteoporosis throughout the remaining portion of the femoral head also may be perceived as a faint subchondral lucent area (not a crescent sign). Perception of this change depends on the geographic pattern of the osteonecrotic segment and the orientation of the x-ray beam (X arrow, Fig. 79–13C,D), and for this reason it cannot be demonstrated in all cases. The emergence of the reactive interface within the previously ischemic zone (with focal cancellous bone resorption, minimal trabecular bone reinforcement, and deposition of ischemic fiber bone within the reactive fibrosis) accounts for the earliest alterations of radiographic density between the infarcted and viable zones.

Phase IV: Remodeling of the Reactive Interface

Phase IV is basically an extension of phase III, with continued repair and remodeling along the entire reactive interface between the viable and osteonecrotic zones. Phase IV is exemplified by a femoral head resected from a 34 year old alcoholic man (Fig. 79–14A). The increasing resorptive activity within the reactive interface also involves the compact subchondral bone wherever the reactive interface intersects with the subchondral bone plate. Therefore, not only is the cancellous bony architecture weakened along the reactive interface because of trabecular bone resorption, but similarly the subchondral bone plate is resorbed and weakened (Fig. 79–14B). Weakening of the existing stress-bearing architecture results in compensatory reinforcement of the trabecular bone in the immediately adjacent viable zone (Fig. 79–14B). The latter response is analogous to bony reinforcement about any lytic bone defect as a mechanism to route stress around nonstress-bearing areas, and it consists primarily of lamellar bone (Fig. 79–14B,D).

Progressive remodeling in the reactive interface results in an unaltered central zone of tissue death (Fig. 79–14A,B,D), surrounded by a slowly inwardly expanding lucent fibroblastic reactive interface, characterized by considerable loss of cancellous bone (Fig. 79–14B) and some ischemic fiber bone formation (Fig. 79–14C). Dystrophic mineralization (deposition of mineral, especially calcium salts, in degenerating or necrotic tissue) of dead fat within the necrotic zone adjacent to the fibrous interface (Fig. 79–14C,D) also is noted. Toward the outer margin of the reactive interface, previously dead cancellous bone may be partially invested by either ischemic fiber or viable lamellar bone (Fig. 79–14D). This area in turn is surrounded by a zone of reinforcing viable trabecular bone (Fig. 79–14B). The latter changes in the outer reactive margin represent a true increase in radiographic density. This sequence of change has classically been referred to as creeping substitution[87, 88] and more recently as creeping apposition.[46, 73]

At this stage, there is no evidence of articular buckling or collapse of the femoral head. The clinical conventional tomogram (Fig. 79–14A) reveals a zone of apparently increased density (osteonecrosis), outlined by a faint radiolucent zone (the internal advancing fibrous reactive interface), in turn surrounded by a dense hypertrophic zone (outer reinforcing reactive margin). The lucent zone represents resorptive (osteoclastic) activity, whereas the hypertrophic zone of increased density is a combination of ischemic fiber bone formation and lamellar reinforcement (osteoblastic activity) of preexisting trabecular bone (Fig. 79–14B–D).

Phase V: The Crescent Sign and Articular Collapse

The supporting bony architecture may become sufficiently weakened by continued resorption of trabecular bone and subchondral bone plate along the reactive interface that the stress of weight-bearing can result in subchondral bone plate fracture with focal articular cartilage buckling and eventual collapse. Continued stress and motion across the subchondral bone plate fracture result in progressive microfracture of the adjacent dead subchondral cancellous trabeculae. Fragmentation and compaction of subchondral bony fracture debris lead to the development of a subchondral lucent area along the fracture line, the crescent sign. This sign frequently is best seen radiographically in a frog-leg view (Fig. 79–15D). In time, flattening of the articular surface becomes apparent (Fig. 79–15A). These find-

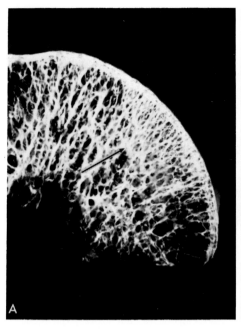

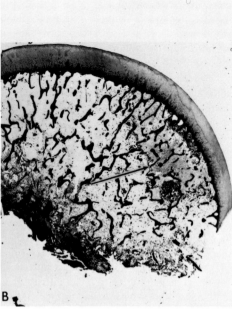

FIGURE 79–12. Fracture of the subcapital femoral neck (2 months).

A Specimen radiograph (2.5×) of the coronally sectioned femoral head segment reveals an intact subchondral bony plate supported in part by a wedge-shaped area of apparently increased radiodensity (arrow). The surrounding cancellous bone trabeculae are coarse but considerably reduced in number.

B Macroscopic section (2.5×) of **A** indicates that the wedge-shaped focus of increased density represents an area of osteonecrosis and ischemic injury (arrow). Note the relative number and size of the cancellous trabeculae in the ischemically injured and necrotic area compared with those in the surrounding osteoporotic viable bone. Considerable reactive change is present along the fracture line.

ings are exemplified by a femoral head resected from a 62 year old man because of persistent hip pain of 9 months' duration (Fig. 79–15A–C). The altered density and early flattening of the femoral head seen in the clinical radiograph (Fig. 79–15A) are better demonstrated in the specimen radiograph (Fig. 79–15B) and macroscopic section (Fig. 79–15C) as subchondral fracture and early articular collapse. The subchondral fracture and reactive interface are perceived only faintly in the standard clinical anteroposterior radiographic view of the hip (Fig. 79–15A). The primary area of collapse in this case appears just superior to the fovea centralis, about which there has been considerable resorption. The lateral extent of the reactive interface is considerably peripheral to the buckled subchondral bone plate. The remaining portion of the femoral head shows the unaltered density of the osteonecrotic zone (Fig. 79–15B,C) and the reactive interface (Fig. 79–15C).

Thus, phase V is characterized primarily by radiographic evidence of early articular flattening (collapse) and subchondral fracture. Recognition of the crescent sign (Fig. 79–15D) as a radiographic indication of infarction and subarticular collapse is important, and this finding must not be confused with the faint subchondral lucent area that occasionally may be seen in the femoral head during the early stage of phase III (X arrow, Fig. 79–13C,D). Once phase V of osteonecrosis is reached, the articular buckling and collapse will be appreciable grossly as an incongruous articular surface that eventually will result in the superimposed degenerative arthritic change.

THE TYPICAL CASE OF ISCHEMIC NECROSIS

Geographic Variation in the Host Response

The cases described previously were selected specifically to illustrate the sequence of histologic and plain film radiographic alterations in the femoral head resulting from the host response to osteonecrosis. In most cases of ischemic necrosis, the host response is not uniform throughout the

involved area; this is true especially in the femoral head. A detailed analysis of a single resected femoral head will be used as an example. The patient, an otherwise healthy 34 year old man, complained of increasing hip pain (Figs. 79–16 to 79–20). The clinical radiograph (Fig. 79–16A) is characterized by a large area of apparent increased radiographic density with some marginal lucency and peripheral reinforcement. A subchondral fracture (the crescent sign) indicates articular buckling and collapse (Fig. 79–16A). The resected femoral head reveals severe buckling of the articular surface with partial collapse anteriorly (Fig. 79–16B). The femoral head was sectioned coronally at four levels (Fig. 79–16C), providing an opportunity to compare the plain, conventional tomographic, and specimen radiographs with the gross appearance, macroscopic sections, and appropriate high power microscopic views illustrating each of the four successive levels (Figs. 79–17 to 79–20).

The sections (Figs. 79–17 to 79–20) portray the full medial and lateral pathologic and radiographic orientation of the osteonecrotic area and the response at each successive level, from the most posterior (Fig. 79–17) to the most anterior level (Fig. 79–20) of involvement.

The most posterior femoral head section (Fig. 79–17) reflects primarily phase III and phase IV morphologic changes. The gross photograph (Fig. 79–17B), the specimen radiograph (Fig. 79–17C), and the macroscopic section (Fig. 79–17D) reveal an intact articular surface and a normal spherical configuration of the femoral head. The slightly opacified area in Figure 79–17B represents the zone of osteonecrosis and is reflected in the specimen radiograph (Fig. 79–17C) as a broad area of increased radiodensity with focal lucent shadows. These lucent areas represent sites of osteoclastic resorption of trabecular bone within the fibrous reactive interface and can be appreciated in the macroscopic and high power microscopic views (Fig. 79–17D–H). The macroscopic section (Fig. 79–17D) indicates the increased radiodensity is due to three factors: a relatively increased density of the osteonecrotic zone because of an extensive vascular-induced osteoporosis in the surrounding viable areas of the femoral head; bone formation

Text continued on page 3476

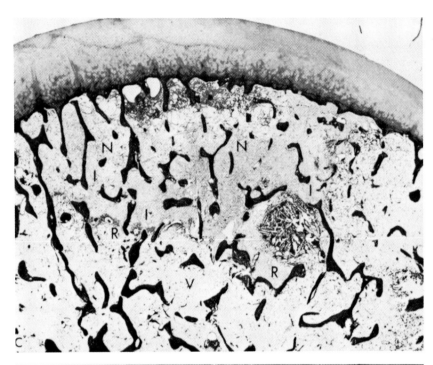

FIGURE 79–12. *Continued*

  C Photomicrograph (8×) reveals an intact articular surface and subchondral plate. Immediately beneath the subchondral plate is an area of necrosis characterized by dissolution of marrow cellular architecture, giving the appearance of basophilic debris (N). The necrotic area is surrounded by a broad area of dead and ischemically injured marrow fat (I). The hemorrhagic cyst is filled with cholesterol crystals from the breakdown of fat cells. Vascular dilation can be seen along the reactive margin (R) between the ischemically injured fat (I) and surrounding viable marrow (V).

  D Photomicrographic view (40×) demonstrates the crystalline appearance of ischemically dead marrow fat cells and spindling of the ischemically injured marrow fat cells. The lower portion of the articular surface above the tidemark is unremarkable. The subchondral plate and underlying cancellous bone, although intact architecturally, are devoid of osteocytic nuclei, indicating bone death. Even the cartilage below the tidemark is devoid of viable cells.

  (Armed Forces Institute of Pathology Neg. Nos. 79-5419, 79-15008, 79-15009, 79-15010.)

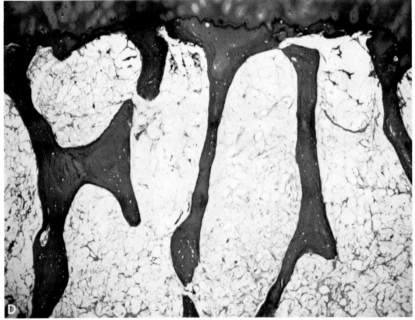

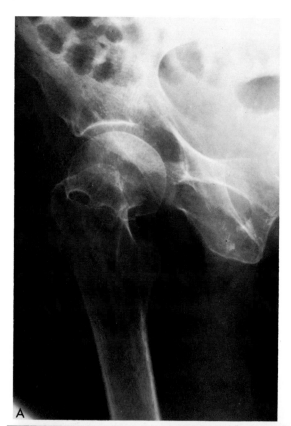

FIGURE 79–13. Fracture of the femoral neck (72 hours with ischemic necrosis of 3 to 6 months' duration).

A Clinical radiograph of a femoral neck fracture that occurred clinically 3 days prior to resection. A slight increase in subchondral bone density beneath the weight-bearing area is seen. The degree of relative osteoporosis above the fracture margin indicates an active process older than 3 days.

B Gross photograph (2.5×) of the coronally sectioned femoral head reveals an opacified area of ischemic necrosis (N). The opacified necrotic area is marginated by a rim of pale reactive tissue (R). The overlying articular surface and subchondral bone are unremarkable. Most of the remaining viable portion of the femoral head (V) has a hyperemic appearance (H). Note the weight-bearing aspect (W).

C Specimen radiograph (2.5×) of the sectioned femoral head reveals an area of subchondral radiodensity beneath the weight-bearing area (W), which corresponds to the area of ischemic necrosis (N). The osteonecrotic segment is surrounded by a faintly perceived reactive margin of variable but focally increased density (R). The remaining viable portion of the femoral head is radiolucent (V) compared with the ischemic area (N). The articular surface and subchondral plate appear intact.

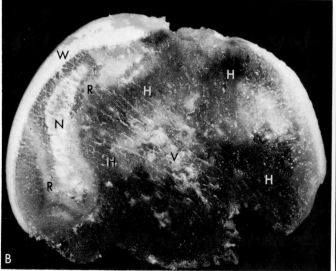

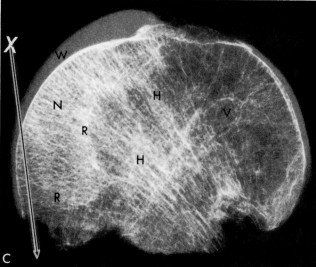

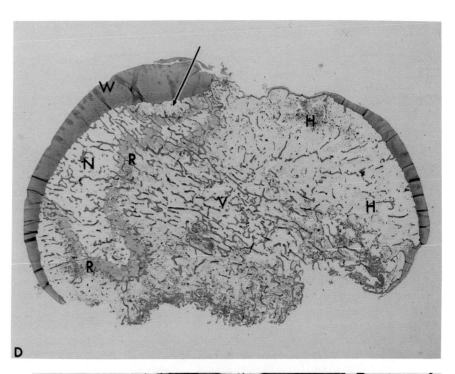

FIGURE 79–13. *Continued*

D Macroscopic section (2.5×, hematoxylin and eosin stain) reveals the area of apparently increased subchondral radiographic density to reflect the unaltered area of ischemic necrosis (N). The subchondral osteonecrotic bone and marrow are surrounded by and separated from the remaining viable portions of the femoral head by a reactive margin of fibrous marrow (reactive interface) (R). Within the reactive interface some osteoclastic resorption of existing cancellous trabeculae and deposition of ischemic fiber bone have occurred. A small focus of previous ischemic necrosis is present immediately superior to the foveal groove, surrounded by a fibrous reactive interface (arrow), subsequently encompassed by a more extensive zone of necrosis. The remaining viable portion of the femoral head (V) shows considerable reactive hyperemia.

E Photomicrograph (8×) of the small subchondral area of previous ischemic necrosis (N1) and reactive margin (R1) surrounded by a second zone of necrosis (N2) and reactive margin (R2) (seen in **D**) indicates extension of a repairing focus of ischemic necrosis.

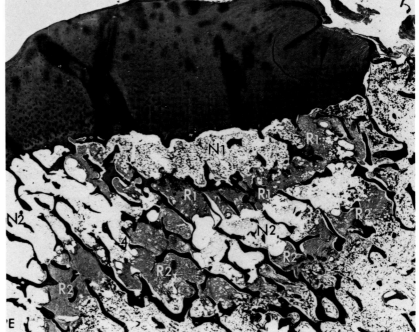

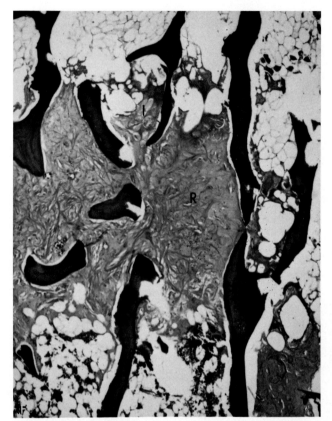 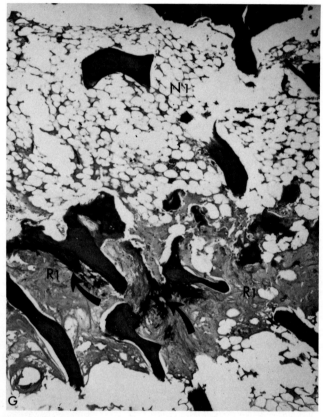

FIGURE 79–13. *Continued*

  F Photomicrograph (40×) of the reactive interface (R) demonstrates the hyalinized appearance of the fibrous modulation of ischemically injured marrow (I).

  G Photomicrograph (40×) of the original area of ischemic necrosis, showing the dead marrow elements and bone (N1) and initial reactive interface (R1) characterized by ischemic fibrous modulation of marrow elements and the formation of atypical ischemic fiber bone between and on the surface of dead cancellous trabeculae (curved arrows). The latter accounts for some of the focal, faintly perceived increase in density along the entire reactive interface in **C.**

  (Armed Forces Institute of Pathology Neg. Nos. 75-10099, 79-15011, 79-15411, 79-15012, 79-15013, 79-1514-1,2.)

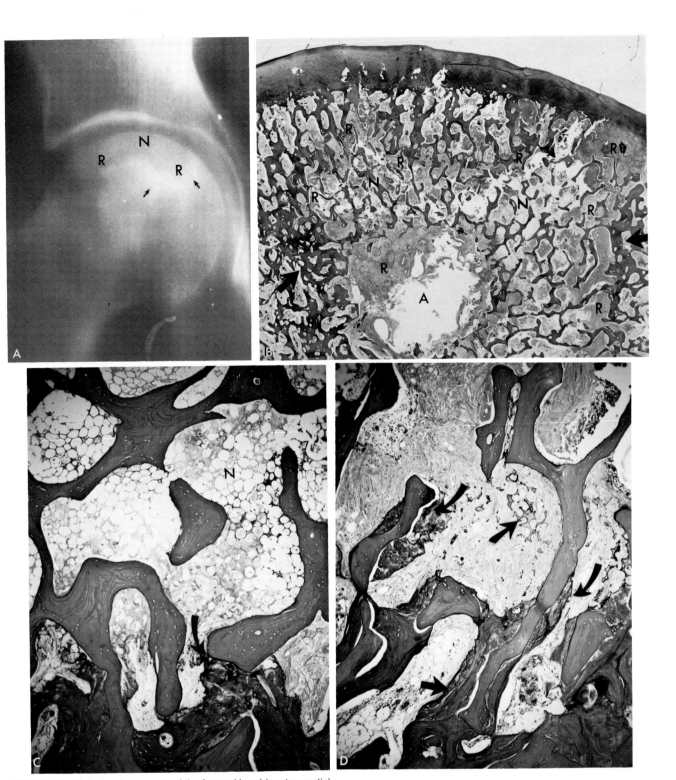

FIGURE 79–14. Ischemic necrosis of the femoral head (nontraumatic).

A Clinical conventional tomographic view demonstrates a spherical femoral head with an unaltered zone of osteonecrosis (N) surrounded by a faint radiolucent margin (R), encompassed by a broadened rim of radiographic density (arrows). The remaining portion of the femoral head and neck shows varying amounts of radiolucency.

B Photomicrograph (8×) of the articular surface and subchondral bone indicates that the radiolucent area is characterized by a broad reactive fibrous interface, within which the bulk of the cancellous bone has been, or is being, resorbed (R). The clear area represents an artifact (A) of tissue processing. The unchanged cancellous bone immediately superior and to the right of the large fibrous defect represents ischemic necrosis (N). The area of necrosis also demonstrates reactive fibrous tissue creeping in from the outer margin (R). There is considerable resorption of the subchondral bony plate where it intersects with the reactive interface (R2 arrow). Bony reinforcement of the adjacent viable trabecular bone (straight arrows) is noted (see Fig. 79–17).

C Photomicrograph (40×) of the osteonecrotic zone and adjacent reactive interface. Note the dead cancellous bone devoid of osteocytic nuclei and dead marrow fat with its ghostlike appearance (N). Considerable ischemic bone formation (curved arrow) is seen as an appliqué on previously dead cancellous bone trabeculae.

D Photomicrograph (40×) of the reactive interface is characterized by the spindled fibrous appearance of the marrow, within which ischemic fiber bone formation (curved arrows) and dystrophic mineralization (tapered arrow) can be identified. Many of the preexisting dead cancellous trabeculae within the reactive interface have been invested by an appliqué of both ischemic (curved arrows) and lamellar (straight arrow) bone. This pattern reflects a receding margin of an infarct.

(Armed Forces Institute of Pathology Neg. Nos. 71-1553-3; 79-15005; 70-15006-1,2.)

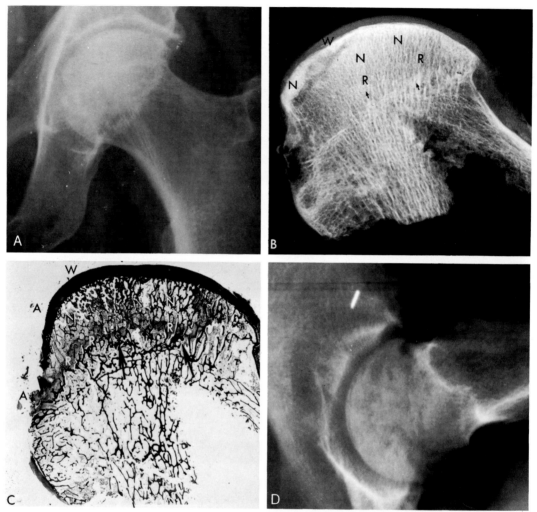

FIGURE 79–15. Ischemic necrosis of the femoral head with subchondral fracture (crescent sign) and early articular buckling.

A Clinical radiograph reveals a slightly dense femoral head with flattening and incongruity of the weight-bearing articular surface.

B Specimen radiograph (2.5×) of the coronally sectioned femoral head shows subarticular bony plate fracture both inferior and superior to the fovea. This has resulted in a subchondral fracture (crescent sign) below the weight-bearing area (see **D**). The cancellous bone immediately subjacent to the fovea shows considerable radiolucency, indicating resorption. The osteonecrotic bone (W) above the subchondral fracture is dense owing to compacted fracture debris. The remaining osteonecrotic subchondral bone demonstrates faint, relatively increased density surrounded by a poorly defined lucent area (R). An equally faint radiodense zone of bony reinforcement (arrows) is noted (see **D**).

C Macroscopic section (2.5×) of the femoral head demonstrates the buckled subchondral plate and subchondral fracture (crescent sign) in the weight-bearing area (W). The subchondral fracture extends from the fovea superiorly to the weight-bearing zone but does not reach the lateral extent of the ischemic segment. The appearance of the subchondral fracture is obscured by a partial artifactual collapse and loss of articular surface about the fovea. Much of the subchondral fracture debris also has been lost in processing. The remaining femoral head is characterized by the unaltered osteonecrotic zone (N), reactive interface that extends to the inferior aspect of the fovea (R), and outer reinforcing bony margin (arrows). The latter microscopic density patterns correlate well with the specimen radiographic appearance in **B**.

D Frog-leg radiographic view from another patient demonstrates the crescent sign, relatively dense necrotic zone, lucent reactive interface, and reinforcing margin in much greater detail.

(Armed Forces Institute of Pathology Neg. Nos. 66-3834-2, 79-5416, 79-14989, 79-5947.)

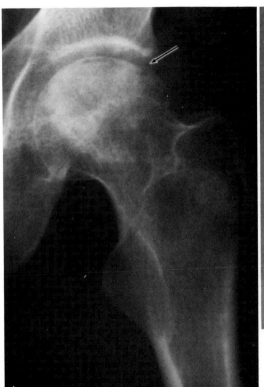

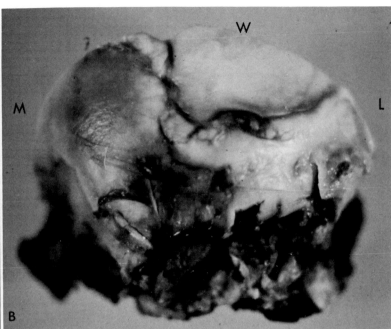

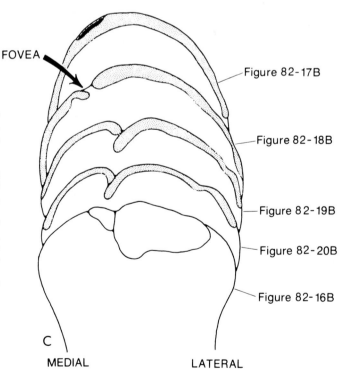

FIGURE 79–16. Typical case of ischemic necrosis.

A Clinical radiograph reveals a broad area of real and apparently increased density involving the anterolateral weight-bearing segment of the femoral head. The crescent sign indicating subchondral fracture is present. Although the joint space appears normal, evidence of articular buckling (arrow) is present.

B Gross photograph (2.5×) of the resected femoral head viewed anteriorly demonstrates severe buckling and collapse of the weight-bearing (W) articular surface. Medial (M) and lateral (L) orientation is noted.

C Schematic drawing indicating the level of each of the four coronal femoral head sections given in Figures 79–17 to 79–20. The most posterior (Fig. 79–17) and most anterior (Fig. 79–20) coronal sections are separated by the intermediate coronal sections (Figs. 79–18 and 79–19).

(Armed Forces Institute of Pathology Neg. Nos. 69-7151-7, 79-14976.)

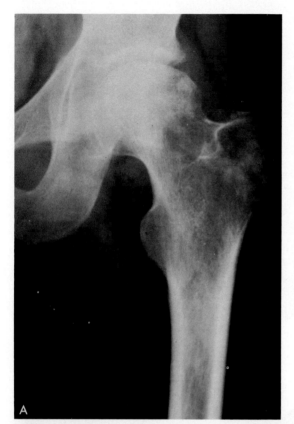

FIGURE 79–17. Posterior coronal section of the femoral head (see Fig. 79–16C).

A Radiograph of the femoral head demonstrating both real and apparent increase in density with some faint peripheral lucency. Articular buckling is noted laterally. (Armed Forces Institute of Pathology Neg. No. 71-10417-1.)

B Gross photograph (2.5×) of posterior level of the coronally sectioned femoral head shows a normal articular surface and spherical configuration. The central osteonecrotic zone (N) appears slightly opacified and is surrounded by a faintly perceived hyperemic margin (R) encompassed by a pale rim (arrows). Note the medial (M), lateral (L), and weight-bearing (W) aspects. (Armed Forces Institute of Pathology Neg. No. 79-14976.)

C Radiograph (2.5×) of the gross specimen in **B** reveals an intact subchondral plate. The central necrotic zone (N) reflects an apparent increase in density surrounded by a faint lucent zone (most pronounced inferiorly) (R) and a rim of increased density (arrows). The remainder of the femoral head appears osteoporotic as a result of active hyperemia (V). (Armed Forces Institute of Pathology Neg. No. 79-5409.)

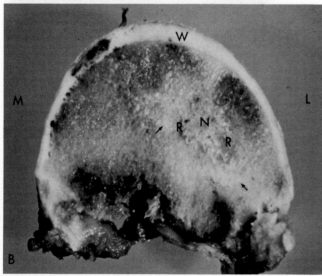

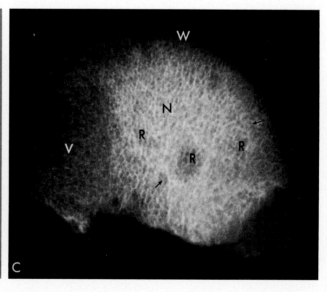

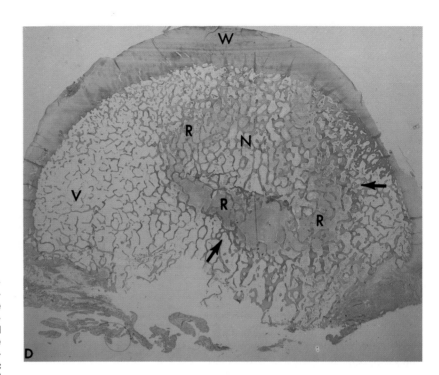

FIGURE 79–17. *Continued*

D Macroscopic section of **B** reflects the essentially normal articular surface and subchondral plate. The central necrotic cancellous bone (N) appears unaltered and is framed by the reactive fibrous interface (R) and a peripheral margin of bony reinforcement (arrows). The thinned cancellous trabeculae in the nonstress-bearing areas have resulted from osteoclastic stimulation by active hyperemia (V). (Armed Forces Institute of Pathology Neg. No. 79-14970.)

E Photomicrograph (8×) demonstrates the unaltered central necrotic cancellous bone (N) surrounded by the fibrous reactive interface (R), in turn surrounded by a compensatory rim of reinforced trabecular bone (arrows). Note the fairly extensive loss of cancellous trabeculae within the reactive interface. (Armed Forces Institute of Pathology Neg. No. 79-14983.)

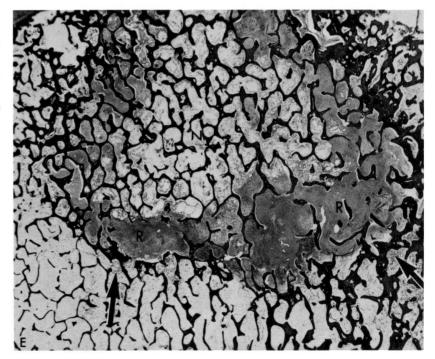

Illustration continued on following page

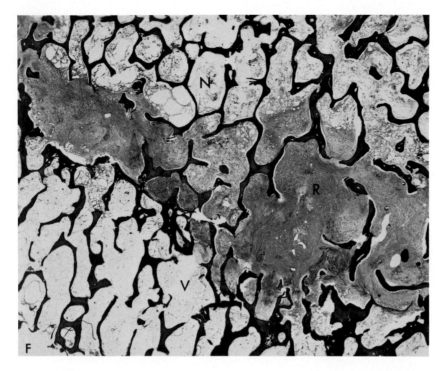

FIGURE 79–17. *Continued*
F Photomicrograph (18×) of the reactive interface (R) separating the central necrotic zone (N) from the surrounding viable tissue (V). Note the loss of cancellous bone and replacement by fibrous tissue. (Armed Forces Institute of Pathology Neg. No. 79-14984.)

(Fig. 79–18) and dystrophic mineralization (Fig. 79–18*F*) accounting for a small but real increase in density within the reactive interface; and the extensive loss of normal trabecular bone resulting from osteoclastic activity within the reactive interface, which is compensated for by reinforcement of the adjacent viable or revitalized trabecular bone along the outer margin of the reactive interface. The loss of stress-bearing capacity due to resorption of the cancellous trabeculae within the fibrous reactive interface (Figs. 79–17*D–H* and 79–18*G*) is accommodated by the adjacent intact trabecular bone. The increased mechanical stress applied to these trabeculae stimulates osteoblastic bony reinforcement primarily by lamellar bone (Figs. 79–17*E,F* and 79–18*H*). Because osteoblastic activity is possible only in areas of bone viability, the bony reinforcement occurs predominantly along the outer margin of the reactive interface and tends to be juxtaposed to areas of maximum bone loss (Figs. 79–17*D–G;* 79–18*D,G,H;* 79–19*D,F;* 79–20*D*).

The next coronal section (Fig. 79–18) is slightly anterior to the section demonstrated in Figure 79–17 (see Fig. 79–16*C*). The clinical conventional tomographic view demonstrates a central dense area surrounded by a lucent zone, which in turn is surrounded by another margin of increased density (Fig. 79–18*A*). This also is seen in the specimen radiograph (Fig. 79–18*C*), gross photograph (Fig. 79–18*B*), and macroscopic section (Fig. 79–18*D*). It is obvious from the specimen radiograph that the excessive vascular-induced osteoporosis of the viable areas accounts for the relatively increased density of an essentially unchanged central necrotic zone (Fig. 79–18*B,D,E*). Excessive bone resorption within the reactive interface (Fig. 79–18*G*), especially along the medial and lateral sides, has weakened the supportive bony architecture and has resulted in microfracture of the subchondral bone plate, with early articular buckling and collapse and subchondral trabecular fracture (Fig. 79–18*B–D*). The latter occurrence produces the clas-

sic crescent sign, well shown in the gross specimen, specimen radiograph, and macroscopic section (Fig. 79–18*B–D*). The pattern of marginal lamellar bone reinforcement (Fig. 79–18*G,H*) around the extent of the broadened reactive fibrous interface (Fig. 79–18*D*) is best appreciated in this level of the specimen (Fig. 79–18*C*). The dense area produced by dystrophic mineralization, entrapped by the slowly advancing fibrous interface (Fig. 79–18*F*), is negligible radiographically at this phase of repair.

The next slightly more anterior coronal section (Figs. 79–16*C*, 79–19) demonstrates extensive resorption within the reactive interface, especially beneath the fovea, resulting in collapse of the articular surface into the substance of the femoral head. At this level (Fig. 79–19*A–E*), the subchondral fracture (crescent sign) is seen to extend from the lateral to the medial area of articular collapse (Fig. 79–19*C*). This zone of extensive resorption within the reactive interface is marginated by a dense reinforced bony rim. The changes in the clinical conventional tomographic view are corroborated in the gross photograph, specimen radiograph, and macroscopic section at a comparable level (Fig. 79–19*A–D*).

In the lateral area of subchondral collapse and weakening, cartilage metaplasia along the fracture line indicates motion (Fig. 79–19*F*). With loss of the subchondral bone plate, articular cartilage proliferation and enchondral bone formation of the overlying articular surface may be seen (Fig. 79–19*F*). Repeated observations in numerous cases of ischemic necrosis indicate one end of the subchondral fracture almost always is in continuity with an area of subarticular bone plate buckling or partial collapse. This location favors the occurrence of subarticular bone plate disruption as a prior event to subchondral fracture. Continued motion across an area of subarticular bone plate fracture likely results eventually in extension of the fracture line into a subchondral location. The immediately peripheral reinforcing bony margin forming in response to the resorbing reac-

Text continued on page 3483

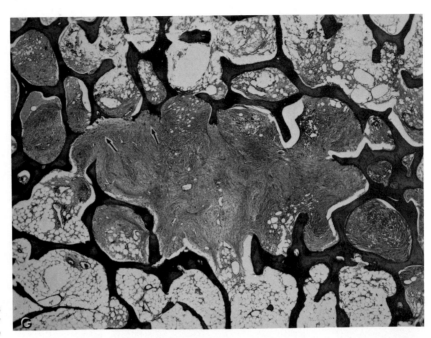

FIGURE 79–17. *Continued*

G Photomicrograph (28×) showing the fibrous reactive interface. Witness the numerous Howship's lacunae and active osteoclastic bony resorption within the reactive fibrous interface (arrows). (Armed Forces Institute of Pathology Neg. No. 79-14986.)

H Photomicrograph (40×) shows active osteoclasts tunneling out a cancellous trabecula within an otherwise moderately cellular reactive fibrous interface. (Armed Forces Institute of Pathology Neg. No. 79-14981.)

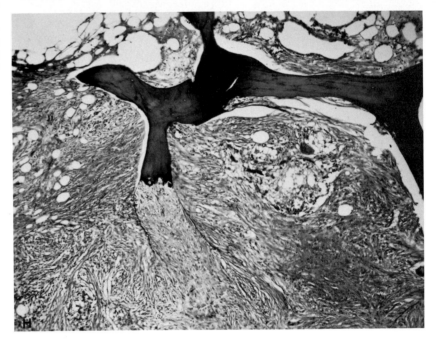

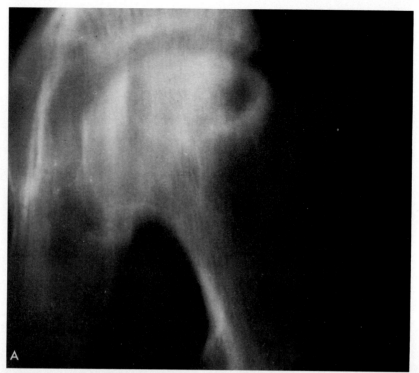

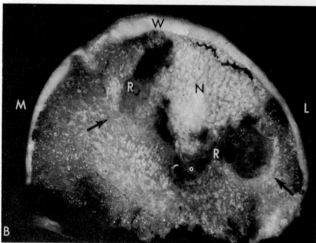

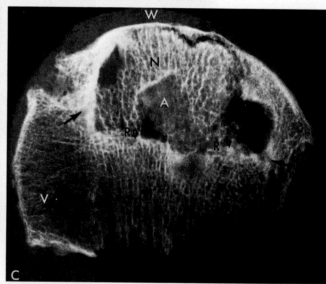

FIGURE 79–18. Posterior intermediate coronal section of the femoral head (see Fig. 79–16C).

A Clinical conventional tomographic view reveals this level of the femoral head to be characterized by a central core of apparently increased density, surrounded by an enlarging radiolucent zone encompassed by a rim of increased density of varying degrees. Note the radiolucent appearance of the inferior medial portion of the femoral head. (Armed Forces Institute of Pathology Neg. No. 71-10417-2.)

B Gross photograph (2.5×) of the femoral head sectioned at approximately the same level and showing the same medial (M), lateral (L), and weight-bearing (W) aspects as the clinical conventional tomogram **(A).** Slight articular buckling is seen over the pale, opacified, wedge-shaped area of osteonecrosis (N), just above the subchondral fracture. Note the clearly defined hyperemic reactive margin (R) about the infarcted area. The sclerotic margin is difficult to perceive in the gross specimen (arrows). (Armed Forces Institute of Pathology Neg. No. 79-14976.)

C Specimen radiograph (2.5×) of the gross section reveals the relatively increased density of the unaltered osteonecrotic segment (N). The central lytic defect is an artifact (A) of surgical removal. The subchondral fracture extends laterally to the extensively resorbed area of the reactive interface. The lucent reactive interface (R1 arrow) corresponds to the hyperemic areas grossly. The peripheral bony reinforcement about the resorptive margin is well defined (straight arrows). Note the radiolucent areas of reflex vascular osteoporosis (V). (Armed Forces Institute of Pathology Neg. No. 79-5409.)

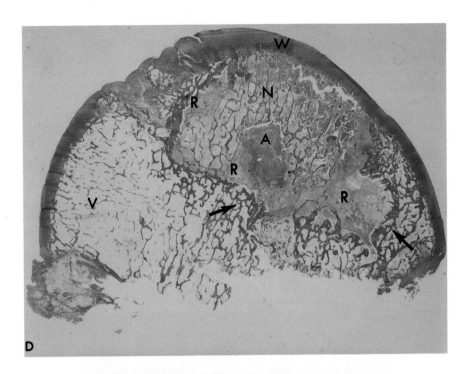

FIGURE 79–18. *Continued*

D Macrosection (2.5×, hematoxylin and eosin stain) of the gross section **(B)** shows the unaltered cancellous bone in the osteonecrotic zone (N), extensive cancellous bone loss within the reactive fibrous interface (R), and marginal bony reinforcement (arrows). These findings correlate well with the radiographic appearance. Note the thinned cancellous trabeculae in the inferior medial portion of the femoral head (V). (Armed Forces Institute of Pathology Neg. No. 79-14973.)

E Photomicrograph (40×) of the osteonecrotic zone, characterized by the unchanged cancellous bone and marrow necrosis. Note the infiltrating margin of revascularized fibrous tissue (R). (Armed Forces Institute of Pathology Neg. No. 79-14980.)

Illustration continued on following page

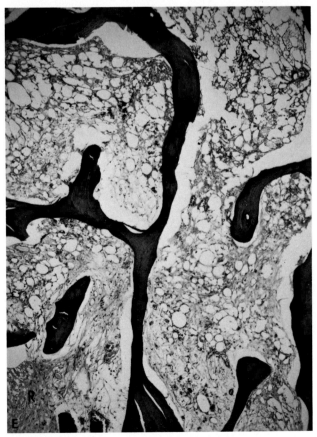

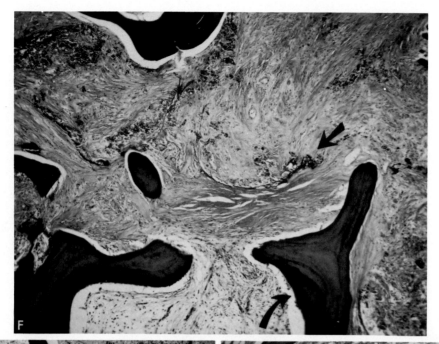

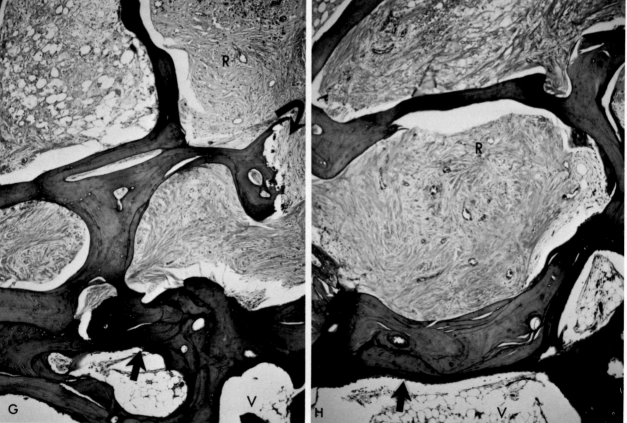

FIGURE 79–18. *Continued*

F Photomicrograph (40×) of the fibrous reactive interface shows dystrophic mineralization (tapered arrow) and trabecular reinforcement (curved arrow). (Armed Forces Institute of Pathology Neg. No. 79-14985.)

G Photomicrograph (40×) of the reactive margin shows active osteoclastic resorption of cancellous bone (curved arrow) within the fibrous portion of the reactive interface (R) and lamellar reinforcement of trabecular bone (straight arrow) in the immediately adjacent viable zone (V).

H Photomicrograph (40×) of the reactive margin. Note the lamellar pattern of trabecular bone reinforcement by osteoblasts (straight arrow) separating the fibrous portion of the reactive interface (R) from the adjacent viable marrow (V). (Armed Forces Institute of Pathology Neg. No. 79-14978.)

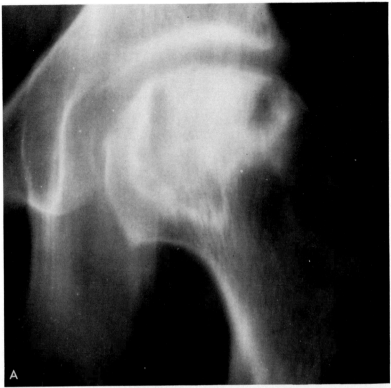

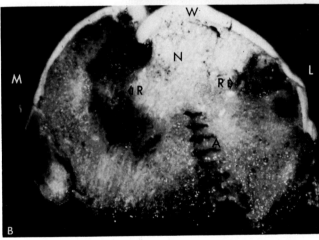

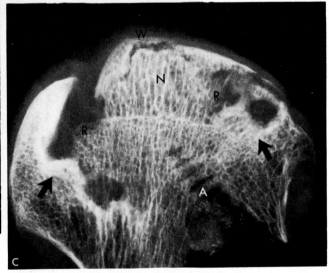

FIGURE 79–19. Anterior intermediate coronal section of the femoral head (see Fig. 79–16C).

A Clinical conventional tomogram demonstrating flattening of the femoral head. Note the reduced central area of relatively increased density and expansion of the lucent reactive margin, especially medially. The peripheral margin of increased density is well defined, but it is most prominent medially. Because of articular flattening, the subchondral fracture is difficult to see. (Armed Forces Institute of Pathology Neg. No. 79-10417-4.)

B Gross photograph (2.5×) of the femoral head sectioned at approximately the same level and showing medial (M), lateral (L), and weight-bearing (W) aspects as in the clinical conventional tomogram **(A).** The most striking feature is the extent of articular collapse into the medial reactive margin (R1 arrow). Subchondral fracture is apparent through the pale osteonecrotic zone (N). Note the articular buckling and resorbed subchondral plate over the lateral reactive margin (R2 arrow). Disregard the artifactual distortion induced during removal (A). (Armed Forces Institute of Pathology Neg. No. 79-14976.)

C Specimen radiograph of the gross section demonstrates extensive bone loss in both the medial and lateral reactive margins (R), which accounts for the articular collapse and buckling, respectively. The subchondral fracture through the unaltered, but relatively dense, osteonecrotic segment (N) extends to both the medial and the lateral resorptive margins. Note the rim of markedly increased density (arrows) peripheral to the resorptive margins, especially along the medial margin. W, Weight-bearing aspect; A, artifact. (Armed Forces Institute of Pathology Neg. No. 79-5409.)

Illustration continued on following page

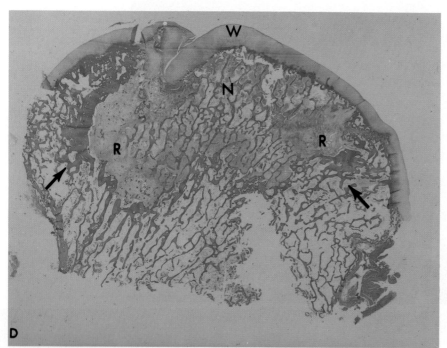

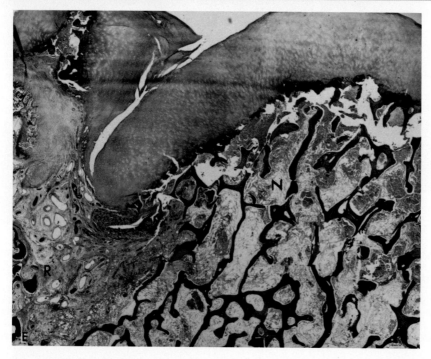

FIGURE 79–19. *Continued*

  D Macroscopic section (2.5×, hematoxylin and eosin stain) of the gross specimen in **B** indicates that articular collapse and buckling have occurred over areas of extensive bone loss within the fibrous reactive interface (R). The subchondral fracture through the unaltered cancellous bone of the osteonecrotic segment (N) extends from the medial to the lateral resorptive margins. Bony reinforcement (arrows) about the reactive interface is especially marked medially and accounts for the peripheral margin of increased density. (Armed Forces Institute of Pathology Neg. No. 79-14972.)

  E Photomicrograph (8×) demonstrates the area of medial articular collapse into the substance of the femoral head. Note the subchondral fracture, unaltered cancellous bone in the necrotic zone (N), and fibrovascular appearance of the resorbed area (reactive interface) (R). (Armed Forces Institute of Pathology Neg. No. 79-14977-1.)

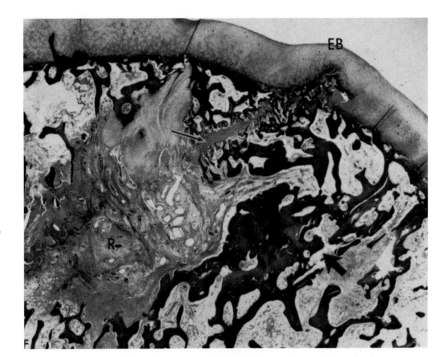

FIGURE 79–19. *Continued*

F Photomicrograph (8×) demonstrates the lateral area of the subchondral plate fracture and articular buckling over the fibrovascular appearing reactive interface (R). The linear area of cartilage metaplasia (thin arrow) along the fracture line extends into an area of endochondral new bone formation within the articular surface (EB). Note the marked bony reinforcement peripheral to the resorptive margin (heavy arrow). (Armed Forces Institute of Pathology Neg. No. 79-14977-2.)

tive interface is sufficiently thick that any extension of the subchondral fracture usually is directed through the dead cancellous bone toward another area of articular collapse (Fig. 79–19*C,D*).

The most anterior coronal section (Fig. 79–16*C*) reveals an extensive area of bone loss (resorption) surrounded by a sclerotic bony margin and complicated by articular collapse and fracture through the osteonecrotic segment (Fig. 79–20). These changes are amplified in the clinical conventional tomographic view (Fig. 79–20*A*) and specimen radiograph (Fig. 79–20*C*). The medial sclerotic margin represents a rim of marked bony reinforcement within the viable portion of the femoral head (Fig. 79–20*D*). The broad zone of bone loss has been replaced by an area of reactive fibrosis. A significant portion of the articular surface and osteonecrotic segment has collapsed (Fig. 79–20*B,D*) into the resorbed (bone-depleted) fibrous area. The degree of articular collapse has resulted in considerable flattening and buckling of the anterolateral portion of the femoral head. This change is best seen in the gross specimen (Figs. 79–16*B*, 79–20*B*).

The radiographic and pathologic features revealed in this sequence of coronal sections from the same femoral head demonstrate the general morphology of ischemic necrosis and underscore the inequality of host response from area to area in the same bone. In this case no morphologic evidence was present to suggest secondary extension of the infarct as an explanation for the variation in host response. It seems likely the availability of a functional circulation is a major factor modifying the repair process. Although the features of this case may be somewhat exaggerated, similar findings usually are seen in most cases of ischemic necrosis examined in this fashion. In this single case of ischemic necrosis, we find both histologic and radiographic evidence of a host response ranging from phase III through late stages of phase V.

LATE COMPLICATIONS OF ISCHEMIC NECROSIS

Fragmentation of the Osteonecrotic Segment

The case illustrated in Figures 79–16 to 79–20 demonstrates fairly extensive resorption and fibrous replacement within the reactive interface. These changes can be so excessive that infraction (i.e., incomplete fracture of bone without displacement of the fragments) may occur along the reactive interface in addition to, or in place of, the more typical subchondral fracture. Therefore, it is possible for either a part or the entire portion of an osteonecrotic segment to become fragmented or functionally separated from the underlying viable area of the femoral head. These changes are exemplified by a femoral head resected from a 44 year old man with a 3 year history of hip pain (Fig. 79–21). The alternating areas of radiolucency and radiodensity in association with flattening of the femoral head in the clinical radiograph (Fig. 79–21*A*) also are seen in the specimen radiograph (Fig. 79–21*B*) and macroscopic section (Fig. 79–21*C*). The prominent bony reinforcement along the outer viable margin of the reactive interface (Fig. 79–21*B,C*) indicates considerable bone loss and fibrous replacement within the reactive interface. This has resulted in an infraction along the entire reactive interface with secondary fractures through the otherwise essentially unaltered osteonecrotic area (Fig. 79–21*B,C*). The resultant motion along the infracted interface has given rise to chondroid metaplasia (Fig. 79–21*D*) similar to that seen in a pseudarthrosis.[181]

Although the femoral head remains intact, partial microscopic fragmentation of the osteonecrotic segment forming bony debris can resemble that seen in a subchondral fracture exposed to continuous motion. Should the articular cartilage surface tear, some of the debris could escape into the joint. This type of change may account for abnormali-

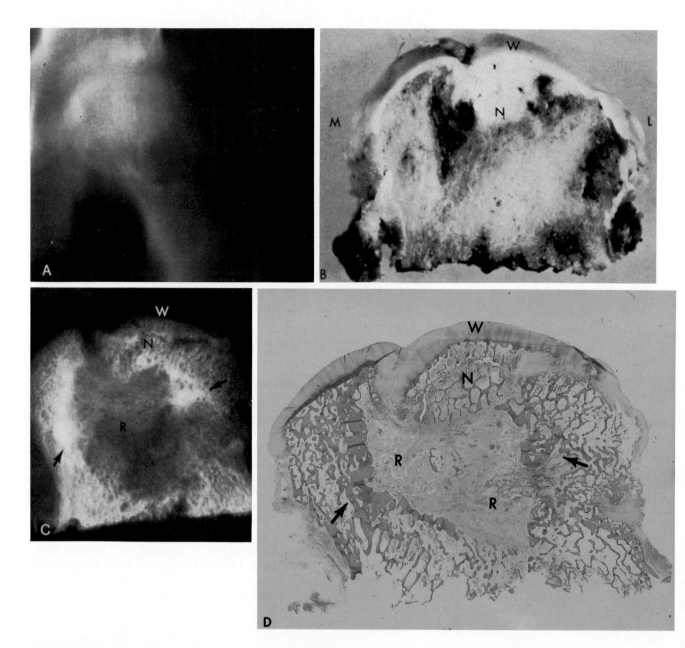

FIGURE 79–20. Anterior coronal section of the femoral head (see Fig. 79–16C).

A Clinical conventional tomographic view reveals the anterior portion of the femoral head to be markedly distorted with areas of both increased and decreased density. The lucent hole in the upper femoral neck below the synovial reflection represents an unusually large area of fibrovascular ingrowth from the periarticular tissues; presumably it is a part of the reparative response. (Armed Forces Institute of Pathology Neg. No. 69-7151-6.)

B Gross photograph (2.5×) of the femoral head sectioned at approximately the same level and showing the same medial (M), lateral (L), and weight-bearing (W) aspects as the clinical conventional tomogram. Marked flattening of the femoral head with articular buckling and collapse is seen. The pale osteonecrotic segment (N) is reduced in size and rimmed by a hyperemic margin. (Armed Forces Institute of Pathology Neg. No. 79-14976.)

C Specimen radiograph (2.5×) reflects the gross distortion and shows extensive bone loss (R) partially surrounded by a sclerotic margin (arrows). The osteonecrotic segment is small and of essentially normal density (N). (Armed Forces Institute of Pathology Neg. No. 79-5409.)

D Macroscopic section (2.5×, hematoxylin and eosin stain) of the gross specimen in **B** demonstrates articular collapse into a large fibrovascular defect. The osteonecrotic zone (N) is reduced in size. The fibrous defect is an extension of the fibrous reactive interface (R) and is enveloped partially by a margin of bony reinforcement (arrows). (Armed Forces Institute of Pathology Neg. No. 79-14971.)

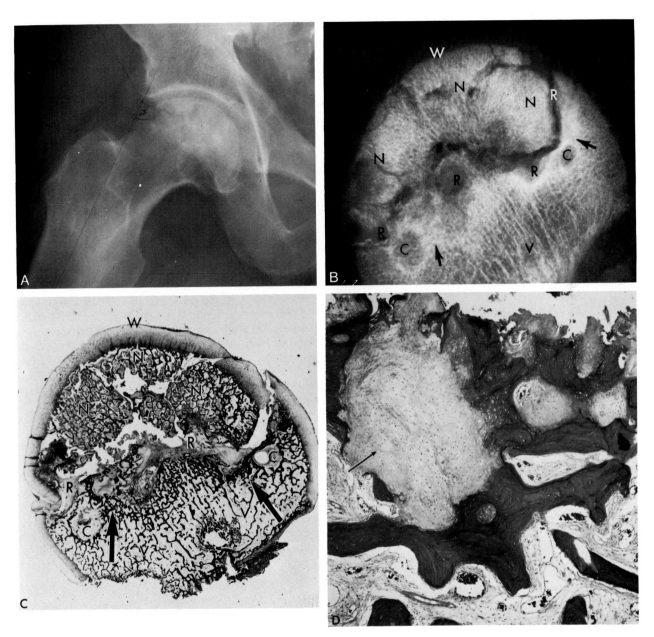

FIGURE 79–21. Ischemic necrosis with fragmentation.

  A Clinical radiograph shows flattening and deformity of the femoral head without evidence of narrowing of the joint space. The altered density patterns indicate infraction through the osteonecrotic segment.

  B Specimen radiograph (2.5×) of the coronally sectioned femoral head reveals the unaltered density of the multiple infracted osteonecrotic segments (N). Marked bone loss is observed along the reactive interface, characterized by a widened radiolucent zone (R). A margin of increased density (reinforced trabecular bone, arrows) is seen in the adjacent viable portion (V) of the femoral head. Circumscribed foci of bone loss are also identified within the sclerotic margin (C).

  C Macroscopic section (2.5×) of the femoral head reveals an infracted reactive interface (R) separating the partially fragmented osteone-crotic segment (N) from the remaining viable portions of the femoral head (V). The marginal sclerosis recognized in **B** is reflected in the macroscopic section as reinforced trabecular bone (arrows) subjacent to the infracted reactive interface. The cysts (radiolucent holes) (C) within the sclerotic margin are analogous to the subchondral cysts that form in degenerative joint disease.

  D Photomicrographic (40×) view of the viable reinforced bony margin adjacent to the reactive interface demonstrates cartilaginous metaplasia (arrow) similar to that seen in a developing pseudarthrosis.

  (Armed Forces Institute of Pathology Neg. Nos. 65-12798, 79-5417, 79-14990, 79-14991.)

ties in a number of patients with ischemic necrosis in whom the resected femoral head demonstrates partial loss of the osteonecrotic bone substance without evidence of having been resorbed.[114]

Superimposed Degenerative Arthritis

Once patients with ischemic necrosis reach phase V (fracture of the subarticular bone plate) and exhibit buckling or partial collapse of the articular surfaces, it usually is only a matter of time until evidence of superimposed degenerative arthritis becomes manifest. The occasional case of secondary ischemic necrosis after primary osteoarthritis should be distinguishable from the foregoing condition in most instances.[169] The articular incongruity resulting from articular buckling or collapse exposes the cartilage surface to shear forces and rapid wear, especially of the noncollapsed portion. The resected femoral head illustrated in Figure 79–22 demonstrating a relatively small area of ischemic necrosis reflects such a sequence. The clinical radiograph reveals evidence of ischemic necrosis with partial loss of joint space in the weight-bearing area (Fig. 79–22A). The resected femoral head was cut and examined in several coronal planes (similar to those in Fig. 79–16C). The most anterior section (Fig. 79–22B–D) reveals the osteonecrotic segment with its overlying articular cartilage. Infraction has occurred along the reactive interface with secondary cyst formation (Fig. 79–22D). Much of the osteonecrotic portion has been removed by osteoclasts (Fig. 79–22B). Both the macroscopic section (Fig. 79–22D) and the specimen radiograph (Fig. 79–22C) indicate the osteonecrotic segment has collapsed into the femoral head, resulting in an incongruous articular surface.

The more posterior coronal section (Fig. 79–22E–G) demonstrates only a minute wedge of residual ischemic necrosis in the gross specimen (Fig. 79–22E). The remaining findings reflect a sizeable area of degenerative arthritic change readily visualized in the gross specimen, specimen radiograph, and macroscopic section (Fig. 79–22E–G). The articular surface shows areas of cartilage fibrillation and eburnated bone (Fig. 79–22D,E,G). Below these areas, the subchondral trabecular bone is reinforced and thickened markedly (Fig. 79–22F,G). This change is the result of stress forces being concentrated on trabecular bone because of the absence of the stress-distributing qualities of the articular cartilage and subchondral bone plate. Early osteophyte formation is seen laterally (Fig. 79–22E–G).

ANCILLARY IMAGING STUDIES

The foregoing segments of this chapter have focused primarily on the pathogenesis and pathologic correlation with sequential plain film radiographic findings in osteonecrosis. Unfortunately, the pathophysiologic findings accounting for the sequential plain film changes in osteonecrosis indicate the reparative process is well established and its eventual consequence (articular collapse in ischemic necrosis) is likely, irrespective of subsequent medical or surgical intervention. Ancillary imaging studies, including angiography, scintigraphy, and MR imaging (Figs. 79–23 and 79–24), offer the opportunity for earlier recognition of osteonecrosis (see Chapter 80).[216, 218, 221] CT scanning, although potentially helpful in establishing the extent of structural alterations in ischemic necrosis and providing data useful in operative planning,[138, 143] is of little additional benefit for early diagnosis.

With regard to imaging techniques, the bone scan is very sensitive in identifying the earliest cellular response to ischemic necrosis.[133, 141, 149, 208] Although not specific in terms of absolute diagnosis, it has proved to be an excellent screening test for probable osteonecrosis in the high risk patient.[155, 157]

MR imaging of the skeleton, especially the femoral head, shows good definition of the marrow space in normal persons as well as in the early and late stages of osteonecrosis.[134, 154, 177, 182, 194, 207] The normal marrow space on spin echo studies with a TR of 500 msec and a TE of 30 msec is of high signal intensity owing to the short T1 and long T2 of the fat and hematopoietic elements. A regional or serpentine-like decrease in signal intensity is seen in osteonecrosis as a result of replacement of the normally high signal intensity produced by fatty marrow. It should be stressed that the decreased signal intensity on MR imaging is not specific for osteonecrosis but is seen in any process altering or replacing fatty marrow with tissue of lower signal intensity.

Preservation of the fat signal on the MR image within the central intramedullary osteonecrotic segments of both bone infarcts and ischemic necrosis is predictable from their respective light microscopic findings. Although the overall distribution of the changes in signal intensity on MR images in the experimental study depicted in Figure 79–24 is not identical to that occurring in vivo in human femoral heads with emerging ischemic necrosis, the sequence and character of the signal alterations are similar and may be perceptible within 10 to 15 days of the initial reactive-reparative response; certainly no longer than 30 days is required for the alterations to be observable.[213, 219]

Assuming the opportunity for prevention has passed, the sooner ischemic necrosis is recognized, the earlier medical or surgical (or both) therapeutic intervention can begin, if indicated. The aforementioned MR imaging changes would appear to represent a more reliable indicator of early ischemic necrosis than the potentially more sensitive but less specific scintigraphic findings.[223]

SUMMARY

Although ischemic necrosis of bone causes cell death, initially little or no change is apparent in bony architecture as a direct result of osteocyte death. It is the progressive reparative host response, both vascular and cellular, that gradually leads to the altered bone density we recognize as characteristic of osteonecrosis. The extent of resorption (removal) and reinforcement (reconstruction) of bone associated with ischemic necrosis, in comparison with metadiaphyseal bone infarcts, would seem to reflect the difference in mechanical requirements at their respective sites and in the amount of bone involved. Because osteonecrosis is three-dimensional the host response initially begins along the peripheral margin of the infarct, rather than uniformly throughout the entire osteonecrotic segment. Why this response tends to remain relatively localized to the outer perimeter is controversial, but it appears related to development of a thick, biologically impenetrable fibrous membrane along the entire reactive interface resulting in virtual

Text continued on page 3491

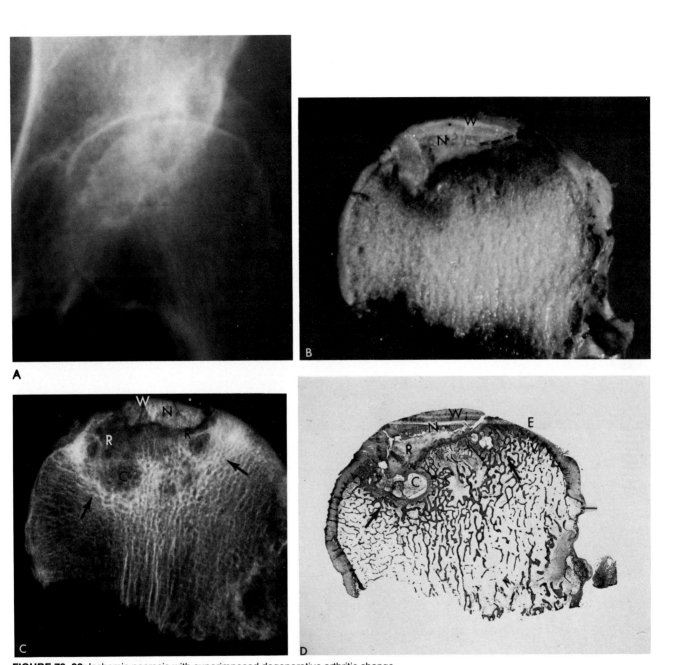

FIGURE 79–22. Ischemic necrosis with superimposed degenerative arthritic change.

A Clinical radiograph demonstrates ischemic necrosis characterized by altered subchondral density and localized articular collapse. Narrowing of the joint space superiorly indicates partial loss of the articular surface.

B Gross photograph (2.5×) of an anterior coronal section of the resected femoral head shows a small zone of osteonecrosis in the weight-bearing area (W) covered by a partially collapsed articular surface. The pale osteonecrotic zone (N) is surrounded by a darkened area of hyperemic reactive tissue.

C Specimen radiographic view of the anterior coronal section in **B** indicates that the small, partially fragmented osteonecrotic zone (N) has collapsed into the extensively resorbed reactive interface (R) with cyst formation (C). The resorbed area is surrounded by a reinforced bony margin (arrows).

D Macroscopic section (2.5×) reflects the histologic basis for the altered density patterns in the specimen and clinical radiographic appearance of the femoral head. Partial loss of the articular cartilage is seen laterally (E) with early osteophyte formation (small arrow). The small residual osteonecrotic segment is surrounded by an infracted reactive interface (R), characterized by fibrous tissue, debris, and cyst formation (C). This region is framed by areas of reinforced (thickened) trabecular bone (large arrows).

Illustration continued on following page

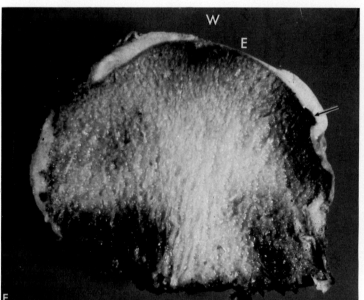

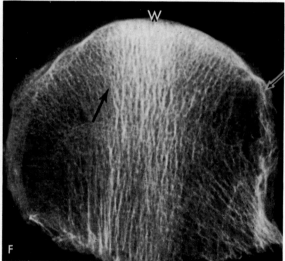

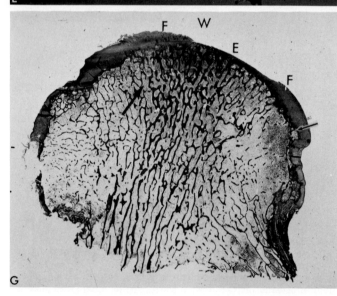

FIGURE 79–22. *Continued*

E Gross photograph (2.5×) of a more posterior coronal section of the femoral head reveals partial loss of the articular surface (E) in the weight-bearing area (W). A minute wedge of preexisting ischemic necrosis, surrounded by a hyperemic border, can be identified subchondrally. Laterally, early osteophyte formation is seen (arrow).

F Specimen radiographic appearance (2.5 ×) of the gross section **(E)** reveals increased density characterized by thickened cancellous bony trabeculae in the subchondral weight-bearing portion of the femoral head (heavy arrow). The lateral subchondral plate appears slightly distorted by osteophyte formation (thin arrow).

G Macroscopic section (2.5 ×) of this level of the femoral head demonstrates complete loss of the articular surface in the weight-bearing area, with eburnated bone (E). Immediately adjacent to the eburnated surface is fibrillated articular cartilage laterally and medially (F). The subchondral bone subjacent to the fibrillated cartilage and eburnated bone reveals marked mechanical reinforcement (heavy arrow) and a hyperemic-appearing reactive marrow. Laterally, the cartilage demonstrates articular endochondral bone formation (thin arrow), representing early osteophyte formation. This accounts for the irregularity of the lateral subchondral plate in the specimen radiograph **(F)** and gross photograph **(E)**.

(Armed Forces Institute of Pathology Neg. Nos. 69-4218-1, 79-15003-1, 79-5410-1, 79-15002-1, 79-15003-3, 79-5410-3, 79-15002-3.)

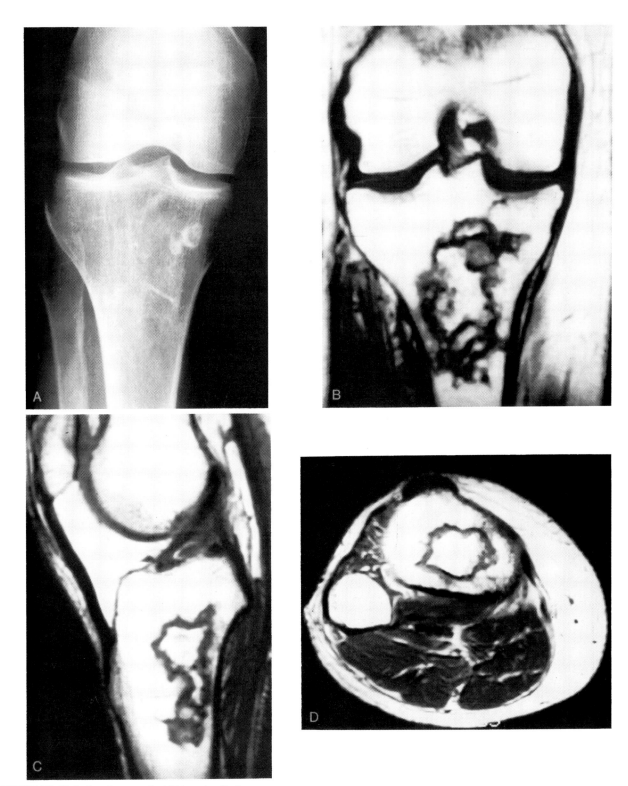

FIGURE 79–23. Ischemic necrosis: MR imaging findings.

A Anteroposterior radiograph of the right knee of a patient with chronic pancreatitis demonstrating a bone infarct involving the proximal portion of the tibia. Note the irregular pattern of focal increased density and extensive area of radiolucency.

B Coronal T1-weighted spin echo MR image of the knee seen in **A.** Observe that the central area of the bone infarct has retained the signal intensity of fat. It is surrounded and encompassed by a hypointense fibroreactive interface or margin.

C Sagittal T1-weighted spin echo MR image of the same knee as in **A** demonstrating signal patterns similar to those seen in **B.**

D Transaxial T1-weighted spin echo MR image through the proximal portion of the tibia in **A.** Again, note that the central area of bone infarction has maintained its hyperintense fat signal, whereas the fibroreactive wall (margin) about the infarct is hypointense. This indicates that little progress in replacing the central infarcted area has occurred despite the long-standing nature of the infarct.

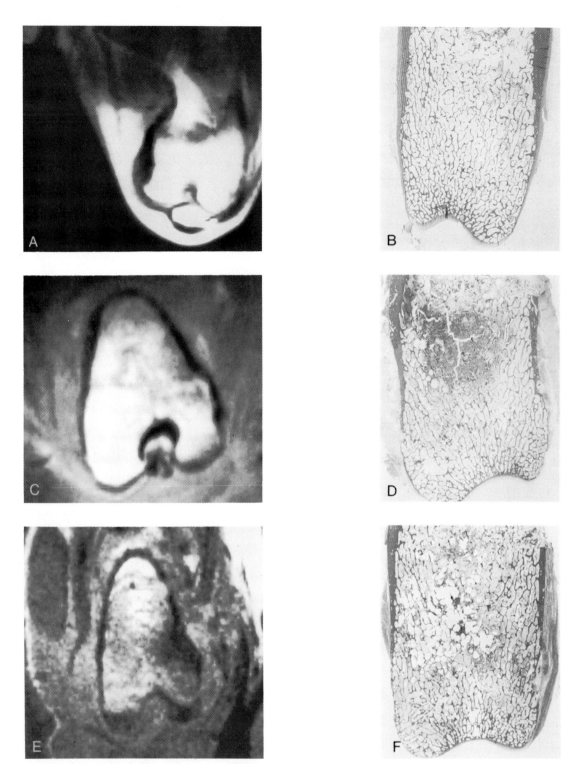

FIGURE 79–24. Ischemic necrosis: MR imaging abnormalities.

   A Coronal T1-weighted spin echo MR image of the distal end of the femur of an untreated or control dog. Note the normal hyperintense marrow signal in the distal part of the femur and patella.

   B Macrosection of the femur in **A.** The cancellous bone and marrow space appear normal. (Hematoxylin and eosin stain, ×2.)

   C Coronal T1-weighted spin echo MR image of the distal end of a treated dog's femur, 16 days after surgical transection (cautery) through the distal metadiaphyseal intramedullary space and stripping of the distal femoral periosteum below the transection site in an attempt to obliterate the vascular supply to the distal femoral metaepiphysis. The initial reparative-inflammatory response replacing and obliterating the normal intramedullary contents is reflected in the MR image by inhomogeneous signal intensity in much of the metaphysis and a residual homogeneous hyperintense signal in one of the femoral condyles.

   D Macrosection of the treated femur in **C.** Note the hemorrhage, altered marrow appearance seen in the metaphysis, and residual osteonecrotic but morphologically intact condylar areas. (Hematoxylin and eosin stain, ×4.)

   E Coronal T1-weighted spin echo MR image of the distal end of the treated dog's femur 30 days after surgical transection (cautery) and periosteal stripping as outlined in **C.** At this time, the reparative-inflammatory response has extended throughout the distal femoral intramedullary space, resulting in inhomogeneous signal intensity.

   F Macrosection of the treated femur in **E.** Note that the normal pale fatty appearance of the marrow space has been altered and replaced by a loose fibroreactive reparative and inflammatory response. (Hematoxylin and eosin stain, ×2.)

mummification of the encased osteonecrotic segment. Within the femoral head and other juxta-articular sites, localized resorption weakens both the cancellous and the subchondral bone along the entire reactive margin, causing eventual articular buckling or collapse in the majority of cases. Once articular buckling or collapse occurs, there is little likelihood reconstruction or repair can restore normal joint continuity or function.

The term "creeping substitution" has been used by many authors to describe the repair of ischemic necrosis. Unfortunately, most of the "creeping" is done along the reactive interface and the bulk of bone substitution occurs along the outer reactive (reinforcing) margin, rather than throughout the entire osteonecrotic segment. Although the term has some basis in fact, from a practical point of view it seems little more than wishful thinking at present. Were the entire infarcted segment to be repaired uniformly at the same time, as perhaps occurs occasionally in patients with femoral neck fracture, it might be possible to circumvent the eventual articular collapse. To this end, the use of vascularized bone grafts, in the hope of accelerating revascularization of the infarcted segment, seems to have met with at least limited, if not universal, success. A multiplicity of precisely drilled parallel holes, traversing the reactive interface and osteonecrotic segment, connecting the viable intramedullary zone to the "involved" subchondral bony plate, could potentially have a similar effect. A final thought based on histologic observations of the evolving fibrous reactive interface suggests that it is the ischemic changes in marrow fat that result in the progressive formation of the thick fibrous membrane, which militates against uniform repair. Selective removal of the ischemically necrotic intramedullary fat in the very early phases of osteonecrosis would provide wide-open channels for immediate revascularization, and at the same time preserve an intact, perfectly placed, autologous-host cancellous bone graft. This suggests that attention be focused not only on the prevention of osteonecrosis in the high risk patient but also on early detection with the hope of effecting repair, without latent articular collapse. Until better preventive and therapeutic measures are established,[145, 151–153, 200] radionuclide studies and MR imaging undertaken to detect impending osteonecrosis in the at-risk patient population and core biopsy decompression in patients with elevated intramedullary pressure in the noncollapsed femoral head continue worthy of consideration.[214, 215, 217]

References

1. Amstutz HA: The hip in Gaucher's disease. Clin Orthop 90:83, 1973.
2. Arkin AM, Schein AJ: Aseptic necrosis in Gaucher's disease. J Bone Joint Surg [Am] 30:631, 1948.
3. Axhausen G: Uber anämische Infarkte am Knochensystem und ihre Bedeutung für dies Lehre von den primären Epiphyseonekrosen. Arch Klin Chir 151:72, 1928.
4. Banks HH: Healing of the femoral neck fracture. In Proceedings of the Conference on Aseptic Necrosis of the Femoral Head. St. Louis, National Institutes of Health, 1964, pp 4–65.
5. Barton CJ, Cockshott WP: Bone changes in hemoglobin SC disease. AJR 88:523, 1962.
6. Boettcher WG, Bonfiglio M, Hamilton HH, et al: Nontraumatic necrosis of the femoral head. Part I. Relation of altered hemostasis to etiology. J Bone Joint Surg [Am] 52:312, 1970.
7. Bohr H, Larsen EH: On necrosis of the femoral head after fracture of the neck of the femur. A microradiographic and histologic study. J Bone Joint Surg [Br] 47:330, 1965.
8. Bohrer SP: Acute long bone diaphyseal infarcts in sickle cell disease. Br J Radiol 43:685, 1970.
9. Boksenbaum M, Mendelson CG: Aseptic necrosis of the femoral head associated with steroid therapy. JAMA 184:262, 1963.
10. Bonfiglio M: Aseptic necrosis of the femoral head. Intact blood supply is of prognostic significance. In Proceedings of the Conference on Aseptic Necrosis of the Femoral Head. St Louis, National Institutes of Health, 1964, p 155.
11. Boyd HB: Avascular necrosis of the head of the femur. Am Acad Orthop Surg Instr Course Lect 14:196, 1957.
12. Boyd HB, Calandruccio RA: Further observations on the use of radioactive phosphorus (P32) to determine the viability of the head of the femur. Correlation of clinical and experimental data in 130 patients with fractures of the femoral neck. J Bone Joint Surg [Am] 45:445, 1963.
13. Brav EA: Traumatic dislocation of the hip: Army experience and results over a twelve-year period. J Bone Joint Surg [Am] 44:1115, 1962.
14. Bravo JF, Herman JH, Smyth CJ: Musculoskeletal disorders after renal homotransplantation. A clinical and laboratory analysis of 60 cases. Ann Intern Med 66:87, 1967.
15. Brown JT, Abrami G: Transcervical femoral fracture. A review of 195 patients treated by sliding nail-plate fixation. J Bone Joint Surg [Br] 46:648, 1964.
16. Caffey J: Pediatric X-ray Diagnosis. 6th Ed. Chicago, Year Book Medical Publishers, 1972, p 1149.
17. Calandruccio RA: The use of radioactive phosphorus to determine the viability of the femoral head. In Proceedings of the Conference on Aseptic Necrosis of the Femoral Head. St Louis, National Institutes of Health, 1964, p 243.
18. Calandruccio RA: Comparison of specimens from non-union of neck of femur with fresh fractures and avascular necrosis specimens. J Bone Joint Surg [Am] 49:1471, 1967.
19. Catto M: A histological study of avascular necrosis of the femoral head after transcervical fracture. J Bone Joint Surg [Br] 47:749, 1965.
20. Catto M: The histological appearances of late segmental collapse of the femoral head after transcervical fracture. J Bone Joint Surg [Br] 47:777, 1965.
21. Catto M: Pathology of aseptic necrosis. In JK Davidson (Ed): Aseptic Necrosis of Bone. Amsterdam, Excerpta Medica, 1976, p 3.
22. Charache S, Page DL: Infarction of bone marrow in the sickle cell disorders. Ann Intern Med 67:1195, 1967.
23. Coleman SS, Compere CL: Femoral neck fractures: Pathogenesis of avascular necrosis, nonunion and late degenerative changes. Clin Orthop 20:247, 1961.
24. Cruess RL, Blennerhassett J, MacDonald RF, et al: Aseptic necrosis following renal transplantation. J Bone Joint Surg [Am] 50:1577, 1968.
25. Dalinka MK, Edeiken J, Finkelstein JB: Complications of radiation therapy: Adult bone. Semin Roentgenol 9:29, 1974.
26. Davidson JK: Dysbaric osteonecrosis. In JK Davidson (Ed): Aseptic Necrosis of Bone. Amsterdam, Excerpta Medica, 1976, p 147.
27. Dickerson RC, Duthie RB: The diversion of arterial blood flow to bone. A preliminary report. J Bone Joint Surg [Am] 45:356, 1963.
28. Diggs, LW: Bone and joint lesions in sickle cell disease. Clin Orthop 52:119, 1967.
29. Diggs LW, Anderson LD: Aseptic necrosis of the head of the femur in sickle cell disease. In WM Zinn (Ed): Idiopathic Ischemic Necrosis of the Femoral Head in Adults. Stuttgart, Georg Thieme, 1971, p 107.
30. Donaldson WF Jr, Rodriguez EE, Shovron M, et al: Traumatic dislocation of the hip joint in children. Final report by the Scientific Research Committee of the Pennsylvania Orthopedic Society. J Bone Joint Surg [Am] 50:79, 1968.
31. Dorfman HD, Norman A, Wolff H: Fibrosarcoma complicating bone infarction in a caisson worker. A case report. J Bone Joint Surg [Am] 48:528, 1966.
32. Dubois EL, Cozen L: Avascular (aseptic) bone necrosis associated with systemic lupus erythematosus. JAMA 174:966, 1960.
33. Edeiken J, Hodes PJ, Libshitz HI, et al: Bone ischemia. Radiol Clin North Am 5:515, 1967.
34. Evans A, Barnard EEP, Walder DN: Detection of gas bubbles in man at decompression. Aerospace Med 43:1095, 1972.
35. Arlet J, Ficat P: Diagnostic de l'ostéo-nécrose fémoro-capitale primitive au stade I (stade pré-radiologique). Rev Chir Orthop 54:637, 1968.
36. Fisher DE: The role of fat embolism in the etiology of corticosteroid-induced avascular necrosis: Clinical and experimental results. Clin Orthop 130:68, 1978.
37. Fisher DE, Bickel WH, Holley KE: Histologic demonstration of fat emboli in aseptic necrosis associated with hypercortisonism. Mayo Clin Proc 44:252, 1969.
38. Fisher DE, Bickel WH: Corticosteroid-induced avascular necrosis. A clinical study of seventy-seven patients. J Bone Joint Surg [Am] 53:859, 1971.
39. Fisher DE, Bickel WH, Holley KE, et al: Corticosteroid-induced aseptic necrosis. II. Experimental study. Clin Orthop 84:200, 1972.
40. Frost HM: In vivo osteocyte death. J Bone Joint Surg [Am] 42:138, 1960.
41. Frost HM: The etiodynamics of aseptic necrosis of the femoral head. In Proceedings of the Conference on Aseptic Necrosis of the Femoral Head. St Louis, National Institutes of Health, 1964, p 393.
42. Gerle RD, Walker LA, Achord J, et al: Osseous changes in chronic pancreatitis. Radiology 85:330, 1965.
43. Gersh I, Hawkinson GE, Rathbun EN: Tissue and vascular bubbles after decompression from high pressure atmospheres. Correlation of specific gravity with morphological changes. J Cell Comp Physiol 24:35, 1944.
44. Gersh I, Still MA: Blood vessels in fat tissue. Relation to problems of gas exchange. Exp Med 81:219, 1945.
45. Ginn HE: Late medical complications of renal transplantation. Arch Intern Med 123:537, 1969.
46. Glimcher MJ, Kenzora JE: The biology of osteonecrosis of the human femoral

head and its clinical implications (3 parts). Clin Orthop *138*:284; *139*:283; *140*:273, 1979.

47. Golding JSR, MacIver JE, Went LN: The bone changes in sickle cell anemia and its genetic variants. J Bone Joint Surg [Br] *41*:711, 1959.

48. Graham J, Wood SK: Aseptic necrosis of bone following trauma. *In* JK Davidson (Ed): Aseptic Necrosis of Bone. Amsterdam, Excerpta Medica, 1976, p 101.

49. Harrelson JM, Hills BA: Changes in bone marrow pressure in response to hyperbaric pressure. Aerospace Med *41*:1018, 1970.

50. Harrison RG, Gossman HH: The fate of radiopaque media injected into the cancellous bone of extremities. J Bone Joint Surg [Br] *37*:150, 1955.

51. Harrington KD, Murray WR, Kountz SL, et al: Avascular necrosis of bone after renal transplantation. J Bone Joint Surg [Am] *53*:203, 1971.

52. Heimann WG, Freiberger RH: Avascular necrosis of the femoral and humeral heads after high-dosage corticosteroid therapy. N Engl J Med *263*:672, 1960.

53. Henard DC, Calandruccio RA: Experimental production of roentgenographic and histological changes in the capital femoral epiphysis following abduction, extension and internal rotation of the hip. J Bone Joint Surg [Am] *52*:600, 1970.

54. Hesse F: Zur pathologischen Anatomie der Schenkelhalsfraktur. Arch Klin Chir *134*:141, 1925.

55. Hill RB Jr: Fatal fat embolism from steroid-induced fatty liver. N Engl J Med *265*:318, 1961.

56. Hook EW, Campbell CG, Weens HS, et al: Salmonella osteomyelitis in patients with sickle cell anemia. N Engl J Med *257*:403, 1957.

57. Hungerford DS: Bone marrow pressure, venography, and case decompression in ischemic necrosis of the femoral head. *In* The Hip, Proceedings of 7th Open Scientific Meeting of the Hip Society, 1979. St Louis, CV Mosby Co (in press).

58. Hungerford DS, Zizic TM: Alcohol associated ischemic necrosis of the femoral head. Clin Orthop *130*:144, 1978.

59. Immelman EJ, Bank S, Krige H, et al: Roentgenologic and clinical features of intramedullary fat necrosis in bones in acute and chronic pancreatitis. Am J Med *36*:96, 1964.

60. Jacobs P: Osteochondrosis (osteochondritis). *In* JK Davidson (Ed): Aseptic Necrosis of Bone. Amsterdam, Excerpta Medica, 1976, p 301.

61. Jaffe HL: Tumors and Tumorous Conditions of the Bones and Joints. Philadelphia, Lea & Febiger, 1958.

62. Jaffe HL: Metabolic, Degenerative and Inflammatory Diseases of Bones and Joints. Philadelphia, Lea & Febiger, 1972.

63. Jaffe HL, Pomeranz MM: Changes in the bones of extremities amputated because of arteriovascular disease. Arch Surg *29*:566, 1934.

64. James NE: Gaucher's disease; report of case. J Bone Joint Surg [Br] *34*:464, 1952.

65. Jee WSS, Arnold JS: Effect of internally deposited radioisotopes upon blood vessels of cortical bones. Proc Soc Exp Biol Med *105*:351, 1960.

66. Jee WSS, Bartley MH, Dockum NL, et al: Vascular changes in bones following bone-seeking radionuclides. *In* CW Mays, et al (Eds): Delayed Effects of Bone Seeking Radionuclides. Salt Lake City, University of Utah Press, 1969, p 437.

67. Johnson LC: Histogenesis of avascular necrosis. *In* Proceedings of the Conference on Aseptic Necrosis of the Femoral Head. St. Louis, National Institutes of Health, 1964, p 55.

68. Jones JP: Alcoholism, hypercortisonism, fat embolism and osseous avascular necrosis. *In* WM Zinn (Ed): Idiopathic Ischemic Necrosis of the Femoral Head in Adults. Stuttgart, Georg Thieme, 1971, p 112.

69. Jones JP, Jr, Jameson RM, Engleman EP: Alcoholism, fat embolism and avascular necrosis (Abstr). J Bone Joint Surg [Am] *50*:1065, 1968.

70. Jones JP, Sakovich L: Fat embolism of bone. A roentgenographic and histological investigation with use of intra-arterial Lipiodol in rabbits. J Bone Joint Surg [Am] *48*:149, 1966.

71. Kahlstrom SC, Burton CC, Phemister DB: Aseptic necrosis of bone. II. Infarction of bones of undetermined etiology resulting in encapsulated and calcified areas in diaphyses and in arthritis deformans. Surg Gynecol Obstet *68*:631, 1939.

72. Kenzora JE, Steele RE, Yosipovitch ZH, et al: Tissue biology following experimental infarction of femoral heads. Part I. Bone studies. J Bone Joint Surg [Am] *51*:1021, 1969.

73. Kenzora JE, Steele RE, Yosipovitch ZH, et al: Experimental osteonecrosis of the apparent head in adult rabbits. Clin Orthop *130*:8, 1978.

74. Kinsell LW (Ed): Adipose Tissue as an Organ: Proceedings (Deuel Conference on Lipids). Springfield, Ill, Charles C Thomas, 1962.

75. Lagier R: Idiopathic aseptic necrosis of the femoral head. An anatomopathological concept. *In* WM Zinn (Ed): Idiopathic Ischemic Necrosis of the Femoral Head in Adults. Stuttgart, Georg Thieme, 1971, p 49.

76. Louyot P, Gaucher A: A propos de 30 observations d'ostéonécroses primitive de la tête fémorale. Rev Rhum Mal Osteoartic *29*:577, 1962.

77. Lynch MJG, Raphael SS, Dixon TP: Fat embolism in chronic alcoholism. Arch Pathol *67*:68, 1959.

78. Lucas PF, Owen TK: Subcutaneous fat necrosis, ''polyarthritis'' and pancreatic disease. Gut *3*:146, 1962.

79. McCollum DE, Mathews RS, Pickett PT: Gout, hyperuricemia and aseptic necrosis of the femoral head (Abstr). Arthritis Rheum *10*:295, 1967.

80. McKay DG: Disseminated Intravascular Coagulation, an Intermediary Mechanism of Disease. New York, Hoeber Medical Division, Harper & Row, 1965.

81. Marshall JH: The retention of radionuclides in bone. *In* CW Mays, et al (Eds): Delayed Effects of Bone Seeking Radionuclides. Salt Lake City, University of Utah Press, 1969, p 7.

82. Middlemiss H: Aseptic necrosis and other changes occurring in bone in the hemoglobinopathies. *In* JK Davidson (Ed): Aseptic Necrosis of Bone. Amsterdam, Excerpta Medica, 1976, p 271.

83. Müssbichler H: Arteriographic findings in necrosis of the head of the femur after medial neck fracture. Acta Orthop Scand *41*:77, 1970.

84. Nachamie BA, Dorfman HD: Ischemic necrosis of bone in sickle cell trait. Mt Sinai J Med *41*:527, 1974.

85. Patterson RJ, Bickel WH, Dahlin DC: Idiopathic avascular necrosis of the head of the femur. A study of fifty-two cases. J Bone Joint Surg [Am] *46*:267, 1964.

86. Perry TT III: Role of lymphatic vessels in the transmission of lipase in disseminated pancreatic fat necrosis. Arch Pathol *43*:456, 1947.

87. Phemister DB: Necrotic bone and the subsequent changes which it undergoes. JAMA *64*:211, 1915.

88. Phemister DB: Repair of bone in the presence of aseptic necrosis resulting from fractures, transplantations and vascular obstruction. J Bone Joint Surg *12*:769, 1930.

89. Phemister DB: Fractures of the neck of femur, dislocations of hip, and obscure vascular disturbances producing aseptic necrosis of head of femur. Surg Gynecol Obstet *59*:415, 1934.

90. Phemister DB: The pathology of ununited fractures of the neck of the femur with special reference to the head. J Bone Joint Surg *21*:681, 1939.

91. Phemister DB: Lesions of bones and joints arising from interruption of the circulation. Mt Sinai J Med *15*:55, 1948.

92. Philp RB, Inwood MJ, Warren BA: Interactions between gas bubbles and components of the blood. Implications in decompression sickness. Aerospace Med *43*:946, 1972.

93. Pourel J. Louyot P, Diebold P, et al: Stéatonécrosis disséminée a déterminations articulaires, osseuses et mésentériques. J Radiol Electrol Med Nucl *51*:423, 1970.

94. Ratcliff RG, Wolf MD: Avascular necrosis of the femoral head associated with sickle cell trait (AS hemoglobin). Ann Intern Med *57*:299, 1962.

95. Riniker P, Huggler A: Idiopathic necrosis of the femoral head. (A further pathoanatomical study). *In* WM Zinn (Ed): Idiopathic Ischemic Necrosis of the Femoral Head in Adults. Stuttgart, Georg Thieme, 1971, p 67.

96. Robbins SL, Angell M: Basic Pathology. 2nd Ed. Philadelphia, WB Saunders Co, 1976, pp 7, 20.

97. Robbins SL, Angell M: Basic Pathology. 2nd Ed. Philadelphia, WB Saunders Co, 1976, p 28.

98. Robbins SL, Angell M: Basic Pathology. 2nd Ed. Philadelphia, WB Saunders Co, 1976, p 184.

99. Rösingh GE, James J: Early phases of avascular necrosis of the femoral head in rabbits. J Bone Joint Surg [Br] *51*:165, 1969.

100. Royzsahegyi I: Die chronische Osteoarthropathie der Caissonarbeiter. Arch Gewerbepath Gewerbehyg *14*:483, 1956.

101. Rourke JA, Heslin DJ: Gaucher's disease. Roentgenologic bone changes over 20 year interval. AJR *94*:621, 1965.

102. Russell J: A Practical Essay on a Certain Disease of Bones Termed Necrosis. Edinburgh, Neill and Co, 1794.

103. Santos JV: Changes in the head of the femur after complete intracapsular fracture of the neck. Their bearing on nonunion and treatment. Arch Surg *21*:470, 1930.

104. Scarpelli DG: Fat necrosis of bone marrow in acute pancreatitis. Am J Pathol *32*:1077, 1956.

105. Sevitt S: Avascular necrosis and revascularisation of the femoral head after intracapsular fracture; a combined arteriographic and histological necropsy study. J Bone Joint Surg [Br] *46*:270, 1964.

106. Sevitt S, Thompson RG: The distribution and anastomoses of arteries supplying the head and neck of the femur. J Bone Joint Surg [Br] *47*:560, 1965.

107. Sherman MS, Phemister DB: The pathology of ununited fractures of the neck of the femur. J Bone Joint Surg *29*:19, 1947.

108. Shin SS: Circulatory and vascular changes in the hip following traumatic hip dislocation. Clin Orthop *140*:255, 1979.

109. Siemsen JK, Brook J, Meister L: Lupus erythematosus and avascular bone necrosis: A clinical study of three cases and review of the literature. Arthritis Rheum *5*:492, 1962.

110. Smith FE, Sweet DE, Brunner CM, et al: Avascular necrosis in SLE. An apparent predilection for young patients. Ann Rheum Dis *35*:227, 1976.

111. Springfield DS, Enneking WJ: Surgery for aseptic necrosis of the femoral head. Clin Orthop *130*:175, 1978.

112. Stein AH: The physiological aspects of circulation to a long bone. *In* Proceedings of the Conference on Aseptic Necrosis of the Femoral Head. St Louis, National Institutes of Health, 1964, p 41.

113. Storey GO: Bone necrosis in joint disease. Proc R Soc Med *61*:961, 1968.

114. Sweet DE: Unpublished data.

115. Todd RM, Keidan SE: Changes in the head of the femur in children suffering from Gaucher's disease. J Bone Joint Surg [Br] *34*:447, 1952.

116. Trueta J: The normal vascular anatomy of the human femoral head during growth. J Bone Joint Surg [Br] *39*:358, 1957.

117. Trueta J, Harrison MHM: The normal vascular anatomy of the femoral head in adult man. J Bone Joint Surg [Br] *35*:442, 1953.

118. Trueta J: Studies of the Development and Decay of the Human Frame. Philadelphia, WB Saunders Co, 1968.

119. Velayos EE, Leidholt JD, Smyth CJ: Arthropathy associated with steroid therapy. Ann Intern Med *64*:759, 1966.

120. Walder DN: A possible explanation for some cases of severe decompression

sickness in compressed-air workers. *In* DJC Cunningham and BB Lloyd (Eds): The Regulation of Human Respiration. Oxford, Blackwell, 1963, p 570.

121. Wang GJ, Sweet DE, Reger SI: Fat cell changes as a mechanism of avascular necrosis of the femoral head in cortisone treated rabbits. J Bone Joint Surg [Am] *59*:729, 1977.

122. Wang GJ, Lennox DW, Reiger SI, et al: Cortisone induced intrafemoral head pressure changes and its response to drilling decompression method. Clin Orthop *159*:274, 1981.

123. Werts MF, Shilling CW: Dysbaric osteonecrosis. An annotated bibliography with preliminary analyses. Washington, DC, Biological Services Communication Project, George Washington University Medical Center, 1972.

124. Woodward HQ, Coley BL: The correlation of tissue dose and clinical response in irradiation of bone tumors and of normal bone. AJR *57*:464, 1947.

125. Woodhouse CF: Anoxia of the femoral head. Surgery *52*:55, 1962.

126. Woodhouse CF: Dynamic influences of vascular occlusion affecting the development of avascular necrosis of the femoral head. Clin Orthop *32*:119, 1964.

127. Anglietti P, Insall JN, Buzzi R, et al: Idiopathic osteonecrosis of the knee. Aetiology, prognosis and treatment. J Bone Joint Surg [Br] *65*:588, 1983.

128. Andresen J, Nielsen HE: Osteonecrosis in renal transplant recipients. Early radiological detection and course. Acta Orthop Scand *52*:475, 1981.

129. Arlet J, Franck JL, Nghiem L, et al: Necroses osseuses multiples et hyperlipémie familiale de type I. A propos d'une observation. Rev Rhum Mal Osteoartic *50*:149, 1983.

130. Arlet J, Marzieres B, Netry C: Osteonecrosis of the femoral head and pregnancy. Clin Rheumatol *1*:95, 1982.

131. Arlot ME, Bonjean M, Chavassieux PM, et al: Bone histology in adults with aseptic necrosis. Histomorphometric evaluation of iliac biopsies in seventy-seven patients. J Bone Joint Surg [Am] *65*:1319, 1983.

132. Baron M, Paltiel H, Lander P: Aseptic necrosis of the talus and calcaneal insufficiency fractures in a patient with pancreatitis, subcutaneous fat necrosis, and arthritis. Arthritis Rheum *27*:1309, 1984.

133. Bassett LW, Gold RH, Webber MM: Radionuclide bone imaging. Radiol Clin North Am *19*:675, 1981.

134. Bluemm RG, Falke THM, Ziedes des Plantes BG Jr, et al: Early Legg-Perthes disease (ischemic necrosis of the femoral head) demonstrated by magnetic resonance imaging. Skel Radiol *14*:95, 1985.

135. Boskely AL, Raggio CL, Bullough PG, et al: Changes in the bone tissue lipids in persons with steroid- and alcohol-induced osteonecrosis. Clin Orthop *172*:289, 1983.

136. Brower AC: The osteochondroses. Orthop Clin North Am *14*:99, 1983.

137. Brown TD, Hild GL: Pre-collapse stress redistributions in femoral head osteonecrosis—a three-dimensional finite element analysis. J Biomech Eng *105*:171, 1983.

138. Brown TD, Mutschler TA, Ferguson AB Jr: A non-linear finite element analysis of some early collapse processes in femoral head osteonecrosis. J Biomech *15*:705, 1982.

139. Casteleyn PP, De Boeck H, Handelberg F, et al: Computed axial tomography and disulphine blue in the evaluation of osteonecrosis of the femoral head. Int Orthop (SICOT) *7*:149, 1983.

140. Chandler FA: Coronary disease of the hip. J Int College Surg *11*:34, 1948.

141. Conklin JJ, Alderson PO, Zizic TM, et al: Comparison of bone scan and radiograph sensitivity in the detection of steroid-induced ischemic necrosis of bone. Radiology *147*:221, 1983.

142. Cruess RL: Steroid-induced osteonecrosis: A review. Can J Surg *24*:567, 1981.

143. Dettoni A, Indemini E, Rossi P, et al: La tomografia assiale computerizzata nella osteonecrosi idiopatica della testa femorale. Chir Organi Mov *67*:615, 1981.

144. De Bastiani G, Bosello O, Magnan B, et al: Metabolic and nutritional factors in the pathogenesis of idiopathic osteonecrosis of the head of the femur (preliminary results of a long-term follow-up investigation). Ital J Orthop Traumatol *10*:85, 1984.

145. Eftekhar NS, Schink-Ascani MM, Mitchell SN, et al: Osteonecrosis of the femoral head treated by pulsed electromagnetic fields (PEMFs): A preliminary report. Hip p 306, 1983.

146. Elmstedt E: Avascular bone necrosis in the renal transplant patient: A discriminant analysis of 144 cases. Clin Orthop *158*:149, 1981.

147. Engel IA, Straus DJ, Lacher M, et al: Osteonecrosis in patients with malignant lymphoma. A review of twenty-five cases. Cancer *48*:1245, 1981.

148. Ergun H, Howland WJ: Postradiation atrophy of mature bone. CRC Crit Rev Diagn Imaging *12*:225, 1980.

149. Esdaile J, Rosenthall L: Radionuclide joint imaging. Compr Ther *9*:54, 1983.

150. Fast A, Alon M, Weiss S, et al: Avascular necrosis of bone following short-term dexamethasone therapy for brain edema. Case report. J Neurosurg *61*:983, 1984.

151. Ficat P, Grijalvo P: Résultats à long terme du forage-biopsie pour les ostéonécroses de la tête fémorale aux stades I et II. A propos de 133 cas revus après un délai moyen de 9 ans 6 mois. Rev Chir Orthop *70*:253, 1984.

152. Ficat RP, Arlet J, Hungerford DS (Eds): *In* Ischemia and Necrosis of Bone. Baltimore, Williams & Wilkins, 1980, p 1.

153. Ficat RP: Treatment of avascular necrosis of the femoral head. Hip p 279, 1983.

154. Fisher MR, Barker B, Amparo EG, et al: MR imaging using specialized coils. Radiology *157*:433, 1985.

155. Franke D: Szintigraphisch nachweisbare Knochenkontusion als Ursache der aseptischen Knochennekrose? Fortschr Med *100*:177, 1982.

156. Garty I, Koren A, Katzumi E: Uncommon sites of bone infarction in a sickle cell anemia patient. Eur J Nucl Med *8*:367, 1983.

157. Gaucher A, Colomb JN, Naoun A, et al: Radionuclide imaging in hip abnormalities. Clin Nucl Med *5*:214, 1980.

158. Gaucher A, Thomas JL, Netter P, et al: Osteomalacia, pseudosacroiliitis and necrosis of the femoral heads in Fanconi syndrome in an adult. J Rheumatol *8*:512, 1981.

159. Gershuni DH: Preliminary evaluation and prognosis in Legg-Calvé-Perthes disease. Clin Orthop *150*:16, 1980.

160. Gold EW, Cangemi PJ: Incidence and pathogenesis of alcohol-induced osteonecrosis of the femoral head. Clin Orthop *143*:222, 1979.

161. Griffiths ID, Maini RN, Scott JT: Clinical and radiological features of osteonecrosis in systemic lupus erythematosus. Ann Rheum Dis *38*:413, 1979.

162. Harper PG, Trask C, Souhami RL: Avascular necrosis of bone caused by combination chemotherapy without corticosteroids. Br Med J *288*:267, 1984.

163. Hely D, Fennell RS III, Petty W, et al: Osteonecrosis of the femoral head and condyle in the post transplantation courses of children and adolescents. Int J Pediatr Nephrol *3*:297, 1982.

164. Houpt JB, Pritzker KP, Alpert B, et al: Natural history of spontaneous osteonecrosis of the knee (SONK): A review. Semin Arthritis Rheum *13*:212, 1983.

165. Hungerford DS: Pathogenetic considerations in ischemic necrosis of bone. Can J Surg *24*:583, 1981.

166. Hungerford DS, Zizic TM: Ischemic bone necrosis in systemic lupus erythematosus II. The treatment of ischemic necrosis of bone in systemic lupus erythematosus. Medicine *59*:143, 1980.

167. Hunter WL Jr, Biersner RJ: Comparison of long-bone radiographs between U.S. Navy divers and matched controls. Undersea Biomed Res *9*:147, 1982.

168. Igarashi M, Hayashi Y, Karube S, et al: An aspect of metabolic bone disease with idiopathic osteonecrosis of the femoral head. Nippon Seikeigeka Gakkai Zasshi *57*:379, 1983.

169. Ilardi CF, Sokoloff L: Secondary osteonecrosis in osteoarthritis of the femoral head. Hum Pathol *15*:79, 1984.

170. Keeley K, Buchanan GR: Acute infarction of long bones in children with sickle cell anemia. J Pediatr *101*:170, 1982.

171. Kindwall EP, Nellen JR, Spiegelhoff DR: Aseptic necrosis in compressed air tunnel workers using current OSHA decompression schedules. J Occup Med *24*:741, 1982.

172. Kleinman RG, Bleck EE: Increased blood viscosity in patients with Legg-Perthes disease: A preliminary report. J Pediatr Orthop *1*:131, 1981.

173. Koren A, Garty I, Katzuni E: Bone infarction in children with sickle cell disease: Early diagnosis and differentiation from osteomyelitis. Eur J Pediatr *142*:93, 1984.

174. Larsen RM: Intramedullary pressure with particular reference to massive diaphyseal bone necrosis: Experimental observation. Ann Surg *108*:127, 1980.

175. Le Parc JM, Paolaggi JB, Lefevre JL, et al: Osteonécroses des "detransplantes renaux" repris en hemodialyse. Comparaison avec une population d'hemodialyses n'ayant pas subi de tentative de transplantation. Ann Med Intern *134*:314, 1983.

176. Lewis VL, Keats TE: Bone end sclerosis in renal osteodystrophy simulating osteonecrosis. Skel Radiol *8*:275, 1982.

177. Littrup PJ, Aisen AM, Braunstein EM, et al: Magnetic resonance imaging of femoral head development in roentgenographically normal patients. Skel Radiol *14*:159, 1985.

178. Macleod MA, McEwan AJ, Pearson RR, et al: Functional imaging in the early diagnosis of dysbaric osteonecrosis. Br J Radiol *55*:497, 1982.

179. McCallum RI: Bone necrosis due to decompression. Phil Trans R Soc Lond *304*:185, 1984.

180. McCarthy EF: Aseptic necrosis of bone. An historic perspective. Clin Orthop *168*:216, 1982.

181. Milgram JW: Reparative cartilaginous callus in subarticular osteonecrosis of bone. A histopathological study of the femoral head. Clin Orthop *186*:272, 1984.

182. Moon KL, Genant HK, Helms CA, et al: Musculoskeletal applications of nuclear magnetic resonance. Radiology *147*:161, 1983.

183. Nixon JE: Avascular necrosis of bone: A review. J R Soc Med *76*:681, 1983.

184. Nixon JE: Early diagnosis and treatment of steroid induced avascular necrosis of bone. Br Med J *288*:741, 1984.

185. Onwubalili JK: Sickle cell disease and infection. J Infect *7*:2, 1983.

186. Oriani G, Balzarini E, Barnini C, et al: Analisi comparative di reperti radiografici di "alterazioni strutturali" ossee in sommozzatori e non sommozzatori. Minerva Med *72*:3573, 1981.

187. Palmer AK, Hensinger RN, Costenbader JM, et al: Osteonecrosis of the femoral head in a family with hyperlipoproteinemia. Clin Orthop *155*:166, 1981.

188. Paolaggi JB, Le Parc JM, Durigon M, et al: Osteonecroses cortisoniques: Acquisitions tirées de l'observation chez l'homme et confrontation avec les resultats de l'experimentation animale. Rev Rhum Mal Osteoartic *67*:719, 1980.

189. Pearson RR, MacLeod MA, McEwan AJ, et al: Bone scintigraphy as an investigative aid for dysbaric osteonecrosis in divers. J R Nav Med Serv *68*:61, 1982.

190. Pellicci PM, Zolla-Pazner S, Rabhan WN, et al: Osteonecrosis of the femoral head associated with pregnancy. Report of three cases. Clin Orthop *185*:59, 1984.

191. Pooly J, Walder DW: Reduction in bone marrow blood flow during simulated dives (Abstr). J Bone Joint Surg [Br] *62*:535, 1980.

192. Prosnitz LR, Lawson JP, Friedlaender GE, et al: Avascular necrosis of bone in Hodgkin's disease patients treated with combined modality therapy. Cancer *47*:2793, 1981.

193. Roux H, Serratrice G, Vovan L, et al: Recherche de globules graisseux circu-

lants par filtrage du serum au cours des osteonecroses primitives de la tête femorale. Rev Rhum Mal Osteoartic *46:*683, 1979.

194. Reiser M, Rupp N, Stettes E: Erfahrungen bei der NMR Tomographie des Skelettsystems. ROFO *139:*365, 1983.

195. Resnick D: Osteonecrosis of metacarpal and metatarsal heads following renal transplantation. Br J Radiol *55:*463, 1982.

196. Roseff R, Canoso JJ: Femoral osteonecrosis following soft tissue corticosteroid infiltration. Am J Med *77:*1119, 1984.

197. Sambrook PN, Hassall JE, York JR: Osteonecrosis after high dosage, short term corticorsteroid therapy. J Rheumatol *11:*514, 1984.

198. Scholz D, Mebel M, Topelmann I, et al: Prevention of osteonecrosis following renal transplantation by using vitamin D2 (ergocalciferol). Proc Eur Dial Transplant Assoc *20:*331, 1983.

199. Shupak R, Bernier V, Rabinovich S, et al: Avascular necrosis of bone with rheumatoid vasculitis. J Rheumatol *10:*261, 1983.

200. Simonnet JH, Aubaniac JM, Vedel F, et al: L'osteotomie intertrochanterienne de flexion dans les osteonecroses aseptiques de la tête femorale de l'adulte. A propos de 52 cas. Rev Chir Orthop *70:*219, 1984.

201. Slichter SJ, Stegall P, Smith K, et al: Dysbaric osteonecrosis: A consequence of intravascular bubble formation, endothelial damage, and platelet thrombosis. J Lab Clin Med *98:*568, 1981.

202. Solomon L: Avascular necrosis of the femoral head: Pre-clinical changes and their bearing on pathogenesis and treatment. J Bone Joint Surg [Br] *61:*126, 1979.

203. Solomon L: Idiopathic necrosis of the femoral head: Pathogenesis and treatment. Can J Surg *24:*573, 1981.

204. Squifflet JP, Pirson Y, van Cangh P, et al: Renal transplantation in children: A comparative study between parental and well-matched cadaveric grafts. Transplantation *32:*278, 1981.

205. Taylor LJ: Multifocal avascular necrosis after short-term high dose steroid therapy. A report of three cases. J Bone Joint Surg [Br] *66:*431, 1984.

206. Thomas IH, Evans A, Walder DN: Saturation of mini-pig bone-marrow with nitrogen during exposure to compressed air. Lancet *2:*127, 1982.

207. Totty WG, Murphy WA, Ganz WI, et al: Magnetic resonance imaging of the normal and ischemic femoral head. AJR *143:*1273, 1984.

208. Tacher FR: Use of radioactive phosphorus in diagnosis of avascular necrosis of the femoral head. J Bone Joint Surg [Br] *32:*100, 1950.

209. Zizic TM, Hungerford DS, Stevens MB: Ischemic bone necrosis in systemic lupus erythematosus. I. The early diagnosis of ischemic necrosis of bone. Medicine *59:*134, 1980.

210. Zolla-Pazner S, Pazner SS, Lanyi V, et al: Osteonecrosis of the femoral head during pregnancy. JAMA *244:*689, 1980.

211. Arlet J: Nontraumatic avascular necrosis of the femoral head. Past, present, and future. Clin Orthop *277:*12, 1992.

212. Atsumi T, Kuroki Y, Yamano K: A microangiographic study of idiopathic osteonecrosis of the femoral head. Clin Orthop *246:*186, 1989.

213. Brody AS, Strong M, Babikian G, et al: John Caffey Award paper. Avascular necrosis: Early MR imaging and histologic findings in a canine model. AJR *157:*341, 1991.

214. Chan TW, Dalinka MK, Steinberg ME, et al: MRI appearance of femoral head osteonecrosis following core decompression and bone grafting. Skeletal Radiol *20:*103, 1991.

215. Colwell CW Jr: The controversy of core decompression of the femoral head for osteonecrosis. Arthritis Rheum *32:*797, 1989.

216. Fordyce MJ, Solomon L: Early detection of avascular necrosis of the femoral head by MRI. J Bone Joint Surg [Br] *75:*365, 1993.

217. Hungerford DS: Response: The role of core decompression in the treatment of ischemic necrosis of the femoral head. Arthritis Rheum *32:*801, 1989.

218. Lafforgue P, Dahan E, Chagnaud C, et al: Early-stage avascular necrosis of the femoral head: MR imaging for prognosis in 31 cases with at least 2 years of follow-up. Radiology *187:*199, 1993.

219. Malizos KN, Quarles LD, Seaber AV, et al: An experimental canine model of osteonecrosis: Characterization of the repair process. J Orthop Res *11:*350, 1993.

220. Matsui M, Saito S, Ohzono K, et al: Experimental steroid-induced osteonecrosis in adult rabbits with hypersensitivity vasculitis. Clin Orthop *277:*61, 1992.

221. Mitchell DG, Steinberg ME, Dalinka MK, et al: Magnetic resonance imaging of the ischemic hip. Alterations within the osteonecrotic, viable, and reactive zones. Clin Orthop *244:*60, 1989.

222. Ohzono K, Takaoka K, Saito S, et al: Intraosseous arterial architecture in nontraumatic avascular necrosis of the femoral head. Microangiographic and histologic study. Clin Orthop *277:*79, 1992.

223. Ruland LJ, Wang GJ, Teates CD, et al: A comparison of magnetic resonance imaging to bone scintigraphy in early traumatic ischemia of the femoral head. Clin Orthop *285:*30, 1992.

224. Saito S, Ohzono K, Ono K: Early arteriopathy and postulated pathogenesis of osteonecrosis of the femoral head. The intracapital arterioles. Clin Orthop *277:*98, 1992.

80

Osteonecrosis: Diagnostic Techniques, Specific Situations, and Complications

Donald Resnick, M.D., and Gen Niwayama, M.D.

Chapter 79 has described in detail the general pathologic and radiologic alterations that accompany osteonecrosis. Although specific changes depend, to some extent, on the precise location and cause of the bone necrosis, the morphologic findings are remarkably similar.

The causes of osteonecrosis are varied. As evidence of this fact, Greenfield[1] lists no fewer than 54 causes of a fragmented femoral head, many of which are related to osseous necrosis. Important etiologic factors include trauma (fracture or dislocation), hemoglobinopathies (sickle cell anemia, sickle variant states), exogenous or endogenous hypercortisolism (corticosteroid medication, Cushing's disease), renal transplantation, alcoholism or pancreatitis, dysbaric conditions (caisson disease), small vessel disease (collagen vascular disorders), Gaucher's disease, gout and hyperuricemia, irradiation, and synovitis with elevation of intra-articular pressure (infection, hemophilia) (Fig. 80–1). In some of these conditions, the exact pathogenesis of osteonecrosis has not been defined despite the accumulation of a great deal of clinical and experimental data. There also is a group of patients in whom no underlying causative disorder can be detected. In this situation, the term primary, idiopathic, or spontaneous osteonecrosis is used.

In this chapter, a review of available diagnostic techniques, specific causes or situations, and complications of osteonecrosis is provided. The reader should refer to Chapter 79 as well as to additional relevant sections of the book for discussion of many of the other systemic disorders that may be associated with osseous necrosis.

DIAGNOSTIC TECHNIQUES

Radiography

The plain film radiographic findings of osteonecrosis of an epiphysis, metaphysis, or diaphysis in a tubular bone or of a flat or irregular bone are so characteristic that additional diagnostic methods frequently are not required. Arc-like subchondral radiolucent lesions, patchy lucent areas and sclerosis, osseous collapse, and preservation of the joint space in an epiphyseal region (Fig. 80–2), lucent shadows with a peripheral rim of sclerosis and periostitis in a diametaphyseal region (Fig. 80–3), and patchy lucent areas and sclerosis with bony collapse in a flat or irregular bone (Fig. 80–4) are typical radiographic signs of osteonecrosis.

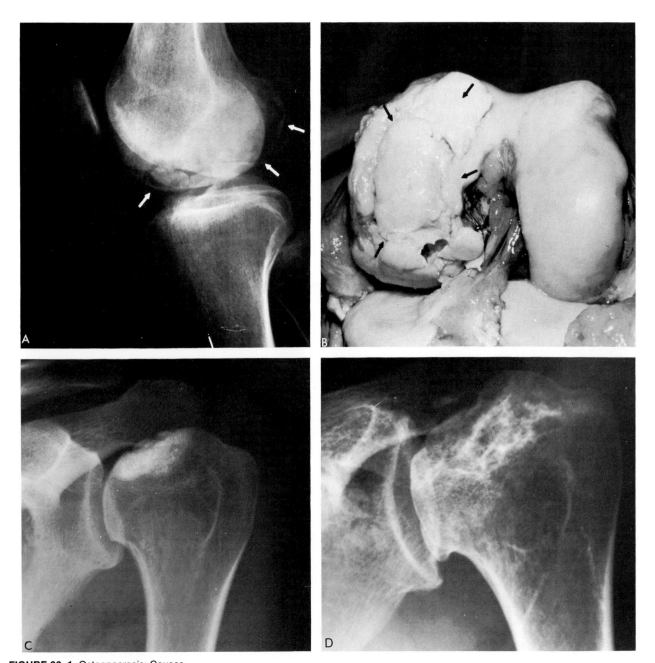

FIGURE 80–1. Osteonecrosis: Causes.

  A, B Exogenous hypercortisolism. Note the extensive osseous fragmentation of the medial femoral condyle (arrows).

  C Renal transplantation. The radiodense ("snow-capped") appearance of the humeral head with associated collapse and fragmentation of bone is typical of osteonecrosis at this site. The joint space is maintained.

  D Alcoholism and pancreatitis. Osteonecrosis of the humeral head is associated with sclerosis and collapse of the articular surface.

Unfortunately, these abnormalities do not appear for several months after the onset of clinical manifestations in many persons and, therefore, do not represent a sensitive indication of early disease (Fig. 80–5). Furthermore, the initial radiographic features of osteonecrosis, especially in the diametaphyseal portions of tubular bones, may lack specificity. Subtle, mottled, poorly defined radiolucent lesions in this situation may simulate the aggressive pattern of bone destruction that accompanies a variety of malignant tumors as well as osteomyelitis.[247] Even in its healing or reparative stage, osteonecrosis may lead to radiographic alterations that resemble those of bone sarcomas.[248]

Radiographs obtained during the application of traction can be useful, especially about the hip.[2] This technique may accentuate the curvilinear radiolucent shadow that is evident in an osteonecrotic epiphysis, perhaps due to the release of gas in the zone of subchondral separation with the induction of a vacuum by traction. A traction force of 30 to 50 lb can be applied manually to each leg for approximately 10 seconds prior to and during the x-ray exposure. It is necessary to fix the patient's position by having him or her grasp the end of the radiographic table or by having an attendant support the patient under the arms. The failure of intra-articular gas to be released during this procedure can indicate the presence of joint fluid.[3]

Conventional Tomography

Conventional tomography occasionally is indicated for the accurate diagnosis of osteonecrosis. In this condition, a radiolucent lesion of an epiphysis with surrounding sclerosis detected on plain film radiography may simulate the appearance of a primary bone tumor, such as a giant cell tumor or chondroblastoma[4]; tomography may indicate angular or wedge-shaped lesional margins and subtle collapse of the osseous surface, allowing a precise diagnosis of bone necrosis (Fig. 80–6). Laminography of a diametaphyseal lesion or one in a flat or irregular bone similarly may define characteristic features of osteonecrosis in difficult cases.

Computed Tomography

CT evaluation of ischemic necrosis of bone (especially in the femoral head) has been accomplished with two goals in mind: to allow early diagnosis of the condition, and to identify the presence and extent of bone collapse—information that guides the orthopedic surgeon in the choice of an appropriate therapeutic procedure.

With regard to the early detection of ischemic necrosis of bone, the advantages of CT over other diagnostic methods are questionable. Although it appears that this technique will delineate subtle alterations of bone necrosis at a time when routine radiographs are normal, it also is apparent that scintigraphy and MR imaging are far more sensitive in this respect (see later discussion).[234, 249] Previous reports indicating the application of CT to the initial diagnosis of osteonecrosis (in the femoral head) underscore the technical necessity of closely spaced transaxial scans and image windows ideal for bone display.[142, 143] Subtle changes in the trabecular architecture are observed, the recognition of which requires knowledge of the normal cross-sectional pattern of trabeculae.

Transaxial CT scans of the normal femoral head demonstrate the principal trabecular groups, which are oriented as arches intersecting one another at roughly right angles. The *primary compressive group* of trabeculae, which extends from the proximal medial cortex of the femoral neck to the superior articular surface of the femoral head in a fanlike, radiating pattern, is seen as a dense interconnecting network of sheets on transaxial images through the upper portion of the femoral head. Inferiorly, these trabeculae blend into the medial femoral cortex. The *primary tensile group* of trabeculae, which arises from the lateral cortex just below the greater trochanter and curves upward and medially across the femoral neck, ending at the inferomedial aspect of the femoral head, along with the *secondary compressive, secondary tensile,* and *greater trochanter groups* of trabeculae, is visualized as an interwoven network of sheets in which individual trabeculae are not so thick or so closely spaced as those of the primary compressive group. The principal and secondary compressive trabeculae and principal tensile trabeculae enclose an area with a relative paucity of trabeculae termed the trigonum internus femoris or Ward's triangle. This triangle is evident on transaxial CT scans as a region of thin, widely spaced trabeculae bordered medially by the primary compressive group and laterally by the primary tensile group. Within the femoral head, the primary compressive trabeculae and the medial portion of the primary tensile group combine to form an area of apparent condensation of bone that, on transaxial images, appears to have a radiating pattern. This pattern is termed the asterisk or star (Fig. 80–7). Alterations in this pattern are considered early evidence of ischemic necrosis of bone (Fig. 80–8).[142, 143]

In patients with more advanced changes of osteonecrosis of the femoral head, transaxial CT scans reveal centrally or peripherally located circular areas of decreased attenuation.[144–146] At this stage, reformation of the CT data in a sagittal or coronal plane is more useful,[225, 249] delineating areas of subchondral fractures and subtle buckling or collapse of the articular surface (Fig. 80–9). The latter finding has therapeutic significance, as the presence of bone collapse, even when minimal, indicates a more advanced stage of the process (Table 80–1) and limits the number of orthopedic procedures (Table 80–2) that can be employed successfully.[147] Further information in assessing the degree of

Text continued on page 3502

TABLE 80–1. Staging of Ischemic Necrosis of the Femoral Head

Stage	Findings
0	Suspected necrosis but no clinical findings and normal radiographs and bone scan
I	Clinical findings, normal radiographs, and abnormal bone scan
II	Osteopenia, cystic areas, and bone sclerosis on radiographs
III	Crescent sign and subchondral collapse without flattening of the femoral head on radiographs
IV	Flattening of the femoral head and normal joint space on radiographs
V	Joint space narrowing and acetabular abnormalities on radiographs

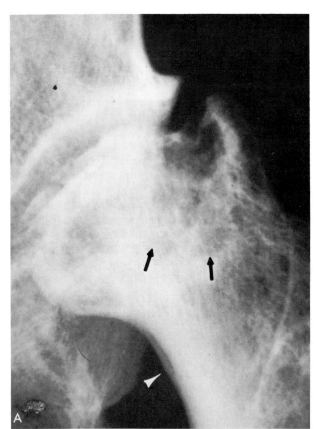

FIGURE 80–2. Osteonecrosis: Epiphysis—radiographic-pathologic correlation.

A The preoperative radiograph outlines extensive collapse of the articular surface of the femoral head with cystic lucent areas (arrows), patchy sclerosis, buttressing (arrowhead), and preservation of joint space.

B, C Sectional radiograph and photograph show displaced cartilage and subchondral bone plate (arrowheads), subjacent osseous resorption (solid arrows), reactive bone formation, and buttressing. Osteophytic lipping is observed (open arrows).

Illustration continued on opposite page

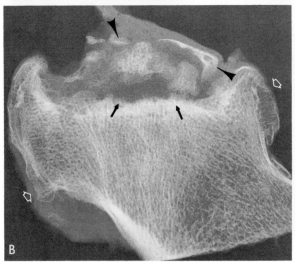

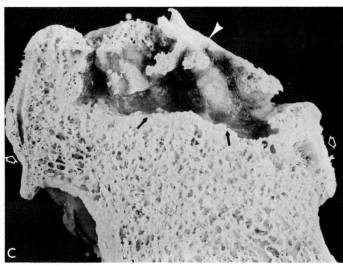

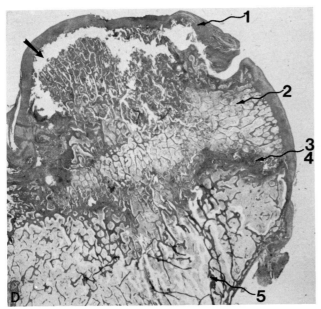

FIGURE 80–2. *Continued*

D A photomicrograph (2×) shows a superficial zone of detached articular cartilage and subarticular trabeculae (1), with subjacent curvilinear area of bony separation (arrow) representing a fracture. Note also a large zone of bone necrosis (2), zones of vascular granulation tissue and new bone formation (3, 4), and deep zone of normal cancellous bone (5).

E A photomicrograph (20×) reveals the superficial zone of detached viable articular cartilage and subarticular trabeculae (1), an area of bony separation or fracture (arrow), and a zone of bone necrosis (2).

F In another area, fibrosis of the marrow space and neovascularization can be identified (20×).

(**A–D,** From Resnick D, et al: AJR *128*:799, 1977. Copyright 1977, American Roentgen Ray Society.)

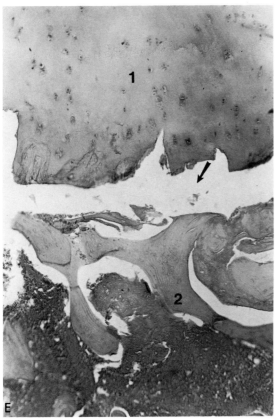

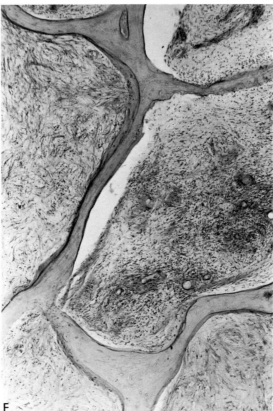

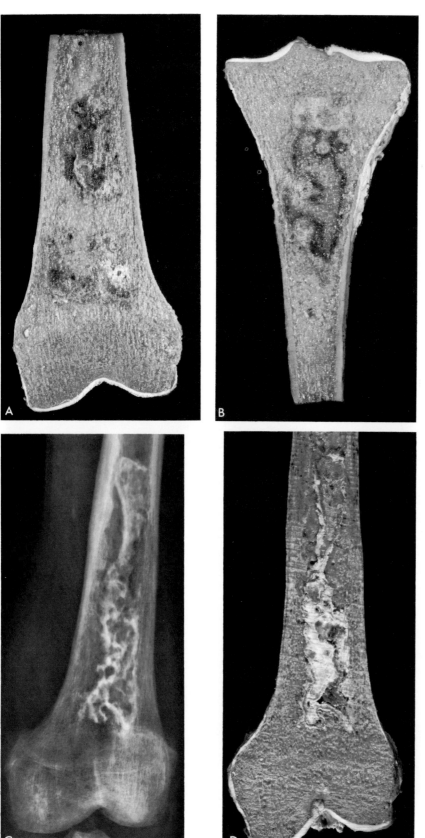

FIGURE 80–3. Osteonecrosis: Diametaphysis—radiographic-pathologic correlation.

A A photograph of the cut surface of the lower part of the left femur removed at autopsy from a 42 year old woman who had had clinical manifestations of systemic lupus erythematosus for about 4 years reveals a relatively large and recent intramedullary infarct in the femoral shaft. This patient had received corticosteroid medications.

B A photograph of the cut surface of the upper part of the tibia shows a large irregularly contoured area of infarction in the shaft. Except in the uppermost portion, where the infarcted area appears whitish, the infarct has a dark peripheral zone of hemorrhagic discoloration.

C A radiograph of the lower half of the left femur of a 69 year old man with intermittent claudication of 4 years' duration demonstrates a bony infarction. Observe the typical shell-like calcification of the lesion.

D A photograph of the cut surface of the lower half of the left femur after amputation of the leg demonstrates necrotic spongy bone and marrow, which are walled off by calcified collagenous fibrous tissue, which varies in thickness from place to place and is serpentine in configuration. In some of the resultant locules, there are residual areas of necrotic spongiosa and fatty marrow.

(From Jaffe HL: Med Radiogr Photogr *45*:58, 1969.)

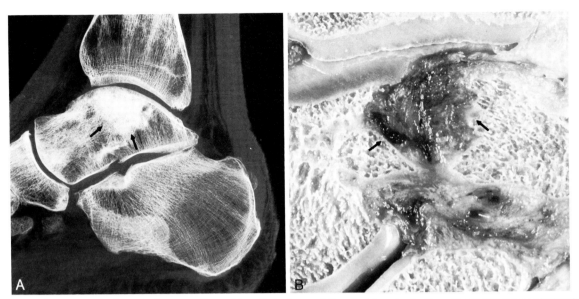

FIGURE 80–4. Osteonecrosis: Irregular bone—radiographic-pathologic correlation. In this patient with corticosteroid-induced ischemic necrosis of bone, observe the sclerotic zone in the talus (as well as the calcaneus), corresponding in position to an irregular hemorrhagic area of infarction (arrows).

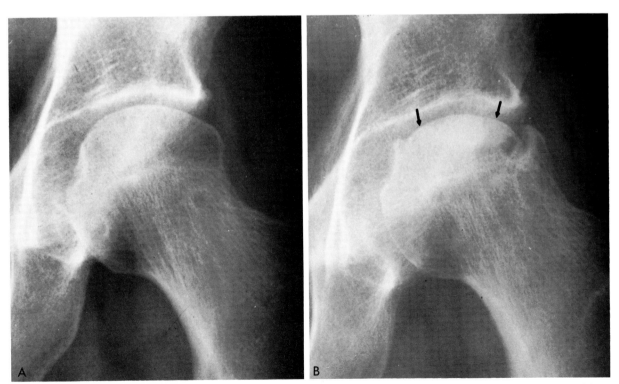

FIGURE 80–5. Osteonecrosis: Inadequacy of radiographic examination. This 35 year old man had had hip pain at the time of his initial radiographic examination, which progressed over the subsequent 6 to 9 months.
  A The initial radiograph was interpreted as normal. A bone scan or MR imaging examination was not accomplished.
  B Seven months later, significant collapse of the superolateral aspect of the femoral head is identified (arrows). The joint is not narrowed.

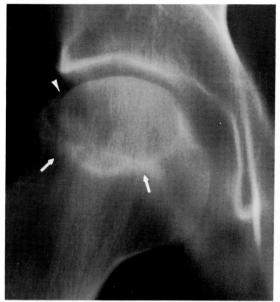

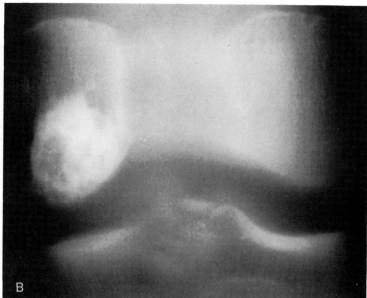

A

FIGURE 80–6. Osteonecrosis: Value of conventional tomography.

A Although the lesion of the femoral head resembles a bone neoplasm, such as a chondroblastoma, typical signs of ischemic necrosis are the curvilinear zone of bone sclerosis (arrows) and the subtle depression of the articular surface (arrowhead). (Courtesy of P. VanderStoep, M.D., Saint Cloud, Minnesota.)

B In a different patient, conventional tomography shows a characteristic appearance of osteonecrosis of the medial femoral condyle, with an irregular sclerotic zone surrounding central radiolucent areas. (Courtesy of P. Kindynis, M.D., Geneva, Switzerland.)

TABLE 80–2. Some Surgical Methods of Treatment of Ischemic Necrosis of the Femoral Head

Method	Rationale
Drilling or forage	Multiple drill holes in the femoral head and neck to establish channels for revascularization
Core decompression	Coring device to create large and small channels from trochanteric region to femoral head, allowing decompression of elevated intraosseous pressure
Free bone grafts with cancellous or cortical bone	Placement of cortical bone (for mechanical support) or cancellous bone (for rapid incorporation) into channels in the femoral head and neck
Vascularized bone grafts with attached muscle pedicle	Same as for free bone grafts except living rather than dead bone is used
Osteochondral allograft	Replacement of collapsed portion of the articular surface with allograft
Osteotomy: Varus or valgus	Shift of femoral head in acetabulum to provide new weight-bearing area
Rotational	Rotation of femoral head in acetabulum to provide new weight-bearing area
Electrical stimulation	Use of electrical current to induce bone formation
Arthroplasty	Replacement of abnormal femoral head (and acetabulum) with prosthesis

osseous involvement in the femoral head is provided by three-dimensional image display of the CT data, a technique that requires a scanning strategy composed of contiguous or overlapping, thin transaxial sections of the involved area. This strategy necessitates a longer examination time, more radiation exposure, and an absence of patient movement (see Chapter 8).

Scintigraphy

The relative insensitivity of radiography in the early detection of osteonecrosis has led to the use of other techniques, including angiography,[5, 6] venography,[7–9] and scintigraphy.[10–12, 130, 131, 133, 148–153, 234, 249–252] Although intraosseous phlebography or pressure readings may reveal elevated intraosseous pressure in the initial stages of osteonecrosis (see later discussion),[132] the radionuclide examination is considered one of the most attractive techniques for early diagnosis of this disorder. Single photon emission computed tomography (SPECT) imaging may further improve the radionuclide sensitivity for such diagnosis.[250] Establishing a correct diagnosis at an initial stage is important, as the success of some of the proposed orthopedic procedures requires their application prior to the appearance of collapse of the articular surface. Scintigraphy may be especially useful in studying the contralateral ''silent'' hip in cases of apparent unilateral osteonecrosis of the femoral head.[129]

Immediately after interruption of the osseous blood supply, scintigraphy with bone-seeking radiopharmaceutical agents can reveal an area of decreased or absent uptake, a ''cold'' lesion. This finding has diagnostic significance, as only a few processes, including infection, plasma cell myeloma, skeletal metastasis, hemangioma, and irradiation, lead to localized regions of diminished radiotracer uptake. After weeks or months, reparative processes in the surrounding

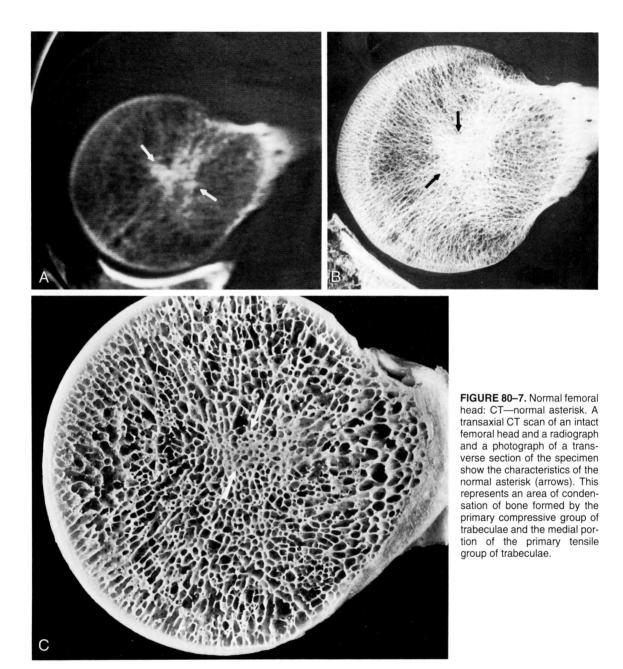

FIGURE 80–7. Normal femoral head: CT—normal asterisk. A transaxial CT scan of an intact femoral head and a radiograph and a photograph of a transverse section of the specimen show the characteristics of the normal asterisk (arrows). This represents an area of condensation of bone formed by the primary compressive group of trabeculae and the medial portion of the primary tensile group of trabeculae.

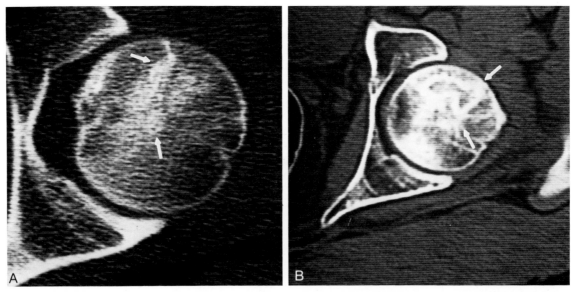

FIGURE 80–8. Osteonecrosis: Value of CT—abnormal asterisk sign. Early **(A)** and later **(B)** stages of ischemic necrosis are characterized by modifications (arrows) of the normal asterisk (compare with Fig. 80–7). The radiodense zone of crossing trabeculae reaches the articular surface of the femoral head and, in **B,** is associated with cystic alterations.

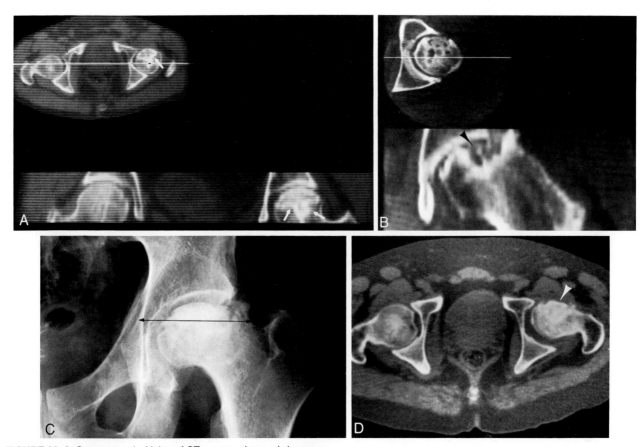

FIGURE 80–9. Osteonecrosis: Value of CT—more advanced changes.

A A transaxial CT scan (top) and a coronal reconstruction (bottom) illustrate a curvilinear zone of sclerosis (arrows) diagnostic of ischemic necrosis of the femoral head. No collapse of the articular surface is evident.

B In similar images from a different patient, observe intraosseous cysts and collapse (arrowhead) of the femoral head. The joint space is narrowed and there is lateral subluxation of the femoral head.

C, D In this patient with advanced ischemic necrosis and considerable deformity of the femoral head, a transaxial CT scan at the approximate level shown in **C** documents the extent of the irregularity of the anterior surface of the bone (arrowhead). Note the forward subluxation of the femoral head and the normal asterisk on the opposite side.

bone are associated with revascularization and increased accumulation of the radioisotope, a "hot" lesion[13, 14] (Fig. 80–10). At some point between these two stages, early in the course of the process, the radionuclide examination can be normal. Even when abnormal, the study is not specific and must be interpreted with knowledge of the radiographic and clinical findings. Furthermore, the scintiscan results, reflecting the absence or presence of regional blood flow, do not evaluate the adequacy or permanency of the vascular supply.[14]

Bone marrow scans with ^{99m}Tc-sulfur colloid also have been used to evaluate osteonecrosis (Fig. 80–11).[15] Normally, after intravenous administration of this agent, approximately 80 to 90 per cent of the substance is phagocytized in the liver and spleen and approximately 10 to 20 per cent is accumulated by phagocytes in the bone marrow.[16] A decrease in accumulation is suggestive of deficient or severely impaired circulation and, as such, may have predictive value regarding the likelihood of subsequent osteonecrosis and the need for surgical intervention. Bone marrow imaging may be more useful than bone imaging in identifying loss of normal vascularity in the femoral head immediately after femoral neck fractures or hip dislocations owing to an earlier loss of function in the marrow cells than in the osteocytes.[152] Investigation with both bone marrow-seeking and bone-seeking agents also may be effective in the assessment of osteonecrosis.[13]

Magnetic Resonance Imaging

The number of scientific publications devoted to the assessment of ischemic necrosis of bone with MR imaging that have appeared in the last decade is extraordinary.[154–156, 230–232, 234–241] To reach firm conclusions regarding the precise role of MR imaging in this assessment, it is appropriate to review briefly some of the more recent and important of these publications. Mitchell and colleagues,[232, 234, 241, 253, 254] in a series of articles in 1986 and 1987, provided some of the initial data examining the sensitivity of MR imaging in patients with osteonecrosis of the femoral head. The results of these studies underscored the superior sensitivity of this method in comparison to radionuclide bone scanning and CT,[234] and indicated the early conversion of hematopoietic marrow to fatty marrow in the proximal portion of the femur in most patients with ischemic necrosis of the femoral head.[241] The authors speculated that such necrosis was indicative of decreased vascularity of the proximal portion of the femur and represented a means of identifying patients with an increased risk for osteonecrosis.[241] In a detailed analysis of the MR imaging appearance of ischemic necrosis of the femoral head, in which the MR imaging features were compared with standard staging methods provided by routine radiography, Mitchell and colleagues[253] emphasized a characteristic double line sign, delineated with T2-weighted spin echo images, in which an outer band of low signal intensity was associated with an inner border of high signal intensity (Fig. 80–12). These investigators classified the signal characteristics of the central portion of the necrotic area into four categories on the bases of the appearances of this region on both T1- and T2-weighted spin echo images: type A pattern was accompanied by high signal intensity on the T1-weighted images and intermediate sig-

nal intensity on the T2-weighted images, a pattern analogous to that of fat; type B pattern was characterized by high signal intensity on both T1- and T2-weighted images, analogous to the appearance of blood; type C pattern was associated with low signal intensity on T1-weighted images and high signal intensity on T2-weighted images, a pattern consistent with the presence of fluid; and type D pattern was accompanied by low signal intensity on both T1- and T2-weighted images, consistent with the presence of fibrous tissue (Fig. 80–13). When the MR imaging patterns were correlated with clinical and radiographic findings, a chronologic sequence appeared to exist in which early osteonecrosis was characterized by retention of normal fat signal throughout the lesion (type A) except for the peripheral rims and advanced osteonecrosis was characterized by low signal intensity throughout the lesion (type D), presumably because marrow fat had been replaced by fibrosis and bone sclerosis.

To investigate the pathogenesis of the double line sign further, Mitchell and coworkers[254] used both conventional and chemical shift MR imaging techniques as well as available pathologic material derived from cadavers and from the femoral heads in patients undergoing total hip replacements. Histologic correlation indicated that the low-intensity outer rim was related to sclerotic bone while the high-intensity inner border was due to granulation tissue or chondroid metaplasia, or to both. Although subsequent studies of the double line phenomenon have indicated other possible causative factors (see later discussion), its value as a specific indicator of osteonecrosis rarely has been challenged.

In 1987, two histopathologic studies of osteonecrotic femoral heads accentuated the complexity of the MR imaging signal characteristics of this process. One of these, that of Bassett and coworkers,[255] was based on the analysis of a single resected specimen that was examined only with T1-weighted spin echo images accomplished with a low field strength (0.3 Tesla) permanent magnet. A subchondral focus of diminished signal intensity was shown to represent saponified fat, consisting also of a transudate of proteinaceous material with probable calcifications. A subjacent region of normal high signal intensity represented mummified fat, and an additional region of diminished signal intensity was composed of fibrous and vascular tissues with histiocytic infiltrates. The second study, that of Takatori and colleagues,[256] was based on an analysis of eight femoral heads derived from six patients with osteonecrosis in whom both T1- and T2-weighted spin echo MR images obtained at 1.5 Tesla were available. Regions of low signal intensity in the femoral heads corresponded to foci of fibrovascular tissue or amorphous necrotic material. Necrotic marrow without revascularization showed high signal intensity. In this same year, the sensitivity of MR imaging in comparison to bone scintigraphy and routine radiography in patients at risk for osteonecrosis was emphasized by Markisz and colleagues,[257] and the specificity of segmental patterns of decreased signal intensity on T1-weighted spin echo MR images in the diagnosis of ischemic necrosis of the femoral head was also emphasized. Conflicting data were presented by Kulkarni and associates,[258] who, using pinhole collimator imaging, indicated a superiority of bone scintigraphy over MR imaging in the diagnosis of osteonecrosis of the

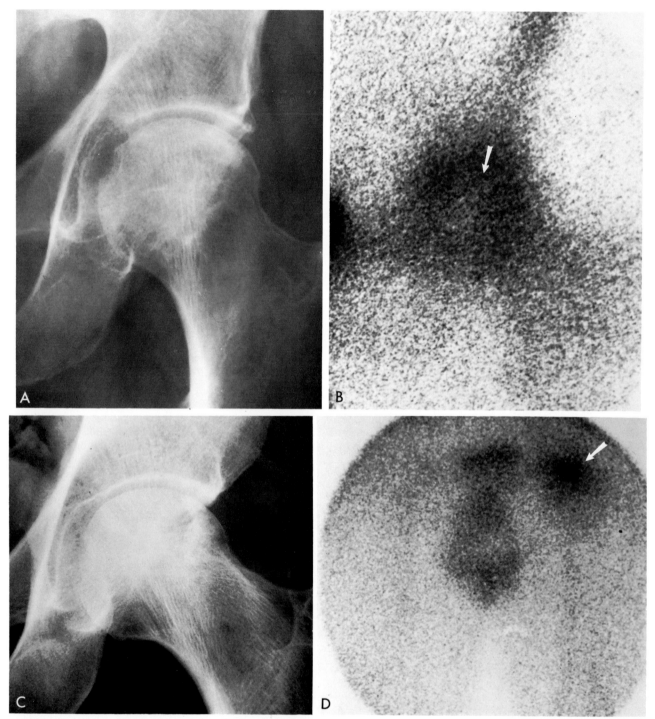

FIGURE 80–10. Osteonecrosis: Value of radionuclide examination—bone scan.

A, B A radiograph of the hip in this 55 year old man reveals a mild degree of patchy sclerosis of the femoral head without collapse of the articular surface. The scan of the hip using technetium pyrophosphate depicts a central area of diminished uptake surrounded by a zone of augmented activity (arrow).

C, D In a different patient with osteonecrosis, the radiograph outlines subchondral resorption and cyst formation without collapse, and the scan with technetium pyrophosphate demonstrates an area of increased uptake of isotope in the left hip (arrow). Note the activity in the bladder.

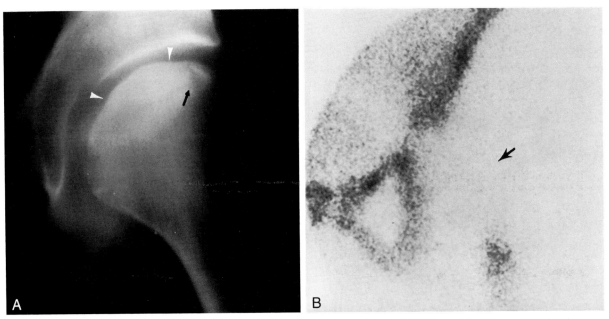

FIGURE 80–11. Osteonecrosis: Value of radionuclide examination—bone marrow scan. In this 50 year old woman, conventional tomography **(A)** shows an area of osseous collapse in the femoral head (arrowheads), bone sclerosis, and a crescent sign (arrow). The sulfur colloid bone marrow scan **(B)** reveals no uptake in the proximal portion of the femur (arrow), indicative of necrosis. (Courtesy of V. Vint, M.D., San Diego, California.)

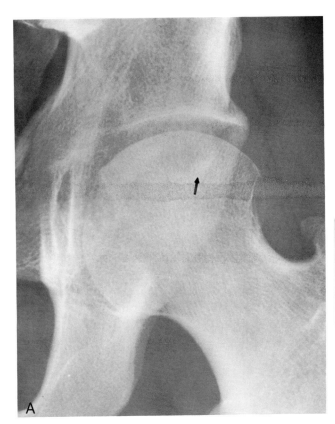

FIGURE 80–12. Osteonecrosis: Value of MR imaging. Double line sign. In this patient with sickle cell anemia, direct radiographic magnification **(A)** reveals a subtle sclerotic zone (arrow), which corresponds in position to an area in **B** characterized by a peripheral region of decreased signal intensity and a central region of increased signal intensity (arrow) on the coronal T2-weighted spin echo display. (Courtesy of L. Rogers, M.D., Chicago, Illinois.)

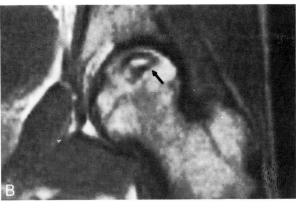

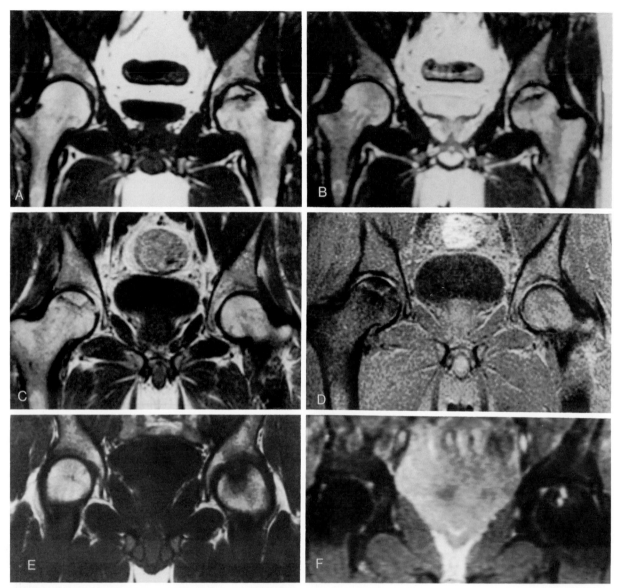

FIGURE 80–13. Osteonecrosis: Value of MR imaging. Classification system.

A, B Type A pattern. Coronal T1-weighted (TR/TE, 600/20) **(A)** and T2-weighted (TR/TE, 2500/70) **(B)** spin echo MR images reveal an area of osteonecrosis in the left femoral head in which a serpentine region of low signal intensity surrounds a central region whose signal characteristics are identical to those of fat.

C, D Type A pattern. Coronal T1-weighted (TR/TE, 600/20) **(C)** and coronal T1-weighted (TR/TE, 650/20) fat suppressed (ChemSat) **(D)** spin echo MR images show osteonecrosis of the right femoral head. In **C,** note the central region displaying signal intensity characteristics of fat surrounded by a curvilinear zone of low signal intensity. In **D,** suppression of the fat signal within the central zone is evident, and a peripheral region of higher signal intensity is seen.

E, F Type C pattern. On the coronal T1-weighted (TR/TE, 600/20) spin echo image **(E),** the area of osteonecrosis in the left femoral head is of low signal intensity. It was of high signal intensity on a T2-weighted image (not shown) and on a short tau inversion recovery (STIR) image (TR/TE, 2200/15; inversion time, 160 msec) **(F).**

femoral heads in two patients with collagen vascular disease in whom the results of venous pressure measurements were used as the gold standard.

In 1988, major articles once again addressed the issues of sensitivity of MR imaging in the diagnosis of osteonecrosis of the femoral head, its diagnostic role versus that of bone scintigraphy, and histopathologic correlation of the MR imaging findings. Coleman and associates,[259] in an assessment of the clinical and imaging records of 24 consecutive patients with ischemic necrosis of the femoral head whose diagnosis was based on established MR imaging criteria and, in some instances, on histologic evaluation of material derived from core decompression, emphasized the ability of MR imaging to allow detection and staging of early osteonecrosis at this skeletal site at a time when the results of routine radiography were negative. These investigators also indicated the superior sensitivity of MR imaging when compared with either radionuclide imaging or CT scanning in this clinical situation, the occurrence of a hip effusion even in the earliest stages of osteonecrosis, and the possible association of clinical manifestations with such fluid. The majority of the early lesions seen with MR imaging revealed a type A pattern with signal characteristics identical to those of fat. Glickstein and coworkers,[260] in an investigation of both ischemic and nonischemic hip disease, observed the high sensitivity of MR imaging in the differentiation of osteonecrosis from normality and from a variety of other disorders, including rheumatoid arthritis, osteoarthritis, and traumatic and neoplastic conditions. A team of five experienced radiologists, in a blinded fashion, used such findings as the double line sign and fluid within subchondral fractures to make this differentiation. Although the studies of Coleman and associates[259] and Glickstein and colleagues[260] indicated the value of MR imaging in the diagnosis of early as well as late osteonecrosis, the results of an investigation by Genez and coworkers[261] were less encouraging. These last investigators used the findings of elevated intramedullary pressure in the femoral head and histologic evidence of osteonecrosis in specimens derived from core decompression procedures as the gold standards for diagnosis, and MR imaging was positive in the assessment of only 5 of 11 femoral heads that, by these standards, were sites of osteonecrosis. The MR images were obtained with either low (0.3 Tesla) or medium (1.0 Tesla) strength magnets using coronal and transaxial spin echo sequences. Although Beltran and coworkers[262] also reported some examples of negative MR images (coronal and transaxial spin echo sequences with T1-, proton density, and T2-weighting) in patients with osteonecrosis of the femoral head proved by positive results of bone marrow biopsy, bone marrow pressure measurements, and bone scintigraphy, these authors concluded that the sensitivity and the specificity of MR imaging in the diagnosis of this condition were superior to those of bone scintigraphy.

Further histopathologic-MR imaging correlative data were provided by Lang and associates[263] in a study of six femoral head specimens with ischemic necrosis. These authors concluded that proton density coronal spin echo MR images helped in the differentiation of necrotic degraded bone marrow with amorphous intertrabecular debris (characterized by low signal intensity) and viable mesenchymal repair tissue (characterized by higher signal intensity) but that more accurate differentiation of viable and necrotic

tissue required correlation of signal intensity data and anatomic and morphologic characteristics of the abnormal regions.

Many of these early reports of MR imaging of the necrotic femoral head were based on results of relatively low resolution, large field of view, coronal images produced with the imager body radiofrequency receiver coils. In 1988, in a prospective study of 30 hips in 15 patients with suspected ischemic necrosis of the femoral head, Shuman and coworkers[264] evaluated the ability of small field of view, sagittal, surface coil images to produce information useful for surgical planning beyond that available on these coronal images (Fig. 80–14). With a high field strength (1.5 Tesla) magnet, 5 mm thick slices, and various combinations of T1-, proton density, and T2-weighted spin echo MR sequences, these investigators concluded that although typical coronal images represented an adequate screening examination for the presence of ischemic necrosis and were preferable for mediolateral localization of focal abnormality, assessment of joint fluid, and detection of fatty conversion of marrow, superior results were obtained with sagittal, small field of view, surface coil images for anteroposterior localization and the detection of joint space narrowing, articular cartilage fracture, and, occasionally, the double line sign.

Additional publications related to MR imaging of osteonecrosis of the femoral head appeared in 1989.[265–270] In general, the results of many of these investigations confirmed those in previous reports, including data that indicated the high sensitivity and specificity of this imaging method in the diagnosis of early (radiographic stages I and II) osteonecrosis,[265, 266, 269] the diagnostic importance of the double line sign,[268] and the value of the MR staging system that had been described initially in 1987.[268] Miller and colleagues[270] compared MR imaging and SPECT in the detection of osteonecrosis of the femoral head in 29 hips with clinical, radiographic, and, in some persons, histologic evidence of such necrosis. Although only T1-weighted MR images in the coronal plane were employed, the authors found that MR imaging was more sensitive in this detection than SPECT.

Almost uniformly, the MR imaging characteristics of osteonecrosis in the previously cited investigations had included focal abnormalities in the head of the femur. The foci were of variable size and had appeared as wedges, bands, lines, rings, or subchondral crescents. Turner and coworkers,[267] however, in an investigation of six painful hips in five patients, reported diffuse marrow abnormalities without focal lesions. The diagnosis of osteonecrosis in these cases was based either on subsequent core biopsies (three cases) or on the later development of focal MR imaging abnormalities previously reported to be highly specific for osteonecrosis (three cases). The diffuse MR imaging pattern, which was characterized by low signal intensity in the femoral head and neck on T1-weighted images and high signal intensity in these same regions on T2-weighted images, was identical to that seen in cases of bone marrow edema occurring in a variety of disorders, such as transient osteoporosis, osteomyelitis, and stress fracture. These results suggested that bone marrow edema may be an early, nonspecific response to an ischemic insult, that the pattern of edema might resolve or be followed by more diagnostic focal abnormalities of osteonecrosis, and that a relationship

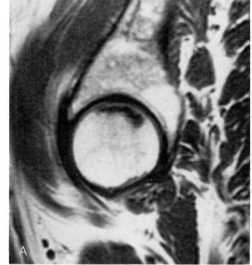

FIGURE 80–14. Osteonecrosis: Value of MR imaging. Sagittal plane.

A A T1-weighted (TR/TE, 966/12) sagittal spin echo MR image shows a characteristic serpentine region of low signal intensity, diagnostic of osteonecrosis of the femoral head.

B, C More advanced changes of osteonecrosis are displayed on coronal T1-weighted (TR/TE, 800/20) **(B)** and sagittal T1-weighted (TR/TE, 600/20) **(C)** spin echo images.

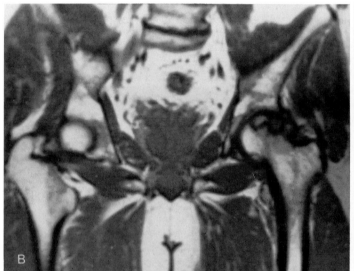

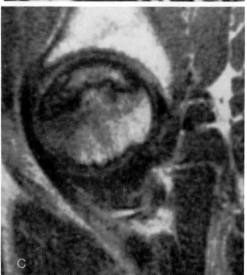

might exist between transient, painful bone marrow edema (or osteoporosis) and ischemic necrosis of the femoral head.

The accumulating data that confirmed the ability of MR imaging to allow detection of osteonecrosis of the femoral head at a time when results of routine radiography as well as bone scintigraphy were normal suggested that this diagnostic technique might be extremely valuable in the identification of those patients with the disease who would benefit from core decompression. Difficulty in determining the precise efficacy of core decompression, however, particularly in asymptomatic patients, has been emphasized as the natural history of the early stages of ischemic necrosis of the femoral head is not clear. In 1991, Kopecky and co-workers[271] investigated the natural history of the MR imaging findings of osteonecrosis of the femoral head in renal allograft recipients, a group at risk for the development of the disease. These investigators reconfirmed the high sensitivity of MR imaging in the detection of osteonecrosis. They found MR imaging abnormalities typical of ischemia and necrosis even in asymptomatic patients. Furthermore, such abnormalities in some of these asymptomatic patients regressed in size and even disappeared over a period of 1 to 2 years with conservative management (Fig. 80–15). The

MR imaging lesions in the asymptomatic patients were smaller than those in the symptomatic persons. Although previous studies had indicated that the likelihood of collapse of the femoral head was less after core decompression of small lesions than after decompression of large lesions,[272] the results of the study by Kopecky and associates[271] suggested that such small lesions may improve spontaneously. Deficiencies of the latter investigation, however, included a limited number of patients and the absence of biopsy proof of the histologic nature of the small lesions.

To define the earliest MR imaging features of osteonecrosis, Brody and coworkers[273] devascularized the distal end of the femur of adult beagle dogs surgically and performed T1-weighted spin echo MR imaging and histologic examinations. The resulting abnormalities were divided into four stages: stage 1 was seen in the first days after operation and revealed homogeneous high signal intensity on MR imaging and only subtle histologic changes of early fat necrosis; stage 2 was apparent within the first week after operation and consisted of linear regions of low signal intensity within the high signal intensity marrow on MR imaging, with fat necrosis and an inflammatory infiltrate found on histologic analysis; stage 3, seen by 16 days after

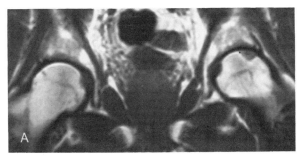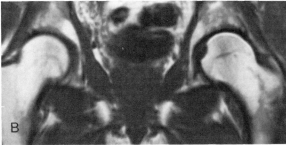

FIGURE 80–15. Osteonecrosis: Value of MR imaging. Spontaneous resolution of abnormalities. In this asymptomatic 40 year old man who had undergone renal transplantation, a coronal T1-weighted (TR/TE, 800/20) spin echo MR image **(A)**, obtained 3 months after transplantation, shows a small focal abnormality in the superior portion of the left femoral head. Fourteen months after transplantation **(B)**, the lesion has disappeared (TR/TE, 800/20). (From Kopecky KK, et al: Radiology *179*:523, 1991.)

operation, showed patchy areas of low signal intensity occupying most of the marrow on MR imaging with a fibrocytic infiltrate on histologic sections; and stage 4, seen by 23 days after operation, showed a more homogeneous low and intermediate signal intensity on MR imaging and histologic findings of more organized fibrocytes and the onset of new bone formation. Although the observations were confined to an animal model and to the avascular zone, the results of this study indicated clearly that MR imaging can show marrow changes as early as 1 week after the onset of ischemic necrosis of bone.

A somewhat similar animal study of osteonecrosis investigated with both MR imaging and scintigraphy was reported by Ruland and colleagues[252] in 1992 with different results. They performed subcapital osteotomies of the femoral neck of rabbits. Bone scintigraphy was found to be more sensitive than MR imaging in the detection of osteonecrosis (which was proved histologically) 3, 5, and 12 days after osteotomy, the radionuclide findings being characterized by decreased uptake of the radiotracer. Despite histologic evidence of necrotic hematopoietic elements in the marrow, MR images remained unremarkable in the first 4 to 6 weeks after operation. Although fat cells generally die within 2 to 5 days after devascularization and MR imaging of bone marrow largely is dependent on the presence and signal characteristics of fat, the results of this study would appear to indicate that MR imaging does not allow effective discrimination between viable and dead fatty marrow. The authors found, however, that MR imaging abnormalities did accompany the reparative process with its associated fibrovascular tissue invasion of the necrotic marrow elements.

More recent studies have confirmed again the sensitivity of MR imaging in the setting of osteonecrosis,[348] its usefulness in the screening for this complication in asymptomatic populations at risk,[274, 349] and its potential role in the prediction of subsequent segmental collapse in osteonecrotic femoral heads.[251, 350, 358] Furthermore, a number of investigations have examined the role of contrast-enhanced MR imaging of the necrotic femoral head. Li and Hiette[275] employed chemical presaturation of fat (ChemSat) as well as the intravenous administration of a gadolinium chelate in combination with spin echo imaging in an analysis of 75 hips in 40 patients with hip pain. Although histologic data were not available in every instance, 18 hips in 11 patients were believed to contain necrotic femoral heads. Three distinct patterns of contrast enhancement were identified, particu-

larly with the use of T1-weighted images combined with fat saturation: a focal area of poorly enhancing tissue surrounded by a brightly enhancing rim; diffuse enhancement of the femoral head and neck; and a combination of the first two patterns of enhancement. The authors concluded that nontraumatic osteonecrosis of the femoral head is associated with hyperemia or an increase in capillary permeability, or both, and that marrow edema is an initial finding of such necrosis. Hauzeur and colleagues[276] used standard and gadolinium contrast-enhanced spin echo MR images of the femoral heads and histologic data derived from core biopsies to correlate the imaging and pathologic findings in a small group of patients with osteonecrosis. Histologic findings that were characterized by trabecular bone necrosis and bone marrow necrosis, accompanied by amorphous eosinophilic debris, were derived from femoral heads that revealed areas of low signal intensity without contrast enhancement on T1-weighted spin echo images and low signal intensity on T2-weighted images. Trabecular bone necrosis associated with mummified fat cells revealed MR imaging characteristics of normal T1- and T2-weighted signal intensity. Trabecular bone necrosis with fibrosis filling the intertrabecular spaces produced low signal intensity on T1-weighted images with enhancement of signal intensity after the intravenous administration of a gadolinium contrast agent. Bands of fibrosis without trabecular bone as seen in fracture zones led to low signal intensity on T1-weighted images that was enhanced with a gadolinium chelate and to high signal intensity on T2-weighted images. Thickened trabecular bone with fibrosis, as seen in the process of creeping substitution, had similar signal intensity characteristics, but the signal intensity was low on the T2-weighted images. In addition to confirming a correlation between histologic and MR imaging data, this study indicated that gadolinium chelates could be employed as an intravenous contrast agent in the identification of foci of fibrosis in the necrotic femoral head.

Nadel and coworkers[277] produced devascularized femoral heads surgically in dogs and then imaged the hips within 3 hours of the devascularization. Standard T1-weighted, T2-weighted, and short tau inversion recovery (STIR) MR sequences were employed, and a series of gradient recalled echo images also was obtained at 6 second intervals for 90 sec synchronously with the intravenous administration of gadolinium contrast agent. The dynamic contrast-enhanced MR images proved to be the most sensitive technique in the differentiation of ischemic and normal bone marrow.

Normal bone marrow was characterized by rapid enhancement of signal intensity; avascular marrow showed persistent lack of such enhancement, although contrast enhancement of signal intensity was observed in the interface between normal and avascular marrow.

Vande Berg and colleagues[278] also used gadolinium-enhanced spin echo as well as fat suppression MR imaging in a study of 15 hips with typical radiographic and MR imaging characteristics of osteonecrosis of the femoral head. Histologic correlation provided by evaluation of six resected femoral heads confirmed that enhanced areas corresponded to sites of viable tissue and nonenhanced areas corresponded to regions of necrotic tissue.

Further investigation of the role of intravenous gadolinium chelates as contrast material in the assessment of the viability of the femoral head was accomplished by Lang and associates.[279] Spin echo and gradient echo MR images were used in a study of 13 patients with acute fracture of the femoral neck, and the gradient echo imaging sequences were repeated after the intravenous administration of gadolinium contrast agent. MR imaging findings were correlated with the results of superselective digital subtraction angiograms of the vessels supplying the femoral head. In patients in whom such angiography showed impaired blood supply to the femoral head, enhanced MR images revealed a femoral head that did not show enhancement of signal intensity and whose resultant signal intensity was lower than that in the enhancing ipsilateral femoral shaft and neck and contralateral femoral head. In patients with persistent perfusion, contrast-enhanced MR images showed a uniform increase in the signal intensity in the ipsilateral femoral head, neck, and shaft. The authors concluded that contrast-enhanced MR imaging may serve as a useful method for evaluation of femoral head perfusion after fracture of the femoral neck.

On the basis of a review of available literature, certain observations can be made with regard to MR imaging in the evaluation of osteonecrosis, particularly that in the femoral head:

1. MR imaging represents a very sensitive method for the early diagnosis of ischemic necrosis of bone. It appears to be more sensitive in this regard than standard bone scintigraphy, although the relative sensitivities of MR imaging and SPECT require further analysis. Standard radiography is an insensitive method for the detection of early osteonecrosis, and CT is best applied to an analysis of the extent of involvement in more advanced cases of ischemic necrosis of bone.

2. Although MR imaging abnormalities occur early in the course of osteonecrosis and, in some situations, may be evident within days after an ischemic event, these abnormalities are somewhat variable in their time of occurrence. They are dependent on alterations of the fat cells in the bone marrow. Ischemic changes first become evident in hematopoietic cells, becoming apparent 6 to 12 hours after the ischemic event, and then are observed in the osteocytes, osteoblasts, and osteoclasts, occurring within 2 days of the ischemic event.[280] Fat cells are more resistant to ischemia, surviving for 2 to 5 days after the insult. Furthermore, initial changes in the fat cells may not lead to an alteration in MR imaging signal characteristics. An inflammatory and hyperemic response in viable tissue adjacent to the devascularized regions produces a reactive interface about the osteonecrotic areas that is associated with increased vascularity, inflammation, granulation tissue, and fibrosis.[280] MR imaging is sensitive to the presence of this reactive interface.

MR imaging may allow the identification of changes that place a femoral head at risk for subsequent osteonecrosis. Two such changes, early conversion of hematopoietic to fatty marrow in the proximal femur and prominent physeal scars that serve to close off the femoral head,[363] have been identified, but neither appears to be a sensitive or specific predictor of disease.

3. Variations in the pattern of MR imaging abnormalities are encountered and are indicative of individual differences in the distribution and extent of involvement and the host response.[281] Focal abnormalities predominate, with some component of diminished signal intensity on T1-weighted spin echo images. The regions of altered signal intensity may be homogeneous or inhomogeneous, however. The most characteristic pattern of involvement is the double line appearance, evident on T2-weighted spin echo MR images at the reactive interface between ischemic and nonischemic bone.[282] On T1-weighted spin echo images, this interface is characterized by a line of low signal intensity reflecting the presence of granulation tissue and, to a lesser extent, sclerotic bone. On T2-weighted spin echo images, a narrower line of low signal intensity, reflecting the presence of bone sclerosis, and an inner zone of high signal intensity, indicating the location of granulation tissue, are apparent, and this combination of findings is designated the double line sign. Chemical shift misregistration artifact appears to contribute to the double line sign.[283, 307, 351] On T2-weighted images, the zone of high signal intensity, representing granulation tissue, typically is shifted slightly so that it is misregistered with respect to a coexisting area of low signal intensity with the same size and shape.[284] Thus, a double line sign may occur in the absence of bone sclerosis, although its diagnostic significance remains the same. The absence of a double line sign does not eliminate the diagnosis of osteonecrosis.

Diffusely distributed MR imaging abnormalities in the femoral head and neck may be encountered in cases of osteonecrosis, and the patterns of signal intensity on T1- and T2-weighted spin echo images in such instances may be indistinguishable from those of transient osteoporosis of the hip and, occasionally, infection and tumor.[341, 352, 353] The probable cause of the diffuse lesions is bone marrow edema, although the relationship of such edema to an ischemic event as well as the relationship of osteonecrosis to the condition of transient painful bone marrow edema requires further investigation.[359] A potential role exists for the intravenous administration of a gadolinium compound to allow differentiation of the edema pattern of osteonecrosis from that seen in the painful bone marrow edema syndrome, but this role is not confirmed.

4. Some correlation exists between the MR imaging characteristics of osteonecrosis and histologic parameters, although the results of numerous investigations on this subject are not consistent. Explanations for such inconsistency include variations in the causes of osteonecrosis that have been studied, attention to different stages of the evolving ischemic process, and the nonspecific nature of the various patterns of signal intensity. Furthermore, the prognostic significance of the changes in signal intensity that occur within

the ischemic zone is not clear. Although the presence of fat within this zone appears to correspond to absent or less dramatic radiographic abnormalities and the presence of fibrous tissue corresponds to more extensive radiographic abnormalities, the value of proposed grading systems of osteonecrosis based on MR imaging features is not yet substantiated. Furthermore, despite the presence of MR imaging alterations in instances of fracture and collapse of subchondral bone in osteonecrosis, the superiority of this imaging method to others, such as CT, in the delineation of such advanced abnormalities is not proved.

5. No uniform agreement exists regarding the choice of imaging plane or specific sequence when MR imaging is applied to the evaluation of osteonecrosis of the femoral head. Most authors use and prefer the coronal plane, perhaps related to the fact that anatomic features of the proximal end of the femur are best recognized in this plane. The coronal plane is ideally suited to the analysis of the subchondral bone of the femoral head, although transaxial images may add supplemental data to this analysis. Sagittal images, particularly when combined with the application of surface coils and small fields of view, appear to increase the sensitivity of MR imaging in the diagnosis of early disease. In the sagittal plane, the fovea centralis of the femoral head, a normal anatomic finding, may be misinterpreted as a site of osteonecrosis, however.

As a significant contribution to the MR imaging changes in osteonecrosis relates to the reparative response of the host and, specifically, to the presence of granulation tissue, imaging sequences designed to detect the water content of such tissue may represent a useful adjunct to the standard T1-weighted and T2-weighted spin echo images. STIR sequences, fat saturation or fat suppression techniques, and heavily T2-weighted fast spin echo sequences with or without fat suppression may be beneficial in the assessment of the presence and extent of ischemic necrosis of bone.[360]

Initial reports of the use of intravenous injection of a gadolinium contrast agent as a means of differentiating between viable and nonviable tissue in cases of osteonecrosis have produced encouraging results, but further investigation is required before contrast-enhanced MR images can be recommended as an important diagnostic technique.

6. Although the application of MR imaging to the detection of ischemic necrosis at skeletal sites other than the femoral head has received far less attention,[247, 285, 286] there is little doubt concerning its efficacy (Fig. 80–16). Ischemic changes in the humeral head, about the knee, in the talus, in the diametaphyseal regions of tubular bones, and in other skeletal locations, whether occurring spontaneously, as a result of trauma, or as a complication of an underlying systemic disease process, can be assessed with MR imaging. The basic MR imaging characteristics in these situations are similar or identical to those seen in cases of osteonecrosis of the femoral head, and the MR imaging examination provides greater sensitivity in diagnosis than routine radiography and bone scintigraphy. Furthermore, in some instances, the MR imaging findings are specific for the diagnosis of osteonecrosis, clarifying the nature of routine radiographic changes that may be misinterpreted as evidence of infection or neoplasm.[247] The MR imaging changes that occur in association with diametaphyseal infarction vary according to the stage of the process. Early infarcts may be of intermediate to high signal intensity on T1-weighted sequences and of high signal intensity on T2-weighted sequences; chronic infarcts typically are of low signal intensity on both T1- and T2-weighted images.[247] In both instances, a serpentine zone of low signal intensity, representing bone sclerosis or fibrosis, may surround the necrotic region. Diagnostic difficulty may be encountered in the detection of infarction in hyperplastic marrow when only T1-weighted spin echo MR images are employed because both may have the same low signal intensity.[280] T2-weighted spin echo MR images and the use of intravenous administration of a gadolinium compound may be helpful diagnostically in this particular situation.[361]

7. MR imaging may be a useful technique in the assessment of the response of the osteonecrotic femoral head to operative intervention, especially core decompression. Considerable controversy exists regarding the efficacy of this therapeutic technique, and opposing points of view have been well summarized by Colwell[342] and Hungerford.[343] The rationale for performing core decompression is based on the belief that the basic causative factor in osteonecrosis of the femoral head is intraosseous hypertension. Therefore, core biopsy might seem a logical and rational therapeutic approach, serving to decompress the bone and thereby improving its blood flow,[343] a procedure that would be more effective in the earlier stages of osteonecrosis, prior to the occurrence of irreversible cellular injury or death. Opponents of this treatment option cite flaws in the basic hypothesis: there is no clear indication that venous stasis plays any major role in ischemic necrosis of the femoral head secondary to trauma; the analogy of metaphyseal bone representing the same type of closed space as a soft tissue compartment is not accurate owing to the presence of intraosseous arteries and veins that allow for significant changes in flow rates mediated by neurologic pathways; multiple disorders of the femoral head, including osteoarthritis, have increased venous pressure as part of their pathologic process, and they have not been treated successfully by core decompression; and it has not been shown that venous pressure that is decreased by core decompression remains decreased for any extended time period.[342] Although proponents of core decompression recognize inconsistent and, sometimes, nonbeneficial results of this procedure in some reported series of patients with osteonecrosis of the femoral head, they cite technical factors involved in the surgery or improper choice of candidates for the procedure, or both, as being responsible for such results. Although many authors have concluded that core decompression may not be effective,[344, 345] the procedure continues to enjoy some popularity.

MR imaging accomplished at variable times after core decompression of osteonecrotic femoral heads occasionally may reveal changing patterns of involvement.[346] Ischemic lesions may decrease in size, although this is not seen uniformly and is more likely to occur when initial lesions are small. Patterns of bone marrow edema also may resolve after surgery. Most typically, however, little change in the MR imaging abnormalities is seen, and the signal intensity characteristics of the necrotic zone remain constant.[346]

Other Techniques

Functional exploration of bone is regarded by some investigators as a simple and safe method that is indispensable for diagnosis in the early stages of ischemic necrosis of

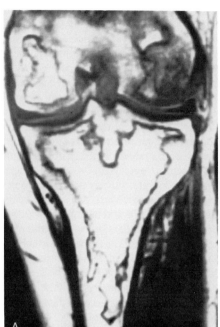
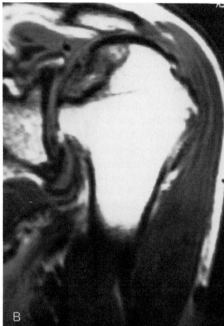
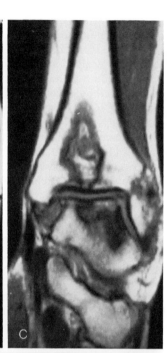
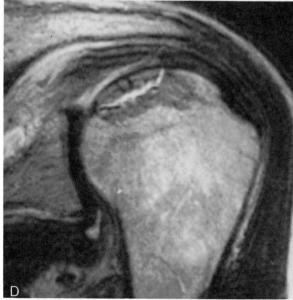

FIGURE 80–16. Osteonecrosis: Value of MR imaging. Involvement of sites other than the femoral head.

A Distal portion of the femur and proximal end of the tibia. A coronal T1-weighted (TR/TE, 600/20) spin echo MR image reveals typical features of osteonecrosis. Note the border of low signal intensity about the ischemic regions.

B Humeral head. A coronal oblique proton density (TR/TE, 1800/20) spin echo MR image shows an irregular region of osteonecrosis in the humeral head. Additional findings include a massive tear of the rotator cuff and a joint effusion.

C Distal portion of the tibia and talus. A coronal T1-weighted (TR/TE, 850/20) spin echo MR image reveals ischemic zones that involve subchondral bone.

(**C,** Courtesy of P. Wilson, M.D., Eugene, Oregon.)

D Humeral head. A coronal oblique T2-weighted (TR/TE, 3600/96) fast spin echo MR image shows classic features of osteonecrosis, including a crescent sign.

(**D,** Courtesy of S. Eilenberg, M.D., San Diego, California.)

bone.[242] This method has been well summarized by Ficat,[157] whose analysis is included here. Measurement of the *pressure in the bone marrow* in the femoral head can be accomplished with the introduction of a cannula placed in the intertrochanteric region under local anesthesia; the normal baseline pressure is approximately 20 mm Hg and values above 30 mm Hg are regarded as abnormal.[157] A stress test used in conjunction with this pressure determination is provided by the injection of 5 ml of isotonic saline solution into the bone; a normal response is an elevation of bone marrow pressure of less than 10 mm Hg above the baseline level.[157] *Oxygen saturation* of greater than 85 per cent in a specimen of blood removed through the cannula is indirect evidence of circulatory failure.[157]

Intramedullary phlebography[7] is accomplished by the injection of contrast material directly into the intertrochanteric region of the femur. The normal venogram is characterized by the absence of pain and the presence of rapid opacification of efferent vessels, especially the ischial and circumflex veins, without any diaphyseal reflux or stasis; in ischemic necrosis of the femoral head, a painful injection is followed by reflux in the diaphysis and intramedullary stasis for 15 min after the procedure.[157]

The final stage of functional exploration of bone is the *core biopsy* (Fig. 80–17), in which a hollow trephine is introduced into the femoral neck from an opening in the

greater trochanter and advanced into the subchondral regions of the femoral head; a second channel is made with a smaller trephine in a different direction.[157] Arlet and Durroux[158] have classified the degrees of histologic alterations in the core biopsy into four types; lesser degrees of involvement are accompanied by necrosis of the hematopoietic or fatty elements, and greater degrees are accompanied by medullary and trabecular necrosis.

The value of some of these tests in the diagnosis of ischemic necrosis of the femoral head, as well as of other sites, has been examined in a number of articles. Robinson and coworkers,[266] in a study of 23 hips that were suspected of having early-stage disease, found that 78 per cent of the femoral heads had MR imaging changes of osteonecrosis, 61 per cent had positive findings by bone marrow pressure studies and intramedullary venography, and 83 per cent revealed histologic evidence of osteonecrosis. In an analysis of 41 patients with known or suspected osteonecrosis of the femoral head, Stulberg and colleagues[250] reported the following values for sensitivity, specificity, positive predictive value, and negative predictive value: bone scintigraphy—83, 83, 96, and 48 per cent; SPECT—91, 78, 94, and 70 per cent; MR imaging—87, 83, 96, and 55 per cent; intraosseous pressure measurements—80, 60, 95, and 25 per cent; and core biopsy—88, 100, 100, and 25 per cent. Zizic and coworkers[287] studied 42 patients with ischemic necrosis of bone about the hip, shoulder, and knee. Hemodynamic studies were performed on the contralateral, asymptomatic joint. Thirty-six of 48 joints had increased bone marrow pressure and of these, 15 (42 per cent) developed histologic or radiographic evidence of osteonecrosis. In none of the 12 bones with normal bone marrow pressure did ischemic necrosis occur. Intraosseous venography also was significantly predictive for ischemic necrosis, both alone and in conjunction with bone marrow pressure measurements.

POSTTRAUMATIC OSTEONECROSIS

After a fracture, bone death of variable extent on either side of the fracture line is common.[17] Necrosis of a large segment of bone after fracture or dislocation, however, generally is restricted to those sites that possess a vulnerable blood supply with few arterial anastomoses; the femoral head, the body of the talus, the humeral head, and the carpal scaphoid represent four such sites.[18] Other locations include the tarsal navicular and carpal hamate and lunate bones. In addition to the peculiarities of blood supply, characteristics common to each of these areas are an intra-articular location of necrotic bone and a limited attachment of soft tissue. In each location, the necrotic portion of the bone may appear radiodense as a result of compression of trabeculae, reactive eburnation as a consequence of the healing process, or lack of participation of the bone in the hyperemia and osteoporosis of neighboring viable bone.[19–23]

Femoral Head

Osteonecrosis of the femoral head is a well-recognized complication of femoral neck fractures and dislocations.[24, 25] Its reported frequency has varied considerably, influenced by many factors, such as the age and sex of the patient, the type and severity of the injury, and the diagnostic techniques and criteria that are employed.[25, 26] Despite this var-

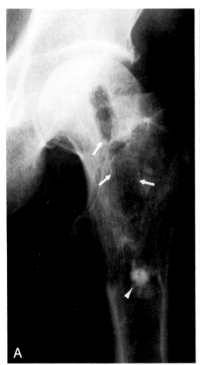
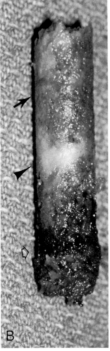

FIGURE 80–17. Osteonecrosis: Value of core biopsy. This 53 year old man had bilateral ischemic necrosis of the femoral heads. Measurement revealed elevation of the intraosseous marrow pressure in the left femoral head, and a subsequent venogram documented intramedullary stasis and diaphyseal reflux of the contrast material.

A The frontal radiograph of the left hip shows a radiodense femoral head, the tract (arrows) left by the hollow trephine, and residual contrast material (arrowhead) from the previous intraosseous venogram.

B The core biopsy shows an avascular zone (solid arrow), sclerotic bone (arrowhead), and a zone of revascularization (open arrow).

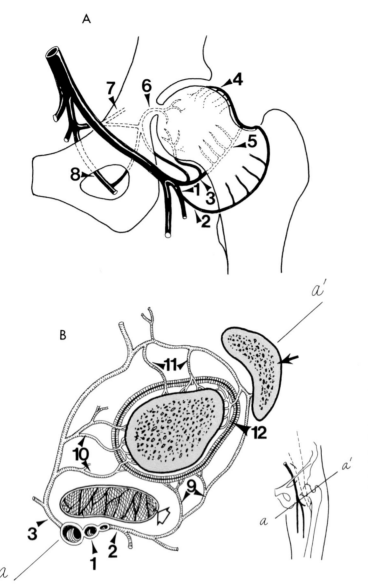

FIGURE 80–18. Femoral head: Vascular supply in adults.

A The major blood supply is derived from the profunda femoris artery (1), from which arise the lateral (2) and the medial (3) circumflex arteries. (The medial and lateral circumflex arteries may arise from the femoral artery rather than the profunda femoris artery in some persons.) As these latter vessels pass anterior and posterior to the femur to anastomose at the level of the trochanters, they send off small branches beneath the capsule of the hip joint. These branches, including the superior retinacular (lateral epiphyseal) arteries (4) and the inferior retinacular (inferior metaphyseal) arteries (5), raise the synovial membrane into folds or retinacula. A second supply of blood is derived from the vessels of the ligamentum teres. Here, the foveal (medial epiphyseal) arteries (6) can be noted. Additional regional vessels are the inferior gluteal artery (7) and the obturator artery (8). (After Graham J, Wood S: In JK Davidson: Aseptic Necrosis of Bone. New York, American Elsevier Publishing Co., 1976, p 101.)

B A cross section of the proximal end of the femur at the base of the neck better delineates the nature of the blood supply. The greater trochanter (arrow) and iliopsoas muscle (open arrow) are indicated. Note the profunda femoris artery (1) and the lateral (2) and medial (3) circumflex arteries. From the lateral circumflex arteries are derived the anterior ascending cervical arteries (9). From the medial circumflex artery are derived the medial (10), posterior (11), and lateral (12) ascending cervical arteries, which, in combination with the anterior ascending cervical arteries, form a subsynovial anastomotic ring on the surface of the femoral neck at the margin of the articular cartilage. The inset shows the plane of section (line a-a'). (After Chung SM: J Bone Joint Surg [Am] 58:961, 1976.)

iation, the importance of the local vascular anatomy in the pathogenesis of osteonecrosis of the femoral head is not questioned.

The principal blood supply to the adult femoral head is via the circumflex femoral branches of the profunda femoris artery[18, 27, 159] (Fig. 80–18). The lateral and medial femoral circumflex arteries pass anterior and posterior to the femur to anastomose at the level of the trochanters, and from these vessels, especially the medial circumflex artery, small branches are derived that pass beneath the capsule of the hip joint and extend in folds or retinacula along the femoral neck, covered by the synovial membrane. They terminate by entering the bone at the cartilaginous margin. The superior (lateral) and the inferior retinacular vessels are the most important structures in this group. A second supply of blood is derived from the vessels of the ligamentum teres. These vascular structures enter the bone of the fovea capitis. A third vascular pathway, the nutrient artery supplying blood to the proximal femoral metaphysis, appears to have an insignificant role in perfusing the femoral head. Despite the presence of anastomoses among the major vessels of

the femoral head in the adult, the connections vary from one person to another and, in many instances, are not functional.[28] It has been established that the superior (lateral) retinacular vessels represent the most important source of blood to the femoral head,[29] whereas the inferior retinacular vessels nourish only a small portion of the head and neck of the femur. A fracture of the femoral neck that traverses the entry site of the superior retinacular vessels into the epiphysis can lead to significant disruption of blood supply and subsequent osteonecrosis.[30] The vessels within the ligamentum teres vary in diameter, and their role in the supply of blood to the femoral head is not defined.[18] Some investigators believe that a prominent vascular supply exists in this area that can anastomose with the lateral epiphyseal vessels and that does not deteriorate with age,[27, 31] whereas other authors maintain that this supply is of little significance.[28] Most reports indicate that the blood flow into foveal areas may provide a source of revascularization when the remainder of the femoral head has been rendered avascular.[18, 29, 32]

The adult pattern of femoral head vascularity, outlined

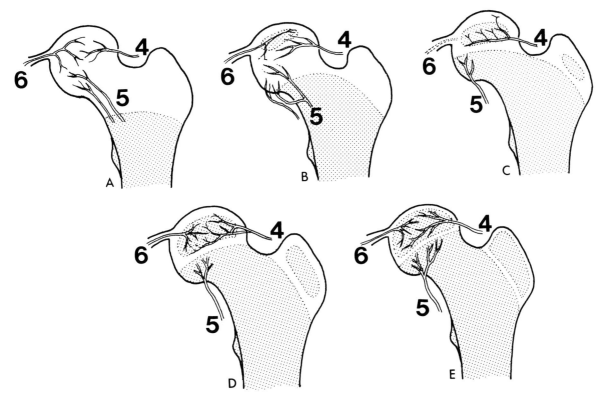

FIGURE 80–19. Femoral head: Vascular supply in the infant, child, and adolescent. Diagrams show the blood supply for the neonate **(A)**, infant and child between 4 months and 4 years of age **(B)**, child between 4 and 7 years of age **(C)**, preadolescent between 7 and 12 years of age **(D)**, and adolescent between 12 years and the time of closure of the growth plate **(E)**. Illustrated are the superior retinacular (4), inferior retinacular (5), and foveal (6) arteries. See text for details. (After Graham J, Wood S: In JK Davidson: Aseptic Necrosis of Bone. New York, American Elsevier Publishing Co, 1976, p 101.)

earlier, usually becomes established with closure of the growth plate at approximately 18 years of age.[18] In infancy and childhood, changing vascular patterns can be noted[33] (Fig. 80–19). In the neonate, three groups of vessels are identified: a superior retinacular or lateral epiphyseal group, an inferior retinacular or inferior metaphyseal group, and a foveal or medial epiphyseal group. With the appearance of ossification, the vasculature of the ligamentum teres gradually disappears, leaving the other two groups as the major suppliers of blood to the proximal portion of the femur. Between the ages of 4 and 7 years, the importance of the lateral epiphyseal vessels is established as the metaphyseal and foveal vessels decrease in extent. After the age of 8 years, a pre-adolescent pattern emerges, consisting of an increased contribution of the foveal vessels. The open growth plate represents an effective barrier, preventing anastomoses between the vessels of the head and the neck. During adolescence, an increased number of the inferior metaphyseal vessels is recognized. As the growth plate closes, the adult pattern appears, with anastomoses between the three arterial systems.[18] It is this influence of age on the pattern of femoral head blood supply that may explain the prevalence of Legg-Calvé-Perthes disease in patients between the ages of 4 and 7 years (see Chapter 81) and the high frequency of osteonecrosis after femoral neck injury in children.[34, 35]

Fractures of the femoral neck in adults (and in children) can be complicated by osteonecrosis of the femoral head (Fig. 80–20). This complication is more frequent in intra-capsular fractures (subcapital, transcervical) than in extra-capsular fractures (intertrochanteric). In the latter situation, the blood supply is not compromised by the fracture line, which lies distal to the capsular insertion on the proximal end of the femur, although, rarely, osteonecrosis does occur after an intertrochanteric fracture, perhaps owing to angulation or deformity of the vascular tree.[29, 160] Ischemic necrosis in fact has been described after isolated trochanteric fractures as well.[161] With transcervical or subcapital fractures, injury to the superior retinacular arteries is frequent, leading to osteonecrosis. Some investigators report that histologic examination of femoral heads after fracture of the neck may indicate necrotic foci in as many as 75 per cent of cases.[36, 37] The frequency of necrosis may increase with displacement and an exaggerated valgus position at the site of fracture, with fractures that involve the superolateral portion of the femoral neck or head,[162] in late reduction, and after use of hardware that is positioned near the fovea, perhaps injuring the blood supply in this region.[18] The radiographic features may include increased density of the necrotic segment (in those cases in which immobilization leads to osteoporosis of viable bone), osseous collapse (usually delayed for a period of 9 months to 1 year after the injury in conjunction with disappearance of the fracture line), flattening, and fragmentation.

As indicated earlier in this chapter, scintigraphy can be useful in the early detection of ischemic necrosis, and the technique frequently has been applied in the patient with a fracture of the femoral neck to assess the viability of the

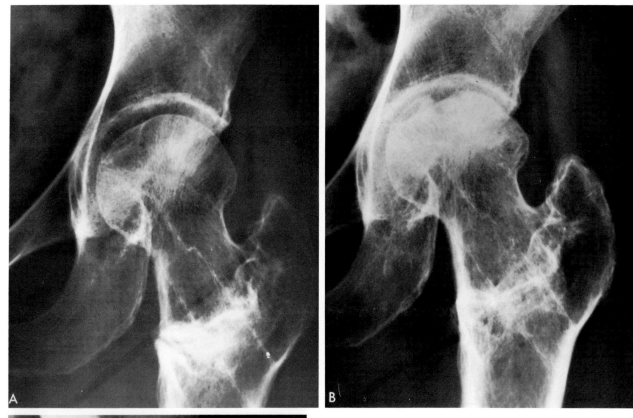

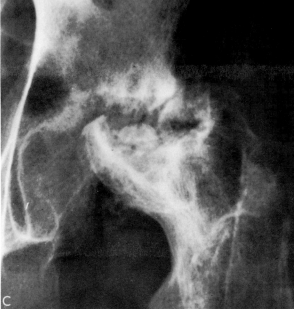

FIGURE 80–20. Posttraumatic osteonecrosis: Femoral head.

A, B Intertrochanteric fracture. Films obtained 2½ years apart reveal evidence of a previous intertrochanteric fracture treated with a Richards nail (that has been removed) and progressive osteonecrosis of the femoral head. This complication is less frequent in intertrochanteric fractures than in subcapital fractures.

C Basicervical fracture. After a fracture of the base of the neck, this patient developed lateral subluxation of the femur and osteonecrosis of the femoral head associated with massive collapse.

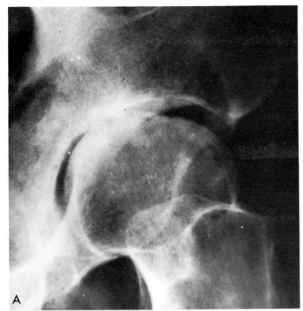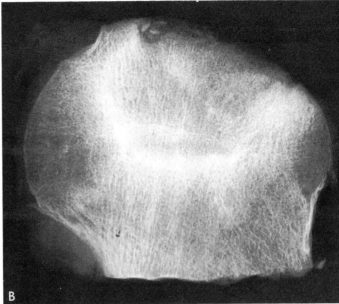

FIGURE 80–21. Posttraumatic osteonecrosis: Femoral head. Posterior dislocation of the hip with acetabular rim fracture. In the period after the injury, this patient revealed collapse of the superolateral aspect of the femoral head. Note the fragmentation of the articular surface and reactive sclerosis about the area of necrosis.

femoral head and to predict the likelihood of delayed collapse of the head.[163–167, 243] Although not uniformly successful,[226] bone scintigraphy allows identification of decreased vascularity in the femoral head shortly after the injury, and such deficient vascular supply indicates a propensity for later osseous collapse. The timing of the examination appears crucial. A preoperative study indicating diminished vascularity to the femoral head correlates with a higher frequency of ischemic necrosis, but a normal preoperative study or one with only minor abnormalities does not necessarily imply a good prognosis; a postoperative radionuclide examination is required, as additional vascular injury may occur at the time of surgery.[168]

As indicated earlier, animal studies also have verified the usefulness of bone scintigraphy[252] and routine[273] and contrast-enhanced[277] MR imaging in the detection of acute ischemia of the femoral head, and contrast-enhanced MR imaging in cases of early ischemia has been shown to be valuable in patients with acute fractures of the femoral neck.[279]

Other traumatic causes of osteonecrosis of the femoral head include dislocation of the hip (Fig. 80–21) and slipped capital femoral epiphysis. The dislocated femoral head may be associated with tears of the vessels in the ligamentum teres and, possibly, injury to the retinacular vessels. Osteonecrosis has been reported in as many as 25 per cent of patients with dislocation, especially if it is complicated by fracture of the acetabulum, a delay in diagnosis and treatment, and early weight-bearing.[38, 39] In children, the resulting radiographic abnormalities resemble those of Legg-Calvé-Perthes disease.[169, 170] After a slipped capital femoral epiphysis, injury to the lateral epiphyseal vessels is more frequent in the presence of severe epiphyseal displacement and manipulative reduction[18]; thus, a frequency rate of osteonecrosis of less than 5 per cent in patients with minimal displacements can rise to 40 per cent in patients with severe

slips in whom aggressive orthopedic manipulations have been undertaken.[40–42] Bone scintigraphy may be used to assess the viability of the femoral head after displacement of the epiphysis.[171]

Osteonecrosis of the femoral head also has been recorded in as many as 68 per cent of patients after developmental dysplasia with dislocation of the hip.[43] The complication appears to be influenced by the method of treatment and the position in which the hip is immobilized.[18] Extreme positions of abduction during immobilization may lead to obstruction of the nearby vascular structures or excessive mechanical pressure on the femoral head.[172, 173] In this regard, it is of interest that osteonecrosis may be observed in the normal hip after immobilization of both sides in cases of unilateral developmental dysplasia with dislocation of the hip, or, rarely, when the opposite dislocated hip has not been treated.[174] In cases in which ischemic necrosis of bone complicates developmental dysplasia of the hip, secondary osteoarthritis may appear later.[137]

Talus

Osteonecrosis of the talus is a recognized and disabling complication of various fractures and injuries. This tarsal bone is covered largely by cartilage, articulating with the tibia and fibula, the calcaneus, and the navicular through a series of joints. Graham and Wood[18] have summarized its vascular anatomy, citing the investigations of Haliburton and coworkers[44] and Mulfinger and Trueta.[45] The talar blood supply is derived mainly from branches of the posterior tibial, peroneal, and dorsalis pedis arteries; the artery of the tarsal sinus and that of the tarsal canal are the two most important branches, which, with their parent trunks, provide the major source of the blood to the bone (Fig. 80–22). The precise intraosseous vascular anatomy varies between the head of the talus and the body of the bone, but

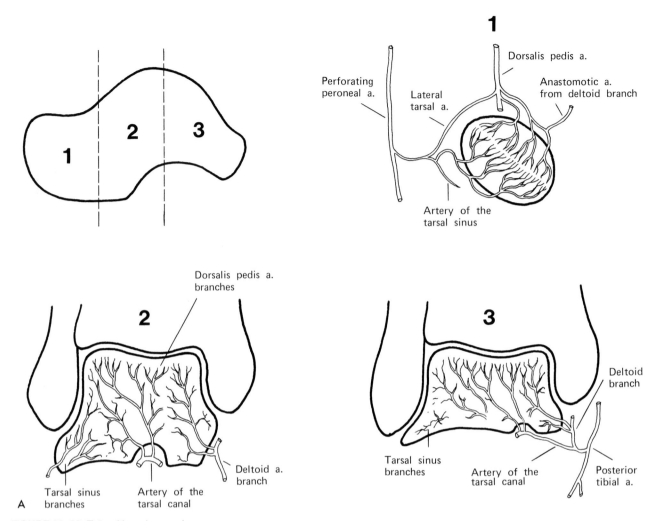

FIGURE 80–22. Talus: Vascular supply.

A Vascular anatomy in coronal sections. 1, Anterior third or head of talus; 2, middle third of talus; 3, posterior third of talus. See text for details.

Illustration continued on opposite page

free anastomoses among the vascular branches exist. Because of these anastomosing channels, a severe soft tissue injury must occur for osteonecrosis to be initiated. The body of the talus is more prone to necrosis than the talar head and neck, and this complication is especially prevalent after fracture of the neck, in which dislocation of the subtalar or ankle joint, or both, also is evident.[46–49] Osteonecrosis of the talus has been reported as a stress injury as well,[288] although the relationship of this finding to osteochondritis dissecans of the talus is not clear.

The radiographic diagnosis of osteonecrosis of the talus can be difficult, and usually it is delayed until osteoporosis of the surrounding viable bone creates a relatively increased density of the talar body. This finding can be apparent within 1 to 3 months after injury and may be combined with collapse of the articular surface (Fig. 80–23). Conversely, the participation of the entire talus in the osteoporosis of immobilization after injury is a good prognostic sign, indicating adequate blood supply to the bone. The presence of a subchondral radiolucent band in the proximal part of the talus, the Hawkins sign, represents bony resorption and can be a useful radiographic sign of an intact vascular supply.[47] This same sign can appear during the revascularization phase after the fracture has united, combined with patchy lucency in the necrotic area of bone. Revascularization appears to be initiated on the medial aspect of the talus and proceeds in a lateral direction, underscoring the importance of the medial blood supply to the bone.[18] The healing process may take several years for completion.

Humeral Head

The blood supply of the head of the humerus is derived from three major sources: a branch of the anterior circumflex humeral artery, the arcuate artery, which enters the bone in the bicipital groove; branches of the posterior circumflex humeral artery, which enter the base of the neck; and vessels in the rotator cuff, which enter at the tendinous insertion to the bone[50, 289] (Fig. 80–24). The vascular supply pierces the bony cortex just distal to the anatomic neck. Osteonecrosis of the humeral head occurs if a fracture leads to loss of blood supply from both the muscular insertions and the arcuate branch of the anterior circumflex humeral artery[18]; this may result after a displaced fracture of the anatomic neck or a severe fracture or fracture-dislocation

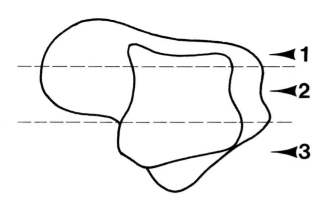

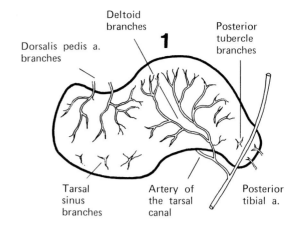

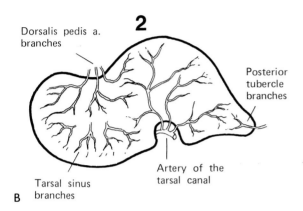

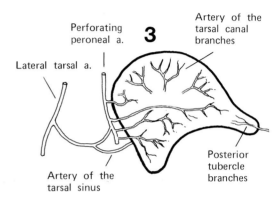

FIGURE 80–22. *Continued*
B Vascular anatomy in parasagittal sections. 1, Medial third of talus; 2, middle third of talus; 3, lateral third of talus. See text for details. (After Mulfinger GL, Trueta J: J Bone Joint Surg [Br] *52*:160, 1970.)

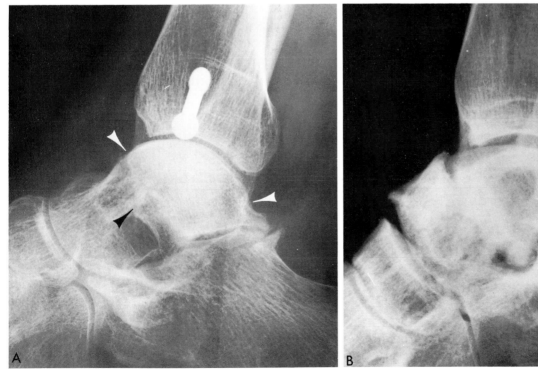

FIGURE 80–23. Posttraumatic osteonecrosis: Talus.
A In this person, who sustained a fracture of the body of the talus as well as of the medial malleolus (which was transfixed with a screw), note the increased radiodensity of the proximal half of the bone (arrowheads).
B In a different person with a nonunion of a midtalar fracture, extensive necrosis is associated with sclerosis and cyst formation.

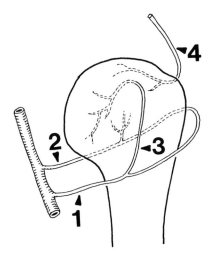

FIGURE 80–24. Humeral head: Vascular supply. Vessels include the anterior circumflex humeral artery (1), the posterior circumflex humeral artery (2), the arcuate artery (3), and the vessels of the rotator cuff (4). (After Graham J, Wood S: In JK Davidson: Aseptic Necrosis of Bone. New York, American Elsevier Publishing Co, 1976, p 101.)

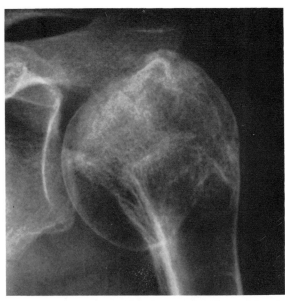

FIGURE 80–25. Posttraumatic osteonecrosis: Humeral head. Although the fracture of the anatomic neck of the humerus is healed, observe the flattened and irregular humeral head, indicative of ischemic necrosis. (Courtesy of J. Schils, M.D., Cleveland, Ohio.)

of the bone.[175] The radiographic findings parallel those in the femoral head, although osseous collapse, common in the femoral weight-bearing area, is less prominent in the humeral head. Patchy lucent shadows and sclerosis, an arc-like subchondral radiolucent area, and depression and fragmentation of the articular surface can be seen (Fig. 80–25).

Scaphoid

Osteonecrosis of the proximal pole of the carpal scaphoid is a well-documented complication after injury to this bone.

Its appearance and characteristics relate to the vascular anatomy of the scaphoid, which has been outlined by Obletz and Halbstein[51] and Taleisnik and Kelly.[52] Three groups of vessels can be identified: a laterovolar group entering the bone distal to the radial articular surface on the flattened volar aspect or on the narrower lateral strip; a dorsal group entering the bone between the radial and trapezoid-trapezium articular surfaces; and a distal group entering in the region of the tubercle[18] (Fig. 80–26). The major intraos-

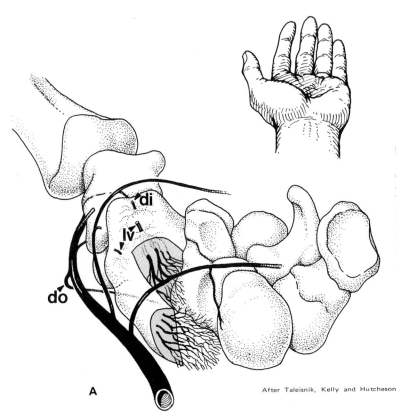

After Taleisnik, Kelly and Hutcheson

FIGURE 80–26. Carpal scaphoid: Vascular supply.

A According to Taleisnik and Kelly: The extraosseous arteries of the scaphoid originate from the radial artery and consist of a laterovolar group (lv), the most important contributor, that enters the scaphoid on the volar aspect and lateral to the radial articular surface, a dorsal group (do) that penetrates the narrow grooved dorsal surface of the scaphoid, and a distal group (di) that supplies a circumscribed zone in the tuberosity. (After Taleisnik J, Kelly PJ: J Bone Joint Surg [Am] *48*:1125, 1966. Courtesy of the Mayo Foundation.)

Illustration continued on opposite page

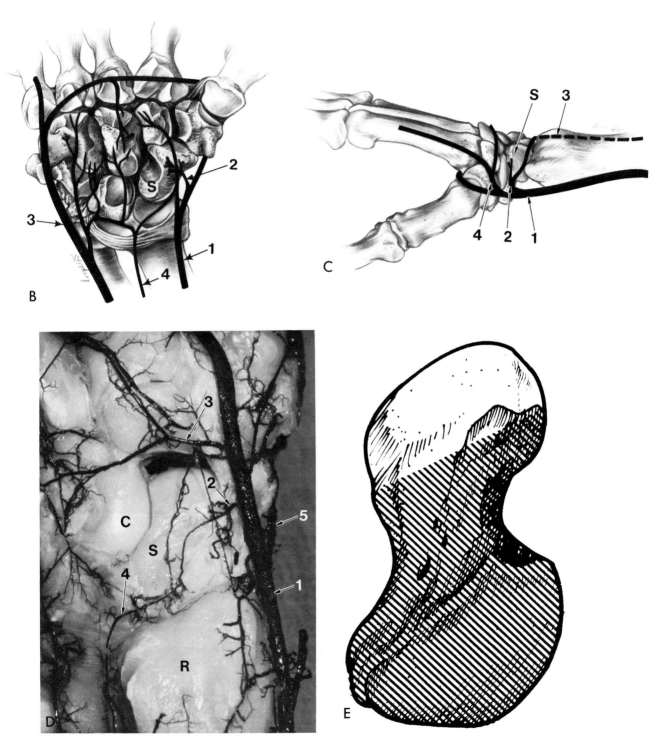

FIGURE 80–26. *Continued*
B–E According to Gelberman and Menon: **B,** A schematic drawing of the volar external blood supply of the scaphoid: S, scaphoid; 1, radial artery; 2, volar scaphoid branches; 3, ulnar artery; 4, anterior division of the anterior interosseous artery. **C,** A schematic drawing of the dorsal blood supply of the scaphoid: S, scaphoid; 1, radial artery; 2, dorsal scaphoid branch; 3, dorsal division of the anterior interosseous artery; 4, intercarpal artery. **D,** Dorsal external blood supply in an injected specimen: S, scaphoid; C, capitate; R, radius; 1, radial artery; 2, dorsal scaphoid branch; 3, intercarpal artery; 4, dorsal division of the anterior interosseous artery; 5, superficial palmar branch of the radial artery. **E,** In a drawing of the scaphoid, note that the proximal 70 to 80 per cent of the bone is supplied by dorsal vessels (shaded area), and the distal 20 to 30 per cent is supplied by volar branches of the radial artery (white area). (From Gelberman RH, Menon J: J Hand Surg 5:508, 1980.)

seous supply is derived from the laterovolar group of vessels.

More recently, Gelberman and Menon[139] studied the vascularity of the scaphoid in 15 fresh cadaveric specimens. They emphasized that the radial artery was the major blood supply to the scaphoid, that the proximal pole and 70 to 80 per cent of the bone received blood from vessels entering the dorsal ridge, that the tuberosity and distal 20 to 30 per cent of the bone were supplied by volar branches of the radial artery and its superficial palmar branch, and that no significant intraosseous anastomoses occurred between dorsal and volar branches. These investigators also noted the excellent collateral circulation to the scaphoid that arose from the dorsal and volar branches of the anterior interosseous artery. On comparing their results with those of Taleisnik and Kelly,[52] Gelberman and Menon concluded that the laterovolar group of vessels in the former study was analogous to their dorsal ridge vessels, and that the distal group of vessels was analogous to their tuberosity vessels.

Osteonecrosis is most likely to occur when a scaphoid fracture involves the proximal pole of the bone; with more distal infractions, the interruption of blood supply is less constant or severe. With rare exceptions,[176] it is the proximal aspect of the bone that undergoes necrosis. The reported frequency of this complication after scaphoid injuries varies with the nature and severity of the fracture or dislocation; a frequency of 11 to 65 per cent has been noted.[53, 54] Ten to 15 per cent seems to be the most common estimated frequency of this complication.[18] The radiographic diagnosis depends on a relative increase in density of the devitalized portion of the scaphoid in comparison with the osteoporotic viable bone (Figs. 80–27 and 80–28), an appearance that is delayed for a period of 4 to 8 weeks and that may be associated with delayed union or nonunion of the fracture, collapse of the necrotic segment, and, eventually, secondary degenerative joint disease of the radiocarpal compartment of the wrist (Fig. 80–29). Scintigraphy with bone-seeking radiopharmaceutical agents may be useful shortly after the injury to identify decreased vascularity of the proximal pole of the scaphoid, manifested as a "cold" area.[177] MR imaging also has been employed as a diagnostic method in the detection of osteonecrosis of the scaphoid (Figs. 80–30 and 80–31) (see Chapter 70).[290]

Although fracture of the ossifying scaphoid bone with subsequent osteonecrosis is uncommon in the child, it may be encountered.[347] Scaphoid fractures in young children require severe trauma and rarely occur as isolated or indirect injuries. Diagnostic difficulty is encountered owing to the presence of unossified portions of the bone (Fig. 80–32).

Capitate

Ischemic necrosis of the capitate occurs in several distinct situations: after accidental trauma in which a fracture

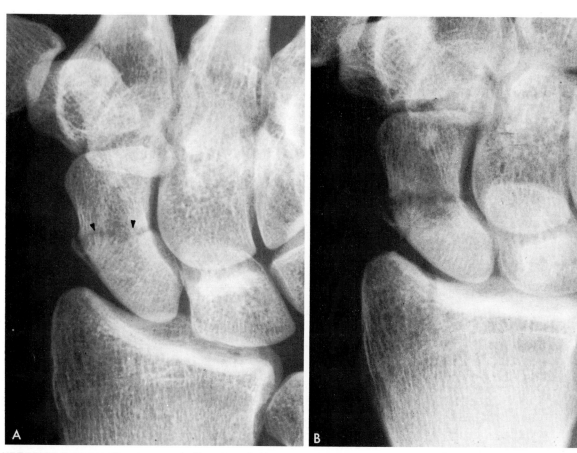

FIGURE 80–27. Posttraumatic osteonecrosis: Carpal scaphoid.
A A film obtained 2 weeks after trauma indicates a scaphoid fracture (arrowheads).
B Six weeks after **A**, increased radiodensity of the proximal half of the scaphoid is accentuated by osteoporosis of the distal half of the bone, indicating the presence of osteonecrosis and reparative bone formation.

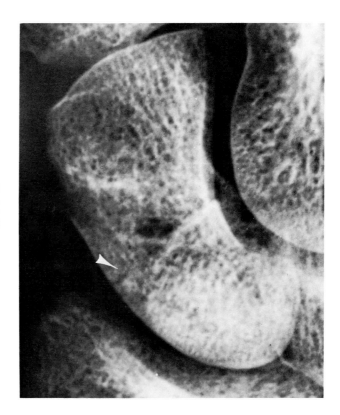

FIGURE 80–28. Posttraumatic osteonecrosis: Carpal scaphoid. Role of magnification radiography. Seven weeks after a scaphoid fracture, a magnification film indicates the persistence of the fracture line (arrowhead) and increased radiodensity of the proximal portion of the scaphoid.

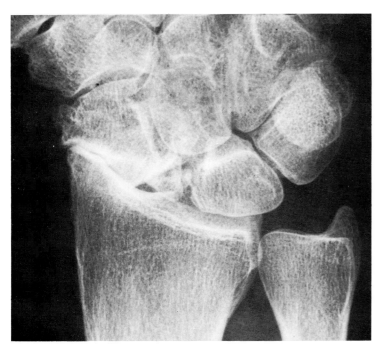

FIGURE 80–29. Posttraumatic osteonecrosis: Carpal scaphoid. Nonunion and secondary degenerative joint disease. A remote fracture of the scaphoid is associated with nonunion, collapse of the necrotic proximal pole, and joint space narrowing, sclerosis, and osteophytes of the radiocarpal and midcarpal compartments. Note that the joint space loss typically occurs between the radius and the distal scaphoid fragment.

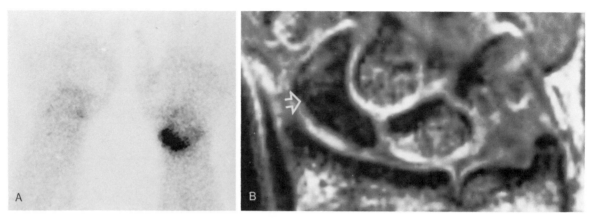

FIGURE 80–30. Posttraumatic osteonecrosis: Carpal scaphoid. MR imaging. In this 25 year old man with a previous fracture of the midportion of the scaphoid bone and persistent pain, a bone scan **(A)** shows increased accumulation of the radionuclide in the scaphoid bone of the left wrist. In a 2 mm thick coronal gradient echo MR image (fast imaging with steady-state precession [FISP]) obtained with volumetric acquisition **(B),** note the abnormally low signal intensity in the proximal portion of the scaphoid, consistent with the diagnosis of osteonecrosis. The site of the previous fracture (which is well healed) is identified (arrow), and the signal intensity in the marrow of the distal portion of the bone appears normal. An old, ununited fracture of the tip of the ulnar styloid process also is evident.

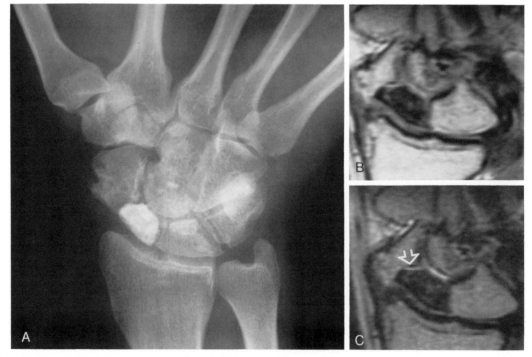

FIGURE 80–31. Posttraumatic osteonecrosis: Carpal scaphoid. MR imaging.
   A Routine radiography reveals typical features of osteonecrosis involving the proximal pole of the bone. No evidence of bone union at the fracture site in the midportion of the scaphoid bone is evident.
   B, C Coronal proton density (TR/TE, 2500/30) **(B)** and T2-weighted (TR/TE, 2500/80) **(C)** spin echo MR images document the abnormally low signal intensity of the marrow in the proximal pole of the bone. In **C,** observe fluid in the midcarpal joint with extension into the fracture gap (arrow).

FIGURE 80–32. Posttraumatic osteonecrosis: Carpal scaphoid. Immature skeleton. A boy of approximately 6 years of age sustained a closed injury resulting in a radiographically evident triquetral fracture. Initially, no abnormality of the developing scaphoid bone was seen. Three months after the injury **(A)**, there is evidence of healing of the triquetral fracture (arrowhead) as well as of sclerosis and cupping of the proximal margin of the ossification center of the scaphoid bone (arrow). Four years after the injury **(B)**, a persistent fracture gap (arrow) is seen. The proximal pole of the scaphoid demonstrates slight increased density. (From Larson B, et al: J Hand Surg [Am] *12*:122, 1987. © 1987, Churchill Livingstone, New York.)

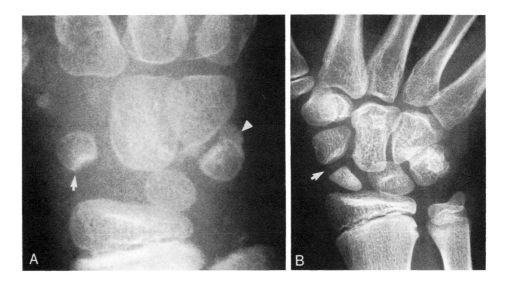

of the capitate is combined with additional fractures and dislocations of the carpal bones; after accidental trauma in which an isolated fracture of the capitate is evident; after repetitive episodes of occupational or recreational stress; and spontaneously in the absence of any type of injury.[291] The occurrence of osteonecrosis in these situations would appear to indicate that the capitate possesses a vulnerable vascular supply, a concept supported by anatomic studies; palmar vessels contribute the majority of the blood supply to the bone, and the proximal pole receives its blood exclusively in a retrograde fashion across the capitate waist analogous to the vascular pattern seen in the scaphoid.[178] It is the proximal pole of the capitate that is the site of ischemic necrosis.

Osteonecrosis of this bone is a recognized complication of a transscaphoid, transcapitate, perilunate fracture-dislocation (scaphocapitate syndrome).[179–181] After a violent blow with the hand typically in a position of dorsiflexion and radial deviation, fractures of the scaphoid and capitate may be combined with perilunate dislocation and, importantly, with 180 degree rotation of the proximal pole of the capitate (Fig. 80–33). As the malpositioned fragment of the capitate commonly lies in the cavity of the fracture site in the parent bone, its abnormal alignment may be overlooked on radiographs, although the rounded proximal articular surface of the capitate now faces distally and the portion of the bone articulating with the lunate has a squared appearance. Delay in diagnosing the nature of the capitate injury with resultant delay in surgical reduction increases the likelihood of subsequent ischemic necrosis as well as of osteoarthritis.

Although infrequent, osteonecrosis of the capitate may occur as a complication of an isolated fracture of this bone,[178] especially if accurate diagnosis of the fracture is delayed. When such injuries are recognized, proper immobilization generally leads to fracture healing and revascularization of the proximal pole.[182]

Ischemic necrosis of the capitate also has been identified in association with chronic stress in those employed in certain occupations (butchers, carpenters, paint sprayers),[183, 184] with sporting activities (gymnasts),[185] or with hypermobility and instability.[186–188] It also may be seen as a delayed complica-

tion after accidental trauma when initial radiographs are normal.[189]

Vertebral Body

In 1891, Kümmell described a posttraumatic osteitis in which painful kyphosis developed in several patients after a symptom-free period of months to years following an injury.[190] Subsequently, Schmorl and Junghanns[191] provided pathologic observations supporting the concept of delayed posttraumatic collapse of vertebral bodies, although the nature of the underlying disease process was not clear. Numerous additional reports of this phenomenon have since appeared,[192–194, 227, 228] and evidence is being accumulated that the vertebral collapse occurs as a consequence of a vascular insult leading to secondary bone necrosis. Such evidence includes the documentation of vascular occlusions using spinal arteriography,[190] the association of delayed vertebral collapse with conditions that predispose to vascular compromise, such as pancreatitis[195] and Gaucher's disease,[194] and the presence of an intraosseous vacuum phenomenon within the collapsed vertebral body,[193, 196, 292, 294] a finding that is suggestive of, although not specific for, ischemic necrosis.[197–203, 229, 244, 293]

The frequency of Kümmell's disease is not known, although probably it is not uncommon. Affected patients generally are middle-aged or elderly men or women, the interval between the acute traumatic episode and the vertebral collapse varies from days to years, and the lower thoracic and upper lumbar vertebral bodies principally are involved (Fig. 80–34). A single vertebra or, more rarely, multiple vertebrae are affected. Spinal cord compression may accompany the vertebral collapse,[295] and gas collections may extend into the adjacent psoas musculature.[296]

MR imaging has been used to study the intravertebral vacuum phenomenon.[293, 297] In reported cases, decreased signal intensity in the area of the vacuum cleft has been observed on T1-weighted spin echo images, and hyperintensity in this region has been evident on T2-weighted images. In the authors' experience, however, low signal intensity, probably related to the gas itself, may be seen on T2-weighted images as well. Indeed, it appears likely that

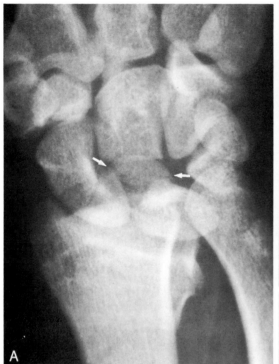

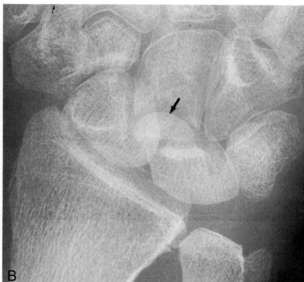

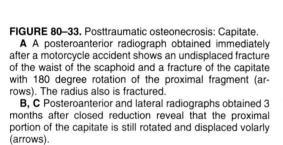

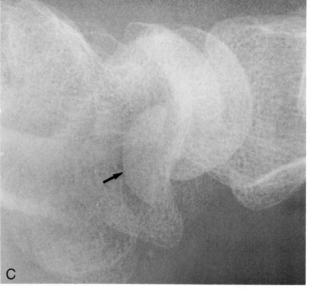

FIGURE 80–33. Posttraumatic osteonecrosis: Capitate.

A A posteroanterior radiograph obtained immediately after a motorcycle accident shows an undisplaced fracture of the waist of the scaphoid and a fracture of the capitate with 180 degree rotation of the proximal fragment (arrows). The radius also is fractured.

B, C Posteroanterior and lateral radiographs obtained 3 months after closed reduction reveal that the proximal portion of the capitate is still rotated and displaced volarly (arrows).

(From Resnik CS, et al: Skel Radiol 9:192, 1983.)

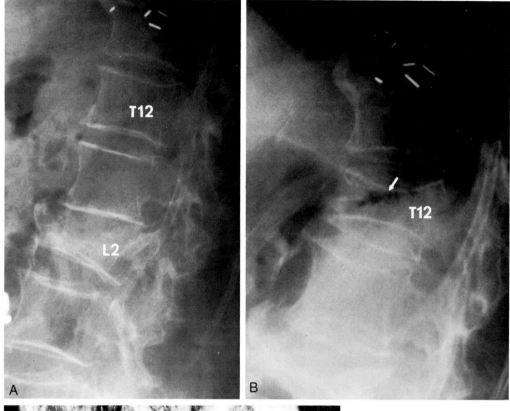

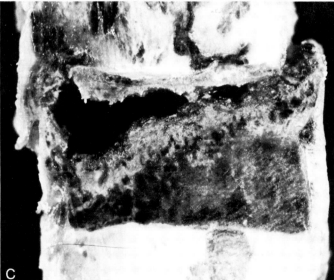

FIGURE 80–34. Posttraumatic osteonecrosis: Vertebral body (Kümmell's disease). This 89 year old woman was involved in a motor vehicle accident approximately 1 year previously. She continued to have back pain.

A An initial lateral radiograph shows an old fracture of the second lumbar vertebra (L2), with considerable collapse of the vertebral body. The remaining vertebral bodies are normal. A bone scan (not shown) revealed increased uptake of the radionuclide not only at the second lumbar level but also in the twelfth thoracic vertebral body (T12).

B Seven days after **A,** a repeat lateral radiograph of the thoracolumbar spine shows a new collapse of the twelfth thoracic vertebral body (T12). Observe the intra-osseous vacuum within the body (arrow), probably indicating ischemic necrosis.

C In a section of a cadaveric spine, an area of bone necrosis has led to an abnormal space within the vertebral body. It is in such a space that the gas, principally nitrogen, collects, producing the intraosseous vacuum phenomenon.

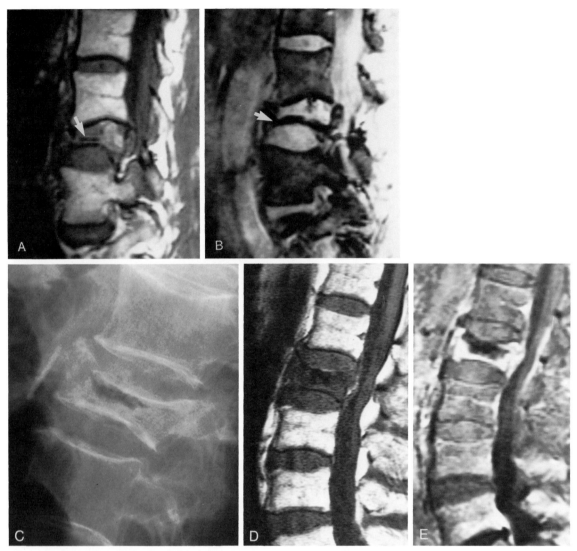

FIGURE 80–35. Posttraumatic osteonecrosis: Vertebral body (Kümmell's disease). MR imaging.

A, B After an injury, delayed collapse of a lumbar vertebral body occurred in this 46 year old woman. A routine radiograph (not shown) revealed a vacuum within the collapsed vertebral body. A sagittal T1-weighted (TR/TE, 600/20) spin echo MR image **(A)** reveals the collapsed vertebral body containing a linear area of low signal intensity (arrow) that corresponded to the site of gas collection. With two-dimensional gradient echo technique (multiplanar gradient recalled, MPGR) (TR/TE, 450/15; flip angle, 30 degrees) **(B)**, low signal intensity again is evident into the involved vertebral body (arrow).

C–E A 71 year old man developed delayed posttraumatic collapse of the second lumbar vertebral body. The radiograph **(C)** shows an intraosseous vacuum at this spinal level. In a sagittal T1-weighted (TR/TE, 300/13) spin echo MR image **(D)**, low signal intensity is seen in this vertebral body. Narrowing of the spinal canal is evident. In a sagittal fat-suppressed T1-weighted (TR/TE, 450/11) spin echo MR image obtained after the intravenous administration of a gadolinium compound **(E)**, low signal intensity persists in the central portion of the vertebral body (consistent with fluid or gas), with enhancement of other portions of the vertebral body.

(C–E, Courtesy of G. Greenway, M.D., Dallas, Texas.)

either low or high signal intensity may appear in the cleft in T2-weighted spin echo MR images, depending on the position of the spine and whether gas or fluid occupies the cleft.[354] In all cases, the linear or bandlike pattern of abnormal signal intensity assumes diagnostic importance (Fig. 80–35).

Gas within a vertebral body is not diagnostic of osteonecrosis. Rarely, gas formation may accompany spinal infections, although its pattern and distribution differ from those of the vacuum phenomenon of vertebral osteonecrosis. Furthermore, focal collections of gas in a vertebral body, most commonly in the cervical spine, may reflect the presence of cartilaginous, or Schmorl's, nodes.[298, 299]

Other Sites

After significant injury or prolonged stress, avascular necrosis can appear at other sites, especially when an osseous fragment loses its soft tissue attachments. Thus, necrosis of the lunate (Fig. 80–36), other carpal bones, tarsal navicular bone, mandibular condyle, patella,[55] glenoid region of the scapula,[204] odontoid process of the axis,[205] and even the metatarsal and metacarpal heads[56] and phalanges[300] can be seen (Figs. 80–37 and 80–38). Precise classification of the alterations is difficult owing to their overlap with changes seen in spontaneous osteonecrosis and in osteochondritis dissecans (Chapter 67) and the osteochondroses (Chapter 81).

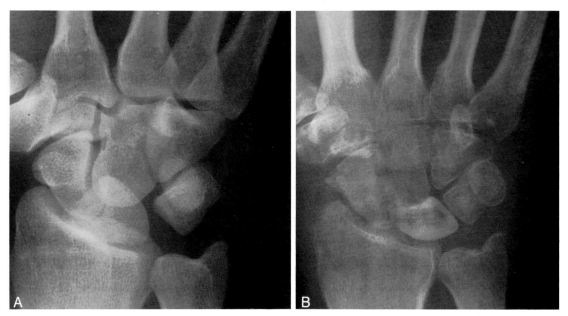

FIGURE 80–36. Posttraumatic osteonecrosis: Lunate. This 24 year old man injured his wrist.

A The initial anteroposterior radiograph demonstrates an abnormal overlap of the lunate and the scaphoid and of the lunate and the capitate, an abnormal relationship between the lunate and the distal surface of the radius, an abnormal interosseous space between the lunate and the triquetrum, and a normal relationship between the scaphoid and the radius. These findings are diagnostic of a lunate dislocation.

B Although the dislocated lunate was reduced immediately, the patient continued to have wrist pain. The radiograph obtained 4 months after **A** shows osteopenia in all of the visualized bones except the lunate, which appears radiodense. This abnormality relates to disruption of the vascular supply to the lunate. Although the midcarpal joint is narrowed, infection was not present.

FIGURE 80–37. Posttraumatic osteonecrosis: Metacarpal head.

A Initial radiograph reveals an unusual fracture-dislocation of the metacarpal head, in which the metacarpal fragment has rotated 180 degrees.

B Follow-up study several months after reduction of the fragment demonstrates increased density of the metacarpal head.

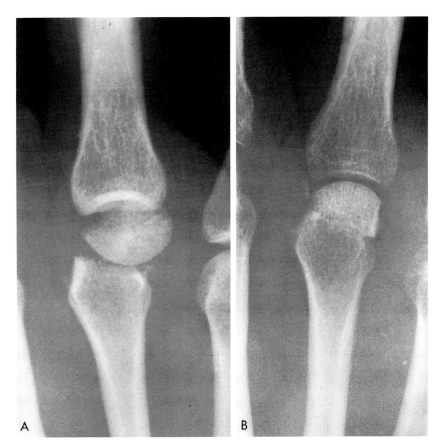

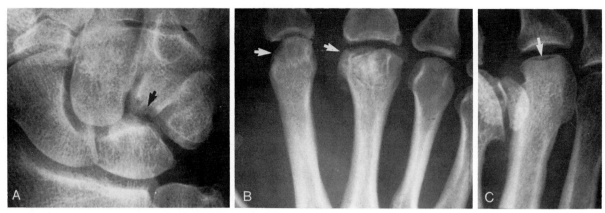

FIGURE 80–38. Posttraumatic versus spontaneous osteonecrosis: Other sites.

A Hamate bone. In this 75 year old man with ulnar-sided wrist pain, spontaneous or stress-related osteonecrosis of the proximal pole of the hamate is seen (arrow). This was confirmed histologically.

B Metacarpal heads. In a 40 year old man, progressive collapse of multiple metacarpal heads (arrows) occurred. The opposite side was affected similarly.

C Metatarsal head. In this 54 year old woman, observe a subchondral radiolucent line in the head of the second metatarsal bone (arrow), consistent with osteonecrosis, and cortical thickening of the shaft of this bone. The abnormalities presumably relate to chronic stress.

(**A, B** Courtesy of G. Greenway, M.D., Dallas, Texas.)

DYSBARIC OSTEONECROSIS

General Features

Recent years have witnessed an increasing exposure of humans to high pressure environments as a result of such factors as the rising popularity of scuba diving and the expanding interest in underwater and space exploration and off-shore oil drilling. A new awareness of and interest in early and late complications of this exposure have appeared. One such late complication is osteonecrosis, which has been designated dysbaric osteonecrosis, caisson disease, pressure-induced osteoarthropathy, and barotraumatic osteoarthropathy.[57]

The term decompression sickness indicates the acute consequences of the liberation of gas bubbles, principally nitrogen, in the blood and the tissues of a person who has undergone decompression too rapidly after a period of exposure to a hyperbaric environment.[58] In a high pressure environment, a person's blood and tissues are saturated with the atmospheric gases, and after rapid return to normal atmospheric pressure, the various gases come out of solution, producing supersaturation of the tissues. Ventilation may allow dispersion of the excess of oxygen and carbon dioxide, but the released nitrogen may produce bubbles within the vascular tree, which act as air emboli that occlude vessels partially or completely at one or more sites, leading to symptoms and signs of vascular insufficiency. Nitrogen accumulation is greatest in tissues rich in fat, and the fatty marrow does not escape this accumulation. Dysbaric osteonecrosis represents one of the late complications of hyperbaric exposure; other long-term effects include paralysis and psychiatric illness.[59]

The association of decompression sickness and dysbaric osteonecrosis is controversial. In general, there appears to be a lack of correlation between these two conditions.[60, 61] Many victims of decompression sickness never develop osteonecrosis and, conversely, bony lesions are discovered in divers and workers who use compressed air who have had no earlier symptoms or signs. Despite this dissociation of findings in the two conditions, it generally is assumed that gas bubbles initiate the manifestations of decompression sickness and that they likely represent the cause of osteonecrosis as well. Experimentally, aseptic necrosis of bone can be produced in animals by exposure to dysbaric environments and artificial emboli with foreign material or lipids.[62–64] The osseous lesions in humans may develop from showers of "silent" embolic bubbles during repeated decompressions in persons in whom the gas tension levels are below those required to produce the acute manifestations of decompression sickness.[61] The frequency of dysbaric osteonecrosis appears to be exaggerated in patients with repeated exposures,[65] exposures to greater pressures, a rapid rate of exposure,[64] and obesity.[61] Lesions may appear or progress even when exposure to hyperbaric pressures no longer exists.[356]

Pathogenesis

Dysbaric osteonecrosis probably represents an ischemic lesion of bone.[245] The exact cause of the ischemia is debated, the various theories being well summarized by Chryssanthou.[61] Embolization of gas bubbles with blockage of vascular channels is considered to be the major factor by many investigators. The presence of intravascular gas bubbles even after asymptomatic decompression has been documented by ultrasonography and other techniques,[61, 65, 66] as well as by light and electron microscopy of various tissues, including bone.[67] This evidence leaves little doubt about the existence of gas in the blood vessels, but the role of this gas in the production of necrosis is not clear. Ischemic changes are influenced by the type of tissue, the duration of the obstruction, the local vascular anatomy, and the size of the affected area.[61, 134] The fatty bone marrow may be especially vulnerable to infarction, particularly in the presence of repeated and sustained gas emboli, because it has an inadequate collateral circulation. Metaphyseal and subchondral regions of tubular bones possess end-arteries, which favor embolic occlusion.

An accessory role of fat embolization in the pathogenesis of dysbaric osteonecrosis also has been suggested.[68] Gas bubbles in fatty marrow and adipose tissue may cause disruption of fat cells with the introduction of potentially embolic lipid material into the circulation. This mechanism may explain the greater risk to obese patients of developing dysbaric osteonecrosis. Alternatively, it is suggested that gas bubbles within the liver may lead to local injury, with extrusion of unstable fats and embolization.[69] This process may be promoted by adhesion of plasma lipids to the blood-gas interface[70] or denaturation of plasma lipoproteins by blood-bubble interface activity, release of lipid moiety, coalescence of liberated lipid, and formation of embolic particles.[61] Thrombotic material also could contribute to embolization in dysbaric osteonecrosis.

The presence of nonembolic ischemic changes in this disorder also has been postulated. Within the rigid osseous tissue, extravascular gas collections might lead to compression of neighboring blood vessels, impairing tissue perfusion; intravascular gas accumulations could initiate injury to the vascular wall, with subsequent stenosis[67]; or release of vasoactive substances could provoke vessel narrowing, with resulting ischemia.[71]

In addition to the ischemic mechanisms that were outlined previously, other hypotheses have suggested that non-ischemic changes are important in the pathogenesis of dysbaric osteonecrosis.[61] Thus, bony abnormalities may be induced by osmotic changes and fluid shifts owing to pressure alterations,[72] increased oxygen tension,[73] or altered immunity and dysproteinemia.

Incidence

The frequency of osseous lesions in patients subjected to high pressure environments depends on the number, length, and severity of exposures and the timing and method of evaluation. In compressed-air workers, the reported frequency has varied from almost zero to 75 per cent,[74, 75, 206] most estimates being in the range of 10 to 20 per cent. As it has been determined that 4 to 12 months usually elapse between the time of exposure and the appearance of radiographic abnormality (an interval that may be considerably longer and influenced by the extent of the necrotic area, the thickness of the overlying tissue, the quality of the radiograph, and the amount of revascularization), radiographic examination shortly after exposure reveals a lower frequency of osseous abnormality.[57]

The reported prevalence of osteonecrosis in divers also has varied, the pertinent literature being summarized by Davidson.[57, 207] Cited are reports from Germany, Norway, Bulgaria, and Japan, in which the frequency of osseous lesions varied from 17 to 65 per cent. This occurrence rate may rise substantially in studies in which long-term follow-up examinations are available. In divers in the British Royal Navy, a lower frequency (4 per cent) has been noted, perhaps owing to stricter surveillance and regulations imposed on these persons.[76] As in the case of compressed-air workers, a delay of at least 6 months or a year between the first exposure to the increased atmospheric pressure and the onset of radiologically evident skeletal alterations is typical in divers.[207] Such alterations are more prevalent in those who have dived to greater depths, those who have had decompression sickness, and those who are older and have more diving experience.[207]

Radiographic and Pathologic Abnormalities

The radiographic and pathologic abnormalities of dysbaric osteonecrosis have been well outlined.[57, 77–85, 340] A popular classification of the bone alterations recognizes two major changes: juxta-articular lesions occurring most frequently in the head of the humerus and femur (Figs. 80–39 and 80–40) and diaphyseal and metaphyseal lesions situated at a distance from the joint (Figs. 80–41 and 80–42).[86] Juxta-articular alterations consist of radiodense areas varying between 3 and 20 mm in diameter, which are slightly less discrete than bone islands (enostoses), spherical segmental opaque areas that eventually may produce a ''snow-capped'' configuration, radiolucent subcortical bands (crescent sign), indicating a fracture of necrotic bone,[233] and osseous collapse and fragmentation; diaphyseal and metaphyseal abnormalities consist of indistinct, poorly defined radiodense foci, irregular calcified areas with a shell-like configuration, and, rarely, radiolucent lesions, perhaps due to sites of necrosis.[57] Debate exists regarding the significance of subtle small opaque lesions and cystic foci in this disorder; similar findings can be seen with equal or lesser frequency in so-called normal persons,[78, 87] diminishing the diagnostic importance of these changes. Thus, care must be exercised in interpreting focal sclerotic or lucent areas, especially if they are few in number and small in size. True osteonecrotic lesions may enlarge, leading to structural failure of the articular surface, or may remain stable for long periods of time.

In compressed-air workers and divers, multiple or single bilateral or unilateral alterations can be seen. The distal shaft of the femur, the humeral head, the femoral head, and the tibial shaft, in descending order of frequency, are the most typical sites of involvement. An infarct that is limited to the shaft of a tubular bone usually is not associated with clinical complaints; when involvement of an epiphysis leads to collapse of the articular surface, pain and swelling can become apparent.

Knowledge of the distribution of the radiologic abnormalities has led to the development of specific radiographic protocols designed to detect the presence of osteonecrosis after caisson disease and to allow its classification on the basis of the extent of involvement.[207] High quality radiographs of the shoulders, hips, shafts of the femora and tibiae, and, perhaps, the knees are suggested.[206, 207] Scintigraphy using bone-seeking radiopharmaceutical agents allows analysis of the distribution of the alterations and is more sensitive than conventional radiography.[208, 209, 355] CT[210] rarely is required.

Pathologic examination reveals necrotic subchondral bone surrounded by collagenous fibrous tissue and thickened, spongy trabeculae. One or more fracture lines can extend through the cartilage, creating osteochondral fragments and an irregular bumpy or grooved articular surface.[58, 83, 88, 89] Chondral changes include brown discoloration, fibrillation, and erosion, but as in all cases of osteonecrosis, these cartilaginous abnormalities are relatively mild in comparison to the severity of the osseous alterations until secondary osteoarthritis supervenes, leading to fragmentation and dissolution of the chondral tissue, osteophytosis, sclerosis, and cyst formation.

Davidson and coworkers[87] described in detail the histologic observations related to the focal sclerotic lesions seen

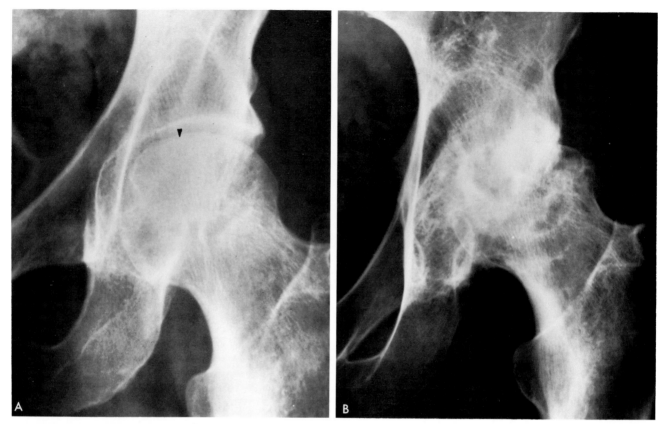

FIGURE 80–39. Dysbaric osteonecrosis: Juxta-articular lesions. This middle-aged man had worked in a decompression chamber for 20 years.
  A An initial film reveals patchy lucency and sclerosis of the femoral head, with subtle flattening of the articular surface, a subchondral radiolucent crescent or fracture (arrowhead), and buttressing of the femoral neck. The opposite hip was affected similarly.
  B Eighteen months after **A,** a considerable increase in the sclerosis associated with obliteration of the joint space can be identified.

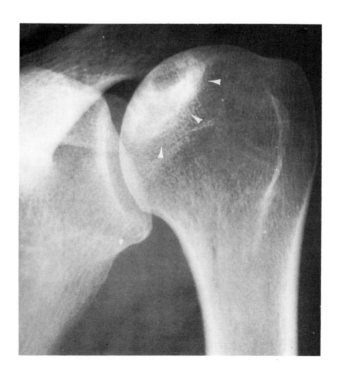

FIGURE 80–40. Dysbaric osteonecrosis: Juxta-articular lesions. The sclerosis or "snow-capped" appearance of the humeral head (arrowheads) is typical of dysbaric osteonecrosis but may be evident in other varieties of necrosis as well.

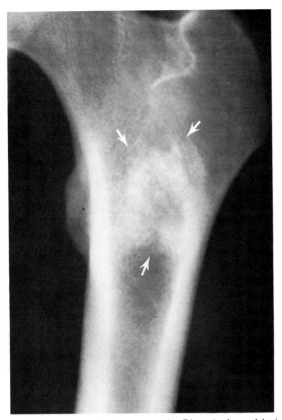

FIGURE 80–41. Dysbaric osteonecrosis: Diametaphyseal lesions. This 28 year old man developed mild discomfort in the hip over a 3 month period without swelling. He was a scuba diver who had made dives to considerable depths. A patchy area of increased sclerosis is evident in the proximal shaft of the femur (arrows). Note the increased density of the periphery of the lesion. Biopsy with histologic evaluation indicated osseous and marrow necrosis compatible with an infarct.

in dysbaric osteonecrosis. The lesions frequently were oriented in the direction of trabeculae and consisted chiefly of lamellar bone that in places was arranged concentrically in haversian systems around small blood vessels. Irregular spikes or thorns were present on the surface of the foci, and necrotic bone was not identified. These histologic observations are identical to those reported in enostoses or bone islands unassociated with dysbaric osteonecrosis, again raising doubt as to the significance of the radiodense foci.

Differential Diagnosis

The radiographic findings associated with dysbaric osteonecrosis generally are indistinguishable from those associated with osteonecrosis of other causes such as sickle cell anemia, Gaucher's disease, and steroid medication. Although diaphyseal calcification in an infarct may simulate that in an enchondroma, a shell-like calcific pattern in infarction differs from the punctate and central calcification in an enchondroma. Small, dense foci in dysbaric osteonecrosis are virtually identical to bone islands and only those that are larger and more numerous may allow accurate diagnosis of this condition. Small cystic areas, as seen in dysbaric osteonecrosis, also can be observed in the femoral neck of normal persons and in periarticular locations in degenerative or posttraumatic conditions. Although conven-

tional tomography may aid in the differential diagnosis of the findings,[85] this technique rarely is indicated.

IDIOPATHIC (PRIMARY OR SPONTANEOUS) OSTEONECROSIS

Osteonecrosis may appear in certain locations in the absence of any recognizable underlying disorder or event. Most characteristically, it is the femoral head or femoral condyles that are involved, although, rarely, spontaneous osteonecrosis can appear at other sites, especially in the metaphyses of long tubular bones[90–92] (Figs. 80–43 to 80–45). Here infarcts often are detected as incidental findings on radiographic examinations accomplished for unrelated reasons, appearing as peripheral rims or shells of calcification in the humerus, the femur, the tibia, or the fibula that must be distinguished from enchondromas. Once recognized, they generally remain unchanged on serial radiographs, although obscuration of a portion of the lesion may reflect disintegration of the central region of the necrotic tissue, liquefaction, and partial absorption.[93]

Spontaneous Osteonecrosis of the Femoral Head in Adults

The first description of idiopathic or spontaneous osteonecrosis of the femoral head in adults appears to be that of

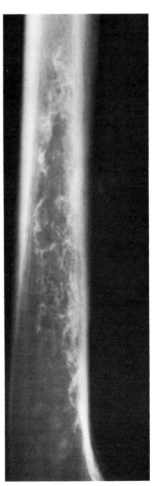

FIGURE 80–42. Dysbaric osteonecrosis: Diaphyseal lesion. In this deep sea diver and astronaut, the irregular calcific deposits in the femur with a shell-like configuration are typical of a bone infarct.

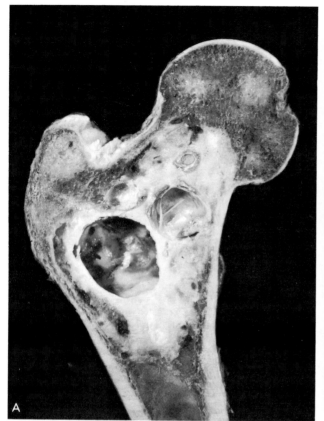

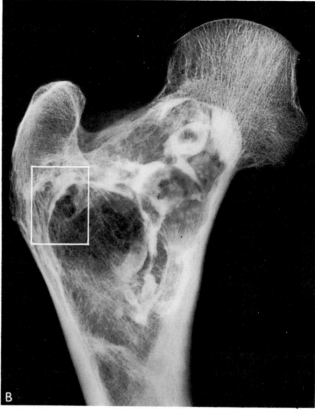

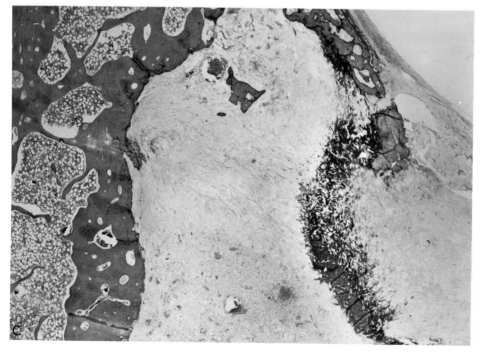

FIGURE 80–43. Idiopathic (primary or spontaneous) osteonecrosis: Proximal portion of the femur.

A A photograph of the cut surface of the upper end of the right femur in a 72 year old man reveals a multilocular cystic area in the femoral neck and the intertrochanteric region. Detailed study of the specimen indicated that in the distant past the area must have been the site of an infarct which in the course of time underwent cystic softening. Neither the gross nor the microscopic appearance was consistent with a lesion of recent origin.

B Radiograph of the sectioned upper end of the femur delineates individual cystic areas that are surrounded by a border of radiopacity, which is thin in some places and thick in others. The radiopaque border may contain some osseous tissue but consists mainly of calcified collagenous connective tissue. The histologic appearance of a portion of the boxed area is shown in **C.**

C A photomicrograph (17×) demonstrates that the inner surface of the cyst, which is on the right side of the photograph, contains a thin lining layer that consists of acellular collagenous tissue, the deeper part of which is calcified. Immediately to the left, there is a zone of nonviable and disintegrating osseous tissue. Farther to the left, there is an area of collagenous tissue, poor in cells and heavily calcified in some places.

(From Jaffe HL: Med Radiogr Photogr *45*:58, 1969.)

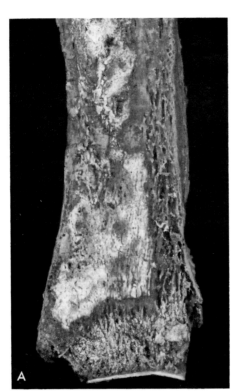

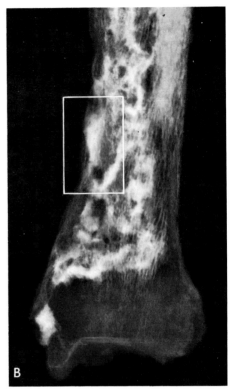

FIGURE 80–44. Idiopathic (primary or spontaneous) osteonecrosis: Distal end of the tibia.

A A photograph of the cut surface of the lower end of the right tibia of a 66 year old woman shows a large area of infarction. This infarct, which is more or less white, was only part of the total lesion, which, occupied almost the entire shaft of the bone.

B A radiograph of the same part of the tibia indicates a vaguely loculated and variegated area of radiopacity, representing the site of infarction. The more intensely radiopaque regions correspond to those areas that are strikingly white in the photographic view.

C Photomicrograph of a part of the boxed area in **B** (25×) indicates the periosteal surface at the upper margin of the illustration. Many of the necrotic spongy trabeculae have undergone disintegration, and the intertrabecular marrow spaces largely are filled with calcified granular detritus, which stains dark.

(From Jaffe HL: Med Radiogr Photogr 45:58, 1969.)

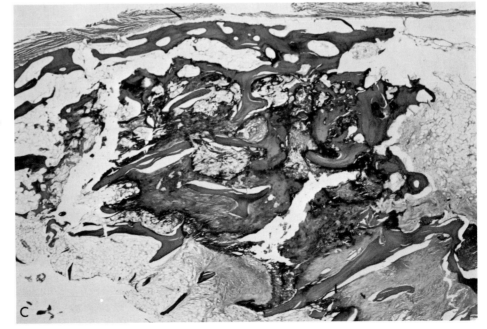

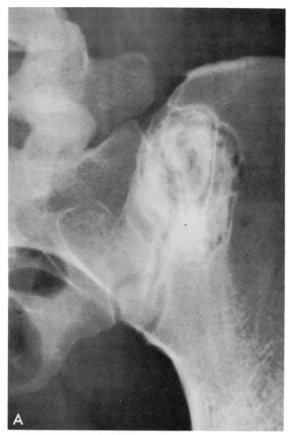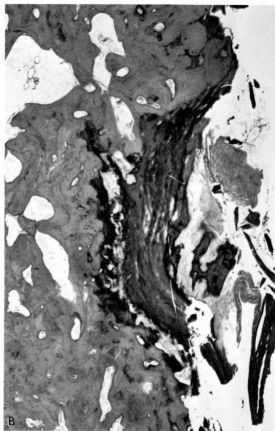

FIGURE 80–45. Idiopathic (primary or spontaneous) osteonecrosis: Ilium.

A A radiograph shows an area of ischemic necrosis in the left iliac bone in the vicinity of the sacroiliac joint of a 33 year old pregnant woman with mild pain involving the lower part of her back. Observe the degree of calcification of the lesion.

B Photomicrograph (25×) shows a fragment of osseous tissue from the posterior or outer cortical wall of the iliac bone in the vicinity of the cystlike space in the interior of the bone in **A.** The darkly discolored area represents osseous tissue that is undergoing granular disintegration. It was white or yellow-white on gross examination. Farther to the left, the disintegrating osseous tissue is lined in part by a thin layer of collagenous connective tissue.

(From Jaffe HL: Med Radiogr Photogr *45*:58, 1969.)

Freund in 1926.[94] Numerous publications later appeared, underscoring the continued interest in this problem, although a specific cause has not been delineated.[95–102, 140, 302] An abnormality of fat metabolism, similar to that occurring in corticosteroid-induced osteonecrosis, leading to marrow infiltration or vascular embolization is the most popular hypothesis.[211, 302, 362] Microangiographic studies have revealed interruption of the superior retinacular arteries, the presence of numerous newly formed vessels arising from the stumps of the interrupted arteries, compensatory hypertrophy of vessels arising from the inferior retinacular arteries and those of the ligamentum teres, and blockage of revascularization about regions of subchondral fracture and collapse.[301, 339] The condition sometimes is designated as Chandler's disease in recognition of the pertinent investigations of Chandler, who referred to spontaneous osteonecrosis of the femoral head as "coronary disease of the hip."[103]

Primary necrosis of the femoral head affects men more frequently than women and usually is seen between the fourth and seventh decades of life. Unilateral or bilateral involvement may be detected; the reported prevalence of bilateral disease has varied from 35 to 72 per cent, influ-

enced predominantly by the method of examination and the length of follow-up.[99] Despite the frequency of bilateral involvement, the condition usually is manifested first as a unilateral symptomatic hip related to osseous collapse in the more severely affected side. The radiographic features vary with the stage of the disorder. Initially, a femoral head of normal osseous contour may reveal mottled radiodense areas scattered throughout its anterosuperior region with a faint curvilinear band of diminished density in the anterior subchondral bone, the crescent sign. As the disease progresses, a focus of increased radiodensity or a lucent zone with a peripheral rim of increased radiodensity is observed. This area may be ovoid, triangular, or wedge-shaped, and although it is diagnostic of osteonecrosis, it is by no means specific for the primary or idiopathic variety. Subtle flattening of the femoral contour adjacent to the sclerotic area can be combined with increased radiodensity of the head, reflecting the presence of revascularization and an attempt at osseous repair. The eventual degree of collapse of the articular surface is variable[303, 304]; experimental data suggest that the degree of structural degradation of the cancellous bone within the main region of infarction is more important than the degree of structural degradation within the subchondral

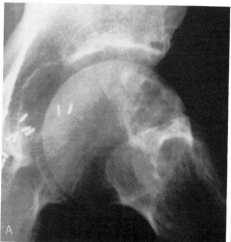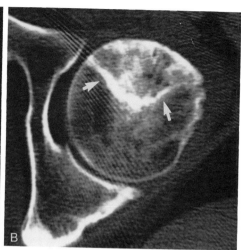

FIGURE 80–46. Spontaneous osteonecrosis of the femoral head: Segmental type.

A In this 55 year old man, a lobulated radiolucent lesion involves the anterior portion of the femoral head. No collapse of bone is evident. Surgical clips are seen.

B Transaxial CT shows a wedge-shaped lesion (arrows) with its base situated on the anterior femoral surface. Note the sclerotic margins of this osteonecrotic region.

bone plate in influencing the time of onset and, perhaps, the degree of femoral head collapse.[305] In some cases, severe disintegration and fragmentation of subchondral bone encourage the superimposition of osteoarthritis, with its typical radiographic features. A rare sequela of this condition is a synovial cyst.[135]

A milder form of osteonecrosis of the femoral head, typically found contralateral to a femoral head revealing classic features of ischemic necrosis, has been designated minimal or segmental osteonecrosis.[306] This type of involvement is not progressive and affects the superficial zone of the femoral head in any of its four quadrants—anterior, superior, medial, or lateral. A wedge shape to the involved area, related to vascular interruption at its apex and a base situated on the articular surface, may be encountered (Fig. 80–46). The resulting radiographic findings are localized to a small portion of the femoral head but otherwise resemble those seen with more extensive osteonecrosis. The pathogenesis of minimal osteonecrosis may relate to a single ischemic event rather than multiple, or repeated, episodes of infarction.

The pathologic findings of idiopathic osteonecrosis of the femoral head are virtually identical to those in other varieties of osteonecrosis (see Chapter 79). On gross examination, the femoral head may appear to have a normal contour, but firm pressure will elicit segmental collapse of the articular surface, the "ping-pong ball" effect. In the area of necrosis, a wedge-shaped zone is seen, which usually is well delineated from the surrounding bone. Microscopic evaluation may reveal a zone of fibrous tissue about the

necrotic bone relatively rich in blood vessels and commonly surrounded by dense sclerotic osseous tissue in the remaining spongiosa of the head and neck.

It should be obvious that the designation of idiopathic osteonecrosis requires elimination of any underlying process that predisposes to such ischemia of the femoral head.[302] These processes include dysbaric osteonecrosis, Gaucher's disease, sickle cell anemia, alcohol abuse, previous corticosteroid treatment, trauma, and hyperuricemia.

Spontaneous Osteonecrosis About the Knee in Adults

Although osteonecrosis about the knee may be observed in association with steroid therapy, sickle cell anemia, other hemoglobinopathies, and renal transplantation, it also may occur in a spontaneous or idiopathic fashion.[104–114, 212–218, 313] This disorder, which sometimes is referred to as Ahlbäck's disease, is distinct from osteochondritis dissecans occurring in adolescence (Table 80–3). It is characterized by the onset, in an older patient (usually over 60 years of age, although children with this disorder[311] have been described) who more frequently is a woman than a man, of abrupt pain in the knee (the patient may be able to recall the exact moment when the pain became apparent), almost always confined to the medial aspect of the joint. The pain typically is worse at night. Localized tenderness and stiffness, an effusion, and restricted motion may be apparent. Unilateral involvement predominates over bilateral involvement. Initially radiographs are normal, and it is not until a period of

TABLE 80–3. Spontaneous Osteonecrosis Versus Osteochondritis Dissecans (About the Knee)

	Spontaneous Osteonecrosis	Osteochondritis Dissecans
Age of onset	Middle-aged and elderly	Adolescent
Symptoms	Pain, tenderness, swelling, restricted motion	Variable; may be lacking
Typical location	Weight-bearing surface of medial femoral condyle	Non–weight-bearing surface of medial femoral condyle
Probable pathogenesis	Trauma, perhaps related to meniscal tear; or vascular insult	Trauma
Sequelae	Degenerative joint disease; intra-articular osteocartilaginous bodies	Intra-articular osteocartilaginous bodies

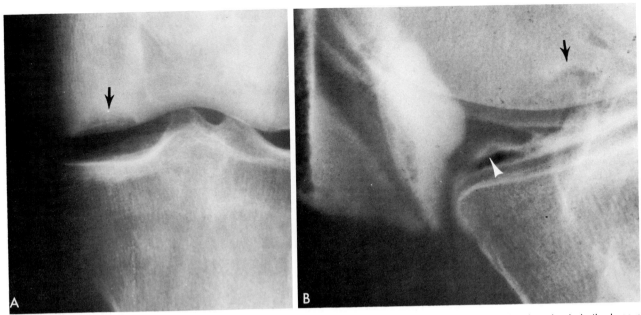

FIGURE 80–47. Spontaneous osteonecrosis about the knee: Medial femoral condyle. This 60 year old man developed pain in the knee of acute onset, which was associated with an effusion. No history of trauma could be elicited, and the patient had not received corticosteroids.

A Two years after the onset of pain, a radiograph reveals flattening of the weight-bearing surface of the medial femoral condyle associated with an osseous excavation (arrow) containing a linear radiodense shadow.

B An arthrogram reveals the site of necrosis (arrow), a tear on the undersurface and tip of the medial meniscus (arrowhead), and a popliteal cyst. It has been suggested that meniscal tears predispose to osteonecrosis of the adjacent femoral condyle (see text).

weeks or months has passed that subtle flattening of the weight-bearing articular surface of the medial femoral condyle is seen (Fig. 80–47) (the lateral condyle is affected infrequently). A narrow zone of increased radiodensity adjacent to the depressed osseous surface may reflect compression of subchondral trabeculae. A radiolucent lesion in the condyle can be detected over the ensuing weeks, which at first is diffuse and irregular in outline and later is more sharply demarcated. Within the lucent area, a radiodense line consisting of cartilage and subchondral bone plate frequently can be identified (Fig. 80–47). If the affected area is small and weight-bearing is avoided, spontaneous healing can occur. If untreated, however, further depression of the bony margin, intra-articular osseous bodies, progressive sclerosis, and periostitis of the distal portion of the femur can be encountered on later examination (Fig. 80–48). Over a period of months or years, joint space narrowing, cyst formation, eburnation, and osteophytosis on apposing margins of the femur and tibia indicate the development of secondary osteoarthritis (Fig. 80–49). Bony collapse, varus deformity, and displacement also can be noted. The eventual radiographic picture may be identical to that of "medial type" osteoarthritis of the knee, and the accompanying degenerative cartilaginous and bony features may obscure the findings of osteonecrosis. In fact, the resemblance of the superimposed degenerative changes in cases of spontaneous osteonecrosis about the knee to those of typical osteoarthritis has led to speculation that a significant number of cases of degenerative joint disease of the knee have their origin in an ischemic event.

The precise distribution of the lesion about the knee represents one of the most important characteristics of spontaneous osteonecrosis. In the vast majority of cases, it is the weight-bearing surface of the medial femoral condyle

that is involved. Atypical cases showing alterations in the non-weight-bearing portion of this condyle are described,[219] although in some instances, such alterations may have resulted from an unrelated process. Spontaneous ischemic necrosis occasionally is observed in the medial portion of the tibial plateau[212, 220, 313] or in the lateral femoral condyle, alone or in combination with changes in the medial condyle of the femur (Fig. 80–50). A similar process has been described even in the lateral portion of the tibial plateau.[220] In instances of tibial involvement, depression of the articular surface and subchondral sclerosis and cyst formation usually occur at the margin of the bone, not on the weight-bearing surface,[212] and may not progress to osteoarthritis.[215]

The delay in the appearance of radiographic findings in this condition has stimulated a search for more sensitive techniques. Scintigraphic examination using bone-seeking radiopharmaceutical agents (Fig. 80–50) has promise in this regard, as focal accumulation of radionuclide can be identified long before radiographic changes appear.[105, 112, 113, 136, 308, 309] Lotke and coworkers[111] described a series of 12 patients with clinical and scintigraphic findings of spontaneous osteonecrosis about the knee without radiographic findings in whom conservative management led to amelioration of symptoms and signs and disappearance of the positive radionuclide findings and in whom radiographic abnormalities never appeared. The use of three-phase bone scintigraphy allows identification of the stages of the process: acute osteonecrosis characterized by focal accumulation of the radionuclide in the region of the medial condyle in the angiographic phase, focal or diffuse hyperemia in the blood pool images, and intense focal uptake in the condyle on the delayed images; subacute osteonecrosis characterized by decreased hyperemia and continued focal accumulation of the radionuclide in the femoral condyle on the

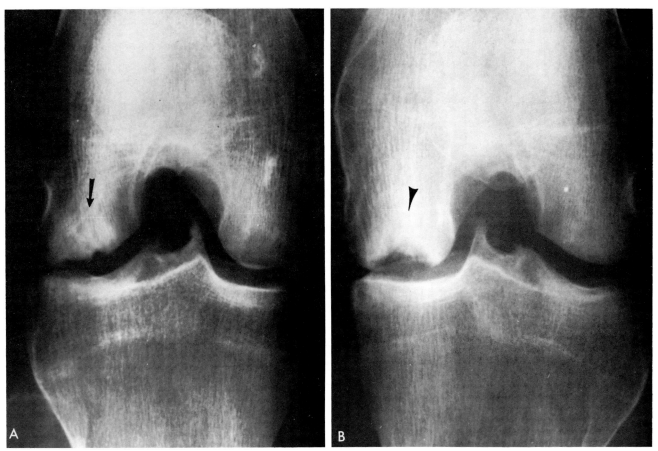

FIGURE 80–48. Spontaneous osteonecrosis about the knee: Medial and lateral femoral condyles. This middle-aged woman developed the spontaneous onset of pain in both knees. She had not received corticosteroids. Observe osseous depression, irregularity, and sclerosis of the lateral condyle of the right femur (arrow) and the medial condyle of the left femur (arrowhead).

delayed scans; and late osteonecrosis characterized by a normal bone scan if the radiographs remain normal or by persistently abnormal activity if the radiographs become positive.[218] Furthermore, the results of both scintigraphy

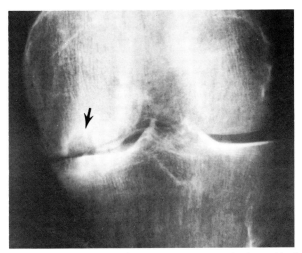

FIGURE 80–49. Spontaneous osteonecrosis about the knee: Medial femoral condyle. An example of spontaneous osteonecrosis with superimposed degenerative joint disease is shown. Joint space narrowing and sclerosis are prominent. Although the appearance simulates that of uncomplicated degenerative joint disease, the degree of bony flattening and the presence of cystic lesions (arrow) in the condyle suggest that osteonecrosis has occurred.

and radiography can be used to group the affected patients into categories reflecting the subsequent clinical course of the disease. Those with scintigraphic abnormalities alone have a good prognosis and respond to conservative treatment; those with positive radionuclide studies and small and stable radiographically evident lesions also do well with conservative therapy; and those with abnormal bone scans and considerable radiographic alterations generally require surgical intervention.[214]

MR imaging also may be employed as a sensitive method in the diagnosis of spontaneous osteonecrosis about the knee (Figs. 80–51 to 80–53).[314, 315] This technique may reveal characteristic abnormalities in a symptomatic patient whose radiographs are normal and bilateral involvement when only one side is symptomatic. Low signal intensity in the affected region is typical on T1-weighted spin echo MR images, and a surrounding area of high signal intensity, probably representing edema, may be evident on T2-weighted images. Additional MR imaging findings include the presence of cystic lesions containing fluid (which are of high signal intensity on the T2-weighted images), bone collapse with buckling of the articular cartilage, and tears or degeneration of the adjacent meniscus.[315] Accurate measurement of the lesion, which appears to have prognostic significance in that larger lesions are associated with a poor clinical outcome, also is possible with MR imaging.

Surgical evaluation of the lesion may identify the depressed osseous surface and articular cartilage and bony

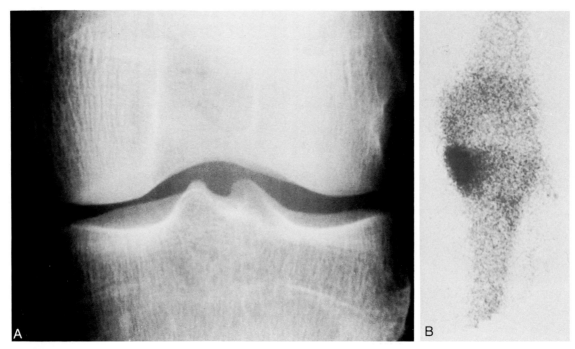

FIGURE 80–50. Spontaneous osteonecrosis about the knee: Medial tibial plateau. This 56 year old man developed the acute onset of severe knee pain. The radiograph **(A)** essentially is normal, but the increased accumulation of the bone-seeking radionuclide **(B)** in the medial aspect of the tibia is consistent with spontaneous necrosis.

fragments that can remain in situ, be slightly displaced, exist free in the articular cavity, or be embedded at a distant synovial site[115] (Fig. 80–54). Microscopy can delineate segmental bony necrosis with cartilaginous irregularity and collapse as well as an adjacent osseous response consisting of histiocytic resorption of necrotic material and formation of granulomatous tissue with surrounding reactive new bone formation.[106] Synovial hypertrophy and fibrosis about bony detritus also can be identified.

The cause and pathogenesis of this condition are not clear. The dominant opinion implicates vascular insufficiency leading to infarction of bone. Elevation of intraosseous pressure in this disorder, similar to that seen in osteonecrosis of the femoral head, supports the presence of an initial ischemic event.[312] A traumatic insult producing microfractures in the subchondral bone plate and overlying osseous and cartilaginous collapse also has been emphasized. Traumatically induced defects in the chondral and bony coat might allow fluid from the cartilage to be expressed into the adjacent marrow space, producing an increase in marrow pressure and pain.[111] A prominent role of meniscal injury in the pathogenesis of spontaneous osteonecrosis also has been proposed.[114] Meniscal tears have been reported in association with this condition, and the impact of the articular surface against a fragmented meniscus during everyday activity could result in local ischemia of the medial femoral condyle. Furthermore, the sudden onset of pain that characterizes spontaneous osteonecrosis about the knee could be related to an acute tear of the meniscus. The appearance of spontaneous osteonecrosis about the knee after meniscal surgery also supports a pathogenetic relationship between this condition and meniscal alterations. Some patients with necrosis do not reveal a torn

meniscus, however, and in others meniscal tears demonstrated on arthrography may reflect the result rather than the cause of the osseous necrosis.[128]

The other entities that enter into the differential diagnosis of the radiographic changes in spontaneous osteonecrosis about the knee are osteonecrosis from additional causes, osteochondritis dissecans, calcium pyrophosphate dihydrate crystal deposition disease, transient osteoporosis, stress fracture, and neuropathic osteoarthropathy. Bone necrosis due to corticosteroids or occurring after renal transplantation produces imaging features that are almost identical to those in spontaneous osteonecrosis (Fig. 80–55). Historical information and involvement of multiple sites in the former two situations are helpful in the correct interpretation of the radiographs, however. Furthermore, steroid-induced osteonecrosis may lead to larger areas of involvement than in spontaneous osteonecrosis,[310] and the lateral femoral condyle commonly is affected. Osteochondritis dissecans affects young patients and classically does not involve the weight-bearing surface of the condyle. Although calcium pyrophosphate dihydrate crystal deposition disease may lead to flattening of the femoral condyles, chondrocalcinosis usually is present in the knee or elsewhere. Transient osteoporosis is associated with increased accumulation of bone-seeking radiopharmaceutical agents but depression of the articular surface is not evident. A stress fracture of the femur or tibia typically occurs at some distance from the joint margin and often is seen in younger and physically active persons. Neuropathic osteoarthropathy can produce fragmentation of the femoral condyles. Generally, the neurologic deficit is obvious, although clinical findings related to certain types of neuropathic joints (e.g., syndromes of congenital insensitivity to pain) may be quite subtle.

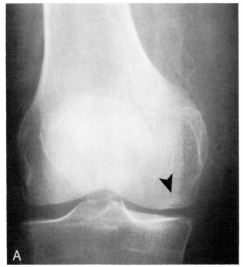

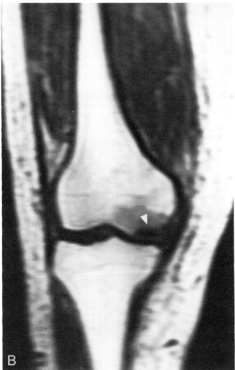

FIGURE 80–51. Spontaneous osteonecrosis about the knee: Medial femoral condyle. MR imaging. In this 81 year old woman with a 1 month history of knee pain, a routine radiograph **(A)** shows a small subchondral radiolucent lesion with a surrounding zone of sclerosis (arrowhead). A coronal T1-weighted (TR/TE, 600/20) spin echo MR image **(B)** reveals a discrete area of low signal intensity in the medial femoral condyle (arrowhead). About this area, more diffuse low signal intensity in the marrow is consistent with edema. (From Pollack MS, et al: Skel Radiol 16:121, 1987.)

Spontaneous Osteonecrosis of the Tarsal Navicular Bone in Adults (Mueller-Weiss Syndrome)

In 1927, Mueller[316] described a condition of the tarsal navicular bone, occurring in adults, that he believed was a chronic deformation related to compression from adjacent bones. Radiographic characteristics included medial or dorsal protrusion of portions of the bone or the entire navicular

bone and a comma-shaped deformity due to collapse of the lateral portion of the bone. Bilateral distribution, asymmetric involvement, and pathologic fractures represented additional findings in the disease. One year later, in a second report, Mueller[317] identified a normal histologic appearance of the tarsal navicular bone in an affected patient and concluded that the condition was congenital and not traumatic. In 1929, Weiss[318] investigated similar abnormalities in adults and proposed osteonecrosis as the primary causative factor. Subsequently, further descriptions of the same disorder, occurring predominantly in women, have appeared, and a variety of names, including bipartite navicular bone and osteopathia deformans, have been used.[319–321]

Bilateral abnormalities are more common than unilateral disease, although unilateral changes may be evident in younger persons. Women are affected more frequently than men, and pes planus and valgus deformity of the ankle are associated features. Initial radiographic alterations include a loss of volume in the lateral aspect of the tarsal navicular bone, which is accompanied by an increase in radiodensity of this portion of the bone (Fig. 80–56). The tarsal navicular assumes a comma-like shape because of lateral compression. Subsequently, dorsal protrusion and fragmentation of the bone may become evident. CT allows precise delineation of the sites of fracture and fragmentation.[321] These fractures generally course in an oblique plane and may be comminuted. MR imaging shows a homogeneous decrease in the signal intensity of the navicular bone on T1-weighted spin echo images.[321] The changes in signal intensity are more variable on T2-weighted images. Effusions in neighboring joints may be observed.

The Mueller-Weiss syndrome certainly is distinct from the well-recognized osteochondrosis of the tarsal navicular bone occurring in children (Köhler's disease). It is a disorder of adults that is characterized by a chronic clinical course, severe and sometimes devastating pain and disability, and progressive deformity. The precise cause of the Mueller-Weiss syndrome is not clear, however. Histologic data generally are lacking. This syndrome probably relates to previous injury or chronic stress. As obesity is a common feature in affected patients, increased loading of the foot may lead to mechanical stress that is most prominent in the tarsal region.[321] The radiographic abnormalities of this syndrome resemble those seen in patients with stress fractures of the tarsal navicular bone.

With regard to differential diagnosis, osteonecrosis of the tarsal navicular bone also may accompany systemic diseases, such as systemic lupus erythematosus, and may complicate corticosteroid administration. Insufficiency fractures of this bone may be evident in patients with rheumatoid arthritis, chronic renal disease, and diabetes mellitus (Fig. 80–57).

Spontaneous Osteonecrosis of the Patella

In 1990, La Prade and Noffsinger[322] described a 16 year old girl with chronic knee pain in whom radiographs revealed a sclerotic defect in the superolateral portion of the patella. At surgery, the lesion appeared to be avascular, with a slightly hyperemic, poorly defined border. Histologic analysis of the excised specimen revealed findings consistent with osteonecrosis. Subsequent to this report, letters appeared in the literature suggesting that the lesion reported

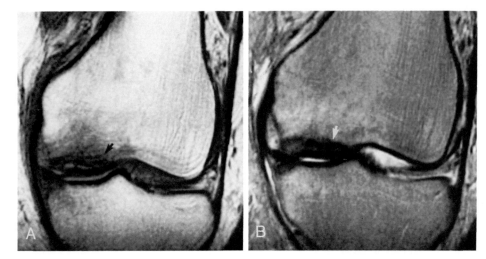

FIGURE 80–52. Spontaneous osteonecrosis about the knee: Medial femoral condyle. MR imaging. In this 67 year old woman with the abrupt onset of knee pain, a coronal proton density (TR/TE, 1000/20) spin echo MR image **(A)** reveals flattening of the medial femoral condyle, with a subchondral zone of low signal intensity (arrow). Broader areas of low signal intensity involve the medial femoral condyle and medial tibial plateau. On a coronal T2-weighted (TR/TE, 3000/76) spin echo image **(B),** the area of necrosis again is evident (arrow). Note the bone marrow edema, with high signal intensity, in the medial femoral condyle and medial tibial plateau. Additional findings include a joint effusion, a torn medial meniscus (not well shown), and subcutaneous edema. (Courtesy of M. Schweitzer, M.D., Philadelphia, Pennsylvania.)

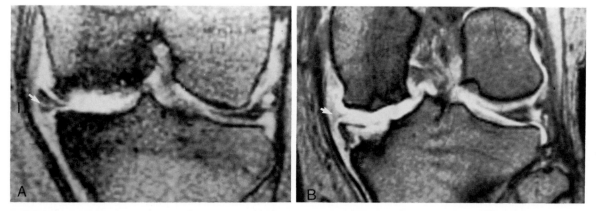

FIGURE 80–53. Spontaneous osteonecrosis about the knee: Medial femoral condyle and medial tibial plateau. MR imaging.

A Medial femoral condyle. A coronal multiplanar gradient recalled (MPGR) MR image (TR/TE, 600/20; flip angle, 45 degrees) shows cartilage loss in both the medial femoral condyle and medial tibial plateau, a subchondral zone of osteonecrosis in the medial femoral condyle, diminished signal intensity in the adjacent tibial plateau consistent with bone sclerosis, a joint effusion, and a tear (arrow) of the medial meniscus. The findings are those of spontaneous osteonecrosis of the medial femoral condyle with secondary osteoarthritis.

B Medial tibial plateau. A similar coronal MPGR image (TR/TE, 600/20; flip angle, 45 degrees) reveals osteonecrosis in the medial tibial plateau with depression and fracture of the articular surface, loss of articular cartilage, sclerosis with low signal intensity in the medial femoral condyle, a joint effusion, and a torn medial meniscus (arrow).

(Courtesy of S. Fernandez, M.D., Mexico City, Mexico.)

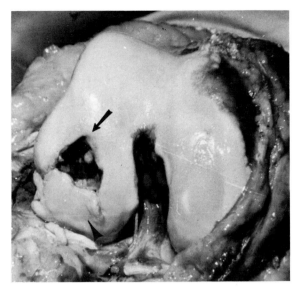

FIGURE 80–54. Spontaneous osteonecrosis about the knee. The surgical findings in this condition include excavation and depression of the weight-bearing osseous surface of the condyle (arrow). Note the bony fragments (arrowhead). (Courtesy of R. Convery, M.D., San Diego, California.)

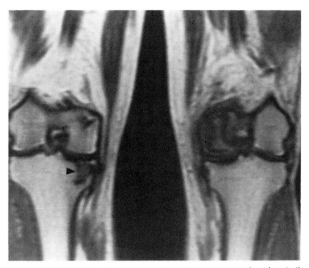

FIGURE 80–55. Corticosteroid-induced osteonecrosis about the knee. In a 47 year old woman receiving corticosteroid therapy for asthma who developed knee pain, a coronal T1-weighted (TR/TE, 600/20) spin echo MR image reveals lesions in the left medial femoral condyle and right medial tibial plateau (arrowhead) consistent with osteonecrosis. (From Pollack MS, et al: Skel Radiol 16:121, 1987.)

by La Prade and Noffsinger most likely represented osteochondritis dissecans[323] or a dorsal defect of the patella.[324]

Despite the presence of a blood supply to the patella that may be vulnerable to injury, as well as reports that indicate that the upper pole of the patella is the typical site of posttraumatic osteonecrosis,[55] the existence of spontaneous osteonecrosis of this bone requires further verification (Fig. 80–58). Ischemic necrosis of the patella, however, is a recognized complication of total knee arthroplasty[325] and corticosteroid therapy.[326, 327]

COMPLICATIONS

Cartilaginous Abnormalities

One of the striking pathologic features of osteonecrosis is the intactness of the chondral surface despite the presence of adjacent severe osseous abnormality (Fig. 80–59A). This finding, which has its radiographic counterpart in preservation of the joint space, supports the commonly held impression that articular cartilage in mature adults derives most, if not all, of its nutrition from synovial fluid and is independent of the subjacent bone. It also is recognized that in those cases in which osteonecrosis leads to significant collapse of the articular surface, incongruities of apposing bony margins may lead to secondary degenerative joint disease.[328] In this situation, cartilaginous fibrillation and erosion may be revealed on radiographs as diminution of the interosseous space (Figs. 80–59B and 80–60). The possibility exists, however, that even in the presence of joint incongruity, the removal of vascular supply to the underlying bone may inhibit the development of osteoarthritic changes in the articular cartilage.[116]

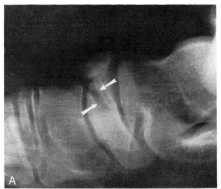
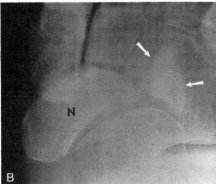
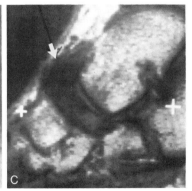

FIGURE 80–56. Spontaneous osteonecrosis of the tarsal navicular bone: Mueller-Weiss syndrome. This 49 year old obese woman had tarsal pain. No evidence of underlying systemic disease was present.
  A A lateral radiograph shows an oblique cleft (arrows), presumably a stress fracture, in the navicular bone. The radiodensity of the bone is increased, with dorsal displacement of the lateral fragment.
  B The frontal radiograph shows medial displacement of a comma-shaped navicular bone (N). The lateral fracture fragment overlies the cuboid and lateral cuneiform bones (arrows).
  C A sagittal T1-weighted (TR/TE, 600/20) spin echo MR image reveals loss of signal intensity in the marrow of a dorsally displaced navicular bone (arrow).
  (From Haller J, et al: AJR 151:355, 1988. Copyright 1988, American Roentgen Ray Society.)

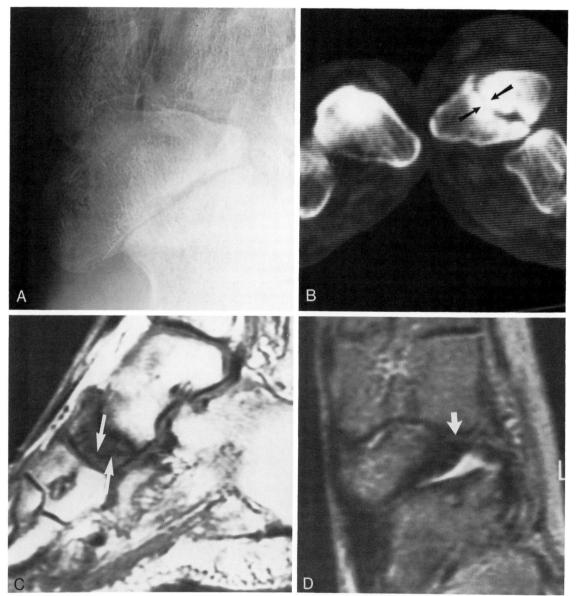

FIGURE 80–57. Insufficiency fracture of the tarsal navicular bone: Chronic renal failure and dialysis. This 62 year old man with chronic renal disease had been on dialysis for 10 years. Tarsal pain began after minor trauma 1 year previously.

A A frontal radiograph shows medial displacement and a comma shape of the navicular bone.

B A coronal CT scan reveals an oblique fracture (arrows) of the bone with adjacent sclerosis.

C A sagittal T1-weighted (TR/TE, 600/20) spin echo MR image shows dorsal protrusion and a decrease in signal intensity of the navicular bone. A fracture is faintly visible (arrows).

D A transverse, or plantar, plane T2-weighted (TR/TE, 2000/70) spin echo MR image shows loss of signal intensity of the compressed lateral portion of the navicular bone (arrow). Regions of high signal intensity in adjacent joints represent effusions.

(From Haller J, et al: AJR *151*:355, 1988. Copyright 1988, American Roentgen Ray Society.)

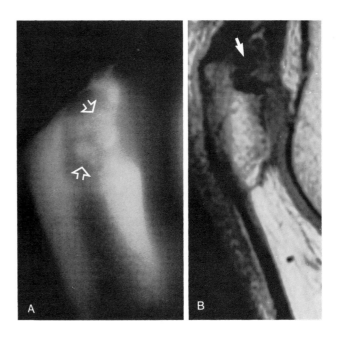

FIGURE 80–58. Spontaneous osteonecrosis of the patella. A 45 year old man developed pain and swelling of the anterior aspect of the knee after a volleyball injury. At arthroscopy, chondromalacia of the superior pole of the patella and normal subchondral bone were observed. Histologic analysis of the lesion confirmed the presence of necrotic bone and cartilage. The differential diagnosis includes osteochondritis dissecans or a dorsal defect of the patella.

A A conventional tomogram in the lateral plane shows irregularity of subchondral bone in the superior portion of the patella with fragmentation (arrows).

B A sagittal T1-weighted (TR/TE, 500/13) spin echo MR image reveals that the lesion (arrow) is of low signal intensity. The integrity of the overlying cartilage cannot be determined.

(Courtesy of G. Greenway, M.D., Dallas, Texas.)

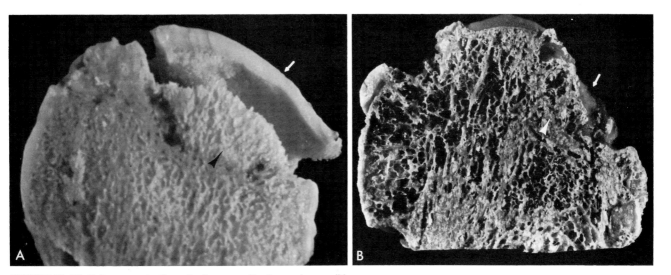

FIGURE 80–59. Osteonecrosis: Complications—cartilaginous abnormalities.

A Cartilage preservation. The viability of the cartilage (arrow) overlying the necrotic bone (arrowhead) is a remarkable feature of osteonecrosis.

B In cases of severe osteonecrosis, secondary degenerative joint disease can lead to fibrillation and erosion of the chondral surface. In this case, much of the cartilaginous surface overlying the necrotic bone (arrowhead) has been eroded (arrow).

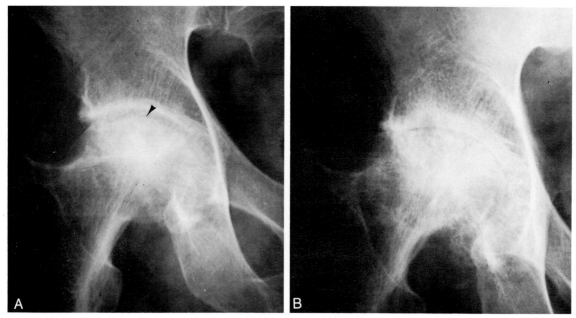

FIGURE 80–60. Osteonecrosis: Complications—cartilaginous abnormalities. Radiographs obtained 6 years apart reveal initially **(A)** collapse of the articular surface of the femoral head (arrowhead) and, subsequently **(B),** secondary osteoarthritis with considerable narrowing of the joint space. In cases such as these, it is difficult to state with certainty that the changes in **B** do not represent osteoarthritis alone unless the sequence of radiographs is available for examination.

An increase in metabolic activity in articular cartilage in immature animals after experimental osteonecrosis has been suggested.[117-120] In addition, radiographs and arthrograms of some patients with Legg-Calvé-Perthes disease have revealed an increased thickness of the chondral surface, perhaps indicating that vascular insufficiency of bone can lead to stimulation of cartilage growth in children. Mankin and coworkers[116] examined the cartilage from nine osteonecrotic femoral heads, however, and were unable to detect significant alterations in histologic characteristics or biochemical and metabolic parameters. No chondrolytic changes could be discovered, although a role for chondrolysis in some cases of osteonecrosis has been proposed. Although such chondrolysis could explain the occasional widespread or diffuse nature of the chondral loss that can be identified on serial radiographs in patients with osteonecrosis, strong evidence for this alteration has yet to be offered. Cartilage cell necrosis usually is not a prominent feature in osteonecrosis, although regional hypocellularity can be seen.[21] Pannus-like material on the chondral surface and fibrocartilaginous replacement of hyaline articular cartilage may be apparent in advanced osteonecrosis,[222] usually in association with osteoarthritic abnormalities.[138]

Intra-articular Osseous Bodies

Infrequently, one or more chondral or osteochondral fragments can appear in osteonecrosis.[121] They may exist free in the articular cavity, in situ in the depressed bony area, or embedded in the synovium at a distant site (Fig. 80–61). In the hip, the foci may produce few or no symptoms, whereas in the knee, symptoms and signs are not unusual. The histologic characteristics of the nidi are consistent with the pathologic nature of this disease, revealing subchondral bone with trabecular reinforcement and relatively normal articular cartilage. In some cases, reattach-

ment of the fragment to the synovial lining results in its partial or complete resorption.[122]

Septic Arthritis

Septic arthritis of the hip has been reported as a complication of osteonecrosis of the femoral head.[334-336] Hematogenous spread of infection from a distant site is the mechanism of contamination of the hip. Accurate diagnosis may be difficult as the clinical features of septic arthritis and an exacerbation of osteonecrosis are similar, and radiographic and scintigraphic features may not be specific.[335]

Pathologic Fracture

Fracture involving an area of osteonecrosis appears to be a rare complication (Fig. 80–62). Marmor[337] reported a patient with spontaneous osteonecrosis of the medial tibial plateau who developed a fracture of the adjacent rim of the tibia, and McGlade and coworkers[338] described two elderly women with ischemic necrosis of the femoral heads in whom unilateral (one patient) or bilateral (one patient) fractures of the femoral neck developed.

Cyst Formation

Cystic degeneration in areas of bone infarction predominates in the diaphyses of tubular bones, especially the tibia (Fig. 80–63) and the humerus.[221] An expanding osteolytic area that erodes the cortex is seen, usually at a single site. As it evolves, the cyst becomes sharply marginated. This feature and the absence of cortical disruption suggest the correct diagnosis, although differentiation of a cyst and malignant degeneration of an osseous infarct may be difficult. With cystic transformation at a site of osteonecrosis, clinical manifestations may be absent or mild and, on

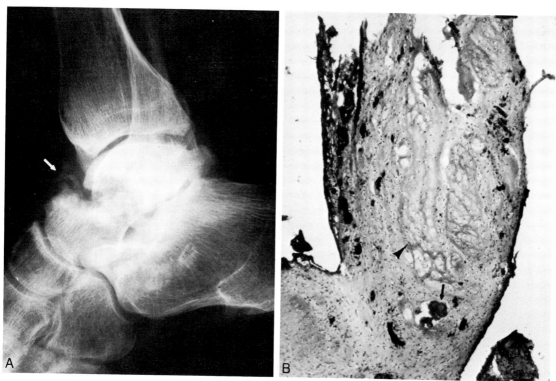

FIGURE 80–61. Osteonecrosis: Complications—intra-articular osseous bodies. This 45 year old man developed a fracture of the talus complicated by ischemic necrosis of the proximal half of the bone. Two years later, he experienced increasing pain and swelling in the ankle.

A An ununited fracture of the midportion of the talus is seen. Note osteonecrosis of the proximal portion of the bone, leading to an increase in radiodensity and multiple osseous fragments in the anterior portion of the joint (arrow).

B Histologic examination of the synovial tissue provided by biopsy shows osseous bodies (arrow) embedded in the synovial membrane and, possibly, chondroid metaplasia (arrowhead). No organisms were recovered from culture of the tissue.

FIGURE 80–62. Osteonecrosis: Complications—pathologic fracture. This patient developed knee pain after a fall.

A A coronal T1-weighted (TR/TE, 600/20) spin echo MR image shows classic features of osteonecrosis involving the distal portion of the femur. Observe the serpentine margin of the lesion with low signal intensity.

B A sagittal T2-weighted (TR/TE, 2000/70) spin echo image shows a fracture (arrow) through the area of osteonecrosis in the medial femoral condyle. Osteonecrosis also involves the adjacent tibial plateau, and a joint effusion is seen.

(Courtesy of S.K. Brahme, M.D., San Diego, California.)

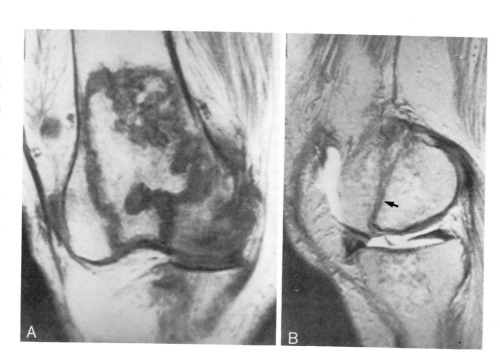

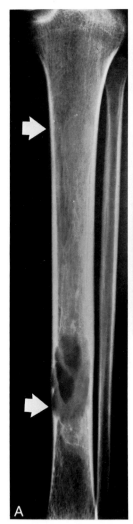

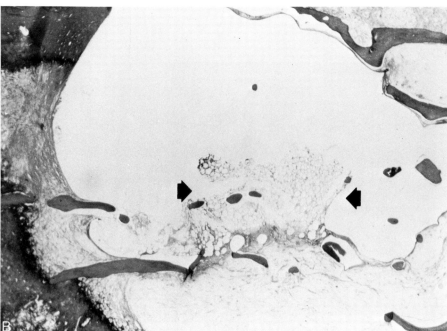

FIGURE 80–63. Osteonecrosis: Complications—cyst formation.

A In this 25 year old black woman, observe a bone infarct (upper arrow) in the shaft of the tibia. A cystic area (lower arrow) has led to erosion of the endosteal margin of the cortex.

B In a different patient with osteonecrosis and cyst formation in the femoral neck, the photomicrograph (12 ×) shows necrotic tissue in the center (arrows), surrounded by a cavity with necrotic marrow and calcification outside the wall of the cyst.

(From Norman A, Steiner GC: Radiology *146*:335, 1983.)

pathologic examination, a hyalinized fibrous wall and dystrophic calcifications are seen.[221] These histologic features as well as radiologic abnormalities that may include an osteolytic focus with internal calcification resemble the characteristics of an intraosseous lipoma, suggesting that the latter may be the result of an ischemic event rather than a tumor (Chapter 83).

Malignant Degeneration

Sarcoma arising in areas of bone infarction has been documented in both idiopathic cases and those related to caisson disease or other disorders.[123–127, 223, 329–332, 357] Men are affected more commonly, and the patient usually is in the fifth to seventh decade of life. Multiple bone infarcts commonly are present. Typically the distal end of the femur (Fig. 80–64) or proximal part of the tibia is the site of neoplasm, although other areas, such as the proximal femur, proximal humerus (Fig. 80–65), or distal tibia, may be altered. Rarely, more than one sarcoma is evident.[223] The lesions may be poorly differentiated, containing fibrous, osteoid, or cartilaginous tissue. They may be interpreted as fibrosarcoma, malignant fibrous histiocytoma,[246] or, more rarely, osteosarcoma, and it is suggested that these tumors arise from some of the cellular elements that are involved

in the repair process. A distinct relationship between infarction and malignant transformation of bone is not accepted by all authorities, particularly because of the very few documented reports that have appeared in the literature. This apparent infrequency may relate to the fact that sarcomatous proliferation may obliterate all evidence of preexistent infarction.[125] Other investigations firmly support a real association between bone infarction and malignancy; however, a long latent period between bone infarction and malignant transformation is evident. It is possible that bone infarction results in a chronic reparative process at the revascularization margins, characterized by histiocyte proliferation. Perhaps, after many years, the histiocyte component may undergo sarcomatous transformation.[127] A similar relationship between the repair process and malignancy has been advocated to explain the occurrence of tumors in areas of bone necrosis adjacent to a prosthesis.[224] Although the prognosis in patients with bone infarction and sarcoma is guarded and disseminated metastasis and death commonly appear in a short period of time, the data in no way justify surgical ablation of infarcts[126] because of the apparent rarity of the complication. The radiographic diagnosis is not difficult, as a soft tissue mass and osseous destruction appear at a site of obvious infarction. MR imaging may be a further useful diagnostic method (Figs. 80–66 and 80–67).[330]

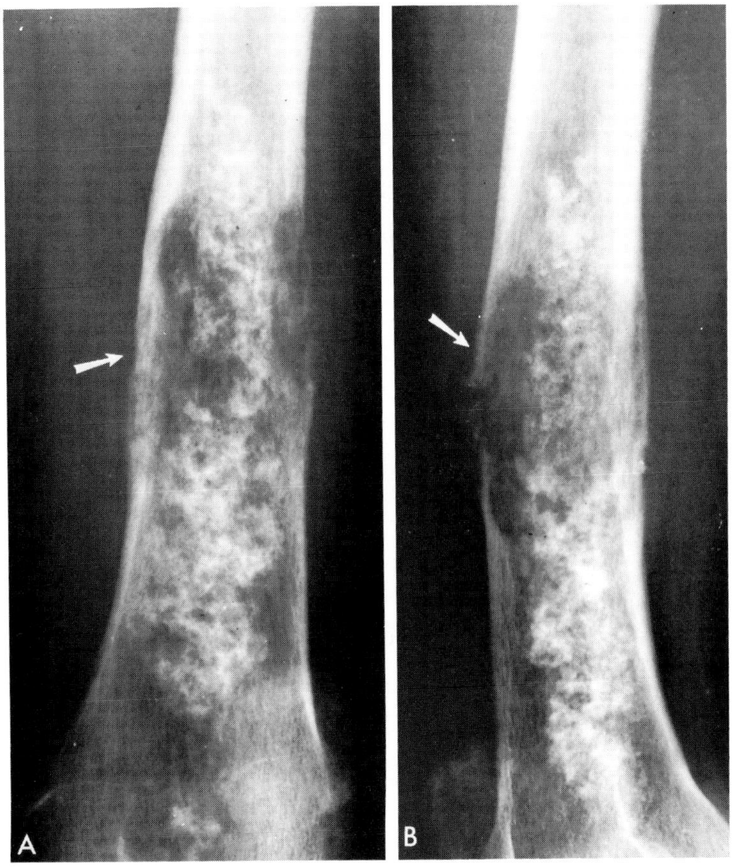

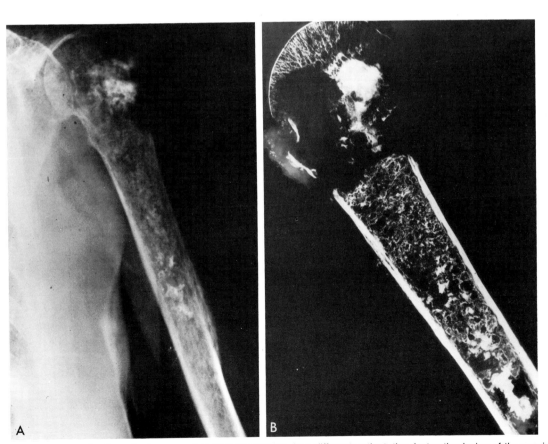

FIGURE 80–64. Osteonecrosis: Complications—malignant degeneration. In this 76 year old woman with bone infarction, a fibrosarcoma developed at the site of bone necrosis in the femur. In addition to the typical calcification of a bone infarct, observe the osteolytic destruction (arrows) with a pathologic fracture representing a fibrosarcoma. (Courtesy of V. Vint, M.D., LaJolla, California.)

FIGURE 80–65. Osteonecrosis: Complications—malignant degeneration. In a different patient, the destructive lesion of the proximal part of the humerus containing calcification in an area of bone infarction represented a sarcoma with fibrous and cartilaginous elements. (Courtesy of R. Freiberger, M.D., New York, New York.)

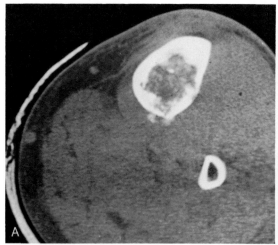

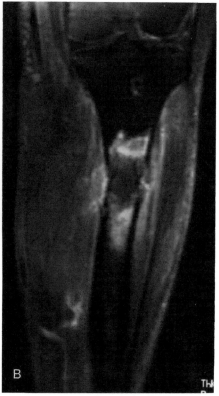

FIGURE 80–66. Osteonecrosis: Complications—malignant degeneration. This 67 year old man developed pain and a mass in his left leg. Routine radiography (not shown) revealed a partially calcified lesion in his proximal tibia, with a pathologic fracture.

A Transaxial CT shows a calcified lesion in the left tibia with cortical erosion and a soft tissue mass.

B A coronal T1-weighted (TR/TE, 600/15) spin echo MR imaging accomplished with chemical presaturation of fat (ChemSat) and after intravenous injection of a gadolinium compound reveals the tibial lesion, pathologic fracture, and soft tissue extension containing regions of enhancement of signal intensity. A smaller lesion is evident in the tibial metaphysis. Further evaluation and biopsy with histologic assessment documented multiple bone infarcts of unknown cause with an associated malignant fibrous histiocytoma of the left tibia.

(Courtesy of G. Bock, M.D., Winnipeg, Manitoba, Canada.)

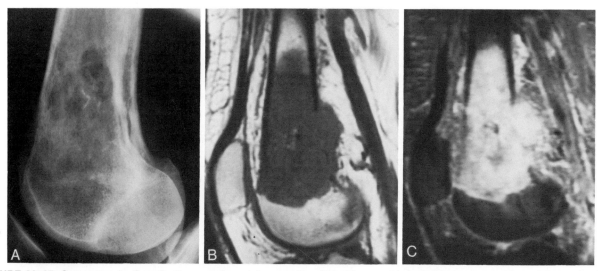

FIGURE 80–67. Osteonecrosis: Complications—malignant degeneration. This 82 year old man with documented bone infarcts developed increasing pain in his knee.

A The routine radiograph shows an osteolytic lesion containing calcification in the distal portion of the femur.

B The lesion is of low signal intensity in a sagittal T1-weighted (TR/TE, 533/16) spin echo MR image, and it extends into the soft tissues posteriorly.

C A sagittal fast short tau inversion recovery (STIR) MR image (TR/TE, 3500/16; inversion time, 160 msec) shows the tumor of high signal intensity, which proved to be an osteosarcoma arising at the site of a bone infarct.

(Courtesy of T. Broderick, M.D., Orange, California.)

Occasionally, the radiographic appearance of dissolution of bone and adjacent calcification may resemble a chondrosarcoma, with or without dedifferentiation, occurring in the absence of osteonecrosis. Rarely, a primary tumor of bone leads to radiographic abnormalities that simulate those of osteonecrosis.[333]

SUMMARY

Osteonecrosis can accompany many diverse disease processes, such as trauma, hemoglobinopathy, exogenous or endogenous hypercortisolism, alcoholism, pancreatitis, dysbaric conditions, and Gaucher's disease. It also may become evident without any recognizable disease or event (primary or spontaneous osteonecrosis). Posttraumatic osteonecrosis is most frequent in the femoral and humeral heads, scaphoid, and talus, although other sites may be affected. Dysbaric osteonecrosis can produce widespread skeletal alterations of epiphyseal, metaphyseal, or diaphyseal segments of tubular bones. Spontaneous osteonecrosis most commonly is recognized about the hip and the knee. Possible complications of bone necrosis are secondary degenerative joint disease, formation of intra-articular osseous and cartilaginous bodies, septic arthritis, pathologic fracture, and cystic or sarcomatous transformation.

References

1. Greenfield GB: Radiology of Bone Diseases. 2nd Ed. Philadelphia, JB Lippincott Co, 1975, p 143.
2. Martel W, Poznanski AK: The effect of traction on the hip in osteonecrosis. A comment on the "radiolucent crescent line." Radiology 94:505, 1970.
3. Martel W, Poznanski AK: The value of traction during roentgenography of the hip. Radiology 94:497, 1970.
4. Gohel VK, Dalinka MK, Edeiken J: Ischemic necrosis of the femoral head simulating chondroblastoma. Radiology 107:545, 1973.
5. Müssbichler H: Arteriographic studies in fractures of the femoral neck and trochanteric region. Angiology 21:385, 1970.
6. Hipp E: Die Gefässes des Hüftkopfes; Anatomie, Angiographie und Klinic. Stuttgart, Enke, 1962.
7. Hulth A, Johansson SH: Femoral-head venography in the prognosis of fractures of the femoral neck. Acta Chir Scand 123:287, 1962.
8. Serre H, Simon L: L'ostéonécrose primitive de la tête fémorale chez l'adulte. Acta Rheumatol Scand 7:265, 1961.
9. Hungerford DS: Early diagnosis of ischemic necrosis of the femoral head. Johns Hopkins Med J 137:270, 1975.
10. Laing PG, Ferguson AB: Iodine-131 clearance-rates as an indication of the blood supply of bone. Nature 183:1595, 1959.
11. Holmquist B, Alffram PA: Prediction of avascular necroses following cervical fractures of the femur based on clearance of radioactive iodine from the head of the femur. Acta Orthop Scand 36:62, 1965.
12. D'Ambrosia RD, Riggins RS, DeNardo SJ, et al: Fluoride-18 scintigraphy in avascular necrotic disorders of bone. Clin Orthop 107:146, 1975.
13. Alavi A, McCloskey JR, Steinberg ME: Early detection of avascular necrosis of the femoral head by 99m-technetium diphosphonate bone scan: A preliminary report. Clin Orthop 127:137, 1977.
14. D'Ambrosia RD, Shoji H, Riggins RS, et al: Scintigraphy in the diagnosis of osteonecrosis. Clin Orthop 130:139, 1978.
15. Meyers MH, Telfer N, Moore TM: Determination of the vascularity of the femoral head with technetium 99m-sulphur-colloid. Diagnostic and prognostic significance. J Bone Joint Surg [Am] 59:658, 1977.
16. Lentle BC, Russell AS, Percy JS, et al: Bone scintiscanning updated. Ann Intern Med 84:297, 1976.
17. McLean FC, Urist MR: Bone. An Introduction to the Physiology of Skeletal Tissue. Chicago, University of Chicago Press, 1955.
18. Graham J, Wood SK: Aseptic necrosis of bone following trauma. In JK Davidson (Ed): Aseptic Necrosis of Bone. Amsterdam, Excerpta Medica, 1976, p 101.
19. Phemister DB: Necrotic bone and subsequent changes which it undergoes. JAMA 64:211, 1915.
20. Catto M: A histological study of avascular necrosis of the femoral head after transcervical fracture. J Bone Joint Surg [Br] 47:749, 1965.
21. Glimcher MJ, Kenzora JE: The biology of osteonecrosis of the human femoral head and its clinical implications. I. Tissue biology. Clin Orthop 138:284, 1979.
22. Glimcher MJ, Kenzora JE: The biology of osteonecrosis of the human femoral

23. Glimcher MJ, Kenzora JE: The biology of osteonecrosis of the human femoral head and its clinical implications. III. Discussion of the etiology and genesis of the pathological sequelae; comments on treatment. Clin Orthop 140:273, 1979.
24. Garden RS: Malreduction and avascular necrosis in subcapital fractures of the femur. J Bone Joint Surg [Br] 53:183, 1971.
25. Barnes R, Brown JT, Garden RS, et al: Subcapital fractures of the femur. A prospective review. J Bone Joint Surg [Br] 58:2, 1976.
26. Coleman SS: Aseptic necrosis of bone due to trauma. Orthop Clin North Am 5:819, 1974.
27. Trueta J, Harrison MHM: The normal vascular anatomy of the femoral head in adult man. J Bone Joint Surg [Br] 35:442, 1953.
28. Sevitt S, Thompson RG: The distribution and anastomoses of arteries supplying the head and neck of the femur. J Bone Joint Surg [Br] 47:560, 1965.
29. Müssbichler H: Arteriographic findings in necrosis of the head of the femur after medial neck fracture. Acta Orthop Scand 41:77, 1970.
30. Claffey TJ: Avascular necrosis of the femoral head. J Bone Joint Surg [Br] 42:802, 1960.
31. Wertheimer LG, Lopes S de L: Arterial supply of the femoral head. A combined angiographic and histological study. J Bone Joint Surg [Am] 53:545, 1971.
32. Sevitt S: Avascular necrosis and revascularisation of the femoral head after intracapsular fractures. A combined arteriographic and histological necropsy study. J Bone Joint Surg [Br] 46:270, 1964.
33. Trueta J: The normal vascular anatomy of the human femoral head during growth. J Bone Joint Surg [Br] 39:358, 1957.
34. McDougall A: Fracture of the neck of femur in childhood. J Bone Joint Surg [Br] 43:16, 1961.
35. Ratliff AHC: Fractures of the neck of the femur in children. J Bone Joint Surg [Br] 44:528, 1962.
36. Phemister DB: Fractures of neck of femur, dislocations of hip, and obscure vascular disturbances producing aseptic necrosis of head of femur. Surg Gynecol Obstet 59:415, 1934.
37. Catto M: A histological study of avascular necrosis of the femoral head after transcervical fracture. J Bone Joint Surg [Br] 47:749, 1965.
38. Brav EA: Traumatic dislocation of the hip. Army experience and results over a twelve-year period. J Bone Joint Surg [Am] 44:1115, 1962.
39. Epstein HC: Posterior fracture-dislocations of the hip. Long-term follow-up. J Bone Joint Surg [Am] 56:1103, 1974.
40. Jerre T: A study in slipped upper femoral epiphysis. With special reference to the late functional and roentgenological results and to the value of closed reduction. Acta Orthop Scand Suppl 6:1, 1950.
41. Wilson PD, Jacobs B, Schecter L: Slipped capital femoral epiphysis: An end-result study. J Bone Joint Surg [Am] 47:1128, 1965.
42. Hall JE: The results of treatment of slipped femoral epiphysis. J Bone Joint Surg [Br] 39:659, 1957.
43. Esteve R: Congenital dislocation of the hip. A review and assessment of results of treatment with special reference to frame reduction as compared with manipulative reduction. J Bone Joint Surg [Am] 42:253, 1960.
44. Haliburton RA, Sullivan CR, Kelly PJ, et al: The extraosseous and intraosseous blood supply of the talus. J Bone Joint Surg [Am] 40:1115, 1958.
45. Mulfinger GL, Trueta J: The blood supply of the talus. J Bone Joint Surg [Br] 52:160, 1970.
46. Morris HD: Aseptic necrosis of the talus following injury. Orthop Clin North Am 5:177, 1974.
47. Hawkins LG: Fractures of the neck of the talus. J Bone Joint Surg [Am] 52:991, 1970.
48. Mindell ER, Cisek EE, Kartalian G, et al: Late results of injuries of the talus. Analysis of forty cases. J Bone Joint Surg [Am] 45:221, 1963.
49. Kenwright J, Taylor RG: Major injuries of the talus. J Bone Joint Surg [Br] 52:36, 1970.
50. Laing PG: The arterial supply of the adult humerus. J Bone Joint Surg [Am] 38:1105, 1956.
51. Obletz BE, Halbstein BM: Non-union of fractures of the carpal navicular. J Bone Joint Surg 20:424, 1938.
52. Taleisnik J, Kelly PJ: The extraosseous and intraosseous blood supply of the scaphoid bone. J Bone Joint Surg [Am] 48:1125, 1966.
53. Mazet R Jr, Hohl M: Fractures of the carpal navicular. Analysis of ninety-one cases and review of the literature. J Bone Joint Surg [Am] 45:82, 1963.
54. Gasser H: Delayed union and pseudarthrosis of the carpal navicular: Treatment by compression-screw osteosynthesis. J Bone Joint Surg [Am] 47:249, 1965.
55. Scapinelli R: Blood supply of the human patella. Its relation to ischaemic necrosis after fracture. J Bone Joint Surg [Br] 49:563, 1967.
56. Gilsanz V, Cleveland RH, Wilkinson RH: Aseptic necrosis: A complication of dislocation of the metacarpophalangeal joint. AJR 129:737, 1977.
57. Davidson JK: Dysbaric osteonecrosis. In JK Davidson (Ed): Aseptic Necrosis of Bone. Amsterdam, Excerpta Medica, 1976, p 147.
58. Jaffe HL: Ischemic necrosis of bone. Med Radiogr Photogr 45:57, 1969.
59. Rószahegyi I: Neurological damage following decompression. In RI McCallum (Ed): Decompression of Compressed Air Workers in Civil Engineering. Proceedings of an International Working Party held at the Ciba Foundation, London, 1965. Newcastle-upon-Tyne, Oriel Press, 1967, p 127.
60. Adams GM, Parker GW: Dysbaric osteonecrosis in US Navy divers. A survey of non-random selected divers (Abstr). Undersea Biomed Res 1:A20, 1974.
61. Chryssanthou CP: Dysbaric osteonecrosis. Etiological and pathogenetic concepts. Clin Orthop 130:94, 1978.

62. Reeves E, McKee AE, Stunkard JA, et al: Radiographic and pathologic studies for aseptic bone necrosis in dogs incurring decompression sickness. Aerospace Med 43:61, 1972.

63. Jones JP Jr, Sakovich L: Fat embolism of bone. A roentgenographic and histological investigation, with the use of intra-arterial Lipiodol in rabbits. J Bone Joint Surg [Am] 48:149, 1966.

64. Chryssanthou CP: Dysbaric osteonecrosis in mice. Undersea Biomed Res 3:67, 1976.

65. McCallum RI, Walder DN, Barnes R, et al: Bone lesions in compressed air workers. With special reference to men who worked in the Clyde tunnels 1958 to 1963. J Bone Joint Surg [Br] 48:207, 1966.

66. Spencer MP, Clarke HF: Precordial monitoring of pulmonary gas embolism and decompression bubbles. Aerospace Med 43:762, 1972.

67. Stegall PJ, Huang TW, Smith KH: The etiology of experimentally induced osteonecrosis (Abstr). Undersea Biomed Res 3:A40, 1976.

68. Amako T, Kawashima M, Torisu T, et al: Bone and joint lesions in decompression sickness. Semin Arthritis Rheum 4:151, 1974.

69. Pauley SM, Cockett ATK: Role of lipids in decompression sickness. Aerospace Med 41:56, 1970.

70. Philp RB, Inwood MJ, Warren BA: Interactions between gas bubbles and components of the blood: Implications in decompression sickness. Aerospace Med 43:946, 1972.

71. Chryssanthou C, Teichner F, Goldstein G, et al: Studies on dysbarism. III. A smooth muscle-acting factor (SMAF) in mouse lungs and its increase in decompression sickness. Aerospace Med 41:43, 1970.

72. Hills BA: Gas-induced osmosis as an aetiologic agent for gouty arthritis and aseptic bone necrosis induced by exposure to compressed air. Rev Subaquatic Physiol Hyperbar Med 2:3, 1970.

73. Sobel H: Oxygen-modified collagen and bone necrosis in divers (Letter to Editor). Lancet 2:1012, 1974.

74. Lewis HE, Paton WDM: Decompression sickness during the sinking of a caisson; a study of some factors in the pathogenesis of caisson disease. Br J Indust Med 14:5, 1957.

75. Bell ALL, Edson GN, Hornick N: Characteristic bone and joint changes in compressed air workers: A survey of symptomless cases. Radiology 38:698, 1913.

76. Elliott DH, Harrison JAB: Bone necrosis—an occupational hazard of diving. J R Nav Med Serv 56:140, 1970.

77. Ohta Y, Matsunaga H: Bone lesions in divers. J Bone Joint Surg [Br] 56:3, 1974.

78. Hauteville D, Esquirol E, Hyacinthe R, et al: Les lésions osseuses latentes des plongeurs. Résultats comparés d'une enquête portant sur 105 plongeurs et 105 sujets témoins. Rev Rhum Mal Osteoartic 43:635, 1976.

79. Horváth F, Rózsahegyi I: Bedeutung der Tomographie für die Diagnose der chronischen Caisson-Osteoarthropathie. ROFO 119:610, 1973.

80. Williams B, Unsworth I: Skeletal changes in divers. Australas Radiol 20:83, 1976.

81. Nellen JR, Kindwall EP: Aseptic necrosis of bone secondary to occupational exposure to compressed air: Roentgenologic findings in 59 cases. AJR 115:512, 1972.

82. Heard JL, Schneider CS: Radiographic findings in commercial divers. Clin Orthop et al: 130:129, 1978.

83. Kawashima M, Torisu T, Hayahi K, et al: Pathological review of osteonecrosis in divers. Clin Orthop et al: 130:107, 1978.

84. Weatherley CR, Gregg PJ, Walder DN, et al: Aseptic necrosis of bone in a compressed air worker. J Bone Joint Surg [Br] 59:80, 1977.

85. Horváth F: Röntgenmorphologie des Caisson-bedingten Knochenmarkinfarktes. ROFO 129:33, 1978.

86. Davidson JK, Griffiths PD: Caisson disease of bone. X-ray Focus 10:2, 1970.

87. Davidson JK, Hanison JAB, Jacobs P, et al: The significance of bone islands, cystic areas and sclerotic areas in dysbaric osteonecrosis. Clin Radiol 28:381, 1977.

88. Swain VAJ: Caisson disease (compressed-air illness) of bone with a report of a case. Br J Surg 29:365, 1942.

89. Kahlstrom SC, Phemister DB: Bone infarcts. Case report with autopsy findings. Am J Pathol 22:947, 1946.

90. Kahlstrom SC, Burton CC, Phemister DB: Aseptic necrosis of bone. II. Infarctions of bone of undetermined etiology resulting in encapsulated and calcified areas in diaphyses and in arthritis deformans. Surg Gynecol Obstet 68:631, 1939.

91. Bullough PG, Kambolis CP, Marcove RC, et al: Bone infarctions not associated with caisson disease. J Bone Joint Surg [Am] 47:477, 1965.

92. Taylor HK: Aseptic necrosis of adults. Caisson workers and others. Radiology 42:550, 1944.

93. Catto M: Pathology of aseptic bone necrosis. In JK Davidson (Ed): Aseptic Necrosis of Bone. Amsterdam, Excerpta Medica, 1976, p 3.

94. Freund E: Zur Frage der aseptischen Knochennekrose. Virchows Arch (Pathol Anat) 261:287, 1926.

95. Chandler FA: Observations on circulatory changes in bone. AJR 44:90, 1940.

96. Serre H, Simon L: Aspects cliniques des necroses parcellaires aseptiques primitives de la tête femorale chez l'adulte. Montpellier Med 56:193, 1959.

97. Mankin HJ, Brower TD: Bilateral idiopathic aseptic necrosis of the femur in adults: "Chandler's disease." Bull Hosp Joint Dis 23:42, 1962.

98. Patterson RJ, Bickel WH, Dahlin DC: Idiopathic avascular necrosis of the head of the femur. A study of fifty-two cases. J Bone Joint Surg [Am] 46:267, 1964.

99. Marcus ND, Enneking WF, Massam RA: The silent hip in idiopathic aseptic necrosis. Treatment by bone-grafting. J Bone Joint Surg [Am] 55:1351, 1973.

100. Kerboul M, Thomine J, Postel M, et al: The conservative surgical treatment of idiopathic aseptic necrosis of the femoral head. J Bone Joint Surg [Br] 56:291, 1974.

101. Inoue A, Ono K: A histological study of idiopathic avascular necrosis of the head of the femur. J Bone Joint Surg [Br] 61:138, 1979.

102. Boettcher WG, Bonfiglio M, Hamilton HH, et al: Non-traumatic necrosis of the femoral head. Part I. Relation of altered hemostasis to etiology. J Bone Joint Surg [Am] 52:312, 1970.

103. Chandler FA: Coronary disease of the hip. J Int Coll Surg 11:34, 1948.

104. Rubens-Duval A, Villiaumey J, Lubetzki D, et al: L'ostéochondrite du genou du sujet âgé. Intérêt de la biopsie synoviale. Rev Rhum Mal Osteoartic 33:638, 1966.

105. Ahlbäck S, Bauer GCH, Bohne WH: Spontaneous osteonecrosis of the knee. Arthritis Rheum 11:705, 1968.

106. Ahuja SC, Bullough PG: Osteonecrosis of the knee. A clinicopathological study in twenty-eight patients. J Bone Joint Surg [Am] 60:191, 1978.

107. Renier JC, Brégeon C, Mazaud J: L'ostéonécrose condylienne du genou de l'adulte et du sujet âgé (étude de 36 observations). Rev Rhum Mal Osteoartic 43:17, 1976.

108. Schauer A: Zur pathologischen Anatomie der spontanen Osteonekrosen. Z Orthop 115:432, 1977.

109. Daumont A, Deplante JP, Bouvier M, et al: L'ostéonécrose des condyles fémoraux chez l'adulte. A propos de 30 cas personnels. Rev Rhum Mal Osteoartic 43:27, 1976.

110. Williams JL, Cliff MM, Bonakdarpour A: Spontaneous osteonecrosis of the knee. Radiology 107:15, 1973.

111. Lotke PA, Ecker ML, Alavi A: Painful knees in older patients. Radionuclide diagnosis of possible osteonecrosis with spontaneous resolution. J Bone Joint Surg [Am] 59:617, 1977.

112. Muheim G, Bohne WH: Prognosis in spontaneous osteonecrosis of the knee. Investigation by radionuclide scintimetry and radiography. J Bone Joint Surg [Br] 52:605, 1970.

113. Bauer GCH: Osteonecrosis of the knee. Clin Orthop 130:210, 1978.

114. Norman A, Baker ND: Spontaneous osteonecrosis of the knee and medial meniscal tears. Radiology 129:653, 1978.

115. Scaglietti O, Fineschi G: La condrite dissecante dell'eta senile. Arch Putti Chir Organi Mov 20:1, 1965.

116. Mankin HJ, Thrasher AZ, Hall D: Biochemical and metabolic characteristics of articular cartilage from osteonecrotic human femoral heads. J Bone Joint Surg [Am] 59:724, 1977.

117. Sanchis M, Zahir A, Freeman MAR: The experimental simulation of Perthes disease by consecutive interruptions of the blood supply to the capital femoral epiphysis in the puppy. J Bone Joint Surg [Am] 55:335, 1973.

118. Rösingh GE, James J: Early phases of avascular necrosis of the femoral head in rabbits. J Bone Joint Surg [Br] 51:165, 1969.

119. Rösingh GE, Steendijk R, van den Hooff A, et al: Consequences of avascular necrosis of the femoral head in rabbits. A histological and radiological study with a statistical analysis of bone-volume ratios. J Bone Joint Surg [Br] 51:551, 1969.

120. Coutts RD, Bradley B, Akeson WH, et al: The effects of avascular necrosis on cartilage of the dog femoral head (Abstr). J Bone Joint Surg [Am] 56:858, 1974.

121. Milgram JW: The classification of loose bodies in human joints. Clin Orthop 124:282, 1977.

122. Milgram JW: The development of loose bodies in human joints. Clin Orthop 124:292, 1977.

123. Furey JG, Ferrer-Torells M, Reagan JW: Fibrosarcoma arising at the site of bone infarcts. A report of two cases. J Bone Joint Surg [Am] 42:802, 1960.

124. Johnson LC, Vetter H, Putschar WGJ: Sarcomas arising in bone cysts. Virchows Arch (Pathol Anat) 335:428, 1962.

125. Dorfman HD, Norman A, Wolff H: Fibrosarcoma complicating bone infarction in a caisson worker. A case report. J Bone Joint Surg [Am] 48:528, 1966.

126. Mirra JM, Bullough PG, Marcove RC, et al: Malignant fibrous histiocytoma and osteosarcoma in association with bone infarcts. Report of four cases, two in caisson workers. J Bone Joint Surg [Am] 56:932, 1974.

127. Mirra JM, Gold RH, Marafiote R: Malignant (fibrous) histiocytoma arising in association with a bone infarct in sickle-cell disease: Coincidence or cause-and-effect? Cancer 39:186, 1977.

128. Hall FM: Osteonecrosis of the knee and medial meniscal tears. Radiology 133:828, 1979.

129. Lee CK, Hansen HT, Weiss AB: The "silent hip" of idiopathic ischemic necrosis of the femoral head in adults. J Bone Joint Surg [Am] 62:795, 1980.

130. Greiff J: Determination of the vitality of the femoral head with 99mTc-Sn-pyrophosphate scintigraphy. Acta Orthop Scand 51:109, 1980.

131. Greiff J, Lanng S, Høilund-Carlsen PF, et al: Early detection by 99mTc-pyrophosphate scintigraphy of femoral head necrosis following medial femoral neck fractures. Acta Orthop Scand 51:119, 1980.

132. Zizic TM, Hungerford DS, Stevens MB.: Ischemic bone necrosis in systemic lupus erythematosus. I. The early diagnosis of ischemic necrosis of bone. Medicine 59:134, 1980.

133. Gregg PJ, Walder DN: Scintigraphy versus radiography in the early diagnosis of experimental bone necrosis. J Bone Joint Surg [Br] 62:214, 1980.

134. Gregg PJ, Walder DN: Regional distribution of circulating microspheres in the femur of the rabbit. J Bone Joint Surg [Br] 62:222, 1980.

135. Leconte PH, Bastien J: Kyste synovial inguinal avec nécrose idiopathique de la tête fémorale. Rev Chir Orthop 65:353, 1979.

136. Rozing PM, Insall J, Bohne W: Spontaneous osteonecrosis of the knee. J Bone Joint Surg [Am] 62:2, 1980.

137. Cooperman DR, Wallenstein R, Stulberg SD: Post-reduction avascular necrosis in congenital dislocations of the hip. J Bone Joint Surg [Am] 62:247, 1980.

138. Jacqueline F, Rabinowicz T: Transformations de la synoviale et du cartilage dans les nécroses post-traumatique et idiopathique de la hanche. In Ficat P, Arlet J: II Symposium International sur la Circulation Osseouse, Toulouse, 1977. Paris, Armour Montagu, 1979, p 355.

139. Gelberman RH, Menon J: The vascularity of the scaphoid bone. J Hand Surg 5:508, 1980.

140. Lee CK, Corcoran SF, Parsons JR: Hyperlipidemia and idiopathic aseptic necrosis of the femoral head in adults. Orthopedics 3:651, 1980.

141. Sugioka Y: Transtrochanteric anterior rotational osteotomy of the femoral head in the treatment of osteonecrosis affecting the hip: A new osteotomy procedure. Clin Orthop 130:191, 1978.

142. Dihlman W: Computed tomography of the hip joint. Medicamundi 28:29, 1983.

143. Dihlmann W: CT analysis of the upper end of the femur: The asterisk sign and ischaemic bone necrosis of the femoral head. Skel Radiol 8:251, 1982.

144. Nebel G: Die Wertigkeit der Computertomographie bei der Diagnose der avaskularen Huftkopfnekrose des Erwachsenen. Akt Rheumatol 7:5, 1982.

145. Heuck FHW, Treugut H: Die "Huftkopfnekrose" bei metabolischen und hormonellen Osteopathien—eine radiologische-morphologische Analyse. Radiologe 24:319, 1984.

146. Casteleyn PP, DeBoeck H, Handelberg F, et al: Computed axial tomography and disulphine blue in the evaluation of osteonecrosis of the femoral head. Int Orthop (SICOT) 7:149, 1983.

147. Steinberg ME, Brighton CT, Steinberg DR, et al: Treatment of avascular necrosis of the femoral head by a combination of bone grafting, decompression, and electrical stimulation. Clin Orthop 186:137, 1984.

148. Kirchner PT, Simon MA: Radioisotopic evaluation of skeletal disease. J Bone Joint Surg [Am] 63:673, 1981.

149. Holder LE: Radionuclide bone-imaging in the evaluation of bone pain. J Bone Joint Surg [Am] 64:1391, 1982.

150. Burt RW, Matthews TJ: Aseptic necrosis of the knee: Bone scintigraphy. AJR 138:571, 1982.

151. Conklin JJ, Alderson PO, Zizic TM, et al: Comparison of bone scan and radiograph sensitivity in the detection of steroid-induced ischemic necrosis of bone. Radiology 147:221, 1983.

152. Turner JH: Post-traumatic avascular necrosis of the femoral head predicted by preoperative technetium-99m antimony-colloid scan. An experimental and clinical study. J Bone Joint Surg [Am] 65:786, 1983.

153. Stromqvist B, Brismar J, Hansson LI: Emission tomography in femoral neck fracture for evaluation of avascular necrosis. Acta Orthop Scand 54:872, 1983.

154. Moon KL Jr, Genant HK, Davis PL, et al: Nuclear magnetic resonance imaging in orthopaedics: Principles and applications. J Orthop Res 1:101, 1983.

155. Moon KL Jr, Genant HK, Helms CA, et al: Musculoskeletal applications of nuclear magnetic resonance. Radiology 147:161, 1983.

156. Totty WG, Murphy WA, Ganz WI, et al: Magnetic resonance imaging of the normal and ischemic femoral head. AJR 143:1273, 1984.

157. Ficat RP: Idiopathic bone necrosis of the femoral head. Early diagnosis and treatment. J Bone Joint Surg [Br] 67:3, 1985.

158. Arlet J, Durroux R: Diagnostic histologique preécoce de l'osteonécrose aseptique de la tête fémorale par le forage-biopsie. In Premier Symposium International de Circulation Osseouse, Toulouse. Paris, Inserm, 1973.

159. Crock HV: An atlas of the arterial supply of the head and neck of the femur in man. Clin Orthop 152:17, 1980.

160. Nielsen PT, Thaarup P: An unusual course of femoral head necrosis complicating an intertrochanteric fracture in a child. Clin Orthop 183:79, 1984.

161. Linhart W, Stampfel O, Ritter G: Posttraumatische Femurkopfnekrose nach Trochanterfraktur. Z Orthop 122:766, 1984.

162. Calandruccio RA, Anderson WE III: Post-fracture avascular necrosis of the femoral head: Correlation of experimental and clinical studies. Clin Orthop 152:49, 1980.

163. Bauer G, Weber DA, Ceder L, et al: Dynamics of technetium-99m methylenediphosphonate imaging of the femoral head after hip fracture. Clin Orthop 152:85, 1980.

164. Lucie RS, Fuller S, Burdick DC, et al: Early prediction of avascular necrosis of the femoral head following femoral neck fractures. Clin Orthop 161:207, 1981.

165. Stromqvist B, Brismar J, Hansson LI, et al: Technetium-99m-methylenediphosphonate scintimetry after femoral neck fracture. A three-year follow-up study. Clin Orthop 182:177, 1984.

166. Stromqvist B: Femoral head vitality after intracapsular hip fracture. Acta Orthop Scand 54(Suppl 250):5, 1983.

167. Brummer R, Hansson LI, Mortensson W, et al: ⁸⁵Sr-scintimetry in femoral neck fracture. Arch Orthop Trauma Surg 101:47, 1982.

168. Stromqvist B, Hansson LI, Ljung P, et al: Preoperative and postoperative scintimetry after femoral neck fracture. J Bone Joint Surg [Br] 66:49, 1984.

169. Barquet A: Avascular necrosis following traumatic hip dislocation in childhood. Factors of influence. Acta Orthop Scand 53:809, 1982.

170. Barquet A: Natural history of avascular necrosis following traumatic hip dislocation in childhood. A review of 145 cases. Acta Orthop Scand 53:815, 1982.

171. Gelfund MJ, Strife JL, Graham EJ, et al: Bone scintigraphy in slipped capital femoral epiphysis. Clin Nucl Med 8:613, 1983.

172. Buchanan JR, Greer RB III, Cotler JM: Management strategy for prevention of avascular necrosis during treatment of congenital dislocation of the hip. J Bone Joint Surg [Am] 63:140, 1981.

173. Thomas CL, Gage JR, Ogden JA: Treatment concepts for proximal femoral ischemic necrosis complicating congenital hip disease. J Bone Joint Surg [Am] 64:817, 1982.

174. Wechsler RJ, Schwartz AM: Ischemic necrosis of the contralateral hip as a possible complication of untreated congenital hip dislocation. Skel Radiol 6:279, 1981.

175. Kofoed H: Revascularization of the humeral head. A report of two cases of fracture-dislocation of the shoulder. Clin Orthop 179:175, 1983.

176. Sherman SB, Greenspan A, Norman A: Osteonecrosis of the distal pole of the carpal scaphoid following fracture—a rare complication. Skel Radiol 9:189, 1983.

177. Bellmore MC, Cummine JL, Crocker EF, et al: The role of bone scans in the assessment of prognosis of scaphoid fractures. Aust NZ Surg 53:133, 1983.

178. Grend RV, Dell PC, Glowczewskie F, et al: Intraosseous blood supply of the capitate and its correlation with aseptic necrosis. J Hand Surg [Am] 9:677, 1984.

179. Vance RM, Gelberman RH, Evans EF: Scaphocapitate fractures. J Bone Joint Surg [Am] 62:271, 1980.

180. Meyers MH, Wells R, Harvey JP Jr: Naviculo-capitate fracture syndrome. Review of the literature and a case report. J Bone Joint Surg [Am] 53:1383, 1971.

181. Resnik CS, Gelberman RH, Resnick D: Transscaphoid, transcapitate, perilunate fracture dislocation (scaphocapitate syndrome). Skel Radiol 9:192, 1983.

182. Rand JA, Linscheid RL, Dobyns JH: Capitate fractures. A long term follow-up. Clin Orthop 165:209, 1982.

183. Rahme H: Idiopathic avascular necrosis of the capitate. Hand 15:274, 1983.

184. James ETR, Burke FD: Vibration disease of the capitate. J Hand Surg [Br] 9:169, 1984.

185. Murakami S, Nakajima H: Aseptic necrosis of the capitate bone in two gymnasts. Am J Sports Med 12:170, 1984.

186. Newman JH, Watt I: Avascular necrosis of the capitate and dorsal dorsiflexion instability. Hand 12:176, 1980.

187. Kimmel RB, O'Brien ET: Surgical treatment of avascular necrosis of the proximal pole of the capitate: Case report. J Hand Surg 7:284, 1982.

188. Bolton-Maggs BG, Helal BH, Revell PA: Bilateral avascular necrosis of the capitate. A case report and a review of the literature. J Bone Joint Surg [Br] 66:557, 1984.

189. Lowry WE Jr, Cord SA: Traumatic avascular necrosis of the capitate bone—case report. J Hand Surg 6:245, 1981.

190. Stojanovic J, Kovac V: Diagnosis of ischemic vertebral collapse using skeletal spinal angiography. ROFO 135:326, 1981.

191. Schmorl G, Junghanns H: The Human Spine in Health and Disease. 2nd American Ed. New York, Grune & Stratton, 1971, p 268.

192. Benedek TG, Nicholas JJ, Reece GJ: Kümmell's disease: A rare cause of posttraumatic back pain. Arthritis Rheum 23:653, 1980.

193. Brower AC, Downey EF Jr: Kümmell disease: Report of a case with serial radiographs. Radiology 141:363, 1981.

194. Hermann G, Goldblatt J, Desnick RJ: Kümmell disease: Delayed collapse of the traumatised spine in a patient with Gaucher type I disease. Br J Radiol 57:833, 1984.

195. Report AC: Vertebral osteonecrosis associated with pancreatitis in a child. J Bone Joint Surg [Am] 60:985, 1978.

196. Bretz GW, Jenkins PG: Gas density in an ununited fracture of a vertebral body. J Bone Joint Surg [Am] 63:1183, 1981.

197. Maldague BE, Noel HM, Malghem JJ: The intravertebral vacuum cleft: A sign of ischemic vertebral collapse. Radiology 129:23, 1978.

198. Michel JL, Bouzat J, Rivoal A, et al: La dissection gazeuse du corps vertébral ou phénomène du vide intrasomatique vertébral. Arguments physiopathologiques. J Radiol 63:479, 1982.

199. Maldague BE, Malghem JJ: Vertebral vacuum phenomenon. Skel Radiol 6:81, 1981.

200. Feldman JL, Menkes CJ, Amor B, et al: L'osteonécrose vertébrale de l'adulte. A propos de 4 cas. Rev Rhum Mal Osteoartic 48:773, 1981.

201. Wendling D, Cassou M, Guidet M: L'image de clarté gazeuse intravertébrale. A propos de 7 nouvelles observations. Rev Rhum Mal Osteoartic 50:607, 1983.

202. Duquesnoy B, Thevenon A, Siame JL, et al: Phénomène du vide intravertébral: Osteonécrose vertébrale ou simple tassement osteoporotique? A propos de quatre cas. Rev Rhum Mal Osteoartic 49:35, 1982.

203. Resnick D, Niwayama G, Guerra JJ Jr, et al: Spinal vacuum phenomena: Anatomical study and review. Radiology 139:341, 1981.

204. Dzioba RB, Quinlan WJ: Avascular necrosis of the glenoid. J Trauma 24:448, 1984.

205. Dove J, Yau ACMC: Avascular necrosis of the dens. A follow-up study. Spine 7:408, 1982.

206. Kindwall EP, Nellen JR, Spiegelhoff DR: Aseptic necrosis in compressed air tunnel workers using current OSHA decompression schedules. J Occup Med 24:741, 1982.

207. Davidson JK: Skeletal and pulmonary radiologic changes in divers. J Soc Occup Med 31:85, 1981.

208. Macleod MA, McEwan AJB, Pearson RR, et al: Functional imaging in the early diagnosis of dysbaric osteonecrosis. Br J Radiol 55:497, 1982.

209. Macleod MA, Pearson RR, McEwan AJB, et al: Bone scintigraphy in dysbaric related osteopathy. Nucl Med Commun 2:236, 1981.

210. Horvath F, Csobaly S: Computertomographie bei der Caissonkrankheit. ROFO 135:16, 1981.
211. Kawai K, Maruno H, Watanabe Y, et al: Fat necrosis of osteocytes as a causative factor in idiopathic osteonecrosis in heritable hyperlipemic rabbits. Clin Orthop 153:273, 1980.
212. Houpt JB, Alpert B, Lotem M, et al: Spontaneous osteonecrosis of the medial tibial plateau. J Rheumatol 9:81, 1982.
213. Koshino T: The treatment of spontaneous osteonecrosis of the knee by high tibial osteotomy with and without bone-grafting or drilling of the lesion. J Bone Joint Surg [Am] 64:47, 1982.
214. Lotke PA, Abend JA, Ecker ML: The treatment of osteonecrosis of the medial femoral condyle. Clin Orthop 171:109, 1982.
215. Houpt JB, Pritzker KPH, Alpert B, et al: Natural history of spontaneous osteonecrosis of the knee (SONK): A review. Semin Arthritis Rheum 13:212, 1983.
216. Aglietti P, Insall JN, Buzzi R, et al: Idiopathic osteonecrosis of the knee. Aetiology, prognosis and treatment. J Bone Joint Surg [Br] 65:588, 1983.
217. Smith DH, Zaphiropoulos GC, Polyzoides AJ: Spontaneous osteonecrosis of the femoral condyle. Rheumatol Rehabil 20:136, 1981.
218. Greyson ND, Lotem MM, Gross AE, et al: Radionuclide evaluation of spontaneous femoral osteonecrosis. Radiology 142:729, 1982.
219. Brucki R, Jager M: Eine atypische juvenile Osteonekrose im medialen Femurkondylus. Z Orthop 120:705, 1982.
220. Lotke PA, Ecker ML: Osteonecrosis-like syndrome of the medial tibial plateau. Clin Orthop 176:148, 1983.
221. Norman A, Steiner GC: Radiographic and morphological features of cyst formation in idiopathic bone infarction. Radiology 146:335, 1983.
222. Vigorita VJ: Pigmented villonodular synovitis-like lesions in association with rare causes of rheumatoid arthritis, osteonecrosis, and advanced degenerative joint disease. Report of five cases. Clin Orthop 183:115, 1984.
223. Heselson NG, Price SK, Mills EED, et al: Two malignant fibrous histiocytomas in bone infarcts. Case report. J Bone Joint Surg [Am] 65:1166, 1983.
224. Bago-Granell J, Aguirre-Canyadell M, Nardi J, et al: Malignant fibrous histiocytoma of bone at the site of a total hip arthroplasty. J Bone Joint Surg [Br] 66:38, 1984.
225. Magid D, Fishman EK, Scott WW Jr, et al: Femoral head avascular necrosis: CT assessment with multiplanar reconstruction. Radiology 157:751, 1985.
226. Drane WE, Rudd TG: Femoral head viability following hip fracture. Prognostic role of radionuclide bone imaging. Clin Nucl Med 10:141, 1985.
227. Nicholas JJ, Benedek TG, Reece GJ: Delayed traumatic vertebral body compression fracture; Part I: Clinical features. Semin Arthritis Rheum 10:264, 1981.
228. Benedek TG, Nicholas JJ: Delayed traumatic vertebral body compression fracture; Part II: Pathologic features. Semin Arthritis Rheum 10:271, 1981.
229. Modena V, Maiocco I, Bosio C, et al: Intravertebral vacuum cleft: Notes on five cases. Clin Exp Rheumatol 3:23, 1985.
230. Jergesen HE, Heller M, Genant HK: Magnetic resonance imaging in osteonecrosis of the femoral head. Orthop Clin North Am 16:705, 1985.
231. Thickman D, Axel L, Kressel HY, et al: Magnetic resonance imaging of avascular necrosis of the femoral head. Skel Radiol 15:133, 1986.
232. Mitchell DG, Rao V, Dalinka M, et al: MRI of joint fluid in the normal and ischemic hip. AJR 146:1215, 1986.
233. Kenzora JE, Glimcher MJ: Pathogenesis of idiopathic osteonecrosis: The ubiquitous crescent sign. Orthop Clin North Am 16:681, 1985.
234. Mitchell MD, Kundel HL, Steinberg ME, et al: Avascular necrosis of the hip: Comparison of MR, CT, and scintigraphy. AJR 147:67, 1986.
235. Bassett LW, Gold RH, Reicher M, et al: Magnetic resonance imaging in the early diagnosis of ischemic necrosis of the femoral head. Preliminary results. Clin Orthop 214:237, 1987.
236. Hartzman S, Reicher MA, Bassett LW, et al: MR imaging of the knee. Part II. Chronic disorders. Radiology 162:553, 1987.
237. Sierra A, Potchen EJ, Moore J, et al: High-field magnetic resonance imaging of aseptic necrosis of the talus. A case report. J Bone Joint Surg [Am] 68:927, 1986.
238. Reinus WR, Conway WF, Totty WG, et al: Carpal avascular necrosis: MR imaging. Radiology 160:689, 1986.
239. Koenig H, Lucas D, Meissner R: The wrist: A preliminary report on high-resolution MR imaging. Radiology 160:463, 1986.
240. Mitchell DG, Kressel HY, Arger PH, et al: Avascular necrosis of the femoral head: Morphologic assessment by MR imaging with CT correlation. Radiology 161:739, 1986.
241. Mitchell DG, Rao VM, Dalinka M, et al: Hematopoietic and fatty bone marrow distribution in the normal and ischemic hip: New observations with 1.5-T MR imaging. Radiology 161:199, 1986.
242. Zizic TM, Marcoux C, Hungerford DS, et al: The early diagnosis of ischemic necrosis of bone. Arthritis Rheum 29:1177, 1986.
243. Wingstrand H, Strömqvist B, Egund N, et al: Hemarthrosis in undisplaced cervical fractures. Tamponade may cause reversible femoral head ischemia. Acta Orthop Scand 57:305, 1986.
244. Kumpan W, Salomonowitz E, Seidl G, et al: The intravertebral vacuum phenomenon. Skel Radiol 15:444, 1986.
245. Gregg PJ, Walder DN: Caisson disease of bone. Clin Orthop 210:43, 1986.
246. Abrahams TG, Hull M: Case report 394. Skel Radiol 15:578, 1986.
247. Munk PL, Helms CA, Holt RG: Immature bone infarcts: Findings on plain radiographs and MR scans. AJR 152:547, 1989.
248. Strecker W, Gilula LA, Kyriakos M: Case report 479. Skel Radiol 17:220, 1988.
249. Lee MJ, Corrigan J, Stack JP, et al: A comparison of modern imaging modalities in osteonecrosis of the femoral head. Clin Radiol 42:427, 1990.
250. Stulberg BN, Levine M, Bauer TW, et al: Multimodality approach to osteonecrosis of the femoral head. Clin Orthop 240:181, 1989.
251. Kokubo T, Takatori Y, Ninomiya S, et al: Magnetic resonance imaging and scintigraphy of avascular necrosis of the femoral head. Prediction of subsequent segmental collapse. Clin Orthop 277:54, 1992.
252. Ruland LJ III, Wang G-J, Teates CD, et al: A comparison of magnetic resonance imaging to bone scintigraphy in early traumatic ischemia of the femoral head. Clin Orthop 285:30, 1992.
253. Mitchell DG, Rao VM, Dalinka MK, et al: Femoral head avascular necrosis: Correlation of MR imaging, radiographic staging, radionuclide imaging, and clinical findings. Radiology 162:709, 1987.
254. Mitchell DG, Joseph PM, Fallon M, et al: Chemical-shift MR imaging of the femoral head: An in vitro study of normal hips and hips with avascular necrosis. AJR 148:1159, 1987.
255. Bassett LW, Mirra JM, Cracchiolo A III, et al: Ischemic necrosis of the femoral head. Correlation of magnetic resonance imaging and histologic sections. Clin Orthop 223:181, 1987.
256. Takatori Y, Kamogawa M, Kokubo T, et al: Magnetic resonance imaging and histopathology in femoral head necrosis. Acta Orthop Scand 58:499, 1987.
257. Markisz JA, Knowles RJR, Althchek DW, et al: Segmental patterns of avascular necrosis of the femoral heads: Early detection with MR imaging. Radiology 162:717, 1987.
258. Kulkarni MV, Tarr RR, Kim E, et al: Potential pitfalls of magnetic resonance imaging in the diagnosis of avascular necrosis. J Nucl Med 28:1052, 1987.
259. Coleman BG, Kressel HY, Dalinka MK, et al: Radiographically negative avascular necrosis: Detection with MR imaging. Radiology 168:525, 1988.
260. Glickstein MF, Burk DL Jr, Schiebler ML, et al: Avascular necrosis versus other diseases of the hip: Sensitivity of MR imaging. Radiology 169:213, 1988.
261. Genez BM, Wilson MR, Houk RW, et al: Early osteonecrosis of the femoral head: Detection in high-risk patients with MR imaging. Radiology 168:521, 1988.
262. Beltran J, Herman LJ, Burk JM, et al: Femoral head avascular necrosis: MR imaging with clinical-pathologic and radionuclide correlation. Radiology 166:215, 1988.
263. Lang P, Jergesen HE, Moseley ME, et al: Avascular necrosis of the femoral head: High-field-strength MR imaging with histologic correlation. Radiology 169:517, 1988.
264. Shuman WP, Castagno AA, Baron RL, et al: MR imaging of avascular necrosis of the femoral head: Value of small-field-of-view sagittal surface-coil images. AJR 150:1073, 1988.
265. Seiler JG III, Christie MJ, Homra L: Correlation of the findings of magnetic resonance imaging and those of bone biopsy in patients who have Stage I or II ischemic necrosis of the femoral head. J Bone Joint Surg [Am] 71:28, 1989.
266. Robinson HJ Jr, Hartleben PD, Lund G, et al: Evaluation of magnetic resonance imaging in the diagnosis of osteonecrosis of the femoral head. Accuracy compared with radiographs, core biopsy, and intraosseous pressure measurements. J Bone Joint Surg [Am] 71:650, 1989.
267. Turner DA, Templeton AC, Selzer PM, et al: Femoral capital osteonecrosis: MR finding of diffuse marrow abnormalities without focal lesions. Radiology 171:135, 1989.
268. Mitchell DG, Steinberg ME, Dalinka MK, et al: Magnetic resonance imaging of the ischemic hip. Alterations within the osteonecrotic, viable, and reactive zones. Clin Orthop 244:60, 1989.
269. Hauzeur JP, Pasteels JL, Schoutens A, et al: The diagnostic value of magnetic resonance imaging in nontraumatic osteonecrosis of the femoral head. J Bone Joint Surg [Am] 71:641, 1989.
270. Miller IL, Savory CG, Polly DW Jr, et al: Femoral head osteonecrosis. Detection by magnetic resonance imaging versus single-photon emission computed tomography. Clin Orthop 247:152, 1989.
271. Kopecky KK, Braunstein EM, Brandt KD, et al: Apparent avascular necrosis of the hip: Appearance and spontaneous resolution of MR findings in renal allograft recipients. Radiology 179:523, 1991.
272. Beltran J, Knight CT, Zuelzer WA, et al: Core decompression for avascular necrosis of the femoral head: Correlation between long-term results and preoperative MR staging. Radiology 175:533, 1990.
273. Brody AS, Strong M, Babikian G, et al: Avascular necrosis: Early MR imaging and histologic findings in a canine model. AJR 157:341, 1991.
274. Tervonen O, Mueller DM, Matteson EL, et al: Clinically occult avascular necrosis of the hip: Prevalence in an asymptomatic population at risk. Radiology 182:845, 1992.
275. Li KCP, Hiette P: Contrast-enhanced fat saturation magnetic resonance imaging for studying the pathophysiology of osteonecrosis of the hips. Skel Radiol 21:375, 1992.
276. Hauzeur J-P, Sintzoff S Jr, Appelboom T, et al: Relationship between magnetic resonance imaging and histologic findings by bone biopsy in nontraumatic osteonecrosis of the femoral head. J Rheumatol 19:385, 1992.
277. Nadel SN, Debatin JF, Richardson WJ, et al: Detection of acute avascular necrosis of the femoral head in dogs: Dynamic contrast-enhanced MR imaging vs spin-echo and STIR sequences. AJR 159:1255, 1992.
278. Vande Berg B, Malghem J, Labaisse MA, et al: Avascular necrosis of the hip: Comparison of contrast-enhanced and nonenhanced MR imaging with histologic correlation. Radiology 182:445, 1992.
279. Lang P, Mauz M, Schörner W, et al: Acute fractures of the femoral neck:

Assessment of femoral head perfusion with gadopentetate dimeglumine–enhanced MR imaging. AJR *160*:335, 1993.

280. Vogler JB III, Murphy WA: Bone marrow imaging. Radiology *168*:679, 1988.

281. Potter HG, Schneider R: Magnetic resonance imaging of the hip. Curr Opinion Orthop *4*:3, 1993.

282. Mitchell DG, Kressel HY: MR imaging of early avascular necrosis. Radiology *169*:281, 1988.

283. Ehman RL, Berquist TH, McLeod RA: MR imaging of the musculoskeletal system: A 5-year appraisal. Radiology *166*:313, 1988.

284. Ehman RL, Berquist TH, McLeod RA: Reply. Radiology *169*:282, 1988.

285. Healy WL: Osteonecrosis of the knee detected only by magnetic resonance imaging. Orthopedics *14*:703, 1991.

286. Patten RM, Shuman WP: MRI of osteonecrosis. MRI Decisions, March/April 1990, p 2.

287. Zizic TM, Lewis CG, Marcoux C, et al: The predictive value of hemodynamic studies in preclinical ischemic necrosis of bone. J Rheumatol *16*:1559, 1989.

288. Travlos J, Learmonth ID: Bilateral avascular necrosis of the talus following strenous physical activity. J Bone Joint Surg [Br] *73*:863, 1991.

289. Gerber C, Schneeberger AG, Vinh T-S: The arterial vascularization of the humeral head. An anatomical study. J Bone Joint Surg [Am] *72*:1486, 1990.

290. Trumble TE: Avascular necrosis after scaphoid fracture: A correlation of magnetic resonance imaging and histology. J Hand Surg [Am] *15*:557, 1990.

291. Milliez PY, Kha HK, Allieu Y, et al: Ostéonécrose aseptique essentielle du grand os. Revue de la littérature à propos de 3 nouveaux cas. Int Orthop (SICOT) *15*:85, 1991.

292. Harverson G: Intravertebral vacuum phenomenon. Clin Radiol *39*:69, 1988.

293. Chevalier X, Wrona N, Avouac B, et al: Thigh pain and multiple vertebral osteonecroses: Value of magnetic resonance imaging. J Rheumatol *18*:1627, 1991.

294. Golimbu C, Firooznia H, Rafii M: The intravertebral vacuum sign. Spine *11*:1040, 1986.

295. Feldmann JL, Alcalay M, Queinnec JY, et al: Spinal cord compression related to vertebral osteonecrosis. Clin Exp Rheumatol *6*:297, 1988.

296. Van Bockel SR, Mindelzun RE: Gas in the psoas muscle secondary to an intravertebral vacuum cleft: CT characteristics. J Comput Assist Tomogr *11*:913, 1987.

297. Naul LG, Peet GJ, Maupin WB: Avascular necrosis of the vertebral body: MR imaging. Radiology *172*:219, 1989.

298. Larsen JL, Smievoll AI: Gas in a cervical vertebral body. A case report with CT confirmation. Eur J Radiol *8*:98, 1988.

299. Ozdoba C, Kurtz B: Case report 474. Skel Radiol *17*:203, 1988.

300. Keats TE, Johnson RR, Fechner RE: Idiopathic punctate necrosis of the phalanges of the feet. Skel Radiol *18*:25, 1989.

301. Atsumi T, Kuroki Y, Yamano K: A microangiographic study of idiopathic osteonecrosis of the femoral head. Clin Orthop *246*:186, 1989.

302. Arlet J: Nontraumatic avascular necrosis of the femoral head. Past, present, and future. Clin Orthop *277*:12, 1992.

303. Ohzono K, Saito M, Takaoka K, et al: Natural history of nontraumatic avascular necrosis of the femoral head. J Bone Joint Surg [Br] *73*:68, 1991.

304. Ohzono K, Saito M, Sugano N, et al: The fate of nontraumatic avascular necrosis of the femoral head. A radiologic classification to formulate prognosis. Clin Orthop *277*:73, 1992.

305. Brown TD, Baker KJ, Brand RA: Structural consequences of subchondral involvement in segmental osteonecrosis of the femoral head. J Orthop Res *10*:79, 1992.

306. Saito S, Ohzono K, Ono K: Minimal osteonecrosis as a segmental infarct within the femoral head. Clin Orthop *231*:35, 1988.

307. Sugimoto H, Okubo RS, Ohsawa T: Chemical shift and the double-line sign in MRI of early femoral avascular necrosis. J Comput Assist Tomogr *16*:727, 1992.

308. Al-Rowaih A, Lindstrand A, Björkengren A, et al: Osteonecrosis of the knee. Diagnosis and outcome in 40 patients. Acta Orthop Scand *62*:19, 1991.

309. Al-Rowaih A, Wingstrand H, Lindstrand A, et al: Three-phase scintimetry in osteonecrosis of the knee. Acta Orthop Scand *61*:120, 1990.

310. Motohashi M, Morii T, Koshino T: Clinical course and roentgenographic changes of osteonecrosis in the femoral condyle under conservative treatment. Clin Orthop *266*:156, 1991.

311. Frizziero L, Tarozzi C, Zizzi F, et al: Atypical spontaneous osteonecrosis of both knees. A case report. Z Rheumatol *45*:129, 1986.

312. Kantor H: Bone marrow pressure in osteonecrosis of the femoral condyle (Ahlbäck's disease). Arch Orthop Trauma Surg *106*:349, 1987.

313. Lotke PA, Ecker ML: Osteonecrosis of the knee. J Bone Joint Surg [Am] *70*:470, 1988.

314. Pollack MS, Dalinka MK, Kressel HY, et al: Magnetic resonance imaging in the evaluation of suspected osteonecrosis. Skel Radiol *16*:121, 1987.

315. Bjorkengren AG, AlRowaih A, Lindstrand A, et al: Spontaneous osteonecrosis of the knee: Value of MR imaging in determining prognosis. AJR *154*:331, 1990.

316. Mueller W: Ueber eine eigenartige doppelseitige Veraenderung des Os naviculare pedis beim Erwachsenen. Dtsch Z Chir *1–2*:84, 1927.

317. Mueller W: Ueber eine typische Gestaltsveraenderung beim Os naviculare pedis und ihre klinische Bedeutung. Fortschr Rongenstr *37*:38, 1928.

318. Weiss K: Ueber die Malacie des Os naviculare pedis. Fortschr Rontgenstr *40*:63, 1929.

319. Brailsford JF: Osteochondritis of the adult tarsal navicular. J Bone Joint Surg [Am] *21*:111, 1939.

320. Volck C: Zwei Faelle von Os naviculare pedis bipartitum. Z Orthop *37*:396, 1937.

321. Haller J, Sartoris DJ, Resnick D, et al: Spontaneous osteonecrosis of the tarsal navicular in adults: Imaging findings. AJR *151*:355, 1988.

322. La Prade RF, Noffsinger MA: Idiopathic osteonecrosis of the patella: An unusual cause of pain in the knee. A case report. J Bone Joint Surg [Am] *72*:1414, 1990.

323. Cella JP: Letter. J Bone Joint Surg [Am] *73*:1574, 1991.

324. Vaishya R: Letter. J Bone Joint Surg [Am] *73*:1574, 1991.

325. Scott RD, Turoff N, Ewald FC: Stress fracture of the patella following duopatellar total knee arthroplasty with patellar resurfacing. Clin Orthop *170*:147, 1982.

326. Oishi Y, Yokota S, Nakagami W, et al: Steroid induced osteonecrosis of the patella. A case report. Acta Orthop Scand *62*:178, 1991.

327. Yamaguchi H, Masuda T, Sasaki T, et al: Steroid induced osteonecrosis of the patella. Clin Orthop *229*:201, 1988.

328. Bullough PG, DiCarlo EF: Subchondral avascular necrosis: A common cause of arthritis. Ann Rheum Dis *49*:412, 1990.

329. Abdelwahab IF, Hermann G, Lewis MM: Transformation of an idiopathic bone infarct into malignant fibrous histiocytoma in a female. A case report. Bull Hosp J Dis *48*:197, 1988.

330. Gaucher AA, Regent DM, Gillet PM, et al: Case report 656. Skel Radiol *20*:137, 1991.

331. Frierson HF Jr, Fechner RE, Stallings RG, et al: Malignant fibrous histiocytoma in bone infarct. Association with sickle cell trait and alcohol abuse. Cancer *59*:496, 1987.

332. Davies AM, Evans N, Grimer RJ: The jockey with a mass in the thigh. Br J Radiol *62*:183, 1989.

333. Greenfield GB, Cardenas C, Dawson PJ, et al: Case report 650. Skel Radiol *20*:67, 1991.

334. Habermann ET, Friedenthal RB: Septic arthritis associated with avascular necrosis of the femoral head. Clin Orthop *134*:325, 1978.

335. Phillips FM, Pottenger LA: Acute septic arthritis in chronic osteonecrosis of the hip. J Rheumatol *15*:1713, 1988.

336. Nuovo MA, Sissons HA, Zuckerman JD: Case report 662. Skel Radiol *20*:217, 1991.

337. Marmor L: Fracture as a complication of osteonecrosis of the tibial plateau. A case report. J Bone Joint Surg [Am] *70*:454, 1988.

338. McGlade CT, Bassett LW, Mirra J, et al: Case report 549. Skel Radiol *18*:322, 1989.

339. Atsumi T, Kuroki Y: Role of impairment of blood supply of the femoral head in the pathogenesis of idiopathic osteonecrosis. Clin Orthop Rel Res *277*:22, 1992.

340. Davidson JK: Dysbaric disorders: Aseptic bone necrosis in tunnel workers and divers. Clin Rheumatol *3*:1, 1989.

341. Mitchell DG: Using MR imaging to probe the pathophysiology of osteonecrosis. Radiology *171*:25, 1989.

342. Colwell CW Jr: The controversy of core decompression of the femoral head for osteonecrosis. Arthritis Rheum *32*:797, 1989.

343. Hungerford DS: Response: The role of core decompression in the treatment of ischemic necrosis of the femoral head. Arthritis Rheum *32*:801, 1989.

344. Hopson CN, Siverhus SW: Ischemic necrosis of the femoral head. Treatment by core decompression. J Bone Joint Surg [Am] *70*:1048, 1988.

345. Saito S, Ohzono K, Ono K: Joint-preserving operations for idiopathic avascular necrosis of the femoral head. Results of core decompression, grafting and osteotomy. J Bone Joint Surg [Br] *70*:78, 1988.

346. Chan TW, Dalinka MK, Steinberg ME, et al: MRI appearance of femoral head osteonecrosis following core decompression and bone grafting. Skel Radiol *20*:103, 1991.

347. Larson B, Light TR, Ogden JA: Fracture and ischemic necrosis of the immature scaphoid. J Hand Surg [Am] *12*:122, 1987.

348. Fordyce MJF, Solomon L: Early detection of avascular necrosis of the femoral head by MRI. J Bone Joint Surg [Br] *75*:365, 1993.

349. Takatori Y, Kokubo T, Ninomiya S, et al: Avascular necrosis of the femoral head. Natural history and magnetic resonance imaging. J Bone Joint Surg [Br] *75*:217, 1993.

350. Lafforgue P, Dahan E, Chagnaud C, et al: Early-stage avascular necrosis of the femoral head: MR imaging for prognosis in 31 cases with at least 2 years of follow-up. Radiology *187*:199, 1993.

351. Duda SH, Laniado M, Schick F, et al: The double-line sign of osteonecrosis: Evaluation on chemical shift MR images. Eur J Radiol *6*:233, 1993.

352. Vande Berg BE, Malghem JJ, Labaisse MA, et al: MR imaging of avascular necrosis and transient marrow edema of the femoral head. RadioGraphics *13*:501, 1993.

353. Hayes CW, Conway WF, Daniel WW: MR imaging of bone marrow edema pattern: Transient osteoporosis, transient bone marrow edema syndrome, or osteonecrosis. RadioGraphics *13*:1001, 1993.

354. Malghem J, Maldague B, Labaisse M-A, et al: Intravertebral vacuum cleft: Changes in content after supine positioning. Radiology *187*:483, 1993.

355. Williams ES, Khreisat S, Ell PJ: Bone imaging and skeletal radiology in dysbaric osteonecrosis. Clin Radiol *38*:589, 1987.

356. Van Blarcom ST, Czarnecki DJ, Fueredi GA, et al: Does dysbaric osteonecrosis progress in the absence of further hyperbaric exposure? A 10-year radiologic follow-up of 15 patients. AJR *155*:95, 1990.

357. Resnik CS, Aisner SC, Young JWR, et al: Case report 767. Skel Radiol *22*:58, 1993.

358. Shimizu K, Moriya H, Akita T, et al: Prediction of collapse with magnetic resonance imaging of avascular necrosis of the femoral head. J Bone Joint Surg [Am] *76*:215, 1994.

359. Richardson ML: Answer. AJR *162*:1244, 1994.

360. Mirowitz SA, Apicella P, Reinus WR, et al: MR imaging of bone marrow lesions: Relative conspicuousness on T1-weighted, fat-suppressed T2-weighted, and STIR images. AJR *162*:215, 1994.

361. Vande Berg B, Malghem J, Labaisse MA, et al: Apparent focal bone marrow ischemia in patients with marrow disorders: MR studies. J Comput Assist Tomogr *17*:792, 1993.

362. Cheras PA, Freemont AJ, Sikorski JM: Intraosseous thrombosis in ischemic necrosis of bone and osteoarthritis. Osteoarthritis Cartilage *1*:219, 1993.

363. Jiang C-C, Shih TTF: Epiphyseal scar of the femoral head: Risk factor of osteonecrosis. Radiology *191*:409, 1994.

81

Osteochondroses

Donald Resnick, M.D.

The designation "osteochondrosis" traditionally has been used to describe a group of disorders that share certain features: predilection for the immature skeleton; involvement of an epiphysis, apophysis, or epiphysioid bone; and a radiographic picture that is dominated by fragmentation, collapse, sclerosis, and, frequently, reossification with re-

constitution of the osseous contour. The radiologic and pathologic features of the osteochondroses initially were interpreted as evidence of a primary impairment of local arterial supply that led to osteonecrosis. With further investigation of these disorders, it became apparent that dissimilarities among them were considerable, and that the osteochondroses were a heterogeneous group of unrelated lesions (Table 81–1). In fact, it now is recognized that osteonecrosis is not apparent on histologic examination in some of the osteochondroses (e.g., Blount's tibia vara, Scheuermann's disease) and that, in others, ischemic necrosis of bone is not a primary event but appears to follow a fracture or other traumatic insult (e.g., Kienböck's disease of lunate bone). Indeed, certain of the osteochondroses are not disorders at all but appear to represent variations in normal ossification (e.g., Sever's phenomenon of the calcaneus). Therefore, it is important to put to rest finally the previously held concept that the osteochondroses are a closely related group of disorders whose basic pathogenesis is vascular insufficiency with osteonecrosis. In reality, the designations of these disorders as (juvenile) osteochondrosis, osteochondritis, osteochondropathy, epiphysitis, apophysitis, or sesamoiditis are inaccurate and should be eliminated.[1, 2]

The heterogeneity of the "osteochondroses" becomes apparent when attempts are made to classify the disorders into more uniform groups. Siffert[228] identified three fundamental types, each associated with disorderly endochondral ossification: articular osteochondroses, nonarticular osteochondroses, and physeal osteochondroses. The *articular osteochondroses* are characterized by initial deformity of the developing epiphysis with the potential for subsequent alteration of the joint itself. The initial epiphyseal deformity, which results from irregularity of endochondral ossification, can be classified further as primary, involving the articular and growth cartilage (e.g., Freiberg's infraction), or secondary to ischemic necrosis (e.g., Legg-Calvé-Perthes disease or Köhler's disease).[228, 229] In both subtypes, chondrogenesis and osteogenesis are affected.

The *nonarticular osteochondroses* involve tendinous and ligamentous attachments to apophyses (e.g., Osgood-Schlatter disease or Sinding-Larsen-Johansson disease) or

TABLE 81–1. Osteochondroses

Disorder	Site	Age (Years)	Probable Mechanism
Legg-Calvé-Perthes disease	Femoral head	4–8	Osteonecrosis, perhaps due to trauma
Freiberg's infraction	Metatarsal head	13–18	Osteonecrosis due to trauma
Kienböck's disease	Carpal lunate	20–40	Osteonecrosis due to trauma
Köhler's disease	Tarsal navicular	3–7	Osteonecrosis or altered sequence of ossification
Panner's disease	Capitulum of humerus	5–10	Osteonecrosis due to trauma
Thiemann's disease	Phalanges of hand	11–19	Osteonecrosis, perhaps due to trauma
Osgood-Schlatter disease	Tibial tuberosity	11–15	Trauma
Blount's disease	Proximal tibial epiphysis	1–3 (infantile) 8–15 (adolescent)	Trauma
Scheuermann's disease	Discovertebral junction	13–17	Trauma
Sinding-Larsen-Johansson disease	Patella	10–14	Trauma
Sever's phenomenon	Calcaneus	9–11	Normal variation in ossification
Van Neck's phenomenon	Ischiopubic synchondrosis	4–11	Normal variation in ossification

miscellaneous sites (Sever's phenomenon); in some instances, they also occur in response to abnormal pressure or chronic stress,[228, 230] which again alters normal chondrogenesis and osteogenesis. The *physeal osteochondroses* (e.g., Blount's disease or Scheuermann's disease) relate to abnormalities of the longitudinal growth plate in either the appendicular or the axial skeleton.

In this chapter, the osteochondroses are grouped according to their probable pathogenesis rather than their site of involvement; however, in certain instances, the exact mechanisms are not yet clear and future investigations may require some adjustment in the manner in which these disorders are classified. Recognizing the diverse nature of these syndromes, the author apologizes for the title of the chapter but believes that the inclusion of the osteochondroses in one place in the textbook has educational benefit.

GENERAL CHARACTERISTICS

Although the individual findings of each of the osteochondroses are unique, certain general characteristics common to most of them can be identified. Many become apparent in the first decade of life at a time when the developing bone still contains a cartilaginous model. With regard to the epiphyseal disorders, the rapidly ossifying central nucleus of bone within the cartilage anlage is especially vulnerable to mechanical pressures superimposed on hormonal or nutritional changes, explaining the appearance of certain of these conditions during the ''midgrowth'' spurt of childhood; others, such as Scheuermann's disease and Osgood-Schlatter disease, occur during the adolescent growth spurt of puberty.[231] Almost all of the osteochondroses are more frequent in boys than in girls. Although a single and unilateral distribution predominates, examples of involvement of multiple and bilateral sites are not uncommon.

The concept that generalized factors may initiate or aggravate some of the osteochondroses is supported by numerous observations, including their occurrence in several members of a single family, in children who are below average in size and have a delay in skeletal maturation, and in those who have congenital anomalies. Furthermore, the changes at some sites resemble those of hypothyroidism and sickle cell anemia. The importance of trauma as an initiating event or common pathway in most of these disorders cannot be denied, however.[232] The development of epiphyseal or apophyseal irregularity and fragmentation in boys at vulnerable periods of accelerated growth and at sites of stress and the existence of experimental evidence documenting that avulsive injuries and fractures can influence endochondral ossification support the causative role of trauma in these syndromes.[232]

Although the radiologic features of the osteochondroses have been well described and documented, the interpretation of the changes in some of the syndromes is debated. As irregularity of endochondral ossification is regarded as a normal variation at certain sites, such as the calcaneus and the tarsal navicular bone, and is believed by some investigators to be compatible with clinical as well as scintigraphic findings, labeling such alterations as diseases or even syndromes[233] may be unwise. Nevertheless, the identification of similar irregularity on radiographs of sites that normally ossify in a uniform fashion and of necrosis, granulation tissue, disorderly ossification, bone absorption, and reparative osteogenesis on histologic inspection[233] supports the belief that some of the osteochondroses should not be regarded as variations of normal. Even in the presence of such uncertainty regarding the significance of the findings, it remains important to be thoroughly familiar with each of the osteochondroses, as many of them are encountered commonly.

DISORDERS CHARACTERIZED BY PRIMARY OR SECONDARY OSTEONECROSIS

Legg-Calvé-Perthes Disease

Background. In 1910, Legg of Boston[3] described an ''obscure affection of the hip joint'' that clinically and radiologically simulated tuberculosis. Independently in the same year, Calvé in France[4] and Perthes in Germany[5] described the same condition, using the designations pseudocoxalgia (Calvé) and arthritis deformans juvenilis (Perthes). In 1913, Perthes[6, 234] introduced the term osteochondritis, and in 1920 Waldenström[7] recognized the flattened femoral head that might occur in this condition, designating the disorder coxa plana, and calling attention to his original description in 1909.[8] Despite the fact that some of the earlier reports falsely attributed the clinical and radiologic manifestations of this affliction to infection, the designations introduced by these investigators are still encountered today, although the term Legg-Calvé-Perthes disease is the most popular.

Clinical Abnormalities. Legg-Calvé-Perthes disease affects children, particularly those between the ages of 4 and 8 years. The mean age of patients with this disorder is 7 years, and the age range of affected patients, almost without exception, is 2 to 12 years. Very rarely, involvement of older adolescents is observed,[361] although permanent sequelae are more frequent in these latter persons. The appearance of Legg-Calvé-Perthes disease in children less than 4 years of age usually is associated with a good prognosis.[11] The disorder is more frequent in boys than in girls, in a ratio of approximately 5 to 1.[377] Either hip can be altered, and bilateral abnormalities are detected in about 10 to 20 per cent of cases, rarely in girls.[378] In those cases in which both hips are involved, the two hips usually are affected successively, not simultaneously (see discussion later in this chapter). Bilateral symmetric fragmentation of the capital femoral epiphyses should suggest the presence of other diseases, such as hypothyroidism. Legg-Calvé-Perthes disease is rare among blacks[9] and is infrequent in native Australians, American Indians, and Polynesians; it occurs most commonly in Japanese, Mongoloid, Eskimo, and Central European populations.[377] A family history of the condition may be detected in approximately 6 per cent of cases.[10]

The principal clinical signs are limping, pain, and limitation of joint motion, particularly abduction and internal rotation of the hip. The pain may be localized to the region of the hip or referred to the thigh or the inside of the ipsilateral knee. These clinical manifestations are neither prominent nor constant and may persist for only a few days or weeks. At other times, more prolonged signs are detected, and atrophy of the soft tissues of the thigh, muscle spasm, and contracture are recognized. A Trendelenburg-type gait usually develops as the disease progresses, and it can persist for several years, even with resolution of the radiographic abnormalities.[378] Occasionally, radiographic changes are noted in patients in whom clinical abnormalities are entirely lacking. A history of trauma can be observed in approximately 25 per cent of cases, with acute onset dating from the time of injury.

These variable clinical manifestations represent a diagnostic challenge to the physician who is examining a child with a painful hip. The possibility of Legg-Calvé-Perthes disease must be considered in a child with acute manifestations in the hip as well as in one with chronic hip complaints.[235]

1. *Acute irritable hip syndrome.* The acute onset of pain in the hip, groin, or knee combined with a limp and limitation of motion in a child of about 3 years, has been referred to as the observation hip, the irritable hip, and transient synovitis of the hip.[236–243, 353, 379–383, 390] Boys are affected more often than girls, and the symptoms and signs usually occur in the spring and summer months.[235] Although the clinical manifestations generally resolve in a period of days with simple bedrest and radiographs usually are normal, reports of more persistent findings and radiologic sequelae (widening of the joint space, coxa magna) have appeared, suggesting that this type of acute syndrome may represent one pattern of clinical presentation of Legg-Calvé-Perthes disease.

The cause of transient synovitis of the hip as well as its relationship to Legg-Calvé-Perthes disease, however, is not clear.[362–364] The accompanying distant infections (tonsillitis, pneumonia, and others) in some instances and the histologic alterations, which include synovial hypervascularity and inflammatory cellular infiltration, are consistent with an infectious or reactive arthritis.[241, 383] Although there is general agreement that a joint effusion[343] and periarticular osteopenia may be identified in this illness, debate exists as to the frequency of subsequent radiologic alterations. Irregularity and flattening of the femoral ossification center[239, 244] and metaphyseal abnormalities in the proximal portion of the femur,[243] which have been identified in 1 to 7 per cent of children following the irritable hip syndrome, are consistent with those seen in Legg-Calvé-Perthes disease, although they may indicate only that synovitis is detrimental to the normal sequence of ossification in the adjacent bone, perhaps owing to vascular compromise, and that synovial inflammation and a joint effusion are common to both conditions. Bone scintigraphy,[384, 385] ultrasonography,[386–388, 481] and MR imaging[389] have been used to examine children with transient synovitis of the hip and, in some cases, to differentiate those with this condition from those who have or will develop Legg-Calvé-Perthes disease. In fact, it is suggested that bone scanning allows differentiation of the two disorders, identifying those children with synovitis (due to Legg-Calvé-Perthes disease) who will later develop osseous abnormalities (Fig. 81–1).[245, 344]

2. *Chronic hip syndrome.* In this pattern of clinical presentation, prolonged pain, stiffness, and a limp are the major manifestations. The pain, which often is worse after rest and on arising from bed in the morning, may be referred to the thigh or knee and is associated with fatigue and an unwillingness to participate in normal activities.[235] Typical radiologic abnormalities usually are apparent.

Radiographic Abnormalities. The radiographic abnormalities have been the subject of a great deal of attention.[12–20, 246–250] The early changes have been summarized by Caffey[15] (Fig. 81–2).

1. *Soft tissue swelling on the lateral side of the articulation.* Capsular bulging with displacement of the capsular fat pad appears to be a more accurate sign of hip disease in children than in adults.[354] Apparently, intra-articular fluid can lead to distortion and obscuration of this fat plane. It is not a specific finding, it is influenced by the position of the leg during radiography, and it usually is accompanied by more obvious radiologic abnormalities.

2. *Smallness of the femoral ossification nucleus.* A diminutive ossification center may be apparent in as many as 50 per cent of patients. The pathogenesis of this finding is not clear. It apparently is unrelated to osseous compression, but may represent an actual retardation of bone growth. Because a decrease in the rate of ossification is not immediately associated with radiographic findings, the detection

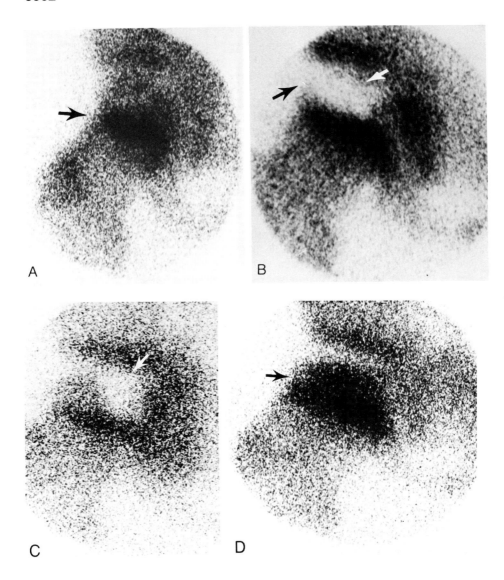

FIGURE 81–1. Acute irritable hip syndrome versus Legg-Calvé-Perthes disease: Scintigraphic abnormalities.

A Acute irritable hip syndrome. As shown here, radionuclide abnormalities usually are characterized by diffusely increased uptake of the bone-seeking radionuclide throughout the femoral head (arrow) without evidence of "cold" areas or a flattened articular surface.

B–D Legg-Calvé-Perthes disease. Typical patterns on bone scintigraphy are "cold" areas (arrows) involving the lateral two thirds of the femoral head **(B)** or, less commonly, the medial or central region (arrow) **(C)**, and diffuse uptake (arrow) in a flattened femoral head **(D)**.

(From Carty H, et al: Skel Radiol *11*:32, 1984.)

of a small ossific nucleus probably indicates that disease has been present for at least several weeks.

3. *Lateral displacement of the femoral ossification nucleus.* Calot[21] and Waldenström[22] have emphasized this early finding in Legg-Calvé-Perthes disease. The ossific nucleus may be displaced laterally 2 to 5 mm, producing an enlargement of the medial portion of the joint space.[23] This change, which has been reported in as many as 85 per cent of cases, has been regarded as an indication of a serious hip problem (even in young children with apparent transient synovitis of the hip) and may account for overloading of the anterosuperior quadrant of the femoral head, with subsequent flattening and compression. It has been suggested that synovitis with intra-articular fluid accumulation could produce such displacement; this might explain a similar appearance seen in pyogenic and tuberculous infection and other synovial disorders.[24] Alternatively, cartilaginous hypertrophy could produce lateral displacement of the femoral head, and arthrography may outline an enlarged medial chondral surface (see discussion later in this chapter).

Lateral movement of the epiphyseal ossification center frequently precedes other radiologic evidence of disease.

Fragmentation and flattening may be absent at this stage, although osteoporosis can be encountered.

4. *Fissuring and fracture of the femoral ossific nucleus.* This is a constant and well-recognized radiographic sign of the disease. It may be detected only on radiographs obtained in the frog-leg position or, at least, is better delineated in this projection (Fig. 81–2*C*). Linear or curvilinear radiolucent shadows are seen, beginning in the anterior margin of the epiphysis and extending posteriorly, and the fracture fragment may remain in situ or be slightly displaced at its peripheral attachment. At this stage, significant displacement or separation and free fragments are not observed. A subchondral location of the infraction is predominant but not invariable, and fracture lines commonly disappear on subsequent examinations. Their appearance and characteristics are similar to those of the subchondral fractures seen in other varieties of osteonecrosis.

5. *Flattening and sclerosis of the femoral ossific nucleus.* Flattening of the epiphyseal nucleus predominates near the fracture lines on the anterolateral superior segment of the femoral head. In almost all cases, this finding is preceded by, or occurs simultaneously with, the development of fissures in the bone, although flattening may later progress as

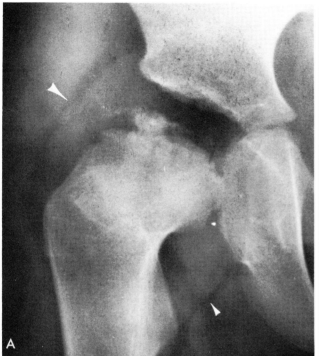

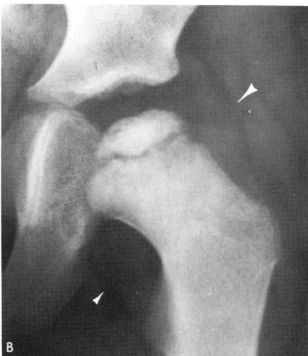

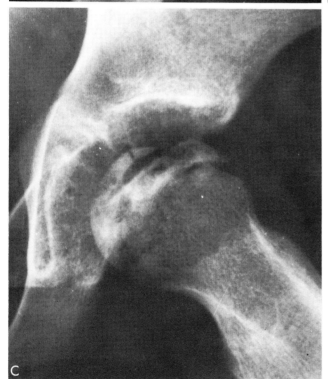

FIGURE 81–2. Legg-Calvé-Perthes disease: Radiographic abnormalities.

A In this child, several of the radiographic changes are demonstrated. Note soft tissue swelling with distortion of the capsular (large arrowhead) and iliopsoas (small arrowhead) fat planes and a small and fragmented femoral ossification nucleus.

B In the same child, a radiograph of the opposite hip reveals soft tissue distortion (arrowheads), a sclerotic femoral ossification center that is laterally displaced and contains radiolucent fissures, and metaphyseal irregularity.

C In a different child, a frog-leg projection delineates the fragmented sclerotic femoral ossification center containing several radiolucent fissures.

the fissure lines disappear. The frog-leg position is optimal for visualizing the degree of bone flattening.

Mild to moderate sclerosis accompanies other radiographic signs of disease. On the anteroposterior view, the entire femoral head may appear radiodense, whereas in the frog-leg position, a segmental and peripheral location is evident. The increased radiodensity of the femoral head generally follows the appearance of fracture and flattening, indicating that sclerosis is a secondary phenomenon due to compression of trabeculae and revascularization, with deposition of new bone on necrotic trabeculae.

6. *Intraepiphyseal gas.* A vacuum phenomenon, caused by release of gas into the clefts and gaps in the subchondral trabeculae, accentuates the exaggerated radiolucent appearance in this area. In most cases, however, this finding is not present, and the radiolucent cleft is due to the fracture line itself. Both the cleft and the vacuum phenomenon are better delineated in the frog-leg view as, in this position, stress enlarges the opening between the osteochondral fragment and the remainder of the femoral head. Gas, presumably nitrogen, flows into the enlarging space.

Although the progression and extent of disease are highly variable (see discussion later in this chapter), further compression, disintegration, fragmentation, and sclerosis of the epiphysis, together with metaphyseal changes, can be seen.

1. *Metaphyseal "cysts."* Radiolucent lesions of the metaphysis are a characteristic part of the radiographic picture of Legg-Calvé-Perthes disease, although their pathogenesis is debated (Fig. 81–3A). Gill[25] considered the lesions to be indicative of primary necrosis of the metaphysis that later spread to the femoral head, and the concept of metaphyseal necrosis was supported by Waldenström.[22] Mindell and Sherman[26] emphasized the late appearance of metaphyseal

defects, their location opposite areas of diminished density in the epiphysis, and their ability to heal in a manner similar to that of the femoral head lesions. Ponseti[27] used trocar biopsies to study the metaphyseal abnormalities, and noted islands or tongues of uncalcified cartilage derived from the growth plate extending into the metaphyseal bone marrow. In a sense, the lesions represented intramedullary enchondromas composed of uncalcified cartilage. According to both Ponseti and others,[15] the metaphyseal cyst was related to a distortion of normal endochondral bone formation in which a disturbance or failure of normal absorption of cartilage was detected. Caffey[15] speculated that fissuring and fibrillation of the growth plate weakened it so that the excessive compression forces on the anterior segment of the femoral head were transmitted through the cartilaginous plate to the anterior segment of the metaphysis, where they compressed capillary loops, preventing normal inflow of arterial blood. This deficiency in vascular supply then reduced the normal resorption of uncalcified cartilage, producing cartilaginous islands in the metaphysis. Caffey emphasized the relatively late appearance of the metaphyseal lesions following the detection of epiphyseal changes and their location in the ventral segment of the metaphysis directly beneath the area of epiphyseal fracture and flattening. Indeed, some observers have suggested that the metaphyseal cysts are not metaphyseal at all but rather relate to the superimposition of the epiphyseal abnormalities on the adjacent metaphysis.[391]

Despite the evidence underscoring a disturbance of endochondral bone formation in the development of metaphyseal lucent areas, support for a necrotic process in the metaphysis still appears.[18] In either case, alterations of vascular supply may represent the primary event, initiating either necrosis or disturbed osseous development. The re-

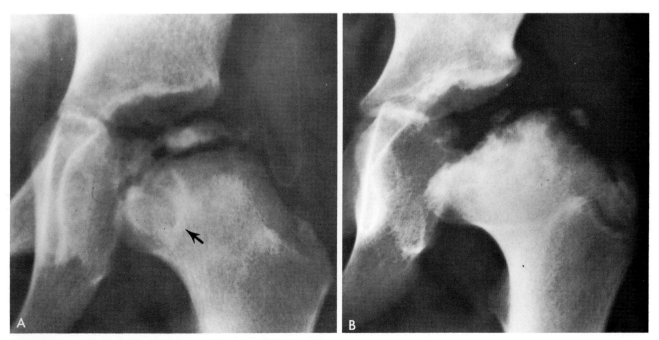

FIGURE 81–3. Legg-Calvé-Perthes disease: Metaphyseal abnormalities.

A Metaphyseal "cysts." Observe the large cystic lesion of the medial metaphysis of the femur (arrow), which is associated with a fragmented, sclerotic, and laterally placed ossific nucleus.

B In another child, note the broad and short femoral neck containing multiple radiolucent lesions. Most of the epiphyseal ossification center is destroyed.

sulting lucency of the metaphysis, which is detected on radiographic examination,[215, 345] may simulate an abscess or tumor. Biopsy is unnecessary, however, if the observer recognizes that such lesions are a definite part of the radiographic appearance in Legg-Calvé-Perthes disease.

2. *Widening and shortening of the femoral neck.* Widening and irregularity of the growth plate and broadening of the metaphysis are additional manifestations of this disorder (Fig. 81–3*B*). Ponseti and Cotton[28] described increased apposition of bone throughout the length of the femoral neck. Edgren[10] attributed the widening of the neck to metaphyseal alterations as well as appositional growth. Robichon and coworkers[19] cited experimental work in animals indicating that diminished blood supply to the femoral head caused not only epiphyseal necrosis but also a decrease in cartilage cell production in the germinal layer of the growth plate, producing a diminution in longitudinal bone growth; appositional growth continued in the metaphysis because of its intact vascular supply. This combination of factors created the short, wide neck that was evident in Legg-Calvé-Perthes disease. Measurements by Robichon and coworkers of the length and width of the femoral neck on radiographs of patients with this disease documented that the degree of shortening and widening of the neck was related to the extent of structural change in the femoral head.

Bowen and collaborators[250] identified two patterns of premature closure of the longitudinal growth plate in the femoral neck in patients with Legg-Calvé-Perthes disease. In both patterns, a bridge of bone formed between abnormal segments in the epiphysis and metaphysis. Centrally located osseous bridges were associated with the development of a short femoral neck, a round femoral head, and a deformed acetabulum; laterally located physeal closure was followed by the development of shortening only in the lateral portion of the femoral neck, lengthening of the medial portion of the femoral neck, an externally tilted femoral head with an oval shape, and a deformed acetabulum. This latter pattern of physeal closure encourages lateral subluxation of the femoral head, whereas medially located osseous bridges, an infrequent pattern, would be expected to be accompanied by deeper seating of the femoral head within the acetabulum.[251]

The greater trochanter possesses a separate blood supply and can continue to develop despite growth disturbance in the adjacent bone. Eventually, it may appear disproportionately large in comparison with the shortened femoral neck.[227, 251, 252]

Pathologic Abnormalities. The fundamental pathologic aberration of the femoral head in this disease is osteonecrosis.[29–33] Necrosis of trabeculae and marrow is observed, which eventually is accompanied by structural failure of the femoral head, resulting in flattening and collapse. In the area of collapse, compression of trabeculae and intertrabecular, amorphous detritus are seen. As in other varieties of osteonecrosis, the chondral surfaces are remarkably well preserved during the early and intermediate stages of Legg-Calvé-Perthes disease. As opposed to the situation in other forms of osteonecrosis, however, separation of articular cartilage and underlying necrotic bone even in late stages of Legg-Calvé-Perthes disease is unusual.[224]

Healing is characterized by revascularization of the necrotic portion of the femoral head. Vessels that contribute to an increase in blood supply to the bone are the periosteal and marrow vessels of the neck and the vessels in the ligamentum teres. Viable bone is deposited on dead trabeculae. Reconstitution of intertrabecular marrow may be accompanied by phagocytic and giant cell activity. Cystic areas containing necrotic trabeculae and detritus can be seen. In some cases, reconstitution of the femoral head almost is complete, although some degree of flattening of the head and shortening and broadening of the femoral neck is not unusual. The healing process appears to be more prominent in those cases in which the disorder begins at a young age,[1] although this is not a constant feature of early-onset Legg-Calvé-Perthes disease.[33]

Course of Disease. The course of Legg-Calvé-Perthes disease is variable. The degree of reconstitution of the ossific nucleus and the ultimate shape of the femoral head depend on the amount of necrosis, its exact location, and the magnitude of forces across the joint. In some instances, the eventual radiographic appearance of the involved head may be indistinguishable from that of its uninvolved counterpart (Fig. 81–4), whereas in others, coxa plana, shortening and widening of the femoral neck, osteochondroma-like lesions of the femoral neck,[255] degenerative joint disease, and intra-articular osseous bodies may be identified (Figs. 81–5 to 81–8). One interesting residual of this disease is a radiodense curvilinear shadow at the base of the femoral neck, termed the sagging rope sign.[248] Although it has been suggested that the presence of this sign implies severe involvement, damage to the physis, and a poor prognosis,[248] its nature is not entirely clear. The sagging rope sign probably represents the radiodense shadow cast by the anterior or lateral edge of a severely deformed femoral head.[256]

In most cases of Legg-Calvé-Perthes disease, changes are isolated to or predominantly involve one hip. In those instances in which bilateral abnormalities are encountered, symmetric involvement is exceedingly rare, a feature that serves to distinguish Legg-Calvé-Perthes disease from other disorders, such as hypothyroidism and epiphyseal dysplasias, that affect the hip.[253] In an extensive review of 147 patients with Legg-Calvé-Perthes disease, Nevelös[221] noted the simultaneous onset of changes in both hips that progressed concurrently in only two patients (approximately 1 per cent of cases). Additionally he observed six patients (approximately 4 per cent) who had simultaneous involvement of both sides but in whom only one side revealed fragmentation. Sixty-two patients (42 per cent) had ''unilateral'' disease with minimal radiographic changes in the opposite hip (irregularities in density or outline of epiphysis or metaphysis); nine patients (6 per cent) had ''unilateral'' disease affecting first one hip and then, after a clear interval, the other hip; and 68 patients (46 per cent) had purely unilateral disease. Other investigators have noted mild radiographic changes in the ''normal'' hip in children with ''unilateral'' Legg-Calvé-Perthes disease.[222, 365] The nature of these changes is unknown, although clinical findings generally are lacking. Their relationship to findings in minimal Legg-Calvé-Perthes disease[223] is unclear.

Although the chondral surface is relatively uninvolved in this disease, joint incongruity can lead to secondary osteoarthritis with cartilaginous fibrillation and erosion.[34] This complication may be more prominent in patients with irregularly healed femoral heads than in those with normal or smoothly flattened heads. Rarely, acute chondrolysis similar

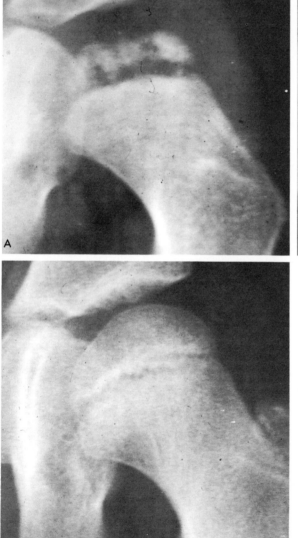

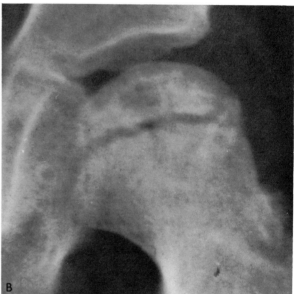

FIGURE 81–4. Legg-Calvé-Perthes disease: Reconstitution of femoral head. Sequential radiographs over a 3½ year period delineate reconstitution of a femoral head involved with this disease.

A The initial radiograph outlines soft tissue swelling and fragmentation of the epiphysis.

B One and one half years later, the epiphysis is smooth, although it demonstrates some lucency and sclerosis, and the metaphysis is widened.

C Two years after **B,** remarkable reconstitution of the femoral head can be seen.

(Courtesy of R. Freiberger, M.D., New York, New York.)

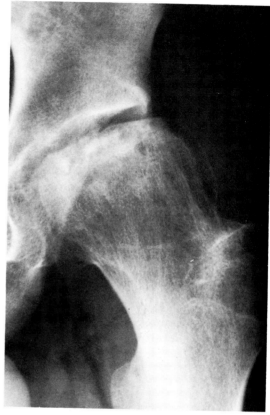

FIGURE 81–5. Legg-Calvé-Perthes disease: Coxa plana and coxa magna. This 14 year old boy with known Legg-Calvé-Perthes disease reveals residual flattening and enlargement of the femoral head with surface irregularity and widening of the femoral neck. The acetabulum is mildly flattened.

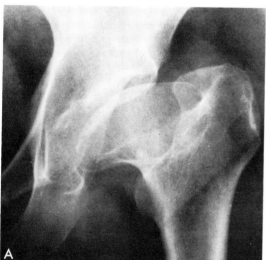
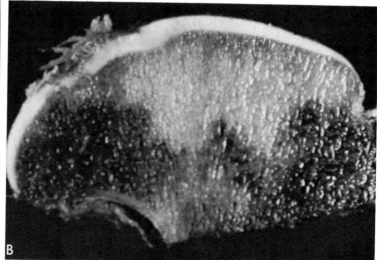

FIGURE 81–6. Legg-Calvé-Perthes disease: Coxa plana and coxa magna. This 53 year old man had had Legg-Calvé-Perthes disease as a child and had experienced pain and tenderness in the left hip.
A Note the smoothly flattened femoral head, the prominent greater trochanter, and the flattened acetabular margin.
B A coronal section of the femoral head following total hip replacement reveals the flattened osseous contour and the remarkable preservation of the chondral surface.

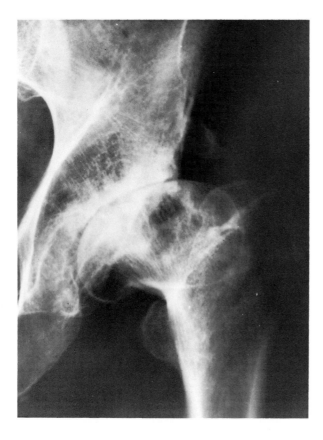

FIGURE 81–7. Legg-Calvé-Perthes disease: Secondary degenerative joint disease. This 60 year old man with a history of Legg-Calvé-Perthes disease developed secondary degenerative joint disease, characterized by articular space narrowing and sclerosis. Note lateral subluxation and cystic lesions of the femoral head and buttressing of the medial portion of the femoral neck.

to that occurring as a complication of a slipped femoral capital epiphysis has been identified in the hips of patients with Legg-Calvé-Perthes disease.[396]

A detached osteochondral fragment (osteochondritis dissecans) can be seen in this disease (Fig. 81–9).[14, 16, 35, 36, 219, 220, 254, 346, 366, 397] The reported frequency of this complication is approximately 2 to 4 per cent, and it is observed almost exclusively in male patients. The risk of developing a persistent, ununited osteocartilaginous fragment appears to increase in patients with a late clinical presentation.[14] Furthermore, the frequency of osteochondritis dissecans in Legg-Calvé-Perthes disease is greater in persons with bilateral involvement. This occurrence rate does not correlate with the degree of deformity of the head or with the length or time of therapy. The average interval between the diagnosis of Legg-Calvé-Perthes disease and the presentation of an intra-articular osteocartilaginous body is about 8 years.

The pathogenesis of osteochondritis dissecans in this condition is not clear; it may be due to persistence of an ununited fragment or to fragmentation of a femoral head that is weakened by revascularization during the healing process. The superolateral aspect of the head is the typical location of the fragment. Usually the osteocartilaginous body remains at its site of origin or becomes depressed into the parent bone. Free intra-articular bodies are unusual, but when present may account for symptoms and signs, including pain, limp, limitation of motion, and secondary degenerative joint disease. Although this complication may be diagnosed on plain films, especially those obtained in a frog-leg position, arthrography (with or without conventional tomography) or CT may further delineate the nature and position of the fragment and the integrity of the overlying cartilage.[14] Furthermore, contrast opacification of the

joint allows identification of purely cartilaginous fragments that cannot be recognized on plain films or conventional tomograms.

Although recurrent episodes of infarction may be essential to the development of Legg-Calvé-Perthes disease, cases demonstrating clinical and radiographic evidence of recurrent disease are unusual.[37–39, 398] In such cases, a second episode of disease occurs 3 to 6 years after the initial attack when the patients are between 6 and 11 years of age. Boys are affected more commonly. Clinical findings of increasing pain, restricted motion, and limp indicate unilateral involvement and are associated with fragmentation of an epiphysis that had partially or completely healed from a previous episode of disease. It is possible that the initial alterations of the proximal capital femoral epiphysis in patients with recurrent disease represent not Legg-Calvé-Perthes disease but Meyer's dysplasia of the femoral head (see discussion later in this chapter).

Classification Systems and Prognosis. It is the variability in the course of Legg-Calvé-Perthes disease that stimulated investigations into the predictive value of certain radiographic or clinical signs in the eventual outcome of the disorder. In general, a better prognosis is observed in boys and in younger patients (below the age of five or six years), perhaps indicating that a longer elapsed time prior to skeletal maturity allows more extensive remodeling and healing of the femoral head. Furthermore, acetabular remodeling seems to occur more predictably during the first eight years of life[378]; osteoporosis of the acetabular roof, irregularity of acetabular contour, premature fusion of the triradiate cartilage, hypertrophy of acetabular articular cartilage, and alterations in acetabular dimensions are more marked in older children and in those with involvement of

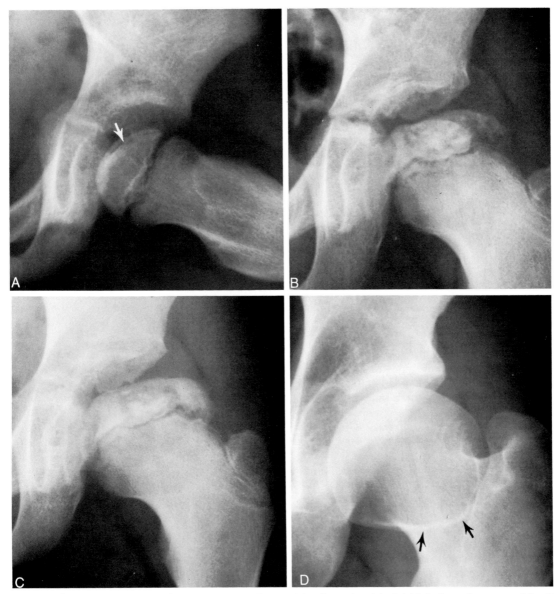

FIGURE 81–8. Legg-Calvé-Perthes disease: Sagging rope sign. Sequential radiographs of the left hip indicate the course of the disease over a 16 year period.

A Age 7 years (phase of disease onset). On this frog-leg view, note the radiolucent crescent sign (arrow).

B Age 8 years (phase of fragmentation). The lateral two thirds of the femoral head is collapsed and fragmented, and the lateral portion of the head is not covered by the acetabulum.

C Age 9 years (phase of healing). The medial aspect of the epiphysis is larger and there is an increase in the amount of bone that is present laterally. The femoral head is not completely covered.

D Age 22 years (residual phase). The femoral head is slightly flattened and large. Note the radiodense curved line, the sagging rope sign (arrows).

(Courtesy of P. VanderStoep, M.D., Saint Cloud, Minnesota.)

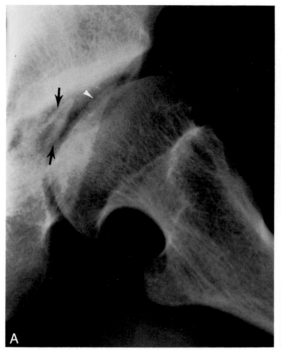
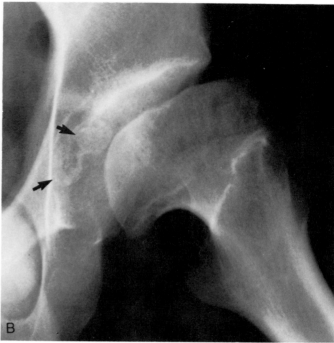

FIGURE 81–9. Legg-Calvé-Perthes disease: Osteochondral fragment.
A In this 27 year old man, a frog-leg view reveals a flattened femoral head, acetabular deformity, and an osseous body (arrows) within the joint, highlighted by the spontaneous release of gas into the articulation. The presence of gas also permits the identification of a thinned cartilaginous surface (arrowhead).
B In a 29 year old man, observe the flattened femoral head and acetabulum and a large intra-articular osseous body (arrows) in the acetabular fossa.

more than half of the femoral epiphysis.[392] Other prognostic signs, including those related to the radiographic characteristics of the disease, are not agreed upon by all orthopedic surgeons. Indeed, there is a lack of uniformity in the classification or grading systems used to describe the radiographic findings in the disease. These systems have been well described by Wenger and coworkers.[378] They can be divided into systems used to classify: (a) the phase of the disease, (b) the extent of the disease, and (c) the end results of the disease.

With regard to the first category, the system of Waldenström generally is employed to determine the phase of healing of Legg-Calvé-Perthes disease. Waldenström emphasized an initial evolutionary period (characterized first by epiphyseal irregularity and density and then by epiphyseal fragmentation); a subsequent healing period in which the epiphysis becomes more homogeneous in its radiographic appearance, with extensive revascularization; and a final period of growth with normal ossification of the deformed femoral head.[378]

The classification of the extent of disease is provided by the systems of Catterall and of Salter and Thompson. Catterall[40, 235] has used four classes or grades of involvement (Table 81–2).

Group I. The anterior part of the epiphysis is the only affected site. Collapse and sequestration are not evident. Metaphyseal changes are unusual in the early stage of the disease but may occur in later stages. Radiographically, the course of the disease is characterized by absorption of the involved segment, followed by regeneration commencing from the periphery.

Group II. Greater involvement is apparent. Collapse and sequestration are followed by absorption and healing. A viable medial and lateral bony segment provides osseous support and maintains epiphyseal height.

Group III. Only a small portion of the epiphysis is not

TABLE 81–2. Grades of Femoral Involvement in Legg-Calvé-Perthes Disease (Catterall Classification)

	Grade			
	I	II	III	IV
Site of epiphyseal involvement	Anterior part	Anterior part	Almost whole epiphysis	Whole epiphysis
Sequestrum	No	Yes	Yes	Yes
Crescent sign	No	Anterior	Anterior and extends posteriorly	Anterior and posterior
Collapse	No	Yes	Yes	Yes
Metaphyseal abnormalities	No	Localized	Diffuse	Diffuse

sequestered. Anteroposterior radiographs reveal a "head within a head" appearance, and collapse of a centrally placed sequestrum is identified. The lateral fragment often is small and osteoporotic, appearing as specks of calcification. From the onset of collapse, this osteoporotic segment and its associated growth plate are displaced in an anterolateral direction, accounting for subsequent broadening of the femoral neck. A small, viable posterior segment may be evident. The course of the disease is similar to that in group II, although metaphyseal changes are more generalized.

Group IV. The whole epiphysis is affected. Total collapse is associated with loss of height between the growth plate and acetabular roof. Epiphyseal displacement can occur anteriorly or posteriorly, and a mushroom-like appearance of the head can be identified. Metaphyseal changes may be extensive.

The purpose of this classification system is to allow identification of the degree of epiphyseal involvement and to relate this involvement to the prognosis of the disease. In general, patients in groups III and IV have a relatively poor prognosis, whereas those in groups I and II do better.[198] These generalizations are not without exception, as some patients in groups III and IV have an unexpectedly good result, whereas others in group II have a poor result. An additional limitation of this classification system is a difficulty in recognizing which pattern is present at an early phase of the disease[226]; at times, patients initially placed in one category will shift to another class on follow-up radiography.[216, 260, 367] Catterall attempted to improve the predictive value of early radiographic changes by identifying four radiologic signs that indicated a capital femoral epiphysis "at risk" for collapse. These findings are (1) Gage's sign (a small, osteoporotic segment that forms a transradiant "V" on the lateral side of the epiphysis); (2) calcification lateral to the epiphysis (reflecting the presence of extruded cartilage); (3) lateral subluxation of the femoral head; and (4) a transverse epiphyseal line. Murphy and Marsh[41] found that these four "head at risk" signs and a fifth, diffuse metaphyseal reaction, correlated better with a poor radiologic result than did the degree of epiphyseal involvement. Dickens and Menelaus[42] observed that the most reliable radiologic factors indicating the prognosis of the disease were the Catterall grouping, the extent of uncovering of the femoral head, the presence of calcification lateral to the outer limit of the acetabulum, and the lateral displacement of the femoral head. Stulberg and associates[258] found that the degree of congruency existing between the femoral head and the acetabulum was the most important prognostic indicator, with aspheric congruency or incongruency being associated with subsequent osteoarthritis. Green and collaborators[259] emphasized epiphyseal extrusion as the principal guide to prognosis, whereas other investigators have stressed the prognostic significance of metaphyseal alterations,[246, 261, 262] coxa plana,[263] subchondral fracture,[264] widening of the medial joint space,[247] and physeal involvement.[265]

Salter and Thompson classified Legg-Calvé-Perthes disease into two groups based on the extent of subchondral fracture and the presence or absence of an intact viable lateral margin of the femoral epiphysis.[378, 393] In group A hips, which correspond to those assigned to Catterall's groups I and II, a subchondral fracture line involves approximately one half of the femoral head; in group B hips,

which correspond to those assigned to Catterall's groups III and IV, no evidence of an intact viable lateral margin of the femoral head is seen on frontal radiographs, and the subchondral fracture extends to the lateral extent of the epiphysis.[378] This system is difficult to apply when the subchondral fracture no longer can be detected.[378]

Classification systems used to judge end results of the disease, as summarized by Wenger and coworkers,[378] are divided into three categories: quantitative uniplanar, quantitative biplanar, and descriptive. The first relies on a determination of the sphericity of the femoral head as delineated on uniplanar anteroposterior radiographs. The second is based on a similar determination of sphericity as delineated on biplanar radiography. The descriptive category is based on a global visual impression of all radiographs. None of these three systems has proved ideal, and interobserver variability in the interpretation of the findings rarely is investigated.[395] Furthermore, newer classification systems continue to be developed,[394] underscoring the lack of confidence that many orthopedic surgeons have in the currently available methods.

It is evident that no simple radiologic observation is indicative of a good or poor result, and that a combination of findings must be used for prognostic accuracy.[257, 266, 399, 400] Most patients are symptom-free 30 to 40 years later, although persistent radiographic alterations usually are evident. Mild limp, leg shortening,[267] and pain can be seen.[43]

Other Diagnostic Methods. *Arthrography* may be used in the evaluation of Legg-Calvé-Perthes disease.[44] In the early stages, contrast opacification of the joint can reveal subtle flattening of the chondral surface at the site of osseous fissuring and an increase in width of both the femoral and the acetabular cartilage. Synovial and soft tissue thickening may[45] or may not[44] be seen. The ligamentum teres may appear swollen.[401] In later stages, arthrography frequently indicates a smooth cartilaginous surface despite the presence of considerable ossific fragmentation (Fig. 81–10). Flattening and lateral extrusion of the chondral coat can be identified in some instances. In late stages of remodeling, the cartilaginous shape generally parallels that of the reconstituted ossification center. A detached or attached osteochondral fragment may be outlined. As arthrography allows identification of the actual size and shape of the abnormal femoral head more accurately than does plain film radiography and, in fact, commonly will allow delineation of a markedly enlarged osteochondral femoral head, it may be a useful guide for the orthopedic surgeon who is interested in knowing what percentage of the head is contained within the acetabulum.[208] In most instances, however, arthrographic findings regarding epiphyseal protrusion parallel those evident on the routine radiographs.[268]

Radionuclide examination with bone-seeking radiopharmaceutical agents allows identification of an area of deficient uptake in the early phase of the disease, owing to varying degrees of impairment of the blood supply.[46–48, 210, 270, 272, 368, 411] This defect is seen most frequently in the anterolateral aspect of a femoral head with partial necrosis and across the entire width of the epiphysis in a head with total necrosis. The scintigraphic abnormality, especially if flow and static images are obtained,[271] antedates radiographic alterations and coincides with the onset of clinical manifestations (Figs. 81–11 and 81–12). It has been suggested that the size and pattern of the radionuclide defect

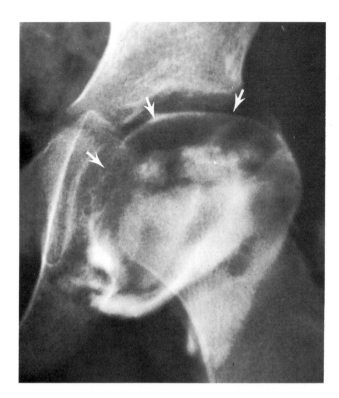

FIGURE 81–10. Legg-Calvé-Perthes disease: Arthrographic abnormalities. This 5 year old boy developed Legg-Calvé-Perthes disease of the left hip. An arthrogram reveals a relatively smooth cartilaginous surface (arrows) despite the presence of extensive ossific irregularity. There is some thickening of the medial chondral surface of the femoral head.

(Courtesy of T. Goergen, M.D., Escondido, California.)

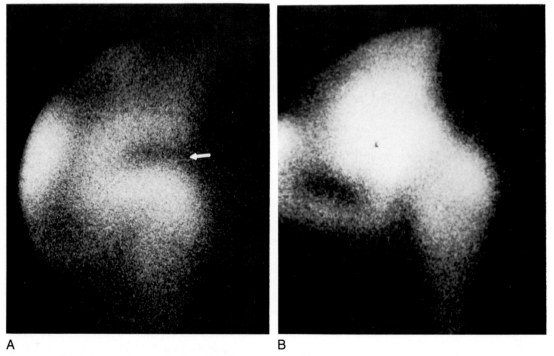

A   B

FIGURE 81–11. Legg-Calvé-Perthes disease: Radionuclide abnormalities.

A An initial radiograph of a painful left hip in this young girl was normal (not shown), but the corresponding bone scan using technetium pyrophosphate reveals a definite area of decreased activity in the left hip (arrow) consistent with early Legg-Calvé-Perthes disease.

B Three months later, the capital femoral epiphysis was slightly dense and flattened, and a metaphyseal lucent area was evident (not shown). A repeat scan reveals increased radionuclide activity in the hip.

(Courtesy of J. Wilcox, M.D., San Diego, California.)

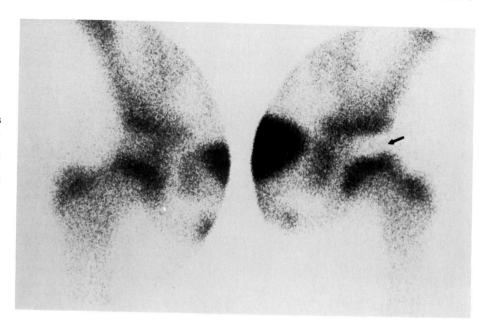

FIGURE 81–12. Legg-Calvé-Perthes disease: Radionuclide abnormalities. In this 9 year old boy, note the characteristic "cold" area (arrow) in the left femoral head on the bone scan. The opposite hip is normal. (Courtesy of V. Vint, M.D., San Diego, California.)

in early stages of the disease may correlate with the ultimate prognosis of the disease,[212] especially if computer processing of the scintigraphic data is used.[211, 218, 269, 271] With the appearance of regeneration and increased vascularity, the photodeficient areas may return to normal or be replaced by areas of augmented activity.[213] A follow-up scan that outlines a focus of deficient activity at a site that was previously normal may indicate a second episode of infarction.

Ultrasonography has been used to define the presence of an effusion and joint space widening in the hips of patients with transient synovitis of the hip or with Legg-Calvé-Perthes disease.[347, 355, 369, 370, 386–388, 412] It also has been employed to define the extent of deformity of the femoral head.[402]

Angiography has been employed as an investigative technique in some patients with Legg-Calvé-Perthes disease.[209] In the early phases of the disease, angiography is not especially useful, although it may demonstrate an interruption of the superior capsular arteries and a generalized decrease of blood flow in the affected hip.[273] Subsequently the procedure may allow identification of the size and the position of sequestered fragments of bone as well as of the distribution of revascularized osseous segments.

Intraosseous venography also has been used to identify venous patterns of drainage[276] and as a means of evaluating the prognosis in patients with Legg-Calvé-Perthes disease.[214]

MR imaging is ideally applied to the evaluation of ischemic necrosis of bone (Chapter 80) and has been used for the identification of infarction of the femoral head in Legg-Calvé-Perthes disease.[274, 348, 403–406] MR imaging is extremely sensitive to the detection of alterations of bone marrow and, therefore, is useful for the assessment of a variety of causes of hip pain in the child, including Legg-Calvé-Perthes disease (Figs. 81–13 and 81–14). Some investigations have documented its superiority to other techniques such as routine radiography and bone scintigraphy in this clinical setting, providing morphologic information regarding the cartilaginous and osseous structures about the hip.[407] In some

children with hip pain, MR imaging may reveal findings consistent with transient bone marrow edema, characterized by decreased signal intensity in the femoral head on T1-weighted spin echo images and normal or increased signal intensity on T2-weighted spin echo images.[389] As such findings in adults occasionally are followed by those of ischemic necrosis of bone, transient bone marrow edema of the femoral head in a child may be a precursor to Legg-Calvé-Perthes disease, although this potential association is not proved. In children with transient synovitis of the hip, MR findings include evidence of a joint effusion; similar findings occur in patients with septic arthritis of the hip.[407]

With regard to the MR imaging characteristics of Legg-Calvé-Perthes disease, Rush and colleagues[408] emphasized the cartilaginous and synovial changes in this disorder. Thickening of both the acetabular cartilage and the cartilage of the femoral head was observed, and loss of containment of the femoral head within the acetabulum was a frequent finding that was variable in extent. A frondlike structure was seen adjacent to the inferomedial portion of the joint space and was believed to represent villous hypertrophy of the synovium within the iliopsoas recess of the hip capsule.

Egund and Wingstrand[404] used MR imaging to evaluate the shape of the cartilaginous femoral head and the adequacy of femoroacetabular containment in 35 children with Legg-Calvé-Perthes disease. These authors judged the information provided by MR imaging to be superior to that obtained with arthrography and, furthermore, they found MR imaging useful in the postoperative assessment of femoroacetabular containment following derotation varus osteotomy.

Egund and associates,[404] as well as other investigators,[403, 405, 406] have indicated the sensitivity of MR imaging in the delineation of areas of bone infarction in children with Legg-Calvé-Perthes disease. The MR characteristics of osteonecrosis in this disease, as in other causes of osteonecrosis, are variable and are addressed in Chapter 80. In Legg-Calvé-Perthes disease, information provided by MR imaging, such as the extent of femoral head infarction, the presence or absence of viable regions of the femoral head,

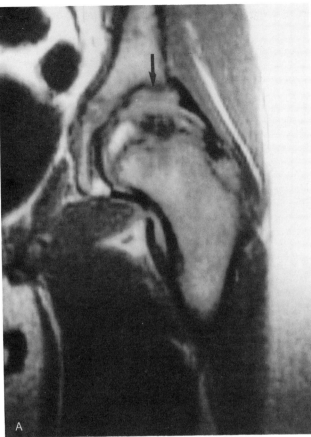

FIGURE 81-13. Legg-Calvé-Perthes disease: MR imaging abnormalities.

A A coronal T1-weighted (TR/TE, 500/28) spin echo MR image of the left hip in an 8 year old child shows low signal intensity in the center of the capital epiphysis; the medial portion of the epiphysis almost is unaffected, while a small lateral fragment demonstrates intermediate signal intensity. The contour of the cartilaginous femoral head is normal, as is the cartilage contour of the acetabulum (arrow).

B, C In a 10 year old child, a coronal T1-weighted (TR/TE, 500/28) spin echo MR image **(B)** reveals low signal intensity of the epiphysis, with a small fragment medially that demonstrates slightly increased signal intensity (small black arrow). Generalized cartilaginous hypertrophy (large black arrow), with a prominence laterally (upper white arrow) and an adjacent defect in the cartilage (arrowhead) is seen. Medially, localized cartilaginous hypertrophy (lower white arrow) surrounded by a synovial recess of lower signal intensity is evident. On an arthrogram **(C),** some of these same structures are indicated.

(From Egund N, et al: Radiology 179:89, 1991.)

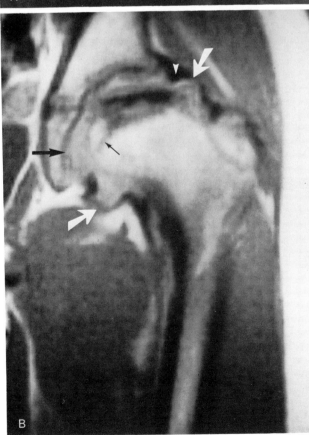

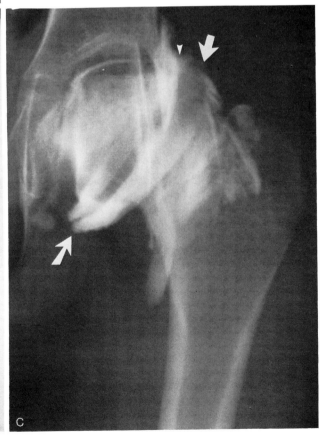

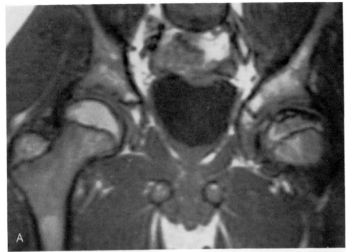

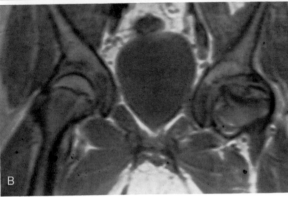

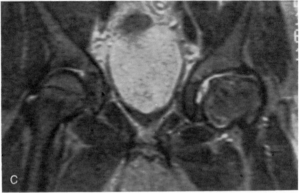

FIGURE 81–14. Legg-Calvé-Perthes disease: MR imaging abnormalities.

A In a 14 year old boy, a coronal T1-weighted (TR/TE, 600/20) spin echo MR image reveals evidence of osteonecrosis of the left femoral head. The ossified portion of the capital epiphysis is flattened and contains superior and lateral regions of abnormal signal intensity. The cartilage surface, of intermediate signal intensity, appears more congruent. The acetabulum is slightly flattened. The opposite hip is normal.

B, C In an 11 year old boy with more extensive involvement of the left hip, coronal portion density (TR/TE, 2000/20) **(B)** and T2-weighted (TR/TE, 2000/70) **(C)** MR images show considerable flattening and irregularity of the femoral head and shallowness of the adjacent acetabulum. A joint effusion is evident. The opposite hip is normal.

and the degree of involvement, if any, of the growth plate, influence the staging of the process and, ultimately, its prognosis.[405]

Etiology and Pathogenesis. It generally is held that vascular insufficiency to the femoral head triggers the radiographic and pathologic findings in Legg-Calvé-Perthes disease, although the factors leading to deficiency of blood supply have not been identified precisely. Trueta's investigations of blood supply to the femoral head during growth identified a vulnerable period between the ages of 4 and 8 years in which the retinacular arteries represented the only important vascular route to the epiphysis, whereas a double vascular supply existed at younger (metaphyseal and retinacular arteries) and older (foveal and retinacular arteries) ages.[49] In adolescence and adulthood, three groups of vessels supply the proximal femur (foveal, retinacular, and metaphyseal arteries). This analysis is interesting, but it does not account for those cases in which infants are affected, nor for the predilection of the disease for boys. Trueta did suggest that a more abundant foveal vascular supply in blacks might explain the relative infrequency of Legg-Calvé-Perthes disease in black persons.

Caffey[15] favored a traumatic cause in which direct compression of the femoral head by the adjacent acetabular roof led to the characteristic radiographic features of the disease, including fracture, flattening, and sclerosis. He emphasized the general retardation of bone development that can be identified in patients with this disease, a finding that has been confirmed by other investigators,[50–52, 199, 275, 371, 409, 410] and suggested that concomitantly retarded supporting connective tissues about the hip might not be able to provide adequate support for the normal heavy stresses in this location. Primary traumatic events producing osseous collapse or traumatic synovitis could lead to compression of adjacent vasculature and secondary osteonecrosis of the femoral head. In addition to arterial insufficiency, disturbed patterns of venous drainage have been identified.[57]

There is experimental evidence suggesting that more than one episode of ischemia and infarction is required for the development of osteonecrosis of the proximal capital femoral epiphysis.[54, 55] Pathologic data in humans underscore the importance of multiple infarctions.[31, 32, 56] The requirement of repeated vascular insults in the production of the disease could explain the chronicity of the disorder, the occurrence of recurrent clinical and radiographic findings, and the eventual appearance of significant growth disturbance.

The role of synovitis and raised intra-articular pressure in the pathogenesis of Legg-Calvé-Perthes disease also has been emphasized. Kemp[58] produced changes in the femoral heads of puppies that simulated those in osteonecrosis by artificially raising the intracapsular pressure for various lengths of time. Other investigators[277, 278, 413] have shown that experimental elevation of intra-articular pressure reduces the blood flow to the femoral head. A synovial effusion of the hip in children with transient synovitis or Legg-Calvé-Perthes disease is associated with such an elevation of intra-articular pressure, particularly with the hip in a position of extension and medial rotation.[414] Legg-Calvé-Perthes disease has been identified in as many as 12 per cent of patients with transient synovitis of the hip.[53] A history of synovitis or the presence of thickening and scle-

rosis of the capsular and synovial tissues on pathologic examination in children with this disease could indicate that the obliteration of blood supply to the femoral head is caused by vascular compression from accumulation of intra-articular fluid.[280] Alternatively, such fluid may represent the initiating event in a chain of events leading to venous obstruction.[279] Abnormal venous patterns, including obstruction of venous outflow from the femoral head, have been demonstrated in Legg-Calvé-Perthes disease[214, 276] and may be associated with an increase in intraosseous pressure in the femoral neck.[279, 281]

Finally, the delayed skeletal maturation of children with this disease and the reported higher frequency of congenital anomalies in extraskeletal sites have suggested to some investigators that genetic and developmental factors may be important.[275, 349] The possibility must be considered that congenital alterations in the blood vessels supplying the femoral capital epiphysis or in the normal development of the acetabulum and femur may lead to vascular or mechanical factors that predispose the child to subsequent osseous collapse; or that Legg-Calvé-Perthes disease is a localized expression of a generalized, transient disorder of epiphyseal cartilage that is responsible for the delay in skeletal maturation.[282] It is obvious that further experimental and clinical data need to be collected before the true cause and pathogenesis of this disease can be identified.[217]

Differential Diagnosis. Fragmentation and collapse of the femoral head (Table 81–3) can be seen in hypothyroidism and in osteonecrosis from other causes (sickle cell anemia, Gaucher's disease, corticosteroid medication). The appearance of femoral head necrosis in a black patient should lead to hemoglobin analysis before the changes are ascribed to Legg-Calvé-Perthes disease. Similarly, bilateral symmetric alterations should be interpreted cautiously, as they are uncommon in the latter disease but may be evident in hypothyroidism, sickle cell anemia, Gaucher's disease, and multiple epiphyseal and spondyloepiphyseal dysplasias.[253, 416]

Meyer's dysplasia of the femoral head (dysplasia epiphysealis capitis femoris)[59] is characterized by retarded skeletal maturation, mild or absent clinical signs, and femoral bony nuclei that appear late and are small and granular. The abnormal femoral head epiphyses usually are apparent by the age of 2 years and gradually are transformed over the ensuing 2 to 4 years by growth and coalescence into enlarging, normal-appearing ossification centers. Sclerosis and metaphyseal changes are not evident in Meyer's dysplasia,

and bilaterality is seen in almost 50 per cent of cases.[415] Residua are unusual, although slight or moderate coxa plana occasionally is recognized. The earlier age of onset, the bilateral nature of the changes, the absence of prominent radiographic abnormalities, and the lack of progression are features that allow differentiation of Meyer's dysplasia from Legg-Calvé-Perthes disease.

A notchlike defect at the vertex of the proximal femoral ossification center has been described as a normal variant in children.[417] Although it may be misinterpreted as evidence of Legg-Calvé-Perthes disease, its location and sharply defined contour allow accurate diagnosis.

Freiberg's Infraction

In 1914, Freiberg[60] described a series of patients with metatarsalgia in whom the metatarsal head appeared to be crushed or collapsed, terming the condition an infraction of bone. Despite the attention that an additional early investigator, Köhler, paid to this condition, Freiberg usually is credited with the first analysis. Both of these men emphasized the typical involvement of the head of the second metatarsal, although it now is recognized that the third and fourth metatarsal heads also can be affected and, in rare instances, perhaps the first metatarsal head as well (see Chapter 39).[1, 61–66, 418] Unilateral changes are characteristic, although bilateral involvement and alterations of more than one digit can be encountered (Fig. 81–15).

Women predominate among patients affected with this disease, the ratio of women to men being approximately 3 or 4 to 1. The disease usually is seen in adolescents between the ages of 13 and 18 years; rare examples of younger or older patients can be uncovered in a review of available literature, and even adults in the fourth to sixth decades of life occasionally first manifest evidence of Freiberg's infraction. Clinical features consist of local pain, tenderness, and swelling and limitation of motion of the corresponding metatarsophalangeal joint. Disabling symptoms and signs can be evident and may require surgical intervention.

Roentgenographic abnormalities include, initially, subtle flattening, increased radiodensity, and cystic lucent lesions of the metatarsal head and widening of the metatarsophalangeal articulation (Fig. 81–16); and, subsequently, an osteochondral fragment with progressive flattening and sclerosis of the metatarsal head and periostitis with increased cortical thickening of the adjacent metaphysis and diaphysis of the bone (Fig. 81–17). Premature closure of the growth plate,[283] intra-articular osseous bodies, deformity and enlargement of the metatarsal head, and secondary degenerative joint disease are recognized complications of the process (Fig. 81–18). The nearby phalangeal base may enlarge and appear irregular. Increased accumulation of bone-seeking radiopharmaceutical agents is evident in the abnormal sites (Fig. 81–19), and MR imaging reveals abnormalities in osseous contour and alterations of signal intensity in the bone marrow (Fig. 81–20).

Pathologic aberrations have been well summarized.[1] Microscopic evidence of necrosis of trabeculae and marrow can be seen at a stage in which the radiographs are entirely normal. Comminution of subchondral trabeculae can be associated with collapse and compression of the articular surface. Revascularization occurs through vascular invasion from the periosteum and metaphyseal regions. Resorption

TABLE 81–3. Some Causes of Femoral Head Irregularity and Collapse in Infants and Children

Disease	Distribution
Legg-Calvé-Perthes disease	Unilateral or bilateral
Meyer's dysplasia	Unilateral or bilateral
Hypothyroidism	Bilateral
Epiphyseal dysplasia	Bilateral
Spondyloepiphyseal dysplasia	Bilateral
Sickle cell anemia	Unilateral or bilateral
Gaucher's disease	Unilateral or bilateral
Infection	Unilateral
Eosinophilic granuloma	Unilateral
Hemophilia	Unilateral or bilateral

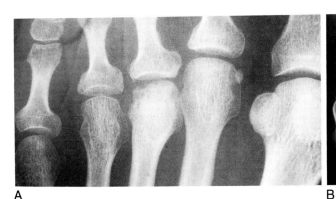 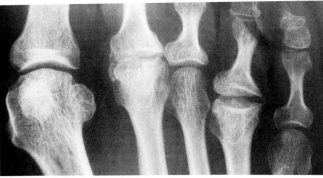

A   B

FIGURE 81–15. Freiberg's infraction: Bilateral involvement. This 48 year old woman complained of pain and tenderness about several metatarsal heads in both feet.

A Note the sclerosis and collapse of the third metatarsal head, with narrowing of the adjacent metatarsophalangeal joint. There is equivocal increased density of the second metatarsal head as well. Adjacent phalangeal new bone formation is seen.

B In the opposite foot, the heads of the second and fourth metatarsal bones are fragmented and flattened. Note the expansion of the corresponding phalangeal bases.

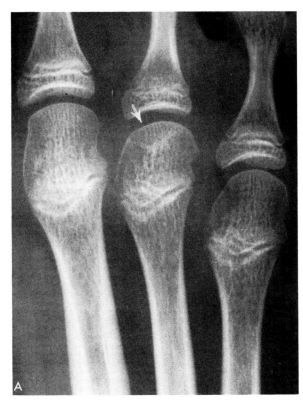 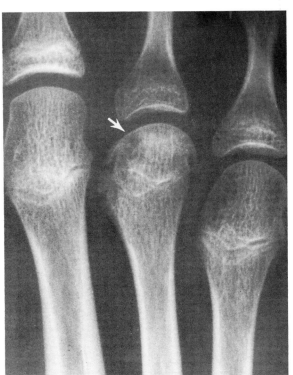

A   B

FIGURE 81–16. Freiberg's infraction: Early radiographic abnormalities. A 14 year old girl developed pain and swelling over the metatarsophalangeal joint. She denied a history of trauma.

A An initial radiograph reveals minimal increased radiodensity of the head of the third metatarsal bone (arrow).

B Approximately four months later, considerable collapse with shortening of the metatarsal bone is evident (arrow).

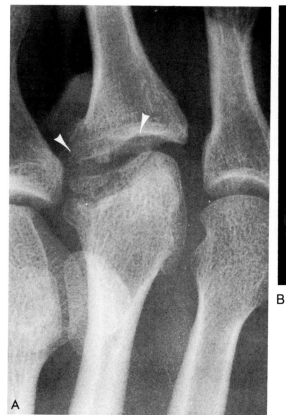

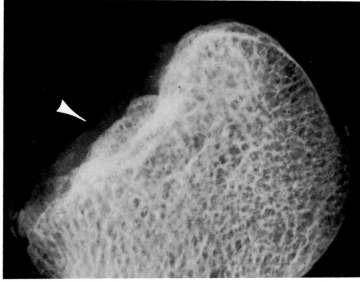

FIGURE 81–17. Freiberg's infraction: Later radiographic abnormalities. This 36 year old man had had pain in his second toe for 12 years. A loose body had been removed from the second metatarsophalangeal joint 2 years prior to his current evaluation.

　A Note the flattened metatarsal head with two osteochondral fragments (arrowheads), osteophytosis, joint space narrowing, and widening of the phalangeal base.

　B A radiograph of a section of the metatarsal head delineates the collapse and irregularity of the bone (arrowhead).

of necrotic trabeculae, osseous regeneration, highly vascular intertrabecular marrow, and cortical thickening related to subperiosteal bony apposition are observed. Complete healing usually is not seen, and even after many years, evidence of previous osteonecrosis exists. Other long-term effects can include osteocartilaginous fragments that remain in situ or are displaced, secondary degenerative joint disease, and proliferative alterations of the base of the neighboring phalanx.

The pathogenesis of the disease process remains speculative. Prevailing opinion suggests that single or multiple episodes of trauma represent the primary event in Freiberg's infraction.[62] Experimental studies have indicated that the epiphysis of the second metatarsal bone is most vulnerable to injury owing to its relative length and firm fixation.[64] The high rate of occurrence of the disorder in women conceivably could be related to the wearing of high-heeled shoes, which creates increased stress on the second metatarsal bone. Repeated injury at this site then may lead to disruption of the articular cartilage, ischemic necrosis of subchondral bone, compression fracture, collapse, and fragmentation.[200]

The radiographic features of Freiberg's infraction are virtually pathognomonic, as they indicate osteonecrosis at a characteristic site, the metatarsal head. Occasionally other disorders, such as systemic lupus erythematosus, can produce bone necrosis at this location. Additional diseases leading to fragmentation of metatarsal heads with articular abnormality include rheumatoid arthritis, calcium pyrophosphate dihydrate crystal deposition disease, diabetes mellitus, and gout, but other radiographic features allow accurate diagnosis. Stress injuries of the matatarsal heads, especially in runners, can produce an appearance simulating that of Freiberg's infraction. Several types of multiple epiphyseal dysplasia may lead to irregularities of ossification of the epiphyses of the metatarsal bones, although other skeletal sites allow accurate radiographic diagnosis. In some persons, a mild degree of normal flattening of the articular surface of the metatarsal head, especially the second, in association with apparent widening of the joint space, can resemble Freiberg's infraction.[419]

Kienböck's Disease

A peculiar affliction of the carpal lunate was described by Peste in 1843[67] and by Kienböck in 1910.[68] Because of the detailed description of the clinical and radiologic features of the disorder offered by the latter investigator, the designation of Kienböck's disease is used most frequently for this condition, although the term lunatomalacia also is encountered.[69–76] Kienböck's disease most commonly is observed in patients between the ages of 20 and 40 years (although it has been identified in children[420] and elderly persons[421]) and has a predilection for the right hand in persons engaged in manual labor; this latter characteristic may indicate that exaggerated use of the dominant hand produces the trauma necessary for the initiation of this condition (see discussion later in this chapter). Bilateral abnormalities occur but are less frequent than unilateral changes.[77, 284, 285]

A history of trauma may be elicited, but this is not a constant feature. Progressive pain, swelling, and disability can be apparent. Radiographic changes are distinctive, although their extent does not appear to correlate closely with the clinical findings.[422] Initially, the lunate may have a normal architecture and density, but a linear or compression

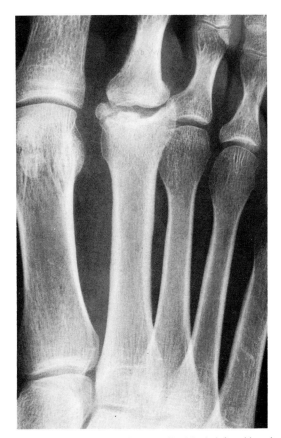

FIGURE 81-18. Freiberg's infraction: Residual deformities. In this 41 year old man, note residual flattening of the second metatarsal head, narrowing of the adjacent joint space, intra-articular osseous bodies, expansion of the phalangeal base, and widening of the second metatarsal with cortical thickening.

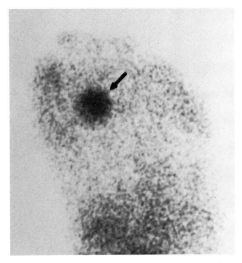

FIGURE 81-19. Freiberg's infraction: Radionuclide abnormalities. Observe the abnormal accumulation (arrow) of the bone seeking radionuclide in the head of the second metatarsal bone. (Courtesy of V. Vint, M.D., San Diego, California.)

fracture can be delineated, especially on tomograms.[69, 78, 79, 201, 356] Subsequently, an increased density of the lunate bone relative to the other carpal bones is noted, followed by evidence of altered shape and diminished size of the bone (Fig. 81–21). Eventually the entire lunate may collapse and

fragment; the degree of fragmentation, particularly that of the posterior surface, can be well shown on lateral tomograms.[72] Complications include disruption of the carpal architecture, scapholunate separation or dissociation, ulnar deviation of the triquetrum, and secondary degenerative joint disease in the radiocarpal and midcarpal compartments of the wrist with articular space narrowing, sclerosis, osteophytosis, and cyst formation.[286, 423] Tendon ruptures, owing to their erosion by the irregular and collapsed lunate, have been reported.[287, 357]

Pathologic descriptions emphasize the occurrence of both fracture and osteonecrosis.[1] An incomplete fracture line can be evident in the subchondral spongiosa of the proximal portion of the lunate associated with osteoclastic resorption, trabecular disintegration and granular detritus, and scar tissue in the intertrabecular marrow. Additional fractures appear, some of which violate the articular cartilage, and necrosis of adjacent trabeculae can be observed. Repair and

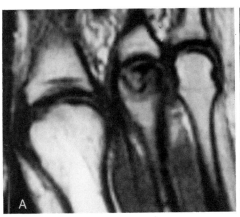
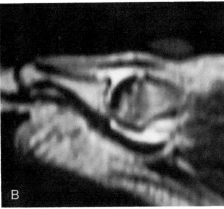

FIGURE 81-20. Freiberg's infraction: MR imaging abnormalities. A 14 year old girl had pain and tenderness about the second metatarsophalangeal joint of the left foot.

A On this T1-weighted (TR/TE, 600/20) spin echo MR image obtained in the plantar plane, abnormal signal intensity in the head of the second metatarsal bone is observed. A serpentine region of low signal intensity outlines the area of necrosis, which contains tissue of signal intensity identical to that of marrow fat. Surrounding bone marrow edema is characterized by intermediate signal intensity, and an effusion has led to distention of the joint capsule.

B A sagittal T2-weighted (TR/TE, 2000/80) spin echo MR image again shows the marrow abnormalities, flat metatarsal head, and joint effusion.

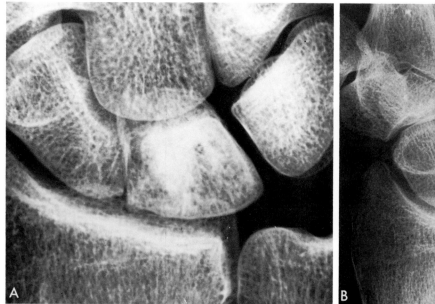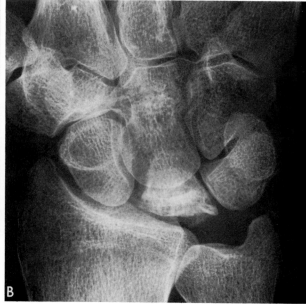

FIGURE 81–21. Kienböck's disease.
A A magnification radiograph demonstrates patchy increased density of the lunate without alterations in the shape of the bone.
B In a different patient, observe the collapse of a sclerotic lunate bone. The ulna is shortened (ulna minus variant).

regeneration are characterized by vascular proliferation and deposition of new bone. Secondary degenerative joint disease is manifested as fibrillation and erosion of cartilage.

The cause and pathogenesis of the condition are not clear. Its occurrence following single or repeated episodes of trauma is a prominent feature in many cases. Certain anatomic and biomechanical features of the lunate may predispose this bone to injury and subsequent osteonecrosis.[1] These features include (1) a vulnerable blood supply arising from vessels that enter the bone on its dorsal or volar aspect, anastomosing within its substance[80, 86, 202] (Fig. 81–22), and (2) a fixed position in the wrist, resulting in substantial forces of various degrees that may be greater than those on neighboring carpal bones.[81] Mechanical forces may be accentuated by the presence of a short ulna (ulnar minus or negative ulnar variance), a finding that can be encountered in as many as 75 per cent of cases.[82–84, 424–426] Clinical, anatomic, and experimental studies have documented that a short ulna is associated with morphologic changes in adjacent structures (such as an increased thickness of the triangular fibrocartilage),[289] that ulnar length influences the manner in which stresses are transmitted across the wrist,[290] and that a short ulna may indicate a propensity to develop carpal ligamentous disruptions.[291] A number of radiographic techniques exist for measurement of ulnar variance,[428] which have been well summarized by Mann and associates.[429] These investigators favor the use of a posteroanterior radiograph of the wrist obtained in a neutral position (with the shoulder abducted 90 degrees, the elbow flexed 90 degrees, and the wrist positioned without ulnar or radial deviation and without palmar flexion or dorsiflexion) and the identification of the long axis of the radius. The ulnarmost point of the articular surface of the radius is found, and a line is drawn perpendicular to the long axis of the radius through this point. Ulnar variance is the distance between this last line and the distalmost point of the dome of the ulna. If the ulna lies proximal to the

radius, an ulnar minus or negative ulnar variance exists. This anatomic arrangement, which might be expected to produce exaggerated contact between the lunate and radius, is not uniformly considered an important finding in patients with Kienböck's disease[85, 288, 427]; furthermore, as Kienböck's disease is rare and ulnar minus variance is not infrequent, other factors must be important in the pathogenesis of the disease.[372]

Many methods, including ulnar lengthening procedures[292, 430] or radial shortening procedures,[430, 431] or both,[356]

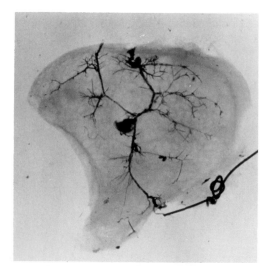

FIGURE 81–22. Lunate bone: Vascular supply.
A lateral view of a preparation of a lunate bone following vascular injection with latex reveals two dorsal vessels and one volar vessel that are anastomosing within the bone. In some cases, two vessels enter the volar aspect of the bone and one vessel enters the dorsal aspect. In either case, a Y pattern of vascularity within the bone is seen, as anastomoses occur in the midportion of the lunate just distal to its center.

(From Gelberman RH, Menon J: J Hand Surg 5:272, 1980.)

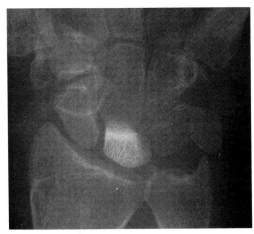

FIGURE 81–23. Osteonecrosis of the lunate. This patient revealed multiple fractures of the distal radius and ulna with lunate dislocation following an injury. A radiograph obtained several months later reveals osteoporosis of the distal radius and distal ulna and carpus, with increased radiodensity of the lunate. This indicates that the injury has disrupted the normal blood supply to the lunate. (Courtesy of V. Vint, M.D., La Jolla, California.)

and lunate replacement,[293, 432] have been used for the treatment of Kienböck's disease. The success of some of them is influenced positively by early diagnosis prior to collapse of bone. In this regard, immobilization in equivocal cases may lead to osteoporosis of normal carpal bones, producing exaggerated radiodensity of an avascular lunate (related to either Kienböck's disease or acute trauma) and allowing accurate diagnosis[69] (Fig. 81–23). Furthermore, MR imaging and scintigraphy may be indicated in some instances.

The role of MR imaging in the analysis of Kienböck's disease is not yet well defined, although preliminary reports have been encouraging in this regard.[373, 433–436] Two patterns of abnormality have been defined, both characterized by loss of signal intensity on T1-weighted spin echo images: focal loss of signal intensity involving the radial half of the lunate; and diffuse loss of signal intensity involving the entire lunate (Fig. 81–24).[434] Whether the first of these patterns is indicative of earlier disease and whether other patterns of distribution of signal loss in the lunate may be encountered in Kienböck's disease are not clear. What is certain is that regions of change of signal intensity in the lunate correspond to sites of osteonecrosis[435, 436] and that MR imaging is more sensitive than radiography and, possibly, bone scintigraphy in the detection of Kienböck's disease.[435] Equally important, MR imaging appears to represent an effective method for eliminating this diagnosis in some patients with wrist symptomatology and, in such cases, may provide evidence of an alternative disease process. Falsely negative MR imaging results in patients with Kienböck's disease have been observed[436] but appear to be infrequent. Indeed, the sensitivity of MR imaging in instances of osteonecrosis in other sites is well established (see Chapter 80). In the wrist, coronal MR images appear to be most beneficial but should be supplemented with sagittal or transaxial images, or both, in some cases. The precise signal characteristics of Kienböck's disease on T2-weighted spin echo and gradient echo images, in common with osteonecrosis in other locations, are variable (Fig. 81–24). Morphologic evidence of this disease, including fracture, collapse, and fragmentation of the lunate, can be delineated with MR imaging in a manner similar to that provided by other tomographic methods, including conventional and computed tomography. In common with abnormalities seen with other imaging methods, MR imaging findings can be used to classify the pattern and extent of involvement of the lunate bone.

With regard to the differential diagnosis of the plain film abnormalities, in cases in which increased radiodensity and collapse of the lunate are observed, the radiographic features easily are differentiated from other conditions affecting the wrist. Osteonecrosis of the lunate may occur, however, in association with complex injuries of the wrist, including lunate dislocations, and, rarely, with corticosteroid therapy.[437]

Köhler's Disease

The relationship of Köhler's disease of the tarsal navicular and osteonecrosis is not defined. Although some investigators regard the condition as a manifestation of normal

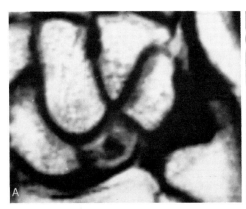
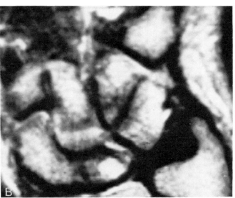

FIGURE 81–24. Kienböck's disease: MR imaging abnormalities.
 A The coronal T1-weighted (TR/TE, 600/20) spin echo MR image demonstrates a central region of low signal intensity in the lunate, and the remaining marrow in this bone is inhomogeneous in signal intensity.
 B With T2 weighting (TR/TE, 1700/80), the central region now demonstrates hyperintensity, and the remaining marrow in the lunate shows regions of high and low signal intensity. The findings are consistent with osteonecrosis, although alternative diagnoses, such as an intraosseous ganglion, could be considered.

or altered ossification, this disorder is discussed here because the predominant theory of its pathogenesis still is one of vascular insufficiency. The disease first was described in 1908 by Köhler[87] as a self-limited condition of the tarsal navicular characterized by flattening, sclerosis, and irregular rarefaction. Köhler's disease is relatively rare, although its exact frequency is difficult to determine because the symptoms and signs may not be of sufficient magnitude to require radiography, and it is impossible to distinguish the radiographic abnormalities from those that occur as a normal variation of growth.

The disorder is more frequent in boys, the ratio of affected boys to affected girls being approximately between 4 and 6 to 1. Complaints most commonly are observed between the ages of 3 and 7 years, occurring at a younger age in girls.[294] Unilateral involvement is evident in approximately 75 to 80 per cent of cases. Clinical manifestations may be quite mild, consisting of local pain, tenderness, swelling, and decreased range of motion.[88–90] The foot may be held in slight varus position so that the patient walks on the outer side of the foot.[1] A history of trauma can be elicited in about 35 per cent of cases. Köhler's disease may occur simultaneously with Legg-Calvé-Perthes disease.[91]

Roentgenograms at an early stage can reveal patchy increase in density, nodularity, and fragmentation with multiple ossific nuclei (Fig. 81–25A, B). Soft tissue swelling may be evident.[203] The bone may be diminished in size and flattened or wafer-like in appearance, yet the interosseous space between the navicular and neighboring bones can be normal, indicating an integrity of the chondral surface (Fig. 81–25C, D). Over a period of 2 to 4 years the bone may regain its normal size, density, and trabecular structure. It is the self-limited and reversible nature of the process that has led to speculation that the "disease," in reality, is an altered sequence of tarsal ossification. Differences in the time of appearance, the degree of maturity, and the size, shape, and radiodensity of the ossifying navicular bone are common in many children, and even in cases of apparent unilateral disease the changes in the asymptomatic extremity may be remarkably similar to those on the symptomatic side. This apparent overlap with normal patterns of ossification leads to considerable difficulty in diagnosis, and two criteria must be used in establishing the presence of Köhler's disease: (1) changes are detected in a previously normal navicular bone; (2) alterations consisting of resorption and reossification must be compatible with those of osteonecrosis.[92] Furthermore, clinical manifestations should be present if the diagnosis is to be considered seriously.[294] Radionuclide examination can further substantiate the diagnosis by revealing diminished uptake of bone-seeking radiopharmaceutical agents during the early stages of the process and accentuated uptake during revascularization.[90]

Pathologic data are meager.[1] A disturbance in endochondral ossification is suggested by the presence of a thickened zone of cartilage about the ossific nucleus.[93, 94] The latter structure may reveal signs of necrosis of both spongiosa and marrow.

There is evidence that Köhler's disease may have a mechanical basis. The location of the tarsal navicular at the apex of the longitudinal arch of the foot may lead to concentration of forces on this bone during normal locomotion. The forces may be concentrated further by the existence of a small space between the distal end of the talus and the first cuneiform, with resulting crowding of the navicular bone.[95] Compression of the bony nucleus at a critical phase of growth could result in altered ossification.[88] Compression forces may occlude vessels in the spongiosa of the bone, producing osteonecrosis.

The only major differential diagnostic consideration in this disease is that of a normal pattern of ossification of the navicular bone in some patients that may result in a fragmented and sclerotic appearance. Differentiation of the normal and abnormal states was discussed previously. Spontaneous or posttraumatic osteonecrosis of the tarsal navicular bone, occurring in adults, is unrelated to Köhler's disease (see Chapter 80).

Panner's Disease

Panner's disease, or osteochondrosis of the capitulum of the humerus, is a rare disease described in 1927 by Panner,[96] who was impressed by its resemblance to Legg-Calvé-Perthes disease. Further descriptions of this disorder have documented that it usually appears between the ages of 5 and 10 years, although it may be seen as early as 4 years and as late as 16 years.[97–102] Boys are affected almost exclusively, and the condition commonly is linked to a history of trauma. It sometimes is termed "little-leaguer's elbow" because of its frequency in young baseball pitchers.[103] Panner's disease also is noted in other athletes, such as gymnasts.[295] Bilateral involvement is rare.

The clinical manifestations typically are mild, and complete recovery is frequent. Pain and stiffness, with restricted range of motion of the elbow (particularly extension), are seen. Local tenderness over the capitulum, synovial thickening and effusion, and flexion contracture can be detected on physical examination. Radiographs reveal fissuring and increased density of the capitulum, decreased size and condensation of bone with increase in the radiohumeral space, fragmentation, and resorption (Fig. 81–26A). These findings usually are more evident if comparison radiographs of the contralateral, uninvolved side are obtained. Regeneration and reconstitution of the capitulum subsequently are observed, and in most cases no residual deformity or disability is seen. Hyperemia can lead to abnormal skeletal maturation of the radial head. The various stages of the process also can be identified with MR imaging (Fig. 81–27).

The detection of a subchondral radiolucent band in the capitulum in the early stages of the disorder is reminiscent of findings in Legg-Calvé-Perthes disease.[104] This abnormality apparently relates to a fracture that in some cases is accompanied by accumulation of gas in the fissure. It probably indicates that osteonecrosis has occurred as a secondary event related to a traumatic insult, with disruption of blood supply to the bone. As indicated by Singer and Roy,[295] Panner's disease occurs at an age when the capitular nucleus is supplied by only one or two discrete and independent vessels whose point of entrance is the posterior surface of the chondroepiphysis. Their location is vulnerable to lateral compression injuries resulting from repetitive valgus stresses. The disease is differentiated from osteochondritis dissecans of the elbow (see Chapter 67) principally on the basis of the age of the patient. Osteochondritis dissecans typically occurs in adolescents or adults at a time

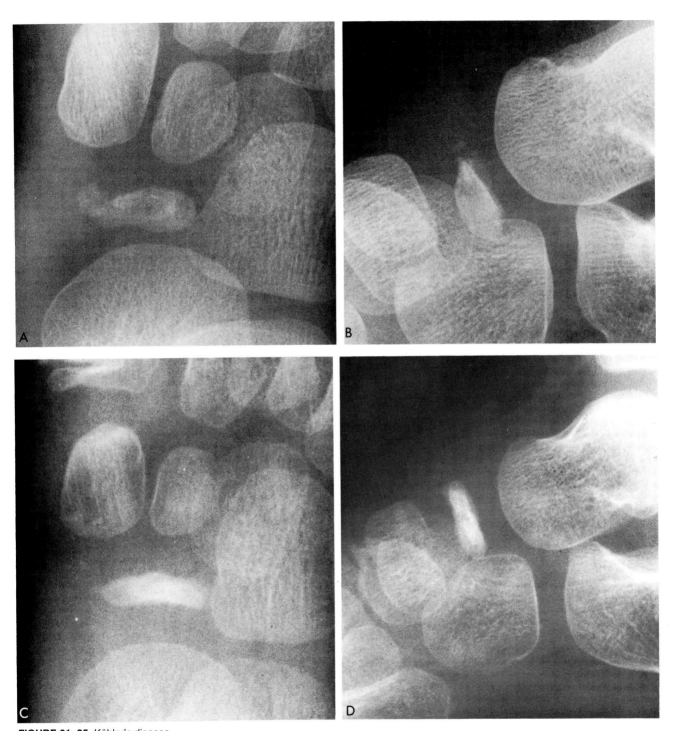

FIGURE 81–25. Köhler's disease.

A, B In this 7 year old boy, anteroposterior and lateral radiographs reveal the small fragmented and slightly dense tarsal navicular bone. The interosseous spaces of the tarsus are not disturbed.

C, D In a 4 year old boy, a wafer-like radiodense tarsal navicular bone is identified. Again, the neighboring joint spaces are not diminished in width.

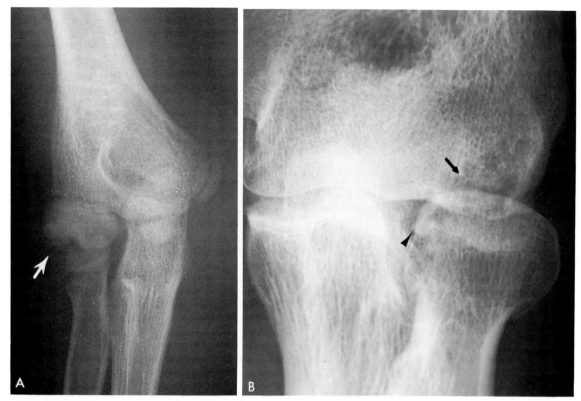

FIGURE 81–26. Panner's disease and osteochondritis dissecans.

A Panner's disease. Findings include fissuring and fragmentation of the capitulum (arrow) and deformity of the adjacent radial head in this child with elbow pain and swelling. (Courtesy of V. Vint, M.D., La Jolla, California.)

B Osteochondritis dissecans. Included in the differential diagnosis of Panner's disease is osteochondritis dissecans, as illustrated here. Observe the radiolucent lesion of the capitulum (arrow). Osteochondritis dissecans about the elbow is observed in adolescents and adults. Osteochondral fragments are not unusual (arrowhead).

when ossification of the capitulum has been completed (Fig. 81–26B).[438]

Thiemann's Disease

In 1909, Thiemann[105] described a teenaged boy with progressive enlargement of the proximal interphalangeal joints of the fingers. Additional reports of this disease have indicated that its principal clinical manifestations are an onset

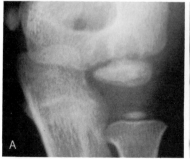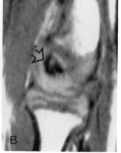

FIGURE 81–27. Panner's disease: MR imaging abnormalities.

A The frontal radiograph shows slight irregularity and increased density of the capitulum.

B A sagittal T1-weighted (TR/TE, 600/20) spin echo MR image demonstrates the abnormal signal intensity (arrow) in the ossified portion of the capitulum. The cartilage about this portion appears normal.

(Courtesy of A. Stauffer, M.D., Mission Viejo, California.)

in the second decade of life, a predilection for boys, painless swelling of proximal interphalangeal articulations, digital shortening, and deformity.[106–109, 296, 297] Involvement of the metacarpophalangeal and tarsometatarsal joints and the interphalangeal articulations of the toes also has been noted in some cases.[358] The disease is familial, probably transmitted as a dominant trait with virtually complete penetrance, although sporadic involvement is reported. A relationship to trauma also has been suggested. Although not fully delineated, the pathogenesis of the disease appears to be an osteonecrosis. In Dessecker's description the histologic features of an involved epiphysis of a proximal interphalangeal joint were characteristic of necrosis, with normal vessels and absent inflammation.[106]

Radiographs reveal irregularity of the epiphyses of the phalanges, especially in the middle fingers. The epiphyses appear sclerotic and fragmented, and may contain medial and lateral osseous excrescences[110] (Figs. 81–28 and 81–29). Eventually, the joint space becomes narrowed, the base of the phalanx thickens, and phalangeal shortening is seen (Fig. 81–30). In some cases, radiographic improvement is seen because of resorption of bone fragments.[296]

Additional alterations that may accompany Thiemann's disease are Legg-Calvé-Perthes disease, bipartite patella, pterygium colli, thyroid enlargement, and diabetes mellitus, but a definite association of this interesting disorder with any of these latter conditions has not been verified.[109]

The differential diagnosis of the phalangeal alterations of Thiemann's disease includes trauma, infection, thermal in-

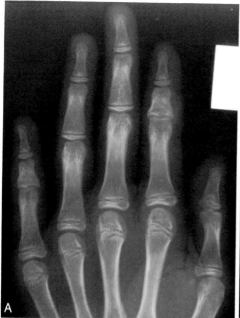
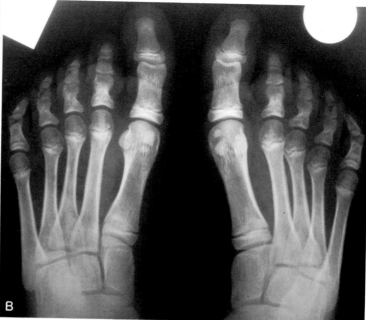

FIGURE 81–28. Thiemann's disease. A 12 year old girl developed pain in the second fingers in both hands at the age of 8 years. Subsequently her fifth fingers were affected and her parents noted that both her hands and her feet had short digits. On physical examination bony protuberances were observed bilaterally at the proximal interphalangeal articulations of the second and fifth fingers.

A A radiograph of the patient's hand shows physeal closure and shortened middle phalanges in the second and fifth fingers. The opposite side was affected similarly.

B A radiograph of the feet reveals short proximal phalanges and premature closure of the physes.

(From Gewanter H, Baum J: J Rheumatol *12*:150, 1985.)

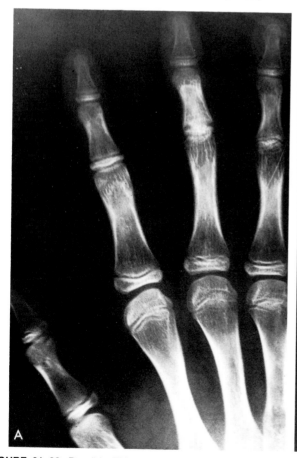
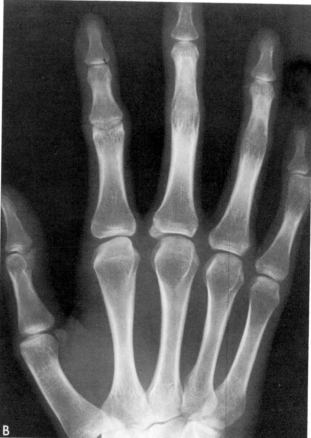

FIGURE 81–29. Possible Thiemann's disease. This 10 year old girl developed pain and swelling of the proximal interphalangeal and metacarpophalangeal joints of the hands. Several family members had had similar abnormalities. Although the diagnosis is not proved and some features are atypical, Thiemann's disease is a prime consideration; juvenile chronic arthritis is another diagnostic possibility, as is familial coalition of joints (Shrewsbury mark).

A Note flattening and increased sclerosis of epiphyses of several metacarpal bones and phalanges, with expansion of the adjacent bony contour. Early fusion of the third and fourth proximal interphalangeal joints can be seen.

B Six years later, bony ankylosis of several proximal interphalangeal joints is observed. The metacarpal heads are irregular.

(Courtesy of L. Goldberger, M.D., La Jolla, California.)

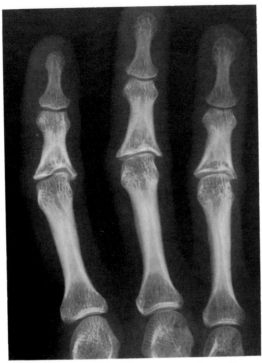

FIGURE 81–30. Thiemann's disease. Residual deformities are seen in this adult. These include shortening of the middle phalanges, broadening of the bases of these phalanges, and narrowing of the interphalangeal joints. The opposite hand was involved similarly. (Courtesy of B. Howard, M.D., Charlotte, North Carolina.)

jury, such as frostbite or burns, juvenile chronic arthritis, other disorders associated with ischemic necrosis of bone, and additional congenital diseases such as acrodysostosis.[359, 439, 440]

DISORDERS RELATED TO TRAUMA OR ABNORMAL STRESS WITHOUT EVIDENCE OF OSTEONECROSIS

Osgood-Schlatter Disease

In 1903, Osgood of Boston[111] and Schlatter of Zurich[112] each described a disorder of the developing tibial tuberosity that they considered to represent a manifestation of trauma. This interpretation was accurate, but some subsequent reports incorrectly emphasized the occurrence of "apophysitis" or osteonecrosis in the pathogenesis of this condition.

Osgood-Schlatter disease occurs in adolescents, usually between the ages of 11 and 15 years, with a younger age of onset in girls than in boys. Boys are affected more frequently than girls, and a history of participation in sports (particularly those that involve kicking, jumping, and squatting[350]) and a rapid growth spurt prior to the onset of symptoms and signs is typical. Although the disease generally is unilateral in distribution, bilateral alterations are detected in approximately 25 per cent of cases.

Clinically, patients usually have local pain and tenderness of variable severity.[1, 113, 114] The pain may be aggravated during activity and ameliorated with rest. Soft tissue swelling and firm masses can be palpated in the involved region, and there is no synovial effusion in the knee.

Although radiographic abnormalities are well known in Osgood-Schlatter disease,[115, 116] technical difficulties may

prevent adequate visualization of the region in some cases. Lateral films should not be overpenetrated, as subtle soft tissue alterations may be missed.[116, 117] In this regard, low kV and xeroradiography may be helpful. Furthermore, as the tibial tuberosity lies slightly lateral to the midline, a lateral projection with the knee in slight internal rotation should be used.[92] Two radiographs obtained in this position, one with bone technique and one with soft tissue technique, should be added to the routine knee radiographs in the evaluation of patients with this disorder.

Interpretation of the radiographs requires knowledge of the normal pattern of ossification of the tibial tuberosity[92, 118, 298] (Fig. 81–31). During initial stages of fetal development, no discrete tuberosity is present and the growth plate of the proximal tibia is oriented transversely. In subsequent stages, an anterior outgrowth occurs from the tibial chondroepiphysis concomitant with fibrovascular ingrowth and vascularization of the chondroepiphysis, and the developing tuberosity is displaced distally by longitudinal growth at the proximal tibial physis. Postnatally, a separate growth plate of the tibial tuberosity develops and coalesces with the primary proximal tibial growth plate. A secondary ossification center develops in the distal portion of the tuberosity and later coalesces with the ossification center of the proximal tibial epiphysis. Finally, closure of the contiguous growth plates of the proximal tibia and tuberosity takes place. On the radiograph, one or more osseous centers in the cartilaginous extension of the tuberosity normally are recognized in girls between the ages of 8 and 12 years and in boys between 9 and 14 years. Thus, the detection of several ossific nodules anterior to the tibial metaphysis must not be misinterpreted as abnormal fragmentation of bone. Also, bony fusion of the tuberosity and tibial metaphysis normally does not occur before the age of 15 years in girls and 17 years in boys.[115]

Radiographic abnormalities in this disease are influenced by the age of the patient. Initially, soft tissue swelling in front of the tuberosity results from edema of the skin and subcutaneous tissue (Fig. 81–32). The margins of the patellar tendon, which attaches to the cartilage of the tibial tuberosity in the child and to the periosteum in the adult, may be indistinct, and increased radiodensity of the infrapatellar fat pad may be identified. If the tuberosity is entirely cartilaginous in structure, no change will be detected in it initially, but examination 3 or 4 weeks later may show single or multiple ossific collections in the avulsed fragment (see discussion later in this chapter)[92] (Fig. 81–33). In the older child in whom the ossification center has begun to develop, one or more foci of radiopacity can be recognized in the vicinity of the tubercle, and the latter protuberance may have surface irregularities marking the sites from which fragments of cartilage and bone have been avulsed.[1] An associated finding is fragmentation of the inferior pole of the patella similar to that occurring in Sinding-Larsen-Johansson disease.[176, 443]

Following the acute stage, soft tissue swelling diminishes, and displaced pieces of bone may increase in size owing to endochondral bone formation and callus formation or may reunite with each other and the underlying tibial tuberosity. Eventually, the radiographic appearance may revert to normal, although persistent ossific fragments frequently mark the site of previous disease (Fig. 81–34). It has been suggested, although not agreed upon uniformly,[486]

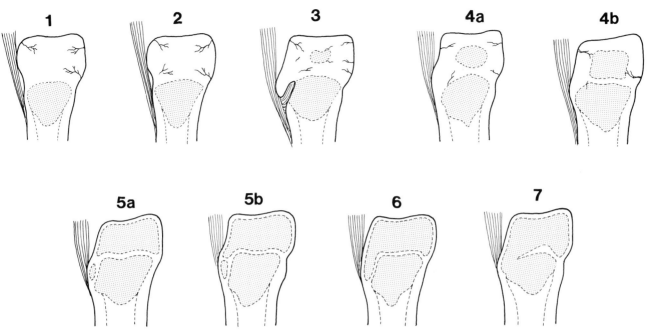

FIGURE 81–31. Tibial tuberosity and proximal tibia: Normal sequence of ossification.

1 Stage 1: Prenatal phase. No tibial tuberosity is present. The growth plate of the proximal tibia is oriented transversely.

2 Stage 2: Prenatal phase. An anterior outgrowth develops from the tibial chondroepiphysis concomitant with fibrovascular ingrowth and vascularization of the chondroepiphysis.

3 Stage 3: Prenatal phase. There is relative distal displacement of the tuberosity by longitudinal growth at the proximal tibial physis, and anatomic separation from the proximal tibial physis takes place by continued fibromesenchymal-vascular ingrowth.

4a, b Stage 4: Postnatal phase. Development of a separate growth plate associated with the tibial tuberosity occurs, and there is subsequent coalescence with the primary proximal tibial growth plate.

5a, b Stage 5: Postnatal phase. A secondary ossification center develops in the distal portion of the tuberosity.

6 Stage 6: Postnatal phase. Coalescence of the ossification center of the tuberosity and the proximal tibial epiphysis occurs.

7 Stage 7: Postnatal phase. Closure of the contiguous growth plates of the proximal tibia and tuberosity takes place.

(After Ogden JA, Southwick WO: Clin Orthop *116*:180, 1976.)

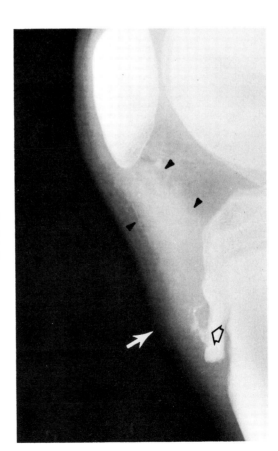

FIGURE 81–32. Osgood-Schlatter disease: Soft tissue abnormalities. Low kV radiography indicates soft tissue edema over the tibial tuberosity (solid arrow). Note indistinctness of the infrapatellar tendon (arrowheads) and osseous irregularity of the tuberosity (open arrow). (Courtesy of J. Weston, M.D., Lower Hutt, New Zealand.)

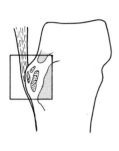
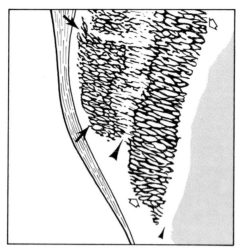
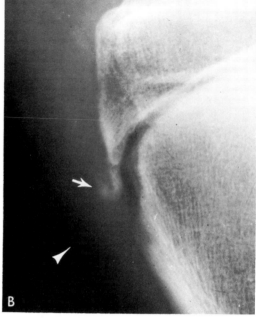

FIGURE 81–33. Osgood-Schlatter disease: Osseous abnormalities.

A A schematic representation of the bony changes in Osgood-Schlatter disease is shown. Inset shows area of bony changes. Avulsion with separation (large arrowhead) of small ossicles (solid arrows) of the developing ossification center of the tibial tuberosity (open arrows) is observed. Note the physis (small arrowhead) and underlying tibia. (After Ogden JA, Southwick WO: Clin Orthop *116*:180, 1976.)

B Observe soft tissue swelling (arrowhead) and an avulsed osseous fragment of the tibial tuberosity (arrow).

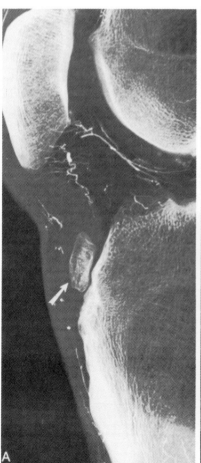
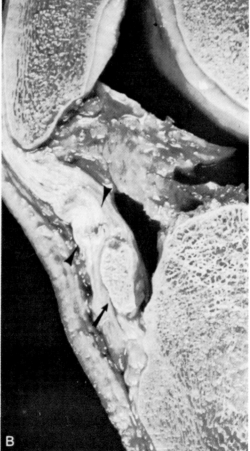

FIGURE 81–34. Osgood-Schlatter disease: Osseous abnormalities. A radiograph **(A)** and photograph **(B)** of a sagittal section of the knee in an adult cadaver show a persistent osseous fragment (arrows) adjacent to the tibial tuberosity consistent with previous Osgood-Schlatter disease. Note the location of the thickened patellar tendon (arrowheads). The opacified vessels on the radiograph relate to an incidental postmortem study.

that the radiographic demonstration of a persistent ossicle at the proximal aspect of the tibial tuberosity may indicate "unresolved" Osgood-Schlatter disease with significant pain and swelling related to bursitis about the mobile ossicle.[204] In addition to a bursa between the ossicle and tibial tuberosity,[441] histologic evaluation may reveal a thin band of scar tissue in these patients with unresolved disease.

Other diagnostic methods that can be used to investigate Osgood-Schlatter disease include ultrasonography[444] and MR imaging (Fig. 81–35).[445] The sonographic picture provides information regarding the development and structure of the ossification center as well as the integrity of the nonossified cartilage and superficial soft tissues. MR imaging reveals evidence of patellar tendinitis, with an abnormally large tendon revealing signal inhomogeneity; and of deep infrapatellar bursitis.

The accurate diagnosis of this condition is based on both the radiographic and the clinical findings. A fragmented tuberosity can occur in other conditions,[119] and, in the absence of current or previous symptoms, may indicate only a normal ossification pattern. Soft tissue swelling is fundamental to the radiographic diagnosis of Osgood-Schlatter disease. In equivocal cases, comparison views of the opposite, uninvolved side may be helpful.

In the past, Osgood-Schlatter disease was considered by some investigators to be an osteonecrosis.[120] More recent studies, however, have indicated that the tibial tuberosity possesses an excellent blood supply[118, 121, 299] and that the pathologic findings in this condition are most consistent with a traumatically induced disruption somewhere along the site of attachment of the patellar tendon to the tibial tuberosity.[1, 122, 123, 298] The appearance of fragmentation of the inferior pole of the patella in some patients with Osgood-Schlatter disease supports the concept of a traumatic insult, as does evidence of patellar tendinitis provided by MR imaging.[445] The mechanical weakness of the patellar tendon-cartilage attachment on the tibial tuberosity favors the occurrence of avulsion of fragments of cartilage and underlying bone.[1] This avulsion can appear at a cartilaginous stage, a chondro-osseous stage, or an osseous stage in the developing ossification center. The normal tuberosity growth plate is not affected because it is well adapted to tensile stress.[118] Thus, premature closure of the physis of the tibial tuberosity with genu recurvatum is rare in this disease.[124, 125, 300] Delayed distal displacement of the developing tuberosity could result in patella alta, whereas excessive displacement could lead to patella baja.[118] Although a relationship between Osgood-Schlatter disease and patella alta has been emphasized in some reports,[351] this has been questioned by other investigators, who cite the difficulty in measuring patellar position accurately in patients with this disease.[204] A small patellar angle created by the junction of two lines, one drawn along the articular surface of the patella and a second from the end of the inferior articular cartilage of the patella to the patellar apex, has been reported in patients with Osgood-Schlatter disease and has been proposed to result in increased tension on the tibial apophysis by the quadriceps muscle.[442]

Reported complications of Osgood-Schlatter disease include nonunion of the bone fragment, patellar subluxation, chondromalacia, avulsion of the patellar tendon,[301] and, as previously noted, genu recurvatum.[124, 125, 300]

Blount's Disease

Blount's disease, tibia vara, or osteochondrosis deformans tibiae is a local disturbance of growth of the medial aspect of the proximal tibial epiphysis, described in 1922 by Erlacher[306] and in 1937 by Blount.[126] The condition generally has been classified into two types, an infantile type in which deformity is noted in the first few years of life, and an adolescent type in which deformity appears in children between the ages of 8 and 15 years (Table 81–4).[448, 483] The infantile type is approximately five to eight times more frequent than the adolescent variety. Recently, the classification of tibia vara has been expanded to include a third type, late onset tibia vara, which typically appears in obese black children between the ages of 6 and 13 years, as well as a fourth condition, focal fibrocartilaginous dysplasia, which leads to abnormalities that may simulate those of classic Blount's disease.[446]

Infantile Tibia Vara. Infantile tibia vara appears to develop when normal physiologic bowing, rather than disappearing progressively to a straight leg or slight valgus position, persists and worsens when the growing child becomes heavier and begins to put weight on the knee joint.[127] In Jamaica, children walk at a relatively early age and have an increased incidence of physiologic bowing, which persists longer than in English children. These two factors apparently contribute to create an unusually high incidence of tibia vara.[128, 130] Other factors leading to increased stress on the medial aspect of the proximal tibia also may be important, as an affinity of this disease with persons of black African stock cannot always be traced to a propensity of affected children to walk at an earlier age.[131] Additional mechanical factors that may contribute to infan-

TABLE 81–4. Infantile Versus Adolescent Tibia Vara

	Infantile	Adolescent
Age of onset	1–3 years	8–15 years
Distribution	Bilateral: 50–75%	Unilateral: 90%
Clinical findings	Obesity	Normal body weight
	Absent pain, tenderness	Pain and tenderness
	Prominent deformity	Mild deformity
	Slight leg shortening	Moderate, severe leg shortening
Etiology or pathogenesis	Trauma	Trauma
	Growth arrest or dysplasia	Growth arrest

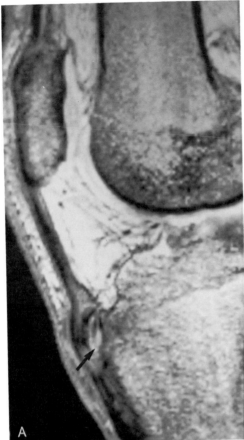

FIGURE 81–35. Osgood-Schlatter disease: MR imaging abnormalities.

A A sagittal gradient echo MR image (fast imaging with steady-state precession [FISP]) (TR/TE, 30/10; flip angle, 40 degrees) in a 21 year old man demonstrates a small ossicle separate from the tibial tuberosity (arrow) and a patellar tendon that is of normal size except for mild thickening distally.

B, C In this 35 year old woman, sagittal T1-weighted (TR/TE, 650/20) **(B)** and T2-weighted (TR/TE, 1800/90) **(C)** spin echo MR images reveal a prominent tibial tuberosity, deep infrapatellar bursitis (arrows), and anterior displacement of the patellar tendon. A large separate ossicle (arrowhead) is seen.

(B, C, Courtesy of H.S. Kang, M.D., Seoul, Korea.)

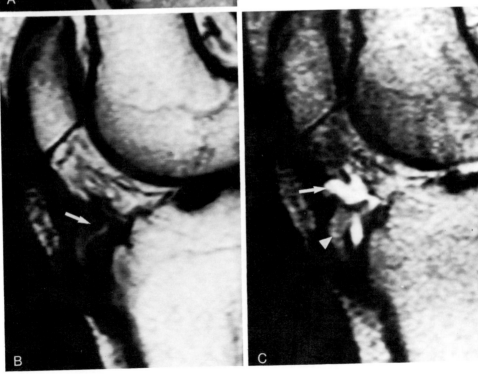

tile tibia vara include excessive body weight, peculiarities in the manner in which children are carried on their mothers' backs, and abnormal articular laxity, but these factors, although possibly important, are not present consistently.[131] Sibert and Bray[132] stressed an autosomal dominant pattern of inheritance with variable penetrance in this condition, and it is possible that infantile tibia vara results from specific environmental agents acting on a genetically predisposed child. The occurrence of this condition in identical twins supports the importance of genetic factors.[447]

Altered mechanical forces in the proximal tibia from various primary causes could increase the mobility of the tibia on the femur, resulting in a change of direction of weight-bearing forces on the upper tibial epiphysis from perpendicular to oblique. This obliquity tends to displace the tibial epiphysis in a lateral direction, overloading the mediodorsal segment of the bone, bending it in a medial and caudal direction. With further longitudinal growth, a vicious circle of events ensues that culminates in progressive varus deformity.[225]

Histologic examination confirms the absence of changes from infection or osteonecrosis. The microscopic findings are consistent with the effects of persistent abnormal pressure on the growth plate; changes predominate in the zone of resting cartilage in the medial part of the proximal tibial growth plate and consist of islands of densely packed and hypertrophied cells, acellular fibrous cartilage, and abnormal groups of capillaries.[129, 133] The medial meniscus may be hypertrophied and hypermobile.

Clinically, affected children may be early walkers and often are obese. Boys and girls are affected equally. Progressive bilateral (60 per cent) or unilateral (40 per cent) bowing of the leg during the first year of life is difficult to differentiate from physiologic changes.[302, 449, 450] The tibia may be angulated acutely inward just below the knee, and a nontender bony protuberance can be palpated along the medial aspect of the proximal tibia. The fibular head also may be prominent. Pain is not evident. Associated findings are obesity, shortening of the leg, tibial torsion, and pronated feet.

Radiographic abnormalities, which never become evident before the age of one year and seldom before the age of two years,[446, 449] simulate those of physiologic bowing but are more severe and can be unilateral or asymmetric in distribution. Furthermore, altered alignment in Blount's disease occurs in the proximal portion of the tibia, not between the femur and the tibia, as seen in physiologic bowing.[304] In Blount's disease, the tibia is in varus position owing to angulation of the metaphysis, and the tibial shaft is ad-

ducted without intrinsic curvature.[92, 205, 303, 305] These alterations in tibial curvature can be identified with a variety of radiographic measurement techniques.[487] A depressed medial tibial metaphysis with an osseous excrescence or outgrowth is seen. The nature and severity of the osseous changes are highly variable. Six stages have been recognized on the radiograph[133–135] (Figs. 81–36 and 81–37).

Stage I (2 to 3 Years). A progressive increase in the degree of varus deformity of the tibia is associated with irregularity of the entire growth plate. The medial part of the metaphysis protrudes with a medial and distal beak.

Stage II (2.5 to 4 Years). A lateromedial depression of the ossification line of the medial portion of the metaphysis and a wedge-shaped medial end of the epiphysis are observed. Complete healing of the lesion is possible at this stage.

Stage III (4 to 6 Years). The cartilage-filled depression in the metaphyseal beak deepens. The medial part of the bony epiphysis remains wedge-shaped and is less distinct. Small calcific foci may be evident beneath the medial border.

Stage IV (5 to 10 Years). With increasing bone maturation, the cartilaginous growth plate is reduced to a narrow plate, and the bony epiphysis occupies an increasing part of the end of the bone. The medial margin of the epiphysis shows definite irregularity. Even at this stage, restoration of a relatively normal epiphysis can occur. In the presence of partial restoration, the resulting radiographic abnormalities may resemble those in the late stages of the adolescent type of tibia vara.

Stage V (9 to 11 Years). The bony epiphysis and the corresponding articular surface are greatly deformed. A "partial double epiphyseal plate" results as the bony epiphysis is separated in two portions by a clear band, extending medially from the lateral portion of the growth plate to the articular cartilage. The triangular area of bone lying between the two branches of the plate generally is considered to be a part of the epiphysis because it possesses a considerable amount of articular cartilage.

Stage VI (10 to 13 Years). The branches of the medially located double growth plate ossify, whereas growth continues in the normal lateral part. Stages V and VI represent phases of irreparable structural damage.

Lateral widening of the growth plate of the proximal tibia and, less frequently, the distal femur has been identified in infantile tibia vara as well as in other conditions associated with bow-leg deformity.[136] This diastasis may result from the chronic stress of the genu varum on the growth plates in the area of the knee; most stress during weight-bearing

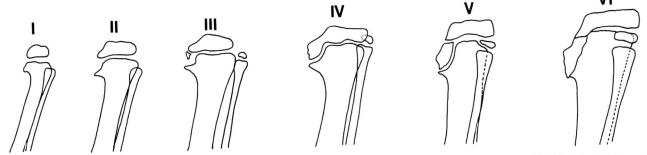

FIGURE 81–36. Blount's disease: Infantile tibia vara. Six stages of the disease (see text for details). (After Langenskiold A: Acta Chir Scand *103*:1, 1952.)

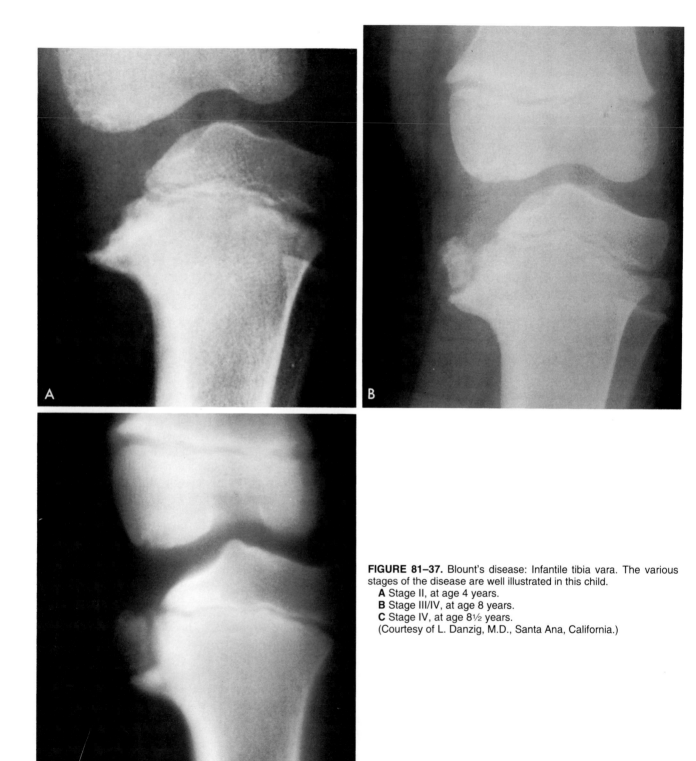

FIGURE 81–37. Blount's disease: Infantile tibia vara. The various stages of the disease are well illustrated in this child.
A Stage II, at age 4 years.
B Stage III/IV, at age 8 years.
C Stage IV, at age 8½ years.
(Courtesy of L. Danzig, M.D., Santa Ana, California.)

on the bowed leg is projected medially, producing distraction or tension force on the lateral aspect of the joint.[137] Similar distraction changes on the medial portion of the growth plate have been noted in association with genu valgum.[138]

Arthrography may be used to investigate infantile tibia vara[92] (see Chapter 13). Findings in initial stages include hypertrophy of the articular cartilage, creating a horizontal joint line despite the presence of angular osseous deformity, and a hypermobile and enlarged medial meniscus. In later stages, angulation of the articular surface may be noted. Similar findings may be depicted with MR imaging (Fig. 81–38).

Adolescent Tibia Vara. The adolescent (or juvenile) form, which is much less frequent than infantile tibia vara, develops in children between the ages of 8 and 15 years. As in infantile tibia vara, involvement of black children is more frequent than whites.[452] The cause is not clear,[482] although an arrest of epiphyseal growth is suspected. A history of trauma or infection occasionally is elicited, and conventional tomography may indicate an osseous bridge between the epiphysis and metaphysis.[133] Alternatively, it has been suggested that adolescent tibia vara is not a disorder distinct from infantile tibia vara and that the deformity occurs not in a limb that has been normally aligned until adolescence but in one that has maintained a mild degree of physiologic bowing.[307, 308] In either case, irregularities of the growth zone with the presence of areas of fibrovascular and cartilaginous repair may be demonstrated on examination of biopsy specimens.[139, 448]

Unilateral alterations occur in approximately 70 to 90 per cent of cases. Leg shortening and mild to moderate varus deformity may be associated with pain and tenderness over the medial prominence of the proximal tibia. Radiographs outline a proximal tibia that is angled about 10 to 20 degrees. The proximal tibial epiphysis reveals medial wedging, and the medial tibial growth plate is diminished in height, but a sharp step-off in the tibial plateau usually is not apparent[92] (Figs. 81–39 and 81–40). Sclerosis on either side of the growth plate, and segmental widening of the lateral portion of the plate of the proximal tibia or distal femur (leading to femoral varus[451]) can be seen. Spontaneous regression of the radiographic abnormalities has been documented but is rare.[446]

Late Onset Tibia Vara. In 1984, Thompson and associates[308] used the term "late onset tibia vara" in a description of the clinical and radiographic characteristics in 11 children between the ages of 6 and 14 years, the majority black, with marked knee deformity. Flattening of the medial aspect of the tibial epiphysis resulting in a wedged shape of the epiphysis and growth plate irregularity were observed radiographically. Histologic abnormalities of involved portions of the tibia resembled those found in infantile tibia vara, suggesting a relationship between the two conditions. Wenger and coworkers[307] indicated that six of seven children with similar clinical and radiologic alterations had significant symmetrical physiologic varus in early childhood that corrected spontaneously, although not completely, on the side that subsequently developed late onset tibia vara.[446] Late onset tibia vara, in common with adolescent tibia vara, is much less frequent than infantile type disease.[484] Owing to overlap in the age of onset of the adolescent type of disease and late onset tibia vara, Thompson and Carter[453] divided late onset disease into two categories: juvenile (previously designated adolescent) and adolescent (the newly described late onset disease). No uniformity currently exists in the use of these terms.

The characteristics of the two types of late onset disease include predominance in blacks and in male children, marked obesity, normal or above normal height, slowly progressive genu varum deformity, pain rather than deformity as the primary initial complaint, no palpable proximal medial metaphyseal beak of the tibia, minimal internal tibial torsion, mild laxity of the medial collateral ligament, and mild discrepancy in length of the lower extremities.[453] The frequency of bilateral involvement in patients with this newly described syndrome of late onset tibia vara is approximately 45 to 50 per cent,[453, 454] and this frequency may be slightly higher in female patients.[454]

Histologic studies of this syndrome reveal findings that are compatible with a traumatic etiology; these include fissuring and clefts in the physis with fibrovascular and cartilaginous repair at the junction of the metaphysis and physis, and are reminiscent of those apparent in cases of slipped femoral capital epiphysis.[454] Foci of necrotic cartilage, with marked disorganization in the degenerative physeal zone, occurring in the medial aspect of the physis, indicate an arrest or partial disturbance of normal endochondral bone formation.[454]

These observations appear to indicate that a spectrum of abnormalities is encountered in patients with tibia vara best categorized according to the age of clinical onset and, there-

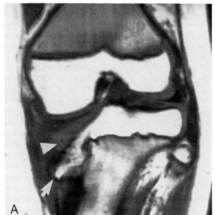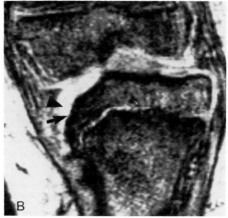

FIGURE 81–38. Blount's disease: Infantile tibia vara. MR imaging abnormalities.

A In this young girl, a coronal T1-weighted (TR/TE, 550/15) MR image shows defective ossification of the medial portion of the tibial epiphysis (arrow) with a slanted bone contour. The unossified epiphyseal cartilage is visible as a region of intermediate signal intensity (arrowhead).

B A coronal gradient echo MR image (FISP) (TR/TE, 30/17; flip angle, 20 degrees) with volumetric acquisition (2.5 mm thick section) reveals the abnormal bone contour (arrow) and the unossified cartilage, appearing as a region of high signal intensity (arrowhead).

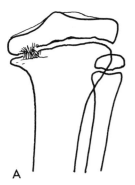
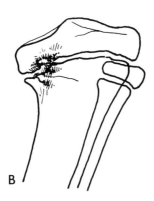

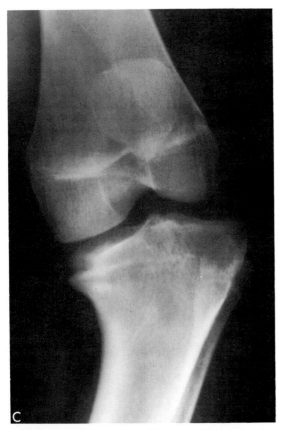

FIGURE 81–39. Blount's disease: Adolescent tibia vara.

A, B Stages of the process. Observe fusion of the medial aspect of the growth plate with progressive sclerosis and varus deformity. (After Langenskiold A: Acta Chir Scand 103:1, 1952.)

C An example of adolescent tibia vara. Note varus deformity, depression of the articular surface of the medial tibial plateau, sclerosis, and osteophyte formation.

fore, to the amount of remaining growth potential.[453] The infantile type of disease is the most likely to lead to the greatest deformity, and the late onset type is least likely to do so. The potential for deformity in the adolescent (or juvenile) type of disease lies between these other two groups. The cause of all three forms of disease appears to be varus stress, growth suppression, and disruption of normal endochondral ossification.[453]

Focal Fibrocartilaginous Dysplasia. One further condition leading to unilateral tibia vara in early childhood first was reported by Bell and colleagues[455] in 1985 and subsequently by Bradish and coworkers[456] in 1988. Other descriptions of this condition soon followed.[457–460] The disor-

der occurs with equal frequency in boys and girls and in the right and left legs. The clinical onset of tibia vara occurs between the ages of 3 and 18 months (with an average of about one year of age), and the child initially presents to the physician at approximately 18 months of age.[459] No instances of bilateral involvement have been reported. In all children with this condition who have not been treated surgically with tibial and fibular osteotomy, spontaneous resolution of the deformity has occurred in a period of 1 to 4 years.[460]

Clinical manifestations include unilateral tibia vara, tibial torsion, and slight shortening of the affected extremity. Routine radiographs are diagnostic, revealing a well-defined, obliquely positioned radiolucent defect in the metadiaphyseal cortex in the proximal and medial portion of the tibia.[460] Endosteal and periosteal thickening of the cortex is an associated finding (Fig. 81–41). CT documents the presence of soft tissue medial to the defect that is indistinguishable from the adjacent muscle and tendon.[460]

On histologic examination, the lesion contains dense hypocellular fibrous tissue resembling tendon with areas of lacuna formation, more like fibrocartilage; this tissue, which occurs close to the insertion site of the pes anserinus tendons, merges with the normal fibrous tissue peripherally.[460]

The cause of focal fibrocartilaginous dysplasia is unknown. It has been suggested that during delivery, trauma may lead to such histologic abnormalities in the medial portion of the tibia.[459] The disorder appears to be distinct from the various forms of Blount's disease.[446]

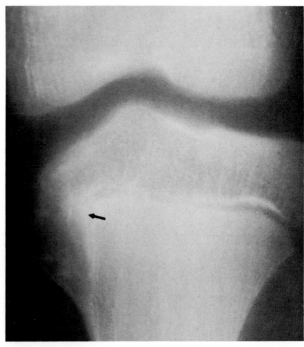

FIGURE 81–40. Blount's disease: Adolescent tibia vara. A 9 year old boy developed pain and tenderness over the medial aspect of the tibia. There was a 30 degree flexion contracture of the knee, and the opposite leg was normal. A conventional tomogram shows a radiolucent area in the medial aspect of the tibial metaphysis, hypoplasia of the medial portion of the epiphysis, an osseous bridge (arrow) extending across the physis, and lateral subluxation of the tibia. (Courtesy of G. Greenway, M.D., Dallas, Texas.)

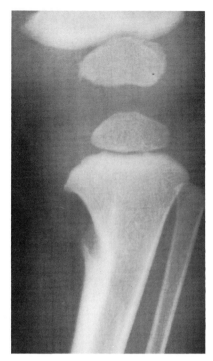

FIGURE 81–41. Focal fibrocartilaginous dysplasia. A 16 month old girl was first noted to have bowing of the left leg at 14 months of age. A radiograph shows a well-defined defect of the metadiaphyseal portion of the medial cortex of the tibia. Note thickening of the cortex adjacent to and below the lesion. (From Herman TE, et al: Radiology *177*:767, 1990.)

Although a number of cortically based lesions, such as juxtacortical chondroma, eosinophilic granuloma and chondromyxoid fibroma, share some radiographic characteristics with focal fibrocartilaginous dysplasia, the associated tibia vara allows accurate diagnosis.[460]

Differential Diagnosis. The radiographic abnormalities in infantile, adolescent, and late onset tibia vara usually are diagnostic. Some difficulty occasionally is encountered in differentiating the infantile type from physiologic bowed legs, and serial radiographs may be necessary (Fig. 81–42). The sharply angular appearance of infantile tibia vara differs from the gradual curve in physiologic bowed legs. Metaphyseal alterations and bowing in Blount's disease also may simulate findings in mild or healing rickets. Additional differential diagnostic possibilities include acute injuries of the proximal tibial growth plate,[461] osteomyelitis, chondrodysplasia punctata,[462] and Ollier's disease.

Scheuermann's Disease

Background. In 1921, Scheuermann[140] described a disorder that led to lower thoracic kyphosis, designating the condition kyphosis dorsalis juvenilis. On the basis of irregularities involving the rims of the vertebral bodies, this investigator concluded that pathologic aberrations had occurred in the region of the growth areas between the vertebral bodies and the ring-like epiphyses, that these changes differed from those in other kyphotic conditions, and that this disease had a close relationship to Legg-Calvé-Perthes disease. Numerous descriptions of juvenile kyphosis followed, and additional terms were introduced, such as vertebral epiphysitis, osteochondrosis juvenilis dorsi, and preadolescent and adolescent kyphosis.[1] Although the predominant involvement of the epiphysis of the vertebral rim initially was interpreted as evidence of osteonecrosis, considerable disagreement as to the cause and pathogenesis of this disorder subsequently developed. Debate also existed regarding the criteria necessary for the diagnosis of Scheuermann's disease. Scheuermann suggested that the radiographic findings were indispensable in establishing the presence of this disorder; in most of his cases, he detected

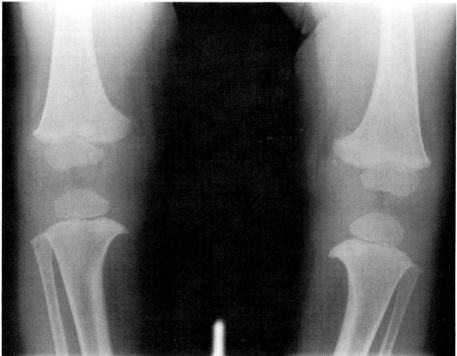

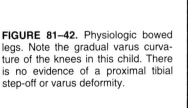

FIGURE 81–42. Physiologic bowed legs. Note the gradual varus curvature of the knees in this child. There is no evidence of a proximal tibial step-off or varus deformity.

three abnormal vertebrae, but later he reported that the number of altered vertebrae might vary from one to five.[141] Currently used criteria frequently require the presence of abnormalities of at least three contiguous vertebrae, each with wedging of 5 degrees or more.[142] Such criteria are not ideal, as they exclude those cases of Scheuermann's disease that are associated predominantly with vertebral irregularity without wedging.[143] Diagnostic criteria based on the presence of clinical findings are inadequate as many patients with this disorder are entirely asymptomatic.

Because of the discrepancies in the criteria used to diagnose juvenile kyphosis, a precise rate of occurrence is difficult to define. The reported frequency during routine examination in military personnel is approximately 4 to 6 per cent,[144, 145] and in industrial workers it is approximately 8 per cent.[142] Most affected persons are between the ages of 13 and 17 years, and the disorder is unusual before the age of 10 years.[146, 147] There is slight predominance of male patients in many series of Scheuermann's disease, although this sex preference is not constant.

Clinical Abnormalities. Clinical manifestations are highly variable. In some persons the disease is totally asymptomatic, being discovered as an incidental finding on lateral radiographs of the chest. In others, prominent symptoms and signs can be seen, commonly appearing around puberty. Most typically, these relate to the middle and lower thoracic spine, although isolated alterations of the lumbar spine (see later discussion) or, more rarely, the cervical spine can be noted.[148–151, 309] Fatigue, defective posture, aching pain aggravated by physical exertion, and tenderness to palpation are encountered. Kyphotic deformity, which may be associated with mild scoliosis, predominates in the thoracic region (75 per cent of patients), although it may be observed in the thoracolumbar (20 to 25 per cent) or lumbar (0 to 5 per cent) segments. A dorsal kyphosis frequently is combined with an exaggerated lumbar and cervical lordosis and a protuberant abdomen.[463] The deformity may be correctable initially, but may become progressively more fixed in position. An angular gibbus deformity is unusual in Scheuermann's disease. Neurologic complaints are not common. Herniation of thoracic intervertebral discs can lead to neurologic manifestations and even paraparesis in occasional cases.[155] Extradural spinal cysts and cord compression at the apex of the abnormal spinal

curvature also have been noted.[156–159, 310, 374, 464] An association of this disease with lumbar disc degeneration and displacement has been suggested.[311, 465]

Radiographic and Pathologic Abnormalities. On radiographs, irregularity of vertebral contours is identified. An undulant superior and inferior surface of affected vertebral bodies is associated with intraosseous radiolucent zones of variable size (cartilaginous or Schmorl's nodes), with surrounding sclerosis (Figs. 81–43 and 81–44). The degree of osseous irregularity is variable, but when severe can be accompanied by loss of intervertebral disc height, particularly in the midportion of the kyphotic curvature. In this same region, wedging or reduction of height of the anterior portion of the vertebral bodies may be seen, a phenomenon that is less striking at the upper and lower limits of the spinal curvature. Small or moderate-sized osteophytes may be evident about the narrowed intervertebral discs and wedge-shaped vertebrae, identical in appearance to the osteophytes of spondylosis deformans.

The degree of thoracic kyphosis also is variable[312]; a kyphotic index can be calculated on a lateral radiograph by measuring the angle at the intersection of two lines, one through the upper endplate of the most craniad vertebra that is involved in the kyphosis, and a second through the lower endplate of the most caudad vertebra. In general, the kyphotic curvature develops slowly unless aggravated by severe physical stress, a factor that may lead to sudden intraosseous displacement of discal material and rapid onset of kyphosis.[152]

Prolapse of large foci of intervertebral disc tissue may be observed anteriorly, and the extruded discal material may extend beneath the apophyseal centers of ossification, appearing submarginally behind the anterior longitudinal ligament.[1] Under these circumstances, a portion of the proximal or distal ring-like apophyseal centers of ossification may be separated from the vertebral body, producing a limbus vertebra (Fig. 81–44B).[313] The subsequent development and ossification of the apophysis can be irregular, creating fragmented ossific radiodense areas that initially were interpreted as evidence of an osteonecrosis of the apophyseal centers. Furthermore, the discal tissue beneath the anterior longitudinal ligament can produce pressure erosion on the adjacent anterior surface of the vertebral body.

Radiographic evidence of healing of the lesions can take

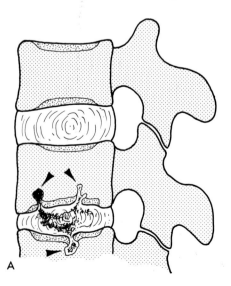

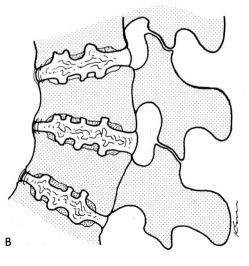

FIGURE 81–43. Scheuermann's disease. The underlying abnormality relates to intraosseous displacement of disc material (cartilaginous nodes) through the cartilaginous endplates (arrowheads). This produces radiolucent lesions of the vertebral bodies with surrounding sclerosis, intervertebral disc space narrowing, and irregularity of vertebral contour. Kyphosis may appear.

A   B

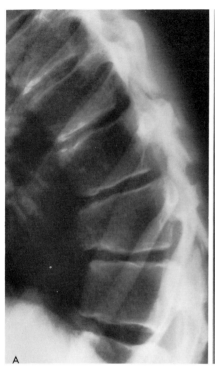
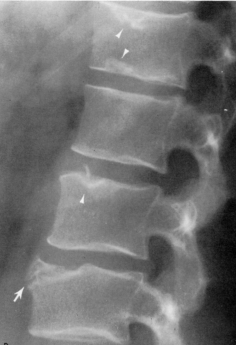
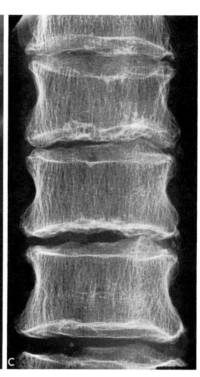
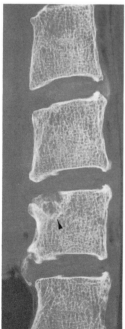
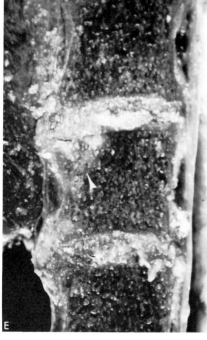

FIGURE 81–44. Scheuermann's disease.

A Thoracic spine. Findings include irregularity of vertebral contour, reactive sclerosis, intervertebral disc space narrowing, anterior vertebral wedging, and kyphosis.

B Lumbar spine. Observe the cartilaginous nodes (arrowheads) creating surface irregularity, lucent areas, and reactive sclerosis. An anterior discal displacement (arrow) has produced an irregular anterosuperior corner of a vertebral body, the limbus vertebra.

C Thoracolumbar spine. A radiograph of a coronal section of a spine delineates the extent of the irregular vertebral contour and intervertebral disc space narrowing.

D, E Cervical spine. A sagittal sectional radiograph and photograph of the cervical spine demonstrate cartilaginous node formation (arrowheads).

several forms (Fig. 81–45). Ossification of the anterior portions of the intervertebral disc can lead to synostosis of one vertebral body with its neighbor[153] (Fig. 81–46). The fusion between the anterior parts of the vertebral bodies may be associated with an unossified but narrowed posterior discal space. This phenomenon can be unaccompanied by symptoms and signs, although a period of discomfort may occur during the ossifying process. If fusion occurs at an early age, persistence of growth of the posterior portions of the vertebrae can accentuate the kyphotic deformity.[153, 154] The resulting anterior contour of the spine can be relatively smooth, although accompanying osteophytes can create surface irregularities.

In addition to the abnormal thoracic kyphosis that characterizes Scheuermann's disease, lateral spinal curvatures depicted on frontal radiographs are identified in this disease. Vertebral body wedging in the coronal plane leads to a scoliosis located at approximately the same level as the kyphosis; this pattern of scoliosis occurs with equal prevalence in boys and girls and is directed equally to the right and the left.[314] A second pattern of scoliosis occurs in regions of compensatory lordosis situated above or, more commonly, below the kyphosis; this type of abnormal spinal curvature is more prevalent in girls than in boys and more often is convex to the right side.[314] Although scoliosis

has received less attention than kyphosis in Scheuermann's disease, some investigators believe that its occurrence suggests a basic relationship between this disease and idiopathic scoliosis,[314] despite the existence of distinct differences in spinal curvature in the two conditions.[315, 316]

The pathologic alterations in Scheuermann's disease involve the intervertebral discs and the vertebral bodies, including the cartilaginous endplates.[1, 152, 160] The intervertebral discs may appear bulged or biconvex in shape, and the neighboring cartilaginous endplates may appear thinner than normal, presumably owing to the pressure of the discal tissue, which deforms the plate, preventing normal endochondral ossification. The cartilaginous endplate then may degenerate, with fissuring, ulceration, and microscopic focal areas of "necrosis."[161] Intraosseous nuclear protrusions occur through the weakened endplates, and the prolapsed disc material becomes surrounded first by a cartilaginous casing, and later by an osseous one.[152] The cartilaginous nodes eventually consist of both nucleus pulposus and anulus fibrosus, and in some cases even the cartilaginous plate itself may be displaced into the vertebral body. Fibrovascular proliferation and narrowing of the intervertebral disc can ensue. This narrowing is maximal on the anterior aspect of the disc, and the resultant pressure on the vertebral bodies in this area may impede normal growth and accentuate

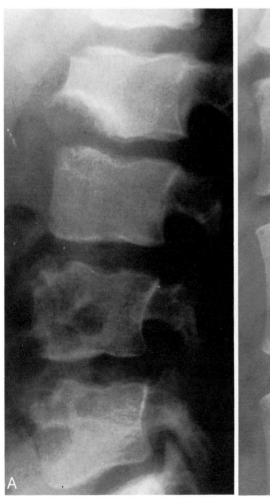
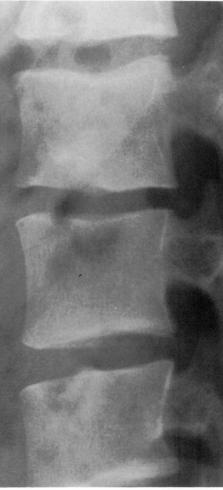

FIGURE 81–45. Scheuermann's disease. Lateral radiographs of the lumbar spine obtained at the ages of 12 years **(A)** and 23 years **(B)** reveal, initially, prominent cartilaginous nodes with vertebral irregularity and, subsequently, healing of most of the lesions with a relatively normal vertebral shape and surface. (Courtesy of G. Greenway, M.D., Dallas, Texas.)

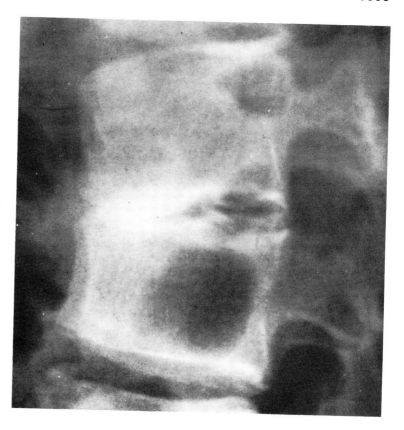

FIGURE 81–46. Scheuermann's disease. Note synostosis of two vertebral bodies owing to ossification of the intervening intervertebral disc. The disc space is narrowed and osteophytosis is present.

the kyphosis. Healing of the discal alterations can result in ossification, with synostosis of vertebral bodies.

Etiology and Pathogenesis. Many concepts of the cause of Scheuermann's disease have been developed and are well summarized by Alexander.[143] Scheuermann's initial assessment stressed the importance of the apophyseal changes, which he attributed to necrosis. This theory has not withstood the test of time, and it is not consistent with the pathologic abnormalities (which do not reveal osteonecrosis) or with the absence of these changes in patients with known ischemic disorders, such as sickle cell anemia. Similarly, the hypothesis that the disorder relates to osteomyelitis, tuberculosis, disproportionate growth between the spine and the sternum, rickets, or endocrine dysfunction has not been verified.[152, 162–164] The possibility that Scheuermann's disease is the product of osteoporosis or some other alteration in bone metabolism has received some support,[165–167, 317, 318] although the absence of osteoporosis in some patients with this disorder[466] and the absence of Scheuermann's disease in some varieties of osteoporosis suggest that other factors are important in the initiation and progression of the spinal deformity.

The importance of genetic factors in the pathogenesis of juvenile kyphosis is supported by the reports of its familial occurrence.[142, 168, 206] Bradford and associates[146] noted a positive family history in approximately one fourth of cases, and Kewalramani and coworkers[169] described the coexistence of Scheuermann's disease and Charcot-Marie-Tooth syndrome in three men of a single family. Halal and colleagues,[168] in a study of five families with juvenile kyphosis, postulated an autosomal dominant pattern of inheritance. These results indicate that heritable factors could be important in this disease, perhaps as a result of genetic influences on the osseous strength of vertebral bodies.

Schmorl[170] and Beadle[171] concluded that cartilaginous node formation is fundamental to the disease process, and that these nodes occurred through congenital indentations of the intervertebral disc in the region of an expanded nucleus pulposus, at which site the cartilaginous endplates were thinner than normal. It was suggested that congenital weakness of the endplates predisposed certain persons to intraosseous discal prolapse during periods of excessive physical stress. This theory is attractive because it is consistent with many of the histologic and histochemical findings in the disease, although the precise nature of the weakened cartilaginous areas has not been clarified.[319, 320, 375] Defects due to vascular channels, ossification gaps, and notochordal remnants have been emphasized, but such sites do not always correspond to areas of node formation, and, in fact, the precise location of discal displacements varies from one person to another. The areas of abnormality in the cartilaginous endplates of patients with Scheuermann's disease are described as large translucent regions of collagen-free tissue[319] or, on chemical analysis, demonstrate alterations in normal collagen synthesis with few glycoproteins and proteoglycans, which are either very abundant or in a different state of aggregation with the other macromolecular components of the matrix, or both.[320]

Alexander[143] has postulated that nuclear expansion represents a traumatically induced growth arrest with secondary nuclear degeneration, and that the cartilaginous node simply is an endplate fracture resulting from failure under dynamic load in compression or shear, at a time when the plate and the metaphysis are vulnerable as a result of rapid growth. This investigator introduced the terms adolescent endplate injury and traumatic spondylodystrophy. In support of this theory, Alexander listed the following observations: (1) Scheuermann's disease and cartilaginous nodes are infrequent in children whose illnesses (e.g., Cushing's disease) preclude normal activity and a normal growth spurt; (2) in the presence of normal activity and growth, osteoporosis appears to predispose the spine to cartilaginous node formation; (3) irregular ossification occurs in conditions in which defects in mucopolysaccharide or other matrix components impair vectoring of chondrocytes (e.g., mucopolysaccharidosis IV, multiple epiphyseal dysplasia); (4) a familial occurrence of the disease may reflect genetically determined defects in vertebral strength; and (5) Scheuermann's disease appears to correlate with other spinal disorders indicative of failure under compression (e.g., intervertebral disc degeneration, spondylolysis).

Analysis of the previously outlined hypotheses and of others[172, 173] indicates that this disorder most likely is a manifestation of cartilaginous node formation. The basis for the nodes is not clear, although stress-induced intraosseous displacements through congenitally or traumatically weakened portions of the cartilaginous endplate appear probable. Such nodes, as well as vertebral body irregularity and wedging, have been identified with increased frequency in athletic adolescents.[467, 468] The radiographic findings reflect the presence of discal material within the vertebral bodies (intraosseous lucent areas) and arrested or abnormal vertebral growth (irregularity of osseous contour), either or both of which can be evident in any one patient with the disease.

Juvenile Lumbar Osteochondrosis. A condition sharing some features with Scheuermann's disease but localized to the lower thoracic and lumbar spine has been described.[469, 470] Affected patients have pain, often severe, in the lower back that appears during adolescence. Boys are involved more commonly than girls, and thoracic deformity, as seen in Scheuermann's disease, is absent. The disorder appears to occur with higher frequency in persons involved in competitive athletics.

Radiographs reveal prominent depressions of the vertebral endplates, with wedging and an increased anteroposterior dimension of affected vertebral bodies. Decreased height of lumbar intervertebral discs, retrolisthesis of lumbar vertebrae, and findings of spinal stenosis may be apparent. Myelography,[470] CT, and MR imaging[465, 471] can be used to confirm the presence of a narrowed spinal canal, and the narrowest portion of the canal typically is at the level of the intervertebral discs (Fig. 81–47).[470] Bone scintigraphy shows mild accumulation of the radionuclide at sites of involvement.[488]

The relationship of this condition to typical Scheuermann's disease is not clear. Of interest in this regard is the occurrence of similar abnormalities of the lumbar spine in patients who have characteristic abnormalities of Scheuermann's disease in the thoracic spine. Clinical manifestations in patients with isolated alterations in the lumbar spine, however, differ from those of classic Scheuermann's disease, suggesting that it may be a distinct disorder.

Differential Diagnosis. Cartilaginous nodes can accompany any disease process that weakens the cartilaginous endplate or subchondral bone of the vertebral body, allowing intraosseous discal displacement. A partial list of such processes includes trauma, neoplasm, metabolic disorders (hyperparathyroidism, osteoporosis, Paget's disease), infection, intervertebral osteochondrosis, and articular disorders (rheumatoid arthritis). Accurate radiographic diagnosis of

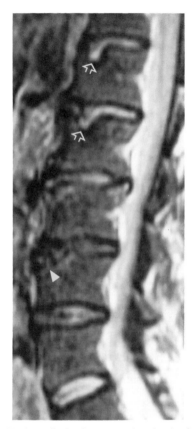

FIGURE 81–47. Juvenile lumbar osteochondrosis. A T2-weighted (TR/TE, 1500/70) sagittal spin echo MR image reveals contour irregularity of multiple lumbar vertebral bodies, with numerous Schmorl's nodes (arrows). A limbus vertebral body (arrowhead) is evident at the fourth lumbar level. Note intervertebral disc degeneration and narrowing of the spinal canal at the levels of the intervertebral discs. (Courtesy of A. Orloff, M.D., San Diego, California.)

these conditions is based on additional spinal and extraspinal manifestations. The combination of kyphosis, cartilaginous nodes, and irregular vertebral outlines is virtually pathognomonic of Scheuermann's disease. Kyphosis of other causes, such as tuberculosis, and postural, osteoporotic, and senile kyphosis, can be eliminated by the absence of these characteristic radiologic findings. Occasionally the spinal abnormalities in certain congenital or inherited disorders, such as the mucopolysaccharidoses and Turner's syndrome, can simulate those of Scheuermann's disease, but additional skeletal alterations ensure accurate diagnosis.

One additional entity that has many radiographic similarities to Scheuermann's disease has been termed progressive noninfectious anterior vertebral fusion.[472] Originally described by Knutsson[473] in 1949 and then by Butler[474] in 1971, this disease develops in early childhood and leads to progressive fusion in the thoracolumbar junction with an acutely angled kyphosis.[472] Clinical manifestations vary considerably; some patients have mild or moderate back pain and stiffness, others have neurologic deficits, and still others are entirely asymptomatic. Initial radiographic abnormalities involve the anterior column of the spine and include erosion and sclerosis of vertebral bodies and narrowing of the intervertebral discs (Fig. 81–48A). At this stage, the findings resemble those of early ankylosing spondylitis. Further obliteration of the intervertebral disc space with bone ankylosis subsequently occurs (Fig. 81–48A,B).

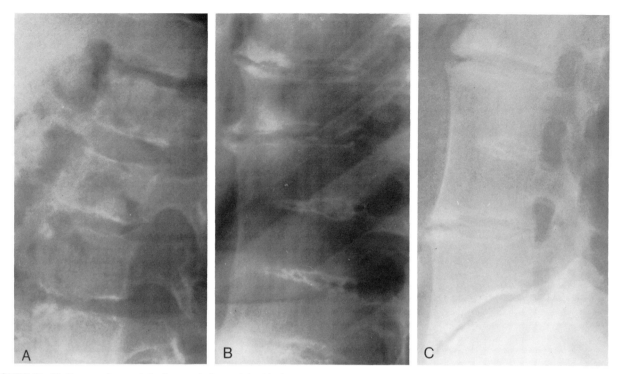

FIGURE 81–48. Progressive noninfectious anterior vertebral fusion.
 A In this young girl, note irregularity of the vertebral margins and disc space loss.
 B, C In the mother of the child in **(A)**, lateral radiographs of the thoracic **(B)** and lumbar **(C)** spine show partial fusion of multiple disc spaces.
 (Courtesy of P. Cockshott, M.D., Toronto, Ontario, Canada.)

Such anterior fusion, when combined with continued growth of the posterior portions of the spine, leads to progressive kyphosis of the thoracolumbar junction. The entire process may evolve over a period of 10 or more years, and kyphotic deformity often exceeds 50 degrees.[472] The cause of noninfectious anterior vertebral fusion is not clear. Clues to potential etiologic factors may be provided by its occasional occurrence in families and the documentation of similar vertebral abnormalities in thalidomide embryopathy (see Chapter 90).[472, 475]

Sinding-Larsen-Johansson Disease

In 1921 and 1922, Sinding-Larsen[174] and Johansson[175] independently described a syndrome that occurred most commonly in the adolescent between 10 and 14 years of age, consisting of tenderness and soft tissue swelling over the lower pole of the patella, accompanied by radiographic evidence of osseous fragmentation. Early reports suggested that the disorder was an "epiphysitis," "apophysitis," or "osteochondritis." It now is recognized that inflammatory changes and osteonecrosis are not fundamental to this condition, but rather that it is traumatic in origin. Its pathogenesis appears to be very similar to that of Osgood-Schlatter disease, and in fact a coexistence of the two disorders has been noted.[176, 443] The lesion probably is related to a traction phenomenon in which contusion or tendinitis in the proximal attachment of the patellar tendon can be followed by calcification and ossification,[177] or in which patellar fracture or avulsion produces one or more distinct ossification sites. The association of fragmentation of the inferior portion of the patella with spastic paralysis[178, 179] is consistent with this

traction phenomenon. Similar findings are observed in athletes, in whom the term "jumper's knee" has been applied[321, 322] and in whom patellar subluxation or dislocation has been advocated as the common mechanism of injury.[322]

In Sinding-Larsen-Johansson disease, pain and tenderness are aggravated by activity. The radiograph reveals small bony fragments adjacent to the distal surface of the patella with overlying soft tissue swelling (Fig. 81–49). The radiodense areas subsequently may coalesce and become incorporated into the patella, eventually yielding a normal radiographic appearance. Ultrasound[444] and MR imaging also may be used to substantiate the diagnosis. The natural duration of the disease is approximately 3 to 12 months.

Patellar fragmentation also may represent a normal variation of ossification or the presence of accessory ossification centers.[180]

"DISORDERS" DUE TO VARIATIONS IN OSSIFICATION

Sever's Phenomenon

Irregularity of the secondary calcaneal ossification center was emphasized in 1912 by Sever,[181] who related the change to an apophysitis of the os calcis that might produce pain and tenderness of the heel. Further support for this concept appeared in subsequent publications[182–184] until, in 1948, Hughes[185] proposed that the condition was a normal variation unrelated to the painful heels of adolescents. It now is generally accepted that fragmentation and sclerosis of the secondary ossification center of the calcaneus can be

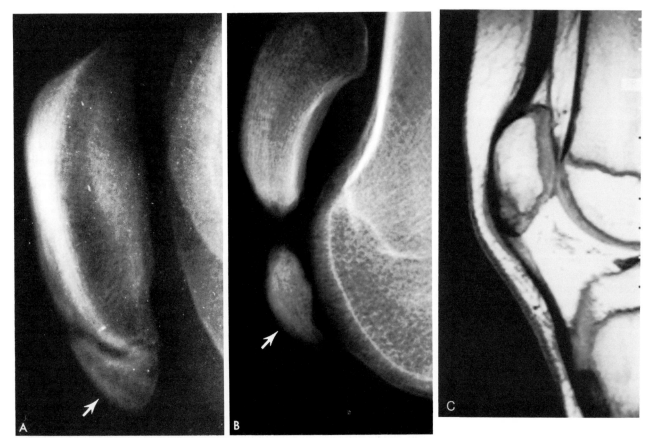

FIGURE 81–49. Sinding-Larsen-Johansson disease.
A In this teen-age boy with painful swelling of the knee, note the extraossific dense area (arrow) adjacent to the inferior pole of the patella.
B In this patient with spastic paralysis, observe fragmentation of the lower pole of the patella (arrow) related to abnormal stress.
C In a 12 year old child, a sagittal T1-weighted (TR/TE, 650/15) spin echo MR image reveals bone irregularity in the lower pole of the patella. (Courtesy of D. Levey, M.D., Corpus Christi, Texas.)

entirely normal (Fig. 81–50) and, in fact, are the result of proper weight-bearing.[186] Such osseous changes may be absent in patients who are immobilized as a result of neurogenic disease or fracture, and may appear with resumption of normal levels of activity.

Ischiopubic Osteochondrosis

A lesion consisting of rarefaction and swelling of the ischiopubic synchondrosis and the neighboring bone was described as an osteochondritis by Van Neck.[187] On the basis of clinical, radiologic, scintigraphic,[324] and pathologic observations, this condition now is regarded as a very common, normal pattern of ossification.[188, 323, 342] This pattern may be unilateral or bilateral in distribution.[476] The time of closure of the synchondrosis is somewhat variable; it usually takes place between the ages of 9 and 11 years. Irregular ossification of the synchondrosis generally is most apparent between the ages of 5 and 8 years (Fig. 81–51).[476]

The differential diagnosis of this normal variant includes a stress fracture, posttraumatic osteolysis, and infection.[325] Diagnostic difficulty arises owing to the occurrence of accumulation of bone-seeking radionuclides about this normal variant. It has been suggested that if such uptake is equal to or greater than that adjacent to the triradiate cartilage, a pathologic process is present.[476]

MISCELLANEOUS DISORDERS

Osteochondroses have been described in almost every epiphysis and apophysis in the body (Table 81–5). In most cases, boys are affected more frequently than girls, altera-

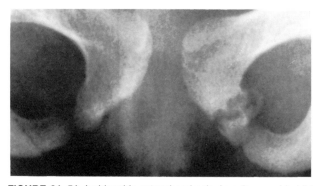

FIGURE 81–51. Ischiopubic osteochondrosis. In a 3 year old child, the ischiopubic synchondrosis on the right side is open with adjacent smooth bone margins; on the left side, irregular ossification is evident. This latter pattern of ossification is within normal limits. (Courtesy of J. Goobar, M.D., Ostersund, Sweden.)

tions rarely develop before the age of 3 years or after the age of 12 years, and developmental irregularities in ossification can be encountered at many of the same skeletal sites. Other sites of osteochondroses include the primary ossification center of the patella,[189] greater trochanter,[190] acetabular roof,[326] proximal tibial epiphysis,[191] distal tibial epiphysis,[192] talus, os tibiale externum, cuneiforms,[193, 327, 352, 476] epiphysis of the fifth metatarsal bone,[194, 376] proximal epiphysis of the hallux,[328] humeral head, trochlea,[329] ulnar olecranon process,[330, 331] distal ulnar epiphysis,[195] heads of the metacarpals,[196, 477] radial head,[197] iliac crest, ischial apophysis, and symphysis pubis. In many instances, the pathogenesis of the osseous fragmentation and sclerosis is

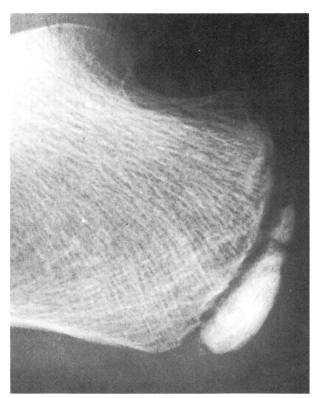

FIGURE 81–50. Sever's phenomenon. An example of sclerosis and fragmentation of the secondary calcaneal ossification center is illustrated. This is a normal consequence of weight-bearing.

TABLE 81–5. Some of the Osteochondroses

Year Reported	Investigator(s)	Location of Lesion
1887	Koenig	Osteochondritis dissecans
1903	Osgood; Schlatter	Tibial tubercle
1908	Köhler	Primary patellar center
1908	Haglund	Os tibiale externum
1908	Köhler	Tarsal navicular
1909	Thiemann	Phalangeal bases
1910	Legg; Calvé; Perthes	Femoral epiphysis
1910	Kienböck	Carpal lunate
1911	Preiser	Carpal scaphoid
1912	Sever	Calcaneal apophysis
1912	Iselin	Fifth metatarsal base
1914	Freiberg	Second metatarsal head
1921	Hass	Head of humerus
1921	Burns	Lower ulna
1921	Scheuermann	Vertebral apophysis
1921	Sinding-Larsen	Secondary patellar center
1922	Mandl	Greater trochanter
1924	Friedrich	Medial end of calvicle
1924	Van Neck	Ischiopubic synchondrosis
1925	Calvé	Vertebral body
1927	Panner	Capitulum of humerus
1927	Mauclaire	Heads of metacarpals
1927	Buchman	Iliac crest
1928	Diaz	Talus
1929	Pierson	Symphysis pubis
1932	Dietrich	Heads of metacarpals
1937	Blount	Medial proximal tibia
1945	Caffey	Entire carpus bilaterally
1950	Liffert and Arkin	Distal tibial center
1953	Milch	Ischial apophysis
1956	Caffey	Tibial spines

(After Brower AC: Orthop Clin North Am *14*:99, 1983.)

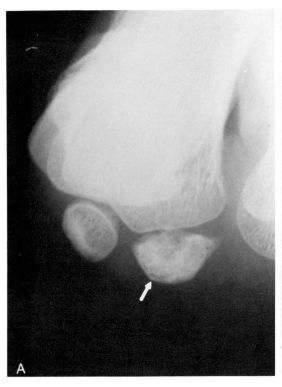

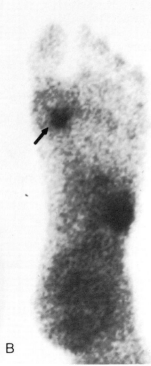

FIGURE 81–52. Sesamoiditis. This 33 year old man developed pain and swelling beneath the great toe. There was no history of recent injury.

A A radiograph shows irregularity and flattening of the lateral sesamoid bone (arrow) beneath the first metatarsal head.

B The bone scan documents increased accumulation of the radionuclide (arrow) in this region as well as laterally in the midfoot.

(Courtesy of V. Vint, M.D., San Diego, California.)

not clear, although alterations due to stress or variations of normal ossification appear likely at certain locations. "Osteochondrosis" of the vertebral body, termed Calvé's disease, leading to flattening and collapse, almost invariably is the result of an eosinophilic granuloma.

Spontaneous osteonecrosis of the carpal scaphoid was first described by Preiser in 1910[332] and usually is referred to as *Preiser's disease.* It subsequently has been reported by other investigators,[207, 333–335, 478] some of whom have interpreted Preiser's original case not as idiopathic ischemic necrosis but as a healing fracture.[335] A history of trauma is frequent in patients who develop Preiser's disease.[485] The fact that few descriptions of this condition exist and that some are regarded as undocumented indicates that Preiser's disease indeed is uncommon.

The initial radiographic appearance is characterized by cystic and sclerotic changes in the carpal scaphoid that are followed by collapse and, in some instances, fracture, especially in the proximal portion of the bone. The findings, which resemble those of Kienböck's disease, usually are observed in adults who may have local pain, tenderness, and decreased strength. Narrowing of the radioscaphoid space, similar to that seen in calcium pyrophosphate dihydrate crystal deposition disease, is an associated finding in some patients.[478] Although accidental trauma is not a constant feature, chronic or repetitive stress (related to occupational or recreational activity) and predilection for involvement of the dominant hand are recorded in many cases. It is possible that Preiser's disease results from a fatigue fracture of the scaphoid.[335]

Osteochondrosis affecting the medial end of the clavicle is termed *Friedrich's disease,* having been described by Friedrich in 1924[336] in two patients with local swelling and tenderness over this portion of the bone. Few additional reports of this condition exist,[337–341, 479, 480] emphasizing how

rare it must be. It is seen in adult women and, less commonly, men and is characterized by radiolucent foci, bone sclerosis, and osteophytosis affecting the inferomedial aspect of the clavicle adjacent to the sternoclavicular joint, generally in a unilateral distribution. The articulation itself may be normal or narrowed, the latter presumably related to secondary osteoarthritis. A history of trauma to the area is encountered in some of the affected patients.

The cause of Friedrich's disease is not known. Although it is believed to represent an ischemic necrosis of the epiphysis of the sternal end of the clavicle, it appears identical to condensing osteitis of the clavicle (Chapter 58), a disorder usually evident in young and middle-aged women. Stress-related alterations of the clavicle, perhaps leading to microfractures and secondary ischemic necrosis, are the most likely cause as bone necrosis was not an early histologic feature in some of the reported cases of Friedrich's disease.[341]

Sesamoiditis is a term applied to irregularity and collapse of one or more of the sesamoid bones, usually in the feet (Fig. 81–52). The existence of such an entity is debated as, in some instances, infection probably is present. In other cases, local trauma may be the initiating event, producing infractions of bone and subsequent interruption of blood supply.[360]

SUMMARY

The osteochondroses are a heterogeneous group of disorders that usually are characterized by fragmentation and sclerosis of an epiphyseal or apophyseal center in the immature skeleton. Reossification and reconstitution of osseous contour can be evident in some cases. These disorders can be divided into three major categories: (1) conditions characterized by primary or secondary osteonecrosis; (2)

conditions related to trauma or abnormal stress, without evidence of osteonecrosis; and (3) conditions that represent variations in normal patterns of ossification. In some cases, a definite pathogenesis has not been identified.

References

1. Jaffe HL: Metabolic, Degenerative and Inflammatory Diseases of Bones and Joints. Philadelphia, Lea & Febiger, 1972, p 565.
2. Jacobs P: Osteochondrosis (osteochondritis). In JK Davidson (Ed): Aseptic Necrosis of Bone. Amsterdam, Excerpta Medica, 1976, p 301.
3. Legg AT: An obscure affection of the hip joint. Boston Med Surg J 162:202, 1910.
4. Calvé J: Sur une forme particulière de pseudo-coxalgie greffée sur des déformations caractéristiques de l'extrémité supérieure du fémur. Rev Chir 30:54, 1910.
5. Perthes GC: Über Arthritis deformans juvenilis. Dtsch Z Chir 107:111, 1910.
6. Perthes GC: Über osteochondritis deformans juvenilis. Arch Klin Chir 101:779, 1913.
7. Waldenström H: Coxa plana. Osteochondritis deformans coxae, Calvé-Perthes'sche Krankheit. Legg's disease. Zentralbl Chir 47:539, 1930.
8. Waldenström H: Der obere tuberkulose Collumherd. Z Orthop Chir 24:487, 1909.
9. Sutro CJ, Pomeranz MM: Perthes' disease. Arch Surg 34:360, 1937.
10. Edgren W: Cox plana: A clinical and radiological investigation with particular reference to the importance of the metaphyseal changes for the final shape of the proximal part of the femur. Acta Orthop Scand Suppl 84:1, 1965.
11. Clarke TE, Finnegan TL, Fisher RL, et al: Legg-Perthes disease in children less than four years old. J Bone Joint Surg [Am] 60:166, 1978.
12. Spragge JW: Legg-Calvé-Perthes disease. In RH Freiberger et al (Eds): Hip Disease of Infancy and Childhood. Curr Probl Radiol 3:30, 1973.
13. Nevelös AE, Colton CL, Burch PRJ, et al: Perthes' disease. A study of radiological features. Acta Orthop Scand 48:411, 1977.
14. Goldman AB, Hallel T, Salvati EM, et al: Osteochondritis dissecans complicating Legg-Perthes disease. A report of four cases. Radiology 121:561, 1976.
15. Caffey J: The early roentgenographic changes in essential coxa plana; their significance in pathogenesis. AJR 103:620, 1968.
16. Kamhi E, MacEwen GD: Osteochondritis dissecans in Legg-Calvé-Perthes disease. J Bone Joint Surg [Am] 57:506, 1975.
17. Somerville EW: Perthes' disease of the hip. J Bone Joint Surg [Br] 53:639, 1971.
18. Katz JF, Siffert RS: Capital necrosis, metaphyseal cyst, and subluxation in coxa plana. Clin Orthop 106:75, 1975.
19. Robichon J, Desjardins JP, Koch M, et al: The femoral neck in Legg-Perthes' disease. Its relationship to epiphyseal change and its importance in early prognosis. J Bone Joint Surg [Br] 56:62, 1974.
20. Zweymüller K, Wicke B: Zur Lateralisation der Oberschenkelkopfes beim M. Perthes. Arch Orthop Unfallchir 75:239, 1973.
21. Calot F: L'orthopédie Indispensable aux Praticiens. 9th Ed. Paris, Maloine, 1926, p 833.
22. Waldenström H: The first stages of coxa plana. J Bone Joint Surg 20:559, 1938.
23. Kemp HS, Boldero JL: Radiological changes in Perthes' disease. Br J Radiol 39:744, 1966.
24. Anderson J, Stewart AM: The significance of the magnitude of the medial hip joint space. Br J Radiol 43:238, 1970.
25. Gill AB: Legg-Perthes disease of the hip: Its early roentgenographic manifestations and its cyclical course. J Bone Joint Surg 22:1013, 1940.
26. Mindell ER, Sherman MS: Late results in Legg-Perthes disease. J Bone Joint Surg [Am] 33:1, 1951.
27. Ponseti IV: Legg-Perthes' disease: Observations on pathological changes in two cases. J Bone Joint Surg [Am] 38:739, 1956.
28. Ponseti IV, Cotton RL: Legg-Calvé-Perthes disease—pathogenesis and evaluation. Failure of treatment with L-triiodothyronine. J Bone Joint Surg [Am] 43:261, 1961.
29. Ferguson AB Jr: The pathology of Legg-Perthes disease and its comparison with aseptic necrosis. Clin Orthop 106:7, 1975.
30. Dolman CL, Bell HM: The pathology of Legg-Calvé-Perthes disease. A case report. J Bone Joint Surg [Am] 55:184, 1973.
31. McKibbin B, Rális Z: Pathological changes in a case of Perthes' disease. J Bone Joint Surg [Br] 56:438, 1974.
32. Jensen OM, Lauritzen J: Legg-Calvé-Perthes' disease. Morphological studies in two cases examined at necropsy. J Bone Joint Surg [Br] 58:332, 1976.
33. Snyder CR: Legg-Perthes disease in the young hip—does it necessarily do well? J Bone Joint Surg [Am] 57:751, 1975.
34. Mose K, Hjorth L, Ulfeldt M, et al: Legg Calvé Perthes disease. The late occurrence of coxarthrosis. Acta Orthop Scand Suppl 169:1, 1977.
35. Stillman BC: Osteochondritis dissecans and coxa plana. Review of the literature with a personal case report. J Bone Joint Surg [Br] 48:64, 1966.
36. Ratliff AHC: Osteochondritis dissecans following Legg-Calvé-Perthes' disease. J Bone Joint Surg 49:108, 1967.
37. Katz JF: Recurrent Legg-Calvé-Perthes disease. J Bone Joint Surg [Am] 55:833, 1973.
38. Bjerkreim I, Hauge MF: So-called recurrent Perthes' disease. Acta Orthop Scand 47:181, 1976.
39. Axer A, Hendel D: Recurrent Legg-Calvé-Perthes' disease. A case report. Clin Orthop 126:170, 1977.
40. Catterall A: The natural history of Perthes' disease. J Bone Joint Surg [Br] 53:37, 1971.
41. Murphy RP, Marsh HO: Incidence and natural history of "head at risk" factors in Perthes' disease. Clin Orthop 132:102, 1978.
42. Dickens DRV, Menelaus MB: The assessment of prognosis in Perthes' disease. J Bone Joint Surg [Br] 60:189, 1978.
43. Gower WE, Johnston RC: Legg-Perthes disease. Long-term follow-up of thirty-six patients. J Bone Joint Surg [Am] 53:759, 1971.
44. Ozonoff MB: Pediatric Orthopedic Radiology. Philadelphia, WB Saunders Co, 1979.
45. Jonsäter S: Coxa plana. A histo-pathologic and arthrographic study. Acta Orthop Scand Suppl 12:7, 1953.
46. Danigelis JA: Pinhole imaging in Legg-Perthes disease: Further observations. Semin Nucl Med 6:69, 1976.
47. Danigelis JA, Fisher RL, Ozonoff MB, et al: 99mTc-polyphosphate bone imaging in Legg-Perthes disease. Radiology 115:407, 1975.
48. Fasting OJ, Langeland N, Bjerkreim I, et al: Bone scintigraphy in early diagnosis of Perthes' disease. Acta Orthop Scand 49:169, 1978.
49. Trueta J: Normal vascular anatomy of the human femoral head during growth. J Bone Joint Surg [Br] 39:358, 1957.
50. Girdany BR, Osman MZ: Longitudinal growth and skeletal maturation in Perthes' disease. Radiol Clin North Am 6:245, 1968.
51. Harrison MHM, Turner MH, Jacobs P: Skeletal immaturity in Perthes' disease. J Bone Joint Surg [Br] 58:37, 1976.
52. Wynne-Davies R, Gormley J: The aetiology of Perthes' disease. Genetic, epidemiological and growth factors in 310 Edinburgh and Glasgow patients. J Bone Joint Surg [Br] 60:6, 1978.
53. Jacobs BW: Early recognition of osteochondrosis of the capital epiphysis of the femur. JAMA 172:527, 1960.
54. Zahir A, Freeman MAR: Cartilage changes following a single episode of infarction of the capital femoral epiphysis in the dog. J Bone Joint Surg [Am] 54:125, 1972.
55. Sanchis M, Zahir A, Freeman MAR: The experimental simulation of Perthes disease by consecutive interruptions of the blood supply to the capital femoral epiphysis in the puppy. J Bone Joint Surg [Am] 55:335, 1973.
56. Inoue A, Freeman MAR, Vernon-Roberts B, et al: The pathogenesis of Perthes' disease. J Bone Joint Surg [Br] 58:453, 1976.
57. Suramo I, Puranen J, Heikkinen E, et al: Disturbed patterns of venous drainage of the femoral neck in Perthes' disease. J Bone Joint Surg [Br] 56:448, 1974.
58. Kemp HBS: Perthes disease: An experimental and clinical study. Ann R Coll Surg Engl 52:18, 1973.
59. Meyer J: Dysplasia epiphysealis capitis femoris. A clinical-radiological syndrome and its relationship to Legg-Calvé-Perthes disease. Acta Orthop Scand 34:183, 1964.
60. Freiberg AH: Infraction of the second metatarsal bone; a typical injury. Surg Gynecol Obstet 19:191, 1914.
61. Panner HJ: A peculiar characteristic metatarsal disease. Acta Radiol 1:319, 1921–1922.
62. Smillie IS: Freiberg's infraction (Koehler's second disease). J Bone Joint Surg [Br] 39:580, 1955.
63. Freiberg AH: The so-called infraction of the second metatarsal bone. J Bone Joint Surg 8:257, 1926.
64. Braddock GTF: Experimental epiphyseal injury and Freiberg's disease. J Bone Joint Surg [Br] 41:154, 1959.
65. Wagner A: Isolated aseptic necrosis in the epiphysis of the first metatarsal bone. Acta Radiol 11:80, 1930.
66. Hoskinson J: Freiberg's disease: a review of long-term results. Proc R Soc Med 67:106, 1974.
67. Peste: Discussion. Bull Soc Anat Paris 18:169, 1843.
68. Kienböck R: Über traumatische Malazie des Mondbeins und ihre Folgezustände: Entartungsformen und Kompressionsfrakturen. Fortschr Geb Roentgenstr Nuklearmed 16:77, 1910–1911.
69. Lichtman DM, Mack GR, MacDonald RI, et al: Kienböck's disease: The role of silicone replacement arthroplasty. J Bone Joint Surg [Am] 59:899, 1977.
70. Cave EF: Kienböck's disease of the lunate. J Bone Joint Surg 21:858, 1939.
71. Therkelsen F, Andersen K: Lunatomalacia. Acta Chir Scand 97:503, 1949.
72. Gentaz R, Lespargot J, Levame JH, et al: La maladie de Kienböck. Approche tomographique. Analyse de 5 cas. Nouv Presse Med 1:1207, 1972.
73. Simmons EH, Dommisse I: The pathogenesis and treatment of Kienböck's disease (Abstr). Clin Orthop 105:300, 1974.
74. Roca J, Beltran JE, Fairen MF, et al: Treatment of Kienböck's disease using a silicone rubber implant. J Bone Joint Surg [Am] 58:373, 1976.
75. Rooker GD, Goodfellow JW: Kienböck's disease in cerebral palsy. J Bone Joint Surg [Br] 59:363, 1977.
76. Rosemeyer B, Artmann M, Viernstein K: Lunatum-malacie. Nachuntersuchungsergebnisse und therapeutische Erwägungen. Arch Orthop Unfallchir 85:119, 1976.
77. Sobel A, Sobel P: Un cas de maladie de Kienboeck bilatérale. J Radiol Electrol Med Nucl 31:13, 1950.
78. Ståhl F: On lunatomalacia (Kienböck's disease). A clinical and roentgenological study, especially on its pathogenesis and the late results of immobilization treatment. Acta Chir Scand Suppl 126:1, 1947.
79. Mouat TB, Wilkie J, Harding HE: Isolated fracture of the carpal semilunar and Kienböck's disease. Br J Surg 19:577, 1932.

80. Lee MLH: The intraosseous arterial pattern of the carpal lunate bone and its relation to avascular necrosis. Acta Orthop Scand 33:43, 1963.
81. Cordes E: Über die Entstehung der subchondralen Osteonekrosen. A. Die Lunatumnekrose. Bruns Beitr Klin Chir 149:28, 1930.
82. Hultén O: Über anatomische Variationen der Handgelenkknochen. Acta Radiol 9:155, 1928.
83. Hultén O: Über die Entstehung und Behandlung der Lunatummalazaie (Morbus Kienböck). Acta Chir Scand 76:121, 1935.
84. Gelberman RH, Salamon PB, Jurist JM, et al: Ulnar variance in Kienböck's disease. J Bone Joint Surg [Am] 57:674, 1975.
85. Chan KP, Huang P: Anatomic variations in radial and ulnar lengths in the wrists of Chinese. Clin Orthop 80:17, 1971.
86. Koken E-W: Anatomische Untersuchungen zum Problem der Blutversorgung des Os lunatum. Z Orthop 113:1022, 1975.
87. Köhler A: Ueber eine häufige bisher anscheinend unbekannte Erkrankung einzelner Kindlicherknochen. Munch Med Wochenschr 55:1923, 1908.
88. Waugh W: The ossification and vascularisation of the tarsal navicular and their relation to Köhler's disease. J Bone Joint Surg [Br] 40:765, 1958.
89. Karp MG: Köhler's disease of the tarsal scaphoid. An end-result study. J Bone Joint Surg 19:84, 1937.
90. McCauley RGK, Kahn PC: Osteochondritis of the tarsal navicular. Radioisotopic appearances. Radiology 123:705, 1977.
91. Froelich R: Des apophysites de croissance. Paris Med 37:430, 1929.
92. Ozonoff MB: Pediatric Orthopedic Radiology. Philadelphia, WB Saunders Co, 1979.
93. Lecène P, Mouchet A: La scaphoidite tarsienne (anatomie pathologique et pathogénie). Rev Orthop 11:105, 1924.
94. Kidner FC, Muro F: Köhler's disease of the tarsal scaphoid or os naviculare pedis retardatum. JAMA 83:1650, 1924.
95. Scaglietti O, Stringu G, Mizzau M: Plus-variant of the astragalus and subnormal scaphoid space, two important findings in Koehler's scaphoid necrosis. Acta Orthop Scand 32:499, 1962.
96. Panner HJ: An affection of the capitulum humeri resembling Calvé-Perthes disease of the hip. Acta Radiol 8:617, 1927.
97. Smith MGH: Osteochondritis of the humerus capitulum. J Bone Joint Surg [Br] 46:50, 1964.
98. Elward JF: Epiphysitis of the capitellum of the humerus. JAMA 112:705, 1939.
99. Klein EW: Osteochondrosis of the capitulum (Panner's disease). Report of a case. AJR 88:466, 1952.
100. Laurent LE, Lindström BL: Osteochondrosis of the capitulum humeri (Panner's disease). Acta Orthop Scand 26:111, 1957.
101. Heller CJ, Wiltse LL: Avascular necrosis of the capitellum humeri (Panner's disease). A report of a case. J Bone Joint Surg [Am] 42:513, 1960.
102. March HC: Osteochondritis of the capitellum (Panner's disease). AJR 51:682, 1944.
103. Adams JE: Injury to the throwing arm. A study of traumatic changes in the elbow joints of boy baseball players. Calif Med J 102:127, 1965.
104. Jacobs P: Osteochondritis dissecans of the hip. Clin Orthop 13:316, 1962.
105. Thiemann H: Juvenile Epiphysenstörungen. Fortschr Geb Roentgenstr Nuklearmed 14:79, 1909.
106. Dessecker C: Zur Epiphyseonekrose der Mittelphalangen beider Hande. Dtsch Z Chir 229:327, 1930.
107. Allison AC, Blumberg BS: Familial osteoarthropathy of the fingers. J Bone Joint Surg [Br] 40:538, 1958.
108. Cullen JC: Thiemann's disease. Osteochondrosis juvenilis of the basal epiphyses of the phalanges of the hand. Report of two cases. J Bone Joint Surg [Br] 52:532, 1970.
109. Rubinstein HM: Thiemann's disease. A brief reminder. Arthritis Rheum 18:357, 1975.
110. Giedion A: Acrodysplasias, cone-shaped epiphyses, peripheral dysostosis, Thiemann's disease, and acrodysostosis. Progr Pediatr Radiol 4:325, 1973.
111. Osgood RB: Lesions of the tibial tubercle occurring during adolescence. Boston Med Surg J 148:114, 1903.
112. Schlatter C: Verletzungen des schnabelförmigen Fortsatzes der oberen Tibiaepiphyse. Bruns Beitr Klin Chir 38:874, 1903.
113. Woolfrey BF, Chandler EF: Manifestations of Osgood-Schlatter's disease in late teenage and early adulthood. J Bone Joint Surg [Am] 42:327, 1960.
114. Stinchfield AJ: The tenosynovitis of Osgood-Schlatter disease. J Bone Joint Surg [Am] 45:1335, 1963.
115. Hulting B: Roentgenologic features of fracture of the tibial tuberosity (Osgood-Schlatter's disease). Acta Radiol 48:161, 1957.
116. Ehrenborg G, Lagergren C: Roentgenologic changes in the Osgood-Schlatter lesion. Acta Chir Scand 121:315, 1961.
117. Scotti DM, Sadhu, VK, Heimberg F, et al: Osgood-Schlatter's disease, an emphasis on soft tissue changes in roentgen diagnosis. Skel Radiol 4:21, 1979.
118. Ogden JA, Southwick WO: Osgood-Schlatter's disease and tibial tuberosity development. Clin Orthop 116:180, 1976.
119. D'Ambrosia RD, MacDonald GL: Pitfalls in the diagnosis of Osgood-Schlatter disease. Clin Orthop 110:206, 1975.
120. Lutterotti M: Beitrag zur Genese der Schlatterschen Krankheit. Z Orthop 77:160, 1947.
121. Ogden JA, Hempton RF, Southwick WO: Development of the tibial tuberosity. Anat Rec 182:431, 1975.
122. Uhry E Jr: Osgood-Schlatter disease. Arch Surg 48:406, 1944.
123. LaZerte GD, Rapp IH: Pathogenesis of Osgood-Schlatter's disease. Am J Pathol 34:803, 1958.
124. Jeffreys TE: Genu recurvatum after Osgood-Schlatter's disease. Report of a case. J Bone Joint Surg [Br] 47:298, 1965.
125. Stirling RI: Complications of Osgood-Schlatter's disease. J Bone Joint Surg [Br] 34:149, 1952.
126. Blount WP: Tibia vara. Osteochondrosis deformans tibiae. J Bone Joint Surg 19:1, 1937.
127. Shopfner CE, Coin CG: Genu varus and valgus in children. Radiology 92:723, 1969.
128. Bateson EM: Non-rachitic bowleg and knock-knee deformities in young Jamaican children. Br J Radiol 39:92, 1966.
129. Golding JSR, McNeil-Smith JDG: Observations on the etiology of tibia vara. J Bone Joint Surg [Br] 45:320, 1963.
130. Bateson EM: The relationship between Blount's disease and bow legs. Br J Radiol 41:107, 1968.
131. Bathfield CA, Beighton PH: Blount disease. A review of etiological factors in 110 patients. Clin Orthop 135:29, 1978.
132. Sibert JR, Bray PT: Probable dominant inheritance in Blount's disease. Clin Genet 11:394, 1977.
133. Langenskiöld A: Tibia vara. Osteochondrosis deformans tibiae. A survey of 23 cases. Acta Chir Scand 103:1, 1952.
134. Langenskiöld A, Riska EB: Tibia vara (osteochondrosis deformans tibiae). J Bone Joint Surg [Am] 46:1405, 1964.
135. Tachdjian MO: Pediatric Orthopedics. Philadelphia, WB Saunders Co, 1972.
136. Currarino G, Kirks DR: Lateral widening of epiphyseal plates in knees of children with bowed legs. AJR 129:309, 1977.
137. Kettelkamp DB, Chao EY: A method for quantitative analysis of medial and lateral compression forces at the knee during standing. Clin Orthop 83:202, 1972.
138. Kilburn P: A metaphysial abnormality: Report of a case with features of metaphysial dysostosis. J Bone Joint Surg [Br] 55:643, 1973.
139. Pitzen P, Marquardt W: O-Beinbildung durch umschriebene Epiphysenwachstumsstörung (Tibia-vara-Bildung). Z Orthop 69:174, 1939.
140. Scheuermann HW: Kyphosis dorsalis juvenilis. Z Orthop Chir 41:305, 1921.
141. Scheuermann H: Kyphosis juvenilis (Scheuermann's Krankheit). ROFO 53:1, 1936.
142. Sørensen KH: Scheuermann's Juvenile Kyphosis. Copenhagen, Munksgaard, 1964.
143. Alexander CJ: Scheuermann's disease. A traumatic spondylodystrophy? Skel Radiol 1:209, 1977.
144. Wassman K: Kyphosis juvenilis Scheuermann—an occupational disorder. Acta Orthop Scand 21:65, 1951.
145. Dameron TE Jr, Gulledge WH: Adolescent kyphosis. US Armed Forces Med J 4:871, 1953.
146. Bradford DS, Moe JH, Montalvo FJ, et al: Scheuermann's kyphosis and roundback deformity. Results of Milwaukee brace treatment. J Bone Joint Surg [Am] 56:740, 1974.
147. Bradford DS, Moe JH, Montalvo FJ, et al: Scheuermann's kyphosis. Results of surgical treatment by posterior spine arthrodesis in twenty-two patients. J Bone Joint Surg [Am] 57:439, 1975.
148. Butler RW: The nature and significance of vertebral osteochondritis. Proc R Soc Med 48:895, 1955.
149. Edgren W, Vainio S: Osteochondrosis juvenilis lumbalis. Acta Chir Scand Suppl 227:1, 1957.
150. Fried K: Die zervikale juvenile Osteochondrose (Scheuermannsche Krankheit). ROFO 105:69, 1966.
151. Lamb DW: Localised osteochondritis of the lumbar spine. J Bone Joint Surg [Br] 36:591, 1954.
152. Schmorl G, Junghanns H: The Human Spine in Health and Disease. Translated by EF Besemann. 2nd Ed. New York, Grune & Stratton, 1971.
153. Butler RW: Spontaneous anterior fusion of vertebral bodies. J Bone Joint Surg [Br] 53:230, 1971.
154. Knutsson F: Fusion of vertebrae following non-infectious disturbance in the zone of growth. Acta Radiol 32:404, 1949.
155. Bradford DS, Garcia A: Neurological complications in Scheuermann's disease. A case report and review of the literature. J Bone Joint Surg [Am] 51:567, 1969.
156. Wise BL, Foster JJ: Congenital spinal extradural cyst. Case report and review of the literature. J Neurosurg 12:421, 1955.
157. Van Landingham JH: Herniation of thoracic intervertebral discs with spinal cord compression in kyphosis dorsalis juvenilis (Scheuermann's disease). Case report. J Neurosurg 11:327, 1954.
158. Adelstein LJ: Spinal extradural cyst associated with kyphosis dorsalis juvenilis. J Bone Joint Surg 23:93, 1941.
159. Cloward RB, Bucy PC: Spinal extradural cyst and kyphosis dorsalis juvenilis. AJR 38:681, 1937.
160. Bradford DS, Moe JH: Scheuermann's juvenile kyphosis. A histologic study. Clin Orthop 110:45, 1975.
161. Laederer R: La dégénérescence juvénile du disque inter-vertebral. (Contribution à la pathogénèse de la maladie de Scheuermann). Schweiz Z Pathol 11:590, 1948.
162. Müller G, Gschwend N: Endokrine Störungen und Morbus Scheuermann. Arch Orthop Unfallchir 65:357, 1969.
163. Simon RS: The diagnosis and treatment of kyphosis dorsalis juvenilis (Scheuermann's kyphosis) in the early stage. J Bone Joint Surg 24:681, 1942.
164. Kemp FH, Wilson DC, Emrys-Roberts E: Social and nutritional factors in adolescent osteochondritis of the spine. Br J Soc Med 2:66, 1948.

165. Mühlbach R, Hahnel H, Cohn H: Zur Bedeutung biochemischer Parameter bei der Beurteilung der Scheuermannschen Krankheit. Med Sport *10*:331, 1970.

166. Gardemin H, Herbst W: Wirbeldeformierung bei der Adoleszentenkyphose und Osteoporose. Arch Orthop Unfallchir *59*:134, 1966.

167. Bradford DS, Brown DM, Moe JH, et al: Scheuermann's kyphosis. A form of osteoporosis? Clin Orthop *118*:10, 1976.

168. Halal F, Gledhill RB, Fraser FC: Dominant inheritance of Scheuermann's juvenile kyphosis. Am J Dis Child *132*:1105, 1978.

169. Kewalramani LS, Riggins RS, Fowler WM Jr: Scheuermann's kyphoscoliosis associated with Charcot-Marie-Tooth syndrome. Arch Phys Med Rehabil *57*:391, 1976.

170. Schmorl G: Die Pathogenese der juvenilen Kyphose. ROFO *41*:359, 1930.

171. Beadle O: The intervertebral disc. Med Res Council Spec Rep Series *161*:1, 1931.

172. Aufdermaur M: Zur Pathogenese der Scheuermannschen Krankheit. Dtsch Med Wochenschr *89*:73, 1964.

173. Aufdermaur M: Die Scheuermannsche Adoleszentenkyphose. Orthopade *2*:153, 1973.

174. Sinding-Larsen MF: A hitherto unknown affection of the patella in children. Acta Radiol *1*:171, 1921.

175. Johansson S: En forut icke beskriven sjukdom i patella. Hygiea *84*:161, 1922.

176. Wolf J: Larsen-Johansson disease of the patella. Seven new case records. Its relationship to other forms of osteochondritis. Use of male sex hormones as a new form of treatment. Br J Radiol *23*:335, 1950.

177. Medlar RC, Lyne ED: Sinding-Larsen-Johansson disease. Its etiology and natural history. J Bone Joint Surg [Am] *60*:1113, 1978.

178. Kay JF, Freiberger RH: Fragmentation of the lower pole of the patella in spastic lower extremities. Radiology *101*:97, 1971.

179. Rosenthal RK, Levine DB: Fragmentation of the distal pole of the patella in spastic cerebral palsy. J Bone Joint Surg [Am] *59*:934, 1977.

180. Green WT: Painful bipartite patella. A report of three cases. Clin Orthop *110*:197, 1975.

181. Sever JW: Apophysitis of the os calcis. NY Med J *95*:1025, 1912.

182. Allison N: Apophysitis of the os calcis. A clinical report. J Bone Joint Surg *6*:91, 1924.

183. Christie AC: Osteochondritis, or epiphysitis: A review. JAMA *87*:291, 1926.

184. Lewin P: Apophysitis of the os calcis. Surg Gynecol Obstet *41*:579, 1925.

185. Hughes ESR: Painful heels in children. Surg Gynecol Obstet *86*:64, 1948.

186. Shopfner CE, Coin CG: Effect of weight-bearing on the appearance and development of the secondary calcaneal epiphysis. Radiology *86*:201, 1966.

187. Van Neck M: Ostéochondrite du pubis. Arch Franco-Belges Chir *27*:238, 1924.

188. Caffey J, Ross SE: The ischiopubic synchondrosis in healthy children: Some normal roentgenologic findings. AJR *76*:488, 1956.

189. Köhler A: Ueber eine häufige, bisher anscheinend unbekannte Erkrankung einzelner kindlicher Knochen. Munch Med Wochenschr *55*:1923, 1908.

190. Mandl F: Die "Schlatter'sche Krankheit" als "Systemerkrankung." Bruns Beitr Klin Chir *126*:707, 1922.

191. Boldero JL, Mitchell GP: Osteochondritis of the superior tibial epiphysis. J Bone Joint Surg [Br] *36*:114, 1954.

192. Siffert RS, Arkin AM: Post-traumatic aseptic necrosis of the distal tibial epiphysis. J Bone Joint Surg [Am] *32*:691, 1950.

193. Meilstrap DB: Osteochondritis of the internal cuneiform, bilateral. Case report. AJR *58*:329, 1947.

194. Iselin H: Wachstumsbeschwerden zur Zeit der Knöchernen Entwicklung der Tuberositas metatarsi quinti. Dtsch Z Chir *117*:529, 1912.

195. Burns BH: Osteochondritis juvenilis of the lower ulnar epiphysis. Proc R Soc Med *24*:912, 1931.

196. Mauclaire P: Epiphysitis der Metakarpusköpfchen mit Hohlbildung der Hand. ROFO *37*:425, 1928.

197. Ellman H: Unusual affections of the preadolescent elbow. J Bone Joint Surg [Am] *49*:203, 1967.

198. Blakemore ME, Harrison MHM: A prospective study of children with untreated Catterall Group 1 Perthes' disease. J Bone Joint Surg [Br] *61*:329, 1979.

199. Bohr HH: Skeletal maturation in Legg-Calvé-Perthes' disease. Int Orthop (SICOT) *2*:277, 1979.

200. Gauthier G, Elbaz R: Freiberg's infraction: A subchondral bone fatigue fracture. A new surgical treatment. Clin Orthop *142*:93, 1979.

201. Beckenbaugh RD, Shives TC, Dobyns JH, et al: Kienböck's disease: The natural history of Kienböck's disease and consideration of lunate fractures. Clin Orthop *149*:98, 1980.

202. Gelberman RH, Bauman TD, Menon J, et al: The vascularity of the lunate bone and Kienböck's disease. J Hand Surg *5*:272, 1980.

203. Weston WJ: Kohler's disease of the tarsal scaphoid. Australas Radiol *22*:332, 1978.

204. Mital MA, Matza RA, Cohen J: The so-called unresolved Osgood-Schlatter lesion. J Bone Joint Surg [Am] *62*:732, 1980.

205. Catonné Y, Pacault C, Azaloux H, et al: Aspects radiologiques de la maladie de Blount. J Radiol *61*:171, 1980.

206. Bjersand AJ: Juvenile kyphosis in identical twins. AJR *134*:598, 1980.

207. Guelpa G, Chamay A, Lagier R: Bilateral osteochondritis dissecans of the carpal scaphoid. Int Orthop (SICOT) *4*:25, 1980.

208. Gershuni DH, Axer A, Hendel D: Arthrography as an aid to diagnosis, prognosis, and therapy in Legg-Calvé-Perthes' disease. Acta Orthop Scand *51*:505, 1980.

209. Théron J: Angiography in Legg-Calvé-Perthes disease. Radiology *135*:81, 1980.

210. Murray IPC: Bone scanning in the child and young adult. Part II. Skel Radiol *5*:65, 1980.

211. Morley TR, Short MD, Dowsett DJ: Femoral head activity in Perthes' disease: Clinical evaluation of a quantitative technique for estimating tracer uptake. J Nucl Med *19*:884, 1978.

212. Fisher RL, Roderique JW, Brown DC, et al: The relationship of isotopic bone imaging findings to prognosis in Legg-Perthes disease. Clin Orthop *150*:23, 1980.

213. Sutherland AD, Savage JP, Paterson DC, et al: The nuclide bonescan in the diagnosis and management of Perthes' disease. J Bone Joint Surg [Br] *62*:300, 1980.

214. Heikkinen E, Lanning P, Suramo I, et al: The venous drainage of the femoral neck as a prognostic sign in Perthes' disease. Acta Orthop Scand *51*:501, 1980.

215. Langenskiöld A: Changes in the capital growth plate and the proximal femoral metaphysis in Legg-Calvé-Perthes disease. Clin Orthop *150*:110, 1980.

216. Kelly FB Jr, Canale ST, Jones RR: Legg-Calvé-Perthes disease. J Bone Joint Surg [Am] *62*:400, 1980.

217. Wynne-Davies R: Some etiologic factors in Perthes' disease. Clin Orthop *150*:12, 1980.

218. Fasting OJ, Bjerkreim I, Langeland N, et al: Scintigraphic evaluation of the severity of Perthes' disease in the initial stage. Acta Orthop Scand *51*:655, 1980.

219. Katz JF, Siffert RS: Osteochondritis dissecans in association with Legg-Calvé-Perthes disease. Int Orthop (SICOT) *3*:189, 1979.

220. Milgram JW: Synovial osteochondromatosis in association with Legg-Calvé-Perthes disease. Clin Orthop *145*:179, 1979.

221. Nevelös AB: Bilateral Perthes' disease. Acta Orthop Scand *51*:649, 1980.

222. Harrison MHM, Blakemore ME: A study of the "normal" hip in children with unilateral Perthes' disease. J Bone Joint Surg [Br] *62*:31, 1980.

223. Herring JA, Lundeen MA, Wenger DR: Minimal Perthes' disease. J Bone Joint Surg [Br] *62*:25, 1980.

224. Inoue A, Ono K, Takaoka K, et al: A comparative study of histology in Perthes' disease and idiopathic avascular necrosis of the femoral head in adults (IANF). Int Orthop (SICOT) *4*:39, 1980.

225. Zayer M: Osteoarthritis following Blount's disease. Int Orthop (SICOT) *4*:63, 1980.

226. Hardcastle PH, Ross R, Hamalainen M, et al: Catterall grouping of Perthes' disease. J Bone Joint Surg [Br] *62*:428, 1980.

227. Barnes, JM: Premature epiphysial closure in Perthes' disease. J Bone Joint Surg [Br] *62*:432, 1980.

228. Siffert RS: Classification of the osteochondroses. Clin Orthop *158*:10, 1981.

229. Omer GE Jr: Primary articular osteochondroses. Clin Orthop *158*:33, 1981.

230. Katz JF: Nonarticular osteochondroses. Clin Orthop *158*:70, 1981.

231. Duthie RB, Houghton GR: Constitutional aspects of the osteochondroses. Clin Orthop *158*:19, 1981.

232. Douglas G, Rang M: The role of trauma in the pathogenesis of the osteochondroses. Clin Orthop *158*:28, 1981.

233. Siffert RS: The osteochondroses. Clin Orthop *158*:2, 1981.

234. Perthes GC: Concerning arthritis deformans juvenilis. Clin Orthop *158*:5, 1981.

235. Catterall A: Legg-Calvé-Perthes Disease. Edinburgh, Churchill Livingstone, 1982.

236. Butler RW: Transitory arthritis of the hip joint in childhood. Br Med J *1*:951, 1933.

237. Lovett RW, Morse JL: A transient or ephemeral form of hip disease, with a report of cases. Boston Med Surg J *127*:161, 1892.

238. Edwards EC: Transient synovitis of the hip joints in children. JAMA *148*:30, 1952.

239. Valderama JAF: The observation hip and its late sequela. J Bone Joint Surg [Br] *45*:462, 1963.

240. Miller OL: Acute transient epiphysitis of the hip joint. JAMA *96*:575, 1931.

241. Vidigal EC, DaSilva OL: Observation hip. Acta Orthop Scand *52*:191, 1981.

242. Sharwood PF: The irritable hip syndrome in children. A long-term follow-up. Acta Orthop Scand *52*:633, 1981.

243. Wolinski AP, McCall IW, Evans G, et al: Femoral neck growth deformity following the irritable hip syndrome. Br J Radiol *57*:773, 1984.

244. Jacobs BW: Synovitis of the hip in children and its significance. Pediatrics *47*:558, 1971.

245. Carty H, Maxted M, Fielding JA, et al: Isotope scanning in the "irritable hip syndrome." Skel Radiol *11*:32, 1984.

246. Smith SR, Ions GK, Gregg PJ: The radiological features of the metaphysis in Perthes disease. J Pediatr Orthop *2*:401, 1982.

247. Haag M, Reichelt A: Widening of the teardrop distance in early stages of Legg-Calvé-Perthes disease compared with the late fate. Arch Orthop Trauma Surg *100*:163, 1982.

248. Apley AG, Wientroub S: The sagging rope sign in Perthes' disease and allied disorders. J Bone Joint Surg [Br] *63*:43, 1981.

249. Catterall A: Legg-Calvé-Perthes syndrome. Clin Orthop *158*:41, 1981.

250. Bowen JR, Schreiber FC, Foster BK, et al: Premature femoral neck physeal closure in Perthes' disease. Clin Orthop *171*:24, 1982.

251. Siffert RS: Patterns of deformity of the developing hip. Clin Orthop *160*:14, 1981.

252. Fernbach SK, Poznanski AK, Kelikian AS, et al: Greater trochanteric overgrowth: Development and surgical correction. Radiology *154*:661, 1985.

253. Crossan JF, Wynne-Davies R, Fulford GE: Bilateral failure of the capital femoral epiphysis: Bilateral Perthes disease, multiple epiphyseal dysplasia,

pseudoachondroplasia, and spondyloepiphyseal dysplasia congenita and tarda. J Pediatr Orthop 3:297, 1983.

254. Osterman K, Lindholm TS: Osteochondritis dissecans following Perthes' disease. Clin Orthop 152:247, 1980.

255. Bowen JR, Schmidt T: Osteochondroma of the femoral neck in Perthes disease. J Pediatr Orthop 3:28, 1983.

256. Clarke NMP, Harrison MHM, Keret D: The sagging rope sign: A critical appraisal. J Bone Joint Surg [Br] 65:285, 1983.

257. Salter RB: The present status of treatment for Legg-Perthes disease. J Bone Joint Surg [Am] 66:961, 1984.

258. Stulberg SD, Cooperman DR, Wallensten R: The natural history of Legg-Calvé-Perthes disease. J Bone Joint Surg [Am] 63:1095, 1981.

259. Green NE, Beauchamp RD, Griffin PP: Epiphyseal extrusion as a prognostic index in Legg-Calvé-Perthes disease. J Bone Joint Surg [Am] 63:900, 1981.

260. Van Dam BE, Crider RJ, Noyes JD, et al: Determination of the Catterall classification in Legg-Calvé-Perthes disease. J Bone Joint Surg [Am] 63:906, 1981.

261. Yucel M: Die Wirkung des metaphysaren Befalls beim Morbus Perthes und seine Bedeutung fur die definitive Huftkopfentwicklung. Z Orthop 118:889, 1980.

262. Danielsson L, Pettersson H, Sunden G: Early assessment of prognosis in Perthes' disease. Acta Orthop Scand 53:605, 1982.

263. Clarke NMP, Harrison MHM: Painful sequelae of coxa plana. J Bone Joint Surg [Am] 65:13, 1983.

264. Salter RB, Thompson GH: Legg-Calvé-Perthes disease. The prognostic significance of the subchondral fracture and a two-group classification of the femoral head involvement. J Bone Joint Surg [Am] 66:479, 1984.

265. Keret D, Harrison MHM, Clarke NMP, et al: Coxa plana—the fate of the physis. J Bone Joint Surg [Am] 66:870, 1984.

266. McAndrew MP, Weinstein SL: A long-term follow-up of Legg-Calvé-Perthes disease. J Bone Joint Surg [Am] 66:860, 1984.

267. Shapiro F: Legg-Calvé-Perthes disease. A study of lower extremity length discrepancies and skeletal maturation. Acta Orthop Scand 53:437, 1982.

268. Gallagher JM, Weiner DS, Cook AJ: When is arthrography indicated in Legg-Calvé-Perthes disease? J Bone Joint Surg [Am] 65:900, 1983.

269. LaMont RL, Muz J, Heilbronner D, et al: Quantitative assessment of femoral head involvement in Legg-Calvé-Perthes disease. J Bone Joint Surg [Am] 63:746, 1981.

270. Bensahel H, Bok B, Cavailloles F, et al: Bone scintigraphy in Perthes disease. J Pediatr Orthop 3:302, 1983.

271. Deutsch SD, Gandsman EJ, Spraragen SC: Quantitative regional blood-flow analysis and its clinical application during routine bone-scanning. J Bone Joint Surg [Am] 63:295, 1981.

272. Kloiber R, Pavlosky W, Portner O, et al: Bone scintigraphy of hip joint effusions in children. AJR 140:995, 1983.

273. De Camargo FP, De Godoy RM Jr, Tovo R: Angiography in Perthes' disease. Clin Orthop 191:216, 1984.

274. Scoles PV, Yoon YS, Makley JT, et al: Nuclear magnetic resonance imaging in Legg-Calvé-Perthes disease. J Bone Joint Surg [Am] 66:1357, 1984.

275. Harrison MHM, Burwell RG: Perthes' disease: A concept of pathogenesis. Clin Orthop 156:115, 1981.

276. Iwasaki K: The role of blood vessels within the ligamentum teres in Perthes' disease. Clin Orthop 159:248, 1981.

277. Lucht U, Bunger C, Krebs B, et al: Blood flow in the juvenile hip in relation to changes of the intraarticular pressure. An experimental investigation in dogs. Acta Orthop Scand 54:182, 1983.

278. Kemp HBS: Perthes' disease: The influence of intracapsular tamponade on the circulation in the hip joint of the dog. Clin Orthop 156:105, 1981.

279. Green NE, Griffin PP: Intra-osseous venous pressure in Legg-Perthes disease. J Bone Joint Surg [Am] 64:666, 1982.

280. Stromqvist B, Wingstrand H, Egund N, et al: Traumatic hip joint tamponade. Two cases with femoral head ischemia. Acta Orthop Scand 56:81, 1985.

281. Launder WJ, Hungerford DS, Jones LH: Hemodynamics of the femoral head. J Bone Joint Surg [Am] 63:442, 1981.

282. Ponseti IV, Maynard JA, Weinstein SL, et al: Legg-Calvé-Perthes disease. Histochemical and ultrastructural observations of the epiphyseal cartilage and physis. J Bone Joint Surg [Am] 65:797, 1983.

283. Sedlin ED: Early epiphyseal fusion in Freiberg's infraction. Foot Ankle 3:297, 1983.

284. Morgan RF, McCue FC III: Bilateral Kienböck's disease. J Hand Surg 8:928, 1983.

285. Steinhauser J, Posival H: Doppelseitige Mondbeinnekrose. Ein Beitrag zur Pathogenese. Z Orthop 120:151, 1982.

286. Razemon JP: La radiologie de la maladie de Kienböck. Ann Radiol 25:353, 1982.

287. Hallett JP, Motta GR: Tendon ruptures in the hand with particular reference to attrition ruptures in the carpal canal. Hand 14:283, 1982.

288. Steinhauser J, Abele H, Schettler G: Anatomisch-morphologische Studien zur sogenannten Minusvariante der Elle am Handgelenk. Z Orthop 111:36, 1973.

289. Palmer AK, Glisson RR, Werner FW, et al: Relationship between ulnar variance and triangular fibrocartilage complex thickness. J Hand Surg [Am] 9:681, 1984.

290. Palmer AK, Werner FW, Eng MM: Biomechanics of the distal radioulnar joint. Clin Orthop 187:26, 1984.

291. Voorhees DR, Daffner RH, Nunley JA, et al: Carpal ligamentous descriptions and negative ulnar variance. Skel Radiol 13:257, 1985.

292. Armistead RB, Linscheid RL, Dobyns JH, et al: Ulnar lengthening in the treatment of Kienböck's disease. J Bone Joint Surg [Am] 64:170, 1982.

293. Stark HH, Zemel NP, Ashworth CR: Use of a hard-carved silicone-rubber spacer for advanced Kienböck's disease. J Bone Joint Surg [Am] 63:1359, 1981.

294. Williams GA, Cowell HR: Köhler's disease of the tarsal navicular. Clin Orthop 158:53, 1981.

295. Singer KM, Roy SP: Osteochondrosis of the humeral capitellum. Am J Sports Med 12:351, 1984.

296. Melo-Gomes JA, Melo-Gomes E, Viana-Queiros M: Thiemann's disease. J Rheumatol 8:462, 1981.

297. Gewanter H, Baum J: Thiemann's disease. J Rheumatol 12:150, 1985.

298. Ogden JA: Radiology of postnatal skeletal development. X. Patella and tibial tuberosity. Skel Radiol 11:246, 1984.

299. Desarnaud M, Lebarbier P, Cahuzac J-P: The arterial blood supply to the tibial tuberosity in the foetus. Anat Clin 3:55, 1982.

300. Zimbler S, Merkow S: Genu recurvatum: A possible complication after Osgood-Schlatter disease. Case report. J Bone Joint Surg [Am] 66:1129, 1984.

301. Bowers KD Jr: Patellar tendon avulsion as a complication of Osgood-Schlatter's disease. Am J Sports Med 9:356, 1981.

302. O'Neill DA, MacEwen GD: Early roentgenographic evaluation of bow-legged children. J Pediatr Orthop 2:547, 1982.

303. Langenskiöld A: Tibia vara: Osteochondrosis deformans tibiae. Blount's disease. Clin Orthop 158:77, 1981.

304. Levine AM, Drennan JC: Physiological bowing and tibia vara. The metaphyseal-diaphyseal angle in the measurement of bowleg deformities. J Bone Joint Surg [Am] 64:1158, 1982.

305. Smith CF: Tibia vara (Blount's disease). J Bone Joint Surg [Am] 64:630, 1982.

306. Erlacher P: Deformierende Prozesse der Epiphysengegend bei Kindern. Arch Orthop Unfallchir 20:81, 1922.

307. Wenger DR, Mickelson M, Maynard JA: The evolution and histopathology of adolescent tibia vara. J Pediatr Orthop 4:78, 1984.

308. Thompson GH, Carter JR, Smith CW: Late-onset tibia vara: A comparative analysis. J Pediatr Orthop 4:185, 1984.

309. Lings S, Mikkelsen L: Scheuermann's disease with low localization. A problem of under-diagnosis. Scand J Rehabil Med 14:77, 1982.

310. Ryan MD, Taylor TKF: Acute spinal cord compression in Scheuermann's disease. J Bone Joint Surg [Br] 64:409, 1982.

311. Cleveland RH, Delong GR: The relationship of juvenile lumbar disc disease and Scheuermann's disease. Pediatr Radiol 10:161, 1981.

312. Montgomery SP, Erwin WE: Scheuermann's kyphosis—long-term results of Milwaukee brace treatment. Spine 6:5, 1981.

313. McCall IW, Park WM, O'Brien JP, et al: Acute traumatic intraosseous disc herniation. Spine 10:134, 1985.

314. Deacon P, Berkin CR, Dickson RA: Combined idiopathic kyphosis and scoliosis. An analysis of the lateral spinal curvatures associated with Scheuermann's disease. J Bone Joint Surg [Br] 67:189, 1985.

315. Dickson RA, Lawton JO, Archer IA, et al: The pathogenesis of idiopathic scoliosis. Biplanar spinal asymmetry. J Bone Joint Surg [Br] 66:8, 1984.

316. Mau H: Die Differentialdiagnose der beginnenden Skoliose beim M. Scheuermann gegenüber der idiopathischen Skoliose. Z Orthop 120:58, 1982.

317. Burner WL III, Badger VM, Sherman FC: Osteoporosis and acquired back deformities. J Pediatr Orthop 2:383, 1982.

318. Bradford DS: Vertebral osteochondrosis (Scheuermann's kyphosis). Clin Orthop 158:83, 1981.

319. Aufdermaur M: Juvenile kyphosis (Scheuermann's disease): Radiography, histology, and pathogenesis. Clin Orthop 154:166, 1981.

320. Ippolito E, Ponseti IV: Juvenile kyphosis. Histological and histochemical studies. J Bone Joint Surg [Am] 63:175, 1981.

321. Hensal F, Nelson T, Pavlov H, et al: Bilateral patellar fractures from indirect trauma. A case report. Clin Orthop 178:207, 1983.

322. Heckman JD, Alkire CC: Distal patellar pole fractures. A proposed common mechanism of injury. Am J Sports Med 12:424, 1984.

323. Sandomenico C, Tamburrini O: Bilateral accessory ossification center of the ischio-pubic synchondrosis. Follow-up over a three year period. Pediatr Radiol 10:233, 1981.

324. Cawley K, Dvorak A, Wilmot M: Normal anatomic variant: Scintigraphy of the ischiopubic synchondrosis. J Nucl Med 24:14, 1983.

325. Jarvis J, McIntyre W, Udjus K, et al: Osteomyelitis of the ischio-pubic synchondrosis. J Pediatr Orthop 5:163, 1985.

326. Niethard FU: Die Osteochondrose und Osteochondronekrose des Huftpfannendaches. Z Orthop 122:94, 1984.

327. Goblyos P: Aseptische-Osteochondronekrose des Os Cuneiform II. ROFO 133:447, 1980.

328. Lyritis G: Developmental disorders of the proximal epiphysis of the hallux. Skel Radiol 10:250, 1983.

329. Clarke NMP, Blakemore ME, Thompson AG: Osteochondritis of the trochlear epiphysis. J Pediatr Orthop 3:601, 1983.

330. Hunter L, O'Connor G: Traction apophysitis of the olecranon. Am J Sports Med 8:51, 1980.

331. Danielsson LG, Hedlund ST, Henricson AS: Apophysitis of the olecranon. A report of four cases. Acta Orthop Scand 54:777, 1983.

332. Preiser G: Eine typische posttraumatische und zur Spontanfraktur fuhrende Ostitis des Naviculare carpi. Fortschr Geb Roentgenstr Nuklearmed 15:189, 1910.

333. Bray TJ, McCarroll HR Jr: Preiser's disease: A case report. J Hand Surg [Am] 9:730, 1984.

334. Ekerot L, Eiken O: Idiopathic avascular necrosis of the scaphoid. Case report. Scand J Plast Reconstr Surg 15:69, 1981.

335. Allen PR: Idiopathic avascular necrosis of the scaphoid. A report of two cases. J Bone Joint Surg [Br] 65:333, 1983.

336. Friedrich H: Über ein Nocht nicht Beschriebenes, der Perthesschen erkrankung Analoges, Krankheitsbild des sternalen Clavikelendes. Dtsch Zeitsch Chir 187:385, 1924.

337. Fischel RE, Bernstein D: Friedrich's disease. Br J Radiol 48:318, 1975.

338. Levy M, Goldberg I, Fischel RE, et al: Friedrich's disease. Aseptic necrosis of the sternal end of the clavicle. J Bone Joint Surg [Br] 63:539, 1981.

339. Schumacher R, Muller U, Schuster W: Seltene lokalisationen juveniler Osteochondrosen. Radiologe 21:165, 1981.

340. Drewes J, Gunther D: Morbus Friedrich. ROFO 136:213, 1982.

341. Jurik AG, DeCarvalho A, Graudal H: Sclerotic changes of the sternal end of the clavicle. Clin Radiol 36:23, 1985.

342. Brower AC: The osteochondroses. Orthop Clin North Am 14:99, 1983.

343. Wingstrand H, Egund N, Carlin NO, et al: Intracapsular pressure in transient synovitis of the hip. Acta Orthop Scand 56:204, 1985.

344. Wingstrand H, Bauer GGC, Brismar J, et al: Transient ischaemia of the proximal femoral epiphysis in the child. Interpretation of bone scintigraphy for diagnosis in hip pain. Acta Orthop Scand 56:197, 1985.

345. Silverman FN: Lesions of the femoral neck in Legg-Perthes disease. AJR 144:1249, 1985.

346. Filipe G, Roy-Camille MY, Carlioz H, et al: L'osteochondrite dissequante de la hanche dans la maladie de Legg-Perthes-Calvé. Rev Chir Orthop 71:55, 1985.

347. Kallio P, Ryöppy S, Jappinen S, et al: Ultrasonography in hip disease in children. Acta Orthop Scand 56:367, 1985.

348. Bluemm RG, Falke THM, Ziedses des Plantes BG Jr, et al: Early Legg-Perthes disease (ischemic necrosis of the femoral head) demonstrated by magnetic resonance imaging. Skel Radiol 14:95, 1985.

349. O'Sullivan M, O'Rourke SK, MacAuley P: Legg-Calvé-Perthes disease in a family: Genetic or environmental. Clin Orthop 199:179, 1985.

350. Kujala UM, Kvist M, Heinonen O: Osgood-Schlatter's disease in adolescent athletes. Retrospective study of incidence and duration. Am J Sports Med 13:236, 1985.

351. Gumppenberg ST, Jakob RP, Engelhardt P: Beeinflubt der M. Osgood-Schlatter die Position der Patella? Z Orthop 122:798, 1984.

352. Leeson MC, Weiner DS: Osteochondrosis of the tarsal cuneiforms. Clin Orthop 196:260, 1985.

353. Wingstrand H: Transient synovitis of the hip in the child. Acta Orthop Scand (Suppl) 219:7, 1986.

354. Rosenborg M, Mortensson W: The validity of radiographic assessment of childhood transient synovitis of the hip. Acta Radiol (Diagn) 27:85, 1986.

355. Adam R, Hendry GMA, Moss J, et al: Arthrosonography of the irritable hip in childhood: A review of 1 year's experience. Br J Radiol 59:205, 1986.

356. Almquist EE: Kienbock's disease. Clin Orthop 202:68, 1986.

357. Miki T, Yamamuro T, Kotoura Y, et al: Rupture of the extensor tendons of the fingers. Report of three unusual cases. J Bone Joint Surg [Am] 68:610, 1986.

358. Schantz K, Rasmussen F: Thiemann's finger or toe disease. Follow-up of seven cases. Acta Orthop Scand 57:91, 1986.

359. Van der Laan JG, Thijn CJP: Ivory and dense epiphyses of the hand: Thiemann's disease in three sisters. Skel Radiol 15:117, 1986.

360. Ogata K, Sugioka Y, Urano Y, et al: Idiopathic osteonecrosis of the first metatarsal sesamoid. Skel Radiol 15:141, 1986.

361. Chacko V, Joseph B, Seetharam B: Perthes' disease in South India. Clin Orthop 209:95, 1986.

362. Vegter J: The influence of joint posture on intra-articular pressure. A study of transient synovitis and Perthes' disease. J Bone Joint Surg [Br] 69:71, 1987.

363. Kallio P, Ryöppy S, Kunnamo I: Transient synovitis and Perthes' disease. Is there an aetiological connection? J Bone Joint Surg [Br] 68:808, 1986.

364. Mukamel M, Litmanovitch M, Yosipovich Z, et al: Legg-Calve-Perthes disease following transient synovitis. How often? Clin Pediatr 24:629, 1985.

365. Arie E, Johnson F, Harrison MHM, et al: Femoral head shape in Perthes' disease. Is the contralateral hip abnormal? Clin Orthop 209:77, 1986.

366. Bowen JR, Kumar VP, Joyce JJ III, et al: Osteochondritis dissecans following Perthes' disease. Arthroscopic-operative treatment. Clin Orthop 209:49, 1986.

367. Christensen F, Soballe K, Ejsted R, et al: The Catterall classification of Perthes' disease: An assessment of reliability. J Bone Joint Surg [Br] 68:614, 1986.

368. Paterson D, Savage JP: The nuclide bone scan in the diagnosis of Perthes' disease. Clin Orthop 209:23, 1986.

369. Egund N, Wingstrand H, Forsberg L, et al: Computed tomography and ultrasonography for diagnosis of hip joint effusion in children. Acta Orthop Scand 57:211, 1986.

370. Rydholm U, Wingstrand H, Egund N, et al: Sonography, arhroscopy, and intracapsular pressure in juvenile chronic arthritis of the hip. Acta Orthop Scand 57:295, 1986.

371. Rayner PHW, Schwalbe SL, Hall DJ: An assessment of endocrine function in boys with Perthes' disease. Clin Orthop 209:124, 1986.

372. Kristensen SS, Thomassen E, Christensen F: Ulnar variance in Kienbock's disease. J Hand Surg [Br] 11:258, 1986.

373. Koenig H, Lucas D, Meissner R: The wrist: A preliminary report on high-resolution MR Imaging. Radiology 160:463, 1986.

374. Klein DM, Weiss RL, Allen JE: Scheuermann's dorsal kyphosis and spinal cord compression: Case report. Neurosurgery 18:628, 1986.

375. Ippolito E, Bellocci M, Montanaro A, et al: Juvenile kyphosis: An ultrastructural study. J Pediatr Orthop 5:315, 1985.

376. Lehman RC, Gregg JR, Torg E: Iselin's disease. Am J Sports Med 14:494, 1986.

377. Thompson GH, Salter RB: Legg-Calvé-Perthes disease. Current concepts and controversies. Orthop Clin North Am 18:617, 1987.

378. Wenger DR, Ward WT, Herring JA: Legg-Calvé-Perthes disease. J Bone Joint Surg [Am] 73:778, 1991.

379. Landin LA, Danielsson LG, Wattsgärd C: Transient synovitis of the hip. Its incidence, epidemiology and relation to Perthes' disease. J Bone Joint Surg [Br] 69:238, 1987.

380. Egund N, Hasegawa Y, Pettersson H, et al: Conventional radiography in transient synovitis of the hip in children. Acta Radiol 28:193, 1987.

381. Lohmander LS, Wingstrand H, Heinegård D: Transient synovitis of the hip in the child: Increased levels of proteoglycan fragments in joint fluid. J Orthop Res 6:420, 1988.

382. Erken EHW, Katz K: Irritable hip and Perthes' disease. J Pediatr Orthop 10:322, 1990.

383. Jones DA: Irritable hip and campylobacter infection. J Bone Joint Surg [Br] 71:227, 1989.

384. Hasegawa Y, Wingstrand H, Gustafson T: Scintimetry in transient synovitis of the hip in the child. Acta Orthop Scand 59:520, 1988.

385. Royle SG, Galasko CSB: The irritable hip. Scintigraphy in 192 children. Acta Orthop Scand 63:25, 1992.

386. Miralles M, Gonzales G, Pulpeiro JR, et al: Sonography of the painful hip in children: 500 consecutive cases. AJR 152:579, 1989.

387. Bickerstaff DR, Neal LM, Booth AJ, et al: Ultrasound examination of the irritable hip. J Bone Joint Surg [Br] 72:549, 1990.

388. Futami T, Kasahara Y, Suzuki S, et al: Ultrasonography in transient synovitis and early Perthes' disease. J Bone Joint Surg [Br] 73:635, 1991.

389. Pay NT, Singer WS, Bartal E: Hip pain in three children accompanied by transient abnormal findings on MR images. Radiology 171:147, 1989.

390. Kallio PE: Coxa magna following transient synovitis of the hip. Clin Orthop 228:49, 1988.

391. Hoffinger SA, Rab GT, Salamon PB: "Metaphyseal" cysts in Legg-Calvé-Perthes' disease. J Pediatr Orthop 11:301, 1991.

392. Joseph B: Morphological changes in the acetabulum in Perthes' disease. J Bone Joint Surg [Br] 71:756, 1989.

393. Salter RB, Thompson GH: Legg-Calvé-Perthes disease: The prognostic significance of the subchondral fracture and a two-group classification of the femoral head involvement. J Bone Joint Surg [Am] 66:479, 1984.

394. Herring JA, Neustadt JB, Williams JJ, et al: The lateral pillar classification of Legg-Calvé-Perthes disease. J Pediatr Orthop 12:143, 1992.

395. Simmons ED, Graham HK, Szalai JP: Interobserver variability in grading Perthes' disease. J Bone Joint Surg [Br] 72:202, 1990.

396. Dominguez R, OH KS, Young LW, et al: Acute chondrolysis complicating Legg-Calvé-Perthes disease. Skel Radiol 16:377, 1987.

397. Rowe SM, Kim HS, Yoon TR: Osteochondritis dissecans in Perthes' disease. Report of 7 cases. Acta Orthop Scand 60:545, 1989.

398. Martinez AG, Weinstein SL: Recurrent Legg-Calvé-Perthes disease. Case review and review of the literature. J Bone Joint Surg [Am] 73:1081, 1991.

399. Sponseller PD, Desai SS, Millis MB: Abnormalities of proximal femoral growth after severe Perthes' disease. J Bone Joint Surg [Br] 71:610, 1989.

400. Ippolito E, Tudisco C, Farsetti P: The long-term prognosis of unilateral Perthes' disease. J Bone Joint Surg [Br] 69:243, 1987.

401. Kamegaya M, Moriya H, Tsuchiya K, et al: Arthrography of early Perthes' disease. Swelling of the ligamentum teres as a cause of subluxation. J Bone Joint Surg [Br] 71:413, 1989.

402. Suzuki S, Awaya G, Okada Y, et al: Examination by ultrasound of Legg-Calvé-Perthes disease. Clin Orthop 220:130, 1987.

403. Pinto MR, Peterson HA, Berquist TH: Magnetic resonance imaging in early diagnosis of Legg-Calvé-Perthes disease. J Pediatr Orthop 9:19, 1989.

404. Egund N, Wingstrand H: Legg-Calvé-Perthes disease: Imaging with MR. Radiology 179:89, 1991.

405. Bos CFA, Bloem JL, Bloem RM: Sequential magnetic resonance imaging in Perthes' disease. J Bone Joint Surg [Br] 73:219, 1991.

406. Rix J, Maas R, Eggers-Stroeder G, et al: M. Legg-Calvé-Perthes. Wertigkeit der MRT in der Frühdiagnostik und Verlaufsbeurteilung. Fortschr Rontgenstr 156:77, 1992.

407. Ranner G, Ebner F, Fotter R, et al: Magnetic resonance imaging in children with acute hip pain. Pediatr Radiol 20:67, 1989.

408. Rush BH, Bramson RT, Ogden JA: Legg-Calvé-Perthes disease: Detection of cartilaginous and synovial changes with MR imaging. Radiology 167:473, 1988.

409. Kristmundsdottir F, Burwell RG, Harrison MHM: Delayed skeletal maturation in Perthes' disease. Acta Orthop Scand 58:277, 1987.

410. Hall AJ, Barker DJP, Dangerfield PH, et al: Small feet and Perthes' disease. A survey in Liverpool. J Bone Joint Surg [Br] 70:611, 1988.

411. Gordon I, Peters AM, Nunn R: The symptomatic hip in childhood: scintigraphic findings in the presence of a normal radiograph. Skel Radiol 16:383, 1987.

412. Marchal GJ, Van Holsbeeck MT, Raes M, et al: Transient synovitis of the hip in children: Role of US. Radiology 162:825, 1987.

413. Vegter J, Lubsen Ch C: Fractional necrosis of the femoral head epiphysis after

transient increase in joint pressure. An experimental study in juvenile rabbits. J Bone Joint Surg [Br] 69:530, 1987.

414. Vegter J: The influence of joint posture on intra-articular pressure. A study of transient synovitis and Perthes' disease. J Bone Joint Surg [Br] 69:71, 1987.

415. Khermosh O, Wientroub S: Dysplasia epiphysealis capitis femoris. Meyer's dysplasia. J Bone Joint Surg [Br] 73:621, 1991.

416. Andersen PE Jr, Schantz K, Bollerslev J, et al: Bilateral femoral head dysplasia and osteochondritis. Acta Radiol 29:705, 1988.

417. Ozonoff MB, Ziter FMH Jr: The femoral head notch. Skel Radiol 16:19, 1987.

418. Fu FH, Gomez W: Bilateral avascular necrosis of the first metatarsal head in adolescence. A case report. Clin Orthop 246:282, 1989.

419. Jensen EL, De Carvalho A: A normal variant simulating Freiberg's disease. Acta Radiol 28:85, 1987.

420. Rasmussen F, Schantz K: Lunatomalacia in a child. Acta Orthop Scand 57:82, 1986.

421. Yoshida T, Tada K, Yamamoto K, et al: Aged-onset Kienböck's disease. Arch Orthop Trauma Surg 109:241, 1990.

422. Mirabello SC, Rosenthal DI, Smith RJ: Correlation of clinical and radiographic findings in Kienböck's disease. J Hand Surg [Am] 12:1049, 1987.

423. Bourne MH, Linscheid RL, Dobyns JH: Concomitant scapholunate dissociation and Kienböck's disease. J Hand Surg [Am] 16:460, 1991.

424. Rasmussen F, Schantz K: Radiologic aspects of lunatomalacia. Europ J Radiol 7:199, 1987.

425. Chen W-S, Shih C-H: Ulnar variance and Kienböck's disease. An investigation in Taiwan. Clin Orthop 255:124, 1990.

426. Almquist EE: Kienböck's disease. Hand Clinics 3:141, 1987.

427. Kristensen SS, Søballe K: Kienböck's disease—the influence of arthrosis on ulnar variance measurements. J Hand Surg [Br] 12:301, 1987.

428. Steyers CM, Blair WF: Measuring ulnar variance: a comparison of techniques. J Hand Surg [Am] 14:607, 1989.

429. Mann FA, Wilson AJ, Gilula LA: Radiographic evaluation of the wrist: What does the hand surgeon want to know? Radiology 184:15, 1992.

430. Werner FW, Murphy DJ, Palmer AK: Pressures in the distal radioulnar joint: Effects of surgical procedures used for Kienböck's disease. J Orthop Res 7:445, 1989.

431. Edelson G, Reis ND, Fuchs D: Recurrence of Kienböck's disease in a twelve-year-old after radial shortening. J Bone Joint Surg [Am] 70:1243, 1988.

432. Kawai H, Yamamoto K, Yamamoto T, et al: Excision of the lunate in Kienböck's disease. Results after long-term follow-up. J Bone Joint Surg [Br] 70:287, 1988.

433. Amadio PC, Hanssen AD, Berquist TH: The genesis of Kienböck's disease: Evaluation of a case by magnetic resonance imaging. J Hand Surg [Am] 12:1044, 1987.

434. Sowa DT, Holder LE, Patt PG, et al: Application of magnetic resonance imaging to ischemic necrosis of the lunate. J Hand Surg [Am] 14:1008, 1989.

435. Trumble TE, Irving J: Histologic and magnetic resonance imaging correlations in Kienböck's disease. J Hand Surg [Am] 15:879, 1990.

436. Desser TS, McCarthy S, Trumble T: Scaphoid fractures and Kienböck's disease of the lunate: MR imaging with histopathologic correlation. Magn Res Imag 8:357, 1990.

437. Culp RW, Schaffer JL, Osterman AL, et al: Kienböck's disease in a patient with Crohn's enteritis treated with corticosteroids. J Hand Surg [Am] 14:294, 1989.

438. Bauer M, Jonsson K, Josefsson PO, et al: Osteochondritis dissecans of the elbow. A long-term follow-up study. Clin Orthop 284:156, 1992.

439. Mooney WR, Reed MH: Growth disturbances in the hands following thermal injuries in children. 1. Flame burns. J Can Assoc Radiol 39:91, 1988.

440. Macnicol MF, Makris D: Acrodysostosis and protrusio acetabuli. An association. J Bone Joint Surg [Br] 70:38, 1988.

441. Høgh J, Lund B: The sequelae of Osgood-Schlatter's disease in adults. Int Orthop (SICOT) 12:213, 1988.

442. Sen RK, Sharma LR, Thakur SR, et al: Patellar angle in Osgood-Schlatter disease. Acta Orthop Scand 60:26, 1989.

443. Traverso A, Baldari A, Catalani F: The coexistence of Osgood-Schlatter's disease with Sinding-Larsen-Johansson's disease. Case report in an adolescent soccer player. J Sports Med Phys Fitness 30:331, 1990.

444. De Flaviis L, Nessi R, Scaglione P, et al: Ultrasonic diagnosis of Osgood-Schlatter and Sinding-Larsen-Johansson diseases of the knee. Skel Radiol 18:193, 1989.

445. Rosenberg ZS, Kawelblum M, Cheung YY, et al: Osgood-Schlatter lesion: Fracture or tendinitis? Scintigraphic, CT, and MR imaging features. Radiology 185:853, 1992.

446. Langenskiold A: Tibia vara. A critical review. Clin Orthop 246:195, 1989.

447. Ikegawa S, Nakamura K, Kawai S, et al: Blount's disease in a pair of identical twins. Acta Orthop Scand 61:582, 1990.

448. Bradway JK, Klassen RA, Peterson HA: Blount disease: A review of the English literature. J Pediatr Orthop 7:472, 1987.

449. Johnston CE II: Infantile tibia vara. Clin Orthop 255:13, 1990.

450. Loder RT, Johnston CE II: Infantile tibia vara. J Pediatr Orthop 7:639, 1987.

451. Kline SC, Bostrum M, Griffen PP: Femoral varus: An important component in late-onset Blount's disease. J Pediatr Orthop 12:197, 1992.

452. Henderson RC, Kemp GJ Jr, Greene WB: Adolescent tibia vara: Alternatives for operative treatment. J Bone Joint Surg [Am] 74:342, 1992.

453. Thompson GH, Carter JR: Late-onset tibia vara (Blount's disease). Current concepts. Clin Orthop 255:24, 1990.

454. Loder RT, Schaffer JJ, Bardenstein MB: Late-onset tibia vara. J Pediatr Orthop 11:162, 1991.

455. Bell SN, Campbell PE, Cole WG, et al: Tibia vara caused by focal fibrocartilaginous dysplasia. Three case reports. J Bone Joint Surg [Br] 67:780, 1985.

456. Bradish CF, Davies SJ, Malone M: Tibia vara due to focal fibrocartilaginous dysplasia. The natural history. J Bone Joint Surg [Br] 70:106, 1988.

457. Husien AM, Kale VR: Tibia vara caused by focal fibrocartilaginous dysplasia. Clin Radiol 40:105, 1989.

458. Olney BW, Cole WG, Menelaus MB: Three additional cases of focal fibrocartilaginous dysplasia causing tibia vara. J Pediatr Orthop 10:405, 1990.

459. Zayer M: Tibia vara in focal fibrocartilaginous dysplasia. A report of 2 cases. Acta Orthop Scand 63:353, 1992.

460. Herman TE, Siegel MJ, McAlister WH: Focal fibrocartilaginous dysplasia associated with tibia vara. Radiology 177:767, 1990.

461. Martinez AG, Weinstein SL, Maynard JA: Tibia vara. Report of an unusual case. J Bone Joint Surg [Am] 74:1250, 1992.

462. Ikegawa S, Nagano A, Nakamura K: Chondrodysplasia punctata mimicking Blount's disease. A case report. Acta Orthop Scand 61:580, 1990.

463. Lowe TG: Scheuermann disease. J Bone Joint Surg [Am] 72:940, 1990.

464. Normelli HCM, Svensson O, Aaro SI: Cord compression in Scheuermann's kyphosis. A case report. Acta Orthop Scand 62:70, 1991.

465. Paajanen H, Alanen A, Erkintalo M, et al: Disc degeneration in Scheuermann disease. Skel Radiol 18:523, 1989.

466. Gilsanz V, Gibbens DT, Carlson M, et al: Vertebral bone density in Scheuermann disease. J Bone Joint Surg [Am] 71:894, 1989.

467. Horne J, Cockshott WP, Shannon HS: Spinal column damage from water ski jumping. Skel Radiol 16:612, 1987.

468. Swärd L, Hellstrom M, Jacobsson B, et al: Back pain and radiologic changes in the thoraco-lumbar spine of athletes. Spine 15:124, 1990.

469. Blumenthal SL, Roach J, Herring JA: Lumbar Scheuermann's. A clinical series and classification. Spine 12:929, 1987.

470. Tallroth K, Schlenzka D: Spinal stenosis subsequent to juvenile lumbar osteochondrosis. Skel Radiol 19:203, 1990.

471. Tertti MO, Salminen JJ, Paajanen HEK, et al: Low-back pain and disk degeneration in children: A case-control MR imaging study. Radiology 180:503, 1991.

472. Smith JRG, Martin IR, Shaw DG, et al: Progressive non-infectious anterior vertebral fusion. Skel Radiol 15:599, 1986.

473. Knutsson F: Fusion of vertebrae following non-infectious disturbance in the zone of growth. Acta Radiol 32:404, 1949.

474. Butler RW: Spontaneous anterior fusion of vertebral bodies. J Bone Joint Surg [Br] 53:2, 1971.

475. Nicholas PJR, Boldero JC, Goodfellow JW, et al: Abnormalities of the vertebral column associated with thalidomide-induced limb deformities. Orthopaedics 1:71, 1968.

476. Mubarak SJ: Osteochondrosis of the lateral cuneiform: Another cause of a limp in a child. A case report. J Bone Joint Surg [Am] 74:285, 1992.

477. Hagino H, Yamamoto K, Teshima R, et al: Sequential radiographic changes of metacarpal osteonecrosis. A case report. Acta Orthop Scand 61:86, 1990.

478. Ferlic DC, Morin P: Idiopathic avascular necrosis of the scaphoid: Preiser's disease? J Hand Surg [Am] 14:13, 1989.

479. Christensen PB, Christensen I: A case of Friedrich's disease of the clavicle. Acta Orthop Scand 58:585, 1987.

480. Féry A: La maladie de Friedrich ou ostéochondrose de l'extrémité sternale de la clavicule. Rev Rhum 55:141, 1988.

481. Zawin JK, Hoffer FA, Rand FF, et al: Joint effusion in children with an irritable hip: US diagnosis and aspiration. Radiology 187:459, 1993.

482. Henderson RC, Greene WB: Etiology of late-onset tibia vara: Is varus alignment a prerequisite? J Pediatr Orthop 14:143, 1994.

483. Greene WB: Infantile tibia vara. J Bone Joint Surg [Am] 75:130, 1993.

484. Henderson RC, Kemp GJ, Hayes PRL: Prevalence of late-onset tibia vara. J Pediatr Orthop 13:255, 1993.

485. Cook DA, Engber WD: Osteochondritis dissecans of the scaphoid: Preiser's disease? Orthopedics 16:705, 1993.

486. Bloom RA, Gomori J, Milgrom C: Ossicles anterior to the proximal tibia with description of an unusually large ossicle probably of traumatic origin. Clin Imaging 17:137, 1993.

487. Feldman MD, Schoenecker PL: Use of the metaphyseal-diaphyseal angle in the evaluation of bowed legs. J Bone Joint Surg [Am] 75:1602, 1993.

488. Mandell GA, Morales RW, Harcke HT, et al: Bone scintigraphy in patients with atypical lumbar Scheuermann disease. J Pediatr Orthop 13:622, 1993.

INDEX

Note: Page numbers in *italics* refer to illustrations; page numbers followed by (t) refer to tables.

I